Contents

Unit I
Foundations for Nursing Practice 3

1 Introduction to Nursing 4
2 Basic Human Needs: Individual, Family, and Community 21
3 Culture and Ethnicity 32
4 Promoting Wellness in Health and Illness 52
5 Theoretical Base for Nursing Practice 65
6 Values and Ethics in Nursing 78
7 Legal Implications of Nursing 95

Unit II
Promoting Wellness Across the Lifespan 113

8 Developmental Theories 114
9 Conception Through Adolescence 128
10 Early, Middle, and Older Adulthood 149

Unit III
Community-Based Settings for Client Care 173

11 Community-Based Healthcare 174
12 Continuity of Care 191
13 Home Healthcare 207

Unit IV
The Nursing Process 221

14 Introduction to Nursing Process 222
15 Core Competencies and Critical Thinking 232
16 Assessing 247
17 Diagnosing 266
18 Planning 281
19 Implementing 300
20 Evaluating 313
21 Documenting, Reporting, and Conferring 329

Unit V
Roles Basic to Nursing Care 357

22 Communicator 358
23 Teacher and Counselor 386
24 Leader, Researcher, and Advocate 411

Unit VI
Actions Basic to Nursing Care 431

25 Vital Signs 432
26 Health Assessment 473
27 Safety 524
28 Asepsis 555
29 Medications 593
30 Perioperative Nursing 669

Unit VII
Promoting Healthy Psychosocial Responses 727

31 Self-Concept 728
32 Stress and Adaptation 754
33 Loss, Grief, and Dying 780
34 Sensory Stimulation 813
35 Sexuality 840
36 Spirituality 882

Unit VIII
Promoting Healthy Physiologic Responses 909

37 Hygiene 910
38 Skin Integrity and Wound Care 972
39 Activity 998
40 Rest and Sleep 1072
41 Comfort 1102
42 Nutrition 1149
43 Urinary Elimination 1211
44 Bowel Elimination 1265
45 Oxygenation 1311
46 Fluid, Electrolyte, and Acid–Base Balance 1366

Fundamentals of Nursing

Carol Taylor
CSFN, RN, MSN, PhD Candidate

Assistant Professor and Ethicist
Holy Family College
Philadelphia, Pennsylvania

Carol Lillis
RN, MSN

Associate Professor
Department of Nursing
Delaware County Community College
Media, Pennsylvania

Priscilla LeMone
RN, DSN

Assistant Professor
Sinclair School of Nursing
University of Missouri—Columbia
Columbia, Missouri

THIRD EDITION

Fundamentals of Nursing

The Art and Science of Nursing Care

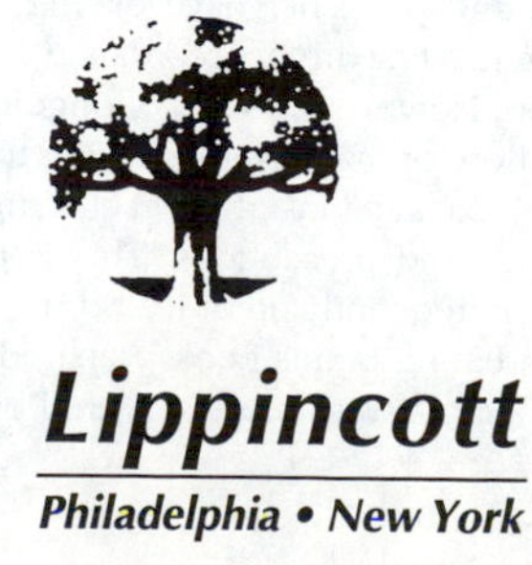

Lippincott
Philadelphia • New York

Acquisitions Editor: Mary Gyetvan, RN, MSN
Developmental Editor: Eleanor Faven
Assistant Editor: Susan M. Keneally
Production Manager/Managing Editor: Helen Ewan/Tom Gibbons
Production Coordinator: Kathryn Rule
Design Coordinator: Kathy Kelley-Luedtke
Indexer: Ann Cassar

3rd Edition

Library of Congress Cataloging-in-Publication Data

Taylor, Carol, CSFN.
Fundamentals of nursing : the art and science of nursing care / Carol Taylor, Carol Lillis, Priscilla LeMone.—3rd ed.
p. cm.
Rev. ed. of: Fundamentals of nursing / [edited by] Carol Taylor, Carol Lillis, Priscilla LeMone, 2nd ed. c1993.
Includes bibliographical references and index.
ISBN 0-397-55278-5 (hardcover : alk. paper)
1. Nursing. I. Lillis, Carol. II. LeMone, Priscilla. III. Title.
[DNLM: 1. Nursing. 2. Nursing Process. 3. Health Promotion. WY 16 T239f 1997]
RT41.F882 1997
610.73—dc20
DNLM/DLC
for Library of Congress 96-17377
CIP

The material contained in this volume was submitted as previously unpublished material, except in the instances in which credit has been given to the source from which some of the illustrative material was derived.

Any procedure or practice described in this book should be applied by the health-care practitioner under appropriate supervision in accordance with professional standards of care used with regard to the unique circumstances that apply in each practice situation. Care has been taken to confirm the accuracy of information presented and to describe generally accepted practices. However, the authors, editors, and publisher cannot accept any responsibility for errors or omissions or for any consequences from application of the information in this book and make no warranty, express or implied, with respect to the contents of the book.

The authors and publisher have exerted every effort to ensure that drug selection and dosage set forth in this text are in accordance with current recommendations and practice at the time of publication. However, in view of ongoing research, changes in government regulations, and the constant flow of information relating to drug therapy and drug reactions, the reader is urged to check the package insert for each drug for any change in indications and dosage and for added warnings and precautions. This is particularly important when the recommended agent is a new or infrequently employed drug.

Materials appearing in this book prepared by individuals as part of their official duties as U.S. Government employees are not covered by the above-mentioned copyright.

9 8 7 6 5 4 3 2 1

With respect, affection, and gratitude, we dedicate the third edition of this text to our developmental editor, **Eleanor Faven**. For 20 years she has played the role of midwife at Lippincott-Raven, expertly coaching authors through both normal and high-risk "births" of nursing texts. New to the world of textbook writing when we began our first edition, we benefited immensely from Eleanor's unique talents. At the time, there was no way we could appreciate the full extent of her giftedness nor comprehend its consequences for us and the world of nursing. Seasoned authors as we complete the third edition, we pause to remedy this deficiency and to introduce this remarkable woman to our readers.

Never afraid of hard work or challenges, Eleanor consistently meets personal and professional challenges with generosity, expertise, commitment, and love. Experienced in all aspects of textbook planning, writing, and production, she is a strong coordinator and somehow manages to elicit everyone's best efforts. She challenges authors to match and exceed her own creativity, hard work, and conscientious attention to detail. When we grew slack, she used her gentle humor (and if all else failed, threatening faxes) to get us back on track. A constant behind-the-scenes force and fierce advocate of excellence, Eleanor is any author's best guarantee that a text will be published on schedule and will faithfully achieve its objectives. Students can be grateful to Eleanor for ensuring that a text is scholarly, user-friendly, consistent in its approach, and chock-full of features to facilitate rapid mastery and application of content.

We salute Eleanor Faven, longtime friend of nursing and now our friend and mentor.

Carol Taylor
Carol Lillis
Priscilla LeMone

To my family and community, whose support enables me to meet each new day with love and courage

Carol Taylor

To Mary Jo Boyer—friend, mentor, and instigator. How boring my life would have been without all your "great ideas"!

Carol Lillis

For family, friends, colleagues, students, and the two Carols—I couldn't do it without you!

Priscilla LeMone

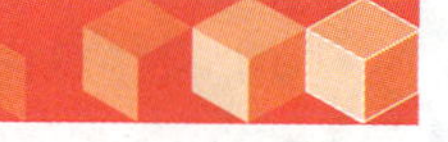

Consultants and Contributors to the Third Edition

Ellen D. Baer, RN, PhD, FAAN, Visiting Professor of Nursing, New York University, New York, New York

Ellen Ellis, RNC, MS, Associate Director, Nursing Education Program, New York State Nurses Association, Latham, New York

Rhonda Gregg, RN, MS, Director Home Care and Hospice, Crozer-Chester Medical Center, Upland, Pennsylvania

Jeannie Langinger, RN, MSN, Maui Community College, Kahului, Hawaii

Susan K. Newbold, RN, MS, PhD, Associate Editor, *Computers in Nursing*

Reviewers for the Third Edition

Janet S. Anderson, RN, MS, Assistant Professor, School of Nursing, University of Rochester, Rochester, New York

Ilene Borze, RN, MSN, CEN, Nursing Faculty, Gateway Community College, Phoenix, Arizona

Debbie Bridgewater, RN, MSN, Instructor, St. Mary's School of Nursing, Huntington, West Virginia

Mary H. Browning, RN, MA Professor, Division of Nursing, Three Rivers Community-Technical College, Norwich, Connecticut

Margaret Conrad, RN, MSN, GNP, Faculty, Department of Nursing, Phoenix College, Phoenix, Arizona

Sandra DeBella, RN, EdD, Chair and Professor of Nursing, Department of Nursing, Sonoma State University, Rohnert Park, California

Lisa Foertsch, RN, MSN, Teaching Specialist, Shadyside Hospital School of Nursing, Pittsburgh, Pennsylvania

Dolores Furlong, PhD, Project Director, BSN Program Expansion, St. Francis Xavier University Department of Nursing, Antigonish, Nova Scotia, Canada

Guadalupe S. Gutierrez, RN, BSN, Nursing Faculty, Pima Community College, Tucson, Arizona

Irene Hatcher, RNC, BSN, Documentation System Specialist, Vanderbilt University Medical Center, Nashville, Tennessee

Esther K. McEvoy, RN, MS, Professor of Nursing and Program Chair, Maria College, Albany, New York

Pat McMahon, RN, MSN, Area Chair Person, Good Samaritan Hospital, School of Nursing, Cincinnati, Ohio

Karen M. Merriman, RN, MSN, Associate Professor, ADN Program Coordinator, University of Charleston, Charleston, West Virginia

Elaine L. Mohn, RN, EdD, Faculty, ADN Program, Chemeketa Community College, Salem, Oregon

M. Carroll Miller, MSN, MA, Associate Professor, Duquesne University School of Nursing, Pittsburgh, Pennsylvania

Paula Nelson-Marten, RN, PhD, DCN, Assistant Professor, Oncology Nursing, University of Colorado School of Nursing, Denver, Colorado

Patsy O'Brien, RN, BSN, Nursing Skills Supervisor, Penn Valley Community College, Kansas City, Missouri

Patricia A. Parsons, MS, MSN, Instructor of Nursing, Austin Community College, Austin, Minnesota

Marilyn Nelson Pase, BS, BSN, MSN, Assistant Professor in Nursing, New Mexico State University, Las Cruces, New Mexico

Sally Phillips, RN, PhD, Associate Professor, Director of Nursing Doctorate Program, University of Colorado School of Nursing, Denver, Colorado

Ann F. Tully, RN, MSN, Nursing Instructor, Highland Community College, Freeport, Illinois

Preface

New efforts to reform healthcare and to guarantee both high-quality and cost-effective care are radically transforming the culture of caregiving. As a result, creative energies have been released and many nurses are newly committed to finding effective means to meet healthcare needs. On the other hand, the "leaner and meaner" system of care that is evolving often seems coldly indifferent to the well-being of those it professes to serve and to its caregivers. Nurses and other healthcare professionals find themselves urged constantly to work harder, smarter, and faster. Although this may evoke the best energies of some, for others it has increased burnout, lowered morale, and harmed the team spirit and sense of camaraderie that make excellence in caregiving possible.

Although nurses need to treasure the essence of nursing and what has traditionally served nursing well, they also need to be responsive to the changing healthcare culture and to radically transformed systems of care. Attempts to "do business as usual" are doomed to failure. Our aim in undertaking this third edition of *Fundamentals of Nursing: The Art and Science of Nursing Care* is to prepare nurses to function competently, enthusiastically, and accountably in this changing system. To fulfill this aim, we have taken the following approaches.

Successful nurses complement their scientific knowledge and technical expertise with a commitment to interpersonal caring and a strong sense of accountability. We demonstrate this holistic approach to care by identifying core competencies of the practicing nurse: cognitive, technical, interpersonal, and ethical/legal. Examples promote human well-being, of significant importance to the client. We refuse to allow caring and trusting nurse–client relationships to become relics of a bygone era.

Today's nurses practice in more nontraditional settings than ever before. We portray nurses meeting the needs of diverse clients in multiple types of settings. Although this concept has always been a strength of this text, the third edition includes a new unit, *Community-Based Settings for Client Care,* and other features dedicated to defining these settings.

An increasing number of people are taking care of seriously ill and dying clients in their homes for long periods of time; they often feel overwhelmed by the burdens of caregiving. On their behalf we include strong teaching, counseling, and advocacy sections. An expanded chapter on loss, grief, and dying has been moved to the clinical unit to introduce students to the responsibilities of nurses as they support people making what are often anguished end-of-life decisions.

A development in healthcare that has been growing through the last several decades was brought about by "consumer" awareness and activity. People are interested in self-care—improving their own health rather than having the healthcare system take care of their illnesses. We emphasize the four aims of nursing: promoting wellness, preventing illness, restoring health, and facilitating coping.

Those new to nursing can quickly become overwhelmed by the demands placed on the nurse's knowledge, technical competence, interpersonal skills, and commitment. Therefore, much care has once again gone into the selection of both the content of this edition and the manner of its presentation. We strive to capture the unique essence of both the art and science of nursing, distilling what the person beginning the study of nursing needs. We invite the beginning practitioner of nursing to identify with the profession, to share in its pride, and to respond to its challenges.

We chose to use the term "client" (rather than "patient") to emphasize respect for the autonomy (self-determination) of the individual and to encourage the nurse to actively involve the client and family as much as possible in care decisions. Care has been taken to communicate that both nurses and clients may be male or female and that they come from every racial and ethnic background and socioeconomic group. Whenever possible, we have tried to avoid male/female distinctions in personal pronouns.

Because our textbook is used by a variety of people throughout North America, we attempted to generalize many statements and use references to Canada throughout the book.

Organization

Fundamentals of Nursing: The Art and Science of Nursing Care is organized into eight units. Ideally, the text is followed sequentially, but every effort has been made to respect the differing needs of diverse curricula and students. Thus each chapter stands on its own merit and may be read independently of others.

Unit I, *Foundations for Nursing Practice,* opens with a description of contemporary nursing. Successive chapters introduce content foundational to nursing practice: human needs (individual, family, and community), culture and ethnicity, wellness, nursing theory, ethics, and law.

Unit II, *Promoting Wellness Across the Lifespan,* provides the basis for understanding growth and development across the lifespan and acknowledges nursing's differing requirements arising from the various developmental stages and abilities to meet developmental tasks.

Unit III, *Community-Based Settings for Client Care,* introduces the multiple settings in which nursing is practiced and prepares students to ensure continuity of care in what could be a fragmented healthcare system. Chapters address the variety of community-based healthcare settings; continuity of care as the client enters a healthcare facility, is transferred within the facility, and discharged into another setting within the community; and care provided within the home.

Unit IV, *The Nursing Process,* offers a detailed step-by-step guide to each component of the nursing process. Practical guidelines and examples are included in each chapter. Separate chapters address the nursing process as a whole, nursing's core competencies, assessing, diagnosing, planning, implementing, and evaluating. A new chapter on documentation, reporting, and conferring highlights these nursing responsibilities.

Unit V, *Roles Basic to Nursing Care,* describes major roles in which nurses function as they interact holistically with clients. Chapters focus on the communicator, teacher and counselor, and leader, researcher, and advocate roles of the nurse as caregiver.

Unit VI, *Actions Basic to Nursing Care,* introduces the foundational skills used by nurses: measuring vital signs, assessing health, promoting safety, maintaining asepsis, administering medication, and caring for surgical clients.

Unit VII, *Promoting Healthy Psychosocial Responses,* explores the nurse's role in helping clients meet basic psychosocial needs: self-concept, stress and adaptation, loss, grief and dying, sensory stimulation, sexuality, and spirituality. In each chapter guidelines are included for assessing and diagnosing unhealthy responses and for planning, implementing, and evaluating appropriate care strategies. Chapters conclude with a client care study illustrating the use of the nursing process and nursing's care competencies to resolve selected nursing diagnoses.

Unit VIII, *Promoting Healthy Physiologic Responses,* uses the same format as Unit VII to focus on the physiologic needs of clients: hygiene, skin integrity, activity, rest and sleep, comfort, nutrition, urinary elimination, bowel elimination, oxygenation, and fluid, electrolyte, and acid–base balance.

Integrated Nursing Process

After the nursing process is introduced in Unit IV, it provides the organizational framework for successive chapters. Chapters in Units VII and VIII, which deal with psychosocial and physiologic responses, begin with a succinct background discussion of the concept, followed by an identification of factors that influence how different individuals respond to these needs. Steps in the nursing process are used to describe related nursing responsibilities.

Assessing. Common elements of both a comprehensive and problem-focused nursing assessment are presented; sample interview questions are included and specific physical assessment techniques described.

Diagnosing. NANDA-approved nursing diagnoses related to the human need being discussed are identified, and tables illustrate the relationship between related factors and the problem statement and provide sample defining characteristics.

Planning. Sample client goals/expected outcomes are suggested based on client strengths.

Implementing. Nursing interventions are clearly explained and are illustrated when this is deemed helpful. Procedures have been streamlined to facilitate mastery, and home health considerations are included. A sufficient variety of nursing interventions is provided to foster the development of a repertoire of nursing actions that makes practicing the art of nursing possible.

Evaluating. Criteria for evaluating the effectiveness of the plan of care are suggested.

Each chapter in Units VII and VIII concludes with a *Nursing Process in Clinical Practice* with the workup of several NANDA diagnoses that demonstrate the comprehensive nursing management of common nursing problems. "Assessment Priorities," "Expected Outcomes," and "Interventions" related to the particular nursing diagnosis are outlined. One diagnosis is further illustrated with a *Client Care Study.* A description of the client precedes a set of *Core Competencies* the nurse needs to provide care for this particular client. Core competencies include *Cognitive, Technical, Interpersonal,* and *Ethical/Legal.* A concluding *Nursing Plan of Care* contributes an additional illustration of the correct use and documentation of the nursing process. As the learner progresses through the text, the nursing process becomes an integral part of nursing care.

Key Features

In this edition we capitalize on the strengths of the first two editions and address new priorities. We further develop or strengthen the following features:

Nursing as an Art and Science. Nursing, as a science, is characterized by a growing body of knowledge that links technical and interpersonal interventions to desired client outcomes; as an art, nursing demands of its practitioners sufficient competency to creatively design individualized strategies to assist clients to reach personal health goals. A unique spirit of caring must prevail always.

Wellness Orientation. A wellness rather than an illness orientation provides a framework for presentation of content. *Promoting Wellness* displays highlight assessment checkpoints for specific components of high-level wellness and include suggestions for designing a self-care prescription. These displays serve a twofold purpose as a self-care model for the learner and an invaluable aid for the individual who is developing the role of client healthcare educator.

The Nurse as Role Model. Nurses, because they are role models for their clients, are directed to assess their own health behaviors before attempting to help clients. Health goals for the nurse are presented in each clinical chapter.

Aims of Nursing. Learners are gradually introduced to the theory, interpersonal skills, and nursing procedures that will enable them to work successfully with clients to promote wellness, prevent illness, restore health, and facilitate coping with altered functioning. Early attention to these broad aims of nursing will prepare learners to meet the needs of clients in diverse healthcare settings.

Basic Human Needs. Common to all people and communities and essential to wellness and survival are basic human needs. The clinical chapters in Unit VII, *Promoting Healthy Psychosocial Responses,* and Unit VIII, *Promoting Healthy Physiologic Responses,* prepare the learner to assist clients and family members in meeting these needs. Learners are encouraged to explore *human responses* to health and illness as indicators of how well an individual is functioning to meet basic human needs.

Holistic Care Across the Lifespan. A holistic orientation to basic human needs exists across the lifespan. This orientation is emphasized through information about growth and development in Unit II, *Promoting Wellness Across the Lifespan;* through developmental considerations and related tables and displays in Unit VII, *Promoting Healthy Psychosocial Responses,* and Unit VIII, *Promoting Healthy Physiologic Responses;* through age considerations in many procedures; and through the diverse ages and needs of clients represented in the client care studies in clinical chapters addressing the lifespan. Wherever appropriate, cultural considerations are included.

Community-Based Care. Clients today spend fewer days in the hospital, are frequently transferred both within the hospital and between healthcare institutions, and need to rely on rapidly proliferating community-based healthcare resources. A new unit III in this edition, *Community-Based Settings for Client Care,* emphasizes the nurse's role in ensuring continuity of care in this system. Because many home health nurses work alone, new features in the book are intended to serve as a mentor to the new nurse. *Home Health Alerts* and displays called *Home Care: Bridging the Gap* throughout the text and *Home Care Considerations* in procedures prepare students to function in nontraditional settings.

Attention to Special Needs of the Older Person. Because the age of the population is increasing, nurses encounter growing numbers of older clients in all practice settings. The section on older adults in Chapter 10, *Early, Middle, and Older Adulthood,* the *Focus on the Older Adult* displays, and general considerations for the older client that appear within the text aim to sensitize students to the special nursing needs of this population.

Personal Accounts. Delighted with the response to the personal accounts of students in the second edition, we invited clients and family caregivers to share their experiences in the third edition. New displays entitled *Through the Eyes of a Student, Through the Eyes of a Client,* and *Through the Eyes of a Family Caregiver* speak eloquently of nursing's power to "make a difference." These personal accounts will evoke smiles, pride, and empathy and will unite nurse caregivers in their struggles to perfect their caregiving skills as they make a difference in the lives of others.

Respect for Client Autonomy. The student is reminded that the nurse does not make decisions for the client and family (significant others). Clients are involved in making decisions regarding their problems, setting expected outcomes, and choosing actions to take to correct problems. Clients and support persons are involved, according to their abilities and motivation, in all aspects of care. At the same time, the text helps the nurse develop concerns for the home caregiver. Family members may suffer from burnout too, and they are the nurses' clients as well as the person who is ill. A new recurrent display, *Helpscan,* provides valuable referral resources for both clients and their professional and nonprofessional caregivers.

Collaborative Dimensions of Care. The client's achievement of health goals is related to the efficient functioning of the healthcare team. The nurse, who possesses unique knowledge of the client, is encouraged to respect the contributions of different members of the healthcare team and work collaboratively with team members.

Critical Thinking. Critical thinking is highlighted in the new chapter on nursing competencies, *Core Competencies and Critical Thinking* (Chapter 15). Recurring displays, *Developing Critical Thinking Skills,* help the student follow the process and develop critical thinking.

Critical thinking situations also are included in other chapters in Unit IV, *The Nursing Process.*

Computer Applications. A nurse computer specialist, through displays called *Computer Applications in Nursing,* highlights some of the ways nurses use computers creatively to link people and resources. Whatever your comfort level with computers, the information highway is here and traffic is brisk.

Nursing Procedures. Procedures are presented in a concise, straightforward, and simplified format that is intended to facilitate competent performance of nursing skills. Scientific rationale accompany each nursing action, and many color photographs and illustrations further reinforce mastery. Special considerations, including modifications and age and home care considerations, are given where appropriate.

Broad Scope of Nursing Practice. The text is written to encompass fundamental skills in a laboratory as well as in actual clinical settings where nurses care for both well and ill clients. To acquaint students of nursing with many exciting career options in nursing, numerous examples are given to illustrate nurses interacting with clients of all ages and backgrounds and in traditional and nontraditional settings.

Nursing Today: Challenges and Solutions. This recurring feature highlights some of today's most pressing issues. Nursing's creative solutions to these problems are described.

Research as a Strength to Practice. Updated *Research in Nursing: Making a Difference* displays, appearing throughout the book, promote the value of research and apply its relevance to nursing practice. Students are challenged to become informed participants in or consumers of clinical research.

Student Instructional Materials Within the Text

A strength of any textbook is its pedagogy. These learning aids have always been a strong feature of *Fundamentals of Nursing: The Art and Science of Nursing Care.* In addition to the elements listed above, the following key features provide instruction for the student of nursing.

Objectives. Each chapter begins with a list of objectives that address the major emphases of the chapter. The student can use them as a basis for outlines or self-testing, or the instructor may use them for evaluating students' knowledge and abilities.

Key Terms and Glossary. Key terms precede the text in each chapter. When these terms are defined in the chapter, they are boldfaced for clarity. A *Glossary* appears at the back of the book for easy studying of these terms.

Key Points. The major points in the text are summarized in *Key Points* at the end of the chapter. They follow the organization of the chapter, and the student may return to the text if further study is necessary.

Bibliography. A *Bibliography* at the end of each chapter helps make the student aware of the variety of resources for information on nursing and gives additional reference materials for instructors or students.

Sample Test Questions. Sample test questions appear at the end of each chapter in Units VI through VIII to facilitate mastery of chapter content. These exercises will assist students who are attempting to improve their objective test-taking skills. New to this edition is a *Self-Study Computer Disk* at the back of the book. Approximately 350 questions may be called up for study and student evaluation.

Historic Precedents. Unit openers give short introductions to historical nursing leaders, their philosophy, and their role in the nursing profession.

Unit Summaries. On unit openers a summary is given of the material covered in that particular unit, its relationship to previous units, and how it fits into the student's preparation for a career in nursing.

Chapter Outlines. Outlines of chapters in the front of the book give an overview of the information in the chapter and, in many cases, its relationship to the nursing process.

Lists of Displays. The displays, or boxed materials, within the text are valuable instructional tools. The student can find these easily through the lists that appear before the text itself.

Summary of New Features

These features have already been discussed, but we list them here so you can see at a glance what is new to the book. In addition to updating all of the chapters in relationship to current healthcare practices, we have made the following additions:

- New four-color design with new art and photos
- New unit III, *Community-Based Settings for Client Care,* focusing on current healthcare trends
- New emphasis on critical thinking and core competencies
- New chapters: 11, *Community-Based Healthcare;* 13, *Home Health Care;* 15, *Core Competencies and Critical Thinking;* 21, *Documenting, Reporting, and Conferring;* and 38, *Skin Integrity and Wound Care.*
- New information regarding eight historical leaders in nursing
- New *Home Health Alert* display, which highlights in-text information to prepare the home healthcare nurse for potential problems

- New displays: *Developing Critical Thinking Skills; Home Care: Bridging the Gap;* and *Helpscan*
- Newest information on *Standard Precautions* from the CDC
- New student interactive computer disk

Teaching/Learning Package

To facilitate mastery of this text's foundational content, a comprehensive teaching/learning package has been developed to assist faculty and students.

Two supplemental books are available for the learner. A *Procedure Checklist* manual includes a checklist for each procedure to facilitate learner evaluation. Foundations of learning developed in the text are augmented in the *Student Study Guide* with practical applications. Chapter-by-chapter exercises enable learners to gain expertise in theory comprehension and application. In addition to developing valuable testing skills, learners using the study guide will find client care presentations in each clinical chapter that facilitate their mastery of nursing process skills. The student works through critical thinking exercises to gain mastery. An *Interactive Self-Study Computer Disk* in the back of the book is new to this edition. It has multiple-choice NCLEX-style questions, with feedback to enhance the student's learning.

Supplemental materials for the faculty member include an *Instructor's Manual,* a printed and computerized *Test Bank,* and *Transparency Acetates*. The Instructor's Manual provides theoretical and clinical resources. Chapter objectives and learning activities encompass a range of cognitive, affective, and psychomotor domains. Critical thinking exercises give learning situations for further teaching. Four-color acetate transparencies enable faculty members to visually enhance their lectures and presentations. A computerized test bank program, *ParTEST,* assists faculty members in testing knowledge attained by learners during the course. Questions are based on material presented in *Fundamentals of Nursing: The Art and Science of Nursing Care*. For the first time, *Lippincott's Clinical Skills Series* (19 VHS videocassettes) and *Lippincott's Clinical Interactive Skills Series* (interactive video disks) are available.

Carol Taylor, CSFN, RN, MSN, PHD(candidate)
Carol Lillis, RN, MSN
Priscilla LeMone, RN, DSN

Acknowledgments

This revision is the work of many talented and committed people, and we wish to gratefully acknowledge the assistance of all who have contributed in any way to the completion of this project. Our first debt of gratitude is to all the nurse educators and students who have adopted the text and shared with us their experiences in using the teaching and learning package. We are deeply grateful for their revision suggestions and trust they will enhance the learning experiences of others.

Our special thanks to the Nursing and Allied Health Editorial Publishing division of Lippincott: to Mary Gyetvan, RN, MSN, Editor, and Susan Keneally, Assistant Editor, both of whom supported our work and provided guidance throughout the project, and Donna L. Hilton, RN, BSN, Vice President and Publisher, who continues to strive for excellence in nursing publishing. To Eleanor Faven, diligent and respected developmental editor of both the first and third editions, but more importantly, *friend, taskmaster,* and *standard of excellence,* we express heartfelt gratitude.

To the members of the production department of Lippincott, who patiently pulled everything together to form a completed book: Tom Gibbons, Project Editor; Kathy Rule, Production Coordinator; and Kathy Kelley-Luedtke, Design Coordinator.

To Susan Blaker, who coordinated the new four-color photo package, which has added to the visual presentation of this edition. The illustration program seeks to communicate the excitement and spirit of the multidisciplined and person-centered character of nursing. The energies and talents of many people contributed to that end. We thank all who generously gave their time, ideas, and resources, and we gratefully acknowledge the special contributions of the following:

- Ken Kasper, Barbara Proud, Gates Rhodes, and Kathy Sloane, photographers
- Maryanne Lieb, Cheryl Meyer, and Cathy Chapley, Delaware County Community College (DCCC) faculty, staff, and administrators, Ed Dubin, RN, and former DCCC student, and the current students who served as models for many of the photos.
- Patty McBride, RN, MSN, CIC coordinator of infection control at Bryn Mawr Hospital, Bryn Mawr, PA, for advising and updating us on changing infection control protocols
- Marie Clark, who developed the math problems and solutions in Chapter 29
- Joan E. Lynaugh, RN, PhD, FAAN, Director, the Center for the Study of the History of Nursing
- Susan Newbold, RN, MS, doctoral student, who created the new Computer Applications in Nursing displays
- Ellen Ellis, RN, who researched the history of nursing for the quotes by and information about some of the many leaders in the profession of nursing

We gratefully acknowledge the influence of our mentors and teachers who have influenced our thoughts and writing; each person we have been privileged to care for as nurses; our students, who continually challenge us to find more effective means to teach nursing; our professional colleagues; and perhaps most importantly, our family and friends, whose love sustained us through the long hours of research and writing.

Finally, we are grateful to the reviewers of this edition and the contributors and reviewers of the previous two editions, whose expertise broadened both the scope and depth of the text.

Carol Taylor
Carol Lillis
Priscilla LeMone

Contents

Unit I
Foundations for Nursing Practice ***3***

1 Introduction to Nursing 4

2 Basic Human Needs: Individual, Family, and Community 21

3 Culture and Ethnicity 32

4 Promoting Wellness in Health and Illness 52

5 Theoretical Base for Nursing Practice 65

6 Values and Ethics in Nursing 78

7 Legal Implications of Nursing 95

Unit II
Promoting Wellness Across the Lifespan ***113***

8 Developmental Concepts 114

9 Conception Through Adolescence 128

10 Early, Middle, and Older Adulthood 149

Unit III
Community-Based Settings for Client Care ***173***

11 Community-Based Healthcare 174

12 Continuity of Care 191

13 Home Healthcare 207

Unit IV
The Nursing Process ***221***

14 Introduction to Nursing Process 222

15 Core Competencies and Critical Thinking 232

16 Assessing 247

17 Diagnosing 266

18 Planning 281

19 Implementing 300

20 Evaluating 313

21 Documenting, Reporting, and Conferring 329

Unit V
Roles Basic to Nursing Care ***357***

22 Communicator 358

23 Teacher and Counselor 386

24 Leader, Researcher, and Advocate 411

Unit VI
Actions Basic to Nursing Care ***431***

25 Vital Signs 432

26 Health Assessment 473

27 Safety 524

28 Asepsis 555

29 Medications 593

30 Perioperative Nursing 669

Unit VII
Promoting Healthy Psychosocial Responses ***727***

31 Self-Concept 728

32 Stress and Adaptation 754

33 Loss, Grief, and Dying 780

34 Sensory Stimulation 813

35 Sexuality 840

36 Spirituality 882

Unit VIII
Promoting Healthy Physiologic Responses ***909***

37 Hygiene 910

38 Skin Integrity and Wound Care 972

39 Activity 998

40 Rest and Sleep 1072

41 Comfort 1102

42 Nutrition 1149

43 Urinary Elimination 1211

44 Bowel Elimination 1265

45 Oxygenation 1311

46 Fluid, Electrolyte, and Acid–Base Balance 1366

Appendices

A. Equivalents 1438

B. Normal Adult Laboratory Values 1441

C. U.S. Recommended Daily Allowances 1448

D. Canadian Recommended Nutrient Intake Range Based on Age and Body Weight Expressed as Daily Rates 1450

Glossary 1451

Index 1469

Expanded Contents

Nursing Procedures, Guidelines, and Techniques *xxxvii*

Nursing Process in Clinical Practice *xli*

Nursing Plans of Care *xliii*

Summary of Special Recurring Displays *xlv*

Unit I

Foundations for Nursing Practice *3*

Chapter 1

Introduction to Nursing *4*

Nursing: An Emerging Profession and Discipline 5
- Historical Background 5
- Nursing in North America 6
- Definitions of Nursing 7
- Nursing: A Profession and a Discipline? 9

Aims of Nursing 9
- Promoting Wellness 10
- Preventing Illness 10
- Restoring Health 10
- Facilitating Coping 11

Educational Preparation for Nursing Practice 11
- Levels of Education 11

Professional Nursing Organizations 15
- National Nursing Organizations 15
- International Nursing Organization 15
- Specialty Nursing Organizations 16

Guidelines for Nursing Practice 16
- Standards of Nursing Practice 16
- Nurse Practice Acts and Licensure 16
- Nursing Process 17

Nursing in Transition 17
- New Directions in Nursing 18
- Changes in Client Needs 18
- Expanded Technology 18
- Increasing Autonomy 18

Chapter 2

Basic Human Needs: Individual, Family, and Community *21*

The Individual 21
- Levels of Needs 21
- The Individual in Health and Illness: Applying Maslow's Theory 24

The Family 24
- What Is a Family? 24
- The Family in Health and Illness 27

The Community 29
- The Community in Health and Illness 29

Chapter 3

Culture and Ethnicity *32*

Concepts of Culture and Ethnicity 33
- Culture 33
- Ethnicity 33
- Race 34
- Cultural Assimilation 34

Factors Affecting Cultural Sensitivity 34

Cultural and Ethnic Influences on Healthcare 35
- Gender Roles 35
- Language and Communication 35
- Orientation to Space and Time 36
- Food and Nutrition 37
- Socioeconomic Factors 37
- Family Support 38
- Physical and Mental Health 38
- Alternative Healing Systems 41

Transcultural Nursing 43
- The Culture of Healthcare 43
- Cultural Imposition and Ethnocentrism 44
- Providing Transcultural Care 44

Chapter 4

Promoting Wellness in Health and Illness *52*

Defining Wellness in Health and Illness 53

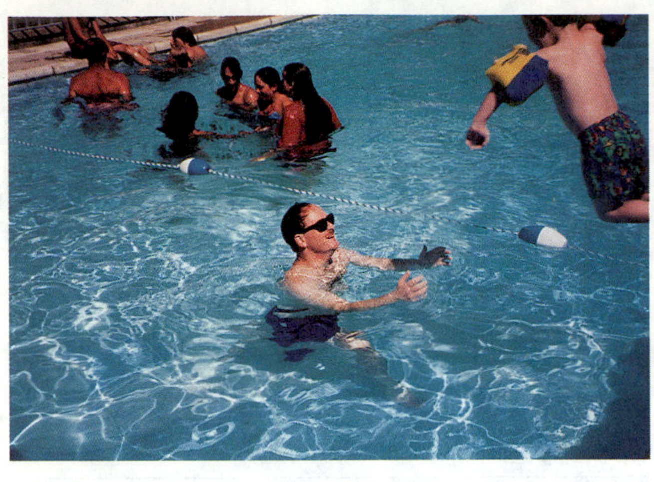

Models of Health and Illness 54
The Health—Illness Continuum 54
High-Level Wellness Model 54
Agent—Host—Environment Model 54
Health-Belief Model 55
Factors Affecting Health and Illness 55
Factors Influencing Health—Illness Status, Beliefs, and Practices 55
Basic Human Needs 57
Self-Concept 58
Promoting Wellness and Preventing Illness 59
Risk Factors 59
Acute and Chronic Illness 59
Effects of Illness on the Family 61
Nursing Care as Preventive Care 61
Levels of Preventive Care 61
Nurse as Role Model 63

Chapter 5

Theoretical Base for Nursing Practice 65

Introduction to Theory 66
Basic Processes in the Development of Nursing Theories 66
Basic Characteristics of Nursing Theory 67
Common Components in Nursing Theories 67
Nursing Theory and Nursing Practice 68
Historical Perspectives and Influences 68
Evolution of Nursing Theory 69
Value of Nursing Theory 69
Conceptual and Theoretical Frameworks for Nursing 69
Dorothy E. Johnson: Behavioral Systems Model 72
Imogene M. King: Open Systems Framework 72
Madeline Leininger: Transcultural Care Diversity and Universality 72
Myra E. Levine: Theory of Nursing 73
Betty Neuman: Healthcare Systems Model 73
Dorothea E. Orem: Self-Care Model 73
Martha E. Rogers: Nursing—A Science of Unitary Man 74
Sister Calista Roy: Roy's Adaptation Model 74
Jean Watson: Nursing—Human Science and Human Care 75
Application of Conceptual and Theoretical Frameworks 75
Client Care Study 75

Chapter 6

Values and Ethics in Nursing 78

Values 79
Development of Values 79
Values Essential to the Professional Nurse 79
Values Clarification 81
Ethics 83
Professional Ethical Conduct 83
Examples of Ethical Problems 86
Nurses and Ethics Committees 92

Chapter 7

Legal Implications of Nursing 95

Legal Concepts 96
Definition of Law 96
Litigation 97
Professional and Legal Regulation of Nursing Practice 97
Credentialing 98
Crimes and Torts 98
Intentional Torts 99
Unintentional Torts 101
Legal Safeguards for the Nurse 104
Contracts 104
Competent Practice 104
Client Education 104
Executing Physician Orders 105
Documentation 106
Adequate Staffing 107
Professional Liability Insurance 108
Risk Management Programs 108
Incident, Variance, or Occurrence Reports 108
Good Samaritan Laws 108
Student Liability 109
Laws Affecting Nursing Practice 109
Occupational Safety and Health 109
National Practitioner Data Bank 109
Reporting Obligations 109
Controlled Substances 109
Discrimination and Sexual Harassment 110
Persons With Disabilities 110
Wills 110
Legal Issues Related to Dying and Death 110

Unit II

Promoting Wellness Across the Lifespan 113

Chapter 8

Developmental Concepts 114

The Nature of Human Growth and Development 115
- Principles of Growth and Development 115

Overview of Developmental Theories 116
- Psychoanalytic Theory: Sigmund Freud 117
- Psychosocial Theory: Erik Erikson 117
- Developmental Tasks: Robert J. Havighurst 119
- Cognitive Development: Jean Piaget 119
- Moral Development: Lawrence Kohlberg and Carol Gilligan 119
- Faith Development: James Fowler 122

Family Influences on Growth and Development 123

Implications for Nursing 124
- Facilitating Effective Family Functioning 124
- Applying Growth and Development Principles 125

Chapter 9

Conception Through Adolescence 128

Environmental and Nutritional Influences 129

Conception and Prenatal Development 129

Neonate (Birth to 28 Days) 130
- Physiologic Development 130
- Common Health Problems 131

Infant: 1 Month to 1 Year 132
- Physiologic Development 132
- Growth Patterns 133
- Cognitive Development 133
- Psychosocial Development 133
- Common Health Problems 133
- Role of the Nurse in Healthcare 134

Toddler: 1 to 3 Years 134
- Physiologic Development 134
- Cognitive Development 136
- Psychosocial Development 136
- Common Health Problems 137
- Role of the Nurse in Healthcare 137

Preschooler: 3 to 6 years 138
- Physiologic Development 138
- Cognitive Development 138
- Psychosocial Development 139
- Moral and Spiritual Development 140
- Common Health Problems 140
- Role of the Nurse in Healthcare 140

School-Age Child: 6 to 12 Years 140
- Physiologic Development 140
- Cognitive Development 140
- Psychosocial Development 140

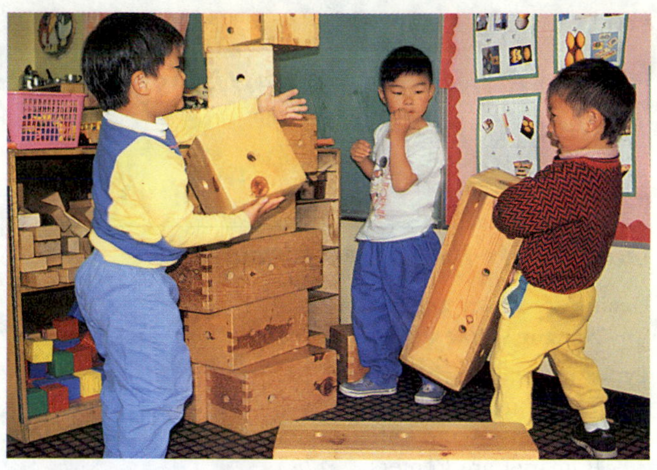

- Moral and Spiritual Development 141
- Common Health Problems 141
- Role of the Nurse in Healthcare 142

Adolescence: 12 to 18 Years 142
- Physiologic Development 142
- Cognitive Development 143
- Psychosocial Development 143
- Moral and Spiritual Development 146
- Common Health Problems 146
- Role of the Nurse in Healthcare 147

Chapter 10

Early, Middle, and Older Adulthood 149

Adult Developmental Theories 150
- Erikson's Developmental Crises 150
- Levinson's Individual Life Structure 150
- Gould's Transformation 150

Early Adulthood: The 20s and 30s 151
- Physiologic Development 151
- Psychosocial Development 151
- Cognitive, Moral, and Spiritual Development 151
- Common Health Problems 152
- The Nurse's Role in Healthcare 153

Middle Adulthood: The 40s and 50s 154
- Physiologic Development 154
- Psychosocial Development 154
- Cognitive, Moral, and Spiritual Development 155
- Common Health Problems 156
- The Nurse's Role in Healthcare 156

Older Adulthood 156
- Physiologic Theories 157
- Cognitive Development 157
- Developmental Theories 160

Paradoxical Aging 163
- The "Graying" Population 163
- An Adaptive Population 163
- Ageism and Common Stereotypes 165

Gerontology and the Healthcare System 166
- Common Health Problems of the Older Adult 166
- The Nurse's Role in Healthcare 168

Unit III

Community-Based Settings for Client Care 173

Chapter 11

Community-Based Healthcare 174

Healthcare Policy and Reform 175
  Nursing's Role in Healthcare Reform 175
Types of Healthcare Settings 175
  The Home Setting 176
  Hospitals: Acute Care Settings 177
  Primary Care Centers 178
  Ambulatory Care Centers and Clinics 178
  Specialized Care Centers 178
  Long-Term Care Facilities 180
  Hospice Services 180
Agencies Providing Care 181
  Voluntary Agencies 181
  Religious Agencies 181
  Government Agencies 181
  Public Health Agencies 182
Frameworks for Care 182
  Managed Care Systems 182
  Case Management 182
  Primary Health Care 183
Collaborative Care 183
Financial Aspects of Healthcare 184
  Federally Funded Healthcare Programs 184
  Group Plans 185
Trends and Issues in Healthcare Delivery 186
  Focus on Self-Care and Wellness 186
  Consumer Movement 187
  Cost Containment 188
  Fragmentation of Care 188
  Changes in Client Care Needs 188
  Healthcare: A Right or a Privilege? 189

Chapter 12

Continuity of Care 191

The Nurse's Role in Providing Continuity of Care 192
Admitting a Client to a Healthcare Setting 192
  Admission to an Ambulatory Healthcare Facility 194
  Admission to the Hospital Unit 194
  Procedure 12-1: *Admitting a Client to a Hospital Unit 196*
Transferring Within and Between Settings 195
Discharging From a Healthcare Setting 200
  Procedure 12-2: *Discharging a Client from a Healthcare Agency 201*
  Leaving the Hospital Against Medical Advice 201

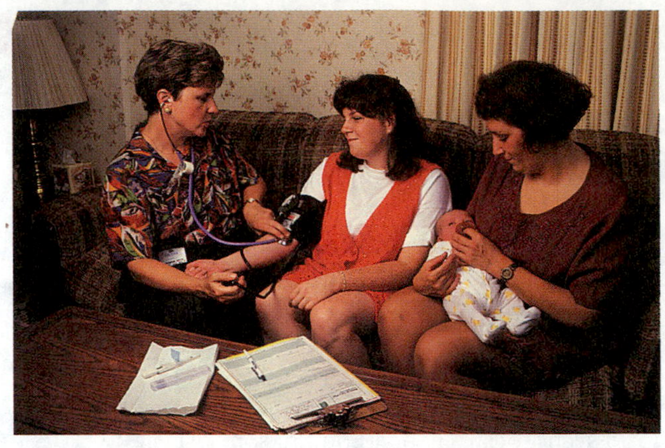

  Discharge Planning 201
Client Care Study 205

Chapter 13

Home Healthcare 207

Definition of Home Healthcare 208
The History of Home Care Nursing 208
Nursing and Home Healthcare 209
  The Unique Role of the Home Care Nurse 210
  Characteristics of the Home Health Nurse 210
  Roles of the Home Health Nurse 211
The Home Visit 213
  The Pre-entry Phase of the Home Visit 213
  The Entry Phase of the Home Visit 213
The Needs of Caregivers in the Home 216
Hospice Nursing in the Home 217
The Future of Home Care 217

Unit IV

The Nursing Process 221

Chapter 14

Introduction to Nursing Process 222

Historical Perspective 223
  Evolution of Nursing Diagnosis 223
Description of Nursing Process 224
  Steps of the Nursing Process 225
  Documenting the Nursing Process 226
Problem Solving and the Nursing Process 226
  Intuitive Problem Solving 227
Characteristics of Nursing Process 228
  Systematic 229
  Dynamic 229
  Interpersonal 229

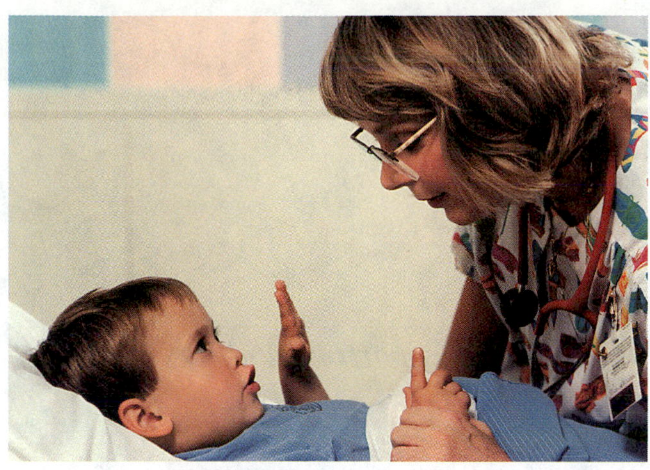

Goal Oriented 229
Universally Applicable 230
Benefits of the Nursing Process 230

Chapter 15

Core Competencies and Critical Thinking 232

Defining the Four Basic Skills 233
Cognitive Competencies 233
Technical Competencies 233
Interpersonal Competencies 233
Ethical/Legal Competencies 235
Developing Cognitive Critical Thinking Competencies 235
Purpose of Thinking 235
Adequacy of Knowledge 236
Potential Problems 236
Helpful Resources 236
Critique of Judgment/Decision 236
Developing Technical Competencies 236
Developing Interpersonal Competencies 238
Promoting Human Dignity and Respect 238
Establishing Caring Relationships 240
Enjoying the Rewards of Mutual Interchange 240
Developing Ethical/Legal Skills 241
Holding Oneself Accountable 241
Reporting Incompetent, Unethical, or Illegal Practices 243
Take the Challenge 244

Chapter 16

Assessing 247

Unique Focus of Nursing Assessment 248
Data Collection 248
Types of Data 248
Characteristics of Data 248
Data Collection Methods 249
Sources of Data 254
Planning Data Collection 260
Comprehensive Versus Focused Data Collection 260
Assessment Priorities 261
Structuring the Assessment 262
Problems Related to Data Collection 262
Data Validation 262
Data Communication 263
Timing 263
Documentation 264

Chapter 17

Diagnosing 266

Unique Focus of Nursing Diagnosis 267
Nursing Diagnosis Versus Medical Diagnosis 267
Nursing Diagnosis Versus Collaborative Problems 267
Data Interpretation and Analysis 269
Recognizing Significant Data 269
Recognizing Patterns or Clusters 269
Identifying Strengths and Problems 270
Reaching Conclusions 272
Formulating and Validating Nursing Diagnoses 273
Writing Nursing Diagnoses 273
What Is Not a Nursing Diagnosis 275
Actual, Potential (High Risk), and Possible Nursing Diagnoses 275
Wellness Diagnoses 275
Validating Nursing Diagnoses 277
Prioritizing Nursing Diagnoses and Documentation 278
Maslow's Hierarchy of Human Needs 278
Client Preference 278
Anticipation of Future Problems 278
Nursing Diagnosis: A Critique 278

Chapter 18

Planning 281

Unique Focus of Nursing Planning 282
Comprehensive Planning 283
Establishing Priorities 284
Writing Goals/Outcomes and Developing Evaluative Strategies 285
Deriving Goals/Outcomes from Nursing Diagnoses 285
Long-Term Versus Short-Term Goals/Outcomes 285
Cognitive, Psychomotor, and Affective Goals 285
Guidelines for Goal/Outcome Writing 286
Common Errors 286
Developing Evaluative Strategy 287
Selecting Nursing Interventions 287
Deriving Nursing Interventions From Nursing Diagnoses 287

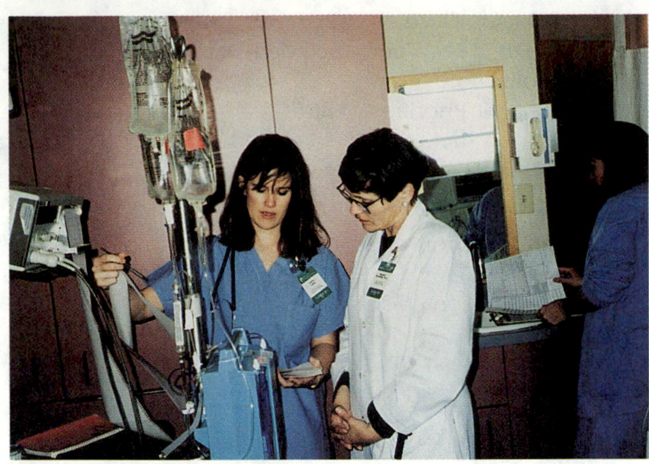

Identifying and Selecting Options 288
Consulting 289
Nursing Orders 289
Writing the Plan of Nursing Care 290
Institutional/Agency Plans of Care 290
Student Plans of Care 291
Problems Related to Planning 296

Chapter 19

Implementing 300

Unique Focus of Nursing Implementation 301
Types of Nursing Interventions 301
The Nursing Interventions Taxonomy Structure 302
Protocols and Standing Orders 302
The Nurse as Coordinator 303
Carrying Out the Plan of Care 303
Prerequisite Core Competencies 304
Determining the Need for Assistance 304
Delegating Nursing Care 304
Promoting Self-Care: Teaching, Counseling, and Advocacy 307
Assisting Clients to Meet Health Goals 307
Responding to the Noncompliant Client 308
Guide for Students 310
Continuing Data Collection 311
Nursing Oneself 311

Chapter 20

Evaluating 313

Unique Focus of Nursing Evaluation 314
Evaluation Criteria and Standards 314
Measuring Client Goal/Outcome Achievement 314
Collecting Evaluative Data 314
Documenting Evaluation 316
Factors That Influence Goal/Outcome Achievement 316
Modifying the Plan of Care 318
Evaluative Programs 322
Quality Assurance 322
From Quality Assurance to Quality Improvement 323
Nursing Audit 324
Self-Evaluation 324
Summary 327

Chapter 21

Documenting, Reporting, and Conferring 329

Documenting Care 330
Guidelines for Effective Documentation 330
Purposes of Client Records 333
Methods of Documentation 333
Formats for Nursing Documentation 337
Potential Legal Problems in Documentation 339
Reporting Care 339
Change-of-Shift Reports 340
Telephone Reports 340
Telephone Orders 341
Transfer and Discharge Reports 341
Reports to Family Members and Significant Others 341
Conferring About Care 341
Consultations and Referrals 341
Nursing Care Conference 342
Nursing Care Rounds 342

Unit V

Roles Basic to Nursing Care 357

Chapter 22

Communicator 358

The Communication Process 359
Forms of Communication 359
Factors Influencing Communication 362
Using Communication in the Nursing Process 364
Using Communication in the Helping Relationship 366
A Helping Relationship Versus a Social Relationship 366
Characteristics of the Helping Relationship 366
Goals of the Helping Relationship 366
Phases of the Helping Relationship 366
Factors Promoting Effective Communication 368
Blocks to Communication 370
Development of Therapeutic Communication Skills 371
Effective Communication Techniques 371
Interpersonal Competencies 375
Assertive Skills 377
Impaired Verbal Communication (NANDA) 377

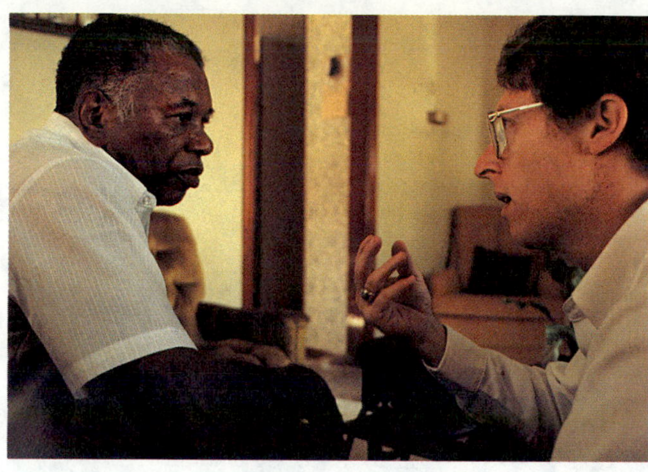

Communicating in Groups 379
Types of Groups 379
Purpose of Groups 382
Roles of Group Members 382

Chapter 23

Teacher and Counselor 386

Aims of Teaching and Counseling 387
Promoting Wellness 387
Preventing Illness 387
Restoring Health 387
Facilitating Coping 387
The Nurse as Teacher 387
Teaching—Learning Process 388
Assessing the Client's Learning Needs 392
Diagnosing the Client's Learning Needs 393
Planning 393
Implementing the Teaching Plan 401
Evaluating Teaching—Learning 402
Documenting 404
The Nurse as Counselor 404
Three Types of Counseling 404

Chapter 24

Leader, Researcher, and Advocate 411

The Nurse as Leader 412
Leadership Dynamics 412
Leadership and Management 416
Models of Client Care Delivery 416
Effecting Change Through Leadership 416
The Nurse Caregiver's Leadership Skills 418
Areas of Leadership 419
Support for Leadership Training 420
The Nurse as Researcher 421
Professionalism 422
Roots of Knowledge 422
Consumerism 423
The Nurse Caregiver's Research Skills 423
The Nurse as Advocate 424
Client's Bill of Rights 425
The Nurse Caregiver's Advocacy Skills 425

Unit VI

Actions Basic to Nursing Care 431

Chapter 25

Vital Signs 432

Frequency of Vital Sign Assessments 433
Body Temperature 433
Regulation of Temperature 434
Normal and Abnormal Body Temperature 435
Equipment 437
Assessment Sites and Methods 439
Procedure 25-1: *Assessing Body Temperature by Oral Method: Glass Clinical Thermometer 440*
Procedure 25-2: *Assessing Body Temperature by Oral Method: Electronic Thermometer 442*
Procedure 25-3: *Assessing Body Temperature by Rectal Method: Glass Thermometer 443*
Procedure 25-4: *Assessing Body Temperature by Axillary Method: Glass Thermometer 447*
Care of Equipment 446
Pulse 446
Regulation of Pulse 446
Normal and Abnormal Pulses 446
Equipment 449
Assessment Sites and Methods 449
Procedure 25-5: *Assessing the Radial Pulse Rate 453*
Procedure 25-6: *Assessing the Apical Pulse Rate 454*
Respiration 455
Regulation of Respiration 456
Normal and Abnormal Respiration 456
Assessment Methods 456
Procedure 25-7: *Assessing the Respiratory Rate 457*
Blood Pressure 456
Physiologic Factors 456
Regulation of Blood Pressure 457
Normal and Abnormal Blood Pressure 458
Equipment 460
Assessment Sites and Methods 461
Procedure 25-8: *Assessing Blood Pressure 463*
Care of Equipment 467
Teaching About Vital Signs for Home Care 468

Chapter 26

Health Assessment 473

Health History 474
Physical Assessment 474

General Guidelines 474
Preparing the Environment 478
Preparing the Client 478
Techniques 478
General Survey 481

Assessment of Body Systems 481

Integument 482
Skin 482
Nails 485
Hair and Scalp 485

Head and Neck 485
Skull 486
Face 486
Eyes and Ears 486
Nose and Sinuses 491
Mouth and Pharynx 492
Neck 493

Thorax and Lungs 495
Inspection 496
Palpation 496
Percussion 496
Auscultation 496

Cardiovascular and Peripheral Vascular Systems 497
Heart 498
Peripheral Vascular System 502

Breasts and Axillae 502
Inspection 503
Palpation 503

Abdomen 503
Inspection 504
Auscultation 506
Percussion 507
Palpation 507

Male and Female Genitalia 507
Female Genitalia 507
Male Genitalia 508

Rectum and Anus 508

Musculoskeletal System 508
Muscles 509

Neurologic System 509
Mental Status 509
Cranial Nerve Function 512
Motor, Sensory, and Reflex Function 514

Documenting the Data 517

The Nurse's Role in Diagnostic Procedures 517

Chapter 27

Safety 524

Factors Affecting Safety 525
Developmental Considerations 525
Lifestyle 527
Mobility 527
Sensory Perception 528
Knowledge 528
Ability to Communicate 528
Health State 528
Psychosocial State 528

Assessing Safety 528
The Client 528
The Environment 529
Specific Risk Factors 529

Diagnosing 533

Planning: Expected Outcomes 534

Implementing 535
Teaching to Prevent Accidents 535
Orienting the Person to Surroundings 539
Preventing Falls 539
Procedure 27-1: *Applying Restraints* *545*
Preventing Fires and Maintaining Fire Safety 543
Preventing Poisoning 544
Preventing Suffocation 548
Preventing Injury From Firearms 548
Preventing Equipment-Related Accidents 549
Preventing Procedure-Related Accidents 550
Filing an Incident Report 551

Evaluating 551

Chapter 28

Asepsis 555

Infection Prevention and Control 556
Infection Cycle 556
Stages of Infection 557
The Body's Defense Against Infection 558
Factors Affecting the Risk of Infection 558
Assessing *559*
Diagnosing *560*
Planning: Expected Outcomes *560*
Implementing *560*
Teaching About Infection Control 560
Using Medical Asepsis 561
Procedure 28-1: *Handwashing* *564*
Controlling Infectious Agents by Sterilization and Disinfection 563

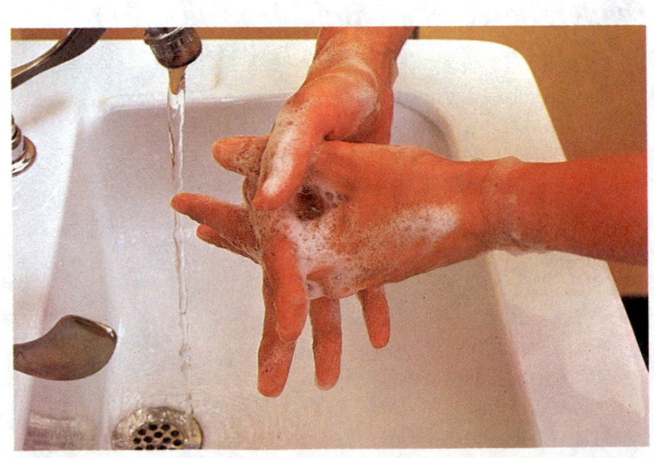

Using Surgical Asepsis 566
Procedure 28-2: *Preparing a Sterile Field 569*
Procedure 28-3: *Donning and Removing Sterile Gloves 573*
Using Isolation and Barrier Techniques for Infection Prevention and Control 571
Procedure 28-4: *Using Personal Protective Equipment 583*
Meeting Psychologic Needs of Clients in Isolation 587
Raising Ethical Concerns About Infection Risks 587
Reporting an Accidental Exposure 588
Using the Infection Control Nurse 589
Evaluating 589

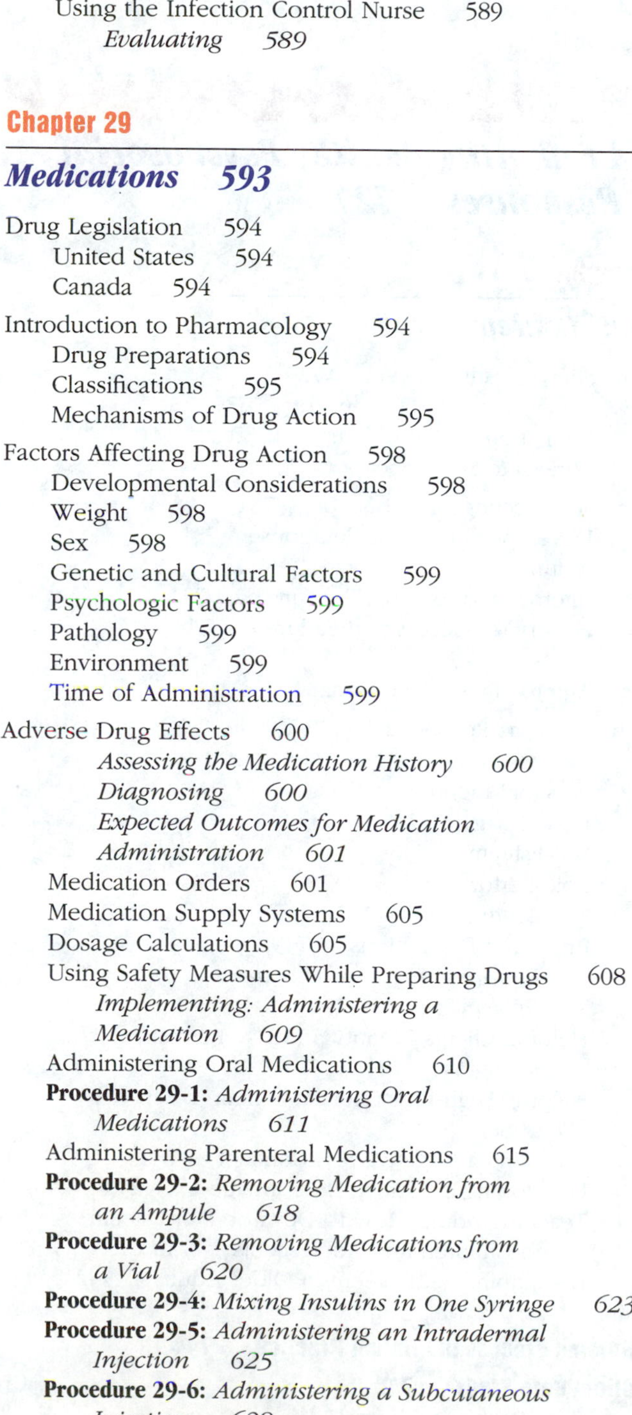

Chapter 29

Medications 593

Drug Legislation 594
United States 594
Canada 594
Introduction to Pharmacology 594
Drug Preparations 594
Classifications 595
Mechanisms of Drug Action 595
Factors Affecting Drug Action 598
Developmental Considerations 598
Weight 598
Sex 598
Genetic and Cultural Factors 599
Psychologic Factors 599
Pathology 599
Environment 599
Time of Administration 599
Adverse Drug Effects 600
Assessing the Medication History 600
Diagnosing 600
Expected Outcomes for Medication Administration 601
Medication Orders 601
Medication Supply Systems 605
Dosage Calculations 605
Using Safety Measures While Preparing Drugs 608
Implementing: Administering a Medication 609
Administering Oral Medications 610
Procedure 29-1: *Administering Oral Medications 611*
Administering Parenteral Medications 615
Procedure 29-2: *Removing Medication from an Ampule 618*
Procedure 29-3: *Removing Medications from a Vial 620*
Procedure 29-4: *Mixing Insulins in One Syringe 623*
Procedure 29-5: *Administering an Intradermal Injection 625*
Procedure 29-6: *Administering a Subcutaneous Injection 628*

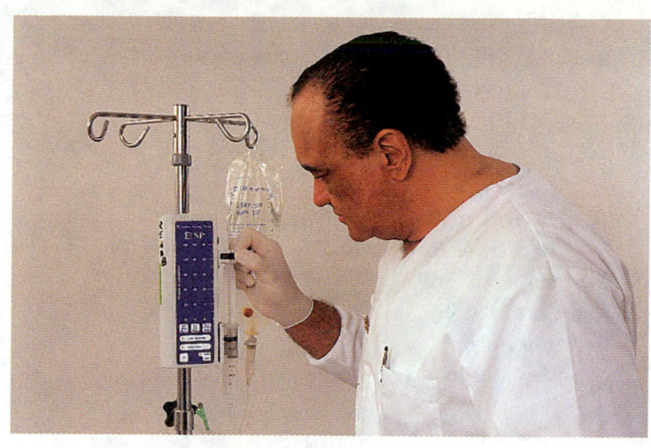

Procedure 29-7: *Administering an Intramuscular Injection 633*
Procedure 29-8: *Adding Medications to an IV Solution Container 638*
Procedure 29-9: *Adding a Bolus IV Medication to an Existing IV 640*
Procedure 29-10: *Administering Medications by IV Piggyback 643*
Procedure 29-11: *Administering IV Medications by Volume-Control Administration Set 645*
Procedure 29-12: *Introducing Drugs Through a Heparin or IV Lock Using the Saline Flush 647*
Administering Topical Medications 642
Procedure 29-13: *Administering an Eye Irrigation 651*
Procedure 29-14: *Administering an Ear Irrigation 654*
Administering Medications by Inhalation 655
Documenting Medication Administration 656
Teaching About Medications and Abuse 661
Evaluating the Client's Response to Medications 662

Chapter 30

Perioperative Nursing 669

The Surgical Experience 670
Phases of the Perioperative Period 670
Classification of Surgical Procedures 670
Anesthesia 671
Informed Consent 672
Ambulatory Surgery 672
Preoperative Nursing Care 673
Assessing 673
Nursing History 673
Physical Assessment 678
Screening Tests 678
Diagnosing 678
Planning: Expected Outcomes 679
Implementing 679
Procedure 30-1: *Preoperative Client Care: Hospitalized Client 680*
Preparing the Client Psychologically 679

Preparing the Client Physically 685
Preparing the Client on the Day of Surgery 685
Evaluating 687

Intraoperative Nursing Care 687
Assessing 687
Diagnosing 687
Planning: Expected Outcomes 687
Implementing 687
Positioning 688
Draping 688
Documenting 688
Transferring to the Postanesthesia Recovery Room 688
Evaluating 688

Postoperative Nursing Care 688
Immediate Postoperative Care 688
Ongoing Postoperative Care 690
Assessing 690
Diagnosing 690
Procedure 30-2: *Postoperative Care When Client Returns to Room 691*
Planning: Expected Outcomes 692
Implementing 693
Preventing Postoperative Complications 694
Promoting a Return to Health 696
Helping the Client Cope 697
Providing Ambulatory Surgery Postoperative Care 697

Wounds and Wound Care 699
Types of Wounds 699
Wound Healing 700
Wound Complications 702
Psychologic Effects of Wounds 703
Assessing the Wound 704
Emergency Wound Assessment and Care 704
Assessing the Surgical Wound 704
Implementing Wound Care 706
Using Dressings 707
Cleaning a Wound and Applying a Clean Dressing 709

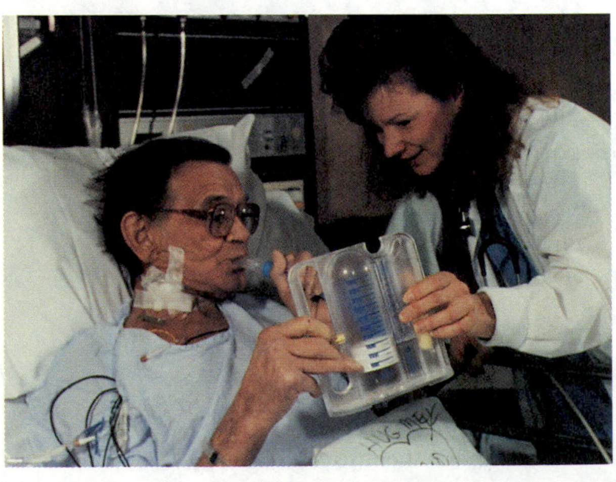

Applying Bandages and Binders 709
Procedure 30-3: *Cleaning a Wound and Applying Clean Dressing 710*
Collecting a Wound Culture 716
Irrigating and Packing a Wound 716
Procedure 30-4: *Collecting a Wound Culture 717*
Documenting Wound Care 716
Changing a Dressing for a Draining Wound 716
Procedure 30-5: *Irrigating a Sterile Wound 718*
Changing Dressings in Special Situations 722
Teaching for Home Care of a Wound 722
Evaluating 723

Unit VII

Promoting Healthy Psychosocial Responses 727

Chapter 31

Self-Concept 728

Overview of Self-Concept 729
Dimensions of Self-Concept 729
Formation of Self-Concept 730
Threats to Self-Concept 731

Factors Affecting Self-Concept 731
Developmental Considerations 731
Culture 731
Internal and External Resources 731
History of Success and Failure 731
Stressors 732
Aging, Illness, or Trauma 733

The Nurse as Role Model 733
Assessing 734
Personal Identity 735
Body Image 736
Self-Esteem 736
Role Performance 737
Diagnosing 737
Important Distinctions 739
Planning: Expected Outcomes 740
Implementing 740
Helping Clients Identify and Use Personal Strengths 741
Helping High-Risk Clients Maintain a Sense of Self 741
Changing a Negative Self-Concept 741
Developing a Positive Body Image 742
Teaching Adults How to Develop Self-Esteem in Children and Adolescents 742
Developing Self-Esteem in Older Adults 742
Evaluating 743

Nursing Process in Clinical Practice 744

Client Care Study 746
Core Competencies 746

Chapter 32

Stress and Adaptation 754

Physiology of Stress and Adaptation 755
Homeostasis 756
Adaptive Responses to Stress 756
Effects of Stress 760
Factors Affecting Stress and Adaptation 763
Sources of Stress 763
Types of Stressors 764
The Nurse as Role Model 764
Assessing Stress 764
Nursing History 765
Physical Assessment 766
Diagnosing 766
Planning: Expected Outcomes 767
Implementing 767
Teaching Healthy Activities of Daily Living 768
Encouraging Use of Support Systems 769
Encouraging Use of Stress Management Techniques 770
Providing Crisis Intervention 770
Addressing Stress in the Nursing Profession 772
Evaluating 772
Nursing Process in Clinical Practice 773
Anxiety 773
Client Care Study 774
Assessment Findings 774
Essential Knowledge and Skills 774
Documentation 775

Chapter 33

Loss, Grief, and Death 780

Loss and Grieving 781
Loss 781
Grieving 781
Dying and Death 782
Responses to Dying and Death 782

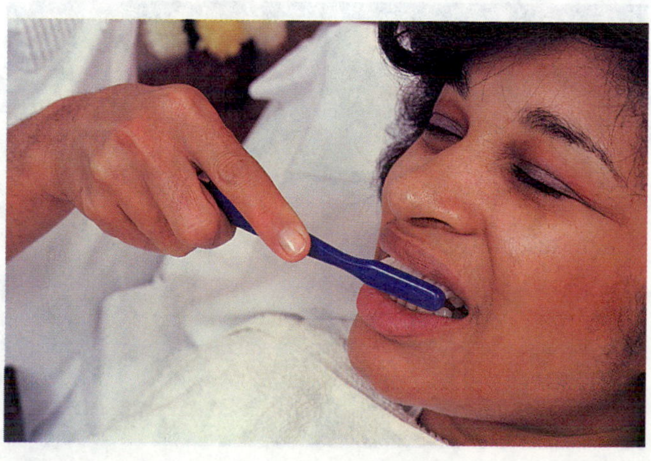

Impact of Terminal Illness 783
Signs of Impending Death 784
Definitions of Death 784
Ethical and Legal Dimensions 784
Factors That Affect Grief and Death 792
Developmental Considerations 792
Family 792
Socioeconomic Factors 792
Cultural Influences 792
Religious Influences 792
Cause of Death 792
The Nurse as Role Model 793
Assessing 794
Diagnosing 794
Response to Loss as the Problem 794
Response to Loss as the Etiology 794
Planning: Expected Outcomes 794
Implementing 797
Developing a Trusting Nurse–Client Relationship 797
Teaching Self-Care and Promoting Self-Esteem 799
Teaching Family Members to Assist in Care 799
Meeting the Needs of Dying Clients 799
Meeting Family Needs 800
Responding to Requests for Suicide Assistance 801
Providing Postmortem Care 801
Evaluating 803
Nursing Process in Clinical Practice 803
Grieving 803
Decisional Conflict 804
Client Care Study 805
Core Competencies 806

Chapter 34

Sensory Stimulation 813

The Sensory Experience 814
Components and Conditions 814
Arousal Mechanism 814
Sensory Alterations 815
Factors Affecting Sensory Stimulation 818
Developmental Considerations 818
Culture 818
Personality and Lifestyle 819
Stress 819
Illness and Medication 819
The Nurse as Role Model 819
Assessing Sensory Functioning 819
Assessing the Sensory Experience 819
Physical Assessment 820
Diagnosing 820
Planning: Expected Outcomes 824
Implementing 825
Preventing Sensory Alteration and Stimulating the Senses 825
Teaching About Sensory Experiences 826

Meeting the Needs of Visually Impaired Clients 826
Meeting the Needs of Hearing Impaired Clients 826
Communicating With a Confused Client 828
Communicating With an Unconscious Client 829
Evaluating 829

Nursing Process in Clinical Practice 830
Sensory Deprivation Related to Inadequate Parenting 830
Chronic Sensory Deprivation Related to Effects of Aging 831

Client Care Study 832
Core Competencies 832

Chapter 35

Sexuality 840

Physiology 841
Female 841
Male 844

Sexual Response Cycle 845
Excitement 846
Plateau 846
Orgasm 846
Resolution 846

Sexual Orientation 846

Sexual Expression 847
Masturbation 848
Sexual Intercourse 848
Oral–Genital Stimulation 848
Celibacy 848
Alternative Forms of Sexual Expression 848

Factors Affecting Sexuality 849
Developmental Considerations 849
Culture 849
Religion 849
Ethics 849
Lifestyle 849
Health State 849
Medications 853

The Nurse as Role Model 855
Sexual Harassment 856
Assessing 857
Sexual History 857
Sexual Dysfunction 859
Physical Assessment 860
Diagnosing 861
Planning: Expected Outcomes 861

Implementing 862
Establishing a Trusting Nurse–Client Relationship 862
Teaching About Sexuality and Wellness 863
Evaluating 863

Nursing Process in Clinical Practice 871
Sexual Dysfunction: Inhibited Sexual Desire 871
Altered Sexuality Patterns: Change in Sexual Expression 872
Knowledge Deficit: Contraceptive Methods 872
Body Image Disturbance Related to Breast Removal 873

Client Care Study 874
Plan of Nursing Care 874

Chapter 36

Spirituality 882

Spirituality and Faith 883
Spirituality and Everyday Living 883
Spirituality, Health, and Illness 884

Major Religions 885
Religions With a Western Philosophy 885
Religions With an Eastern Philosophy 887
Native American Religions 887

Religion and Law, Ethics, and Medicine 889

Factors Affecting Spirituality 889
Developmental Considerations 889
Family 889
Ethnic Background 889
Formal Religion 890
Life Events 890

The Nurse as Role Model 890
Assessing Spirituality 890
Nursing History 890
Nursing Observation 890
Diagnosing 891
Planning: Expected Outcomes 891
Implementing 892
Offering Supportive Presence 892
Facilitating the Client's Practice of Religion 894
Nurturing Spirituality 895
Praying With a Client 895
Counseling the Client Spiritually 895
Contacting a Spiritual Counselor 896
Resolving Conflicts Between Spiritual Beliefs and Treatments 896
Evaluating 897

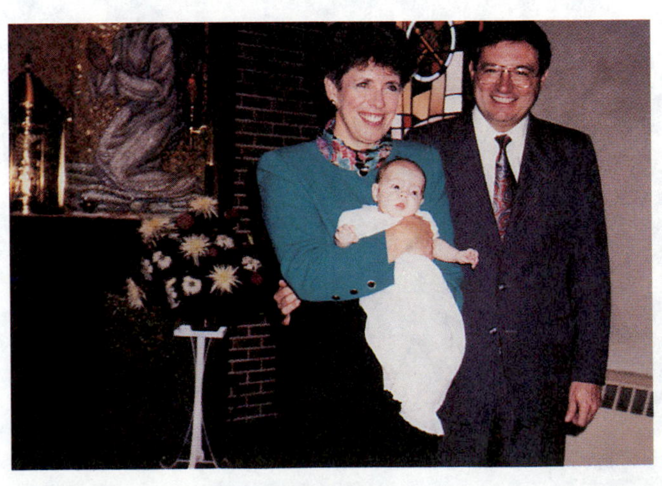

Nursing Process in Clinical Practice 898
Spiritual Distress 898
Client Care Study 899
Assessment Findings 899
Core Competencies 900

Unit VIII

Promoting Healthy Physiologic Responses 909

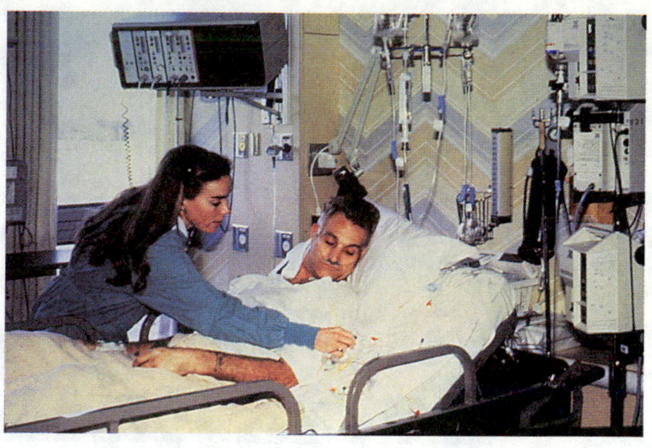

Chapter 37

Hygiene 910

Physiology of the Skin and Its Appendages 911
Functions of Skin and Mucous Membranes 912
Principles of Skin Care 912
Factors Affecting Skin Condition and Personal Hygiene 913
Skin Condition 913
Personal Hygiene 913
The Nurse as Role Model 914
Basic Skin Care and Personal Hygiene 915
Assessing 915
Nursing History 915
Physical Assessment 916
Diagnosing 916
Planning: Expected Outcomes 918
Implementing 918
Providing Scheduled Hygienic Care 918
Helping With Bathing 919
Procedure 37-1: *Giving a Bed Bath 921*
Assisting With Antiembolism Stockings 927
Procedure 37-2: *Applying Antiembolism Stockings 928*
Applying Intermittent Pneumatic Compression Stockings 930
Massaging the Back 930
Bedmaking 930
Procedure 37-3: *Making an Unoccupied Bed 931*
Procedure 37-4: *Making an Occupied Bed 936*
Providing Environmental Care 930
Teaching Clients About Skin Care 940
Evaluating 942
Oral Care 942
Assessing 942
Nursing History 942
Physical Assessment 942
Diagnosing 944
Planning: Expected Outcomes 944
Implementing 944
Administering Oral Hygiene 945
Procedure 37-5: *Assisting the Client With Oral Care 946*
Procedure 37-6: *Providing Oral Care for the Dependent Client 948*
Teaching Oral Hygiene 945
Evaluating 950
Care of the Eyes, Ears, and Nose 950
Assessing 950
Nursing History 950
Physical Assessment 950
Diagnosing 951
Planning: Expected Outcomes 952
Implementing 952
Cleaning the Eyes 952
Caring for the Unconscious Client's Eyes 953
Providing Care of Eyeglasses 953
Providing Care of Contact Lenses 953
Providing Care of an Artificial Eye 954
Providing Ear Care 954
Providing Nose Care 954
Evaluating 954
Hair Care 954
Assessing 954
Nursing History 954
Physical Assessment 955
Diagnosing 956
Planning: Expected Outcomes 956
Implementing 956
Grooming the Hair 956
Shampooing the Hair 956
Caring for Beards and Mustaches 957
Shaving 957
Evaluating 958
Nail and Foot Care 958
Assessing 958
Nursing History 958
Physical Assessment 958
Diagnosing 958
Planning: Expected Outcomes 958
Implementing 959
Providing Care of Fingernails 959
Providing Foot Care 959
Providing Foot Care for the Diabetic Client 960
Evaluating 960

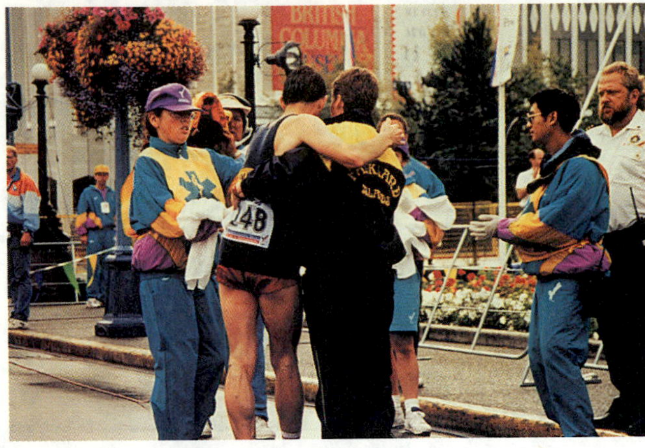

Perineal and Vaginal Care 960
Assessing 960
Nursing History 960
Physical Assessment 962
Diagnosing 962
Planning: Expected Outcomes 962
Implementing 963
Providing Perineal Care 963
Providing Vaginal Care 964
Evaluating 964

Nursing Process in Clinical Practice 965
Bathing/Hygiene Self Care Deficit 965
Altered Oral Mucous Membrane 965

Client Care Study 966
Core Competencies 966

Chapter 38

Skin Integrity and Wound Healing 972

Development of Pressure Ulcers 973
Mechanisms of Development 973
Staging of Pressure Ulcers 974
Factors Affecting Skin Integrity 975
Mobility and Immobility 975
Nutrition and Hydration 975
Moisture on the Skin 975
Mental Status 977
Age 977
Assessing Skin Integrity 977
Nursing History 977
Physical Assessment 979
Assessment Measures 981
Diagnosing 982
Planning: Expected Outcomes 982
Implementing 985
Preventing Pressure Ulcers 985
Treating Pressure Ulcers 985
Evaluating 990

Nursing Process in Clinical Practice 990
Impaired Skin Integrity Related to Presence of Mechanical Factors 990
Assessment Priorities 991
Expected Outcomes 991
Interventions 991

Client Care Study 992
Core Competencies 992

Chapter 39

Activity 998

Physiology of Movement 999
Skeletal System 999
Muscular System 1003
Nervous System 1003
Body Mechanics 1003

Factors Affecting Body Alignment and Mobility 1006
Developmental Considerations 1006
Physical Health 1006
Mental Health 1010
Lifestyle Variables 1010
Attitude and Values 1015
Fatigue and Stress 1016
External Factors 1016

Exercise 1016
Types of Exercise 1016
Effects of Exercise and Immobility on Major Body Systems 1017
Role of Exercise in Preventing Illness and Promoting Wellness 1022
Risks Related to Exercise 1022

The Nurse as Role Model 1023
Assessing 1023
Nursing History 1023
Physical Assessment 1024
Diagnosing 1029
Planning: Expected Outcomes 1031
Implementing 1031
Positioning Clients 1031
Assisting With Range-of-Motion Exercises 1037
Procedure 39-1: *Turning a Client in Bed 1038*
Moving and Lifting the Client 1039
Procedure 39-2: *Moving a Client Up in Bed (One Nurse) 1041*
Procedure 39-3: *Transferring a Client From Bed to Stretcher 1042*
Procedure 39-4: *Transferring a Client From Bed to Stretcher (Three-Carrier Lift) 1044*
Procedure 39-5: *Assisting a Client to Transfer From Bed to Chair 1046*
Logrolling a Client 1048
Using a Hydraulic Lift 1048
Helping Clients Ambulate 1048
Procedure 39-6: *Transferring a Dependent Client From Bed to Chair (Two Nurses) 1049*
Designing Exercise Programs 1056
Teaching Exercise Benefits to Populations at Risk 1058
Evaluating 1059

Nursing Process in Clinical Practice 1059
Activity Intolerance 1059
Impaired Physical Mobility 1060
Risk for Injury: Complications of Immobility 1061
Altered Health Maintenance: Lack of Exercise Program 1061
Client Care Study 1062
Core Competencies 1062

Chapter 40

Rest and Sleep 1072

Physiology of Sleep 1073
Circadian Rhythms 1074
Stages of Sleep 1074
Sleep Cycle 1075
Sleep Requirements and Patterns 1075
Factors Affecting Sleep 1076
Developmental Considerations 1076
Physical Activity 1076
Psychologic Stress 1076
Motivation 1076
Cultural Implications 1076
Diet 1080
Alcohol Intake 1080
Common Sleep Disorders 1081
The Nurse as Role Model 1081
Assessing Rest and Sleep 1083
Sleep History 1083
Sleep Diary 1084
Physical Assessment 1086
Diagnosing 1086
Planning: Expected Outcomes 1088
Implementing 1089
Preparing a Restful Environment 1089
Promoting Bedtime Rituals 1089
Offering Appropriate Bedtime Snacks and Beverages 1090
Promoting Relaxation 1090
Promoting Comfort 1091

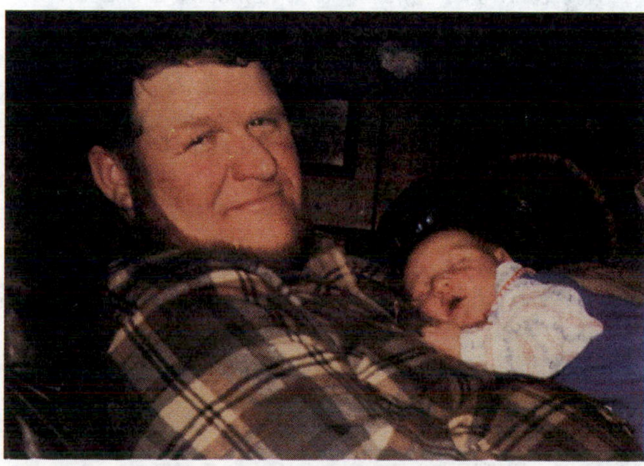

Respecting Normal Sleep–Wake Patterns 1091
Scheduling Nursing Care to Avoid Unnecessary Disturbance 1091
Using Medications to Produce Sleep 1091
Teaching About Rest and Sleep 1091
Evaluating 1091
Nursing Process in Clinical Practice 1093
Sleep Pattern Disturbance: Insomnia 1093
Sleep Pattern Disturbance: Sleep Deprivation 1094
Client Care Study 1095
Core Competencies 1096

Chapter 41

Comfort 1102

The Pain Experience 1103
Definition 1103
Origins of Pain 1103
Transmission of Pain Stimuli 1104
Perception of Pain 1107
Modulation of Pain 1108
Duration, Severity, Quality, and Periodicity of Pain 1108
Responses to Pain 1108
Acute Versus Chronic Pain 1109
Factors Affecting the Pain Experience 1109
Culture 1109
Religious Beliefs 1112
Environment and Support People 1112
Anxiety and Other Stressors 1112
Past Pain Experience 1112
The Nurse as Role Model 1113
Assessing the Pain Experience 1113
Misconceptions 1114
Components of Pain Assessment 1115
Diagnosing 1119
Planning: Expected Outcomes 1122
Chronic Pain 1122
Implementing 1122
Establishing a Trusting Nurse–Client Relationship 1122
Manipulating Factors Affecting the Pain Experience 1122
Initiating Nonpharmacologic Relief Measures 1123
Procedure 41-1: *Giving a Back Massage 1126*
Managing Pharmacologic Relief Measures 1127
Reviewing Additional Pain Control Measures 1137
Considering the Ethical/Legal Responsibility to Relieve Pain 1137
Teaching the Client About Pain 1138
Evaluating 1138
The Pain Experience 1138
Treatment Modalities 1139
Client and Family Response 1139
Nursing Process in Clinical Practice 1139
Pain: Acute Postoperative 1140
Chronic Pain: Malignant 1140

Client Care Study 1142
Core Competencies 1142

Chapter 42

Nutrition *1149*

Principles of Nutrition 1150
Energy Balance 1150
Energy Nutrients 1152
Regulatory Nutrients 1157
How to Choose an Adequate Diet 1158
Food Guide Pyramid 1161
Recommended Dietary Allowance and Recommended Nutrient Intakes 1161
Dietary Recommendations 1162
Food Labeling 1163
Factors Affecting Nutrition 1163
Physiologic Factors That Influence Nutrient Requirements 1163
Sociocultural and Psychologic Factors 1169
Decreased Food Intake 1169
The Nurse as Role Model 1169
Assessing Nutritional Status *1170*
Dietary Data 1171
Medical–Socioeconomic Data 1173
Anthropometric Data 1173
Clinical Data 1174
Biochemical Data 1174
Diagnosing *1175*
Wellness Diagnosis 1176
Planning: Expected Outcomes *1176*
Implementing *1177*
Teaching Nutritional Information 1178
Monitoring Nutritional Status 1179
Stimulating Appetite 1179
Assisting With Eating 1180
Providing Nutrition in Special Situations 1186
Providing Enteral Nutrition 1181
Procedure 42-1: *Inserting a Nasogastric Tube* *1183*
Procedure 42-2: *Administering a Tube Feeding* *1188*
Providing Parenteral Nutrition 1193
Procedure 42-3: *Removing a Nasogastric Tube* *1194*
Procedure 42-4: *Irrigating a Nasogastric Tube Connected to Suction* *1195*
Procedure 42-5: *Monitoring the Blood Glucose Level* *1197*
Evaluating *1198*
Nursing Process in Clinical Practice 1199
Altered Nutrition: More Than Body Requirements—Obesity 1199
Altered Nutrition: Less Than Body Requirements—Iron Deficiency Anemia 1201
Knowledge Deficit—New Therapeutic Diet 1202
Client Care Study 1202
Assessment Findings 1202
Core Competencies 1203

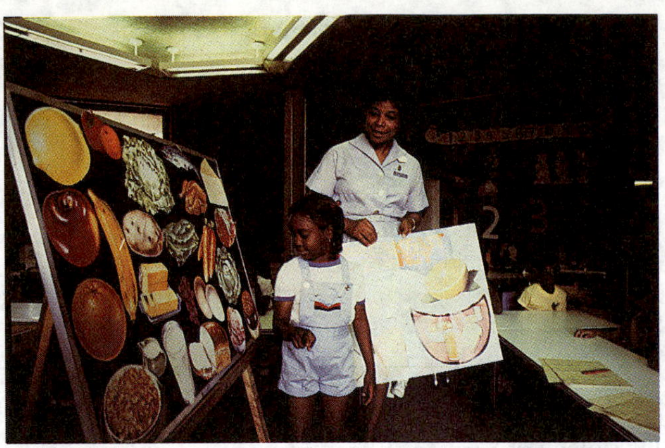

Chapter 43

Urinary Elimination *1211*

Physiology 1212
Kidneys and Ureters 1212
Bladder 1212
Urethra 1212
Act of Micturition 1213
Factors Affecting Micturition 1214
Developmental Considerations 1214
Food and Fluid 1214
Lifestyle 1214
Psychologic Variables 1215
Activity and Muscle Tone 1215
Pathologic Conditions 1216
Medications 1216
The Nurse as Role Model 1216
Assessing *1216*
Nursing History 1216
Physical Assessment 1217
Assessment Measures 1218
Diagnosing *1225*
Planning: Expected Outcomes *1225*
Implementing *1225*
Promoting Normal Urination 1228
Caring for an Incontinent Client 1230
Procedure 43-1: *Offering and Removing a Bedpan or Urinal* *1231*
Catheterizing the Client's Bladder 1235
Procedure 43-2: *Catheterizing the Female Urinary Bladder (Straight and Indwelling)* *1239*
Procedure 43-3: *Catheterizing the Male Urinary Bladder (Straight and Indwelling)* *1243*
Procedure 43-4: *Irrigating the Catheter Using the Closed System* *1246*
Procedure 43-5: *Giving a Continuous Bladder Irrigation* *1247*
Assisting With Urinary Diversions 1251
Procedure 43-6: *Applying a Condom Catheter* *1252*
Evaluating *1253*
Procedure 43-7: *Changing a Stoma Appliance on an Ileal Conduit* *1254*

Nursing Process in Clinical Practice 1255
Altered Urinary Elimination Related to Dysuria 1255
Altered Urinary Elimination Related to Maturational Enuresis 1256
Urinary Retention Related to Varying Etiologies 1256
Risk for Infection Related to Indwelling Catheter 1257
Client Care Study 1258
Core Competencies 1258

Chapter 44

Bowel Elimination 1265

Physiology 1266
Large Intestine 1266
Anal Canal and Anus 1268
Act of Defecation 1268
Normal Defecation 1268
Factors Affecting Bowel Elimination 1268
Developmental Considerations 1268
Daily Patterns 1269
Food and Fluid 1270
Activity and Muscle Tone 1270
Lifestyle 1270
Psychologic Variables 1270
Pathologic Conditions 1270
Medications 1270
Diagnostic Tests 1271
Surgery and Anesthesia 1271
The Nurse as Role Model 1272
Assessing 1272
Nursing History 1272
Physical Assessment 1272
Assisting With Diagnostic Studies 1274
Diagnosing 1277
Planning: Expected Outcomes 1282
Implementing 1282
Promoting Regular Bowel Habits 1282
Teaching About Cathartics, Laxatives, and Antidiarrheals 1285
Decreasing Flatulence 1287
Emptying the Colon of Feces 1287
Procedure 44-1: *Administering a Cleansing Enema 1290*
Managing Fecal Incontinence 1293
Designing and Implementing Bowel Training Programs 1294
Meeting Needs of Clients With Bowel Diversions 1295
Procedure 44-2: *Changing or Emptying an Ostomy Appliance 1298*
Providing Comfort Measures 1301
Evaluating 1301

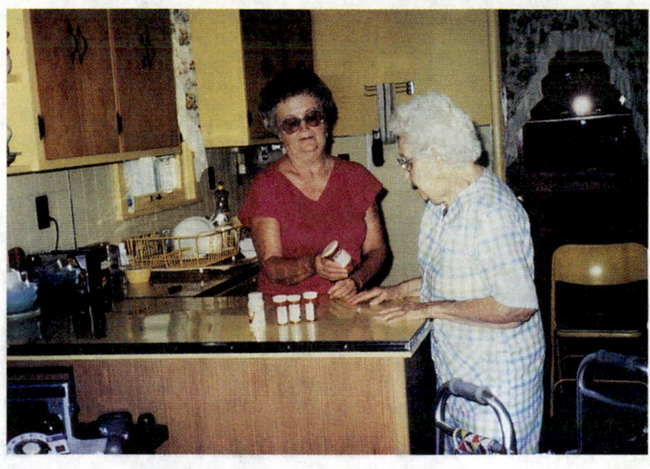

Nursing Process in Clinical Practice 1301
Constipation 1301
Bowel Incontinence 1302
Diarrhea 1303
Client Care Study 1304
Core Competencies 1304

Chapter 45

Oxygenation 1311

Physiology of Respiration 1312
The Respiratory System 1312
Pulmonary Ventilation 1313
Alveolar Gas Exchange 1314
Transport of Respiratory Gases 1315
Control of Respirations 1315
Developmental Variations 1316
Factors Affecting Respiratory Functioning 1316
Levels of Health 1316
Development 1316
Opioids (Narcotic Analgesics) 1317
Lifestyle 1317
Environment 1317
Psychologic Health 1318
The Nurse as Role Model 1318
Assessing Respiratory Functioning 1318
Nursing History 1318
Physical Assessment 1319
Common Methods to Assess Respiratory Functioning 1321
Diagnosing 1324
Procedure 45-1: *Using a Pulse Oximeter 1326*
Planning: Expected Outcomes 1327
Implementing 1328
Teaching About Pollution-Free Environments 1328
Establishing a Trusting Nurse–Client Relationship 1329
Promoting Proper Breathing 1329
Promoting and Controlling Coughing 1331
Promoting Comfort 1332

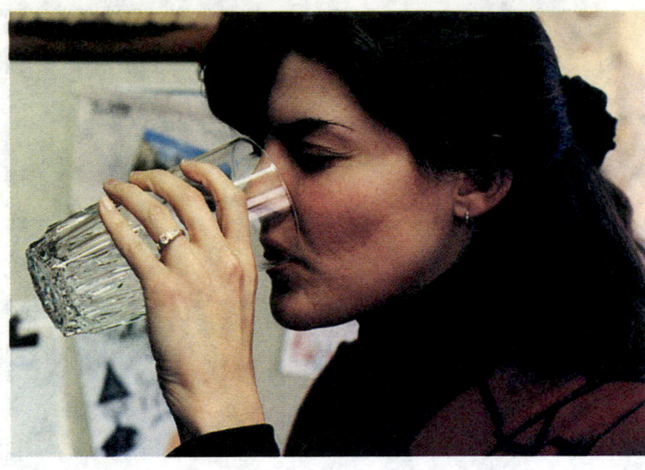

Using Nebulizers 1335
Providing Supplemental Oxygen 1335
Procedure 45-2: *Administering Oxygen by Nasal Cannula 1341*
Procedure 45-3: *Administering Oxygen by Mask 1342*
Using Artificial Airways 1344
Procedure 45-4: *Administering Oxygen by Tent 1345*
Assisting Ventilation 1348
Procedure 45-5: *Suctioning the Nasopharyngeal and Oropharyngeal Areas 1349*
Procedure 45-6: *Suctioning the Tracheostomy 1352*
Clearing an Obstructed Airway 1354
Procedure 45-7: *Providing Tracheostomy Care 1355*
Administering Cardiopulmonary Resuscitation 1358
Hyperbaric Oxygen Therapy 1358
Evaluating 1359

Nursing Process in Clinical Practice 1359
Impaired Gas Exchange 1359
Ineffective Breathing Pattern 1360
Ineffective Airway Clearance 1360

Client Care Study 1361
Core Competencies 1361

Chapter 46

Fluid, Electrolyte, and Acid–Base Balance 1366

Physiology 1367
Body Fluids 1367
Electrolytes 1368
Fluid and Electrolyte Movement 1371
Fluid Balance 1373
Acid–Base Balance 1374
Disturbances in Fluid, Electrolyte, and Acid–Base Balance 1377
Fluid Imbalances 1377
Electrolyte Imbalances 1379
Acid–Base Imbalances 1386
The Nurse as Role Model 1388
Assessing 1388
Nursing History 1389
Physical Assessment 1389
Diagnosing 1396
Planning: Expected Outcomes 1397
Implementing 1398
Preventing Fluid Imbalances 1399
Developing a Dietary Plan 1399
Modifying Fluid Intake 1400
Administering Medications 1402
Administering Intravenous Therapy 1402
Procedure 46-1: *Starting an Intravenous Infusion 1405*
Procedure 46-2: *Regulating IV Flow Rate 1413*
Procedure 46-3: *Changing IV Solution and Tubing 1416*
Procedure 46-4: *Monitoring an IV Site and Infusion 1418*
Procedure 46-5: *Changing an IV Dressing 1421*
Replacing Blood and Blood Products 1423
Procedure 46-6: *Converting a Primary Intravenous Access to a Heparin or Saline Lock 1424*
Procedure 46-7: *Administering a Blood Transfusion 1425*
Giving Total Parenteral Nutrition 1429
Evaluating 1429

Nursing Process in Clinical Practice 1430
The Surgical Client 1430
The Oncology Client 1431

Client Care Study 1432
Core Competencies 1432

Appendices 1438

A. Equivalents 1438
B. Normal Adult Laboratory Values 1441
C. U.S. Nutritional Tables 1447
D. Canadian Nutritional Tables 1449

Glossary 1450

Index 1469

Nursing Procedures, Guidelines, and Techniques

This list includes procedures, boxed displays called *Guidelines for Nursing Care,* and lists of interventions within the text. It does not include interventions and techniques described in paragraphs within the text.

Chapter 3 Culture and Ethnicity

Techniques for practicing transcultural care 44

Chapter 8 Developmental Concepts

Guidelines for Nursing Care: Growth and Development 124

Chapter 10 Early, Middle, and Older Adulthood

Guidelines for Nursing Care: Older Adult 169

Chapter 12 Continuity of Care

Guidelines for Nursing Care: Nurse–Client Relationship 193
Procedure 12-1: Admitting a Client to a Hospital Unit 196
Guidelines for Nursing Care: Height and Weight 200
Procedure 12-2: Discharging a Client From a Healthcare Agency 201

Chapter 17 Diagnosing

Guidelines for writing nursing diagnoses and statements 273

Chapter 18 Planning

Guidelines for Nursing Care: Writing Goals/Outcomes 287
Guidelines for Nursing Care: Developing the Plan of Nursing Care 290

Chapter 19 Implementing

Guidelines for Nursing Care: Implementation 307
Guidelines for Nursing Care: Student Responsibilities 310

Chapter 21 Documenting, Reporting, and Conferring

Guidelines for Nursing Care: Documentation 332
Guidelines for Nursing Care: Safe Computer Charting 337

Chapter 22 Communicator

Guidelines for Nursing Care: Clients of Different Cultures 376
Guidelines for Nursing Care: Communicating in Special Circumstances 381

Chapter 23 Teacher/Counselor

Guidelines for Nursing Care: Teaching–Learning Process 389

Chapter 24 Leader/Researcher/Advocate

Techniques to overcome resistance to change 417

Chapter 25 Vital Signs

Procedure 25-1: Assessing Body Temperature by Oral Method: Glass Clinical Thermometer 440
Procedure 25-2: Assessing Body Temperature by Oral Method: Electronic Thermometer 442
Procedure 25-3: Assessing Body Temperature by Rectal Method: Glass Thermometer 443
Technique for assessing temperature by tympanic membrane 445
Procedure 25-4: Assessing Body Temperature by Axillary Method: Glass Thermometer 447
Technique for obtaining apical pulse 452
Technique for obtaining apical-radial pulse 452
Procedure 25-5: Assessing the Radial Pulse Rate 453
Procedure 25-6: Assessing the Apical Pulse Rate 454
Procedure 25-7: Assessing the Respiratory Rate 557
Procedure 25-8: Assessing Blood Pressure 463
Technique for teaching self-assessment of temperature, pulse, or blood pressure 468

Chapter 26 Health Assessment

Technique for general palpation 479
Technique for assessing pupils 487
Technique for using Weber and Rinne's tests 491
Technique for palpating the thyroid gland 493
Technique for inspecting the cervix and vagina 507

Chapter 27 Safety

Guidelines for Nursing Care: Restraints 543
Guidelines for Nursing Care: Alternatives to Restraints 544
Procedure 27-1: Applying Restraints 545
Guidelines for Nursing Care: Decreasing Equipment-Related Accidents 550

Chapter 28 Asepsis

Teaching about medical asepsis in the home 561
Guidelines for Nursing Care: Medical Asepsis 562
Procedure 28-1: Handwashing 564
Techniques for cleaning equipment 566
Guidelines for Nursing Care: Surgical Asepsis 567
Procedure 28-2: Preparing a Sterile Field 569
Procedure 28-3: Donning and Removing Sterile Gloves 573
Guidelines for Nursing Care: Preventing Needlestick Injuries 578
Procedure 28-4: Using Personal Protective Equipment 583

Chapter 29 Medications

Procedure 29-1: Administering Oral Medications 611
Interventions for administering medications to children 610
Interventions for administering medications to older clients 614
Interventions for administering medications through a nasogastric tube 615
Procedure 29-2: Removing Medication From an Ampule 618
Interventions for mixing medications in one syringe 617
Procedure 29-3: Removing Medications From a Vial 620
Procedure 29-4: Mixing Insulins in One Syringe 623
Procedure 29-5: Administering an Intradermal Injection 625
Procedure 29-6: Administering a Subcutaneous Injection 628
Interventions to reduce discomfort in subcutaneous or intramuscular administrations 636
Procedure 29-7: Administering an Intramuscular Injection 633
Procedure 29-8: Adding Medications to an IV Solution Container 638
Procedure 29-9: Adding a Bolus IV Medication to an Existing IV 640
Procedure 29-10: Administering Medications by IV Piggyback 643
Procedure 29-11: Administering IV Medications by Volume-Control Administration Set 645
Procedure 29-12: Introducing Drugs Through a Heparin or Intravenous Lock Using the Saline Flush 647
Guidelines for Nursing Care: Applying Transdermal Drug Patches 649
Guidelines for Nursing Care: Instilling Eyedrops 650
Procedure 29-13: Administering an Eye Irrigation 651
Guidelines for Nursing Care: Instilling Ear Drops 653
Procedure 29-14: Administering an Ear Irrigation 654
Guidelines for Nursing Care: Instilling Nose Drops 655
Guidelines for Nursing Care: Inserting Vaginal Suppositories or Cream 656
Interventions when medication errors occur 661

Chapter 30 Perioperative Nursing

Procedure 30-1: Preoperative Client Care: Hospitalized Client 680
Interventions for meeting psychologic needs 679
Teaching effective deep-breathing exercises 683
Teaching effective coughing 684
Technique for using incentive spirometry 684
Teaching client leg exercises 684
Preparing the client the day of surgery 685
Procedure 30-2: Postoperative Care When Client Returns to Room 691
Interventions to prevent/monitor cardiovascular complications 694
Interventions for the client in shock 694
Interventions for the client who is hemorrhaging 694
Interventions for the client with thrombophlebitis 694
Interventions for the client with pulmonary embolus 695
Interventions to prevent/monitor respiratory complications 695
Interventions for the client with pneumonia 695
Interventions for the client with atelectasis 696
Interventions to prevent/monitor wound complications 696
Assessments and interventions for bowel elimination 696
Assessments and interventions for urinary elimination 696
Assessments and interventions for nutritional and fluid needs 696
Interventions to provide comfort and rest 697
Interventions to facilitate coping 697
Guidelines for Nursing Care: Emergency Assessment/Care of Specific Wounds 705
Guidelines for Nursing Care: Removing Staples and Sutures 707
Procedure 30-3: Cleaning a Wound and Applying Clean Dressing 710
Procedure 30-4: Collecting a Wound Culture 717
Procedure 30-5: Irrigating a Sterile Wound 718
Techniques for wounds with purulent drainage 722

Chapter 31 Self-Concept

Interventions for a positive body image 742

Chapter 32 Stress and Adaptation

Guidelines for Nursing Care: Reducing Anxiety in Client Entering Healthcare Setting 762
Interventions to reduce the nurse's stress 772

Chapter 34 Sensory Stimulation

Guidelines for Nursing Care: Stimulating the Senses 821
Interventions for communicating with the visually impaired client 826
Interventions for communicating with clients with hearing deficits 826
Interventions for communicating with the confused client 828
Interventions for communicating with the unconscious person 829

Chapter 36 Spirituality

Interventions to facilitate normal spiritual practices in an unfamiliar environment 894

Chapter 37 Hygiene

Interventions for shower and tub baths 919
Interventions for bed self-bathing 920
Procedure 37-1: Giving a Bed Bath 921
Interventions for giving a towel bath 920
Interventions for applying antiembolism stockings 927
Procedure 37-2: Applying Antiembolism Stockings 928
Procedure 37-3: Making an Unoccupied Bed 931
Procedure 37-4: Making an Occupied Bed 935
Procedure 37-5: Assisting the Client With Oral Care 946
Procedure 37-6: Providing Oral Care for the Dependent Client 948
Interventions for flossing the teeth 945
Interventions for cleaning the eyes (encrusted or discharge) 952
Interventions for shampooing hair of client on bedrest 956
Interventions for shaving clients 957
Interventions for fingernail care 959
Interventions for foot care 959
Interventions for foot care for the diabetic client 960
Interventions for perineal care 963
Interventions for therapeutic vaginal douche 964

Chapter 38 Skin Integrity and Wound Care

Guidelines for Nursing Care: Preventing Pressure Ulcers 986
Interventions in wound cleansing 985
Interventions for dressing wounds 986
"No-touch technique" for dressing change 988

Chapter 39 Activity

Interventions for range-of-motion exercises 1037
Interventions for moving and lifting clients 1037
Procedure 39-1: Turning a Client in Bed 1038
Procedure 39-2: Moving a Client Up in Bed (One Nurse) 1041
Procedure 39-3: Moving a Client From Bed to Stretcher 1042
Procedure 39-4: Transferring a Client From Bed to Stretcher (Three-Carrier Lift) 1044
Procedure 39-5: Assisting a Client to Transfer From Bed to Chair 1046
Interventions for logrolling 1048
Interventions for quadriceps drills 1048
Procedure 39-6: Transferring a Dependent Client From Bed to Chair (Two Nurses) 1049
Interventions for dangling 1050
Interventions for clients with walker, cane, brace, or crutches 1053
Interventions for measuring for axillary crutches 1055
Interventions in developing an individualized exercise plan 1056

Chapter 41 Comfort

Interventions to guide the client to use imagery 1124
Procedure 41-1: Giving a Back Massage 1126
Interventions for effective individualized pain management 1130
Guidelines for Nursing Care: Epidural Opioids 1133
Interventions in home care use of oral morphine 1137

Chapter 42 Nutrition

Interventions for diet instructions 1158
Interventions for stimulating appetite 1179
Interventions for assisting with eating 1180
Interventions to provide comfort for NPO clients 1181
Interventions for aspirating fluid from small-bore tubes 1182
Procedure 42-1: Inserting a Nasogastric Tube 1183
Guidelines for Nursing Care: Checking Placement of Feeding Tube 1187
Procedure 42-2: Administering a Tube Feeding 1188
Interventions contributing to successful tube feeding 1191
Guidelines for Nursing Care: Preventing Complications in Enteral Feeding 1191
Interventions in parenteral nutrition therapy 1193
Procedure 42-3: Removing a Nasogastric Tube 1194
Procedure 42-4: Irrigating a Nasogastric Tube Connected to Suction 1195
Procedure 42-5: Monitoring the Blood Glucose Level 1197

Chapter 43 Urinary Elimination

Interventions for measuring urine output when the client has an indwelling catheter 1219
Interventions for obtaining a clean-catch midstream urine specimen from a female client 1220
Interventions for obtaining a clean-catch midstream urine specimen from a male client 1222
Interventions to stimulate urination 1228
Procedure 43-1: Offering and Removing a Bedpan or Urinal 1231
Interventions for inserting an indwelling catheter 1237
Procedure 43-2: Catheterizing the Female Urinary Bladder (Straight and Indwelling) 1239
Procedure 43-3: Catheterizing the Male Urinary Bladder (Straight and Indwelling) 1243

Procedure 43-4: Irrigating the Catheter Using the Closed System 1246
Interventions to care for the client with an indwelling catheter 1246
Procedure 43-5: Giving a Continuous Bladder Irrigation 1247
Interventions for removing the indwelling catheter 1250
Procedure 43-6: Applying a Condom Catheter 1252
Procedure 43-7: Changing a Stoma Appliance on an Ileal Conduit 1254

Chapter 44 Bowel Elimination

Guidelines for Nursing Care: Testing for Fecal Occult Blood 1276
Interventions for removing fecal impaction digitally 1289
Procedure 44-1: Administering a Cleansing Enema 1290
Guidelines for Nursing Care: Inserting a Rectal Suppository 1293
Interventions in a bowel training program 1294
Interventions in ileostomy and colostomy care 1295
Procedure 44-3: Changing or Emptying an Ostomy Appliance 1298
Teaching the ostomy client about medications 1301

Chapter 45 Oxygenation

Procedure 45-1: Using a Pulse Oximeter 1326
Guidelines for Nursing Care: Using an Incentive Spirometer 1330
Interventions for percussing by cupping 1332
Interventions in vibration 1333
Interventions for postural drainage 1333
Guidelines for Nursing Care: Using a Nebulizer Device 1337
Precautions for oxygen administration 1338
Guidelines for Nursing Care: Transporting a Client With a Portable Oxygen Cylinder 1339
Procedure 45-2: Administering Oxygen by Nasal Cannula 1341
Procedure 45-3: Administering Oxygen by Mask 1342
Procedure 45-4: Administering Oxygen by Tent 1345
Guidelines for Nursing Care: Inserting an Oropharyngeal Airway 1346
Procedure 45-5: Suctioning the Nasopharyngeal and Oropharyngeal Areas 1349
Procedure 45-6: Suctioning the Tracheostomy 1352
Procedure 45-7: Providing Tracheostomy Care 1355

Chapter 46 Fluid, Electrolyte, and Acid–Base Balance

Guidelines for Nursing Care: Measuring Fluid Intake and Output 1397
Interventions in preventing fluid imbalance 1399
Interventions for increasing fluids 1400
Interventions for restricting fluids 1401
Procedure 46-1: Starting an Intravenous Infusion 1405
Guidelines for Nursing Care: Caring for a Client With a PICC 1410
Interventions in selecting an IV site 1411
Procedure 46-2: Regulating IV Flow Rate 1413
Procedure 46-3: Changing IV Solution and Tubing 1416
Procedure 46-4: Monitoring an IV Site and Infusion 1418
Procedure 46-5: Changing an IV Dressing 1421
Procedure 46-6: Converting a Primary Intravenous Access to a Heparin or Saline Lock 1424

Nursing Process in Clinical Practice

Nursing care is developed around the following nursing diagnoses in clinical chapters of this book. Nursing diagnoses used in Nursing Plans of Care are shown in the next list.

Chapter 31 Self-Concept

Self-Concept Disturbance 738

Chapter 32 Stress and Adaptation

Stress 767

Chapter 33 Loss, Grief, and Dying

Grieving 796
Decisional Conflict 804

Chapter 34 Sensory Stimulation

Sensory Deprivation 830
Chronic Sensory Deprivation 831

Chapter 35 Sexuality

Sexual Dysfunction 871
Altered Sexuality Patterns 872
Knowledge Deficit 872
Body Image Disturbance 873

Chapter 36 Spirituality

Spiritual Distress 873

Chapter 37 Hygiene

Bathing/Hygiene Self-Care Deficit 965
Altered Oral Mucous Membrane 965

Chapter 38 Skin Integrity and Wound Care

Impaired Skin Integrity 990

Chapter 39 Activity

Activity Intolerance 1059
Impaired Physical Mobility 1060
Risk for Injury 1061
Altered Health Maintenance 1061

Chapter 40 Rest and Sleep

Sleep Pattern Disturbance: Insomnia 1093
Sleep Pattern Disturbance: Sleep Deprivation 1094

Chapter 41 Comfort

Pain: Acute Postoperative Pain 1140
Chronic Pain: Malignant 1140

Chapter 42 Nutrition

Altered Nutrition: More Than Body Requirements 1199
Altered Nutrition: Less Than Body Requirements 1201
Knowledge Deficit 1202

Chapter 43 Urinary Elimination

Altered Urinary Elimination (related to dysuria) 1255
Altered Urinary Elimination (related to maturational enuresis) 1256
Urinary Retention 1256
Risk for Infection 1257

Chapter 44 Bowel Elimination

Constipation 1301
Bowel Incontinence 1302
Diarrhea 1303

Chapter 45 Oxygenation

Impaired Gas Exchange 1359
Ineffective Breathing Pattern 1360
Ineffective Airway Clearance 1360

Chapter 46 Fluid, Electrolyte, and Acid–Base Balance

Fluid Volume Deficit 1430
Fluid Volume Excess 1430

Nursing Plans of Care

Nursing Plans of Care have been developed to accompany a Client Care Study at the end of each clinical chapter. The Plans of Care are based on the following nursing diagnoses:

Chapter 31 Self-Concept

Situational Low Self-Esteem 747

Chapter 32 Stress and Adaptation

Anxiety 775

Chapter 33 Loss, Grief, and Dying

Caregiver Role Strain 806

Chapter 34 Sensory Stimulation

Sensory/Perceptual Alteration 833

Chapter 35 Sexuality

Knowledge Deficit 874

Chapter 36 Spirituality

Spiritual Distress 900

Chapter 37 Hygiene

Self-Care Deficit 967

Chapter 38 Skin Integrity and Wound Care

Impaired Skin Integrity 992

Chapter 39 Activity

Impaired Physical Mobility 1060

Chapter 40 Rest and Sleep

Sleep Pattern Disturbance 1093

Chapter 41 Comfort

Ineffective Individual Coping 1143

Chapter 42 Nutrition

Altered Nutrition: Less Than Body Requirements 1199

Chapter 43 Urinary Elimination

Functional Incontinence 1259

Chapter 44 Bowel Elimination

Diarrhea 1303

Chapter 45 Oxygenation

Ineffective Airway Clearance 1360

Chapter 46 Fluid, Electrolyte, and Acid–Base Balance

Fluid Volume Deficit 1430

Summary of Special Recurring Displays

Special displays (referred to as boxes) recur throughout the text. The following are helpful to the student of nursing. Another special display, *Guidelines for Nursing Care,* is included in the list of interventions and procedures.

Chapter 1 Introduction to Nursing

Computer Applications in Nursing 12

Chapter 2 Basic Human Needs: Individual, Family, and Community

Research in Nursing: Making a Difference 25
Examples of Nursing Diagnoses 26

Chapter 3 Culture and Ethnicity

Through the Eyes of a Student 34
Nursing Today: Challenges and Solutions 36
Examples of Nursing Diagnoses 39
Research in Nursing: Making a Difference 40
Developing Critical Thinking Skills 42
Focused Assessment 45

Chapter 4 Promoting Wellness in Health and Illness

Nursing Today: Challenges and Solutions 58
Focus on the Older Adult 60

Chapter 6 Values and Ethics in Nursing

Helpscan 91

Chapter 7 Legal Implications of Nursing

Computer Applications in Nursing 101

Chapter 8 Developmental Theories

Research in Nursing: Making a Difference 124

Chapter 9 Conception Through Adolescence

Nursing Today: Challenges and Solutions 130
Examples of Nursing Diagnoses 134
Examples of Nursing Diagnoses 146

Chapter 10 Early, Middle, and Older Adulthood

Examples of Nursing Diagnoses 154
Research in Nursing: Making a Difference 158
Focus on the Older Adult 159
Through the Eyes of a Student 163
Example of Nursing Diagnoses 167

Chapter 11 Community-Based Healthcare

Nursing Today: Challenges and Solutions 187
Computer Applications in Nursing 187

Chapter 13 Home Healthcare

Examples of Nursing Diagnoses 215
Focused Assessment Guide 216
Through the Eyes of the Family Caregiver 215

Chapter 14 Introduction to Nursing Process

Through the Eyes of a Client 224
Through the Eyes of a Client 229
Computer Applications in Nursing 230

Chapter 15 Essential Knowledge and Skills in Nursing

Through the Eyes of a Student 235
Through the Eyes of a Student 236
Developing Critical Thinking Skills 237

Chapter 16 Assessing

Through the Eyes of a Student 251
Through the Eyes of a Student 261

Chapter 18 Planning

Computer Applications in Nursing 297

Chapter 19 Implementing

Through the Eyes of the Family Caregiver 306
Developing Critical Thinking Skills 309
Through the Eyes of a Student 310
Computer Applications in Nursing 311

Chapter 20 Evaluating

Computer Applications in Nursing 324

Chapter 21 Documenting, Reporting, and Conferring

Computer Applications in Nursing 342

Chapter 22 Communicator

Research in Nursing: Making a Difference 363
Through the Eyes of a Student 365
Through the Eyes of a Client 372
Computer Applications in Nursing 382

Chapter 23 Teacher and Counselor

Research in Nursing: Making a Difference 391
Computer Applications in Nursing 401
Computer Applications in Nursing 403
Examples of Nursing Diagnoses 409

Chapter 24 Leader, Researcher, and Advocate

Computer Applications in Nursing 419
Computer Applications in Nursing 424

Chapter 25 Vital Signs

Focus on the Older Adult 434
Through the Eyes of a Student 448
Helpscan 468

Chapter 26 Health Assessment

Focus on the Older Adult 479
Focus on the Older Adult 482
Focused Assessment Guide 489

Chapter 27 Safety

Research in Nursing: Making a Difference 527
Promoting Wellness 529
Helpscan 536
Home Care: Bridging the Gap 540
Focus on the Older Adult 549
Home Care: Bridging the Gap 549

Chapter 28 Asepsis

Focus on the Older Adult 559
Promoting Wellness 579
Helpscan 586
Through the Eyes of a Student 587
Nursing Today: Challenges and Solutions 588

Chapter 29 Medications

Focus on the Older Adult 598
Focused Assessment Guide 601
Research in Nursing: Making a Difference 597
Through the Eyes of a Student 595
Promoting Wellness 602
Helpscan 662

Chapter 30 Perioperative Nursing

Focus on the Older Adult 675
Research in Nursing: Making a Difference 677
Through the Eyes of a Student 689
Developing Critical Thinking Skills 698
Focus on the Older Adult 703

Chapter 31 Self-Concept

Research in Nursing: Making a Difference 730
Promoting Wellness 733
Focused Assessment Guide 735
Nursing Diagnoses for Common Problems 738
Home Care: Bridging the Gap 740
Helpscan 742
Focus on the Older Adult 744

Chapter 32 Stress and Adaptation

Helpscan 758
Promoting Wellness 765
Focused Assessment Guide 765
Focused Assessment Guide 766
Nursing Diagnoses for Common Problems 767
Research in Nursing: Making a Difference 768
Through the Eyes of a Student 769
Developing Critical Thinking Skills 771

Chapter 33 Loss, Grief, and Dying

Computer Applications in Nursing 785
Promoting Wellness 793
Focused Assessment Guide 795
Nursing Diagnoses for Common Problems 796
Research in Nursing: Making a Difference 798
Helpscan 800
Home Care: Bridging the Gap 801
Through the Eyes of a Student 802

Chapter 34 Sensory Stimulation

Research in Nursing: Making a Difference 820
Focused Assessment Guide 821
Nursing Diagnoses for Common Problems 823
Helpscan 825
Focus on the Older Adult 829

Chapter 35 Sexuality

Research in Nursing: Making a Difference 847
Developing Critical Thinking Skills 852
Promoting Wellness 857
Focused Assessment Guide 858
Focus on the Older Adult 859
Nursing Diagnoses for Common Problems 862
Through the Eyes of a Student 863

Helpscan 864
Home Care: Bridging the Gap 869

Chapter 36 Spirituality

Promoting Wellness 891
Focused Assessment Guide 892
Nursing Diagnoses for Common Problems 893
Helpscan 896
Research in Nursing: Making a Difference 897

Chapter 37 Hygiene

Focus on the Older Adult 914
Focused Assessment Guide 915
Through the Eyes of a Student 919
Research in Nursing: Making a Difference 943
Helpscan 952
Through the Eyes of a Student 959
Promoting Wellness 961

Chapter 38 Skin Integrity and Wound Care

Research in Nursing: Making a Difference 978
Focused Assessment Guide 981
Helpscan 988
Home Care: Bridging the Gap 990

Chapter 39 Activity

Research in Nursing: Making a Difference 1020
Focus on the Older Adult 1022
Promoting Wellness 1024
Focused Assessment Guide 1025
Nursing Diagnoses for Common Problems 1030
Helpscan 1031

Chapter 40 Rest and Sleep

Promoting Wellness 1084
Focused Assessment Guide 1085
Nursing Diagnoses for Common Problems 1087
Focus on the Older Adult 1089
Research in Nursing: Making a Difference 1090
Developing Critical Thinking Skills 1092
Helpscan 1093

Chapter 41 Comfort

Research in Nursing: Making a Difference 1111
Promoting Wellness 1113
Focused Assessment Guide 1116
Nursing Diagnoses for Common Problems 1121
Through the Eyes of the Client 1124
Focus on the Older Adult 1135
Helpscan 1139

Chapter 42 Nutrition

Focus on the Older Adult 1165
Promoting Wellness 1171
Focused Assessment Guide 1174
Nursing Diagnoses for Common Problems 1178
Helpscan 1179
Research in Nursing: Making a Difference 1180
Through the Eyes of a Student 1182

Chapter 43 Urinary Elimination

Research in Nursing: Making a Difference 1215
Promoting Wellness 1217
Focused Assessment Guide 1218
Home Care: Bridging the Gap 1223
Nursing Diagnoses for Common Problems 1227
Focus on the Older Adult 1229
Developing Critical Thinking Skills 1233
Through the Eyes of a Student 1236
Helpscan 1250

Chapter 44 Bowel Elimination

Research in Nursing: Making a Difference 1271
Promoting Wellness 1272
Focused Assessment Guide 1273
Nursing Diagnoses for Common Problems 1283
Helpscan 1284
Focus on the Older Adult 1285
Through the Eyes of a Student 1288

Chapter 45 Oxygenation

Research in Nursing: Making a Difference 1317
Promoting Wellness 1318
Focused Assessment Guide 1320
Nursing Diagnoses for Common Problems 1328
Focus on the Older Adult 1329
Helpscan 1359

Chapter 46 Fluid, Electrolyte, and Acid–Base Balance

Promoting Wellness 1389
Focused Assessment Guide 1390
Nursing Diagnoses for Common Problems 1398
Focus on the Older Adult 1399
Research in Nursing: Making a Difference 1401
Helpscan 1412

Nursing is both an art and a science. It is a profession that uses specialized skills and knowledge to give care to the whole person in both health and illness and in a variety of practice settings. Unit I introduces concepts necessary to provide nurses with the foundations for nursing practice by defining nursing as a whole. Chapters in this unit introduce the profession of nursing; basic needs of individuals, their families, and the community; culture and ethnicity; promotion of wellness in both health and illness; the theoretical base for nursing; and values, with their ethical and legal implications for nursing practice.

Historical perspectives, educational preparation, professional organizations, and guidelines for professional nursing practice serve as a base for understanding what nursing is and how it is organized. An understanding of basic human needs and the individualized definitions of wellness and illness prepare the nurse to integrate the human dimensions—the physical, intellectual, emotional, sociocultural, spiritual, and environmental aspects of each person—into the care given to promote wellness, prevent illness, restore health, and facilitate coping with altered function or death. Knowledge of the varied methods of care delivery is necessary in today's complex healthcare system.

Nursing theories provide a base for nursing practice, defining the rationale for nursing actions and offering a focus for nursing care. An understanding of the influence of values on human behavior and of the ethical dimensions of nursing practice is essential to responsible and accountable client care. Finally, sensitivity to the legal implications of professional nursing practice is imperative in today's culture.

Unit I explores the foundations for nursing practice from the perspective of the nurse and a holistic understanding of the client. Students of nursing are introduced to a challenging and rewarding profession, and are provided with a knowledge base to ground the development of caregiving skills and professional relationships and behaviors.

Foundations for Nursing Practice

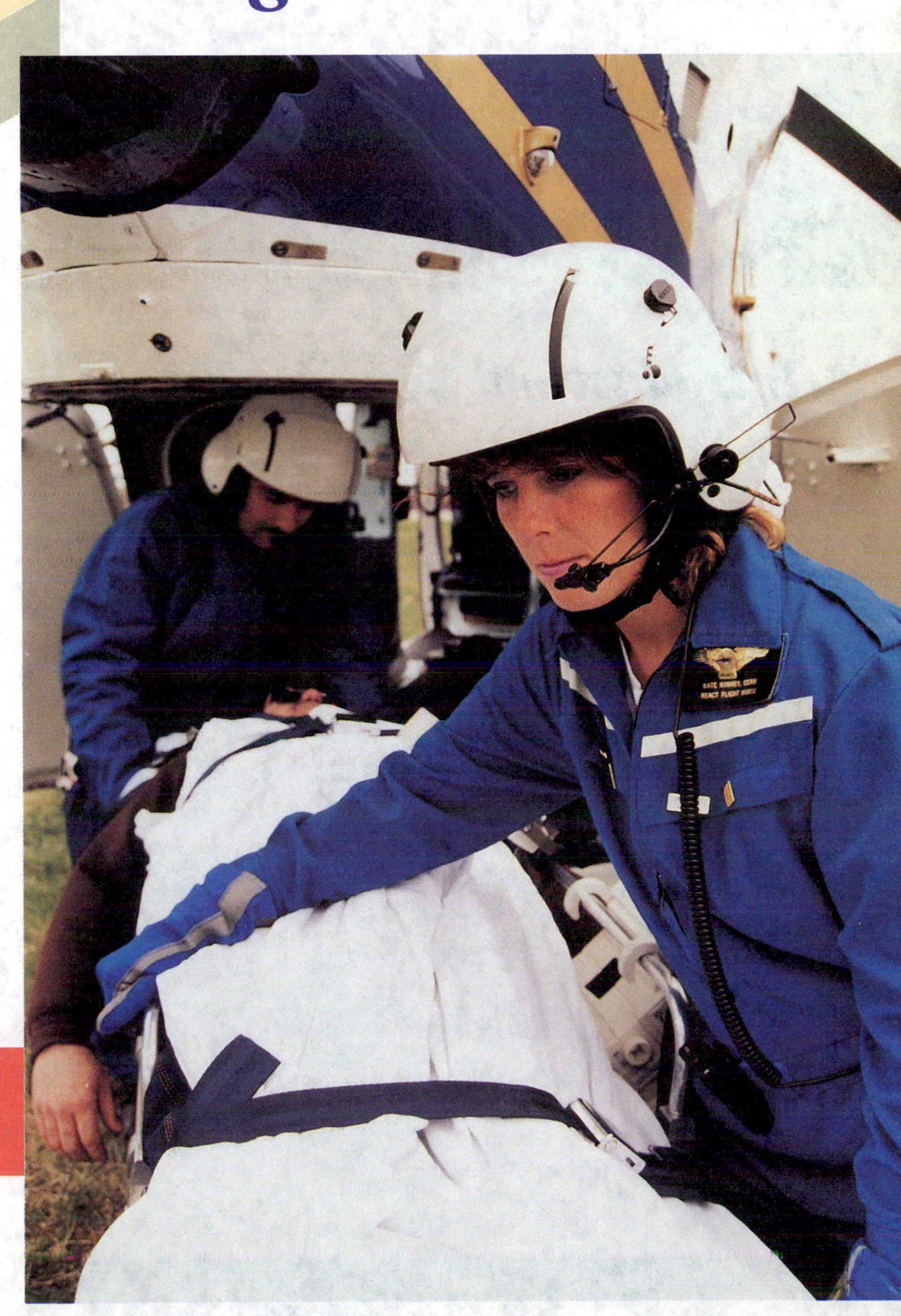

"Basic to any philosophy of nursing seems to be these three concepts: (1) reverence for the gift of life; (2) respect for the dignity, worth, autonomy, and individuality of each human being; (3) resolution to act dynamically in relation to one's beliefs."

Ernestine Wiedenbach (1900–)
a faculty member at Yale University School of Nursing, where she developed her model of nursing from years of experience in various nursing positions

Unit I

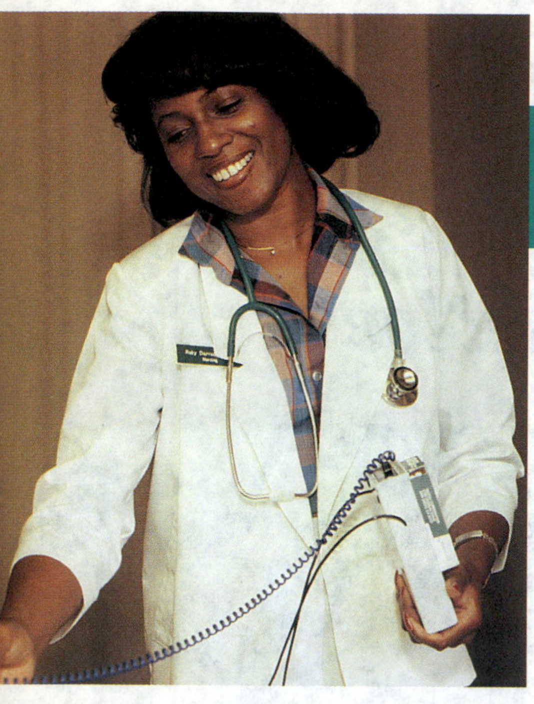

Chapter 1

Introduction to Nursing

Objectives

After studying this chapter, the learner should be able to:

Define key terms used in the chapter.

Describe the historical background, the definitions of nursing, and the status of nursing as a profession and as a discipline.

Identify the aims of nursing as they interrelate to facilitate maximum function and quality of life for clients.

Describe the various levels of educational preparation in nursing.

Discuss the effect of nursing organizations, standards of nursing practice, nurse practice acts, and the nursing process on the practice of nursing.

Identify current trends in nursing.

Key Terms

continuing education
dependent nursing actions
discipline
independent nursing actions
in-service education
interdependent nursing actions
licensure
nurse practice act
nursing
nursing process
profession
standards
wellness

What is *nursing*? Consider the following examples of who nurses are and what they do:

- Delton Nix, RN, graduated from an associate degree nursing program 3 years ago and is now working full-time in a hospital medical unit while he attends school part-time toward a baccalaureate degree in nursing; his goal is to become a nurse anesthetist.
- Mary Cunningham, RN, graduated from a diploma program 20 years ago and has been the director of nurses at a nursing home in a small rural town since graduation.
- Jeiping Wu, RN, FNP, is a graduate of a master's program in nursing, specializing as a family nurse practitioner. She has an independent practice in a rural primary health clinic.
- Samuel Cohen, LPN, decided to follow his life's dream to become a nurse after 20 years as a postal worker. After examining all his options and goals, he completed a practical nursing program and is now a member of an emergency ambulance crew in a large city.
- Amy Orlando, RN, BSN, graduated from a baccalaureate in nursing program 2 years ago and recently began a new job in an urban community health service.
- Roxanne McDaniel, RN, PhD, has a doctorate in nursing; she teaches and conducts research at a large university.

These examples illustrate how difficult it is to describe nursing clearly. If your class were asked to complete the sentence, "Nursing is . . . ," many different responses would be given, because each person would provide an answer based on his or her own personal experience and knowledge of nursing at that time. As you progress toward graduation and as you practice nursing after graduation, those definitions will change, reflecting changes within yourself as you learn about and experience nursing.

Most basically defined, **nursing** is the care of others. That care may involve any number of activities, ranging from carrying out complicated technical procedures to something as seemingly simple as holding a hand. All nursing actions focus on the person receiving care and are a blend of the art and the science of nursing. The *science* of nursing is the knowledge base for the care that is given, and the *art* of nursing is the skilled application of that knowledge to help others reach maximum function and quality of life.

This chapter introduces you to nursing as a whole, including a brief history of nursing from its beginnings to the present, and to definitions of nursing formulated by nursing leaders and nursing organizations. Educational preparation, professional organizations, and guidelines for professional nursing practice serve as a base for understanding what nursing is and how it is organized. Because nursing is a part of an ever-changing society, a brief discussion of current trends in nursing is also included.

Nursing: An Emerging Profession and Discipline

Historical Background

From the beginning of time, the nurse has been regarded as a caregiver. This role has traditionally been defined by groups, communities, and societies in which nursing was practiced. Healthcare and nursing as we currently know it are based on what has happened in the past.

In early civilizations, humans believed that illness had supernatural causes. The theory of animism was developed in an attempt to understand the cause of the mysterious changes in bodily functions. This theory was based on the belief that everything in nature was alive with invisible forces and endowed with power. Good spirits brought health; evil spirits brought sickness and death. The roles of the physician and the nurse were separate and distinct. The physician was the medicine man who treated disease by chanting, inspiring fear, or opening the skull to release evil spirits (Dolan, Fitzpatrick, & Herrmann, 1983). The nurse usually was the mother who cared for her family during sickness by providing physical care and herbal remedies. This nurturing and caring role of the nurse has continued to the present.

As tribes became civilizations, temples became the centers of medical care because of the belief that illness was caused by sin and the gods' displeasure (ie, disease literally means "dis-ease"). Priests were highly regarded as physicians, but neither human life nor women were valued by society; the nurse was viewed as a slave, carrying out menial tasks based on the orders of the priest–physician. In contrast, during the same period, the ancient Hebrews proposed rules for ethical human relationships, mental health, and disease control through the Ten Commandments and the Mosaic Health Code. Nurses cared for sick people in the home and the community and also practiced as nurse–midwives (Dolan, Fitzpatrick, & Herrmann, 1983).

With the beginning of Christianity, nursing began to have a formal and more clearly defined role. Led by the belief that love and caring for others were important, women called *deaconesses* made the first organized visits to sick people, and members of male religious orders gave nursing care and buried the dead. Both male and female nursing orders were founded during the Crusades. Hospitals were built to care for the enormous number of pilgrims needing healthcare, and nursing became a respected vocation. The early Middle Ages ended in chaos, but nursing had developed purpose, direction, and leadership.

At the beginning of the 16th century, society changed from one with a religious orientation to one that emphasized warfare, exploration, and expansion of knowledge. Many monasteries and convents closed, leading to a tremendous shortage of people to care for the sick. To meet this need, women who had committed crimes were recruited into nursing in lieu of serving jail sentences. Along with a poor reputation, nurses received low pay and worked long hours in unfavorable conditions.

From the middle of the 18th century to the 19th century, social reforms changed the roles of nurses and of women in general. It was during this time that nursing, based on many of the beliefs and examples of Florence Nightingale, began as we currently know it. Florence Nightingale was born in 1820 to a wealthy family. She grew up in England and was well educated and traveled extensively. Despite strong opposition from her family, Nightingale received nurse's training at age 31 years. The outbreak of the Crimean War and a request by the British to organize nursing care for a military hospital in Turkey gave Nightingale an opportunity for achievement (Kalish & Kalish, 1995). Because she was able to overcome enormous difficulties successfully, Nightingale challenged prejudices against women and elevated the status of all nurses. After the war, she returned to England, where she established a training school for nurses and wrote books about healthcare and nursing education.

Florence Nightingale's contributions are numerous and far-reaching:

- Identifying personal needs of the client and the role of the nurse in meeting those needs
- Establishing standards for hospital management
- Establishing a respected occupation for women
- Establishing nursing education
- Recognizing the two components of nursing—health and illness
- Believing that nursing is separate and distinct from medicine
- Recognizing that nutrition is important to health
- Instituting occupational and recreational therapy for sick people
- Stressing the need for continuing education for nurses
- Maintaining accurate records that are recognized as the beginnings of nursing research

Florence Nightingale elevated the status of nursing to a respected occupation, improved the quality of nursing care, and founded modern nursing education. Florence Nightingale and other images of nursing care in the 19th century are shown in Figure 1-1.

Nursing in North America

The work of Florence Nightingale and the care provided for battle casualties during the Civil War focused attention on the need for educated nurses in both Canada and the United States. Schools of nursing were founded in connection with hospitals, but although these schools were established on the beliefs of Nightingale, the training they provided was based more on apprenticeship than on educational programs. Hospitals saw an economic advantage in having their own school, and most hospital schools were organized to provide more easily controlled and less expensive staff for the hospital. This resulted in the loss of clear guidelines separating nursing service and nursing education. As students and as graduates, female nurses were under the control of male hospital administrators and physicians. The lack of educational standards, the male dominance of healthcare, and the pervading Victorian belief that women depended on men combined to contribute to several decades of slow progress toward professionalism in nursing (Kalish & Kalish, 1995).

World War II had an enormous effect on nursing. For the first time, large numbers of women worked outside the home. In the process, they also became more independent and assertive. These changes in women and in society resulted in an increased emphasis on education. The war itself had identified a need for more nurses and had resulted in a knowledge explosion in medicine and technology, which broadened the role of nurses. After World War II, efforts were directed at upgrading nursing education. Schools of nursing were based on educational objectives and were increasingly developed in university and college settings, leading to degrees in nursing for both men and women.

Since the 1950s, nursing has broadened in all areas, including practice in a wide variety of healthcare settings, the development of a body of knowledge specific to nursing, the conduct and publication of nursing research, and the recognition of the role of nursing in promoting wellness. Increased emphasis on the importance of nursing knowledge as the base for nursing practice has led to the growth of nursing as a profession and as a discipline. Table 1-1 summarizes the contributions of people important to the development of nursing as a profession.

Florence Nightingale, initiator of major reforms in health care and nursing training in England

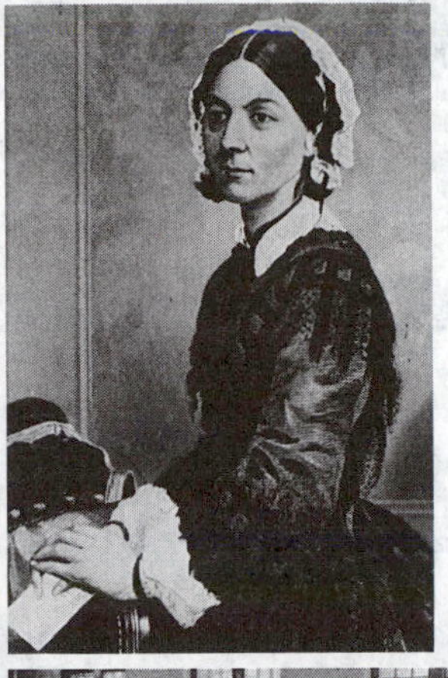

Clara Barton, founder of the American Red Cross in 1882

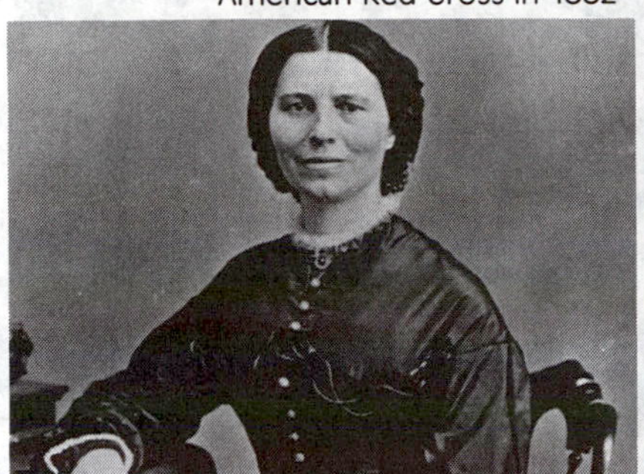

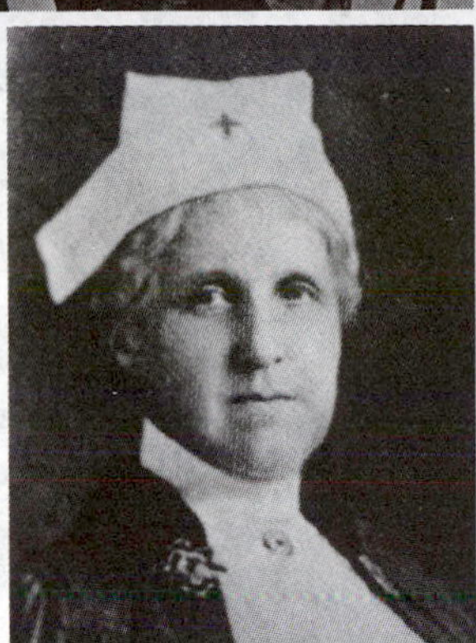

Jane Delano, an Army nurse, instrumental in the organization of the Red Cross Nursing Service in the early 1900 s

Vassar training camp classroom, 1918

Vassar training camp faculty, 1918

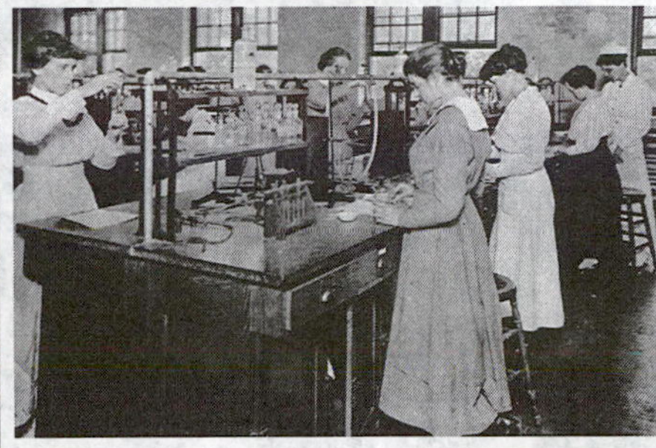

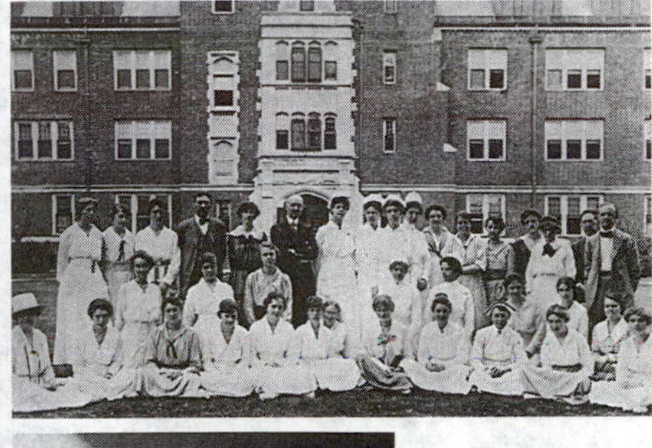

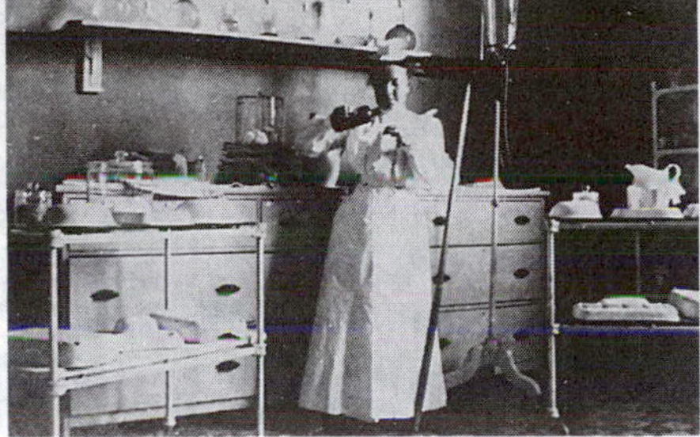

Philadelphia General Hospital nurse, late 1800 s

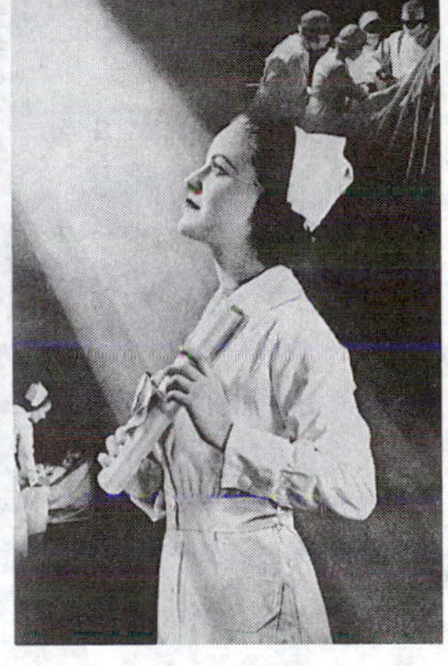

Post-WWII nursing school poster

Figure 1-1
Images of nurses spanning more than 100 years of service. (Courtesy of The Center for the Study of the History of Nursing, University of Pennsylvania.)

Definitions of Nursing

The word *nurse* originated from the Latin word *nutrix*, meaning to nourish. Definitions of nurse and nursing are based on this word origin to describe the nurse as a person who nourishes, fosters, and protects; a person prepared to take care of sick, injured, and aged people. However, the expanding roles and functions of the nurse in today's society have made any one definition too limited. As described by Ellis and Hartley (1995), one can no longer say "a nurse is a nurse is a nurse" (p. 5). This section offers several definitions that provide a broad perspective of nursing. Chapter 5 offers further definitions of nursing by specific nursing theorists.

International Council of Nurses. The following definition was written by Virginia Henderson and adopted by the International Council of Nurses (ICN) in 1973:

> The unique function of the nurse is to assist the individual, sick or well, in the performance of those activities contributing to health or its recovery (or to peaceful death) that he would perform unaided if he had the necessary strength, will, or knowledge. And to do this in such a way as to help him gain independence as rapidly as possible.

American Nurses Association. In 1965, the American Nurses Association (ANA) Committee on Education issued a position paper that broadly defined nursing as an independent profession. The statement said:

> Nursing is a helping profession and, as such, provides services which contribute to the health and well-being of people. Nursing is a vital consequence to the individual receiving services; it fills needs which cannot be met by the person, by the family, or by other persons in the community.

Table 1-1
People Important to the Development of Nursing

Person	Contribution
19th Century	
Clara Barton	Volunteered to care for wounds and feed Union soldiers during the Civil War; served as the supervisor of nurses for the Army of the James, organizing hospitals and nurses; established the Red Cross in the United States in 1882.
Dorothea Dix	Superintendent of the Female Nurses of the Army during the Civil War; was given the authority and the responsibility for recruiting and equipping a corps of army nurses; she was a pioneering crusader for the reform of the treatment of the mentally ill.
Mary Ann Bickerdyke	Organized diet kitchens, laundries, an ambulance service, and supervised nursing staff during the Civil War.
Louise Schuyler	A nurse during the Civil War, she returned to New York and organized the New York Charities Aid Association; this organization worked to improve care of the sick in Bellevue Hospital; one recommendation was to have standards for nursing education.
Linda Richards	The first trained nurse in the United States; a graduate of the New England Hospital for Women and Children in Boston, Massachusetts in 1873. She became the night superintendent of Bellevue Hospital in 1874 and began the practice of keeping records and writing orders.
Jane Addams	Provided social services within a neighborhood setting; a leader for women's rights; recipient of the 1931 Nobel Peace prize.
Lillian Wald	Established a neighborhood nursing service for the sick poor of the lower East Side in New York City; the founder of public health nursing.
Mary Elizabeth Mahoney	Graduated from the New England Hospital for Women and Children in 1879 as America's first black nurse.
Harriet Tubman	A nurse and an abolitionist, she was active in the underground railroad movement before joining the Union Army during the Civil War.
Nora Gertrude Livingston	Established a training program for nurses at the Montreal General Hospital (the first 3-year program in North America).
Mary Agnes Snively	Director of the nursing school at Toronto General Hospital and one of the founders of the Canadian Nurses Association).
Sojourner Truth	A nurse who not only provided care to soldiers during the Civil War, but also worked for the women's movement.
Isabel Hampton Robb	A leader in nursing and nursing education, she organized the nursing school at Johns Hopkins Hospital where she initiated policies that included limiting the number of hours in a day's work and wrote a textbook to help student learning; was the first president of the Nurses Associated Alumnae of the United States and Canada (which later became the American Nurses' Association).
20th Century	
Mary Adelaide Nutting	As a member of the faculty of Teachers' College, Columbia University, she became the first professor of nursing in the world and, with Lavinia Dock, published the four-volume *History of Nursing.*
Elizabeth Smellie	A member of the original Victorian Order of Nurses for Canada (a group who provided public health nursing); organized the Canadian Women's Army Corps during World War II.
Lavinia Dock	A nursing leader and women's right activist who was instrumental in the Constitutional amendment giving women the right to vote.
Mary Breckenridge	Established the Frontier Nursing Service and one of the first midwifery schools in the United States.

The essential components of professional nursing are care, cure, and coordination. The care aspect is more than "to take care of"; it is "caring for" and "caring about," as well. It is dealing with human beings under stress, frequently over long periods. It is providing comfort and support in time of anxiety, loneliness, and helplessness. It is listening, evaluating, and intervening appropriately.

The promotion of health and healing is the cure aspect of professional nursing. It is assisting clients to understand their health problems and helping them to cope. It is the administration of medication and treatments. And it is the use of clinical nursing judgment in determining, on the basis of clients' reactions, whether the plan for care needs to be maintained or changed. It is knowing when and how to use existing and potential resources to help clients toward recovery and adjustment by mobilizing their own resources.

Professional nursing practice is this and more. It is sharing responsibility for the health and welfare of all those in the community, and participating in programs designed to prevent illness and maintain health. It is coordinating and synchronizing medical and other professional and technical services as these affect clients. It is supervising, teaching, and directing all those who give nursing care.

These concepts and beliefs were expanded by ANA in 1980 in *Nursing: A Social Policy Statement,* which defined *nursing practice* as "the diagnosis and treatment of human responses to actual or potential health problems" (p. 9). This definition further legitimized the assessment and analysis of signs and symptoms and the use of nursing knowledge to implement and evaluate nursing actions taken to meet needs for potential or actual health problems. The social policy statement is currently under revision to meet the challenge of defining nursing as we move into the next century.

Canadian Nurses Association. The Canadian Nurses Association (CNA) made the following philosophic statement about nursing:

> The nursing professional exists in response to a need of society and holds ideals related to man's health throughout his life span. Nurses direct their energies toward the promotion, maintenance, and restoration of health, the prevention of illness, the alleviation of suffering and the ensuring of a peaceful death when life can no longer be sustained. Nurses value a holistic view of man and regard him as a biopsychosocial being who has the capacity to set goals and make decisions and who has the right and responsibility to make informed choices congruent with his own beliefs and values. Nursing, a dynamic and supportive profession guided by its code of ethics, is rooted in caring, a concept evident throughout its four fields of activity—practice, education, administration, and research. (1989, p. iii)

In all of the definitions, the central focus is the person receiving care (who may be called either the patient or the client), and includes the physical, emotional, social, and spiritual dimensions of that person. Nursing is no longer considered to be primarily concerned with illness care; the concepts and definitions have expanded to include the prevention of illness, the promotion of wellness, and the maintenance of health for individuals, families, and communities.

Nursing: A Profession and a Discipline?

As definitions of nursing have expanded to describe more clearly the roles and actions of nurses, increased attention has focused on the question of nursing as a profession and as a discipline. Nursing is gaining recognition as a **profession,** based on the criteria that a profession must have

- A well-defined body of knowledge
- A strong service orientation
- Recognized authority by a professional group
- A code of ethics
- A professional organization that sets standards
- Ongoing research
- Autonomy

A **discipline** has a specific and unique body of knowledge that uses existing and new knowledge to solve problems creatively and meet human needs within ever-changing boundaries. To be considered a discipline, certain criteria must be met:

- An impressive body of lasting works
- Suitable techniques
- Concerns that are relevant to human activities
- Relevant traditions that inspire future knowledge development
- Considerable scholarly recognition and achievement

Nursing involves specialized skills and application of knowledge based on education that has both theoretical and clinical components. Nurses uphold standards set forth by professional organizations and follow an established code of ethics. The concerns of nursing focus on human responses to actual or potential health problems and are increasingly focused on wellness, an area of caring that encompasses nursing's unique knowledge and abilities. Nursing is rich in tradition. Furthermore, nursing is increasingly being recognized as scholarly, with academic qualifications, research, and publications specific to nursing becoming more widely accepted and respected.

Nursing has evolved through history from a technical service to a person-centered process that affects the lives of others to allow maximizing of potential in all human dimensions. This has been an active process, as the profession and the discipline of nursing has developed by using lessons from the past to gain knowledge for practice in the present and in the future.

Aims of Nursing

The following four broad aims of nursing practice can be identified from the definitions of nursing:

- To promote wellness
- To prevent illness
- To restore health
- To facilitate coping

To meet these aims, the nurse uses knowledge and skills to give care in a variety of traditional and expanding nursing roles. The primary role of the nurse as caregiver is given shape and substance by the interrelated roles of communicator, teacher, counselor, leader, researcher, and advocate. These roles, as well as expanded career roles and functions of nurses, are defined in Tables 1-2 and 1-3 and fully discussed in Unit IV. Activities within the roles are carried out by the nurse in many different settings, including hospitals, nursing homes,

Table 1-2
Roles and Functions of Nurses

Role	Function
Caregiver	The provision of care to clients that combines both the art and the science of nursing in meeting physical, emotional, intellectual, sociocultural, and spiritual needs. As a caregiver, the nurse integrates the roles of communicator, teacher, counselor, and leader, researcher, advocate to promote wellness through activities that prevent illness, restore health and facilitate coping with disability or death. The role of caregiver is the primary role of the nurse.
Communicator	The use of effective interpersonal and therapeutic communication skills to establish and maintain helping relationships with clients of all ages in a wide variety of healthcare settings.
Teacher	The use of communication skills to assess, implement, and evaluate individualized teaching plans to meet learning needs of clients and their families.
Counselor	The use of therapeutic interpersonal communication skills to provide information, make appropriate referrals, and facilitate the client's problem-solving and decision-making skills.
Leader	The assertive, self-confident practice of nursing when providing care, effecting change, and functioning with groups.
Researcher	The participation in or conduct of research to increase knowledge in nursing and improve client care.
Advocate	The protection of human or legal rights and the securing of care for all clients based on the belief that clients have the right to make informed decisions about their own health and lives.

clinics, offices, mobile units, and the home. Of these settings, care is increasingly provided out of the hospital and in the community. These activities are directed toward maximizing wellness for the client and his or her family.

Promoting Wellness

Wellness is a state of human functioning that may be defined as the achievement of one's maximum attainable potential. The American Hospital Association (1980) further described wellness as follows:

> The objective of wellness is not merely to avoid illness or to prolong life; rather, its objective is to enhance the quality of a person's life through activities that are designed to continually improve the state of his physical, mental, emotional and spiritual well being . . . wellness is as achievable by the aged, the chronically ill, or the handicapped as by anyone else.

Nurses promote wellness by maximizing strengths that are specific and individualized within each person. Wellness is an essential part of each of the other aims of nursing, with identification and analysis of client strengths a component of preventing illness, restoring health, and facilitating coping with disability or death. Every client, no matter how ill, has strengths. The nurse identifies and uses these strengths to help the client reach maximum function and quality of life or meet death with dignity.

Wellness promotion is the framework for nursing activities. The client's self-awareness, health awareness, wellness skills, and use of resources are all considered as the nurse provides care. Through knowledge and skill, the nurse

- Facilitates decisions about lifestyle that enhance the quality of life and encourages acceptance of responsibility for one's own health
- Increases health awareness by assisting in the understanding that health is more than just not being ill and by teaching that certain behaviors and factors can contribute to or diminish wellness
- Teaches wellness skills by promoting decision making so that self-care activities maximize achievement of goals that are realistic and attainable, and by serving as a role model
- Encourages the use of wellness resources by providing information and referrals

Preventing Illness

The objectives of illness-prevention activities are to reduce the risk of illness, to promote good health habits, and to maintain the individual's optimal functioning. Nurses primarily promote health by teaching and by personal example. Such activities include the following:

- Educational programs in areas such as prenatal care for pregnant women, smoking-cessation programs, and stress-reduction seminars
- Community programs and resources that encourage healthy lifestyles, including aerobic exercise classes, swimnastics, and physical fitness programs
- Literature and television information on diet, exercise, and the importance of good health habits
- Health assessments in institutions, clinics, and community settings that identify areas of strength and the potential for illness

Restoring Health

Activities to restore health encompass those most traditionally considered to be the nurse's responsibility. This area focuses on the individual with an illness but ranges from early detection of a disease to rehabilitation and teaching during recovery. Activities include

Table 1-3
Expanded Career Roles and Functions of Nurses

Title	Description
Clinical nurse specialist (eg, enterostomal therapist, geriatrics, infection control, medical–surgical, maternal–child, oncology, quality assurance, nursing process)	A nurse with an advanced degree, education, or experience who is considered to be an expert in a specialized area of nursing; carries out direct client care, consultation, teaching clients, families, and staff, and conducting research
Nurse practitioner	A nurse with an advanced degree, certified for a special area or age of client care; works in a variety of healthcare settings or in independent practice to make health assessments and deliver primary care
Nurse anesthetist	A nurse who completes a course of study in an anesthesia school; carries out preoperative visits and assessments, administers and monitors anesthesia during surgery, and evaluates postoperative status of clients
Nurse midwife	A nurse who completes a program in midwifery; provides prenatal and postnatal care and delivers babies to women with uncomplicated pregnancies
Nurse educator	A nurse, usually with an advanced degree, who teaches in educational or clinical settings; teaches theoretical knowledge and clinical skills; conducts research
Nurse administrator	A nurse who functions at various levels of management in healthcare settings; responsible for the management and administration of resources and personnel involved in giving client care
Nurse researcher	A nurse with an advanced degree who conducts research relevant to the definition and improvement of nursing practice and education
Nurse entrepreneur	A nurse, usually with an advanced degree, who may manage a clinic or health-related business, conduct research, provide education, or serve as an adviser or consultant to institutions, political agencies, or businesses

- Providing direct care of the person who is ill, by such measures as providing physical care, administering medications, and carrying out procedures and treatments
- Performing diagnostic measurements and examinations (eg, taking blood pressure, measuring blood sugars) that detect an illness
- Referring questions and abnormal findings to other healthcare providers as appropriate
- Planning, teaching, and carrying out rehabilitation for illnesses such as heart attacks, arthritis, and strokes
- Working in mental health and chemical-dependency programs

Facilitating Coping

Although the major focus of healthcare is promoting, maintaining, or restoring health, these goals cannot always be met. Nurses also facilitate client and family coping with altered function, life crisis, and death. **Altered function** results in a decrease in an individual's ability to carry out activities of daily living and expected roles. Nurses can facilitate an optimal level of function through maximizing strengths and potentials, teaching, and knowledge of and referral to community support systems. Nurses provide care to both clients and families during the terminal illness, and they do so in hospitals, long-term nursing facilities, and homes. Nurses are also becoming more active in hospice programs, which assist individuals and their families in preparing for death and in living as comfortably as possible until death occurs.

Educational Preparation for Nursing Practice

Levels of Education

Educational preparation for nursing practice currently involves several different types of programs. Students may choose to enter a practical nursing program and be licensed as a licensed practical nurse (LPN) or licensed vocational nurse (LVN), or they may enter a diploma, an associate degree, or a baccalaureate program to be licensed as a registered nurse (RN). State laws in the United States and in some provinces of Canada recognize both the LPN or LVN and RN as having the proper credentials to practice nursing, although the responsibilities are different for the two levels. Graduate programs are also available in nursing, providing master's and doctoral degrees.

A major issue in nursing involves educational preparation. The multiple educational preparations are confusing to institutions employing nurses, to consumers of healthcare services, and to nurses themselves. Nursing organizations are working hard to answer questions such as, "What is technical nursing?" and "What is professional nursing?" as well as, "Should graduates of all programs take the same kind of licensing examination and have the same title?" These questions should be resolved during your nursing career.

This section discusses education for LPNs and RNs, as well as graduate nursing education, continuing education for nurses, and in-service education.

Practical and Vocational Nursing Education

Practical nursing was established to teach graduates to give bedside nursing care to clients. Schools for practical nursing programs are located in such varied settings as high schools, technical or vocational schools, community colleges, or independent agencies. Most programs are 1-year programs divided into one-third classroom and two-thirds clinical laboratory hours. On completion of the program, graduates are eligible to take the National Council Licensure Examination (NCLEX-PN) for licensure as a licensed practical nurse (LPN) or licensed vocational nurse (LVN). In Canada, some provinces offer a similar program for practitioners called registered nursing assistants.

LPNs work under the direction of a physician or RN to give direct care to clients, focusing on meeting healthcare needs in hospitals, nursing homes, and home health agencies.

Registered Nursing Education

Three primary types of educational programs lead to **licensure** as an RN. In the United States, these types are (1) diploma, (2) associate degree, and (3) baccalaureate programs. Canada has nursing education in (1) 2-year community college, (2) 3-year hospital-based diploma, and (3) university baccalaureate programs. Graduates of all types of programs take the same RN licensing examination. In the United States, graduates take the NCLEX-RN examination, and graduates of Canadian schools take the Canadian Nurses Association Testing Service examination. Although both are national examinations, they are administered by, and the nurse is licensed in, each state or province. It is illegal to practice nursing unless one has a license verifying completion of an accredited (by the state or province) program in nursing and has passed the licensing examination. Nurses gain legal rights to practice nursing in another state or province by applying to that state's or province's board of nursing and receiving reciprocal licensure.

Computer Applications in Nursing

The National Council Licensure Examination for Nurses

Since April 1994, the National Council of State Boards of Nursing Examination, known as the National Council Licensure Examination (NCLEX), has been administered via computer. Previously, graduate nurses in all states took a paper-and-pencil examination that was offered only twice a year within a 2-day period. Now graduates may take the examination year-round at their convenience in a 1-day time frame. The NCLEX is administered at more than 200 locations nationwide, which is a four-fold increase over the previous examination sites.

The test is written using the computerized adaptive testing (CAT) method, which uses computer technology and measurement theory. Standard multiple-choice questions are used, but each candidate's test is different. Questions are answered and the computer calculates a competence index based on all this and earlier answers. Subsequent questions are selected by the computer based on previous answers. The examination continues until a pass or fail decision is made. Some graduates may take a minimum of 75 questions and pass the test whereas others may take as many as 265 questions. The graduate has up to 5 hours (including rest breaks) to complete the examination.

Candidates may not skip questions or return to previous questions because of the adaptive branching testing. Once an answer is given, the next questions are given based on that answer. NCLEX candidates need not be skilled in computer use before taking the examination. A keyboard tutorial and practice exercise are given before the examination. The space bar and the enter key are the only two keys needed to take the examination.

The results of the examination are transmitted electronically on a daily basis to the National State Board Educational Testing Service. Pass/fail reports will be sent to the State Boards of Nursing for distribution to the candidate. Results may be known within 1 month; previously, resting results were not known until 3 months.

The examination tests the knowledge, skills, and abilities needed to demonstrate the safe and effective practice of entry-level nursing. The test questions are written by nursing professionals and reviewed by a national panel of nursing experts.

Diploma in Nursing. Many nurses practicing in the United States received their basic nursing education in 3-year, hospital-based diploma schools of nursing (Ellis & Hartley, 1995). The first schools of nursing established to educate nurses were diploma programs, and until the 1960s, they were the major source of graduates. In recent years the number of diploma programs has greatly decreased.

Current graduates of diploma programs have a sound foundation of the biologic and social sciences, with a strong emphasis on clinical experience in direct client care. Graduates work in acute, long-term, and ambulatory healthcare facilities (Ellis & Hartley, 1995).

Associate Degree in Nursing. Associate degree nursing education is based on a research project carried out by Dr. Mildred Montag in the 1950s. At that time, a shortage of nurses existed, and the project was created to meet the needs of society by preparing nurses in less time than was required in diploma programs. The emphasis of this type of program was education instead of service.

Currently, most associate degree programs are in community junior colleges. These 2-year educational programs attract more men, more minorities, and more nontraditional students than do the other types of programs. Associate degree education prepares nurses to give care to clients in structured settings, including hospitals, long-term care, and home health. Graduates of these programs are technically skilled and well prepared to carry out nursing roles and functions. Competencies of the associate degree nurse on entry into practice, as defined by the National League for Nursing (NLN), are listed in the accompanying box.

Baccalaureate in Nursing. The first baccalaureate nursing programs were established in the United States and Canada in the early 1900s. However, the number of programs and the number of enrolling students did not increase markedly until the 1960s. (Most graduates receive a bachelor of science in nursing [BSN] degree and, hence, are referred to having a BSN throughout this section.)

Educational Outcomes of Associate Degree Nursing Programs: Competencies at Graduation

On graduation, the associate degree nurse demonstrates the following competencies:

Role as Provider of Care

Assessment

- Obtains data through assessment of the client
- Collects additional data relative to the client from family, significant others, health records, health care team members, and other resources.
- Identifies changes in health status that affect the client's ability to meet needs.
- Contributes the information to a data base.

Diagnosis

- Identifies actual or potential health care needs on the basis of assessment.
- Selects nursing diagnoses on the basis of analysis and interpretation of data.

Planning

- Participates with the client, family, significant others, and members of the health care team to establish the client-centered goals directed toward promoting and restoring the client's optimal level of health, preventing illness, and providing rehabilitation.
- Establishes priorities for care with recognition of client's diagnoses and needs.
- Develops care plan incorporating data related to the client's cultural and spiritual beliefs and physiologic, psychosocial, and developmental needs and strengths.
- Collaborates with other health care workers in the development of individualized teaching plans that include health counseling, discharge planning, and implementation of a therapeutic regimen.
- Supports client's right to make decisions regarding care.

Implementation

- Implements a care plan according to priority of goals.
- Initiates nursing interventions in response to client's needs.
- Adjusts priorities for nursing interventions in response to client's needs.
- Uses current technology to enhance client care.
- Demonstrates safe performance of nursing skills.
- Provides for physical safety of the client.
- Promotes an environment conducive to maintenance or restoration of the client's ability to carry out activities of daily living.
- Promotes the rehabilitation potential of the client.
- Administers and monitors the prescribed medical regimen for the client undergoing diagnostic tests and/or therapeutic procedures.
- Promotes psychologic safety of the client.
- Demonstrates caring behavior in providing nursing care.
- Uses communication techniques that assist the client, family, and significant others to cope with and resolve problems.
- Communicates verbally and in writing client behaviors, responses to nursing interventions, and responses to medical regimen.
- Implements teaching plans that are specific to the client's level of development, knowledge, and learning needs.

(continued)

Educational Outcomes of Associate Degree Nursing Programs: Competencies at Graduation *(continued)*

- Provides for continuity of care in the management of chronic health care needs.
- Makes referrals on the basis of identified client needs and knowledge of available resources.

Evaluation

- Determines the effects of nursing interventions on the status of the client.
- Participates with the client, family, significant others, and members of the health care team in the evaluation of client's progress toward goals
- Revises care plan as needed.

Role as Manager of Care

- Establishes priorities for nursing care for a group of clients.
- Delegates aspects of nursing care to other health care workers commensurate with their education preparation and experience.
- Is accountable for nursing care delegated to other workers.
- Assists other nursing personnel to develop skills in providing nursing care.
- Interacts with other members of the health care team in a collegial manner.
- Uses appropriate channels of communication to accomplish goals related to delivery of client care.
- Provides for continuity of care within the employing institution.
- Serves as an advocate for clients.
- Seeks assistance from other members of the healthcare team when the situation encountered is beyond the nurse's knowledge and experience.
- Uses current technology to increase efficiency of management of client care and resources.
- Practices in a cost-effective manner.

Role as Member Within the Discipline of Nursing

- Practices within the ethical and legal framework of nursing.
- Maintains confidentiality of information regarding clients.
- Communicates truthfully in verbal and written form the client's behavior and responses to interventions.
- Reports concerns regarding quality of care to the appropriate person.
- Values nursing as a career and values own practice.
- Supports peers and other workers in the delivery of client care.
- Recognizes and reports ethical dilemmas encountered in practice.
- Serves as a role model to members of the nursing team.
- Uses information from current literature to provide safe nursing care.
- Recognizes the importance of nursing research in advancing nursing practice.
- Uses resources for continuous learning and self-development.
- Uses constructive criticism and suggestions for improving nursing practices.

(National League for Nursing. [1990]. *Educational outcomes of associate degree nursing programs: Roles and competencies* [Pub. No. 23-2348]. New York: NLN, Council of Associate Degree Programs.)

The increase in number of programs and student enrollment is the result of recommendations made by ANA, NLN, and CNA that the entry level for professional practice be at the baccalaureate level. Although nurses with a BSN practice in a wide variety of settings, the 4-year degree is required for many administrative, managerial, and community health positions.

In BSN programs, the major in nursing is built on a general education base with concentration on nursing at the upper level. Students acquire knowledge of theory and practice related to nursing and other disciplines, provide nursing care to individuals and groups, work with members of the healthcare team, use research to improve practice, and have a foundation for graduate study. Nurses who graduate from a diploma or associate degree program and wish to complete requirements for a BSN may choose to enroll in an RN to BSN program or may complete requirements through an external degree program. The accompanying box describes the characteristics of the graduate of the baccalaureate program in nursing as defined by NLN.

Graduate Education in Nursing

The two levels of graduate education in nursing are the master's and doctoral degrees. A master's degree in nursing prepares the graduate to function in educational settings, in managerial roles, as clinical specialists, and as nurse practitioners. Nurses with doctoral degrees meet requirements for academic advancement and are prepared to carry out research necessary to advance nursing theory and practice.

Continuing Education

The ANA (1994) *Standards for Nursing Professional Development: Continuing Education and Staff Development* defines **continuing education** as those professional development experiences designed to enrich the nurse's contribution to health. Formal continuing education through courses, seminars, and workshops is offered by colleges, hospitals, voluntary agencies, and private groups. In some states, continuing education is required to maintain licensure.

Characteristics of the Graduate of the Baccalaureate Program in Nursing

The graduate of the baccalaureate program in nursing is able to

- provide professional nursing care, which includes health promotion and maintenance, illness, care, restoration, rehabilitation, health counseling, and education based on knowledge derived from theory and research
- synthesize theoretical and empirical knowledge from nursing, scientific, and humanistic disciplines with practice
- use the nursing process to provide nursing care for individuals, families, groups, and communities
- accept responsibility and accountability for the evaluation of the effectiveness of their own nursing practice
- enhance the quality of nursing and health practices within practice settings through the use of leadership skills and a knowledge of the political system
- evaluate research for the applicability of its findings to nursing practice
- participate with other health care providers and members of the general public in promoting the health and well-being of people
- incorporate professional values as well as ethical, moral, and legal aspects of nursing into nursing practice
- participate in the implementation of nursing roles designed to meet emerging health needs of the general public in a changing society

(National League for Nursing. [1987]. *Characteristics of baccalaureate education in nursing* [Pub. No. 15-1758]. New York: NLN.)

In-Service Education

Many hospitals and healthcare agencies provide education and training for employees of their institution or organization. This is called **in-service education** and is designed to increase the knowledge and skills of the nursing staff. Programs might involve learning a nursing skill or how to use new equipment.

Professional Nursing Organizations

One of the criteria of a profession is having a professional organization that sets standards for practice and education. Nursing meets this criterion. Professional organizations also are concerned with current issues in nursing and healthcare, and influence healthcare legislation. The benefits of belonging to a professional nursing organization include networking with colleagues, having a voice in the legislation affecting nursing, and keeping current with trends and issues in nursing.

National Nursing Organizations

North America has three major professional organizations for nurses: (1) ANA, (2) CNA, and (3) NLN. The ANA is the professional organization for RNs in the United States. Founded in the late 1800s, its members are state nurses' associations, with individual nurses belonging to the state organization. ANA establishes standards of practice, encourages research to advance nursing practice, represents nursing through legislative actions, and supports the National Student Nurses' Association (NSNA).

CNA is the national nursing association for RNs in Canada. CNA has provincial organizations, supported by local districts. CNA supports the same goals as ANA—to improve standards of health, to foster high standards of nursing, and to promote the professional development and welfare of nurses. CNA has also been active in nursing education, licensing, and registration for nurses.

NLN is an organization open to all people interested in nursing, including nurses, nonnurses, and agencies. Established in 1952, its objective is to foster the development and improvement of all nursing services and nursing education. The following are the major activities of NLN:

- Conducts one of the largest professional testing services in the United States, including pre-entrance testing for potential students and achievement testing to measure student progress
- Sponsors continuing education workshops and seminars nationwide
- Serves as the primary source of research data about nursing education; conducts annual surveys of schools and new RNs
- Provides voluntary accreditation for educational programs in nursing

The national organizations for student nurses are NSNA in the United States and the Canadian University Nursing Student Organization in Canada. Members are students enrolled in nursing education programs. Programs and activities focus on professional development and healthcare.

International Nursing Organization

The ICN, founded in 1899, was the first international organization of professional women, with nurses from both the United States and Canada among the charter members. By sharing a commitment to maintaining high standards of nursing service and nursing education and by promoting ethics, ICN provides a way for national nursing organizations to work together. The ICN (1973) *Code for Nurses* stated "The need for nursing is universal. Inherent in nursing is respect for life, dignity and rights of man. It is unrestricted by considerations of nationality, race, creed, color, age, sex, politics, or social status."

Specialty Nursing Organizations

A wide variety of nursing organizations currently are available to nurses. These organizations provide information on specific areas of nursing, often have publications directed toward the specialty area of nursing, and may be involved in certification activities. The following examples illustrate the variety of organizations:

American Association of Critical Care Nurses
Association of Operating Room Nurses
American Indian Nurses' Association
Canadian Gerontological Nursing Association
National Black Nurses' Association, Inc.
Nurses' Christian Fellowship
American Public Health Association

Guidelines for Nursing Practice

As previously described, nursing continues to evolve and change to meet the needs of society. The ANA Congress for Nursing Practice (1973) stated that a profession must control its practice to guarantee the quality of its service to the public and that "a profession that does not maintain the confidence of the public will soon cease to be a social force." Nursing controls and guarantees its practice through standards of practice, nurse practice acts and licensure, and use of the nursing process. Each of these will guide your nursing education as a student and your nursing practice after graduation.

Standards of Nursing Practice

The ANA (1991) *Standards of Clinical Nursing Practice* defines the activities of nurses that are specific and unique to nursing. **Standards** allow nurses to carry out professional roles, serving as protection for the nurse, the client, and the institution where healthcare is given. Each nurse is accountable for his or her own quality of practice and is responsible for the use of these standards to ensure knowledgeable, safe, and comprehensive nursing care. The standards, outlined in the accompanying box, apply to the practice of all RNs and lay the foundation for the practice of professional nursing in all settings. The CNA (1987) publication *A Definition of Nursing Practice: Standards for Nursing Practice* provides a parallel purpose in Canada, although some provinces have opted to write their own standards. These standards are outlined in the accompanying box.

American Nurses Association Standards of Clinical Nursing Practice

Standards of Care

Assessment: The nurse collects client health data.

Diagnosis: The nurse analyzes the assessment data in determining diagnoses.

Outcome identification: The nurse identifies expected outcomes individualized to the client.

Planning: The nurse develops a plan of care that prescribes interventions to attain expected outcomes.

Implementation: The nurse implements the interventions identified in the plan of care.

Evaluation: The nurse evaluates the client's progress toward attainment of outcomes.

Standards of Professional Performance

Quality of care: The nurse systematically evaluates the quality and effectiveness of nursing practice.

Performance appraisal: The nurse evaluates his or her nursing practice in relation to professional practice standards and relevant statutes and regulations.

Education: The nurse acquires and maintains current knowledge in nursing practice.

Collegiality: The nurse contributes to the professional development of peers, colleagues, and others.

Ethics: The nurse's decisions and actions on behalf of clients are determined in an ethical manner.

Collaboration: The nurse collaborates with the client, significant others, and health care providers in providing client care.

Research: The nurse uses research findings in practice.

Resource use: The nurse considers factors related to safety, effectiveness, and cost in planning and delivering client care.

(American Nurses Association. [1991]. *Standards of clinical practice.* Kansas City, MO: ANA. Copyright © 1991, ANA.)

Nurse Practice Acts and Licensure

Nurse practice acts are laws established in each state (United States) and province (Canada) to regulate the practice of nursing. They are broadly worded and vary among jurisdictions, but all of them have certain elements in common. In general, they

- Are designed to protect the public by defining the legal scope of nursing practice, excluding untrained or unlicensed people from practicing nursing
- Create a state board of nursing or regulatory body having the authority to make and enforce rules and regulations concerning the nursing profession
- Define important terms and activities in nursing, including legal requirements and titles for RNs and LPNs
- Establish criteria for the education and licensure of nurses

The board of nursing for each state or province is given legal authority to approve taking the licensing examination to graduates of approved schools of nursing. The individual who successfully meets the requirements for licensure is then given a license to practice nursing in the state or province. The license, which must be renewed annually, is valid during the life of the holder and

Canadian Nurses Association Standards for Nursing Practice

Standard I

Nursing Practice Requires That a Conceptual Model for Nursing Be the Basis of That Practice

1. Nurses are required to have a clear idea or conception of the *distinct goal of nursing.*
2. Nurses are required to have a clear idea or conception of the *client.*
3. Nurses are required to have a clear idea or conception of their *role* in response to the health needs of society.
4. Nurses are required to have a clear idea or conception of the *source of client difficulty.*
5. Nurses are required to have a clear idea or conception of the *focus and modes of nursing intervention.*
6. Nurses are required to have a clear idea or conception of the expected *consequences* of nursing activities.

Standard II

Nursing Practice Requires the Effective Use of the Nursing Process

1. Nurses are required to *collect data* in accordance with their conception of the client.
2. Nurses are required to *analyze data* collected in accordance with their conception of the goal of nursing, their role, and the source of client difficulty.
3. Nurses are required to *plan* their nursing actions based upon the identified actual and potential client problems, in accordance with their conception of the focus and modes of intervention.
4. Nurses are required to perform nursing actions which *implement* the plan.
5. Nurses are required to *evaluate* all steps of the nursing process in accordance with their conceptual model for nursing.

Standard III

Nursing Practice Requires That the Helping Relationship Be the Nature of the Client–Nurse Interaction

1. Nurses are required to initiate interaction in a way that increases the likelihood that the client will perceive the health service experience as understandable, manageable, and meaningful at the onset.
2. Nurses are required to set mutually agreed upon expectations as a means of increasing the likelihood that the client will perceive the health service experience as understandable, manageable, and meaningful.
3. Nurses are required to ensure a successful termination of the helping relationship.

Standard IV

Nursing Practice Requires Nurses to Fulfill Professional Responsibilities

1. Nurses are required to respect *statutes and policies* relevant to the profession and the practice setting.
2. Nurses are required to comply with the *Code of Ethics* of their profession.
3. Nurses are required to function as members of a *health team.*

is registered in the state or province. The license and the right to practice nursing can be denied, revoked, or suspended for professional misconduct (eg, incompetence, negligence, chemical impairment, or criminal actions).

As nursing roles continue to expand, and as issues in nursing are resolved, nurse practice acts will reflect those changes. It is essential that nurses are knowledgeable of the specific nurse practice act under which they practice.

Nursing Process

The nursing process, fully described in Unit IV, is one of the major guidelines for nursing practice. The roles of the nurse are implemented through the **nursing process,** which integrates both the art and the science of nursing. That is, the implementation of the nursing process is nursing made visible.

The nursing process allows the nurse to identify healthcare needs and strengths of the client, to establish and carry out a plan of care to meet those needs, and to evaluate the effectiveness of the plan. The nursing process allows the nurse to focus on the client as an individual and to define those areas of client care that are within the domain of nursing (Carpenito, 1995).

Nursing in Transition

Nursing changes constantly in response to the needs and resources of society as a whole. Nursing also changes in response to factors such as definitions of nursing, aims of nursing, educational levels of nursing, and expanded practice roles. Current issues and trends in nursing briefly discussed in this section are new directions in nursing, changes in client needs, expanded technology, and increasing autonomy. These are complex subjects and the information provided is only intended to serve as an introduction. Many of these trends and issues also are discussed in other chapters.

New Directions in Nursing

Currently there is a shortage of nurses prepared at advanced levels (ie, master's and doctoral degrees) and those with the knowledge and skills to meet the complex needs of the client in the home setting. Various factors have been identified as responsible for this shortage, including a change in the healthcare needs of clients, economic conditions affecting the setting in which care is given, and career mobility.

Individuals requiring care are more acutely ill but spend less time within the hospital setting as a result of healthcare reimbursement plans (see Chapter 11). This has resulted in an increased demand for nursing care in community settings. With advanced education and expanded roles, nurses are taking advantage of career mobility to move into management, educational, and community settings. In addition, nurse practitioners are increasingly establishing independent practices where they diagnose and treat illnesses. Nurses also have increased autonomy (ie, freedom to regulate their work behavior) in making decisions about the care of others and are being better paid for their knowledge and skill.

Changes in Client Needs

Changes such as the trend toward shorter hospital care have created new client needs, and thus new opportunities for nursing (Fig. 1-2). Client education is an important aspect of care—teaching clients and their families how to care for the clients after dismissal from the hospital often begins before or on admission. Consideration of the healthcare needs of the client and the family in the home setting is a major component of planning client care. It is essential to maintain continuity in care between the nurse in the hospital and the nurse in the home setting. In addition, clients who require hospital care are increasingly older and/or acutely ill. The complex needs of the client during the acute stage of illness or injury while in the hospital setting requires nursing knowledge and skill to provide not only "high-tech" but also "high-touch" care.

Another aspect of changes in client needs is the increasing population of older people who require both wellness promotion and health restoration. This issue is discussed in Chapters 4 and 10. Other changes in client needs that require nursing consideration involve the homeless, indigent, and people with acquired immunodeficiency syndrome. These groups, as well as others, require innovative nursing care to meet special needs.

Expanded Technology

Both technologic advances and increased autonomy affect nursing practice today. It is impossible to visit a health setting of any type without being aware of the rapid advances that have been made in technology. Diagnostic procedures, inpatient and outpatient surgical procedures, intensive care units, and client care units are all heavily based on high-tech concepts and machines. These machines often go home with the client, where ventilators, kidney dialysis machines, intravenous fluids, and a wide variety of monitors are becoming more common. The nurse must continually update knowledge and skills to use the technology to give safe, individualized care. In addition, computerization in a wide variety of applications has become commonplace in healthcare, providing more accurate assessments, monitoring infusion rates, and providing documentation and care plan capabilities.

Increasing Autonomy

Nursing interventions—the activities nurses carry out as caregivers—are also in transition. Nursing autonomy has increased and the special role of the nurse in providing care has been recognized. It is important to realize that with authority to carry out actions also comes responsibility for one's actions. Even if an action is carried out on the direct order of a physician, the nurse is still re-

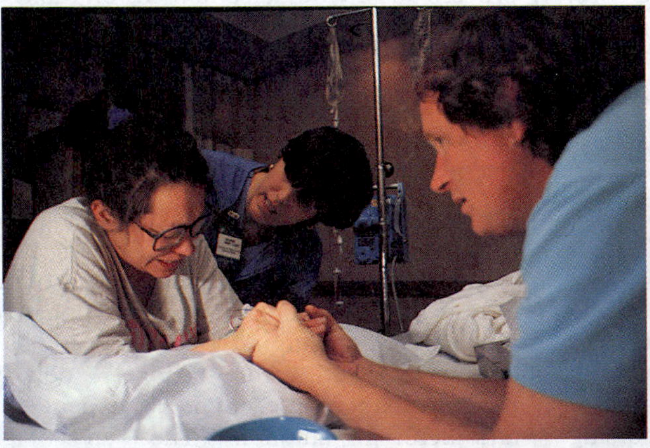

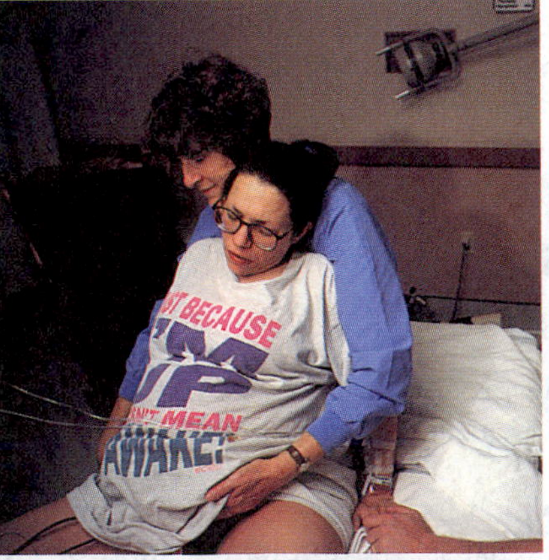

Figure 1-2
Growing numbers of women's health centers staffed with certified nurse practitioners and nurse midwives provide affordable health maintenance care. (Photo by B. A. Rupert.)

sponsible for using critical thinking based on knowledge to provide safe care.

Traditionally, nursing actions have been divided into three categories:

Dependent nursing actions: Those activities that the nurse does based on physician orders. Even dependent actions (eg, administering prescribed medications) require knowledge and skill, as well as the legal responsibility to question any order that is inappropriate.

Interdependent or collaborative nursing actions: Those activities that the nurse carries out in collaboration with other members of the healthcare team. Examples include monitoring the client for the side effects of medications or for changes in the results of diagnostic tests, and reporting findings that indicate increased risk for illness to the appropriate person.

Independent nursing actions: Those activities that the nurse orders and carries out based on assessments, knowledge, and judgment. A wide range of activities are included in this area, including health assessments, nursing diagnoses and care plans, teaching, and counseling.

The distinctions between these categories are blurring as nurses increase educational levels and legal authority to diagnose and treat illnesses. A major trend is toward nurse practitioners establishing practices in which they, in collaboration with a physician, independently provide care for clients of all ages. While hospital-based nursing care is often primarily dependent on physician orders, home-based care is more independent and collaborative in meeting client healthcare needs.

Regardless of the type of intervention, independent nursing judgment is required as the intervention is carried out.

As nurses continue to define their own practice, the special and distinctive role of nursing in caring for others will become increasingly recognized.

Key Points

- Nursing has always involved caring; the role of the nurse as caregiver has been present since early civilization.
- Definitions of nursing have changed and expanded through time in response to societal needs and the social and political structure in which nursing has existed.
- The base for nursing practice and nursing education as we currently know it was established by Florence Nightingale, who positively influenced healthcare standards, nursing practice, nursing education, and women's rights.
- Nursing education in North America has changed from service-oriented hospital training schools to educational programs primarily offered in colleges and universities.
- The roles, functions, and professional status of nursing have been defined and described by ICN, ANA, and CNA. In all definitions, the central focus of nursing is the person receiving care.
- Nursing is an emerging profession and discipline. It is a practice that applies knowledge through specialized skills, upholds standards developed by and for the profession, develops theories and conducts research, and uses the nursing process to give individualized and holistic care.

Bibliography

Alfaro, R. (1994). *Applying nursing diagnosis and nursing process: A step-by-step process* (3rd ed.). Philadelphia: Lippincott.

American Hospital Association. (1980). Wellness: What is it? *Promoting Health, 1*(1), 1–5.

American Nurses Association. (1973). *Standards: Nursing practice. Developed by the Congress for Nursing Practice.* Kansas City, MO: ANA.

American Nurses Association. (1980). *Nursing: A social policy statement.* Kansas City, MO: ANA.

American Nurses Association. (1991). *Standards of clinical nursing practice.* Kansas City, MO: ANA.

American Nurses Association. (1994). *Standards for professional development: Continuing education and staff development.* Washington, DC: ANA.

American Nurses Association, Committee on Education. (1965). *A position paper.* New York: ANA.

Anderson, C. (1994). Advanced practice: The options. *Nursing Outlook, 42*(6), 253–254.

Backer, B. (1993). Lillian Wald: Connecting caring with activism. *Nursing and Healthcare, 14*(3), 122–129.

Bulechek, G. M., & McCloskey, J. C. (1992). *Nursing interventions: Treatments for nursing diagnoses* (2nd ed.). Philadelphia: Saunders.

Canadian Nurses Association. (1987). *A definition of nursing practice: Standards for nursing practice.* Ottawa, Canada: CNA.

Carpenito, L. J. (1995). *Nursing diagnosis: Application to clinical practice* (6th ed.). Philadelphia: Lippincott.

Condon, E. (1992). Nursing and the caring metaphor: Gender and political influences on an ethics of care. *Nursing Outlook, 40*(1), 14–19.

Curtin, L. L. (1990). Designing new roles: Nursing in the '90s and beyond. *Nursing Management, 21*(2), 7–8.

Deloughery, G. (1995). *Issues and trends in nursing.* St. Louis: Mosby.

Diers, D. (1990). The art and craft of nursing. *American Journal of Nursing, 90*(1), 65–66.

Dolan, J. A., Fitzpatrick, M. L., & Herrmann, E. K. (1983). *Nursing in society: A historical perspective*. Philadelphia: Saunders.

Drugge, S. (1991). The essence of nursing. *Canadian Nurse, 87*(10), 28.

Ellis, J., & Hartley, C. (1995). *Nursing in today's world: Challenges, issues, trends* (5th ed.). Philadelphia: Lippincott.

Fryback, P., & Reinert, B. (1993). Facilitating health in people with terminal diagnoses by encouraging a sense of control. *MEDSURG Nursing, 2*(3), 197–201.

Grindel, C., & McGuffin, B. (1992). Standards of clinical nursing practice. *MEDSURG Nursing, 1*(1), 23–28.

Hammond, M. (1990). Is nursing a semi-profession? *Canadian Nurse, 86*(2), 21–23.

Hupcey, J. (1993). Factors and work settings that may influence nurse practitioner practice. *Nursing Outlook, 41*(4), 181–185.

International Council of Nurses. (1973). *1973 code for nurses*. Geneva: Impimeries Populaires.

Kalish, P., & Kalish, B. (1995). *The advance of American nursing* (3rd ed.). Philadelphia: Lippincott.

Kelly, L. Y. (1992). *The nursing experience: Trends, challenges, and transitions* (2nd ed.). New York: McGraw-Hill.

Lindberg, J., Hunter, M., & Kruszewski, A. (1994). *Introduction to nursing: Concepts, issues and opportunities* (2nd ed.). Philadelphia: Lippincott.

McCloskey, J., & Grace, H. (1994). *Current issues in nursing* (4th ed.). St. Louis: Mosby.

Mitchell, P., & Grippando, G. (1993). *Nursing perspectives and issues* (5th ed.). Albany, NY: Delmar.

Moccia, P. (1992). In 1992: A nurse in every school. *Nursing and Health Care, 13*(1), 14–18.

National League for Nursing. (1987). *Characteristics of baccalaureate education in nursing* (Pub. No. 23-1758). New York: NLN.

National League for Nursing. (1990). *Educational outcomes of associate degree nursing programs: Roles and competencies* (Pub. No. 23-2348). New York: NLN, Council of Associate Degree Programs.

Nightingale, F. (1859). *Notes on nursing: What it is and what it is not.* Commemorative Edition. Philadelphia: Lippincott.

Swanson, K. (1993). Nursing as informed caring for the well-being of others. *IMAGE: Journal of Nursing Scholarship, 25*(4), 352–357.

Utz, S. (1993). Beating a path to nursing's door: Scientific support for holistic practice. *MEDSURG Nursing, 2*(4), 290–293.

Chapter 2

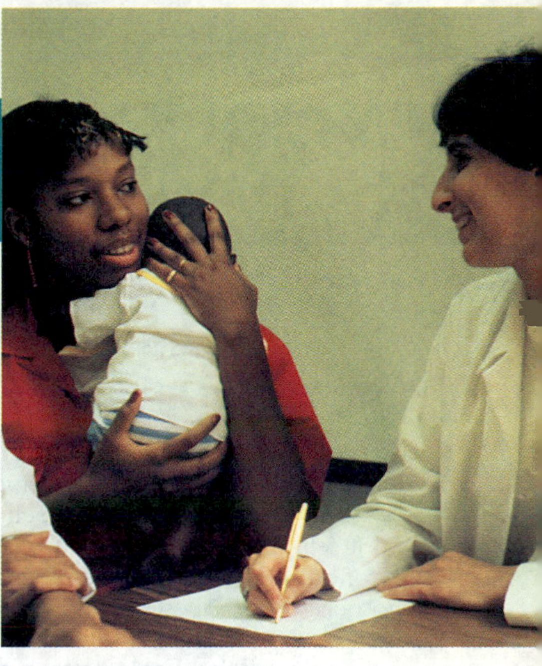

Basic Human Needs: Individual, Family, and Community

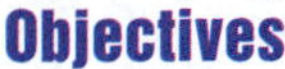

Objectives

After studying this chapter, the learner should be able to:

Define key terms used in the chapter.

Describe each level of Maslow's hierarchy of basic human needs.

Discuss nursing actions necessary to meet needs for each level of Maslow's hierarchy.

Discuss family concepts, including family roles, structures, functions, developmental stages, tasks, and health risk factors.

Identify aspects of the community that affect individual and family health.

Describe nursing interventions to promote and maintain wellness in the individual as a member of a family and as a member of the community.

Key Terms

basic human needs
blended family
community
extended family
family
hierarchy of basic needs
love and belonging needs
nuclear family
physiologic needs
safety and security needs
self-actualization needs
self-esteem needs
step family
traditional family

Humans are complex organisms, influenced by and responsive to both internal and external environments. Our behaviors, our feelings about self and others, our values, and the priorities we set for ourselves are all the result of physiologic and psychosocial needs. These needs are common to all people and are essential to the health and survival of all people, so they are labeled **basic human needs**. Basic human needs are met or unmet in a variety of ways. Some needs are met independently, but most require relationships and interactions with other people for partial or complete fulfillment. Need satisfaction largely depends on an individual's social environment, especially a person's family and community.

Holistic nursing care, which is based on the consideration of all of the dimensions affecting basic human needs in health and in illness, allows the nurse to provide care that is person centered and wellness oriented. Chapter 3 provides an introduction to the cultural dimension, and Chapter 4 discusses the dimensions of the whole person and the interaction of basic human needs with those dimensions. This chapter discusses how basic human needs affect the individual, the family, and the community.

The Individual

In nursing, we are concerned with the physical and psychologic needs of each individual client. Abraham Maslow (1968) developed a **hierarchy of basic human needs** (Fig. 2-1) that is used to determine the needs of the client that are the most important at any given time. Certain needs are more basic or essential than others and must at least be minimally met before other needs can be considered.

Levels of Needs

Maslow's hierarchy of basic needs is useful in understanding the relationships of basic human needs and in establishing priorities of care. The hierarchy is based on the theory that something is a basic need if:

- Its absence results in illness
- Its presence prevents illness or signals health
- Meeting an unmet need restores health
- It is preferred over other satisfactions if unmet
- There is a feeling of something missing when the need is unmet
- There is a feeling of satisfaction when the need is met

Maslow arranged the hierarchy of basic human needs to illustrate that certain needs are more basic than other needs. Although all of the needs are present within each person all of the time, the person strives to meet certain of the needs (at least to a minimal level) before attending to other needs. The five levels of needs, with physiologic needs being the most basic, are as follows:

Level 1: Physiologic needs
Level 2: Safety and security needs
Level 3: Love and belonging needs
Level 4: Self-esteem needs
Level 5: Self-actualization needs

Nursing care is often directed toward meeting unmet needs. Maslow's hierarchy provides a framework for nursing assessment and for understanding the needs of clients at all levels so that interventions to meet needs become a part of the plan of care. For example, in caring for a person coming into the emergency department with a heart attack, the nurse's immediate concern would be the client's physiologic needs (ie, oxygen and pain relief). However, at the same time, safety needs (eg, following proper precautions with oxygen use and ensuring the person does not fall off the examining table) and love and belonging needs (eg, letting a family member stay with the person, if possible) are major considerations.

The nursing activities that you will learn as you progress through your education are aimed at meeting basic human needs of clients. The following discussion describes each level of need.

Physiologic Needs

Physiologic needs, located at the base of the hierarchy of needs, are the most essential to life and therefore have the highest priority. **Physiologic needs**—oxygen, food, water, temperature, elimination, sexuality, physical activity, and rest—must be minimally met to maintain life. Most healthy children and adults meet their physiologic needs

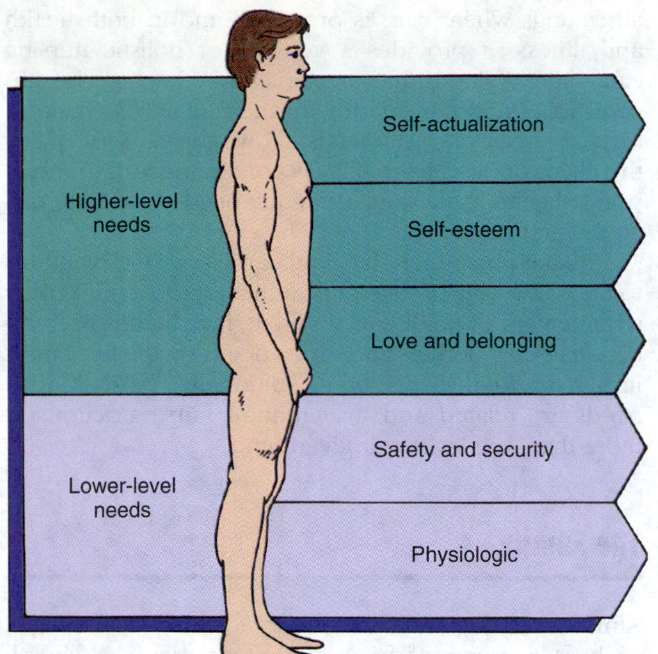

Figure 2-1
Maslow's hierarchy of basic human needs.

through self-care, but physiologic needs are often a major part of the nursing care plan for young, old, disabled, and ill people who require assistance in meeting them.

Oxygen is the most essential of all needs; all body cells require oxygen for survival. Oxygenation of body cells is carried out primarily by the respiratory and cardiovascular systems, and any alteration in their structure and function can result in increased need for oxygen. This need may be acute (necessitating cardiopulmonary resuscitation) or chronic (requiring special positioning, treatments, and teaching). Nurses evaluate oxygen needs by assessing skin color, vital signs, and mental responsiveness of clients.

Physical activity and rest are also basic physiologic needs. Physical activity is accomplished by intact and functioning neuromuscular and bony systems. Immobility, with disuse of muscles and bones, affects all other basic needs. Rest and sleep allow time for the body to rejuvenate and be free of stress. Individual requirements for rest and sleep vary widely, but the effects of deprivation have been well documented. Factors that influence sleep are age, environment, exercise, stress, and drug use. Clients entering the healthcare setting often need increased rest and sleep but are unable to meet these needs without or because of the nurse's interventions.

Safety and Security Needs

Safety and security needs come next in priority and involve both physical and emotional components. **Physical safety** means protecting a person from potential or actual harm. Nurses carry out a wide variety of activities to meet clients' physical safety needs, for example:

- Handwashing and using sterile techniques to prevent infection
- Using electrical equipment properly
- Administering medications knowledgeably
- Using skill moving and ambulating clients
- Teaching parents about household chemicals that are dangerous to children

Emotional safety and security involves trusting others and being free of fear, anxiety, and apprehension. Clients entering the hospital often fear the unknown and may have increased emotional security needs. Nurses can meet such needs by encouraging religious practices that are a source of strength and support, allowing as much independent decision making and control as possible, and carefully explaining new and unfamiliar procedures and treatments.

Love and Belonging Needs

All humans have a basic need for love and belonging. Following physiologic and safety and security needs, this is the next priority of need and is often called a higher level need. **Love and belonging needs** include the understanding and acceptance of others in both giving and receiving love, and the feeling of belonging to others—friends, peers, families, neighborhoods, and communities.

People who perceive that their love and belonging needs are unmet often have a sense of loneliness and isolation. They may withdraw physically and emotionally, or they may become overly demanding and critical. Often these behaviors are a signal (or cue) that unmet love and belonging needs are present. Nurses should always consider love and belonging needs in their care plan. Some nursing interventions to meet this need are as follows:

- Including family and friends in the care of the client (Fig. 2-2)

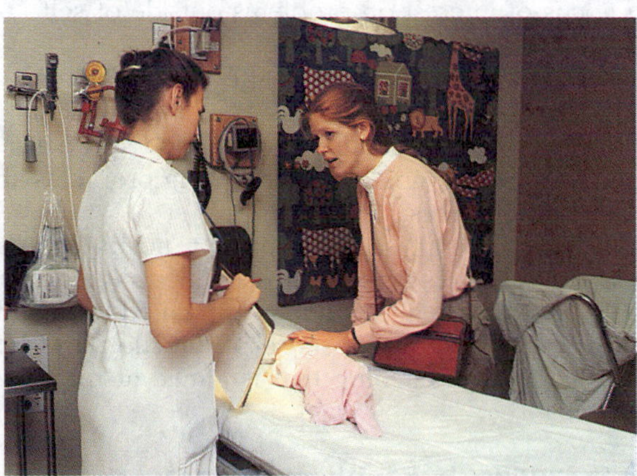

Figure 2-2
By teaching the mother to care for her infant, the nurse is helping to fulfill the need for love and belonging of both mother and child.

- Establishing a nurse–client relationship based on mutual understanding and trust (by demonstrating caring, encouraging communication, and respecting privacy)
- Referring clients to groups that focus on problems (such as cancer support groups or AA)

Self-Esteem Needs

The next highest priority on the hierarchy is the **self-esteem need**—the need for a person to feel good about himself or herself, to feel pride and a sense of accomplishment, and to believe that others also hold one in high regard. Self-esteem gives the individual confidence and independence.

Many factors affect self-esteem. When a person's role changes (eg, through job loss or through loss of a child who has just moved out of the home), self-esteem can be seriously altered because responsibilities and relationships have also changed. Other changes that may affect self-esteem are a change in body image, such as a gain in, or loss of, weight; an injury; or a growth spurt during puberty. Nurses must remember that the person's perception of the change—rather than the actual change itself—is what affects that individual's self-esteem.

Nurses can meet clients' self-esteem needs by accepting values and beliefs, encouraging clients to set attainable goals, and facilitating support by family or significant others. These actions will promote a sense of worth and self-acceptance.

Self-Actualization Needs

The highest level on the hierarchy of needs is the **self-actualization need**—the need for an individual to reach his or her potential through full development of the individual's unique capabilities. In general, each lower level of need must be met to some degree before this need can be satisfied. The process of self-actualization is one that continues throughout life. Maslow lists the following qualities that indicate achievement of one's potential:

- Acceptance of self and others as they are
- Focus of interest on problems outside of self
- Ability to be objective
- Feelings of happiness and affection for others
- Respect for all people
- Ability to discriminate between good and evil
- Creativity as a guideline for solving problems and pursuing interests

To meet clients' self-actualization needs, the nurse must focus on strengths and possibilities, rather than on problems. Nursing interventions are aimed at providing holistic care; providing a sense of direction and hope; and engaging in teaching that is aimed at maximizing potentials.

The Individual in Health and Illness: Applying Maslow's Theory

Maslow's hierarchy of basic needs can be applied to the assessment, planning, implementation, and evaluation of client care. The hierarchy can be used with all ages, in all settings where care is provided, and in both health and illness. It provides a vehicle for holistic nursing care—identifying unmet needs as they become health-care needs and considering all the human dimensions. The hierarchy of basic needs allows the nurse to place the client on the health–illness continuum and to incorporate health models into meeting needs (these are discussed in Chapter 4).

As the nurse identifies and carries out interventions to meet needs, he or she must remember that this is only a framework or guideline, and that, in actuality, each individual sets priorities and meets needs on the level most important to that person. Additionally, basic human needs are related and may require nursing actions at more than one level at a given time.

The Family

Almost every person is a member of a number of groups, such as a group of friends, a work group, a church group, or a school group. Each of these groups is concerned with a specific part of the person's life and is important to the person. However, only one group is concerned with all parts of a person's life and with meeting his or her physical, emotional, and social needs. That group is the family.

What Is a Family?

A **family** can be simply defined as any group of people who live together. Families exist in all sizes and configurations and are essential to the health and survival of the individual family members, and to society as a whole. The family serves as a buffer between the needs of the individual family member and the demands and expectations of the society in which it exists. The role of the family is to meet the needs of its members while also meeting the needs of society (Friedman, 1992).

Duvall (1977) defined family as two or more people who are related through blood, marriage, adoption, or birth. Friedman (1992) expanded that definition by describing a family as comprising two or more people who are emotionally involved with each other and live close together. This definition includes more of the different types of current family structures in which members may be unrelated either biologically or legally.

Family Structures

No single, commonly accepted form of family structure currently exists. The following discussion briefly introduces the many different types of family structures.

Traditional Family. The **traditional family** comprises a father, a mother, and their children (Fig. 2-3). The father and mother are married, and all members of the family live in the same house until the children leave home as young adults. The traditional family may com-

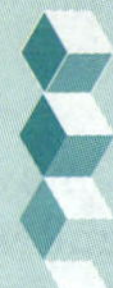

Research in Nursing: Making a Difference

Basic Human Needs: Individual, Family, Community

Basic human needs are met largely through family relationships and interactions. Nursing interventions are planned and implemented to meet not only individual needs, but also needs of the family. Research to identify the most effective way to meet individual and family needs is ongoing, providing knowledge from which to individualize and personalize care.

Related Research

Brewer, N., & Warren, M. (1994). Altered Family Processes related to an ill family member: A validation study. *Nursing Diagnosis, 5*(3), 115–120.
The purpose of this study was to validate defining characteristics for the nursing diagnosis *Altered Family Processes* related to an ill family member. A list of characteristics defined by the North American Nursing Diagnosis Association and the literature was evaluated by practicing registered nurses, and the results were analyzed. Included in the findings were the defining characteristics of denial of family member's illness, failure of family members to maintain own health, financial concerns, inability to accept medical diagnosis, and problems in communication within the family and with healthcare providers. As care for clients increasingly moves into the community setting, knowledge of altered family responses to illness is essential.

Reinhard, S. (1994). Perspectives on the family's caregiving experience in mental illness. *IMAGE: Journal of Nursing Scholarship, 26*(1), 70–74.
The trend toward community-based care for mentally ill adults means that most people with a serious mental illness have family members who assist them. This paper describes the factors that have increased families' caretaking responsibilities. These factors include a lack of skills necessary to live independently, leading to long-term family responsibilities for monitoring and controlling its members behaviors. In addition, many parents of mentally ill adults are older and worry about the future when they are no longer able to provide care. Conclusions are that increased collaboration between healthcare providers and family members is essential so that education and support is available and provided. By learning about mental illness and gaining problem-solving techniques, family members are better able to cope and to provide needed care. The authors suggest that curricular changes and practicum experiences are necessary to prepare nurses to work collaboratively with families.

Jones, E. (1995). Deaf and hearing parents' perceptions of family functioning. *Nursing Research, 44*(2), 102–105.
This study was conducted to compare deaf and hearing parents' perceptions of family functioning. This is an area of family life of the hearing impaired that has had little research. The Feetham Family Functioning Survey was used to survey information from 40 deaf parents and 40 hearing parents. Findings of the study were that there were more similarities than differences in perceptions of family functioning between the two groups, with both groups perceiving similar satisfaction with overall family functioning. Both groups also placed high value on spousal relationships and spending time with their children. One area of difference was that the deaf parents placed a higher value on leisure and recreational activities. Authors of the study suggest that nurses caring for deaf-parented families view them within a broad cultural context rather than focusing on their hearing impairment.

Summary

These studies examined family functioning and concerns of families with physically ill members, mentally ill members, and hearing impairments. The current trend toward decreasing institutional care and increasing community-based care means that nurses must now, more than ever, include family members in every aspect of care. The needs of each individual are often inseparable from the needs of the family and community, and each aspect must be considered when planning and providing nursing care. Continued research will provide the knowledge base for providing individualized, holistic, family-centered care.

prise biologic parents and children, adoptive parents and children, surrogate parents and children, or stepparents and children.

Fitting within the traditional family definition are couples without children and couples with grown children who no longer live at home. The **blended family** is also a traditional family, although it comprises family units who join together to form a new family structure. Children in a blended family live most often with one birth parent and one non–birth parent in a unit called a **step family**.

In the traditional **nuclear family**, the father is the family member who goes to work, providing economic security, while the mother stays at home, providing physical and emotional safety and security. This family group usually lives in close geographic proximity to rel-

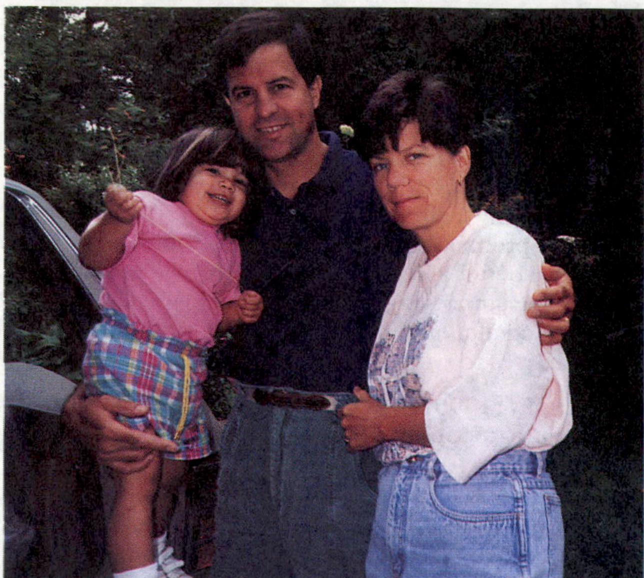

Figure 2-3
A traditional nuclear family.

atives, such as aunts, uncles, and grandparents, who are a part of the **extended family**.

The traditional family unit still has the same form (ie, mother, father, and children), but the roles of the members have changed considerably. Two major factors have caused this change: (1) increased education and career opportunities for women and (2) changes in the U.S. economy requiring that families earn additional income to maintain a desired standard of living. As a result, two-career families, in which both parents work outside the home, have become the norm instead of the exception. When both parents work, there is usually a blending of tasks, with the father taking a more active role in housework and child care and the mother contributing to economic support.

With changes in the traditional family structure have come other influences on the needs of family members. Considerations for the family, and for nursing care, include support systems (in our mobile society, family members may live hundreds or thousands of miles away), availability of child care, time for leisure and recreation, and changing role models.

Single-Parent Families. Single parents may be never married, separated, divorced, or widowed. Most often, the single parent is divorced or widowed, but increasing numbers of never-married men and women are choosing to become parents. The single-parent family is most often headed by a woman. It is estimated that more than one-half of all children in North America live in single-parent families. Single parents have many special problems and needs, including financial concerns, role shifts (ie, being both father and mother, remarriage or relationships with the opposite sex), and social stigma. These problems are important considerations when planning and implementing nursing care (Friedman, 1992).

Other Family Structures. Some families do not meet the definition of traditional or single-parent families but do meet the criteria previously outlined. It is critical for nurses to remember that there are no absolute "rights" or "wrongs," and that one individual's values must not be imposed on another person. Acceptance of family members and relationships is essential to holistic, individualized client care. Other family structures include the following:

Cohabiting families: This form includes those individuals who choose to live together for a variety of reasons—relationships, financial need, or changing values. Cohabiting families include unmarried adults living together, communal or group marriages, and gay and lesbian families.

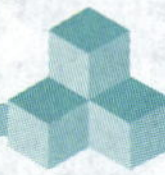

Examples of Nursing Diagnoses

The Family

The following nursing diagnoses are examples of those that might be appropriate for the family as client.

- Risk for Infection related to presence of active tuberculosis in two family members
- Risk for Injury related to homeless state of family members (mother and infant)
- Risk for Poisoning related to living in old house with peeling lead-based paint
- Altered Parenting related to parental lack of knowledge about child care
- Altered Family Processes related to traumatic injury and long-term hospitalization of father of the family
- Caregiver Role Strain related to long-term care for husband with Alzheimer's disease
- Altered Family Processes related to inability of members to communicate effectively
- Parental Role Conflict related to mother's verbalization of inability to provide care for chronically ill child in the home
- Ineffective Family Coping: Disabling related to abandonment of child with AIDS
- Ineffective Management of Therapeutic Regimen: Families related to parental disregard for need for ongoing treatment for child with cystic fibrosis

Single adults: Although the single person is not living with others, he or she is part of a family of origin, usually has a social network with significant others, or may even regard a pet as family. Most single adults living alone are found in two age groups: (1) the young adult who achieves independence and enters the work force and (2) the older person left alone through death of a spouse.

Family Functions

The family provides a set of functions important to the needs of the individual family members and to society as a whole. The family provides the individual with the necessary environment for development and social interactions; it also provides new and socialized members for society. Five major functions of the family are as follows:

Physical: The family provides a safe, comfortable environment necessary to growth, development, and rest or recuperation.

Economic: The family provides financial aid to family members and also meets monetary needs of society.

Reproductive: The family gives birth to children.

Affective and coping: The family provides emotional comfort to members. It also helps members establish an identity and maintain that identity during times of stress.

Socialization: The family teaches; transmits beliefs, values, attitudes, and coping mechanisms; provides feedback; and guides problem solving (Friedman, 1992).

Developmental Tasks of Families

Duvall (1977) identified both critical family developmental tasks and stages of the family life cycle. Duvall's theory, based on Erikson's theory of psychosocial development (defined in Chapter 8), states that all families have certain basic tasks for survival and continuity, and also have specific tasks related to each stage of development throughout the life of the family. The basic tasks defined in the accompanying box are closely related to the functions of the family. They are included here because they expand those functions previously discussed.

These family developmental tasks are related to sequential stages in the life of a family. Seven stages and related developmental tasks are identified in Table 2-1. If developmental tasks are not met, societal disapproval and intervention may occur in areas such as child abuse, police actions, welfare agencies, or health departments (Edelman & Mandle, 1994). The successful mastery of each developmental stage is important to adaptation and family growth through successive stages.

Tasks for Family Survival and Continuity

- Providing shelter, food, clothing, and healthcare
- Allocating resources (money, time, space) according to each member's needs
- Determining individual roles and responsibilities in the support, management, and care of the home and family members
- Ensuring socialization of members through the internalization of increasingly mature roles in the family and in society
- Establishing socially acceptable ways of interacting, communicating, and expressing feelings (eg, affection, aggression, sexuality)
- Rearing children (natural, adopted) and then releasing them appropriately
- Relating to the community (school, church, work, neighborhood) and establishing rules for relatives, guests, friends
- Maintaining morale and motivation, rewarding achievement, meeting personal and family crises, setting attainable goals, and developing family loyalties and values

(Duvall, E. [1977]. *Marriage and family development* [5th ed.]. © 1977 by Harper & Row Publishers, Inc. Reprinted by permission of HarperCollins Publishers, Inc.)

The Family in Health and Illness

Healthcare activities, health beliefs, and health values are learned as part of a family. In health and illness, as well as in other areas of life, the individual reflects behaviors learned as a family member. When a person enters the healthcare system, he or she brings his or her own personal behaviors and needs, but the person also brings (in a sense) his or her family, too. Friedman (1992) has clearly identified the importance of family-centered nursing care, based on the following rationale:

- The family comprises interdependent members who affect one another. If some form of illness occurs in one member, all other members become a part of the illness. Nursing assessment and interventions must consider the whole family in a holistic approach.
- A strong relationship exists between the family and the health status of its members; therefore, the role of the family is essential in every level of nursing care.
- The level of wellness of the family and, in turn, each member, can be significantly improved through health promotion activities.
- Illness of one family member may indicate the same problem in other members; through assessment and intervention, the nurse can assist in improving the health status of all family members.

Risk Factors

Family patterns of behavior and the environment provided by the family, the environment in which the fam-

Table 2-1
Family Stages and Tasks

Stage	Task
Beginning family	Establishing a mutually satisfying marriage
	Planning to have or not have children
Childbearing family	Having and adjusting to infant
	Supporting needs of all three members
	Renegotiating marital relationship
Family with preschool children	Adjusting to costs of family life
	Adapting to needs of preschool children to stimulate growth and development
	Coping with parental loss of energy and privacy
Family with school-age children	Adjusting to the activity of growing children
	Promoting joint decision making between children and parents
	Encouraging and supporting children's educational achievements
Family with adolescents and young adults	Maintaining open communication among members
	Supporting ethical and moral values within the family
	Balancing freedom with responsibility for teenagers
	Releasing young adults with appropriate ritual and assistance
	Strengthening marital relationship
	Maintaining supportive home base
Postparental family	Preparing for retirement
	Maintaining ties with older and younger generations
Aging family	Adjusting to retirement
	Adjusting to loss of spouse
	Closing family home

(Family stages and tasks from Duvall, E. [1977]. *Marriage and family development* [5th ed.]. © 1977 by Harper & Row Publishers, Inc. Reprinted by permission of HarperCollins Publishers, Inc.; and Aldous, J. [1975]. *The developmental approach to family analysis.* Minneapolis: University of Minnesota Press.)

ily lives, and genetic factors can place family members at risk for health problems. It is important for nurses to assess these factors before developing nursing care plans or plans for health promotion. Typical questions that should be included in a family assessment are as follows:

- What is the family structure?
- What is the socioeconomic level?
- What is the ethnic background and religious affiliation of family members?
- Who cares for children if both parents work?
- What health practices are common (eg, type of foods eaten, times eaten, immunizations, bedtime, exercise)?
- What habits are common (eg, do any family members smoke, drink to excess, or use drugs)?
- How does the family cope with stress?
- Do close friends or family members live nearby, and can they help if necessary?

When conducting a health assessment for a family, the nurse should consider the risk factors for altered health described below and listed by family developmental level in the accompanying box.

Lifestyle

- Lack of knowledge about sexual and marital roles, leading to teenage marriage and pregnancy; divorce; sexually transmitted diseases; child, spouse, or elder abuse; and lack of prenatal or child care
- Alterations in nutrition, either more or less than body requirements at any age
- Chemical dependency, including the use of alcohol, drugs, and nicotine
- Inadequate dental care and hygiene
- Unsafe or unstimulating home environment

Psychosocial Factors

- Inadequate child care resources when both parents work, both for preschool and school-age children
- Inadequate income to provide safe housing, food, clothing, and healthcare
- Conflict between family members

Environmental Factors

- Lack of knowledge or finances to provide safe and clean living conditions
- Work or social pressures, which add to stress
- Air, water, or food pollution

Developmental Factors

- Families who have new babies, especially if support systems are unavailable
- Older people, especially those living alone or on a fixed income
- Unmarried, adolescent mothers who lack personal, economic, and educational resources

Biologic Factors

- Birth defects
- Mental retardation
- Genetic predisposition to certain diseases, including cardiovascular diseases and cancer

Nursing Actions to Promote Wellness

The role of the nurse in reducing risk factors focuses on activities that promote health for all family members at any level of development. Each person has a personal definition of health, based on family beliefs and values about health and illness. By providing interventions that emphasize wellness, the nurse assists both the individ-

Risk Factors for Alterations in Family Health Based on Family Developmental Level

Couple and Childbearing Couple

- Inadequate knowledge about contraception and family planning
- Inadequate knowledge about sexual and marital roles
- Lack of knowledge about child health and safety
- Unsafe home environment
- Inadequate resources for child care if working
- Child abuse or neglect
- First pregnancy before age 16
- Inadequate nutrition, obesity
- Abuse of nicotine, drugs, alcohol
- Low socioeconomic status
- Sexually transmitted diseases
- Rubella

Family With Adolescents

- Racial and ethnic family of origin
- Family values of aggressiveness, dependence on social welfare
- Low socioeconomic status
- Inadequate knowledge to teach problem-solving skills
- Conflict between parents and children
- Sexual abuse
- Use of nicotine, drugs, and/or alcohol
- Sexually transmitted diseases

Family With Middle-Aged Adults

- Diet high in fat, sugar, salt
- Obesity
- Use of nicotine and alcohol
- Physical inactivity
- Depression
- Environmental exposure to sunlight, radiation, asbestos, and pollution

Family With Older Adults

- Increasing age with loss of physical function
- Depression
- Chronic illnesses
- Poor nutrition
- Lack of exercise
- Death of spouse
- Limited income
- Past lifestyle

Adapted from *Healthy people: The Surgeon General's report on health promotion and disease prevention.* (1982). Health and Human Services Pub. No. 79-55071, Washington, DC: US Government Printing Office; and A. Sugars, E. O'Neil, & J. Bader. (1991). *Healthy people 2000: National health promotion and disease prevention objectives.* Durham, NC: The Pew Health Professions Commission.

ual and the family to meet basic human needs. Examples of nursing interventions to promote wellness in the family are shown in Table 2-2. Nurses may carry out the activities or may refer the individual or family to groups for additional education.

The family is the primary educational and support structure for the individual. The family, as a social unit, provides the environment and relationships necessary to meet basic human needs. Health beliefs and practices are learned within the family context and are strongly influenced by the family's developmental level. Health promotion activities and nursing actions can reduce the risk of illness and facilitate healthy behaviors at any age within the family life cycle.

The Community

A person, as an individual and as a member of a family, also belongs to a community. The community environment affects the ability of the individual to meet basic human needs. This section of the chapter discusses the community as it relates to basic human needs, including influences on health and illness.

A **community** can be defined in a variety of ways, but the most basic definition is that a community is a specific population (or group of people) living in a specified geographic area under similar regulations and having common values, interests, and needs. Within a community, people interact and share resources.

The Community in Health and Illness

The community has a strong influence on the health promotion and illness prevention of its individuals and families (Fig. 2-4). Just as the family has risk factors for the health of individual members, so does the community have risk factors involving resources, economics, and services. Nursing assessments and interventions would not be comprehensive and individualized if the community influence were not also considered.

Risk Factors

It is not within the scope of this book to discuss community health nursing as a whole. However, because the community provides the environment affecting health and illness, it is important to discuss environmental factors influencing the safety and security of the individuals within that community. The following are examples of community factors affecting health:

- Number and availability of healthcare institutions and services
- Housing codes and police and fire departments
- Nutritional services for low-income infants, mothers, school lunch programs, and older people

Table 2-2
Nursing Interventions to Promote Family Health and Wellness

Family Developmental Level	Nursing Interventions and Referrals
Couple and child-bearing family	Family planning clinics Prenatal classes Immunization information Poison-prevention programs
Family with school-age children	Vision and hearing screenings Dental health information Parent support groups Communicable disease control
Family with adolescents	Alcohol and drug abuse information Accident prevention programs Sex education Nutrition support groups Mental health programs
Family with middle-aged adults	Blood pressure screenings Exercise classes Stress reduction programs Specific support groups (stop smoking, Alcoholics Anonymous, coping with grief)
Family with older adults	Screening for chronic diseases (hypertension, glaucoma, diabetes) Retirement information Home safety programs Pharmacology information

- Zoning regulations separating residential and industrial areas
- Waste disposal services and locations
- Air and water pollution regulations
- Food sanitation guidelines
- Health education services and dissemination
- Recreational opportunities
- Prevalence of violent crimes or drug use

To illustrate how the community can affect individual and family needs, consider the following examples:

- Maria, age 20, lives in an inner-city, two-room apartment with her 6-month-old baby girl. The apartment lacks adequate heat and plumbing. Maria has no family living nearby, and her husband has left her. Maria rarely leaves her apartment because she fears the street gangs and drug addicts. She has never taken her baby to a local clinic for checkups because she does not want to ask her neighbors for directions.
- Anne, age 22, lives in a small house in a rural area. She is married and has a 2-year-old son. Her husband works at a local factory, and Anne works part-time at a clothing store. Both Anne and her husband have family members who live nearby, and they see them often. Anne, her husband, and her son all have regular health assessments.

These two different examples are given to demonstrate that the community plays a major role in the health of the people who live within it. Maria and her infant are at much greater risk for illness than are Anne and her family. Even if the two women had identical healthcare needs, a plan of care would reflect different interventions because of their community environments.

Nursing in the Community

Nurses carry out a variety of activities that involve community health, designed to promote wellness and prevent illness. Nurses promote wellness as individuals, as caregivers within institutional settings, and as community-based healthcare providers.

As individuals, nurses provide community services as volunteers in health-related activities (eg, screenings, educational programs, or blood drives) and as role models for health practices and lifestyles. Nurses working in healthcare institutions include community influences in developing individualized nursing care plans and in making referrals to community agencies and support groups. Community-based nurses are employed in many different kinds of health-related practice settings, including home healthcare, community health centers, school nursing, occupational nursing, and independent nursing practice. Community-based care is discussed in Chapter 11.

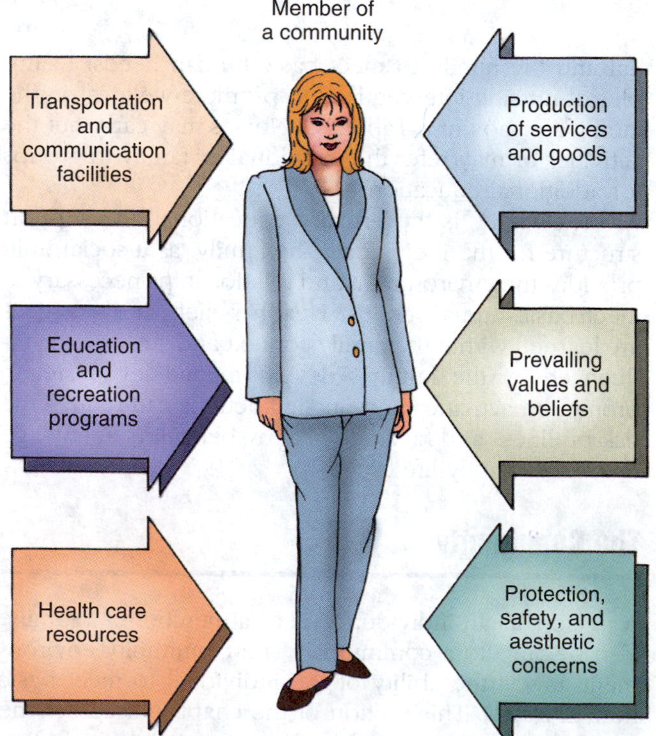

Figure 2-4
Many characteristics of a community influence the health of its members. This diagram shows six categories of characteristics that influence the health of a member of a community

Key Points

- Basic human needs are common to all people and are essential to health and survival. Many needs are met through a person's social environment, specifically the person's family and community.
- Maslow's hierarchy of basic human needs describes five levels of needs: (1) physiologic, (2) safety and security, (3) love and belonging, (4) self-esteem, and (5) self-actualization.
- Physiologic needs have the highest priority and are the base of the hierarchy. These needs include oxygen, food, water, temperature, elimination, sexuality, physical activity, and rest.
- Safety and security needs include a physical component, involving protection from potential or actual harm, and an emotional component, including trust and freedom from fear.
- Love and belonging needs include both giving and receiving love, and having a sense of belonging to others.
- Self-esteem needs focus on a person's feeling good about himself or herself and believing that others also hold that person in high regard.
- Self-actualization needs are the highest level of need and are met when a person achieves his or her potential.
- The family, the basic social unit of society, serves as a buffer between the needs of society and the needs of individual members. Many different family structures (or forms) exist, but all families carry out the same functions—physical, economic, reproductive, affective and coping, and socialization.
- The family life cycle has definite stages and developmental tasks.
- Family-centered nursing care incorporates basic human needs, family concepts, and risk factors into nursing interventions to promote wellness.
- The community provides an environment that is an integral component of individual needs and family functions. Holistic nursing care integrates community risk factors and influences in all types of healthcare settings.

Bibliography

Aldous, J. (1975). *The developmental approach to family analysis.* Minneapolis: University of Minnesota Press.

Anderson, K. H., & Tomlinson, P. S. (1992). The family health system as an emerging paradigmatic view for nursing. *IMAGE: Journal of Nursing Scholarship, 24*(1), 57–63.

Brewer, N., & Warren, M. (1994). Altered family processes related to an ill family member: A validation study. *Nursing Diagnosis, 5*(3), 115–120.

Cetinski, G., & Milne, R. (1991). Family caregivers. *Canadian Nurse, 87*(1), 33–34.

Chez, N. (1994). Helping the victim of domestic violence. *American Journal of Nursing, 94*(7), 32–37.

Danielson, C. B., Hamel-Bissel, B. P., & Winstead-Fry, P. W. (1992). *Families, health, and illness: Perspectives on coping and interventions.* St. Louis: Mosby–Year Book.

Duvall, E. (1977). *Marriage and family development* (5th ed.). Philadelphia: Lippincott.

Edelman, C., & Mandle, C. (1994). *Health promotion throughout the lifespan* (3rd ed.). St. Louis: Mosby–Year Book.

Friedman, M. (1992). *Family nursing: Theory and assessment* (3rd ed.). Norwalk, CT: Appleton & Lange.

Healthy people: The Surgeon General's report on human promotion and disease prevention (abridged). (1990). Washington, DC: American Public Health Association.

Jones, E. (1995). Deaf and hearing parents' perceptions of family functioning. *Nursing Research, 44*(2), 102–105.

Kelley, S. (1993). Caregiver stress in grandparents raising grandchildren. *IMAGE: Journal of Nursing Scholarship, 25*(4), 331–337.

Leahey, M., Stout, L., & Myrah, I. (1991). Family systems nursing. *Canadian Nurse, 87*(2), 31–33.

Lundeen, S. (1992). Health needs of a suburban community: A nursing assessment approach. *Journal of Community Nursing, 9*, 235–244.

Maslow, A. (1968). *Toward a psychology of being* (2nd ed.). New York: Van Nostrand–Reinhold.

Meierhoffer, L. L. (1992). Nurses battle family violence. *American Nurse, 24*(4), 1, 7–8.

Pender, N. (1987). *Health promotion in nursing practice* (2nd ed.). Norwalk, CT: Appleton-Century-Crofts.

Reinhard, S. (1994). Perspectives on the family's caregiving experience in mental illness. *IMAGE: Journal of Nursing Scholarship, 26*(1), 70–74.

Smith, M., & Martin, F. (1995). Domestic violence: Recognition, intervention, and prevention. *MEDSURG Nursing, 4*(1), 21–25.

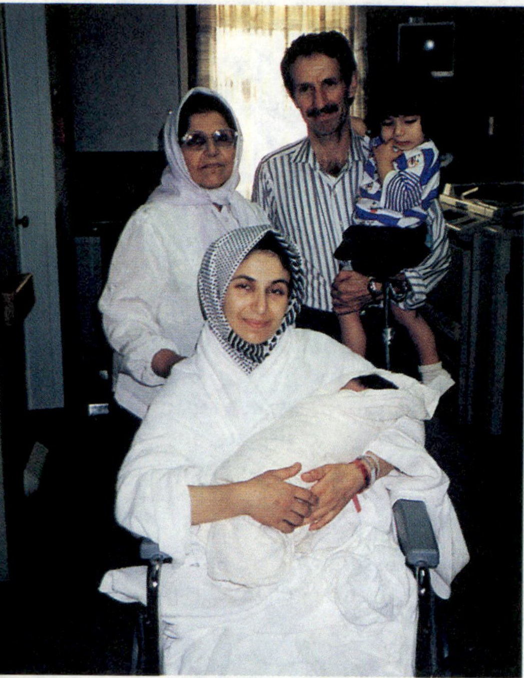

Chapter 3

Culture and Ethnicity

Objectives

After studying this chapter, the learner should be able to:

Define key terms used in the chapter.

Discuss the concepts of culture and ethnicity.

Describe cultural and ethnic characteristics that influence healthcare, including gender roles, language and communication, orientation to space and time, food and nutrition, socioeconomic factors, importance of family, physical and mental characteristics, spiritual characteristics, and perceptions of illness and health.

Compare and contrast the culture of the healthcare system with the broad concept of culture.

Identify the factors that affect the interaction of the nurse and the client in terms of culturally different healthcare values.

Discuss the guidelines that are useful in practicing transcultural nursing care.

Use knowledge of specific cultural and ethnic factors in providing holistic, individualized, culture-sensitive nursing care to clients.

Key Terms

cultural assimilation
cultural imposition
cultural blindness
culture
culture conflict
culture shock
dominant group
ethnicity
ethnocentrism
minority group
personal space
race
stereotyping
subculture
transcultural nursing

We live in a society that is made up of widely diverse groups of people. The groups include people of different racial and ethnic backgrounds, people with different sexual orientations, and people from different socioeconomic backgrounds. These groups and subgroups are called *cultures.* The number of cultural groups within the population continues to increase; by the year 2080, over half of the population of the United States will be part of groups that have traditionally been considered minorities (U.S. Bureau of the Census, 1990). As people of different societies and cultures emigrate to North America, this pattern of change will continue.

Culture is an integral component of both health and illness because of genetic characteristics and the values and beliefs we learn from our families and communities. In order to provide holistic care to people from diverse cultural backgrounds, nurses must be sensitive to the cultural needs, characteristics, and values of individuals, families, and groups.

This chapter focuses on the concepts of culture and ethnicity, including definitions of terms and a discussion of various characteristics that are culturally based and influence nursing care. It also provides a broad introduction to the major cultural and ethnic groups, and examines the importance of integrating transcultural nursing concepts into one's daily practice of nursing.

Concepts of Culture and Ethnicity

Culture

All people have culture, made visible by the attitudes and institutions unique to their particular group. **Culture,** broadly defined, is a view of the world, as well as a set of values, beliefs, and traditions that are handed down from generation to generation. Culture includes the beliefs, habits, likes and dislikes, and customs and rituals learned from one's family (Boyle & Andrews, 1995; Spector, 1991). As described by Leininger (1990), "culture includes all human activities taking material and nonmaterial forms and expressions . . . the political, economic, social, religious, educational, philosophical, technological, and environmental contexts in which human beings live and function" (p. 535). The characteristics of culture include the following:

- Culture guides behavior into acceptable ways for the people in a specific group. It is shared by, and provides an identity for, all members of the same cultural group.
- Culture is learned by each new generation through both formal and informal life experiences. Language is the primary means of transmitting culture.
- The practices of a particular culture often arise because of the group's social and physical environment.
- Cultural practices and beliefs are adapted over time, but they mainly remain constant as long as they satisfy needs.
- Culture influences the way people of a group view themselves, have expectations, and behave in response to certain situations. Because a culture is made up of individuals, differences within cultures as well as across cultures are found.

Within a culture are subgroups, or subcultures. A **subculture** is a large group of people who are members of a larger cultural group but have certain ethnic, occupational, or physical characteristics that are not common to the larger culture. For example, nursing is a subculture of the larger healthcare system culture, and teenagers and older adults are regarded as subcultures in North America.

Cultures have dominant groups and minority groups. A **dominant group** is the group within the culture that has the authority to control the value system and determine the rewards of the system. The dominant group usually is (but does not have to be) the largest group in a society (for example, white middle-class people are the dominant group in North America). A **minority group** usually has some physical or cultural characteristic (such as race, religious beliefs, or occupation) that identifies the people within it as different.

Ethnicity

Ethnicity is the sense of identification of a collective cultural group, largely based on the group's common heritage. One belongs to a specific ethnic group either through birth or through adoption of characteristics of that group. People within an ethnic group share com-

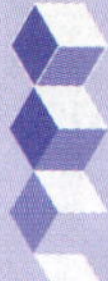

Through the Eyes of a Student

I was doing my maternity rotation, and was assigned to labor and delivery. I was assigned a woman who spoke no English—she and her husband were from Central America and had been in the United States for only 2 months.

When I arrived at 7 AM, the night nurse was giving a report about my patient to the day nurse. The night nurse was frantic—no one understood the couple, all efforts to locate a translator had come up empty, and, quite frankly, she had no idea exactly what condition this woman was in.

I quickly began to think back on my 2 years of Spanish. Could I be of any help to this couple? I wondered. Would I remember enough to communicate with them about giving birth? Then I decided that any little bit of communication at this point was better than none, so I spoke up. I told both nurses that I spoke some Spanish, and asked if I could be of any help. The night nurse literally hugged me!

I began by telling the expectant couple that I was a nursing student and that I spoke some Spanish. We exchanged introductions and then I asked the woman some assessment questions. Nothing I said was complicated—all of my sentences were short and simple, but who needed more than that?

Then the couple asked me some questions. They had heard about "cutting open the stomach" to deliver a baby. I naturally assumed that they meant a cesarean delivery. They looked so afraid, but I had to be honest. They wanted to know how it was done and why. The words I could not remember or did not know I acted out. They looked so relieved when I was finished.

The man said that they thought *all* babies were born this way in our country. He said that they had never heard of this procedure until coming to the United States. No wonder they were so frightened!

The doctor came in, examined the woman, and said she was fully dilated. The doctor asked if I could teach a crash course in Lamaze breathing to the woman. She also asked me if I would stay throughout the delivery because she would need assistance in translating directions to the woman. Of course I said yes.

The woman was terrified. I told her that it was normal to be afraid, and that I would be with her during the delivery. She took my hand and whispered, "Muchas gracias." I never felt more useful than I did at that moment.

—A. Kelly Gaylor, Holy Family College, Philadelphia

mon and unique cultural and social beliefs and behavior patterns, including language and dialect, religious practices, literature, folklore, music, political interests, food preferences, and employment patterns. Ethnicity largely develops through day-to-day life with family and friends within the community.

Race

Although ethnicity often is used interchangeably with race, these terms are not the same. Classifying people by **race** is a way of categorizing them into subgroups according to specific physical characteristics, such as skin pigmentation, body stature, facial features, and hair texture. Although there has been a blending of physical characteristics through the centuries, the three major classifications by race are Caucasian, Negroid, and Mongoloid.

Cultural Assimilation

Because minority groups live within the dominant group, many of their members lose the cultural characteristics that made them different. This process is called **cultural assimilation** or *acculturation*. Assimilation occurs when one value is dropped and a value of the dominant culture is picked up. When people immigrate, their values are on one end of the spectrum and the values of the dominant culture are on the other end. As immigrants go to work, go to school, move out of the community, and learn the dominant language, they move closer to the dominant culture. The process and the rate of assimilation are individualized. Because the degree of assimilation is so variable, nurses cannot assume characteristics based on ethnic groups.

Mutual cultural assimilation does occur, with some characteristics of both groups being traded. For example, when the Vietnamese came to the United States they learned to speak English, and Americans learned to cook with the vegetables preferred by the Vietnamese. In this way, almost all of us gain from the many cultures with which we live. Although we seldom think about it, the clothes we wear, the foods we eat, the music we enjoy, the slang we use, and the leisure activities we practice are all areas in which we have become acculturated.

Factors Affecting Cultural Sensitivity

A variety of factors may negatively affect culturally sensitive care. When one assumes that all members of a culture or ethnic group act alike, **stereotyping** is at work. Common stereotypic beliefs are that all Italians are emotional, that all Germans are stoic, that men never cry, and that the elderly are senile. Stereotyping may be positive or negative. Negative stereotyping includes racism, ageism, and sexism. These are beliefs that certain races, ages, or genders are inherently superior to others, leading to discrimination against those considered inferior. Stereotyping often is done by members of the dominant group about the minority group in a culture (Fig. 3-1).

Cultural blindness occurs when one ignores differences and proceeds as though they do not exist. This is a common practice in the healthcare system, especially in regard to what are considered nontraditional methods of care. **Cultural imposition** is the belief that everyone should conform to the majority belief system. When this does not happen, the person may experience **culture conflict** and ridicule the beliefs and traditions of others in an effort to make his or her own values more secure (Boyle & Andrews, 1995).

Cultural and Ethnic Influences on Healthcare

North America is multicultural and multiethnic. As such, there is a wide diversity of people in almost every populated area. This means that it is important for us, as nurses, to be aware of and sensitive to the needs of a culturally diverse client population. This section deals with general considerations in transcultural care; specific values and behaviors of different groups are discussed later in the chapter.

Gender Roles

In many cultures, the male is the dominant figure. In cultures where this is true, males make decisions for other family members as well as for themselves. For example, if approval for medical care is needed, the man gives it, no matter which family member is involved. In cultures where the male is dominant, the female usually is passive. In African-American families, however, as well as in many Caucasian families, the female often is dominant.

Knowledge of the dominant member of the family is an important consideration in planning nursing care. If the dominant member is ill and can no longer make decisions, the whole family probably is anxious and confused. If a nondominant family member is ill, he or she may require help in verbalizing needs, particularly if they differ from those the dominant member perceives as being important.

Language and Communication

When people from another part of the world move to North America, they may speak their own language fluently, but have difficulty speaking the language of their new country. This is especially true of the women in the family (many of whom do not work outside the home), of the older generation, and of groups of people who live in proximity to others who speak the same language. Children usually assimilate more rapidly and learn the language of the dominant culture quickly because they leave home each day, go to school, and make new friends of the dominant culture. Wage earners also tend to learn a new language more quickly from the work setting. Assimilation is slower for people who stay at home, especially if they live in communities of their ethnic culture. Language acquisition is thus tied to necessity and assimilation rather than to degree of difficulty.

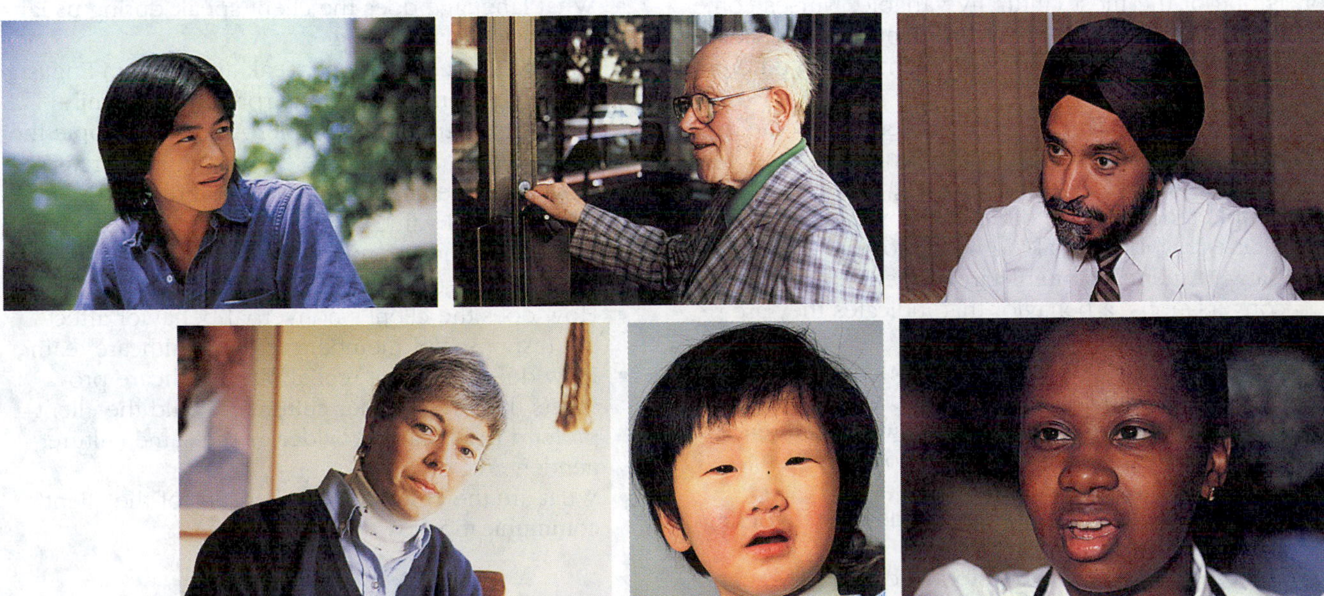

Figure 3-1
Identifying one's own prejudices is the first step toward eliminating them. Think about the assumptions you make about the people in these images.

Nursing Today: Challenges and Solutions

Promoting Cultural Diversity in Nurses

A program called Project Linc (Ladders in Nursing Careers) is being used to promote career advancement and cultural diversity in nursing. This project was developed for healthcare employees who are unable to pursue careers in nursing because of financial, educational, or other barriers. The focus is on minorities, because so few—actually only about 10% of all nurses—are non-whites. The project was initially developed by the Greater New York Hospital Foundation to increase the racial and cultural diversity of nursing while also increasing the numbers of nurses in the area, and has been successful since its inception in 1989. The Robert Wood Johnson Foundation is replicating the program at other sites across the nation.

Participants in the program attend nursing school full-time and work part-time at their hospital jobs while receiving full-time pay and benefits. Financial support is available for tuition, lab fees, books, and some supplies. Participants must agree to pay back the loan by working at the hospital 18 months for every year they are in Project LINC. Since its inception, 435 employees from 58 hospitals and nursing homes have enrolled in RN or LPN programs and more than 97% of the graduates are now licensed.

Source: Cassetta, R. (1993). Cultural diversity promoted through "Ladders" program. *American Nurse, 25*(1), 16.

Most Americans do not learn a second language. As a result, communication problems can arise during healthcare activities. This problem is not unique to non–English-speaking clients; even in different regions of the United States, certain dialects or word meanings can cause differences in understanding. Consider how difficult it must be to describe symptoms or give a personal health history when you do not understand the questions being asked. Something as simple as showing the nurse where you hurt is impossible if you do not know what is being said. In addition, clients may forget English words or revert to a more familiar language in the stress of an injury or illness.

Eye contact, as a nonverbal communication behavior, is one of the most culturally variable. Nurses come from a culture that emphasizes eye contact while speaking, but other cultures regard this behavior in different ways. For example:

- Direct eye contact may be considered impolite or aggressive by Asians, Native Americans, Indochinese, Arabs, and Appalachians; these groups of people tend to avoid direct eye contact and avert their eyes while speaking with another.
- Native Americans often stare at the floor during conversations, a behavior that indicates they are carefully listening.
- Some African Americans may roll their eyes at what are considered to be ridiculous questions.
- Hispanic Americans look downward in deference to age, gender, social position, economic status, and authority.
- Muslim-Arab women indicate modesty by avoiding eye contact with males.
- Hasidic Jewish males tend to avoid direct eye contact with women (Boyle & Andrews, 1995).

Nurses who work in an area that has a high population of residents who speak a language other than English need to learn pertinent words and phrases in that language. Many agencies have a qualified interpreter, or one can be found in the community. Sometimes a family member or friend can translate for the nurse. It is important to select an interpreter who has knowledge of the healthcare system to avoid misinterpretation of questions and answers. Many family members are protective and may not be the most reliable means of transferring information. Nurses may find themselves talking in a louder tone of voice to a client who does not understand what is being said; it is important to remember that this is a communication problem, not a hearing problem. Considerations for transcultural assessment of communication follow, adapted from Boyle and Andrews (1995), and Chapter 22 provides information on communicating with non–English-speaking clients.

- What language does the client speak during usual activities of daily living?
- How well does the client speak and write in English?
- Does the client need an interpreter? Are family members or friends available? Are there people the client would not want to serve as an interpreter?
- How does the client prefer to be addressed?
- What cultural values and beliefs of the client may vary techniques of communication and care (such as eye contact, space, or social taboos)?
- How does the client's nonverbal behavior affect the responses of members of the healthcare team?
- How does the client feel about healthcare providers that are of other cultures; would the client prefer a healthcare provider of the same culture, gender, and/or age?
- What are the cultural characteristics of the client's communications with others?

Orientation to Space and Time

Personal space is the area surrounding a person that is regarded as part of the person. This area, individualized to each person and to different cultures and ethnic groups, is the distance maintained from others during personal interactions. When one's personal space is not taken into consideration, one may become uncomfortable or even angry. With nursing care, which involves physical contact and close communications, it is important to know cultural personal space preferences. As examples, people of Arabic and African origin commonly sit and stand close to one another when talking, whereas people of Asian and European descent are more comfortable talking with some distance between themselves and others.

Most people and almost all institutions in North America value promptness and punctuality. When arriving for an appointment, doing a job, or carrying out an activity, being on time and getting the job done are viewed as important. This is not true in some other cultures. For example, in some South Asian cultures, being late is considered a sign of respect. In addition, although most of middle-class North America is future-oriented (including activities that promote health not only in the present but also in the future), other cultures are more concerned with the present or the past. This means that client teaching may have to be adapted; as an example, if a client is to take a medication twice a day at home, the teaching plan should focus on taking the pill twice a day (for example, one in the morning and one in the evening) rather than at 9 AM and 9 PM.

Food and Nutrition

The way foods are prepared and the foods that are eaten often are culturally related. Certain food groups serve as staples of the diet based on culture, and remain so even when members of that culture are living in a different country. For example, rice and vegetables are the staples of Asians and Chinese, and pasta is a staple of Italians. Mexican Americans favor beans and tortillas, whereas Puerto Ricans try to eat a balance of hot, cold, and cool foods (the classification is based on type of foods and not temperature of foods). These are only examples and should not be used to select client foods; the nurse should always ask the client about food preferences.

Clients in the hospital setting often do not have much of a choice of foods. This means that people with cultural food preferences may not be able to select appealing foods and thus may be at risk for less than adequate nutrition. When assessing the cause of decreased appetite in clients, the nurse should determine if the problem is one of culture. It may be possible for family or friends to bring in foods that satisfy nutritional needs and still meet dietary restrictions. Culturally sensitive assessment of nutrition considers the following questions, with examples of differences:

1. Which foods are considered edible and which are not?

   In France corn is considered animal feed, whereas corn is a commonly eaten vegetable in the United States.

   Religious beliefs prohibit some Jewish, Muslim, and Seventh-Day Adventist clients from eating pork.

   Clients who follow a vegetarian diet do not eat pork, beef, or chicken.

2. What times and types of food are considered meals?

   Anglo-Americans typically eat three meals a day, with foods such as bacon and eggs or cereal for breakfast, sandwiches and soup for lunch, and meat with potatoes and vegetables for dinner. In contrast, soup is often eaten for every meal by Vietnamese, beans are a staple for every meal among Mexican people, and people from Middle Eastern countries often eat cheese and olives for breakfast.

   Native American and Latin American people usually eat two meals a day.

   Rural southern African Americans often eat large amounts of food on weekends and less food at meals during the week.

   Holy days or religious holidays influence food choices for almost all cultures.

3. With whom is the food eaten?

   Men and women eat separately in some Middle Eastern cultures; this tradition has significance for group dining in settings such as mental health institutions and long-term care facilities.

   Dietary teaching must be individualized according to cultural values about the social significance and sharing of food.

Socioeconomic Factors

The amount of money a person or family has or does not have affects the way the person or family meets basic needs and maintains health. Poverty is a major problem in North America. Poverty leads to other problems concerning healthcare financing, care of infants and children, and homelessness. All these areas are of concern to nursing.

The Culture of Poverty

There has been much debate over the true definition of poverty. In terms of economics, a person or family whose income falls below the poverty line is considered poor. The U.S. Bureau of the Census designates a family as poor if it falls short of the pretax money income needed to purchase a minimum amount of goods and services. On the other hand, it has been stated that poverty is a relative term that reflects a judgment made on the basis of standards prevailing in the community. The standards change in time and place; what is judged poverty in one community might be regarded as wealth in another (Spector, 1991). No matter how poverty is defined, it is an increasingly devastating epidemic—one that has evolved into a culture of its own. At highest risk are families headed by single mothers, older people, and future generations of those now living in poverty.

The so-called feminization of poverty threatens to raise the number of people who are living at poverty level. The number of female-headed households is increasing as a result of divorce, abandonment, unmarried motherhood, and changes in abortion laws. Because many households depend on two incomes for economic survival, a single woman supporting a household is at a financial disadvantage. The number of single-parent families headed by women is closely associated with the increasing number of children living in poverty and the number of homeless families with children.

The expanding population of older people has contributed to problems with poverty. Most older people live on fixed incomes, which often do not keep up with inflation, and many (particularly widows) are on the borderline of poverty or have already slipped into the poverty culture. Socioeconomic status differs by the cultural group of the older adult. For example, Pacific/Asian, African-American, Native American, and Hispanic people generally have lower incomes than do majority populations. The work history of the cultural group, especially those who have worked all their lives as agricultural workers, often means an individual has no Social Security or Medicare benefits.

In some cases the culture of poverty is passed from generation to generation. This seems to be especially true in such groups as migrant farm workers, families living on welfare, and people who live in isolated areas of Appalachia. Poverty cultures have the following characteristics:

- Feelings of despair, resignation, and fatalism
- Day-to-day attitude toward life with no hope for the future
- Unemployment and need for financial or government aid
- Use of escape valves such as alcohol and drugs
- Unstable family structure with abusiveness and abandonment
- Decline in self-respect and retreat from community involvement

Effects of Poverty on Healthcare

Poverty has long been a barrier to healthcare. It prevents many people from adequately meeting their basic human needs. Lack of affordable or adequate housing is a problem frequently experienced by poor people. When low-income housing is available, it often is associated with low-cost maintenance, sometimes resulting in the absence of such necessities as running water, heat, and electricity. To stretch their available money and to pool resources, many poor people live in crowded conditions, with several families living together in one household.

Research has demonstrated that crowded living conditions foster depersonalization, correlate with higher crime rates, and lead to psychologic problems, such as schizophrenia, alienation, and feelings of worthlessness (Spector, 1991). They also contribute to an increased incidence of disease and illness because of the proximity of people, the sharing of utensils and belongings, poor sanitation, and other poor health habits. The health effects of such conditions include a higher incidence and severity of illness in poor people than in people of higher-income groups.

Access to healthcare facilities frequently necessitates transportation, which many times is neither affordable nor available to poor people. Their access to health insurance also is frequently limited, and commonly a choice must be made between purchasing food and purchasing healthcare. In 1963, Canada introduced a national health insurance program aimed at ensuring Canadian citizens equal access to healthcare regardless of age, economic status, creed, or ethnic origin. Despite this program and a high-quality healthcare system, people's health remains directly related to their economic status. Those in the upper-income group live longer and are freer of disability than those in the lower-income group. Other barriers to healthcare include isolation, language or communication difficulties, seasonal occupations, migration patterns, depersonalization, and institutional prejudice (Spector, 1991).

Family Support

In many cultural and ethnic groups, people have large, extended families and consider the needs of any family member to be equal to or greater than their own, and are unwilling to share with those outside the family (including healthcare providers) private information about family members. Other cultural groups have great respect for the elders in the family, and would never consider institutional care for them. Including the family in planning care for any client is a major component in nursing care to meet individualized needs, especially if those needs can be met only through consideration of all members of the family.

Physical and Mental Health

Differences and similarities in physiologic and psychologic characteristics are found among cultural and ethnic groups. These characteristics influence the health and illness status of group members.

Physiologic Characteristics

Researchers theorize that past generations slowly adapted to their surrounding environment. Dark-skinned people developed lighter skin as early populations moved to colder northern climates where there is less sunlight throughout the year compared with equatorial climates. Lighter skin is better able to use vitamin D from sunlight than darker skin. It also is theorized that a person's nose shape and size evolved according to the climate in which the person lived (Henderson & Primeaux, 1981). From a scientific and anthropologic point of view, these adaptations were logical changes necessary for improving the lives and well-being of human beings. Some of these biologic variations were

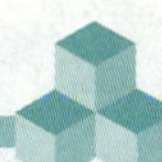

Examples of Nursing Diagnoses

Culture and Ethnicity

The following nursing diagnoses are examples of those that might be appropriate for providing holistic transcultural care:

- Impaired Verbal Communication related to inability to speak English and interpreter unavailable
- Impaired Social Interaction related to recent move away from neighborhood and friends of same ethnic group
- Altered Parenting related to use of culturally based discipline considered inappropriate or abusive by current country of residence
- Spiritual Distress related to inability to regularly take part in significant culturally based rituals
- Family Coping: Potential for Growth related to request for information about child care
- Ineffective Management of Therapeutic Regimen (Individual) related to mistrust of traditional healthcare personnel
- Relocation Stress Syndrome related to recent move from country of origin
- Situational Low Self Esteem related to language difficulties and inability to secure employment
- Powerlessness related to inability to make healthcare providers understand the importance of dietary and social values and beliefs

effective adaptations for a particular period or for living in a certain environment.

Once a person is removed from the environment that encouraged the biologic variation, the variation could have a detrimental effect on health and well-being. The results of various studies have shown that certain ethnic groups have particular characteristics that make them more prone to developing specific diseases and conditions. These conditions may be acquired as a result of environmental factors, or they may be inherited. Some of the variations are discussed in the next section.

Keloid Formation. Keloids result from the overgrowth of connective tissue that occurs during the healing process after an injury, surgery, or other type of connective tissue damage. People of African heritage are much more likely to develop keloids. Rather than healing level with the surrounding skin tissue, the wound of a person with a tendency toward keloid formation heals with a rough, lumpy, or elevated scar.

Lactase Deficiency. Milk and many milk products contain lactose, a sugar. The enzyme lactase must be present in the body to break down lactose during digestion. Without lactase, the lactose ferments in the intestines, resulting in gas (flatus), diarrhea, and abdominal bloating and cramping. Lactase deficiency and lactose intolerance are more common in Hispanic women and in both men and women of African, Chinese, and Thai ancestry (Boyle & Andrews, 1995).

People with a lactase deficiency have to obtain their calcium and protein requirements from other sources because they are not able to tolerate regular milk products. Special milk and milk products are available but are more expensive. Sharp cheeses (aged more than 60 days) and fermented milk products, such as yogurt, buttermilk, and sour cream, may be tolerated.

Sickle Cell Anemia. Sickle cell anemia is most common in people with African or Mediterranean ethnic backgrounds. The sickle cell trait originally served as a protective mechanism against malaria. People with sickle cell anemia have sickle-shaped red blood cells (RBCs) that break down more rapidly than normal-shaped RBCs. The sickle shape also prevents the RBCs from moving easily through the smaller vessels in the body. This factor can lead to the smaller vessels being clogged by the RBCs, which can cause many potentially serious problems. Sickle cell carriers can be identified by a blood test.

Tay-Sachs Disease. People of Eastern European Jewish descent may carry a gene for a hereditary disorder called Tay-Sachs disease. A child born with this progressive disease has a short life span, usually less than 2 years. There is no cure or treatment for this devastating disease. Carriers of the disease can be identified by serum analysis.

G6PD Deficiency. Glucose-6-phosphate dehydrogenase is an enzyme normally found in RBCs. G6PD deficiency affects about 10% of the African-American population. The deficiency is sex-linked and carried on the X female chromosome. A person with this deficiency has RBCs that are unable to maintain a cell membrane. Without this protective membrane, RBCs are easily destroyed (hemolyzed) by various oxidant drugs, such as aspirin, ascorbic acid, probenecid, sulfa drugs, and vitamin K, and by fava beans (also called horse or broad beans). This destruction results in anemia, which may be severe and life-threatening, and in elevated bilirubin levels (a result of the hemolyzed RBCs), which causes jaundice (yellowing of the skin and sclerae).

Thalassemia. Thalassemia, a genetic disorder, affects the hemoglobin in the RBCs. The production of the alpha or beta globin chains is defective, and disrupts RBC function. This disorder is most commonly found in people of Mediterranean, Asian (especially Chinese), and African origin.

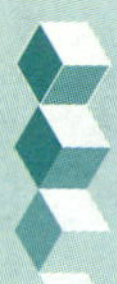

Research in Nursing: Making a Difference

Transcultural Nursing Care

People requiring nursing care to promote health and prevent illness may be citizens of any part of the world. To meet the individualized needs of these people, nurses must be familiar with and provide care from a framework recognizing values and cultures that may differ from their own. Individualized assessments and interventions can be made only if cultural and ethnic influences and factors are integrated into planning for holistic care. In addition, a variety of ethnically and racially diverse nurses are needed to meet the needs of an increasingly multicultural client population. The studies described here are examples of this critical element of nursing practice.

Related Research

Ahijevych, K., & Bernhard, L. (1994). Health-promoting behaviors of African American women. *Nursing Research, 43*(2), 86–89.
The purpose of this study was to identify health-promoting lifestyle behaviors of African-American women. The subjects of the sample were 187 women between the ages of 18 and 69. Findings were compared to other published reports. The results illustrated that the African-American women in this study tended to rank lower on healthy behaviors. Factors believed to influence healthy behaviors in this population include lower income, employment status, medical problems, readability and possible middle-class bias of the instrument used in the research, and lack of control over living arrangements. The sample did have a higher performance on health responsibility than most other groups. Implications of the study include the importance of assessing and enhancing health-promoting behaviors in African-American women.

Frye, B., & D'Avanzo, C. (1994). Cultural themes in family stress and violence among Cambodian refugee women in the inner city. *Advances in Nursing Science, 16*(3), 64–77.
Cambodian refugee women living in American inner cities frequently face the cumulative trauma of war experience and cultural adaptation. The qualitative study was conducted to investigate cultural beliefs, coping strategies, and management of family stress among this population. Findings from interviews identified that nonconfrontation and withdrawal were primarily used to manage stressful and violent events. These methods of coping are hypothesized as culturally based. Further research with this high-risk population is recommended to develop culturally sensitive care.

Reiskin, H., & Haussler, S. (1994). Multicultural students' perceptions of nursing as a career. *IMAGE: Journal of Nursing Scholarship, 26*(1), 61–64.
The purposes of this study included an exploration of the perceptions of nursing by racially and ethnically diverse high school students. The sample, composed of 276 students beginning their junior year in high school, agreed that nurses worked with their hands, worked very hard, and were very busy. However, the students of all ethnic and racial groups did not see nursing as their ideal career. African-American and Latino students had the most positive perceptions of nurses in terms of making money, working in safe places, and being appreciated by others. These same qualities were ranked the lowest by Asian students. Authors of the study recommend that nurse educators gear recruitment efforts toward ethnic minorities, correct inaccurate perceptions, and provide mentoring activities. These activities will help increase the number of students and nurses who are not only culturally diverse but also culturally sensitive.

Summary

Cultural diversity in clients and in nurses themselves is increasingly recognized as an essential consideration in nursing care. No matter the age group or population, nursing interventions to meet the needs of the client and the family must be planned and implemented within a framework of cultural values and orientation. As nursing advances into the next century, this component of nursing care must become an integral part of both nursing practice and nursing education.

Sarcoidosis. Much more prevalent in the African-American population, sarcoidosis involves the formation of multiple tubercles or nodules on various parts of the body, most commonly the lymph nodes, liver, spleen, lungs, skin, eyes, and small bones of the feet and hands. These nodules eventually form into fibrous tissue. Skeletal muscle involvement can result in muscle atrophy (wasting). If the myocardium is involved, major cardiac problems can result.

Gout. Gout is most commonly found in men, especially those of Puerto Rican or Filipino descent. Excessive quantities of uric acid are found in the blood and may be deposited in joints and cartilage. The deposition of uric acid results in swelling, inflammation, and pain in the affected area. The uric acid crystals eventually may permanently damage the joints. These crystals also predispose the person to the formation of renal calculi (kidney stones).

Psychologic Characteristics

In most situations, a person relates the behaviors of another person to her or his own familiar culture. This process usually is multidirectional; for example, in a healthcare setting, the client evaluates the attitudes and actions of the healthcare provider at the same time the healthcare provider makes perceptions about the behavior of the client. It is important to remember that what may seem reasonable and important to a client may seem ridiculous and irrelevant to a nurse. The reverse perception also is true: practices a nurse perceives as logical and effective may seem senseless, incompetent, or even dangerous to a client.

Most mental health norms have been based on research and observations made of white, middle-class people. Many ethnic groups have their own norms or acceptable patterns of behavior concerning psychologic well-being and psychologic reactions to certain situations. For example, most Hispanic people deal with problems within the family and telling problems to a stranger is not within their value system; however, psychotherapy can be effective as long as the therapist integrates the value system of the client into the treatment plan. Many traditional Chinese people consider mental illness a stigma; therefore, seeking psychiatric help is a disgrace to the family. Traditionally, Chinese people prefer to avoid or minimize any type of conflict, so the use of any direct confrontation during psychotherapy may not work as well as expected. Also, Chinese people traditionally have been taught that the expression of strong emotions results in disharmony and imbalance between the body's energy forces (*yin and yang*) and is considered a sign of weakness. As a result of this belief, therapy involving the venting of strong feelings and emotions may be unacceptable to the client. In situations of extreme stress or high anxiety, some Puerto Ricans may demonstrate hyperkinetic seizure activity known as *ataques*. This behavior is a culturally accepted reaction.

Culture Shock. **Culture shock,** or the feelings a person experiences when placed in a different culture that is perceived as strange, may result in psychologic discomfort or disturbances. The patterns of behavior a person found acceptable and effective in his or her own culture often are not adequate in the new one. The person may then feel foolish, fearful, incompetent, inadequate, embarrassed, humiliated, and inferior. These feelings eventually can lead to frustration, anxiety, and loss of self-esteem.

Reaction to Pain. Healthcare researchers maintain that the expressions and behaviors exhibited by people in pain are culturally prescribed. Some cultures allow and even encourage the open expression of emotions experienced by a person in pain, whereas other cultures frown on the open and free expression of emotions. The main concern of nurses in this area of cultural expression is the categorization of clients as the ideal client. A client who quietly and stoically deals with pain may have her pain reduction needs ignored by nurses. It often is assumed that a client who does not complain of pain is not experiencing any great degree of pain. Nurses should be sensitive to other signals of discomfort, such as holding or applying pressure to the painful area, self-restriction of activities that intensify the pain, and uncontrollable, spontaneous expressions of discomfort, such as facial grimacing and moaning. Clients who freely express their discomfort should not be classified as constant complainers whose requests for pain relief sometimes seem excessive. Pain is a warning from the body that something is wrong, and every complaint of pain should be carefully assessed.

Nursing care for the client in pain is always individualized (see Chapter 41), but important culture-sensitive considerations include:

- Recognize that culture is an important component of individuality and that each person holds (and has the right to hold) various beliefs about pain.
- Respect the client's right to respond to pain in whatever manner is culturally and individually appropriate.
- Never stereotype a client's perceptions or responses to pain based on culture.

Alternative Healing Systems

Values and beliefs about illness, health, and illness care are developed as a direct result of cultural and ethnic influences. Folk medicine classifies illnesses as natural or unnatural. Natural illnesses are caused by dangerous agents, such as cold air or impurities in the air, water, or food. Unnatural illnesses are punishments for failing to follow God's rules, resulting in evil forces or witchcraft causing physical or mental health problems.

Folk Healers. In some cultures the power to heal is thought to be a gift from God bestowed on certain people. It is believed that these special people, healers, know what is wrong with a client through divine intervention and experience. A client who is familiar with such healers may perceive modern healthcare providers as incompetent because they have to ask many questions before they can treat an illness. A folk healer may prescribe boiled herbal tea as a treatment. Someone who is accustomed to this type of treatment may find it difficult to take a succession of pills that are not even steeped in hot water. Folk healers traditionally are less expensive, usually more accessible, and more understanding of the client's cultural and personal needs, and they speak the client's language.

Traditional Folk Medicine. Having knowledge and understanding of traditional folk remedies used by culturally different clients greatly improves and enhances effective nursing care and facilitates a safe return of the client to a state of wellness or health.

Developing Critical Thinking Skills

Situation

Your friend, Amy Chang, confides to you that she is very worried about her grandmother. When you meet Mrs. Chang she demonstrates many of the assessment findings related to congestive heart failure. Although her family has entreated her to seek medical attention, Mrs. Chang insists on relying on herbal teas and traditional Chinese remedies. Now 88 years old, Mrs. Chang came to America from mainland China when she was 14. While raising a family that is thoroughly Americanized, Mrs. Chang has resisted embracing her new culture and now wants nothing to do with "American medicine." Amy, who is also a nursing student, loves her grandmother dearly and is frustrated by her stubborn refusal to see an internist. Both of you have reason to believe that she could be helped by medical attention. What do you do?

1. ***Identify Goal of Thinking***
   Clarify your thinking about alternative medicine so that you can decide how you ought to respond to Mrs. Chang's worsening physical condition.

2. ***Assess Adequacy of Knowledge***
   Pertinent circumstances: While you have strong reason to believe that Mrs. Chang is suffering from congestive heart failure, she has not been medically diagnosed and you lack definitive knowledge about her medical condition and the likelihood that she would respond to treatment. You do know that she places a high value on traditional Chinese culture and strongly believes that if she is to be healed, the healing will result from herbal teas and traditional Chinese remedies. She has no confidence in American medicine. Her family describe her as being extremely strong-willed and very lovable.

   Prerequisite knowledge: In order to decide how you should respond in this situation, you need to know that traditional Western medicine is not the only beneficial system of medicine. It would be very helpful for you and Mrs. Chang's family to learn more about Chinese medicine and the probability of its benefiting her (as well as the possibility of its harming her) in her present condition. You will also need to learn more about what is essential to Mrs. Chang's well-being. How much value does she place on physical health? How important is it for her to live (and possibly die) within the familiar and comforting boundaries of her culture? You will want to assess what teaching, counseling, and support Mrs. Chang needs to reach an informed and voluntary decision that is right for her.

   Room for error: Since Mrs. Chang's life may literally be at stake, there is not much room for error in the manner you and her family choose to respond. Even if her condition is not life-threatening, her sense of well-being may be severely threatened if she feels forced to pursue treatment that is alien and frightening.

   Time constraints: Although you are uncertain about the seriousness of her condition, you understand that the sooner she receives effective therapy the better. Unless her condition suddenly deteriorates this is not a decision that needs to be made within the next 24 hours.

3. ***Address Potential Problems***
   The most serious obstacle to critical thinking in this situation would be an inability to weigh the respective merits of alternative healing systems. Cultural bias may result in the untested assumption that American medicine is necessarily superior to all other systems of healing and that it would be morally wrong to support a choice for anything else. The love of Mrs. Chang's family and their desire to do everything possible to keep her well may interfere with their ability to allow her the freedom to make the choice that is right for her.

4. ***Consult Helpful Resources***
   Your first challenge will be to learn more about traditional Chinese medicine and you will want to consult with local authorities as well as available literature. The National Institutes of Health have now established an Office of Alternative Medicine, which may provide helpful information. Your most important resource may be Mrs. Chang herself, and it will be important to try to learn from her as much as you can about what she values and what her goals are at this point in her life.

5. ***Critique Judgment/Decision***
   After getting to know Mrs. Chang better, you realize that she is firmly committed to her ways and adamant about not going to an American doctor or into a hospital at this point of her life. You (with her family) thus have only two options: to force her to see an internist against her will, possibly deceiving her in order to get her to the internist's office, or to support her choice to rely on familiar remedies, which may or may not successfully resolve her problems. The first alternative may save her life, and her family can see no other choice. You realize that by making this choice the family is imposing its values on Mrs. Chang and violating her autonomy, her right to determine the course of her life. You decide to support her and to try to explain to her family the importance of doing this. You understand that if her condition is serious and her traditional remedies prove ineffective her death may be hastened, but she accepts this consequence and prefers it to embracing an alien and frightening culture.

A common mode of treatment in many cultures is the use of herbs. In fact, many medications used today have a basis in herbs or other plant sources that have been used for centuries to cure illnesses. A problem may arise when a client is being cared for by both an herbalist and a physician. The herbalist may be prescribing an herb and the physician a drug, both of which have the same action. The client may be overmedicated or undermedicated because of the double prescription.

The nurse should not discourage the client's use of traditional folk medicine unless it is harmful to the client's health and well-being or decreases the effectiveness of the nursing and medical care planned. Incorporating the client's traditional healthcare beliefs into the care plan is an effective way to gain trust and cooperation. For example, if a client traditionally drinks an herbal tea to alleviate symptoms of an illness, there is no reason why both the herbal tea and the medications prescribed by the physician cannot be used as long as the tea is safe to drink and the ingredients do not interfere with or exaggerate the action of the medication.

Other types of alternate therapies include the use of cutaneous stimulation, therapeutic touch, acupuncture, and acupressure. Cutaneous stimulation by massage, vibration, heat, cold, or nerve stimulation reduces the intensity of the sensation of pain. Therapeutic touch is an intentional act that involves an energy transfer from the healer to client to stimulate the client's own healing potential. Acupuncture, long used in China, is a method of preventing, diagnosing, and treating pain and disease by inserting special needles into the body at specified locations. Acupressure involves a deep-pressure massage of appropriate points of the body; it may be self applied.

Transcultural Nursing

Madeleine Leininger (1978), whose theory of transcultural care is described in Chapter 5, defines **transcultural nursing** as follows:

> Transcultural nursing is a formal area of study and practice focused on a comparative study of human cultures with respect to discovering universalities (similarities) and diversities (differences) as related to nursing phenomena of care (caring), health (wellness), or illness patterns within a cultural context and with a focus on cultural values, beliefs, and lifeways of people and institutions, and using this knowledge to provide culture-specific or universal care practices.

When the nurse provides transcultural nursing care, it means that the care is planned and implemented in a way that is sensitive to the needs of individuals, families, and groups representing the diverse cultural populations within society. When cultural diversity is recognized and respected, cultural sensitivity is present and nursing care is provided that accepts the significance of cultural factors in health and illness. To provide transcultural care, the nurse must be aware that the healthcare system itself is a culture, and that cultural imposition and ethnocentrism must be avoided.

The Culture of Healthcare

The healthcare system (described in Chapter 11) is a culture with customs, rules, values, and a language of its own. As you progress through your education, you will be acculturated into the culture of the healthcare system and will develop values of health and healthcare. Many of the customs and rules are typical of the society in which we live; for example, cleanliness and punctuality are valued behaviors. The accompanying box outlines some common cultural norms of the healthcare system.

Nursing is the largest subculture of the healthcare system. Most nurses are members of, and have the same value systems as, the dominant middle class in North America. According to Boyle and Andrews (1995), the typical American nurse is "white, middle-class, Anglo-

Cultural Norms of the Healthcare System

Beliefs

- Standardized definitions of health and illness
- Omnipotence of technology

Practices

- Maintenance of health and prevention of illness
- Annual physical examinations and diagnostic procedures

Habits

- Charting
- Frequent use of jargon
- Use of a systematic approach and problem-solving methodology

Likes

- Promptness
- Neatness and organization
- Compliance

Dislikes

- Tardiness
- Disorderliness and disorganization

Customs

- Professional deference and adherence to the pecking order found in autocratic and bureaucratic systems
- Use of certain procedures attending birth and death

Rituals

- Physical examination
- Surgical procedure
- Limiting visitors and visiting hours

Saxon, Protestant, female, and socialized into a subculture labeled 'healthcare professional, subdivision nurse' " (p. 37). When the nurse, with a particular set of cultural values about health, interacts with a client who has his or her own particular set of cultural values about health, the following factors affect the interaction:

- The cultural background of each participant
- The expectations and beliefs of each about healthcare
- The cultural context of the encounter (for example, hospital, clinic, home)
- The degree of agreement between the two persons' sets of beliefs and values (Boyle & Andrews, 1995)

Cultural Imposition and Ethnocentrism

Cultural imposition, described by Leininger (1991) as "one of the most serious problems in the health field" (p. 36), is the tendency for health personnel to impose their beliefs, practices, and values on people of other cultures because they believe that their ideas are superior to those of another person or group. When health professionals assume that they have the right to make choices and decisions for clients, clients respond in the same way that minority cultures respond to dominant cultures: by becoming passive, resistive, angry, or noncompliant.

Closely related to cultural imposition is **ethnocentrism,** the belief that one's own ideas, beliefs, and practices are the best, superior, or most preferred to other lifeways (Leininger, 1978). To overcome this practice, the nurse must carefully and critically examine his or her own values and beliefs and be willing to understand health and illness from the cultural viewpoint of the client receiving care.

Providing Transcultural Care

A major theme of transcultural nursing care is to focus on the caring practices of various cultures. Caring is a universal phenomenon, even though the forms and manifestations may vary among cultures. Caring practices are the protecting and assisting activities related to health and performed as part of a culture.

Nursing care can become complicated when the client and the nurse have distinctly different cultural norms. The nurse's role is to understand the client's needs and to adapt care to meet those needs. Unless the nurse is willing to examine carefully and clarify his or her own attitudes and values and to be sensitive to others who are "different," the use of cultural concepts to provide holistic care will be unsuccessful.

Sometimes a nurse is placed in a cultural bind: the nurse's cultural upbringing influences values and beliefs, and the nurse is expected to adopt the customs of the nursing profession and at the same time accommodate the folkways and norms of individual clients. A careful merging of modern and traditional cultural beliefs is a necessary prerequisite for safe, considerate, and successful nursing care of all clients.

Once cultural awareness and sensitivity in planning client care have been attained, it is easier to recognize the client's use of traditional folk medicine and its importance. When caring for a client who subscribes to such practices, the nurse takes this circumstance into account during assessment and planning.

Cultural Assessment

The most effective way to identify specific factors that influence behavior is to do a cultural assessment of the client. The primary informant should be the client, if possible. If the client is not able to respond to the questions, a family member or a friend can be consulted.

Client differences in values, religion, dietary practices, family lines of authority, family life patterns, and beliefs and practices related to health and illness can be anticipated. Research has made it possible to obtain this anticipatory information before initiating contact with the client, with the reminder that information about specific cultures is general in content and must be individualized according to each client once interaction has begun. One part of the Andrews/Boyle Transcultural Nursing Assessment Guide (1995) is illustrated in the accompanying box.

Holistic Healthcare

A rationale for transcultural nursing is offered by the fact that the nursing profession values holistic and comprehensive approaches to providing care. Holistic healthcare takes into consideration the whole person interacting with the environment. When applying a philosophy of holistic healthcare, the knowledge and use of cultural factors cannot be ignored because a person's culture is an integral part of his or her life and, therefore, of holistic nursing care. A client can be placed in jeopardy if a healthcare professional lacks cultural awareness or sensitivity.

Considerations for Transcultural Care

Table 3-1 lists cultural factors that affect nursing care for specific cultures. The following guidelines are useful in practicing transcultural nursing care:

- Become aware of the role of cultural influences in your own life. Objectively examine your own beliefs, values, practices, and family experiences. As you become more sensitive to the importance of these factors, you also will become more sensitive to cultural influences in others' lives.
- Identify biases in your own life. How do they affect your feelings about others? How could they affect your nursing care of others?
- Learn as much as possible about the belief system and practices of people in your community and, specifically, of clients in the area in which you work. Cultural practices and beliefs are deeply rooted and must be considered in planning and implementing health teaching and care.

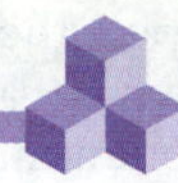

Focused Assessment Guide

Transcultural Assessment: Health-Related Beliefs and Practices

1. To what cause(s) does the client attribute illness and disease (eg, divine wrath, imbalance in hot/cold or yin/yang, punishment for moral transgressions, hex, soul loss, pathogenic organism)?
2. What are the client's cultural beliefs about the ideal body size and shape? What is the client's self-image compared to the ideal?
3. What name does the client give to his or her health-related condition?
4. What does the client believe promotes health (eating certain foods; wearing amulets to bring good luck; sleep; rest; good nutrition; reducing stress; exercise; prayer; rituals to ancestors, saints, or intermediate deities)?
5. What is the client's religious affiliation (eg, Judaism, Islam, Pentacostalism, West African voodooism, Seventh-Day Adventism, Catholicism, Mormonism)? How actively involved in the practice of this religion is the client?
6. Does the client rely on cultural healers (eg, curandero, shaman, spiritualist, priest, minister, monk)? Who determines when the client is sick and when the client is healthy? Who influences the choice/type of healer and treatment that should be sought?
7. In what types of cultural healing practices does the client engage (use of herbal remedies, potions, massage; wearing of talismans, copper bracelets, or charms to discourage evil spirits; healing rituals, incantations, prayers)?
8. How are biomedical/scientific healthcare providers perceived? How does the client and his or her family perceive nurses? What are the expectations of nurses and nursing care?
9. What comprises appropriate "sick role" behavior? Who determines what symptoms constitute disease/illness? Who decides when the client is no longer sick? Who cares for the client at home?
10. How does the client's cultural group view mental disorders? Are there differences in acceptable behaviors for physical versus psychologic illnesses?

Source: Andrews, M., & Boyle, J. (1995). *Transcultural concepts in nursing care.* (2nd ed.). Philadelphia: Lippincott.

- Practice techniques of observation and listening to acquire knowledge of beliefs and values of clients to whom care is being given. Some people, especially those of minority cultures, may have been belittled and subjected to ridicule and insults, and may be hesitant to discuss their beliefs and practices. The topic must be approached carefully. If the nurse is motivated by sincerity, respect, and concern, his or her attitude conveys this, and most clients respond positively. On the other hand, if the nurse is motivated by curiosity and has a condescending attitude, most clients respond negatively.
- Incorporate factors from the client's cultural background into healthcare whenever possible and when the practices are not considered harmful to health. To ignore or contradict the client's background may result in refusal of care or noncompliance with prescribed therapy.
- Keep in mind that health practices are part of the overall culture and that changing them may have widespread implications for the person. An accurate understanding of these implications is essential before such a change is implemented. The nurse also needs to provide the necessary support and reinforcement for the client if a change in a health practice with a cultural basis is considered necessary.
- Do not force the client to participate in care that conflicts with his or her values. If the client is forced to accept it, the care may become harmful because resulting feelings of guilt and alienation from a religious or cultural group are likely to threaten the client's well-being.
- Accommodate the cultural dietary practices of clients as much as possible. Dietary departments in many hospitals supply clients with meals that are consistent with special dietary practices. Families may be encouraged to bring food from home for clients with particular preferences when this practice does not violate hospital policy. Teaching clients and families about therapeutic diets also can be done within the framework of particular cultural practices.
- Take into consideration the cultural role of the family member who makes most of the important decisions. In some cultures, it is the husband or father, whereas in others it is the grandmother or another respected elder. To disregard this fact or to proceed with nursing care that is not approved by this person can result in conflict or in disregard for what has been taught. The nurse should be careful to involve this person in the nursing care planning.
- Seek assistance of a respected family member, member of the clergy, or folk medicine practitioner as indicated so that the client is more likely to ac-

cept familiar healthcare services. Acknowledging the role of the person's folk medicine practitioner can be an important way of building trust. If invited, folk medicine practitioners can work closely with professional health practitioners in the interest of the client and family. Such efforts promote mutual understanding, respect, and cooperation.

- Modify care to include folk practices and practitioners as much as possible, and be an advocate for clients from diverse cultural groups.
- Use past transcultural experiences as a guide, but never as the solution to all transcultural solutions.
- Learn from your mistakes and do not repeat them. All nurses make mistakes at some time when caring for culturally different clients. Inadvertent mistakes are just that, but repeated mistakes are careless and disrespectful; they adversely affect the nurse's interaction with clients and coworkers.
- Treat each person as an individual. What was true of one person will not be true of another, even if they are from the same cultural background. View each person as an individual with rights, and help the client retain dignity.

(text continues on page 50)

Table 3-1
Cultural Factors That Affect Nursing Care

White Middle Class

Family
- Nuclear family is highly valued.
- Elderly family members may live in a nursing home when they can no longer care for themselves.

Folk and Traditional Health Care
- Self-diagnosis of illnesses
- Use of over-the-counter drugs (especially vitamins and analgesics)
- Dieting (especially fad diets)
- Extensive use of exercise and exercise facilities

Values and Beliefs
- Youth is valued over age.
- Cleanliness
- Orderliness
- Attractiveness
- Individualism
- Achievement
- Punctuality

Common Health Problems
- Cardiovascular diseases
- Gastrointestinal diseases
- Some forms of cancer
- Motor vehicle accidents
- Suicides
- Mental illness
- Chemical abuses

Nursing Considerations
- Careful assessment of client's use of over-the-counter medications (observe for signs and symptoms of toxic medication levels, especially fat-soluble vitamins)
- Nutritional assessments of dietary habits

African American

Family
- Close and supportive extended-family relationships
- Develop strong kinship ties with nonblood relatives from church or organizational and social groups
- Family unity, loyalty, and cooperation are important.
- Usually matriarchal

Folk and Traditional Health Care
- Varies extensively and may include spiritualists, herb doctors, root doctors, conjurers, skilled elder family members, voodoo, faith healing

Values and Beliefs
- Present oriented
- Members of the African-American clergy are highly respected in the black community
- Frequently highly religious

Common Health Problems
- Hypertension (precise cause unknown, may be related to diet)
- Sickle cell anemia
- Skin disorders; inflammation of hair follicles, various types of dermatitis and excessive growth of scar tissue (keloids)
- Lactose enzyme deficiency resulting in poor toleration of milk products
- Higher rate of tuberculosis
- Diabetes mellitus
- Higher infant mortality rate than in the white population

(continued)

Table 3-1 *(continued)* Cultural Factors That Affect Nursing Care

Nursing Considerations
- Many African-American families may still use various folk healing practices and home remedies for treating particular illnesses.
- Special care may be necessary for the hair and skin.
- Special consideration should be given to the sometimes extensive and frequently informal support networks of clients (ie, religious and community group members who offer assistance in a time of need).

Asian

(Beliefs and practices vary, but most Asian cultures share some characteristics.)

Family
- Welfare of the family is valued above the person.
- Extended families are common.
- A person's lineage (ancestors) is respected.
- Sharing among family members is expected.

Folk and Traditional Health Care
- Theoretical basis is in Taoism, which seeks a balance in all things.

Folk and Traditional Health Care (continued)
- Good health is achieved through the proper balance of yin (feminine, negative, dark, cold) and yang (masculine, positive, light, warm).
- An imbalance in energy is caused by an improper diet or strong emotions.
- Diseases and foods are classified as hot or cold and a proper balance between them will promote wellness (eg, treat a cold disease with hot foods).
- Many Asian health care systems use herbs, diet, and the application of hot or cold therapy. Also, many Asians believe that there are points on the body that are located on the meridians or energy pathways. If the energy flow is out of balance, treatment of the pathways may be necessary to restore the energy equilibrium.

  Acumassage—Technique of manipulating points along the energy pathways
  Acupressure—Technique for compressing the energy pathway points
  Acupuncture—Technique by which fine needles are inserted into the body at energy pathway points

Values and Beliefs
- Strong sense of self-respect and self-control
- High respect for age
- Respect for authority
- Respect for hard work
- Praise of self or others is considered poor manners.
- Strong emphasis on harmony and the avoidance of conflict

Common Health Problems
- Tuberculosis
- Communicable diseases
- Malnutrition
- Suicide
- Various forms of mental illness
- Lactose enzyme deficiency

Nursing Considerations
- Some members of Asian cultures may be upset by the drawing of blood for laboratory tests. They consider blood to be the body's life force, and some do not believe that it can be regenerated.
- Some members believe that it is best to die with the body intact, so they may refuse surgery except in dire circumstances.
- Members of many Asian cultures seldom complain about what is bothering them. Therefore, the nurse must carefully assess the client for pain or discomfort by observing for nonverbal signs of discomfort, such as facial grimacing or wincing and holding of the painful area.
- Some Asians consider it polite to give a person the responses the person is expecting. Therefore, misinformation may be transmitted to the questioner in an effort, on the client's part, to be respectful.
- Some members may move from physician to physician in an attempt to be cured of an illness, but to avoid insulting or embarrassing a physician, they will not inform him or her that they are going to another physician. This can result in confusion, inaccuracies, and overmedication.
- Some Asians may refuse to have diagnostic studies done because they believe that a skilled and competent physician can diagnose an illness solely through a physical examination.

(continued)

Table 3-1 *(continued)*
Cultural Factors That Affect Nursing Care

- Some members may have a difficult time understanding the importance of taking a regimen of medications because many of their folk treatments involve the ingestion of one dose of herbal mixtures.
- Dietary counseling may be necessary if the client is on a salt-restricted diet because many Asian foods have a high salt content related to the use of soy sauce.

Hispanic, Mexican American

Family
- Familial role is important.
- *Compadrazgo:* special bond between a child's parents and his or her grandparents
- Family is the primary unit of society.

Folk and Traditional Health Care
- *Curanderas(os):* frequently folk healers who base treatments on humoral pathology—basic functions of the body are controlled by four body fluids or "humors":
  Blood—hot and wet
  Yellow bile—hot and dry
  Black bile—cold and dry
  Phlegm—cold and wet
- The secret of good health is to balance hot and cold within the body; therefore, most foods, beverages, herbs, and medications are classified as hot (*caliente*) or cold (*fresco, frio*) (a cold disease will be cured with a hot treatment).

Values and Beliefs
- Respect is given according to age (older) and sex (male).
- Roman Catholic Church may be very influential.
- God gives health and allows illness for a reason; therefore, may perceive illness as a punishment from God. An illness of this type can be cured through atonement and forgiveness.

Common Health Problems
- Diabetes mellitus and its complications
- Poverty and resultant problems, such as poor nutrition, inadequate medical care, poor prenatal care
- Lactose enzyme deficiency

Nursing Considerations
- It may be difficult to convince an asymptomatic client that he or she is ill.
- Special diet considerations are necessary if the client believes in the hot/cold theory of treating illnesses.
- Diet counseling may be necessary at times because many members have a normal diet that is high in starch.

Hispanic, Puerto Rican

(Since the Jones Act of 1917, all Puerto Ricans are American citizens.)

Family
- *Compadrazgo*—same as in Mexican-American culture

Folk and Traditional Health Care
- Similar to that of other Spanish-speaking cultures

Common Health Problems
- Parasitic diseases, such as dysentery, malaria, filariasis, and hookworms
- Lactose enzyme deficiency

Values and Beliefs
- Place a high value on safeguarding against group pressure to violate a person's integrity (may be difficult for Puerto Ricans to accept teamwork)
- Close-mouthed about personal and family affairs (psychotherapy may be difficult to achieve at times because of this belief)
- Proper consideration should be given to cultural rituals such as shaking hands and standing up to greet and say goodbye to people.
- Time is a relative phenomenon; little attention is given to the exact time of day.
- *Ataques*—culturally acceptable reaction to situations of extreme stress, characterized by hyperkinetic seizure activity

Nursing Considerations
- It may be difficult to teach Puerto Rican clients to follow time-oriented actions (eg, taking medications, keeping appointments).

(continued)

Table 3-1 *(continued)*
Cultural Factors That Affect Nursing Care

Native American

(Each tribe's beliefs and practices vary to some degree.)

Family

- Families are large and extended.
- Grandparents are official and symbolic leaders and decision makers.
- A child's namesake may become the same as another parent to the child.

Folk and Traditional Health Care

- Medicine men (shaman) are heavily used.
- Heavy use of herbs and psychologic treatments, ceremonies, fasting, meditation, heat, and massages

Common health problems

- Alcoholism
- Suicide
- Tuberculosis
- Malnutrition
- Communicable diseases
- Higher maternal and infant mortality rates than in most of the population
- Diabetes mellitus
- Hypertension
- Gallbladder disease

Values and Beliefs

- Present oriented. Taught to live in the present and not to be concerned about the future. This time consciousness emphasizes finishing current business before doing something else.
- High respect for age.
- Great value is placed on working together and sharing resources.
- Failure to achieve a personal goal frequently is believed to be the result of competition.
- High respect is given to a person who gives to others. The accumulation of money and goods often is frowned on.
- Some Native Americans practice the Peyotist religion in which the consumption of peyote, an intoxicating drug derived from mescal cacti, is part of the service. Peyote is legal if used for this purpose. It is classified as a hallucinogenic drug.

Nursing Considerations

- The family is expected to be part of the nursing care plan.
- Note taking often is taboo because it is considered an insult to the speaker because the listener is not paying full attention to the conversation. Good memory skills often are required by the nurse.
- Indirect eye contact is acceptable and sometimes preferred.
- It often is considered rude or impolite to indicate that a conversation has not been heard.
- A low tone of voice often is considered respectful.
- A Native American client may expect the caregiver to deduce the problem through instinct and not through asking many questions and history taking. If this is the case, it may help to use declarative sentences rather than direct questioning.

Hawaiian

Family

- Familial role is important.
- 'Ohana, or extended families, are jointly involved in child-rearing.
- Hierarchy of family structure; each gender and age have specific duties.
- Closely knit families in small, isolated communities

Folk and Traditional Health Care

- Kahuna La'au Lapa'au is the ancient Hawaiian medical practitioner.
- View patient's illness as part of the whole.
- Relationships between the physical, psychologic, and spiritual
- Emphasis on preventative medicine
- Treatment uses over 300 medicinal plants and minerals

Values and Beliefs

- Aloha: a deep love, respect and affection between people and the land
- Respect, given to people and land
- Christian gods replaced the myriad of Hawaiian gods.
- Lifestyle more revered than compliance with healthcare issues
- Present oriented, less initiative and drive than that of direction and achievement
- Death seen as part of life and not feared

Common Health Problems

- Diabetes mellitus and its complications
- Hypertension (unknown cause; perhaps related to diet)
- Gout (perhaps related to diet)
- Respiratory disorders: asthma, allergies, tuberculosis
- Skin disorders: bacterial, fungal, cancer
- Obesity
- Smoking, alcoholism, drug abuse

(continued)

Table 3-1 *(continued)*
Cultural Factors That Affect Nursing Care

Nursing Considerations
- Many Hawaiians may still use folk healing practices and home remedies.
- Special consideration given to the extensive family network during hospitalization
- Acceptance from healthcare practitioners of current health practices and lifestyle

Appalachian

Family
- Intense interpersonal relations
- Family is cohesive, and several generations often live close to each other.
- Elderly are respected as providers.
- Tend to live in rural, isolated areas

Folk and Traditional Health Care
- "Granny" woman, or folk healer, provides care and may be consulted even if receiving traditional care.
- Various herbs, such as foxglove and yellow root, are used for common illnesses such as malaise, chest discomfort, heart problems, and upper respiratory infections.
- Elderly may have had only limited contact with healthcare providers and be skeptical of modern healthcare.

Values and Beliefs
- Independence and self-determination
- Isolation is accepted as a way of life.
- Person-oriented
- May be fatalistic about losses and death
- Belief in a divine existence rather than attending a particular church

Common Health Problems
- Cardiovascular disorders
- Respiratory disorders
- Nutritional disorders
- Smoking, alcoholism

Nursing Considerations
- Treat each person with regard for personal dignity.
- Allow family members to remain with client as support system.
- Acceptance from healthcare providers of current health practices and lifestyle
- Allow clients to make decisions about care.

Key Points

- Culture is the set of values, beliefs, and traditions held by a specific social group that is learned and handed down from generation to generation.
- One's culture guides behavior, is primarily transmitted through language, and can be adapted over time.
- Ethnic groups are made up of people who share common and unique cultural and social beliefs and social patterns.
- Stereotyping, which occurs when the assumption is made that all members of a culture or ethnic group act alike, often is practiced by the dominant group about a minority group in a culture.
- As members of a minority group live within a dominant group, cultural characteristics often are lost through assimilation.
- A wide variety of cultural and ethnic characteristics affect transcultural nursing care. These characteristics include family member roles, communications, nutrition, and income levels.
- Poverty has a major influence on health and illness, affecting health-related behaviors. This issue is made even more complex because of the increased number of families headed by single women, of older people, and of homeless families.
- Certain physiologic and psychologic characteristics that are found in specific cultural and ethnic groups are risk factors for illness.
- The healthcare system is a culture, with nursing being the largest subculture.
- As part of the healthcare system, which has its own values and behaviors, nurses must be aware of the tendency of healthcare professionals toward cultural imposition and ethnocentrism.
- Guidelines for transcultural nursing care help the nurse accept the values, beliefs, and behaviors of others. Holistic nursing care requires that cultural influences and factors be integral components of an individualized plan of care.
- When nurses provide transcultural care, they demonstrate cultural sensitivity by recognizing and respecting cultural diversity.

Bibliography

Adams, R., Briones, E. H., & Rentfro, A. (1992). Cultural considerations: Developing a nursing care delivery system for a Hispanic community. *Nursing Clinics of North America, 27*(1), 107–117.

Ahijevych, K., & Bernhard, L. (1994). Health-promoting behaviors of African American women. *Nursing Research, 43*(2), 86–89.

American Nurses Association. (1991). *Philosophical statement on ethics and human rights*. Kansas City, MO: ANA.

American Nurses Association. (1991). *Position statement on cultural diversity in nursing practice*. Kansas City, MO: ANA.

Andrews, M.M., & Boyle, J.S. (1995). *Transcultural concepts in nursing care*. (2nd ed.). Philadelphia: Lippincott.

Bernal, H. (1993). A model for delivering culture-relevant care in the community. *Public Health Nursing, 10*(4), 228–232.

Boston, P. (1992). Understanding cultural differences through family assessment. *Journal of Cancer Education, 7*(3), 261–266.

Casimir, G., & Morrison, B. (1993). Rethinking work with "multicultural populations." *Community Mental Health Journal, 29*(6), 547–559.

Cassetta, R. (1993). Cultural diversity promoted through "Ladders" program. *American Nurse, 25*(1), 16.

Diaz-Gilbert, M. (1993). Caring for culturally diverse patients. *Nursing 93, 23*(10), 44–45.

Frye, B., & D'Avanzo, C. (1994). Cultural themes in family stress and violence among Cambodian refugee women in the inner city. *Advances in Nursing Science, 16*(3), 64–77.

Groce, N., & Zola, I. (1993). Multiculturalism, chronic illness, and disability. *Pediatrics, 91*(5 part 2 Suppl), 1048–1055.

Haggar, V. (1994). Cultural challenge. *Nursing Times, 90*(15), 71–72.

Henderson, G., & Primeaux, M. (1981). *Transcultural health care*. Menlo Park, CA: Addison-Wesley.

Huggins, M. (1994). Intercultural communication. *Plastic Surgical Nursing, 14*(1), 47–49.

Juarbe, T. (1995). Access to healthcare for Hispanic women: A primary healthcare perspective. *Nursing Outlook, 43*(1), 23–28.

Leininger, M. (1978). *Transcultural nursing: Concepts, theories, and practices*. New York: Wiley & Sons.

Leininger, M. (1990). Transcultural nursing: A worldwide necessity to advance nursing knowledge and practice. In J. McClosky & H. Grace (Eds.). *Current issues in nursing* (3rd ed.). St. Louis: Mosby.

Leininger, M. (1991). Becoming aware of types of health practitioners and cultural imposition. *Journal of Transcultural Nursing, 2*(2), 32–39.

Leininger, M. (1994). Quality of life from a transcultural nursing perspective. *Nursing Science Quarterly, 7*(1), 22–28.

Lillington, L., Royce, J., Novak, D., Ruvalcaba, M., & Chlebowski, R. (1995). Evaluation of a smoking cessation program for pregnant minority women. *Cancer Practice, 3*(3), 157–163.

McCubbin, H., Thompson, E., Thompson, A., McCubbin, M., & Kaston, A. (1993). Culture, ethnicity, and the family: Critical factors in childhood chronic illnesses and disabilities. *Pediatrics, 91*(5 part 2 Suppl), 1063–1070.

Meleis, A. I., Lipson, J. G., & Paul, S. M. (1992). Ethnicity and health among five Middle Eastern immigrant groups. *Nursing Research, 41*(2), 93–103.

Reiskin, H., & Haussler, S. (1994). Multicultural students' perceptions of nursing as a career. *IMAGE: Journal of Nursing Scholarship, 26*(1), 61–64.

Secundy, M. G. (Ed.). (1992). *Trials, tribulations, and celebrations: African-American perspectives on health, illness, aging, and loss*. Yarmouth, ME: Intercultural Press.

Spector, R. E. (1991). *Cultural diversity in health and illness*. (3rd ed.). New York: Appleton & Lange.

U.S. Bureau of the Census. (1990). *Current population reports: Money income and poverty status of families and persons in the United States*. Washington, DC: U.S. Government Printing Office.

Yoshimura, R. (1993). Cultural diversity in the workplace. *Imprint, 40*(4), 48, 50.

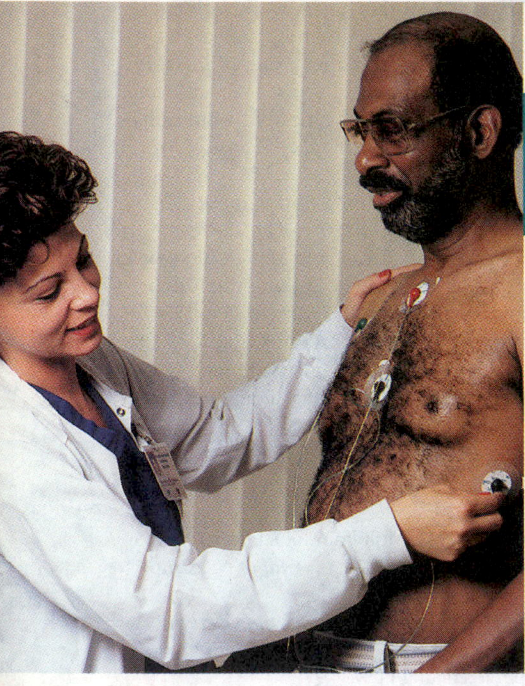

Chapter 4

Promoting Wellness in Health and Illness

Objectives

After studying this chapter, the learner should be able to:

Define key terms used in the chapter.

Describe wellness, health, and illness.

Identify the factors influencing health and illness, including the human dimensions, basic human needs, and self-concept.

Compare and contrast acute illness and chronic illness.

Summarize the role of the nurse in promoting wellness based on knowledge of risk factors for illness, illness behaviors, and the effects of illness on the family.

Describe the levels of preventive care.

Key Terms

acute illness
agent–host–environment model
chronic illness
client
disease
health
health-belief model
health–illness continuum
high-level wellness
illness
primary preventive care
risk factor
secondary preventive care
tertiary preventive care
wellness

The primary role of the nurse as caregiver is to prevent illness, to restore health, and to facilitate coping so as to maximize wellness in clients of all ages, in any setting, and in both health and illness. **Wellness** is more than just good health; it is an active process in which an individual progresses toward maximum potential possible, regardless of current state of health. Wellness is influenced by a variety of factors, including the environment, basic human needs, and one's culture. This chapter discusses how the practice of nursing is influenced by the **client**—the person receiving care. To give holistic care, the nurse must understand and respect each person's individualized definition of wellness and response to illness. A knowledge base of health and illness, as well as a philosophy of wellness, is even more important to nursing care in view of the continuing trends of providing most care in the home, increasing numbers of older persons, and an increasing incidence of chronic illnesses.

Defining Wellness in Health and Illness

Wellness is defined by each person relative to his or her own values and beliefs. The perception of one's degree of wellness is also influenced by the family, community, and society in which a person lives. Consider the following examples:

- Sally Tong, age 4 years, was born with a heart defect. However, the defect was repaired when Sally was a baby, and she is an active member of her pre-school class, takes gymnastics lessons, and wants to be a doctor when she grows up.
- Angela Doss is 34, married, and has two school-age children. She has chronic rheumatoid arthritis and is in a wheelchair. Angela takes care of her house and family and uses a specially designed car to get to her part-time job.
- Judson Carle is 67 years old. He was diagnosed with diabetes and high blood pressure last year, and takes medications for both health problems. Judson is retired but volunteers 3 days weekly in a local hospital as a transport technician.

Would Sally, Angela, and Judson be defined as well? Although they have a physical condition that would allow them to define themselves as being ill, they are all productive members of their society and would say they are healthy.

Wellness and health are more than the absence of illness. Health must be defined by each person and must consider the dimensions of that person—the physical, intellectual, emotional, sociocultural, spiritual, and environmental aspects that compose the whole person. Equal consideration of all these interrelated and interdependent components of the whole person serves as the basis for holistic nursing care (Fig. 4-1).

Because health is individualized to each person and is affected by so many factors, definitions are difficult. The most widely accepted definition of **health,** which includes the concept of wellness, was made in 1947 by the World Health Organization: Health is a state of complete physical, mental, and social well-being, not merely the absence of disease or infirmity (p. 1). This definition has been expanded since the 1940s (see Models of Health and Illness). In contrast to definitions from the scientific community, most individuals describe and define health by how they feel ("I feel really sick"); by the absence or presence of symptoms of illness ("I have a terrible pain in by stomach"); or their ability to carry out their normal activities of daily living ("I felt so much better that I got up and cooked supper").

Definitions of illness are also individualized to each person who experiences an alteration in health. Illness is also difficult to define, because the terms *disease* and *illness* are often used to mean the same process. **Disease** is a medical term, meaning that there is a pathologic change in the structure or function of the body or mind. It is a condition that has specific symptoms and boundaries, whereas health and illness are individualized perceptions and definitions of oneself. An **illness** is the response the person has to a disease; it is an abnormal process in which the person's level of functioning is changed compared with a previous level. The response is different for each person, and is influenced by self-perceptions; others' perceptions; the effects of changes in body structure and function; the effects of those changes on roles and relationships; and cultural and spiritual values and beliefs. It is important to remember that a person may have a disease, and consider himself or herself to be ill, but still achieve maximum functioning and quality of life, which is wellness.

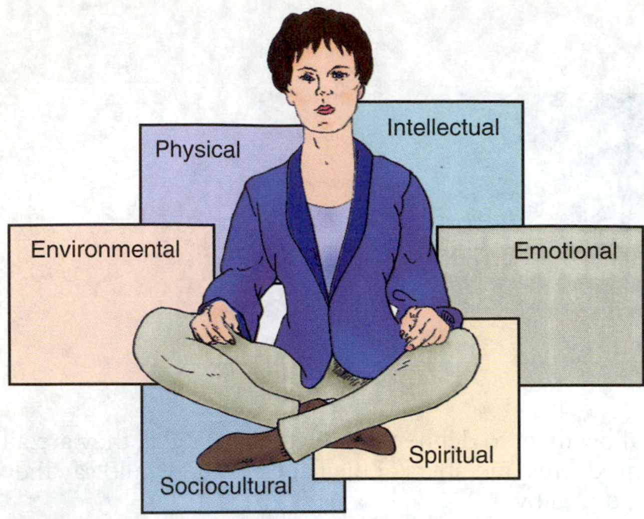

Figure 4-1
The human dimensions. All of these interdependent parts compose the whole person.

Models of Health and Illness

Because definitions of health and illness are not specific, health models (examples developed to give a visual impression of something that cannot be observed directly) have been developed to help describe the concepts and relationships involved in health and illness. The models described in this chapter are the health–illness continuum, the high-level wellness model, the agent–host–environment model, and the health-belief model.

The Health–Illness Continuum

One way to measure a person's level of wellness is to use the **health–illness continuum.** According to this model, health is a constantly changing state, with high-level wellness and death being on opposite ends of a graduated scale, or continuum (Fig. 4-2). The nurse must be aware that a client with a chronic illness may place himself or herself at different points on the continuum at any given time, depending on how well the client believes he or she is functioning for the illness.

High-Level Wellness Model

Halbert Dunn (1961) described his model of **high-level wellness** as functioning to one's maximum potential while maintaining balance and purposeful direction in the environment. The concept of high-level wellness can be applied to the individual, family, community, environment, and society. This discussion focuses on Dunn's model as it applies to the individual.

Dunn differentiates "wellness" from "good health," believing that good health is a passive state wherein the person is not ill. Wellness, on the other hand, is a more active state, oriented toward maximizing the potential of the individual, regardless of the state of health. Dunn also defined processes that help a person know who and what he or she is. These processes are *being* (recognizing self as separate and individual); *belonging* (being part of a whole); *becoming* (growing and developing); and *befitting* (making personal choices to befit the self for the future).

Dunn's model is holistic, allowing the nurse to care for the total person with regard for all dimensional factors affecting the person's state of being as he or she strives to reach maximum potential. For example, when planning and giving care to a young male college student paralyzed after a diving accident, the nurse would include nursing activities to meet his educational needs (intellectual dimension); incorporate friends and family (sociocultural dimension); provide or refer for counseling (emotional dimension); and ask the hospital chaplain to visit (spiritual dimension).

Agent–Host–Environment Model

The **agent–host–environment model** of health and illness, developed by Leavell and Clark (1965), was developed to describe health in a community but it is also useful when examining the causes of disease in an individual. The model is actually more useful in predicting illness than in promoting wellness, although recognition of risk factors resulting from interaction of agent–host–environment is important in the promotion and maintenance of health.

The three variables involved are defined as follows:

Agent: A factor that must be present or absent for an illness to occur. It may be biologic, chemical, physical, mechanical, or psychosocial.

Host: Living beings (ie, human or animal) capable of being infected or affected by an agent. Host reaction is influenced by family history, age, and health habits.

Environment: Everything external to the host that makes illness more or less likely. Examples of environmental factors are air pollution and sound (noise) levels.

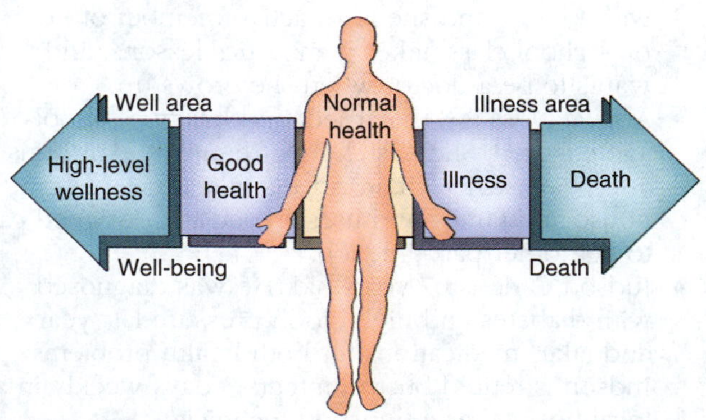

Figure 4-2
The health–illness continuum.

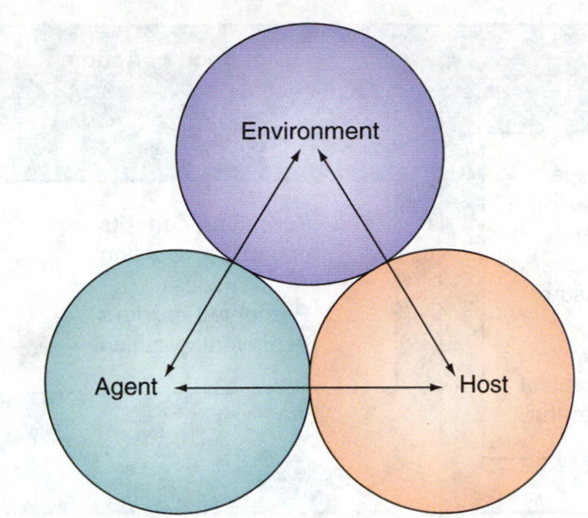

Figure 4-3
The agent–host–environment triangle.

The triangle in Figure 4-3 shows that each of the agent–host–environment factors affects and is affected by the others. The factors are constantly interacting, and a combination of factors increases the possibility of illness. When the variables (agent–host–environment) are balanced, health is maintained; when they are out of balance, disease occurs. Thus, health is an ever-changing state.

Health-Belief Model

In the United States and Canada, free or low-cost screenings and information are available to help in the early detection of disease and to educate about healthy living to prevent illness. Why then don't more people take advantage of these services or change their lifestyles? This question can be answered through the widely used health-belief model, which describes health behavior.

The **health-belief model** (Rosenstock, 1974) is based on what people perceive, or believe, to be true about themselves in relation to health. This model is based on three components: (1) perceived susceptibility to a disease, (2) perceived seriousness of a disease, and (3) perceived value of action.

Perceived susceptibility to a disease is an individual's belief that he or she either will or will not contract a disease. Perceived susceptibility may range from being afraid of contracting a disease to complete denial that certain behaviors will result in illness. For example, the person who smokes cigarettes may believe he or she is at danger for lung cancer and may stop smoking, or the person may believe smoking will pose no serious threat and, hence, will continue to smoke.

Perceived seriousness of a disease involves two factors: (1) seriousness of the disease and (2) its perceived effect on the person's lifestyle. This component is based on how much the person knows about the disease and can result in a change in health behavior. If the person who smokes believes that lung cancer could lead to physical disability or death and would affect his or her ability to work and care for the family, the person is more likely to stop smoking. Both perceived susceptibility to a disease and perceived seriousness of a disease are part of beliefs about the threat of disease.

Perceived value of action is concerned with how effective the individual believes preventive measures will be in preventing illness. It is influenced by two factors: (1) conviction that carrying out a recommended action will prevent or modify the disease and (2) the person's perception of the cost and unpleasant effects of performing the health behavior (compared with not taking any action). Based on this component, the person may believe that stopping smoking will prevent future breathing problems and that the initial withdrawal symptoms can be overcome, and therefore will stop smoking.

Figure 4-4 illustrates the component health-belief perceptions and modifying factors. This model is useful in teaching individuals about health and illness. The nurse can identify the client's health beliefs and then structure goals to realistically meet client needs. Teaching and wellness-promotion activities are ineffective unless the client believes they are important and necessary.

Factors Affecting Health and Illness

As the preceding models of health and illness illustrate, many factors influence a person's health status. These factors may be internal or external to the individual, and may or may not be under conscious control. However, they do affect client responses to nursing care. To plan and give holistic care, the nurse must understand how these factors influence behavior in both healthy and ill clients.

This section addresses factors that affect health and illness, including factors influencing health–illness status, beliefs, and practices; basic human needs; and self-concept. This section provides only an introduction to these concepts; other chapters in the book fully discuss each topic.

Factors Influencing Health–Illness Status, Beliefs, and Practices

The factors influencing health–illness status, health beliefs, and health practices are described as they relate to the person in terms of the human dimensions previously discussed (see Fig. 4-1). Each person is a composite of these human dimensions, and each dimension influences the behaviors of the person receiving care. As you care for clients, consideration of these dimensions is an integral part of the nursing process (Fig. 4-5).

Physical Dimension. Genetic makeup, age, developmental level, race, and sex are all part of an individual's physical dimension and strongly influence health status and health practices. Examples are as follows:

- The adolescent male who is prone to take risks while driving, increasing the possibility of an accident

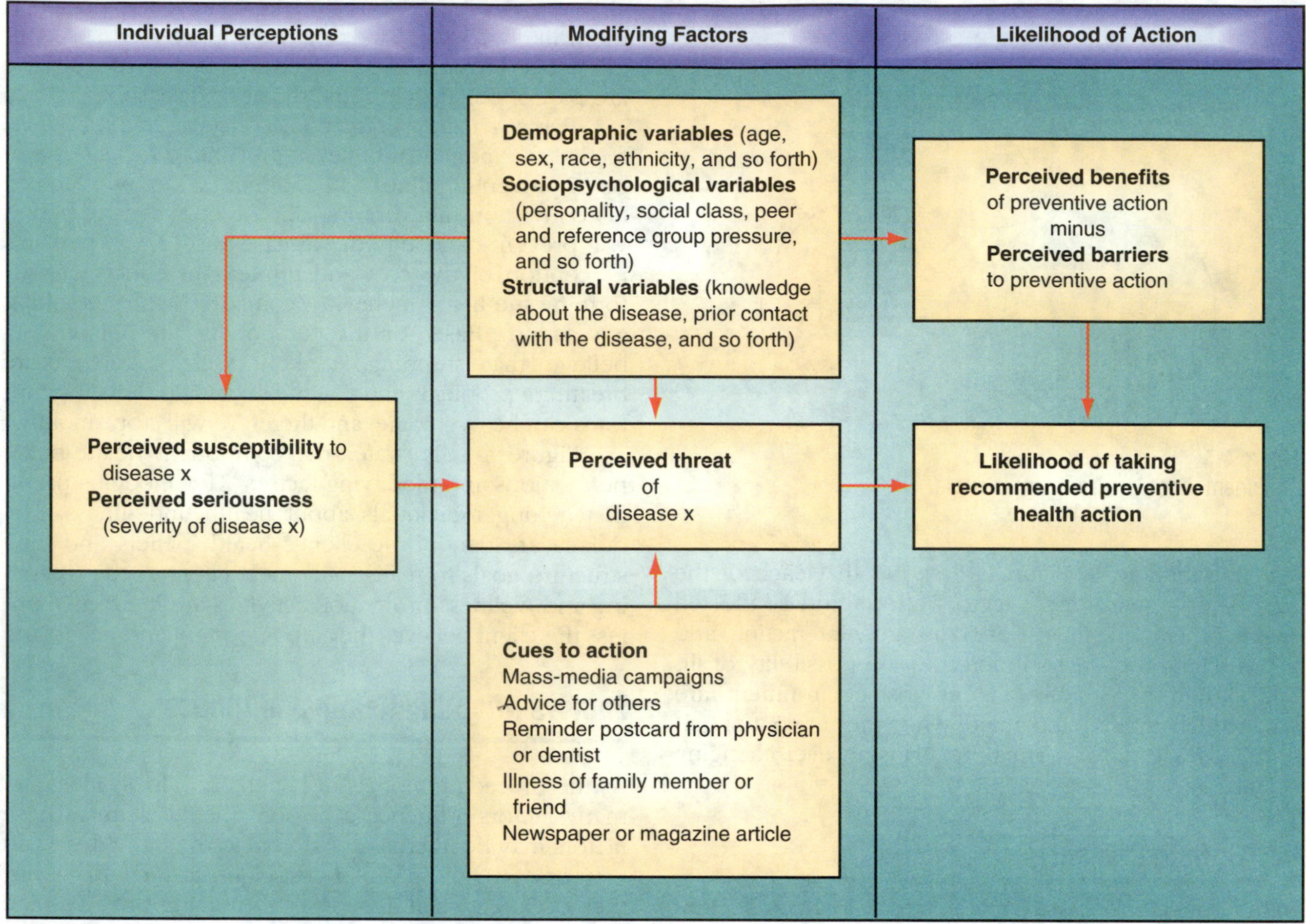

Figure 4-4
Health belief model. (Becker, M. [Ed.]. [1974]. *The health belief model and personal health behavior.* Thorofare, NJ: Charles B. Slack.)

- The young woman who has a family history of breast cancer and diabetes and therefore is at higher risk to develop these conditions
- The middle-aged African American man who is more prone to develop high blood pressure
- The older adult who has increased risk for one or more chronic illnesses

Emotional Dimension. How the mind and body interact to affect body function and to respond to body conditions also influences health. Long-term stress affects the body systems and anxiety affects health habits; conversely, calm acceptance and relaxation can actually change body responses to illness. Consider the following:

- Before a test, a student always has diarrhea.
- Worried about her teenage son, a mother chain smokes.
- The adolescent with poor self-esteem begins to experiment with drugs.
- Using relaxation techniques, a young woman reduces her pain during the delivery of her baby.
- After learning biofeedback skills, a man reduces his previously elevated blood pressure.

Intellectual Dimension. The intellectual dimension encompasses cognitive abilities, educational background, and past experiences. These influence a client's responses to teaching about health and reactions to nursing care during illness. They also play a major role in health behaviors. Examples of situations involving this dimension include the following:

- An older woman who only completed the fifth grade and needs to be taught how to give herself injections
- A young college student with diabetes who follows a diabetic diet but continues to drink beer and eat pizza with friends several times a week
- A middle-aged man who quits taking his high blood pressure medication after developing unpleasant side effects

Environmental Dimension. The environment has many influences on health and illness. Housing, sanitation, cli-

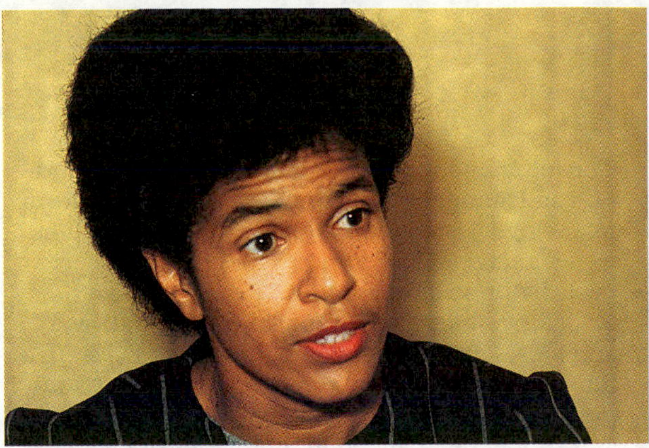
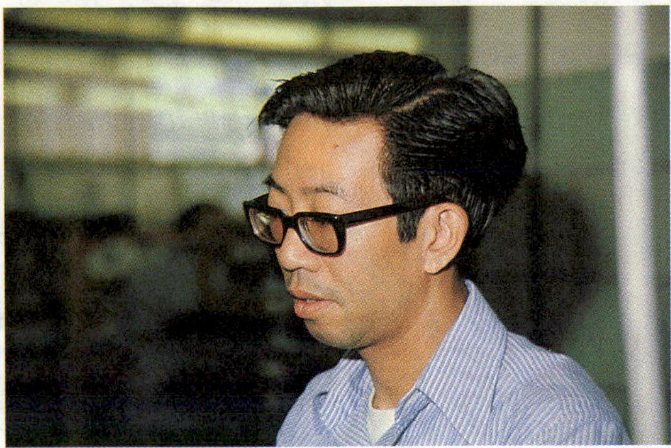

Figure 4-5
Each client has his or her own set of physical, emotional, intellectual, environmental, sociocultural, and spiritual dimensions that become part of the nurse's concerns in giving care. Consider the different dimensions presented by these persons.

mate, and pollution of air, food, and water are aspects of the environmental dimension. There are many examples of environmental causes of illness, including these selected few:

- Deaths, especially among older adults, resulting from inadequate heating and cooling
- Increased incidence of asthma and respiratory problems in large cities with smog
- Increased incidence of skin cancer in people who life in hot, sunny areas of the world
- Food poisoning
- Drowning

Sociocultural Dimension. Health practices and beliefs are strongly influenced by a person's economic level, lifestyle, family, and culture. Low-income groups are less likely to seek medical care to prevent or treat illness; high-income groups are more prone to stress-related habits and illness. The family and the culture to which a person belongs determine patterns of living and values about health and illness that are often unalterable. All of these factors are involved in personal care, patterns of eating, lifestyles, and emotional stability. Violence is an ever-increasing risk for injury or death in our society, as outlined in the accompanying box. Examples of other sociocultural factors that influence health and illness are:

- The adolescent who sees nothing wrong with smoking or drinking because his parents smoke and drink
- The parents of a sick infant who do not seek medical care because they have no money
- The single parent, abused as a child, who in turn physically abuses her own small son
- The person of Asian descent who uses herbal remedies and acupuncture to treat an illness

Spiritual Dimension. Spiritual and religious beliefs and values are important components of how a person behaves in health and illness. It is important that the nurse respect these values and understand their importance to the individual client. Included in this dimension are the following examples:

- Roman Catholics require baptism for both live births and stillborn babies.
- Orthodox and Conservative Jews may observe kosher laws, prohibiting the intake of pork or shellfish.
- Jehovah's Witnesses are opposed to blood transfusions.

Basic Human Needs

All of us are familiar with the following occurrences:

- A drink of water "goes the wrong way" and you experience a sense of panic until you can take a breath.
- You are too busy to eat breakfast and are "starving to death" by lunch.
- As you start your first college class, your thoughts are filled with questions about how you will react to the new experience.
- You plan to spend a part of each weekend with your family.
- A neighbor has emergency surgery and you volunteer to care for her children.

These actions—and many more like them—are the result of needs. As defined in Chapter 2, a *need* is something that is *essential* to the emotional and physiologic health and survival of humans. Basic human needs are essential and are common to all people. All people strive to meet basic needs; at any given time, an individual's needs may be met, partially met, or unmet. A person whose needs are met may be considered to be healthy, and a person with one or more unmet needs is at increased risk for illness or health alterations in one or more of the human dimensions.

Nursing Today: Challenges and Solutions

Handgun Violence: America's Public Health Epidemic

The number one public health problem today is violence, primarily from the use of handguns in violent acts. Children take guns to school, innocent victims die of drive-by shootings, and the healthcare costs from injuries are enormous. Consider the following statistics:

- Every year, more than 24,000 Americans die as homicides, suicides, or accidents from handguns.
- A child dies every 2 hours from a gunshot.
- Every 6 hours an adolescent commits suicide with a gun.
- At least $1 billion is spent every year on hospital costs associated with the treatment and care of people who have been shot.
- Firearm injuries result in $14.4 billion in lifetime costs (medical care and loss of productivity) per year.

Nurses and other healthcare providers can slow this ever-increasing trend. Providers can implement preventive efforts through legislation, client screening and intervention, and client and community education. The American Nurses Association recently supported efforts to include gun control in healthcare legislation by signing on to a letter from Public Citizen, Ralph Nader's group. The letter encouraged Congress to include handgun and ammunition tax in the healthcare reform financing legislation to increase revenue devoted to healthcare delivery and to reduce healthcare costs by preventing injuries.

Nurses are also working at the federal, state, and local levels to enact gun control policies. In addition, asking clients about accessibility to handguns should be a part of every family assessment and should be included in interviews of clients who are depressed or suicidal. Educational materials about the storage of handguns to prevent children's access are also important in reducing injury or death from guns.

The University of Maryland Medical Center has a Violence Intervention Project, working with victims of intentional violence. This program considers cultural and community effects on the victim's lives, and includes individual, family, and group counseling to keep participants from being repeat clients. Handgun violence often occurs because a handgun is available, or because young people do not know how to resolve conflicts appropriately. Counseling and education are used as interventions in this project to reduce the risk of injury and death and to reduce the economic cost of care for victims of violence.

Source: Cassetta, R. (1994). Handgun violence: America's public health epidemic. *American Nurse, 26*(9), 1, 16.

Needs are an integral part of each person's human dimensions.

Physical needs involve all of the body's physiologic processes, including breathing, the intake and output of food and fluids, temperature, circulation, and movement.

Emotional needs are concerned with the feelings of a person, such as fear, happiness, sadness, and loneliness.

Intellectual needs are focused on processes such as thinking, learning, problem solving, and decision making.

Environmental needs deal with our physical surroundings as they affect safety and security, and include housing, neighborhood, climate, and atmosphere.

Sociocultural needs relate to the relationships and communications a person has with others, such as friends, a sense of belonging to a group or community, and being loved by others.

Spiritual needs concern a person's values and beliefs as they relate to a higher being and to the performance of activities to help others.

The nursing procedures and actions that you will learn as you progress through your education are aimed at meeting your clients' basic human needs.

Self-Concept

Another variable influencing health and illness is self-concept, which incorporates both how a person feels about self (*self-esteem*) and the way the person perceives his or her physical self (*body image*). Self-concept has both physical and emotional aspects, and is an important factor in the way each individual reacts to stress and illness, follows self-care health practices, and interrelates with others. For example, the adolescent who has anorexia nervosa and is dangerously thin may still perceive herself as being overweight and refuse to eat. In contrast, the person who is overweight may feel that nothing will change the way others see him or her or will have an effect on the person's acceptance by others. Thus, the person refuses to follow a diet and exercise program.

A person's self-concept is the product of a variety of past experiences, interpersonal interactions, physical and cultural influences, and education. It includes a person's perceptions of his or her own strengths and weaknesses. Illness can alter self-concept as it affects roles, independence, and relationships with important others. Chapter 31 fully discusses self-concept.

Promoting Wellness and Preventing Illness

This section discusses the client at risk for illness and the client who becomes ill. Nurses often care for clients entering the healthcare system because of an illness (the causes of illness are outlined in the accompanying box). Therefore, illness behavior and the effects of illness on the family are discussed. Acute and chronic illness are defined to serve as a base for learning about different kinds of illnesses. The levels of healthcare activities carried out by nurses to promote health and prevent illness are included to illustrate the expanded role of nurses in society.

Risk Factors

A **risk factor** is a factor in a person's human dimensions that increases that person's chance for illness or injury. Risk factors can be categorized into six major areas. These areas, with examples, are listed in Table 4-1.

As with other components of health and illness, risk factors are often interrelated; as the number of risk factors increases, so does the possibility of disease. For example, the overweight executive, under pressure to increase sales, smokes and drinks alcohol in excess. These factors, combined with a family history of heart disease, place this person at higher risk for illness. The older adult is also at risk for illness or injury (see the accompanying box).

A health-risk appraisal is an assessment of the total person. The "picture" of the individual that is made from the assessment indicates areas of risk of disease or injury, as well as areas that support health. There are a variety of forms used to perform the assessment, but all of them take a broad approach to health, focusing on lifestyle and health behaviors. Such an appraisal appears in the box, Health-Style: A Self-Test, near the end of the chapter.

Certain practices are supportive of health:

- Sleeping regularly, 7 to 8 hours per night
- Eating breakfast
- Eating regular meals, with few snacks
- Maintaining ideal body weight
- Using alcohol in moderation, if at all
- Not smoking
- Maintaining positive mental health and self-concept

As the number of health practices increases, so does the level of wellness.

Table 4-1
Major Areas of Risk Factors

Risk Factor	Example
Age	School-aged children are at high risk for communicable diseases.
	After menopause, women are more likely to develop cardiovascular disease.
Genetic	A family history of cancer or diabetes predisposes a person to developing the disease.
Physiologic	Obesity increases the possibility of heart disease.
	Pregnancy places increased risk on both the mother and the developing fetus.
Health habits	Smoking increases the probability of lung cancer.
	Poor nutrition can lead to a variety of health problems.
Lifestyle	Multiple sexual relationships increase the risk of sexually transmitted diseases (eg, gonorrhea or AIDS).
	Events that increase stress (eg, divorce, retirement, work-related pressure) may precipitate accidents or illness.
Environment	Working and living environments (such as hazardous materials and poor sanitation) may contribute to disease.

Causes of Diseases

- Inherited genetic defects
- Developmental defects resulting from exposure to such factors as virus or chemicals during pregnancy
- Biologic agents or toxins
- Physical agents such as temperature, chemicals, radiation
- Generalized tissue responses to injury or irritation
- Physiologic and emotional reactions to stress
- An excessive or insufficient production of body secretions (hormones, enzymes, and so forth)

Acute and Chronic Illness

Illnesses are classified as either acute or chronic. A person may be acutely and chronically ill at the same time—for example, the adult with diabetes (a chronic illness) who has appendicitis (an acute illness). Each of these broad classifications of illness is discussed in the following section.

Acute Illness

An **acute illness** has a rapid onset of symptoms and lasts only a limited, relatively short time. Although acute

Focus on the Older Adult

Accident Prevention in the Home and Community

- Have good lighting in all rooms of the house, including the bedrooms, stairs, and basement. Avoid going from very bright light to darker areas, or give your eyes time to adjust.
- Do not sit or stand up rapidly, but rather rise slowly. If dizziness occurs, remain in one position until the dizziness is gone and ask for help.
- Install hand-rails by the commode and in the shower or tub.
- Do not use throw rugs.
- Install smoke alarms, heat sensors, and carbon monoxide detectors as appropriate. Be sure some alarm system is located on every floor of the house.
- Never step into a tub or shower without first checking the temperature of the water.
- Always wear corrective lenses and/or hearing aids when driving.
- Always wear seat belts.
- Do not drive a car after taking medicine that causes sleepiness or dizziness.

illnesses may be life threatening, many do not require medical attention. If medical intervention is required, specific treatment with medications (eg, antibiotics for pneumonia) or surgical procedures (eg, an appendectomy for appendicitis) will return the person to normal functioning. With self-treatment and use of over-the-counter (OTC) medications, simple acute illnesses such as the common cold or diarrhea do not usually require medical treatment.

Illness Behaviors. When a person becomes acutely ill, certain illness behaviors, described by Suchman (1965), may occur in identifiable stages. These behaviors are the way people cope with the alterations in function caused by the disease. Illness behaviors are highly individualized and are influenced by age, gender, family values, economic status, culture, educational level, and mental status. Although these stages of illness may be seen in the chronically ill person, they are much more typical of acute illness.

There are no specific timetables for the stages of illness behaviors. The stages may occur rapidly or slowly. The nursing roles throughout the stages remain constant. In all stages, the nurse accepts the client as an individual, gives nursing care based on priority of needs, and facilitates recovery through physical care, emotional support, and health education.

Stage 1: Experiencing Symptoms. How do people define themselves as "sick"? The first indication of an illness is usually the recognition of one or more symptoms that are incompatible with one's personal definition of health. Although pain is the most significant symptom indicating illness, other common symptoms include a rash, fever, bleeding, or a cough. If the symptoms last for a short time or are relieved by self-management, no further action is taken. However, if the symptoms continue the person enters the next stage.

Stage 2: Assuming the Sick Role. The person now defines himself or herself as being sick, seeks validation of this experience from others, gives up normal activities, and assumes a "sick role." At this stage, most people center on their symptoms and bodily functions. Depending on individual health beliefs and practices (and on the variables discussed previously), the person may choose to do nothing, buy over-the-counter medications to relieve symptoms, or seek care from a healthcare provider for diagnosis and treatment. In this society, an illness becomes truly legitimate when the diagnosis and prescribed treatment are determined by a healthcare provider. When help from the healthcare provider is sought, the person becomes a client and enters the next stage.

Stage 3: Assuming a Dependent Role. This stage is characterized by the decision to accept the diagnosis and follow the prescribed treatment plan. This stage of illness is complex and involves all of the human dimensions and basic human needs. By seeking medical care, a person conforms to the opinions of others, often requires assistance in carrying out activities of daily living, and needs emotional support through acceptance, approval, physical closeness, and protection.

It is at this stage that the client may enter the hospital. To facilitate adherence to treatment plans, the hospitalized client needs effective relationships with caregivers, knowledge about the illness, and an individualized plan of care. The responses of the client to care depend on a variety of factors, including the seriousness of the illness, the degree of fear about the disease, the loss of roles, the support of others, and previous experiences with illness care. The client is expected, by both caregivers and family, to get well and resume normal roles.

Stage 4: Achieving Recovery and Rehabilitation. Recovery and rehabilitation may begin in the hospital and conclude at home or may be totally concluded at a rehabilitation center or at home. As hospitals become increasingly centered on acute care, more and more clients will complete this final stage of illness behavior at home. In this stage, the person is expected to give up the dependent role and resume normal activities and responsibilities. If the plan of care included health education, the individual may return to health at a higher level of functioning and wellness than was present before the illness.

Chronic Illness

Chronic illness is a broad term, encompassing many different physical and emotional alterations in health, with one or more of the following characteristics:

- It is a permanent change.
- It causes, or is caused by, irreversible alterations in normal anatomy and physiology.
- It requires special client education for rehabilitation.
- It requires a long period of care or support.

Chronic illnesses usually have a slow onset and commonly have periods of *remission* (when the disease is present, but the person does not experience symptoms) and *exacerbation* (the symptoms reappear). With exacerbation, the person is in the acute phase of the chronic illness. Examples of common chronic illnesses are heart problems, diabetes mellitus, lung diseases, and arthritis.

Chronic illnesses are the leading health problem in the world. Current trends supporting further increase in chronic illnesses include diseases of aging, diseases of lifestyle, environmental factors, and the AIDS epidemic (Shugars, O'Neil, & Bader, 1991). More nursing care of clients with chronic illnesses will be required as we advance into the 21st century. Although not all people with a chronic illness require care, there are certain needs that all people who are chronically ill must meet to be able to live with the illness on a day-to-day basis for the rest of their lives:

- Living as normally as possible, despite the symptoms and treatment that make an individual feel different from others
- Learning to modify activities of daily living, relationships, and self-care activities
- Maintaining a positive self-concept and sense of hope
- Grieving over losses in physical structure and function, financial income, status, role, and dignity
- Learning how to live with chronic discomfort
- Following the prescribed medical therapy
- Maintaining a feeling of being in control
- Confronting the inevitability of death (Miller, 1983; Pollock, 1986)

As a nurse, you will care for individuals of all ages who have a chronic illness, and you will provide that care in all types of settings, including homes, hospitals, clinics, nursing homes, and institutions. Whatever the age of the client, the effects and demands of the illness, or the setting, the nurse must make every effort to promote wellness in the client with a chronic illness, with a focus of care that emphasizes what is possible rather than what can no longer be.

Effects of Illness on the Family

Most of your nursing care will be given to clients with some form of support system. The system usually comprises family members but also may include, or comprise, significant others, peers, and friends. When an illness occurs, roles change for both the client and the family. The following are examples of family reactions to, and influences on, illness of a member.

- A chronic illness creates stress for the client and family because it may require lifelong alterations in roles or lifestyle, frequent hospitalizations, economic problems, and decreased social interactions among members.
- Parents of a sick child often react with blame, overprotection, and severe anxiety.
- Family members of clients requiring intensive care often feel alone and frightened. They may also feel guilty and imagine the worst possible outcome.
- The reactions of family members to the hospital experience will vary; some want to be there all the time, whereas others avoid visiting.
- Family members need information about the client's care and health status, both in the hospital and at home. They often rely on the nurse for answers, for emotional support, and for feeling a part of the care given.

Nursing Care as Preventive Care

Levels of Preventive Care

The current focus of healthcare is on preventive care. Leavell and Clark (1965) describe the three levels of preventive care as primary, secondary, and tertiary.

Primary Level. Primary preventive care is directed toward health promotion and specific protection against illness. Activities at this level may focus on individuals or groups. Examples of primary-level activities are immunizations, family planning services, dental care teaching, poison-control information, and accident prevention education.

Secondary Level. Secondary preventive care focuses on health maintenance for clients experiencing health problems or on prevention of complications or disabilities. Examples of activities for this level are carrying out nursing actions for hospitalized clients (eg, providing skin care, giving medications, or exercising arms and legs); assessing children for normal growth and development; teaching breast self-examination; and encouraging regular medical and dental screenings and care.

Tertiary Level. Tertiary preventive care is aimed at helping rehabilitate clients and restore them to a maximum level of functioning after an illness. Nursing activities on a tertiary level include teaching a client with diabetes how to recognize and prevent complications or referring a woman to a support group after removal of a breast due to cancer.

Health-Style: A Self-Test

All of us want good health. But many of us do not know how to be as healthy as possible. Health experts now describe *lifestyle* as one of the most important factors affecting health. In fact, it is estimated that as many as seven of the ten leading causes of death could be reduced through common-sense changes in lifestyle. That's what this brief test, developed by the Public Health Service, is all about. Its purpose is simply to tell you how well you are doing to stay healthy. The behaviors covered in the test are recommended for most Americans. Some of them may not apply to people with certain chronic diseases or disabilities, or to pregnant women. Such people may require special instructions from their physicians.

Cigarette Smoking

If you never smoke, enter a score of 10 for this section and go the next section on *Alcohol and Drugs.*

	almost always	sometimes	almost never
1. I avoid smoking cigarettes.	2	1	0
2. I smoke only low tar and nicotine cigarettes *or* I smoke a pipe or cigars.	2	1	0

Smoking score: ______

Alcohol and Drugs

	almost always	sometimes	almost never
1. I avoid drinking alcoholic beverages *or* I drink no more than one or two drinks a day.	4	1	0
2. I avoid using alcohol or other drugs (especially illegal drugs) as a way of handling stressful situations or the problems in my life.	2	1	0
3. I am careful not to drink alcohol when taking certain medicines (for example, medicine for sleeping, pain, colds, and allergies), or when pregnant.	2	1	0
4. I read and follow the label directions when using prescribed and over-the-counter drugs.	2	1	0

Alcohol and drugs score: ______

Eating Habits

	almost always	sometimes	almost never
1. I eat a variety of foods each day, such as fruits and vegetables, whole grain breads and cereals, lean meats, dairy products, dry peas and beans, and nuts and seeds.	4	1	0
2. I limit the amount of fat, saturated fat, and cholesterol I eat (including fat on meats, eggs, butter, cream, shortenings, and organ meats such as liver).	2	1	0
3. I limit the amount of salt I eat by cooking with only small amounts, not adding salt at the table, and avoiding salty snacks.	2	1	0
4. I avoid eating too much sugar (especially frequent snacks of sticky candy or soft drinks).	2	1	0

Eating habits score: ______

Exercise and Fitness

	almost always	sometimes	almost never
1. I maintain a desired weight, avoiding overweight and underweight.	3	1	0
2. I do vigorous exercises for 15 to 30 minutes at least three times a week (examples include running, swimming, brisk walking).	3	1	0
3. I do exercises that enhance my muscle tone for 15 to 30 minutes at least three times a week (examples include yoga and calisthenics).	2	1	0
4. I use part of my leisure time participating in individual, family, or team activities that increase my level of fitness (such as gardening, bowling, golf, and baseball).	2	1	0

Exercise/fitness score: ______

Stress Control

	almost always	sometimes	almost never
1. I have a job or do other work that I enjoy.	2	1	0
2. I find it easy to relax and express my feelings freely.	2	1	0
3. I recognize early, and prepare for, events or situations likely to be stressful for me.	2	1	0
4. I have close friends, relatives, or others whom I can talk to about personal matters and call on for help when needed.	2	1	0
5. I participate in group activities (such as church and community organizations) or hobbies that I enjoy.	2	1	0

Stress control score: ______

Safety

	almost always	sometimes	almost never
1. I wear a seat belt while riding in a car.	2	1	0
2. I avoid driving while under the influence of alcohol and other drugs.	2	1	0
3. I obey traffic rules and the speed limit when driving.	2	1	0
4. I am careful when using potentially harmful products or substances (such as household cleaners, poisons, and electrical devices).	2	1	0
5. I avoid smoking in bed.	2	1	0

Safety score: ______

(continued)

Health-Style: A Self-Test *(continued)*

What Your Scores Mean to You

Scores of 9 and 10

Excellent! Your answers show that you are aware of the importance of this area to your health. More important, you are putting your knowledge to work for you by practicing good health habits. As long as you continue to do so, this area should not pose a serious health risk. It's likely that you are setting an example for your family and friends to follow. Because you got a very high test score on this part of the test, you may want to consider other areas where your scores indicate room for improvement.

Scores of 6 to 8

Your health practices in this area are good, but there is room for improvement. Look again at the items you answered with "Sometimes" or "Almost never." What changes can you make to improve your score? Even a small change can often help you achieve better health.

Scores of 3 to 5

Your health risks are showing! Would you like more information about the risks you are facing and about why it is important for you to change these behaviors? Perhaps you need help in deciding how to successfully make the changes you desire. In either case, help is available.

Scores of 0 to 2

Obviously, you were concerned enough about your health to take the test, but your answers show that you may be taking serious and unnecessary risks with your health. Perhaps you are unaware of the risks and what to do about them. You can easily get the information and help you need to improve, if you wish. The next step is up to you.

Where Do You Go from Here

Start by asking yourself a few frank questions: *Am I really doing all I can to be as healthy as possible? What steps can I take to feel better? Am I willing to begin now?* If you scored low in one or more sections of the test, decide what changes you want to make for improvement. You might pick that aspect of your lifestyle where you feel you have the best chance for success and tackle that one first. Once you have improved your score there, go on to other areas.

If you already have tried to change your health habits (to stop smoking or exercise regularly, for example), don't be discouraged if you haven't yet succeeded. The difficulty you have encountered may be due to influences you've never really thought about—such as advertising—or to a lack of support and encouragement. Understanding these influences is an important step toward changing the way they affect you.

There's help available. In addition to personal actions you can take on your own, there are community programs and groups (such as the YMCA or the local chapter of the American Heart Association) that can assist you and your family to make the changes you want to make. If you want to know more about these groups or about health risks, contact your local health department or the National Health Information Clearinghouse. There's a lot you can do to stay healthy or to improve your health—and there are organizations that can help you. Start a new "health-style" today!

For assistance in locating specific information on these and other health topics, write to the National Health Information Clearinghouse:

National Health Information Clearinghouse
P.O. Box 1133
Washington, DC 20013

(Reprinted with permission of the National Health Information Clearinghouse.)

Nurse as Role Model

Nurses, as role models for health and wellness, must take care of their own health to be able to give effective nursing care to others. Not only does good personal health enable nurses to practice more efficiently, it also enables them to serve as health models for clients and their families. Nurses can help clients acquire new health behaviors by modeling the very behaviors that are important to the clients' well-being.

It is difficult for nurses to be sincerely attentive to the needs of clients when their own needs are not being met. Because no one is perfectly healthy all of the time, it is important that as nurses prepare for professional practice they spend time getting to know themselves. From this self-knowledge should come a commitment to actively pursue holistic health. To help you begin your self-knowledge, take the self-test in the accompanying box. As you mutually develop care with clients, you may want to use this self-test to help your clients learn a new health-style.

In Units VII and VIII, a list of healthcare goals for the nurse, under the heading Nurse as Role Model, precedes text and explores how nurses can help clients. The wellness promotion guides highlighted throughout the text may be useful to you as well as to your clients. These guides can be used to assess and identify both strengths and increased risk for alterations in health. The guides can also serve as the basis for teaching self-care to clients.

Key Points

- Health and illness are relative processes, defined by each person. Wellness, or the achievement of maximum function and strength, is possible even when a person has been diagnosed as being ill.
- Health and illness relationships and interactions can be described by the use of models such as the health–illness continuum, high-level wellness model, agent–host–environment model, and health-belief model.
- Wellness levels are influenced by the dimensions that compose the whole person, by needs, and by self-concept. These factors are interrelated and affect actual and potential health–illness status and behaviors.
- People at risk for an illness can be identified through a health-risk appraisal. If a person is identified at risk for illness, nurses can promote lifestyle practices that support health.
- Acute illnesses occur rapidly, have a relatively short time span, and may be either self-treated or require medical intervention. The person with an acute illness progresses from the onset of symptoms to recovery through certain definite stages.
- Chronic illnesses more often have a slow onset, cause permanent change, and require long-term medical care. The increasing number of older adults, accompanied by an increase in chronic illnesses, means that nursing care of the chronically ill will become even more important in the 21st century.
- Nursing care for clients in both health and illness must include their family members. Illness results in altered expectations and reactions from family members.
- Nurses carry out wellness promotion activities on primary, secondary, and tertiary levels.

Bibliography

Alford, D., & Futrell, M. (1992). Wellness and health promotion of the elderly. *Nursing Outlook, 40*(5), 221–226.

American Public Health Association. (1990). *Healthy people 2000: National health promotion and disease prevention objectives.* Washington, DC: APHA.

Braden, C. (1990). A test of the self-help model: Learned response to chronic illness experience. *Nursing Research, 39*(1), 42–47.

Brewer, N., & Warren, M. (1994). Altered Family Processes related to an ill family member: A validation study. *Nursing Diagnosis, 5*(3), 115–120.

Cassetta, R. (1994). Handgun violence: America's public health epidemic. *American Nurse, 26*(9), 1, 16.

Dunn, H. (1961). *High-level wellness.* Arlington: Beathy.

Edelman, C., & Mandle, C. (1994). *Health promotion throughout the life span* (3rd ed.). St. Louis: Mosby.

Fryback, P., & Reinert, B. (1993). Facilitating health in people with terminal diagnoses by encouraging a sense of control. *MEDSURG Nursing, 2*(3), 197–201.

Hymovich, D., & Hagopian, G. (1992). *Chronic illness in children and adults: A psychosocial approach.* Philadelphia: Saunders.

Jensen, L., & Allen, M. (1993). Wellness: The dialectic of illness. *IMAGE: The Journal of Nursing Scholarship, 25*(3), 220–223.

Leavell, H., & Clark, E. G. (1965). *Preventive medicine for the doctor in the community* (3rd ed.). New York: McGraw-Hill.

Maslow, A. (1968). *Toward a psychology of being* (2nd ed.). New York: Van Nostrand Reinhold.

Miller, J. F. (1983). *Coping with chronic illness: Overcoming powerlessness.* Philadelphia: Davis.

Murray, R. B., & Zentner, J. P. (1993). *Nursing assessment and health promotion through the lifespan* (5th ed.). Norwalk, CT: Appleton & Lange.

Pender, N., Barkauskas, V., Hayman, L., Rice, V., & Anderson, E. (1992). Health promotion and disease prevention: Toward excellence in nursing practice and education. *Nursing Outlook, 40*(3), 106–112, 120.

Pollock, S. E. (1986). Human responses to chronic illness: Physiologic and psychosocial adaptation. *Nursing Research, 35*(2), 90–95.

Robert Wood Johnson Foundation Annual Report. (1993). *Chronic health conditions.* Princeton, NJ: The Robert Wood Johnson Foundation.

Rosenstock, I. (1974). Historical origin of the health belief model. *Health Education Monographs, 2,* 334.

Schultz, A. (1995). What is health promotion? *Canadian Nurse, 91*(7), 31–34.

Shugars, D. A., O'Neil, E. H., & Bader, J. D. (Eds.). (1991). *Healthy American: Practitioners for 2005—An agenda for action for U.S. health professional schools.* Durham, NC: Pew Health Professions Commission.

Suchman, E. (1965). Stages of illness and medical care. *Journal of Health and Human Behavior, 6,* 114.

Travis, J., & Ryan, R. (1988). *Wellness workbook* (2nd ed.). Berkeley, CA: Ten Speed Press.

World Health Organization. (1947). *Constitution.* Geneva: WHO.

Chapter 5

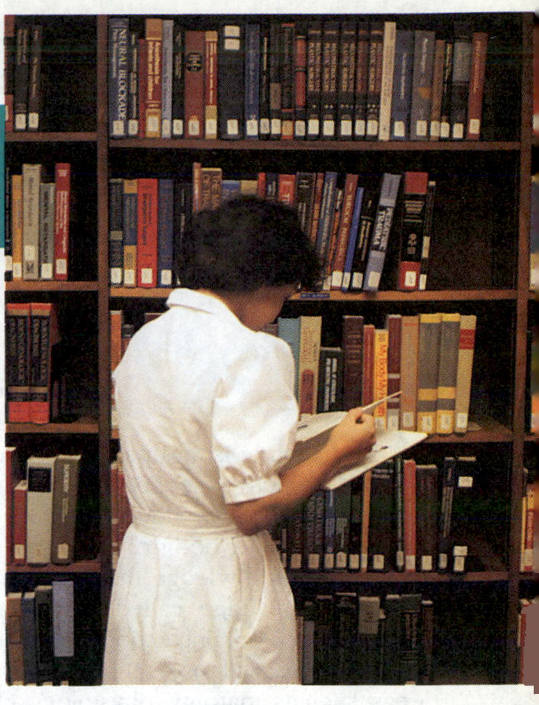

Theoretical Base for Nursing Practice

Objectives

After studying this chapter, the learner should be able to:

Define key terms used in the chapter.

Describe the underlying processes and characteristics of nursing theory.

Define the four common components of nursing theory.

Summarize the historical background, cultural influences, and value of nursing theory.

Discuss selected nursing theories, including definitions, assumptions, beliefs, and applications to nursing practice.

Key Terms

adaptation
adaptation theory
concept
conceptual framework or model
deductive reasoning
developmental theory
general systems theory
inductive reasoning
nursing theory
philosophy
process
theory

Nursing is a unique healthcare discipline in which a service, based on knowledge and skill, is provided to others. Nursing therefore has two parts—a body of knowledge and the application of that knowledge through nursing practice. The body of knowledge, called a *knowledge base*, provides a rationale for nursing actions. As you learn and practice nursing, you will use rationales from many different areas, such as anatomy, physiology, chemistry, nutrition, psychology, and sociology. You will also use a knowledge base developed specifically for nurses, allowing you to know what nursing care is and why and how it is given. This chapter discusses how nursing knowledge—also known as nursing theory—has been developed and how it is used to give safe and knowledgeable nursing care.

Introduction to Theory

Each individual collects, organizes, and arranges facts to build a knowledge base that defines his or her personal reality. A similar organization and a structure of facts and events are present in large bodies of knowledge, through philosophies, concepts, theories, and processes.

Philosophy is the study of wisdom, fundamental knowledge, and the processes used to develop and construct our perceptions of life. Philosophy both provides a viewpoint and implies a system of values and beliefs. Each individual develops a personal philosophy to give meaning to experiences and to direct behavior and attitudes. Personal philosophies are developed by learning from interpersonal relationships, through formal and informal educational experiences, through religion and culture, and from the environment.

The philosophy of each nurse and the philosophies of schools of nursing and of healthcare institutions form the basis of giving nursing care. As nurses give care, teach, and work with others, they reflect both a personal and a professional philosophy through values and beliefs about concepts such as goodness, wellness, health, illness, accountability, and ethics. In the same way, nursing education and nursing practice settings provide education or client care based on philosophic beliefs about humans, health, teaching and learning, and quality client care.

Concepts can be compared with ideas: they are abstract impressions from the environment organized into symbols of reality. Concepts describe objects, properties, and events, and the relationships among them. A group of concepts that follows an understandable pattern makes up a **conceptual framework or model.** Concepts can be thought of as the individual bricks and boards used to build a house, with the conceptual framework being the blueprint that specifies where each brick and board should go.

A **theory** is a group of concepts that form a pattern of reality. A theory is a statement that explains or characterizes a process, an occurrence, or an event, and is based on observed facts but lacks absolute or direct proof. Theories arrange a group of related statements or concepts so that they give meaning to a series of events. Theories can be tested, changed, or used to guide research or to provide a base for evaluation. They are derived through two principal methods: (1) **deductive reasoning,** in which one examines a general idea and then considers specific actions or ideas, and (2) **inductive reasoning**, in which the reverse process is used—one identifies a specific idea or action and then makes conclusions about general ideas. Nursing theorists use both of these methods.

A **process** is a series of actions, changes, or functions that bring about a desired result. During a process, one takes systematic and continuous steps to meet a goal and uses both assessments and feedback to direct actions to meet the goal. A particular theory or conceptual framework with its own specific definitions directs the way in which these actions are carried out. The delivery of nursing care within the nursing process (described in Unit IV) is directed in an institution by specific conceptual frameworks and theories.

Basic Processes in the Development of Nursing Theories

Nursing theory, as defined by Barnum (1994), "attempts to describe or explain the phenomenon (process, occurrence, or event) called nursing." Nursing theory differentiates nursing from other disciplines and activities in that it serves the purposes of describing, explaining, predicting, and controlling desired outcomes of nursing care practices.

Nursing theories are often based on and influenced by other broadly applicable processes and theories. The ideas and principles of the theories that follow are basic to many nursing concepts and are a part of the nursing literature. It is important that nurses understand these theories and terminologies so they can develop their own knowledge base in nursing. The following is a brief description of the major points of each theory.

General Systems Theory. **General systems theory** has been used by a wide range of disciplines since it emerged in the 1920s. Its primary theorist, Ludwig von Bertalanffy, developed the theory so that it could be universally applied. This theory explains the breaking of whole things into parts and then learning how the parts work together in "systems." It includes the relationship between the whole and the parts and defines how the parts will function and behave. These concepts may be applied to different kinds of systems, for example, to molecules in chemistry, cultures in sociology, organs in anatomy, and health in nursing.

Key points in general systems theory are as follows:

- A system is a set of interacting elements, all serving the common purpose of contributing to the overall goal of the system; the whole system is always greater than the sum of its parts.
- Systems are hierarchical in nature and comprise interrelated subsystems that work together in such a way that a change in one element could affect other subsystems as well as the whole.
- Boundaries separate systems both from each other and from their environments.
- A system communicates with and reacts to its environment through processes that enter the system (input) or are transferred to the environment (output).
- An open system allows energy, matter, and information to move freely between systems and boundaries, whereas a closed system does not allow input from or output to the environment (no known closed systems exist in reality).
- To survive, open systems maintain balance through feedback.

Stress/Adaptation Theory. **Adaptation theory** defines **adaptation** as the adjustment of living matter to other living things and to environmental conditions. Adaptation is a dynamic or continuously changing process that effects change and involves interaction and response. Human adaptation occurs on three levels—the internal (self), the social (others), and the physical (biochemical reactions). See Chapter 32 for more information on stress and adaptation.

Developmental Theory. **Developmental theory** outlines the process of growth and development of humans as orderly and predictable, beginning with conception and ending with death. Although the pattern is one of definite stages, the progress and behaviors of an individual within each stage are unique. The growth and development of an individual are influenced by heredity, temperament, emotional and physical environment, life experiences, and health status.

Several theorists are important to developmental theory, but only two are mentioned briefly because their work is often used to develop nursing theory and to organize nursing practice. Eric Erikson based his theory of psychosocial development on the process of socialization, emphasizing how individuals learn to interact with the world. Erikson recognized the role of social, biologic, and environmental factors in development and defined specific tasks or conflicts to be accomplished or overcome during what he defined as the eight stages of life. See Chapter 8 for more information on developmental theory.

Abraham Maslow divided his theory of human needs by the physical and psychosocial needs considered essential to human life, rather than by chronologic age, as Erikson did. Maslow defined five levels of need (physiologic well-being; physical safety; affection, love, and relationships; self-esteem; and self-actualization) existing in a hierarchy, with several needs being able to exist simultaneously. See Chapter 2 for more information on the theory of human needs.

As you continue in your nursing education and practice, you will learn how systems, adaptation, and developmental theories are used in planning and giving holistic care to clients. The discussion of specific nursing theories will enable you to better understand the knowledge base used to develop the concepts unique to nursing.

Basic Characteristics of Nursing Theory

Nursing theories identify and define interrelated concepts specific to nursing and clearly state the relation between these concepts. Nursing theories must be logical in nature; they should use orderly reasoning and describe relations that are developed using a logical sequence. Theories must also be consistent with the basic assumptions used in their development. Nursing theories should be simple and general; simple terminology and broadly applicable concepts ensure their usefulness in a wide variety of nursing practice situations. Nursing theories should also increase the nursing profession's body of knowledge by generating research. Furthermore, nursing theory should guide and improve practice.

Nursing theory is valuable in research, education, and practice. In addition, nursing theory guides nurses by providing a knowledge base, organizing concepts, providing guidelines for practice, and identifying nursing care goals (Chinn & Jacobs, 1991; Torres, 1990).

Common Components in Nursing Theories

Four concepts common to nursing theory that influence and determine nursing practice are (1) person, (2) environment, (3) health, and (4) nursing. Each of these concepts is defined and described by a nursing theorist, and although these concepts are common to all nursing theories, both the definitions and the relations among them may differ greatly from one theory to another. Of the four concepts, the most important is that of the person. The focus of nursing, regardless of definition or theory, is the person (Fig. 5-1).

Nursing Theory and Nursing Practice

Historical Perspectives and Influences

Nightingale's Definition and Belief. Florence Nightingale, the nurse who established the theoretical base of nursing, developed and published a philosophy and a theory of health and nursing that has served as a solid foundation for the nursing profession (Fig. 5-2). Her contributions to nursing theory include identifying the role of the nurse in meeting the client's personal needs; recognizing the importance of environmental influences on the care of sick people; and elevating the standards and acceptance of nursing by developing sound principles of nursing education. Nightingale also influenced nursing knowledge and practice by demonstrating efficient and knowledgeable nursing care, defining nursing practice as separate and distinct from medical practice, and differentiating between health nursing and illness nursing (Dolan, Fitzpatrick, & Herrmann, 1983).

Cultural Influences on Nursing. Certain cultural influences have affected nursing as we currently know it. Although since the beginning of time both men and women have given comfort and assistance to sick people, nursing essentially had been considered "women's work" until the last two decades. In the 18th and 19th centuries, women were viewed as subservient and inferior to men. However, after Nightingale established an acceptable occupation for educated women and facilitated improved attitudes toward nursing, the role of the woman as nurse became more favorably accepted.

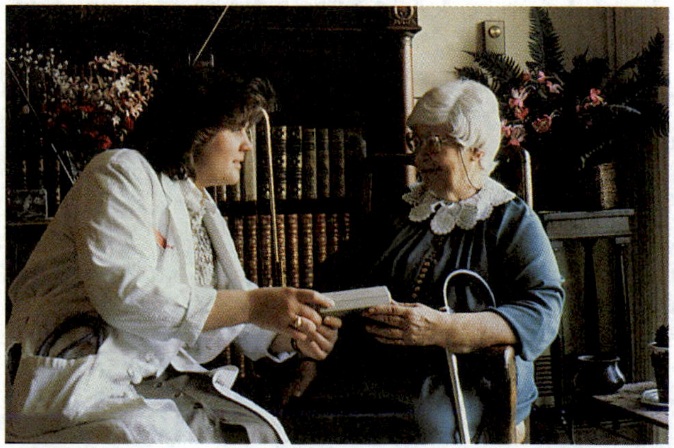

Figure 5-1
Four concepts common to all nursing theories are person, environment, health, and nursing. The most important concept, and the focus of nursing, is the person. (Photo by Gates Rhodes, courtesy of School of Nursing, University of Pennsylvania.)

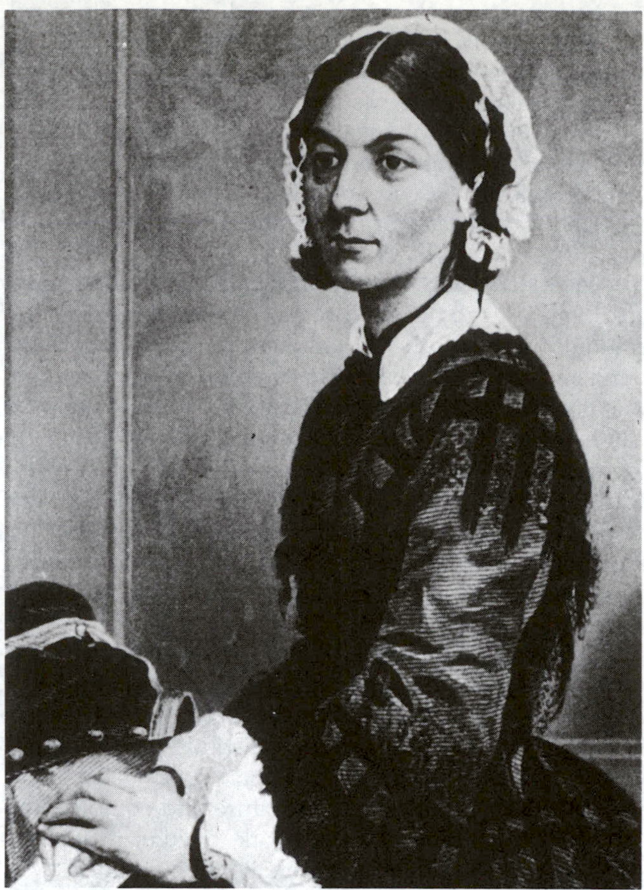

Figure 5-2
Florence Nightingale developed and published a philosophy and theory of health and nursing that has served as a solid foundation for the nursing profession. (Photo courtesy of the Center for the Study of the History of Nursing, University of Pennsylvania.)

Despite Nightingale's belief in the uniqueness of nursing, the training of nurses was initially carried out under the direction and control of the medical profession (Kalish & Kalish, 1995). Because the conceptual and theoretical basis for nursing practice came from outside the profession, nursing has struggled for years to establish its own identity and to receive recognition for its significant contributions to healthcare.

Nursing in the United States

Influences of Educational Frameworks. Most schools of nursing established in the United States were adapted from Nightingale's model. There was no planned educational curriculum; rather, learning came from lectures by physicians and by practical experience acquired through caring for sick people in the hospital (Dolan, Fitzpatrick, & Herrmann, 1983). This service orientation for nursing education remained the strongest influence on nursing practice until the 1950s. Rather than developing a body of knowledge specific to nursing, nursing care was carried out under the control and direction of the hospital administration and the physicians practicing in that hospital. Nursing care was based on traditional ideas about following orders, as well as on common wisdom about caring for others based on either "common sense" or widely accepted scientific principles (Chinn & Jacobs, 1991). It is no wonder that nursing knowledge remained undeveloped and fragmented for so long.

Development of a Scientific Base for Nursing. During the first half of the 20th century, a change in the structure of society resulted in a change of roles for women and, in turn, in nursing. As a result of World Wars I and II, women increasingly entered the work force, became more independent, and sought higher education. At the same time, nursing education began to focus on education instead of on training, and nursing research was conducted and published. As women became more assertive, nursing's need for a clearly defined identity of unique contributions to the healthcare system emerged. In the 1950s, the idea of nursing as a science became more generally accepted, and philosophic beliefs and a knowledge base for nursing practice began to evolve. Today's nursing practice focuses on giving holistic client care based on sound rationales from nursing knowledge.

Evolution of Nursing Theory

Research and Publishing in Nursing. Beginning in the 1950s, as great advances were made in technology and medical research, nursing leaders realized that research about the practice of nursing was necessary to meet the health needs of modern society. Increasing numbers of nurses began to conduct nursing research and write articles telling other nurses how to carry out nursing research. Two major developments in nursing theory were made during the 1950s: (1) the first research journal, *Nursing Research*, was published in 1950 (and continues today), and (2) as ideas were published, they served as a basis for theory development (Chinn & Jacobs, 1991; Kalish & Kalish, 1995).

Educational Advances in Nursing. Beginning in the 1960s, baccalaureate programs in nursing began to increase in both number and enrollment. At the same time, master's and doctoral programs in nursing were established. This upward trend in education for nurses was reflected in the nursing literature; more attention was given to the consideration and formulation of knowledge specific to nursing.

Value of Nursing Theory

Broad Goals of Nursing Theory. Nursing theory provides a rational and knowledgeable reason for nursing actions, based on organized, written descriptions of what nursing is and what nurses do. Additionally, nursing theory gives nurses the knowledge base necessary for acting and responding appropriately in nursing care situations; provides a base for discussion; and, ideally, provides resolution of current nursing issues. Furthermore, nursing theory allows the nurse who knows and practices theory to have better problem-solving skills, so that nursing actions are organized, considered, and purposeful. Nursing theory also prepares the nurse to question assumptions and values in nursing, thus further defining nursing and increasing the knowledge base.

Applying Theory to Practice. Nurses have difficulty agreeing on what nursing really is; however, if theory-based nursing is practiced, direction is provided that allows nurses to work toward a common goal, with the ultimate outcome being improved client care.

Improving and Facilitating Communication. Nursing is based on communication with others—clients, other healthcare team members, community members—as well as with nurses practicing in a variety of specialty settings. Because concepts are both abstract and highly individualized, verbal communication with others can be interpreted in many ways. As ideas are developed and words are defined, nurses build a knowledge base and a common terminology to use in communicating with other professionals.

Improving Autonomy of Nursing. The term *autonomy* means independence and self-governance. As a discipline, nursing is in the process of defining its own independent functions and contributions to healthcare. The development and use of nursing theory provide autonomy in the practice of nursing:

- Having a body of knowledge specific to the discipline allows members of that discipline to be viewed by others as experts; this, in turn, gives nurses authority to carry out actions.
- Actions carried out and based on sound rationale are trusted and respected.
- Nursing theory makes nursing care visible, leading to increased internal control by nurses.
- As nurses demonstrate that nursing care does indeed make a difference and that nursing services are valuable, the discipline becomes more independent.

Conceptual and Theoretical Frameworks for Nursing

The theories and conceptual models included in this section have been selected because they represent different approaches to defining the reality of nursing and because they are used in a variety of educational, research, and practice settings. They are arranged in alphabetical order as a means of organization only. Accompanying each theory or model is a brief summary of the central theme, basic assumptions, definitions, and applications in nursing. The information is summarized in Table 5-1. Students who find a particular framework relevant and

(text continues on page 72)

Table 5-1
Theorists and Their Conceptual Models

Theorist	Central Theme	Definitions			
		Person	*Environment*	*Health*	*Nursing*
Johnson's behavioral systems model	The human as a behavioral system	Humans with two major systems: biologic and behavioral	Society as the environment in which an individual exists, influencing the individual's behavior	Purposeful, adaptive responses (physical, mental, emotional, social) to internal and external stimuli to maintain balance and comfort	Primary goal is to foster balance within an individual, specific to the behavioral system, when illness occurs
King's open systems framework and theory of goal attainment	Interrelationships of concepts and the process of human interactions	Humans are open systems who are social, rational, perceiving, controlling, purposeful, and action and time oriented	Not specifically defined	Dynamic life experience of a human, implying continuous adjustment to stressors in the internal and external environment through optimal use of one's resources to achieve maximum potential for daily living	A process of human interactions between nurse and client whereby each perceives the other and the situation, and, through communication, together set goals, explore means, and agree on means to achieve goals
Leininger's transcultural care model	A model that provides culturally specific care consistent with nursing science and knowledge	Caring beings capable of being concerned about, holding interest in, or having regard for other people's needs, well-being, and survival	The culture of each individual, group, or society	A state of well-being that is mainly known and expressed in cultural meanings and ways	A learned humanistic art and science that focuses on personalized care behaviors and processes that are directed toward promoting and maintaining health behaviors or recovery from illness. These behaviors and processes have physical, psychocultural, and social significance or meaning.
Levine's theory of nursing	Conservation, the holistic person	A living being who continually interacts with his or her environments and adapts to change	The healthcare system, including the nurse	Maintenance of the unity and integrity of the client	A discipline that focuses on the human and the complexity of his or her relationships with the environment; the essence of nursing is human interaction

(continued)

Table 5-1 *(continued)*
Theorists and Their Conceptual Models

Theorist	Central Theme	Definitions			
		Person	*Environment*	*Health*	*Nursing*
Neuman's healthcare systems model	A healthcare systems model for a total person approach to client problems	Each human is a total person as a client system and is a composite of biologic, psychologic, sociocultural and developmental variables	Those internal and external forces that surround humans and with which they constantly interact	Views health as levels of wellness or stable lines of defense	A unique profession, concerning itself with all the variables affecting human response to stressors, with a primary concern for the total person
Orem's self-care model	Nursing and self-care activities	Humans with physical, psychologic, interpersonal, and social components, meeting self-care needs through learned behavior	Modern society's values and expectations	Wellness in the integrity of the individual; illness results in the person's inability to maintain self-care	The giving of direct assistance to a person who is unable to meet his or her own self-care needs, developed through nursing education and experiences
Rogers' science of unitary mean [sic]	Unitary human and his or her life processes; nursing science	Humans who are unified beings with individuality, in continuous exchange of energy with the environment	All of the patterns that exist external to the individual	Not specifically defined	An art and a science directed toward the unitary human and concerned with the nature and direction of human development
Roy's adaptation model	The person in constant interaction with a changing environment	A biopsychosocial being that is basically good	All the conditions, circumstances, and influences surrounding and affecting the development of organisms	A state or process of being or becoming an integrated and whole person	A theoretical system in which knowledge prescribes a process of analysis and action related to the care of the ill or potentially ill person
Watson's theory of caring	Nursing as a human science and human care	A person who is in need of the caring process to attain or maintain health or die a peaceful death; the person has personal, internal, and mental-spiritual mechanisms to allow the self to be healed.	Human life—the spiritual–mental–physical being in the world, which is continuous in time and space	The unity and harmony within the mind, body, and soul; the degree of congruence between the self as perceived and the self as experienced	An art and science of a human-to-human care process with a spiritual dimension; nuring comprises knowledge, thought, values, philosophy, commitment, and action

useful are encouraged to explore the literature to learn more about the theory or model and the theorist.

Dorothy E. Johnson: Behavioral Systems Model

Dorothy Johnson believes that nursing care is directed toward caring for the whole client to facilitate effective and efficient behaviors necessary to prevent illness. Her behavioral systems model integrates systems, developmental, and needs theories into a specific nursing focus. Johnson believes the four goals of nursing are to assist the person:

- Whose behavior is commensurate with social demands
- Who is able to modify his or her behavior in ways that support biologic imperatives
- Who is able to benefit, to the fullest extent during illness, from the physician's knowledge and skill
- Whose behavior does not give evidence of unnecessary trauma as a result of illness

Johnson views nursing as being separate from medicine in that medicine focuses on pathologic changes in the ill person, whereas nursing focuses on the behaviors of the person. She sees the nursing role as being complementary to the medical role. Nurses, giving care, supply functional requirements to the client through protection, nurturance, and stimulation. She views humans as individuals who act in ways that make up an individualized behavioral system. Within this behavioral system are seven interrelated subsystems. Changes in one subsystem affect all the others. The seven subsystems are as follows:

Attachment or "affiliative": This is the first behavioral subsystem to develop, initially allowing the infant to attach (bond) to a significant caregiver and continuing through life with other individuals. These attachments provide a sense of security.

Dependency: The behaviors in this subsystem precipitate nurturing by others and result in approval, attention, and physical assistance.

Ingestive: Behaviors surrounding the intake of food belong in this subsystem, including social and cultural factors.

Eliminative: The behaviors in this subsystem are involved with the excretion of waste products from the body and also relate to physical control and social situations.

Sexual: The behaviors in this subsystem are cultural and gender behaviors related to procreation and gratification.

Aggressive: In this subsystem, the behaviors are concerned with protection and self-preservation.

Achievement: Behaviors that attempt to control the environment, including intellectual, physical, creative, mechanical, and social skills, belong in this subsystem.

Johnson believes that both the internal and external environments of the system need to be orderly and predictable to maintain balance. If the subsystems are out of balance, "tension" and disequilibrium result. Nursing, as part of the external environment, can help the client return to a state of balance.

Imogene M. King: Open Systems Framework

Imogene King developed both a conceptual framework (open systems) and a theory of goal attainment derived from the framework. She used many sources to develop these bodies of knowledge. Some assumptions basic to this framework are:

- The focus of nursing is the care of humans.
- The nursing goal is the health of individuals and healthcare for groups.
- Humans are in constant interaction with their environment.

Within the framework are three interacting systems, each of which is defined and has relevant concepts:

Personal systems: Each individual is a personal system. The concepts defined in personal systems are perception, self, growth and development, body image, space, and time.

Interpersonal systems: Interpersonal systems are formed as humans interact. The concepts are interaction, communication, transaction, role, and stress.

Social systems: Social systems include families, religious groups, educational systems, work systems, and peer groups. The concepts are organization, authority, power, status, and decision making.

King developed her conceptual framework based on the belief that individuals actively interact with others and objects in the environment and are changed as a result of the experiences. King describes her theory of goal attainment as the interpersonal system in which two people come together in a healthcare organization to help or be helped to maintain a state of health that permits functioning in roles. A nurse (having special knowledge and skills) and a client (with self-knowledge and personal problems) interact to identify problems and to establish and achieve goals. Based on this theory, King offers several propositions, including the following:

- If perceptual accuracy is present in nurse–client interactions, transactions will occur.
- If nurse and client make transactions, goals are attained.
- If goals are attained, effective nursing care will occur.
- If nurses with special knowledge and skills communicate appropriate information to clients, mutual goal setting and goal attainment will occur.

Madeline Leininger: Transcultural Care Diversity and Universality

Leininger's theoretical/conceptual model of nursing is based on the belief that nursing is a transcultural care profession, with care being the central area of concern for nursing. Nursing is believed to be an art and a science that provides culture-specific care to individuals and groups to promote or maintain health behaviors or recovery from illnesses. Within the model are the following three types of culturally based nursing actions:

Cultural care preservation (maintenance): Those culturally based actions that help the individual preserve or maintain favorable health and caring lifeways.

Cultural care accommodation (negotiations): Those culturally based actions that reflect ways to adapt, negotiate, or adjust to the health and caring lifeways of others.

Cultural care repatterning (reconstruction): Those reconstructed or altered actions designed to help clients change meaningful health or life patterns.

The model is based on a substantial number of propositions and assumptions. A selected sample is as follows:

- Culture is the blueprint for thought and action and is the dominant force in determining health–illness caring patterns and behaviors.
- Cultural values vary among all humans and groups of humans.
- Human caring is a universal phenomenon that is expressed differently in all cultures.
- Caring unifies the intellectual and practical dimensions of nursing.

Myra E. Levine: Theory of Nursing

Myra Levine based her theory of nursing on the belief that the essence of nursing is human interaction. Assumptions that define the theory are as follows:

Condition: Clients entering the healthcare system are in a state of illness or altered health.

Responsibilities: The nurse is responsible for recognizing the client's organismic response (ie, changes in behavior or level of body function) as the client adapts or attempts to adapt to the environment (environment equals illness and nurse). The four levels of response are (1) fear, (2) stress, (3) inflammatory, and (4) sensory.

Functions: Nursing functions include interventions to promote adaptation to illness and evaluation of interventions as supportive or therapeutic. Supportive interventions help maintain the present health state and prevent further illness. Therapeutic interventions promote healing and restore health.

The foundation for all nursing intervention, as defined by Levine, consists of four conservation (meaning to maintain balance) principles that support the goal of nursing, which is to maintain or restore a person to a state of health:

Conservation of energy: Balancing energy intake and output to avoid excessive fatigue (rest, nutrition, exercise)

Conservation of structural integrity: Maintaining or restoring the structure of the body (promoting healing)

Conservation of personal integrity: Maintaining or restoring a sense of identity and self-worth (recognition of unique qualities)

Conservation of social integrity: Recognizing the client as a social being (especially with significant others)

Levine's theory is focused on one person—the client. This theory has major implications in acute-care settings, where nursing interventions are supportive or therapeutic.

Betty Neuman: Healthcare Systems Model

Neuman's model, the *total person approach,* can be used to provide an organized approach to a variety of nursing problems and for understanding humans and their environment. The model focuses on the client system's reaction to stress and the factors of reconstitution or adaptation. The person is an open system interacting with the environment. Surrounding each person are internal and external factors that are stressors. Over a lifetime, the person becomes a "normal line of defense" who uses biologic, psychologic, sociocultural, and developmental skills to deal with stressors. Stressors cause the line of defense to react or respond as the total person. The stressors may be extrapersonal, interpersonal, or intrapersonal. The effect of the stressors on the system is individualized and depends on such variables as the number of stressors, how long they last, and the system's coping skills.

Nursing interventions can be carried out on three preventive levels. When the stressor is identified but no reaction has occurred, interventions can decrease the degree of reaction or increase the line of defense. This is called *primary prevention.* When the reaction has already happened, *secondary prevention* is carried out, with interventions aimed at treating symptoms and reducing reactions. After active treatment, *tertiary prevention* strengthens the lines of defense through education and uses the system's total resources to prevent further occurrences.

Dorothea E. Orem: Self-Care Model

The nursing model of Dorothea Orem is based on the belief that the individual has a need for self-care actions and that nursing can assist in meeting that need to maintain life, health, and well-being. The model is widely used in all areas of nursing. *Self-care,* as defined by Orem, consists of the activities that individuals carry out on their own behalf. These actions are deliberate, have pattern and sequence, and are developed from day-to-day living. The ability of the individual to perform self-care is called *self-care agency* and is usually carried out by adults. Infants and children, as well as aged, ill, and disabled people require complete care or help with self-care activities. Three categories of *self-care requisites* (the purposes of actions directed toward the provision of self-care) follow:

Universal self-care requisites: These are common to all humans and are associated with maintaining life, health, and well-being. They include air, water, food, elimination, activity and rest, solitude and social interaction, prevention of hazards, and promotion of human functioning.

Developmental self-care requisites: These include maintaining conditions to support life and human development.

Health deviation self-care: This is required in illness, injury, or as a result of medical tests or treatments to correct a condition.

Orem suggests that a person needs nursing when the person has a health-related self-care deficit. The areas of nursing practice are:

- Entering into and maintaining nurse–client relationships with individuals, families, or groups
- Determining if and how clients can be helped through nursing
- Responding to clients' requests and needs
- Giving direct help to clients and families
- Coordinating and integrating nursing with the client's daily living, other healthcare activities, and social or educational services required

Orem has defined three nursing systems on the premise that the nursing system depends on the self-care needs and abilities of the client. In the first system (wholly compensatory), the nurse gives total care to meet all needs. In the second (partly compensatory), both the nurse and the client perform care measures. In the third (supportive–educative), the client can carry out self-care activities but requires assistance.

Martha E. Rogers: Nursing—A Science of Unitary Man

Martha Rogers has written a complex theory of nursing. The goal of this theory is to develop a science of nursing that would provide a growing body of theoretical knowledge applicable in nursing practice to the achievement of meaningful service to humanity.

Rogers' theory is built on a knowledge base of the history of humanity and of the universe (anthropology, sociology, astronomy, religion, philosophy, history, and mythology). Based on the belief that humans are the center of nursing's purpose, Rogers' theory considers the total individual, describing the human life process and explaining and predicting the nature and direction of human development. Both systems and developmental theories are a part of Rogers' theory.

Rogers' basic assumptions about humans are as follows:

- Humans are unified wholes who are more than a sum of their parts.
- Humans are constantly interacting with their environment.
- Anything that occurs in life is unique because no two things in life can ever be repeated in an identical manner or under identical circumstances.
- Humans develop patterns of behaving, and their behavior becomes predictable.
- Humans are distinctive in their capacity for abstract thought, imagery, and emotion.

Nursing concepts are derived and nursing science principles are identified from these basic assumptions. Based on these assumptions, Rogers identifies four building blocks:

Energy fields: Both the human and the environment are viewed as energy fields; there is a constant exchange of energy between the two that is essential to life.

Openness: This is based on the belief that the universe consists of open systems.

Pattern and organization: These are identifying characteristics of the energy field that is undergoing continuous change.

Four-dimensionality: This is a characteristic of both human and environmental fields.

Sister Calista Roy: Roy's Adaptation Model

Sister Calista Roy (1984) developed the adaptation model of nursing. This model is widely used as a philosophic base and conceptual model in nursing education. The adaptation model is essentially a systems model. The assumptions basic to this model are as follows:

- Each person is a biophysical being and an integrated whole. All body systems are balanced to produce a functioning person with biologic, psychosocial, and social needs. Constant interaction with the changing environment of the modern world subjects the person to continual changes and stressors.
- Each person uses both innate and acquired mechanisms to cope with changes and adapt individually, with either positive or negative responses. The adaptation level reached is the result of three classes of stimuli—the primary cause of the change, other situational factors, and beliefs and past experiences shaping the response.
- Each person responds to needs (requirements within the individual stimulating a response to maintain integrity) in one or more of four modes—physiologic, self-concept, interdependent behaviors, and role-function.
- Each person's position on the health–illness continuum changes in relation to the effectiveness of coping to maintain an adaptive state.

As defined by Roy, response to a decrease in body integrity creates a need state, and the individual responds with an act or behavior. The physiologic mode involves oxygenation and circulation, fluid and electrolyte balance, nutrition, rest and activity, and regulation of temperature, hormones, and sensory function. The self-concept mode is concerned with the perception of one's physical self and personal self, including personality, moral and ethical beliefs, and values. The interdependence mode involves social relationships, including both the need to be interdependent and the need for support by others. The role-function mode involves the behaviors of a person in each role taken on in life.

In Roy's model, all nursing activity is aimed at promoting the individual's adaptation to health and illness in all four adaptive modes. This model guides the nurse in using observation and interviewing skills to make an individualized assessment of each person, and serves as a guide in planning and carrying out nursing actions.

Jean Watson: Nursing—Human Science and Human Care

Jean Watson's theory and philosophy of caring is based on the values of kindness, concern, love of self and others, and respect for the spiritual dimension of the person. In nursing as a human science (Watson, 1988), *human caring in nursing* is defined as an art and a science in which caring is a human-to-human process demonstrated through a therapeutic interpersonal interaction. The basic assumptions of Watson's theory of nursing are as follows:

- A person's mind and emotions are windows to the soul. Although nurses give physical care and carry out procedures, the nurse's presence in the relationship transcends the physical and material world, facilitating the client to develop a higher sense of self.
- Although a person's body is confined in time and space, the mind and soul transcend time and space and may be an indicator of the spiritual evolution of humans.
- A nurse may have access to a person's inner self, provided the physical body is not perceived and treated as separate from the mind, emotions, and sense of self.
- People need each other in a caring, loving way. Love and caring are needs that are often overlooked. We need to love, respect, and care for ourselves with dignity before we can respect, love, and care for others and treat them with dignity. (Watson, 1988, pp. 50–51)

Within the theory, optimal health is the attainment of all needs, but even when the scientists in medicine believe that nothing can be done for a client, the nurse can provide care by providing comfort measures and instilling hope. Caring is the mechanism by which nurses help individuals and groups reach self-actualization, maintain or attain health, or die a peaceful death. Holistic, individualized care is given through transpersonal caring, which is a human art, a human science, and the moral ideal of nursing.

Application of Conceptual and Theoretical Frameworks

The aims of nursing, described in Chapter 1, are the same for all nursing theorists, but the values, assumptions, and beliefs individualize each framework when giving nursing care. The brief client care study that follows illustrates how the conceptual and theoretical frameworks discussed in this chapter apply to an individual requiring nursing care.

Client Care Study

Julie Smith is an 18-year-old college freshman. She has an academic scholarship and is active in music and art activities. When Julie came home for winter vacation, her parents were alarmed to see how much weight she had lost. Her mother cooked all of Julie's favorite foods, but Julie refused to eat more than a few bites, saying that she was "too fat." Her mother finally convinced Julie to go to the doctor. The examination showed that Julie weighed only 85 pounds; she had lost more than 20 pounds in 4 months. After tests showed no disease process, the doctor diagnosed anorexia nervosa (an eating disorder).

Based on Johnson's model, nursing care for Julie initially focuses on ineffective functioning within or between the behavioral subsystems. The nurse plans and implements to give Julie the external support necessary to modify her behaviors, return to a state of equilibrium, and regain effective functioning of her whole system.

Based on King's theory, nursing care for Julie uses communications and mutual participation in the plan of care. The nurse and Julie mutually interact to identify problems, set goals, and carry out planned activities. An effective plan of care results in Julie's self-fulfillment and health maintenance.

A nursing plan of care for Julie, when using Leininger's model as a framework, is based on Julie's cultural values, beliefs, and health practices. Using that knowledge, the nurse provides nursing interventions that have physical, psychocultural, and social significance for Julie. If Julie's cultural practices are different from those of the nurse, it is important for the nurse to remember that nurses should not value the healthcare practices of their own culture to the exclusion of the client's culture.

Levine's theory emphasizes the nurse's interventions necessary to help Julie adapt to and reach a state of health. A holistic assessment of Julie provides information about strengths and weaknesses to support a nursing diagnosis. The plan of care includes supportive or therapeutic interventions that are evaluated in terms of their effect on Julie's health status.

Using Neuman's model, the plan of care for Julie is based on a total person approach. Assessments and interventions focus on Julie's perceptions, responses, and resources relative to stressors in her environment and to the variables affecting her responses. Goals and interventions are mutually designed for all three levels of preventive nursing care: (1) strengthening the flexible line of defense, (2) facilitating wellness, and (3) maintaining a maximum level of wellness. Nursing interventions reduce the degree of Julie's reaction to stressors.

Using Orem's framework, the nurse first assesses and analyzes Julie's ability to maintain therapeutic self-care and then identifies deficits to determine why nursing is needed. Based on this information, the nurse designs a system that will be most effective in overcoming the self-care deficits. The nurse then will implement the system to help Julie change conditions in herself or in her environment, and meet her self-care requirements.

When planning and giving nursing care to Julie using Rogers' theory, the nurse becomes an integral part of the environment that is focused on Julie as a whole person, working toward achieving optimal health. The plan of care is based on an analysis of Julie's interactions with the environment, including past and present experiences as well as behavioral patterns and developmental level. Nursing activities are directed toward modifying variations in the behavior patterns and life processes so that Julie can reach her total potential as a human.

Using Roy's model, the nurse focuses on promoting Julie's adaptive responses to improve health. A nursing process is used first to assess behaviors affecting Julie's health and then to make a nursing diagnosis, stating the desired adaptive behaviors. The goals of the nursing care plan are derived through mutual agreement with Julie. The nursing interventions planned and carried out are aimed at altering the environmental stimuli so that an adaptive response could be made, or at increasing Julie's coping ability to make healthy adaptive responses.

The care of Julie, based on Watson's theory, is based in participative, interpersonal experiences between Julie and her nurse. The nurse will pass on to Julie feelings that have been lived through, realized, or learned. As Julie experiences these same feelings, she will be able to facilitate self-healing and discover inner power and control.

The application of conceptual and theoretical frameworks of nursing provides a focus for nursing care activities. The person receiving care is the central theme, but the way each theorist defines that person, the environment, health, and nursing gives the methodology of nursing a unique focus specific to a particular theory or model. The ultimate goal of each framework, however, is holistic client care, individualized to meet needs, prevent illness, and promote wellness.

Key Points

- Nursing is a combination of a body of knowledge and the application of that knowledge through nursing practice.
- Large bodies of knowledge organize and structure both facts and events into philosophies, concepts, and theories. These bodies of knowledge are then put into action by a process. In nursing, this is the nursing process.
- Nursing theories define concepts and relations specific to nursing, using orderly reasoning and logical sequence. They should be both understandable and widely applicable.
- Nursing theories provide for the improvement of nursing practice through nursing research.
- Florence Nightingale's philosophy and theory of nursing provided the base for modern nursing.
- Nursing theory describes or explains nursing and usually includes the concepts of person, environment, health, and nursing.
- Nursing theories are often based on other processes and theories, including general systems, adaptation, and human development.
- Changes in society during the 20th century led to improvement and advances in nursing education, nursing research, and nursing practice.
- Nursing theory provides rationale for nursing actions, gives direction to all aspects of nursing, improves communications, and provides autonomy for the profession of nursing.
- Individual theories and conceptual models provide an organizing framework that can be applied to nursing practice.

Bibliography

Barnum, B. (1994). *Nursing theory: Analysis, application, evaluation* (4th ed.). Philadelphia: Lippincott.

Chapman, J., Mitchell, G., & Forchuk, C. (1994). A glimpse of nursing theory-based practice in Canada. *Nursing Science Quarterly, 7*(3), 104–112.

Chinn, P., & Jacobs, M. (1991). *Theory and nursing: A systematic approach* (3rd ed.). St. Louis: Mosby.

Dolan, J. A., Fitzpatrick, M. L., & Herrmann, E. K. (1983). *Nursing in society: A historical perspective.* Philadelphia: Saunders.

George, J. (Ed.). (1990). *Nursing theories: The base for professional practice* (3rd ed.). Norwalk, CT: Appleton & Lange.

Hekton, L. M. (1989). Martha E. Rogers: A life history. *Nursing Science Quarterly, 2*(2), 63–73.

Johnson, D. (1959). The nature of a science in nursing. *Nursing Outlook, 7*(5), 291–294.

Kalish, P., & Kalish, B. (1995). *The advance of American nursing* (3rd ed.). Philadelphia: Lippincott.

King, I. (1971). *Toward a theory for nursing: General concepts of human behavior.* New York: Wiley.

Leininger, M. M. (1978). *Transcultural nursing: Concepts, theories, and practices.* New York: Wiley.

Levine, M. (1973). *Introduction to clinical nursing* (2nd ed.). Philadelphia: Davis.

Malenski, V. M. (1986). *Explorations on Martha Roger's science of unitary human being.* Norwalk, CT: Appleton-Century-Crofts.

Marriner-Tomey, A. (1994). *Nursing theorists and their work.* St. Louis: Mosby.

Meleis, A. I. (1991). *Theoretical nursing: Development and progress* (2nd ed.). Philadelphia: Lippincott.

Neuman, B. (1989). *The Newman systems model.* Norwalk, CT: Appleton & Lange.

Nevin-Haas, M. (1992). Checking the fit. *Canadian Nurse L'Infirmiere, 88*(2), 33–34.

Orem, D. (1995). *Nursing: Concepts of practice* (5th ed.). St. Louis: Mosby–Year Book.

Rogers, M. (1970). *The theoretical basis of nursing.* Philadelphia: Davis.

Roy, C. (1984). *Introduction to nursing: An adaptation model* (2nd ed.). Englewood Cliffs, NJ: Prentice-Hall.

Roy, C., & Andrews, H. (1991). *The Roy adaptation model: The definitive statement.* Norwalk, CT: Appleton & Lange.

Torres, G. (1990). The place of concepts and theories within nursing. In J. B. George (Ed.). *Nursing theories: The base for professional practice* (pp. 1–12). Norwalk, CT: Appleton & Lange.

Watson, J. (1988). *Nursing: Human science and human care: A theory of nursing* (Pub. No. 15-2236). New York: National League for Nursing.

Weiss, M., Hastings, W., Holly, D., & Craig, D. (1994). Using Roy's adaptation model in practice: Nursing perspectives. *Nursing Science Quarterly, 7*(4), 153–157.

Woods, E. (1994). King's theory in practice with elders. *Nursing Science Quarterly, 7*(2), 65–69.

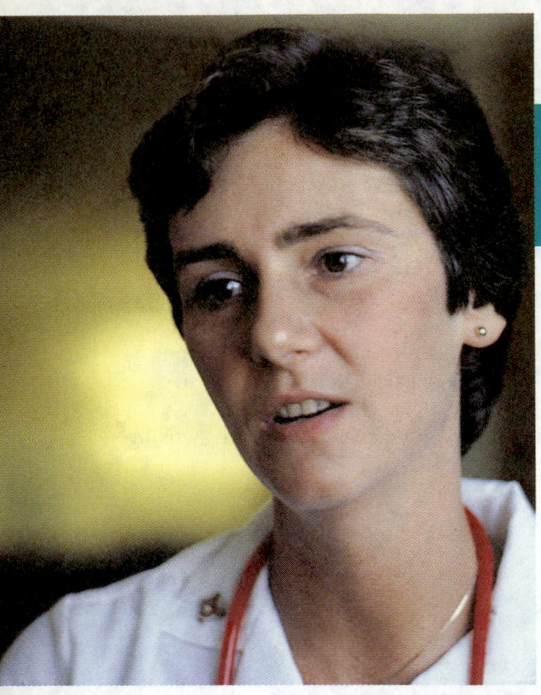

Chapter 6

Values and Ethics in Nursing

Objectives

After studying this chapter, the learner should be able to:

Define key terms used in the chapter.

List five common modes of value transmission.

Describe seven steps in the valuing process.

Use values clarification strategies in clinical practice.

Compare and contrast the principle- and care-based approaches to bioethics.

Describe three typical concerns of the nurse advocate.

Describe nursing practice that is consistent with the code of ethics for nursing.

Recognize ethical issues as they arise in nursing practice.

Use an ethical framework and decision-making process to resolve ethical problems.

Identify four functions of institutional ethics committees.

Key Terms

advocacy
attitude
autonomy
beliefs
beneficence
care-based approach
confidentiality
deontologic
ethics
fidelity
justice
morals
nonmaleficence
paternalism
principle-based approach
utilitarian
value
value system
values clarification
veracity

The unique nature of nursing places nurses at the bedside and in groups of professionals where critical decisions are being made about the best way to treat injury and illness and to solve healthcare problems. Often the question confronting the nurse is not, "How do I do this?" but rather, "Should I do this?" The more science and technology increase the options available to clients and healthcare professionals, the more frequently nurses will find themselves asking, "We can do this, but *should we,* here and now, for this client?" The answer to this and other ethical questions is important for quality care. Nurses need to examine their intuitions, opinions, and convictions about what is morally right and wrong and monitor how these influence their nursing care.

This chapter explores the influence of values on human behavior and the ethical dimensions of nursing practice. Chapter 14 describes specific ethical skills that are essential to nursing practice. Nurses who understand how clients' values and their own values shape nurse–client interactions and who continually develop sensitivity to the ethical dimensions of nursing practice are best able to provide quality care.

Values

A **value** is a personal belief about worth that acts as a standard to guide one's behavior. A **value system** is an organization of values in which each value is ranked along a continuum of importance; a value system often operates as a personal code of conduct.

Because attitudes and beliefs also influence human behavior, it is important to distinguish them from values. An **attitude** is a feeling or an emotion, generally including positive or negative judgment, toward people, objects, or ideas. **Beliefs** refer to a special class of intellectual attitudes based primarily on faith as opposed to fact.

A person's values influence beliefs about human needs, health, and illness; the practice of health behaviors; and human responses to illness. Nurses who work effectively with clients are sensitive to how a client's values and their own values influence their interactions.

Development of Values

An individual is not born with values; rather, values are formed over a lifetime from information from the environment, family, and culture. As children observe actions, they quickly learn what has high and low value for family members. If the parents spend a good portion of each day cooking and the family spends a long time eating and talking at the table, the children learn to value food and the good times it represents. Similarly, children learn helpfulness is a good and respected quality if praised when helping parents, grandparents, and siblings.

Common modes of value transmission include the following:

Modeling: Children learn what is of high or low value by observing parents, peers, and significant others. Thus, modeling may lead to socially acceptable or unacceptable behavior.

Moralizing: Children are taught a complete value system by parents or an institution (eg, church or school) that allows little opportunity for them to weigh different values.

Laissez-faire: Children are left to explore values (no one set of values is presented as best for all) and to develop a personal value system. This approach is often accompanied by little or no guidance and can lead to confusion and conflict.

Rewarding and punishing: Children are rewarded when demonstrating values held by parents and punished when demonstrating unacceptable values.

Responsible choice: Children are encouraged to explore competing values and to weigh their consequences. Support and guidance are offered as children develop a personal value system.

Values Essential to the Professional Nurse

In 1985, the American Association of Colleges of Nursing undertook a project that included the identification of values essential to the practice of professional nursing. The group identified seven values (aesthetics, altruism, equality, freedom, human dignity, justice, and truth) and related attitudes and personal qualities. These values are defined, and examples given, in the accompanying box.

Value Neutrality

In an effort to encourage healthcare professionals to respect and accept the individuality of clients, some educators have advised that professionals be "value neutral" and "nonjudgmental" in their professional roles. Thus the nurse has a "commitment to clients whether or not the nurse and the clients hold the same values. The nurse does not assume that personal values are right and should not judge the client's values as right or wrong depending on their congruence with the nurse's personal

Essential Values of the Professional Nurse, With Examples of Attitudes and Personality Qualities*

Aesthetics

Qualities of objects, events, and people that provide satisfaction

Appreciation Creativity Imagination Sensitivity	• Adapts the environment so it is pleasing to the client • Creates a pleasant work environment for self and others • Presents self in a manner that promotes a positive image of nursing

Altruism

Concern for the welfare of others

Caring Commitment Compassion Generosity Perseverance	• Gives full attention to the client when providing care • Assists other personnel in providing care when they are unable to do so • Expresses concern about social trends and issues that have implications for health care

Equality

Having the same rights, privileges, or status

Acceptance Assertiveness Fairness Self-esteem Tolerance	• Provides nursing care based on the client's needs irrespective of personal characteristics† • Interacts with other providers in a nondiscriminatory manner • Expresses ideas about the improvement of access to nursing and health care

Freedom

Capacity to exercise choice

Confidence Hope Independence Openness Self-direction Self-discipline	• Honors individual's right to refuse treatment • Supports the rights of other providers to suggest alternatives to the plan of care • Encourages open discussion of controversial issues in the profession

Human Dignity

Inherent worth and uniqueness of an individual

Consideration Empathy Humaneness Kindness Respectfulness Trust	• Safeguards the individual's right to privacy • Addresses others as they prefer to be addressed • Maintains confidentiality of clients and staff • Treats others with respect regardless of ground

Justice

Upholding of moral and legal principles

Courage Integrity Morality Objectivity	• Acts as a healthcare advocate • Allocates resources fairly • Reports incompetent, unethical, and illegal practice objectively and factually

Truth

Faithfulness to fact and reality

Accountability Authenticity Honesty Inquisitiveness Rationality Reflectiveness	• Documents nursing care accurately and honestly • Obtains sufficient data to make sound judgments before reporting infractions of organizational policies • Participates in professional efforts to protect the public from misinformation about nursing

*Values are listed in alphabetic rather than priority order.

† From American Nurses' Association. (1976) *Code for nurses.* Washington, DC: ANA

(*Essentials of college and university education for professional nursing.* [1986]. Washington, DC: American Association of Colleges of Nursing.)

value system" (Steele & Harmon, 1983, p. 27). This kind of thinking enables a nurse to care for a client with different values. For example, a nurse who strongly believes that any premarital or extramarital sex is wrong may offer competent and compassionate nursing care to a young female prostitute with active herpes lesions. On the other hand, if the same client, following education, indicates that she is unconcerned about whom she might infect in future sexual encounters, the nurse has a moral obligation to protect the client and others from the harm the client's values may cause.

Values Clarification

Values clarification is a process by which people come to understand their own values and value system. "It is a process of discovery and allows the person to discover through feelings and analysis of behavior what choices to make when alternatives are presented, and to identify whether or not these choices are rationally made or are the result of previous conditioning" (Steele & Harmon, 1983, p. 13). Values clarification has a beneficial application to nursing.

Values theorists most often describe the process of valuing as having seven steps centered on three main activities: (1) choosing, (2) prizing, and (3) acting (Raths, Simon, & Harmin, 1978; Simon, 1972). When one values something, one:

Chooses

- Freely
- From alternatives
- After careful consideration of the consequences of each alternative

Prizes

- With pride and happiness
- With public affirmation

Acts

- With incorporation of the choice into one's behavior
- With consistency and regularity on the value

Values Clarification by the Nurse

For example, if respect for human dignity is a value that characterizes your nursing practice, you:

Choose

- Freely choose to believe in the worth and uniqueness of each individual
- Realize that you have other options (that you could treat with dignity only those people who are most like you)
- Believe that respecting each person's human dignity yields the best consequences for you and for all of society

Prize

- Feel proud and happy with your choice (you especially enjoy when clients let you know they appreciate your care and when nursing colleagues and supervisors compliment you on interpersonal skills)
- Are able to defend this value when someone's human dignity is being ignored

Act

- Incorporate this value into your practice
- Attempt consistently to respect human dignity in both your personal and professional life

As you become more conscious of this value, you will be sensitive to those of your actions that are inconsistent with it. You may feel uncomfortable after gossiping with other nurses during break about a client no one likes; you realize that this behavior contradicts your basic respect for human dignity. Thus, values clarification is a "process by which we increase the likelihood that our living in general, and a decision in particular [to respect human dignity], will, first, have a positive value for us, and, second, for the society we serve" (Kirschbaum, 1977).

Steele and Harmon (1983) offer numerous exercises for nurses seeking to clarify their personal and professional values. Uustal (1978) describes 10 strategies to increase self-awareness and appreciation and to explore selected values conflicts and ethical dilemmas in nursing.

Clinical Applications

Unless the nurse is comfortable with change and believes that health is important enough to merit learning a new treatment regimen, client education is doomed to failure. The accompanying box illustrates how the steps in the valuing process can be used to assist a client with high blood pressure take charge of his health and manage his medications. Other clinical examples follow.

Client Places Low Value on Health and Health Behaviors. You become frustrated when repeated attempts to teach or counsel a 26-year-old pharmaceutical salesperson meet with failure. Although hospitalized with a serious duodenal ulcer, all he can talk about is his job and meeting his sales quota.

Values Clarification. First help this client identify his basic life values. Ask him, "What three things are most important to you in life?" or have him rank the following behaviors in terms of how he would most likely spend an unexpected free day:

______ Enjoy some quiet time alone (eg, thinking, reading, listening to music)

______ Spend time with family, friends

______ Do something active (eg, hiking, playing ball, swimming)

______ Watch television

______ Volunteer time and energy to help someone else

______ Use time for my job

______ Other

Discuss what these rankings indicate about his values. Determine whether his rankings would be different

Steps in the Valuing Process

Case: A male client with high blood pressure.

Choosing

1. Freely
Rehospitalized for high blood pressure after abruptly stopping his antihypertensive medication, the client decides from now on to take his medication as prescribed.

2. From Alternatives
After a teaching–learning session with a nurse, the client understands he has basically three options:

- Comply with prescribed treatment regimen.
- Refuse to take the medication but try harder to control his blood pressure through diet, exercise, and stress management.
- Refuse to take his medication and assume a "we'll see" attitude.

3. After Consideration of the Consequences
The client understands the *probable* consequences of these options:

- Compliance with the treatment regimen will yield the best control of high blood pressure (but may cause some annoying side effects).
- Diet, exercise, and stress management may reduce his blood pressure somewhat but did not yield sufficient control in the past.
- High blood pressure may result in serious complications such as stroke, kidney disease, or impaired vision.

Prizing

4. With Pride and Happiness
The client states, "Now that I understand high blood pressure better and know what I can do to control it, I feel more in charge of my life—and I like that!"

5. With Public Affirmation
The client states to his wife, "I guess I was wrong to stop taking that medicine when I blamed it for how lousy I was feeling. You can bet that won't happen again. If you ever hear me complaining about my pills, remind me to see my doctor right away."

Acting

6. With Incorporation of the Choice Into One's Behavior
After discharge from the hospital, the client takes the medication as prescribed.

7. With Consistency and Regularity on the Value
The client seeks to understand any new medication he is prescribed (ie, reason for the medication, possible side effects, consequences of the noncompliance) and successfully manages the treatment regimen; he feels proud of his new knowledge and self-care abilities.

if he were asked how he *wished* he would spend the free day versus how he would *most likely* spend it.

Choosing. After exploring with this client how values might affect other aspects in his life (ie, long-term effects of stress related to his present preoccupation with job performance), counsel him to choose his key values freely. It would be a positive sign if health were among these values, but it might not be.

Prizing. Use affirmation to reinforce the client's wellness-promoting values and, when possible, enlist the support of family members. For example: "Your wife seemed so happy yesterday when you told her you decided to quit smoking. You can see how much she loves you and values your health."

Acting. Assist the client to plan new behaviors consistent with the values he has chosen and to think of ways those behaviors can be incorporated into his life. "Once you get home, how will your life be different?" "You said you wanted to begin to take time for yourself—how are you going to do this?"

Values of Client and Family Members Conflict. You sense a growing tension while counseling the young parents of a child with asthma. Questioning ("You seem uncomfortable with what I'm saying now. Is there something wrong?") reveals that the wife is a confirmed smoker and cat lover who has told her husband that even if these behaviors are hurting their child, she is unwilling to give them up.

Values Clarification. Suggest that both parents complete the following exercise and then talk about their different responses.

Where do you stand on the following issues? (Indicate your responses in the following manner: SA, strongly agree; A, agree; D, disagree; SD, strongly disagree; U, undecided.)

_______ A parent's primary obligation is to meet the needs of his or her child.

_______ Each member of a family is entitled to pursue personal pleasures—even if these are not in the best interest of all.

_______ Pleasure is more important than health.

_______ The choices one family member makes can dramatically affect other family members (positively and negatively).

This exercise will help the parents to evaluate their basic values, explore areas of conflict, and, perhaps, move toward joint choosing, prizing, and acting on several health-promoting values.

Ethics

Ethics is systematic inquiry into the principles of right and wrong conduct, of virtue and vice, and of good and evil as they relate to conduct. Many people use the term *ethics* when describing the professional ethics incorporated into a code of professional conduct, such as nursing codes of ethics. **Morals,** although similar in meaning to ethics, usually refer to personal standards of right and wrong. It is important to distinguish ethics from religion, law, custom, and institutional practices. For example, the fact that an action is legal or customary does not in itself make the action morally right.

As nurses assume increasing responsibility for managing care, it is critical that they be prepared to recognize the ethical dimensions of their practice and to participate competently in ethical decision making. Seventy-nine percent of the 934 nurses surveyed by the American Nurses Association Center for Ethics and Human Rights at the ANA Convention in 1994 reported confronting ethical issues in practice daily (43%) or weekly (36%). Over 50% of the nurses identified the following four issues as the most frequent: cost-containment issues that jeopardize patient welfare; end-of-life decisions; breaches of patient confidentiality; and incompetent, unethical, or illegal practices of colleagues. Pain management, use of advance directives, informed consent for procedures, access to healthcare, issues in the care of HIV/AIDS persons, and providing "futile" treatment completed the list of 10 (Scanlon, 1994).

Professional Ethical Conduct

Nurses committed to high-quality care base their practice on professional standards of ethical conduct. The study of professional ethical behavior begins in nursing school, continues in formal and informal discussions with colleagues and peers, and culminates when nurses "try on" and make their own the behaviors of role models who practice professional nursing that is consistent with high ethical standards. Where do nurses learn the standards for professional ethical behavior? At the very least nurses should understand the ethical theories which dictate and justify professional conduct, be familiar with codes of professional ethics, standards of practice, and client bills of rights; and be skilled in using a model of ethical decision making to resolve ethical problems.

Theories of Ethics

Ethical theories are systems of reflection that attempt to explain how we ought to live and why. These theories may be broadly categorized as action-guiding theories that answer the question, "What ought I to do?" or character-guiding theories that answer the question, "What kind of person ought I to be?" Action-guiding theories fall into two main categories:

Utilitarian: The rightness or wrongness of an action depends on the consequences the action produces.

Deontologic: An action is right or wrong independent of the consequences it produces.

Nursing ethics, which is a subset of bioethics, is the formal study of the ethical issues that arise in the practice of nursing and of the analysis used by nurses to make ethical judgments. Nurse ethicists frequently use two popular theoretical and practical approaches to doing bioethics: the principle-based approach and the care-based approach.

Principle-Based Approach. The principle-based approach to doing bioethics offers specific action guides for practice. The Beauchamp/Childress four-principles approach to biomedical ethics (1994) directs that we ought to act so as to respect the decision-making capacity of autonomous persons (**autonomy**); avoid causing harm (**nonmaleficence**); provide benefits and balance these benefits against risks and harms (**beneficence**); and distribute benefits, risks, and costs fairly (**justice**). Ethical dilemmas arise when fidelity to these principles suggests two conflicting courses of action. A mother demands costly, aggressive treatment for her child who is born without a brain and who will never be able to enjoy simple human pleasures. Autonomy demands respect for this mother's treatment preferences, but justice dictates that the public monies involved be used for other infants more able to benefit from aggressive treatment. Sadly, there is no foolproof method for identifying which principle is most important when there is conflict among competing principles. Popularized versions of the principle-based approach to bioethics have too frequently resulted in a type of "quandary ethics" that diminishes in importance the everyday ethical concerns of nurses and misleadingly suggests that how ethical dilemmas are resolved is unimportant, so long as one can justify one's recommendation with recourse to a principle.

Care-Based Approach. Dissatisfaction with the principle-based approach to bioethics led many nurses to look to care as the foundation for nursing's moral obligation. The nurse–client relationship is central to the care-based approach, which directs attention to the "particulars" of individual clients who are viewed within the context of their life narrative. The care perspective directs that how I choose to be each time I encounter a client or colleague is a matter of ethical significance. Ethics is not reduced to a decision to withhold or withdraw life-sustaining treatment. Characteristics of the care perspective include:

- Centrality of the caring relationship
- Promotion of the dignity and respect of clients as people

- Attention to the particulars about individual clients
- Cultivation of responsiveness to others and professional responsibility
- A redefinition of fundamental moral skills to include virtues like kindness, attentiveness, empathy, compassion, reliability (Taylor, 1993)

Advocacy

Nursing has traditionally held that its primary commitment is to the client, and more recently has claimed client advocacy as a legitimate nursing role. **Advocacy**, which is discussed in Chapter 24, is the protection and support of another's rights. As a distinct moral obligation for nurses, it finds justification in both the principle- and care-based approaches to nursing ethics. Nurses who wish to practice in this tradition:

- Make sure that their loyalty to an employing institution or colleague does not compromise their primary commitment to the client
- Give priority to the good of the individual client rather than to the good of society in general
- Carefully evaluate the competing claims of autonomy (self-determination) and client well-being

When respecting autonomy, the nurse respects and supports the client's right to make decisions. Informed consent is described in Chapter 7. When promoting client well-being, the nurse acts in the best interests of the client. Ideally, both autonomy and client well-being are promoted in each nurse–client interaction; however, conflicts sometimes arise. For instance, if an older male client with a serious chronic lung disease who understands well the danger of smoking asks the nurse to get him a pack of cigarettes, the nurse must decide whether to respect his autonomy and follow his wishes or to promote his medical well-being. Nurses sensitive to the need to promote both client autonomy and well-being may often experience conflict, but they are more likely than other nurses to succeed in securing the client's genuine best interests.

Nursing Codes of Ethics

A professional code of ethics provides a framework for making ethical decisions and sets forth professional expectations. Nursing codes of ethics inform both nurses and society of the primary goals and values of the profession. Reflected in the codes are universal moral principles such as respect for persons; autonomy (self-determination); beneficence (doing good); nonmaleficence (avoiding harm); **veracity** (truth-telling); **confidentiality** (respecting privileged information); **fidelity** (keeping promises); and justice (treating people fairly). These principles should be compatible with the nurse's personal value system and moral code. Other functions of professional nursing codes include the following:

- Indicating nursing's acceptance of the responsibility and trust with which it has been invested by society
- Providing guidance for conduct and relationships in carrying out nursing responsibilities consistent with the ethical obligations of the profession and with high quality in nursing care
- Providing a means for the exercise of professional self-regulation (American Nurses' Association, 1985, pp. i–iv)

Codes are effective in accomplishing their goals only to the extent that they are upheld by members of the profession. Code requirements may exceed legal requirements. Although violations of the law subject a nurse to civil or criminal liability (see Chapter 7), violations of the code of ethics may result in reprimands, censure, suspension, and expulsion.

Codes of ethics for nursing include the International Council of Nurses (ICN) *ICN Code for Nurses* (adopted in 1953 and revised in 1965 and 1973); the ANA *Code for Nurses With Interpretive Statements* (adopted in 1950 and revised in 1968, 1976, and 1985); and the Canadian Nurses Association (CNA) *Code of Ethics for Nursing* (adopted in 1980 and revised in 1991). These are highlighted in the accompanying box.

Nursing Standards of Practice

When the American Nurses Association revised its Standards of Clinical Nursing Practice in 1991, it developed standards of professional performance as well as standards of care. The fifth standard of professional performance describes the nurse's ethical obligations.

> Standard V. Ethics: The nurse's decisions and actions on behalf of clients are determined in an ethical manner.
>
> ***Measurement Criteria***
>
> 1. The nurse's practice is guided by the *Code for Nurses.*
> 2. The nurse maintains client confidentiality.
> 3. The nurse acts as a client advocate.
> 4. The nurse delivers care in a nonjudgmental and nondiscriminatory manner that is sensitive to client diversity.
> 5. The nurse delivers care in a manner that preserves/protects client autonomy, dignity, and rights.
> 6. The nurse seeks available resources to help formulate ethical decisions. (1991, p. 15)

A Patient's Bill of Rights

The American Hospital Association developed *A Patient's Bill of Rights* in 1972 (revised in 1992; see the accompanying box). The bill of rights includes the rights and responsibilities of the client while receiving care in the hospital. A number of other bills of rights have emerged recently, such as the Pregnant Patient's Bill of Rights, the Indian Patient's Bill of Rights, a Nursing Home Bill of Rights, and the Veterans Administration Code of Patient Concern. Each of these bills of rights emphasizes a specific aspect of client rights within a particular health agency. These bills of rights imply a code of ethics the nurse observes professionally.

Three Codes of Ethics for Nurses

*International Council of Nurses Code for Nurses**

The fundamental responsibility of the nurse is fourfold—to promote health, to prevent illness, to restore health, and to alleviate suffering.

The need for nursing is universal. Inherent in nursing is respect for life, dignity, and rights of humans. It is unrestricted by considerations of nationality, race, creed, age, sex, politics or social status.

Nurses render health services to the individual, the family, and the community and coordinate their services with those of related groups.

Nurses and People

The nurse's primary responsibility is to those people who require nursing care.

The nurse, in providing care, promotes an environment in which the values, customs, and spiritual beliefs of the individual are respected.

The nurse holds in confidence personal information and uses judgment in sharing this information.

Nurses and Practice

The nurse carries personal responsibility for nursing practice and for maintaining competence by continual learning. The nurse maintains the highest standards of nursing care possible within the reality of a specific situation.

The nurse uses judgment in relation to individual competence when accepting and delegating responsibilities.

The nurse, when acting in a professional capacity, should at all times maintain standards of personal conduct that reflect credit on the profession.

Nurses and Society

The nurse shares with other citizens the responsibility for initiating and supporting action to meet the health and social needs of the public.

Nurses and Coworkers

The nurse sustains a cooperative relationship with coworkers in nursing and other fields. The nurse takes appropriate action to safeguard the individual when his or her care is endangered by a coworker or any other person.

Nurses and the Profession

The nurse plays the major role in determining and implementing desirable standards of nursing practice and nursing education.

The nurse is active in developing a core of professional knowledge.

The nurse, acting through the professional organization, participates in establishing and maintaining equitable social and economic working conditions in nursing.

American Nurses Association Code for Nurses†

1. The nurse provides services with respect for human dignity and the uniqueness of the client unrestricted by considerations of social or economic status, personal attributes, or the nature of health problems.
2. The nurse safeguards the client's right to privacy by judiciously protecting information of a confidential nature.
3. The nurse acts to safeguard the client and the public when health care and safety are affected by the incompetent, unethical, or illegal practice of any person.
4. The nurse assumes responsibility and accountability for individual nursing judgments and actions.
5. The nurse maintains competence in nursing.
6. The nurse exercises informed judgment and uses individual competence and qualifications as criteria in seeking consultation, accepting responsibilities, and delegating nursing activities to others.
7. The nurse participates in activities that contribute to the ongoing development of the profession's body of knowledge.
8. The nurse participates in the profession's efforts to implement and improve standards of nursing.
9. The nurse participates in the profession's efforts to establish and maintain conditions of employment conducive to high quality nursing care.
10. The nurse participates in the profession's effort to protect the public from misinformation and misrepresentation and to maintain the integrity of nursing.
11. The nurse collaborates with members of the health professions and other citizens in promoting community and national efforts to meet the health needs of the public.

Canadian Nurses Association Code of Ethics for Nursing Clients‡§

I. A nurse treats clients with respect for their individual needs and values.

II. Based on respect for clients and regard for their right to control their own care, nursing care reflects respect for the right of choice held by clients.

III. The nurse holds confidential all information about a client learned in the health care setting.

IV. The nurse is guided by consideration for the dignity of clients.

V. The nurse provides competent care to clients.

VI. The nurse maintains trust in nurses and nursing.

(continued)

Three Codes of Ethics for Nurses *(continued)*

VII. The nurse recognizes the contribution and expertise of colleagues from nursing and other disciplines as essential to excellent health care.
VIII. The nurse takes steps to ensure that the client receives competent and ethical care.
IX. Conditions of employment should contribute in a positive way to client care and the professional satisfaction of nurses.
X. Job action by nurses is directed toward securing conditions of employment that enable safe and appropriate care for clients and contribute to the professional satisfaction of nurses.
XI. The nurse advocates the interests of clients.
XII. The nurse represents the values and ethics of nursing before colleagues and others.
XIII. Professional nurses' organizations are responsible for clarifying, securing, and sustaining ethical nursing conduct. The fulfillment of these tasks requires that professional nurses' organizations remain responsive to the rights, needs, and legitimate interests of clients and nurses.

*Adapted from International Council of Nurses. (1973). ICN *Code for nurses: Ethical concepts applied to nursing.* Geneva, Imprimeries Populaires.

† From American Nurses Association. (1985). *Code for nurses.* Kansas City, MO: ANA.

‡ This represents only one element of the code—values. Obligations, which provide more specific direction for conduct than do values by spelling out what a value requires under particular circumstances, and limitations, which describe exceptional circumstances in which a value or obligation cannot be applied, are provided with each value in the publication.

§ From Canadian Nurses Association. (1991). *Code of ethics for nursing.* Ottawa, Ontario: CNA.

Ethical Decision Making

Two types of moral and ethical problems commonly faced by nurses are moral dilemmas and moral distress. In a *moral dilemma* two (or more) clear moral principles apply but support mutually inconsistent courses of action. In *moral distress* the nurse knows the right thing to do but institutional constraints make it nearly impossible to pursue the right actions (Jameton, 1993, p. 542). Nurses need sound analytic skills and the ability to engage in moral reasoning to resolve moral dilemmas and moral distress. Every nurse needs to be confident in using a process of ethical decision making. The accompanying client care study illustrates a five-step model of ethical decision making that is based on the nursing process.

1. Assess the situation (gather data)
2. Diagnose (identify) the ethical problem
3. Plan: Identify options and explore the probable consequences of each; use ethical reasoning to decide upon a course of action which you can justify
4. Implement your decision
5. Evaluate your decision

Examples of Ethical Problems

Ethical problems commonly arise between nurses and clients, nurses and physicians, nurses and other nurses, and nurses and their employing institutions. Moreover, nurses are often most conflicted when good practice seems to require acting against their personal moral convictions. As you read through the mini-cases that follow, try to determine your response. The above process of ethical decision making should prove helpful. Resources for ethical decision making are highlighted in the accompanying box.

Nurses and Clients

Troublesome nurse–client situations that can result in ethical distress for nurses include **paternalism** (acting for clients without their consent to secure good or prevent harm), deception, confidentiality, allocation of scarce nursing resources, informed consent, and conflicts between the client's and nurse's values and interests.

Paternalism. An alert older resident who lives in a nursing home and who is now at high risk for falls refuses to call the nurse for assistance when getting out of bed. The nurse must decide whether to obtain an order to restrain the client. Does preventing potential harm justify violating the client's right to autonomy and make it acceptable for the nurse to act as a "parent" and choose an action the client does not want because it is believed to be in the client's best interest?

Deception. A postoperative client asks the student nurse, who is about to administer an intramuscular injection for pain, "Is this your first shot?" It is the student's first injection and the student is anxious. Would the student's intent to decrease the client's anxiety justify telling the client, "No, I've given several before"?

Confidentiality. A nurse asks a middle-aged woman who is crying quietly, "Would you like to share what's troubling you?" The woman tells the nurse she has no idea how she will pay for this clinic visit because she entered the country illegally 2 months ago and is trying to earn enough money to help her family back home. She begs the nurse not to tell anyone. If the nurse believes this anxiety is interfering with the client's ability to obtain needed healthcare, would it be ethical to break the woman's confidence to obtain help for her?

A Patient's Bill of Rights

Introduction

Effective health care requires collaboration between patients and physicians and other health care professionals. Open and honest communication, respect for personal and professional values, and sensitivity to differences are integral to optimal patient care. As the setting for the provision of health services, hospitals must provide a foundation for understanding and respecting the rights and responsibilities of patients, their families, physicians, and other caregivers. Hospitals must ensure a health care ethic that respects the role of patients in decision making about treatment choices and other aspects of their care. Hospitals must be sensitive to cultural, racial, linguistic, religious, age, gender, and other differences as well as the needs of persons with disabilities.

The American Hospital Association presents *A Patient's Bill of Rights* with the expectation that it will contribute to more effective patient care and be supported by the hospital on behalf of the institution, its medical staff, employees, and patients. The American Hospital Association encourages health care institutions to tailor this bill of rights to their patient community by translating and/or simplifying the language of this bill of rights as may be necessary to ensure that patients and their families understand their rights and responsibilities.

*Bill of Rights**

1. The patient has the right to considerate and respectful care.
2. The patient has the right to and is encouraged to obtain from physicians and other direct caregivers relevant, current, and understandable information concerning diagnosis, treatment, and prognosis.

   Except in emergencies when the patient lacks decision-making capacity and the need for treatment is urgent, the patient is entitled to the opportunity to discuss and request information related to the specific procedures and/or treatments, the risks involved, the possible length of recuperation, and the medically reasonable alternatives and their accompanying risks and benefits.

   Patients have the right to know the identity of physicians, nurses, and others involved in their care, as well as when those involved are students, residents, or other trainees. The patient also has the right to know the immediate and long-term financial implications of treatment choices, insofar as they are known.
3. The patient has the right to make decisions about the plan of care prior to and during the course of treatment and to refuse a recommended treatment or plan of care to the extent permitted by law and hospital policy and to be informed of the medical consequences of this action. In case of such refusal, the patient is entitled to other appropriate care and services that the hospital provides or transfer to another hospital. The hospital should notify patients of any policy that might affect patient choice within the institution.
4. The patient has the right to have an advance directive (such as a living will, health care proxy, or durable power of attorney for health care) concerning treatment or designating a surrogate decision maker with the expectation that the hospital will honor the intent of that directive to the extent permitted by law and hospital policy.

   Health care institutions must advise patients of their rights under state law and hospital policy to make informed medical choices, ask if the patient has an advance directive, and include that information in patient records. The patient has the right to timely information about hospital policy that may limit its ability to implement fully a legally valid advance directive.
5. The patient has the right to every consideration of privacy. Case discussion, consultation, examination, and treatment should be conducted so as to protect each patient's privacy.
6. The patient has the right to expect that all communications and records pertaining to his/her care will be treated as confidential by the hospital, except in cases such as suspected abuse and public health hazards when reporting is permitted or required by law. The patient has the right to expect that the hospital will emphasize the confidentiality of this information when it releases it to any other parties entitled to review information in these records.
7. The patient has the right to review the records pertaining to his/her medical care and to have the information explained or interpreted as necessary, except when restricted by law.
8. The patient has the right to expect that, within its capacity and policies, a hospital will make reasonable response to the request of a patient for appropriate and medically indicated care and services. The hospital must provide evaluation, service, and/or referral as indicated by the urgency of the case. When medically appropriate and legally permissible, or when a patient has so requested, a patient may be transferred to another facility. The institution to which the patient is to be transferred must first have accepted the patient for transfer. The patient must also have the benefit of complete information and explanation concerning the need for, risks, benefits, and alternatives to such a transfer.
9. The patient has the right to ask and be informed of the existence of business relationships among

(continued)

A Patient's Bill of Rights *(continued)*

the hospital, educational institutions, other health care providers, or payers that may influence the patient's treatment and care.

10. The patient has the right to consent to or decline to participate in proposed research studies or human experimentation affecting care and treatment or requiring direct patient involvement, and to have those studies fully explained prior to consent. A patient who declines to participate in research or experimentation is entitled to the most effective care that the hospital can otherwise provide.
11. The patient has the right to expect reasonable continuity of care when appropriate and to be informed by physicians and other caregivers of available and realistic patient care options when hospital care is no longer appropriate.
12. The patient has the right to be informed of hospital policies and practices that relate to patient care, treatment, and responsibilities. The patient has the right to be informed of available resources for resolving disputes, grievances, and conflicts, such as ethics committees, patient representatives, or other mechanisms available in the institution. The patient has the right to be informed of the hospital's charges for services and available payment methods.

The collaborative nature of health care requires that patients, or their families/surrogates, participate in their care. The effectiveness of care and patient satisfaction with the course of treatment depend, in part, on the patient fulfilling certain responsibilities. Patients are responsible for providing information about past illnesses, hospitalizations, medications, and other matters related to health status. To participate effectively in decision making, patients must be encouraged to take responsibility for requesting additional information or clarification about their health status or treatment when they do not fully understand information and instruction. Patients are also responsible for ensuring that the health care institution has a copy of their written advance directive if they have one. Patients are responsible for informing their physicians and other caregivers if they anticipate problems in following prescribed treatment.

Patients should also be aware of the hospital's obligation to be reasonably efficient and equitable in providing care to other patients and the community. The hospital's rules and regulations are designed to help the hospital meet this obligation. Patients and their families are responsible for making reasonable accommodations to the needs of the hospital, other patients, medical staff, and hospital employees. Patients are responsible for providing necessary information for insurance claims and for working with the hospital to make payment arrangements, when necessary.

A person's health depends on much more than health care services. Patients are responsible for recognizing the impact of their lifestyle on their personal health.

Conclusion

Hospitals have many functions to perform, including the enhancement of health status, health promotion, and the prevention and treatment of injury and disease; the immediate and ongoing care and rehabilitation of patients; the education of health professionals, patients, and the community; and research. All these activities must be conducted with an overriding concern for the values and dignity of patients.

*These rights can be exercised on the patient's behalf by a legally designated surrogate or proxy decision maker if the patient lacks decision-making capacity, is legally incompetent, or is a minor.

Allocation of Scarce Nursing Resources. A nurse has just been pulled from your unit, leaving it understaffed. Among your clients are a 33-year-old man recovering from a heart attack who is being discharged in the morning (he tells you he still has many questions); an older client who is close to death; and a woman with cancer who has been vomiting all day and who is in severe pain. You know you cannot meet everyone's needs well. How do you "distribute" your nursing care? (You really *like* the client who is going home in the morning.)

Informed Consent. A resident is attempting to perform a spinal tap on an adolescent who you know dislikes the resident. After one failed attempt, the adolescent tells the resident to stop. The resident asks you to administer an antianxiety medication to the client so the resident can get the spinal tap done quickly. Should you administer the medication knowing the client no longer consents to the procedure?

Conflicts Between the Client's and Nurse's Interests. Home health nurses are taking turns being assigned to care for new clients who test positive for the human immunodeficiency virus. One nurse, who is nursing her 8-month-old infant, refuses to take her turn, fearing she will transmit the disease to her baby. The other nurses tell her she must accept the assignment of this HIV-positive client because none of them is willing to take her turn. Is a nurse ever justified in refusing to nurse a client assigned to his or her care?

Client Care Study Using a Five-Step Process for Resolving the Ethical Problem

Jean W. is a labor and delivery room nurse in a small community hospital that serves both private clients and clinic clients. Jean has always felt that certain members of the obstetrics–gynecology medical staff have treated these two groups of clients differently. On this particular morning, Jean is caring for a woman who is scheduled for an elective cesarean delivery. The woman (who is a clinic client) has made it very clear that she wants to be awake for the delivery and has requested epidural or spinal anesthesia. Jean is dismayed when the anesthesiologist enters the delivery room because the anesthesiologist's success rate with epidural anesthesia is poor. The anesthesiologist unsuccessfully attempts to perform an epidural block. After waiting 20 minutes for results, the obstetrician is growing impatient and instructs the anesthesiologist to put the client to sleep. Jean feels the rights of this client are being violated but is unsure of what her response should be.

Step 1: Assess the Situation (Gather Data)

Describe the situation that gives rise to the problem: main people involved (their views and interests); client's overall nursing, medical, and social situation; relevant legal, administrative, and staff considerations.

The client is in stable medical condition (elective cesarean delivery, not an emergency) and has made it very clear that she wishes to be awake for the delivery. The client is not a private paying client of the obstetrician. The nurse believes her role is to promote/protect the client's interests; she knows of no reason in this case why the client's preferences should be disregarded.

The anesthesiologist has a poor success record with epidural anesthesia.

The obstetrician seems to want to complete delivery quickly. In the past, he has seemed to give more weight to following wishes of private clients as opposed to clinic clients. He is the head of the obstetrics–gynecology department; he believes nurses should obey physicians unquestioningly.

Nurses have in the past expressed dissatisfaction with the different levels of care being provided to private and clinic clients, but no one to date has formally addressed the concern.

Step 2: Diagnose (Identify) the Ethical Problem

State the problem clearly: unsure of ethical issue; two or more moral principles are in conflict; object to proposed course of action.

Jean W. objects to the obstetrician's intent to disregard the client's wish to be awake for her delivery; she is aware of no good reasons justifying this course of action.

Identify your relationship to the decision.

The nurse will be a participant in carrying out the decision.

Identify time parameters.

The decision for this case must be made immediately; it would be helpful to plan to avoid situations like this in the future.

Step 3: Plan

a. Identify Options

Identify all the possible courses of action open to you and weigh the outcomes of each; consider immediate consequences to the people involved as well as long-term consequences to the institution and society.

The nurse can say nothing to the obstetrician and help with the delivery. If asked by the client later why she needed to be put to sleep, the nurse can (1) tell the truth, (2) refer her to the obstetrician, (3) express sympathy that she could not be awake, or (4) say nothing. *Outcome:* The client's wishes are disregarded; delivery occurs in record time and the obstetrician is happy; the nurse fulfills obligation to physician and hospital but feels she has betrayed the client's trust. *Long-term outcome:* There is a good probability the same problem will happen again.

Or

(continued)

Client Care Study Using a Five-Step Process for Resolving the Ethical Problem *(continued)*

The nurse can remind the obstetrician that the client was adamant about wanting to be awake and suggest that a different anesthesiologist be called in. If the obstetrician agrees, the client may get her wish and everyone is satisfied with the outcome (the nurse must still decide how to prevent recurrence of this dilemma). If the obstetrician refuses and insists that the client be put to sleep, the nurse can (1) refuse to participate (if another nurse is unavailable or unwilling to replace her, the nurse has abandoned the client and harm may ensue); or (2) participate and proceed as above or resolve to speak to the obstetrician in a "cool moment" after the delivery to see how to avoid this problem in the future. If the nurse does not get satisfaction with the obstetrician, then she must decide whether to move through the proper administrative channels. Depending on the institution and people involved, the nurse may be affirmed or censored for this move. *Long-term outcome:* Future clients may be helped by the nurse following through with her concerns.

Or

The nurse can say nothing and assist with this delivery, believing it to be the wisest course of action for the time being, but resolve to take the steps above to correct the perceived injustice. *Outcome:* There is no benefit for the present client but potential benefit to future clients.

b. Think the Ethical Problem Through

See if conventional principles of professional ethics address and resolve the problem; if not, see if broader ethical principles and theories clarify and resolve the problem. Rely on those principles you judge most important and of which you feel most sure.

Basic moral principles: The good of clients (beneficence) should be the nurse's primary concern; this strongly suggests that the nurse should act, but it does not address the nurse's obligation to do so if she feels it would jeopardize her own good (job security).

Respect for persons would suggest that the client's autonomy (right to self-determination) should be respected unless there is strong justification for not doing so.

Justice would suggest that whether a client pays the obstetrician privately should have no bearing on the quality of care received.

Care-based ethics would obligate Jean to serve as an effective advocate for her client, respecting the nurse's commitment to be faithful to the nurse–patient relationship.

c. Make a Decision

Choose a course of action that best reflects your considered judgment; consultation with an institutional ethics committee or other staff may be helpful.

Jean W. feels from past interactions with this obstetrician that her speaking up will not influence his decision to have the client put to sleep. She decides to speak with the obstetrician after the delivery and follow up with whatever approach is necessary to avoid recurrence.

Steps 4–5: Implement and Evaluate Your Decision

Act and compare the actual outcome with what you considered and hoped for in advance. How can you improve the decision process next time?

Jean W. will never know if speaking up would have resulted in the client's wishes being respected. Although she is dissatisfied with the outcome of this case, she hopes to prevent this from happening to other clinic clients in the future. In this instance, a hospital committee was formed to study the problem and make recommendations. If Jean W. had been told to "mind her own business" unless she wanted trouble, she would have to make a decision weighing client benefit on one hand with potential personal risk or harm on the other.

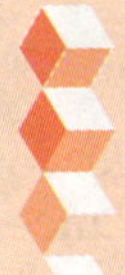

Helpscan

The following are ethical resources for healthcare professionals:

- American Nurses Association Center for Ethics and Human Rights
  600 Maryland Avenue, SW
  Suite 100 West
  Washington, DC 20024-2571
  (202) 651-7055

  Publishes the *Ethics and Human Rights Communique,* which provides an ongoing vehicle of communication for nurses facing ethical and human rights dilemmas in practice. *Communique* informs readers about important upcoming events and resources of interest such as bibliographies, surveys, grants, ANA conferences, ethical continuing education offerings and new ANA publications.

- National Reference Center for Bioethics Literature
  Kennedy Institute of Ethics
  Georgetown University
  Washington, DC 20057
  800-MED-ETHX

  A specialized collection of library resources concerned with contemporary biomedical issues in the fields of ethics, philosophy, medicine, nursing, science, law, religion, and the social sciences. Call for bioethics information; BIOETHICSLINE searches (computerized data base); search strategies; reference help; publication orders.

- The Hastings Center
  255 Elm Road
  Briarcliff Manor, NY 10510
  914-762-8500

  A nonprofit, nonpartisan organization that carries out educational and research programs on ethical issues in medicine, the life sciences, and the professions. Publishes *The Hastings Center Report.*

Nurses and Physicians

Nurse–physician situations can also result in ethical distress for nurses. Common problems include disagreements about the proposed medical regimen, conflicts regarding the scope of the nurse's role, and physician incompetence.

Disagreements About the Proposed Medical Regimen. In the nursing home where you work, any client who loses a significant amount of weight (more than 10% of usual body weight) is automatically subjected to an exhaustive battery of tests (including a complete gastrointestinal [GI] series) to determine whether there are any physical causes for the weight loss (eg, tumor). You strongly object to one client being put through these tests because she has made it clear that she wants to die and will starve herself to death if that is the only way she can do it. The medical director insists that the client undergo the diagnostic studies because there is a long history of client family dissatisfaction with the medical care. The director wants to avoid causing further dissatisfaction. Are you responsible for preparing the client for these diagnostic studies and scheduling them? Are there grounds for refusing to participate?

Conflicts Regarding the Scope of the Nurse's Role. A young woman needing surgery that will result in a permanent colostomy tells the nurse how afraid she is and how much she dreads getting used to "the thing." The nurse is certain this client would benefit greatly from the help of the young staff enterostomal therapist (ET), who also has a colostomy. However, when this suggestion is mentioned to the surgeon, the surgeon tells the nurse that he does his own teaching and counseling for all his clients and does not "believe" in ETs. He points out that the nurse's duty here is to carry out his orders. Does it fall within the scope of nursing to recommend the ET to the woman? Is the nurse morally obligated to make this recommendation to the client?

Physician Incompetence. A nurse who works in the operating room notices that a pediatric surgeon who has been on the staff for several years and done excellent work seems all of a sudden not to be concentrating during surgery and to be making more mistakes than usual. Rumors have been circulating about a problem with cocaine abuse following the surgeon's divorce. The parents of one pediatric client dissatisfied with the progress the client is making ask the nurse for an opinion about the surgeon. Should the nurse voice personal concerns? Is the nurse morally obligated to report the physician to the proper hospital authority for investigation?

Nurses and Other Nurses

Some of the most difficult ethical problems nurses encounter result from nurse–nurse interactions and may be complicated by obligations of friendship. Problems include claims of loyalty and nurse incompetence.

Claims of Loyalty. A nurse working the 11 PM to 7 AM shift tells the other nurse on the unit, "I just made rounds and everyone is OK. Please cover for me while I catch an hour of sleep. I had an awful day." She neglects to tell the nurse who is covering that it was mentioned in report that one client needed special monitoring. This client dies unexpectedly while the nurse sleeps. When she wakes up and discovers the death, she begs the other nurse, her friend, never to tell anyone she was sleeping. "The client could have died anyway between my rounds."

Nurse Incompetence. When you make your morning rounds, a client tells you that one of the nurses fondled her body and made suggestive remarks during the previous night shift. You suspect that the client may simply be trying to cause trouble and because you like the nurse in question, find it hard to believe the client. What should you do?

Nurses and Institutional and Public Policy

As nurses assume increased responsibility for decision making at all levels of care, the institutional and public policy arenas offer unique dilemmas. Two current examples are short-staffing and healthcare rationing.

Short-Staffing. Restructuring has resulted in chronic understaffing on the unit where you work. You believe that clients are now at risk because there simply are not enough nurses to provide quality care. Some nurses are talking about forming a union and going on strike. Because yours is the only major hospital in a rural area, you are unsure if striking is a morally legitimate option. What do you do?

Healthcare Rationing. In the United States, as many as 42 million people are uninsured or underinsured and have limited access to healthcare. Whether each person has a "right" (is entitled to) basic healthcare continues to be the subject of debate. There are plans for rationing healthcare that could limit the options available to the elderly, the poor, the terminally ill, and to those in society whom many view as having limited "social value." What moral obligation do you have to contribute to this debate? How might you ensure that your voice and the nursing viewpoint are heard?

Nurses' Personal Moral Convictions and Practice Demands

Assisted Suicide. You are the nurse case manager for a woman with a history of breast cancer whose cancer recurred (metastasis to the spine) after she was cancer free for 7 years. She frequently tells you when you come to visit her at home that she is unwilling to fight anymore and wants to die with some dignity while she is still in control. She begs you to get her something that will "put her gently to sleep once and for all before her pain gets worse." You believe that this is her sincere wish, not depression speaking, and honestly believe that she would be better off spared the last stage of her illness. Your religious beliefs, however, tell you that assisted suicide is wrong under any circumstances. How do you reconcile your desire to help this woman with your religious conviction that what she is asking for is intrinsically evil?

Nurses and Ethics Committees

An increasing number of healthcare institutions have developed ethics committees whose chief functions include education, policy making, case review, and consultation. These committees are uniquely equipped to deal with the complexities of modern healthcare because they are multidisciplinary and provide a forum where radically divergent views can be aired without fear of repercussion. Nurses bring an important voice to the ethics committee. When cases are being reviewed, nurses can help to ensure that the technical facts are understood, that the appropriate decision makers have been identified, that the client's medical and overall best interests have been identified, and that the course of action selected from the alternatives is justified by sound ethical principles. The nurse's strong background in interpersonal communications has the potential to contribute unique knowledge of the client and family to the discussion and to facilitate the ethics committee's group dynamics.

Nurses also play an important role in policy making. They are frequently able to identify what policies are needed to address recurring ethical concerns and to suggest needed modifications of existing policies.

Key Points

- Knowing whether to perform a nursing action ("should I?") is often as important as knowing how to perform the action.
- A value is a belief about worth that acts as a standard to guide behavior. Values influence beliefs about human needs, health and illness, the practice of health behaviors, and human responses to health and illness.
- Values are formed over a lifetime from information a person receives from the environment and from the family and culture. Common modes of value transmission are modeling, moralizing, laissez-faire, rewarding and punishing, and responsible choice.
- The American Association of Colleges of Nursing identified altruism, aesthetics, equality, freedom, human dignity, justice, and truth as essential values for the practicing nurse.

- Although it is important for nurses to respect the value orientations of others, not all values are equal. Nurses may find themselves morally obligated to respond to client values likely to cause harm to the client or others.
- Values clarification is a process by which people come to understand their own values and value system. The process of valuing is centered on choosing, prizing, and acting.
- Ethics offers the nurse a means to look at and evaluate alternative courses of right action using basic moral concepts and principles. It reduces the likelihood that nursing actions to resolve ethical problems will be based solely on intuition, opinions, and self-interest.
- Theories of ethics offer moral guides to action and to character. Nursing ethics is a distinct subset of bioethics. Nurse ethicists frequently use two popular theoretical and practical approaches to ethics, the principle-based approach and the care-based approach.
- Nurse advocates who are sensitive to the need to promote both client autonomy (self-determination) and client well-being may experience ethical conflict, but are more likely than other nurses to be successful in securing the client's genuine best interests.
- The nursing codes of ethics (ICN, ANA, CNA) provide a framework for making ethical decisions and set forth professional expectations. They inform both nurses and society of the profession's primary goals and values. Codes are effective only when upheld by members of the profession.
- Ethical problems faced by nurses include moral dilemmas and moral distress.
- One of several processes for resolving ethical problems in nursing is the following five-step process: (1) assess the situation (gather data); (2) diagnose (identify) the ethical problem; (3) plan: identify options and explore the probable consequences of each, use ethical reasoning to decide upon a course of action which you can justify; (4) implement your decision; and (5) evaluate your decision.
- Nurses often serve on institutional ethics committees whose chief functions include education, policy formation, case review, and consultation.

Bibliography

Aiken, T. D., & Catalano, J. T. (1994). *Legal, ethical, and political issues in nursing.* Philadelphia: Davis.

American Association of Colleges of Nursing. (1986). *Essentials of college and university education for professional nursing.* Washington, DC: AACN.

American Nurses Association. (1985). *Code for nurses with interpretive statements.* Kansas City, MO: ANA.

American Nurses Association. (1988). *Ethics in nursing: Position statements and guidelines.* Kansas City, MO: ANA.

American Nurses Association. (1991). *Standards of clinical nursing practice.* Washington, DC: ANA.

Beauchamp, T. L., & Childress, J. F. (1994). *Principles of biomedical ethics* (4th ed.). New York: Oxford University Press.

Benjamin, M., & Curtis, J. (1992). *Ethics in nursing* (3rd ed.). New York: Oxford University Press.

Bishop, A. H., & Scudder, J. R. (1990). *The practical, moral, and personal sense of nursing.* Albany: State University of New York Press.

Canadian Nurses Association. (1991). *Code of ethics for nursing.* Ottawa, Ontario: CNA.

Council on Ethical and Judicial Affairs, American Medical Association. (1993). Caring for the poor. *JAMA, 269*(19), 2533–2537.

Donley, R. (1993). Ethics in the age of health care reform. *Nursing Economics, 11*(1), 19–24, 51.

Edwards, B. S. (1993). When the physician won't give up. *American Journal of Nursing, 93*(9), 34–37.

Edwards, B. S. (1994). When the family can't let go. *American Journal of Nursing, 94*(1), 52–56.

Eriksen, J. (1993). Putting ethics into education. *Canadian Nurse, 89*(5), 18–20.

Fry, S. T. (1989). The role of caring in a theory of nursing ethics. *Hypatia, 4*(2), 88–103.

Fry-Revere, S. (1994). Ethics consultations: An update on accountability issues. *Pediatric Nursing, 20*(1), 95–98.

Hughes, T. L., & Smith, L. L. (1994). Is your colleague chemically dependent? *American Journal of Nursing, 94*(9), 31–35.

Husted, G. L., & Husted, J. H. (1991). *Ethical decision making in nursing.* St. Louis: Mosby.

International Council of Nurses. (1973). *ICN code for nurses: Ethical concepts applied to nursing.* Geneva: Imprimeries Populaires.

Jameton, A. (1993). Dilemmas of moral distress: Moral responsibility and nursing practice. *AWHONN's Clinical Issues in Perinatal and Women's Health Nursing, 4*(4), 542–551.

Kirschbaum, H. (1977). *Advanced values clarification.* La Jolla, CA: University Associates.

Noddings, N. (1984). *Caring: A feminine approach to ethics and moral education.* Berkeley, CA: University of California Press.

Oddi, L. F., & Cassidy, V. R. (1990). Participation and perceptions of nurse members in the hospital ethics committee. *Western Journal of Nursing Research, 12*(3), 307–317.

Pence, T., & Cantrall, J. (Eds.). (1990). *Ethics in nursing: An anthology.* New York: National League for Nursing.

Raths, L. E., Simon, S. B., & Harmin, M. (1978). *Values and teaching* (2nd ed.). Columbus: Charles E. Merrill.

Rodney, P., & Starazomski, M. (1993). Constraints on the moral agency of nurses. *Canadian Nurse, 89*(9), 23–26.

Royal College of Nursing of the United Kingdom. (1980). *Guidelines on confidentiality in nursing.* London: Author.

Rozovsky, L. E. (1980). *The Canadian patient's book of rights.* Toronto: Doubleday Canada.

Scanlon, C. (1994). Survey yields significant results. *American Nurses Association Center for Ethics and Human Rights Communique, 3*(3), 1–3.

Silva, M. C. (1984). The American Nurses' Association code for nurses: Purposes, content, and enforceability. *Health Matrix, 2*(2), 55–63.

Simon, S. B. (1972). *Values clarification.* New York: Hart.

Steele, S. M., & Harmon, V. M. (1983). *Values clarification in nursing* (2nd ed.). Norwalk, CT: Appleton-Century-Crofts.

Taylor, C. (1993). Nursing ethics: The role of caring. *AWHONN's Clinical Issues in Perinatal and Women's Health Nursing, 4*(4), 552–560.

Uustal, D. B. (1978). Values clarification in nursing: Application to practice. *American Journal of Nursing, 78*(12), 2058–2063.

Zink, M. R., & Titus, L. (1994). Nursing ethics committees—Where are they? *Nursing Management, 25*(6), 70–76.

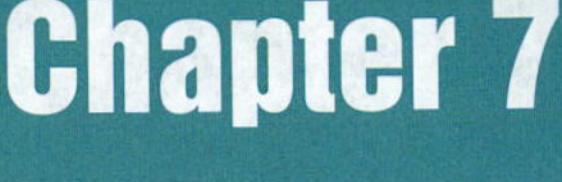

Chapter 7

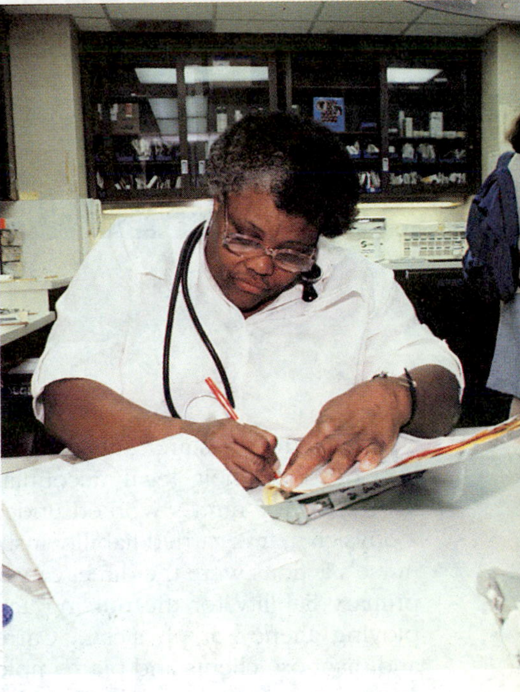

Legal Implications of Nursing

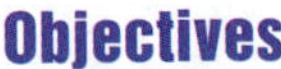

Objectives

After studying this chapter, the learner should be able to:

Define key terms used in the chapter.

Define law and describe its four sources.

Describe the professional and legal regulation of nursing practice.

Identify the purpose of credentialing, using as examples accreditation, licensure or registration, and certification.

Identify grounds for suspending or revoking a license or registration.

Differentiate intentional torts (assault and battery, defamation, invasion of privacy, false imprisonment, fraud) and unintentional torts (negligence).

Evaluate personal areas of potential liability in nursing.

Describe the legal procedure once a plaintiff files a complaint against a nurse for negligence.

Describe the roles of the nurse as defendant, fact witness, and expert witness.

Use appropriate legal safeguards in nursing practice.

Explain the purpose of incident reports.

Describe laws affecting nursing practice.

Key Terms

accreditation
assault
battery
certification
common law
credentialing
crime
defamation of character
expert witness
fact witness
felony
fraud
liability
litigation
malpractice
misdemeanor
negligence
plaintiff
statutory law
tort

As the roles and duties of nurses expand, so too does their legal accountability. In the past, many nurses worked under the supervision of a physician, few carried liability insurance, and even if a nurse's actions were the direct cause of harm to a client, primary liability for the nursing action fell on the employing agency or physician. Currently, nurses assess and diagnose clients and plan, implement, and evaluate nursing care independently. Full legal responsibility and accountability for these nursing actions rest with the nurse. A steadily increasing number of nurses are being named as litigants in negligence cases and being brought to court to defend their practice.

While many nurses continue to work in traditional settings like hospitals and nursing homes, more nurses are working in nontraditional community settings such as home care agencies, clinics, day-care centers, and nurse-managed health centers. Advanced practice nurses may have independent practices. It has never been more crucial for nurses to document their actions carefully and take part in other malpractice prevention practices. Nurses who wish to avoid legal conflicts must develop trusting nurse–client relationships (satisfied clients rarely sue); practice within the scope of their competence; and identify potential liabilities in their practice and develop prevention strategies.

Legal Concepts

Definition of Law

A *law* is a standard or rule of conduct established and enforced by the government of a society. Laws are intended chiefly to protect the rights of the public. *Public law* is a law in which the government is directly involved. It regulates the relationships between individuals and the government. An important body of public law describes the powers of the government in authority. Private law, also called *civil law*, regulates the relationships among people. Civil law includes laws relating to contracts, ownership of property, and the practice of nursing, medicine, pharmacy, and dentistry.

Sources of Laws

Four sources of law exist at both the federal and state (provincial) level—constitutions, statutes, administrative law, and common law.

Constitutions. Federal and state constitutions indicate how their governments are created and given authority and state the principles and provisions for establishing specific laws. Although they contain relatively few laws (called constitutional laws), they serve as guides to legislative bodies.

Statutes. A **statutory law** is enacted by a legislative body. In the United States, statutory laws must be in keeping with the federal constitution and with the constitution of the state as well. Nurse practice acts are an example of statutory laws.

Administrative Law. Executive officers (eg, the President of the United States or Prime Minister of Canada, state governors or provincial premiers, or city mayors) administer various agencies that, among other functions, are responsible for law enforcement. These agencies have power to make administrative rules and regulations, in conformity with enacted law, which act as laws and are enforceable. Boards of nursing are administrative agencies at the state level. Rules and regulations they adopt are administrative laws. One example of a municipal administrative agency is a city's board of health.

Common Law. The government provides for a judiciary system, which is responsible for reconciling controversies. It interprets legislation at the local, state (province), and national levels as it has been applied in specific instances and makes decisions concerning law enforcement. A body of law known as **common law** has evolved from these accumulated judiciary decisions. Common law is thus court-made law. Most law in the area of malpractice is court-made law. The exception is in the province of Quebec, where a civil law system is in effect.

Common law is based on the principle of *stare decisis,* or "let the decision stand." After a decision has been made in a court of law, that decision becomes the rule to follow when other cases involving similar circumstances and facts arise. The case that first sets down the rule by decision is called a *precedent.* Court decisions can be changed but only when strong justification exists. Common law helps prevent one set of rules from being used to judge one person and another set to judge another person in similar circumstances.

Litigation

A lawsuit is a legal action in a court. **Litigation** is the process of a lawsuit. The person or government bringing suit against another is called the **plaintiff**. The one being accused of a crime or tort (defined later) is called the *defendant.* The defendant is presumed innocent until proved guilty of a crime or tort.

The two levels of courts in the United States are (1) trial court and (2) appellate court. The trial court, the first-level court, hears all the evidence in a case and makes decisions on facts, usually through a jury. The appellate court only hears cases questioning a point of law decided by the trial court. No witnesses testify at the appellate court level. The opinions of appellate judges are published and become common law.

Professional and Legal Regulation of Nursing Practice

Nurses who engage in the safe practice of their profession respect both the voluntary and legal controls that map the boundaries of nursing practice. Both these controls are designed to provide quality healthcare and to protect society from unsafe nursing practice (Fig. 7-1).

Voluntary standards, developed and implemented by the nursing profession itself, are not mandatory but are used as guidelines for peer review. Professional nursing organizations continually reassess the functions, standards, and qualifications of their members. The organizations are guided by their own assessment of soci-

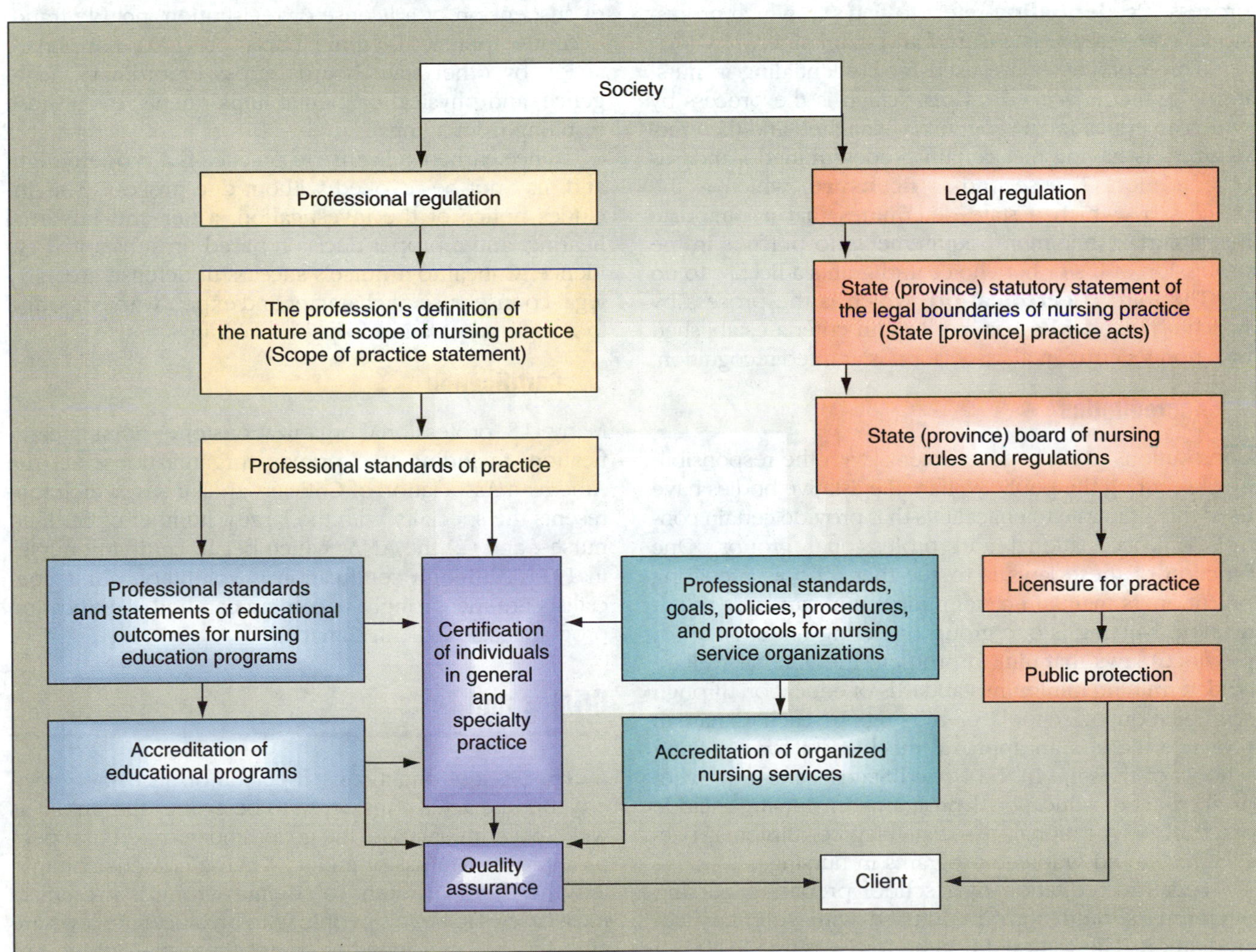

Figure 7-1
Diagram of proposed professional and legal regulation of nursing practice showing the separation of and parallels between professional and legal regulatory processes. (American Nurses' Association. [1987]. *The scope of nursing practice.* Kansas City, MO: ANA, p. 5.)

ety's need for nursing and by the public's expectations of nursing. Examples of voluntary standards include the American Nurses Association (ANA) and Canadian Nurses Association (CNA) standards of practice (see Chapter 1), professional standards for the accreditation of education programs and service organizations, and standards for the certification of individual nurses in general and specialty areas of practice.

Legal standards are developed by legislative action and are implemented by authority granted by the state (or province) to determine minimum standards for the education of nurses, to set requirements for licensure or registration, and to decide when a nurse's license may be suspended or revoked. Examples of legal standards include state and province nurse practice acts and rules and regulations of nursing.

Credentialing

Nursing has taken several steps to ensure the competence of its practitioners, including the credentialing process. **Credentialing** refers to ways in which professional competence is ensured and maintained.

Three processes are used for credentialing in nursing. The first is **accreditation**, which is the process by which an educational program is evaluated and then recognized as having met certain predetermined standards of education. The second is **licensure**, which is the process by which a state determines that a candidate meets certain minimum requirements to practice in the profession of his or her choice and grants a license to do so. The third is **certification**, which is the process by which a person who has met certain criteria established by a nongovernmental association is granted recognition.

Accreditation

Constitutions provide governments with the responsibility of securing the public welfare. Legislative bodies have used this principle to enact laws that provide certain controls on occupational and professional groups. One function of these laws is to see that schools preparing practitioners maintain certain minimum standards of education. Nursing is one group operating under state (or province) laws that aim to promote the general welfare by determining minimum standards of education through accreditation of schools of nursing. In each Canadian province there is an approval mechanism for certifying schools of nursing. In the United States, state-approved, or accredited, educational programs in nursing include practical or vocational, associate degree, diploma, baccalaureate, and graduate programs in nursing.

Legal accreditation of a school preparing nursing personnel should not be confused with voluntary accreditation. The National League for Nursing (NLN) is a voluntary agency that accredits schools when they meet certain criteria established by NLN. Most schools choose to seek this voluntary accreditation, and many prospective students prefer selecting a school that has been accredited by NLN. Accreditation by NLN of educational programs to prepare nurses is not a legal requirement for a school to exist. State accreditation is a legal requirement.

Licensure and Registration

Licensure is a specialized form of credentialing that has a legal basis in laws passed by a legislative body. A *license* is a legal document that permits a person to offer to the public skills and knowledge in a particular jurisdiction, where such practice would otherwise be unlawful without a license. Licensure and registration are mandatory in Canada. Both must be renewed periodically. Licensure and registration are discussed in Chapter 1.

Licensure or Registration Revocation. The State Board of Nurse Examiners in the United States (or the registering body in Canada) may revoke or suspend a nurse's license or registration for drug or alcohol abuse (currently the most frequent reason). Other reasons for revocation or suspension of a license or registration include fraud, deceptive practices, criminal acts, previous disciplinary action by other state boards, gross or ordinary negligence, and physical or mental impairments, even those resulting from aging.

Once earned, a license to practice is a property right and may not be revoked without due process. This includes notice of the investigation, a fair and impartial hearing, and a proper decision based on substantial evidence. Critical to a nurse's successful defense are early legal counsel, use of character and expert witnesses, and thorough preparation for all proceedings.

Certification

Many U.S. professional organizations offer nursing certification, including two primary organizations: (1) the American Association of Critical-Care Nurses, which represents the specialty with the largest number of certified nurses, and (2) the ANA, which began certifying nurses in 1974. Although certification is voluntary, nurse specialists are increasingly becoming certified. Certification programs also exist in Canada.

Crimes and Torts

A **crime** is a wrong against a person or his or her property, but the act is considered to be against the public as well. In a criminal case, the government, called "the people," prosecutes the offender. When a crime is committed, the factor of intent to commit wrong is present in most cases. However, people who break certain laws are guilty of a crime, whether or not there was intent. For example, failure to observe the Federal Food, Drug, and Cosmetic Act may constitute a crime.

In most cases, criminal law is statutory law and only infrequently common law. Crimes are classified as felonies or misdemeanors. A **misdemeanor** is a less serious crime than a felony. Misdemeanors are commonly punishable with fines or with imprisonment for less than 1 year, or with both, or with parole. A **felony** is punishable by imprisonment in a state or federal penitentiary for more than 1 year.

A **tort** is also a wrong committed by a person against another person or his or her property. Torts generally result in civil trials. In most instances, the court in a civil case will settle damages with money but rarely by imprisonment. Torts may be intentional or unintentional acts of wrongdoing. Some of the intentional torts for which nurses may be held liable include assault and battery, defamation of character, invasion of privacy, false imprisonment, and fraud. A person committing an intentional tort is considered to have knowledge of the permitted legal limits of his or her words or acts. Violating these limits is grounds for prosecution. Unintentional torts are referred to as **negligence**.

An act generally considered a tort may, because of its severity, be classified as a crime. For example, gross negligence that demonstrates the offender is guilty of complete disregard for another's life may be tried as both a civil and criminal action. It is then prosecuted under criminal as well as civil law. By its very nature, a wrong tried as a crime implies a more serious offense with more legal implications than a tort.

Intentional Torts

Assault and Battery

Assault is a threat or an attempt to make bodily contact with another person without that person's consent. **Battery** is an assault that is carried out and includes every willful, angry, and violent or negligent touching of another person's body or clothes or anything attached to or held by that other person. Forcibly removing a client's clothing, administering an injection after the client has refused it, and shoving a client into a chair are all examples of battery. When a nurse needs to defend himself or herself or others from an assaultive client, only those actions necessary for self-protection or the aid of another are permitted.

Every individual has the right to be free from invasion of his or her person, and the adult client who is alert and oriented has the right to refuse any aspect of treatment. The fact that treatment is desirable does not allow the nurse or physician to proceed without the consent of the client or to go beyond the limits to which the person has consented.

Informed Consent. Every person is granted freedom from bodily contact by another person unless consent has been granted. In all healthcare agencies an informed and voluntary consent is needed upon admission (for routine treatment); for each specialized diagnostic procedure or medical or surgical treatment; and for experimentation involving clients. The consent must be written, be signed by the client or person legally responsible for the client, and be for the procedure performed. A signed consent is not needed in an emergency if there is an immediate threat to life or health, experts agree that it is an emergency, and the client is unable to consent and the legally authorized person cannot be reached. Although some value informed consent as a protection against lawsuits, the central values underlying informed consent include the promotion of a client's well-being and respect for the client's self-determination (President's Commission for the Study of Ethical Problems in Medicine and Biomedical and Behavioral Research, 1982). Elements of informed consent include disclosure, comprehension, competence, and voluntariness (see the accompanying box).

Obtaining an informed consent is the responsibility of the person who will execute the diagnostic or treatment procedure or conduct the research study. The nurse's role is to confirm that a signed consent is in the client's chart and to respond to any questions the client has about the consent. In some instances, the nurse may be responsible for having the client sign the consent form after the physician has explained to the client the procedure, its risks and benefits, and alternative treatments. The documentation of the consent process through the use of a printed consent form should not be confused with the actual explanation given to the client and the informed consent itself. When documenting consent, the nurse should assess if the client understands what he or she is signing and report to the physician any problems. Having clients describe in their own words what they understand they are consenting to is the best means to assess adequacy of understanding. Nurses often find themselves in a position in which they question the client's understanding of the proposed procedure and its risks or the client's ability to voluntarily consent to the procedure. Impediments include effects of anxiety, pain, medication, depression, and temporary or permanent states of disorientation and confusion. Unless a nurse is actually obtaining consent for a nurse-prescribed and initiated intervention, the nurse signs the consent form as a witness to having seen the client sign the form, not to having obtained the consent (Fig. 7-2).

Consequences of not obtaining a valid consent include charges of battery against the nurse, doctor, and healthcare agency (the agency has a duty to protect clients and is responsible for its employees' actions). A client's refusal to sign a consent should be documented, and the client should be informed of the possible consequences of the refusal. The client should sign a release form indicating his or her refusal to consent and releasing the nurse, physician, and agency from responsibility for outcomes of this act. This statement should be witnessed.

Defamation

Defamation of character is an intentional tort in which one party makes derogatory remarks about another, di-

Checklist to Ensure Informed Consent

Disclosure

1. Patient has been informed of current medical status and course of treatment.
2. Patient has been informed of the risks and benefits of various treatment alternatives.
3. Patient has been told that no outcomes can be guaranteed.
4. Patient has been given a professional opinion as to the best alternative.

Comprehension

5. The nurse has been innovative in transmitting information to aid understanding.
6. Interior impediments to comprehension (eg, anxiety, pain, and medication) have been assessed.
7. Exterior impediments to comprehension (eg, transcultural barriers, terminology, and speed of presentation) have been assessed.

Competence

8. The nurse has assessed competence in terms of the abilities of the client, considering age, education, and emotional stability.
9. The nurse has assessed the requirements of the task.
10. The nurse has assessed the possible deleterious effects of the client's decision.
11. The client possesses a set of values and goals that make possible reasonably consistent choices.
12. The client is able to communicate and understand the information presented.
13. The client has the ability to reason and deliberate.

Voluntariness

14. The nurse had determined that the client has not been forced to consent.
15. The nurse has been careful to avoid coercive influences by herself/himself or others.
16. The nurse has been careful to avoid subtle manipulation of the client by herself/himself or others.

(Taylor, C., & Hobaugh, R. [1986]. *Dimensions in Critical Care Nursing, 5*[2], 98–105.)

minishing the other party's reputation. *Slander* is an untruthful oral statement about a person that subjects that person to ridicule or contempt. *Libel* is written defamation. Defamation of character is grounds for an award of civil damages. Damages are awarded on the basis of the degree of harm done to the plaintiff. Nurses who make false statements about their clients or coworkers run the risk of being sued for slander or libel. A person charged with slander or libel may not be liable if it can be proved that the statement was made not to injure another but for a nonmalicious, justifiable purpose (eg, proof of consent, truth, privilege, or fair comment).

Invasion of Privacy

The U.S. Supreme Court has interpreted the right against invasion of privacy as inherent in the federal constitution. It holds that the Fourth Amendment protects citizens by giving them the right of privacy and the right to be left alone. Disclosure of confidential information whenever a client's problem is inappropriately discussed with a third party may be construed as invasion of privacy and may subject the nurse to liability. The nurse's intimate knowledge of the client increases legal risk in this regard.

No uniformity exists in Canadian laws dealing with the right to privacy, although two provinces have statutory laws that protect the right to privacy (Storch, 1982).

Certain acts by nurses could constitute invasion of privacy, as the following examples illustrate:

- Unnecessary exposure of clients while moving them through health-agency corridors or while caring for them in rooms they share with others
- Talking with clients in rooms that are not soundproof
- Discussing information concerning clients with people not entitled to the information (eg, with the client's employer or the press)
- Pressing the client for information not necessary for care planning
- Interacting with the client's family in ways not authorized by the client
- Using tape recorders, dictating machines, computer banks, and the like without taking precautions to ensure the client's confidentiality
- Preparing written or oral class assignments about clients without concealing their identity
- Carrying out research without taking proper precautions to ensure the anonymity of clients

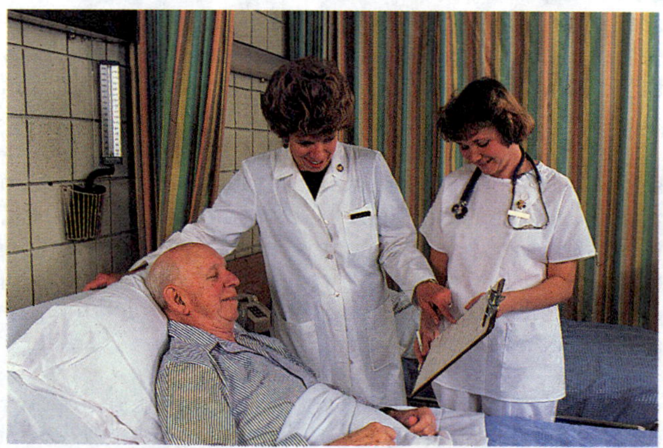

Figure 7-2
Elements of informed consent include disclosure, comprehension, competence, and voluntariness. The documentation of the consent process through the use of a printed consent form does not substitute for the actual explanation given to the client and the informed consent itself. (Photo © B. Proud.)

At times an individual's right to privacy may conflict with other rights such as the public's right to information. When in doubt about disclosing confidential information, the nurse should consult the nursing supervisor, ethics committee, or public relations department of the institution.

False Imprisonment

Unjustified retention or prevention of the movement of another person without proper consent can constitute false imprisonment. For example, only a reasonable amount of restraint should be used in circumstances that warrant it. The indiscriminate and thoughtless use of restraints on a client can constitute the act of false imprisonment.

A person cannot be legally forced to remain in a health agency, such as a hospital, if he or she is of sound mind, even when health practitioners believe the person should remain for additional care. Health agencies have special forms to use when a client insists on being discharged against medical orders. The person's signature indicates that the agency cannot be held responsible for any harm that may result from the client's leaving. People who are mentally ill may be committed to a psychiatric institution for treatment without their consent (involuntary commitment) only when it can be proved that they are harmful to themselves or others.

Fraud

Fraud is willful and purposeful misrepresentation that could cause, or has caused, loss or harm to a person or property. Misrepresentation of a product is a common fraudulent act. In nursing, people fraudulently misrepresenting themselves to obtain a license to practice may be prosecuted under nurse practice acts. Also, misrepresenting the outcome of a procedure or treatment may constitute fraud.

Unintentional Torts

Negligence and Malpractice

Negligence is defined as performing an act that a reasonably prudent person under similar circumstances would not do, or conversely, failing to perform an act that a reasonably prudent person under similar circumstances would do. As the definition implies, an act of negligence may be an act of omission or commission. **Malpractice** is the term generally used to describe negligence of professional personnel.

Elements of Liability. **Liability** consists of four elements that must be established to prove that malpractice or negligence has occurred—duty, breach of duty, causation, and damages. *Duty* refers to an obligation to use due care (what a reasonably prudent nurse would do) and is defined by the standard of care appropriate for the nurse–client relationship. *Breach of duty* is the failure to meet the standard of care. *Causation*, the most difficult element of liability to prove, links the failure to meet the standard of care (breach) to actually causing the injury. *Damages* are the actual harm or injury resulting to the client. Examples of these four elements are presented in Table 7-1.

Computer Applications in Nursing

Privacy and Confidentiality of Healthcare Records

The American Nurses Association Code for Nurses (1950) states, "The nurse safeguards the client's right to privacy by judiciously protecting information of a confidential manner." It addresses the client's right to privacy, protection of information, and access to records.

Security measures that a nurse can be aware of, particularly when using computerized healthcare records, include the following:

- Authorized users of an automated information system should have individual passwords and identification codes that are changed frequently.
- Terminals, including those at the point of care, should have key locks as an additional measure to prevent unauthorized access to data.
- The computer system should "time out" when not in use for a specific period of time. The authorized user would need to re-enter the password and identification code to regain access.
- Temporary employees, such as traveling nurses, should have temporary passwords assigned.
- Employees who leave the organization should have their passwords and IDs terminated.
- The system should be able to track which users viewed, deleted, or updated client information.
- Some information, such as results of AIDS testing, should not be stored on a computer.
- Computer printouts must be discarded appropriately as they may contain sensitive data about a client.
- Your organization should have a policy regarding the use of client data in research. Client identifiers should be removed before the data are analyzed.
- Every nurse must be aware of the laws and statutes that protect the confidentiality of medical records. Most states have guidelines on the sharing of medical information. Your State Board of Nursing may revoke your license for serious breaches of client confidentiality.

Protecting the privacy and confidentiality of healthcare records is the duty of every nurse (McMullen & Philipsen, 1996).

Table 7-1
Examples of Elements of Liability

Element	Example
Duty	Hospital staff nurses are responsible for • Accurate assessment of clients assigned to their care • Alerting responsible health care professionals to changes in a client's condition • Competent execution of safety measures for clients
Breach of duty	• Failure to note and report that an elderly client assessed as alert on admission is exhibiting periods of confusion • Failure to execute and document use of appropriate safety measures (eg, upper and lower bedside rails, use of restraints if necessary, assisted ambulation)
Causation	• Failure to use appropriate safety measures; this failure causes the client to fall while attempting to get out of bed, resulting in a fractured left hip
Damages	• Fractured left hip, pain and suffering, lengthened hospital stay, and need for rehabilitation

Standards of Care. To determine negligence, a standard of care is devised by deciding what a reasonably prudent person would or would not have done under similar circumstances.

Each nurse is responsible for following the standards of care for his or her particular area of practice. For example, the labor and delivery nurse must understand how standards for nursing practice differ from those for medical obstetric practice (nurse practice act); be familiar with specific standards for obstetric nursing (eg, Standards of the Nurses' Association of the American College of Obstetricians and Gynecologists); and execute the nursing responsibilities detailed in the hospital's policies and procedures and in the job description. If hospital policy dictates an assessment of each woman in the early stages of labor every 30 minutes, the nurse must adhere to this standard unless he or she documents a reason for doing otherwise.

Table 7-2 lists areas of potential liability associated with each of the ANA standards of clinical nursing practice. Although any nurse can make an error, nursing errors can result in serious outcomes for the client, as is illustrated in the table.

Malpractice Litigation

When a client believes that he or she has been injured through the negligence of a nurse or other healthcare professional and pursues legal action, one of three outcomes usually ensues:

- All parties concerned work toward a fair settlement.
- The case is presented to a malpractice arbitration panel (in the United States).
- The case is brought to trial court.

The steps involved in malpractice litigation, in which the case is brought to the trial court, are shown in Figure 7-3. The nurse may be involved in legal proceedings as a defendant, a fact witness, or an expert witness.

Nurse as Defendant. When a nurse is named a defendant, it is important to work closely with an attorney while preparing the defense. The attorney representing the nurse's interests will be secured either by the nurse (if carrying personal liability insurance) or by the employing agency. Recommendations for the nurse defendant include the following:

- Do not discuss the case with anyone at your agency (in the United States, the nurse may discuss the case with the risk manager).
- Do not discuss the case with the plaintiff.
- Do not discuss the case with the plaintiff's lawyer.
- Do not discuss the case with anyone testifying for the plaintiff.
- Do not discuss the case with reporters.
- Do not alter the client's records. Tampering with a chart is the worst mistake you can make—you may well ruin your defense.
- Do not hide any information from your lawyer.
- Do not go to the witness stand unprepared.
- Do not be discourteous on the witness stand.
- Do not volunteer any information. (Mandell, 1986)

Nurse as Fact Witness. A nurse who has knowledge of the actual incident prompting the legal case may be called on by either attorney to testify as a **fact witness**. It is critical that fact witnesses, who are placed under oath, base their testimony only on first-hand knowledge of the incident and not on assumptions. The nurse will be asked if the testimony is based on independent recollection of the incident or on documentation in the client record. The nurse may testify, "I do not remember Ms. Jones but I see from review of her record that I cared for her on the evenings of June 10, 13, 14, and 17." When in doubt about the facts of the incident, the nurse should simply testify, "I do not remember that." New research into memory is showing that people often remember things differently from the way they were and challenges the value of the eyewitness memory. Thus, accurate documentation remains the nurse's best defense.

Nurse as Expert Witness. The role of a nurse called on by either attorney to testify as an **expert witness** is to explain to the judge and jury what happened based on the client's record and to offer an opinion whether the nursing care met acceptable standards. Nurse expert witnesses need a solid educational background and strong clinical experience comparable with those of the nurse defendant. An understanding of the legal aspects of nursing and malpractice liability and knowledge of the state (or province) nurse practice act and the standard of nursing care where the incident occurred are also necessary.

Table 7-2
Areas of Potential Liability for Nurses

Standards of Care*	Areas of Potential Liability	Examples
Standard I: Assessment		
The nurse collects client health data.	• Incomplete data base obtained (occurs frequently when client is too ill at admission to respond to questions) • Significant omissions or errors in recording data base • Failure to note in the client's plan of care (and to execute) need for more frequent nursing assessments • Failure to recognize and to report significant changes in the client's condition	• Child too weak to be weighed on admission; chart contains no record of client's weight; dosage of postoperative antibiotic therapy (which should be calculated on child's weight) too small to prevent infection; abscess develops • Nurse fails to detect and report observable signs that an older client is at risk of abuse in her home from her granddaughter • Previously alert client was exhibiting periods of confusion; found beating roommate with a hairbrush • Mother's labor is failing to progress, nurses unaware of signs of fetal distress; obstetrician not informed; irreversible cerebral damage to fetus • Healthy client making slower than usual postanesthesia recovery; signs of developing cerebrovascular accident (slurred speech, difficulty moving extremities, falling to one side) present and unnoted
Standard II: Diagnosis		
The nurse analyzes the assessment data in determining diagnoses.	• Failure to identify priority nursing diagnosis critical to the client's care • Nursing diagnosis incorrectly developed and "labels" the client negatively	• Nowhere in the resident's plan of care was it noted that the client had a history of choking on food ("impaired swallowing") and that close supervision was indicated during meals; client aspirated brussel sprout and died • Homosexual male client without AIDS admitted for gallbladder surgery questions the few interactions he has with staff, nursing diagnosis on cardex reads "High Risk for Violence: Directed at Others (AIDS), related to homosexuality"
Standard III: Outcome Identification		
The nurse identifies expected outcomes individualized to the client.	• No indication in nursing care plan that nurses were aware of and sensitive to the client's health care priorities	• Obese client with a history of impaired circulation continually refuses to ambulate after major abdominal surgery; client dies following a massive pulmonary embolism; plan of care showed no concern or attempt to compensate for client's lack of mobility; family states no nurse consulted them to encourage mobility
Standard IV: Planning		
The nurse develops a plan of care that prescribes interventions to attain expected outcomes.		
Standard V: Implementation		
The nurse implements the interventions identified in the plan of care.	• Client's record contains no documentation of attempts to teach appropriate self-care measures to client and family • Nursing interventions deviate from usual standard of care (understaffing, indifference on part of nurse, inexperience of nurse, faulty or scarce equipment or resources)	• Male client discharged from short-procedure unit on crutches; falls first day home, refracturing leg; alleges his not receiving instructions for crutch-walking caused fall; client record contains no documentation of client education • Skin breakdown on frail, older homebound client worsens with eventual muscle deterioration; sepsis; nurses seem confused about treatment regimen for pressure ulcers; treatment is inconsistent

(continued)

Table 7-2 *(continued)*
Areas of Potential Liability for Nurses

Standards of Care*	Areas of Potential Liability	Examples
Standard VI: Evaluation		
The nurse evaluates the client's progress toward attainment of outcomes.	• No evidence in plan of care and nursing notes that nurses evaluated whether the client achieved target goals • Client discharged before key goals are met and without follow-up instruction	• Male client newly started on insulin therapy discharged without understanding the relationship among food, exercise, and insulin and after giving himself the insulin only once—no referral made to visiting nurse; client readmitted after 2 weeks with dangerously low blood sugar following overdose with insulin

*From American Nurses Association. (1991). *Standards of clinical nursing practice.* Kansas City, MO: ANA.

Legal Safeguards for the Nurse

Contracts

A *contract* may be defined as the exchange of promises between two parties. The law of contracts provides a remedy for a breach of contract so that the person who suffers from a broken contract may be compensated for any resulting loss. For a contract to be legally enforceable, it must contain real consent of the parties, a valid consideration, a lawful purpose, competent parties, and the form required by law (Creighton, 1986, p. 35).

Practicing nurses enter into legally valid and binding contracts with both their employers and their clients. It is thus important that they understand and are able to fulfill the terms of their agreement before giving consent.

Competent Practice

Competent practice remains the nurse's most important and best legal safeguard (Fig. 7-4). Each nurse is responsible for making sure that educational background and clinical experience are adequate to fulfill the nursing responsibilities described in the job description. Legal safeguards include the following:

- Respecting legal boundaries of practice
- Following institutional procedures and policies
- "Owning" personal strengths and weaknesses; seeking means of growth, education, supervised experience, and discussions with colleagues
- Evaluating proposed assignments; refusing to accept responsibilities for which the nurse is unprepared
- Keeping current
- Respecting client rights and developing rapport with clients
- Keeping careful documentation
- Working within the agency to develop and support management policies

Competent practice includes developing sensitivity to common sources of client injury, such as falls, use of restraints, and malfunctioning equipment, and then taking specific measures to prevent client injury. The accompanying box lists the most frequent allegations against nurses and related prevention tips.

Client Education

U.S. courts affirm the client's right to know and view client education as the legal duty of the nurse. Standards for client education are derived from national professional standards and from state nurse practice acts in the United States and provincial nurse practice acts in Canada, as well as the local standards described in agency policies, procedure manuals, and job descriptions. Special forms for documenting the nurse's assessment of the client's learning needs and for subsequent teaching are available at some agencies. Failure to conduct or document the assessment of learning needs and teaching may later be construed as negligence.

General guidelines for the nurse wishing to execute client education responsibilities competently include the following:

- Determine in your practice setting what specific aspects of client education are the responsibility of nursing. Consult your job description and be familiar with agency policies regarding client education and its documentation.
- Remember that an important aim of nursing is to assist clients in managing their own care. Discuss the nursing plan of care with the client and family and identify their learning needs and learning readiness. Document the teaching plan as part of the nursing plan of care. Document all nursing efforts to educate the client and family about healthcare management and also document the client's response. If a client refuses health education or refers the nurse to a family member (eg, "Talk to my wife about my pills, she'll be giving them to me at home"), document this on the client's record. If client education greatly increases the client's anxiety and the client requests not to be given any more information, the nurse should doc-

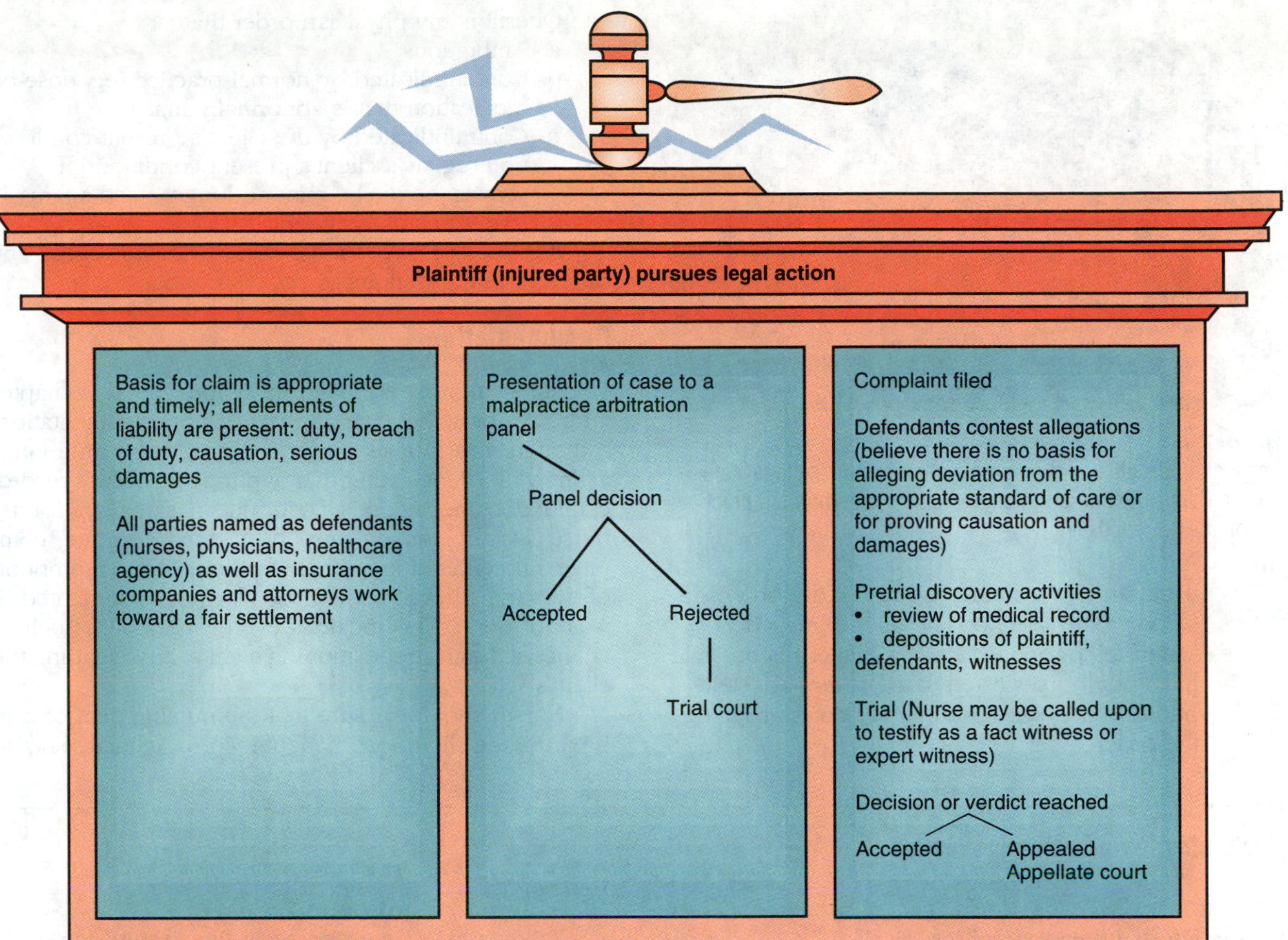

Figure 7-3
Civil legal procedure in malpractice litigation.

ument the client's initial response to teaching, the client's request that it be stopped, and, if the nurse complied, the reason for doing so.

- Because lack of time is a frequently offered reason for failing to document client education, nurses should assess what type of client documentation is routinely offered. If possible, they should develop forms or checklists that will facilitate rapid documentation. For example, preoperative checklists have greatly facilitated the recording of preoperative teaching and are often introduced as evidence in court that preoperative teaching was done. Other successful models include forms for documenting diabetic teaching, teaching after a myocardial infarction, and teaching postpartal and baby care to mothers. The teaching role of the nurse is discussed in Chapter 23.

Executing Physician Orders

Nurses are legally responsible for carrying out the orders of the physician in charge of a client unless an order is one that would lead a reasonable person to anticipate injury if it were carried out. Guidelines when executing orders follow:

1. Be familiar with the parties, designated in your nurse practice act, who can legally write orders for the nurse to execute (in many states, a physician's assistant cannot legally write orders for the nurse).
2. Be familiar with your institutional/agency policy regarding physician orders.
3. Attempt to have all physician's orders in writing. Verbal and telephone orders should be countersigned within 24 hours. To eliminate errors caused by telephone orders:
   a. Limit telephone orders to true emergency situations in which there is no alternative.
   b. Designate the nurses who may take telephone orders (those who have more education and experience, such as a primary nurse).
   c. Repeat a telephone order back to the physician.
   d. Document the order, its time and date, the situation necessitating the order, the physician prescribing and reconfirming the order as it is read

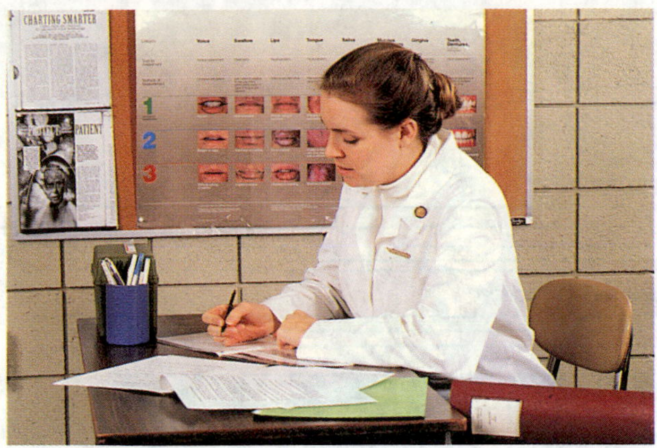

Figure 7-4
Competent practice is the nurse's most important legal safeguard. Careful documentation is the key to competent practice. (Photo © B. Proud.)

back, and your name; indicate if the order is a VO (verbal order) or TO (telephone order).

e. When telephone extensions make this possible, have two nurses listen to a questionable telephone order, with both nurses countersigning the order.

4. Question any physician order that is:
   a. Ambiguous
   b. Contraindicated by normal practice (eg, dose of medication that is abnormally high)
   c. Contraindicated by the client's present condition (eg, as a client's present condition improves, he or she may no longer need aggressive forms of treatment)

It is good practice for the nurse to double check any order a client questions.

Documentation

Documentation is discussed in Chapter 21; this chapter addresses only the legal implications of documentation. Although most nurses prefer to spend their time interacting with clients rather than writing in a client's record, careful documentation is a critical legal safeguard for the nurse. Documentation must be factual, accurate, complete, and entered in a timely fashion. The presumption of the law is that if something was not documented, it was not done. This includes even routine acts such as taking vital signs, repositioning clients, and ensuring the client's safety.

Nurses should be sure that the nursing plan of care is part of the client's permanent record. Agencies should

Nursing Malpractice Prevention

Most Frequent Allegations Against Nurses and Related Prevention Tips

1. **Failure to ensure client safety**
   Monitor clients in a timely manner. Assess and document potential for injury. Incorporate safety needs into plan of care.
   Clearly define criteria for use of restrictive devices. Ensure that the use of restrictive devices is consistent with agency policy. Use the least restrictive devices which will be effective in preventing injury.
   Update knowledge on client safety and new interventions to prevent and reduce injury.
   Evaluate whether or not clients at high risk for injury are routinely being identified before injury results.
2. **Improper treatment or performance of treatment**
   Question treatments you believe are improper. Know your agency's policy for questioning a problematic order.
   Use proper techniques when performing procedures and follow agency procedures.
   Seek assistance when unsure of a new procedure. Never perform an intervention until you know what you are doing, why you are doing it, and your ongoing assessment and teaching responsibilities.
   Update your clinical skills through continuing education classes, conferences, and workshops.
3. **Failure to monitor and report**
   Follow physician orders regarding monitoring of clients unless changes in the client's condition necessitate a change in the frequency of monitoring; report need for change to the physician.
   Report any requested information or significant changes in a client's condition. If unsure of the significance of an observed change, consult with an experienced colleague.
   Perform appropriate and timely nursing assessments.
   Ensure that the nurse–client ratio is adequate.
4. **Medication errors and reactions**
   Verify any questionable medical orders.
   Verify client's name before administering medication.
   Listen to client's objections regarding medication and investigate client concerns *before* administering the medication.
   Refer to a drug reference for any questions on appropriate dosages, side effects, and reactions.
   Know your agency's policies on verbal and written medication orders and on medication administration.
   Update your knowledge of medications and new medication administration protocols.

(continued)

Nursing Malpractice Prevention *(continued)*

5. **Failure to follow agency procedure**
   Know your agency's procedures. Ensure that your orientation to new responsibilities familiarizes you with pertinent policies and procedures.
   If you must deviate from a procedure, discuss the incident with your supervisor and decide on appropriate action.
   Advise the appropriate person of procedures that need to be revised.
6. **Documentation**
   Document significant information about your clients objectively and factually.
   Know and follow the agency's documentation policies.
   Be time specific about the information, such as when you performed actions, made observations, or performed client assessments.
   Document legibly when writing, spell correctly, and use only agency-approved abbreviations.
   Be sensitive to privacy considerations when documenting on a computer.
   Routinely evaluate the quality of documentation and update your knowledge of new documentation methodologies.
7. **Equipment use**
   Learn how to operate equipment in a safe and appropriate manner. *Never* operate equipment with which you are unfamiliar.
   Use predetermined procedures when teaching clients how to use equipment and ensure that all the nurses involved in client education are teaching the same procedures.
   Provide home care clients with the telephone number of a 24-hour backup hospital or home care service available in case of emergency.
   Have clients demonstrate their competence with equipment before allowing them to use it.
   Attend orientations and in-services on the use of new or modified equipment.
8. **Adverse incidents**
   When adverse incidents occur, complete the appropriate documentation and report the incident to the designated individual following agency policy.
   Do not assume, voice, or record any blame for the incident.
   Know the institutional chain of command for reporting instances where client care is at issue.
   Support agency loss prevention programs that identify potential liabilities, guard against client injuries, and maximize the defense of the agency and its employee nurses.
9. **Clients with HIV**
   Be conscious of actions that could result in a lawsuit:
   Discrimination in treatment
   Nosocomial (in hospital) transmission of virus
   Breach of confidentiality
   Participation in testing a client for HIV without first obtaining informed consent.
   Know and follow agency policies and procedures for the care of clients with infectious diseases.
   Update your knowledge of HIV infection; be familiar with national standards (such as those established by the Centers for Disease Control) and pertinent state/province laws.

Adapted in part from *American Nurse,* June 1989, p. 28.

have flow sheets or some type of documentation form that enables nurses to check off routine aspects of care rapidly and completely. The nurse should write a comprehensive nursing note for each client problem the nurse addressed during his or her time of duty. The note should include the current nature of the problem, how the nurse intervened, the client's response, and, when appropriate, future priorities for care. Once a problem is noted, nursing documentation should evidence continuity of care until the problem is resolved.

A common problem reported by nurses is not knowing how to document an incident, for example, when the nurse believes the client needs medical attention and intervention but the responsible physicians are not responding to calls for assistance. In this case, the best legal safeguard for the nurse is to document the facts of the incident, being careful not to make incriminatory statements such as, "Anyone could see we were losing this client rapidly" or "Once again, Dr. Jones was unavailable when her client needed her." The note should document the time the physician was called, the time of response or lack of response, and the subsequent nursing response (eg, nursing supervisor notified). Such a note documents that the nurse is carefully assessing the client, recognizing significant cues, and reporting them appropriately. The nursing supervisor should write the next note after reviewing the case and choosing a course of action. Client noncompliance with the therapeutic regimen should also be documented along with the nurse's attempts to increase compliance.

Adequate Staffing

Understaffing is a problem that results in reduced quality of nursing care and may jeopardize client safety. Temporary management solutions to understaffing, such as floating nurses from one unit to another or asking nurses to work overtime or double (back-to-back) shifts, are ineffective because they further jeopardize client safety. A nurse in an understaffed agency will be held to a professional standard of judgment with respect to accepting responsibility for work and for delegating nursing responsibilities to others. If client injury results, the agency and nurse employee will most likely be named as codefendants.

Professional Liability Insurance

Although a nurse's best legal safeguard is always competent practice, the increasing number of malpractice claims naming nurses as defendants make it wise for nurses to carry their own liability insurance. Nurses may obtain this insurance through ANA, through provincial nursing associations in Canada, and through other sources.

Reasons ANA (1990) lists for purchasing a personal professional liability insurance policy are as follows:

Protection of the nurse's best interests: If the nurse is named defendant in a malpractice action along with the agency, a conflict of interest could arise between the nurse and the agency. Nurses have no assurance of their best interest being represented unless they have their own coverage, which provides their own attorney.

Limitations of employer's coverage: Most healthcare facilities carry "claims made" insurance, which means if the nurse is no longer working there or the facility closes, the nurse is not covered when a claim is filed.

Care or advice given outside of work: An employer's policy only covers the nurse within the confines of the work setting.

Risk Management Programs

In the hope of reducing malpractice claims, many healthcare agencies have initiated risk management programs designed to identify, analyze, and treat risks. Elements of a comprehensive risk management program include:

Safety program: The aim is to provide a safe environment in which the basic safety needs of clients, employees, and visitors are met.

Products safety program: The aim is to ensure safe and adequate equipment; this involves ongoing equipment evaluation and maintenance.

Quality assurance program: The aim is to provide quality healthcare to clients; this involves ongoing evaluation of all systems used in the care of the client.

Nurses with legal questions will often find risk managers a helpful resource.

Incident, Variance, or Occurrence Reports

An incident report, also termed variance or occurrence report, is a tool used by healthcare agencies to document the occurrence of anything out of the ordinary that results in or has the potential to result in harm to a client, employee, or visitor. These reports are used for quality improvement and should not be used for disciplinary action against staff members. They are a means of identifying risks. More harm than good results from ignoring mistakes. Incident reports improve the management and treatment of clients by identifying high-risk patterns and initiating in-service programs to prevent future problems. These forms also make all the facts about an incident available to the agency in case of litigation.

The nurse responsible for a potentially or actually harmful incident or who witnesses an injury is the one who fills in the incident form. This form should contain the complete name of the person or people involved and the names of all witnesses; a complete factual account of the incident; the date, time, and place of the incident; pertinent characteristics of the person or people involved (eg, alert, ambulatory, asleep) and of any equipment or resources being used; and any other variables believed to be important to the incident. A physician completes the incident form with documentation of the medical examination when there has been actual or potential injury to a client, employee, or visitor.

In some states, the incident report may be used in court as evidence. The nurse documenting a client incident should include a complete account of what happened in the client's record; additionally, the nurse should prepare the incident report. However, documentation on the client record should not include the fact that an incident report was filed. In Canada, incident reports are on file in the institution.

Good Samaritan Laws

Good Samaritan laws are designed to protect health practitioners when they give aid to people in emergency situations. For example, a physician at the scene of an automobile accident may give emergency care without fear of legal suit if such care appears necessary, unless care is given in a grossly negligent manner.

Forty-eight states and the District of Columbia have Good Samaritan laws, although the laws vary considerably. Nurses are covered in some states but not in others. Good Samaritan legislation exists in four Canadian provinces and covers both physicians and nurses. So far, there appears to be no common law resulting from decisions based on these statutes.

No person has a legal obligation to help another, and a health practitioner, as any other person, may choose to help or to leave the scene of an emergency. However, in many situations, there would appear to be an ethical responsibility to assist. When health practitioners assist a person in an emergency situation and consent for the care is impossible, they are expected to use good judgment in determining whether an emergency exists and to give care that a reasonably prudent person with a similar background and in a similar circumstance would give.

Student Liability

Student nurses are responsible for their own acts of negligence if these result in client injury. Moreover, they are held to the same standard of care that would be used to evaluate the actions of a registered nurse. Legal responsibilities of student nurses include careful preparation for each new clinical experience and a duty to notify their clinical instructor if they feel in any way unprepared to execute a nursing procedure. For no reason should a student attempt a clinical procedure if unsure of the correct steps involved in its application. The student nurse is responsible for being familiar with agency policies and procedures.

A hospital may also be held liable for the negligence of a student nurse enrolled in a hospital-controlled program because the student is considered an employee of the hospital. The status of students enrolled in college and university programs is less clear, as is the liability of the educational institution in which they are enrolled and the healthcare agency offering a site for clinical practice.

Nursing instructors may share a student's responsibility for damages in the event of client injury if the student's assignment called for clinical skills beyond the student's competency or the instructor failed to provide reasonable and prudent clinical supervision. Because the status of clients can change rapidly, especially in an acute-care setting, students should notify their instructor or a staff member of any significant changes in the client's condition, even if they are unsure of the meaning of these changes.

Most nursing programs require students to carry personal professional liability insurance. School policies provide coverage only for clinical nursing done for educational purposes. Moreover, student nurses who work as nursing assistants or in some other healthcare role are legally permitted to offer only the services contained in their job description. Even if they feel confident with medication administration, catheter insertion, and other professional nursing acts, they risk disciplinary action when they perform these procedures outside the supervised clinical practice setting.

Laws Affecting Nursing Practice

Occupational Safety and Health

The Occupational Safety and Health Act of 1970, commonly known as OSHA, set legal standards in the United States in an effort to ensure safe and healthful working conditions for men and women. The act, which is intended to reduce work-related injuries and illnesses, has affected healthcare agencies and has increased certain responsibilities for many nurses. In December 1991, OSHA published a rule establishing safety standards for workers who may be exposed to bloodborne pathogens in the course of their employment. Occupational health and safety acts are provincial statutes in Canada. The following examples illustrate situations that could violate standards, if care is not taken, because of the potential threat to worker safety:

- Use of electrical equipment
- Use of isolation techniques for clients with infectious diseases and the management of contaminated equipment and supplies
- Use of radiation, such as infrared or ultraviolet radiation; sound or radio waves; and laser beams
- Use of chemicals, such as those that are toxic or flammable

The law, which continues to be updated, is specific concerning its applications, and fines can be severe when infractions are noted. Nurses can assist in implementing this law by promoting health and safety precautions wherever they work. Nurses employed in industrial settings have a particularly important role in conforming to the law's requirements. The United States Labor Department created a new Office of Occupational Health Nursing at the Occupational Safety and Health Administration to underscore the major role such nurses play in striving for safe and healthful workplaces.

National Practitioner Data Bank

The Health Care Quality Improvement Act of 1986 was enacted to encourage healthcare practitioners to identify and discipline practitioners who engage in unprofessional conduct and restrict the ability of incompetent practitioners to move from state to state without disclosure of the practitioner's previous performance. When a state licenses, certifies, or registers practitioners they become subject to the National Practitioner Data Bank requirements. The Act contains two major provisions: (1) immunity from civil damages for peer review and (2) establishment of the National Practitioner Data Bank as an information clearinghouse. Nurses may be reported to the National Practitioner Data Bank for medical malpractice payments, adverse licensure actions, or adverse professional actions.

Reporting Obligations

The unique nature of nurse–client interactions frequently results in the nurse's having knowledge (eg, of child abuse, rape, or a communicable disease) that a state (or province) requires to be reported. Legislation varies in this regard, and the nurse is responsible for knowing what needs to be reported in the local area and to what authority.

Controlled Substances

Both the United States and Canada have special laws governing the distribution and use of controlled substances (drugs with abuse potential), such as narcotics, depressants, stimulants, and hallucinogens. Drug abuse laws are specific and violations are considered criminal acts. Nursing responsibilities for controlled substances include their storage in special locked compartments and documentation responsibilities.

Discrimination and Sexual Harassment

Title VII of the Civil Rights Act of 1964 protects employees from discrimination based on race, color, religion, sex, or national origin, and provides that pregnant women receive the same protection as other employees and applications. The Equal Employment Opportunity Commission (EEOC), which enforces Title VII, defines sexual harassment as "unwelcome sexual advances, requests for sexual favors, and other verbal or physical conduct of a sexual nature" occurring in the following circumstances:

- Submission to sexual advances is implicitly or explicitly considered a condition of employment.
- Submission to sexual advances is used as a basis for employment decisions.
- Sexual harassment interferes with job performance even if it only creates an intimidating, offensive, or hostile atmosphere. (EEOC, 1980, sections 3950.10-3950.11)

Persons With Disabilities

Observing that there are at least 43 million Americans with physical or mental disabilities and that discrimination against such individuals persists in such critical areas as employment, housing, public accommodations, education, transportation, communication, and health services, Congress passed the Americans With Disabilities Act of 1990. The Act provides a very broad definition of "disability"; it covers any individual who has a physical or mental impairment that substantially limits one or more major life activities or who has a record of such impairment. In addition to covering persons who have impairments that have traditionally been perceived as disabilities, the Act also specifically protects persons who have communicable diseases such as AIDS or HIV, persons who are recovering from drug or alcohol addiction, and persons who are regarded as being disabled, whether or not they are in fact disabled. The Act imposes two requirements on businesses covered by the Act. First, it prohibits such entities from discriminating against disabled persons. Second, it requires covered entities to "reasonably accommodate" individuals who are protected by the Act.

Wills

State and provincial laws regulate requirements for a will. The person who makes a will is called the *testator*. A will describes intentions a testator wishes carried out upon his or her death. A person who receives money or property from a will is called a *beneficiary*. Nurses are occasionally asked to witness a testator's signing of his or her will and should be familiar with the following guidelines.

- The witness should feel sure that the testator is of sound mind, that is, the testator knows what he or she is doing and is free of the influence of drugs that could likely distort his or her thinking.
- The witness should feel sure that the testator is acting voluntarily and is not being coerced in any way concerning the terms of his or her will.
- Witnesses should watch the testator sign his or her will and they should sign in the presence of each other. State law indicates how many witnesses must acknowledge the testator's signature on a will. Two or three witnesses are most commonly required.
- Witnesses to the signature on a will do not need to read it, but they should be sure that the document being signed is a will and not some other type of document.
- In most states, a person who is a beneficiary in a will is disqualified to act as a witness to the testator's signature.

Legal Issues Related to Dying and Death

Legal responsibilities for the dying or deceased client are discussed in Chapter 33. Topics addressed include advance directives, do-not-resuscitate orders, assisted suicide, direct voluntary euthanasia, organ donation, autopsy, and inquest.

Key Points

- As the roles and duties of the nurse have expanded, so too has the legal accountability of the nurse.
- Laws are standards or rules of conduct established and enforced by the government of a society to protect the rights of the public. Laws may be constitutional, statutory, administrative, or common.
- Voluntary standards regulating nursing practice are developed and implemented by the nursing profession itself. These standards include the ANA and CNA standards of practice, professional standards for the accreditation of education and service programs, and certification standards.
- Legal standards are mandatory and are developed by legislative action controlling professional conduct. They include the nurse practice acts and rules and regulations of nursing.

- Credentialing is the process of ensuring and maintaining professional competence. Credentialing involves accreditation, licensure or registration, and certification.
- A nurse whose license is suspended or revoked because the nurse engaged in drug and alcohol abuse or other acts of unprofessional conduct is entitled to due process of law.
- Intentional torts for which the nurse may be liable include assault and battery, defamation of character, invasion of privacy, false imprisonment, and fraud.
- Every individual has the right to be free from invasion of person, and thus consent is needed for all diagnostic, treatment, or research procedures. The person performing the procedure is responsible for obtaining informed consent. Documenting the informed consent may be delegated to nursing.
- Negligence is defined as performing an act that a reasonably prudent person under similar circumstances would not do or as failing to perform an act.
- Legal safeguards for the nurse include understanding and fulfilling the terms of contracts with employers and employees, competent practice, thorough client education, safe execution of physician orders, careful documentation, professional liability insurance, and participation in risk management programs.
- The client's record should never be tampered with in an attempt to prepare a better defense.
- Competent practice includes respecting legal boundaries of nursing, following institutional procedures and policies, owning personal strengths and being aware of weaknesses, evaluating proposed assignments, keeping current, respecting client rights and developing rapport with clients, providing careful documentation, and working with nursing management to develop and implement programs to improve quality care and decrease risks of client injury.
- Student nurses are legally responsible for their own acts of negligence resulting in client injury. They are held to the same standard of care that would be used to evaluate the actions of an RN.
- Nurses need to be knowledgeable about specific laws affecting nursing practice. These include laws regulating occupational health and safety, the National Practitioner Data Bank, reporting obligations, controlled substances, discrimination/sexual harassment, persons with disabilities, wills, and legislation related to dying and death.

Bibliography

Aiken, T. D., & Catalano, J. T. (1994). *Legal, ethical and political issues in nursing*. Philadelphia: Davis.

American Nurses Association. (1990). *Liability prevention and you: What nurses and employers need to know*. Washington, DC: ANA.

American Nurses Association. (1994). *Guidelines on reporting incompetent, unethical or illegal practices*. Washington, DC: ANA.

Calder, K. (1994). Beyond informed consent. *Canadian Nurse, 90*(11), 23–26.

Calfee, B. E. (1995a). Going before the board: How to prepare yourself. *Nursing, 25*(3), 56–58.

Calfee, B. E. (1995b). Was it really wrongful termination? *Nursing, 25*(4), 65.

Calfee, B. E. (1996). Labor laws: Working to protect you. *Nursing, 26* (2); 34–40.

Creighton, H. (1986). *Law every nurse should know* (5th ed.). Philadelphia: Saunders.

Editors of *Nursing 94*. (1994). Confronting sexual harassment. *Nursing, 24*(10), 4850.

Fickeissen, J. L. (1990). 56 ways to get certified. *American Journal of Nursing, 90*(3), 50–57.

Fiesta, J. (1988). *Law and liability for nurses* (2nd ed.). Albany: Delmar Publishers.

Grant, A. (1994). Instructor, students and the law. *Canadian Nurse, 90*(10), 53.

Lammer, M. (1994). Nurses alert! Nurses and the Good Samaritan act. *Concern, 23*(2), 8–9.

Mandell, M. (1986). Ten legal commandments for nurses who get sued. *Nursing Life, 6*(3), 18–21.

McMullen, P. C., & Philipsen, N. C. (1996). Confidentiality: Computer security and data protection. In B. R. Heller, M. E. Mills, & C. A. Romano (Eds.). *Information management in nursing and health care*. Springhouse, PA: Springhouse.

Moore, G. M. (1993). Surviving a malpractice lawsuit. *Nursing, 23*(10), 55–57.

Need for liability protection keeps growing: An interview with Pat McLean, manager, Canadian Nurses Protective Society. (1992). *RN*, April/May, 8–10.

Phillips, E. (1994). Accountability, responsibility, liability. *Canadian Nurse, 90*(4), 51–52.

President's Commission for the Study of Ethical Problems in Medicine and Biomedical and Behavioral Research. (1982). *Making healthcare decisions: A report* (vol. 1). Washington, DC: U. S. Government Printing Office.

Sorich, M. P. (1994). Nursing malpractice litigation: A personal journey. *MCN, 19*(5), 249–252, 254.

Storch, J. (1982). *Patient's rights: Ethical and legal issues in healthcare and nursing*. Toronto: McGraw-Hill Ryerson.

Taylor, C., & Hobaugh, R. (1986). The role of the critical care nurse in developing informed consent. *Dimensions of Critical Care Nursing, 5*(2), 98–105.

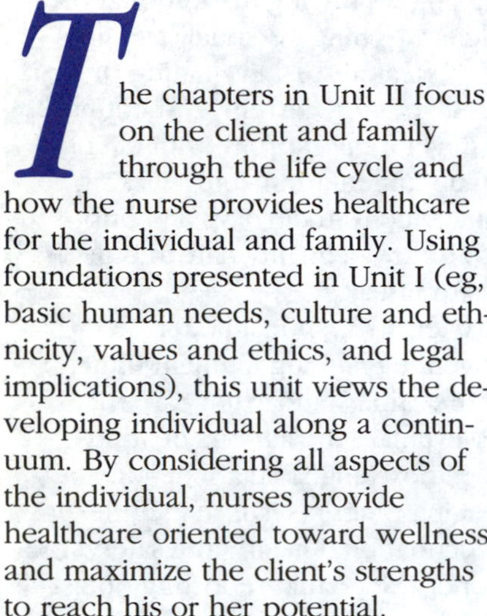

The chapters in Unit II focus on the client and family through the life cycle and how the nurse provides healthcare for the individual and family. Using foundations presented in Unit I (eg, basic human needs, culture and ethnicity, values and ethics, and legal implications), this unit views the developing individual along a continuum. By considering all aspects of the individual, nurses provide healthcare oriented toward wellness and maximize the client's strengths to reach his or her potential.

The unit begins with developmental concepts and principles necessessary to understanding growth and development across the lifespan. A section on developmental theories gives an overview of major theorists and their contributions to the understanding of psychosocial, physical, cognitive, moral, and faith development. The influence of the family on the individual's growth and development are studied. The application of these concepts and theories to effective nursing care is pursued.

The individual is followed through the various phases of development from conception through adolescence. Common health problems of each age group and the role of the nurse for that particular age group are considered.

The adult years are broken down into early, middle, and older adult stages. Again developmental theories are followed as the adult continues in the life cycle. Common health problems and the nurse's role in healthcare for the adult continue through older adulthood. The unit ends with a look at the paradigm of aging and stereotypes common to the older adult. Gerontology and the healthcare system related to this field are discussed.

Promoting Wellness Across the Lifespan

"The concern of nursing is with man in his entirety, his wholeness. Nursing's body of scientific knowledge seeks to describe, explain, and predict about human beings."

Martha Rogers (1914–1994)
a nationally renowned nurse theoretician, author, lecturer, and consultant whose "theory of man" inspired tremendous creativity, research activity, and intellectual growth in the nursing profession

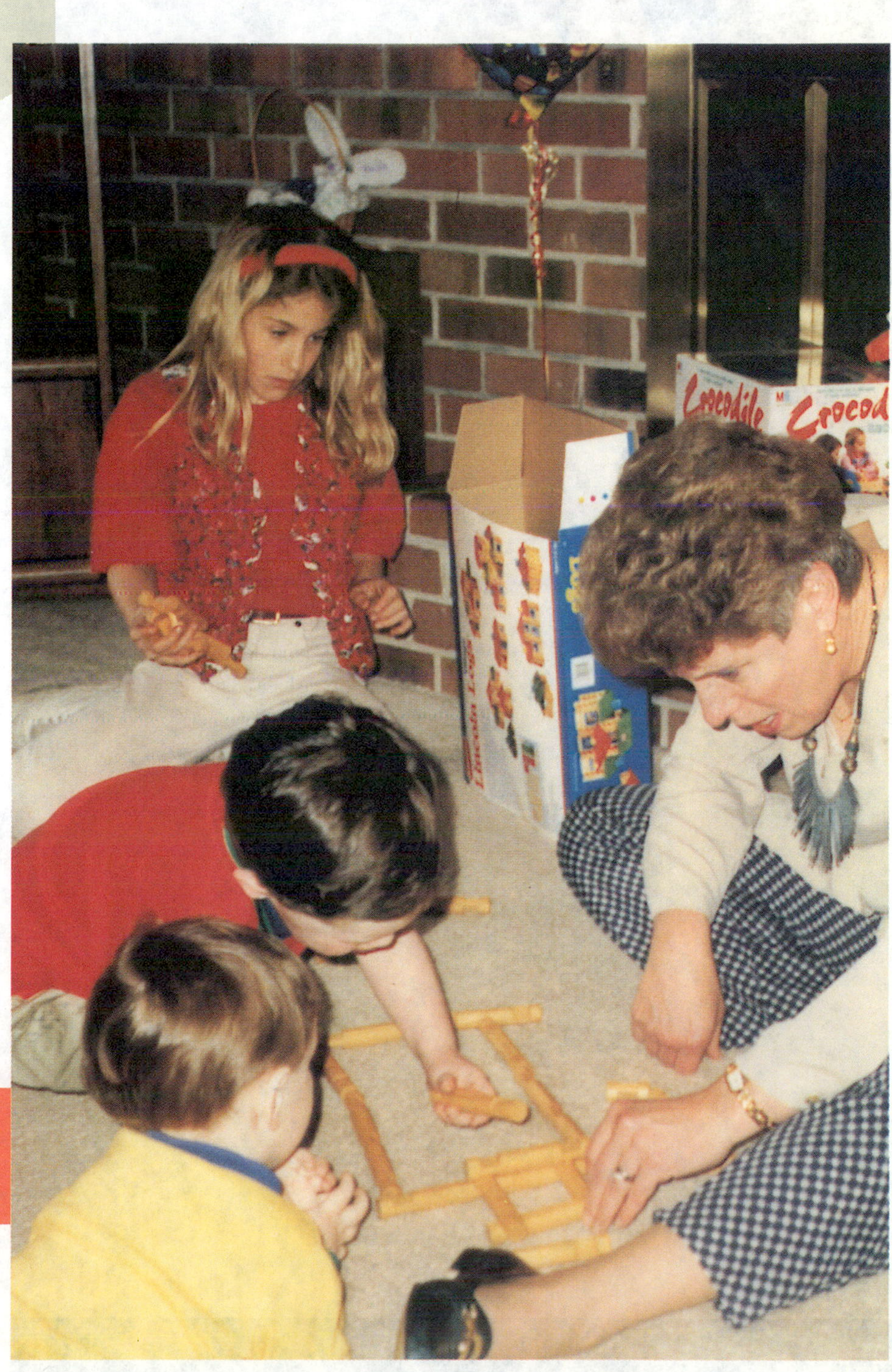

Unit II

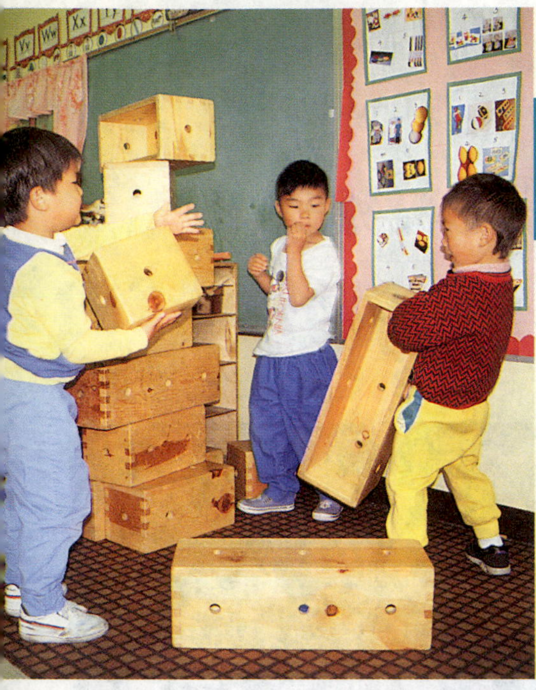

Chapter 8

Developmental Concepts

Objectives

After studying this chapter, the learner should be able to:

Define key terms used in the chapter.

Summarize basic principles of growth and development.

Discuss the theories of Freud, Erikson, Havighurst, Piaget, Kohlberg, Gilligan, and Fowler.

Describe the importance of incorporating theories of growth and development in assessing and planning nursing care for individuals and families.

Describe the role of the family in growth and development.

List implications for nursing practice that uses a knowledge base of growth and development.

Key Terms

accommodation
assimilation
cognitive development
developmental task
faith
growth and development
moral development
psychosocial theory

As caregivers, nurses promote health and wellness for people from birth to death. All people, regardless of age, have unique healthcare needs that result from the physical, emotional, intellectual, social, spiritual, and cultural aspects of their developmental level. To plan and give holistic and individualized care, the nurse must understand typical growth and development characteristics, tasks, and needs for clients of all ages.

Physical development has a predetermined genetic base because of inheritance patterns carried on chromosomes. Thus, the unborn child begins life with specific physical attributes, either properly formed or malformed. Environmental factors from birth through the early years of growth provide initial psychologic and social contact through positive or negative parenting experiences. As environmental influences expand beyond the immediate caregivers or family, psychosocial experiences increase and affect development. Cognitive, moral, and spiritual growth are fostered through contact within families, schools, and communities. Information derived from multiple theories of human and family development assist the nurse in perceiving these interrelated variables at designated stages throughout life.

This chapter presents basic principles of growth and development to serve as a foundation for understanding the human being at various life stages. Major theories examining cognitive, psychosocial, spiritual, and moral development are discussed. In addition to reviewing theories specific to the individual's development, the family and its influence on personal development are briefly discussed.

The Nature of Human Growth and Development

The human processes of **growth and development** are the result of two interrelated factors—heredity and environment. Humans simultaneously grow and develop in physical, cognitive, psychosocial, moral, and spiritual dimensions, with each dimension being an essential part that makes up the whole person. Development is a dynamic and continuous process, characterized by a series of ascents, plateaus, and declines as one proceeds through life. Each phase of development also has a period of disequilibrium, when adjustment to internal and external demands are more difficult, and a period of equilibrium, when adjustment to demands is more easily made (Erikson, 1963; Mussen, Conger, & Kagan, 1974). If adjustments are not made in the appropriate level of development, one may have difficulties during a later stage of life.

Principles of Growth and Development

Although growth and development in each of the dimensions are individualized, certain generalizations can be made about the nature of human development. These generalizations form the principles that serve as guidelines for understanding growth and development. The broad generalizations are as follows:

Growth and development are orderly and sequential as well as continuous and complex. All humans experience the same growth patterns and developmental levels. As these patterns and levels are individualized, a wide variation in biologic and behavioral changes is considered normal. Within each developmental level, certain milestones are identified, for example, the time the infant rolls over, crawls, walks, and begins to say his or her first words.

Growth and development follow regular and predictable trends. Cephalocaudal (proceeding from head to tail) development is the first trend, with the head and brain developing first, followed by the trunk, legs, and feet. Photographs of an infant in utero show the large size of the head compared with the rest of the body (Fig. 8-1). The second trend is proximodistal development, which means that growth progresses from gross motor movements (such as learning to lift one's head) to fine motor movements (such as learning to pick up a toy with the fingers). The last trend is symmetrical development of the body, with both sides of the body developing equally.

Growth and development are both differentiated and integrated. As nerve pathways develop, they become more specialized, allowing the growing child to respond to different stimuli. Throughout the life span, each new learned activity builds on

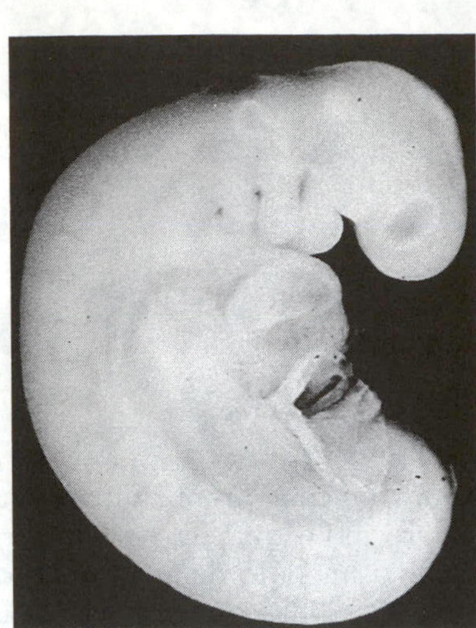
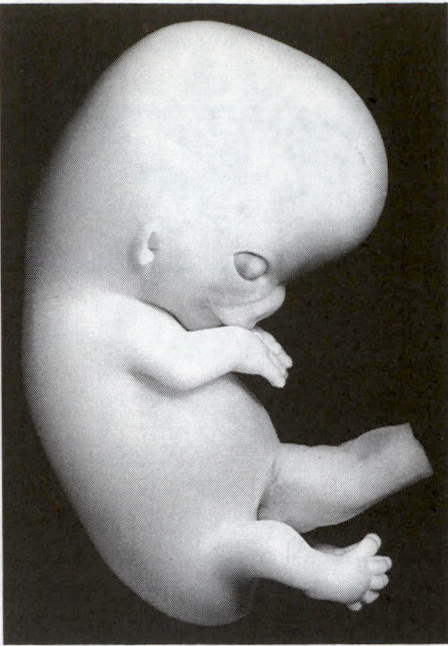
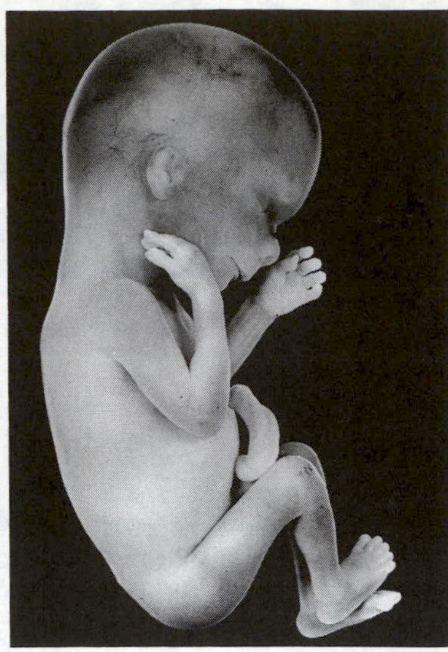

Figure 8-1
Three stages of human development in utero—at about 4, 8, and 16 weeks—showing the development first of the head and then the trunk and limbs. (Courtesy of the Carnegie Institute, Washington, DC.)

previous learning and abilities, so that increasingly complex tasks can be accomplished. For example, the toddler learning to use a spoon combines motor skills, hand–eye coordination, cognitive patterning, and social imitation from watching others to repeat an act when appropriate. As children grow and develop, the task of learning to use a spoon becomes basic, forming the foundation for learning more advanced skills that require manual dexterity.

Different aspects of growth and development occur at different stages and at different rates, and can be modified. For example, muscles and bones both grow most rapidly during the first year of life; during the toddler and preschool years, bone growth slows but muscle fibers increase in size and strength. The most intense period of speech development is between ages 3 and 5 (Fig. 8-2). Sexual maturity begins during the preadolescent years and progresses into the adult years, but is based on gender and sex role identity established from birth. Many factors can modify growth and development, including nutrition, love and affection from caretakers, and illnesses.

The pace of growth and development is specific for each person. Both physical and psychologic skills and maturation vary among people. For example, while learning to walk, a child may concentrate energies on the task and temporarily slow down in language development. Cultural variations also may be seen; Oriental and Asian children tend to be smaller than Caucasian children of the same age. In addition, one's genetic heredity places restrictions on the upper limits that can be achieved in growth and development.

Overview of Developmental Theories

Researchers have studied human development and behavior since the beginning of the 20th century, and have developed classic theories to explain human responses that are expected at certain ages during life. Although a

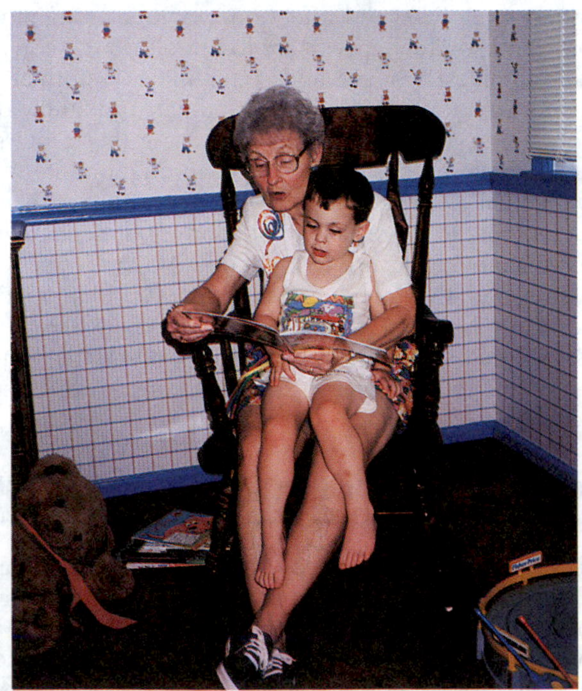

Figure 8-2
Speech development is greatest between the ages of 3 and 5 years; it is fostered by interaction and communication with caregivers.

psychologic approach is common to all developmental theories, each theory focuses on a different influence. The theories discussed in this section examine cognitive, social, and instinctual influences on human growth and development.

Psychoanalytic Theory: Sigmund Freud

Freud's theory (1923) stressed the impact of instinctual human drives on determining behavior. The primary concepts of the theory are the unconscious mind, the id, the ego, the superego, and stages of development based on sexual motivation. Freud identified the underlying stimulus for human behavior as sexuality, which he called libido. Libido was defined as general pleasure-seeking instincts rather than purely genital gratification.

Major Components of Freud's Theory

Unconscious mind: Contains memories, motives, fantasies, and fears that are not accessible to recall but directly affect behavior.

Id: Part of the psyche concerned with self-gratification by the easiest and quickest available means.

Ego: Conscious part of the psyche that serves as a mediator between the desires of the id and the constraints of reality so that one may live effectively within one's social, physical, and psychologic environment. The ego includes one's intelligence, memory, problem solving, separation of reality from fantasy, and incorporation of experiences and learning into future behavior. Development of the ego in the first year of life allows the infant, by 6 months of age, to view self as separate from others and to begin to alter behaviors in response to cues. Ego development continues throughout life.

Superego: Part of the mind that represents one's conscience and develops from the ego during the first year of life as the child learns praise versus punishment for actions. The ego represents the internalization of rules and values so that socially acceptable behavior is practiced.

A further contribution of Freud's theory was the description of defense mechanisms, which are means of unconscious coping when the id's impulses cannot be satisfied so as to reduce stress in the conscious mind. Defense mechanisms are discussed in Chapter 32. In addition, Freud described a series of developmental stages through which all people must pass (Table 8-1).

Freud's Stages of Development

Oral stage (ages 0 to 18 months): The infant's pleasures center around gratification by using the mouth for sucking and satisfying hunger.

Anal stage (ages 8 months to 4 years): This stage begins when neuromuscular control is developed to allow control of the anal sphincter. Toilet training is a crucial issue that requires delayed gratification as the child compromises between enjoyment of bowel function and limits set by social expectations.

Table 8-1
Freud's Stages of Psychosexual Development

Stage	Age	Sexual Activity
Oral	0–18 months	Sucking, swallowing, chewing, biting
Anal	8 months–4 years	Expulsion and retention of waste products
Phallic	3–7 years	Masturbation
Latent	5–12 years	—
Genital (adult sexuality)	12–20 years	Masturbation, sexual intercourse, feelings for others

(Data from Fong, C., & Resnick, R. [1980]. *The child: Development through adolescence.* Menlo Park, CA: Benjamin/Cummings)

Phallic stage (ages 3 to 7 years): The child has increased interest in gender differences, one's own gender, and conflict and resolution of that conflict with the parent of the same sex (named the Oedipus complex in boys and the Electra complex in girls when intimate sexual possessiveness of the opposite-sex parent is shown). Curiosity about the genitals and masturbation increases.

Latency stage (ages 7 to 12 years): This stage marks the transition to the adult sexuality or genital stage during adolescence. Increasing sex role identification with the parent of the same sex prepares for adult roles and relationships.

Genital stage (ages 12 to 20 years): At this stage, sexual interest can be expressed in overt heterosexual relationships. Sexual pressures and conflicts cause turmoil as the adolescent makes adjustments in relationships.

Psychosocial Theory: Erik Erikson

Erikson's (1963) developmental theory was based on work by Freud, but was expanded to include cultural and social influences in addition to biologic processes. **Psychosocial theory** is based on four major organizing concepts: (1) stages of development, (2) developmental goals or tasks, (3) psychosocial crises, and (4) the process of coping (Newman & Newman, 1975). Erikson believed that development is a continuous process made up of distinct phases characterized by the achievement of developmental goals that are affected by the social environment and significant others.

Erikson identified eight stages that progress from birth to old age and death (Table 8-2). Each stage is characterized by a developmental crisis that has to be mastered, with polarities that indicate the possibility of successful or unsuccessful resolution of the crisis. Unsuccessful resolution at any one stage may delay progress through the next stage, but mastery can occur later.

Table 8-2
Erikson's Stages of Psychosocial Development

	Developmental Crisis	Stage
Stage I	Trust vs mistrust	Infancy
Stage II	Autonomy vs shame and doubt	Toddler years
Stage III	Initiative vs guilt	Preschool years
Stage IV	Industry vs inferiority	School-age years
Stage V	Identity vs role confusion	Adolescence
Stage VI	Intimacy vs isolation	Young adulthood
Stage VII	Generativity vs stagnation	Middle adulthood
Stage VIII	Ego integrity vs despair	Later adulthood

Erikson's Stages of Development

Trust versus mistrust—infancy: The infant learns to rely on caregivers to meet basic needs of warmth, food, and comfort so that trust in others is formed. Mistrust is the result of inconsistent, inadequate, or unsafe care (Fig. 8-3).

Autonomy versus shame and doubt—toddler (ages 1 to 3): As motor and language skills develop, the toddler learns from the environment and gains independence through encouragement from parents to feed, dress, and toilet self. If the parents are overprotective or have expectations that are too high, shame and doubt, as well as feelings of inadequacy, may develop in the child.

Initiative versus guilt—preschool (ages 4 to 6): Confidence gained as a toddler allows the preschooler to have initiative in learning, so that new experiences are actively sought out and the how and why of activities are explored. If restrictions or reprimands for seeking new experiences and learning are experienced, guilt results, and the child becomes hesitant to attempt more challenging skills in motor or language development.

Industry versus inferiority—school-age: Focusing on the end result of achievements, the school-age child gains pleasure from finishing projects and receiving recognition for accomplishments (Fig. 8-4.) If the child is not accepted by peers or cannot meet parental expectations, a feeling of inferiority and lack of self-worth may develop.

Identity versus role confusion—adolescence: As many changes occurs in his or her body, the adolescent is in transition from childhood to adulthood. Hormonal changes produce physiologic growth of secondary sex characteristics and mood swings. Trying on roles and even rebellion are considered normal behaviors in acquiring a sense of who one is and what direction one will take in life. Role confusion occurs when the adolescent is unable to establish identity and a sense of direction.

Intimacy versus isolation—young adulthood: The tasks for the young adult are to unite self-identity with identities of friends and to make commitments to others (Fig. 8-5). Fear of such commitments results in isolation and loneliness.

Generativity versus stagnation—middle adulthood: The middle adult years are a time of concern for the next generation as well as involvement with friends and community. There is a desire to make a contribution to the world. If this task is not met, stagnation results, and the person becomes self-absorbed and obsessed with her or his own health needs or regresses to an earlier level of coping.

Ego integrity versus despair—later adulthood: As one enters one's older years, reminiscence of life events provides a sense of fulfillment and purpose. If one believes that one's life has been a series of failures or missed directions, a sense of despair may prevail.

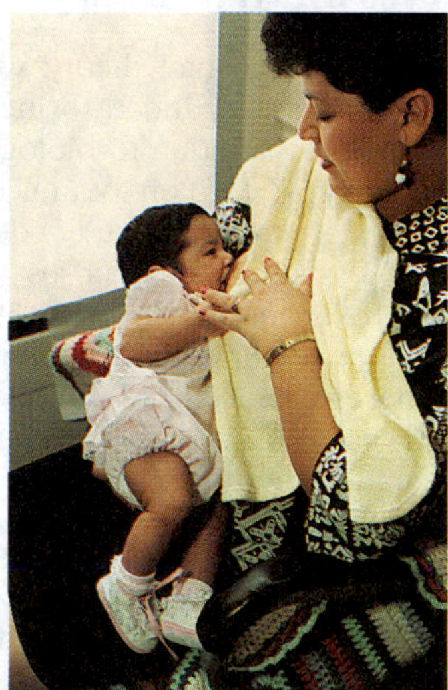

Figure 8-3
Infants develop a sense of trust and security as they learn that they can rely on their caregivers to fulfill their needs. (Photo © Kathy Sloane.)

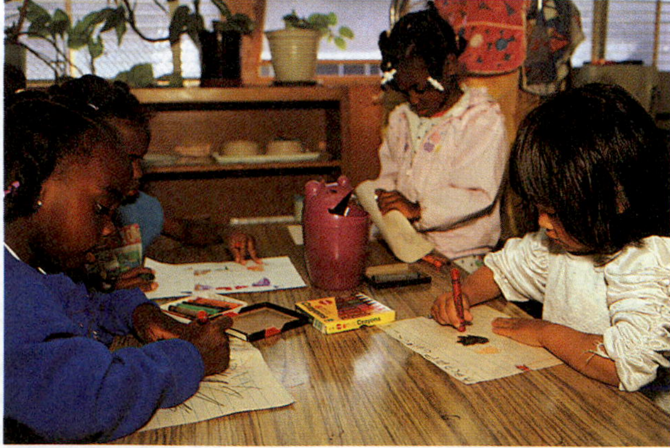

Figure 8-4
School-age children focus on the end results of accomplishments—recognition and praise from family, teachers, and peers—developing a sense of competition and industry. (Photo © Kathy Sloane.)

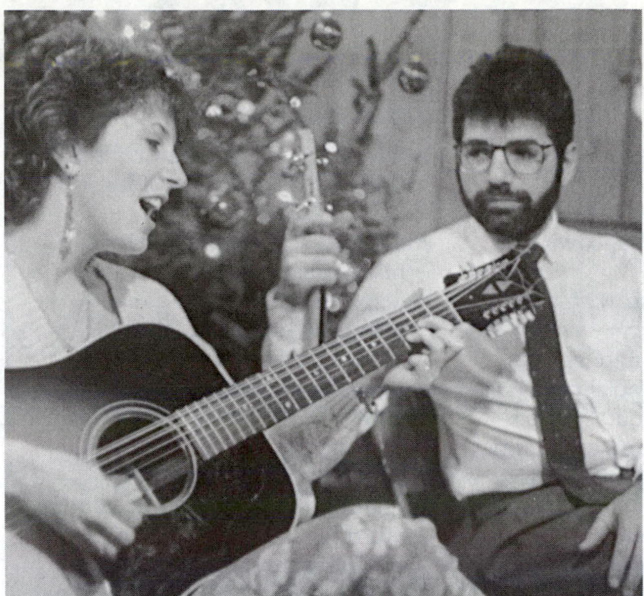

Figure 8-5
Establishing intimacy in young adulthood involves integrating self-identity and identities of others, and establishing relationships based on commitment, which necessitates self-sacrifice and compromise. (Photo by Tracy Baldwin.)

Developmental Tasks: Robert J. Havighurst

Havighurst (1972) believed that living and growing are based on learning, and that a person must continuously learn to adjust to changing societal conditions. He described learned behaviors as **developmental tasks** that occur at certain periods in life. Successful achievement leads to happiness and success in later tasks, whereas unsuccessful achievement leads to unhappiness, societal disapproval, and difficulty in later tasks. The developmental tasks arise from maturation, personal motives and values that determine occupational and family choices, and civic responsibility. The accompanying box summarizes the developmental tasks described by Havighurst.

Cognitive Development: Jean Piaget

Piaget, a Swiss psychologist, developed a theory of **cognitive development** from infancy through adolescence. Piaget believed that learning occurred as a result of the internal organization of an event, which formed a mental schemata, and served as a base for further schemata as one grew and developed. Intellectual growth, as described by Piaget, was a continual restructuring of knowledge to progress to higher levels of problem solving and critical thinking. Two continual processes of assimilation and accommodation stimulate intellectual growth in the child. **Assimilation** is the process of integrating new experiences into existing schemata; **accommodation** is an alteration of thought processes to correlate more complex information (Piaget & Inhelder, 1969). Four stages of cognitive development were described by Piaget (Table 8-3).

Piaget's Stages of Cognitive Development

Sensorimotor stage (birth to 24 months): During this period, the child progresses through a series of developmental stages, for example:
- 0 to 1 month—demonstrates basic reflexes, such as sucking (Fig. 8-6)
- 1 to 4 months—discovers enjoyment of random behaviors (such as smiling or sucking thumb) and repeats them
- 4 to 8 months—relates own behavior to change in environment, such as shaking a rattle to hear the sound (Fig. 8-7)
- 8 to 12 months—coordinates more than one thought pattern at a time to reach a goal, such as repeatedly throwing an object on the floor; only objects in sight are considered permanent
- 12 to 18 months—recognizes the permanence of objects, even if out of sight; can understand simple commands
- 18 to 24 months—begins to develop reasoning and can anticipate events

Preoperational stage (ages 2 to 7): This stage is characterized by the beginning use of symbols, through increased language skills and pictures, to represent the preschooler's world (Fig. 8-8). This stage is divided into two parts: the preconceptual stage (ages 2 to 4) and the intuitive stage (ages 4 to 7). Play activities during this time allow the child to better understand life events and relationships.

Concrete operational stage (ages 7 to 11): During this time, children learn by manipulating concrete or tangible objects, and can classify articles according to two or more characteristics. Logical thinking is developing with an understanding of reversibility, relations between numbers, and loss of egocentricity. Another characteristic of this stage is the ability to incorporate another's perspective.

Formal operational stage (age 11 or older): This stage is represented by the use of abstract thinking and deductive reasoning. General concepts are related to specific situations and alternatives are considered. The world is evaluated by testing beliefs in an attempt to establish values and meaning in life (Fig. 8-9).

Moral Development: Lawrence Kohlberg and Carol Gilligan

Lawrence Kohlberg. Kohlberg (1969) developed a theory of **moral development** with levels that closely follow Piaget's theory of cognitive development. Each level is further divided into two separate stages:

Preconventional level: This level follows intuitive thought, and is based on external control as the child learns to conform to rules imposed by authority figures. At stage 1, *punishment and obedi-*

Developmental Tasks Described by Robert J. Havighurst

Infancy and Early Childhood

- Learning to walk
- Learning to take solid foods
- Learning to talk
- Learning to control the elimination of body wastes
- Learning sex differences and sexual modesty
- Forming concepts and learning to describe social and physical reality
- Getting ready to read

Middle Childhood

- Learning physical skills necessary for ordinary games
- Building wholesome attitudes toward oneself as a growing organism
- Learning to get along with age-mates
- Learning an appropriate masculine or feminine social role
- Developing fundamental skills in reading, writing, and calculating
- Developing concepts necessary for everyday living
- Developing conscience, morality, and a scale of values
- Achieving personal independence
- Developing attitudes toward social groups and institutions

Adolescence

- Achieving new and maturer relations with age-mates of both sexes
- Achieving a masculine or feminine social role
- Accepting one's physique and using the body effectively
- Achieving emotional independence from parents and other adults
- Preparing for marriage and family life
- Preparing for an economic career
- Acquiring a set of values and an ethical system as guide to behavior—developing an ideology
- Desiring and achieving socially responsible behavior

Early Adulthood

- Selecting a mate
- Learning to live with a marriage partner
- Starting a family
- Rearing children
- Managing a home
- Getting started in an occupation
- Taking on civic responsibility
- Finding a congenial social group

Middle Age

- Assisting teenage children to become responsible and happy adults
- Achieving adult social and civic responsibility
- Reaching and maintaining satisfactory performance in one's occupational career
- Developing adult leisure-time activities
- Relating oneself to one's spouse as a person
- Accepting and adjusting to the physiologic changes of middle age
- Adjusting to aging parents

Later Maturity

- Adjusting to decreasing physical strength and health
- Adjusting to retirement and reduced income
- Adjusting to death of a spouse
- Establishing an explicit affiliation with one's age-group
- Adopting and adapting social roles in a flexible way
- Establishing satisfactory physical living arrangements

Havighurst, R. J. (1972). *Developmental tasks and education* (3rd ed.).

ence orientation, the motivation for choices of action is fear of physical consequences of authority's disapproval. As a result of the consequences, a perception of goodness or badness develops. At stage 2, *instrumental relativist orientation,* the thought of receiving a reward overcomes fear of punishment, so actions that satisfy this desire are selected.

Conventional level: This level is obtained when the person becomes concerned with identifying with significant others and shows conformity to their expectations. Values and ideals supported by family and friends are respected, regardless of consequences. Stage 3, *"good boy–good girl" orientation,* is when the person strives for approval in an attempt to be viewed as "good." Stage 4, *"law and order" orientation,* is when behavior focuses on following social or religious rules as a respect for authority. In his later work, Kohlberg maintained that many adults are at this stage because they think abstractly and view themselves as members of society (Duska & Whelan, 1975).

Postconventional level: This level is associated with moral judgment that is rational and internalized into one's standards or values. Stage 5, *social contract, utilitarian orientation,* supports correct behavior as defined by the legal rights of society. Laws can be changed, however, to meet society's needs, while maintaining respect for self and others. Stage 6, *universal ethical principle orientation,*

Table 8-3
Jean Piaget's Theory of Cognitive Development

Stage	Age
Sensorimotor	0–24 months
Reflective	0–1 month
Primary circular reactions	1–4 months
Secondary circular reactions	4–8 months
Coordination of secondary schemata	8–12 months
Tertiary circular reactions	12–18 months
Invention of new means through mental combinations	18–24 months
Preoperational	2–7 years
Preconceptual	2–4 years
Intuitive	4–7 years
Concrete operational	7–11 years
Formal operational	11+ years

represents the person's concern for equality for all human beings, which is guided by personal opinions and standards, regardless of those set by society or laws. Justice may be internalized at an even higher level than society. Few adults ever reach this stage of development.

Kohlberg recognized that moral development is influenced by cultural effects on perceptions of justice in interpersonal relationships. The beginnings of moral development are witnessed in parent and child communications during the early childhood years, as the young child tries to please his or her parents. The concept of morality emerges as a subset of a person's beliefs or values and governs choices made throughout life. Rules and regulations established by society eventually are challenged and evaluated as a person either accepts societal rules into his or her own internal set of values or rejects them.

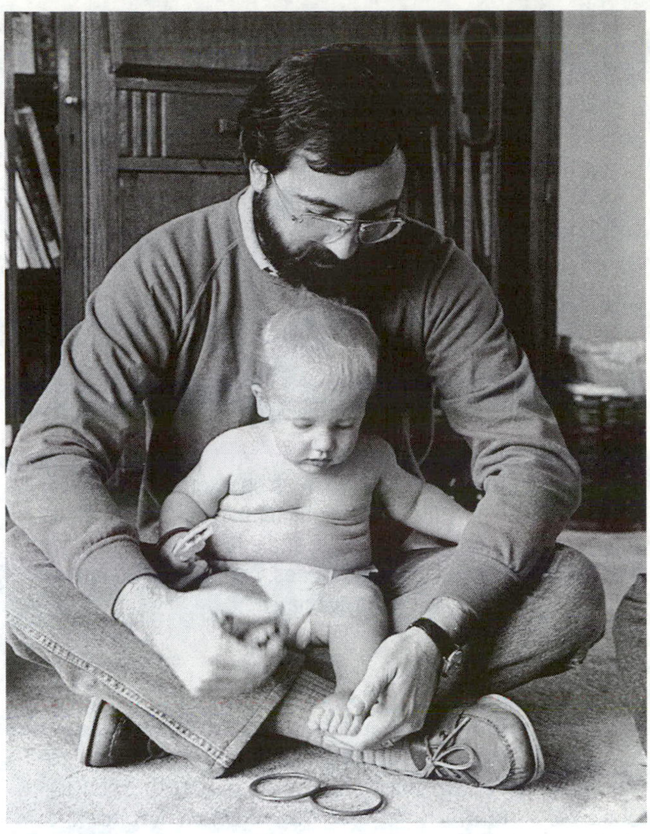

Figure 8-7
From about age 4 months, infants can begin to relate their own behavior as causing a change in the environment, and from about age 8 months, can integrate more than one thought pattern to obtain a purposeful goal. (Reeder, S. J., & Martin, L. L., [1991]. *Maternity nursing* [17th ed.]. Philadelphia: Lippincott.)

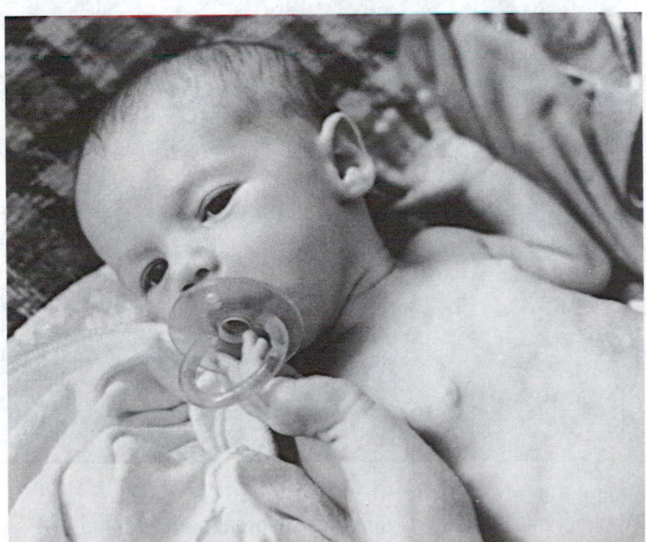

Figure 8-6
During the first month of life, the infant has no understanding of the environment and can respond only by exercising basic reflexes such as sucking.

Carol Gilligan. Gilligan (1977, 1982) originally worked with Kohlberg. As she listened to women discuss their own real-life moral conflicts, she recognized that there was a conception of morality from the female viewpoint that was not represented in Kohlberg's work.

In Gilligan's theory, males and females have different ways of looking at the world. Males are more likely to associate morality with obligations, rights, and justice. Females are more likely to see moral requirements emerging from the needs of others within the context of a relationship. This moral orientation of females is called the *ethic of care,* which develops through three levels. Each level ends with a transitional period—a time when the female considers new approaches to moral considerations and moves to a new level.

Level 1—Selfishness: In the first level, the focus is on needs of the self. "Should" and "would" are the

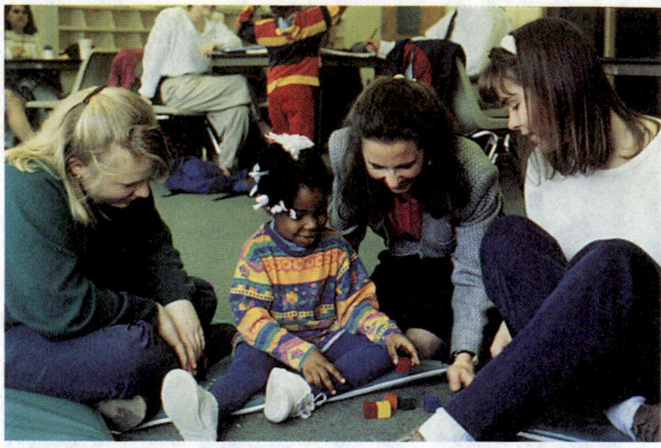

Figure 8-8
The preschool child's development is characterized by the beginning use of symbols through language and pictures, an ability to learn simple sequences, and a basic ability to categorize objects. (Photo by Gates Rhodes, courtesy of School of Nursing, University of Pennsylvania.)

same. Morality is seen as sanctions by society. Relationships often are disappointing, and as a result, a woman may choose to isolate herself to avoid getting hurt. The transition that follows this level is characterized by the move from selfishness to responsibility—a move that integrates the responsibility to care for self with the desire to care for others.

Level 2—Goodness: Moral judgment is based on shared norms and expectations, and societal values are adopted. Acceptance by others becomes critical, and the ability to protect and care for others is seen as the defining characteristic of female goodness. This characteristic is upheld through beliefs that one is responsible for the actions of others but that others are responsible for the choices that are made. As self-sacrifice is examined, the second transition occurs, with the woman asking if her own needs are not also important. A shift from goodness to truth (as well as a new conception of goodness) takes place.

Level 3—Nonviolence: A changed understanding of self and a redefinition of morality allow the woman to reconcile selfishness and responsibility. Nonviolence (the injunction against hurting) governs all moral judgments and actions. Care becomes a universal obligation toward self and toward others. Moral problems usually are considered within the context of maintaining relationships and response, and of promoting the welfare or preventing the harm of others.

Gilligan developed a theory of moral development that views females as developing a morality of response and care and males as developing a morality of justice. Research will facilitate further development of this theory and increase knowledge about human development.

Faith Development: James Fowler

Fowler (1981) has developed a developmental theory of the spiritual identity of humans, based on work by Piaget, Kohlberg, and Erikson. He describes **faith** as follows (1981, p. 4):

> Faith is not always religious in its content or context. . . . Faith is a person's or group's way of moving into the force field of life. It is our way of finding coherence in and giving meaning to the multiple forces and relations that make up our lives. Faith is a person's way of seeing him or herself in relation to others against a background of shared meaning and purpose.

Faith, therefore, is not necessarily religious, but it comprises the reasons one finds life worth living.

Fowler's theory is composed of prestage and six stages of faith development. The age when a certain stage exists varies, but the sequence does not. Equilibrium, or the plateau of faith development, can occur at any stage, beginning with stage 2.

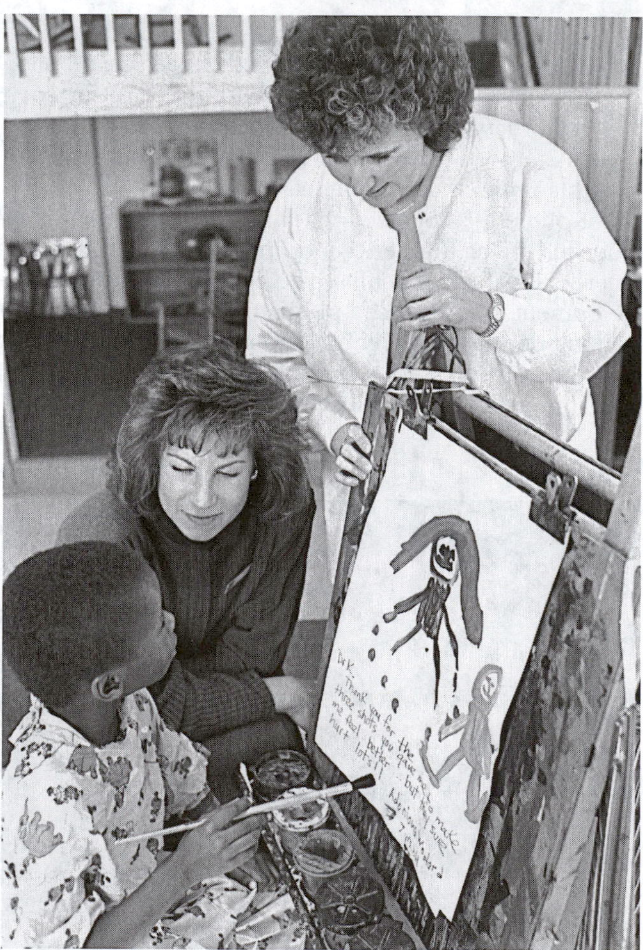

Figure 8-9
Abstract reasoning is required for children to understand that painful medical treatments given now will make them feel better later. A child who is not old enough to have reached the formal operational stage, in which abstract reasoning develops, may require special attention from the health care staff to understand the uncomfortable experiences of the hospital stay. (Photo by Don Walker, courtesy of Thomas Jefferson University Hospital.)

In the organization of the stages of faith development, Fowler explained a triadic relationship between self, shared causes or values, and others, which is the unifying factor in all stages and is based on trust. During the prestage, called *undifferentiated faith,* trust, courage, hope, and love compete with threats of abandonment and inconsistencies in the infant's environment. The strength of faith in this stage is based on the relationship with the primary caregiver. The stages, listed in Table 8-4, are:

Stage 1—Intuitive–projective faith: This stage is most typical of the 3- to 7-year-old child. Children imitate religious gestures and behaviors of others, primarily their parents. They follow parental attitudes toward religious or moral beliefs without a thorough understanding of them. Imagination in this stage leads to long-lived images and feelings that must be questioned and reintegrated in later stages (Fig. 8-10).

Stage 2—Mythical–literal faith: This stage predominates in the school-age child with increased social interaction. Stories represent religious and moral beliefs, and existence of a deity is accepted. Perspectives of others can be appreciated, as well as the concept of reciprocal fairness.

Stage 3—Synthetic–conventional faith: This is the characteristic stage for many adolescents. As the person experiences increasing demands from work, school, family, and peers, the basis for identity is complex. An ideology has emerged but has not been closely examined until now. The person begins to question some of the life-guiding values or religious practices in an attempt to stabilize his or her own identity.

Stage 4—Individuative–reflective faith: This stage is critical for older adolescents and young adults because the responsibility for their commitments, beliefs, and attitudes becomes their own. Many adults do not construct this stage, and for some people it does not emerge until they are in their 30s or 40s. Searching for self-identity no longer defined by the boundaries of faith compositions of significant others is a primary concern.

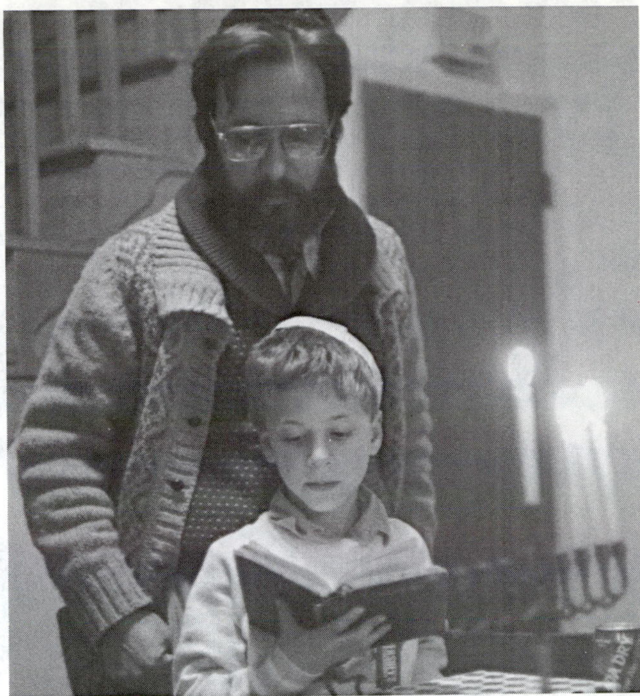

Figure 8-10
In the earliest stage of faith development, the child imitates religious gestures and behaviors of parents and others. Images and feelings experienced in early years will be reevaluated and reintegrated in later stages.

Table 8-4
Comparison of Psychosocial and Faith Stages

Erikson's Psychosocial Stages	Fowler's Faith Stages
Trust vs mistrust	Undifferentiated (infancy)
Autonomy vs shame and doubt	Intuitive-projective (early childhood)
Initiative vs guilt	
Industry vs inferiority	Mythical-literal (school years)
Identity vs role confusion	Synthetic-conventional (adolescence)
Intimacy vs isolation	Individuative-reflective (young adulthood)
Generativity vs stagnation	Conjunctive (midlife)
Ego integrity vs despair	Universalizing

(Data from Fowler, J. W. [1981]. *Stages of faith: The psychology of human development and the quest for meaning.* New York: Harper & Row.)

Stage 5—Conjunctive faith: This stage integrates other viewpoints about faith into one's understanding of truth. One is able to see the paradoxical nature of the reality of one's own beliefs. Along with this realization, the divisions of faith development among people become apparent.

Stage 6—Universalizing faith: This stage involves overcoming paradoxes noted in stage 5, and makes tangible the values of absolute love and justice for humankind. The faith relationship noted in stage 6 is characterized by total trust in the principle of being and the existence of the future, whether derived from the Judeo-Christian image of faith or otherwise.

Family Influences on Growth and Development

The family is mentioned in this chapter because the study of growth and development would not be complete without noting the interrelationship between an individual and the family (see the accompanying box). Family dynamics, a major environmental influence, begin with conception and continue throughout life. The functions, structures, and developmental tasks of the

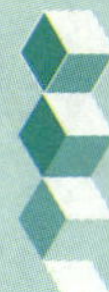

Research in Nursing: Making a Difference

Growth and Development

Knowledge of the theories of normal growth and development, as well as the influences of the family on growth and development, are essential components of nursing care of clients of all ages. Nurses use the knowledge base in this area to recognize normal patterns and to identify variations from normal. Although this is important for any age client, it is especially important in the care of children.

Bossert, E. (1994). Factors influencing the coping of hospitalized school-age children. *Journal of Pediatric Nursing: Nursing Care of Children and Families, 9*(5), 299–306.
This study was conducted to identify factors influencing the coping process in hospitalized children. The sample of 82 children, who were hospitalized in an acute care pediatric unit of six hospitals, ranged in age from 8 to 11. The effects of health status (being either chronically ill or acutely ill), gender, and level of anxiety were assessed through interviews and scales. Findings of the study were that children who were acutely ill perceived their coping to be more effective than did children with chronic illnesses. In addition, children who had low anxiety were more likely to perceive their coping as more effective than did children with high anxiety.

Murata, J. (1994). Family stress, social support, violence, and sons' behavior. *Western Journal of Nursing Research, 16*(2), 154–168.
The literature commonly links the low-income, inner-city family who is single-parent and female headed with child behavior problems. This study examined the relationships among family stress, social support, mothers' conflict resolution patterns, and sons' behavior in a group of primarily African-American, single women who lived alone with their children in the inner city. Findings were compared to a nationally representative group of white, Anglo-Saxon, Protestant families. Although the sample of inner-city mothers reported more family stress and less social support, the family violence rates did not differ in the two groups. Thirty-nine percent of sons from the inner-city group were reported to have behavior problems. The author recommended family stress as the best focus of nursing interventions in these high-risk families.

Walker, L., & Montgomery, E. (1994). Maternal identity and role attainment: Long-term relations to children's development. *Nursing Research, 43*(2), 105–110.
Much has been written about the importance of the maternal role in the first year of infancy. However, little is known about how the features of the early maternal role affect children as they grow and develop. The purpose of this study was to examine the relationship of early maternal role indicators to children's competence and adjustment during the school-age period. Data was collected from 124 mother–infant pairs at five time periods within nine years. Although maternal identity and perceived and demonstrated role attainment were measured, only maternal identity was found to be a significant predictor of children's socioemotional outcomes. Despite limited findings, the authors recommend that nurses continue to be sensitive to the emerging maternal identity and to helping with parenting when caring for new mothers.

Summary

As evidenced by these studies, many different factors influence the growth and development of children; in these examples, factors range from illness to single-parent families to maternal identity. Recognizing the importance of growth and development principles and using those principles as a base for individualized nursing interventions are essential. Nursing research, conducted to describe and explore experiences from a developmental framework, can provide increased knowledge and more effective nursing care.

family are discussed with human needs in Chapter 2; the establishment of a family is discussed in Chapter 10 in the section dealing with the young adult.

The family plays a vital role in wellness promotion and illness prevention. Family values and one's ethnic or cultural heritage influence interpretation of illness. A health problem or developmental crisis of any family member can affect the remainder of the unit. Health practices, whether positive or negative, often are shared in the family, being learned by younger members. Sometimes the family may even be the cause of illness of individual members. Alterations in coping and communication patterns may predispose families to dysfunctional means of relating to one another.

Implications for Nursing

Facilitating Effective Family Functioning

The nurse has a responsibility to assess not only the health needs of individual members of the family but also the demands placed on the total family in meeting every member's needs. The nurse can then function as a catalyst in planning appropriate interventions and teaching, and as a collaborator with other healthcare professionals (social workers, psychologists, physicians, clergy) in achieving optimal family wellness.

Nurses plan and implement activities to facilitate effective family functioning so that growth and development is enhanced. The nurses role is primarily through teaching, with the following areas emphasized (each stage of growth and development in the following chapter includes nursing actions to promote wellness):

- Information about risk factors within individual family members, such as drinking alcohol, smoking cigarettes, or using illegal drugs
- Knowledge and skills to increase health promotion and coping behaviors
- Family strengths that foster individual and family development
- Risk factors in the home environment, such as open containers of cleaning solutions or open stairways
- Prevention of illness, injury, abuse, and neglect

These broad categories of teaching must be individualized to the needs of each family. The adolescent who is a single mother requires knowledge different from that of a family seeking information on childproofing their home. Both individual developmental tasks and family developmental tasks are essential considerations in providing holistic nursing care.

Applying Growth and Development Principles

The complex and interrelated elements that contribute to the phenomenon of human development constitute not only biophysical factors but also factors of personality development. The theories presented from Freud, Erikson, Havighurst, Piaget, Kohlberg, Gilligan, and Fowler give knowledge of the evolution of cognitive, psychosocial, moral, and spiritual development. In relating to the whole person, all the components of development need to be evaluated to understand certain life events or concerns.

Although these theorists have brought a great deal of insight into the process of human development, some limitations exist in each theory. Therefore, in planning holistic nursing care for clients with diverse needs, backgrounds, and ages, nurses should assess the client and support decisions for interventions on rationale from multiple theories of development so as to provide comprehensive health promotion. Guidelines for incorporating principles and theories of growth and development are listed in the accompanying box. A few examples are discussed here.

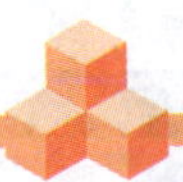

Guidelines for Nursing Care

Incorporating Principles and Theories of Growth and Development

General guidelines for incorporating principles and theories of growth and development and family dynamics into daily practice of nursing care are listed below. They are provided as suggestions for working with clients of all ages.

- Be knowledgeable about the various stages of cognitive, psychosocial, moral, and spiritual development and prepared to support developmental stages typical of certain ages.
- Maintain flexibility in assessing people, and respect the uniqueness of each person. Although the literature describes development typical of a particular age, not everyone fits into an exact mold.
- Anticipate possible regression during difficult periods or times of crisis, accepting and supporting a person's return to a forward progression in development.
- Become cognizant that environmental and cultural influences have a strong effect on development, especially psychosocial development. A deprived environment can be detrimental, whereas an enriched environment enhances development.
- Assess each person with an awareness that within each stage of development, a person may retain some behaviors of a previous stage, attain goals of the current stage, and begin to exhibit behaviors of the next stage. There is a time of transition to the next stage with no definite beginning or ending to the particular stage of development.
- Remember that clients are members of families and that the family unit can have both positive and negative influences on the development of individual members. Attempt to support good family relationships and healthy environments that assist members to reach their greatest potential for growth. Provide client teaching to individuals and their families to aid in their understanding of periods of development.
- Be ready to provide healthcare to clients who are ill or who fail to meet developmental goals. Collaborate with other members of the healthcare team in providing care to prevent or minimize disruption of development and to promote optimal wellness throughout life.
- Provide environments and experiences that are developmentally challenging.

1. While interviewing a young mother with her first child, the nurse senses a frustrated single parent as the mother reviews the task of rearing her 14-month-old child alone. Based on Freud, the nurse can relate the behaviors typical of the oral stage of development for the infant. Havighurst and Erikson support the stage of gaining independence in learning to walk for the toddler. Recognizing that the mother may be limited in her support system, the nurse may need to assess further to identify problems with intimacy and a feeling of generativity. In planning care for this young mother, the nurse anticipates needed emotional support and health teaching about the normal toddler years. The mother's anxiety level and the child's attempts to investigate the environment through locomotion and oral exploration place them at risk for injury from falls or aspiration. The nurse has a primary role in prevention through client education based on astute observation and knowledge of child development.
2. A 16-year-old girl is admitted to the nursing unit after having sustained multiple injuries in a motor vehicle accident. The injuries include several deep facial lacerations and a fractured femur. The young woman is stabilized, medicated for pain, and placed in traction. The nurse notices the girl crying quietly in her room. Realizing the importance of self-identity for the adolescent (Erikson, 1963), the nurse approaches the girl and asks if she would like to talk. Initially seeming hesitant, the girl is able to discuss her fears of scar formation on her face and comments from her friends. The nurse can assist by allowing the girl to share her feelings and by encouraging her to talk with her physician to find out the possible outcome after healing occurs.
3. A 70-year-old man fell and fractured his hip while repairing the exterior of his home. Having been the traditional head of his household, he now is troubled by needing others, including his wife, to care for him. He appears withdrawn, refusing to talk and eating poorly. Reflecting on Havighurst's and Erikson's theories, the nurse knows that the man may be fluctuating between feelings of non-adjustment and acceptance of declining health and a sense of ego integrity.

These situations demonstrate the application of growth and development theories to the practice of nursing. Healthcare needs change quickly as a person grows and passes through life. These needs are unique for each person but include certain similarities at specific periods. The nurse is faced with the dynamic tasks of planning care based on both general and unique health needs of a client and continually revising aspects of care in the evolution of the growth process or alteration in health status.

Key Points

- Nurses provide care to all ages in the life continuum; this care involves both individuals and their families.
- Growth and development theories, taken together, involve all aspects of life: physiologic, cognitive, psychosocial, moral, spiritual, and family dimensions.
- Principles of growth and development state that the processes are (1) orderly and sequential, (2) continuous and complex, (3) specific for each person, (4) influenced by environmental factors, (5) directed by regular trends, and (6) quantitative and qualitative, and that they (7) become integrated, (8) have vulnerable periods, (9) have rates and patterns that can be modified, and (10) occur at different stages and at different rates.
- Freud's psychosexual theory explains ego development through predictable id–superego conflicts.
- Erikson identifies personality development in a series of stages from birth to later adult years, when critical tasks must be mastered.
- Havighurst focuses on the concept of learning in order to understand growth and development.
- Piaget's theory describes cognitive development from infancy through adolescence based on assimilation, accommodation, and formation of schemata.
- Kohlberg presents a theory of moral judgment of reasoning that begins in early childhood years. Gilligan developed a theory of moral development in females that is based on caring and responsibility.
- Fowler defines faith or spirituality as comprising meaning for life, which includes values, beliefs, and, possibly, religious affiliation.
- Each developmental theory explains a portion of the process of development and provides part of the nurse's understanding of the total being and coping abilities. Such theories are limited by their specific focus and the theorist's beliefs about growth and development.
- The family plays a vital role in promoting wellness and preventing illness. Both positive and negative health practices are shared in the family and learned by younger members. Health problems affect the family unit.

Bibliography

Billingham, K. A. (1982). *Developmental psychology for the healthcare professions*. Boulder: Westview.

Bossert, E. (1994). Factors influencing the coping of hospitalized school-age children. *Journal of Pediatric Nursing: Nursing Care of Children & Families, 9*(5), 299–306.

Coles, R. (1990). *The spiritual life of children*. Boston: Houghton & Mifflin.

DeMaio-Esteves, M. (1990). Mediators of daily stress and perceived health status in adolescent girls. *Nursing Research, 39*(6), 360–363.

Duska, R., & Whelan, M. (1975). *Moral development: A guide to Piaget and Kohlberg*. New York: Paulist.

Erikson, E. H. (1963). *Childhood and society* (2nd ed.). New York: Norton.

Flanagan, O., & Jackson, K. (1987). Justice, care, and gender: The Kohlberg–Gilligan debate revisited. *Ethics 97,* 622–637.

Fong, B. C., & Resnick, M. R. (1980). *The child: Development through adolescence*. Menlo Park, CA: Benjamin/Cummings.

Fowler, J. W. (1981). *Stages of faith: The psychology of human development and the quest for meaning*. New York: Harper & Row.

Fowler, J. W. (1991). *Weaving the new creation: Stages of faith and the public church*. San Francisco: Harper Collins.

Freud, S. (1923/1974). *The ego and the id*. London: Hogarth.

Friedman, M. M. (1992). *Family nursing: Theory and assessment* (3rd ed.). Norwalk, CT: Appleton & Lange.

Gilligan, C. (1977). In a different voice: Women's conceptions of the self and of morality. *Harvard Educational Review, 47,* 481–517.

Gilligan, C. (1982). *In a different voice*. Cambridge, MA: Harvard University Press.

Havighurst, R. J. (1972). *Developmental tasks and education*. New York: David McKay.

Janes, B., & Morse, J. (1990). Adolescent girls' perceptions of and preparation for menarche. *Canadian Journal of Nursing Research, 22*(2), 47–58.

Kempe, H., & Helfer, R. E. (1968). *The battered child*. Chicago: University of Chicago Press.

Klaus, M. H., & Kennell, J. H. (1982). *Parent–infant bonding*. St. Louis: Mosby.

Kohlberg, L. (1969). Stage and sequence: The cognitive–developmental approach to socialization. In D. Gaslin (Ed.). *Handbook of socialization: Theory and research* (pp. 347–380). Chicago: Rand McNally.

Mott, S. R., Fazekas, N. F., & James, S. R. (1990). *Nursing care of children and families: A holistic approach* (2nd ed.). Menlo Park, CA: Addison-Wesley.

Murata, J. (1994). Family stress, social support, violence, and sons' behavior. *Western Journal of Nursing Research, 16*(2), 154–168.

Mussen, P. H., Conger, J. J., & Kagan, J. (1974). *Child development and personality* (4th ed.). New York: Harper & Row.

Newman, B. M., & Newman, P. R. (1975). *Development through life: A psychosocial approach*. Homewood, IL: Dorsey.

Parker, R. S. (1990). Measuring nurse's moral judgments. *Image: Journal of Nursing Scholarship. 22*(4), 213–218.

Piaget, J., & Inhelder, B. (1969). *The psychology of the child*. New York: Basic Books.

Sorenson, E. S. (1990). Children's coping responses. *Journal of Pediatric Nursing, 5*(4), 259–267.

Walker, L., & Montgomery, E. (1994). Maternal identity and role attainment: Long-term relations to children's development. *Nursing Research, 43*(2), 105–110.

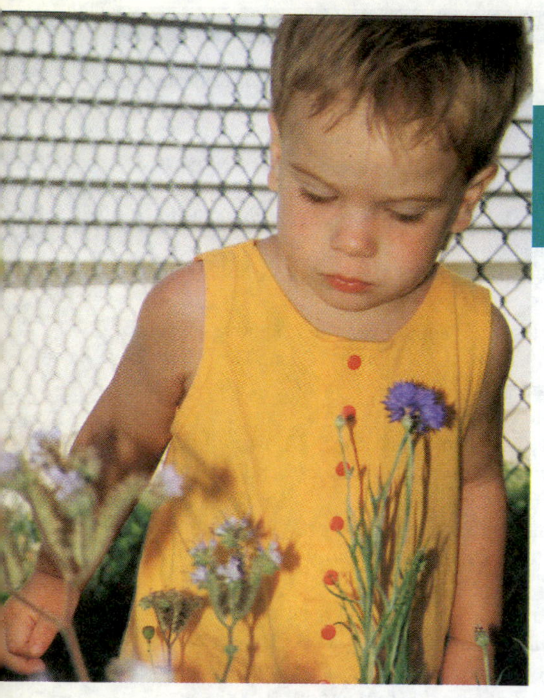

Chapter 9

Conception Through Adolescence

Objectives

After studying this chapter, the learner should be able to:

Define key terms used in the chapter.

Summarize major physiologic, cognitive, psychosocial, moral, and spiritual developments from conception through adolescence.

List common health problems of each age period from conception through adolescence.

Describe nursing actions to promote wellness at each developmental level.

Key Terms

adolescence
attachment
bonding
child abuse
colic
failure to thrive
infant
negativism
neonate
preschooler
puberty
regression
school-age child
separation anxiety
sexually transmitted disease
sudden infant death syndrome
temperament
toddler

Growth and development occur throughout each person's life. Knowledge of sequential growth and developmental milestones provides the base for planning and implementing holistic, individualized nursing care for clients and their families.

This chapter continues the discussion of theories of development introduced in Chapter 8, with specific information relating to various stages of growth and development. Included are the sequential developmental stages that occur from conception to adolescence. Developmental stages of the young, middle, and older adult are discussed in Chapter 10. The period from conception to adolescence is divided into different stages, but the term *childhood* encompasses the entire period. Included within this time span are prenatal development, the neonate, the infant, the toddler, the preschooler, and the school-age child. Each of these stages is discussed in this section, including physiologic, psychosocial, and cognitive development; common health problems; and the nurse's role in meeting healthcare needs.

Although developmental milestones are briefly presented, the chapter focuses primarily on providing information that is necessary as the nurse promotes optimal functioning, growth, and wellness for clients of any age. Nursing's focus on wellness for the child is described in the accompanying box.

Environmental and Nutritional Influences

Environmental and nutritional factors influence all stages of development. The effect of each can occur independently, but they are more likely to be interrelated. The following examples illustrate these interrelations:

- Infants who are malnourished in utero develop fewer brain cells than do infants who have had adequate prenatal nutrition.
- Substance abuse by the mother during pregnancy increases the risk of congenital anomalies, low birth weight, and prematurity in neonates.
- Federally sponsored school meal programs support the belief that learning is enhanced when nutrition is adequate.
- Failure to thrive, a condition of early infancy, has been linked to both nutritional and emotional deprivation.
- Child abuse is an extreme example of physical and emotional harm or deprivation, leading to deficits in physical or psychosocial development, or both.
- Substance abuse among adolescents is associated with an increased incidence of teenage pregnancy, violence, accidents, and suicide. Abuse of alcohol (as well as abuse of other drugs) is more prevalent in teens who have poor family relationships, low self-esteem, and poor social skills.

Conception and Prenatal Development

Human growth and development begin at the moment the ovum is fertilized by the sperm. The fertilized ovum, or *zygote,* contains the full complement of genetic information provided by each parent that determines gender and influences personality, intellect, and physical and psychologic traits. The growth and development of the fetus are orderly and continuous, and proceed in three stages:

1. The *preembryonic stage* lasts for about 3 weeks. The zygote implants in the uterine wall, and has three distinct cell layers:

   The *ectoderm,* the outer cell layer, which becomes the brain, spinal cord, nervous system, and outer body parts (skin, hair, nails)

   The *endoderm,* the inner cell layer, which becomes the respiratory system, the digestive system, the liver, and the pancreas

   The *mesoderm,* which becomes the skeleton, connective tissue, cartilage, and muscles and the circulatory, lymphoid, reproductive, and urinary systems
2. The *embryonic stage* occurs from the 4th through the 8th week. Rapid growth and differentiation of the germ cell layers take place, and by the end of this period, all basic organs have been established, the bones have begun to ossify, and some human features are recognizable. Because this is a period of such rapid growth and change, the fetus is especially vulnerable to any factor that might cause congenital anomalies (such as maternal use of alcohol, nicotine, or drugs of any kind).

Nursing Today: Challenges and Solutions

Children: A Community in Crisis

Although the United States is one of the wealthiest nations in the world, each year thousands of children do not receive adequate healthcare. Problems that contribute to this lack of healthcare for children include lack of prenatal care, poor immunization rates, poverty, lack of education among parents, violence, and HIV/AIDS. Consider the following examples:

- Less than 40% of all 2-year-old children are fully immunized against major childhood disease.
- Of every 1000 infants, 9 die before the age of 1; this mortality rate is higher than 19 other nations.
- One-fourth of all children age 10 to 16 experience some sort of violent assault each year.
- An estimated 20% of the 31 million adolescents have at least one serious health problem, such as asthma, heart disease, depression, hearing and vision impairments, or psychologic difficulties arising from abuse or other maltreatment.

Nurses are meeting the challenge to improve the health of the nation's children in many different ways. Examples are:

- Nurses at Egleston Children's Hospital at Emory University in Atlanta have developed a children's advocacy program that focuses on family-centered education to prevent injuries. Aspects include health and safety fairs, media campaigns, and school programs to teach about car seats, safe homes and playgrounds, fire safety, nutrition, and conflict resolution.
- The Wisconsin HIV Primary Care Support Network for Children, Adolescents, and Their Families, located at the Children's Hospital of Milwaukee, Wisconsin, is an organization of healthcare providers that works with primary care providers, HIV/AIDS services, and families to coordinate care for children with HIV/AIDS. Nurses link children and their families with the community to provide information, provide emotional support, and coordinate community resources.
- More than 26,000 school nurses around the country provide health screenings, emergency care, immunizations, and other mandated services to children. In some states, school nurse practitioners are licensed to write prescriptions.

Source: Cassetta, R. (1994). Children: A community in crisis. *American Nurse, 26*(10), 1, 20, 21; Staff (1994). School-based nursing fills gaps in adolescent healthcare. *American Nurse, 26*(10), 20, 37.

3. The *fetal stage* is from 9 weeks to birth. Continued growth and development of all body organs and systems take place. By the time birth occurs, the average neonate weighs 7½ lb (3.4 kg) and is 20 inches (50.8 cm) long.

Neonate (Birth to 28 Days)

At birth, the neonate must adapt to extrauterine life, and must make several significant physiologic adjustments to do so. Although these adjustments occur in all body systems, the most important occur in the respiratory and circulatory systems. Assessment of the neonate is done immediately after birth. There are several measurement scales, but the Apgar is the one most commonly used. The Apgar rating scale is applied to neonates at 1 minute and 5 minutes after birth. Each category (Table 9-1) is rated as 0, 1, or 2. The rating for each category is then totaled to a maximum score of 10. Normal neonates score between 7 and 10. Neonates who score between 4 and 6 require special assistance; those who score below 4 are in need of immediate life-saving support.

Physiologic Development

The physical characteristics of the neonate include those shown in Figure 9-1 and the following:

Table 9-1
Apgar Scoring Chart

Sign	0	1	2
Heart rate	Absent	Slow (less than 100 beats/min)	Over 100 beats/min
Respiratory effort	Absent	Slow, irregular	Good, crying
Muscle tone	Flaccid	Some flexion of extremities	Active motion
Reflex irritability	No response	Weak cry or grimace	Vigorous cry
Color	Blue, pale	Body pink, extremities blue	Completely pink

Figure 9-1
Reflexes and behaviors of the neonate. (Reeder, S. J., & Martin, L. L. [1991]. *Maternity nursing* [17th ed.]. Philadelphia: Lippincott.)

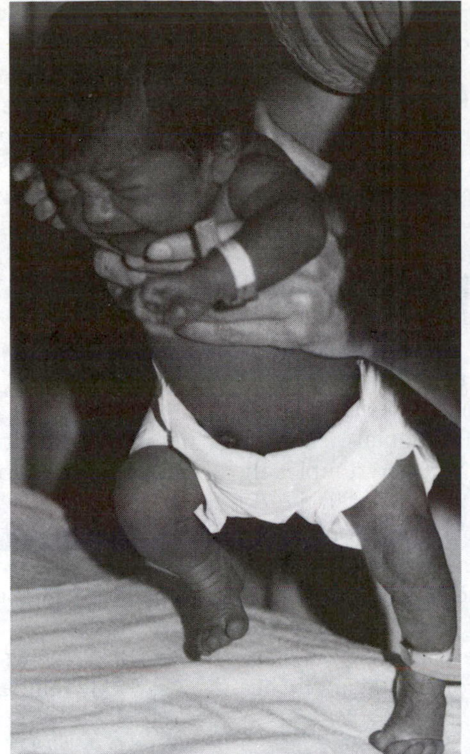

Stepping reflex

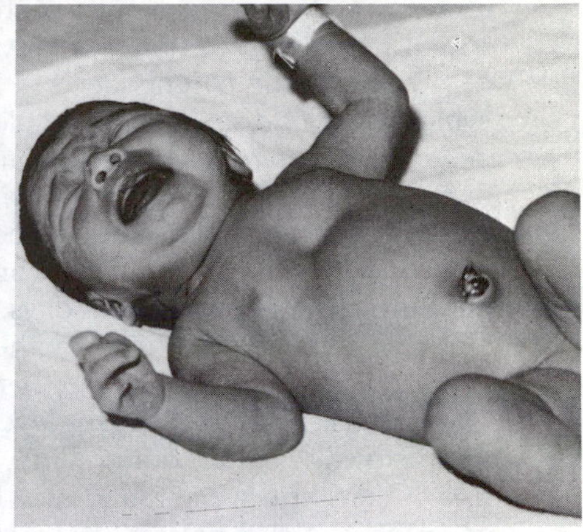

Active crying state

Moro reflex

Quiet alert state

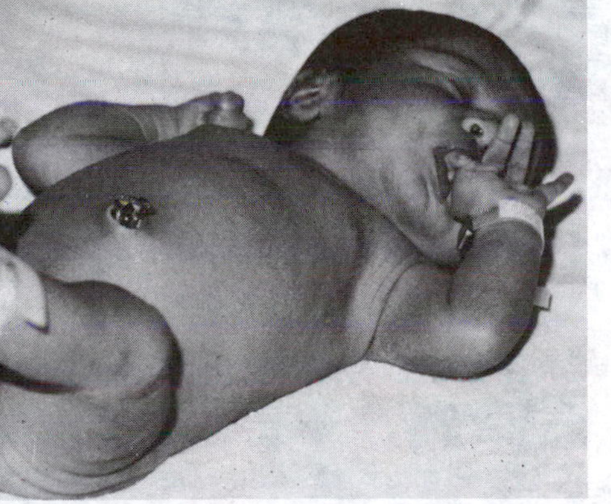

Hand-to-mouth and sucking activity

- Has reflexes that allow sucking, swallowing, blinking, sneezing, and yawning
- Has labile temperature control that responds quickly to environmental temperatures
- Is alert to the environment, sees color and form, hears and turns toward sound, can smell and taste, and is sensitive to touch and pain
- Can eliminate both stool and urine
- Will drink breast milk, glucose water, and plain water

The neonate also inherits a transient immunity from infections as a result of immunoglobulins that cross the placenta. Breast-feeding provides further protection against bacterial and viral infections through immunoglobulins and leukocytes in breast milk. The high lactose content in breast milk, combined with limited protein, promotes an acid environment that is unsuitable for bacterial growth. Antibodies secreted in breast milk help to control some viral infections.

Common Health Problems

Particular difficulties related to the birth process, the transition to extrauterine life, or *congenital anomalies* may necessitate intervention by healthcare personnel. Breathing difficulties may occur, especially if the neonate has been sedated by drugs given to the mother during labor and delivery. The premature neonate is vulnerable to *respiratory distress syndrome* because of the relative immaturity of lung function. The neonate delivered by cesarean birth is at risk for respiratory difficulties because of excess mucus in the lungs. Therefore, frequent suctioning is common in the cesarean-delivered neonate.

Incompatibility between the blood group of the mother and that of the neonate requires prompt care at birth. Congenital malformations, such as cleft palate and cleft lip, spina bifida, and Down syndrome, present profound and long-term health problems. Birth traumas, which may result in temporary symptoms, are of concern because the parents need to be reassured that the symptoms will disappear. Examples include *caput succedaneum*, *molding*, bruises from the use of forceps during delivery, and *subconjunctival hemorrhage*. Parents also need help to understand the nonthreatening nature of *physiologic jaundice*, which commonly is present during the neonate's first days.

The neonate born to a mother who smokes cigarettes, drinks alcohol, or uses drugs is of special concern. These substances may cause developmental deficits as well as complications during birth. Nicotine doubles the risk of low birth weight, and may be a factor in the development of cleft palate. Fetal alcohol syndrome in the neonate of the mother who drinks is believed to be a leading cause of birth defects, including growth retardation, developmental delay, and impaired intellectual ability. The maternal use of cocaine, crack-cocaine, and heroin increases the probability of congenital anomalies, prematurity, low birth weight, and withdrawal syndromes (Bennett & Woolf, 1991).

Cocaine or crack-cocaine use brings about abrupt changes in the mother's blood pressure, resulting in numerous small strokes in the developing fetus. When "crack babies" are born, they are lethargic, hypersensitive to noise or stimuli, and unable to focus visually, and they have diarrhea. The number of neonates born with this syndrome, which may last for 2 to 3 weeks after birth, is increasing. The long-term effects are not fully known.

Infant: 1 Month to 1 Year

At the end of the first month, the neonate becomes an **infant** and is so until the first birthday (Fig. 9-2).

Physiologic Development

The physical characteristics of the infant include the following:

- Brain grows to about half the adult size.
- Body temperature stabilizes.

As the infant enters the second half of his first year, play will begin to involve manipulation of objects and the environment.

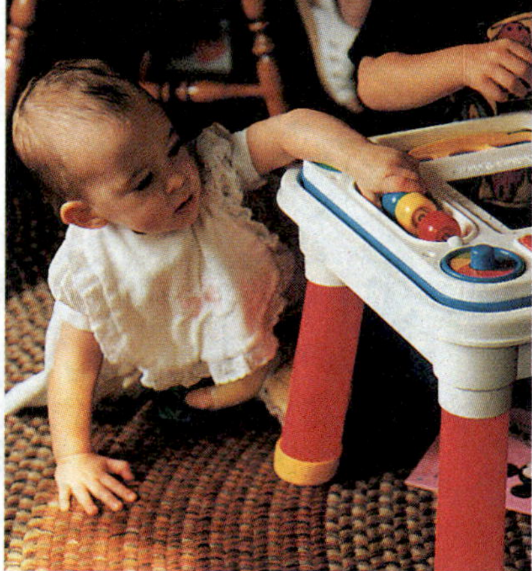

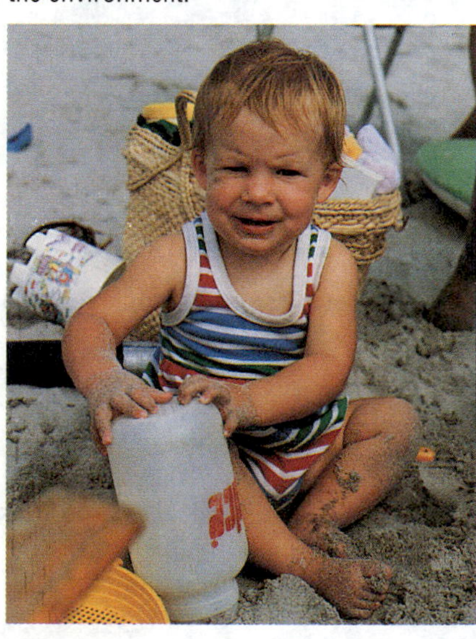

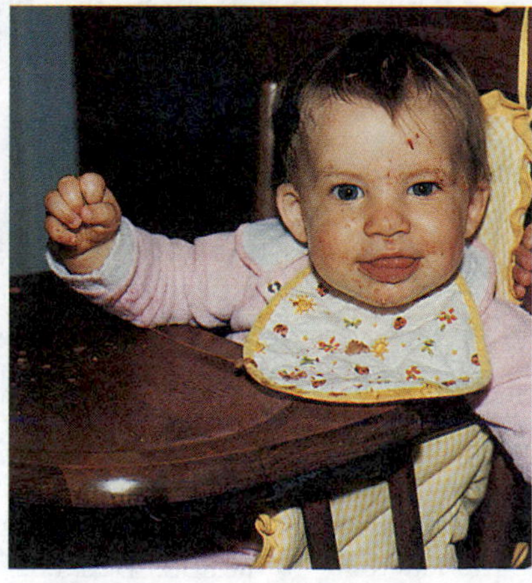

Developmental tasks of the first year include taking solid food.

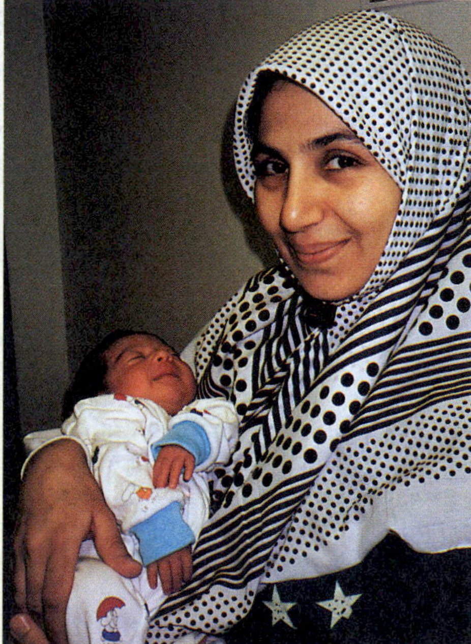

Bonding may occur in the first few hours after birth or later in the first few months and is necessary for later attachment.

Figure 9-2
Development in the infant.

- Motor abilities develop to allow using building blocks, trying to feed self, crawling, and walking.
- Eyes begin to focus and fixate.
- Heart doubles in weight; the heart rate slows and blood pressure rises.
- Deciduous teeth begin to erupt at 4 to 6 months.
- Birth weight usually triples by 1 year; at 1 year, the average male baby weighs 22 lb (10 kg) and the average female baby weighs 21 lb (9.5 kg). Length increases by 50%.

Growth Patterns

The adequacy of rate and totality of growth in the infant and toddler is assessed by comparison with standardized growth charts. Several such charts are available; each is gender specific because the growth rates of boys and girls differ. Care should be taken in making comparisons for the following reasons:

- Each child has individual variations and short-term spurts and lags in growth.
- Atypical infants, such as those who are premature or have low birth weight, are not addressed.
- Growth charts may be ethically and socioeconomically weighted in favor of white, middle-class children.

The Denver Developmental Screening Test (DDST) is commonly used as a screening test for quickly and inexpensively determining atypical developmental patterns in infants and children. The following critical areas of development are assessed in the DDST:

- Gross motor behavior and skills
- Fine motor behavior and skills
- Language acquisition
- Personal and social interaction

The test isolates problem areas that require more precise assessments. The student is referred to pediatric textbooks for further information about this test.

Cognitive Development

The infant from birth to 1 year is in the sensorimotor stage of development described by Piaget. Language development is in the prelinguistic phase. Babies begin to coo and make pleasurable sounds soon after birth, and by age 12 months they can convey wishes through a few key words. Language development has several consistent characteristics, regardless of the specific language being learned. They are as follows:

- Use of syllable repetition (such as ma-ma, da-da, bye-bye)
- Identical early phonetic expressions (babbling sounds)
- Imitation of sounds and intonations spoken by caregivers

Psychosocial Development

Based on the developmental theories discussed in Chapter 8, the infant has the following characteristics:

- Is in the oral stage (Freud), striving for immediate gratification of needs and having a strong sucking need
- Develops trust (Erikson) when the caregiver can be counted on to provide food when the infant is hungry; trust also is facilitated by diaper-changing, warmth, and comforting
- Meets developmental tasks (Havighurst) by learning to take solid food, walk, and talk

Other components of psychosocial development in the neonate and infant include attachment, play, and temperament.

Attachment is an active, affectionate, reciprocal relationship between two people. It can be differentiated from bonding. **Bonding**, described by Klaus and Kennell (1982), occurs during a sensitive period in the first few hours after birth (although bonding also may occur later in the first few months) and is necessary for later attachment. Bonding may be considered the initial fusing of two persons, and attachment the long-term maintenance and strengthening of the fused state.

Play allows the infant and child to discover the environment and begin to learn how to control it. Beginning as soon as the baby is aware of sensations and the pleasure they produce, play progresses from self-pleasure to interaction with others. The two dimensions of play are social play and cognitive play. Social play is motivated by a desire for fun, pleasure, and relationships with others. Cognitive play is motivated by the desire to learn.

Temperament is primarily inborn, although it is influenced by environment. Characteristics of temperament allow description of a baby and child as "easy," "slow to warm," and "difficult" (Thomas, Chess, & Birch, 1968). The "easy" infant sleeps, eats, and eliminates easily; smiles spontaneously; and cries in response to significant needs. The "slow to warm" infant is more passive and distant. The "difficult" infant has volatile and labile responses, often is a restless sleeper, is highly sensitive to noises, and eats poorly. These traits remain fairly consistent throughout one's life. The behavior of caregivers as they care for the baby can influence both positively and negatively the degree to which temperament will dictate behavioral style.

Common Health Problems

Various health problems in infancy may require the intervention of healthcare personnel. Gastroenteritis and food allergies are common. Skin disorders, such as diaper dermatitis (diaper rash), seborrheic dermatitis (infant dandruff), prickly heat rash, and thrush (infection of the oral mucous membrane by the fungus *Candida albicans*), also are common.

Safety concerns must be addressed during infancy. The relative immobility of the infant makes susceptibility to suffocation a possibility. The swallowing reflex matures progressively from birth, but until it is fully developed, aspiration is a risk. As the infant becomes more

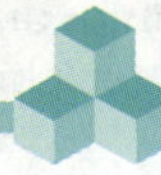

Examples of Nursing Diagnoses

Infancy Through School Age

The following are examples of nursing diagnoses that might be appropriate for the child from infancy through school age:

- Risk for Infection related to exposure to other children in childcare and at school
- Diarrhea related to milk intolerance
- Fluid Volume Deficit related to severe case of vomiting and diarrhea
- Risk for Suffocation related to parents' lack of knowledge of safety precautions
- Disorganized Infant Behavior related to environmental overstimulation
- Risk for Poisoning related to parents' lack of knowledge of proper storage of hazardous liquids
- Risk for Injury related to lack of knowledge about proper use of skates, bicycles, roller blades, and trampolines
- Self Esteem Disturbance related to physical abuse by caregiver

mobile, the risk of falls increases. Preventive measures against such safety hazards must be taught to new parents. In addition, the use of special car safety seats and restraints for infants is mandated by law in most states.

Several health problems in infancy are significant enough for further discussion. These are infant colic, failure to thrive, sudden infant death syndrome, and abuse.

Infant Colic. **Colic** is acute abdominal pain caused by spasmodic contractions of the intestine during the first 3 months of life. The exact cause of colic is not known, but the following factors have been associated with this problem: swallowing excess air, feeding too rapidly, overfeeding, ingestion of excess carbohydrates, overexcitement, allergies, emotional distress in the infant, and anxiety in the primary caregiver.

Failure to Thrive. **Failure to thrive** results in severely inadequate physiologic development (particularly height and weight) in an infant. This condition is thought to be related to disturbed infant–primary caregiver interaction. Although this relation appears to be present in most instances, underlying physical causes must first be ruled out. If the cause is deemed to be psychosocial, then the dynamics commonly involve inadequate nutritional intake related to caregiver ignorance and lack of concern for emotional nurturing. Specialized health intervention usually is warranted.

Sudden Infant Death Syndrome. **Sudden infant death syndrome** (SIDS) is the sudden death of an infant or a young child, unexpected by history, in which a post mortem examination fails to reveal a cause of death. The general risk is 2 out of every 1000 live births, with SIDS causing about one-third of all deaths between ages 1 week and 1 year. The highest incidence occurs in the 3rd and 4th months of life. Increased risk is found in families who are poor or live in crowded housing, during cold months of the year, and during infant sleep periods. Maternal health, smoking, and nutrition are all being investigated as contributing factors. It is now recommended that infants sleep on their side or back (rather than the stomach); this practice has reduced the number of deaths from SIDS.

Child Abuse. The incidence of reported cases of child abuse has increased dramatically and is a cause of national concern. Healthcare workers are in an excellent position to recognize families at risk and offer interventions.

Home Healthcare Alert

A child who has repeated or unreported injuries (abrasions, burns, swollen tissues, hematomas, dislocations, fractures) may be the victim of child abuse.

Role of the Nurse in Healthcare

The most essential role of the nurse in meeting healthcare needs of the infant is the prevention of illness and the promotion of wellness through teaching family members. Teaching may range from providing basic information about prevention of diaper rash to facilitating grieving in parents who have lost a baby to SIDS. Examples of specific areas of preventive teaching for parents of infants are given in Table 9-2.

Immunization against contagious diseases begins during the first year of life and should follow a regular schedule, as outlined in Table 9-3.

Toddler: 1 to 3 Years

From 1 to 3 years the child is considered a **toddler** (Fig. 9-3).

Physiologic Development

Physiologic development continues steadily during the toddler years, but the pace is considerably slower than that during infancy. Growth and development include the following:

Child Abuse

Child abuse is the "intentional nonaccidental physical or sexual abuse of a child by a parent or other caregiver entrusted with his or her care" (Freiberg, 1992, p. 176). Most child abuse begins in infancy. More than 1 million cases of child neglect or abuse are reported each year. When serious physical abuse that results in permanent injury or death occurs, the term battered child syndrome is used; fatal battering most often occurs in children under age 5. Sexual abuse accounts for about 20% of all reported child abuse, with 25% of sexual abuse being done to preschoolers.

Although abuse occurs in all ethnic groups and in all levels of society, certain factors increase the potential for abusive behavior:

- Parents under stress from unemployment, depression, poor social and marital relationships, substance abuse, or health problems
- Children who cry frequently, have sleep difficulties, wet the bed, are hyperactive or aggressive, who have difficult temperaments, or who have physical, emotional, or cognitive disabilities
- Lack of knowledge about parenting and normal behaviors of children
- Lack of family and social support for the caregivers

Health care professionals must recognize and report abuse of children and provide interventions for high-risk families. In some states, education about child abuse is mandated for nurses and other health care providers. In Canada, there is mandatory reporting of child abuse and maltreatment. The long-term treatment of abused children and their families is complex and multidisciplinary. A team approach may be used, most often using community health nurses, social workers, early childhood educators, and mental health professionals. Specific resources by state may be found in the publication (for purchase) *The National Directory of Children and Youth Services* from:

American Association for Protecting Children of the American Humane Society
9725 East Hampden Avenue
Denver, CO 80231

Table 9-2
Promoting Wellness in Infancy

Areas of Concern	Preventive Teaching
Accident prevention	• Associate common accidents to developmental abilities of the infant. • Encourage relaxed, slow feeding and regular "bubbling" (burping) to prevent aspiration. • Emphasize that bottles should not be propped and left with an unattended infant. • Emphasize the use of bumper pads and keeping crib sides up at all times to prevent injury related to bumping or falling. • Teach the correct usage of infant car seats. • Emphasize never leaving an infant unattended on a table, chair, or regular bed. • Teach proper positioning of infant for sleeping, and discourage the use of pillows to prevent suffocation.
Nutrition and feeding methods	• Assist the mother with the initiation and maintenance of breastfeeding. • If bottle feeding, provide information on the preparation of formula at feeding, expulsion of air from the bottle, nipple type and hole size, and positioning for an effective feeding experience. • Emphasize the significance of emotional nurturing during feeding. • Discuss the age at which solid foods are needed (ie, 5 to 6 months). • Discuss the sequence of solid foods (ie, cereals, vegetables, fruits, meats, and protein products).
Infections	• Encourage prompt attention for infections. • Encourage completion of required immunizations of infancy.
Hygiene and skin care	• Teach proper infant bathing techniques (ie, washing eye from inner to outer canthus, washing genitals last, umbilical cord care). • Discuss the proper use of creams, oils, and powders. • Describe the nature of infant skin and its susceptibility to disturbance. • Teach diapering and hygienic practices related to the disposal of products of elimination. • Teach care related to hair, nails, and genitals (particularly circumcised males).
Developmental performance	• Provide accurate information about development norms. This can prevent unrealistic expectations in caregivers and assist in isolating and treating developmental delays earlier.
Emotional attachment	• Encourage intimate child–caregiver contact in the crucial period immediately after birth. • Provide information about the sequence of normal attachment behaviors in infants. • Reassure concerned caregivers that attachment feelings occur at different rates for different caregivers and infants.

Table 9-3
Recommended Childhood Immunization Schedule: United States*

Vaccine	Age: Birth	2 mo	4 mo	6 mo	12[5] mo	15 mo	18 mo	4–6 yr	11–12 yr	14–16 yr
Hepatitis B[1]	HB-1									
		HB-2		HB-3						
Diphtheria, Tetanus, Pertussis[2]		DTP	DTP	DTP	DTP or DTaP at 15+ mo			DTP or DTaP	Td	
H. influenzae type b[3]		Hib	Hib	Hib	Hib					
Polio		OPV	OPV	OPV				OPV		
Measles, Mumps, Rubella[4]					MMR			MMR	or MMR	

*Vaccines are listed under the routinely recommended ages. *Shaded bars* indicate range of acceptable ages for vaccination.

[1] *Infants born to HBsAg-negative mothers* should receive the second dose of hepatitis B vaccine between 1 and 4 months of age, provided at least 1 month has elapsed since receipt of the first dose. The third dose is recommended between 6 and 18 months of age.

Infants born to HBsAg-positive mothers should receive immunoprophylaxis for hepatitis B with 0.5 mL hepatitis B immune globulin (HBIG) within 12 hours of birth, and .5 mL of either Merck & Co. vaccine (Recombivax HB) or SmithKline Beecham vaccine (Engerix-B) at a separate site. In these infants, the second dose of vaccine is recommended at 1 month of age and the third dose at 6 months of age. All pregnant women should be screened for HBsAg in an early prenatal visit.

[2] *The fourth dose of DTP* may be administered as early as 12 months of age, provided at least 6 months have elapsed since DTP3. Combined DTP-Hib products may be used when these two vaccines are to be administered simultaneously. DTaP (diphtheria and tetanus toxoids and acellular pertussis vaccine) is licensed for use for the 4th and/or 5th dose of DTP vaccine in children 15 months of age or older and may be preferred for these doses in children in this age group.

[3] *Three* H. Influenzae *type b conjugate vaccines* are available for use in infants: HbOC [HibTITER] (Lederle Praxis); PRP-T [ActHIB; OmniHIB] (Pasteur Mérieux, distributed by SmithKline Beecham; Connaught); and PRP-OMP [PedvaxHIB] (Merck & Co.). Children who have received PRP-OMP at 2 and 4 months of age do not require a dose at 6 months of age. After the primary infant Hib conjugate vaccine series is completed, any licensed Hib conjugate vaccine may be used as a booster dose at age 12 to 15 months.

[4] *The second dose of MMR vaccine* should be administered either at 4 to 6 years of age or at 11 to 12 years of age.

[5] *Vaccines recommended in the second year of life* (12 to 15 months of age) may be given at either one or two visits.

Approved by the Advisory Committee on Immunization Practices (ACIP), the American Academy of Pediatrics (AAP), and the American Academy of Family Physicians (AAFP), 1995.

- Rapid brain growth; increase in length of long bones of the arms and legs; growth of muscles
- Can use fingers to pick up small objects
- Can walk forward and backward, run, kick, climb stairs, and ride a tricycle
- Drinks from a cup and uses a spoon
- At age 2, is typically four times the birth weight, averaging 30 to 35 lb (13.6 to 15.9 kg) and 23 to 37 inches (58.4 to 94 cm) in height
- Is able to have bladder control during the day and sometimes during the night (2½ to 3 years)
- Can turn pages in a book and, by age 3, can draw stick people

Cognitive Development

The toddler is in Piaget's last two stages of sensorimotor development, thereby beginning to understand object permanence, following simple commands, and anticipating events. The toddler is able to understand self as separate from others, and the perception of body image begins. As part of body image development, several body parts can be identified and named, and gender identity is present.

Language begins at about age 1, with the use of single or bisyllable sounds. Around age 2, children begin to use short sentences.

Psychosocial Development

Based on psychosocial theories, the toddler has the following characteristics:

- Is in Freud's anal stage, as increased muscle development and sphincter control encourage the child to focus on the pleasure of sphincter contraction and relaxation. Freud believed that caregiver fixation on toilet training could result in adults who were either excessively messy or excessively clean.

Toddlers enter a stage of autonomy, promoting exploration.

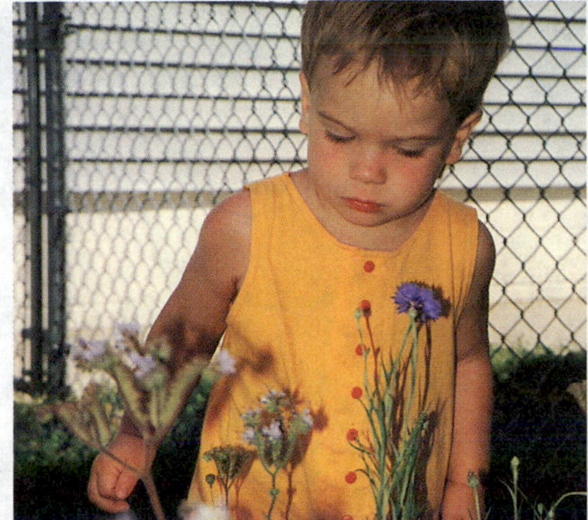

Play in toddlerhood may be solitary or parallel.

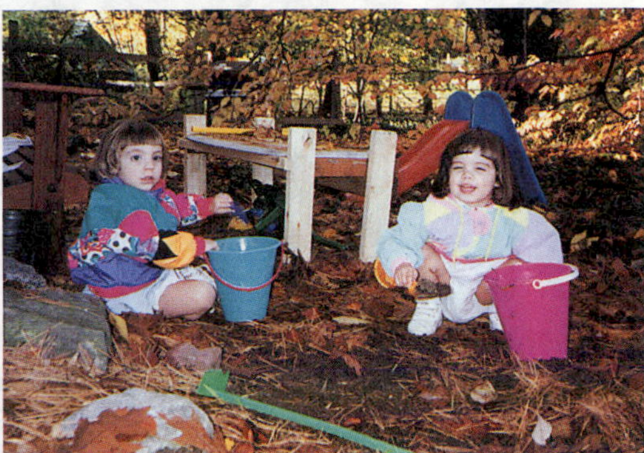

Toddlers start to see themselves as separate from others.

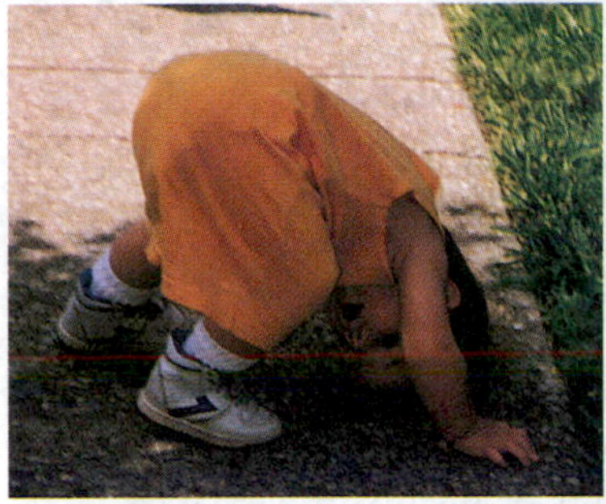

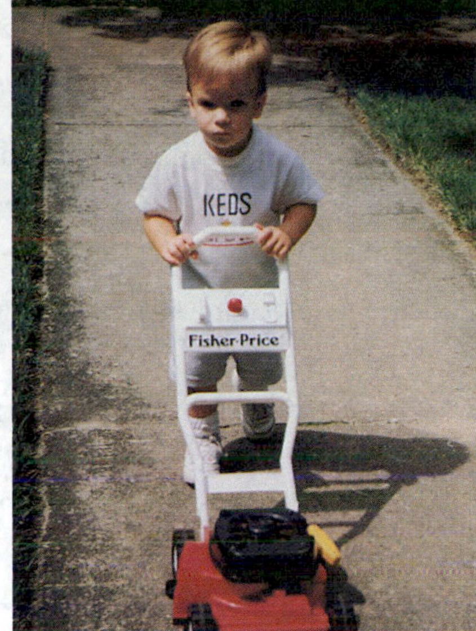

Cognitive development can be promoted by allowing the toddler the opportunity to observe and imitate.

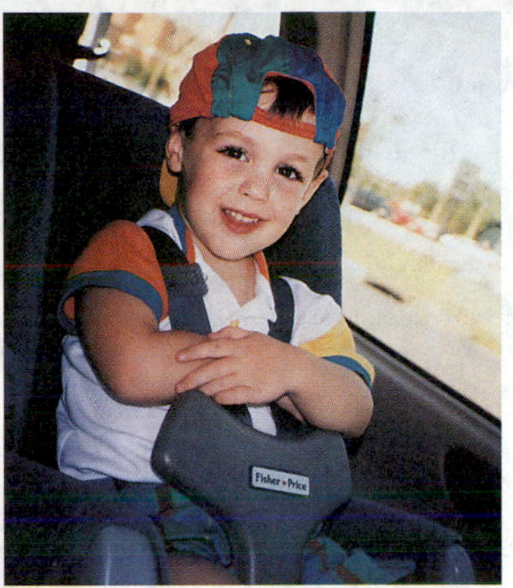

Safety becomes a common concern for caregivers.

Figure 9-3
Development in the toddler.

- Enters Erikson's stage of autonomy versus shame and doubt. Independence in feeding, walking, dressing, and toileting as well as the ability to verbally express wishes facilitate autonomy. Children who do not feel autonomous may be reluctant to explore and fearful of activities and people.
- Has the developmental task (Havighurst) of learning to control the elimination of urine and feces; begins to learn sex differences, form concepts, learn language, and distinguish right from wrong.

Toddlers may exhibit separation anxiety, negativism, and regression. **Separation anxiety** occurs when a child is afraid of being sent away from those people who are loved and serve as security. **Negativism** (characteristically expressed by saying no) is the result of the toddler's effort to have some measure of control over the environment. **Regression**, or behavior that is more characteristic of a younger age, can occur at any time in response to stressful circumstances. The most common regressive behaviors are excessive clinging to caregivers, loss of control over elimination, and the use of more infantile speech patterns.

Common Health Problems

Accidents, such as motor vehicle accidents, poisonings, burns, drownings, aspiration, and falls, remain the major cause of death in toddlerhood. Dental problems can occur, especially if the toddler is allowed to go to sleep with a bottle of milk or sweetened liquid in his or her mouth. Respiratory tract and middle ear infections are common. Some surgeries, such as repair of a cleft lip and palate, may be done in the toddler years. Surgery to repair most congenital anomalies is not done until later childhood.

Role of the Nurse in Healthcare

The role of the nurse in wellness promotion continues, as shown by the examples in Table 9-4. A significant part of teaching is in helping caregivers find the means of

Table 9-4
Promoting Wellness in Toddlerhood

Areas of Concern	Preventive Teaching
Accident prevention	• Explain how the autonomy needs of the toddler need to be met with an eye to safety. • Suggest locking poisons out of child's reach. • Suggest safety plugs for electric outlets. • Advise to block stairs with a gate and then help the child learn how to maneuver stairs. • Advise not allowing toddler to have small, hard food items, such as popcorn, peanuts, raw carrots, or hard candy, or balloons, which may cause aspiration. • Discourage the toddler from running with food in his or her mouth. • Encourage the proper use of car seats. • Advise never to leave the child unattended near water. • Suggest teaching toddler of dangers in clear, simple terms (eg, stove hot). • Advise against tossing child into the air or swinging child by the arms.
Toilet training	• Explain developmental tasks necessary for toilet training. • Correct misconceptions about mastery of this task. • Suggest some helpful literature for caregivers.
Negativism	• Help caregivers understand the normality of negativism in toddlerhood and its meaning from the child's point of view.
Feeding and nutrition	• Suggest that food be provided in forms the toddler can manipulate independently. • Advise caregivers to not be concerned about the messiness of toddler eating habits because the independence gained by the child is more important. • Provide soft finger foods that the child can eat while playing. • Reassure caregivers that short anorexic periods are common in toddlerhood.
Hygiene and dental care	• Emphasize the teaching of good hygiene habits (eg, handwashing after toileting or before eating). • Suggest teaching the toddler how to brush teeth (with assistance). • Encourage caregivers to take the toddler with them for dental appointments as an observer. Many dentists encourage this.
Infections	• Encourage caregivers to attend to respiratory tract infections promptly because of the high correlation between such infections and otitis media. • Encourage the completion of initial immunization schedule and any necessary boosters.
Play habits	• Encourage the selection of toys that emphasize gross motor skills and creativity. • Advise parents that sharing is not likely to occur and that parallel play is an important precursor to interactive play.

helping their toddler through encouraging health independence while setting firm limits.

Home Healthcare Alert

If toddlers or small children are in the house, ensure that all household cleaners are stored in areas the child cannot reach.

Preschooler: 3 to 6 years

At around age 3, the chubby toddler begins to give way to the leaner and better coordinated **preschooler**. Although growth and development are slower than in infancy and toddlerhood, they are still steady (Fig. 9-4).

Physiologic Development

The physical characteristics of the preschooler include the following:

- Head is close to adult size by age 6.
- Motor abilities include skipping, throwing and catching a ball, copying figures, and printing letters and numbers.
- Full set of 20 deciduous teeth is present, but baby teeth begin to fall out and are replaced by permanent teeth.
- Average weight at ages 5 to 6 is 45 lb (20.4 kg), with boys being slightly heavier than girls.

Cognitive Development

The preschooler is in Piaget's preoperational stage of development. Passing through the preconceptual and the intuitive phases, the child demonstrates the following transitional changes:

- Egocentrism decreases as socialization with other children increases and ability to express self verbally improves.
- Play is more related to real-life events (rather than fantasy).
- Basic curiosity results in constant questions and improved reason is more related to real-life events (rather than fantasy).

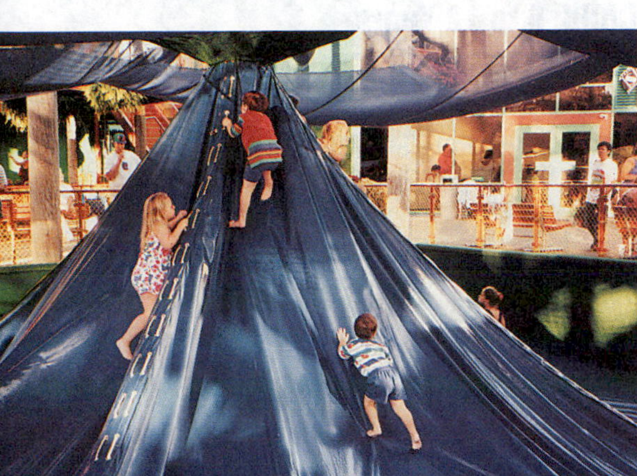

Preschooler play is associative and cooperative in its social dimension and cognitive development is demonstrated in constructive and pretend play.

Basic curiosity results in questioning and an improved reasoning ability in the preschooler.

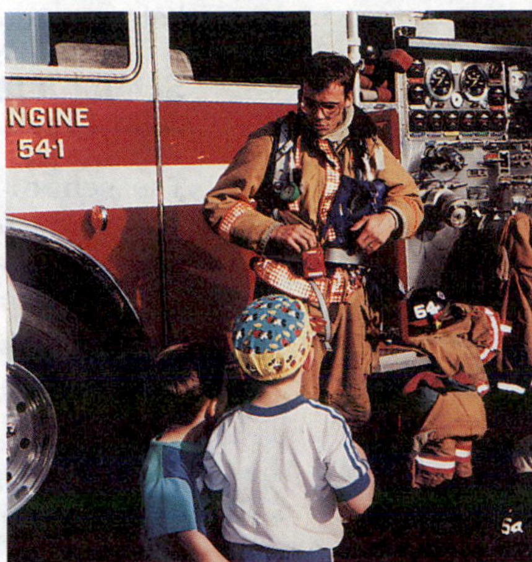

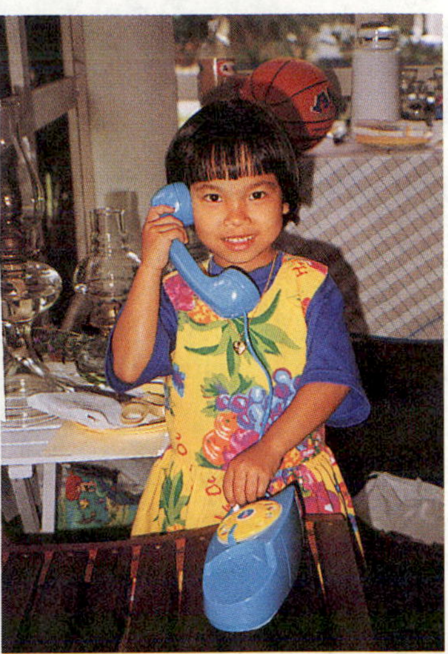

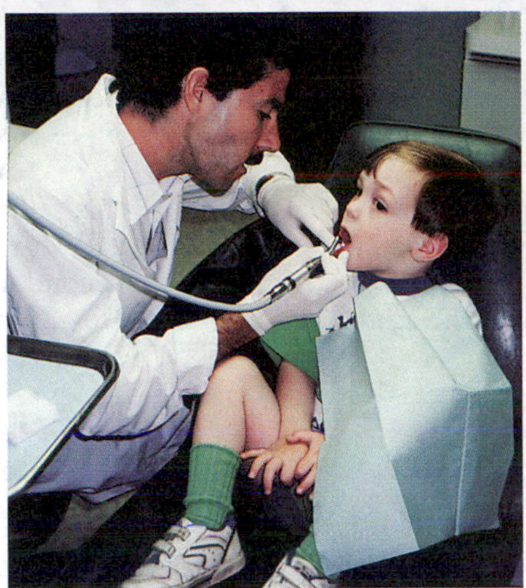

A visit to the dentist is useful for teaching dental hygiene and helps the preschooler overcome the fear of the unknown.

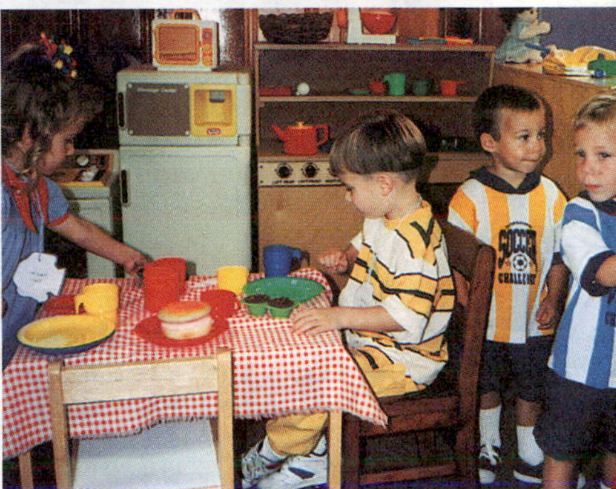

Symbolic play gradually becomes more related to real-life events.

Figure 9-4
Development in the preschooler.

- Basic curiosity results in constant questions and improved reasoning ability.

Language development is seen in more elaborate and grammatically correct sentences, with 6- to 18-word sentences becoming common by age 6. The incessant use of "why?" increases the child's knowledge, encourages further conversations, and develops language abilities.

Preschoolers clearly identify themselves as male or female, can understand basic body functions, and have a curiosity about sex differences. This curiosity often leads to "playing doctor," which is normal behavior for the age. Many children in this age-group want to look special or dressed up, and gain increased self-esteem through compliments about appearance.

Psychosocial Development

Based on psychosocial theories of growth and development, the preschooler has the following characteristics:

- Is in Freud's phallic stage, with the biologic focus primarily genital. The child has a sexual desire for the opposite-sex parent but, as a means of defense, strongly identifies with the same-sex parent; as a result of this conflict resolution, the superego and conscience begin to develop.
- Is in Erikson's stage of initiative versus guilt. Inner turmoil is created when natural curiosity is pitted against a constant examination of the propriety of one's actions by a rigid conscience. Realistic self-limits are learned through social interactions.
- Has four developmental tasks (Havighurst): to learn sex differences and modesty, to describe social and physical reality through concept formation and language development, to get ready to read, and to learn to distinguish right from wrong.

The preschooler often has fears. The primary task of becoming more socially oriented can cause many fears, with shyness and fear of new places common. Two other common fears during the preschool years are fear of the dark and fear of having nightmares, which often are made worse by the child's own fertile imagination and ability to fantasize. Support and validation of feelings by caregivers are essential.

Moral and Spiritual Development

Kohlberg's preconventional phase of moral reasoning dominates this age. The focuses of this stage for the preschooler are obeying rules to avoid punishment and obeying them because it is in one's self-interest to do so—for example, a reward will be forthcoming.

The cognitive, psychosocial, and moral development of the preschooler provide the base for spiritual development, as described by Fowler. The preschooler attends activities at church or synagogue with the family but does not understand the religious concepts. The concept of a deity is literal, with God being viewed as a human male. Imagination of concepts such as heaven, hell, and holy spirits is incomprehensible but often frightening.

Home Healthcare Alert

Lead poisoning is a risk for abnormal growth and development. Be alert for chipping and flaking paint, especially in older homes. Suggest an annual test for lead for every child between the ages of 6 months and 6 years.

Common Health Problems

Preschoolers continue to have health problems that are common in toddlerhood. Communicable diseases and respiratory tract infections are frequent, especially with increased interaction with other children at nursery schools and day care. Preschoolers are prone to accidents because of their increased curiosity about the world. Some congenital disorders, such as hypospadias, inguinal hernias, and cardiac anomalies, will require surgery at this time. Dental caries become common if teeth are neglected. As language becomes more sophisticated, speech disorders may become apparent.

Role of the Nurse in Healthcare

Table 9-5 provides examples of areas of concern and preventive teaching in promoting wellness in preschoolers. When caring for the preschool child who is scheduled for surgery or requires hospitalization, the nurse must recognize that fear of pain and body mutilation as well as separation anxiety are important considerations.

The nurse can allay some fears by explaining procedures in language the child can understand and by being honest about how much pain a procedure will cause. Many healthcare institutions and agencies have preprocedure visits for the child having surgery so that he or she can become familiar with the setting and with the activities that will be done. Allowing the child to practice procedures on a doll and encouraging the child to express feelings openly also are beneficial. Encouraging caregivers to take an active role in the child's care helps to reduce fear and separation anxiety.

School-Age Child: 6 to 12 Years

The **school-age child** from 6 to 12 years is sturdy, strong, and usually lean. Physical growth during this time is relatively slow but continues steadily, with both refinement and subtle changes taking place (Fig. 9-5).

Physiologic Development

Physiologic development of the school-age child includes the following:

- Brain reaches 90% to 95% of adult size; by age 12, the nervous system is almost completely matured, resulting in coordinated body movements.
- Motor abilities progress from the ability to hold a pencil and print words at age 6 to the ability to write in script and in sentences at age 12.
- Sexual organs grow but are dormant until late in this period, when hormonal changes begin.
- All permanent teeth are present, except for the second and third molars, by age 12.
- Height increases 2 to 3 inches (5.1 to 7.6 cm) and weight increases 3 to 6 lb (1.4 to 2.7 kg) a year.

Cognitive Development

The school-age child is at Piaget's concrete operational stage of development, organizing facts about the environment to use for problem solving. During this period, the child has the following characteristics:

- Thinks logically and develops concepts of mass, volume, weight, and measurement
- Deals best with actual objects and people, but relates concepts and compares events
- Uses inductive reasoning to solve new problems
- Generalizes about people, places, and things
- Develops classification systems
- Develops an awareness and understanding of other people's feelings and points of view
- Understands reversal of events

The school-age child has well-developed language skills, using language in a more sophisticated manner. The ability to store information in long-term memory and retrieve it in the remembering (recall) process is more efficient.

Body image, self-concept, and sexuality are interrelated. Sexual development results in a strong need to understand body function clearly and to have accurate information about sexuality.

Psychosocial Development

The psychosocial development of the school-age child is as follows:

Table 9-5
Promoting Wellness in Preschoolers

Area of Concern	Preventive Teaching
Accident prevention and safety	• Advise that preschoolers, now out of car seats, need to learn how to use seat belts. • Advise that clear boundaries regarding where tricycles or bicycles can be ridden need to be given. • Teach simple road safety (eg, looking both ways before crossing the street). • Encourage education of children regarding strangers and block parent programs. • Encourage education about sexual abuse (ie, explaining to child what is and is not appropriate touching by an adult). • Swimming lessons can begin and basic water safety taught. • Teach the dangers of matches, and practice home fire safety drills.
Infections	• Advise that these are an inevitable result of increased socialization. • Advise teaching children sound hygiene practices such as handwashing after toileting, correct disposal of tissues after use, nonsharing of items like eating utensils. • Keep immunizations current.
Sleep disorders	• Explain to caregivers the commonality of this problem among preschoolers. • Suggest that relaxed bedtime rituals and a night light can help. • Advise that comforting and warm reassurance are needed when a child is awakened by nightmares.
Dental hygiene	• Teach that preschoolers should be brushing their teeth and flossing with caregiver assistance. • Advise that a dental visit at this time is useful for teaching dental hygiene and overcoming fear of the unknown.
Play habits	• Advise caregivers that make-believe play and imaginary friends are common and normal in the preschool years. • Encourage caregivers to promote socialization through neighborhood play groups and nursery school.
Self-esteem	• Encourage caregivers to provide opportunities to make new discoveries and gain a sense of autonomy by experiencing neighborhood and preschool activities. • Advise to avoid frequent criticism and overprotectiveness. • Teach caregivers the importance of providing opportunities for the child to plan and carry out activities, and giving appropriate praise for accomplishments.

- Is in the latency stage of Freud's theory, with psychosocial energies being channeled toward strong identification with own sex
- Is in the industry versus inferiority stage of Erikson's theory, illustrated by the focus of the child on learning useful skills and thereby developing positive self-esteem. A sense of identity begins to emerge and values are integrated. The emphasis is doing, succeeding, and accomplishing.
- Has the following developmental tasks (Havighurst):
    - Learning physical game skills
    - Learning appropriate masculine or feminine social role
    - Developing fundamental skills in reading, writing, and calculating
    - Developing concepts necessary for everyday living
    - Achieving personal independence
    - Developing conscience, morality, and a scale of values

Peer relationships become the major gauge for determining status, skill, and personableness. Peer groups in middle childhood help prepare the child for getting along in the larger world and teach appropriate sex role behavior. They also act as transition modes for the child as he or she leaves the total caregiver influence and heads toward adult independence.

Moral and Spiritual Development

Most of the middle childhood years are spent in the conventional phase of moral development. Behavior is based on familial and peer group beliefs, and conformity to the norm is common. Following school regulations, respecting teachers, and viewing justice as a means of fair play are all important.

In Fowler's theory, school-age children view religious faith as a relationship that involves reciprocal fairness. They take part in rituals of their faith with a basic understanding of the rituals' significance. The importance of spiritual beliefs and the possibility of life after death are accepted, even if not totally understood.

Common Health Problems

Accidents continue to be common in the school-age child. With increased interactions with other children in school, communicable conditions such as scabies, impetigo, and head lice are more prevalent. Drug and alcohol abuse, although not as common as in adolescence, has been documented in children as young as age 8 (Salkind & Ambron, 1990).

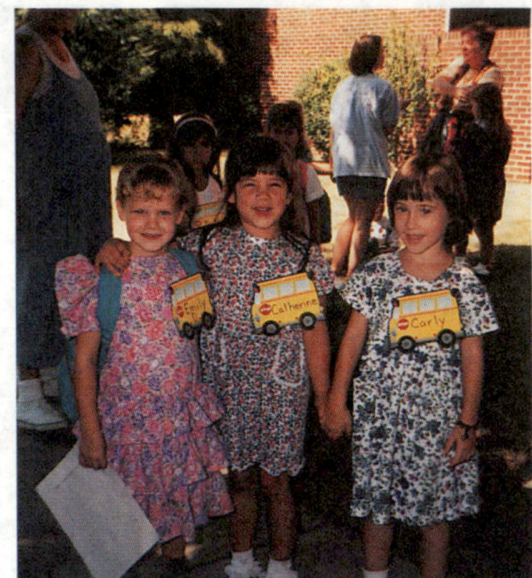

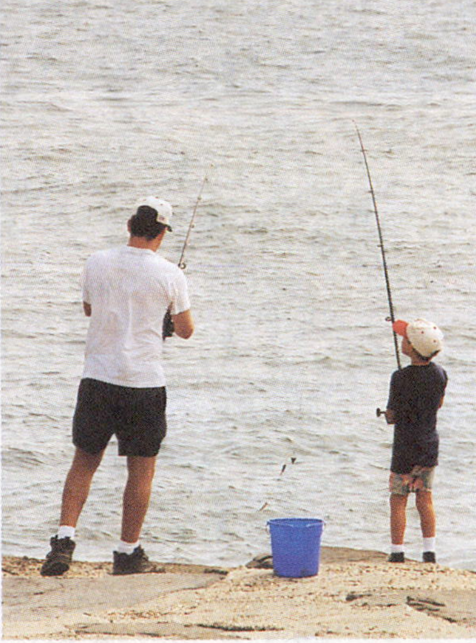

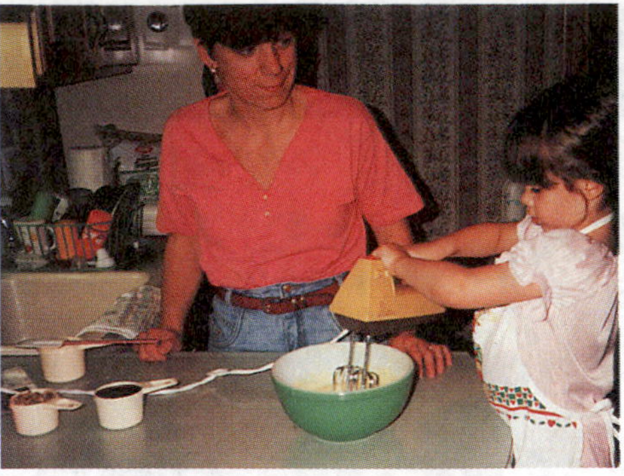

The school-age child has limited interest in members of the opposite sex, and strong identification with one's own sex is dominant.

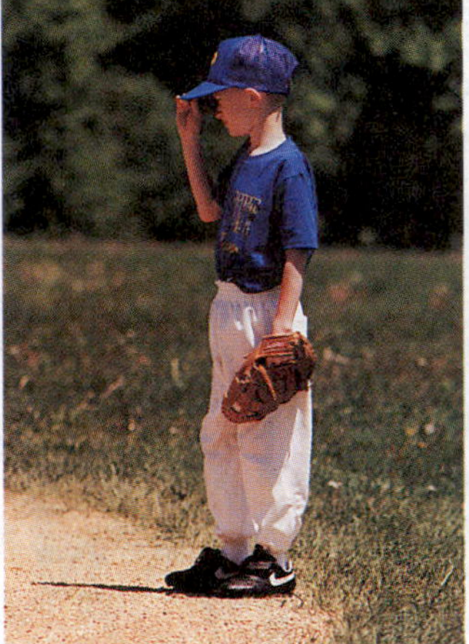

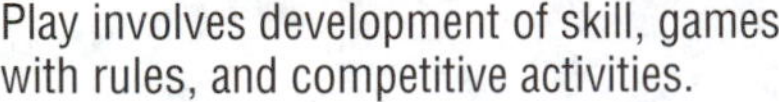

Play involves development of skill, games with rules, and competitive activities.

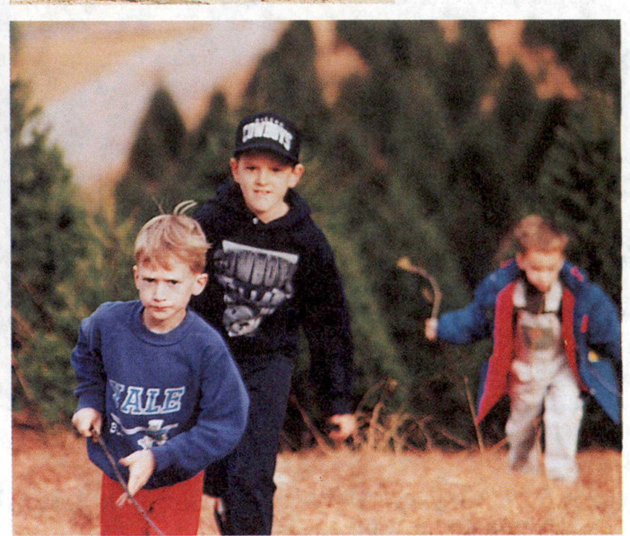

Figure 9-5
Development in the school-age child.

Role of the Nurse in Healthcare

The nurse's role in promoting wellness for the school-age child involves individual and family teaching, which may be conducted by the school nurse. Table 9-6 provides examples of nursing activities specific to this age-group.

Adolescence: 12 to 18 Years

The adolescent years are, among other things, a time of rapid physical growth, reproductive maturity, and emotional development (Fig. 9-6). This is a time of change as the child becomes an adult. Although a time span is defined, each person is different. Some people enter **adolescence** at age 11 or 12 and go on into the middle or late 20s; others enter at age 14 and end within a year (Freiberg, 1992). Physical, cognitive, and social factors are critical in determining the length of the adolescent period.

Physiologic Development

The changes that take place in the adolescent's body transform him or her from a child to an adult in appearance. The physiologic development includes the following:

- The feet, hands, and long bones grow rapidly, accompanied by an increase in muscle mass (especially in males).
- Primary and secondary development occurs, with maturation of the genitalia (Fig. 9-7); presence of body hair (Fig. 9-8); breast development (Fig. 9-9) and menstruation in females; facial hair growth, voice changes, and spermatogenesis in males.
- *Puberty* begins at age 10 or 11 for girls (with menstruation usually beginning between ages 11 and 14) and at age 12 or 13 for boys.
- Sebaceous and axillary sweat glands become active.
- Full adult size is reached, although some males may continue to grow into the 20s.

Table 9-6
Promoting Wellness in School-Age Children

Area of Concern	Preventive Teaching
Accident prevention	• Emphasize traffic safety. • Encourage the use of seat belts. • Emphasize bicycle, skateboard, and scooter safety. • Teach children to take water safety programs.
Communicable conditions	• Encourage proper hygiene habits, including not sharing personal items like combs. • Home visit may be required to discuss home health practices if a child has a communicable condition like pediculosis. • Advise of common treatment methods for conditions like scabies, impetigo, and pediculosis. • Teach about STDs, including AIDS.
Substance abuse	• Early preventive teaching about alcohol, nicotine, and street drugs that includes guidance for families is essential.
Sexuality	• Sex education needs to begin as early as age 7 or 8. • Families need encouragement to talk about sex at home. • Caregivers need encouragement to answer questions honestly and correctly. • Menstruation needs to be discussed by at least age 8 because some girls menstruate as young as age 9.
Mental health concerns: School phobia Depression and suicide	• Nurse needs to work with teachers and families so that they learn to recognize behavior that indicates mental health difficulties. • Nurse can provide referral for specialized assistance.
Physical fitness	• Teach good food choices that are lower in fat, salt, and sugar, but avoid strenuous dieting if child is overweight. An estimated 25% of all children are obese. • Emphasize the importance of physical activity: Children should exercise nonstop for at least 20 to 25 minutes three times a week.
Self-esteem	• Teach caregivers to encourage independent activities and social interactions, and to be sure that successes are greater in number than failures. • Provide the child with positive statements that demonstrate being valued, important, and loved.

A true assessment of adolescent development would be incomplete without an expansion of the profound changes in reproductive functioning. **Puberty**, which is the period of life when the ability to reproduce begins, can be divided into the following three stages:

Prepubescence: Secondary sex characteristics begin to develop but the reproductive organs do not yet function.

Pubescence: Secondary sex characteristics continue to develop and ova and sperm begin to be produced by the reproductive organs.

Postpubescence: Reproductive functioning and the development of secondary sex characteristics reach adult maturity.

The developmental occurrences at each stage are described in Table 9-7.

Cognitive Development

According to Piaget, adolescence is the stage when the cognitive development of formal operations is developed. Deductive, reflective, and hypothetical reasoning are possible, and abstract concepts can be handled. Long-term goals can be set as the concept of time, its passage, and the future become real. These abilities can make problem solving difficult for the adolescent, and challenging the decision making of adults is common. Egocentrism returns, and imaginary audiences and daydreaming are used.

Psychosocial Development

Based on developmental theories, the adolescent has the following characteristics:

- Is in Freud's genital stage. The libido reemerges in a mature, adult form. Freud believed that this new state upsets the delicate balance of the id, ego, and superego, so that intellectualization becomes the common mechanism used to justify behavior.
- Tries out different roles, personal choices, and beliefs, according to Erikson, in the stage called identity versus role confusion. Self-concept is being stabilized, with the peer group acting as the influential body.
- Has the following developmental tasks, defined by Havighurst:
  - Achieving new and maturer relationships with both males and females of the same age
  - Achieving a masculine or feminine social role

The prom is an opportunity to practice formal adult social skills among one's peers.

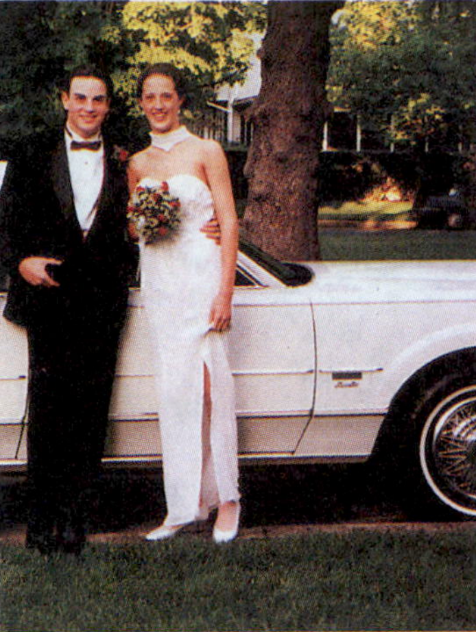

The development of self-identity in adolescence involves "trying out" different roles and self-images.

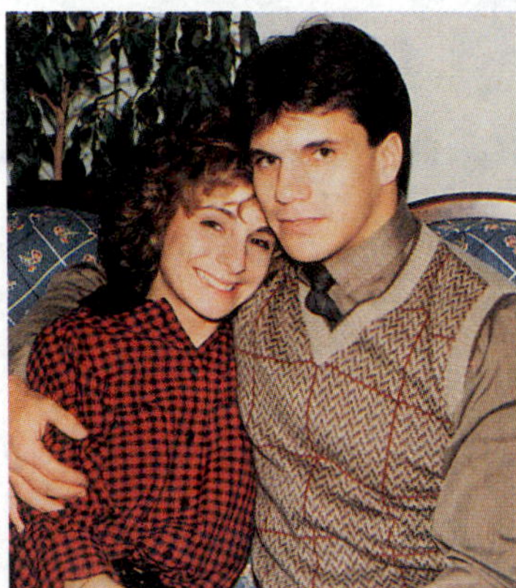

A primary developmental task of adolescence is to achieve new and more mature relationships with peers of both sexes.

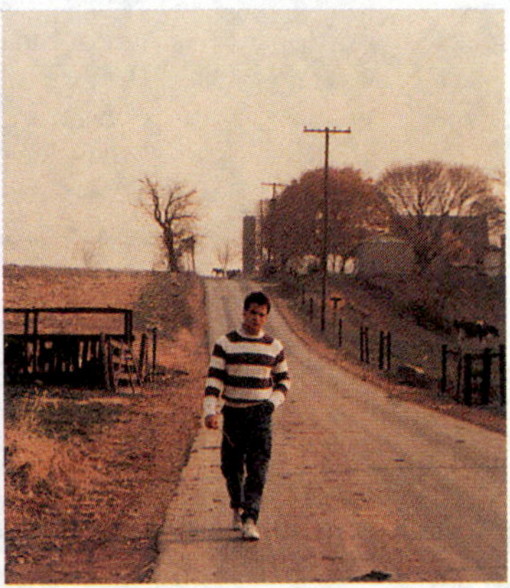

Athletic activities and skills are important in adolescence.

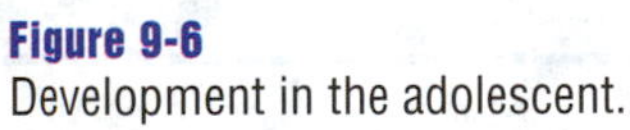

Figure 9-6
Development in the adolescent.

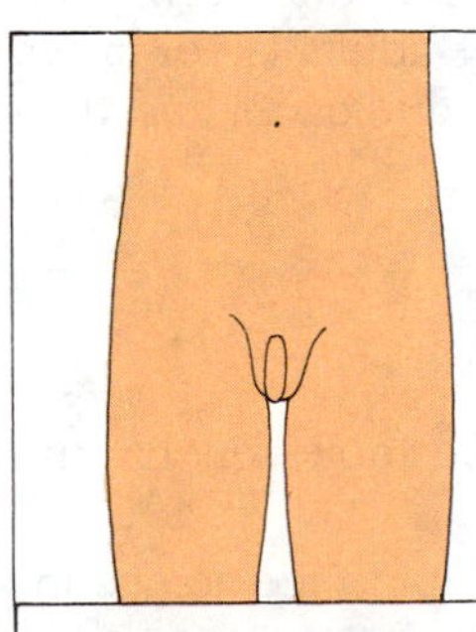	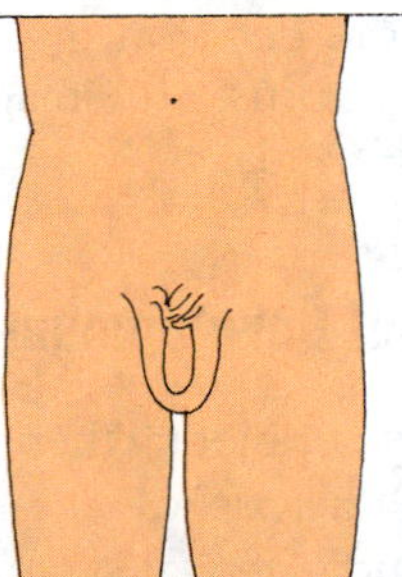	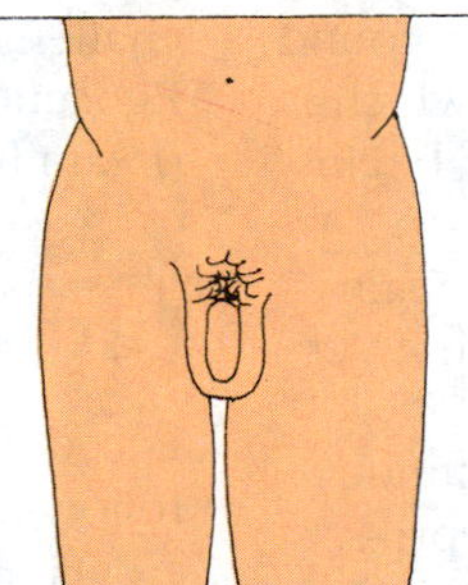	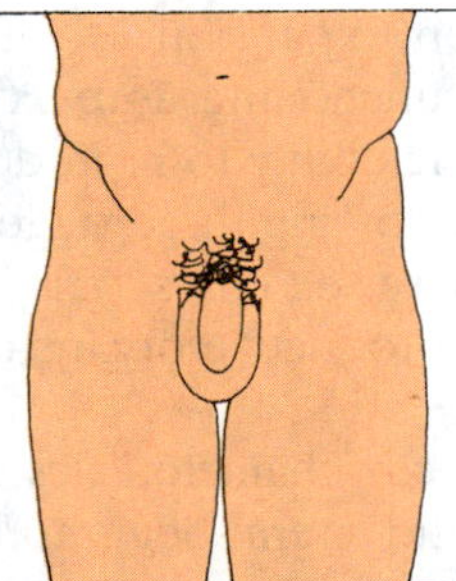	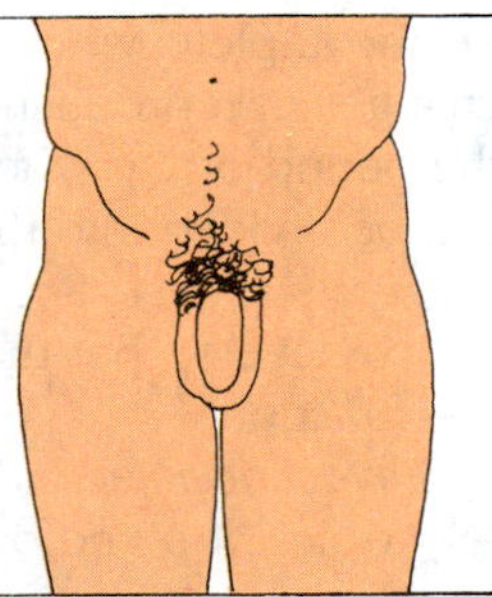
Stage 1 Preadolescent; genitals are the same size and proportion as childhood No pubic hair	Stage 2 Enlargement of scrotum and testes, but not penis; scrotal skin reddens and changes texture Sparse growth of downy, straight, slightly dark hair, chiefly at base of penis	Stage 3 Penis enlarges in length; further growth of scrotum and testes Darker, coarse, curly hair, beginning to spread out	Stage 4 Penis increases in breadth and growth of glands; darkening of scrotal skin Hair adult in type, but area covered smaller than in adult	Stage 5 Genitals adult in size and shape Hair adult in quantity and distribution

Figure 9-7
Maturational stages of male genital development.

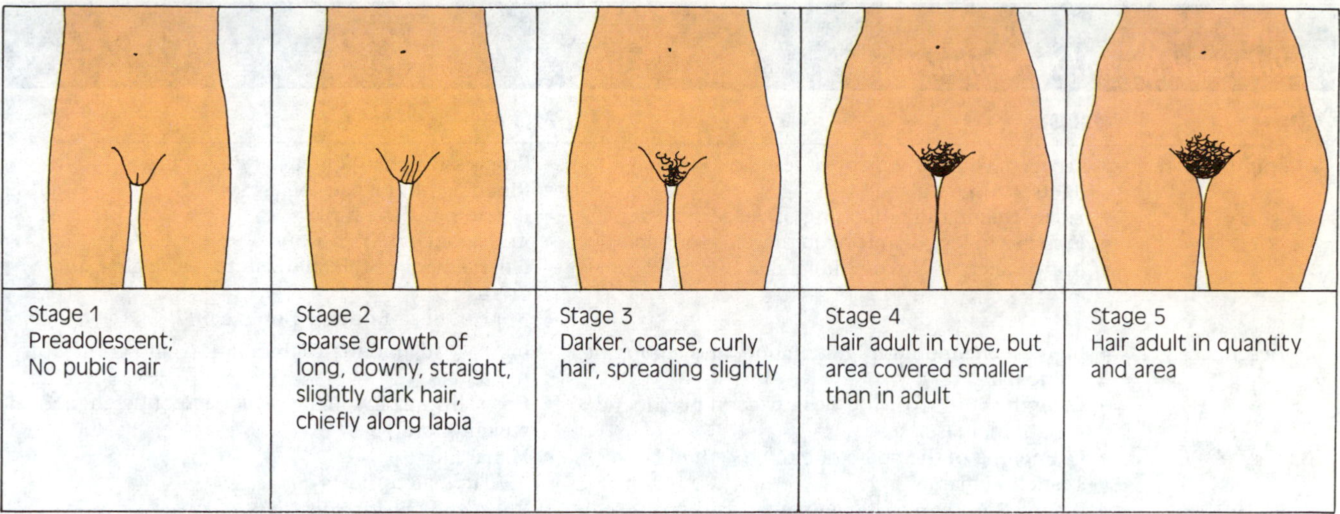

Figure 9-8
Maturational stages of female pubic hair development.

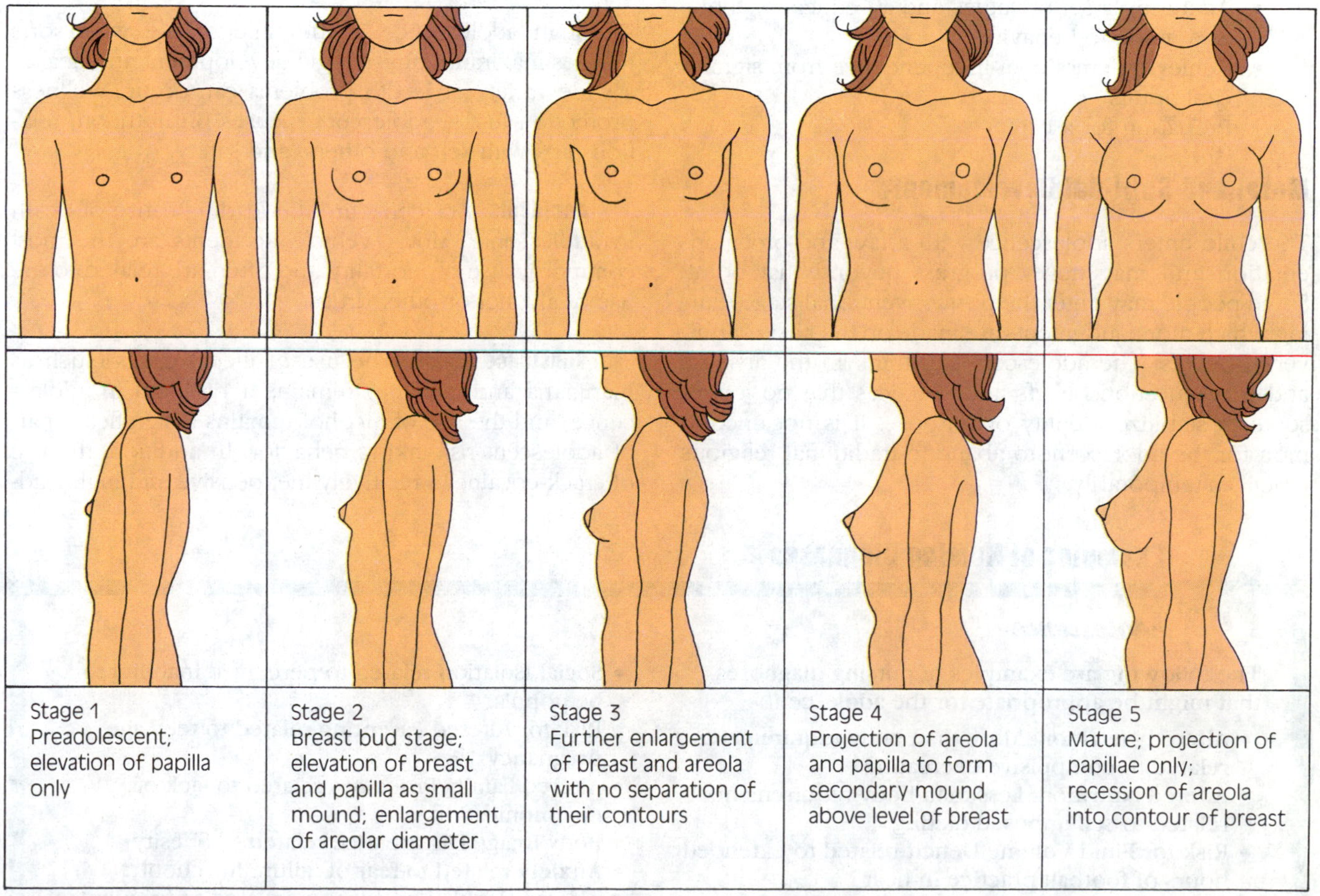

Stage 1	Stage 2	Stage 3	Stage 4	Stage 5
Preadolescent; elevation of papilla only	Breast bud stage; elevation of breast and papilla as small mound; enlargement of areolar diameter	Further enlargement of breast and areola with no separation of their contours	Projection of areola and papilla to form secondary mound above level of breast	Mature; projection of papillae only; recession of areola into contour of breast

Figure 9-9
Maturational stages of female breast development.

Table 9-7
Adolescent Sexual Development

Stage	Males	Females
Prepubescence	• Progressive enlargement of testicles, seminal ducts, prostate gland • Enlargement and reddening of the scrotal sac • Increase in length and circumference of penis • Appearance of downy pubic hair	• Progressive enlargement of the ovaries • Ripening of graafian follicles • Rounding of the hips • Appearance of breast buds • Enlargement of the fallopian tubes, vagina, and uterus • Appearance of downy pubic hair
Pubescence	• Increase in amount, pigmentation, and curling of pubic hair • Growth spurt involving peak pace of height and weight increase • Deepening of the voice due to growth of larynx • Testicles enlarge • Scrotum grows and its pigmentation increases • Penis grows in length and circumference • Spermatogenesis begins	• Increase in amount, pigmentation, and curling of pubic hair • Growth spurt involving peak pace of height and weight increase • Menarche • Axillary hair appears • Vulva and clitoris enlarge • Breast tissue develops • Ovulation begins
Postpubescence	• Completion of sexual growth and development • Fertility	• Completion of sexual growth and development • Fertility

- Accepting one's personal appearance
- Acquiring a set of values and an ethical system as a guide to behavior
- Achieving emotional independence from significant adults
- Preparing for a career

Moral and Spiritual Development

The child enters adolescence with a law-and-order orientation and may never progress beyond that point. Some people may enter the postconventional stage, during which moral judgments are made on the basis of universal beliefs. The adolescent can think in the abstract and may question beliefs and practices that no longer serve to stabilize identity or purpose. It is not uncommon for the adolescent to abandon traditional religious practices temporarily.

Common Health Problems

Although adolescence is the time of life when one reaches maximum physiologic development and health, a wide variety of health problems can occur. Wellness promotion in the adolescent focuses on nutrition, relationships with self and others, and safety.

Accidents. Accidents are the leading cause of death in adolescents. Motor vehicle accidents are the most common cause of mortality and often are related to the use of alcohol or other drugs.

Substance Abuse. The use of illegal drugs (such as marijuana and cocaine) remains a problem in adolescence, and the use of alcohol remains a significant part of adolescent risk-taking behavior. In addition, the use of crack-cocaine, a relatively inexpensive and highly ad-

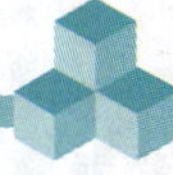

Examples of Nursing Diagnoses

Adolescence

The following are examples of nursing diagnoses that might be appropriate for the adolescent:

- Altered Nutrition: More than body requirements related to compulsive overeating
- Altered Nutrition: Less than body requirements related to self-imposed dieting
- Risk for Fluid Volume Deficit related to extended hours of football practice in heat
- Risk for Injury related to risk-taking behavior while driving
- Risk for Trauma related to lack of knowledge about water safety
- Social Isolation related to perceived inability to be popular
- Risk for Altered Parenting related to teen-age pregnancy
- Altered Family Processes related to lack of communication
- Body Image Disturbance related to obesity
- Anxiety related to fear of failure in school
- Altered Health Maintenance related to frequent use of alcohol and drugs

dictive drug, has reached epidemic proportions in many areas of North America.

Suicide. The suicide rate in adolescents has increased drastically over the past 30 years, with suicide being more prevalent in adolescents than in any other age-group. Suicide is the third leading cause of death in adolescence. Although girls attempt suicide more often than boys, boys are more likely to complete it. Depression is a possible contributing factor.

Home Healthcare Alert

Do not ignore verbal or nonverbal indicators of suicide in an adolescent. Make an immediate referral to someone trained in suicide intervention.

Pregnancy. The United States leads the developed countries in the number of pregnancies among adolescents aged 15 to 19 (Murray & Zentner, 1993). These pregnancies are physically, psychologically, and economically costly for the adolescent mother, the infant, the family, and society. Most adolescent mothers are poor, do not complete high school, and are at high risk for complications involving the pregnancy and the infant.

Nutritional Difficulties. Fad dieting and socialization that involves fast foods are common among adolescents. For those adolescents who are obsessed with body image (particularly females), severe eating disorders can result. The most common are anorexia nervosa (compulsive dieting to the point of self-starvation) and bulimia (a destructive cycle of binge eating followed by self-induced vomiting in an effort to prevent weight gain). The psychodynamics of these conditions are complex but almost always involve a negative self-concept. Although these disorders were once considered uncommon, 1 out of every 100 women and girls report symptoms of anorexia, and bulimia seems to be even more prevalent.

Sexually Transmitted Diseases. Adolescents who engage in sexual intercourse are at a higher risk for contracting **sexually transmitted diseases** (STDs) and their complications than are adults. Lack of knowledge, lack of psychosocial maturity, embarrassment, and the denial of the need to plan ahead and use condoms are the most common reasons for this increased risk. Gonorrhea is the most prevalent STD among adolescents of both sexes. Trichomonal and monilial infections, as well as human papillomavirus, are common in adolescent girls. Chlamydial infections occur in both sexes, as does syphilis and herpes simplex type II (genital herpes).

None of these STDs have such serious implications for individuals and society as a whole as acquired immune deficiency syndrome (AIDS) does. Although AIDS can be transmitted through means other than sexual contact (eg, blood transfusions and intravenous drug use), transmission is primarily through sexual intercourse. AIDS is a major cause of death in the world and its incidence is predicted to increase.

Role of the Nurse in Healthcare

Areas of concern in adolescence and preventive teaching activities are found in Table 9-8. Teaching often is done by the school nurse. Perhaps one of the more significant activities of the nurse during this period is that of facilitating healthy family relationships. Mutual respect, open communications, and accurate information exchange among family members pave the road for a healthy transition from adolescence to adulthood.

Table 9-8
Promoting Wellness in Adolescents

Area of Concern	Preventive Teaching
Substance abuse	• Advise adolescents of statistics about substance abuse. • Discuss the risks of substance abuse. • Discuss the physical consequences of substance abuse. • Discuss the psychosocial consequences of substance abuse. • Assist in preparing strategies for saying no to substance use.
Motor vehicle accidents	• Encourage driver education classes for adolescents. • Discuss the relation of alcohol consumption and motor vehicle accidents.
Suicide	• Assist teachers and caregivers to identify risk factors and data indicative of suicide risk (eg, decreased school performance, social withdrawal). • Advise adolescents with depression where to seek help (eg, psychiatrist, community clinics, crisis centers)
Nutrition	• Discuss healthy eating habits. • Discuss dangers of excessive or nutritionally unsound dieting. • Help caregivers and teachers recognize "risk" students. • Advise adolescents who legitimately need to lose weight to consult a physician or respected weight loss organization (eg, Weight Watchers).

(continued)

Table 9-8 *(continued)*
Promoting Wellness in Adolescents

Area of Concern	Preventive Teaching
Sex education	• Provide factual information about physical and psychosexual development. • Discuss the nature and prevention of STDs. • Discuss safe sex practices in relation to STDs, particularly AIDS. • Assist with developing strategies for saying no to sexual activity for those who wish. • If adolescent is or intends to become sexually active, discuss responsible sexual behavior and birth control. • Provide assistance to pregnant adolescents by: Discussing options Encouraging medical care Encouraging psychosocial counseling
Self-esteem	• Teach caregivers that normal behavior includes belonging to a peer group, the desire to be like everyone else, and trying on different roles (which may include hairstyles, clothing, and jewelry). • Keep lines of communication open. • Encourage caregivers to facilitate independence while providing love and consistent rules.

Key Points

- Heredity dictates an individual child's growth potential, whereas environment and nutrition influence the degree to which that potential will be reached.
- Growth and development in childhood begin rapidly, increase at a slower, steady pace in the middle, and end rapidly.
- The development of higher levels of moral and spiritual reasoning is directly related to higher levels of cognitive ability.
- The family is an integral part of a child's growth and development.
- Healthy development occurs if the tasks of each stage are completed before entering the next stage.
- The nurse's role in child healthcare is focused on preventive teaching.
- An understanding of childhood development is essential to understanding adulthood.

Bibliography

Bennett, E. G., & Woolf, D. (Eds.). (1991). *Substance abuse* (2nd ed.). Albany: Delmar.

Bhagat, R., & Shuster, S. (1995). Preschool health fairs. *Canadian Nurse, 91*(7), 49–50.

Bobak, I. M., Jensen, M. D., & Zalar, M. K. (1994). *Maternity and gynecologic care: The nurse and the family* (5th ed.). St. Louis: Mosby.

Cassetta, R. (1994). Children: A community in crisis. *American Nurse, 26*(10), 1, 20, 21.

Chambers, M. (1993). Play as therapy for the hospitalized child. *Journal of Clinical Nursing, 2*(6), 349–353.

Engle, W. (1973). The development from sound to phenome in child language. In C. A. Ferguson & D. I. Slobin (Eds.). *Studies of child language development*. New York: Holt, Rinehart, & Winston.

Erikson, E. (1963). *Childhood and society*. New York: Norton.

Freiberg, K. L. (1992). *Human development: A lifespan approach* (4th ed.). Boston: Jones & Bartlett.

Fuller, J., & Schaller-Ayers, J. (1994). *Health assessment: A nursing approach* (2nd ed.). Philadelphia: Lippincott.

Grindler, J., Hadler, S., Strebel, P., & Watson, J. (February 1995). Recommended childhood immunization schedule. United States—1995. *Clinical Pediatrics*, 66–72.

Klaus, M. H., & Kennell, J. H. (1982). *Parent–infant bonding*. St. Louis: Mosby.

Martin, L., Reeder, S., & Koniak, D. (1992). *Family, newborn and women's healthcare* (17th ed.). Philadelphia: Lippincott.

May, K. A., & Mahlmeister, L. R. (1994). *Comprehensive maternity nursing: Nursing process and the childbearing family* (3rd ed.). Philadelphia: Lippincott.

McCaleb, A., & Edgil, A. (1994). Self-concept and self-care practices of healthy adolescents. *Journal of Pediatric Nursing: Nursing Care of Children and Families, 9*(4), 233–238.

Murray, R., & Zentner, J. (1993). *Nursing assessment and health promotion: Strategies through the life-span* (5th ed.). Norwalk, CT: Appleton & Lange.

Myers, N., & Perlmutter, M. (1978). Memory in the years from 2 to 5. In P. Ornstein (Ed.). *Memory development in children*. Hillsdale, NJ: Erlbaum.

Nelson, K. (1973). *Structure and strategy in learning to talk*. Monographs of the Society for Research in Child Development, 38.

Quinn, A. (1993). Commentary on Erik Erikson: Ages, stages, and stories. *AWHONN's Women's Health Nursing Scan, 7*(6), 4.

Salkind, N., & Ambron, S. (1990). *Child development* (6th ed.). New York: Holt, Rinehart & Winston.

Sorensen, E. (1994). Daily stressors and coping responses: A comparison of rural and suburban children. *Public Health Nursing, 11*(1), 24–31.

Staff. (1994). School-based nursing fills gaps in adolescent healthcare. *American Nurse, 26*(10), 20, 37.

Struck, C. (1994). Women and children: Infant mortality, urban programs, and home care. *Nursing Clinics of North America, 29*(3), 395–408.

Thomas, A., Chess, S., and Birch, H. G. (1968). Temperament and behavior discussed in children. New York: New York University Press.

Waley, L., & Wong, D. (1995). *Nursing care of infants and children* (5th ed.). St. Louis: Mosby.

Chapter 10

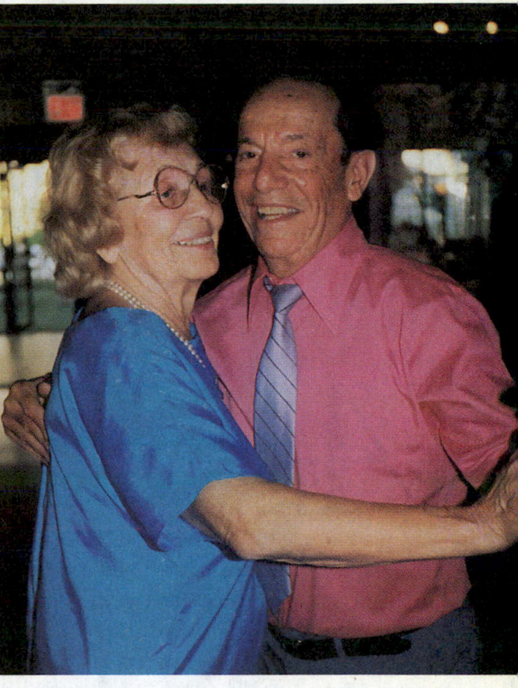

Early, Middle, and Older Adulthood

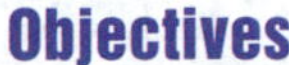

Objectives

After studying this chapter, the learner should be able to:

Define key terms used in the chapter.

Discuss the adult development theories of Gould, Levinson, and Erikson.

Discuss developmental tasks of the older adult, as described by Erikson and Havighurst.

Summarize major physiologic, cognitive, psychosocial, moral, and spiritual developments of early, middle, and older adulthood.

Compare physiologic and functional changes that occur with normal aging.

Identify socioenvironmental factors in our society that may inhibit the older adult from meeting needs and realizing potentials.

Discuss nursing implications concerning the continued growth and development of the adult.

Describe common myths and stereotypes that perpetuate ageism.

Describe the healthcare needs of the older adult in terms of chronic illnesses, accidental injuries, and acute care needs.

List family and community resources that can be used to maintain the health and independence of the older client.

Key Terms

ageism
alternative care
Alzheimer's disease
dementia
frail-old
functional health
gerontologic nursing
gerontology
life review
middle adult
older adult
old-old
reality orientation
reminiscence
social isolation
sundowning syndrome
young adult

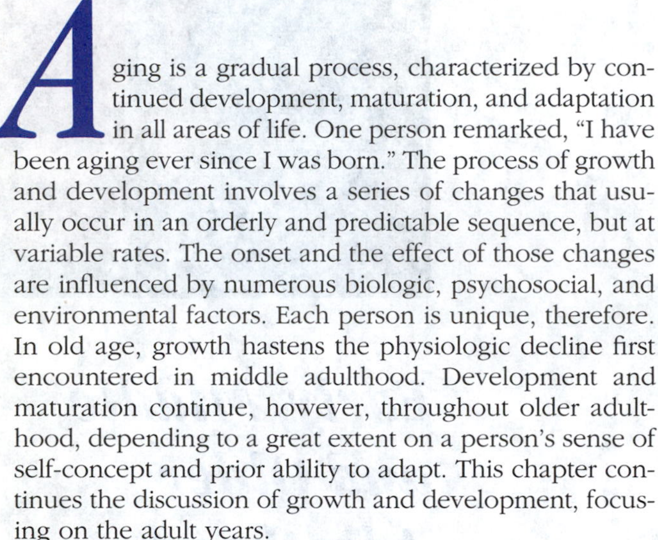

Aging is a gradual process, characterized by continued development, maturation, and adaptation in all areas of life. One person remarked, "I have been aging ever since I was born." The process of growth and development involves a series of changes that usually occur in an orderly and predictable sequence, but at variable rates. The onset and the effect of those changes are influenced by numerous biologic, psychosocial, and environmental factors. Each person is unique, therefore. In old age, growth hastens the physiologic decline first encountered in middle adulthood. Development and maturation continue, however, throughout older adulthood, depending to a great extent on a person's sense of self-concept and prior ability to adapt. This chapter continues the discussion of growth and development, focusing on the adult years.

Adult Developmental Theories

Theories have been developed to describe adult growth and development. Included here is a summary of the theories most commonly used for the young and the middle adult.

Erikson's Developmental Crises

Erikson (1963) describes two major crises, with related tasks, for the early and the middle adult. They are summarized in Table 10-1. If the developmental tasks are not accomplished and the crisis is not resolved, the young adult becomes isolated and self-absorbed; the middle adult experiences a sense of stagnation and loss. Adults who do not achieve the tasks satisfactorily tend to focus on themselves, becoming overly concerned with their physical and emotional health needs.

Levinson's Individual Life Structure

Levinson and coworkers (1978) based their theory on what they call "individual life structure," centered around the belief that the pattern of life at any point in time is formed by the interaction of three components—the self (values, motives), the social and cultural aspects of one's life (family, religion, career, ethnic background), and the particular set of roles in which one participates (eg, husband, daughter, friend, student). When anything changes in one component, the whole life structure must then reorganize. According to Levinson, the major periods in young and middle adult life are as follows:

Early adult transition (ages 18 to 22): The major concerns are to break away from one's family, make initial career choices, establish intimate relationships, and select personal values, goals, and lifestyle.

Entering the adult world (ages 22 to 28): The person now builds on previous choices; there may be a transient quality to occupational choices and friendships.

Settling down (ages 30 to 40): The person invests energies in those areas of life most important personally (family, work, community) and strives to gain status, respect from others, and a sense of authority.

Midlife transition (ages 40 to 45): At this time of life, there is a reappraisal of goals and values. The person may choose to either continue or reorganize and change the established lifestyle.

Pay-off years (ages 45 to 65): This is a time of maximum influence, self-direction, and self-approval.

Gould's Transformation

Gould (1972) believes that a central theme for the adult years is "transformation," with specific beliefs and developmental phases. According to this theory, adults exhibit the following characteristics:

Ages 18 to 22: They believe that they have established control of themselves but could be pulled back into the family.

Ages 22 to 28: They feel established as adults and separate from the family but believe that they must demonstrate their competence as independent adults to their parents. They want to enjoy the present but also build for the future.

Ages 29 to 34: They no longer perceive the need to prove themselves and become more accepting of self. Marriages and careers are well established, but questions about life in general are present.

Table 10-1
Developmental Tasks of Early and Middle Adulthood

Young Adult (20–30 years)	Middle Adult (40–60 years)
Stage/Crisis	
Intimacy versus isolation	Generativity versus stagnation
Tasks	
• Selecting a life partner • Choosing an occupation or a career • Establishing independence from parents • Establishing intimate relationships • Establishing a social network • Forming a personal philosophic and ethical structure	• Establishing and guiding the next generation • Accepting middle-age changes • Adjusting to the needs of aging parents • Being comfortable with spouse • Reevaluating goals and accomplishments

Ages 35 to 43: They continually look inward and question self, values, and life. They see time as having an end, and believe that there is little time left to shape the behavior of adolescent children.

Ages 43 to 50: They believe their personalities are set. They accept life span as having definite boundaries. They have a special interest in spouse, friends, and community.

Ages 50 to 60: They have decreased negativism and increased feelings of self-satisfaction. Spouses become valued companions. There is a realization of mortality and a concern for health.

Although theorists divide adult life into various age-groups by developmental stages and tasks, it is fairly common to use two major adult age-groups. The remainder of the chapter deals with the young adult (ages 20 to 40) and the middle adult (ages 40 to 60). Changes and special needs of older adults are discussed later.

Early Adulthood: The 20s and 30s

The young adult is considered to have reached maturity—to have completed physical growth and to have developed internal and external controls and values acceptable to society. There are no specific measurements of maturity of the average adult person. Each person is an individual, and a wide range of normal values and behaviors are considered healthy.

Physiologic Development

The young adult has well developed and coordinated organ systems, functioning at peak efficiency. Although some normal changes begin to take place during the latter part of the period, for the most part, physical changes are minimal. The major exception is in the pregnant woman. Table 10-2 compares the physical development of the early adult with that of the middle adult.

Psychosocial Development

Although physical growth and development are minimal, there are major psychosocial developmental requirements for the young adult. Included in psychosocial development are the major tasks of vocational and relationship choices (Fig. 10-1).

Choosing a Vocation. The decision to enter the world of work is strongly influenced initially by the need to become independent of one's family and to be self-sufficient. The choice of an occupation or a career also is guided by the desire to get married, to raise a family, and to become part of the community.

Occupational and career choices are largely tied to educational choices. Many careers necessitate education beyond high school level. Adults learn from both informal and formal experiences, and are largely goal-directed learners. If the identified goals are to increase career opportunities, maintain financial stability, and pursue upward mobility, the adult will be motivated to learn and change. The major factor in achieving satisfaction with one's vocational choice is the belief that one is functioning to capacity and making a contribution to society.

Choosing Relationships. The developmental tasks of the young adult are centered on choosing a mate and establishing a family. In today's society, an increasing number of young adults choose to remain single or to live together in heterosexual or homosexual relationships. The accepted societal norm is still to fall in love with a member of the opposite sex, get married, and establish a family.

Cognitive, Moral, and Spiritual Development

The young adult has the ability to solve problems and carry out logical reasoning. The ability to learn is enhanced throughout adult life by educational and life experiences. The young adult, as compared with the adolescent, is creative in thought, objective, realistic, and less self-centered. Although learning takes place in var-

Table 10-2
Physiologic Development: Early and Middle Adult

Assessment	Early Adult	Middle Adult
General body structure	• Weight evenly distributed (wide normal individual variations)	• Fatty tissue redistributed; men tend to develop abdominal fat, women thicken through the middle • Weight gain
Skin and hair	• Skin smooth with decreased acne • Hair resilient and evenly distributed	• Dry skin • Wrinkle lines appear on the face • Gray hair appears • Men may begin to lose hair on the head
Cardiovascular	• Well developed with peak efficiency	• Cardiac output starts to decrease • Increased fatigue
Musculoskeletal	• Maximum tone, strength, coordination	• Gradual decrease in muscle mass, strength, and agility • Loss of calcium from bones, especially in postmenopausal women
Sensory	• Normally full visual and hearing acuity	• Changes in visual acuity, especially for near vision (presbyopia) • Diminished hearing acuity, especially for high-pitched sounds
Reproductive	• Fully developed • Females have regular menstrual cycles • Males' sexual maturity remains at a peak	• Decreasing hormone production resulting in menopause or andropause

ious settings, the young adult often actively seeks formal educational opportunities, both as a post–high school choice and as a means of changing directions in careers.

Young adults who have satisfactorily mastered previous levels of moral development (as defined in Chapter 8) enter the conventional level. At the conventional level, the person is concerned with maintaining expectations, and values conformity, loyalty, and social order. An estimated 80% of adults do not move beyond this stage or do so only as middle adults (Murray & Zentner, 1993).

Spiritually, the young adult focuses on reality and may ask questions about spirituality. This individuating–reflective period (as defined by Fowler) brings discovery of the meaning of values as they relate to the achievement of social purposes and to the acceptance of the value systems of others.

Common Health Problems

The 20s and 30s normally are a time of good health, but physical and emotional problems can result from lifestyle, developmental, or situational crises; family history; and the environment. Even if an illness does not appear at this age, the person is at increased risk later in life.

Lifestyle Risks. Various risk factors are present in the way a young adult chooses to live. Some actual and potential health hazards of lifestyle are as follows:

Violent death: Accidents are the leading cause of death in young adults; suicide ranks third. Alcohol is associated with most motor vehicle accidents.

Relationships: Sexual experimentation and changing social values may result in unwanted pregnancy or STDs. STDs include genital herpes, gonorrhea, syphilis, and AIDS.

Drug abuse: Drug abuse is a major threat to the health of young adults. Prolonged use of various substances can cause death, physical and emotional problems, and disease. Commonly abused substances are nicotine, alcohol, marijuana, amphetamines, and cocaine.

Diet and exercise: Young adults require fewer calories than adolescents because growth is completed. Fast foods and busy lifestyles often are a way of life, resulting in increased caloric intake and minimal exercise. As a result, obesity can become a health problem.

Developmental or Situational Stressors. The young adult has to deal with many stressors as a result of choices about lifestyle, occupation, and relationships. Family-centered stressors may be related to both positive and negative factors: marriage, divorce, parenthood, death of a parent. The increased stress may precipitate mental or physical health problems, aggravated by ineffective coping mechanisms such as substance abuse, child abuse, spouse abuse, decreased nutrition and rest, and risk-taking behavior. Problem areas for the young adult include the following:

- An increasing number of men and women are choosing to remain single. This singlehood status has advantages and disadvantages. Being single gives one the freedom to come and go as one chooses, to have more autonomy, and to spend money and time as one wishes. On the other hand, external pressures to marry and the desire for love,

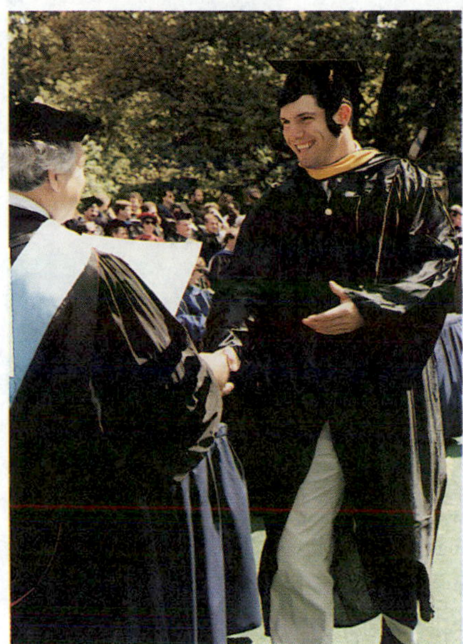

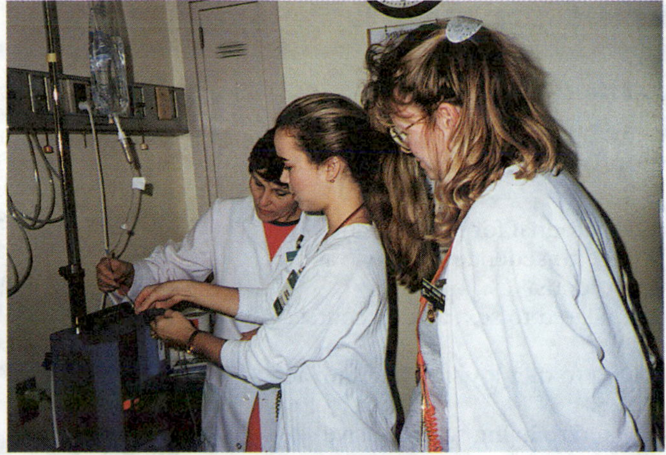

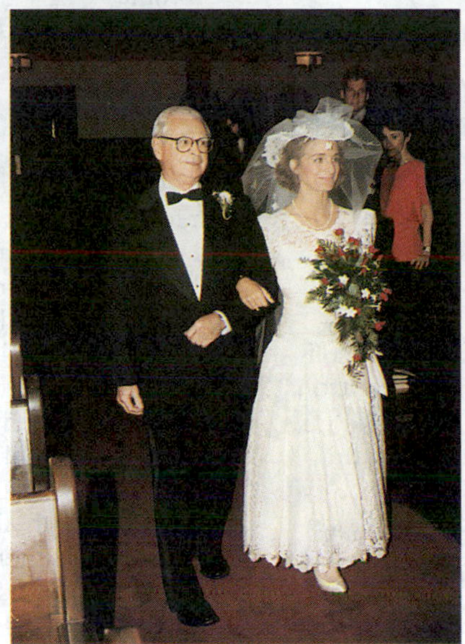

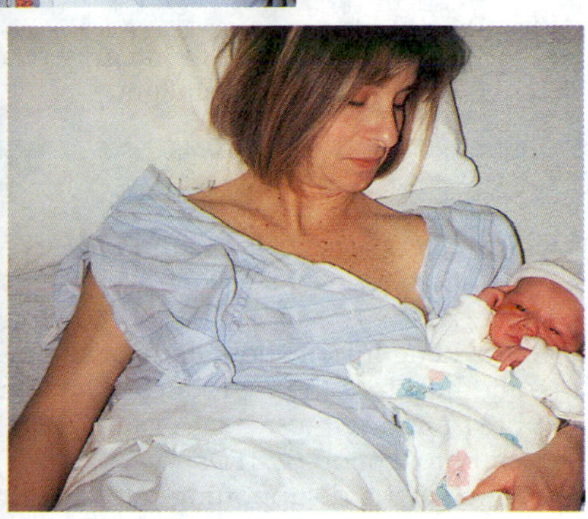

Figure 10-1
Developmental tasks of the young adult center on establishing intimate relationships and a home and getting started in an occupation.

to belong, and to raise a family may make the young adult question the decision to remain single.

- The decision by young married couples to have children may be delayed until careers are established, or there may be no children by choice. If children are desired, infertility (the inability to conceive after 1 year of coitus without contraception) may add even more stress.
- Divorce is common in our society, with rates being highest for those marrying young, having low income, and having low educational levels. It separates children from their families, has long-term emotional costs, and increases the number of single-parent families headed by women.
- Women who are married, have a job or career, and have a family must contend with multiple roles. The desire to be superwoman and do all things well is physically and emotionally exhausting. Women who have postponed having children may realize in their middle to late 30s that their so-called biologic clock is winding down; an increasing number of women in this age group are having a first child.

Family History. A family history of chronic diseases such as hypertension, heart disease, and diabetes increases a person's risk of developing the disease.

Environment. The young adult may be exposed to environmental pollutants at work. There is an increased risk of becoming ill or injured because of economic difficulties, poor housing and hygiene, and increased probability of accidents. Additionally, the young adult, actively spending leisure and work time in contact with others, increases his or her exposure to acute infectious disease.

The Nurse's Role in Healthcare

Many activities that promote health are discussed in Chapter 2. As with any client, the nurse must consider each young adult as an individual, taking a holistic view of special needs and influences on health maintenance. Nursing considerations specific to the young adult are as follows:

- Teaching the need for regular physical examinations and dental care, including screenings for diseases most common to this age

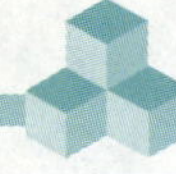

Examples of Nursing Diagnoses

Young to Middle Adult

The following are examples of nursing diagnoses that might be appropriate for the young to middle adult:

- Altered Nutrition: Potential for More Than Body requirements related to sedentary lifestyle and primary diet of fast foods
- Risk for Infection related to sexual intercourse without condom use
- Constipation related to diet low in fiber and lack of exercise
- Risk for Injury related to living with abusive person
- Risk for Impaired Skin Integrity related to frequent exposure to sunlight
- Altered Role Performance related to loss of job
- Sexual dysfunction related to abuse of alcohol and drugs
- Caregiver Role Strain related to constant care of aging parents
- Ineffective Denial related to continued use of nicotine despite family history of lung cancer
- Situational Low Self Esteem related to recent divorce
- Post-trauma Response related to recent rape trauma
- Fear related to diagnosis of cancer

- Teaching preventive health practices related to nutrition, rest, substance use, and stress-related illnesses
- Providing information about sexuality, pregnancy, and health of the reproductive system through self-breast and self-testicular examination, birth control, and prevention of STDs
- Providing and supporting safety education in the workplace and in activities of daily living

Acute illness in the young adult is more of an annoyance than of serious consequence. If the young adult is hospitalized, motivation to recover and to resume normal activities is strong. The nurse must remember that independence and self-sufficiency are important to the young adult; the dependent sick role is not easily accepted. Healthcare will be facilitated if the young adult is informed and involved in decisions about care.

Although chronic illnesses are less common, their occurrence in the young adult can lead to delayed development, loss of independence, and permanent changes in personal and career goals.

Middle Adulthood: The 40s and 50s

The middle adult years are a time of change in both physical and psychosocial dimensions. The changes are gradual and individualized. As the normal life span increases, most people in this age-group still consider themselves young in relation to the older population. Visible signs of aging and an awareness of time left to live, however, make the middle adult evaluate achievement of goals and influence adaptation to older age.

Physiologic Development

The early years of this period of life are marked by maximum physical development and functioning. As time passes, gradual physiologic changes—both internal and external—occur. These are not pathologic changes, but rather normal changes that result from aging. Self-image and self-concept must be altered to adapt successfully to and accept these normal changes. The physical development of the middle adult is outlined in Table 10-2.

The hormonal changes that take place in midlife affect men and women differently. Women undergo a change called menopause, a gradual decrease in ovarian function, with subsequent depletion of estrogen and progesterone. This change usually occurs between ages 40 and 55. With the cessation of ovulation, menstrual periods stop (either gradually or abruptly); many women also experience hot flashes, mood swings, and fatigue. The whole process lasts for several years, and on completion, the woman is no longer able to become pregnant. Men do not have physical symptoms from the decreased levels of hormones, called andropause. Androgen levels diminish slowly; the man may have some loss of sexual potency but is still capable of reproduction.

Psychosocial Development

The middle adult years usually are a time of increased personal freedom, economic stability, and social relationships. They also are a time of increased responsibility and an awareness of one's own mortality (Fig. 10-2). One is faced with the realization that half of one's life is over and many things are still undone. This realization can lead to developmental crises and situational stressors.

Role Transition. Various changes can take place during the middle years. These changes include changes in relationships within a marriage, with children who are becoming adults, and with aging parents.

Relationships with one's spouse may go through contrasting changes. Although this usually is a time of security and stability, with stronger emotional commitment and sharing, it also may be a time of disenchantment. The husband or wife may develop negative, critical feelings and attitudes as a result of changes in physical appearance, energy levels, and sexual needs and abilities. Dis-

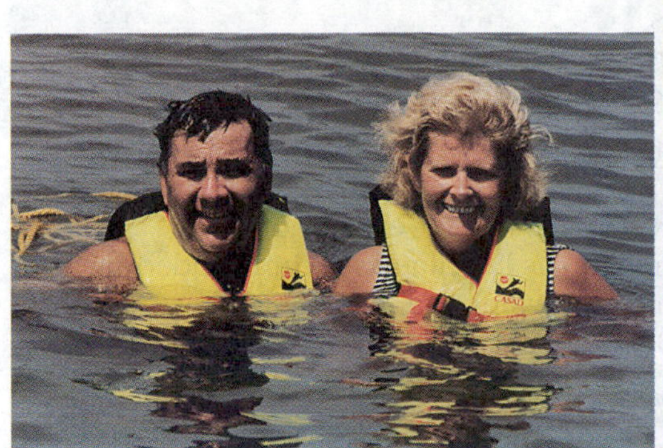

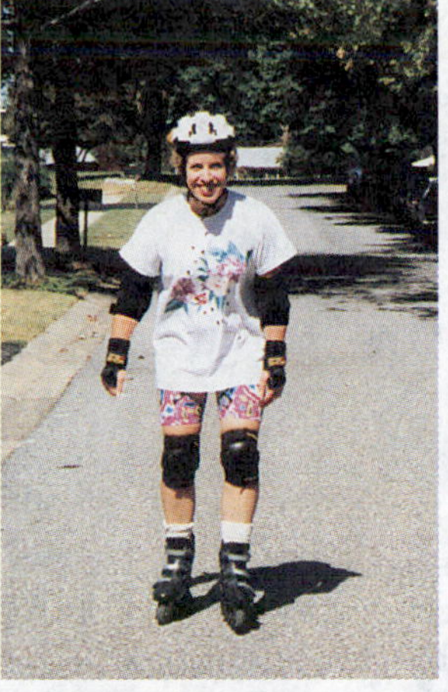

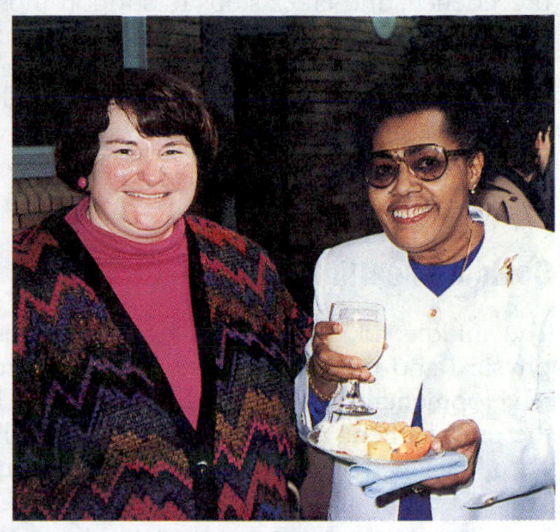

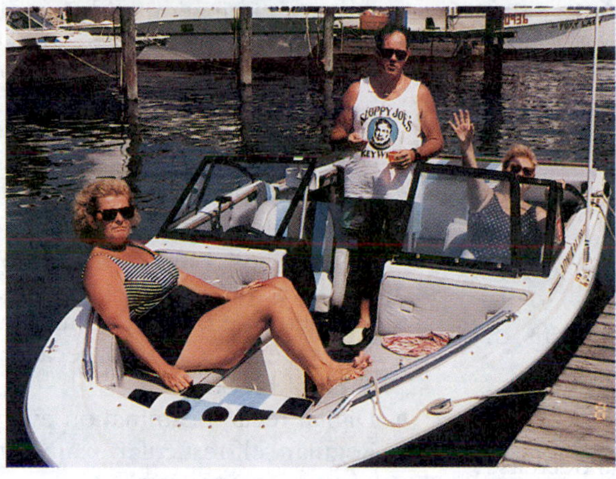

Figure 10-2
The middle adult years are characterized by greater expendable wealth, renewed relationship with one's spouse, and expanded social relationships.

satisfaction with achievement of career and family goals contributes to the stresses placed on the marriage. Extramarital affairs and divorce may be the result.

Widowhood (the status change resulting from the death of a husband or wife) may take place in the middle years. The loss of a spouse is a major crisis and a threat to self-concept, as well as a major role change. A multitude of changes may occur, including reduced income, changes in lifestyle and social relationships, and the need for help to work through the loss and grief.

The middle-aged adult is caught in a "generation sandwich." Children often are independent and married, with children of their own. Although much has been written about the *empty-nest syndrome* (resulting from the last child leaving home), most middle-aged parents welcome the space, time, and independence when freedom from parenting occurs. As involvement in and responsibility for children are decreasing, there may be an increasing need to become involved in caring for aging parents and other family members. The physical aging or death of a parent makes one's own aging and inevitable death a reality.

Midlife Transition. This phenomenon seems to occur in both men and women in their late 30s to early 40s. The transition involves changes in physiology, work, and family relationships. The following areas of one's life may be questioned:

- Women may choose to go to school, get a job, or change their career. Conversely, women who have been immersed in a career may decide in their early 40s to have children and stay at home.
- Men may become workaholics, spending little time with family or in leisure activities. Many men may choose to make a career change, often with increased emphasis on job satisfaction.
- As the 50s approach, questions about retirement and economic security become more prevalent, with increased interest in examining benefits of financial and retirement plans.
- Although one may not feel that one is aging, the realization that others consider the middle adult years as being older can be stressful.

Cognitive, Moral, and Spiritual Development

Cognitive and intellectual abilities of the middle adult change little from those of the young adult. There often is increased motivation to learn, especially if the knowledge gained can be immediately applied and has personal relevance. Problem-solving abilities remain throughout adulthood, although response time may be slightly longer. This is due not to a decrease in ability but rather to a longer memory search of increased amounts of material and to a desire to think a problem through before responding.

Morally, the middle adult may either remain at the conventional level or move to the postconventional level, especially if the person has had sustained responsibility for the welfare of others and has consistently applied ethical principles developed in adolescence. At this level, the adult believes that the rights of others take precedence, and takes steps to support those rights.

As with moral development, not all adults progress to Fowler's paradoxical–consolidative state of spiritual development. Fowler believes that only some people reach this stage, and only after age 30. Most middle adults are less rigid in beliefs and have increased faith and trust in spiritual strength.

Common Health Problems

The middle adult, like the young adult, is subject to physical and emotional health problems from lifestyle, developmental or situational crisis, family history, and the environment. Both acute and chronic illnesses may occur, but with increased age recovery time is longer. This is a result of slower and more prolonged responses to stressors, more pronounced reactions to an illness, and the possibility of more than one illness being present at a time.

The leading causes of death in the middle adult years are motor vehicle accidents, occupational accidents, suicide, and chronic disease (cancer in women and heart attacks in men). Major health problems are cardiovascular and pulmonary diseases, cancer, rheumatoid arthritis, diabetes mellitus, obesity, alcoholism, and depression.

The risk of developing these common health problems often is a result of the combination of lifestyle and aging. As one gets older, energy requirements decrease. The middle adult tends to maintain eating patterns and caloric intake while, at the same time, having less physical activity. This trend can result in obesity and atherosclerosis, with increased risk for high blood pressure, coronary artery disease, renal failure, and diabetes. Additionally, smoking and alcohol consumption put the person at greater risk for developing lung cancer, chronic respiratory problems, liver disease, and peptic ulcer disease.

Chronic illness in the middle adult has a major impact on self-concept and may precipitate changes in life structure. For example, after a serious heart attack, a man may face changes in his family role, his earning capacity, and his social relationships. All of these changes are a source of great stress.

Middle age does not automatically result in physical and emotional health problems. Many men and women remain healthy throughout their lives, but knowledge of proper preventive healthcare and the special needs of this age group can lead to improved quality and quantity of life.

The Nurse's Role in Healthcare

The nurse plays a major role in promoting health in the middle adult by teaching, serving as a role model, and encouraging self-care responsibilities.

The following health promotion activities are recommended:

Adults Aged 20 to 40

- Breast self-examination every month
- Breast examination by a healthcare provider every 3 years
- Baseline mammogram as recommended by a healthcare provider

Adults Aged 40 or Older

- Breast examination by a healthcare provider yearly
- Self-breast examination every month
- Mammogram as baseline as recommended by healthcare provider and then every year past age 50

All Women

- If age 18 or older and for sexually active people, pelvic examination and Papanicolaou test yearly
- After three or more consecutive normal annual tests, Pap tests may be done less frequently at the provider's discretion

All Middle Adults

- Complete physical examination every 2 years
- Annual dental examination
- Eye examination every 1 to 2 years, including a test for glaucoma
- Maintenance of current immunizations
- Annual examination of fecal material for the presence of blood
- Digital rectal examination every year
- Regular self-testicular examination and regular prostate examinations
- Cancer screening for women, as recommended by the American Cancer Society

The middle adult should be taught the importance of proper nutrition, rest, and exercise, as well as the dangers of substance abuse. Referrals to support groups and individual counseling may be necessary to strengthen the coping mechanisms and allow acceptance of personal and family changes.

Although the young and middle adult years are a time of change, they also are the period of life when a person is at optimal physical and psychosocial functioning. Having successfully met developmental tasks, the adult is ready to enjoy the rest of life. A sense of continuity and adaptability, achieved from the beginning of the 20s to the end of the 50s, is essential to satisfactorily meeting developmental tasks of aging and to the enjoyment of one's remaining years.

Older Adulthood

Our society has arbitrarily labeled the **older adult** as one over age 65. The population of North America is growing older, with residents over age 65 constituting 12% of the total census (U. S. Department of Health and Human Services, 1991). With this shift in age come increased healthcare needs. As the healthcare system changes to meet these needs, the nurse will care for more older adults—both well and ill—in various settings. It is essential, therefore, that nurses understand the concepts of growth and development as they relate to older adults. Illness, functional disabilities, and hospitalization cause major disruptions in the growth and development of any person, but they can be particularly devastating to an older person.

It is the nurse's role to promote wellness, prevent illness, restore health, and facilitate coping with life experiences and to assist the client to challenge and complete developmental tasks successfully to reach individual's potential as a unique human being. These functions of nursing care are just as important to the care of the older adult as they are to people of any age.

Physiologic Theories

Growth refers to biologic processes that result in physical change. In older adulthood, the process of aging becomes progressively more rapid. There are numerous theories that describe how and why aging occurs, but none is universally accepted. The *genetic theory* of aging holds that life span depends to a great extent on genetic factors. Genes within the organism control "genetic clocks" that determine the occurrence and rate of metabolic processes, including cell division. According to the *wear-and-tear* theory, organisms wear out from increased metabolic functioning and cells become exhausted from continual energy depletion in adapting to stressors (Sorenson & Thorson, 1995). There is no agreement as to why some people, even within families or similar environments, age much more rapidly than others. Although internal processes may in part predetermine aging, other factors, such as drugs, nutrition, and smoking, also may play a role.

Physiologic Status

In the older adult, all organ systems undergo some degree of decline in overall functioning, and the body becomes less efficient. (Normal physiologic changes in structure and function of the body with aging are outlined in the accompanying box.) Body functions that require integrated activity of several organ systems are affected the most. For example, aging of the heart muscles causes fluid retention in both peripheral tissues and the lungs, causing swelling of the legs and making breathing more difficult. The most commonly encountered chronic disorders are cardiovascular disorders such as hypertension and strokes, cancers, and skeletal disorders such as arthritis and osteoporosis.

Functional Status

There is growing evidence that aging is not synonymous with disease and disability. Although 80% of older adults have one or more chronic disorders, their ability to adapt determines whether they are ill or healthy. Most continue their activities from middle age and adapt intuitively to gradual limitations of aging. It may take longer to complete any given activity, or the activity may need to be modified. An older adult with arthritis may need to use an electric can opener rather than a manual one; a person with heart disease may need 3 hours to mow the lawn, with intermittent rest periods, rather than 1 hour (Fig. 10-3).

The greatest threat to the health of older adults is that the physiologic reserve of the various organ systems is gone. When illness occurs, increased physical and emotional stress places an older adult at risk for complex reactions. An older adult is more likely to develop complications and to require longer to recover. For instance, an older client with a hip fracture is at high risk for pneumonia and skin breakdown because of immobility, decreased ability to expel pulmonary secretions, and thinner, more fragile skin. The nurse knows that the older client has less reserve, and works to maintain normal functioning. Complications are prevented by careful assessment of the symptoms and by assisting the client to cough and deep breathe, turn, and carry out personal hygiene.

Cognitive Development

The term *cognition* is used to indicate cerebral functioning, including the ability to perceive and understand one's world. Cognition does not change appreciably with aging. An older adult continues to learn and problem solve, and intelligence and personality remain consistent (see the accompanying box). It is normal for an older adult to take longer to respond and react, particularly in new or unfamiliar surroundings. Knowing this, the nurse should slow the pace of care and allow the older client extra time to ask questions or complete activities. Mild short-term memory loss is common, but can be remedied by an older adult with the use of notes, schedules, and calendars.

When serious mental impairment occurs, the effect on the client and family can be devastating. **Dementia** describes various organically caused disorders that progressively affect cognitive functioning. Of the dementias that affect older adults, **Alzheimer's disease** is the most common. It affects brain cells, and is characterized by patchy areas of the brain that degenerate, or break down. A person with Alzheimer's disease faces a progressively serious and ultimately fatal disorder. At first, forgetfulness and impaired judgment may be evident. Over a period of several years, the person becomes progressively more confused, forgetting family and becoming disoriented in familiar surroundings. When the ability to perform simple activities of daily living is lost, the person requires constant supervision and care, often in a nursing home. There is no effective medical treatment for Alzheimer's disease, which is the leading cause of cognitive impairment in old age. Comprehensive and empathetic nursing care are important. The nurse directs nursing care to ensure the client's safety and to meet basic needs of nutrition and fluids, elimination, and hygiene. Both the client and family need emotional sup-

(text continues on page 160)

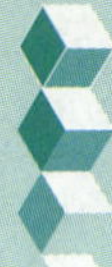

Research in Nursing: Making a Difference

The Older Adult

As the population of North America continues to age, the health promotion and healthcare needs of the older adult are increasingly a focus of nursing research. The studies summarized here illustrate that nursing recognizes that older adults require interventions tailored to meet needs in both health and illness.

Related Research

Porter, E. (1994). Older widow's experience of living alone at home. *IMAGE: Journal of Nursing Scholarship, 26*(1), 19–24.
This qualitative study was conducted by interviewing seven older widows living alone. Analysis of the data identified four areas of importance to these women: *making aloneness acceptable, going my own way, reducing my risks,* and *sustaining myself. Aloneness* was made acceptable through sharing with families or pets and by leaving and returning home. *Going my own way* was facilitated by carrying out tasks and responsibilities of living alone, such as care of the house and financial negotiations. Concerns for safety were met by activities that would prevent falls or doing too much. *Sustaining myself* meant that the women did what was necessary to continue to live at home; this area included maintaining health and enjoying pleasurable experiences. The women who provided information stressed that they intended to continue to live at home as long as possible. Continued research is suggested to identify and provide interventions necessary to assisting this population in maintaining independent living.

Lierman, L., Young, H., Powell-Cope, G., Georgiadou, F., & Benoliel, J. (1994). Effects of education and support on breast self-examination in older women. *Nursing Research, 43*(3), 158–163.
The purpose of this study was to determine the effects of an educational program and structured support on breast self-examination (BSE) frequency, proficiency, and perceived skill in middle-aged and older women. Following an educational program, 157 women were interviewed at 6 months and 12 months. The women were randomly divided into three groups: no-support group, selected partner support group, and peer support group. A significant correlation was noted between self-ratings of proficiency and BSE frequency in all groups; however, no significant differences were found between support groups. It is suggested that the strong educational program, combined with the women's motivation, may have reduced the need for a support partner. Older women are willing and able to change their behavior and conduct regular BSE when provided with the necessary information and skills.

Moloney, M. (1995). Older women's stories of being strong. *IMAGE: Journal of Nursing Scholarship, 27*(2), 104–109.
As people live longer, it becomes increasingly important to identify and explore those factors that make women strong. This study was conducted to discover some of the possible meanings of inner strength in older women's lives. The sample consisted of seven Caucasian and five African-American women over the age of 65. Data were collected through unstructured interviews, and were analyzed to identify themes that constituted a pattern. The three patterns that emerged from the data were *surviving, finding strength,* and *gathering the memories . . . seeing the patterns. Surviving* included the themes of living with loss, living through hard times, being different, and putting it behind you. *Finding strength* was described as a quality that developed out of life experiences. *Gathering the memories . . . seeing the patterns* was enabled through telling their stories, a process that allowed reflection and finding meaning in what had happened during their lives. The findings of this study can be used by nurses as they view themselves and their female clients. Seeing women as strong and helping women verbalize that strength may potentiate health.

Summary

Research aimed at promoting wellness and optimal functioning at all levels of health and illness in the aging population is critical to nursing. Although these studies were about older women, findings can be applied to older men who live alone, require health education, and use strengths. Focusing on independent self-care that promotes physical and psychologic health and developing specific nursing assessments and interventions to meet health care needs of the older adult provides direction for future health promotion and illness prevention strategies.

Focus on the Older Adult

Normal Physiologic Changes of Older Adulthood

General Status

- Progressively decreasing efficiency of physiologic processes results in a fragile balance and hinders the body's ability to maintain homeostasis.
- Physical or emotional stressors cause the older adult to be more vulnerable because of decreased physiologic reserves.
- The older adult may continue to engage in all activities of middle age but intuitively adjusts to a modified pace and more frequent rest periods.

Integumentary

- Wrinkling and sagging of skin occur with decreased skin elasticity; dryness and scaling are common.
- Balding becomes common in men, and women experience thinning of hair also; hair loses pigmentation.
- Skin pigmentation and moles are common, although the skin may become pale because of loss of melanocytes.
- Nails typically thicken and become brittle and yellowed.

Musculoskeletal

- Decreases in subcutaneous tissue and weight commonly are found in the old-old.
- Muscle mass and strength decrease.
- Bone demineralization occurs, and bones become porous and brittle.
- Joints tend to stiffen and lose flexibility, and range of motion may decrease.
- Overall mobility commonly slows and posture tends to stoop. Height decreases slightly.

Neurologic

- The central nervous system responds more slowly to multiple stimuli. Hence, the cognitive and behavioral response of the older adult may be delayed.
- Rate of reflex response decreases.
- Temperature regulation and pain perception become less efficient.
- The sense of balance declines, and fine movements may become more difficult.
- Sleep at night typically shortens and the older adult may awaken more easily. Cat naps become common.

Special Senses

- Diminished visual acuity (*presbyopia*) occurs, with increased sensitivity to glare and decreased ability to adjust to darkness. Cataracts may further obscure vision.
- Diminished hearing acuity (*presbycusis*) occurs, particularly diminished pitch discrimination in the presence of environmental noises.
- The senses of taste and smell are decreased.

Cardiopulmonary

- Blood vessels become less elastic and often rigid and tortuous. Venous return becomes less efficient. Fatty plaque deposits continue to occur in the linings of the blood vessels. Lower-extremity edema and cooling may occur, particularly with decreased mobility.
- The body is less able to increase heart rate and cardiac output with activity.
- Pulmonary elasticity and ciliary action decrease so clearing of the lungs becomes less efficient. Respiratory rate may increase, accompanied by diminished depth.

Gastrointestinal

- Digestive juices continue to diminish and nutrient absorption decreases.
- Malnutrition and anemia become more common.
- With reduced muscle tone and decreased peristalsis, constipation and indigestion are common complaints.

Dentition

- Tooth decay and loss continue for most older adults.
- Eating habits may change, particularly if the older adult lacks teeth or has ill-fitting dentures.

Genitourinary

- Blood flow to the kidneys decreases with diminished cardiac output.
- The number of functioning nephron units decreases by 50%; waste products may be filtered and excreted more slowly.
- Fluids and electrolytes remain within normal ranges, but the balance is fragile.
- Bladder capacity decreases by 50%. Voiding becomes more frequent; two or three times a night is usual. A decrease in bladder and sphincter muscle control may result in stress incontinence or incomplete bladder emptying.
- About 75% of men over age 65 experience hypertrophy of the prostate gland; surgery may be required if urinary retention occurs.
- There is atrophy, decrease of secretions, and thinning of the older woman's genital tract.

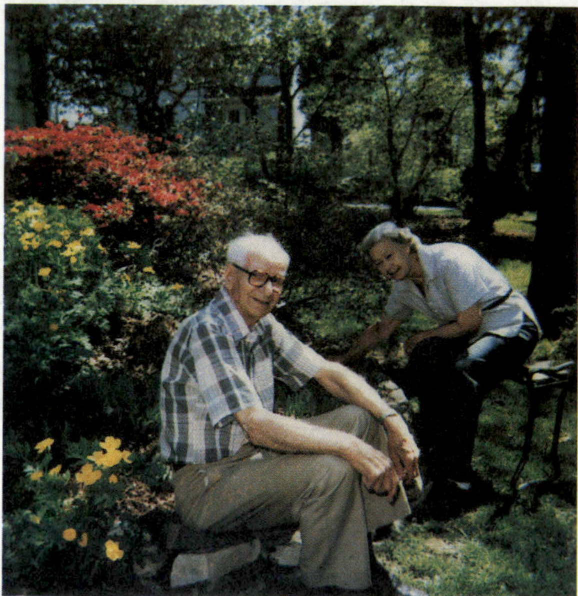

Figure 10-3
This couple, married 61 years, enjoys gardening together. They've found that they can continue most activities of middle age with only minor adjustments.

port and teaching, and may benefit from community resources that can ease the family's burden.

Sometimes confusion and depression in an older adult are mistaken for permanent dementias. Drug interactions, circulatory or metabolic problems, or even nutritional deficiencies are likely to be the real cause. An older adult also may become confused when too many changes or losses occur at one time or when she or he is moved to a radically different environment. Sometimes a type of confusion called **sundowning syndrome** occurs, in which an older adult habitually becomes confused with darkness. The nurse can assist other members of the health team in determining the cause of the client's confusion and in helping to reorient the client. For example, the nurse uses **reality orientation** to redirect the client's attention to what is real in the environment. Nursing interventions include the use of calendars and clocks, calling the client by name, and talking about the client's family and the season. The client also is encouraged to make decisions, to promote a sense of control over the environment. The nurse must remember that many older adults have hearing and visual impairments. These impairments can be counteracted by speaking clearly and slowly, looking directly at the client, and repeating instructions. The environment should be well lighted but without glare.

Cognitive Status of the Older Adult

- Intelligence increases into the 60s, and learning continues throughout life.
- Cognitive functioning is related to use. Reasoning ability and abstract thought remain astute, particularly for usual situations and familiar experiences.
- Processing and reaction times increase and may be evident in slower and seemingly more deliberate responses.
- There is a decreased capacity for adaptation, especially in stressful or unfamiliar environments and with impaired senses.
- Recent memory loss may occur, but long-term memory remains intact.

Developmental Theories

In developmental theories, new tasks associated with older adulthood are identified, and new behavioral patterns emerge. An early controversial psychosocial theory, called the *disengagement theory*, maintained that an older adult withdraws from societal interactions because it is mutually desired and satisfying for both the individual and society. Later studies have shown that isolation is not desired or acceptable, and that as societal interactions decrease, a healthy older adult increases close relationships with family and friends. According to the *activity theory*, successful aging involves the ability to maintain high levels of activity and functioning. An older adult may substitute activities but does not slow down or disengage from society. The *identity–continuity theory* assumes that healthy aging is related to the ability of the older adult to continue similar patterns of behavior that existed in young to middle adulthood.

Most theorists agree that a person's self-concept is relatively stable throughout adult life. An older adult who has developed a strong sense of self-identity and has successfully met challenges earlier in life will probably continue to do so. This person substitutes new roles for old roles and perhaps continues former roles in a new context. For example, the business manager, on retirement, may continue to use leadership talents in community organizations. Older adults with a strong self-concept typically describe themselves as being healthier than others or "young for my years." On the other hand, events that accompany aging can threaten a person's self-concept. Depending on the person's outlook on life and past ability to cope, events such as retirement, loss of health or income, and isolation can be devastating. For example, the retired teacher whose sense of identity was closely tied to career may suddenly find that friends, income, and sense of accomplishment are lost and, consequently, may feel a great loss of control and self-identity.

Erikson: Psychosocial Development

Erikson identifies ego integrity versus despair and disgust (Erikson, 1963) as the last stage of human development, which begins around age 60. The older adult continues to look forward but now also looks back and begins to

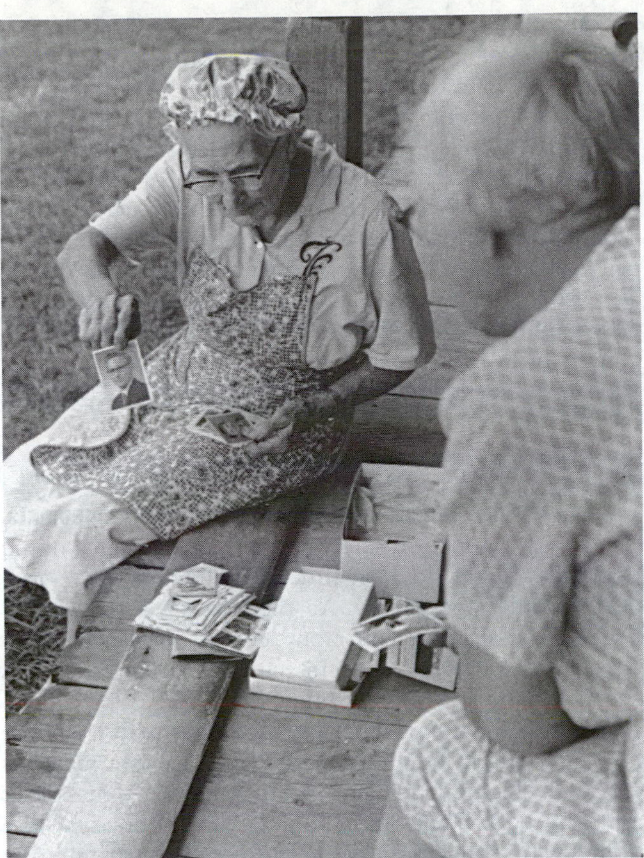

Figure 10-4
Reminiscing is a culturally universal phenomenon of aging. It is a way for the older adult to reasses life experiences and further develop a sense of accomplishment, fulfillment, and reward in life. (Photo by Karen Baldwin.)

reflect on his or her life. It is a time for realization of a "wholeness" perspective, with an inner search for meaning and order of the life cycle. The older adult searches for emotional integration and acceptance of the past and present, as well as acceptance of physiologic decline without fear of death. The nurse is familiar with older adults who like to retell stories or past events. This phenomenon is called **life review** or **reminiscence** and has been identified worldwide. In a sense, it is a way for an older adult to relive and restructure life experiences and is part of achieving ego integrity (Fig. 10-4).

As with other developmental stages identified by Erikson, ego integrity is facilitated when the older adult has successfully accomplished tasks earlier in life. It can be a time to look backward with pride and without regrets and forward with optimism and enthusiasm. A person who regrets the past and sees current problems as insurmountable may despair. This person may view life as a series of unresolved problems and missed opportunities and feel worthless or hopeless. The despairing person may want to do things over but fears the lack of time before death.

Tasks of midlife continue or resurface. The older adult still strives to guide the coming generations and to leave something behind (generativity versus stagnation). The need for love and closeness continues (intimacy versus isolation), as does a strong sense of who one is in relation to family and community (identity versus role diffusion). Because of physical and social changes associated with aging, the older adult is repeatedly faced with the need to adapt and to again face already completed tasks.

Havighurst: Developmental Tasks

According to Havighurst, the major tasks of old age are primarily concerned with the maintenance of social contacts and relationships. Successful aging depends on a person's ability to be flexible and adapt to new age-related roles. The person must find new and meaningful roles in old age while maintaining reasonable comfort within the social customs of our times (Ebersole & Hess, 1991). The developmental tasks that, according to Havighurst, are associated with "later maturity" (Havighurst, 1972) are listed in the accompanying box. Also, a discussion of each task follows.

Adjusting to Declining Physical Strength and Health. As stated earlier, most older adults gradually modify their lifestyles to accommodate for declining vigor and strength. Rest periods become more frequent; at the same time, continued activity is important for maintaining all physiologic functions. An older adult is at high risk for accidents and falls and may need to curtail driving or use a cane or other aid to remain mobile. Modification in diet and prescribed medications may be necessary, and because of chronic illness an older adult may need to adjust to living with pain. With severe illness, loss of independence over oneself and one's environment can occur. The loss of health is difficult to adjust to because it affects every aspect of life.

Adjusting to Retirement and Reduced Income. Retirement brings a change in a person's concept of time. An older adult must learn to occupy leisure time in a way that maintains self-esteem and is personally satisfying. Retirement is considered the hallmark of old age, and

Havighurst's Developmental Tasks of Later Maturity

- Adjusting to declining physical strength and health
- Adjusting to retirement and reduced income
- Adjusting to changes in health of one's spouse
- Establishing an explicit affiliation with one's age-group.
- Adopting and adapting social roles in a flexible way
- Establishing satisfactory physical living arrangements

satisfaction with retirement is closely tied to income and the relationships one has outside of work. Most older adults manage on smaller incomes after retirement, but about 27% live at or below the poverty level (USDHHS, 1991). Lack of finances can affect an older adult's ability to meet all needs, from adequate medical care and housing to social and creative interests.

Adjusting to Changes in the Health of One's Spouse. When one's spouse becomes ill or dies, numerous and difficult adjustments must be made. An older adult may face new roles for the first time. A husband may begin to cook meals; a wife may learn to handle family finances. These role changes come at a time when stress is already high. Physical care can be overwhelming if the other spouse also is in poor health. Adaptations may occur in living conditions and lifestyle, and the spouse may need to plan social and recreational events alone.

The need for love and belonging does not diminish with age, and may become acute with the loss of one's spouse. We are sexual beings, and our sexual behavior does not necessarily stop in old age. Sexuality encompasses who we are, and older adults are no exception. Like younger adults, older adults need to express intimacy physically by touching and emotionally by sharing joys, sorrows, ideas, and values.

Establishing an Explicit Affiliation With One's Age-Group. With an aging population, social organizations for older adults are becoming more numerous. For example, most communities have senior citizens' centers that offer meals, social and informational programs, and other activities for a nominal fee. Other organizations offer the opportunity for travel, cultural events, and political involvement. Affiliation with other people of the same age allows older adults to share common interests and concerns and find status among their peers. It should not be assumed, however, that older adults want to associate only with others of the same age (Fig. 10-5).

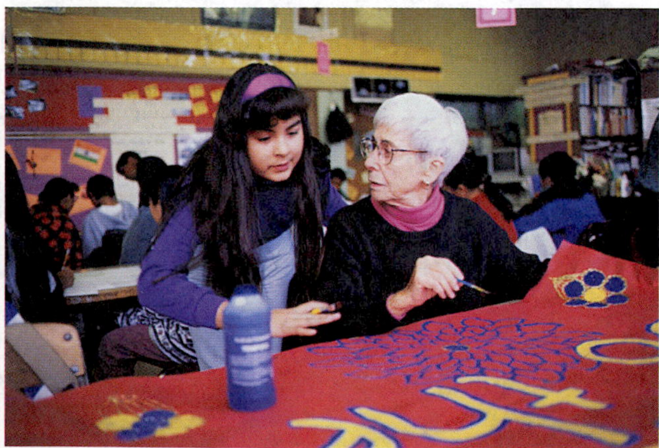

Figure 10-5
Social relationships and satisfying leisure activities remain important throughout life. This older adult volunteers in art class with 6th-grade Asian and Latina girls. (Photo © Kathy Sloane.)

Adopting and Adapting Social Roles in a Flexible Way. Social roles change with the developmental tasks and adjustments of older adulthood, but the need to feel valued, useful, and productive continues. An older adult may develop new hobbies or increase involvement in community, church, or family affairs. He or she may do volunteer work or even launch into a new career. If an older adult cannot adjust and form new relationships, social isolation can become a problem. **Social isolation** is a sense of being alone and lonely because of fewer meaningful relationships. It may occur because of declining health or income, transportation problems, or ageism. Whatever the cause, prolonged social isolation has been correlated to declining health and higher mortality (Berkman, 1983).

Establishing Satisfactory Physical Living Arrangements. The ability to function safely and independently at home depends a great deal on functional health, transportation, income, and family. An older adult, for example, may need assistance with home repairs, housecleaning, or grocery shopping. Architectural barriers, such as steps, may need to be modified. Easy access to medical and recreational facilities and churches may become more important. In urban areas, fear of crime may necessitate changes in living arrangements. Many older adults in poor health may be able to continue living at home with some assistance from visiting community nurses or with the aid of other services, such as home-delivered meals and senior transportation.

Home Healthcare Alert

If an older adult is losing weight, ask yourself: "Is income sufficient to buy food? Does this person have transportation to buy food? Is there adequate storage for food?"

Most older adults prefer to live in their own homes. It is difficult to move from one's home. Moving in with adult children creates changes in roles and authority. When moving to an extended-care facility, such as a nursing home, the loss of one's home and, sometimes, possessions and the need to conform to the routines of institutional living can be traumatic for the client and family. Some people, however, choose to move for convenience, social relationships, or needed healthcare.

Retirement centers and senior citizens' housing have recently flourished. For those who need healthcare, alternative methods of care have become available. Examples of alternative care are respite care facilities, which allow the family a needed rest by temporarily housing and caring for an ailing older family member, and day-care centers, which provide a safe, stimulating environment during the day, when family members must work. The nurse must be knowledgeable about which healthcare and social services are available in the client's community so that the client and family can be informed. Thus, the nurse can effectively work with other members of the healthcare team to ensure that the client gets needed services.

Paradoxical Aging

The "Graying" Population

Based on information compiled by the U. S. Senate Special Committee on Aging (U. S. Department of Health and Human Services, 1991), about 31 million people are age 65 or older in the United States. It is projected that by the year 2040, about 22% of the total population will be age 65 or older. In addition, the older population is living longer; it is estimated that there were 61,000 people over the age of 100 and that there will be over 100,000 people over the age of 100 by the year 2000. These shifts in population are the result of an increased life expectancy and a decrease in birth rates. On the average, North American women can now expect to live to age 78 and men to age 71. The predicted life expectancy in 2030 is 82.3 years for women and 75.4 years for men.

Old-old and **frail-old** are terms used to identify people over age 75; this group is the fastest-growing segment in the population. The population age 85+ is expected to more than triple in size between 1980 and 2030 and to be nearly 7 times larger in 2050 than in 1980. The old-old have special significance for nursing care because they are more likely to need help with mobility and basic activities of daily living. They may need increasing assistance to maintain a safe and comfortable living environment. The older the person, the more likely that he or she needs family and community support to maintain functional health.

This age shift in the population is influencing all of society and helping to shape social, political, and healthcare issues. Older adults are emerging as a strong social and political force: consider such examples as Mother Theresa and Maggie Kuhn (founder of the Gray Panthers).

An Adaptive Population

The older adult population is the most unique and diversified group in today's society because its members have lived the longest and have participated in and adapted to complex societal changes. Within the life span of the older adult, society has developed from a rural agricultural base, through industrialization, into a service-oriented, high-technology base (Fig. 10-6). Consider that in 1900, a 20-mile trip meant an all-day undertaking—probably in a horse-drawn wagon. Today a person can fly across the continent in less time and with considerably less effort. Lighting has progressed from kerosene lamps to electricity. Information that once took weeks or months to be received now is instantaneous as a result of computers. Most older adults have lived through the trauma of one or two world wars. Most had parents with strong ethnic ties to another country, and many were immigrants themselves. The older adult has lived through the Great Depression of the 1930s and developed self-sufficiency. Major societal changes, such as the enactment of Social Security and Medicare, necessitated adaptations and helped to shape the values and lifestyles of older adults.

Further adaptations become necessary with advancing age because of physical or mental limitations, retirement, loss of a spouse or family members, or changing income. The older adult is faced with numerous role changes that may be directly related to chronologic age

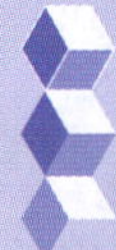

Through the Eyes of a Student

The first and most difficult client I ever encountered as a student was an older man who had chronic obstructive pulmonary disease. I entered his room to introduce myself and to explain that I would be his student nurse for the day. The client told me that the last thing he needed or wanted was a student nurse to "bother him all day." He went on to explain that he had already told his "real nurse" this and that I should go and "find another patient."

After leaving the room, the last thing I wanted to do was to enter it ever again. I went to the instructor and related to her what the client had said. She decided that it would be an educational experience for me to deal with this client and to remain his nurse. I took a few minutes to think about how I would explain this to the client, remain calm, and avoid bursting into tears.

I went back to the client's room. I told him that I was still his student nurse for the day, but I would come into his room only when I had to perform a task essential to his care. I then reassured him that his regular nurse also would be in to take care of him. The client appeared reassured and stopped mumbling under his breath.

I kept my promise and entered the room only when there was a purpose. The client remained terse and unfriendly the entire day, but when I told him I would be leaving for the day, he did say, "Thank you for everything. It wasn't as bad as I thought it was going to be." As I left for the day, I thought the same thing.

—Stacy A. Maillie,
Delaware County Community College,
Media, Pennsylvania

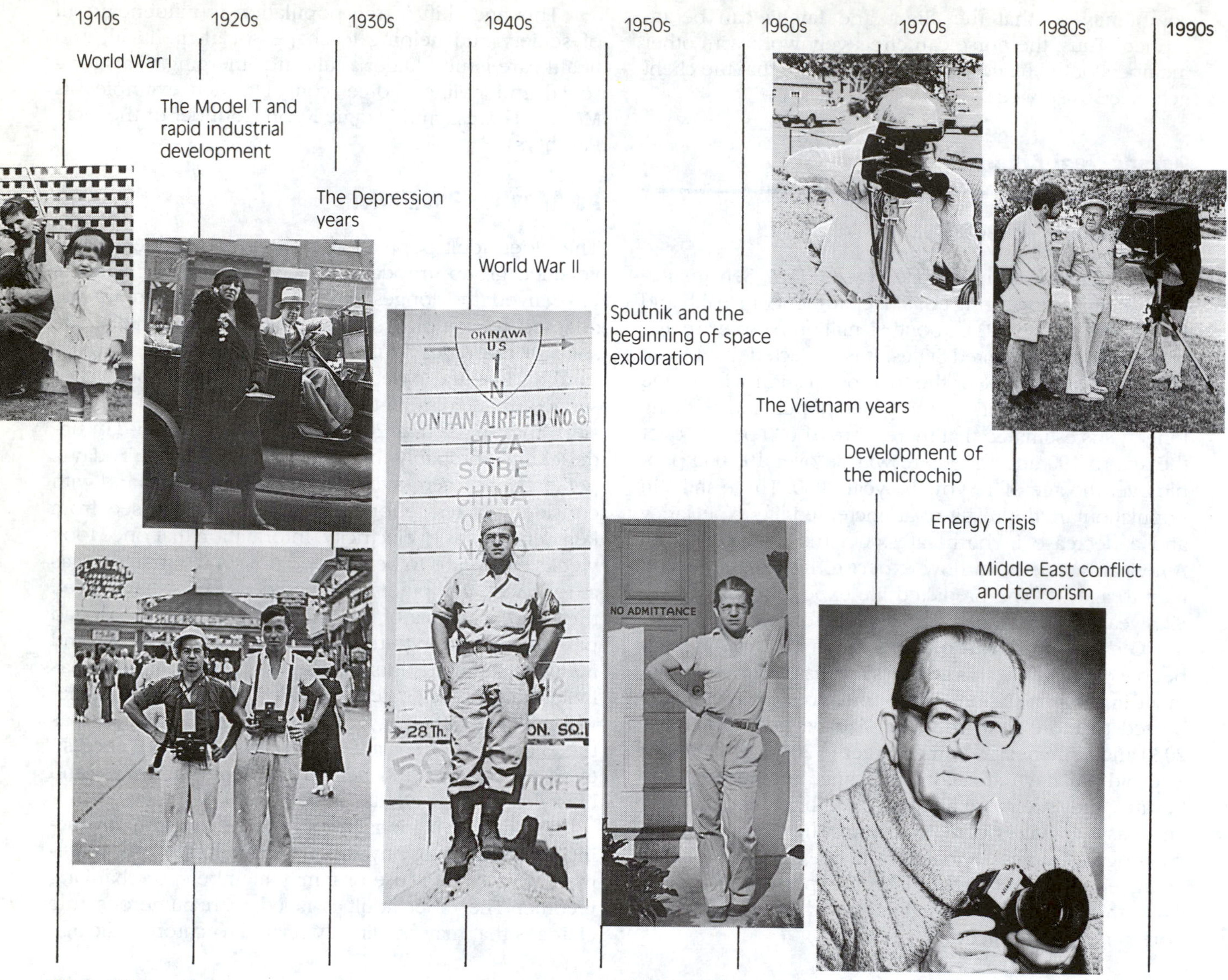

Figure 10-6
The older adult population is a unique group with vast and diverse experience. Images from one man's life highlight some of the social events and change that this population group has experienced.

or health status. Lost roles must be replaced with new roles and activities that are acceptable and satisfying to the person.

Older people, thus, are living in a world that requires change and adaptation. It is a time to reach one's potential and to satisfy long-range goals that may have been delayed because of other responsibilities. It also can be a time to turn over to others "productive" tasks such as career or community leadership. Research has shown that most older adults do adjust and adapt to new roles and most are satisfied with their lives and with what they have. Depending on the older adult's adaptability and supportive resources, older adulthood may promote feelings of happiness, peace, and understanding or of sorrow, conflict, and confusion.

Functional Health Versus Disease. Most older adults regard themselves as healthy and deny severe limitations in activities. Most are never institutionalized, nor do they suffer the effects of senility. *Healthy*, however, does not necessarily mean without disease. More than 4 out of 5 older adults suffer from at least one chronic illness. Like younger adults, they define their health in relation to how well they function—that is, whether or not they can engage in their usual and desired daily activities. This **functional health** definition includes a person's ability to remain self-reliant, to "make do," and to maintain a sense of control and independence over self and environment. There is a trend toward increasing independence and self-care in older adults with activities of daily living; in 1990 32% lived with a spouse, 35% lived with other people, and 33% lived alone. These living arrangements are expected to remain constant over the next 30 years. Those who live alone are at greatest risk for loss of independence and increased need for long-term care.

Family and Role Reversal. Spouse and other family members are natural support systems who help the older adult maintain functional health and independence and meet developmental tasks of old age. Supportive assistance may include the provision of transportation, food, shelter, social interactions, and even complex medical and nursing treatments. Significant others, such as close friends and neighbors, also may take on tasks formerly assumed to be the responsibilities of the traditional family.

Not all families can assist an aged member satisfactorily because of such factors as geographic distance, low income, poor health, strained marital relationships, and infringement on career or lifestyle. Adult children may feel "sandwiched" between responsibilities for their own children and careers and the needs of older parents. It can be a guilt-ridden and emotionally draining time for all involved when physical or emotional illness reverses roles and strains family resources.

The nurse must recognize that the whole family is the client and assess the family for capabilities and limitations in assisting the aged member. The nurse can help ease the strain by listening to client and family concerns and by validating the importance of family needs. The nurse assists the client and family to find workable solutions, and may refer the family to community support services.

Ageism and Common Stereotypes

Sometimes the older adult is the victim of ageism. **Ageism** is a form of prejudice, like racism, in which older adults are stereotyped by characteristics found in only a few members of their group. Fundamental to ageism is the view that older people are different from *me* and will remain different from *me*; therefore, they do not experience the same desires, needs, and concerns. Industrialism and technologic advances have placed a high priority on productivity, so that retired people may be said to have "outlived their usefulness." Along with this, the younger generations often have lost ties to the older generation because of increased mobility of the nuclear family and thus lack experiences with older relatives and their friends. Common myths compared with reality are outlined in Table 10-3.

Older people may be *incorrectly* depicted as being rigid or narrow-minded, unable to learn, unreliable because of memory loss, too old to enjoy sexual pleasure, or childlike and dependent. Many people fear advancing age because of the pervasive views that older people are poor, lonely, in frail health, and able to look forward only to institutionalization in a nursing home. These descriptors are not true for most older adults (Fig. 10-7).

Most older adults are satisfied with their lives, finding retirement and old age more enjoyable than they had

Table 10-3
Myths and Realities: The Older Adult

Myth	Reality
Old age begins at 65.	The decision to set 65 as the age of eligibility for Social Security payments was made in the 1930s, based on the labor market needs and the economy of the country at that time. The age of 65 became synonymous with old age by accident.
Most older adults are ill and institutionalized.	Only about 5% of older adults live in institutions.
Old age means inevitable mental deterioration.	Personality is not changed by chronologic aging.
Most older adults are lonely and socially isolated.	Loneliness comes as a result of death of loved ones, departure of friends from the community, or other losses. This does not mean that older adults are lonely for social contact, but rather that they feel deeply about the losses in their lives.
Intelligence declines with age.	As long as the older adult remains intellectually active, there is no decline in intelligence. Processing information may require increased time to respond.
Interest in sexual activity is inappropriate for older adults.	The frequency of sexual activity may decrease, but the ability to perform and enjoy sexual activity lasts well into the 90s in healthy older adults.
Body image is of little concern.	Older adults are concerned about how they look and want to be attractive to others.
Bladder problems are a normal part of being old.	Incontinence is not a normal part of aging. It is an abnormal condition and requires medical treatment.
Older adults do not deserve aggressive treatment for disease conditions.	Older adults deserve aggressive treatment if they want aggressive treatment.

Source: Birchenall, J., & Streight, M. (1993). *Care of the older adult* (3rd ed.). Philadelphia: Lippincott, p. 6.

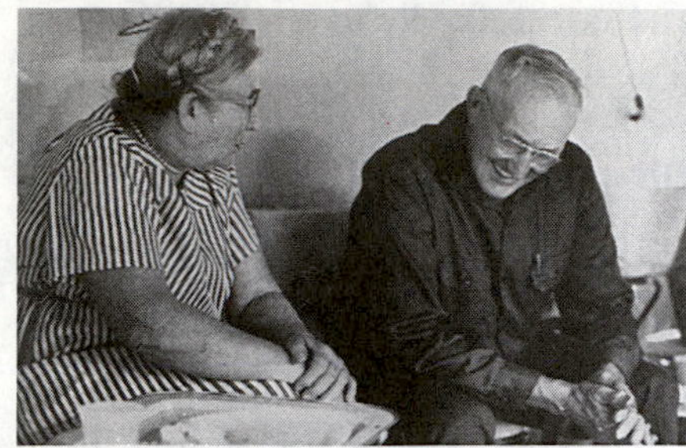
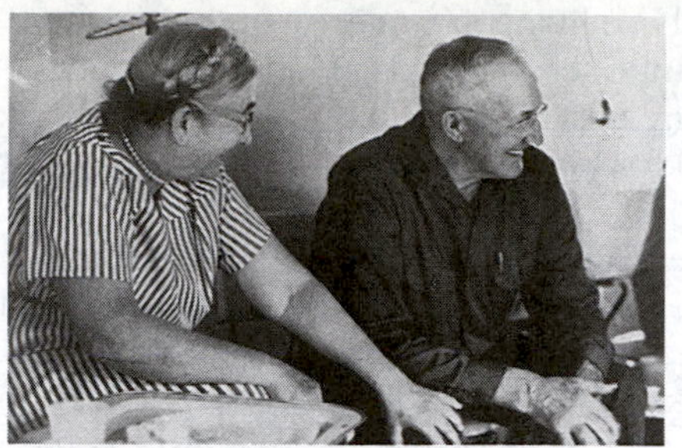
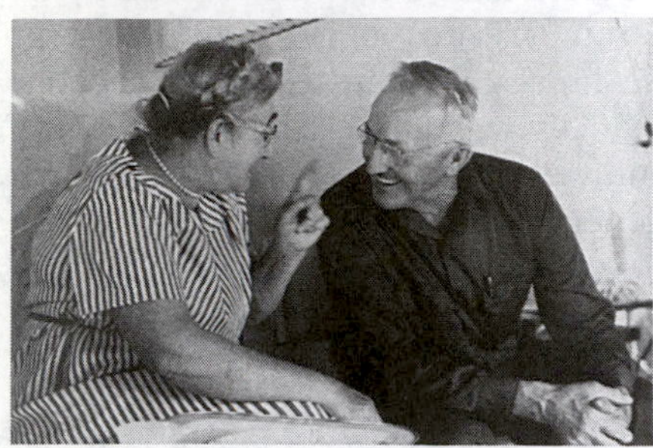
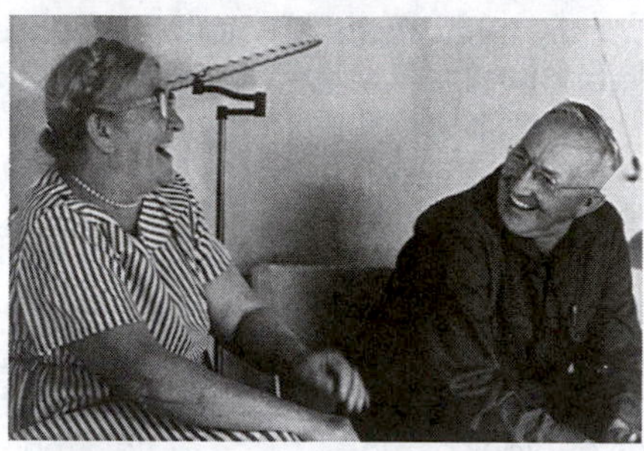

Figure 10-7
Stereotypical images of the older adult as narrow-minded, forgetful, sexless, and dependent are untrue for most of the older adult population. This couple exhibits the vitality, sensuality, joy, and playfulness of a young couple. (Photos by Karen Baldwin.)

anticipated. Three fourths live in their own homes, and one third of these live alone. Most older adults maintain close ties with their families and have incomes above the poverty level (USDHHS, 1991).

Gerontology and the Healthcare System

Knowledge of aging has increased dramatically in the past 40 years. **Gerontology** is the scientific and behavioral study of all aspects of aging and its consequences. Normal changes that occur with aging are the result of complex interactions among genetics, biologic systems, and physical and social environments. Disease complicates a person's ability to adapt and maintain functional health (the ability to carry out usual and desired daily activities). Mental or physical decline in the older adult often may not be directly related to the aging process, but rather result from the absence of supportive care and services that could prevent disease and maintain the older adult's ability to function.

The increasingly aging population has greatly strained a healthcare system that has traditionally focused on cures and acute disease processes. For the older client with chronic disorders, the focus of care should include the client's and family's goals and promote functional health and independent living to the greatest extent possible. Gerontologic, or gerontic, nursing does just that. **Gerontologic nursing** combines basic knowledge and skills of nursing with a specialized knowledge of aging in both illness and health (Fig. 10-8).

Common Health Problems of the Older Adult

As the population of older adults increases, nurses will increase the amount of time they spend providing care for this population. The older adult who requires care to prevent illness and promote wellness is found in all types of healthcare settings, including hospitals, long-term care facilities, emergency departments, outpatient surgeries, and homes. The nursing care that is planned and implemented for the older adult should be based on the following factors:

- Most older people are not impaired but are functional in the community, thereby benefiting from wellness-oriented interventions.
- Older people are more vulnerable to physical, emotional, and socioeconomic problems than people in other age groups, and may require special attention to health promotion and maintenance.

This section provides a broad introduction to the healthcare needs of the older adult in terms of chronic illness, accidental injuries, and acute illness (see the accompanying box).

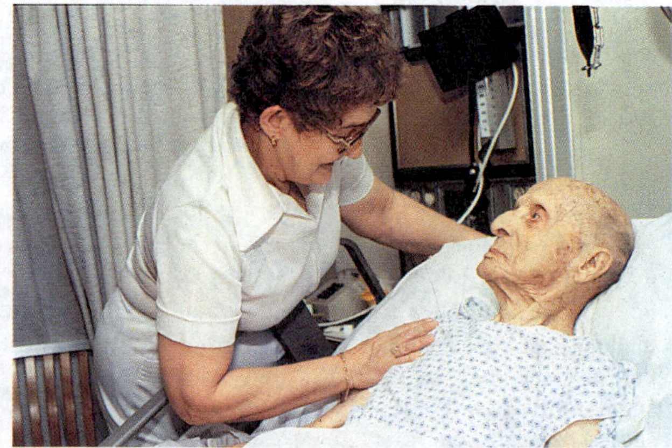

Figure 10-8
The hospitalized older adult requires nursing interventions to prevent complications and to promote wellness. (Photo © Kathy Sloane.)

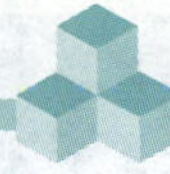

Examples of Nursing Diagnoses

Older Adult

The following are examples of nursing diagnoses that might be appropriate for the older adult:

- Risk for Infection related to dry, thin skin
- Risk for Altered Body Temperature related to very high environmental temperatures and lack of air-conditioning or fans
- Risk for Injury related to unstable gait and decreased vision from cataracts
- Risk for Loneliness related to death of spouse
- Ineffective Individual Coping related to diagnosis of chronic illness
- Impaired Physical Mobility related to severe arthritic changes in legs
- Impaired Home Maintenance Management related to recent surgery
- Impaired Memory related to cognitive impairment from onset of Alzheimer's disease
- Anxiety related to increase of crime and violence in neighborhood

Chronic Illness. The probability and incidence of a person becoming ill increases with age. The most common chronic illnesses in the older adult are arthritis, hypertension, hearing impairments, and heart disease. Other causes of illness or disability include acute illnesses such as fractures and pneumonia, motor vehicle accidents, and falls. These acute illnesses or accidents may cause chronic health problems. The leading causes of death in the elderly, accounting for 7 of every 10 deaths, are heart disease, cancer, and stroke.

Although illness affects all dimensions of a person, no matter what age, older adults have to contend with a variety of problems as they live with chronic illness. Although aging is a normal process and chronic illness is a pathologic process, both often occur at the same time. The problems of aging and the problems of chronic illness interrelate to increase problems in all areas of one's life, including—but not limited to—self-care, lifestyle, economics, social factors, and living arrangements. Consider the following:

- Chronic illness limits activities in about 15% of the population, but almost 50% of adults over age 65 have limitations as a result of one or more chronic illnesses.
- Meeting the expense of healthcare often is difficult for older adults and their families. Medication costs with chronic illness continue for the rest of a person's life, with multiple medications being the rule rather than the exception. Hospitalization costs continue to rise, and the price of high-quality, long-term care may well be beyond the client's or family members' ability to pay. In addition, special diets, special equipment, or medical supplies increase economic difficulties.
- Family members must learn how to cope with the needs of the ill person. Included are personal hygiene, medication administration, special diets, elimination, activities of daily living, and recognition of symptoms that necessitate medical attention. Family members also must adapt to psychologic stressors in the form of changes in communications, changes in roles (for example, the older mother in effect becomes the child), and changes in their own lifestyle as they become the caregivers.

Accidents and Injuries in the Older Adult. As described by Myers and Sharpe (1990), injuries that occur in the older adult "are a serious problem in terms of mortality, morbidity, changes in level of self-care, suffering, length of hospitalization, costs, and quality of life" (p. 109). An older adult is at increased risk for accidental injury because of changes in vision and hearing, loss of mass and strength of muscles, slower reflexes and reaction time, and decreased sensory ability. In addition, the effects of chronic illness and medication may make an older adult more prone to accidental injuries.

The older population of North America, with reduced income, may live in inadequate housing situated in neighborhoods with heavy traffic and high crime rates. They may be isolated from family members, and many live alone. Combined with normal changes of aging and the effects of any illness, older people not only are at increased risk, but also have a more difficult time regaining health after an injury.

The most serious threats are injuries that result from falls. Falls may occur in the home, community, or healthcare institution. Hip fracture is the most common consequence of a fall, with surgery to repair the hip the most common surgery for people over age 75. Hip fracture and the resultant surgery mean that the person must be hospitalized, has increased risk for disability and death, and often has permanent limitations, even after recovery.

Age-Related Needs. An older adult who requires surgery or medical treatment for chronic or acute illness has special, age-related needs no matter what the setting for care. Nursing care to meet age-related needs in any setting are outlined in Table 10-4, using functional health patterns as a framework.

Home Healthcare Alert

Ensure that floors are clear of throw rugs and clutter to prevent falls in the older adult.

Table 10-4
Meeting Healthcare Needs of the Older Adult

Area of Concern	Nursing Actions
Health Perception and Health Management	
Health concerns	• Review with client perceptions of current health status, health problems, and medications taken.
Safety practices	• Age-related sensory deficits (eg, sight, hearing) and slower response times may require special safety practices to prevent injury, such as leaving a light on at night.
Nutrition and Metabolism	
Chewing ability	• Check to see if client has lost or damaged teeth; if dentures are present, check if they fit well and are available. Be sure that food is appropriate to client's ability to chew.
Dietary intake	• Assess height, weight, eating patterns, and food choices. The older adult is at risk for alterations in nutrition (either as excess weight or as malnutrition).
Elimination	
Bladder elimination	• Ask about frequency of urine elimination; reduced bladder capacity with aging can result in more frequent need to empty bladder. • Provide assistance as necessary, and ensure that floor is uncluttered, that toilet is easily accessible, and that lighting is sufficient. • The inability to control urine is not a normal age-related change. If client is incontinent of urine, perform further assessments.
Bowel elimination	• Changes in diet and activity, the effects of medications and surgery, and loss of privacy can all contribute to changes in bowel elimination. • Know client's normal time for bowel elimination. • Ensure that diet (staying within ordered dietary guidelines) has necessary fluid and fiber content to promote normal elimination. If client does not eat well or complains of lack of appetite, assess for constipation.
Activity and Exercise	
Impaired activity	• Assess ability to walk; consider normal activity levels and any impairment from illness or surgery. If client uses a walker or cane, be sure assistive device is available. • Consider effects of illness, surgery, and medications on strength and motor function. Changes in nutrition, fluids, and electrolytes may increase fatigue and loss of strength (already decreased by age-related changes in cardiac output, lung changes, and degenerative changes in the musculoskeletal system).

(continued)

The Nurse's Role in Healthcare

Although specific nursing care adapted to the needs of the older client is described throughout this text, general implications for care are included here. The nurse must recognize physiologic and psychosocial interrelationships and view the older client holistically.

Illness can severely disrupt an older adult's ability to function independently. The ill client is under increased physical and emotional stress, which increases the risk for complications because of the lack of physiologic reserves. When a client is hospitalized or institutionalized, family and community interactions are severely inhibited. The acute-care environment itself adds new stressors, such as diagnostic tests, treatments, and surgery. In the face of new and unfamiliar routines and sensory stimulation, prior coping skills may not work, and an older client probably feels less able to understand and control the new environment. An older client is more likely than a younger client to suffer multisystem dysfunctions, *iatrogenic* complications (those caused by medications or treatments), accidents such as falls, and increasing dependence and confusion.

Home Healthcare Alert

The older adult's ability to feel changes in heat and cold is impaired. Ensure that the client knows how to prevent hyperthermia or hypothermia.

Major nursing care goals are to assist the older client to function as independently as possible and to continue to develop individual potentials. The nurse collaborates with the family and other disciplines to prevent complications of illness, to secure a safe and comfortable environment, and to promote the client's return to wellness. General guidelines for nursing care are outlined in the accompanying box.

Table 10-4 *(continued)*
Meeting Healthcare Needs of the Older Adult

Area of Concern	Nursing Actions
Cognition and Perception	
Cognitive abilities	• Slow down pace of activity and wait for responses; although intellectual ability is not affected with age, reaction and response times often are. • Repeat teaching as many times as necessary, especially if short-term memory is impaired. • Assess levels of vision and hearing. If client wears glasses or hearing aid, be sure it is used. Ensure that glass lenses are clean and that hearing aid batteries are strong.
Sleep and Rest	
Sleep pattern changes	• Assess normal time of going to bed and getting up, bedtime rituals, number of hours slept, and nap schedule. Sleep may be impaired as a result of pain, anxiety, and the effect of medications. • Encourage activity and exercise within ordered limits during the daytime. Discourage excessive naps.
Sexuality	
Perceptions of self as male or female	• One's sexual self-concept includes feelings about self as an attractive man or woman. Assist as necessary with hygiene, hair care, oral care, makeup, and clean bedclothes. Be sure environment is clean and odor-free.
Love and belonging	• Provide interventions that demonstrate genuine caring; ask preferred name, listen carefully, show respect for belongings, provide touch in various ways.
Coping and Stress	
Response to stress	• Be aware that illness and hospitalization are major stressors and may further impair the ability to recover from illness or injury. • Assess client's sources of strength and ensure that (as much as possible) those are available; include cultural and spiritual values and needs. • Encourage use of support systems, including family, friends, pets.
Self-Concept	
Altered self-concept	• Carry out interventions to maintain or improve physical function, and to maintain appearance. Illness, pain, and changes in grooming and dress can all lower self-esteem. • Encourage display of small photographs or personally relevant items that provide familiar components of one's life or lifestyle. • Set mutual goals with client as progress toward wellness is made. • Facilitate client's role as an active decision maker.

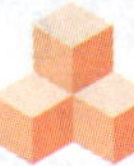

Guidelines for Nursing Care

Caring for the Older Adult

- Maintain the client's physiologic reserves. Carefully assess the client so that complications are discovered early.
- Prevent multisystem complications. Include nursing care that maintains physical integrity and function, such as skin care and planned rest and activity times. Teach client and family members what symptoms to report to the healthcare provider.
- Provide a safe and uncluttered environment with comfortable temperatures and good lighting. If the environment is unfamiliar, orient the client to routines and equipment. Teach safety measures in the home, such as using a nightlight, avoiding throw rugs, and having safety bars around the tub and commode.
- Slow your pace of care. Allow the client extra time to carry out activities, particularly those that require physical coordination, such as grooming and eating.
- Encourage independence. Teach the family to allow the client to provide self-care independently as much as possible.
- Beware of the stereotype of ageism. Treat each client as a unique person. Although many older clients have similar needs, factors such as background, interests, capabilities, values, culture, and lifestyle may differ greatly.

(continued)

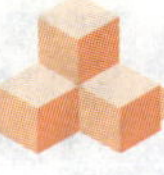

Guidelines for Nursing Care *(continued)*

Caring for the Older Adult

- Promote continued development. Assist the client and family to accept physical limitations. Work with them to adapt the environment so that functional health is maintained. Ask yourself the following questions:
  - Does the client have obvious developmental lags that need to be further identified?
  - Is the client or family deprived of normal needs or activities because of institutionalization or isolation?
  - Is the client deprived of normal learning experiences because of physical or sensory limitations?
  - How can we help the client or family find creative alternatives to accomplish developmental tasks?
- Be familiar with the resources available in the community. Collaborate with the healthcare team to provide information and referrals for resources for the client and family.

Key Points

- Growth and development continue as a sequence of predictable patterns throughout the adult life span.
- Erikson, Levinson, and Gould have described major developmental stages and tasks for the young and the middle adult.
- The young adult has reached optimal physical development, but major psychosocial adaptation centers on choosing a vocation and defining relationship choices.
- During the middle adult years, visible signs of aging and an awareness of mortality appear. Various role changes may occur, and midlife crisis may precipitate changes in lifestyle.
- Both young and middle adults are generally healthy, but increased risk for illness results from lifestyle, developmental or situational crises, family history, and the environment.
- Nursing considerations to promote health and prevent illness in early and middle adulthood focus on teaching self-care activities and the importance of regular physical examinations.
- According to Erikson, the older adult continues to look forward but also reflects back on life experiences to find meaning and acceptance. Havighurst views the major tasks of older adulthood to be primarily concerned with social relationships and roles.
- In older adulthood, physiologic aging becomes more rapid, with all organ systems showing decline in efficiency. The lack of physiologic reserves places the older client at risk for multisystem complications.
- The older adult continues to learn and problem solve; intelligence and personality remain consistent after middle age.
- Most older adults adjust well to aging and continue to live active, independent, and productive lives. Although chronic illness is common, most older adults regard themselves as healthy.
- Ageism is a form of prejudice in which the older adult is incorrectly stereotyped as being different from other members of society. Also, aging is not synonymous with disease.
- Gerontologic nursing is a specialty field within the nursing profession, with specialized knowledge of aging in both health and illness that can benefit all nurses.
- A major goal of nursing care is to help the client regain and maintain functional health; the nurse does this by collaborating with the client, family, and healthcare team.

Bibliography

Badger, T. (1993). Physical health impairment and depression among older adults. *IMAGE: Journal of Nursing Scholarship, 25*(4), 325–330.

Bennett, E. G., & Woolf, D. (Eds.). (1991). *Substance abuse* (2nd ed.). Albany: Delmar.

Berkman, L. F. (1983). The assessment of social networks and social support in the elderly. *Journal of the American Geriatric Society, 31*(12), 228–232.

Berry, A. L., & Davignon, D. R. (1991). Changes with age. In M. Patrick, S. Woods, R. Craven, R. Rokosky, & P. Bruno (Eds.). *Medical–surgical nursing: Pathophysiological concepts* (2nd ed.). Philadelphia: Lippincott.

Birchenall, J., & Streight, M. (1993). *Care of the older adult* (3rd ed.). Philadelphia: Lippincott.

Boynton, P. R. (1989). Health maintenance alteration: A nursing diagnosis of the elderly. *Clinical Nurse Specialist, 3*(1), 5–10.

Burgener, S., & Chiverton, P. (1992). Conceptualizing psychological well-being in cognitively-impaired older persons. *IMAGE: Journal of Nursing Scholarship, 24*(3), 209–213.

Burke, M. M., & Walsh, M. B. (1992). *Gerontologic nursing: Care of the frail elderly.* St. Louis: Mosby–Year Book.

Dychtwald, K. (1986). *Wellness and health promotion for the elderly.* Rockville, MD: Aspen.

Ebersole, P., & Hess, P. (1991). *Toward healthy aging: Human needs and nursing responses* (3rd ed.). St. Louis: Mosby.

Eliopoulos, C. (1990). *Caring for the elderly in diverse care settings.* Philadelphia: Lippincott.

Eliopoulos, C. (1993). *Gerontological nursing.* Philadelphia: Lippincott.

Eliopoulos, C. (1995). *Manual of gerontologic nursing.* St. Louis: Mosby.

Erikson, E. (1963). *Childhood and society* (2nd ed.). New York: Norton.

Freiburg, K. L. (1992). *Human development: A lifespan approach* (4th ed.). Boston: Jones & Bartlett.

Fuller, J., & Schaller-Ayers, J. (1994). *Health assessment: A nursing approach* (2nd ed.). Philadelphia: Lippincott.

Gould, R. (1972). The phases of adult life: A study in developmental psychology. *American Psychiatry, 129,* 33–43.

Hardy, M. A. (1990). A pilot study of the diagnosis and treatment of impaired skin integrity: Dry skin in older persons. *Nursing Research, 1*(2), 57–63.

Havighurst, R. J. (1972). *Developmental tasks and education* (3rd ed.). New York: Longman.

Hawranik, P., & Walker, J. (1995). Targeting seniors. *Canadian Nurse, 91*(7), 35–39.

Hendricks, J., & Hendricks, C. D. (1986). *Aging in mass society: Myths and realities* (3rd ed.). Boston: Little, Brown.

Lenihan, A. A. (1988). Identification of self-care behaviors in the elderly: A nursing assessment tool. *Journal of Professional Nursing, 4*(4), 285–288.

Levinson, D. J., Darrow, C. N., Klein, E. B., Levinson, M. H., & McKee, B. (1978). *The seasons of a man's life.* New York: Knopf.

Lien-Gieschen, T. (1993). Validation of social isolation related to maturational age: Elderly. *Nursing Diagnosis, 4*(1), 37–44.

Lierman, L., Young, H., Powell-Cope, G., Georgiadou, F., & Benoliel, J. (1994). Effects of education and support on breast self-examination in older women. *Nursing Research, 43*(3), 158–163.

Matteson, M. A., & McConnell, E. S. (1988). *Gerontological nursing: Concepts and practice.* Philadelphia: Saunders.

Mattice, M., & Mitchell, G. J. (1990). Caring for confused elders. *Canadian Nurse, 86*(11), 16–18.

Murray, R., & Zentner, J. (1993). *Nursing assessment and health promotion: Strategies through the life-span* (5th ed.). Norwalk, CT: Appleton & Lange.

Myers, A. H., & Sharpe, A. (1990). Risks and prevention. In C. Eliopoulos (Ed.). *Caring for the elderly in diverse care settings* (pp. 110–145). Philadelphia: Lippincott.

Nolan, M. (1994). Geriatric nursing: An idea whose time has gone? A polemic. *Journal of Advanced Nursing, 20*(6), 989–996.

Porter, E. (1994). Older widow's experience of living alone at home. *IMAGE: Journal of Nursing Scholarship, 26*(1), 19–24.

Rosen, S. (1994). Managing delirious older adults in the hospital. *MEDSURG Nursing, 3*(3), 181–189.

Seymour, M. (1991). Too old for care. *Canadian Nurse, 87*(11), 26–27.

Sorenson, H., & Thorson, J. (1995). Biological theories of aging. *Journal of Subacute Care, 1*(3), 35–39.

Stolley, J. (1994). When your patient has Alzheimer's disease. *American Journal of Nursing, 94*(8), 34–41.

Tappen, R., & Beckerman, A. (1993). A vulnerable population: Multiproblem older adults in acute care. *Journal of Gerontological Nursing, 19*(11), 38–42.

U. S. Department of Health and Human Services. (1991). *Aging America: Trends and projections.* Prepared by the U. S. Senate Special Committee on Aging, the American Association of Retired Persons, the Federal Council on Aging, and the U. S. Administration on Aging. Washington, DC: US Department of Health and Human Services (DHHS Pub. No. [FcoA] 91-28001).

Valente, S. (1994). Recognizing depression in elderly patients. *American Journal of Nursing, 94*(12), 18–25.

Nurses care for clients in a wide variety of settings within the community. As the healthcare environment changes, nurses increasingly provide care to promote wellness and restore health outside the traditional hospital setting. The chapters in Unit III provide information about the different community-based settings in which nursing care is provided. The chapters in this unit provide an introduction to types and methods of community-based healthcare delivery, roles of members of the healthcare team in providing collaborative interdisciplinary care, activities to provide continuity of care as clients move between and among healthcare settings, and the care provided by nurses for clients in their homes.

Community-based healthcare is provided in settings that range from very large public hospitals to one-room apartments. For example, clients may receive healthcare services as in-patients or ambulatory out-patients in a hospital, through voluntary or public health agencies, in day-care centers and schools, in offices and clinics, or through crisis intervention centers. Care is often provided by a team of healthcare providers to meet physical, psychologic, sociocultural, economic, and spiritual needs. Healthcare services may be financed through federal funding, health maintenance organizations, or private insurance. All of these factors, combined with increasing concern about healthcare provision, have raised questions about cost containment, consumer rights, fragmentation of care, and changing client populations and needs.

As clients enter, leave, and move between healthcare settings, the nurse is most often the member of the healthcare team responsible for coordinating care and teaching so that continuity of care is maintained. Information is provided in this unit about admitting clients to hospital and ambulatory settings, transferring clients between healthcare settings, and providing discharge planning to clients and their families. Because more and more healthcare is provided to clients in their own homes, Chapter 13 provides a base for understanding what home health care is and what the nurse does when providing care in the client's home. Characteristics and roles of the home health nurse are described, and components of the home visit are discussed.

Unit III provides information necessary to the provision of client care within a variety of community-based settings. This information enables the nurse to work within the healthcare system to meet individualized client needs and provide holistic, client-centered care.

Community-Based Settings for Client Care

". . . a realization that the call to the nurse is not only for the bedside care of the sick, but to help in seeking out the deep-lying basic causes of illness and misery, that in the future there may be less sickness to nurse and to cure."

Lillian Wald (1867–1940)
a visionary humanitarian who initiated child labor law revision, improved housing conditions in tenements, supported education for the mentally handicapped, originated public health nursing, and founded the Visiting Nurse Service at the Henry Street Settlement House, New York City

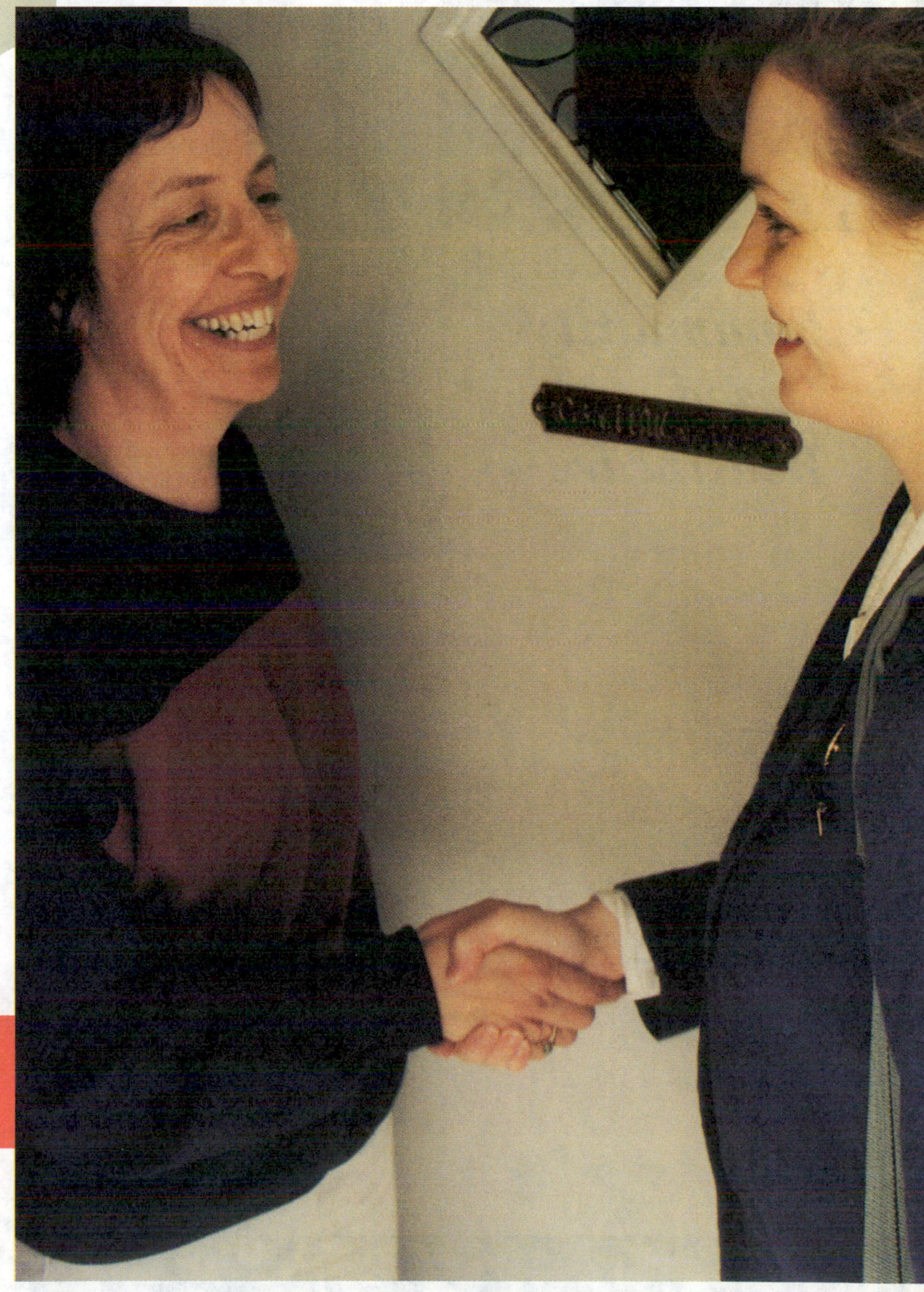

Unit III

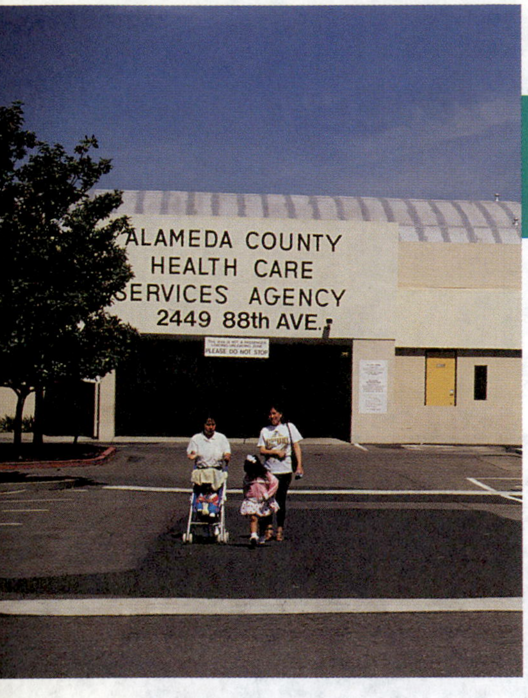

Chapter 11

Community-Based Healthcare

Objectives

After studying this chapter, the learner should be able to:

Define key terms used in the chapter.

Describe the role of nursing in meeting the challenges of healthcare reform.

Compare and contrast the different community-based settings in which healthcare is provided.

Describe community-based healthcare agencies and services.

Discuss the elements of managed care, case management, and primary healthcare.

Describe the roles of members of collaborative healthcare teams.

Discuss various methods of financing healthcare in the United States and Canada.

Discuss trends and issues affecting healthcare delivery.

Key Terms

ambulatory care
case management
community-based healthcare
consumer
day-care centers
diagnosis-related groups
health maintenance organization
inpatient
long-term care
managed care
Medicaid
Medicare
National Medical Care
outpatient
preferred provider organization
primary health care
public health agencies
Public Health Service
rehabilitation centers
voluntary agencies

The healthcare system comprises all the institutions, agencies, policies, payment plans, providers, and individual clients and families involved in healthcare. This chapter provides an introduction to community-based healthcare, including healthcare policy and reform, healthcare agencies, healthcare settings, frameworks for care, collaborative care, financial aspects, and selected trends and issues affecting the healthcare system as we near the year 2000. The following two chapters provide more information about community-based healthcare: Chapter 12 discusses continuity of care as clients move among healthcare settings, and Chapter 13 discusses care of the client in the home setting.

Healthcare Policy and Reform

Many questions are being asked about the healthcare system as it currently exists. The primary areas being questioned are access to healthcare, the quality of healthcare, and the cost of healthcare. These questions are debated at the local, state, and federal level as well as by healthcare providers and consumers of healthcare services. Healthcare reform plans have been proposed at both the federal and state levels, but as yet no one plan has been accepted.

The changes taking place in healthcare provide opportunities for nurses to shape healthcare for the future. Although it is impossible to predict exactly what the practitioner of the future will be doing, projections have been made that outline competencies for the year 2005 (Pew Health Professions Commission, 1991). The competencies are outlined in the accompanying box. These projections, coupled with the national health promotion and disease prevention objectives outlined in *Healthy People 2000* (American Public Health Association, 1990), emphasize the importance of nursing's role in improving access to care, quality of care, and cost of care. Examples of the objectives in *Healthy People 2000* are outlined in the accompanying box.

Nursing's Role in Healthcare Reform

The goals of healthcare reform are cost containment and improved healthcare for all citizens through universal access to services. Where do nurses fit into the reform movement? First, nurses are becoming a stronger voice in protesting the health-related problems in our nation. Second, nurses in greater numbers are increasing their education and becoming advanced practice nurses (APNs). As such, nurse practitioners are providing primary healthcare services in areas and to people long neglected—the elderly, women and infants, the poor, and those living in rural areas. Nurses incur one quarter of the training costs to become primary care providers, then consume only one half of the salary of providers at a similar level (Mundinger, 1994). In addition, the focus of nursing care provided by all nurses is on holistic care essential to illness prevention and health promotion.

Nursing's Agenda for Healthcare Reform, published by the American Nurses Association in 1991, made recommendations for a restructuring of the healthcare system to focus on the healthcare needs of the consumers not only for the population in general, but also in schools, homes, the community, and the workplace. The document further recommended that the care provided focus on wellness and care, not illness and cure. Major topics of the document include:

- A restructured healthcare system
- A federally defined standard package of essential healthcare services available to all U.S. citizens and residents
- A phase-in of essential services
- Planned change to anticipate health service needs that correlate with changing national demographics
- Steps to reduce healthcare costs

Types of Healthcare Settings

Community-based healthcare is care that is provided to people who live within a defined geographic region or have common needs. It is holistic, considering all dimensions of the individual in both health and illness. Community-based healthcare is designed to meet needs of people as they move between and among healthcare settings. Figure 11-1 shows some of the settings for healthcare.

It has been estimated that there are more than 7000 hospitals, 4000 community health agencies, and 26,000 long-term care facilities in the United States (Ellis & Hartley, 1995). When one considers that only clients who re-

Competencies for Healthcare Practitioners for 2005

Practitioners for 2005 should:

- Care for the community's health
- Expand access to effective care
- Provide contemporary clinical practice
- Emphasize primary care
- Participate in coordinated care
- Ensure cost-effective and appropriate care
- Practice prevention
- Involve patients and families in the decision-making process
- Promote healthy lifestyles
- Access and use technology appropriately
- Improve the healthcare system
- Manage information
- Understand the role of the physical environment
- Provide counseling on ethical issues
- Accommodate expanded accountability
- Participate in a racially and culturally diverse society
- Continue to learn

Pew Health Professions Commission. (1991). *Healthy America: Practitioners for 2005.* Durham, NC: The Pew Health Professions Commission

quire complex surgery, who are acutely ill or seriously injured, or who are having babies are hospitalized—and then only for a minimum period of time—it is apparent that the vast majority of healthcare services are provided in settings outside the hospital. Consideration of the client's needs for health restoration and health promotion throughout the lifespan make nursing provided within a community-based healthcare framework essential.

Community-based healthcare is provided within many different types of settings. Healthcare services are provided in community-based settings such as clinics, hospitals, homes, schools, and day-care centers for children and older people. Other community-based settings include crisis intervention centers, mental health centers, drug and alcohol rehabilitation programs, store-front clinics, and churches. Some community-based healthcare agencies provide immunizations for infants and children; screenings for sexually transmitted diseases (STDs) or tuberculosis; and verification of need and voucher distribution for milk and food for women and children with low incomes through the Women, Infants, and Children (WIC) program. Community-based healthcare may also focus on special needs, such as the older adult or terminally ill clients.

Nurses are involved in caring for clients and families in all of these settings and more. The accompanying box lists examples of nursing activities in different types of community-based healthcare settings.

People requiring care are often categorized as either inpatients or outpatients. When people enter a healthcare setting such as a hospital and stay for more than 24 hours, they are said to be **inpatients**. Along with this acute care focus has come a proliferation of services offered for the **outpatient**—the person who requires healthcare services but does not need to stay in an institution for those services. Individuals who do not require inpatient care can receive treatment, care, and education on an outpatient basis. Examples of services provided on an outpatient basis include surgical procedures, diagnostic tests, medications, physical therapy, counseling, and health education. Outpatient services are rapidly expanding and are provided by hospitals, healthcare providers offices, ambulatory care centers, and clinics. A form of outpatient care provided by hospitals is in short-stay units, where clients having diagnostic tests or surgery enter the hospital, have the procedure, and then return to the hospital room for a brief (from 1 to 6 hours) recovery period before going home.

The Home Setting

Home care is one of the most rapidly growing areas of the healthcare system. (See Chapter 13 for a full discussion of this type of community-based nursing care.) Care for clients may be provided in their homes through com-

Healthy People 2000

National Health Promotion and Disease Prevention Objectives: Tobacco

- Reduce the rise in deaths from chronic obstructive pulmonary disease to achieve a rate of no more than 25 per 100,000 people.
- Reduce cigarette smoking to a prevalence of no more than 15 percent among people aged 20 and older.
- Reduce the initiation of cigarette smoking by children and youth so that no more than 15 percent have become regular cigarette smokers by age 20.
- Increase to at least 50 percent the proportion of cigarette smokers aged 18 and older who stopped smoking cigarettes for at least one day during the preceding year.
- Increase smoking cessation during pregnancy so that at least 60 percent of women who are cigarette smokers at the time they become pregnant quit smoking early in pregnancy and maintain abstinence for the remainder of their pregnancy.
- Reduce to no more than 20 percent the proportion of children aged 6 and younger who are regularly exposed to tobacco smoke in the home.
- Reduce smokeless tobacco use by males aged 12 through 24 to a prevalence of no more than 4 percent.

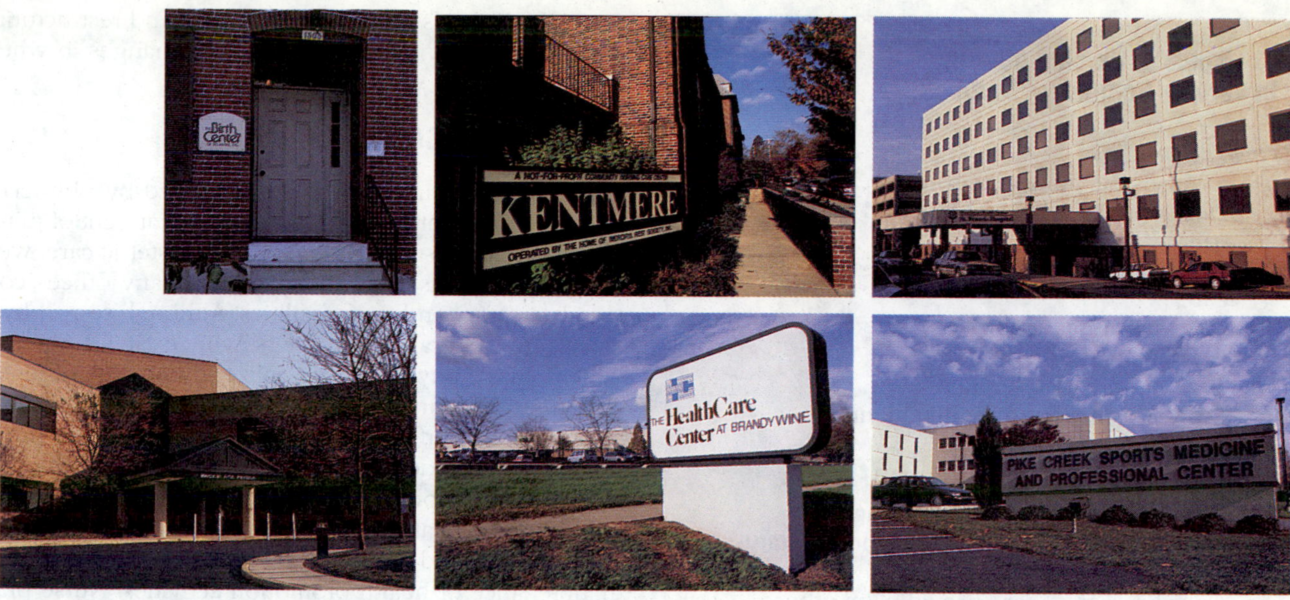

Figure 11-1
In recent years, the number and variety of health care settings have increased dramatically. (Photos © B. Proud.)

munity health departments, visiting nurses' associations, hospital-based case managers, and home health agencies. These agencies provide many different health-related services, including skilled nursing assessment, teaching and support of clients and family members, and direct care for clients.

The importance of home healthcare is evidenced by many factors, including the following:

- The prospective payment system of reimbursement (DRGs), which encourages early discharge from the hospital, has created a new, acutely ill population that needs skilled care at home.
- There are increasing numbers of older people living longer with multiple chronic illnesses who are not institutionalized.
- With more sophisticated technology, people can be kept alive and relatively comfortable in their own homes.
- Healthcare consumers demand that services be humane and that provisions be made for a dignified death at home.

Nurses who work in this type of setting make assessments and provide physical care, administer medications, teach, and support family members. They also collaborate with other healthcare providers such as physicians, physical therapists (PTs), occupational therapists, and respiratory therapists (RTs) to plan and provide client care.

Hospitals: Acute Care Settings

Hospitals have been the traditional setting for providing care for people who were too ill to care for themselves at home, who were severely injured, who required surgery or complicated treatments, or who were having babies. These individuals were admitted to the hospital and were not discharged until they were fully recovered or had used all of the services available within the hospital. As a result of federal regulations and other healthcare reimbursement policies, this is no longer true. With the trend toward discharging clients earlier in their hospital stay, hospitals now focus more often on the acute care needs of the client.

Hospital size ranges from as few as 20 beds to large medical centers with hundreds of beds. Various services are provided, depending on the size and location of the hospital. Most hospitals provide emergency care, inpatient care, surgery, diagnostic tests, and client education. Other services provided within the hospital setting might include intensive care units, obstetrical care, social services, outpatient clinics and surgery, educational programs, and long-term skilled nursing facilities. Hospitals may provide care for all types of illnesses and trauma, or may specialize. Specialty hospitals, or special units in general hospitals, meet the varied needs of clients, including children, clients needing rehabilitation, clients requiring psychiatric or drug dependency care, and clients with severe burns.

Hospitals are classified as public or private and as for-profit or not-for-profit. Public hospitals, which are not-for-profit institutions, are financed and operated by local, state, or national agencies. Many clients admitted to a public hospital do not have health insurance, and services are provided at no cost or little cost to the client. The cost is covered by taxes or public funds. Private hospitals may be for-profit or not-for-profit and are operated by communities, churches, businesses or corporations, and charitable organizations. Many clients cared for in private hospitals have some type of personal health insurance or healthcare plan.

Canadian hospitals receive funding from federal and provincial sources. Clients have basic health insurance

Examples of Nursing Activities in Various Healthcare Settings

Client's Home
- Assesses the home environment and the client
- Develops the relationship based on mutual trust
- Plans, implements, and evaluates the plan of care
- Provides direct care
- Coordinates care of others
- Teaches client and family
- Provides support for family members
- Makes referrals

Hospitals
- Serves as administrator or manager
- Assesses and monitors client's health status
- Provides direct care
- Coordinates the care provided by others
- Teaches clients and families
- Plans, implements, and evaluates the plan of care
- Provides staff information
- Coordinates discharge planning to ensure continuity of care
- Provides specialized care
- Makes referrals

Ambulatory Care
- Makes assessments of health status of clients
- Assists (or is) the primary care provider
- Provides direct client care
- Coordinates care provided by others
- Teaches clients and family
- Plans, implements, and evaluates the plan of care
- Serves as a client advocate

Long-Term Care
- Serves as administrator
- Coordinates the care provided by others
- Provides direct care
- Teaches clients and families
- Plans, implements, and evaluates the plan of care
- Makes referrals

specific to the province in which they reside. In addition, some clients have private health insurance plans or health plans through employment that provide extended coverage and additional benefits.

Although trends are changing, hospitals still employ more nurses than any other type of facility, as shown in Figure 11-2. Nurses employed in the hospital setting have many roles. Although many nurses are direct care providers, other roles include manager of other members of the healthcare team that provides client care, administrator, nurse practitioner, clinical nurse specialist, client educator, in-service educator, and researcher. The current emphasis on cost containment and restructuring has made and will continue to make changes in where and how nurses work.

Primary Care Centers

Primary healthcare services are provided by physicians in their offices through diagnosis and treatment of minor illnesses, minor surgical procedures, obstetric care, well-child care, counseling, and referrals. Many offices contain laboratory and x-ray facilities. Although some physicians are general practitioners who treat all types of illness, many physicians specialize in one type of illness or surgery. A nurse in a physician's office makes health assessments, performs technical skills, assists the physician, and provides health education. Some offices include a nurse practitioner or clinical nurse specialist, who works collaboratively with the physician to make assessments and care for clients who require health maintenance or health promotion activities. Nurse practitioners are also establishing offices and clinics to provide primary care and treatment to clients and only refer complex health problems to a physician.

Ambulatory Care Centers and Clinics

Ambulatory care centers and clinics may be located in hospitals, may be provided as a freestanding service by a group of physicians who work together, or may be run by a nurse practitioner. Ambulatory care centers and clinics are often located in areas that are most convenient for people, such as shopping malls or other community settings. Many ambulatory care centers and clinics offer walk-in services so that appointments are unnecessary, and they are also open at times other than traditional office hours. Nurses in ambulatory care centers and clinics provide technical skills (such as administering medications), determine the priority of care needs among clients, and provide teaching about all aspects of care. A special type of ambulatory care center is an urgent-care center, which provides walk-in emergency care services. Ambulatory surgical centers, discussed in Chapter 30, are another form of ambulatory care center.

Specialized Care Centers

Specialized care centers provide services for a specific population or group. They are usually located in easily accessible locations within a community.

Day-Care Centers. Day-care centers have a variety of purposes. Some centers care for infants and children who are healthy but need care while parents work; some also care for children with minor illnesses. Elder-care centers and senior citizen centers provide a place for older adults to socialize and to receive care while family members work. Some daycare centers provide health-related services and care to people who do not need to be in a healthcare institution but cannot be at home alone. Such centers include centers for older people;

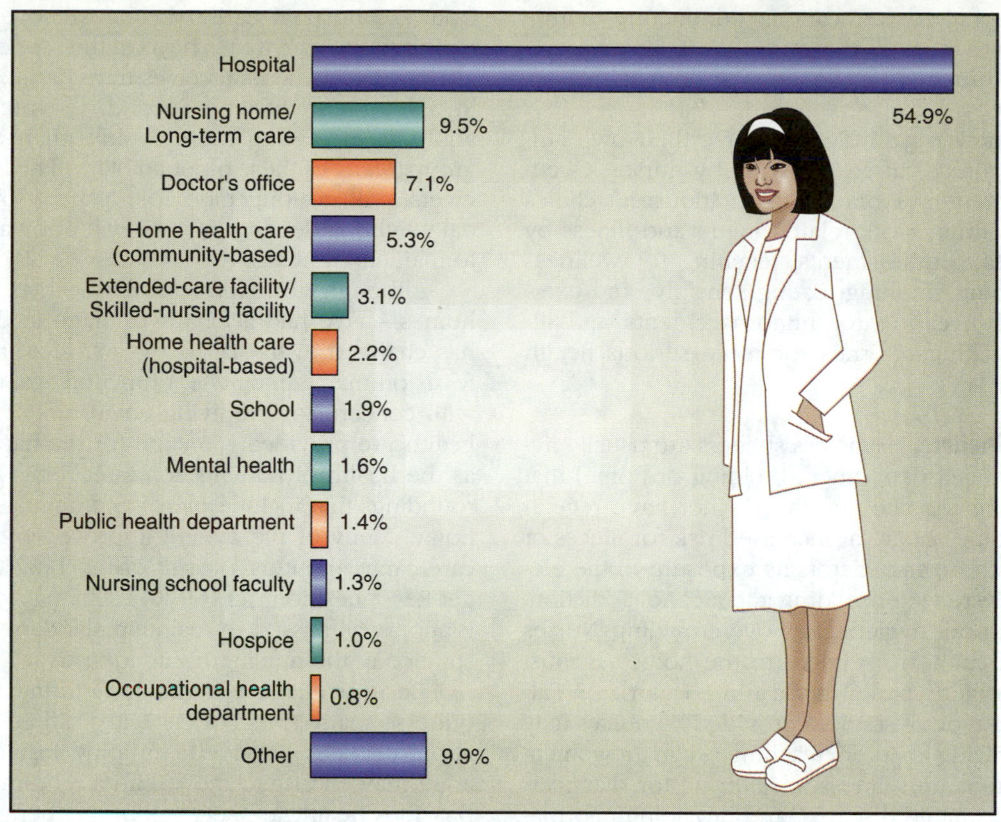

Figure 11-2
Settings in which nurses work. Most nurses are employed in hospitals. Nursing homes, long-term care facilities, and physician's offices are the next most popular settings. (Data: 1994 survey of the nurse universe. Harvey Research Organization, Inc. 1994.)

clients requiring physical rehabilitation; clients with special needs (eg, cerebral palsy); clients who are in drug and alcohol programs; and clients requiring mental health services. Nurses who work in day-care centers administer medications and treatments, conduct health screenings, teach, and counsel.

Mental Health Centers. Mental health centers may be associated with a hospital or may provide services as an independent agency. The services provided may be crisis centered, or may involve long-term counseling. Clients receive outpatient care through a variety of interventions, including individual and group counseling, prescription of medications, and assistance with independent living. Crisis intervention centers are also mental health centers. They typically provide 24-hour services and hot lines for people who are suicidal, who are abusing drugs or alcohol, and who require psychologic or psychiatric counseling. These centers also provide information and services for victims of rape and abuse. Nurses who work in mental health centers must have strong communication and counseling skills, and must be thoroughly familiar with community resources specific to the needs of clients being served.

Rural Health Centers. Rural health centers are often located in geographically remote areas. These centers developed as a result of federal funding for healthcare facilities in areas with a low economic base and few healthcare providers. Many rural health centers are run by nurse practitioners, who serve as the client's primary health provider for the care of minor acute illnesses as well as chronic illness care. Clients who are seriously ill or injured are given emergency care and then transported to the nearest large hospital. Nurses who practice independently do so in collaboration with a physician who approves protocols for care. Many rural hospitals, physicians, and nurse practitioners now have immediate access to information about diagnosis and treatment of illness through telecommunication and computers.

Schools. Although schools are not traditionally considered to be a healthcare setting, school nurses are often the major source of health assessment, health education, and emergency care for the nation's children. The role of the school nurse reflects changes in society itself: children in schools today are from many different racial and ethnic groups, have varying socioeconomic backgrounds, and have more complex disabilities requiring expert knowledge and skills for management during school hours (Harrison, Faircloth, & Yaryan, 1995). School nurses provide many different services, including maintaining immunization records, providing emergency care for physical and mental illnesses, administering prescribed medications, conducting routine health screenings (such as those for vision, hearing, and scoliosis), and providing information about health.

Industry. Many large industries have their own ambulatory care clinic, staffed primarily by nurses. Occupational health nurses practicing in industrial clinics focus on preventing work-related injury and illness by conducting health assessments, teaching for wellness (such as stopping smoking, eating sensibly, and exercising regularly), caring for minor accidents and illnesses, and making referrals for more serious health problems.

Homeless Shelters. Homeless shelters are usually living units (such as an apartment building or home) that provide housing for people who do not have regular shelter. The homeless are at increased risk for illness or injury from such diverse factors as exposure to the elements, exposure to violence, drug and alcohol addiction, poor nutrition, poor hygiene, and overcrowding. Nurses who provide healthcare services to the homeless must be sensitive, nonjudgmental, and caring (Ugarriza & Fallon, 1994). The type of services provided by nurses may include immunizing children, teaching pregnant women, treating infections and illnesses, referring for diagnosis of sexually transmitted diseases, and providing information about maintaining health.

Rehabilitation Centers. **Rehabilitation centers** specialize in services for clients requiring physical or emotional rehabilitation and for treatment of any type of drug dependency. The centers may be freestanding or may be associated with a hospital. The goal is to return clients to optimal health and to the community as productive members of society. Centers that focus on rehabilitation use a healthcare team composed of different members such as physicians, nurses, physical therapists (PTs), OTs, and counselors. The role of the nurse includes direct care, teaching, and counseling. The practice of rehabilitation nursing is based on a philosophy of encouraging independent self-care within the client's capabilities.

Long-Term Care Facilities

Long-term care facilities provide healthcare and help with activities of daily living for people of any age who are physically or mentally unable to care for themselves independently. The care may extend for periods ranging from days to years. Settings that provide long-term care are usually independent facilities, but may be associated with a hospital. Included are facilities that provide transitional subacute care, intermediate and long-term care, and skilled care; nursing homes; retirement centers; and residential institutions for mentally and developmentally or physically disabled clients of all ages.

Long-term care facilities have proliferated, primarily because of two factors. First, clients are being discharged from the hospital earlier in their recovery period and often require care that is beyond the scope of home care. This group of clients receives transitional, subacute care in a long-term facility. Second, the number of older adults is increasing more rapidly than any other age group. Many of these older adults will not have any caregivers, will no longer be able to carry out activities of daily living independently, or will not want to continue to maintain a home.

Although long-term facilities—especially nursing homes—have had a negative image in the past, much has changed in the last 10 years. Most nursing homes focus on maintaining client function and independence, with concern for the living environment as well as the healthcare provided. Concern for the happiness as well as the health of nursing home residents has led to surroundings that include plants and animals as part of the home. Many of the overall improvements in long-term care came about as a result of the 1987 Omnibus Budget Reconciliation Act (OBRA); as a part of that act, legislation was passed to maintain standards of quality assurance in the nursing home industry.

Because clients entering long-term care facilities require so many levels of care, it is difficult to generalize about services provided. In some instances, an older adult may choose to move into a retirement center that provides healthcare services only when needed. Other people who enter a nursing home may require complete care for as long as they live. Those individuals entering convalescent centers only remain until they are considered recovered. The nurse's roles in a long-term care facility may be as a provider of direct care, supervisor, administrator, and teacher. Because most clients are older, increasing numbers of gerontology nurse specialists are contributing their knowledge and expertise to the care of these clients. Almost all long-term care facilities require that skilled nursing care be available at all times. Hence, the care given to clients can only be performed by or under the direct supervision of a licensed nurse.

Hospice Services

Hospices are special services available to terminally ill individuals and their families. The hospice agency may be public or private and may provide both inpatient and home care. These agencies are committed to maintaining quality of life and dignity for the dying person by providing an environment that encourages open communication, symptom management, and comfort measures for the client, and that supports the family during and after death of the client. Many hospice agencies are developed and supervised by nurses but use trained volunteers to supply emotional and physical support, assist with transportation and household care, serve as liaison between client and healthcare providers, and provide short-term respite care for family members who are primary caregivers.

Agencies Providing Care

Many different types of agencies provide healthcare services within a community. Those discussed here are voluntary agencies, religious agencies, and government agencies.

Voluntary Agencies

Community agencies are often not-for-profit **voluntary agencies**. These agencies are financed by private donations, grants, or fundraisers (although some may charge minimal fees). Examples of volunteer agencies are Meals on Wheels, which supplies meals to older and homebound people; transportation services for older and physically disabled people; hearing contact people for hearing impaired clients; and shopping or housecleaning services. Other types of not-for-profit voluntary community agencies found in the United States and Canada include such agencies as the Heart Association and the Lung Association. Physicians and nurses are often active members of these organizations and provide health screenings and educational programs.

Voluntary agencies may also provide the setting for support groups. These groups are designed to provide education and a support system for clients who wish to adjust to health problems. Members of the support groups have experienced the same type of problem. By sharing problems, members learn to solve problems in dealing with a stressful or crisis situation. Examples of support groups are:

- Alcoholics Anonymous, an international organization for recovering alcoholics. The purpose of the support group is to help individuals stop drinking and remain sober. Meetings are held in an accessible community location such as a church or hospital.
- Cancer support groups, which focus on support and solving problems experienced by people diagnosed with cancer. Most cancer support group meetings are held at a hospital.
- Reach to Recovery is a support group for women who have had a breast removed for cancer or have had breast reconstruction surgery. Among other activities, members visit women prior to surgery, teach exercises to prevent muscle atrophy, and provide information about prostheses and clothing.

Other voluntary agencies in which nurses may work are recreational events. For instance, nurses may volunteer time for sports events, such as the one shown in Figure 11-3.

Religious Agencies

Parish nursing is an area of community-based nursing practice that emphasizes holistic healthcare, health promotion, and disease prevention activities. Parish nursing is based on the belief that health promotion means reaching people before they are sick. Activities are often volunteer services and are based within a church. Parish nurses function as health educators, resource and referral persons, and facilitators of lay volunteer and support groups. Parish nurses reach out to those most vulnerable—the elderly, those who have suffered a loss or change, single parents, and children.

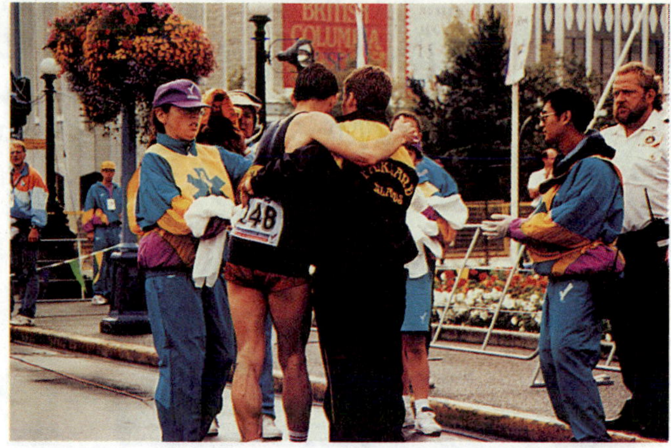

Figure 11-3
Two nurses assist a runner at the completion of the men's marathon during the Victoria Commonwealth Games, Canada. (Photo by Paul Jonson, courtesy of Sandy Gilmour.)

Government Agencies

Government agencies are financed by national, state, local, or provincial taxes. City taxes help support city hospitals and public health clinics; state and provincial taxes help support state mental health hospitals; and national taxes aid in financing national health and welfare programs such as the Canadian Department of Health and Welfare.

Veterans Administration and Military Agencies

Veterans Administration (VA) hospitals and military hospitals all come under the umbrella of government-supported and government-operated healthcare. VA hospitals provide healthcare services to veterans and military hospitals provide care to members of the armed forces and their immediate families.

Public Health Service

The **Public Health Service** (PHS) is a federal health agency that falls under the direction of the U.S. Department of Health and Human Services. A similar health service is provided by the Department of Health and Welfare in Canada. PHS is a multifaceted program that covers a wide range of services. It is the medical branch of the U. S. Coast Guard and the principal source of Native American healthcare through the Indian Health Services. The amount of direct client care provided by

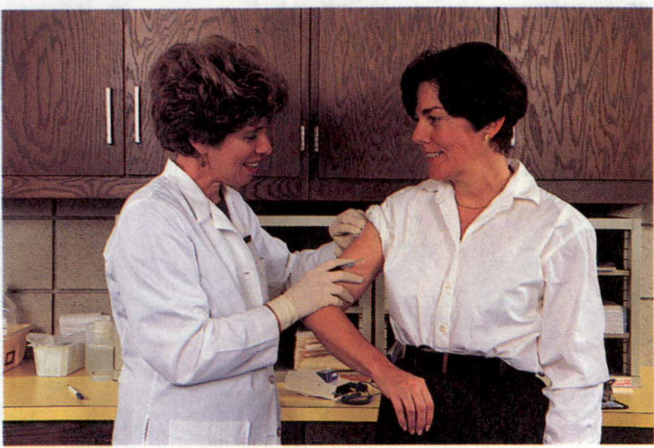

Figure 11-4
Administering an immunization at a public health clinic. (Photo © B. Proud.)

PHS is more limited than in the past. PHS supplies funds to health centers that provide care to migrant workers and to community agencies that supply healthcare to the poor or uninsured. The principal budget of PHS goes to grant programs for poor and uninsured individuals.

The Centers for Disease Control (CDC) in Atlanta and the National Institutes of Health (NIH) are both part of PHS. CDC focuses on the epidemiology, prevention, control, and treatment of communicable diseases such as STDs. NIH is engaged in various health research activities.

PHS also supplies healthcare professionals (eg, nurses, physicians, dentists, and pharmacists) to the U. S. Department of Justice to provide care in federal prisons. The service is also involved to varying degrees in drug and alcohol abuse and mental health programs within the state. PHS activities vary from area to area. In most cases, they focus on community needs and attempt to meet those needs whenever possible.

The types of governmental healthcare services and agencies available in Canada are similar to those in the United States. The major difference between the two systems is the way that healthcare is financed. The Canadian healthcare system is financed by healthcare plans within each province. These plans cover all Canadian residents for most of their necessary hospital care and physicians' fees. These provincial health insurance plans are financed by federal and provincial taxes, employers, or personal policies.

Public Health Agencies

Public health agencies are local, state or provincial, or federal agencies that provide public health services to members of various sizes of communities (ie, local, county, provincial, state, or federal). Public health departments are usually funded by taxes and often have administrators that are elected or appointed. Local agencies provide services and programs to prevent illness and promote health, such as tuberculosis screening, immunizations (Fig. 11-4), and sexually transmitted disease screening. Public health agencies work collaboratively with state and local departments to ensure health through activities such as inspections of restaurants and water supplies. They also provide educational programs, and may provide direct care services for low-income people or people living in rural, isolated areas. Nurses who practice in public health agencies focus on prenatal care, well-child care, screening programs, education, and outreach into the community.

Frameworks for Care

There are different methods for ensuring continuity of care and cost-effective care as a client moves through the healthcare system. These methods include managed care systems, case management, and primary health care.

Managed Care Systems

Managed care is an organized system of healthcare that influences the selection and use of healthcare services of a population that is high-quality and cost-effective (Federa & Camp, 1994). The care of the individual is carefully planned and monitored from the initial contact to discharge from a healthcare episode. Planning and monitoring activities are conducted to ensure that standards are followed and costs are minimized. More and more, health maintenance organizations and insurance companies are changing to managed care systems. A form of managed care is proposed as a national healthcare plan; in general, large umbrella organizations will provide all aspects of care and will compete for the business of the consumer of services. Choice will occur only between managed care organizations and not between individual healthcare providers (Ellis & Hartley, 1995).

Case Management

Case management is a process of coordinating an individual client's healthcare for the purpose of maximizing positive outcomes and containing costs (Ellis & Hartley, 1995). Although there are several different forms of case management, all focus on enhancing continuity of care and effectively using healthcare resources. The primary objective in many case management systems is to identify specific protocols and timetables for care and treatment in a format called a critical pathway. Critical pathways incorporate independent and collaborative nursing interventions to reach desired client outcomes within a specific timeframe.

In the past 5 years, nursing case management has emerged as an important method of coordinating care, controlling costs, and improving access to healthcare.

The nurse case manager is responsible for these goals and may follow the client from diagnosis of an illness to hospitalization and then back to home care. During the healthcare episode, the nurse case manager is responsible for managing the client's interactions with the entire healthcare system. Other areas of nurse case management include:

- Coordinating care within a managed care system to effectively meet consumer healthcare needs and organization cost-containment needs
- Working with clients within a health insurance system to approve high-cost items such as diagnostic tests and hospital admission
- Working within a hospital system to make admission procedures more timely and to coordinate services while the client is hospitalized
- Establishing wellness programs in corporations
- Establishing a private practice to focus on a specific group of clients, such as the older adult

Nurses who are case managers do not give direct care; rather they coordinate the care provided by others. In this role, nurse case managers have increased autonomy and power within the healthcare system.

Primary Health Care

Primary health care was originally conceptualized in 1978 by the World Health Organization (WHO) and the United Nations International Children's Emergency Fund (UNICEF). The concept was developed based on decreases in illness and death in member countries that were achieved by simple, local, inexpensive solutions to health problems, especially when combined with economic and social development. Further discussion led to the Alma-Ata declaration, which focused on a global health strategy called primary health care. Primary health care is defined as essential health care based on practical, scientifically sound, and socially acceptable methods and technology, made universally accessible to individuals and families in the community through their full participation and at a cost the community can afford. It brings health care as close as possible to where people live and work (Barnes et al., 1995).

Primary health care differs from primary care. Primary care is the delivery of health care services, including the initial contact and ongoing care. Included in primary care is the responsibility for referral to other providers based on client needs. Both physicians and nurse practitioners provide primary care, which has an individual client, provider-directed focus. In contrast, primary health care has a community-based philosophical base that emphasizes universal access and affordability of health care, health of the population, and consumer involvement. However, it is important to remember that primary care, as well as case management, can be practiced within a primary health care philosophy.

Collaborative Care

No matter what the type of setting or framework for care, the nurse works with a variety of professionals as client care is planned, provided, and evaluated (Fig. 11-5). For example, the nurse may request a consult with a dietitian for a client who is not eating well or for one who needs to lose weight. After the dietitian talks with the client and mutually determines a plan of care, the nurse can reinforce the plan and evaluate its effectiveness. Collaboration between and among nurses is also an essential part of holistic client care. The primary goal of each member of the healthcare team is to promote wellness and restore health. Included in this section is a discussion of each member of the healthcare team (other than nurses) with whom you will be working most often.

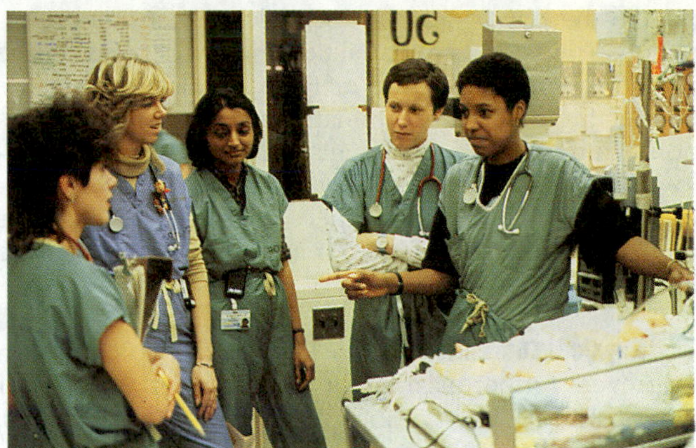

Figure 11-5
Collaboration by all members of the healthcare team facilitates quality care. (Photo by Gates Rhodes, courtesy of School of Nursing, University of Pennsylvania.)

Physician. The physician is primarily responsible for the diagnosis of illness and the medical or surgical treatment of that illness. Physicians are granted the authority to admit clients to healthcare settings by a healthcare agency or institution itself (eg, by the board of a hospital) and to practice care within that setting through such actions as writing orders, interpreting the results of laboratory and diagnostic tests, performing procedures and surgery, and working collaboratively with other professionals. Individuals become physicians after extensive education and clinical practice, and by passing a licensing examination. Depending on the curriculum completed, a physician may graduate from a medical school and become a Doctor of Medicine (MD) or may graduate from a college of osteopathy and become a Doctor of Osteopathy (DO). Both the MD and DO have almost exactly the same type of education and areas of practice, but osteopathic medicine places emphasis on the study of mechanical changes in tissues as a cause of illness and on treatment that involves manipulation of body structures. Physicians may choose to be general practitioners, or may choose to specialize in the treatment of one type of illness (such as a cardiologist) or a specific type of surgery (such as an orthopedic surgeon).

Physician's Assistant (PA). A PA has completed specific courses of study as preparation for providing support to the physician, but does take a licensing examination. The PA's responsibilities usually depend on the physician supervising the activities, and might include conducting physical examinations and suturing lacerations. In most states, a nurse is not legally bound to follow a PA's orders unless they are cosigned by a physician. This is an important aspect to investigate if PAs are employed by hospitals in your area. PAs do not practice in Canada.

Physical Therapist (PT). A PT seeks to restore function or prevent further disability in a client after an injury or illness. The PT uses various techniques to treat clients, including massage, heat, cold, water, sonar waves, exercises, and electrical stimulation. Most PTs are also educated in the use of psychologic strategies to motivate clients.

Respiratory Therapist (RT). An RT has been trained in techniques that improve pulmonary (lung) function and oxygenation. RTs may also be responsible for administering a variety of tests that measure lung functioning and for educating the client about the use of various devices and machines prescribed by the physician.

Occupational Therapist (OT). An OT assists the physically challenged client to adapt to limitations. The OT uses a variety of adaptive devices and strategies to aid a client in carrying out activities of daily living.

Speech Therapist. A speech therapist is trained to help hearing-impaired clients speak more clearly, to assist a client who has had a stroke to relearn how to speak, and to correct or modify a variety of speech disturbances in children and adults. Speech therapists also diagnose and treat swallowing problems in clients who have had a head injury or a stroke.

Dietitian. Generally, a registered dietitian (RD) is responsible for managing and planning for the dietary needs of clients. The RD is knowledgeable about all aspects of nutrition and its effects on the body. An RD can adapt specialized diets for the individual needs of clients, counsel and educate individual clients, and supervise the dietary services of the entire facility.

Pharmacist. A pharmacist is licensed to formulate and dispense medications. The pharmacist is also responsible for keeping a running file of all client medications and for informing the physician when a potential or actual medication error in prescribing has occurred or when prescribed drugs may interact adversely. The pharmacist is an excellent resource for both clients and nurses for any information related to medications.

Social Worker. A social worker counsels clients and family members and also informs them of and refers them to various community resources. The role of the social worker encompasses many activities, such as counseling, reporting suspected drug addiction or abuse, assisting with decisions about life-sustaining treatments, adopting children, and placing clients in long-term care facilities.

Chaplain. Most agencies employ a chaplain to give spiritual support and guidance to clients and their families. The chaplain may also refer a client to a priest, minister, or rabbi of the client's own religious denomination.

Financial Aspects of Healthcare

Healthcare is very expensive, with costs continuing to increase. Few citizens can afford to pay for healthcare from personal resources. The costs of healthcare are often covered by the federal government and private organizations through federally funded programs, prepaid plans, and private insurance.

Federally Funded Health care Programs

The federally funded healthcare programs are primarily through Medicare and Medicaid in the United States and the National Medical Care Insurance program in Canada.

United States

The history of federally funded healthcare, legislated by the federal government, is summarized as follows:

- The 1965 **Medicare** amendments to the Social Security Act established national and state health insurance programs for the elderly under Title 18. Within a decade, almost all citizens over the age of 65 held Medicare insurance for hospital care, extended care, and home healthcare. The primary provisions of Medicare are summarized in Table 11-1.
- In 1965, **Medicaid** was also established under Title 19 of the Social Security Act. This program is a federally funded public assistance program for people with low incomes. The primary provisions of Medicaid are summarized in Table 11-1.
- In 1972, Medicare coverage was increased to include permanently disabled workers and their dependents if they also qualified for Social Security benefits.
- In 1983, Medicare converted to a prospective payment plan called **diagnosis-related groups** (DRGs). This plan pays the hospital a predetermined, fixed amount that is determined by the medical diagnosis or specific procedure rather than by the actual cost of hospitalization and care. DRGs were implemented by the federal government in an effort to control rising healthcare costs. The plan pays only the amount of money preassigned to a diagnosis (eg, an appendectomy); if the cost for hospitalization is greater than that assigned, the hospital must absorb the additional

cost. However, if costs are less than that assigned, the hospital makes a profit.

- In 1988, Medicare was again expanded to include catastrophic care costs and expensive medications.

Medicare and Medicaid are contrasted in Table 11-1. People who receive Medicare pay both a deductible cost and a monthly premium for full insurance coverage. Part A of Medicare, which pays most inpatient hospital costs, is paid by the federal government. Part B of Medicare, which is voluntary, is paid by monthly premium; it covers most outpatient costs for physician visits, medications, and home health services. The full cost of some services is not covered by Medicare; it is recommended that clients subscribe to supplemental insurance policies offered by private insurance companies. Also, because Medicare is federally funded, benefits may change annually according to decisions made concerning the federal budget.

Current budgetary considerations are forcing state and federal agencies to trim Medicaid expenditures. The rapid growth of an aging population and an increase in the number of poor people, many of whom are women and children, are draining the Medicaid budget. For survival, the Medicaid programs are implementing reforms such as reduced benefits, or are placing clients into managed care programs.

Canada

The 1958 Canadian National Hospital Insurance program and the 1968 **National Medical Care** Insurance program provide health insurance for every Canadian citizen, funded through taxes. The 1984 Canada Health Act clarifies and defines the conditions of Canadian health insurance—universality, accessibility, comprehensiveness, and portability among provinces. The organization and services vary among provinces, with incentives for programs that promote health promotion, community services, and home care. The law provides hospital care for all citizens without cost; medical care costs are partially funded through employers or individuals through an annual fee.

Group Plans

Group plans for financing healthcare in the United States include health maintenance organizations (HMOs), preferred provider organizations (PPOs), and private insurance. Enrollment in these plans is voluntary. An individual pays a fixed rate on either a monthly or annual plan and, in turn, receives financial coverage for all the healthcare necessary to maintain wellness and treat illness.

Because group plans such as HMOs and PPOs assume the financial loss or gain of the healthcare services used by their clients, they encourage preventive healthcare to avoid the higher costs of illness and hospitalization. For the same reason, these plans carefully monitor the quality and quantity of the healthcare delivered to clients. They also place limitations on the use of high-cost procedures and require certain guidelines to be followed when a higher-cost procedure is recommended by a physician. Some people do not like these plans because they use a selective contracting approach, mandating subscriber use of specific institutions and healthcare providers. Some consumers dislike the lack of control they have in making decisions relating to personal or family health.

Table 11-1
Medicare and Medicaid: Who and What Do They Cover?

	Medicare	Medicaid
Who does it cover?	• All persons 65 years and older • People who have kidney failure • People with approved disabilities • Dependents of people who are disabled	• People with low income of any age • Beneficiaries of Aid to Families with Dependent Children (AFDC) • Elderly, blind, and disabled people covered by supplemental security benefits
What does it cover?	• Hospitalization, home care, and hospice care for people 65 and older and those who are disabled (Part A) • Part B, which is voluntary and must be paid by the client, provides partial coverage for physician services to client eligible for Part A	• (Coverage depends on state regulations)
What doesn't it cover?	• Routine physical examinations • Dental care or dentures • Hearing tests or hearing aids • Eyeglasses	• Inpatient and outpatient hospital care • Physician and nurse midwife services • Home health care • At-risk pregnancy care • Therapy for persons who have speech, hearing, and language disorders • Prescription medications • Dental, chiropractic, and vision care • Hospice care

Health Maintenance Organizations

Health maintenance organizations (HMOs) are prepaid group healthcare plans that allow enrollees to receive all the medical services they require through a group of affiliated providers. There are often no additional out-of-pocket costs, or the enrollees may pay only a small fee, called a co-pay. An HMO may employ all its providers (including physicians) or may be formed by a group of physicians in alliance who provide care as independent practitioners (an independent practice association or IPA). In most HMO structures, the client does not have a choice about healthcare providers, and receives all services from physicians associated with or part of the HMO. HMOs are becoming more popular, especially with large employers, as they do support the concept of managed care.

Preferred Provider Organizations

Preferred provider organizations (PPOs) allow a third-party payer (such as a health insurance company) to contract with a group of healthcare providers to provide services at a lower fee in return for prompt payment and a guaranteed volume of clients and services. However, clients have more choices: although they are encouraged to use specific providers, they may also seek care outside the panel without referral and pay additional out-of-pocket expenses. A form of this type of insurance plan is the preferred provider arrangement (PPA). In a PPA, the contract is made with an individual healthcare provider rather than with a group of providers. Similarly, a point-of-service (POS) plan encourages the use of specified physicians and services, but pays a portion of expenses if referrals are made to physicians outside the organization.

Private Insurance

Personal healthcare can be financed by private insurance; through large, nonprofit, tax-exempt organizations; or through smaller, private, for-profit insurance companies. To be insured, members pay monthly premiums either by themselves or in combination with their employer. These plans are called third-party payers because the insurance company pays all or most of the cost of care. The premiums on private insurance plans tend to be higher than with HMOs, but the client can choose the physician and services desired.

Long-Term Care Insurance

A recent development in the healthcare insurance market is the growing interest in long-term care (LTC) insurance. In general, a minimal amount of LTC is paid for by private insurance. Most LTC (about 90%) is paid for by Medicaid and out-of-pocket spending. Medicare pays for a small percentage of LTC. The steady increase in the population of people aged 65 years and older has become a major concern within the healthcare financing area.

Some commercial insurance companies offer LTC benefits. Promoters of LTC insurance have developed models of plans that would cover a variety of services such as nursing home care and home care as well as other services that would help prevent the institutionalization of older, debilitated, and chronically ill people. Adult day-care centers and respite care would also fall under these types of services and would be covered by benefits.

Trends and Issues in Healthcare Delivery

A few of the issues that influence trends in healthcare are discussed in this section. In your career as a nurse, you may find that some questions are answered, but you will also discover that more challenges arise. As a nurse, it will be important for you both personally and professionally to be knowledgeable about all the aspects of the healthcare delivery system.

Focus on Self-Care and Wellness

Health awareness and the desire for personal involvement in one's own healthcare has strongly influenced the delivery of healthcare services in society. People are becoming convinced that it is better to remain healthy than it is to neglect one's health and then treat a resulting illness or injury. This belief has far-reaching influences on the way we live. Stress management programs, nutritional awareness, exercise and fitness programs, and antismoking and antidrug campaigns are all examples of this trend (Fig. 11-6). Equally as important in the health of all members of society are measures such as promoting the wearing of seat belts, promoting automobile and airplane safety, controlling smog, control of handguns, and eliminating hazardous wastes.

A public interest in self-care has evolved into a strong force in terms of the education and services provided by healthcare professionals. Consumers of healthcare are often better educated about health, prefer to control and make decisions about their own personal

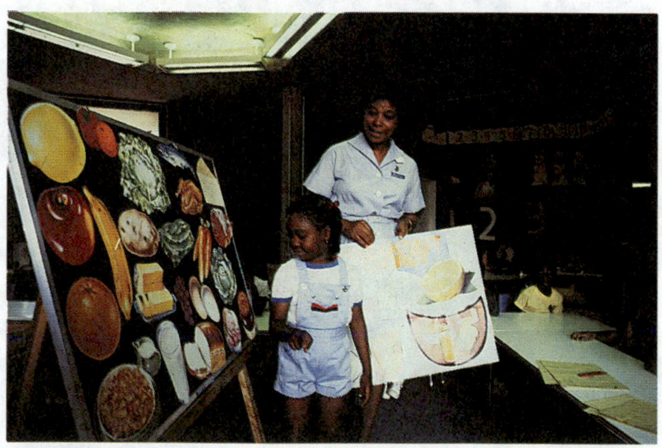

Figure 11-6
Young children in school, community centers, and other community groups can be taught the importance of eating healthful foods.

Nursing Today: Challenges and Solutions

The Future of Nursing

Many changes are taking place in the healthcare system, and all of the changes affect nurses and nursing care. Words such as career security, restructuring, managed care, and workforce redesign—once little considered as important by nurses—are now common topics. The American Nurses Association believes that the work life of the nurse will probably change as dramatically as other components of the healthcare delivery system. Predictions for change include:

- Increased acuity in hospital and long-term care settings
- Less hospital care and more community care
- More care delivered in organized systems that manage quality and cost across multiple sites
- An increased focus on primary healthcare and prevention
- An increased need for health services with a constricted resource base

Nurses have always provided continuity of care and a continuum of services for patients, their families, and the community in both health and illness. However, if nursing is to become an integral element of the healthcare system as changes become a reality, they must define their professional future to ensure that nurses are valued, valuable, and essential providers in all practice settings.

Source: Betts, V. (1995). Defining our future, dividing our resources. *American Nurse, 27*(3), 5.

health, and want to be active participants in planning and implementing their own healthcare.

Consumer Movement

A **consumer** is someone who uses a commodity or service. Consumers of healthcare services have become better educated about the services they require and the services that are available. They also have become concerned about access to services and the cost of those services. Consumers have questioned escalating costs and the proliferation and duplication of services. Consumers have become actively involved in the administration of healthcare agencies and have helped develop standards for care, client rights, and cost-containment measures as protection for clients when they enter a healthcare setting. On the other hand, the consumer movement has led to an increase in malpractice lawsuits, resulting in

Computer Applications in Nursing

Community-Based Healthcare

The computer is used in the community setting for administrative and practice support. The administrator can use the computer to gather epidemiologic and administrative statistics, for billing and payroll, and to make appointments. The community nurse uses the computer for client assessment and data gathering, home care management plans, physiologic monitoring, and documentation. The home care nurse can use portable computers, notebooks, or handheld devices to improve communication and the quality of client care.

The home health nurse no longer has to start the day in the office. Rather, information can be downloaded from the agency's main office into a laptop computer via a telephone line. The nurse can access client information, the agency's policy and procedure manual, a database with medication teaching materials, and a program to analyze potential drug interactions. Electronic mail can be exchanged with the office, other health professionals, and clients. Clients can participate in support groups, for example, people with AIDS and caregivers of people with Alzheimer's.

Advantages of using information technology in the community include the speed of communication; the ability to retrieve, compile, and summarize data; and the ability to present data legibly and attractively. Standard care plans can be stored and adapted to fit the individual client. Automated care plans save time on the part of the nurse and reduce errors, omissions, and misunderstandings between caregivers and clients. Continuity and consistency of care is supported by the use of automated care plans.

Future uses of technology in the home care environment include the use of high-speed telecommunications and laptops to transmit x-rays, magnetic resonance imaging, computer tomography images, electrocardiograms, electroencephalograms, and a complete medical history (Hannah, Ball, & Edwards, 1994; Hassett & Farver, 1995).

high malpractice insurance rates (especially for physicians) and the necessity to carefully document care given. The increased paperwork often serves to take the nurse away from actual client care.

Cost Containment

The healthcare system is experiencing a financial crisis. Health costs have increased dramatically, and some analysts believe that cost-containment measures have been implemented too late to effectively reverse the current upward swing in health costs. The actual short-term and long-term results of these cost-containment measures remain to be seen.

Historically the healthcare system and the financial arrangements for paying for healthcare encouraged the use of expensive and sometimes inappropriate or ineffective health services. Many insurance plans paid for inpatient hospital care but not for ambulatory outpatient care. Therefore, to receive payment, clients were often hospitalized unnecessarily. Healthcare has also focused on the treatment of illnesses instead of on their prevention because preventive strategies often were not covered by a client's health insurance policy. Third-party reimbursement effectively insulated clients from knowing the actual cost of their healthcare. Because the insurance company was responsible for paying the incurred bills, the client was often bypassed in this process and seldom saw the bills for the care received.

The increased competition among hospitals further fueled the increase in health costs. Technologically, amazing advances have been made, but as new machines and more advanced and expensive procedures are developed and used, clients' expectations of hospital resources will also increase. The media are constantly informing the public of new and innovative treatment modalities. As a result, consumers expect these services to be available in "their" hospital. To attract clients, hospitals invest huge sums of money in technologically advanced equipment. Supporters of cost-containment measures are encouraging hospitals to cooperate with one another and share resources rather than compete. Other efforts at cost containment include hospital restructuring and multiple hospitals joining together as one system.

Fragmentation of Care

Increased healthcare research has resulted in an upward spiral of technology and knowledge. In effect, this means that healthcare providers can no longer keep up with all of the advances made, so that specialization has become almost the rule rather than the exception. What does this mean for the client?

A physician who is a general practitioner diagnoses and treats a variety of common health problems. However, a client who requires diagnosis and treatment for a more complex problem is usually referred to a physician who is a specialist. For example, a client with diabetes and a heart condition may be cared for by the family physician, a cardiologist, and an endocrinologist. The hospitalized client not only comes in contact with many different healthcare providers (eg, registered nurses, licensed practical nurses, nursing assistants, nurse specialists, physical therapists, dietitians, and students) but also is frequently seen by other physician specialists called in on consultation or to do surgery. It is no wonder that the client becomes confused about care and treatments. This fragmentation of care can result in the loss of continuity of care, resulting in conflicting plans of care, too much or too little medication, and higher healthcare costs (Fig. 11-7).

Changes in Client Care Needs

This topic is a major issue in healthcare delivery. The older adult, and particularly those over age 70, are the most rapidly growing segment of our population. As people age, there is an associated increase in chronic illnesses. This presents two problems. First, these clients require more healthcare in both inpatient and outpatient settings. As a result, hospitals are increasingly filled with older men and women who are in the acute or terminal stages of one or more chronic illnesses. Second, these clients need additional doctor's visits, more medications, and more health-related supplies, but they often have difficulty affording these needs, especially if they are on a fixed income. This problem may be further compounded by a lack of transportation, a scarcity of family members or support systems, and a desire for independence that interferes with compliance with healthcare regimens. Many of these needs are also found in the growing number of people with AIDS and the homeless.

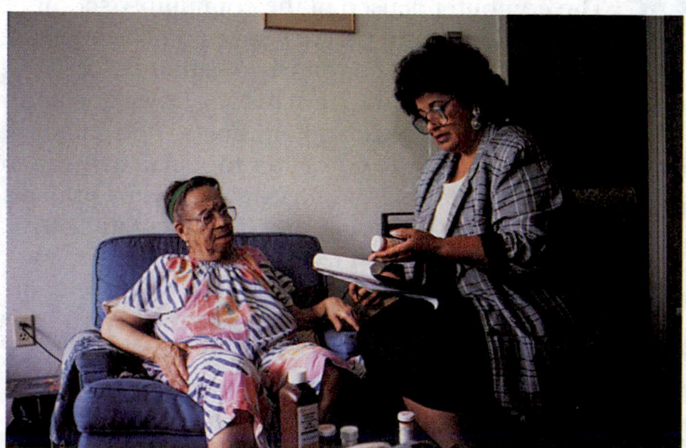

Figure 11-7
The nurse who visits in the home has a responsibility to assess the amount and types of medications the client is taking and whether the client understands when and how to take the medications. Reports are made or prescriptions questioned through the physician. (Photo © Kathy Sloane.)

Healthcare: A Right or a Privilege?

Two major factors that influence healthcare provision in the United States are (1) the ability to pay and (2) location of facilities. Poor or uninsured people, minorities, residents of rural areas and older people often are faced with inadequate access to healthcare services. In the United States, 37 to 39 million people currently have no or inadequate insurance. Although many people assume that all people have a right to healthcare, consider these questions that pose ethical dilemmas:

Do uninsured people who do not take care of themselves deserve the same healthcare as the employed person with insurance?

Who provides funds for the healthcare needs of the homeless population?

Is the person who goes on national television asking for an organ donation for his or her child any more deserving than the person who has been waiting months for just such a transplant?

Are you willing to pay increased insurance premiums so that the drug addict who overdoses can have intensive care?

If 20 people need a heart transplant and only one heart is available, who decides who gets another chance at life?

These are only a few of the questions being raised, and there are no easy answers. The issue of who gets healthcare and, in turn, who pays the bills, will be of major importance to society as we move into the 21st century. These issues present both challenges and opportunities for the nurse of the future.

Key Points

- Healthcare policy and reform issues are creating changes in healthcare that provide nurses with opportunities to shape healthcare for the future.
- Community-based healthcare is care that is provided in all types of healthcare settings, is provided to people who live in a defined geographic area with common needs, is holistic, and is designed to meet the needs of people as they move between and among healthcare settings.
- Community-based heathcare is provided in homes, hospitals, primary care centers, ambulatory care centers, specialized care centers, rehabilitation centers, long-term care facilities, hospices, and agencies. Nurses care for clients in all these settings and more.
- Healthcare services provided to clients in their homes include skilled nursing assessment, teaching and support of clients and family members, and direct care.
- Hospitals provide a wide variety of inpatient and outpatient services and are classified as either private or public, for-profit or not-for-profit. Care within the hospital setting is focused on the acute care needs of clients.
- Primary healthcare services are provided in offices by physicians and nurse practitioners.
- Ambulatory care centers are often located in convenient areas, may offer walk-in services, and are open for a longer period than offices. Urgent-care centers provide emergency care services and ambulatory surgical centers are sites for surgical procedures and care.
- Specialized care centers provide services for a specific population or group; they include day-care centers, mental health centers, rural health centers, schools, industry, and the homeless.
- Long-term care centers provide care and support for physically and mentally challenged people of any age. Care, which may range from only a few days to years, includes transitional subacute care, intermediate and long-term care, and skilled care. Settings for long-term care include hospitals, nursing homes, retirement centers, and residential institutions.
- Hospices provide special services for terminally ill clients and their families.
- Agencies that provide community-based healthcare services include voluntary agencies, religious agencies, and government agencies. Veterans hospitals, the Public Health Service, and public health agencies are also agencies that provide care and services to clients.
- Methods of ensuring continuity of care and cost-effective care include managed care systems, case management, and primary health care.
- Members of the healthcare team collaborate to promote client wellness and to restore health to clients who require healthcare services.
- Healthcare costs are financed through federally funded programs, group plans, and private healthcare insurance.
- Medicare is a federal health insurance program in the United States for people aged 65 years or older, people with permanent kidney failure, and certain physically challenged individuals. Medicaid is a federally funded health insurance program for people with low incomes.
- The National Medical Care insurance program provides hospital care to all citizens of Canada.
- Current societal issues influencing healthcare delivery focus on wellness promotion, changes in client care needs, cost containment, and consumer rights. Clients are better educated about health matters, prefer more control and more participation in decision making about personal health, and are becoming active participants in planning and implementing healthcare.

Bibliography

Allen, S. (1994). Medicare case management. *Home Healthcare Nurse, 12*(3), 21–27.

American Nurses Association. (1991). *Nursing's agenda for healthcare reform.* Washington, DC: ANA.

American Public Health Association. (1990). *Healthy People 2000: National Health promotion and disease prevention objectives.* Washington, DC: Author.

Barnes, D., Eriges, C., Juarbe, T., Nelson, M., Proctor, S., Sawyer, L., Shaul, M., & Meleis, A. (1995). Primary health care and primary care: A confusion of philosophies. *Nursing Outlook, 43*(1), 7–16.

Betts, V. (1995). Defining our future, dividing our resources. *American Nurse, 27*(3), 5.

Buerhaus, P. (1994). Managed competition and critical issues facing nurses. *Nursing & Healthcare, 15*(1), 22–26.

Buzath, J., Lievaart, B., & Schow, E. (1992). Political action: Choice or obligation? *Canadian Nurse, 88*(2), 35–36.

Dee-Kelly, P., Heller, S., & Sibley, M. (1994). Managed care: An opportunity for home care agencies. *Nursing Clinics of North America, 29*(3), 471–481.

Drew, J. C. (1990). Health maintenance organizations: History, evolution, & survival. *Nursing and Healthcare, 11*(3), 145–149.

Ellis, J., & Hartley, C. (1995). *Nursing in today's world: Challenges, issues, and trends.* Philadelphia: Lippincott.

Federa, R., & Camp, T. (1994). The changing managed care market. *Journal of Ambulatory Care Management, 17*(1), 1–7.

Gale, B. J., & Steffl, B. J. (1992). The long-term care dilemma: What nurses need to know about Medicare. *Nursing and Healthcare, 13*(1), 34–41.

Gilmour, S., & Hitesman, A. (1995). Nursing meets sports medicine. *Canadian Nurse, 91*(5), 32–36.

Hannah, K. J., Ball, M. J., & Edwards, M. J. A. (1994). *Introduction to nursing informatics.* New York: Springer-Verlag.

Harrison, B., Faircloth, J., & Yaryan, L. (1995). The impact of legislation and litigation on the role of the school nurse. *Nursing Outlook, 43*(2), 57–61.

Hassett, M. M., & Farver, M. H. (1995). Information management in home care. In M. J. Ball, K. J. Hannah, S. K. Newbold, & J. V. Douglas (Eds.). *Nursing informatics: Where caring and technology meet* (2nd ed.). New York: Springer-Verlag.

Hull, M. M. (1991). Hospice nurses: Caring support for caregiving families. *Cancer Nursing, 14*(2), 63–70.

Jordan, P. (1994). Healthcare reform: Current and proposed approaches. *Oncology Nursing Forum, 21,* 1215–1220.

King, J. (1993). Coalition building between public health nurses and parish nurses. *Journal of Nursing Administration, 23*(2), 27–31.

King, M. L. (1992). Care management. *Canadian Nurse, 88*(4), 15–17.

Kongstvedt, P. (1993). *The managed healthcare handbook* (2nd ed.). Gaithersburg, MD: Aspen.

Lamb, G., & Stempel, J. (1994). Nurse case management from the client's view: Growing as insider-expert. *Nursing Outlook, 42*(1), 7–13.

LeFort, S. (1993). Shaping healthcare policy. *Canadian Nurse, 89,* 23–27.

Mikulencak, M. (October 1992). The satisfying role of parish nursing. *American Nurse,* 10.

Mundinger, M. (1994). Healthcare reform: Will nursing respond? *Nursing & Healthcare, 15*(1), 28–33.

Pew Health Professions Commission. (1991). *Healthy America: Practitioners for 2005.* Durham, NC: The Pew Health Professions Commission.

Rozovsky, L. (1979). *Canadian hospital law* (2nd ed.). Ottawa: Canadian Hospital Association.

Sandhu, B. K., & Duquette, A., & Kerouac, S. (1992). Care delivery modes. *Canadian Nurse, 88*(4), 18–20.

Schorr, T. (1993). The term is "healthcare." *Nursing & Healthcare, 14*(6), 294–295.

Shalala, D. (1993). Nursing & Society: The unfinished agenda for the 21st century. *Nursing & Healthcare, 14*(6), 289–291.

Shortridge, L. (1993). Establishing a nurse-managed health center: Getting started. *Nurse Practitioner Forum, 4*(3), 133–142.

Sprayberry, L. (1993). Nursing's dual role in healthcare policy. *Nursing & Healthcare, 14*(5), 250–254.

Storch, J. (1985). The Canadian healthcare delivery system: Policies, programs, services. In M. Stewart et al. (Eds.), *Community health nursing in Canada* (pp. 33–48). Toronto: Gage.

Ugarriza, D., & Fallon, T. (1994). Nurses' attitudes toward homeless women: A barrier to change. *Nursing Outlook, 42*(1), 26–29.

Uphold, C., & Graham, M. (1993). Schools as centers for collaborative services to families: A vision for change. *Nursing Outlook, 41*(5), 204–211.

Witek, J., & Hostage, J. (1994). Medicaid managed care: Problems and promises. *Journal of Ambulatory Care Management, 17*(1), 61–69.

Chapter 12

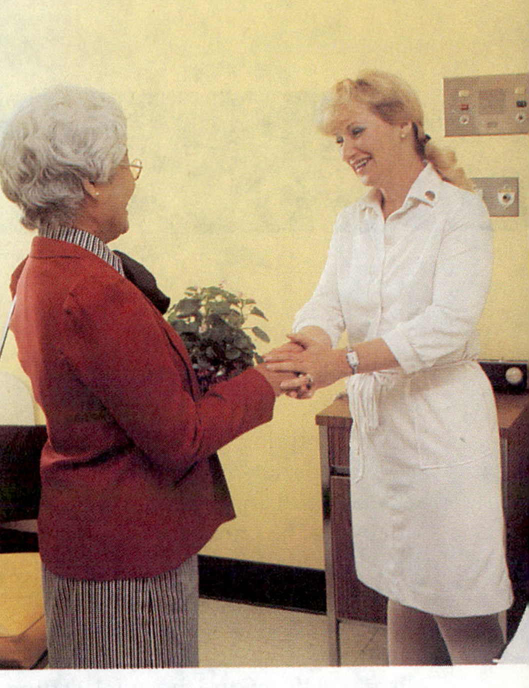

Continuity of Care

Objectives

After studying this chapter, the learner should be able to:

Define key terms used in the chapter.

Describe the role of the nurse in ensuring continuity of care between and among client care settings.

Discuss considerations for establishing an effective nurse–client relationship when admitting a client to a healthcare setting.

Compare and contrast admission of a client to an ambulatory setting and a hospital setting.

Discuss transfer of clients within and among healthcare settings.

Describe the components of discharge planning in providing continuity of care.

Key Terms

ambulatory facilities
compliance
continuity of care
discharge planning

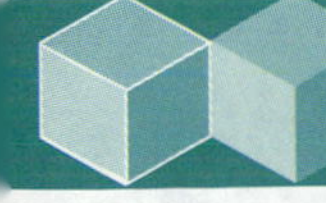

Entering and leaving a healthcare setting are experiences that produce anxiety for the client and for family members. Equally anxiety producing is the care that must be provided at home after the client leaves the healthcare setting. The nurse is most often the person who is responsible for helping the client make a smooth transition from one type of care setting to another. This chapter discusses admission and dismissal from the hospital setting, transfer from one type of setting to another, and discharge planning in preparation for home care. The focus of the discussion is on the client's needs and the nurse's role in providing continuity of care.

The Nurse's Role in Providing Continuity of Care

Most individuals were born in a hospital; thus, they became consumers of healthcare from the first day of life. They continue to require services of some type until they die. Although many different healthcare providers and settings will be a part of that care (see Chapter 11), the nurse is often the primary person responsible for communicating needs; teaching self-care; and, in many instances, providing needed care. As a result, one of the primary responsibilities of the nurse as caregiver is ensuring continuity of care.

Continuity of care refers to the coordination of services provided before a person enters a healthcare setting, during the time they are in the setting, and after they leave the setting. Continuity of care ensures a smooth transition between ambulatory or hospital care and home care or other types of community-based care. Coordination provides a client-focused and individualized continuum of healthcare. Such a practice reduces anxiety and facilitates the client in reaching optimal functioning or wellness.

Continuity of care is essential in the current healthcare delivery system. The emphasis on wellness and prevention of illness makes teaching for individuals of all ages critical components of client care. To provide continuity of care, the nurse must do the following:

- Include discharge planning in the care of any person admitted to any type of healthcare setting
- Collaborate with other members of the healthcare team in meeting physical, psychologic, sociocultural, and spiritual needs of the client and family in all settings and at all levels of health
- Involve the client and the client's family in the planning process

The purpose of planning for continuity of care, which is more commonly referred to as **discharge planning**, is to ensure that client and family needs are consistently met as the client moves from one level of care to another. Discharge planning is described in detail later in the chapter, but basically it involves the following:

- Assessing the strengths and limitations of a client and strengths and limitations of the family or support person and the environment
- Planning for continuity in healthcare from one setting to another, including the home
- Implementing and coordinating the plan of care, considering individual client needs as well as individual, family, and community resources
- Evaluating the effectiveness of care

This chapter is intended to be only an introduction to the different ways in which clients enter a healthcare setting and move from one type of setting to another. Discharge planning is discussed primarily in relation to the care of the client at home; this aspect of care will become increasingly common as the nursing profession moves into the 21st century.

Admitting a Client to a Healthcare Setting

People enter the healthcare setting to become consumers of healthcare services (clients) for many different reasons. Consider the following examples:

Joe Sol, aged 5 years, has been having increasing numbers of throat infections, and his tonsils are badly infected. Joe's pediatrician has decided that Joe must have a *tonsillectomy* (removal of tonsils) in a hospital, entering the morning of surgery and going home that afternoon.

Jane Yee, aged 38 years, has had heavy menstrual periods. As a diagnostic procedure, her doctor schedules her for a dilation of the cervix and curettage of the uterus (*D & C*) at a community ambulatory surgery center.

Tom Valiz, aged 28 years, injured his back while working at his construction job. After diagnostic studies, he has been going to a community health center each day for heat therapy and exercises.

Sarah Hale, aged 16 years, has been brought to the hospital emergency room for acute alcohol intoxication. After treatment, she is admitted to the hospital's chemical dependency unit for observation.

Sadie Aird, aged 78 years, has had congestive heart failure for the past 10 years. She is cared for at home by her daughter, with the help of a home health nurse and aide.

Jim Zamba, aged 28 years, is admitted to the hospital through the emergency room, sent to surgery, and then placed in the intensive care unit (ICU) for treatment of severe head injuries following a motorcycle accident. After recovery from the acute phase of care, Jim will go to a special rehabilitation center.

Although all of these individuals require care, they will not all have the same kind of needs nor will they be alike as clients. Some of them will be admitted and discharged on the same day, some of them will remain in the acute-care setting only as long as acute care is needed, and some will require long-term care.

For years, hospitals have been the primary method of delivering care to people who were too ill to be cared for at home or required surgery. However, because of increasing costs and a healthcare cost reimbursement program that is prospective instead of retrospective, hospital admissions for many surgical procedures and lengths of hospital stay are decreasing. Increasing numbers of clients are having surgery, diagnostic tests, and emergency care in ambulatory care settings or on an outpatient basis. Even clients who are admitted may stay for fewer than 24 hours, may be admitted the morning of the surgery, or may go home during an interim period between diagnosis and care.

All people who enter a healthcare setting must take on a new role. They must add to their already established roles (eg, spouse, parent, sibling, student) the role of client. In addition to adding a new role, they also enter an environment in which they are surrounded by strangers and in which they encounter different sounds, sights, and smells.

All people who become healthcare clients have needs that require attention. In meeting these needs during admission of the client, the nurse is providing holistic care while establishing the base for the way in which the client will respond to and evaluate the remainder of his or her stay. The accompanying box describes nursing guidelines for establishing an effective nurse–client relationship to ensure that each client is considered as an individual in any type of setting.

During the admission process, the nurse acts not only as a practitioner but also as a person concerned about the welfare of client and family. The admission period corresponds to the orientation phase of the helping relationship described in Chapter 22. In addition, regulatory guidelines provide direction for both continuity of care and quality of care. For example, the standards for admission and discharge, established by the Joint Commission on Accreditation of Healthcare Organizations, include the following:

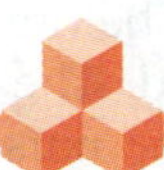

Guidelines for Nursing Care

Establishing an Effective Nurse–Client Relationship Respectful of Client Individuality

- **Recognize and take necessary steps to reduce anxiety. Anxiety is a natural reaction to the unknown. Anxiety reduction can be facilitated through therapeutic communications, teaching, and acceptance. Some common concerns that cause anxiety follow:**

  Will I have pain?
  Who will take care of my family if I die?
  Will strangers be looking at my body?
  How much will this cost?
  What if I can't keep my job?
- **Remember that the medical or surgical condition for which the client is being treated is only one part of the client's life. Although it may be the primary concern for the client, other concerns include family needs, financial status, and the future.**
- **Communicate with the client as an individual so that he or she can maintain his or her own identity. Ask clients how you should address them—some people would prefer Mr., or Mrs., Ms. [last name]; others would rather be called by their first name. Do not lump all older adults as "Grandma" or "Grandpa." Be sure that you do not refer to Mr. Jones, admitted to room 2218 for treatment of a ruptured appendix, as "the appendix in 2218."**
- **Take time to learn *who* the client being admitted is, including the client's cultural and religious background. Respect the client's values and beliefs even though they may differ from yours.**
- **Provide for client-family participation and decision making in all aspects of care.**

- Each client's need for nursing care related to admission is assessed by a registered nurse.
- Each client's assessment includes consideration of biophysical, psychosocial, environmental, self-care, educational, and discharge planning factors.
- The client and family are involved in care as appropriate.
- Nursing staff members collaborate, as appropriate, with physicians and members of other clinical disciplines to make decisions regarding the client's need for nursing care.
- In preparation for discharge, continuing care needs are assessed and referrals for such care are documented in the client's medical record.

Admission to an Ambulatory Healthcare Facility

An individual may require care in many different kinds of ambulatory facilities, including physician offices, clinics, outpatient services, emergency rooms, and same-day surgery centers. **Ambulatory facilities** are those in which the client receives healthcare services but does not remain overnight. The goal of such facilities is to keep ambulatory those clients under care or to enable those clients who are able to provide self-care at home with assistance as necessary from healthcare providers. Individuals go to ambulatory settings for wellness promotion, health maintenance, or for medical or surgical treatment.

In most ambulatory settings, clients enter a reception area, where they are asked to complete a short health history. They then go to an examination room and a physical assessment is completed. Depending on their needs, diagnostic tests may be done, immunizations given, medications prescribed, or minor surgery performed. All clients require teaching, which should include written instructions about care at home, health promotion activities, and how to contact someone for further questions. Referrals to community agencies, support groups, or other types of healthcare settings may be necessary.

Admission to ambulatory or same-day surgery facilities is somewhat different. Screening tests, teaching, and admission procedures usually are completed before clients enter the setting. They arrive at the setting, have the procedure, and go home when recovery is satisfactory (see Chapter 30). If clients have surgery in the hospital setting, the regular admission procedures are completed on arrival; in most instances, screening tests and teaching are done before the day of surgery. It is the nurse's responsibility to assess what has been done and individualize the care plan to clients' needs.

Admission to the Hospital Unit

In most hospitals, admission begins in the admitting office. Staff obtain information about clients and print that information on an admission sheet. This admission sheet becomes part of a client's permanent record, and includes the following information:

Full name
Address
Date of birth
Name of admitting physician
Gender
Marital status
Nearest relative
Occupation and employer
Financial status for healthcare payment
Religious preference
Date and time of admission
Identification number
Admitting diagnosis

The identification number, as well as the client's name and physician's name (and any other information required by a specific institution), becomes a part of the identification bracelet that is placed on the client's wrist. This bracelet is an important safety component during the client's treatment because it is the means of accurate identification for many procedures and treatments, including medication administration, diagnostic tests, and surgery. The bracelet is essential for identifying clients who are irrational, comatose, or young.

After the necessary forms have been completed in the admitting office, clients are usually taken to the unit to which they have been assigned. Because of cost-containment measures, laboratory studies and x-rays as well as the admitting office procedures may be completed on an outpatient basis before the day of admission.

Preparing the Room for Admission

The admitting office should notify the unit before the client's arrival so the room can be prepared. The following activities should be carried out by the nurse in anticipation of the client's arrival:

- Position the bed. For the ambulatory client, the bed should be in its lowest position. Place the bed in its highest position if the client will arrive on a stretcher. Ensure furniture in the room has been arranged to allow easy access to the bed (Fig. 12-1).
- Open the bed. Fold back the bedspread, top blanket, and top sheet.
- Assemble necessary equipment and supplies. A hospital admission pack (which contains such items as a bath basin, water pitcher, drinking glass, tissues, soap, and lotion) is placed in the room. A hospital gown or pajamas should be in the room, although the client may choose to wear personal pajamas or gowns. Equipment for taking vital signs (ie, stethoscope, sphygmomanometer, or thermometer) and height and weight should be in the room or readily available. If lab work has not been done previously, a container for a clean urine specimen should also be available.

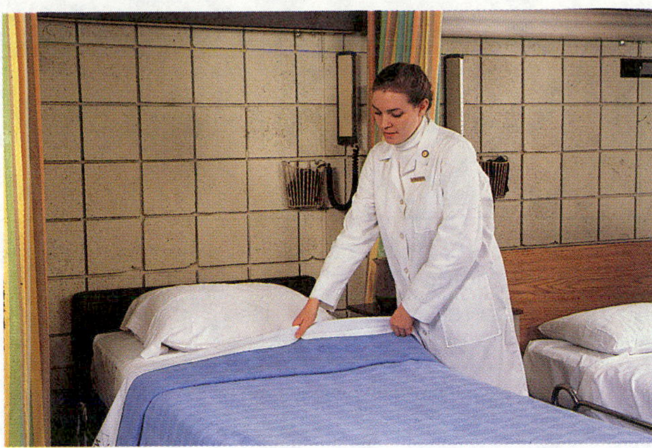
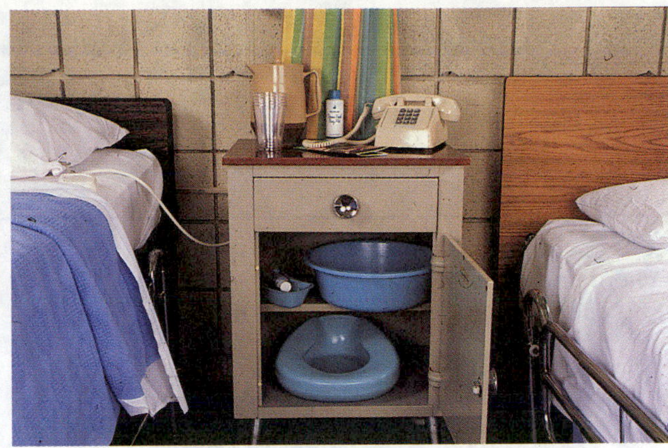

Figure 12-1
In anticipation of the client's arrival, the nurse should open the bed, position the bed, and assemble necessary equipment and supplies. (Photos © B. Proud.)

- Assemble special equipment and supplies. The client may require oxygen therapy, cardiac monitoring, or suction equipment. The nurse ensures equipment is functioning properly and is ready for the client's use on arrival.
- Adjust the physical environment of the room. This may include turning on lights and setting the room temperature.

Welcoming the Client to the Unit

Although other members of the healthcare team may assist in the admitting procedure, it is the nurse who is responsible for the comfort and well-being of the client on arrival to the unit as outlined in Procedure 12-1. The nurse makes the admission assessment and documents the information on the admission data base. A sample form illustrates typical information that is collected and documented. Each agency has its own form. The information on the form is used to develop the nursing care plan for the client and also is used as a data base for discharge planning and home care.

The client should be welcomed to the unit in the same courteous manner that would be used in welcoming a guest into one's own home. In most instances, the client is accompanied by family members who may either remain with the client to provide support and information or be asked to wait in the waiting room during the admission procedure. The nurse needs to assess the needs of the client and family and decide which should be done.

Obtaining the client's weight and height is a part of the admission procedure in both inpatient and outpatient settings. The box Guidelines for Nursing Care describes the procedure for obtaining weight and height. Table 12-1 provides a height and weight table for use as a standard reference. This table, composed by the Metropolitan Life Insurance Company, represents survey results of Americans who purchased life insurance, and is adjusted according to height and frame size for adults between the ages of 25 and 59.

Transferring Within and Between Settings

Although little has been written about the transfer of clients, it is common for some type of move to be made within settings as well as among settings. For example:

- Clients often are moved within the hospital setting from emergency room to hospital room, from ICU to hospital room (and vice versa), from one floor to another, or from one room to another room on the same floor.
- Clients are transferred to and from acute-care settings to long-term settings.
- Clients are transferred from acute-care settings to rehabilitation centers.
- Clients are transferred from ambulatory-care settings to acute-care settings.

All of these examples demonstrate how often a client may be transferred. Often the transfer meets the needs of the setting rather than the needs of the client.

When a transfer occurs, the client must readjust to new surroundings, new roommates, new routines, and new people providing care. If the transfer is to a higher level of care, as in a move to ICU, the client experiences unfamiliar sights and sounds. A transfer to a long-term facility may be one that is not desired but has become necessary if family members cannot provide care at home or if no other support people are available. All of these factors cause stress and anxiety.

The nurse may not be responsible for the actual physical move but is responsible for ensuring that the comfort, safety, and knowledge needs of the client and family are met. Although documentation and procedures differ depending on the institution and type of transfer,

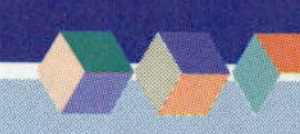

PROCEDURE 12-1

Admitting a Client to a Hospital Unit

Action	Rationale
1. Check the client's identification band. Greet the client and relatives by name. Introduce yourself to the client and the client to his or her roommate.	Calling the client by name, extending common courtesies, and welcoming the client and relatives often helps them to feel at ease and less frightened.

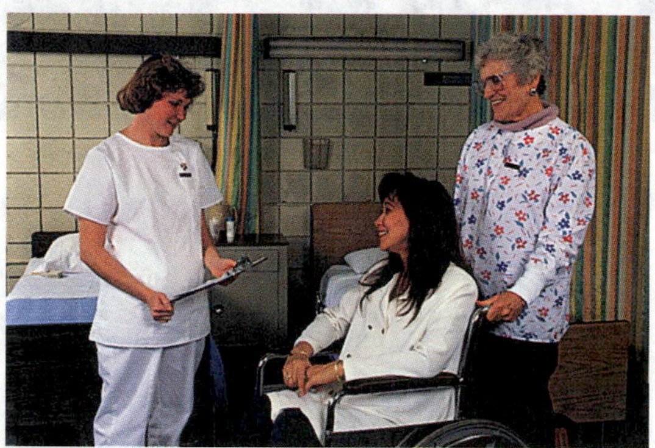

Action 1: Greeting the client.

Action	Rationale
2. Explain use of the bathroom and equipment, such as the call system, bed controls, television, telephone, and lights. Explain agency routines, such as meal times, visiting hours, and so on. Explain what space and territory belongs to the client.	Explaining agency routines and how to use equipment helps put the client at ease. Knowing how to use equipment also decreases the risk of accidents. Explaining space and territory allows the client a sense of control over the environment.
3. Place the signal device and other equipment so that they will be convenient for the client to use.	Being unable to call for help is unsafe and can result in accidents. When equipment is handy for clients, accidents, such as falling, are less likely to occur.
4. Obtain the client's temperature, pulse and respiratory rates, and blood pressure. Obtain a urine specimen at a convenient time.	Obtaining these signs and a specimen is an important part of the client's physical examination on admission and is the nurse's responsibility.
5. Provide for privacy. Ask relatives to leave unless they will assist with undressing the client.	Providing privacy shows respect and interest in the client.
6. Help the client to undress, if indicated, and assist the client into a comfortable position in bed.	Assisting the client to undress and get into bed conserves strength, helps prevent accidents, and prepares the client for care. Allow a client with no functional limitations to change alone.

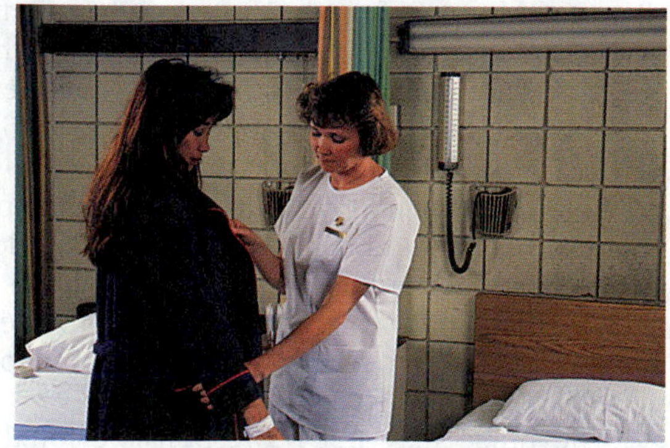

Action 6: Helping the client change into sleepwear.

Action	Rationale
7. Take care of the client's clothing and valuables. Follow agency procedure.	Losing items is upsetting to the client and can result in legal problems.

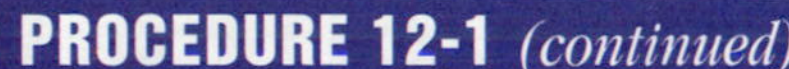

PROCEDURE 12-1 *(continued)*

Admitting a Client to a Hospital Unit

Action	Rationale
8. Indicate to family members that they may return to the client's bedside. Answer any questions or make referrals as appropriate.	The worries and fears of family and significant others should be considered during the admission process.
9. Carefully explain to the client what will be happening and what to expect. Elicit questions about the admission process and answer questions honestly.	Not knowing what will happen is stressful. This explanation may help decrease anxiety. Therapeutic communications help to establish a sense of trust and rapport.

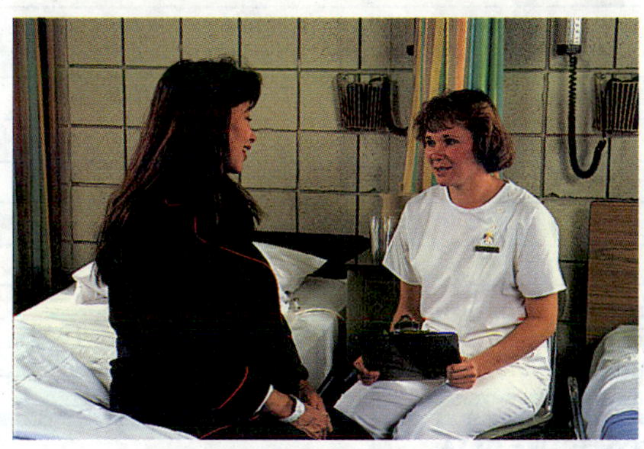

Action 9: Talking to the client about what to expect.

Action	Rationale
10. Do necessary recording on client's record, following agency policy. Begin the nursing history and assessment—it may or may not be advisable to have the family in the room.	The information is an important part of the client's permanent record. Presence of family may inhibit the responses of the client.
11. If the client is an adult, continue the history and assessment. If the client is an infant, child, elderly person, or is confused, collect necessary data from family or significant others before they leave.	The client may divulge important information that is not shared with family members. If the client cannot provide information, consultation with secondary sources may be necessary.

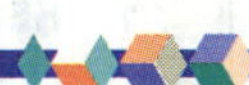

client needs are always a priority in ensuring a smooth transition and ensuring continuity of care.

Transfer Within the Hospital Setting

Considerations for transfer within the hospital setting include the following:

- In some situations in which a client moves from room to room on the same floor, the furniture (eg, bed or bedside table) is moved as well.
- The client's personal belongings must be moved and put up in the new room. Every effort must be made to ensure that belongings are not misplaced or lost.
- If the client is moved to ICU, it may be necessary for family members to take home personal belongings and flowers.
- The client's chart, Kardex, care plan, and medications must be correctly labeled for the new room, and other hospital departments (eg, dietary, pharmacy, or physical therapy) must be notified as appropriate.
- If the client is transferred to another floor or to (or from) ICU, the nurse at the original area gives a verbal report about the client to the nurse at the new area. Care priorities are identified and the existence of advance directives is noted. Accurate and complete communications are essential in ensuring continuity of care.

Transfer to a Long-Term Care Facility

Considerations for transfer to a long-term care facility include the following:

- All of the client's belongings are carefully packed and sent to the facility with the client. Prescriptions and appointment cards for return visits to the physician's office also may be sent with the client.
- The client is discharged from the hospital setting, but a copy of the chart may be sent to

(text continues on page 200)

Admission Data Base

DATE 1-16-97 TIME 0900

ADMISSION ☐ **OBSERVATION**

☒ AMBULATORY ☐ WHEELCHAIR ☐ STRETCHER

☐ CORRECT INDENTIFICATION BAND

ADMITTED FROM. ☒ HOME ☐ NURSING FACILITY

☐ EMERGENCY ROOM ☐ OTHER ______

INFORMATION GIVEN BY: ☐ FAMILY MEMBER ☐ FRIEND ☒ PATIENT

☐ UNABLE TO TAKE HISTORY · PATIENT UNRESPONSIVE/CONFUSED/ NOT ACCOMPANIED BY FAMILY OR FRIEND

☐ PREVIOUS MEDICAL RECORD

ORIENTATION TO ROOM

☒ VISITING HOURS ☒ CALL LIGHT IN REACH: ☒ EXPLAINED

☒ OPERATION OF BED AND SIDE RAILS ☒ USE OF PHONE

☒ VALUABLES SENT HOME ☐ IN SAFE ☐ IN POSSESSION

SPECIFY ______

☒ PATIENT HANDBOOK ☒ INTRODUCED TO ROOMMATE

MEDICAL HISTORY

ADMITTED MEDICAL DIAGNOSIS Peptic Ulcer

PAST HOSPITALIZATIONS AND/OR ILLNESS: (MEDICAL, SURGICAL, EMOTIONAL PROBLEMS) 1986 - Appendectomy

WHAT IS REASON FOR ADMISSION? (PATIENT'S OWN WORDS) "My doctor says I have An ulcer"

***SUBJECTIVE DATA:**

1. HEALTH PERCEPTIONS/HEALTH MANAGEMENT PATTERN

GENERAL HEALTH Excellent

USE OF: ☐ TOBACCO: HOW MUCH/HOW LONG? No

☐ ALCOHOL: HOW MUCH/HOW LONG? NO

☐ OTHER DRUGS TYPE(s) None

2. NUTRITIONAL/METABOLIC PATTERN

DIET/RESTRICTIONS/SUPPLEMENTS: Regular diet

☐ INSTRUCTED IN DIET PREVIOUSLY BY: ______

TIME OF LAST P.O. INTAKE: 0700

FLUID INTAKE (AMOUNT/DAY) 5-6 glasses

WEIGHT: ☐ NO PROBLEMS ______

☐ GAIN ______ ☒ LOSS/HOW MUCH/HOW LONG 10 lbs / 1 month

☒ SKIN NORMAL ☐ HEALING PROBLEMS

☐ COLOR CHANGE OF SKIN

☐ SKIN LESIONS/RASH ______

3. RESPIRATION/CIRCULATION PATTERN

HISTORY OF: ☐ COUGH ☐ SPUTUM ______

☐ SHORTNESS OF BREATH ☐ WITHOUT EXERCISE ☐ WITH EXERCISE

HISTORY OF: ☐ PACEMAKER ☐ RATE ______

☐ BLOOD CLOTS ☐ CHEST PAIN ☐ PEDAL EDEMA

☒ CHECK BOX IF DATA IS PERTINENT

*SEE NURSES NOTES FOR FURTHER NOTATIONS OR ANY CHANGES.

NURSING ADMISSION DATA

CURRENT MEDICATIONS, SUPPLEMENTS, NON-PRESCRIPTION DRUGS:

NAME	DOSE/FREQUENCY	LAST DOSE
Aspirin	2 prN	1 month
Maalox	prN	this Am

☐ MEDICATION TO PHARMACY ☐ MEDICATION SENT HOME

ALLERGEN: (DRUGS, FOOD, TAPES, DYES, OTHERS)

ALLERGEN	SYMPTOMS
Penicillin	rash

LEGAL GUARDIAN (NAME/PHONE) ______

CONTACT PERSON (NAME/PHONE) Mrs. Solle, 335-4001

PHYSICIAN NOTIFIED ✓ TIME 0830

PRIMARY CARE PHYSICIAN Dr. Wills

***OBJECTIVE DATA:**

1. CLINICAL DATA

AGE 36 HEIGHT 5'6"

WEIGHT 122 ☒ BEDSCALE ☐ STANDING APPROXIMATE ______

TEMP: 98.4 PULSE: 118 RESPIRATIONS 16

BLOOD PRESSURE (RIGHT ARM) 120/68 (LEFT ARM) 122/70

☒ SITTING ☐ LYING

N.T./N.A. INITIALS O.B.

2. NUTRITIONAL/METABOLIC PATTERN

ORAL MUCOSA: ☒ HEALTHY COLOR ______

☐ MOIST ☐ DRY ☐ LESIONS ______

TEETH: ☒ NO PROBLEM CONDITION: ______

☐ DENTURES ☐ UPPER ☐ LOWER ☐ PARTIAL

☐ MISSING TEETH ☐ CAPS/CROWNS

☒ WELL NOURISHED ☐ OBESE ☐ EMACIATED

SKIN: ☒ TURGOR NORMAL ☐ OTHER ______

☒ INTACT ☐ OTHER ______

TEMP warm COLOR brown ☐ DIAPHORESIS

☐ TUBES ______

3. RESPIRATION/CIRCULATION PATTERN

BREATH SOUNDS Clear

LIP COLOR pink ☐ USE OF ACCESSORY MUSCLES

COUGH: ☐ NON-PRODUCTIVE ☐ PRODUCTIVE SPUTUM COLOR ______

APICAL RATE 120 RHYTHM: ☒ REGULAR ☐ IRREGULAR

ABNORMAL HEART SOUNDS NOTED NO

NECK VEIN DISTENTION AT 45 DEGREES: ☐ PRESENT ☒ ABSENT

☐ EDEMA: LOCATION ______

RIGHT DORSALIS PEDAL PULSE: ☒ STRONG ☐ WEAK ☐ ABSENT

LEFT DORSALIS PEDAL PULSE: ☒ STRONG ☐ WEAK ☐ ABSENT

CALF TENDERNESS ☒ NO ☐ YES ☐ N/A

EXTREMITIES COLOR brown

TEMP warm

4. ELIMINATION PATTERN

ABDOMEN: ☒ SOFT ☐ FIRM

☐ NON-TENDER ☐ TENDER

☐ NON-DISTENDED ☐ DISTENDED ______ Girth

☐ OSTOMIES/TUBES: TYPE ______

☐ NORMAL BOWEL SOUNDS ☐ HYPOACTIVE ☒ HYPERACTIVE ☐ ABSENT

(Courtesy of Southeast Missouri Hospital, Cape Girardeau, Missouri.)

(continued)

Admission Data Base *(continued)*

***SUBJECTIVE DATA (Cont'd)** LBM______

4. ELIMINATION PATTERN

BOWEL HABITS: STOOLS/DAY 2 COLOR dk. brown ☒ SOFT/FORMED
☐ CONSTIPATION: ☐ LAXATIVE ☐ ENEMA
☐ DIARRHEA ☐ INCONTINENCE

BLADDER HABITS: URINATES/DAY 5-6 ☒ NO PROBLEM ☐ SELF-CATH
☐ URGENCY ☐ FREQUENCY ☐ NOCTURIA
☐ DYSURIA ☐ HEMATURIA ☐ INCONTINENCE

5. SEXUALITY/REPRODUCTIVE PATTERN (IF APPROPRIATE)

LAST MENSTRUAL PERIOD 1-10-97 MENSTRUAL PROBLEMS ☐ YES ☐ NO ☒
BIRTH CONTROL MEASURES None # PREGNANCIES 2
COMPLICATIONS OF PREGNANCIES None
HX VENEREAL DISEASE No
SEXUAL CONCERNS: None

6. ACTIVITY/EXERCISE PATTERN

ENERGY LEVEL: ☐ TIRES EASILY ☐ AVERAGE ☒ HIGH/ENERGY
ABLE TO: ☒ FEED SELF ☒ BATHE SELF
☐ BATHE/FEED SELF WITH ASSISTANCE
☒ AMBULATE ☒ CLIMB STAIRS
☒ CAN DO HOUSEHOLD CHORES
AIDS: ☐ CANE ☐ WALKER ☐ WHEELCHAIR ☐ OTHER ______
GAIT: ☐ STEADY ☐ UNSTEADY ☐ LIMP ☐ UNABLE TO WALK
PROTHESIS ______

7. SLEEP/REST PATTERN

DO YOU FEEL RESTED AFTER SLEEP? ☒ YES ☐ NO ☐ NO PROBLEM
SLEEP PROBLEMS: ☐ TROUBLE FALLING ASLEEP ☐ EARLY AM WAKING
☐ OTHER ______

8. COGNITIVE/PERCEPTUAL PATTERN

HEARING: ☒ NORMAL ☐ IMPAIRED ☐ LEFT EAR ☐ RIGHT EAR ☐ AID
VISION: ☐ NORMAL ☐ IMPAIRED ☒ GLASSES ☐ PROTHESIS
☐ FARSIGHTED ☐ NEARSIGHTED
OTHER PROBLEMS ______
COMMUNICATION: LANGUAGE SPOKEN English
UNDERSTANDS ______ UNABLE TO: ☐ READ ☐ WRITE
ABLE TO: ☒ READ ☒ WRITE ☐ LIP READ
COGNITION: ☒ NO PROBLEMS ☐ RECENT MEMORY CHANGE
☐ DIFFICULTY LEARNING
DISCOMFORT/PAIN: ☐ NO ☒ YES DESCRIBE Epigastric
HOW DO YOU MANAGE YOUR PAIN? Bland food, Maalox

9. COPING/STRESS TOLERANCE PATTERN

SPECIAL CONCERNS REGARDING HOSPITALIZATION? ☐ NO ☒ YES
Care of Children

10. SELF-PERCEPTION/SELF-CONCEPT PATTERN

CONCERNS ABOUT HOW YOUR ILLNESS AFFECTS YOU? ☐ NO ☒ YES
Concerned about health

11. ROLE/RELATIONSHIP PATTERN

MARITAL STATUS: ☐ MARRIED ☐ SINGLE ☐ WIDOWED ☒ DIVORCED
CHILDREN (#) 2 OTHER DEPENDENT(S) 0
OCCUPATION Secretary
RESIDENCY (TYPE) apartment
WHO LIVES AT HOME WITH YOU? Children
SUPPORT SYSTEM (CLOSE FRIEND/FAMILY MEMBER) Yes
FAMILY CONCERNS ABOUT HOSPITALIZATION? Yes

12. VALUE/BELIEF PATTERN

RELIGIOUS AFFILIATION Baptist
RELIGIOUS RESTRICTIONS Ø
☐ WOULD LIKE CHAPLAIN TO VISIT (IF YES, NOTIFY CHAPLAIN)

☒ WOULD LIKE FAMILY MINISTER TO VISIT
NAME Mr. Ame PHONE 314-6000
RELIGIOUS ACTIVITIES IMPORTANT TO YOU Bible
SUBJECTIVE DATA SIGNATURE P. LeMone RN (Nurse)

6. ACTIVITY/EXERCISE PATTERN

ROM: ☒ FULL ☐ OTHER ______
BALANCE AND GAIT: ☒ STEADY ☐ UNSTEADY ☐ LIMP ______
HAND GRASPS: ☒ EQUAL ☒ STRONG
☐ WEAKNESS/PARALYSIS ☐ RIGHT ☐ LEFT
LEG MUSCLES: ☒ EQUAL ☒ STRONG
WEAKNESS/PARALYSIS ☐ RIGHT ☐ LEFT

8. COGNITIVE/PERCEPTUAL PATTERN

LEVEL OF CONSCIOUSNESS: ☒ ALERT ☒ RESPONDS TO PAIN
ORIENTED TO: ☒ TIME ☒ PLACE ☒ PERSON
MOOD: ☒ CALM ☐ SAD ☐ ANGRY
☐ WITHDRAWN ☐ OTHER ______
PUPILS: ☒ EQUAL ☒ REACTIVE ☐ OTHER ______
COGNITION: ☒ ABLE TO FOLLOW SIMPLE COMMANDS
☒ RESPONDS APPROPRIATELY TO QUESTIONS
☐ UNABLE TO FOLLOW COMMANDS
☐ OTHER ______
HEARING: ☒ NORMAL ☐ OTHER ______
VISION: ☒ NORMAL ☐ OTHER ______
MANIFESTATIONS OF PAIN ______

10. SELF-PERCEPTION/SELF-CONCEPT PATTERN

EYE CONTACT: ☒ APPROPRIATE ☐ DOWNCAST ☐ STARING
BODY POSTURE: ☒ RELAXED ☐ STOOPED ☐ RIGID
BEHAVIOR: 1 (2) 3 4 5 (CIRCLE)
RELAXED — NERVOUS
OTHER ______

11. ROLE/RELATIONSHIP PATTERN

BEHAVIOR: (1) 2 3 4 5 (CIRCLE)
PASSIVE — ASSERTIVE — AGGRESSIVE
INTERACTION WITH FAMILY/SIGNIFICANT OTHER: ☐ N/A
☒ RELAXED ☐ TENSE ☐ ANGRY ☐ WITHDRAWN ☐ OTHER ______

COMMENTS:
Worried about effect of illness and possible surgery on care of children, job, and income. Has strong support of family.

SIGNATURE P LeMone, RN ______ (Nurse)

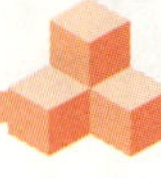

Guidelines for Nursing Care

Obtaining Height and Weight With an Upright Balance Scale

Obtaining Height

- Ask client to remove shoes.
- Raise L-shaped sliding arm on the measuring device attached to the scale somewhat higher than the client's approximate height.
- Ask the client to step on the platform of the scale and stand erect with the back to the measuring device and the heels together
- Lower the L-shaped sliding arm until it rests on top of the client's head.
- Read the height in inches and record.
- Ask the client to step down from the platform.

Obtaining Weight

- Balance the scale on zero.
- Ask client to remove shoes (and coat, if appropriate) and step onto the platform.
- Move the sliding indicator to the left until the scale balances.
- Read the weight in pounds and record.
- Ask the client to step down from the platform.
- Return the scale weight indicator to zero.
- Considerations: Daily weights should be obtained at the same time each day (usually early morning), with the client wearing the same clothing, and using the same scale.

the long-term facility (depending on physician preference and agency protocol). The original chart, being a legal document, remains at the hospital.

- In most instances, a detailed assessment and care plan is sent from the hospital to the long-term facility. In addition, verbal communications from the nurse at the hospital to the nurse at the long-term facility are used to ensure continuity of care.

Discharging From a Healthcare Setting

In meeting the needs of the client on discharge from a healthcare agency, the nurse must consider that the person may be expecting to change from a dependent role to a more independent self-care role. Although discharge is almost always a welcome event, it can also be one that causes anxiety and fear. The procedure for discharge is outlined in Procedure 12-2.

Table 12-1
Metropolitan Life Insurance Company Height and Weight Table

	Weight (lb) Men*				Weight (lb) Women†		
Height	*Small Frame*	*Medium Frame*	*Large Frame*	**Height**	*Small Frame*	*Medium Frame*	*Large Frame*
5′ 2″	128-134	131-141	138-150	4′ 10″	102-111	109-121	118-131
5′ 3″	130-136	133-143	140-153	4′ 11″	103-113	111-123	120-134
5′ 4″	132-138	135-145	142-156	5′ 0″	104-115	113-126	122-137
5′ 5″	134-140	137-148	144-160	5′ 1″	106-118	115-129	125-140
5′ 6″	136-142	139-151	146-164	5′ 2″	108-121	118-132	128-143
5′ 7″	138-145	142-154	149-168	5′ 3″	111-124	121-135	131-147
5′ 8″	140-148	145-157	152-172	5′ 4″	114-127	124-138	134-151
5′ 9″	142-151	148-160	155-176	5′ 5″	117-130	127-141	137-155
5′ 10″	144-154	151-163	158-180	5′ 6″	120-133	130-144	140-159
5′ 11″	146-157	154-166	161-184	5′ 7″	123-136	133-147	143-163
6′ 0″	149-160	157-170	164-188	5′ 8″	126-139	136-150	146-167
6′ 1″	152-164	160-174	168-192	5′ 9″	129-142	139-153	149-170
6′ 2″	155-168	164-178	172-197	5′ 10″	132-145	142-156	152-173
6′ 3″	158-172	167-182	176-202	5′ 11″	135-148	145-159	155-176
6′ 4″	162-176	171-187	181-207	6′ 0″	138-151	148-162	158-179

*Weights at ages 25 to 59 are based on lowest mortality. Weight in pounds are according to frame (in indoor clothing weighing 5 lb, shoes with 1-inch heels).

†Weights at ages 25 to 59 are based on lowest mortality. Weight in pounds are according to frame (in indoor clothing weighing 3 lb, shoes with 1-inch heels).

(Courtesy of Statistical Bulletin, Metropolitan Life Insurance Company.)

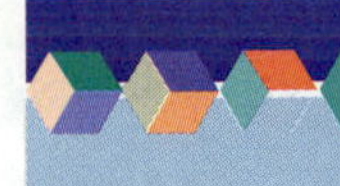

PROCEDURE 12-2

Discharging a Client From a Healthcare Agency

Action	Rationale
1. Check to see that the client has a discharge order.	It is the physician's responsibility to discharge a client.
2. Make sure the client or support person has had discharge instructions (ie, regarding diet, medications) and signs that he or she understands these instructions.	The client or a support person should be able to continue with necessary care after discharge when properly instructed.
3. Have all necessary equipment and supplies ready for the client.	Having equipment and supplies ready saves time and the annoyance of having to wait for them when the client is ready to leave.
4. Check to see that proper financial arrangements have been made by the client or support person. Obtain valuables. Observe agency policies.	These actions help to avoid legal problems.
5. Assist the client to dress and pack belongings. Make sure the client has all personal belongings.	Assisting the client conserves client strength. Time and trouble are saved when the client leaves with all belongings.
6. If the client needs reimbursement for future home visits, be sure the physician has given a written order for all services.	There must be a physician's order for reimbursement by Medicare and other third-party payers.
7. Transport the client and belongings to a car and assist the client into the car as necessary.	Assisting the client conserves client strength. Such assistance is courteous and helps the client feel that personnel are interested in the client's welfare.
8. Make necessary recordings on the client's records and complete the discharge summary.	It is important legally and for hospital records to complete the client's permanent record.

Special Considerations If the client is leaving without a physician's consent, check to see that the proper form has been completed. If the client refuses to sign the form, document your explanation to the client and consequent refusal to sign release form; notify the physician. Because a person cannot be held legally in an institution against his or her wishes, a properly signed form releases the agency and physician from responsibility should problems arise because the client refused further care.

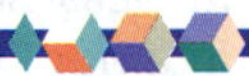

Leaving the Hospital Against Medical Advice

A client will sometimes decide to leave the hospital *against medical advice* (AMA). Although the client is legally free to do so, this choice does carry a risk of increased illness or complications. If a client decides to leave AMA, a form must be signed that releases the physician and healthcare institution from any legal responsibility for the client's health status. The client is informed of any possible risk before signing the form. The signature of the client must be witnessed, and the form becomes part of the client's record.

Discharge Planning

Planning the discharge actually begins on admission, when information about the client is collected and documented. **Discharge planning** is a systematic process of preparing the client to leave the healthcare agency and for maintaining continuity of care. The key to successful discharge planning is an exchange of information among the client, the caregivers, and those responsible for care both while the client is in the institution and after the client returns home. The coordination of care is usually the nurse's responsibility, but some hospitals have a nurse whose primary responsibility is discharge planning.

With earlier discharge, clients often are still acutely ill when they go home, and many require complicated treatment and care by family members. It is no longer unusual for family members to change sterile dressings, monitor intravenous medications, give complete physical care, and prepare special diets. If they are unprepared for these interventions, the client may have an exacerbation of the illness or experience complications that would require readmission to the hospital. The nurse must ensure that family members are taught the necessary knowledge

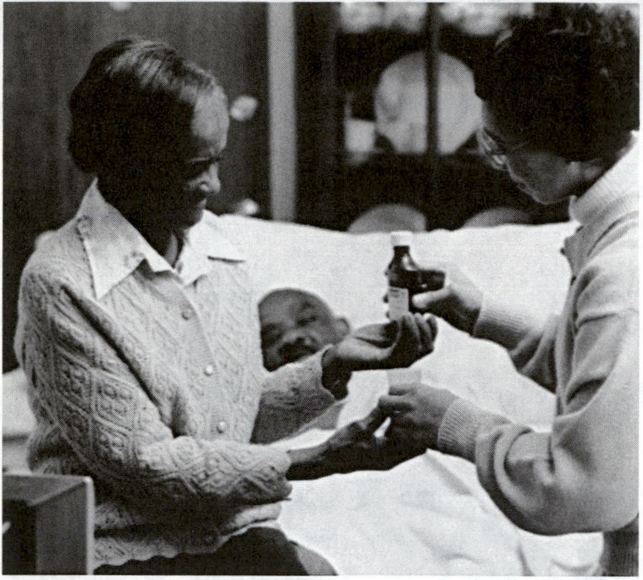

Figure 12-2
Clients or caregivers must be taught special skills such as medication administration, diet planning, or feeding so that they can care for themselves when nursing services are no longer provided. (Photo by Robert Coldwell, courtesy of Community Home Health Services of Philadelphia.)

and skills (Fig. 12-2) and that referrals are made to such agencies as home healthcare or social services to provide support and assistance during the recovery period. Home care is discussed in Chapter 13.

Discharge planning is virtually the same as the nursing process. It is a process by which a multidisciplinary team anticipates and plans for the needs of a client and family after discharge from a healthcare facility. The ultimate goal in assisting the client and family is the achievement of an optimal level of wellness. Effective discharge planning also guarantees continuity of care in the least stressful manner. Discharge planning can occur in a number of ways. Each institution has its own organizational structure to which it must adhere. Discharge planning must:

- Be coordinated
- Be interdisciplinary
- Be initiated as early as possible
- Be carefully planned
- Involve the client, family, or significant others who are caregivers

Initiation of the process involves identifying clients who need discharge planning. All clients need this service, but certain clients are at higher risk for specific needs and services. The nurse who conducts the initial nursing assessment is in the best position to determine these special needs. The following characteristics have been identified to indicate the need for a formal discharge plan and referral to another agency:

- Lack of knowledge of the treatment plan
- Social isolation
- Newly diagnosed chronic disease
- Major surgery
- Radical surgery
- Prolonged recuperation from major surgery or illness
- Emotional or mental instability
- Complex home-care regimen
- Financial difficulties
- Lack of available or approximate referral sources
- Terminal illness

Discharge planning is also indicated when a client is to be placed in a nursing home or other continued care setting.

Assessing

Assessment involves collecting and organizing data about a client. (Assessment and interviewing are covered in detail in Chapters 16 and 26.) When assessing the client for discharge, the family is included as the unit of care. The client and family must be actively involved in the discharge process if the transition from hospital to home is to be effective.

Important elements of a discharge planning assessment are listed in the accompanying box. Whatever assessment tool is used, it must be a holistic assessment that encompasses all aspects of the client or family life. The medical record and physician orders must also be consulted for the exact medication and treatment plan before a nursing care plan can be developed.

Diagnosing

Nursing diagnoses, based on the discharge planning assessment, are developed that recognize the needs of both the client and the family. The family, which is the unit of care, is affected by the health status of the member requiring care. Examples of nursing diagnoses for a client being discharged from the healthcare setting are:

- Self-Care Deficit related to inability to bathe or dress self secondary to right-sided weakness following a left-brain cerebrovascular accident (stroke)
- Anxiety related to uncertain outcome of treatment of cancer by chemotherapy
- Ineffective Family Coping related to lack of financial or personal support systems
- Impaired Home Maintenance Management related to chronic respiratory illness (emphysema) that limits ability to shop for food and clean the home

It is important to determine whether the problems are actual or potential. For example, the client with chronic respiratory problems may have assistance from a member of the family who has come to stay for 1 month, but the client will be alone at home after that time. In this case, the problem is not currently an actual problem but has the potential to become one unless planning is done to meet needs in 1 month.

Planning: Expected Outcomes

The sample data base form, including information for discharge planning, follows Gordon's (1982) organizing

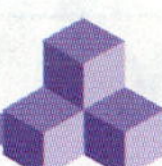

Focused Assessment Guide

Discharge Planning

Factors to Assess	Questions and Approaches
Health data	Establish the following data base: age; sex; height; weight; medical diagnosis; past medical history; current health problems; surgery; and functional limitations (eg, amputations, wheelchair or walker use, impaired hearing or sight).
Personal data	"How do you feel about being discharged?" (Note specifically if client appears anxious or frightened.) "What are your expectations for recovery?" (Unrealistic expectations require additional teaching.) "What personal coping methods do you use? Are these effective or ineffective? What language do you speak and understand?"
Caregivers	Establish who the caregivers are and ask the following of them: "What are your expectations and fears about providing care at home? What do you believe about health and illness? Do you live with the client?"
	Establish the caregivers' age, sex, relationship to the client, past experience with this treatment or illness, and values, beliefs, and cultural practices that may affect client care.
Environment	Assess both the home and the community: Are there barriers that will inhibit function (eg, narrow stairs if the client requires a wheelchair)? Are there assistive devices in the bathroom? Are hot water, heat, and space needed for supplies available? Is the community rural or urban? Is health care accessible and readily available? Is transportation available? Are there any known hazards in the environment?
Financial and support services	Complete a financial profile, to include expenses for care after discharge (consider medications, special foods, equipment, supplies).
	What resources are available to assist in caring for the client? (Consider all available resources, including Medicaid, food stamps, meal services to the home.) If the client will be living alone, what support services are available and how can they be obtained?

framework based on functional health patterns. The expected outcomes of the plan of care must be mutually set and realistic if they are to be met. When goals are established with the client, **compliance** (the act of completing what is expected of one) with the treatment regimen is more likely. Outcomes that are not mutually agreed on or not based on a complete assessment of the client's needs most often result in noncompliance. For example, a client may have been taught about a special diet but does not follow the diet after discharge because of financial problems, lack of transportation, and lack of refrigeration for food storage.

There are important elements of teaching that must be included in the nursing care plan for the client and must be implemented before discharge. These elements include the following:

Medications: Drug name, dosage, purpose, effects, times to be taken, and possible side effects. The information specific to medications should be given both verbally and in writing. It is often helpful to make a large clock face and write the names of the medications in the correct time slot.

Procedures and treatments: All steps of the procedure (eg, dressing changes) should be demonstrated, practiced, and given in writing. The caregiver should then demonstrate the procedure or treatment. It is important that caregivers understand the purpose of what is being done and have information about how to get supplies.

Diet: The purpose of the diet as well as expected outcomes should be clearly described. Examples of written diet plans and meals are helpful. It is also helpful for the caregiver to plan diets while the client is in the hospital and to save any menu or meal forms to use as a reference at home.

Referrals: Often appointments are made from the hospital for the first visit to a physician or agency. Whether this is done or not, the client and family members should be instructed on how to make contact with providers of follow-up care, as well as who to call if they have questions or problems. Information about referrals should be based on knowledge of the client's economic situation, access to transportation, support systems, and home environment.

Health promotion: All aspects of the illness or effects of treatment should be clearly described with verbal and written materials. Many sources of written information are available to give to clients; these sources range from printed organizational literature (eg, from the American Heart Association) to teaching materials developed by the institution. The client should be able not only to discuss verbally the physical and emotional effects of the illness but also to describe what will be done to achieve the highest level of wellness possible.

Discharge Summary

Nursing Services
DISCHARGE SUMMARY
(This side to be filled out by nursing staff)

1) HEALTH MANAGEMENT PATTERN

Follow-up Care, Appointments:
Physician: Dr. Wills Date 1-29-97 Time 1300
Date ____ Time ____
Outpatient Appt: ____ Date ____ Time ____

2) NUTRITIONAL/METABOLIC PATTERN

Diet - Order at Discharge Soft - Regular as tolerated
Dressings ☒ Not Applicable ☐ Reach to Recovery Referral
Wound Care ____

Written Instructions given ☒ Diet Instructor Signature P LeMone RN

4) ELIMINATION PATTERN: ☐ Incontinent: Management ____
LBM 1-28-97
Urinary - Catheter Care: ____
Written instructions given ☐ Instructor Signature ____

6) ACTIVITY/EXERCISE PATTERN

Activity at Discharge: ☒ as tolerated ☐ with assist ☐ bed rest
Pt ☐ Significant other ☐ Instructed on: ____
☐ surgical limitation (explain) ____
☐ other limitation (explain) ____

8) COGNITIVE/PERCEPTUAL PATTERN

Medications - Instructions: ☒ Pt ☒ Significant other
Preadmission meds returned ☐ initials ____

Continued Home Meds	Instruct. Sheet #	New Prescriptions	Instruct. Sheet #
		Tagamet 150mg BID	

Discharge Assessment Discharged to home with family members. States pain is relieved and verbalizes reduction of concerns. Understands diet (to avoid foods that cause distress) and importance of continuing medications.

Date 1-29-97 Departure Time 1100 Transported by WC / Volunteer
Via: ☒ w/c ☐ ambulatory ☐ ambulance ☐ child carried by ____ ☐ AMA

Signature of Discharging Nurse P. LeMone, RN

(Courtesy of Southeast Missouri Hospital, Cape Girardeau, Missouri.)

Client Care Study

The following example demonstrates consideration of all dimensions of the person in planning and coordinating discharge planning. Mr. Smith is a 55-year-old married man with a diagnosis of cerebrovascular accident (stroke) with left hemiparesis (weakness). He has difficulty communicating verbally and has a history of hypertension for 10 years. He is to be discharged from the hospital in 3 days if his blood pressure remains stable. He will be going home with four new medications, an indwelling urinary catheter, and a feeding tube. After reviewing the medical record, the nurse interviews Mr. and Mrs. Smith. The assessment reveals Mr. Smith is limited in his ability to transfer from bed to chair. Both Mr. and Mrs. Smith are fearful of discharge, but Mr. Smith believes he will be able to return to work as an accountant in 3 weeks, and Mrs. Smith thinks he'll never work again. They have never faced a life-threatening illness in the past, but he has had severe hypertension and has not complied with diet or medication regimens. Mr. Smith believes he will be fine soon and hates the thought of being an invalid at his age. The Smiths are both Roman Catholic. They have no strong cultural preferences in terms of diet. They have two adult children who live out of state with their own families. Mrs. Smith does have a younger sister who lives nearby. They are both college educated. The Smiths live in a suburban area in a two-story home with narrow stairs leading to two baths and three bedrooms on the second floor. They have adequate plumbing but no assistive devices. Their doctor's office is about 1 mile away, and shopping is nearby.

Mrs. Smith does not believe she can manage care of the feeding tube and indwelling catheter. She also needs instruction in the new medication and diet regimen. She is terrified that she may be unable to handle an emergency in the middle of the night. Financially, this two-income family has quickly become a one-income family and shortly will have no income. Mr. Smith is not 65 years old and thus is not yet eligible for Medicare.

How would the nurse coordinate this discharge plan? The physician must be consulted for diet, medication, and other treatment orders. Physical therapy has already been initiated at the hospital. Occupational therapy needs to evaluate Mr. Smith's ability to perform activities of daily living and to fit him with assistive devices. The nutritionist needs to counsel the Smiths on the low-sodium diet (1 g) and on creative ways to prepare low-salt meals. The social worker has been called for financial assessment to determine exactly what services the Smiths can expect to have reimbursed by their insurance carrier, and how they will manage their out-of-pocket expenses. The nurse begins to formulate a teaching plan for medications and treatment. Mrs. Smith must learn about the Foley catheter and feeding tube before discharge to feel more in control. It is hoped some of the Smiths' fears are addressed and new coping strategies developed. The nurse also makes a referral to a home health agency to continue physical therapy and nursing care.

Teaching Plan. The teaching plan is discussed in detail in Chapter 23. Review of the sample teaching plan in Chapter 23 aids in understanding the steps and strategies of discharge planning. All aspects of teaching may not be completed in the hospital, and referral to a home care agency may be necessary for follow-up care and teaching.

Implementing

Implementation is the actual carrying out of the teaching plan and referrals (Fig. 12-3). All teaching should be documented in the nurse's notes and the discharge summary. Written instructions are given to the client. Return demonstrations must be satisfactory. The client and caregiver must have exposure to and practice with the equipment they will be using at home.

The home-care referral is made before the client is actually discharged. As much information as possible about the client and the hospitalization should be given to the agency. Such information includes the kind of surgery; medication (including need for intravenous fluids at home); the client's physical and mental status; significant social factors (eg, frail caregiver with health problem, no caregiver); and expected needs of the family. Transportation should be arranged at this time.

For a home-care referral to be made and subsequent home visits to be reimbursed, there must be a written order by the physician for all services. Clients must meet

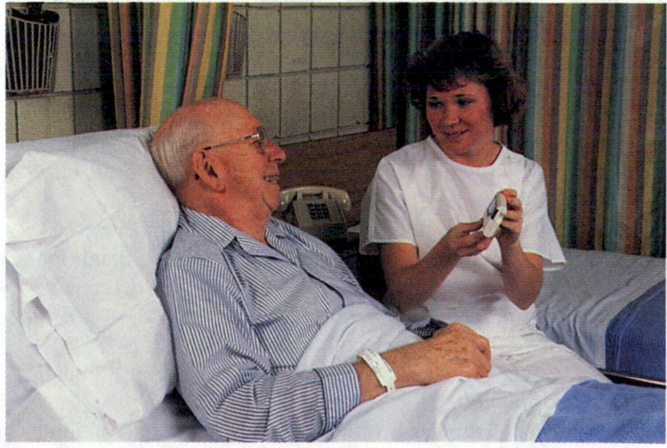

Figure 12-3
Written instructions for continuing self-care at home should be given to the client. In addition, the nurse reviews the instructions with the client to ensure that the client clearly understands the instructions. (Photo © B. Proud.)

certain criteria to have home-care services reimbursed by Medicare and other third-party payers.

Evaluating

Evaluation of the discharge plan is crucial in making the discharge planning process work. Planning and referrals must be scrutinized to ensure quality and appropriateness of services. Evaluation is ongoing, and the need for revision of plans also changes.

Further evaluation of the discharge process is usually conducted a few weeks after the client has been home. It may be carried out by way of a telephone call, a questionnaire, or a home visit.

Key Points

- The nurse is the primary person responsible for ensuring continuity of care as clients move from one type of healthcare setting to another.
- Continuity of care is the coordination of services provided to clients; it ensures a smooth transition between ambulatory or hospital care and home care or other types of community-based care.
- Continuity of care is provided by including discharge planning as a part of the care plan from admission, collaborating with other members of the healthcare team, and involving the client and family in planning.
- Anxiety about the unknown can be reduced by establishing a therapeutic nurse-client relationship on admission to a setting that provides healthcare.
- Although admission and dismissal from ambulatory and hospital settings differ, the focus is on meeting client needs and providing individualized care. The nurse is responsible for assessments, teaching, and developing a care plan with the client and family.
- Transfer of a client from one level of care or setting to another is common. The nurse provides care to meet comfort, safety, and knowledge needs of the client and family, ensuring continuity of care.
- Discharge planning is a systematic process of preparing the client to leave a healthcare agency and for maintaining continuity of care. This process is coordinated and multidisciplinary and is carried out with consideration of each client's needs when moving to a different level of care or setting. Information about medications, diet, procedures and treatments, referrals, and health promotion activities may be included in the teaching plan for discharge.

Bibliography

Bagis-Smith, J., & McKeehan, K. M. (1990). Continuity of care across hospital-community boundaries. In J. C. McCloskey & H. K. Grace (Eds.), *Current issues in nursing* (pp. 181–186). St. Louis: Mosby.

Beddar, S., & Aikin, J. (1994). Continuity of care: A challenge for ambulatory oncology nursing. *Seminars in Oncology Nursing, 10*(4), 254–263.

Bostrom, J., Tisnado, J., Zimmerman, J., & Lazar, N. (1994). The impact of continuity of nursing care personnel on patient satisfaction. *Journal of Nursing Administration, 24*(10), 64–68.

Bulachek, G. M., & McClosky, J. C. (1992). *Nursing interventions: Treatments for nursing diagnoses.* (2nd ed.). Philadelphia: Saunders.

Carpenito, L. J. (1995). *Nursing diagnosis: Application to clinical practice* (6th ed.). Philadelphia: Lippincott.

Cary, A. (1992). Promoting continuity of care: Advocacy, discharge planning, and case management. In M. Stanhope & J. Lancaster, *Community health nursing: Process and practice for promoting health* (3rd ed.) (pp. 681–706). St. Louis: Mosby–Year Book.

Eliopolos, C. (1993). *Gerontological nursing* (3rd ed.). Philadelphia: Lippincott.

Gillan, J. (1994). Familiar problem . . . patients need continuity of care. *Nursing Times, 90*(27), 54.

Gordon, M. (1982). *Nursing diagnosis: Process and application.* New York: McGraw-Hill.

Kammer, C. (1994). Stress and coping of family members responsible for nursing home placement. *Research in Nursing & Health, 17*(2), 89–98.

Krol, M. (1993). Strategies to improve continuity of care and decrease rehospitalization of cancer patients: A review. *ONS Nursing Scan in Oncology, 2*(6), 13.

Lumsdon, K. (1993). Bridging the gap: Home- and community-based programs integrate acute and long-term care. *Aging Today, 76*(23), 44, 48.

Magilvy, J., Congdon, J., & Martinez, R. (1994). Circles of care: Home care and community support for rural older adults. *Advances in Nursing Science, 16*(3), 22–33.

Malone-Rising, D. (1994). The changing face of long-term care. *Nursing Clinics of North America, 29*(3), 417–430.

McIntosh, J., & Worley, N. (1994). Beyond discharge: Telephone follow-up and aftercare. *Journal of Psychosocial Nursing & Mental Health Services, 32*(10), 21–27.

Mitchell, S. (1994). Facilitating transitions across care settings. *Canadian Oncology Nursing Journal, 4*(2), 104–106.

Smith, L. (1994). Continuity of care through nursing case management of the chronically ill child. *Clinical Nurse Specialist, 8*(2), 65–68.

Trella, R. (1994). From hospital to nursing home: Bridging the gaps in care. *Geriatric Nursing—American Journal of Care for the Aging, 15*(6), 313–316.

Warner, L. (1994). Changing ideas . . . continuity of care for clients . . . staff changes are making it difficult to achieve this. *Nursing Times, 90*(46), 42.

Young, H., & Hegyvary, S. (1993). Progress report on a "continuum of care" partnership: An experiment in linking up long-term care services. *Nursing Homes, 42*(9), 29.

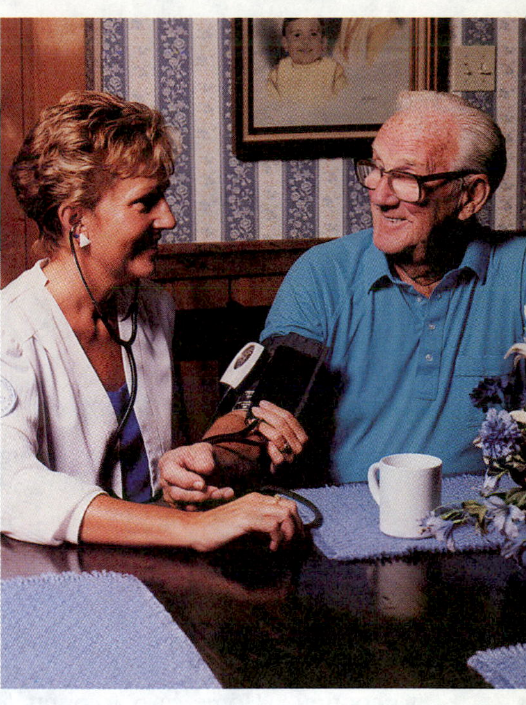

Chapter 13

Home Healthcare

Objectives

After studying this chapter, the learner should be able to:

Define home healthcare.

Outline the history of home healthcare.

Describe the characteristics and roles of the home health nurse.

Identify the essential components of the pre-entry and entry phase of the home visit.

Compare the role of the family in home care to hospital-based care.

Describe the purpose of hospice nursing.

Key Terms

entry phase

home healthcare

pre-entry phase

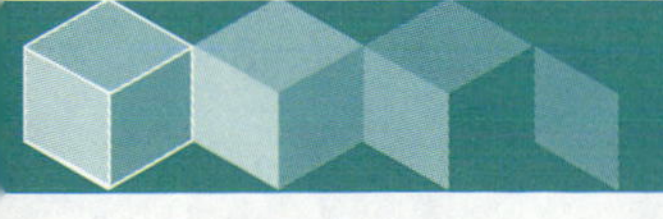

The past 5 years have brought many changes in the healthcare industry, and as a result, changes in the settings in which nurses provide care. One of these changes has been the shift from hospital-based settings to community-based care. Home care has experienced an unprecedented rate of growth because of this shift. Managed care has had a major effect on the move from hospital to home and this trend is expected to continue. Home care accounts for only a small portion of the total national healthcare expenditures and is considered one of the fastest growing areas of healthcare today. In order to provide care in the home, it is projected that more than 8,000 registered nurses over the number now employed in home healthcare will be needed by the year 2000 (U. S. Department of Health and Human Services, 1991).

Settings and agencies providing community-based care were discussed in Chapter 11; this chapter focuses on the care provided by nurses in the home.

Information in this chapter provides a base for understanding what home healthcare is and what the nurse does when providing care in the client's home.

Definition of Home Healthcare

Home healthcare is care provided in the client's home. It encompasses care to all ages of clients with both chronic and acute healthcare needs. Home healthcare is defined by McNamara (1982) as:

> That component of comprehensive healthcare where services are provided to individuals and families in their places of residence for the purpose of promoting, maintaining, or restoring health or minimizing the effects of illness and disability. Service appropriate to the needs of the individual client and family are planned, coordinated, and made available by an agency or institution, organized for the delivery of healthcare through the use of employed staff, contractual arrangement, or a combination of administrative patterns. (p. 61)

When providing home healthcare, nurses integrate community health principles focusing on environmental, socioeconomic, cultural, and personal health factors that affect the individual's and family's health (Humphrey & Milone-Nuzzo, 1991). The essential components of home healthcare are the client, the family, healthcare professionals from various disciplines, and goals to facilitate the client in reaching maximum independence and health status. The role of each member of the healthcare team is outlined in Table 13-1.

Healthcare providers are accustomed to the hospital client who conforms to the hospital routine and to the hospital's schedule for eating, bathing, taking medications, and visiting with their families. Home care nursing is unique because once the nurse crosses the threshold of the client's home, care must be adapted to the client's schedules, customs, and needs. The hallmark of a home care nurse is the ability to blend clinical skills with flexibility to provide quality client care.

The History of Home Care Nursing

Home healthcare began in the 1800s. The birthplace of the modern concept of home care nursing was Liverpool, England. Mr. William Rathbone, a wealthy philanthropist, had a wife who was dying. He hired nurses who cared for her at home until she died. Because of his personal experience, he organized a system of visiting nurses that could help others with the same needs. In 1859, Dr. Rathbone and Florence Nightingale started a school to train home care nurses. After graduation, nurses were qualified to care for sick clients who were confined to their homes (Clemen-Stone, Eigsti, & McGuire, 1987).

The late 1800s brought a large influx of immigrants into America and a rapid growth in population in most cities. Home nursing agencies began to emerge in New York, Boston, and Philadelphia to meet the health needs of the residents in these areas. In 1885, a home care agency was established in Buffalo, New York, which provided home healthcare to the sick. Lillian Wald and Mary Brewster opened the Henry Street Settlement House in New York City in 1893. Visiting nurses from this agency were used to care for poor residents living in tenements. Eventually, these providers of home care became known as Visiting Nurse Associations (VNAs), which focused on providing personal care to the sick and health teaching to families. Public health nursing

Table 13-1
Collaborative Roles of Members of the Home Healthcare Team

Member	Role
Physician	Certifies that the client has a health problem to receive home healthcare. Prescribes and certifies a plan of care for treatment for the client receiving home healthcare.
Nurse	Provides direct care to clients and families. Teaches client and family self-care. Conducts research to ensure cost effectiveness and quality of care. May be administrator of home health agency, and serve as consultant to staff. Coordinates services of other healthcare providers.
Physical Therapist	Provides direct care, such as muscle strengthening exercises, gait training, and massage. Teaches client and family to promote self-care.
Occupational Therapist	Evaluates the client's functional level and teaching activities to promote self-care in activities of daily living. Assesses the home for safety and provides adaptive equipment as necessary.
Speech Pathologist	Provides direct care services to clients with speech, language, or hearing needs. Teaches client and family to facilitate speech and language ability as well as eating and swallowing.
Social Worker	Assists client and family in dealing with the social, emotional, and environmental factors that affect their well-being. Makes referrals to appropriate community resources. Provides assistance with securing equipment and supplies, and for healthcare finances.
Home Health Aide	Implements the plan of care designed by the nurse. Assists clients with hygiene. May carry out light housekeeping.

emerged at the turn of the century and focused on the health of the community at large. These nurses primarily visited the poor and immigrants, attempting to improve the general health status of these groups (Harris, 1994).

Prior to World War II, physicians often made home care visits to treat the sick. During the war, physicians experienced a shift in practice from the home to the hospital and office setting. Nurses began to provide most of the home care visits during this time (Mundinger, 1983). VNAs began to be developed in most major cities and in urban areas throughout the country. Hospital-based home care agencies began to develop as hospitals looked for ways to expand services to their communities. The availability of extensive resources from the hospital enabled these agencies to provide broader services in increased amounts.

Home care services expanded to include the older population in the mid-1960s. The 1965 Social Security Act provided program coverage for home healthcare to older adults participating in Medicare. Not long after, Medicaid home health benefits were initiated. The Medicare and Medicaid programs, discussed in Chapter 11, provide the structure for most home health agencies today (National Association for Home Care, 1994).

There are many reasons for the increase in community-based home care. As the American population continues to age, home care services are increasing and expanding to the over-65 age group. The introduction of diagnosis related groups (DRGs) in the hospital setting created an earlier discharge from the hospital than clients previously experienced. Many of these clients are still in need of skilled professional care once they return home. As a result, home care visit volume has rapidly grown. Additionally, third-party payers began looking for an effective way to reduce the escalating costs of healthcare through use of managed care programs.

Nursing and Home Healthcare

Prior to the late 1980s, home care nurses were considered generalists. Recently, many home care nurses have begun to specialize in advanced practice skills to meet the growing demands encountered in caring for the acutely ill client at home. Some of these specialties include enterostomal therapy, cardiac care, mental healthcare, and maternal/child healthcare (Fig. 13-1). Specialized nursing knowledge and skills, combined with more sophisticated technology, means that many clients with acute and chronic healthcare needs can be treated safely and effectively in the home.

The nursing profession has its roots in home care. During the past several decades, most of nursing practice has taken place in the hospital setting. As the home

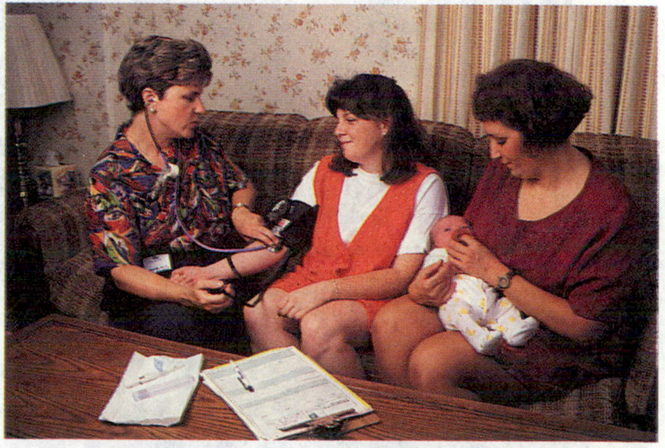

Figure 13-1
The nurse providing care in the home integrates knowledge and skills to implement family-centered specialized care.

care industry continues to grow, the practice of nursing is coming full circle and is moving back to the home.

The Unique Role of the Home Care Nurse

Home care nursing is unique in that care is provided in a setting that is unfamiliar to the nurse but familiar and comfortable to the client. For most people, the home is a place of safety and security, having meaning and given value because of ownership, family relationships and memories, independence, control, and protection. Home care is provided to the client in a setting that is controlled by the client and family. Instead of the client coming to the nurse, the nurse goes to the client. Clients or their caregivers must give permission for the nurse to enter the practice setting because the nurse is a guest in their home. The nurse is not able to regulate the setting where care is provided, but rather must essentially adapt to the client's environment instead of the client adapting to the hospital environment.

Characteristics of the Home Health Nurse

Nurses choose to practice home health nursing for various reasons. Many nurses enjoy practicing in an autonomous setting where they can use their expertise in an expanded role. Others enjoy the ability to manage their time independently and appreciate the satisfaction derived from clients as they welcome them into their home and into their life. Home care nurses find satisfaction in networking with other community agencies to provide individualized care. Home health nursing provides a channel through which nurses can use creativity in their delivery of care.

Knowledge and Skill

Nurses who provide care in the home setting must be knowledgeable and skilled. They must be able to practice independently and be accountable for their actions. Effective communication is essential and clinical skills are very important (Fig. 13-2). Physical assessment skills are necessary to identify positive and negative changes in healthcare status. Procedures such as administering intravenous fluids, changing complex wound dressings, caring for ostomies, and providing ventilator care are often required. One recent study (Caie-Lawrence, Peploski, & Russell, 1995) found that practicing home health nurses identified the following areas of knowledge as being most important in home care: legal regulations, physical assessment, body mechanics, nursing diagnoses, and infection control.

Independence

Nurses providing care in the home make independent decisions and assume responsibility for their decision making. Home care nurses are generally alone while providing care, and consultation with other professionals is not readily available. There is no one to turn to and say "What does this look like to you?" Therefore, the nurse must be able to make decisions related to the client's care independently. Combining a sound theoretical foundation with clinical skills and creative problem solving enables the nurse to make appropriate decisions related to client care.

Accountability

Accountability is another important characteristic of the role of the home health nurse. In a hospital setting, the

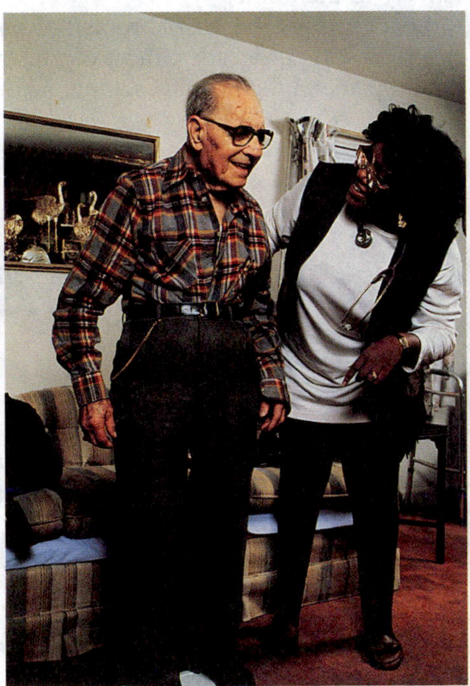

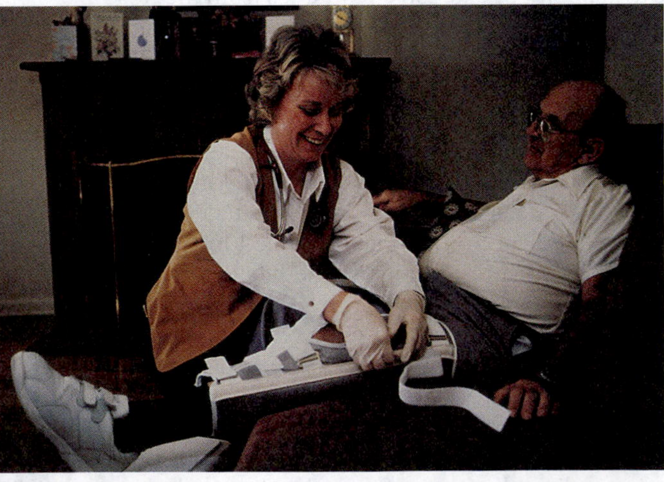

Figure 13-2
Home health nurses combine effective communication skills with a sound clinical knowledge base when caring for clients.

nurse generally works a shift and reports to the next shift nurse who then continues to care for the client. The home care nurse generally does not have a next shift to report to, but must rely on caregivers to continue the care. If there is no caregiver, the nurse returns to face the same issues at the next visit. The nurse is accountable to the client, the family, and the primary healthcare provider. Increased autonomy may increase legal risk. Suggestions for decreasing that risk are listed in Table 13-2; legal aspects of nursing are discussed in Chapter 7.

Roles of the Home Health Nurse

In addition to having the skills necessary as a caregiver, the nurse providing care in the home is a client advocate, coordinator of services, and client/family educator. These roles are briefly described here; further information is found in Unit V.

Client Advocate

Advocacy—the protection and support of another's rights—is an important role of the home health nurse. Clients may need help with negotiating through complex health systems or with handling insurance problems or state and federal regulations that affect their care and their living environment. For example, the nurse may have to convince the client's insurance carrier of the need for continued home health services. Clients may need help understanding complex billing issues related to their care. Home care nurses can often mobilize services needed to improve the client's living environment. The nurse plays an advocacy role when communicating with the client's physician or primary healthcare provider. The physician may not be aware of the home environment and may be ordering treatments that cannot be accomplished in this client's home setting. Communicating the client's needs to the physician enables the nurse to implement the appropriate treatments that fit into the client's lifestyle.

Coordinator of Services

The home care nurse is generally the coordinator of all other healthcare providers visiting the client, including physical therapy, occupational therapy, speech therapy, medical social workers, and home health aides. The nurse is the primary source for communicating with and coordinating the client's care with the primary healthcare provider. The nurse must use effective communication skills with other healthcare providers while coordinating services for the client. The accompanying samples of forms indicate how the home healthcare nurse coordinates services among other healthcare providers and teaches a client's wife to assist in care.

The home care nurse is also responsible for coordinating community resources needed by the client. Having a sound knowledge base of the role of various community resources and disciplines enables the nurse to provide comprehensive services to the client. For example, the nurse must understand the role of a social

Table 13-2
Decreasing Legal Risk in Home Healthcare Nursing

What to Know?	Questions to Ask
Chain of command in an emergency	1. Whom do I call if the client's physician is not available? 2. Is it appropriate to call the hospital for assistance? 3. When, if ever, should I call the medical director of the home health agency? 4. When should I call an ambulance or 911?
Care of nonclinical situations	1. What should I do if a family member is acutely ill? 2. What should I do if a family member threatens me? 3. What if my client is alone without food or medicine?
Equipment and procedures	1. How do I learn how to operate specialized equipment or perform advanced procedures? 2. How do I refuse an assignment if I do not feel comfortable with the client's needs? 3. What is the most effective way of ensuring and documenting that family members know how to operate equipment? 4. How do I get written approval to use my own stethoscope and blood pressure cuff? 5. How and to whom do I report malfunctioning equipment? 6. How do I document malfunctioning equipment?
Informed consent	1. How do I document informed consent for procedures if it has not already been obtained? 2. Is the client fully aware of the Patient Self-Determination Act? How do I document the client's decisions about treatment?
Accountability for other healthcare providers	1. What type of written parameters should I provide for providers, such as home health aides? 2. How do I ensure that other healthcare providers are knowledgeable of the plan of care and documentation of that care?

Adapted from Sullivan, G. (1994). Home care: More autonomy, more legal risks. *RN, 57*(5), 63–64, 67–69. Reprinted by permission.

HOME HEALTH CERTIFICATION AND PLAN OF TREATMENT

Patient's HI Claim No.	2. Start Of Care Date	3. Certification Period		4. Medical Record No.	5. Provider No.
777-88-7788A	100394	From: 100394	To: 120394	S2521	78-9999

Patient's Name and Address
Smythe, Samuel A.
25952 North Hawthorne Lane
Sky City, WI 50000

7. Provider's Name, Address and Telephone Number
BHC Home Care
2001 Oak Lane
Sky City, WI 50000

8. Date of Birth 021719 — 9. Sex [X] M [ ] F

ICD-9-CM	Principal Diagnosis	Date
1. ICD-9-CM 890.1	Open wound, left hip	100194
2. ICD-9-CM	**Surgical Procedure**	**Date**
79.35	Open reduction, left femur	092794
3. ICD-9-CM	**Other Pertinent Diagnoses**	**Date**
820.9	Fracture, left femur	092694
428.0	Congestive heart failure	090594
715.09	Osteoarthritis	030094
250.00	NIDDM	010090

10. Medications: Dose/Frequency/Route (N)ew (C)hanged
Cephradine 250 mg. Q 6 hrs. PO x 21 days
DC p̄ 10 AM dose 102494 (N)
Tolectin 400 mg. TID PO
Furosemide 40 mg. Q AM PO (C)
KCl 10 mEq. Q AM PO (C)
Digoxin 0.125 mg. Q AM PO
Vitamin-mineral supplement 1 cap. QD PO
Acetaminophen tabs. 2 Q 4 hrs. PRN PO - pain(N)

4. DME and Supplies: Wheelchair, walker

15. Safety Measures: Proper footwear, clear pathways when ambulating. O_2 precautions.

6. Nutritional Req. 1800 calorie ADA, 2 gm. Na

17. Allergies: No known allergies

8.A. Functional Limitations
1 [ ] Amputation; 2 [ ] Bowel/Bladder (Incontinence); 3 [ ] Contracture; 4 [ ] Hearing; 5 [ ] Paralysis; 6 [X] Endurance; 7 [X] Ambulation; 8 [ ] Speech; 9 [ ] Legally Blind; A [ ] Dyspnea With Minimal Exertion; B [X] Other (Specify) Occasional orthopnea

18.B. Activities Permitted
1 [ ] Complete Bedrest; 2 [ ] Bedrest BRP; 3 [ ] Up As Tolerated; 4 [X] Transfer Bed/Chair; 5 [X] Exercises Prescribed; 6 [ ] Partial Weight Bearing; 7 [ ] Independent At Home; 8 [ ] Crutches; 9 [ ] Cane; A [X] Wheelchair; B [X] Walker; C [ ] No Restrictions; D [ ] Other (Specify)

9. Mental Status: 1 [X] Oriented; 2 [ ] Comatose; 3 [ ] Forgetful; 4 [ ] Depressed; 5 [ ] Disoriented; 6 [ ] Lethargic; 7 [ ] Agitated; 8 [ ] Other

0. Prognosis: 1 [ ] Poor; 2 [ ] Guarded; 3 [X] Fair; 4 [ ] Good; 5 [ ] Excellent

1. Orders for Discipline and Treatments (Specify Amount/Frequency/Duration)

Wound care Ⓛ hip daily: Irrigate with normal saline, pack with saline-soaked 4x4s, cover with ABD. O_2 2L PRN HS per cannula - orthopnea.

Skilled Nursing: Daily for 62 days. Assess wound, S/S fluid retention. Perform wound care. Teach diet, O_2 precautions; new/changed medications.

Physical Therapy: One visit first week, 3 times a week for 8 weeks. Evaluation, therapeutic exercises, gait training. Teach use of walker, transfer technique. Establish home program.

Home Health Aide: 3 times a week for 9 weeks. Personal care. Assist with transfers, home exercise program.

2. Goals/Rehabilitation Potential/Discharge Plans

Anticipate daily visits to end 010395. Rehab potential good for patient to ambulate independently with walker by 120394. Will be compliant with diet, medications, therapeutic regimen. Plan discharge to care of wife when wound complications resolved.

3. Nurse's Signature and Date of Verbal SOC Where Applicable: Jane Dayes, RN 100394

25. Date HHA Received Signed POT: OCT 13 1994

4. Physician's Name and Address
Albert Richard, MD
1641 Pine Circle
Sky City, WI 50000

26. I certify/recertify that this patient is confined to his/her home and needs intermittent skilled nursing care, physical therapy and/or speech therapy or continues to need occupational therapy. The patient is under my care, and I have authorized the services on this plan of care and will periodically review the plan.

27. Attending Physician's Signature and Date Signed: Albert Richard MD 10/10/94

28. Anyone who misrepresents, falsifies, or conceals essential information required for payment of Federal funds may be subject to fine, imprisonment, or civil penalty under applicable Federal laws.

Form HCFA-485 (U-4) (02-94)

(Sample data © 1995 Beacon Health Corporation, Mequon WI. Used with permission.)

worker or physical therapist to decide the need for these services. Community resources such as Meals on Wheels, the American Cancer Society, services for clients who are visually or hearing impaired, and local services for the aging may be used. As the coordinator of care, the nurse directs the various services toward a common goal of improving the client's health and promoting independence.

Educator

Nurses providing home care find that the majority of their time is spent in teaching clients and families about the disease process, nutrition, medications, or treatment and care of wounds. The nurse identifies learning needs and mutually develops goals for teaching the necessary information to promote wellness.

The nurse provides essential information necessary to keep the client safe until the next visit, using what works best in the home. The goal is to facilitate clients' and caregivers' ability to care for themselves (Stulginsky, 1993a). The teaching-learning process is fully described in Chapter 23.

The Home Visit

As described by Stulginsky (1993b), "few families understand why people are sent home from the hospital 'still sick.' Even fewer understand what home care is. All they know is that the nurse is coming to help" (p. 477). Home care clients often feel frightened, in pain, and abandoned. Family members face challenges in handling equipment, in providing care that is totally unlike anything they have ever done for a loved one, and in dealing with unfamiliar and often terrifying sounds, odors, and substances. Even family members who are themselves nurses may find providing care at home very different from providing care to others in the hospital. The accompanying box describes one such experience.

The Pre-entry Phase of the Home Visit

During the referral process, the home care agency is contacted by the physician or discharge planner of a hospital and a brief past medical history is obtained, along with indications for home health services. The referral nurse at the home care agency should collect as much information as possible about the client's diagnoses, past surgical experience, socioeconomic status, and treatments ordered. This phase of the home care visit can be defined as the **pre-entry phase**. The nurse is assigned the case, reviews the information, and calls the client to make an initial contact and schedule the visit. During this conversation the nurse can gather information to determine if the client's caregivers can answer questions related to their needs. It may be possible to determine the client's cognitive abilities, orientation, and caregiver status through the conversation. All information is important to the nurse as the first visit is planned. The home care nurse must develop a trusting relationship with the client and family during the first introductory visits.

Supplies that the nurse may need for the client are gathered during the pre-entry phase. Wound care products, dressings, or educational materials are organized to take with the nurse on the first visit. The home care nurse uses a "field chart" to document the assessment and care provided to the client. This chart is carried with the nurse on subsequent visits.

Safety is an important aspect that the nurse must assess before making the visit. Evaluating the safety of the area where the client lives is important. The nurse may need to arrange the visit so that it is at a time when it is safe to be in that area. The nurse should always know the destination before arriving for the visit. In some unsafe areas, the nurse may be accompanied by police or security officers.

Home Healthcare Alert

Be prepared for random acts of violence. Post your itinerary; make sure that someone in your agency knows where you are. Use a cellular phone programmed with emergency numbers. Have a code phrase to signal that you are in danger and need help. Attempt to schedule visits with potentially combative clients when a family member or neighbor can be present. Although mace or pepper spray can disable an attacker temporarily, it can also be used against you (Morrison, 1995).

The Entry Phase of the Home Visit

The second phase of the visit is the **entry phase**. During the entry phase, the nurse develops rapport with the client and family, mutually determines desired outcomes, makes assessments, plans and implements prescribed care, and provides teaching. The nurse must remember that he or she is a guest in the client's home and is offering services that the client may choose to accept or reject. Important considerations in making home care visits include negotiating and honoring visit times, establishing rapport with the client and family, defining what nursing care will be provided, and teaching to promote independence in self-care (Stulginsky, 1993b).

The nurse must gain the trust of the client and family and must recognize and respect the values of the client. Acceptance of the client's living conditions is necessary even though they may differ from that of the nurse. It is important for the nurse to ask permission prior to using the client's home for activities such as handwashing. Often the nurse believes the client's home or sick room may need the furniture rearranged to make it more accessible to equipment and to remove safety hazards. The client should give permission before any changes are made.

Controlling Infection

Infection control techniques are practiced to prevent the spread of infection from one client's home to the next. Home care nurses carry routine equipment in a bag, and appropriate bag technique is used to prevent the spread of infection. The basic premises behind bag technique are:

- The nurse's hands are washed before accessing supplies from the bag.
- Anything that the nurse takes out of the bag is cleaned before returning it to the bag.

SKILLED NURSING VISIT NOTE

Patient Samuel Smythe

DATE 061394 TIME 11:00-11:45	No S/S fluid retention. Wound measures 9x5x3 cm. Small amount of purulent drainage. Wound bed 70% slough, 30% granulation tissue. Wound care performed: irrigated with normal saline, packed with wet to dry 4x4s, covered with ABD. Surrounding skin intact. Expresses discomfort during procedure. Taught use of pain med 1 hr. before procedure. Reports occasional constipation. Observed aide transfer patient. Uses safe technique. Patient satisfied with care. Can demonstrate exercises but reluctant to do alone. Taught wife how to assist.
VISIT FREQUENCY Daily ☐ Change ☐ Patient informed	
BP 140/86 Standing (Sitting) Lying	
TEMPERATURE 98.2°	
PULSE 80, regular (Apical) Radial	
RESPIRATIONS 26	
LUNG SOUNDS Clear	
DIET/APPETITE 1800 cal. Taught fiber sources.	
ACTIVITY LEVEL Weak. Transfers with 1.	
AIDE SUPERVISION Observed K. Jackson	
PHYSICIAN CONTACT/APPT. Appt. 061594	
CARE COORDINATION Reviewed PT program with aide.	
CONFERENCE	
☐ PROGRESS NOTE	SIGNATURE *Susan Jackson RN*

SKILLED NURSING VISIT NOTE

Patient Samuel Smythe

DATE 091994 TIME 7:30-8:20	Venipuncture for FBS – Ⓛ antecubital. Verbalizes routine for blood, urine testing. Still has difficult performing finger stick. Doe not get enough blood strip for accurate reading. Demonstrated procedure for finger stick. Using Ⓡ side abdomen for all injections. Taught need to rotate sites. Developed rotation schedule.
VISIT FREQUENCY Weekly. Aide dc'd 0913 ☐ Change ☒ Patient informed	
BP 132/76 Standing (Sitting) Lying	Change in insulin dose on 0919; blood sugar 175-225. SN taught insulin administration. Feeling more comfortable about performing care.
TEMPERATURE 97.6°	
PULSE 70, regular (Apical) Radial	
RESPIRATIONS 22	
LUNG SOUNDS Clear	
DIET/APPETITE 1800 cal. ADA "Good appetite"	
ACTIVITY LEVEL Ambulates 30' – walker No longer uses wheelchair.	
AIDE SUPERVISION	
PHYSICIAN CONTACT/APPT. Appt. 092394	
CARE COORDINATION	
CONFERENCE	
☒ PROGRESS NOTE 090594-091994	SIGNATURE *Susan Jackson RN*

Home Healthcare Alert

The nurse must wash his or her hands before and after treating the client. According to recent Standard Precautions Guidelines from the CDC, gloves should be worn when touching blood, body fluids, secretions, excretions, and contaminated items. Clean gloves should be put on just before touching mucous membranes and nonintact skin.

- Anytime the nurse needs to access the bag, handwashing must take place first.
- The bag should be placed on a liner before setting it down in the client's home.

Assessing

The ability to assess the client accurately is an important skill for the home care nurse. The nurse must be skilled not only in physical assessment but also in psychologic,

Through the Eyes of the Family Caregiver

"I'm So Glad to Have You Home, But What Do I Do Now?" (and this is just the first day. . . .)

I am a nurse, and have been a nurse for 30 years. I have a diploma in nursing, a baccalaureate in nursing, a master's in counseling, and a doctorate in nursing. I have taught others how to be nurses for over 25 years. Nothing in all my educational and practice experiences prepared me to care for the complex needs of my husband, Jacque, when he had surgery two years ago. Following diagnosis of metastatic thyroid cancer, a large lower thoracic spinal cord tumor (which put pressure on the spinal nerves, causing leg weakness and bladder malfunction) and the thyroid gland were removed surgically and steel rods were implanted almost the entire length of the spine. After 30 days in the hospital for diagnosis, surgery, and recovery, Jacque came home—unable to do more than move from the bed to a chair, and with a catheter in his bladder that was attached to a drainage bag.

Before he came home I got a hospital bed with electric controls, a bedside commode, and a bedside table. I cleared out the family room furniture, got a friend to put the television up on a table (so it could be seen from the hospital bed), and thought I was all ready to give my husband expert care. The first challenge came when he got up in a chair to eat his dinner—we had no chairs with a high enough seat or a straight enough back to allow use of the bedside table. I ran up and down stairs to look at chairs, and finally decided the antique arm chair in the living room would work, and it did. Now another problem—where to hang the catheter drainage bag? And how best to move so it didn't pull when he moved? And remember to empty the bag before he gets up!

I fixed a wonderful homecoming meal for this man I love, and he could only eat a few bites. Now back to bed and a new problem. He got out of the bed and into the chair just fine, but now he can't get out of the chair and into the bed, because his legs are still so weak. What did I do wrong—it worked in the hospital. It took me two days to realize that I forgot to lower the bed height so Jacque wouldn't have to push up so hard to get his bottom on the bed.

Then, after finally literally hauling him back in bed, I realized that I did not know how to move him up in bed. The physical therapist had taught him how to get up in a chair, but not how to move himself up in bed (they always did it for him in the hospital). This is a 250-pound man we are talking about. I could turn him from side to side, but I couldn't physically move him up in bed and he couldn't stay where he was. After a lot of trials, we figured out that he could wiggle one side of his body at a time and slowly inch up in bed. Now he was exhausted and in pain, and I felt totally incompetent. Thank goodness the home health nurse is coming to visit tomorrow.

If I felt this way, how must family members feel who know nothing about caring for someone who is sick or in pain? I have such respect for all those family members who provide such wonderful care, and for the nurses who provide home care that calms the fears and answers the questions.

Priscilla LeMone

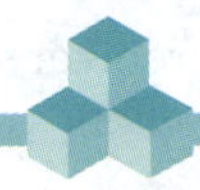

Examples of Nursing Diagnoses

Home Healthcare

The following nursing diagnoses are examples of those that might be appropriate for the client in the home setting:

- Risk for Infection related to large draining wound and lack of clean living environment
- Constipation related to lack of bulk in diet and immobility
- Risk for Injury related to weakness and cluttered home environment
- Risk for Impaired Skin Integrity related to inability to move self in bed
- Impaired Social Interaction related to inability to take part in family and community celebrations
- Altered Family Processes related to chronic illness of head of the family
- Caregiver Role Strain related to complex health needs
- Spiritual Distress related to inaccessibility of traditional folk medicine practitioner
- Ineffective Individual Management of Therapeutic Regimen related to living alone and having limited income
- Impaired Physical Mobility related to paralysis following automobile accident
- Impaired Home Maintenance Management related to fatigue and pain
- Knowledge Deficit related to availability of community resources
- Anxiety related to care of complex medical regimen at home

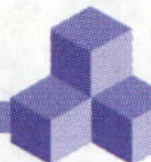

Focused Assessment Guide

Cultural Considerations in Home Care

Factors to Assess	Areas
Family and kinship	Ethnic or cultural identity Roles and responsibilities of family members Family structure and decision makers Communication patterns Age and gender of all members Personal space
Social network	Friends and significant others Celebration of important events Sources of support
Daily living	Work Leisure time activities Nutritional practices Cultural or religious beliefs and taboos followed
Health practices and beliefs	Cause of illness Treatment of illness Use of traditional folk medicine and practitioners Culturally appropriate responses to physical and emotional effects of illness

Adapted from Andrews, M., & Boyle, J. (1995). *Transcultural concepts in nursing care* (2nd ed.). Philadelphia: Lippincott.

socioeconomic, environmental, spiritual, and cultural assessment. The accompanying box outlines factors to assess in cultural considerations. Most of the initial assessment will take place during the first home visit. Ongoing assessment will occur during subsequent visits as the nurse uses various skills in collecting the data needed.

In addition to client assessment, the family is assessed, taking into account the various role that each family member plays and how this contributes to the health status of the client. The nurse determines whether the client and family understand and are agreeable with the plan of care that is established. It is important to determine if the caregivers are cognitively able to understand the instructions provided and are capable of providing care. The nurse must be able to asses an overall view of the family unit and how the client fits into this unit.

Home care nurses use direct observation during visits to decide if lifestyle, cleanliness, and family interactions are potential problems in the home. For example, the nurse may note that there is no food in the refrigerator or in the kitchen cupboards. A referral for services such as "Meals on Wheels" may be necessary to provide adequate nutrition for the client. Home care nurses frequently encounter safety hazards such as throw rugs or clutter that could easily cause falls. Other hazards identified may include those related to infection control, such as unclean homes with rodent or insect infestations or lack of running water. The nurse may determine that caregivers have an alcohol or drug problem that impairs their ability to care for the client. All of these aspects are taken into consideration if they could interfere with the client's health and safety.

Teaching

Since home care is meant to be short-term and intermittent, the nurse includes the family and friends in the teaching process so they may learn how to care for the client once home care is no longer indicated. Teaching is designed and implemented based on the following considerations:

- Teaching is geared to the client's and caregiver's readiness to learn and is adapted to the client's physical and emotional status.
- Major problem areas are identified, and information that is essential to keep clients safe until the next home visit is the major focus.
- Teaching is adapted to what works best in the home.
- Incentives to learn include knowledge of serious consequences as well as positive benefits of carrying through with certain behaviors (Stulginsky, 1993b).

The Needs of Caregivers in the Home

Traditionally, when a client enters the hospital the family plays a minor role in actual care. Families and friends visit with the client and sometimes even stay overnight. However, they are generally not involved in the direct care of the client. The hospital staff provides personal care for the client and administers medications and treatments. Once the client is discharged, the responsibility for the burden of care is shifted to the caregiver, who may or may not be physically or mentally able to handle this responsibility. Upon discharge, the family is given a multitude of instructions within a limited time frame and is expected to carry out this care at home.

As healthcare continues to shift from the hospital setting to community-based care, families will bear the burden associated with this change. Clients are discharged sooner and with a higher acuity level than in previous decades. Chronically ill clients will need continued long-term personal care at home that is not covered by the current Medicare benefit. The financial burden associated with this care is more than many families can afford.

The home care nurse plays an important role in easing the burden of care by facilitating client and family access to community resources to assist the family in meeting various needs. The nurse determines when a caregiver is becoming overwhelmed with the care and attempts to provide resources to relieve the burden. The nurse also supports family decisions about complex treatments. The following questions may be used for discussion (Zerwekh, 1995, p. 14):

What is most important to you?
What do you want for your life and that of your family?
How do you want to live?
How is this technology supporting and not supporting what you want?

Hospice Nursing in the Home

Hospice nursing provides care to clients who are dying from a terminal illness. This care is most often provided in the home setting. Hospice care usually begins when the client has 6 months or less to live and ends with the family 1 year after the death. This continuation of care for the family after the death is bereavement care. Nurses providing hospice care work with an interdisciplinary team of other health professionals such as social workers, pastoral counselors, home health aides, and volunteers to provide comprehensive palliative care.

The American hospice movement was originally led by volunteers (many of whom were nurses) who wanted to make life better for those who were dying. These devoted volunteers promoted the dignity of clients during their death and decreased their institutionalization. In 1969, Dr. Elizabeth Kübler-Ross published the book *On Death and Dying,* which identified the five stages that many terminally ill clients experience. She promoted the use of home care as a more effective means of providing support and care to dying clients and their families.

In 1986, Congress passed the Medicare Hospice Benefit and also gave states the option of including hospice services in their Medicaid programs. Since then, clients who are dying of cancer or any other terminal illness may receive hospice care in the comfort of their homes with their families nearby.

The hospice nurse must combine all of the skills of the home care nurse with the ability to provide daily emotional support to dying clients and their families. Hospice nurses are especially skilled in pain and symptom management. Their focus is on improving quality of life and preserving dignity for the client in death. After the death, the nurse continues to care for the client's family during the bereavement period for up to 1 year. Nurses use this time to help families work through the grief process after their loss.

Most hospice care is delivered to clients in their home. Some hospices also have an inpatient (hospital) setting where clients can receive short-term care, as a respite for caregivers, or long-term palliative care. In whatever setting, hospice care provides terminally ill clients a humane option of dying with dignity.

The Future of Home Care

The 1990s have been a time of transition, growth, and specialization for the home care industry. By 2000, more complex services will be provided at home. Acuity levels of clients will rise owing to earlier discharges from the hospital setting. Increasing numbers of surgical procedures are being performed on an outpatient or short-stay basis; thus families and friends will have more responsibility for providing care for loved ones at home. Specialization will continue to expand in the areas of cardiac care, wound care, and intravenous therapy services. The role of prevention will continue to grow in home care through use of health screening, immunization, and community education programs. Keeping people healthy will be a goal to prevent illness and resultant admissions to the inpatient setting. Home care nurses will need to expand their knowledge and skill continually to meet the challenge of providing preventative, acute, and chronic care to clients in their homes.

Key Points

- Home healthcare is a rapidly expanding component of the healthcare system.
- Home healthcare is care provided in the client's home, encompassing the care of clients of all ages and with both chronic and acute healthcare needs.
- Home healthcare began in England, emerged in the United States in the 1880s, and expanded to the older population in the 1960s.
- Nurses who provide home healthcare are increasingly specializing to implement the technology and meet client needs.

- Home healthcare nurses provide care that adapts to the client's environment. They must have knowledge and skill, be independent, and accountable.
- Home health nurses are providers of care, and also are a client advocate, coordinator of services, and educator.
- The home visit has two phases: pre-entry and entry. During pre-entry, the nurse collects client information, gathers supplies, and ensures personal safety. During entry, the nurse develops rapport with the client and family, mutually determines outcomes, makes assessments, implements care, and provides teaching.
- Caregiver needs are also an important consideration in home healthcare.
- Hospice nursing (care for the dying client) is often provided in the home, with a focus on improving quality of life and preserving dignity in death.

Bibliography

Andrews, M., & Boyle, J. (1995). *Transcultural concepts in nursing care* (2nd ed.). Philadelphia: Lippincott.

Boston, P. (1992). Understanding cultural differences through family assessment. *Journal of Cancer Education, 7*(3), 261–266.

Buls, P. (1995). The effects of home visits on anxiety levels of the client with a coronary artery bypass graft and the family. *Home Healthcare Nurse, 13*(1), 22–29.

Caie-Lawrence, J., Peploski, J., & Russell, J. (1995). Training needs of home healthcare nurses. *Home Healthcare Nurse, 13*(2), 53–61.

Clemen-Stone, S., Eigsti, D., & McGuire, S. (1987). *Comprehensive family and community health nursing* (2nd ed.). New York: McGraw-Hill.

Ellenbecker, C., & Shea, K. (1994). Documentation in home healthcare practice: Evidence of quality care. *Nursing Clinics of North America, 29*(3), 495–506.

Frisch, N. (1993). Home care nursing and psychosocial-emotional needs of clients: How nursing diagnosis helps to direct and inform practice. *Home Healthcare Nurse, 11*(2), 64–65, 70.

Gurfolino, V., & Dumas, L. (1994). Hospice nursing: The concept of palliative care. *Nursing Clinics of North America, 29*(3), 533–546.

Harris, M. (1994). *Handbook of home healthcare administration.* Gaithersburg, MD: Aspen.

Humphrey, C., & Milone-Nuzzo, P. (1991). *Home care nursing: An orientation to practice.* Norwalk, CT: Appleton & Lange.

McNamara, E. (1982). Hospitals discover comprehensive home care. *Hospital, 56*, 60–66.

Morrison, B. (1995). Home health care: Staying safe in dangerous times. *Nursing, 25*(10), 49–51.

Mundinger, M. (1983). *Home care controversy: Too little, too late, too costly.* Rockville, MD: Aspen.

National Association for Home Care. (1994). *Basic statistics about home care 1994.* Washington, DC: National Association for Home Care.

Stulginsky, M. (1993a). Nurses' home health experience. Part I: The practice setting. *Nursing & Healthcare, 14*(8), 402–407.

Stulginsky, M. (1993b). Nurses' home health experience. Part II: The unique demands of home visits. *Nursing & Healthcare, 14*(9), 476–485.

Sullivan, G. (1994). Home care: More autonomy, more legal risks. *RN, 57*(5), 63–64, 67–69.

U. S. Department of Health and Human Services. (1991). *Health personnel in the U.S., eighth report to Congress* (DHHS No. HRS-P-00-92-1). Rockville, MD: U. S. Government Printing Office.

Varricchio, C. (1994). Human and indirect costs of home care. *Nursing Outlook, 42*(4), 151–157.

Yost, L. (1995). Cancer patients and home care. *Cancer Practice, 3*(2), 83–87.

Zerwekh, J. (1995). High-tech home care for nurses. *Home Healthcare Nurse, 13*(1), 9–14.

The nursing process is a systematic, client-centered, goal-oriented method of caring that provides a framework for nursing practice. Unit IV discusses each of the five steps of the nursing process—assessing, diagnosing, planning, implementing, and evaluating. It also describes the core competencies nurses need to use the process to promote client well-being and concludes with a chapter on documentation, reporting, and conferring.

The steps of the nursing process are not actually separate items but rather are parts of a whole, used to identify needs, establish priorities of care, maximize strengths, and resolve actual or potential alterations in human responses to health and illness, thereby promoting wellness to the highest level possible for each client.

Assessment, the systematic and continuous collection and communication of data, allows analysis of data to identify problems and strengths of clients. During planning, the nurse and client mutually set goals and agree on nursing interventions necessary to meet the expected outcomes. The nurse implements the plan of care, adapting to each individual, and documents nursing actions and client responses. After implementation, the nurse and client evaluate the effectiveness of the plan, based on achievement of goals, and determine if the plan should be continued, modified, or terminated.

The nursing process is nursing practice in action. Unit IV provides the information necessary for the beginning application of the nursing process; as core competencies are learned and practiced (both as students and as nurses), the process becomes an integral component of each nurse–client interaction. The outcome is comprehensive and individualized nursing care.

The Nursing Process

". . . the nursing process is educative and therapeutic when nurse and patient can come to know and to respect each other, as persons who are alike, and yet different, as persons who share in the solution of problems."

Hildegarde Peplau (1909–)
an active participant in ANA and NLN and a leader in developing the significance of interpersonal relationships in psychiatric nursing, whose landmark book integrated theory into her model at a time when nursing theory was in its infancy

Unit IV

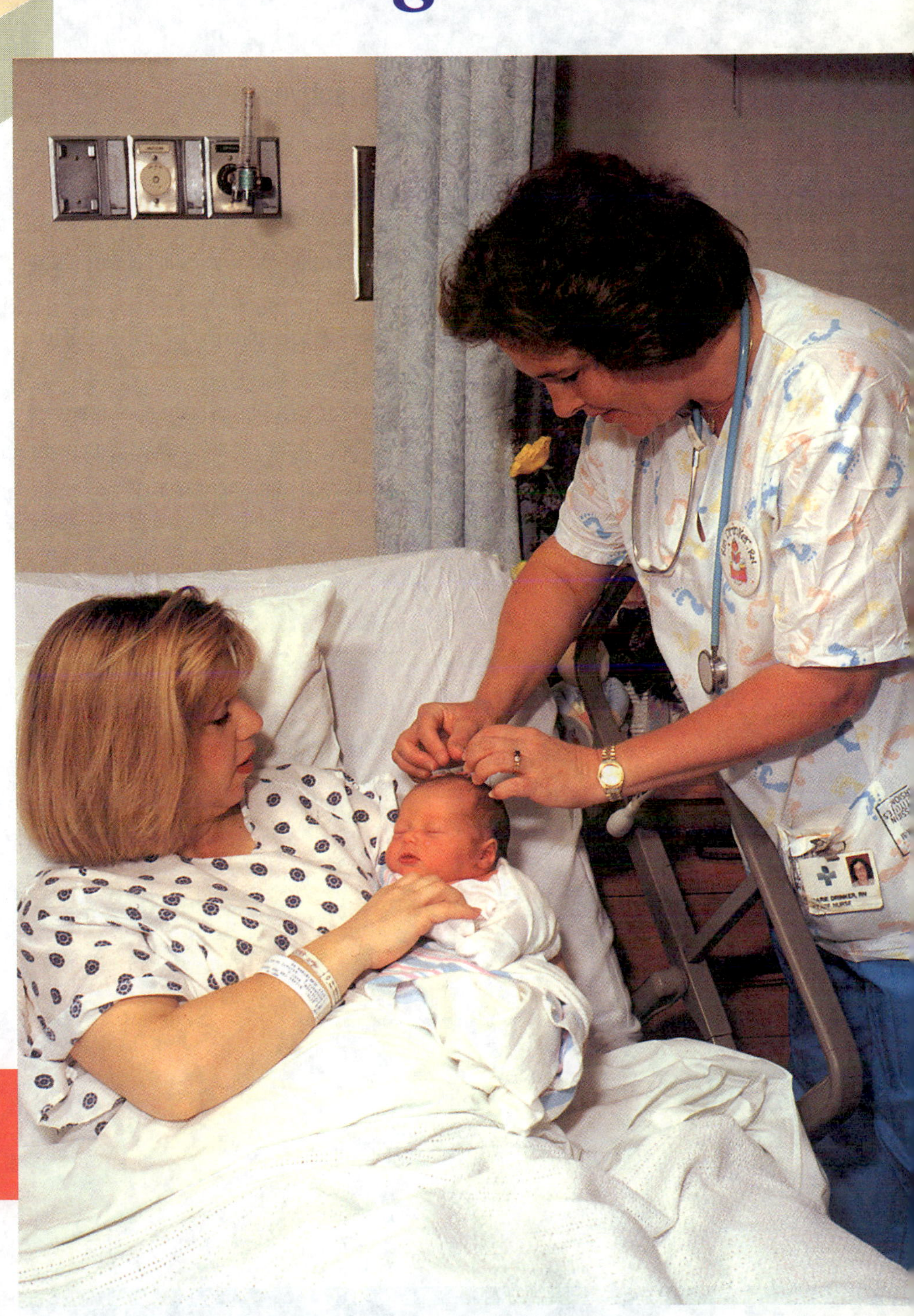

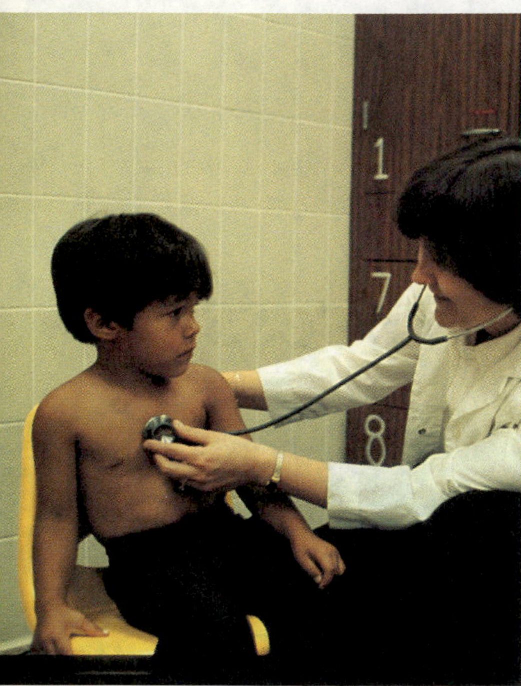

Chapter 14

Introduction to Nursing Process

Objectives

After studying this chapter, the learner should be able to:

Define key terms used in the chapter.

Describe the historic evolution of the nursing process.

Describe the nursing process and each of its five steps.

List five characteristics of the nursing process.

List three client and three nursing benefits of using the nursing process correctly.

Key Terms

assessing
diagnosing
evaluating
implementing
intuitive problem solving
nursing process
planning
scientific problem solving
trial-and-error problem solving

Traditionally, nurses have prided themselves on comforting those who are ill and on executing with precision such tasks as dressing wounds, administering medications, and bathing, feeding, and ambulating clients. Many of these tasks were ordered by physicians, and few nurses in the past would have characterized their "work" as being independent, scientifically based, or creative.

The healthcare delivery system has changed, and nursing has changed with it. Nurses now work with well and ill clients in both private and institutional settings. In addition to their role as caregiver, nurses fill specialized roles as care managers–coordinators, teachers, counselors, advocates, and researchers. Nurses are responsible for a unique dimension of healthcare, "the diagnosis and treatment of human responses to actual or potential health problems" (American Nurses Association, 1980), and as such are knowledgeable, competent, and independent professionals who work collaboratively with other healthcare professionals to design and deliver holistic care.

As the practice of nursing became more complex, nurses began to study the *process* of nursing to both understand and improve the means nurses use to accomplish their aims.

Historical Perspective

Since the term *nursing process* was first used by Hall in 1955, many nurses have struggled to define exactly what constitutes the "work of nursing" and what makes nurses successful. In the 1960s, nursing theorists began to describe nursing as a distinct entity among the healthcare professions, and also delineated specific steps in a process approach to nursing practice. In 1967, Yura and Walsh published the first comprehensive book on nursing process, in which they described four steps in the nursing process—assessment, planning, intervention, and evaluation. They viewed the element of nursing diagnosis as the logical conclusion of the assessment phase, whereas Gebbie and Lavin (1974) made nursing diagnosis a separate step in the process. These and other studies led to the development of the five-step nursing process commonly used today—assessment, diagnosis, planning, implementation, and evaluation.

The steps of the nursing process were legitimized in 1973, when the American Nurses Association Congress for Nursing Practice developed *Standards of Practice* to guide nursing performance. These standards were revised in 1991 and appear in Chapter 1. The standards for nursing practice were quickly reflected in revised nurse practice acts in many states.

The Joint Commission on Accreditation of Healthcare Organizations requires that care be documented according to the nursing process, and the National League for Nursing mandates that educational programs incorporate the nursing process as their cognitive process. In 1982, the state board examinations for professional nursing practice underwent major revisions. One of the organizing concepts used in the revisions was nursing process. The revised examinations are structured to test the practitioner's ability to assess clients; to diagnose health problems amenable to nursing therapy; and to plan, implement, and evaluate nursing care. The examinations had previously organized content on a medical model, structured according to medical specialties—medicine, surgery, maternity, pediatrics, and psychiatry.

Evolution of Nursing Diagnosis

The term *nursing diagnosis* first appeared in the literature in the 1950s. In 1976, Aspinall described nursing diagnosis as "the weak link" in nursing process. As early as 1966, Hammond wrote that nurses need both to be competent in information-seeking strategies and to have a good background of theoretical knowledge with which to conduct the search for cues and evaluate evidence—all resulting in accurate diagnosing. Key elements in the evolution of nursing diagnosis as an integral component of nursing process include the following:

- In 1972, the New York State Nurse Practice Act identified diagnosing as part of the legal domain of professional nursing; practice acts in many other states have been revised similarly since then.
- In 1973, the American Nurses Association's *Standards of Practice* included diagnosing as a function of professional nursing.

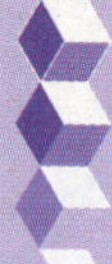

Through the Eyes of a Client

"Push!" coached the nurse. I was minutes away from giving birth to my son. I didn't want to bear down, even though I knew that if I pushed harder it would soon be over. It hurt too much. The doctor, nurse, and my husband were encouraging me, but I just couldn't push well. Then the door to my room opened and another nurse came in. She was someone I've worked with and knew well. When I heard her voice, somehow I became more focused. What she said, but more importantly, *how she said it,* made a difference. Soon after that my son Michael was born.

As a perinatal nurse I have attended to many women as they experienced childbirth. Now I was on the receiving end of nursing care. I was glad to have the first nurse, because as a coworker she had always impressed me as a "good" nurse. She seemed to be well organized, efficient, and knowledgeable. Regarded highly by her peers, she was also a kind person. As I awaited contractions, I noticed that indeed she was very efficient. She had her paperwork completed and organized even though I had arrived only a short time ago. Sadly, when it came time for me to push, she was ineffective in eliciting my cooperation. It took a different nurse with a different quality of presence to make me push.

Afterwards I wondered, was I a "client" for the first nurse, someone for whom she would plug the appropriate information into proper slots? Or was I a real *person* (someone she knew and cared about)? Why was the second nurse able to transcend her "duties," the necessary tasks at hand? She understood that the priority at the time was not the paperwork. Her care and concern shot through the mechanics of the situation and helped to decimate the anguish of that moment. Is this the "ethic of care"? If so, then perhaps even the "best" nurses sometimes lack an understanding of its necessity in their own therapeutic relationships, their own professional ethos.

—Joan W. Kiely, RN, MA

- Also in 1973, Gebbie and Lavin of St. Louis University called the First National Conference on Classification of Nursing Diagnoses, beginning a national effort to identify, standardize, and classify health problems treated by nurses. Conferences are held every 2 years, and much progress has been made in defining, classifying, and describing nursing diagnoses.

At its first meeting in 1973, the National Group, since renamed the North American Nursing Diagnosis Association (NANDA), appointed a task force to accomplish the following goals:

- Gather information and disseminate it through the Clearinghouse for Nursing Diagnosis.
- Encourage educational activities at regional and state levels to promote the implementation of nursing diagnoses. These activities include conferences to organize nurses to identify additional diagnostic labels and workshops to teach nurses about nursing diagnoses.
- Promote and organize activities to continue the development, classification, and scientific testing of nursing diagnoses. These activities include planning national conferences, identifying criteria for accepting diagnoses, surveying current research activities, and exploring varied methods for classification.

Description of Nursing Process

The **nursing process** is a systematic method that directs the nurse and client as they together (1) determine the need for nursing care, (2) plan and implement the care, and (3) evaluate the results. The steps in this client-centered, goal-oriented process are interrelated; each of the five steps depends on the accuracy of the steps preceding it. The process provides a framework that enables the nurse and client to do the following:

- Systematically collect client data (assessing)
- Clearly identify client strengths and problems (diagnosing)
- Develop a holistic plan of individualized care that specifies the desired client goals and related outcomes and the nursing interventions most likely to assist the client to meet those expected outcomes (planning)
- Execute the plan of care (implementing)
- Evaluate the effectiveness of the plan of care in terms of client goal achievement (evaluating)

In each step of the process, the nurse and client work together as partners; the client's health state and resources influence the client's level of participation. When the client is an infant, unconscious, or uncooperative, the steps of the process are worked through with the help of a family member or support person.

The primary purpose of the nursing process is to help the nurse manage each client's care scientifically, holistically, and creatively (Fig. 14-1). To do this successfully, the nurse needs many intellectual, technical, interpersonal, and ethical/legal competencies, as well as the willingness to use them creatively when working with clients to promote wellness, to prevent disease or illness, to restore health, and to facilitate coping with altered functioning. Many of these skills are described in the units that follow.

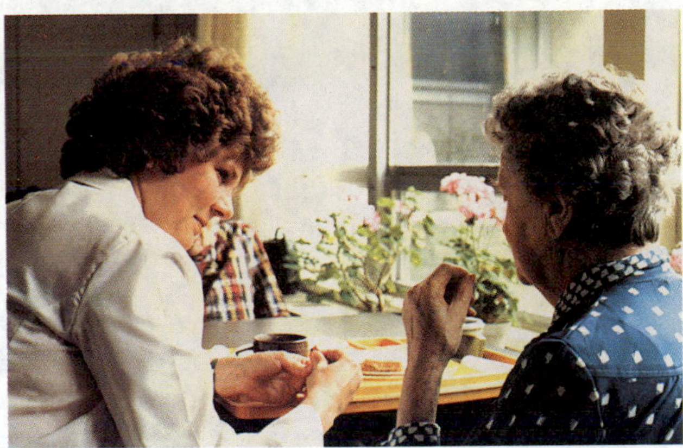

Figure 14-1
The nursing process achieves for the client scientifically based, holistic, individualized care; the chance to work collaboratively with nurses; and continuity of care. (Photo by Gates Rhodes, courtesy of School of Nursing, University of Pennsylvania.)

Steps of the Nursing Process

The five steps of the nursing process are shown in Figure 14-2. Each step is briefly described here and discussed in greater detail in the chapters that follow. Those who want to study nursing process or any of its steps in greater detail should consult one of the nursing texts that deals exclusively with nursing process (eg, Alfaro, 1994; Atkinson & Murray, 1990; Christensen & Kenney, 1994; Iyer, Taptich, & Bernocchi-Losey, 1991; LaMonica, 1985; Marriner, 1983; Pinnell & de Meneses, 1986; and Yura & Walsh, 1988).

Assessing

The first step in the nursing process, **assessing**, is the systematic and continuous collection, validation, and communication of client data. Data collection guidelines reflect the nursing theory of the particular institution. (Nursing theory is discussed in Chap. 5.) In general, nurses are concerned with how human functioning is enhanced by health promotion and compromised by illness and suffering. The remaining steps of the nursing process depend on complete, accurate, and relevant data.

During the assessment step of the nursing process, the nurse does the following:

- Establishes the data base, which includes nursing history, physical assessment, review of the client record and nursing literature, and consultation with the client's support people and healthcare professionals
- Continuously updates the data base
- Validates data
- Communicates data

Diagnosing

Diagnosing is analysis of client data to identify data clusters that indicate actual or potential health problems, factors that contribute to or cause these problems, and coping patterns or strengths of the client.

The nurse next determines if each health problem is best treated by nursing or by another health discipline. When data analysis reveals an actual or potential health problem that nursing intervention can prevent or resolve, the problem is termed a *nursing diagnosis.* During the diagnosis step of the nursing process, the nurse does the following:

- Interprets and analyzes client data
- Identifies client strengths and client health problems
- Formulates and validates nursing diagnoses
- Develops a prioritized list of nursing diagnoses

Planning

Planning is the establishment of client goals/outcomes by the nurse, working with the client, that prevent, reduce, or resolve problems identified in the nursing diagnoses, and the determination of related nursing interventions most likely to assist the client in achieving these goals. In addition, a comprehensive plan of care also specifies (1) the nursing assistance needed by the client to meet human needs, and (2) the nursing interventions dictated by the plan of medical care. During the planning step of the nursing process, the nurse does the following:

- Establishes priorities
- Writes client goals/expected outcomes and develops an evaluative strategy
- Selects nursing interventions
- Communicates the plan of nursing care

Implementing

Implementing involves the carrying out of the plan of care. It includes all interventions performed by nurses to promote wellness, prevent disease or illness, restore health, and facilitate coping with altered functioning. During the implementing step of the nursing process, the nurse does the following:

- Carries out the plan of nursing care
- Continues data collection and modifies the plan of care as needed
- Documents care

Evaluating

Evaluating is the measuring of the extent to which client goals have been met. The nurse and the client together measure how well the client has achieved goals/outcomes specified in the plan of care, and nurse and client identify factors that either positively or negatively influenced goal/outcome achievement. Client response to the plan of care determines whether nursing care should be continued as is, modified, or terminated. If evaluation points to a need to modify nursing care, then the accuracy, completeness, and relevance of the assessment data, as well as the appropriateness of client diagnoses, goals, and nursing interventions, should all be carefully reviewed and modified. During the evaluation step of the nursing process, the nurse does the following:

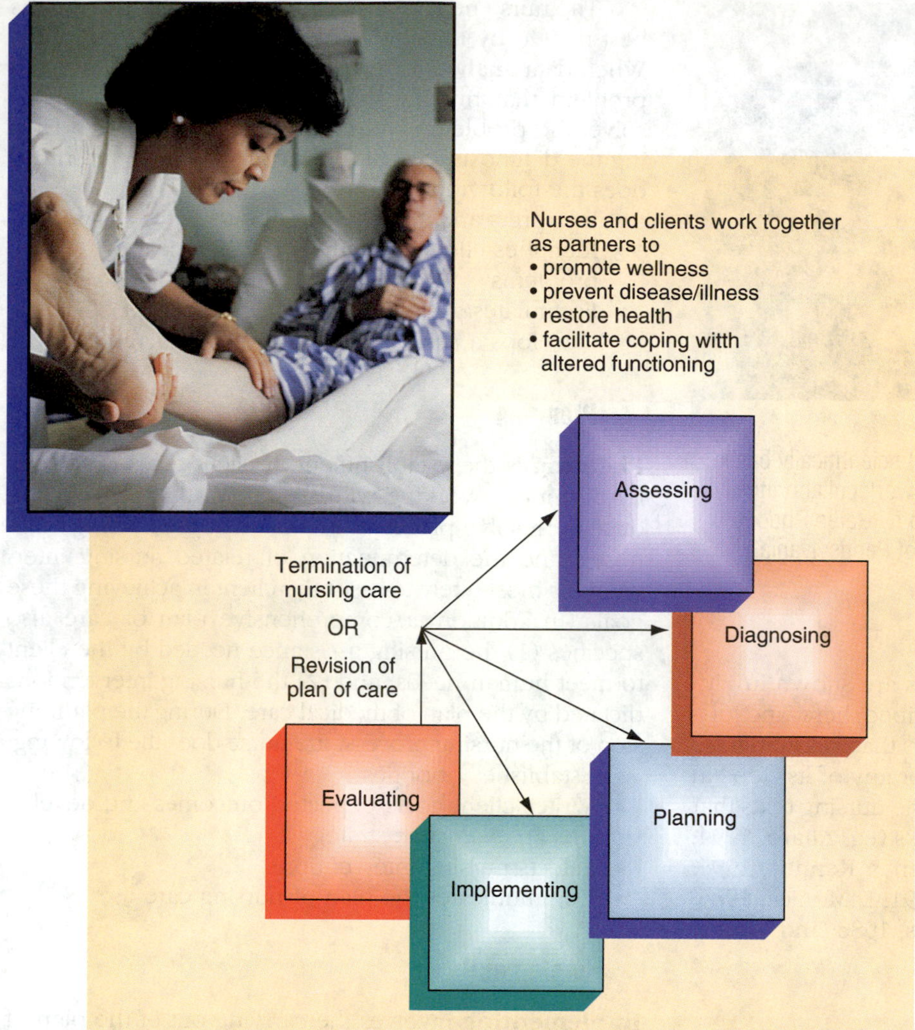

Figure 14-2
The nursing process. The nursing process is a systematic method that directs the nurse and client as, together, they determine the need for nursing care (assessing and diagnosing), and then plan, implement, and evaluate care. The steps in this client-centered, goal-oriented process are interrelated, and each of the five steps depends on the accuracy of the step preceding it. Evaluation, the fifth step in the process, leads either to the termination of nursing care or to revision of the plan of care after each preceding step in the process has been evaluated.

- Measures the client's achievement of desired goals/outcomes
- Identifies factors that contribute to the client's success or failure
- Modifies the plan of care, if indicated

An overview of the steps of the nursing process is presented in Table 14-1; the accompanying box gives examples of each of the steps.

Documenting the Nursing Process

More than ever before, nurses are aware of the need to document nursing care. Legally speaking, a nursing action not documented is a nursing action not performed. Each chapter in this unit offers specific documentation guidelines for nursing process activities; Chapter 21 discusses documentation in general. It is helpful to practice documentation while learning any given nursing activity; like any other nursing skill, documentation improves with practice. Examples of nursing documentation, nursing assessments, plans of care, and notes are provided throughout this text.

Problem Solving and the Nursing Process

One of the strengths of the nursing process is that it is based on a methodology that is familiar to most nursing students—problem solving. Problem solving is a basic life skill; identifying a problem and then taking steps to resolve it is a matter of common sense. Different approaches to problem solving yield different results, some of which are more successful than others.

The **trial-and-error method** of problem solving involves testing any number of solutions until one is found that works for that particular problem. This method is not efficient for the nurse and can be dangerous to the client; it is, therefore, not recommended as a guide for nursing practice.

The **scientific method** of problem solving is a systematic, seven-step problem-solving process that involves (1) problem identification, (2) data collection, (3) hypothesis formulation, (4) plan of action, (5) hypothesis testing, (6) interpretation of results, and (7) evaluation, resulting in conclusion or revision of the study. This method is used most correctly in a controlled laboratory

Table 14-1
Overview of the Nursing Process

Component	Description	Purpose	Activities
Assessing	Collection, validation, and communication of client data	Make a judgment about the client's health status, ability to manage his or her own health care, and need for nursing Plan individualized holistic care that draws on client strengths and is responsive to changes in the client's conditions	1. Establish the data base • Nursing history • Physical assessment • Review of client record and nursing literature • Consultation with client's support people and health care professionals 2. Continuously update the data base 3. Validate data 4. Communicate data
Diagnosing	Analysis of client data to identify client strengths and health problems that independent nursing intervention can prevent or resolve	Develop a prioritized list of nursing diagnoses	1. Interpret and analyze client data 2. Identify client strengths and health problems 3. Formulate and validate nursing diagnoses 4. Develop prioritized list of nursing diagnoses
Planning	Specification of (1) client goals/outcomes to prevent, reduce, or resolve the problems identified in the nursing diagnoses; and (2) related nursing interventions	Develop an individualized plan of nursing care	1. Establish priorities 2. Write goals/outcomes and develop an evaluative strategy 3. Select nursing interventions 4. Communicate plan of nursing care
Implementing	Carrying out the plan of care	Assist clients to achieve desired goals—promote wellness, prevent disease and illness, restore health, facilitate coping with altered functioning	1. Carry out the plan of care 2. Continue data collection and modify the plan of care as needed 3. Document care
Evaluating	Measuring the extent to which the client has achieved the goals specified in the plan of care, identifying factors that positively or negatively influenced goal achievement; revise the plan of care if necessary	Continue, modify, or terminate nursing care	1. Measure how well the client has achieved desired goals/outcomes 2. Identify factors that contribute to the client's success or failure. 3. Modify the plan of care (if indicated)

setting, but is closely related to the more general six-step problem-solving process commonly used by healthcare professionals as they work with clients. The relation between these methods and the nursing process is shown in Table 14-2.

Intuitive Problem Solving

For years, nurse theorists and educators have argued that clinical judgments should be based on data alone (the scientific method), in an attempt to establish nursing as a science, worthy of the respect of other professions. Controversy has recently been sparked by nurses both studying and writing about the role of **intuitive problem solving** in clinical decision making. Many veteran nurses can describe situations in which an "inner prompting" led to a quick nursing intervention that saved a client's life. Benner (1984, p. 295) describes intuition as "direct apprehension of a situation based upon a background of similar and dissimilar situations and embodied intelligence or skill." Schraeder and Fischer (1986, p. 161) credit to intuitive perception "a wide range of experience, from the sudden, inexplicable feeling that 'something is wrong,' to recognizing the teaching moment, when to offer encouragement, and when it is most helpful simply to listen."

Advocates of intuition recommend the following:

- Welcoming flashes of intuition as additions to logical reasoning, rather than disruptions

Example of the Steps of the Nursing Process

Assessing

You are checking on a client who had abdominal surgery yesterday and hear that the client has considerable pain. "It kept me up all night." The client has been reluctant to ask for any pain medication, fearing effect of the drug. "I don't want to become a junkie." The client's blood pressure and pulse rate are slightly elevated.

Diagnosing

You analyze the data above and write the nursing diagnosis: *Pain related to a fear of taking pain-relieving medications.* The client agrees that this is becoming a problem.

Planning

You decide to work with the client to achieve the goal: *By 3:00 PM client reports sufficient relief of pain to enable him to rest and to get out of bed to go to the bathroom.* The client wants to accomplish the goal. You identify teaching as the primary nursing intervention.

Implementing

After asking the client about his experiences with pain-relieving medications, you explain that although many of these drugs are addictive when abused, there is no harm if they are taken as prescribed postoperatively. You also explain that it is important for him to experience enough pain relief to be able to cough and deep breathe, ambulate, and do other things important to his recovery. You suggest that the medication will be most effective if taken before his pain peaks and becomes intense. You administer the prescribed medication for pain when the client indicates that he is willing to give it a try.

Evaluating

After enough time has elapsed for the medication to take effect, you check back with the client to evaluate whether or not he has obtained relief and met his goal. If the client is satisfied and you both feel comfort is no longer a problem, you terminate the plan of care for this diagnosis. If the client still feels pain or is dissatisfied with the medication, each of the preceding steps of the nursing process is reevaluated, and necessary changes are made in the plan of care.

- Validating intuitions: when an intuition cannot be validated (eg, when the nurse senses that something is wrong with the client, although there are no clinical signs), careful monitoring of the client should be initiated
- Furthering nursing research to help find ways to (1) cultivate intuition and its typical results (accurate, early diagnosis; vigilant monitoring; better client care) and (2) document the information intuition supplies (Rew, 1987)

Beginning nurses must use nursing knowledge and scientific problem solving as the basis of care they give; intuitive problem solving comes with years of practice and observation. If the beginning nurse has an intuition about a client, the information should be discussed with the supervisor.

Characteristics of Nursing Process

Various words and phrases have been used to describe the nursing process; key descriptors include *systematic, dynamic, interpersonal, goal-oriented,* and *universally applicable.*

Table 14-2
Comparison of Steps in the Problem-Solving Process, the Scientific Method, and the Nursing Process

Problem-Solving Process	Scientific Method	Nursing Process
1. Problem encountered	1. Problem identification	1. Assessing
2. Data collection	2. Data collection	
3. Exact nature of problem specified	3. Hypothesis formulation	2. Diagnosing
4. Plan of action determined	4. Plan of action developed to test hypothesis	3. Planning
5. Plan of action carried out	5. Hypothesis testing	4. Implementing
6. Outcomes of the plan evaluated and the plan continued, modified, or terminated	6. Interpretation of results	5. Evaluating
	7. Evaluation resulting in conclusion or revision of the study	

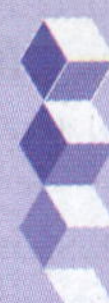

Through the Eyes of a Client

I recently spent 2 months in a university teaching hospital while doctors tried to find a way to regulate my heart beats. Many of the days were filled with tests, some of which were frightening. I was given many drugs—most of which turned out not to be helpful. I was a 2-hour car ride away from my home, family, and friends—which meant there wasn't always a familiar face at my bedside.

I quickly learned I could judge what kind of day I was going to have as soon as I saw my nurse each morning. There were basically three types of nurses.

All of them brought my medicines and helped with the treatment plan. With some nurses, however, I also experienced the comfort and security of knowing that my expressed needs would be promptly and respectfully tended to. If I needed help getting up to the bathroom or asked for something for pain, I could count on help coming quickly. And finally there were those few with whom I knew I was going to have a great day because they would "make it happen" no matter how sick I was feeling. These were the nurses who offered a hug with their medicines, who had a moment to sit and listen, who teased about the "fashion statements" I was making with my nightgowns, and who "walked me through" new tests so that at least I felt better prepared to face the unknown. Most often it wasn't what they did but how they did it.

I wish all nurses understood the power they have to influence a patient's basic sense of wellbeing. A hospital can be a pretty scary, lonely place. Nurses can make all the difference!

—Mildred Taylor, Pine Grove, PA

Systematic

A quick look at the many and varied activities of any nurse on a busy day might lead one to conclude that nursing is little more than the execution of countless haphazard tasks. A closer look will reveal that each nursing task is part of an ordered sequence of activities. Moreover, each activity depends on the accuracy of the activity that precedes it, and influences the actions that follow it. Without a complete and accurate data base, the nurse cannot identify client strengths and problems; lacking knowledge of these, it is impossible for the nurse and client to develop a plan of care based on realistic and valued client goals. Unless the goals/outcomes are well written, nursing actions and evaluation will be meaningless. The nursing process directs each step of nursing care in a sequential, ordered manner.

Dynamic

Although the nursing process is presented as an orderly progression of steps, in reality there is great interaction and overlapping among the five steps. No one step in the nursing process is a one-time phenomenon; each step is fluid and flows into the next step. In some nursing situations, all five stages occur almost simultaneously. When a nurse discovers that a client is choking on food and cannot speak or breathe, the nurse quickly identifies the problem and takes steps to dislodge the food particle blocking the airway—all the while evaluating the effectiveness of the intervention. In other instances—for example, child abuse—the nursing team may labor over each step of the nursing process as nurses work with the family to resolve complex problems. As well as being dynamic, the nursing process is continually open to change; at any point, new client data may cause the plan of care to proceed in an entirely different direction.

Interpersonal

Always at the heart of nursing is the human being. Nursing exists as a profession because some people require assistance as they respond to health and illness. The nursing process ensures that nurses are client-centered rather than task-centered (Fig. 14-3). Rather than simply approaching a client to take vital signs, the nurse thinks: "How is Mr. Barclay today? Any new data that indicate a need to modify his plan of care? Are our nursing actions helping him to achieve his goals? How can we better help him?"

The nursing process encourages nurses to work together to help clients use their strengths to meet all their human needs. This is different from viewing the client as a "problem to be solved" and interacting mechanically to provide the solution. Working intimately with clients helps nurses to explore their own strengths and limitations and to develop themselves personally and professionally.

Goal Oriented

Countless good things can be accomplished for most clients, ranging from improving their oral hygiene to helping them cope with the demands of being a new parent, recover from an acute medical illness, live with chronic pain, or prepare for death. Likewise, it would take hundreds of pages to list and describe all the nursing actions a nurse might perform for a client. Moreover, nurses and clients often differ in the importance they attach to selected goals. The nursing process offers a means for nurses and clients to work together to iden-

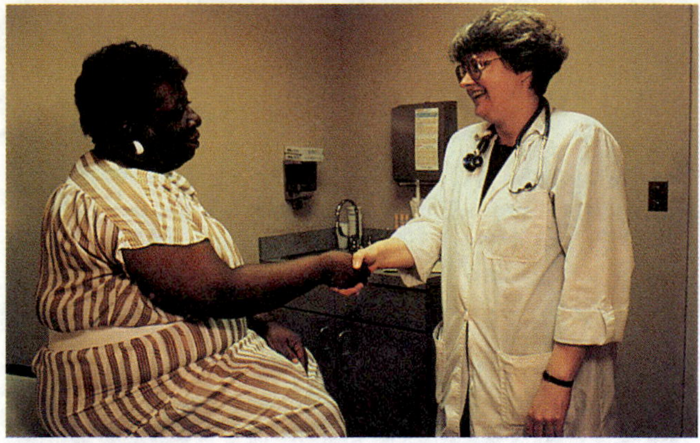

Figure 14-3
One characteristic of the nursing process is that it ensures that nursing is client centered rather than task oriented. (Photo by Gates Rhodes, courtesy of School of Nursing, University of Pennsylvania.)

tify specific goals related to wellness promotion, disease and illness prevention, health restoration, and coping with altered functioning, which are most important to the client, and to match them with the appropriate nursing actions. Once these are recorded in the plan of care, each nurse can quickly determine the client's priorities and begin nursing with a clear sense of how to proceed. The client benefits from continuity of care, and each nurse's care moves the client closer to goal achievement.

Universally Applicable

The one constant in healthcare is change. Once nurses have a working knowledge of the nursing process, they find that they can practice nursing with well or ill people, young or old, in any type of practice setting. Efforts made by the student nurse to master nursing process will result in the student's possession of a valuable tool that can be used with ease in any nursing situation.

What should be clear from the preceding discussion on nursing process is that it provides a framework for all the nurse's activities. With each nurse–client interaction, it is important to assess the client, note any significant alterations in health status, determine if the nursing action is helping the client achieve his or her goals, and modify the plan of care as necessary. Thus, the nurse who feeds a pediatric client through a special tube as ordered by a physician continually assesses how the child is responding to the feeding and if the child or family will be able to manage the feedings independently when the child is discharged. Depending on the results of the nursing assessment, new nursing diagnoses may be needed, as may additions to the plan of care. The nursing process offers direction for *all* the activities carried out by the nurse when caring for clients.

Benefits of the Nursing Process

When used properly, the nursing process achieves for the client scientifically based, holistic, individualized care; the opportunity to work collaboratively with nurses; and continuity of care. Nurses who use the nursing process in a thoughtful and systematic way achieve a clear and efficient plan of action by which the entire nursing team can achieve results for clients; the satisfaction that they are making an important "difference" in the lives of their clients; and the opportunity to grow professionally as nurses evaluate the effectiveness of interventions and variables that contribute positively or negatively to the client's goal achievement.

Computer Applications in Nursing

Computer Use in the Clinical Practice of Nursing

Currently nurses use computers to assist with practice in clinical settings. In a hospital setting, computers are used by nurses to:

- Enter orders and retrieve results from various ancillary departments
- Document client progress using critical pathways or other methodologies
- Track medication administration
- Enter client assessments
- Monitor clients
- Initiate discharge planning
- Support decisions
- Determine client acuity level
- Educate clients
- Conduct quality assurance audits
- Conduct interdepartmental communications
- Graphically display client data

Some nurses input and access data by way of hand-held or point-of-care terminals that allow them to provide care and chart it immediately. Benefits of automated charting include:

- Accurate, timely, complete, and legible documentation
- Reduced medication errors
- Increased time with the client
- Improved communication with all client care departments
- Improved nurse satisfaction
- Better access to information
- Improved quality of care

These benefits will serve to help the nurse, the organization, and ultimately the client.

Key Points

- The nursing process is a systematic method that directs the nurse and client as they together determine the need for nursing care (assessing and diagnosing) and then plan, implement, and evaluate care.
- The primary purpose of the nursing process is to help the nurses manage each client's nursing care scientifically, holistically, and creatively.
- In each step of the nursing process, the nurse and client work together as partners. The client's health state and resources influence his or her level of participation.
- Assessment is the systematic and continuous collection, validation, and communication of client data.
- Diagnosing is the analysis of client data to identify (1) data clusters that indicate actual or potential problems in the way the client is responding to health or illness, (2) factors that contribute to or cause these problems, and (3) coping patterns or other strengths the client can draw on to prevent or resolve the problem.
- During the planning step of the nursing process, the nurse, working with the client, (1) develops client goals/expected outcomes that, if achieved, prevent, reduce, or eliminate the problems specified in the nursing diagnoses and (2) identifies the nursing interventions most likely to achieve these goals/outcomes.
- Implementation is simply the carrying out of the plan of nursing care. It includes all the actions performed by the nurse to promote wellness, prevent disease and illness, restore health, and facilitate coping with altered functioning.
- During evaluation, the nurse and client measure how well the client has achieved the goals/outcomes specified in the plan of care and identify factors that positively or negatively influenced goal achievement. Client responses to the plan of care determine if nursing care is to be continued without change, modified, or terminated.
- Underlying the science and art of nursing is a successful blend of the scientific problem-solving method and the intuitive method.
- The nursing process is systematic, each step depending on the accuracy of the previous step and influencing the steps that follow. The steps of the nursing process are interrelated; each step is fluid and moves into the next.
- The nursing process is an interpersonal process that is always client-centered rather than task-centered. As nurses help clients to use their strengths to meet all their human needs, nurses themselves grow personally and professionally.
- A goal-oriented process, the nursing process offers a means for nurses and clients to work together to identify the specific health goals that are most important to the client—and to match these with the appropriate nursing interventions.

Bibliography

Alfaro, R. (1994). *Application of nursing process: A step-by-step guide* (3rd ed.). Philadelphia: Lippincott.

American Association of Colleges of Nursing. (1986). *Essentials of college and university education for nursing.* Washington, DC: AACN.

American Nurses Association. (1980). *Nursing: A social policy statement.* Washington, DC: ANA.

American Nurses Association Congress for Practice. (1973; revised 1991). *Standards of practice.* Washington, DC: ANA.

Aspinall, M. J. (1976). Nursing diagnosis: The weak link. *Nursing Outlook, 24*(7), 433–436.

Atkinson, J., & Murray, M. E. (1990). *Understanding the nursing process* (4th ed.). New York: Macmillan.

Benner, P. (1984). *From novice to expert.* Menlo Park, CA: Addison-Wesley.

Christensen, P. J., & Kenney, J. W. (1994). *Nursing process: Application of conceptual models* (4th ed.). St. Louis: Mosby.

Fonteyn, M. E., & Cooper, L. F. (1994). The written nursing process: Is it still useful to nursing education? *Journal of Advanced Nursing, 19*(2), 315–319.

Gebbie, K., & Lavin, M. A. (1974). Classification of nursing diagnosis. *American Journal of Nursing, 74,* 250–253.

Hall, L. E. (1955). Quality of nursing care. Address given at the Department of Baccalaureate and Higher Degree Programs of the New Jersey League for Nursing. *Public Health News* (June). New Jersey: New Jersey State Department of Health.

Hammond, K. R. (1966). Clinical inference in nursing: A psychologist's point of view. *Nursing Research, 15,* 27–38.

Hill, L., & Smith, N. (1990). *Self-care nursing: Promotion of health* (2nd ed.). East Norwalk, CT: Appleton & Lange.

Iyer, P., Taptich, B., & Bernocchi-Losey, D. (1991). *Nursing process and nursing diagnosis* (2nd ed.). Philadelphia: Saunders.

Joint Commission on Accreditation of Healthcare Organizations. (1995). *Accreditation manual for hospitals.* Oakbrook Terrace, IL: JCAHO.

LaMonica, E. (1985). *The humanistic nursing process.* Monterey, CA: Wadsworth.

Marriner, A. (1983). *The nursing process: A scientific approach to nursing* (3rd ed.). St. Louis: Mosby.

Mauksch, I. G., & David, M. (1972). Prescription for survival. *American Journal of Nursing, 72*(12), 2189–2193.

McHugh, M. K. (1987). Has nursing outgrown the nursing process? *Nursing, 17*(8), 50–51.

McHugh, M. K. (Ed.). (1987). Nursing process. *Holistic Nursing Practice, 1*(3).

Pinnell, N., & de Meneses, M. (1986). *The nursing process.* Norwalk, CT: Appleton-Century-Crofts.

Renz, M. C. (1993). Learning from intuition. *Nursing, 23*(7), 44–45.

Rew, L. (1987). Nursing intuition: Too powerful—and too valuable—to ignore. *Nursing, 17*(7), 43–45.

Schraeder, B. D., & Fischer, D. K. (1986). Using knowledge to make clinical decisions. *MCN, 11,* 161–163.

Yura, H., & Walsh, M. B. (1988). *The nursing process: Assessing, planning, implementing, evaluating* (5th ed.). Norwalk, CT: Appleton-Century-Crofts.

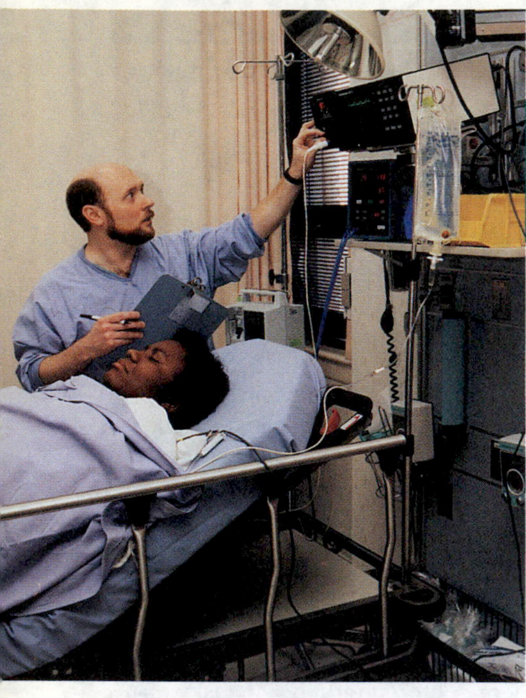

Chapter 15

Core Competencies and Critical Thinking

Objectives

After studying this chapter, the learner will be able to:

Define key terms used in the chapter.

Describe the four core competencies essential to nursing practice.

Use a model of critical thinking when making clinical judgments and decisions.

Identify four habits which assist in the development of technical competencies.

Describe a personal plan to develop the interpersonal competencies essential to quality care.

Explain the relationship between a nurse's sense of accountability and client well-being.

Identify personal strengths and weaknesses in light of nursing's essential knowledge and competencies.

Key Terms

cognitive competencies
critical thinking
ethical/legal competencies
interpersonal competencies
technical competencies
whistleblowing

The first comprehensive text on the nursing process identified three types of skills essential to nursing practice: intellectual, interpersonal, and technical (Yura and Walsh, 1967). More recently, Alfaro-LeFevre (1994) writes that effective use of the nursing process requires "*manual* skills to complete technical procedures, *intellectual* skills to solve problems and make decisions, and *interpersonal* skills to establish good interpersonal relationships with clients, significant others, and co-workers" (p. 16). The unique challenges now confronting nurses in our rapidly changing healthcare delivery system demand these three types of skills plus *ethical/legal* skills.

In a recent review of the literature, Johnson (1994) states that nursing art includes at least five separate nursing abilities. They are the nurse's ability to (1) grasp meaning in patient encounters, (2) establish a meaningful connection with the patient, (3) skillfully perform nursing actions, (4) rationally determine an appropriate course of nursing actions, and (5) morally conduct his or her nursing practice.

Before you continue in more depth your study of each step of the nursing process, it is useful to look at the competencies essential to nursing practice. Understanding them will help you consciously plan to develop them as you begin your mastery of nursing process. Few nurses excel naturally in all four of these skills and even experienced nurses struggle to grow more proficient in the skills which lead to excellence.

Defining the Four Core Competencies

Cognitive Competencies

Cognitive competencies enable nurses to reason about the nature of things sufficiently to "make sense" of their world and to conceptually grasp what is necessary to achieve valued goals. Nurses skilled cognitively are able to:

- Offer a scientific rationale for each element in a client's plan of care (prerequisite sciences include nursing and medical science, as well as basic sciences such as chemistry, microbiology, anatomy, physiology, psychology, sociology, and anthropology)
- Select those nursing interventions which are most likely to yield desired outcomes
- Use critical thinking to problem-solve creatively

Critical thinking is defined as "a systematic way to form and shape one's thinking. It functions purposefully and exactingly. It is thought that is disciplined, comprehensive, based on intellectual standards, and, as a result, well-reasoned" (Paul, 1993, p. 20). Cognitively skilled nurses are critical thinkers. The four domains of critical thinking—elements of thought, abilities, affective dimensions, and standards—are highlighted in Table 15-1.

Technical Competencies

Technical competencies enable nurses to manipulate equipment skillfully, in a manner that produces a desired goal. They involve everything from manual dexterity and good eye–hand coordination to an ability to troubleshoot when equipment malfunctions, based upon an understanding of the technical workings of the equipment. Nurses who are skilled technically are able to:

- Use technical equipment with sufficient competence and ease to achieve goals with minimal distress to involved participants
- Creatively adapt equipment and technical procedures to the needs of particular clients in diverse circumstances

Interpersonal Competencies

Interpersonal competencies enable nurses to establish and maintain caring relationships that facilitate the achievement of valued goals while simultaneously affirming the worth of participants in the relationship. Nurses skilled in interpersonal relations are able to:

- Use interactions with clients, their significant others, and colleagues to affirm the worth of involved participants
- Elicit the personal strengths and abilities of clients and their significant others to achieve valued health goals
- Provide the healthcare team with knowledge about the client's valued goals and expectations

Table 15-1
The Four Domains of Critical Thinking

I. Elements of Thought: The Basic Building Blocks of Thinking

Element	*Fundamental Standard*	*Potential Problems*	*Principle*
Purpose	1. Clarity of purpose 2. Significance of purpose 3. Achievability of purpose 4. Consistence of purpose	1. Unclear purpose 2. Trivial purpose 3. Unrealistic purpose 4. Contradictory purposes	All reasoning has a purpose.
Question at issue or central problem	1. Clarity of question 2. Significance of question 3. Answerability 4. Relevance	1. Unclear 2. Insignificant 3. Not answerable 4. Irrelevant	To settle a question you must understand what it requires.
Point of view	1. Flexibility in point of view 2. Fairness of point of view 3. Clarity of point of view 4. Breadth of point of view	1. Restricted 2. Biased 3. Unclear 4. Narrow	Reasoning is better when multiple, relevant points of view are sought out, articulated clearly, empathized with fairly and logically, applied consistently and dispassionately.
Empirical dimension	1. Clear evidence 2. Relevant information 3. Fairly gathered and reported evidence 4. Accurate data 5. Adequate evidence 6. Consistently applied data	1. Unclear 2. Unfairly or self-servingly gathered 3. Inaccurate 4. Insufficient	Reasoning can only be as sound as the evidence it is based on.
Concepts and ideas	1. Clarity of concepts 2. Relevance of concepts 3. Depth of concepts 4. Neutrality of concepts	1. Unclear 2. Irrelevant 3. Superficial 4. Biased	Reasoning can only be as clear, relevant, and deep as the concepts which shape it.
Assumptions	1. Clarity of assumptions 2. Justifiability of assumptions 3. Consistency of assumptions	1. Unclear 2. Unjustified 3. Contradictory	Reasoning can only be as sound as the assumptions it makes.
Implications and consequences	1. Significance of implications 2. Realistic nature of implications 3. Clarity of articulated implications 4. Precision of articulated implications 5. Completeness of articulated implications	1. Unimportant 2. Unrealistic 3. Unclear 4. Imprecise 5. Incomplete	To reason through an issue or decision, you must understand the implications and consequences that follow from it.

II. Abilities: The Skills Essential to Higher-order Thinking

- Ability to evaluate the credibility of sources of information
- Ability to analyze arguments, interpretations, beliefs, or theories
- Ability to clarify the meaning of words and phrases
- Ability to transfer insights into new contexts
- Ability to generate and assess possible solutions
- Ability to develop criteria for evaluation: clarify values and standards
- Ability to read, listen, write, and speak critically

III. Affective Dimensions: The Attitudes, Dispositions, Passions, and Traits of Mind Essential to Higher-order Thinking in Real Settings

- Thinking independently
- Exercising fair-mindedness
- Developing insight into egocentricity and sociocentricity
- Developing intellectual humility and suspending judgment
- Developing intellectual courage
- Developing intellectual good faith and integrity
- Developing intellectual perseverance
- Developing confidence in reason
- Developing intellectual curiosity

IV. Intellectual Standards: The Standards Used to Critique Higher-order Thinking

clear	precise
specific	accurate
relevant	plausible
consistent	logical
deep	broad
complete	significant
adequate (for purpose)	fair

Content from Paul, R. W. (1993). *Critical thinking: How to prepare students for a rapidly changing world.* Santa Rosa, CA: Foundation for Critical Thinking, pp. 123–132.

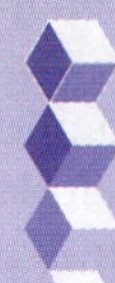

Through the Eyes of a Student

It was a gorgeous day, the kind of day when weather alone can boost one's spirits. The leaves were glistening with morning dew as I entered the hospital parking lot eagerly awaiting the day's assignment. Although it was early in my first semester of nursing school, I felt confident in my abilities to provide the expected level of care, because I had 13 years of previous clinical experience as a registered dietician.

My professor, a woman who exuded professionalism, had assigned me to a terminal cancer patient on "no code" orders. The look in my professor's eyes and the tone in her voice as she handed me the patient's chart should have been a warning about the gravity of his condition. Unfortunately, nothing was going to squash my enthusiasm.

The patient, a 72-year-old retired bishop, had been in the hospital for the past 3 weeks and he had full mental capacity. A review of his chart showed that medical care was limited to comfort measures, primarily pain control. Of further significance, there were no family members: he was facing an imminent death alone.

I found him sitting on the side of his bed waiting for assistance to the bathroom. The patient detailed the plans for his morning care, which included nothing more than the usual bath and linen change. Probably sensing my upbeat attitude, he stressed his need for a slow pace and reiterated this need throughout the morning. To the best of my abilities I complied with his request—all the while maintaining a cheerful disposition. As the morning progressed I detected that he was becoming increasingly distant, no matter what I did to improve his comfort level.

At the end of my shift I felt that something was terribly missing in the care I provided. I felt inadequate and disappointed that I had failed my patient. My spirits were leveled to ground zero. Pondering the events over and over in my mind did not reveal my obvious deficiency. A few weeks went by before I finally realized what I had done wrong. During a postclinical conference a classmate related a similar experience with a young, terminally ill woman. In response to my classmate's upbeat disposition, the patient bluntly told her that her positive attitude "was not respectful or supportive of her state of health." And all of a sudden I realized that I had failed the bishop by my inability to emphathize with him and with what he was experiencing. The focus of my care had not been on the feelings of my patient. What a painful realization.

Subsequent class lectures and readings on nursing as an interpersonal process have captured my attention. Striving to improve my ability to apply that process in the therapeutic use of self is what sets nursing apart from other care providers. To me, it is what defines the essence or art of nursing science.

—Jane J. Miller, RN, RD,
Georgetown University, Washington, DC

- Work collaboratively with the healthcare team as a respected and credible colleague to secure valued goals

Ethical/Legal Competencies

Ethical and legal competencies enable nurses to conduct themselves in a manner that is consistent with their personal moral code and professional role responsibilities. Nurses skilled in ethical/legal competence are able to:

- Be trusted to act in ways which advance the interests of clients
- Be accountable for their practice to themselves, the clients they serve, the care-giving team, and society
- Act as effective client advocates
- Mediate ethical conflict among the client, significant others, healthcare team, and other interested parties
- Practice nursing faithful to the tenets of professional codes of ethics
- Use legal safeguards which reduce the risk of litigation

Cognitive and technical competencies equip nurses to manage the clinical problems stemming from the client's changing health or illness state. Interpersonal and ethical competencies are essential, however, if nurses are concerned about broader notions of client well-being.

Developing Cognitive Competencies: Critical Thinking

Nurses who wish to develop the critical thinking competencies essential to quality nursing practice will find it helpful to work methodically through a set of five types of considerations when posed with a thinking challenge. These include purpose of thinking, adequacy of knowledge, potential problems, helpful resources, and critique of judgment/decision.

Purpose of Thinking

The first step when trying to think critically about a situation is to identify the purpose or goal of your thinking. This helps to discipline thinking by keeping all thoughts directed to the goal. The purpose of critical thinking may be to make a judgment about a particular client or situation or to make a decision about how best to intervene.

Adequacy of Knowledge

At the outset of critical thinking, it is important for you to judge if the knowledge available to you is accurate, complete, and relevant. If you reason with false information or lack important data, it is impossible to draw a sound conclusion. You will also want to be sure that you understand all the details relevant to the issue under consideration. What is at stake? How much time do you have to make a decision? How much room is there for error?

Potential Problems

As you become skilled in critical thinking, you will learn to "flag" and remedy pitfalls to sound reasoning. Common problems include working with untested or faulty assumptions; accepting an unproven claim or line of argument; allowing bias to color your thinking; and reasoning illogically, eg, making generalizations on the basis of a single experience or case, or allowing emotion to rule reason. The more familiar you are with these common impediments to critical thinking, the easier it will be to detect them in your own thinking.

Helpful Resources

Wise professionals are always quick to recognize their limits and to seek help in remedying their deficiencies. Experienced clinicians know that learning is continuous and expect practice to confront them with challenges that demand new knowledge. Critical thinkers know what help they need to assist their reasoning and know what resources to tap. Key resources include experienced clinicians, texts and journals, institutional policies and procedures, and professional groups and writings.

Critique of Judgment/Decision

Ultimately you must identify alternative judgments or decisions, weigh the merits of each, and reach a conclusion. It is helpful to try to predict the consequences of your major options before concluding your reasoning. You will also want to evaluate the alternative you selected as your decision begins to influence your actions.

The accompanying box illustrates the use of these five considerations to facilitate critical thinking about a client care dilemma experienced by a student new to clinical practice. The merits of thinking critically about which of the options is most likely to meet the client's needs are readily apparent. Since nurses literally hold the well-being of clients in their hands, sloppy reasoning is both dangerous and inexcusable—even for someone new to clinical practice.

Developing Technical Competencies

Some people are naturally "good with their hands" and quickly master intricate procedures that involve working with technical equipment. Others have to practice

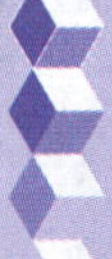

Through the Eyes of a Student

My first experience with an open wound was with a woman who had a stage four sacral decubitus. I needed to do a dressing change with packing. I was fearful of what the wound would look like. I thought for sure I was going to be "grossed out," and I was—not by the appearance of the wound, but by the odor. The stench was awful! I started to feel queasy, and I began to sweat, and I thought I was going to pass out and fall right over on the patient. While I was packing the wound I kept thinking that I was never going to get out of that room. I looked over at my clinical instructor and searched her face for approval of my technique, and I wondered if she also smelled anything and if it was making her feel sick too!

After the procedure was over and I left the room, I asked my instructor if all wounds smell that awful and would the smell always make me feel sick. Her response was that sometimes an odor will be really bad and it might make me feel sick. With this kind of reassurance I thought this is it; I never want to smell that again and no way do I want to be a nurse. Later I realized that I had forgotten there was someone else in that room: the patient. She had to stay in there with that wound and its odor. It was for this reason I changed my mind about leaving nursing. I remembered that it was wanting to help patients to deal with their wounds that made me decide to be a nurse in the first place.

—Barbara L. Dlugosz, Holy Family College, Philadelphia, PA

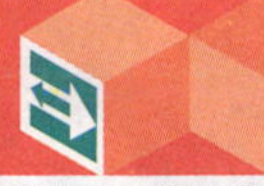

Developing Critical Thinking Skills

Situation

Mrs. Mitchell is an 82-year-old nursing home resident who was admitted to a community hospital for treatment of dehydration secondary to pneumonia. Convalescing well, she is now allowed short periods of assisted ambulation and may sit up as tolerated. On the morning you first meet her she is awake and demanding angrily to have her vest restraint removed so that she can walk independently to the bathroom. You remove her restraint, help her to the bathroom, and wonder whether or not to reapply the restraint as you get her back into bed. She seems clear headed and tells you she has no idea why she is being tied to the bed since she knows enough to use her light to get help when she needs it. She demands you to take the restraint away and pulls back angrily when you attempt to place it over her head. You don't remember any mention of a restraint order when you read her chart the previous day and have not yet gotten report from the charge nurse. Your options are to leave her unrestrained while you clarify the need for the restraint or incur her wrath and forcibly restrain her until you can ascertain the need. You like Mrs. Mitchell and feel sorry that anyone should have to be restrained and are reluctant to wrestle with an 82-year-old woman.

1. ***Goal of Thinking***

   Short term: Reach a prudent decision about the need to restrain Mrs. Mitchell until you can clarify the need for the restraint with the charge nurse. **Long term:** Evaluate the merits of restraining clients in different types of situations to facilitate future decision making.

2. ***Adequacy of Knowledge***

   Pertinent circumstances: In her weakened condition, this client may be at high risk for falls, and should she attempt to get out of bed unassisted a fall is a real possibility. You feel sympathetic to her plight of being tied in bed against her will and wonder if violating client dignity and liberty is something nurses are routinely expected to do. You are unsure of your legal risk but feel fairly certain that you are responsible for keeping her safe and that not to do so could be grounds for negligence. No other students or staff nurses are in the room and you cannot clarify the order without leaving the client unattended.

   Prerequisite knowledge: In order to make a decision in this situation you need knowledge about the client's need to be restrained and the benefits and risks of restraining and not restraining her. Given the situation of conflicting goods—preserving her dignity and liberty versus maintaining safety—you need to know how to determine which good ought to triumph in this situation. You should be familiar with the hospital's restraint policy and understand your moral and legal obligations. For example, failure to restrain her may be construed as negligence, while restraining her against her will may be assault and battery.

   Room for error: Given the significant risks you are incurring by choosing either option—potential fall versus assault to human dignity—there is little room for error. Until you know what her risk for fall is you should err on the side of caution.

   Time constraints: You may have time to wait with the client until another nurse comes into the room who can stay with the client until you clarify her need to be restrained. If this is not an option, you will need to decide quickly in order to be attentive to other priorities: getting report, beginning client care, etc.

3. ***Potential Problems***
   - Sincere desire to do the right thing but great anxiety about not knowing what this is
   - Untested, intuitive sense that restraining an alert, uncooperative client is wrong under any circumstances
   - Fear that if you don't restrain her and she falls, you will be legally responsible
   - Fear of making a wrong clinical decision which will jeopardize your clinical grade
   - Hope that your good interpersonal skills may save the day and buy you the time you need to get help

4. ***Helpful Resources***

   Key resources include experienced colleagues, nursing instructor, charge nurse, hospital policy, professional literature on restraint use, hospital risk manager, client bill of rights.

(continued)

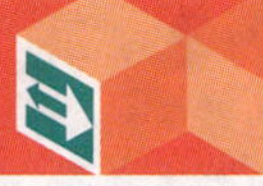

Developing Critical Thinking Skills *(continued)*

5. ***Critique of Judgment/Decision***
   There are basically two options: to restrain or not restrain Mrs. Mitchell until you can clarify the need for a restraint. If you restrain her and there is no need, you run the risk of increasing her agitation and violating her dignity. If you fail to restrain her and the restraint is needed, she may fall and suffer a concussion or fractured hip. You decide to reapply the restraint carefully after explaining to Mrs. Mitchell that you are a student nurse and need to check the order for the restraint before leaving it off. Given all your uncertainties, you decide that maintaining the client's safety ought to be your first priority until you determine if there are overriding considerations. Mrs. Mitchell is not happy with your decision but seems to understand your reasoning and does not fight you when you reapply the vest restraint. You promise to return quickly and keep your promise.

   When you talk with the charge nurse she tells you that there is no need for Mrs. Mitchell to be restrained and that the night nurse tends to be overzealous about protecting elderly clients. You happily return to Mrs. Mitchell and remove the restraint. You later meet with your instructor to see what you can do to ensure that Mrs. Mitchell and other clients on the unit are not restrained for inappropriate reasons. Your instructor compliments you for reasoning well about what was in this client's best interests. She remarks that had there been a need to restrain the client you may have jeopardized her safety by unthinkingly following your sympathetic instinct to leave her unrestrained.

procedures many times before they feel competent handling equipment and performing clinical activities independently. Whatever your natural technical skill, you can help yourself master the manual skills essential to quality nursing process by developing the following habits.

- When a procedure demands manual dexterity, practice the necessary skill until you feel confident in its execution before attempting to perform it with a client.
- Take time to familiarize yourself with new equipment before using it in a clinical procedure. Understand how it works and what supplies are needed to ensure optimal functioning. If possible, anticipate problems and know how to remedy them.
- Identify nurses who are technical experts and ask them to share their secrets. Many experienced clinicians have developed quality, time-saving techniques which they are willing to share.
- Never be ashamed to seek assistance when feeling unsure of how to perform a procedure or manage equipment. Never forget that client well-being, and sometimes a client's life itself, literally depend upon your technical competence.

Many nursing procedures are described in the clinical chapters in this text. Performance checklists are available which break each procedure down into its component parts, allowing you to evaluate your performance of each step of the procedure. This type of self-knowledge will enable you to quickly identify and remedy recurrent deficiencies in technical skills.

Developing Interpersonal Competencies

Characteristics of interpersonal caring that are essential to the practice of nursing include:

- Promotion of the dignity and respect of clients as people
- Centrality of the caring relationship
- Mutual enrichment of both participants in the nurse–client relationship

Promoting Human Dignity and Respect

Nurses committed to respecting the human dignity of clients will find it helpful to reflect on the following questions.

What about clients obligates me to respect their human dignity? Must all clients be respected equally? Are some clients more deserving of respect? Can a client ever forfeit the right to be respected?

What does it mean to respect the dignity of clients? What are five concrete ways I demonstrate respect?

What are my strengths and deficiencies when it comes to respecting clients?

In what ways must I change (if any) if I wish to be faithful to the duty of respecting the dignity of clients?

What clients most challenge my ability to care for clients respectfully? How do I respond to this challenge? What does this teach me for the future?

Nurses often underestimate their power to heal simply by the quality of their respectful and caring presence. Each time a nurse walks into a room, he or she communicates one of three messages to the person encountered: (1) "Drop dead," (2) "You are nothing to me," or (3) "You are precious and I care about you." Even a 60-second nurse–client interaction can enhance or jeopardize human well-being. It is important for nurses to be sensitive to what their looks, speech, and touch communicate to clients and colleagues. The more vulnerable the client and the more threatened the client's sense of self, the more powerful the nurse's message to affect the recipient's sense of worth and well-being.

The learning activity in the accompanying box was developed for nurses caring for older clients in a nursing home. You may want to try the suggested learning activities with a friend. Take turns being both the nurse

Learning Experience

Human Dignity: How Who I Am As a Caregiver Affects Others

Description

The purpose of this exercise is to explore the notion of "therapeutic use of self." You will be challenged to reflect upon the effect your looks, speech, and touch have on other people. Role play and guided discovery will be used to enable you to experience the affirming and negating influences of different means of human relating.

Objectives

Upon conclusion of this exercise you will be able to:

1. Demonstrate how looks, words, and touch can be used to harm or benefit others.
2. Describe how the way you approach others enhances or diminishes their well-being.
3. Identify one care behavior you plan to modify to improve your nursing practice.

Learning Activities

Invite an experienced nurse to demonstrate how looks, words, and touch can be used to communicate three different messages to others: "Drop dead." "You are nothing." "You are precious and I care about you." After the demonstration, team up with another student and experience giving and receiving these messages. Share the feelings you both experienced. After these preliminary exercises, role play the suggested nursing situations (or others of your choosing) and once again process the experience. Talk about the relevance of this experience to human interaction in general and conclude the exercise by writing a goal for your practice.

Worksheet

A. Practice looking at a colleague three different ways:
   1. "Drop dead" look
   2. "You are nothing" look
   3. "You are precious and I care about you" look

B. Practice speaking to a colleague in three different ways:
   1. Angry: "I don't care if it's my turn. It's your resident so you answer the light. She's probably messed."
   2. Indifferent: "Your resident, your light."
   3. Helpful: "I think Mrs. Jones' light is on again. Do you need help?"

C. Practice touching a colleague in three different ways:
   1. Violent: Stand and face your colleague. Grab your colleague's upper arms and forcibly push her/him into a chair.
   2. Indifferent: Pick up your colleague's wrist and feel for a pulse.
   3. Using warm lotion, massage your colleague's hands.

D. Talk about how each of the above looks, words, and touches made you feel. Talk about how you think they make clients or residents feel.

E. Role play each of the situations below three different ways, trying to incorporate looks, words, and touches which communicate:

   First time: Drop dead.
   Second time: You are nothing.
   Third time: You are precious and I care about you.

   1. Student feels overwhelmed by client care assignment and approaches clinical instructor to discuss her options.
   2. Student walks into client's room to begin morning care.
   3. Student assists elderly client to stand and ambulate around room.
   4. Student brings medication to client.
   5. Student approaches another student and asks for help changing the bed linens of an obese client who is on complete bed rest.

F. Name one thing you have decided to try and do differently when you take care of your clients as a result of this session.

G. Does what you experienced today have any implications for who you are when you are not nursing?

and the older adult and talk about how different types of nursing presence make you feel.

Establishing Caring Relationships

Increasingly, nurses are reporting that new systems of care and the demand to "work harder, faster, and smarter" to keep up in today's competitive healthcare arena are rendering traditional nurse–client relationships obsolete. As you begin your practice you will want to ask yourself what priority you assign to caring. Nurses who accept the claim that there can be no excellence in nursing in the absence of this relationship commit themselves to finding creative means to establish caring relationships. Obviously, many variables will influence the quality of relationships which are possible, not the least of which is the acuity level of the client and the client's length of stay. Helpful reflection questions include the following:

Do I know my clients well enough to promote anything more than the well-being of their body?

If asked to describe a client, would I be able to report on anything other than the client's physical condition?

Is the care I routinely provide *really* holistic, individualized, prioritized according to medical need *and* the client's interests, and continuous? Do my care plans reflect this?

What does the content of the client report and nursing documentation communicate about nursing's priorities in my practice setting?

What are my strengths and deficiencies in creating caring relationships?

In what ways (if any) must I change to better establish caring relationships?

Nurses committed to caring relationships routinely use opportunities for conversation to communicate genuine interest in who the client is and what the client is experiencing in order to provide meaningful nursing assistance. For example, rather than allow a talkative older adult to "chatter" aimlessly, a nurse skilled in developing caring relationships will direct the conversation. Leading statements or questions that are often successful in eliciting useful information from older clients include the following.

"Tell me something about your life at home. What do you miss most now that you are here?"

"What family members and friends do you see most often? Who do you think knows you best and would you trust to be able to speak for you if you were ever unable to speak for yourself?"

"Most of us have some goal or dream that keeps us going. It might be owning our own home, seeing some relationship patched up, or being reunited with a deceased loved one. What is your dream?"

"When you've had troubles in the past, what did you draw on for strength? What keeps you going?"

"Looks like you've got a lot of time for thinking these days . . . would you like to share what's been on your mind?"

"Looks like we'll be spending some time together . . . what would you like to do with this time? How may I help you?

Nurses who are sensitive to the well-being of their clients will find many ways to communicate caring. Happily, most caring is mutually enriching and nurses who care find themselves reenergized for the more demanding aspects of their practice.

Enjoying the Rewards of Mutual Interchange

In any helping profession, but especially in nursing, countless opportunities exist to interact with others. Those committed to interpersonal caring enrich everyday interactions by investing them with something of themselves and, in turn, receive something of the other, as shown in Figure 15-1. Remember your last nurse–client encounter. Whether you were administering a medication, checking vital signs, or preparing a client for discharge, you had the choice of merely accomplishing the given task, or of accomplishing the task while simultaneously communicating a personal gift of support, caring, strength, and peacefulness. Frequently overlooked, these interpersonal gifts may contribute to a client's healing as significantly as medical interventions. And rather than deplete their giver, these inter-

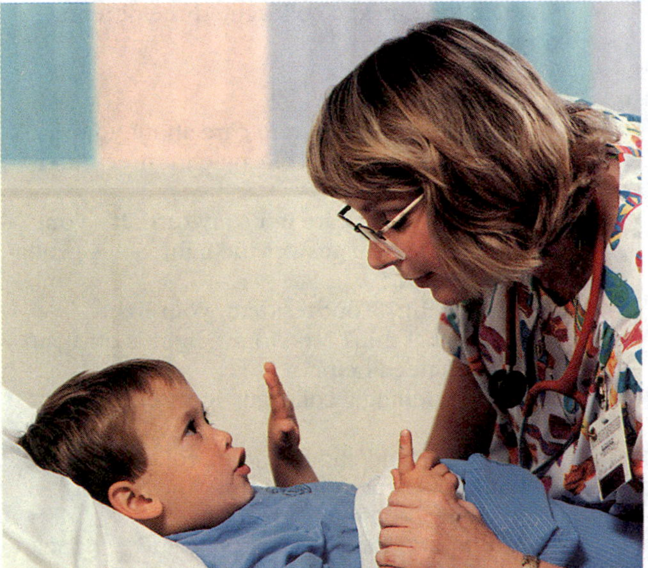

Figure 15-1
Interpersonal caring enriches the lives of everyone participating, providing a mutual exchange of giving and receiving. (Photo by Einrosia; courtesy of Shore Memorial Hospital and Nursing Spectrum.)

personal gifts invite similar gifts from the recipient which return to enrich the caregiver. Nothing causes burnout faster than a practice that is reduced to the performance of multiple tasks stripped of their human significance. When a client is given care in a way that "makes a difference" in terms of his or her well-being, the client's gratitude, even when unspoken verbally, finds a way to renew the nurse's energy. Too seldom do we stop our busy practices long enough to reflect on how who we are that day is influencing the well-being of those receiving our care. It is helpful to question:

To what extent am I conscious of how my mood influences the well-being of others?

Have I ever consciously tried to transmit strength, peace, support, or joy to another? What were the results?

Am I aware of any situation where my fatigue, anxiety, frustration, or negativity was communicated to a client in a manner that negatively influenced his or her well-being?

Am I conscious of ways in which clients enrich me personally or enrich my practice?

In what ways is my practice different when I am attuned to the interpersonal dimensions of nurse–client interactions?

In what ways must my practice change if I am to better facilitate healing by willing something of my essence to clients?

Developing Ethical/Legal Competencies

Nurses who prize their role in securing client well-being are sensitive to the ethical and legal implications of nursing practice. Chapters 6, 7, and 24 describe essential components of ethical and legal competence for nurses. While it can take years to master effective client advocacy skills and to become proficient in mediating ethical conflict, even nurses new to practice are responsible for certain basic ethical skills. One of the greatest challenges students of nursing face is balancing the competing demands of home life, school, and the hospital or practice setting. Learning to be true to oneself, to the clients for whom one is responsible, to the caregiving team, and to the profession and society is an ongoing struggle. Examining one's sense of accountability is critical as one assumes professional responsibilities.

Holding Oneself Accountable

Nurses committed to interpersonal caring hold themselves accountable for the human well-being of clients entrusted to their care. Being accountable means being attentive and responsive to the healthcare needs of individual clients. It means that my concern for the client transcends whatever happens during my shift, and that I ensure continuity of care when I leave a client. In today's system of increasingly fragmented care, clients often find themselves unable to point to any one caregiver who knows their overall situation and is capable and willing to coordinate the efforts of the healthcare team. Being responsive and responsible earns a client's trust that "all will be well" as simple to complex healthcare needs are addressed. Nurses committed to responsible caring will reflect on the following.

To what extent does my commitment to securing the human well-being of those in my care dictate my work priorities?

How comfortable am I in voicing unmet client needs to other members of the healthcare team?

Do other caregivers listen when I present client concerns because of my successful track record of client advocacy?

What system variables need to change for us to meet the human needs of our clients adequately?

In what ways must I change in order for my clients to be able to count on me to respond in a responsible way to their needs?

Nurses who are sensitive to the legal dimensions of practice are careful to develop strong senses of both ethical and legal accountability. Competent practice is a nurse's best legal safeguard. Nurses seeking to develop legal competence may find it helpful to ask the following questions:

Do I know the legal boundaries of my practice?

Am I familiar with pertinent institutional procedures and policies?

Do I "own" my personal strengths and weaknesses and seek assistance as needed?

Am I careful to never accept responsibility for an assignment for which I am unprepared?

Am I knowledgeable about, and respectful of, client rights?

Does my documentation provide a legally defensible account of my practice?

When working to develop ethical and legal accountability, nurses must recognize that both deficiencies *and excesses* of responsible caring are problematic. While it is reasonable to hold oneself accountable for securing the human well-being of my clients, nurses can err by setting for themselves unrealistic standards of responsiveness and responsibility. Prudence is always necessary to balance responsible self-care with care of others. Inexperienced nurses may feel totally responsible for effecting client outcomes beyond their control and become frustrated and sad when unable to produce the desired outcome. Conversations about what it is reasonable to hold one another and ourselves accountable for are always helpful. The sample learning activity in the accompanying box was designed to explore accountability issues.

Learning Experience

Accountability

Description
The purpose of this exercise is to explore the issue of accountability. You will be challenged to reflect upon whether or not your everyday nursing practice demonstrates a commitment to ensuring the human well-being of those in your care. Individual patterns of responding to human need and responsible caring will be critiqued. Roleplaying and guided discovery will be used to invite you to experience the effects of both responsible caring and the indifferent provision of services.

Objectives
Upon conclusion of this session you will be able to:

1. Describe how the way you respond (or fail to respond) to the needs of clients influences their general sense of well-being.
2. Critique the amount of responsibility you and other nurses accept for the well-being of individual clients.
3. Describe one way your practice will change in order for you to be more accountable to yourself, your clients, the nursing profession, and society.

Learning Activities
Choose another student and work through exercises 1 to 4. Begin by describing your own positive and negative experiences of being cared for and draw parallels to how clients feel when they believe they can count on their caregivers to recognize and respond to their needs. Then develop and discuss a list of personal, client, and system variables that either facilitate or impede responsible caring. Finally, role play the given scenarios and focus discussion on how different nursing responses influence client well-being. End the discussion by developing a goal for your practice that will help you to be accountable to yourself, clients, the nursing profession, and society.

Worksheet

Objective
To critique our responsiveness to client need and the amount of responsibility we each assume to secure client well-being.

Exercise One
Take a moment to reflect on a recent experience when you felt vulnerable (eg, new role responsibilities: first clinical rotation, new job, new spouse, new parent; car breaks down; major purchase). Share with a colleague how the conduct of the one(s) you expected to be sensitive and responsive to your need influenced your overall sense of well-being. Draw parallels to nursing.

Exercise Two
List all the *personal* variables that enable you to care for your clients responsibly (eg, coming to work rested, honestly caring about clients) and which impede your ability to do this (eg, you come to work but are mentally and emotionally back home with some other problem, such as difficulties with spouse, sick child).

Positive Personal Variables	Negative Personal Variables

Next list all the *system* variables that enable you to care for your clients responsibly (eg, client assignments are matched to your developing level of expertise, good team spirit among caregivers and their willingness to work together to meet complex client needs) and which impede your doing this (eg, student assignments are unrealistic, chronic understaffing results in staff being unavailable to direct students, sense in the healthcare institution that management has "given up" and is no longer concerned about quality: bottom line is always money).

Positive System Variables	Negative System Variables

Finally list *client* variables which positively and negatively influence your ability/willingness to care for your clients responsibly (eg, client looks like me, client is pleasant and makes few demands, client has strong potential for complete recovery, or client is homeless, has a history of self-abuse).

(continued)

Learning Experience *(continued)*

Positive Client Variables	Negative Client Variables

Talk about how you plan to address the negative variables that interfere with your ability to care for clients responsibly. What does it mean to be accountable to yourself, your clients, the nursing profession, and society?

Exercise Three

Role play each of the scenarios below and discuss how the nurse responds (or fails to respond) is likely to influence the client. It would be helpful to discuss how you think nurses on your unit *would* respond to this type of situation and how you think they *should* respond. If these differ, discuss why.

1. You are doing a postpartal exam when the woman being examined tells you the following: "I don't know what my husband and I are going to do. We've only been married five years and this is our fourth baby. We're both Catholic and I guess shouldn't use any contraceptives. But I worry all the time about Ted getting laid off. We're just about managing as it is."
2. You suspect from the blood pressure reading you just obtained that the elderly clinic client you are examining is not taking his medication or complying with other aspects of the treatment plan. "I try to take 'em but sometimes I forgets." The clinic is understaffed and you have many more clients to see, some of whom have waited for over an hour.
3. You tell the resident that you don't think the pain medication one woman with metastatic cancer is receiving is adequate and the resident tells you that it's a more than adequate dose that will not get her addicted to morphine.
4. Another nurse tells you that he's utterly frustrated because Dr. Braxton refuses to talk with a client about advance directives because, "It might depress her." You share this nurse's belief that the client wants to participate in decision making and that it is very possible that she will lose the ability to do this soon.
5. One of the clients on your surgical unit has been hospitalized for over 3 months following an unsuccessful attempt to resect a lung tumor. He has had one complication after another, is unable to be weaned from the ventilator, and is now developing kidney failure. His prognosis is poor. A quiet man, he makes no demands on his family or the staff. Care has basically revolved around treating each new complication and now dialysis is being considered. His wife asks you, "Why are we doing all this?"
6. You are making a home visit to a 32-year-old man with end-stage AIDS. He tells you that he is tired of fighting, has no money, and no longer wants to be a bother to his friends. He asks you what he can do to end his life.

Exercise Four

Review each of the above six situations and discuss with your colleague the legal implications of being accountable. What legal safeguards would you recommend?

Exercise Five

Name one thing about your practice that you have decided to change as a result of this session.

Reporting Incompetent, Unethical, or Illegal Practices

Each employing institution/agency providing nursing services has an obligation to establish a process for the reporting and handling of practices by individuals or by healthcare systems that jeopardize client health or safety. The American Nurses Association Code for Ethics obligates nurses to report professional conduct that is incompetent, unethical, or illegal. For nurses, incompetent practice is measured by nursing standards, unethical practice is evaluated in light of professional codes of ethics, and illegal practice is identified in terms of violations of law. Parameters for evaluating each are highlighted in the accompanying box.

Whistleblowing is a term generally used to refer to employees who report their employers' violation of the law to appropriate law enforcement agencies outside the employers' facilities. Citing the inadequacies of current laws to protect whistleblowers, the American Nurses Association offers the following caution: "because of the limits of current law, nurses should be advised that they may not be protected against retaliation for reporting

Parameters for Evaluating Incompetent, Unethical, or Illegal Practice

Parameters of Competent Nursing Practice

1. State Nurse Practice Acts and Regulations
2. The Scope of Practice
3. Professional Standards of Nursing Practice
   a. Clinical (including specialty practice)
   b. Administration
   c. Education
4. Practice Guidelines
5. Protocols

Parameters of Ethical Nursing Practice

1. Professional Codes of Ethics

Parameters of Legal Nursing Practice

1. Federal and State Health Regulations
2. Pharmacy Laws (state)
   a. Uniform Controlled Substances Act (state)
   b. Controlled Substances Act (federal)
3. OSHA Standards and Regulations (state and federal)
4. Medical Records and Communicable Disease Laws (state)
5. Environmental Laws
   a. Hazardous Waste Regulations
   b. Air Quality Regulations
   c. Water Quality Regulations
6. Centers for Disease Control Guidelines
7. Anti-Discrimination Laws (eg, AIDS)
8. Service Facility Regulations (state)
9. Clinical Laboratory Improvement Act (CLIA/state)
10. JCAHO Regulations

American Nurses Association. (1994). *Guidelines on reporting incompetent, unethical or illegal practices.* Washington, DC: ANA, 5–7.

the incompetent, unethical or illegal practices of their employers" (1994, p. 12).

Take the Challenge

This chapter concludes with an assessment tool you can use to assess your proficiency in the competencies essential to competent use of the nursing process (see the accompanying box). After completing the exercise, share your self-evaluation with a trusted colleague or clinical instructor and see if your assessments of your abilities agree. Celebrate your natural and developed strengths. Begin now to plan a strategy to boost those competencies in which you are deficient. This may sound trite, but it is true: your clients will be grateful you cared enough to be your best.

Take the Challenge

Read the professional behaviors below and circle the number that best reflects the proficiency you now have in each of these essential nursing competencies.

1 = no skills   3 = moderately skilled   5 = excellent skills
2 = somewhat skilled   4 = well skilled

Cognitive Competencies

1 2 3 4 5 • offer a scientific rationale for each element in a client's plan of care

1 2 3 4 5 • select those nursing interventions that are most likely to yield desired outcomes

1 2 3 4 5 • use critical thinking to creatively problem solve

Technical Competencies

1 2 3 4 5 • use technical equipment with sufficient competence and ease to achieve goal with a minimum of distress to involved participants

1 2 3 4 5 • creatively adapt equipment and technical procedures to the needs of particular clients in diverse circumstances

(continued)

Take the Challenge *(continued)*

Interpersonal Competencies

1 2 3 4 5 • creative use of look, speech, and touch to communicate respect and enhance sense of worth

1 2 3 4 5 • skilled use of presence and conversation to demonstrate empathy and to obtain sufficient knowledge about the client to personalize care and serve as an effective advocate

1 2 3 4 5 • responsible, competent attentiveness to the holistic needs of clients such that trust is built and clients experience comfort of security

1 2 3 4 5 • value mutual enrichment of both participants in the nurse–client relationship

Ethical/Legal Competencies

1 2 3 4 5 • self-motivated to act in ways that advance the interests of clients (consistently trustworthy)

1 2 3 4 5 • accountable for practice to self, clients served, the caregiving team, and society

1 2 3 4 5 • consistently serve as effective client advocate

1 2 3 4 5 • skilled in mediating ethical conflict among the client, significant others, healthcare team, and other interested parties

1 2 3 4 5 • practice nursing faithful to the tenets of professional codes of ethics

1 2 3 4 5 • use legal safeguards that reduce the risk of litigation

Key Points

- The unique challenges now confronting nurses demand that nurses be proficient in cognitive, technical, interpersonal, and ethical/legal competencies.
- Cognitive competencies enable nurses to "make sense" of their world and to grasp conceptually what is necessary to achieve valued goals. It is impossible to practice nursing successfully without using critical thinking skills.
- Nurses wishing to develop critical thinking skills will find it helpful to work through five sets of considerations when posed with a thinking challenge: (1) purpose of thinking, (2) adequacy of knowledge, (3) potential problems, (4) helpful resources, and (5) critique of judgment/decision.
- Technical competencies enable nurses to use equipment and procedures with sufficient competence and ease to achieve goals with minimal distress to the involved participants.
- Interpersonal competencies enable nurses to establish and maintain caring relationships which facilitate the achievement of valued goals while affirming the worth of participants in the relationship.
- Ethical and legal competencies enable nurses to conduct their lives in a manner that is consistent with their personal moral code and professional role responsibilities.
- Professional codes of ethics obligate nurses to report professional conduct that is incompetent, unethical, or illegal.

Bibliography

Aiken, T. D., & Catalano, J. T. (1994). *Legal, ethical, and political issues in nursing.* Philadelphia: Davis.

Alfaro-Lefevre, R. (1994). *Applying nursing process: A step-by-step guide* (3rd ed.). Philadelphia: Lippincott.

Alfaro-LeFevre, R. (1995). *Critical thinking in nursing: A practical approach.* Philadelphia: Saunders.

American Nurses Association. (1990). *Liability prevention and you: What nurses and employers need to know.* Washington, DC: ANA.

American Nurses Association. (1994). *Guidelines on reporting incompetent, unethical or illegal practices.* Washington, DC: ANA.

Aroskar, M. A. (1993). Incompetent, unethical or illegal practice—teaching students to cope. *Journal of Professional Nursing, 9*(3), 130.

Benner, P. (1984). *From novice to expert.* Menlo Park, CA: Addison-Wesley.

Benner, P., & Wrubel, J. (1989), *The primacy of caring in health and illness.* Menlo Park, CA: Addison-Wesley.

Brooks, K. L. (1993). Critical thinking in clinical practice. *Holistic Nursing Practice, 7*(3), vi-80.

Chafree, J. (1990). *Thinking critically* (3rd ed.). Boston: Houghton Mifflin.

Davies, E. (1995). Reflective practice: A focus for caring. *Journal of Nursing Education, 34*(4), 167–174.

Ennis, R. H. (1996). *Critical thinking*. Upper Saddle River, NJ: Prentice-Hall.

Fiesta, J. (1994). Failure to act like a professional. *Nursing Management, 25*(7), 15–17.

Fitzpatrick, J. M., While, A. E., & Roberts, J. D. (1992). The role of the nurse in high quality care: A review of the literature. *Journal of Advanced Nursing, 17*(10), 1210–1219.

Geissler, E. M. (1990). Nurturance flows two ways. *American Journal of Nursing, 90*(4), 72–74.

Gendron, D. (1994). The tapestry of care. *Advances in Nursing Science, 17*(1), 25–30.

Heinrich, K., & Killeen, M. E. (1993). The gentle art of nurturing yourself. *American Journal of Nursing, 93*(10), 41–44.

Jacono, B. J., & Jacono, J. K. (1995). A holistic approach to teaching responsibility and accountability. *Nurse Educator, 20*(1), 20–23.

Jenks, J. M. (1993). The pattern of personal knowing in nurse clinical decision making. *Journal of Nursing Education, 32*(12), 399–405.

Johnson, J. (1994). A dialectical examination of the nursing art. *Advances in Nursing Science, 17*(1), 1–14.

Kataoka-Yahiro, M. (1994). A critical thinking model for nursing judgment. *Journal of Nursing Education, 33*(8), 351–356.

Kolcaba, K. Y. (1995). The art of comfort care. *IMAGE: Journal of Nursing Scholarship, 27*(4), 287–289.

Locsin, R. C. (1995). Machine technologies and caring in nursing. *IMAGE: Journal of Nursing Scholarship, 27*(3), 201–203.

Miller, M. A., & Babcock, D. E. (1996). *Critical thinking applied to nursing*. St. Louis: Mosby.

Paul, R. W. (1993). *Critical thinking: How to prepare students for a rapidly changing world*. Santa Rosa, CA: Foundation for Critical Thinking.

Phillips, E. (1994). Accountability, responsibility, liability. *Canadian Nurse, 90*(4), 51–52.

Rubenfeld, M. G., & Scheffer, B. K. (1995). *Critical thinking in nursing: An interactive approach*. Philadelphia: Lippincott.

Schick, T., & Vaughn, L. (1995). *How to think about weird things*. Mountain View, CA: Mayfield Publishing Co.

Stark, J. (1995). Critical thinking: Taking the road less traveled. *Nursing, 25*(11), 53–56.

Taylor, C. (1995). Rethinking nursing's basic competencies. *Journal of Nursing Care Quality, 9*(4), 1–13.

Wilkinson, J. (1992). *Nursing process in action: A critical thinking approach*. Redwood City, CA: Addison-Wesley Nursing.

Yura, H., & Walsh, M. (1967). *The nursing process: Assessing, planning, implementing, evaluating*. Norwalk, CT: Appleton-Century-Crofts.

Chapter 16

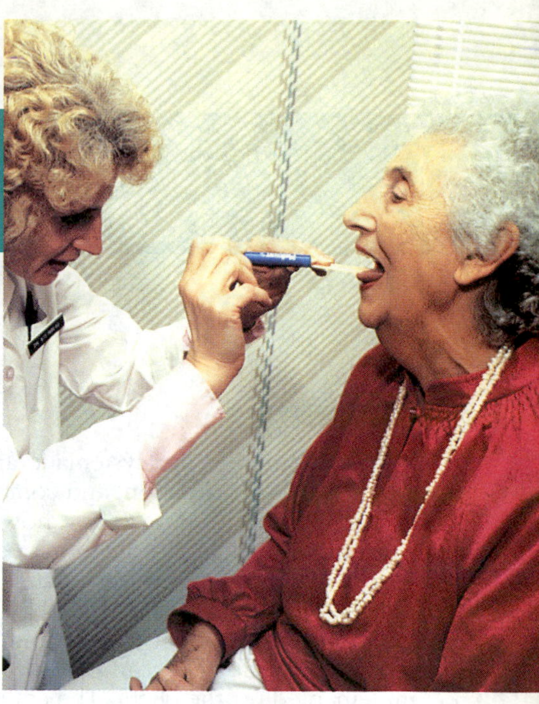

Assessing

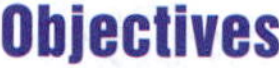

Objectives

After studying this chapter, the learner should be able to:

Define key terms used in the chapter.

Describe the purpose of the initial nursing assessment and of ongoing nursing assessments.

Differentiate a nursing assessment from a medical assessment.

Differentiate objective and subjective data.

Describe the purpose of nursing observation, interview, and physical assessment.

Obtain a nursing history using effective interviewing techniques.

Identify five sources of client data useful to the nurse.

Differentiate comprehensive admission assessments from focused assessments.

Plan client assessments by identifying assessment priorities and structuring the data to be collected systematically.

Identify common problems encountered in data collection, noting their possible cause.

Explain when data need to be validated and several ways to accomplish this.

Describe the importance of knowing when to report significant client data and of proper documentation.

Obtain complete, accurate, factual, and relevant client data.

Key Terms

assessing
data
data base
focused assessment
interview
nursing history
objective data
observation
physical assessment
subjective data
validation

Assessing is the systematic and continuous collection, validation, and communication of client data; these **data** reflect how health functioning is enhanced by health promotion or compromised by illness. A **data base** (or baseline data) includes all the pertinent client information collected by the nurse and other healthcare professionals; as such, it enables a comprehensive and effective plan of care to be designed and implemented for the client. The collection of client data is a vital step in the nursing process because the remaining steps depend on complete, accurate, factual, and relevant data.

The initial comprehensive nursing assessment results in a data base that enables the nurse to make a judgment about a client's health status, ability to manage his or her own healthcare, and need for nursing; refer the client to a physician or other healthcare professional, if indicated; and plan and deliver individualized, holistic nursing care that draws on the client's strengths. In addition to an initial assessment of the client, ongoing assessments are made by the nurse. Ongoing nursing assessment alerts the nurse to changes in the client's responses to health and illness and suggests necessary changes in the plan of nursing care or care offered by other healthcare professionals.

During the assessment step of the nursing process, the nurse establishes the data base by interviewing the client to obtain a nursing history; the nurse may also perform a nursing examination to collect data. Other sources of client information used by the nurse include the client's support people, the client record, the client's healthcare professionals, and nursing and other healthcare literature. After the nurse has established the data base, data about the client are collected continuously because the client's health status can change quickly. Questionable data are verified (validated) as part of the assessment step of the nursing process. All pertinent data are recorded and, when appropriate, verbally communicated to the responsible person, so that the data can best benefit the client (Fig. 16-1).

Unique Focus of Nursing Assessment

When nurses make nursing assessments, they do not duplicate medical assessments. Medical assessments target data pointing to pathology whereas nursing assessments focus on client responses to health problems. Is there, for example, interference with meeting basic human needs? Can the client perform activities of daily living? Although the findings of a nursing assessment may contribute to the identification of a medical diagnosis, the unique focus of nursing assessments is on the client's responses to actual or potential health problems. The accompanying box highlights the nursing knowledge and skills needed to assess clients.

Data Collection

Types of Data

There are two types of data—objective and subjective. **Objective data** are information perceived by the senses; data observed by one person can be verified by another person observing the same client. Examples of objective data are an elevated temperature reading (101°F), skin that is moist, and refusal to look at or eat food. Objective data also are called signs or overt data.

Subjective data are information perceived only by the affected person; these data cannot be perceived or verified by another person. Examples of subjective data are feeling nervous, nauseated, or chilly and experiencing pain. Subjective data also are called symptoms or covert data (Table 16-1).

Characteristics of Data

When collecting and recording client data, it is important to be complete, accurate, factual, and relevant.

Complete. To the extent that it is possible, all the client data needed to understand a client health problem and develop a plan of care to maximize wellness should be identified. For example, knowing that a client has lost weight is meaningless until the nurse discovers (1) if the weight loss was intentional or unintentional, (2) if it was related to a change in eating or exercise patterns or to some underlying pathology, and (3) how the client views and is responding to the weight loss.

Factual and Accurate. Both the client and the nurse may intentionally or unintentionally misrepresent or dis-

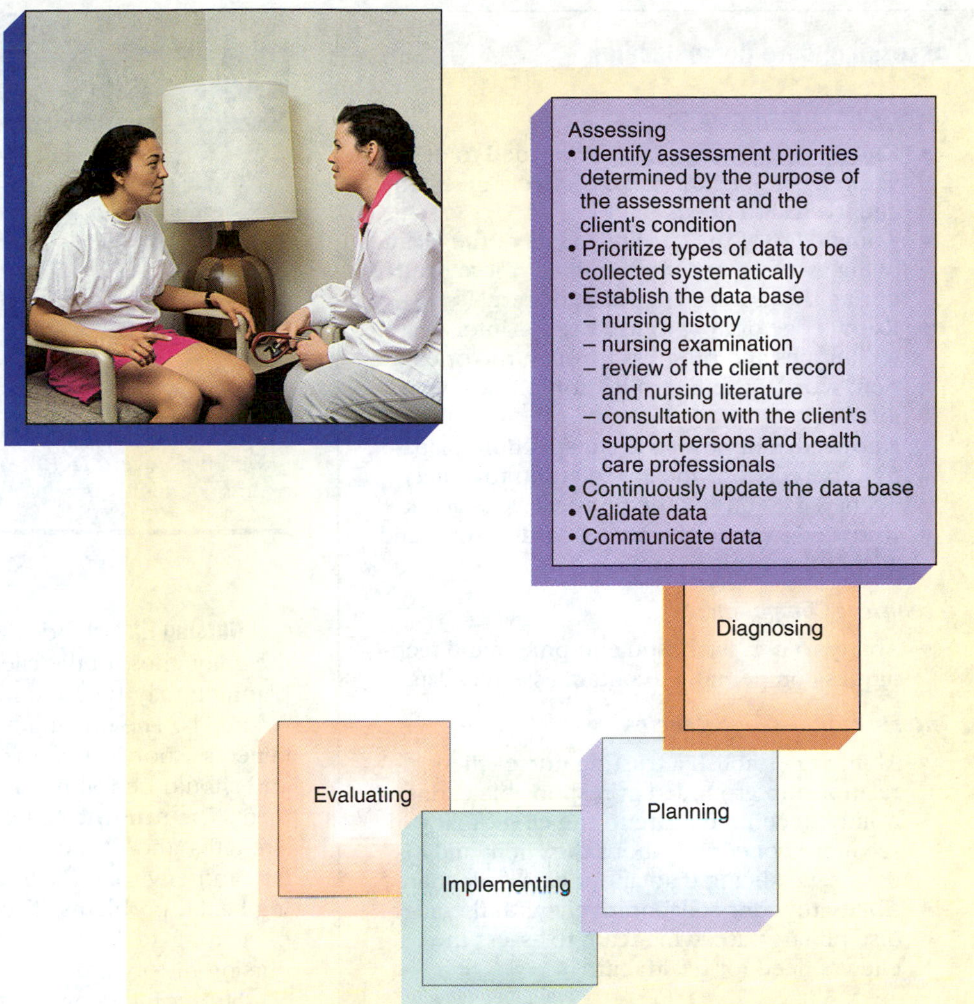

Figure 16-1
Assessing. The primary source of client information is the client. Resources include the client's support people, the client record, information from other healthcare professionals, and information from nursing and healthcare literature.

tort client information. For example, a client who values being thin may describe a weight gain of several pounds as the onset of obesity. Nurses concerned with accuracy and fact continually verify what they hear with what they observe using other senses and validate all questionable data. When nurses suspect that personal bias or stereotyping is influencing their data collection, it is appropriate for them to consult with another nurse. It also is best to describe observed behaviors rather than the interpretation of the behavior. Such a description may read: "Client frequently is observed lying with his face to the wall. Attempts to engage him in conversation fail. He refused lunch today and ate only soup for dinner." "Client is depressed," conversely, is the nurse's interpretation of the client's behavior; it is not a factual statement. Recording the client's behaviors factually allows other healthcare professionals to explore causes of the behavior with the client.

Relevant. Because recording comprehensive data can become an endless task, one challenge facing nurses is to determine *what type* of data and *how much* data to collect for each client. This chapter describes ways to do this. The aim is to record concisely all pertinent data. Often only experience teaches nurses what data are needed in specific cases.

Learning how to collect, validate, and communicate data that are complete, accurate, factual, and relevant is the focus of the remainder of this chapter.

Data Collection Methods

Common methods used in the collection of data in nursing include observation, interview, and physical assessment.

Observation

Observation is the conscious and deliberate use of the five physical senses to gather data. The skilled nurse uses each nurse–client interaction to observe and interpret meaningful stimuli (data). Student nurses can develop such observation skills by training themselves to carefully observe the following each time they encounter a client:

- What are the client's current responses (physical and emotional) to his or her situation? Be alert to

Assessing: Core Competencies

Cognitive Competencies

- Knowledge of what data are needed to develop a plan of care that effectively meets the client's health needs
- Knowledge of the specific needs of the client being assessed and ways to meet these needs during the assessment phase of care
- Knowledge of how to use various interview techniques and progress through the orientation, working, and termination phases of an interview
- Knowledge of how to use inspection, palpation, percussion, and auscultation to collect needed data during the physical assessment
- Knowledge of pertinent standards of care and agency/institutional policies

Technical Competencies

- Ability to use diagnostic equipment and techniques competently to obtain essential data

Interpersonal Competencies

- Ability to establish a trusting nurse–client relationship grounded in responsible caring
- Ability to communicate to the client that you are more concerned about the client and his or her well-being than about data collection
- Ability to work collaboratively with the interdisciplinary caregiving team to assess the client's need for health care

Ethical/Legal Competencies

- Commitment to do whatever is necessary to obtain and document an adequate data base
- Ability to serve as a trusted and effective client advocate

signs of distress—difficulty breathing, bleeding, pain, heightened anxiety—as well as to anything out of the ordinary—sudden eruption of rash, changes in levels of consciousness, and so forth.

- What is the client's current ability to manage his or her care (need for additional information or nursing assistance)?
- What is the immediate environment? Consider the safety of the environment as well as the functioning of equipment (intravenous therapy, oxygen, drains). Who are the people in the room? What are the temperature and odor of the room?
- What is the larger environment (hospital or community)?

Interview

An **interview** is a planned communication. During the assessment step of the nursing process, the nurse interviews the client to obtain a nursing history.

Table 16-1
Comparison of Objective and Subjective Data

Objective Data	Subjective Data
32-year-old man Height: 5′8″ Weight: 9/18/97—224 lb 2/4/98—202 lb	"I'm beginning to feel better about myself now that I'm losing weight and I seem to have more energy."
Posterior, left midcalf is warm and red.	"My leg hurts when I walk."
Client observed fidgeting with bed covers; facial features are tightly drawn.	"I'm so afraid of what they might find when they cut me open tomorrow."

Nursing History. Ideally, the nursing history captures the uniqueness of the client and records this, so that care planning may be patterned to meet the client's individual needs. The nursing history should, therefore, be obtained as soon as possible after a client presents for care, and should be followed by the nursing physical assessment. The **nursing history** should clearly identify client strengths and weaknesses, health risks such as hereditary and environmental factors, and potential and existing health problems. The focus of the nursing history is on getting to know the *person*. Data included in the nursing history are listed in the accompanying box.

Strong interviewing skills are needed to obtain the necessary client data and to communicate concern for the client. A brief discussion of the work of each phase of the interview follows.

Phases of the Interview. The four phases in the nurse–client interview are the preparatory phase, introduction, working phase, and termination. More detailed information on interviewing techniques can be found in Chapter 22.

Preparatory Phase. Before initiating the interview, the nurse prepares to meet the client by reading current and past records and reports, when available. During this phase it is important not to let stereotypes and prejudices predetermine the nurse–client relationship. If the nurse is aware of personal prejudices, they can be dealt with constructively. Professional nurses learn to approach clients with open minds and to be sensitive to the human needs that underlie diverse behaviors.

During the preparatory phase, the nurse should ensure that the environment in which the interview is to be conducted is private and relaxed. Unless the client wants to have family members or friends present during the interview, the nurse should interview the client alone, either in the client's room or in a quiet office.

Both the seating arrangement and the distance between nurse and client are important (Fig. 16-2). Chairs placed at right angles to each other and about 3 to 4 ft

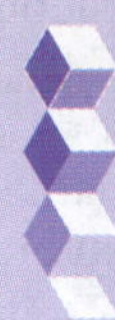

Through the Eyes of a Student

During my chronic medical–surgical rotation, my clinical group was placed on an oncology floor. My first thought was, "Oh no, not the cancer floor!" The word *fear* didn't even begin to describe how I felt. These clients had enough problems without some "green" nursing student aggravating them all day. I kept thinking these people are extremely ill and won't want to be bothered by my intruding questions.

Nonetheless, I knew I had to do it. Not only did I have to take care of this client all day, I had to develop a data base and plan of care. I knew I would have to do a lot more than give him his morning care and leave him alone. I would have to carry on an extended conversation with this patient to get all the information I needed.

As if all of this wasn't enough to make me throw in the white flag, when my client assignment was given, I discovered my client was a male and only 1 year older than me. A 28-year-old man with terminal cancer—this was too scary!

Clinical day came, as I knew it would, and I was shaking. I walked in that room and together the client and I planned his care. I explained to him the things I needed to talk about with him and I couldn't believe it—he didn't tell me to go away! We talked at length about his disease process and how it had affected his plans and goals. He opened up to me about his spirituality, his relationships with friends and family, and other personal subjects. Periodically he would cringe, and I could tell it was time for a break. He was hurting too badly to go on at that time.

At the end of that day, my viewpoint was totally different than it had been that morning. I walked away from that room and off that floor feeling like I had made a difference for this person. We had shared a lot and he seemed so appreciative for the time I took to talk with him. The amazing part was that all I had to do was just be myself and allow him to do the same and our day flowed smoothly. The lesson I learned here was important for me: Keep calm and hold on to compassion and nursing offers many rewards!

—Nancy E. Driskill,
Southeast Missouri State University,
Cape Girardeau, Missouri

(0.9 to 1.2 m) apart facilitate an easy exchange of information. If the client is in bed, placing a chair at a 45-degree angle to the bed is helpful. If the nurse stands at the foot or side of the client's bed and physically talks or looks down at the client, a superior–inferior relationship is communicated and can defeat the purpose of the interview. Whenever possible it is best to communicate with clients at eye level.

The interview should be scheduled when both the nurse and the client are free of concerns and distractions, so they can concentrate on the task. Ten to 15 minutes may be all that is necessary in some circumstances, whereas an hour or more may be required in others. Information can be gathered in several meetings, especially if the nurse notices that the client is tiring or is in pain.

Critical Thinking Exercise 16-1

Working with another student, together interview clients in both home and institutional settings. Make a list of the objective and subjective data you gather on each client interviewed and compare your data lists. Explore the reasons for the differences you discover among clients, between home and residential settings, and between what you and your partner decide to record.

Introduction. The interview's introduction is critical because it sets the tone not only for the remainder of the interview, but also for every nurse–client interaction that follows. At the end of this phase of the interview, the client should know the name of the primary nurse and what he or she can expect of nursing, should sense that the nurse is competent and cares about him or her, and should know what is expected of him or her in terms of developing the plan of care and participating in its execution.

The nurse initiates the interview by stating his or her name and status, identifying the purpose of the interview, and clarifying the roles of nurse and client. A typ-

Components of a Nursing History

- Client's profile: name, age, sex, marital status, religion, occupation, education
- Client's reason for seeking health care
- Client's normal health habits and patterns and any need for nursing assistance
- Client's current state of health, functioning of body systems, and past medical and surgical history
- Meaning client attributes to health and illness and characteristic response or coping patterns
- Client's developmental history, family history, environmental history, and psychosocial history
- Client's and family's expectations of nursing and of the healthcare team
- Client's and family's ability and willingness to participate in the plan of care
- Client's personal resources and deficits

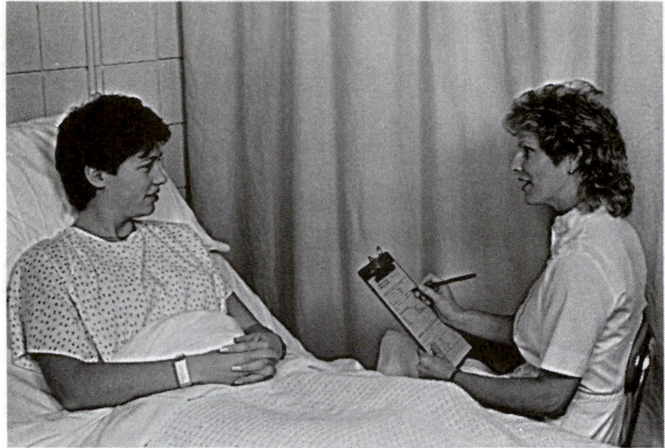

Figure 16-2
In the interview, both the seating arrangement and the distance from the client are important in establishing a relaxed and comfortable environment for data collection. (Photo © Ken Kasper.)

ical introduction might run like this: "Good afternoon, Miss LeBon. My name is Lisa Gray, and I'll be your nurse case manager. Right now I'd like to ask you a few questions about yourself so that we can plan your nursing care together. Feel free to respond only to those questions you feel comfortable answering, and know that your responses will be treated confidentially by the staff. This will take about 20 minutes. Is this time convenient for you? Do you need anything before we start?"

The initial impression the nurse creates is critical, especially with clients who are new to the healthcare environment. All nurses that the client encounters in the future may be judged in light of this first impression. When the nurse communicates respect and genuine concern for the client, the client is then encouraged to discuss health concerns and problems freely. The interpersonal qualities of a respectful presence, professionalism, and caring invite the client's confidence and inspire hope that help is available.

During the introduction, it is important for the nurse to assess the client's comfort and ability to participate in the interview. It also is appropriate to discuss confidentiality. The client should know where the data being recorded are stored, how they will be used, and who has access to them. Some nurses record data on the appropriate form while with the client, whereas other nurses take notes and complete the form later. Bedside computers are facilitating quick documentation. Documenting data should not interfere with the sharing of information during the interview. If a contractual agreement which clearly identifies the responsibilities of both client and nurse is indicated, terms are discussed at this time.

Working Phase. During the working phase of the interview, the nurse gathers all the information needed to form the subjective data base. The accuracy, completeness, and relevance of the data base depend on the nurse's use of the interviewing and basic communication techniques discussed in Chapter 22. The communication techniques highlighted below are important ingredients of a successful interview.

- Focus on the client during the interview, demonstrating interest and concern: use the client's name of choice, use eye contact appropriately, and avoid rushing the client.
- Listen to the client attentively; use reflection and paraphrase to communicate to the client that he or she is being understood.
- Ask about the client's main problem first using terminology the client understands; save personal or delicate questions for when a rapport is established. Defer less important questions until a later interview if the client is too ill or upset to communicate easily.
- Pose questions and comments to the client in the manner best suited to produce the desired communication (see Chapter 22):
  - Closed questions elicit specific information.
  - Open-ended questions allow the client to verbalize freely.
  - Reflective questions encourage the client to elaborate on thoughts and feelings.
  - Direct questioning may be used to validate information, to clarify information, or to place events into a meaningful sequence.
- Avoid comments and questions that impede communication (see Chapter 22)—cliches, questions that require a yes or no answer only, intimidating why or how questions, probing questions, giving advice, using judgmental comments, changing the subject, giving false assurance.
- Use silence and touch appropriately.

Many client variables can positively or negatively affect the outcome of an interview. Table 16-2 identifies client variables that can negatively influence an interview unless the nurse responds appropriately.

Termination. The successful interview is concluded carefully. A client should be advised that the interview is coming to an end. It is helpful to recapitulate the interview, highlighting key points. Both the client and the nurse should be satisfied that the important data are recorded. A helpful strategy is to ask the client after the summary: "Is there anything else you would like us to know that will help us plan your care?" This gives the client an opportunity to add data the nurse did not think to include.

Before leaving the client, it is helpful to alert the client as to what he or she can expect. The client also should know when the nurse will reestablish contact, for example, "Thank you for answering these questions, Miss LeBon. Please feel free to keep us informed of anything you think we should know. I'll be leaving soon, but when I return tomorrow morning, I'll discuss your plan of care. This afternoon will be busy for you: some blood tests and a chest x-ray have been ordered. Your evening will probably be quiet. Do you have any questions? Is there anything else I can do for you before I leave?"

Table 16-2
Client Variables That Can Negatively Influence an Interview and Suggested Nursing Responses

Client Variables	Effect on Interview	Nursing Response
High anxiety	Client may speak rapidly or incoherently and may jump from one topic to another; client may deny or misrepresent what he is experiencing.	Normalize anxiety: "Many people find it difficult to talk about their health and become anxious"; approach client gently, speak slowly and softly; underscore importance of the client sharing what he or she is experiencing so nurses can help.
Pain	Client offers clipped responses and yes or no answers whenever possible; overriding concern is pain relief.	Do everything possible to make client comfortable before the interview, including obtaining an order for and administering pain medication; if pain persists, obtain only vital data and defer remainder of interview until client is more comfortable.
Language difficulty (client not fluent in nurse's language because speaks a different language, has a limited education, or fears saying the "wrong thing")	Vital client data will not be communicated; client may mistakenly be labeled "indifferent" or "noncommunicative."	Speak clearly (do not raise voice) using simple language; whenever possible obtain the assistance of an interpreter (family member may help but if client data are confidential a stranger may be preferable).
Previous negative experience with nurses or healthcare delivery system	Client is aloof, unwilling to participate in interview; general attitude: "Why should I waste my time telling you anything . . . it won't do me any good."	"I know other people who have had a tough time with nurses or the system . . . life isn't perfect . . . but how about giving us a chance this time to show you what nurses can do?" Communicate respect for the client and competence.
Unrealistic expectations of healthcare professionals	Client expects nurses and other healthcare professionals to magically know everything about him or her and to "take care" of him or her; "surrenders" himself or herself to the system—"you know best" attitude.	Communicate clearly that no one knows or understands the client like the client does, and invite him or her to become involved in his or her care; "No two persons are alike and unless you tell me a little more about yourself and how you are feeling, there is no way we'll be able to plan good care."

Physical Assessment

Physical assessment is the examination of the client for *objective data* that may better define the client's condition and help the nurse in planning care. The physical assessment normally follows the nursing history and interview and may verify data gathered during the history or yield new data. There has been a great deal of controversy about nursing's role in the physical assessment of the client, caused by concern that this is a duplication of medicine's role. Physicians traditionally have performed the intake physical assessment, which commonly is the mechanism of entry into the healthcare delivery system as well as the basis for medical treatment. Some nurses in expanded roles are performing comprehensive intake physical assessments, which identify health and illness states, and are then recommending or prescribing appropriate follow-up care. In any case, all nurses conduct selected aspects of physical assessment for nursing purposes.

Unlike the physical assessment performed by the physician to identify pathology and its cause, the nursing physical assessment focuses primarily on the client's functional abilities. If a neurologic deficit is present, the nurse is concerned with identifying how this deficit affects the client's reasoning and sensorimotor abilities. For example, the client who has had a cerebrovascular accident (stroke) is examined to determine ability to comprehend and communicate information and execute the tasks of everyday life.

Purposes of the nursing physical assessment include the appraisal of health status, the identification of health problems, and the establishment of a data base for nursing intervention (Fig. 16-3).

Nurses practicing in different settings may use different physical assessment techniques for different purposes. Nurses in the coronary care unit use sophisticated, high-technology assessment techniques, whereas nurses in a rehabilitation center use a wide range of physical assessment skills that focus on identifying functional and nonfunctional response patterns to disabilities.

The nursing physical assessment involves the examination of all body systems in a systematic manner; a head-to-toe format commonly is used. These data may

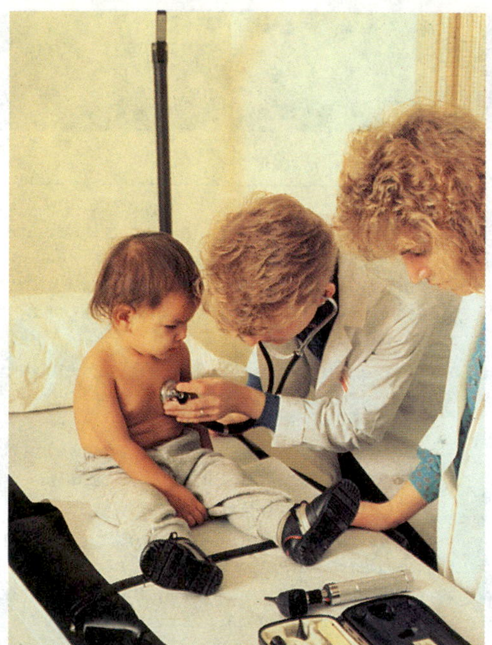

Figure 16-3
Two nurses provide a physical examination of a First Nations infant in a clinic. No matter what the setting or the age of the client, the physical examination should include appraisal of health status, identification of health problems, and the establishment of a data base for nursing intervention. (Photo courtesy of Medical Services Branch, Health Canada.)

be documented on a separate nursing physical assessment tool, or incorporated into a combined data base assessment form, as shown on pages 255 to 259. Nurses also may use physical assessment skills to evaluate selected systems.

Techniques. Four methods are used to collect data during a physical assessment—inspection, palpation, percussion, and auscultation. These techniques and the basic skills the student must learn to perform physical assessment are described in Chapter 26.

Sources of Data

Client

The client is the primary and usually the best source of information. Unless specified otherwise, it is assumed that the data recorded in the nursing history have been collected from the client. Most clients are willing to share information when they know it will be helpful in planning their care. Although data collected from the client usually are accurate, the nurse should be alert to certain difficulties. For example, a client who is acutely ill may not be able to communicate adequately if her pain is severe or her consciousness is altered in any way. An emotionally upset client may distort information: a client who is fearful because he thinks that the illness may threaten his work or life may deny certain symptoms or deliberately give misleading facts. If the nurse becomes aware that the client's report of symptoms differs from physical findings or data obtained from other sources, it is important to note this and to explore the cause of the discrepancy. The client with limited mental capacity or a very young client cannot be relied on to report accurately. Children, older people, and people with decreased mental capacity or impaired verbal ability should be encouraged to respond to interview questions as best they can. Bypassing these clients and automatically turning to a family member, friend, or caregiver for information communicates powerfully that the nurse either has no time for the client to express his or her needs or mistakenly doubts the client's ability to communicate these needs.

Support People

Family members, friends, and caregivers are especially helpful sources of data when the client has limited capacity to share information with the nurse or when the client is a child. Husbands and wives can supply information concerning their spouses. Friends may accompany a client to a health agency, and often can supply useful information. Care must be taken to determine that the client does not object to data being gathered from friends and that the friends want to participate. Also, the nurse is cautioned that there should be a clear understanding by the client, family, and friends of the confidentiality of the data collected. Whenever data are gathered from support people, this should be indicated in the nursing history.

Client Record

Records prepared by different members of the healthcare team provide information essential to comprehensive nursing care. The nurse should review records early when gathering data—in some instances, before the first contact with the client. Such a review helps to focus the nursing assessment and to confirm and amplify information obtained from other sources.

The client's health record or chart, which lists such information as age, sex, occupation, religious preference, next of kin, and financial status, is one type of record. The health record includes information entered by various healthcare professionals, such as the physician, social worker, dietitian, physiotherapist, and laboratory technicians. Nurses who want their care to be supportive of the client as he or she responds to changes in health status must be familiar with the many sections of the client record other than the documentation of the nursing plan of care and nursing notes. The following are important sources of data for the nurse.

Medical History, Physical Examination, and Progress Notes. These sources record the findings of physicians as they assess and treat the client; they focus on identifying

(text continues on page 260)

BRONSON METHODIST HOSPITAL
Kalamazoo, Michigan

Medical/Surgical-Critical Care Admission Assessment

A. DEMOGRAPHIC DATA

Name: Margaret Tembra
Prefers to be called: Mrs. Tembra Age: 72
Date: 9/2/97 Time of arrival to unit: 2:00 pm
Mode of admission: wheelchair
I.D. bracelet on and coincides with addressograph: ☑ Yes ☐ No Information given by: patient and her daughter Lisa
If unable to reach next of kin/legal guardian, contact: Barbara Tembra Phone: 634-5221
Valuables (list and state disposition): eye glasses (at bedside); purse taken home by daughter Lisa; no other valuables
Admitted from: ☑ Home ☐ Nursing Home ☐ Assisted Living ☐ Foster Care ☐ Senior Citizens' Apartments ☐ Other
Facility Name: Adm. Medical Diagnosis: T.I.A.

B. VITAL SIGNS

Ht: 5′ 2″ Wt: 63.6 Kg
Temp: 98.2°F ☑ Oral ☐ Ax. ☐ Rectal
Pulse: 88 ☐ Reg. ☑ Irreg.
Resp.: 18 ☑ Reg. ☐ Irreg.
BP: Left: 184/120
☑ Lying ☐ Sitting ☐ Standing
Right: 180/120
☑ Lying ☐ Sitting ☐ Standing

C. ORIENTATION TO UNIT

(The following have been explained):

Call system/bed-bathroom	☑ Yes	☐ N/A	Floor restrictions	☑ Yes	☐ N/A
Bed operation/siderails	☑ Yes	☐ N/A	Visitation Policy	☑ Yes	☐ N/A
Bathroom/bedpan-urinal	☑ Yes	☐ N/A	Lounge	☑ Yes	☐ N/A
TV/CH2/telephone	☑ Yes	☐ N/A	Newspaper/mail	☑ Yes	☐ N/A
Meal/cafeteria hours	☑ Yes	☐ N/A	Siderails policy	☑ Yes	☐ N/A
Smoking policy	☑ Yes	☐ N/A	Chaplain services	☑ Yes	☐ N/A

Signature: Margaret Tembra

D. **Health Patterns Assessment:** Complete information, **including patient's words.** Indicate N/A if non-applicable. Circle, code, or check all other findings as appropriate.

1. HEALTH PERCEPTION/HEALTH MANAGEMENT

Reason for hospitalization/chief complaint: "I fell in the kitchen this morning and couldnt move my left leg for awhile; I've also been having 'headaches'."
Recent illness/exposure to communicable disease: —
Previous hospitalizations/surgeries: about 1970 gall bladder surgery; hospitalized for high blood pressure 1989
What other health problems have you had? —
Things done to manage health: "I drink lots of water, eat fruit and avoid fried foods. I try not to worry so much."
Statement of patient's general appearance (include condition of hair, skin, nails): Alert, medium-built, well-nourished female; appears anxious about hospitalization: voice low, grabs daughter's hand; neat appearance; skin pale, cool and dry; gray hair-thin; scalp clean; thick nails; adequate cappillairy refill.
Tobacco use: ☐ Yes ☑ No ☐ Used to smoke:
EtOH use: none
Allergies: ☐ Yes (list with reaction experienced) ☑ No
Food: —
Medications/anesthetics: —
Other (e.g., wool, tape, pollens): regular soaps cause skin to be excessively dry

FORM 102 (Revised 10/84) — Page 1

(continued)

Patient's Name: Tembra, Margaret Hospital No.: 4629 F Date: 9/2/97

Medications: (e.g., prescript., non-prescript.) ☑ Yes ☐ No Did you bring? ☐ Yes ☑ No Taken home? ☐ Yes ☐ No ☐ N/A

NAME	DOSE	SCHEDULE	REASON	PRESCRIBING PHYSICIAN
hydralazine	?	OD	high blood pressure	Dr. Skomar
aspirin	ⅱ	PRN	headaches	—
metamucil	1 Tbsp	PRN	constipation	—

Have you been taking your medication(s) as prescribed? yes

OTHER PERTINENT DATA: —

SCT initials

2. NUTRITION/METABOLIC

Special diet? — Supplements: —

Pattern of daily food/fluid intake: Drinks at least 5-6 glasses H_2O daily + juices + tea; ↓ fried, fatty foods; likes baked or broiled meat, vegetables + fruit, "sweet tooth."

Appetite: "very good" Wt. loss/gain: —

Nausea/Vomiting: —

GI pain: —

Condition of oral mucous membranes: pink, moist

Dental condition: dentures clean Dentures: ☑ Upper ☑ Lower ☐ Partial ☐ N/A

Skin: ☐ Warm ☑ Dry ☑ Cool ☐ Moist ☐ Other: pale

Turgor: ☑ Supple ☐ Firm ☐ Fragile ☐ Dehydrated ☐ Other:

Color: ☐ Pink ☑ Pale ☐ Dusky ☐ Cyanotic ☐ Jaundiced ☐ Mottled ☐ Other:

Edema: +1 ankles

Wounds/drains/dressings: —

Skin problems (description and location): skin on legs and upper arms dry + scaley; scratch marks; reddened area under left breast – skin intact.

I.V.'s: — ☐ N/A

OTHER PERTINENT DATA: —

SCT initials

3. ELIMINATION

Abd. tenderness/guarding/distention: —

Bowel sounds: present all 4 quadrants Stoma (type): —

Any problems with hemorrhoids/involuntary stool? hx hemorrhoid 2° straining/constipation

Usual bowel pattern (frequency, character, consistency, etc.): stools tend to be hard and dry -- q 2-3 days Date of last BM: 9/1/97

If problem, describe: occasional (1x/wk) constipation

Use of anything to manage bowels (e.g., laxatives, enemas, suppositories, "home remedies", anti-diarrheals): ↑ fluids, ↑ fruit, metamucil; dislikes bran

Usual urinary pattern (frequency, character, amount, incontinence, nocturia, etc.): 5-6 x per day; up once at night to void

Last void (time): "this AM"

If problem, describe: —

Perspiration/nocturnal sweats: —

OTHER PERTINENT DATA: —

SCT initials

FORM 102 (Revised 10/84) — Page 2

(continued)

4. ACTIVITY / EXERCISE

CARDIO-VASCULAR STATUS

Peripheral pulses: palpable, strong

☐ N/A

Neurovascular check (e.g., capillary refill): ↓ sensation (hot/cold, sharp/dull) L leg; rapid capillary refill

Chest pain/radiation: —

Jugular vein distention: ☐ Yes ☑ No

Hx of murmur: ☐ Yes ☑ No

Pacemaker: ☐ Yes ☑ No

Presence of A-V Shunt: — ☑ No

Arterio-venous bruit: ☑ N/A

Tembra, M., 4269 F

Monitor/rhythm: ☑ N/A

Hemodynamic monitoring: — ☑ N/A

RESPIRATORY STATUS

Respiratory pattern: ☑ No problem ☐ Dyspnea ☐ Nocturnal Dyspnea ☐ S.O.B. at rest ☐ S.O.B. on exertion: — ☐ Other: —

Lung sounds: clear

Use of accessory muscles? ☐ Yes ☑ No

Cough/production: —

O_2 supplement: — ☑ N/A

Resp. tubes (e.g., ET, trach, chest/describe secretions/drainage): — ☑ N/A

Ventilatory assistance: ☑ N/A

ACTIVITIES OF DAILY LIVING/MOBILITY STATUS

Use the **Activity Level Code** below to assess admission statuses:

Activity Level Code	ADL Status		Mobility Status
0-total independence	Feeding set up tray	Meal Preparation —	Bed mobility 2
1-assist with device	Bathing 2	Cleaning —	Cart transfer bedrest
2-assist with person	Dressing 0	Shopping —	Chair/toilet transfer bedrest
3-assist with device & person	Grooming 0	Laundry —	Ambulation bedrest
4-total dependence	Toileting 1	Other —	R.O.M. 2

Handedness: ☑ Right ☐ Left

Able to use? ☑ Yes ☐ No

Reasons for ADL/Mobility limitations: Bedrest ordered during diagnostic work-up; At present able to move all 4 extremities ☐ N/A

Devices used for assist: Bed pan ☐ N/A

Do you need assistance with transportation? ☐ Yes ☐ No If "Yes", specify: —

Where do you plan to be discharged? home

Will you need assistance? ☐ Yes ☑ No

If "Yes", describe:

OTHER PERTINENT DATA: —

SCT initials

5. COGNITIVE / PERCEPTUAL

Level of consciousness: Alert

Oriented to: ☑ Person ☑ Place ☑ Time

Behaviors (describe): Face reflects concern about 's morning's paralysis + hospitalization

Hx of epilepsy/seizures/Parkinson's, etc.: —

REFLEXES

Reflexes: ☑ No problem ☐ Problem (If "No problem", do not complete this section.)

Eyes: Pupil size: r O l O Equal? ☑ Yes ☐ No Reaction to light: r ✓ l ✓

Accommodation: r ✓ l ✓ Deviation:

Handgrasp: r ✓ l ✓ Gag: ✓ Swallow: ✓

Movement of extremities: ↓ strength and ↓ movement left lower extremity

SENSORIUM

Eyes/sight:	☐ No problem ☑ Deficit:	"blurry vision" at times	Aid: eyeglasses
Ears/hearing:	☐ No problem ☑ Deficit:	"hard of hearing" Ⓛ ear	Aid: none
Nose/smell:	☑ No problem ☐ Deficit:		
Tongue/taste:	☑ No problem ☐ Deficit:		
Skin/touch:	☑ No problem ☐ Deficit:		
Numbness/tingling:	☐ No problem ☑ Deficit:	left leg "feels queer—pins and needles"	
Dizziness:	☐ No problem ☑ Deficit:	feels "slightly dizzy—unsteady"	

FORM 102 (Revised 10/84) — Page 3

(continued)

Patient's Name: Tembra, M. Hospital No.: 4269 F Date: 9/2/97

COGNITIVE/PERCEPTUAL

PAIN

Pain: ☐ No problem ☑ Problem (If "No problem", do not complete this section.)

If "Problem", describe location, type, intensity, onset, duration: headaches – began about 6 months ago – of increasing frequency and severity; at present occur 1-2×/wk, last 1-2 days

Methods of pain management: Asprin, other OTC extra strength pain relievers only helps "a little"

COGNITION

Primary language: English Speech deficit: — Aid: —

Any learning difficulties? —

OTHER PERTINENT DATA: —

SCT initials

6. SLEEP/REST

Usual sleep/rest pattern: 11 pm – 7 am

Adequate? ☑ Yes ☐ No Factors affecting sleep/rest: gets up to void once during night

Methods to promote sleep: —

Hx of sleep disturbances: —

OTHER PERTINENT DATA: —

SCT initials

7. SELF-PERCEPTION SELF-CONCEPT

Are there any ways you feel differently about yourself since you've been ill/hospitalized? "never questioned my health" expresses fear

Description of non-verbal behaviors: quiet speech, wrinkled brow, wants daughter near

OTHER PERTINENT DATA: daughter reports mother has been very independent, strong woman – rarely ill

SCT initials

8. ROLE/RELATIONSHIP

Marital status: Widowed Children: 3

Do you live? ☐ Alone ☑ With family ☐ Other: lives with daughter Lisa + her family

Family feelings regarding hospitalization: Concern

Who are the people that will help you most at this time? 2 daughters: Lisa, Barbara

Are you presently employed? ☐ Yes ☑ No Occupation: ☐ N/A

Are you presently in school? ☐ Yes ☑ No Will illness/hospitalization interfere? ☐ N/A

Upon discharge, if necessary, will you be able to afford?

Medications: ☑ Yes ☐ No Supplies: ☑ Yes ☐ No Medical Care: ☑ Yes ☐ No

OTHER PERTINENT DATA: Husband died 8 months ago – moved in with daughter 6 months ago after selling family home – High Stress

SCT initials

9. SEXUALITY/REPRODUCTIVE

Female: ☐ N/A Menopausal: ☑ Yes ☐ No Menstrual pattern: ☐ N/A

Problems/changes: —

Date of L.N.M.P. ☑ N/A Possibly pregnant? ☐ Yes ☐ No ☐ N/A

Pregnancy history: G3 P3

Use of birth control measure ☐ Yes ☐ No ☑ N/A Type:

Any problems with use?

Monthly self-breast exam? ☐ Yes ☑ No ☐ N/A

Vaginal discharge/bleeding/lesions: —

Receiving medical attention? ☐ Yes ☑ No ☐ N/A

OTHER PERTINENT DATA: —

SCT initials

Male: ☑ N/A Prostate problems?

Monthly self-testicular exam? ☐ Yes ☐ No ☐ N/A

Penile discharge/bleeding/lesions:

Receiving medical attention? ☐ Yes ☐ No ☐ N/A

OTHER PERTINENT DATA:

initials

FORM 102 (Revised 10/84) — Page 4

(continued)

Tembra, M. 4269F

COPING/STRESS

10. Have you experienced any recent stressful situations in addition to your illness/hospitalization? ☑ Yes ☐ No

If "Yes", please describe briefly: *In past year:*
death of husband
sale of family home
relocation with daughter

Are there any ways we can be of assistance? *"can't think of any"*

How do you usually manage stresses? *talk with friends, pray*
"I used to share everything with my husband"

What do you do for relaxation? *used to crochet, watch TV*

Support groups/counselling resources used: *—*

Were they helpful? ☐ N/A

OTHER PERTINENT DATA: *misses husband very much*

SCT	initials

VALUE/BELIEF

11. Will illness/hospitalization interfere with any of the following?

Spiritual or religious practices? ☐ Yes ☑ No

Cultural beliefs or practices? ☐ Yes ☑ No

Familial traditions? ☐ Yes ☑ No

If "Yes", to any of the above, please describe briefly:

Would you like your clergy or hospital chaplain to be contacted? ☑ Yes ☐ No ☐ N/A *daughter will contact minister*

OTHER PERTINENT DATA:

SCT	initials

IMPRESSIONS

E. Include: a. Possible nursing diagnostic concept labels to consider for care planning.
b. Possible referral resources to consider for discharge planning needs.
c. Other pertinent information

a. Diagnostic labels: Colonic Constipation, High Risk for Impaired Physical Mobility, High Risk for Altered Health Maintenance Related to Knowledge Deficit: TIA ⟶ stroke management, disturbance in self-concept, skin integrity impairment

b. Social Service Referral
referral to home minister

	initials

DATE	TIME	INITIALS	SIGNATURES	
9/2/97	*2:00 pm*	*SCT*	*S. Carol Taylor, RN*	(1st Adm. R.N.)
				(2nd Adm. R.N.)
				(3rd Adm. R.N.)
				(4th Adm. R.N.)

FORM 102 (Revised 10/84) — Page 5

pathology and its cause and on determining the medical regimen that will best treat the problem.

Consultations. The client's physicians may invite specialists to assess and work with the client; the focus is on documenting findings that help establish a medical diagnosis or on planning and executing the treatment regimen.

Reports of Diagnostic Studies. Reports of laboratory studies and other diagnostic tests, such as x-rays, offer the nurse objective data that can either confirm or conflict with data collected during the nursing history or examination. Results of diagnostic studies are helpful to physicians in establishing a diagnosis and in monitoring the client's response to treatment. The results of these same studies also may be helpful to nurses in evaluating the success of nursing interventions.

Reports of Therapies by Other Healthcare Professionals. Other healthcare professionals who interact with the client also record their findings and note any progress the client is making in their specific areas—for example, nutrition, physical therapy, or speech therapy. These reports help the nurse to better assess the client's progress in general and are useful when determining the client's ability to return home and manage care independently.

Records of previous admissions for healthcare and records from other health agencies, such as a social service agency or a home healthcare agency, also are valuable sources of data. They contain information about the client's previous medical or surgical problems and response patterns, which may be important determinants of the current plan of care.

Other Healthcare Professionals

Nurses can learn a great deal about a client's normal health habits and patterns and her or his response to illness by talking with other nurses, physicians, social workers, and other members of the healthcare team (Fig. 16-4). Although such communication is always important, it can be critical when clients are transferred from home to institution, from institution to institution, or from one hospital to another. The only way to ensure continuity of care is to make special efforts to share pertinent information.

Nursing and Other Healthcare Literature

To obtain a comprehensive client data base, it may be necessary to consult the nursing and related literature on specific health problems. For example, if a nurse has not cared for a client with Paget's disease before, it is important for him or her to read about the clinical manifestations of the disease and its usual progression in order to know what to look for when assessing the client. In addition to information concerning the medical diagnoses, treatment, and prognosis, a literature review

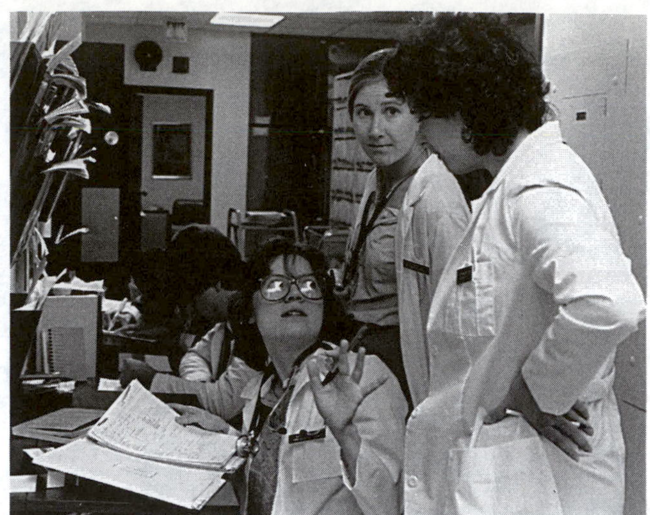

Figure 16-4
Nurses can learn a great deal about a client's normal health habits and patterns and responses to illness by talking with other nurses, physicians, social workers, and other members of the healthcare team. This exchange of information is particularly important when clients transfer from one healthcare setting to another or to home.

offers the nurse important information about nursing diagnoses, developmental norms, and psychosocial and spiritual practices that is helpful when assessing clients.

Planning Data Collection

Comprehensive Versus Focused Data Collection

Nursing assessments include both the comprehensive admission assessment (data base assessment) and the focused assessment. *Data base assessment* usually is performed during the nurse's initial contact with the client. The nurse collects data concerning *all aspects* of the client's health, establishing priorities for ongoing, focused assessments. A data base nursing assessment structured according to Gordon's 11 functional health patterns appears in the box in this chapter under "Structuring the Assessment." In a **focused assessment** the nurse gathers data about a *specific problem* that has already been identified (Alfaro, 1994, p. 36). A focused assessment may be done during the initial assessment if client health problems surface, but it is routinely part of ongoing data collection.

Critical Thinking Exercise 16-2

Allow another student to perform a comprehensive nursing assessment (interview and physical assessment) on you. Reflect on what you experienced. Offer the student feedback about which of her or his behaviors were helpful, comforting, distressing. Change roles and talk about what you learned from this experience.

Assessment Priorities

Before beginning to collect data on any client, the nurse should have a good sense of the type of data needed to best develop a satisfactory plan of care. Client data of interest to the nurse include the following:

- Client profile (name, address, age, sex, race, culture, religion, education, occupation)
- Client's developmental stage and ability to meet developmental tasks
- Family, psychosocial, and environmental histories
- Health beliefs, habits, patterns (how client meets basic human needs)
- Client's responses (physical and emotional) to health and illness (functioning of each major body system)
- Meaning client attaches to health and illness
- Presence of risk factors
- Client resources—internal (eg, coping strengths) and external (eg, support people, adequate finances, availability of healthcare)
- Client's expected and preferred modes of treatment (past experiences with healthcare professionals)

The purpose for which the assessment is being performed offers the best guidelines as to what type and how much data to collect. Assessment priorities are influenced by the client's health orientation, developmental stage, and need for nursing.

Health Orientation. Wellness assessments, such as Health-Style: A Self-Test in Chapter 4, may be used by nurses to assist clients to identify potential and actual health risks and to explore habits, behaviors, beliefs, attitudes, and values that influence levels of wellness (Pinnell & de Meneses, 1986). Hill and Smith (1990) offer nurses who are interested in wellness a variety of specialized assessment tools that focus on relationships; psychologic, environmental, and physical self-care; relaxation; spirituality; humor and play; movement and exercise; sleep and dreams; nutrition; and sexuality. These assessments are very different from the comprehensive admission assessments of clients being hospitalized for treatment in terms of the type of client data gathered.

Developmental Stage. Nursing assessments are modified according to the developmental needs of clients. For example, when assessing an infant, special attention is given to weight gain and physical growth, feeding and elimination problems, sleep–activity cycles, and the parenting skills of caregivers. When children are hospitalized, it is similarly important to note how independent the child is with basic care measures (toileting, hygiene, dressing, eating), what words the child uses to indicate the need to void and defecate, play preferences, and so forth.

Need for Nursing. Whether nurses will be interacting with the client for a short or a long period (same-day surgery versus surgery that necessitates a long recovery in an intensive care unit) and the nature of nursing care needed by the client (assistance with the birth of a baby versus support and care throughout a terminal illness) powerfully influence the type of data the nurse collects. A general guideline when assessing clients is to gather only data that are helpful when planning and delivering care. Thus it would be inappropriate to collect a detailed sexual history on a client admitted to the hospital overnight after a slight concussion. Conversely, the nurse who fails to ask a pregnant woman admitted to the hospital for observation because of bleeding during her first trimester whether she has any questions about resuming sexual activity once she gets home is doing the client a great disservice.

Practical Considerations. Data already collected from the client and communicated in the client record should

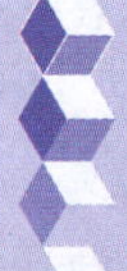

Through the Eyes of a Student

As a first-year nursing student, I often questioned myself on my technique in assessing a client. Sure, I understood what my instructors taught me, but was I doing it right? So I find my client has an elevated temperature, or perhaps urinary output is scanty—but what does it all mean? I often wondered if I would be able to make sense of all this information, and would I *really* be able to detect a problem should one develop. Well, it works! Keep assessing, recording, and reporting.

During my second year (first semester), I realized how an assessment can aid in saving your client's life. A continuous assessment for 2 days saved my 91-year-old client. I detected early signs of pulmonary edema and congestive heart failure, and was able to notify appropriate medical personnel and immediately implement life-saving procedures. Sure it was scary, but how proud I felt when the nursing staff congratulated me on a job well done! I realized how significant my assessment was for my client, when as I stood with her in the x-ray department she looked up at me from her stretcher and thanked me for taking good care of her. Knowing my client was aware of what I had done for her meant the world to me, and at this point, I realized why I had chosen the nursing profession.

—Delores (Dee) C. Pascale,
Delaware County Community College,
Media, Pennsylvania

not be repeatedly sought from the client unless there is a need to validate this data. Repetitious questioning can be annoying to the client and may cause the client to wonder about the lack of communication among health-care professionals. A careful review of the client record before interviewing the client avoids this problem.

Before meeting a new client, it is helpful to take a minute to think carefully about the type of data needed to plan quality care. After the comprehensive nursing assessment has been completed, client health problems dictate assessment priorities for future nurse–client interactions.

Structuring the Assessment

Having now studied the different types of data about clients that nurses collect, it is easy to see the need to structure data collection systematically. Using systematic guidelines specifically developed for a nursing assessment ensures that comprehensive, holistic data are collected for each client and lead easily to the formulation of nursing diagnoses. Once the nurse internalizes the assessment guidelines, it is easier for her or him to focus on the client during the assessment rather than worry about what to assess next.

Most schools of nursing and healthcare institutions have developed their own structured assessment guidelines, many of which are based on a selected nursing theory. One example is based on Gordon (1987), who proposes a standardized structure for delineating the basic areas of assessment that is applicable to all clients and compatible with all nursing theories. This framework (see box) identifies 11 functional health patterns and organizes client data into these patterns.

Functional Health Patterns

Health-perception–health-management pattern: Describes client's perceived pattern of health and well-being and how health is managed

Nutritional–metabolic pattern: Describes pattern of food and fluid consumption relative to metabolic need and pattern indicators of local nutrient supply

Elimination pattern: Describes patterns of excretory function (bowel, bladder, and skin)

Activity–exercise pattern: Describes pattern of exercise, activity, leisure, and recreation

Cognitive–perceptual pattern: Describes sensory–perceptual and cognitive pattern

Sleep–rest pattern: Describes patterns of sleep, rest, and relaxation

Self-perception–self-concept pattern: Describes self-concept pattern and perceptions of self (eg, body comfort, body image, feeling state)

Role–relationship pattern: Describes pattern of role-engagements and relationships

Sexuality–reproductive pattern: Describes client's patterns of satisfaction and dissatisfaction with sexuality pattern; describes reproductive patterns

Coping–stress-tolerance pattern: Describes general coping pattern and effectiveness of the pattern in terms of stress tolerance

Value–belief pattern: Describes patterns of values, beliefs (including spiritual), or goals that guide choices of decisions

Gordon, M. (1987). *Nursing diagnosis: Process and application* (2nd ed.). New York: McGraw-Hill, p. 93.

Problems Related to Data Collection

Common problems encountered during data collection include inappropriate organization of the data base, omission of pertinent data, irrelevant or duplicate data, erroneous or misinterpreted data, too few data acquired from the client, recording of interpretation of data rather than observed behavior, and failure to update data base. Table 16-3 lists these problems and describes possible causes and remedies.

Data Validation

Validation is the act of confirming or verifying. The purpose of validating is to keep data as free from error, bias, and misinterpretation as possible. Validation is an important part of assessment because invalid information can lead to inappropriate nursing care.

Validation of all data is neither possible nor necessary; the nurse needs to decide which items need verification. For example, data needs to be verified when there are discrepancies: a client tells the nurse he is fine and has no concerns, but the nurse notes that he demonstrates tense body musculature and seems curt in his responses. There is a discrepancy between what the person is saying and what the nurse is observing, and so validation is necessary to determine accuracy. Validation in this instance may take the form of the nurse saying, "You tell me you feel fine, but right now your body and behaviors are telling me something else. I wonder why this is?"

Data also need verification when they lack objectivity. For example, a nurse suspects that the client hears from one ear but does not seem to hear well from the other. The nurse should validate the data before proceeding, and should determine whether the client does indeed have a hearing problem. Suspicions are not objective. In this instance, the nurse needs to test the client's hearing in both ears. Speaking toward the ear that is suspected to hear well, the nurse explains, "It seems to me that you hear better out of one ear than the other. I would like to test this. I'll bring a watch slowly toward your right ear first and then toward your left. Please look straight ahead and tell me when you first hear the watch ticking." The nurse then records how far

Table 16-3
Common Problems of Data Collection, Possible Causes, and Suggested Remedies

Problem	Possible Causes	Suggested Remedies
Data base inappropriately organized	Failure to plan for the assessment by identifying needed data; use of inappropriate tools for data collection	Review the guidelines for specifying pertinent data. Consider modifying tool for data collection or select an alternative tool.
Pertinent data omitted	Not following up on cues during data collection; inappropriate guidelines	Identify potentially relevant factors in advance of collection. Practice interview strategies.
Irrelevant or duplicate data collected	Failure to identify specific purpose of data collection; failure to review available client records; use of inappropriate tools for data collection	Determine specific purpose of data collection for each client. Consider existing data before initiating collection. Consider modifying data collection tool or selecting alternative.
Erroneous or misinterpreted data collection	Failure to observe carefully or validate during data collection; interviewer prejudices or stereotypes	Sharpen observation skills by independently observing the same situation with a peer and compare notes afterward. Role play several validation techniques.
Too little data acquired from client	Failure to establish sufficient rapport or use appropriate communication techniques with client; failure to know what information is wanted	Review and practice communication techniques discussed in Chapter 22. Role play several explanations of purpose of data collection. Identify general data desired before collection.
Interpretation of data is recorded rather than the observed behavior	Nurse jumps to hasty conclusion about client's behavior and deprives others of exploring with the client possible causes of the behavior; deficient validation	Review the distinction between data and interpretation of data. Practice documenting observed client behavior concisely.
Failure to update the data base	Erroneous belief that assessment is concluded once the initial data base is recorded; low priority attached to ongoing data collection	Recollect that it is impossible to give quality, individualized care without knowledge of changes in the client's status. Ongoing data collection is critical to the deletion or modification of old problems and the identification of new problems.

the watch was from each ear when the client first heard it ticking.

The nurse may validate data as they are collected or at the end of the data-gathering process. When it is clear that the data are correct, the nurse is ready to analyze the data and formulate nursing diagnoses—the next step of the nursing process.

Data Communication

The client data collected by the nurse, both initially and as client contact continues, are of no benefit to the client and the healthcare team unless they are appropriately communicated. Appropriate communication involves correct timing and proper documentation.

Timing

Immediate verbal communication of data is indicated whenever assessment findings reveal a critical change in the client's health status that necessitates the involvement of other nurses or healthcare professionals (Fig. 16-5). The nurse who observes an elevated temperature of 103.2°F (39.5°C) in a client scheduled for surgery that morning must report this to the charge nurse and to the surgeon, who will probably cancel surgery. Failure to communicate this finding could result in the client's receiving preoperative sedation, being taken to the operating room, and even having the surgery performed under less than optimal conditions. Similarly, a nurse who hears a client making suicidal remarks must communicate this information to the healthcare team, so that all are alerted to the client's danger and suicide precautions may be taken immediately.

Legal Alert

Nurses are responsible for alerting the appropriate healthcare professional whenever assessment data differ significantly from the client's baseline, indicating a potentially serious problem. Interventions for which the nurse may be legally responsible include increasing the frequency of assessments and initiating necessary changes in the treatment regimen.

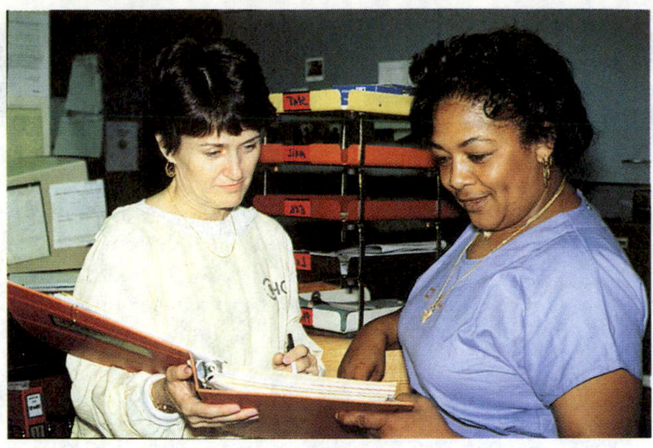

Figure 16-5
Immediate verbal communication of data is indicated whenever assessment findings reveal a critical change in the client's health status. (Photo by Gates Rhodes, courtesy of School of Nursing, University of Pennsylvania.)

The nurse who is unsure of the significance of a particular finding is well advised to consult with another nurse. In some situations, years of experience are needed to accurately distinguish significant from nonsignificant findings. Neither ignorance nor the fear of appearing less than competent justifies failure to report critical data.

Documentation

The initial data base should be entered into the computer or recorded in ink, using the designated agency forms, the same day the client is admitted to the agency. If, for any reason, important data cannot be obtained during the initial assessment, this needs to be documented so that it is obtained as soon as possible. Objective and subjective client data should be summarized and written, so that data communicate a unique sense of the client and are comprehensive, concise, and easily retrievable. The data should be written legibly, and good grammar and only standard medical abbreviations should be used. To facilitate quick data retrieval, data should be presented under clearly marked headings.

Critical Thinking Exercise 16-3
Collect several different forms for recording the initial comprehensive nursing assessment (hospital, nursing home, home care, and school of nursing forms). Identify and explain the differences you see. Experiment with using the different forms and make a list of features which help you to get all the data you need in the easiest way possible.

Whenever possible, subjective data should be recorded using the client's own words. Quotation marks should be used: "I feel tired from the moment I first get up in the morning. Any more it seems I have no energy at all." Client reports also may be paraphrased: Client reports feeling dyspneic, "hard to catch my breath" when walking one flight of stairs.

The tendency to record data using nonspecific terms that are subject to individual definition or interpretation—adequate, good, average, normal, poor, small, large—should be avoided. One nurse's sense of what constitutes an average fluid intake may be very different from that of another nurse. It is important to be specific. Chapter 21 offers general documentation guidelines.

Key Points

- Assessing is the systematic and continuous collection, validation, and communication of client data. A data base is all the pertinent client information collected by the nurse and other healthcare professionals that enables a comprehensive and effective plan of care to be designed and implemented for the client.
- Ongoing nursing assessment alerts the nurse to changes in the client's responses to health and illness and suggests necessary changes in the plan of care.
- Unlike medical assessments, whose primary purpose is to define the existence of medical problems and identify the underlying pathology, nursing assessments are focused primarily on client responses to health problems.
- Objective data are perceptible to the senses and verifiable by another person observing the same data. Subjective data can only be perceived by the affected person and cannot be perceived or verified experientially by another.
- Common methods used for collecting data in nursing are observation, interview, and physical assessment. Observation is the conscious and deliberate use of the five senses to gather data. Skilled nurses observe clients for significant data during each nurse–client interaction.
- Strong interviewing skills are needed by the nurse to obtain a comprehensive nursing history that captures the unique qualities and characteristics of the client in a way that makes individualized care planning possible.
- During the nursing physical assessment, the nurse assesses the client for objective data to better define the client's condition and help the nurse in planning care. The nursing examination focuses primarily on the client's functional abilities.
- The primary source of client data is the client. Unless otherwise specified, it is assumed that the data recorded in the nursing history are from the client. Other important sources of client data are the client's support people, the client record,

other healthcare professionals, and the nursing and related healthcare literature.

- A data base nursing assessment is done during the nurse's initial contact with the client, and involves collecting data about all aspects of the client's health. A focused assessment may be done during any nurse–client interaction. Its purpose is to gather data about a specific problem.
- Before beginning to collect data, the nurse should have a good sense of the type of data needed to develop a satisfactory plan of care. Assessment priorities are influenced by the client's health orientation, developmental stage, and need for nursing.
- Using systematic assessment guidelines specifically developed for a nursing assessment ensures that comprehensive, holistic data are collected for each client and that those data easily lead to the formulation of nursing diagnoses.
- Problems related to data collection include inappropriate organization of data base, omission of pertinent data, irrelevant or duplicate data, erroneous or misinterpreted data, too little data acquired from the client, recording of interpretation of data rather than observed behavior, and failure to update data base.
- Validation is the act of confirming or verifying. The purpose of validation is to keep data as free from error, bias, and misinterpretation as possible. Data need to be verified when they contain discrepancies and lack objectivity.
- Client data collected by the nurse, both initially and as client contact continues, are of no benefit to the client and the nursing and healthcare teams unless they are appropriately communicated. It is important to learn when significant data need to be communicated verbally immediately and how to document data.
- Client data should be summarized and written so that they communicate a unique sense of the client and are comprehensive, concise, and easily retrievable.

Bibliography

Alfaro, R. (1994). *Applying the nursing process: A step-by-step guide* (3rd ed.). Philadelphia: Lippincott.

American Nurses Association. (1980). *Nursing: A social policy statement.* Washington, DC: ANA.

Barkauskas, V. H., Stoltenberg-Allen, K., Ciofu-Baumann, L., & Darling-Fisher, C. (1994). *Health and physical assessment.* St. Louis: Mosby.

Bates, B. (1995). *A guide to physical examination* (6th ed.). Philadelphia: Lippincott.

Braverman, B. G. (1990). Eliciting data from the patient who is difficult to interview. *Nursing Clinics of North America, 25*(4), 743–750.

Catherman, A. (1990). Biopsychosocial nursing assessment: A way to enhance care plans. *Journal of Psychosocial Nursing, 28*(6), 31–33.

Cormier, L. S., Cormier, W. H., & Weisse, R. J. (1984). *Interviewing and helping skills for health professionals.* Monterey, CA: Wadsworth.

Davis, A. J. (1984). *Listening and responding.* St. Louis: Mosby.

Domarad, B. R., & Buschmann, M. T. (1995). Interviewing older adults: Increasing the credibility of interview data. *Journal of Gerontological Nursing, 21*(9), 14–20.

Gordon, M. (1987). *Nursing diagnosis: Process and application* (2nd ed.). New York: McGraw-Hill.

Hill, L., & Smith, N. (1990). *Self-care nursing: Promotion of health* (2nd ed.). East Norwalk, CT: Appleton & Lange.

Hogstel, M. O., & Keen-Payne, R. (1993). *Practical guide to health assessment through the lifespan.* Philadelphia: Davis.

Laschinger, H. S. (1990). Helping students apply a nursing conceptual framework in the clinical setting. *Nurse Educator, 15*(3), 20–24.

McPhetridge, L. M. (1968). Nursing history: One means to personalize care. *American Journal of Nursing, 68*(1), 68–75.

Milholland, D. K. (1994). Privacy and confidentiality of patient information: Challenges for nursing. *JONA, 24*(2), 19–24.

Parish, L. (1986). Communicating with hospitalized children. *Canadian Nurse, 82*(1), 21–24.

Parker, K. (1986). Health works: An adolescent assessment tool. *Canadian Nurse, 82*(1), 28–31.

Pinnell, N., & de Meneses, M. (1986). *The nursing process.* Norwalk, CT: Appleton-Century-Crofts.

Rubenfeld, M. G., & Scheffer, B. K. (1995). *Critical thinking in nursing: An interactive approach.* Philadelphia: Lippincott.

Simonsen, S. M. (1996). *Telephone health assessment: Guidelines for practice.* St. Louis: Mosby.

Stewart, C. J., & Cash, W. B. (1991). *Interviewing principles and practice* (6th ed.). Dubuque: Brown.

Vessey, J. A., & Richardson, B. L. (1993). A holistic approach to symptom assessment and intervention. *Holistic Nursing Practice, 7*(2), 13–21.

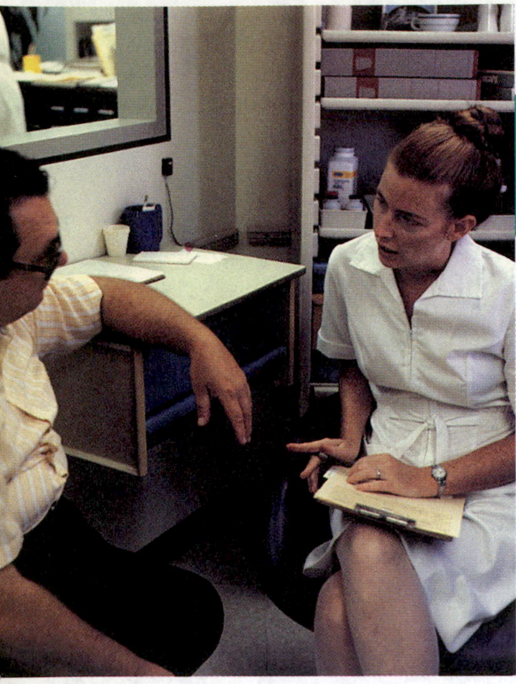

Chapter 17

Diagnosing

Objectives

After studying this chapter, the learner should be able to:

Define key terms used in the chapter.

Describe the term nursing diagnosis, distinguishing it from a collaborative problem and a medical diagnosis.

Describe the four steps involved in data interpretation and analysis.

Use the guidelines for writing nursing diagnoses when developing diagnostic statements.

Describe means to validate nursing diagnoses.

Develop a prioritized list of nursing diagnoses using identifiable criteria.

Describe the benefits and limitations of nursing diagnoses.

Key Terms

actual problem
collaborative problem
cue
data cluster
diagnosing
health problem
medical diagnosis
nursing diagnosis
possible problem
potential problem
wellness diagnosis

Once the nurse has collected and recorded the client data, the work of diagnosing begins—the second step in the nursing process. The purpose of diagnosing is to identify (1) actual and potential problems in the way the client responds to health or illness, (2) factors that contribute to or cause the problems (etiologies), and (3) strengths the client can draw on to prevent or resolve the problems.

During the diagnosing step of the nursing process, the nurse interprets and analyzes data gathered from the nursing assessment. These data help the nurse identify client strengths and health problems. A **health problem** is a condition related to health that necessitates intervention if disease or illness is to be prevented or resolved, and if coping and wellness are to be promoted.

When health problems are identified, the nurse must decide which healthcare professional can best treat the problem. Actual or potential health problems that can be prevented or resolved by independent nursing intervention are termed **nursing diagnoses**. The nurse formulates and validates nursing diagnoses, and lists these nursing diagnoses by priority (Fig. 17-1).

A brief history of the evolution of nursing diagnosis can be found in Chapter 14. Now an accepted and essential step in the nursing process, nursing diagnosis was initially confused with medical diagnosis, and this sparked great controversy. Although the confusion has been resolved, many nurses have been slow to understand and accept the "work" of diagnosing. Several books have been written to describe the relation of diagnosing to the other steps in the nursing process (see Bibliography).

Unique Focus of Nursing Diagnosis

During the diagnosing step of the nursing process, the nurse identifies what it is about the client that is nursing's unique concern (ie, what it is about the client that gives rise to the need for nursing, as opposed to the need for medicine or for physical therapy). Nursing diagnoses are, therefore, written to describe client problems that nurses can treat independently. As nurses interpret and analyze client data, they may identify health problems that are better treated by physicians (medical diagnoses) or by nurses working with other healthcare professionals (collaborative problems). In such a case, the nurse reports the findings to the physician or other appropriate healthcare professional and works collaboratively with him or her on resolving the problem (Fig. 17-2). Core competencies essential to nursing diagnosis are highlighted in the box on page 270.

Nursing Diagnosis Versus Medical Diagnosis

Medical diagnoses identify diseases, whereas nursing diagnoses focus on identifying human responses to health and illness. Medical diagnoses describe problems for which the physician directs the primary treatment, as opposed to nursing diagnoses, which describe problems treated by nurses within the scope of independent nursing practice. A medical diagnosis remains the same for as long as the disease is present; a nursing diagnosis may change from day to day as the client's responses change. These distinctions are in keeping with the differing foci of medical and nursing practices.

Critical Thinking Exercise 17-1

Recall a client who is newly diagnosed with AIDS. List possible medical and nursing diagnoses and collaborative problems. Explain the differing purposes of medical and nursing diagnoses and collaborative problems. State nursing's ***diagnostic contribution*** *to the interdisciplinary caregiving team.*

Nursing Diagnoses Versus Collaborative Problems

Nursing diagnoses also must be distinguished from collaborative problems. Together, nursing diagnoses and collaborative problems constitute the range of responses that nurses treat, and as such define the unique nature of nursing (see Fig. 17-2). Carpenito defines **collaborative problems** as "certain physiologic complications that nurses monitor to detect onset or changes in status. Nurses manage collaborative problems using physician-prescribed and nursing-prescribed interventions to minimize the complications of the event" (1995, p. 29).

Unlike medical diagnoses, collaborative problems represent situations that are the primary responsibility of nurses. Unlike nursing diagnoses, collaborative prob-

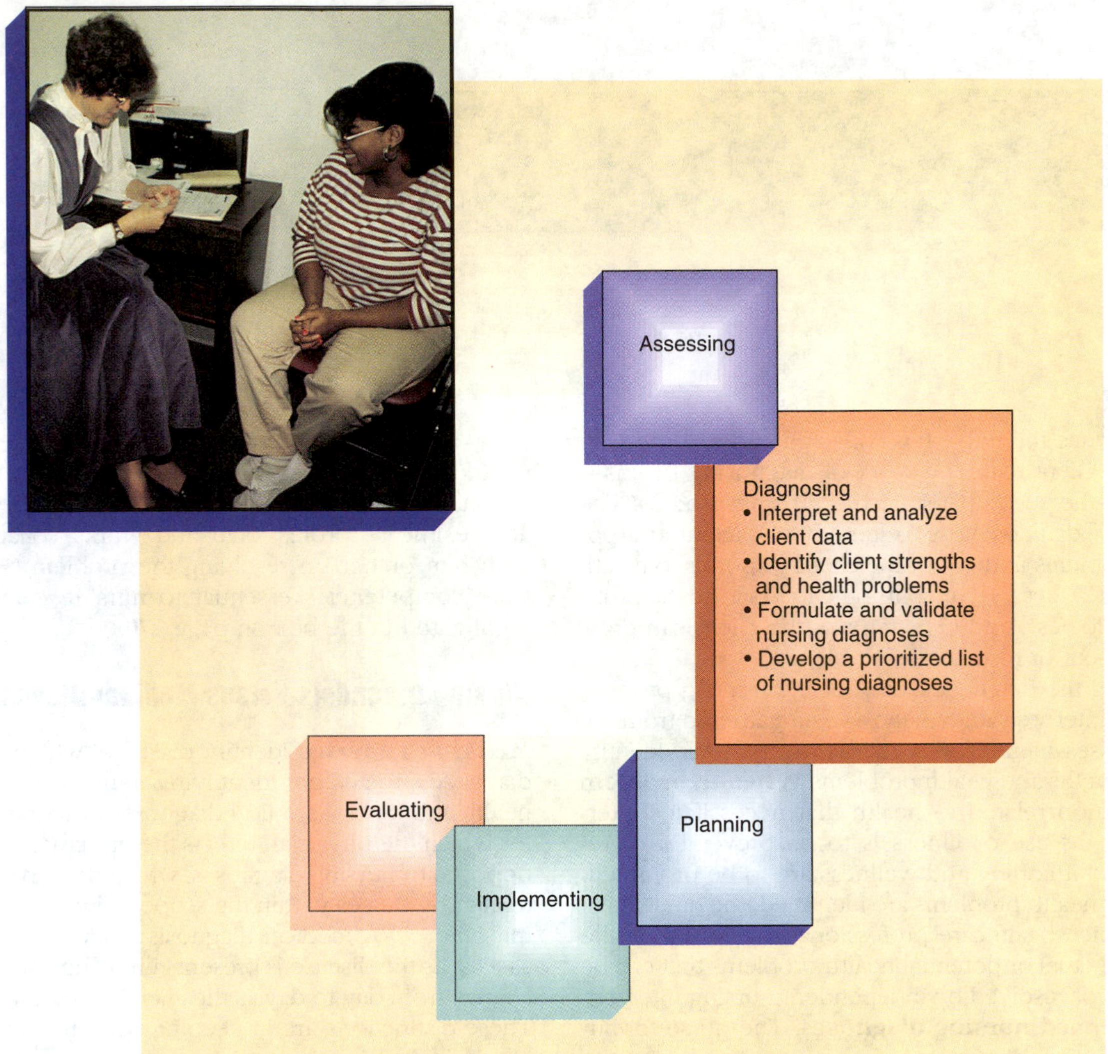

Figure 17-1
Diagnosing. Diagnosing is the interpretation and analysis of client data to identify client strengths and health problems that independent nursing intervention can prevent or resolve. Nursing diagnoses may change from day to day as the client's responses to health and illness change. (Photo by Gates Rhodes, courtesy of School of Nursing, University of Pennsylvania.)

lems represent situations in which the prescription for definitive treatment comes from both nursing and medicine. "When the nurse writes client outcomes that require delegated medical orders for goal achievement, the situation is not a nursing diagnosis but a collaborative problem" (Carpenito, 1995, p. 33). Because collaborative problems deal with potential complications, it is important that they be identified early so that the related nursing care, which is preventive, can be instituted early. Figure 17-3 shows collaborative problems identified by a nurse caring for a client with ovarian cancer. These problems are related to a medical disease, a medical treatment, and a diagnostic study. To write a diagnostic statement for a collaborative problem, remember Alfaro's rule:

> If you need to write a diagnostic statement for a collaborative problem, focus on the **potential complications** of the problem. Use "PC" (for potential complication), followed by a colon, and list the complications that might occur. For clarity, link the potential complications and the collaborative problem by using "related to." **Example**: PC: pneumothorax related to fractured ribs (1994, p. 115).

Table 17-1 shows how nurses successfully interpreted different clusters of data that led to the identification of a nursing diagnosis, collaborative problem, and medical diagnosis. In the first example, a nursing diagnosis was identified and successfully treated. In the next example, the nurse identified a collaborative problem and initiated intervention within the scope of her practice. When this failed to resolve the problem, a physician was contacted to order medication or a catheterization. In the last example, the nurse's early detection and reporting of the problem to the physician led to the physician's prompt medical diagnosis of cystitis and successful antibiotic therapy.

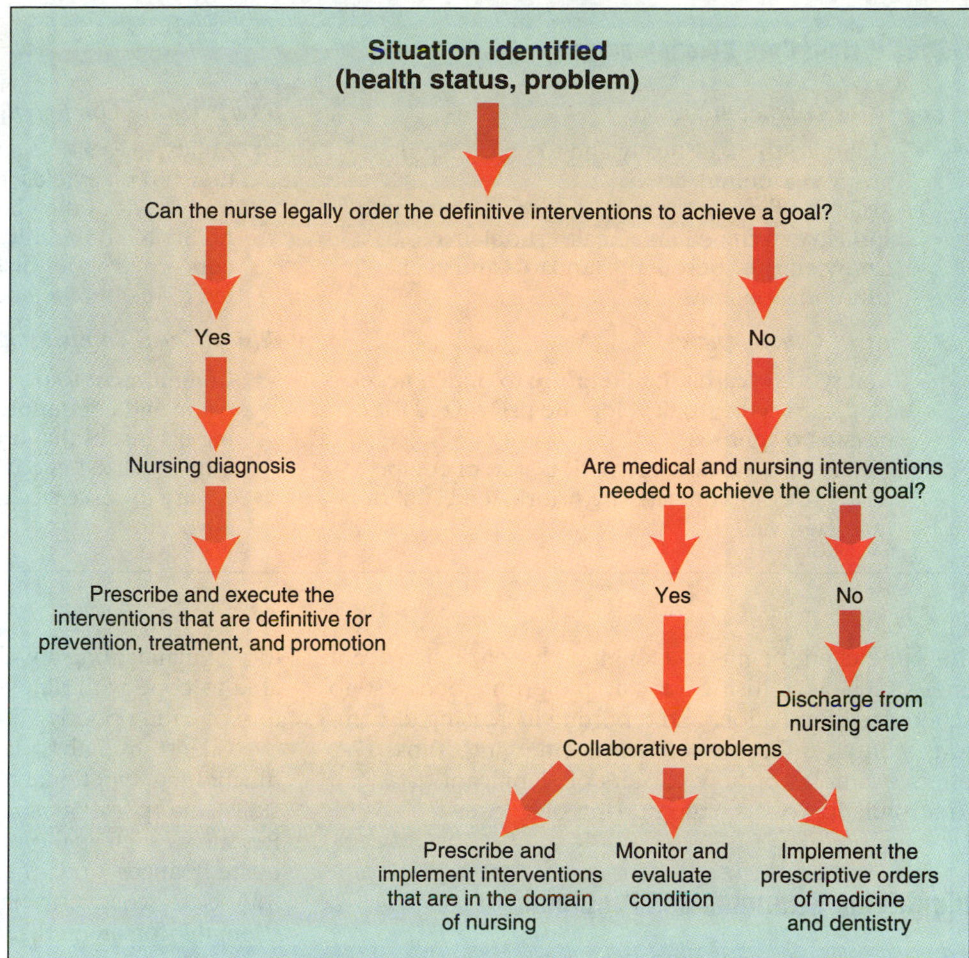

Figure 17-2
Differentiation of nursing diagnoses from collaborative problems. (©1990, 1988, 1985. Lynda Juall Carpenito. Used with permission. Carpenito, L. J. [1995]. *Nursing diagnosis: Application to clinical practice* [6th ed., p. 33]. Philadelphia: Lippincott.)

Data Interpretation and Analysis

Most experienced nurses begin the work of interpreting and analyzing data while they are still collecting (assessing) it. The term **cue** often is used to denote significant data or data that influence decisions. Such significant data should raise a red flag for the nurse, who then looks for patterns or clusters of data that signal an actual, potential, or possible nursing diagnosis.

Recognizing Significant Data

Sorting out *healthy* client responses from those that are *not healthy* is not as clear-cut as it may seem. To avoid erroneously labeling selected client health patterns as unhealthy while failing to detect actual unhealthy behavior, nurses must be familiar with comparative standards to be used in data interpretation and analysis.

Comparing Data With Standards. A standard or a norm is a generally accepted rule, measure, pattern, or model that can be used for comparing data in the same class or category. For example, when determining the significance of a client's blood pressure reading, appropriate standards include normative values for the client's age-group, race, and illness category. The client's own normal range, if known, is an important standard. A pressure of 150/90 may be high for someone whose pressure normally is 120/70, but it may be normal for a person with hypertension. Examples of how standards may be used to identify significant cues follow below (Gordon, 1994):

- Changes in a client's usual health patterns that are unexplained by expected norms for growth and development
- Deviation from an appropriate population norm
- Behavior that is nonproductive in the whole-person context
- Behavior that indicates a developmental lag or evolving dysfunctional pattern

Recognizing Patterns or Clusters

A **data cluster** is a grouping of client data or cues that points to the existence of a client health problem. Nursing diagnoses should always be derived from clusters of significant data, rather than from a single cue. The danger of deriving a nursing diagnosis from a single cue is illustrated in the following example. The nurse who diagnoses a woman recovering from gallbladder surgery with ineffective coping may have misinterpreted the client's use of tears as a healthy release of emotion. If

Diagnosing: Core Competencies

Cognitive Competencies

- Ability to think critically and to engage in diagnostic reasoning
- Ability to develop nursing diagnoses that are responsive to the client's health problems
- Knowledge of pertinent standards and agency/institutional policies

Technical Competencies

- Ability to research the literature to obtain necessary knowledge to develop the prioritized list of nursing diagnoses
- Ability to use a documentation system competently to communicate the prioritized list of nursing diagnoses

Interpersonal Competencies

- Ability to establish a trusting nurse–client relationship that yields knowledge of the individualized needs of the client
- Ability to communicate to the client that you are concerned about his/her priorities and committed to his/her well-being

Ethical/Legal Competencies

- Commitment to do whatever is necessary to develop and communicate a prioritized list of nursing diagnoses that are responsive to the client's individualized needs
- Ability to serve as a trusted and effective client advocate

the same client begins to exhibit a cluster of significant cues, such as refusing to eat, preferring bed rest to scheduled ambulation, and reporting increasing discomfort, then an unhealthy pattern is emerging. Table 17-2 offers examples of how clusters of significant data lead to formulation of accurate nursing diagnoses.

Identifying Strengths and Problems

The next step in analyzing data is to determine client strengths and problems.

Determining the Client's Strengths

If a client appears to meet a standard, the nurse then concludes that the client has a strength in that particular area, and that this strength contributes to the client's level of wellness. For example, a person who has a history of maintaining a well-balanced diet usually is better able to cope with illness than a person who has a history of eating poorly.

Client strengths may include healthy physiologic functioning, emotional health, cognitive abilities, coping skills, interpersonal strengths, and spiritual strengths. Resources such as the presence of support people, adequate finances, and a healthy environment may all contribute to client strengths. Many people take their strengths for granted, and may not know how to use them effectively when responding to illness. Discussing observed strengths with clients and counseling clients about ways to develop and use their strengths are important nursing measures.

Determining the Client's Problem Areas

A person who does not meet a certain health standard probably has a limitation in this aspect of health status,

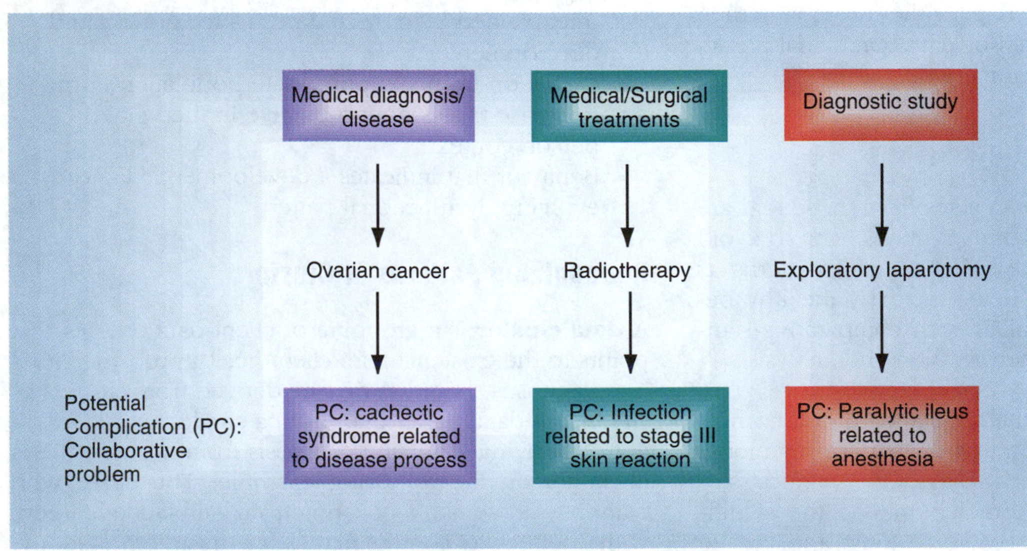

Figure 17-3
Collaborative problems.

Table 17-1
A Comparison: Nursing Diagnosis, Collaborative Problem, Medical Diagnosis

	Nursing Diagnosis	Collaborative Problem	Medical Diagnosis
Definition	A nursing diagnosis is a clinical judgment about individual, family, or community responses to actual or potential health problems or life processes. Nursing diagnosis provides the basis for selection of nursing interventions to achieve outcomes for which the nurse is accountable (NANDA)	Certain physiologic complications that nurses monitor to detect onset of changes in status (Carpenito)	Traumatic or disease condition or syndrome validated by medical diagnostic studies
Focus	Monitoring human responses to actual and potential health problems	Monitoring pathophysiologic responses of body organs or systems	Correcting or preventing pathology of specific organs or body systems
Sample data cluster	56-year-old mother of seven; 5′4″, 167 lb; "Whenever I sneeze lately, I dribble urine. This is embarrassing."	42-year-old woman; 1 hour after delivery; spinal anesthesia; 1500 mL fluid infused in past 4 hours without client voiding; unable to void	"Whenever I have to urinate it burns terribly. I also feel like I have to go all the time—real bad." Small, frequent voidings, cloudy urine; T—100.8°F
Diagnostic statement	Stress Incontinence related to degenerative changes in pelvic muscles and structural supports associated with advanced age, obesity, gravid uterus	Potential complication: urinary retention related to fluid overload and effects of anesthesia	Cystitis
Select nursing responses	Teach Kegel exercises to increase muscle tone; explore client's willingness and motivation to pursue weight reduction and exercise program; evaluate need for bladder-training program	Monitor for signs of increasing urine retention; offer bedpan and encourage voiding with running water, warm water dripped over perineum, etc; if no result, administer physician-prescribed medication; if no result, perform physician-prescribed catheterization	Report signs and symptoms to physician; obtain urine culture; report results to physician; administer appropriate physician-prescribed antibiotic

and may profit from professional services. For example, a person who has a long history of constipation is probably in need of care to help overcome this problem. As stated previously, the nurse makes a decision about whether the data represent a nursing diagnosis or a collaborative problem, or whether they should be reported to the physician because they might contribute to the identification of a medical diagnosis.

Determining Problems the Client Is Likely to Experience

It is important for the nurse to identify potential health problems. For example, the nurse notes that a client has signs of a wound infection, but laboratory test results show that the client's white blood cell count has not increased, as is usual when such an infection is present. The nurse concludes that the body apparently is not building up normal defenses to combat the infection. The nurse then predicts the problems this client is likely to encounter, such as a longer than normal healing period. This prediction has implications for nursing care, such as measures related to the client's diet, fluid intake, urine output, and mobility.

When determining strengths and problems, it is helpful to determine if the client agrees with the nurse's identification of a problem and is motivated to work toward its resolution.

Critical Thinking Exercise 17-2

Try to interview two clients with the same medical diagnosis. Develop a prioritized list of nursing diagnoses for both and reflect on the differences. Compare and contrast the strengths of both clients. If you can do this exercise with another student, explore why there are differences between the lists of nursing diagnoses and client strengths you and your partner develop.

Table 17-2
Diagnosing

Data Interpretation and Analysis		Formulation of Tentative Nursing Diagnosis	Validation of Nursing Diagnosis
Significant Cues	*Sample Data Clusters*		
Change in a client's usual health patterns that is unexplained by expected norms for growth and development	• "I guess I lost about 20 to 30 pounds over the last 6 months—I think I've just been too busy to eat." • Height: 5′8″ • Weight: 102 lb • 35-year-old mother of 4-year-old twin boys; returned to work (executive secretary) for first time since delivery of twins 7 months ago	Altered Nutrition: Less Than Body Requirements, related to stress of new job; role conflict and demands	Accurate diagnosis: Client validates this diagnosis, agreeing with contributing factors
Deviation from an appropriate population norm	• Teacher notices and reports frequency of bruises on third-grade boy who is repeatedly observed alone during recess periods and who is withdrawn in classroom • In conversation with the school nurse, one parent remarks: "That boy brings out the worst in me! I don't know why but I often have to smack him hard to make him listen."	High Risk for Violence (Child Abuse) related to ? etiology (deficient parenting skills?)	Incomplete diagnosis: Additional data collection yields new information: • Father out of work for past 18 months • Father was abused as a child Diagnosis restated: High Risk For Violence (Child Abuse) related to increased family stress and father's history of being abused
Behavior that is nonproductive in the whole-person context	• Fiancé abruptly terminated relationship 3 months before established wedding date • Noticeable change in physical appearance; frequently wears same clothes; makeup, jewelry, hair-styling are absent; strong body odors present • No desire to be with others; goes home (lives alone) immediately after work • Stopped attending aerobics classes	Self-Esteem Disturbance related to feeling rejected by fiancé	Premature diagnosis resulting from incomplete data collection. Client has a long history of major depressive states, one of which may have resulted in the breakup of this relationship. Medical diagnosis and treatment indicated. Changes in appearance are indicative of depressive state. Need to explore related nursing diagnoses.
Behavior indicating developmental lags or evolving dysfunctional patterns	• Admitted to nursing home 2 months ago • "I have nothing to live for anymore . . . why don't I die?" • Wishes to remain in room seated in chair—will only ambulate with great urging • Anything requiring movement has become "too much bother." • Decreased muscle mass, tone, and strength; reduced joint mobility	Impaired Physical Mobility related to difficult transition to nursing home	Accurate but routinized diagnosis that may result in staff's acceptance of status quo unless a more specific cause is identified

Reaching Conclusions

The nurse reaches one of four basic conclusions after interpreting and analyzing the client data. Different nursing responses are possible for each conclusion:

- No problem
  - No nursing response indicated
  - Reinforce client's health habits and patterns
  - Initiate health promotion activities to prevent disease or illness or to promote a higher level of wellness
  - Wellness diagnosis may be indicated
- Possible problem
  - Collect more data to confirm or disconfirm suspected problem

Actual or potential nursing diagnosis
- Unable to treat because client denies problem and refuses treatment (make sure client understands possible outcomes of this stance)
- Begin planning, implementing, and evaluating care designed to prevent, reduce, or resolve the problem

Clinical problem other than nursing diagnosis
- Consult with appropriate healthcare professional and work collaboratively on problem
- Refer to appropriate healthcare professional

Formulating and Validating Nursing Diagnoses

Writing Nursing Diagnoses

NANDA List of Nursing Diagnoses

Those just beginning to write nursing diagnoses may find it helpful to consult the list of health problems accepted by the North American Nursing Diagnosis Association (NANDA) for testing and study. The accompanying box lists the current nursing diagnoses from NANDA. The NANDA list is a beginning list of suggested terms for health problems that may be identified and treated by nurses. Each of the diagnostic category labels accepted by NANDA consists of three components: (1) the title or label that provides a name for the diagnosis that is a concise description of the health problem, (2) causative and contributing factors, and (3) defining characteristics. There are distinct advantages to nurses' use of common terminology when formulating nursing diagnoses.

Pocket-sized handbooks of NANDA-approved nursing diagnoses are available, and may be of great help to the student who is unfamiliar with this grouping of problem statements. Nurses who encounter different health problems within the scope of their practices that they believe to be nursing diagnoses may submit these to the NANDA Diagnosis Review Committee.

Two- and Three-Part Statements

Once the nurse recognizes a cluster of significant client data indicating a health problem that can be treated by independent nursing intervention, it is time to write the nursing diagnosis. Most nursing diagnoses are written either as two-part statements listing the client's problem and its cause or as three-part statements that also include the problem's defining characteristics (Table 17-3).

Problem. The purpose of the problem statement is to describe the health state or health problem of the client as clearly and concisely as possible. Because this section of the nursing diagnosis identifies what is unhealthy about the client and what the client would like to change in his or her health status, it suggests client goals. NANDA recommends use of the following quantifiers when writing the problem statement: altered, impaired, depleted, deficient, excessive, dysfunctional, disturbed, ineffective, decreased, increased, acute, chronic, and intermittent.

Etiology. The etiology identifies the physiologic, psychologic, sociologic, spiritual, and environmental factors believed to be related to the problem as either a cause or a contributing factor. Because the etiology identifies the factors that are maintaining the unhealthy client state and preventing the desired change, the etiology directs nursing intervention. Unless the etiology is correctly identified, nursing actions may be inefficient and ineffective. For example, a diabetic client who is frequently admitted to the hospital with hyperglycemia and who has a poor history of dietary and pharmacologic management is diagnosed to be noncompliant. Assuming that the noncompliance is related to a knowledge deficit and then channeling all nursing activities and energies into teaching the client how to manage the diabetes is useless if the noncompliance is actually a result of the client's decreased will to live.

Defining Characteristics. The subjective and objective data that signal the existence of the actual or potential health problem are the third component of the nursing diagnosis. NANDA has identified defining characteristics for each accepted nursing diagnosis, and familiarity with these characteristics assists nurses in recognizing clusters of significant data. Table 17-3 defines the three components of a nursing diagnosis statement and shows how they affect client goals, nursing measures, and evaluation. Other examples of nursing diagnosis statements are found throughout the book.

Guidelines for Writing Nursing Diagnoses

The following guidelines will help the student nurse learn to write nursing diagnoses and statements:

1. Phrase the nursing diagnosis as a client problem or alteration in health state rather than as a client need.
2. Check to make sure that the client problem precedes the etiology and that the two are linked by the phrase *related to.*
3. Defining characteristics, when included in the nursing diagnosis, should follow the etiology and be linked by the phrase *as manifested by.*
4. Write in legally advisable terms.
5. Use nonjudgmental language.
6. Be sure the problem statement indicates what is unhealthy about the client or what the client wants to change (enhance).
7. Avoid using defining characteristics, medical diagnoses, or something that cannot be changed in the problem statement.
8. Reread the diagnosis to make sure the problem statement suggests client goals and that the etiology will direct the selection of nursing measures.

...g Diagnoses

Activity Intolerance
Activity Intolerance, Risk for
Adaptive Capacity: Intracranial, Decreased
Adjustment, Impaired
Airway Clearance, Ineffective
Anxiety
Aspiration, Risk for
Body Image Disturbance
Body Temperature, Risk for Altered
Breastfeeding, Effective
Breastfeeding, Ineffective
Breastfeeding, Interrupted
Breathing Pattern, Ineffective
Caregiver Role Strain
Caregiver Role Strain, Risk for
Communication, Impaired Verbal
Community Coping, Ineffective
Community Coping, Potential for Enhanced
Confusion, Acute
Confusion, Chronic
Constipation
Constipation, Colonic
Constipation, Perceived
Decisional Conflict (Specify)
Decreased Cardiac Output
Defensive Coping
Denial, Ineffective
Diarrhea
Disorganized Infant Behavior
Disorganized Infant Behavior, Risk for
Disuse Syndrome, Risk for
Diversional Activity Deficit
Dysfunctional Grieving
Dysfunctional Ventilatory Weaning Response
Dysreflexia
Energy Field Disturbance
Environmental Interpretation Syndrome, Impaired
Family Coping: Compromised, Ineffective
Family Coping: Disabling, Ineffective
Family Coping: Potential for Growth
Family Process: Alcoholism, Altered
Family Processes, Altered
Fatigue
Fear
Fluid Volume Deficit
Fluid Volume Deficit, Risk for
Fluid Volume Excess
Functional Incontinence
Gas Exchange, Impaired
Grieving, Anticipatory
Grieving, Dysfunctional
Growth and Development, Altered
Health Maintenance, Altered
Health Seeking Behaviors (Specify)
Home Maintenance Management, Impaired
Hopelessness
Hyperthermia
Hypothermia
Incontinence, Bowel
Incontinence, Functional
Incontinence, Reflex
Incontinence, Stress
Incontinence, Total
Incontinence, Urge
Individual Coping, Ineffective
Infant Feeding Pattern, Ineffective
Infection, Risk for
Injury, Risk for
Knowledge Deficit (Specify)
Loneliness, Risk for
Management of Therapeutic Regimen: Community, Ineffective
Management of Therapeutic Regimen: Families; Ineffective
Management of Therapeutic Regimen: Individual, Effective
Management of Therapeutic Regimen (Individuals), Ineffective Noncompliance (Specify)
Memory, Impaired
Nutrition: Less than body requirements, Altered
Nutrition: More than body requirements, Altered
Nutrition: Potential for more than body requirements, Altered
Oral Mucous Membrane, Altered
Organized Infant Behavior, Potential for Enhanced
Pain
Pain, Chronic
Parent/Infant/Child Attachment, Risk for Altered
Parental Role Conflict
Parenting, Altered
Parenting, Risk for Altered
Perioperative Positioning Injury, Risk for
Peripheral Neurovascular Dysfunction, Risk for
Personal Identity Disturbance
Physical Mobility, Impaired
Poisoning, Risk for
Post-Trauma Response
Powerlessness
Protection, Altered
Rape-Trauma Syndrome
Rape-Trauma Syndrome: Compound Reaction
Rape-Trauma Syndrome: Silent Reaction
Relocation Stress Syndrome
Role Performance, Altered
Self Care Deficit
  Bathing/Hygiene
  Feeding
  Dressing/Grooming
  Toileting
Self Esteem, Chronic Low
Self Esteem, Situational Low
Self Esteem Disturbance
Self-Mutilation, Risk for
Sensory/Perceptual Alterations (Specify) (visual, auditory, kinesthetic, gustatory, tactile, olfactory)
Sexual Dysfunction
Sexuality Patterns, Altered
Skin Integrity, Impaired
Skin Integrity, Risk for Impaired
Sleep Pattern Disturbance
Social Interaction, Impaired
Social Isolation
Spiritual Distress
Spiritual Well-Being, Potential for Enhanced
Suffocation, Risk for
Sustain Spontaneous Ventilation, Inability to
Swallowing, Impaired
Thermoregulation, Ineffective
Thought Processes, Altered
Tissue Integrity, Impaired
Tissue Perfusion, Altered (Specify Type) (Renal, cerebral, cardiopulmonary, gastrointestinal, peripheral)
Trauma, Risk for
Unilateral Neglect
Urinary Elimination, Altered
Urinary Retention
Violence, Risk for: Self-directed or directed at others

North American Nursing Diagnosis Association (1994). NANDA nursing diagnoses: Definitions and classification, 1995–1996. Philadelphia: NANDA.

Table 17-3
Formulation of Nursing Diagnosis Statements

	Definition	Purpose	Example
Problem	Identifies what is unhealthy about the client, indicating the need for change (clear, concise statement of the client health problem)	Suggests the client goals (expectations for change)	Bathing/Hygiene Self-Care Deficit ↓ related to ↓
Etiology	Identifies the factors that are maintaining the unhealthy state or response (contributing or causative factors)	Suggests the appropriate nursing measures	Fear of falling in the tub and obesity ↓ as manifested by ↓
Defining characteristics	Identify the subjective and objective data that signal the existence of the problem (cues that reflect the existence of a problem)	Suggest evaluative criteria	Strong body and urine odor, unclean hair: "I'm afraid I'll fall in the tub and break something." (5′4″, 170 lb)

Examples:

Two-part diagnostic statement: Bathing/Hygiene Self-Care Deficit related to fear of falling in tub and obesity

Three-part diagnostic statement: Bathing/Hygiene Self-Care Deficit related to fear of falling in tub and obesity, as manifested by strong body and urine odor, unclean hair, statement of fearing fall in tub, and height and weight: 5′4″, 170 lb

Common errors in writing nursing diagnoses are shown in Table 17-4, along with suggestions for correcting them.

What Is Not a Nursing Diagnosis

The nursing diagnosis statement is written in terms of a client problem, alteration in health state, or client strength *for which nursing provides the primary therapy.* The following are not nursing diagnoses: medical diagnoses, medical pathology, diagnostic tests, treatments, or equipment. Similarly, although all the following need to be considered when identifying nursing diagnoses, they do not belong as such in the diagnosis statement: therapeutic client needs, therapeutic client goals, a single sign or symptom, or an *unvalidated* nursing inference. Examples of these items, frequently and erroneously placed in nursing diagnoses, appear in Table 17-5. Illustrations are derived from clients with diabetes mellitus.

Actual, Potential (Risk), and Possible Nursing Diagnoses

Client health problems may be **actual** (problem is present), **potential** (problem may occur), and **possible** (problem may be present).

A potential nursing diagnosis is written when the health problem is likely to occur unless the nurse intervenes in a particular way. NANDA-approved diagnoses once designated as "potential" were labeled "high risk" in 1992 and changed to "risk" in 1994. NANDA's definition of a risk nursing diagnosis is as follows (NANDA, 1994):

> [Risk nursing diagnoses] describe human responses to levels of wellness in an individual, family, or community that have a potential for enhancement to a higher state.

A possible nursing diagnosis is written when the nurse suspects that a health problem exists but needs to gather more data to confirm the diagnosis (Carpenito, 1995, p. 16).

An actual nursing diagnosis for a client who has experienced vomiting, diarrhea, and excessive diaphoresis for 3 days is *Fluid Volume Deficit related to abnormal fluid loss.* If the diarrhea persists and weakness interferes with the client's normal perineal hygiene, he or she may be at risk for skin breakdown. This is written as the potential diagnosis *Risk for Impaired Skin Integrity.* If the nurse suspects that a disturbance of self-concept also is present but lacks the necessary data (defining characteristics) to confirm this, it can be written as a possible diagnosis: *Possible Disturbance in Self-Concept.* This alerts other nurses to the need to collect more data about the client's self-concept.

Wellness Diagnoses

A persistent critique of nursing diagnoses that focus exclusively on client health problems is their limited applicability in nursing settings that primarily deal with healthy clients. To remedy this concern, **wellness diag-**

Table 17-4
Common Errors in Writing Nursing Diagnoses and Recommended Corrections

Error	Example	Correction	Example
Writing the diagnosis in terms of needs and not response	Needs assistance with bathing related to bed rest	Write the diagnosis in terms of response rather than need	Self-Care Deficit: Bathing related to immobility
Making legally inadvisable statements	Noncompliance due to hostility toward nursing staff (the words *due to* imply a direct cause-and-effect relationship)	Use "related to" rather than "due to" or "caused by" to link the etiology to the problem statement	Noncompliance related to hostility toward nursing staff (denotes a relation between the problem and etiology but not necessarily a causal relation)
	Spouse Abuse related to husband's immaturity and violent temper	Write diagnosis in legally advisable terms: statements that may be interpreted as libel or that imply nursing negligence are legally hazardous to all the nurses caring for the client	High Risk for Violence: Spouse Abuse related to husband's reported inability to control behavior.
	Impaired Skin Integrity related to client's lying on back all night		Impaired Skin Integrity related to mobility deficit
Identifying as a problem a client response that is not necessarily unhealthy	Mild Anxiety related to impending surgery	Include in the problem statement of the nursing diagnosis only client responses that are unhealthy or that the client wants to change	No need for nursing diagnosis: mild anxiety before surgery is a healthy response that motivates preoperative self-care behavior
Identifying as a problem signs and symptoms of illness	Cough related to long history of smoking	Avoid including signs and symptoms of illness in the problem statement of the nursing diagnosis	Ineffective Airway Clearance related to 20-year history of smoking
Identifying as a client problem or etiology what cannot be changed	Alterations in Bowel Elimination: Permanent Colostomy related to cancer of bowel	Express the problem statement and etiologic factors in terms that can be changed; otherwise, nursing energies are being directed to a hopeless task	Self-Care Deficit: Care of Colostomy, related to severe anxiety about cancer and feelings of powerlessness
	Grieving related to death of spouse		Dysfunctional Grieving related to inability to accept death of spouse
Identifying environmental factors rather than client factors as a problem	Cluttered Home related to inability to discard anything	Express the problem statement in terms of unhealthy client responses rather than environmental conditions	High Risk for Injury related to cluttered home (inability to discard anything)
Reversing clauses	Knowledge Deficit related to alteration in parenting	Avoid reversing the problem statement and etiologic statement	Altered Parenting related to knowledge deficit: Child growth and development, discipline
Having both clauses say the same thing	Alteration in Comfort related to pain (pain *is* the comfort alteration—what is contributing to the pain?)	Be sure that the *two* parts of the diagnosis do not mean the same thing	Unrelieved Incisional Pain related to fear of addiction
Including value judgments in the nursing diagnosis	Poor Home Maintenance Management related to laziness	Write the diagnosis without value judgments; avoid words such as poor, inadequate, abnormal, unhealthy	Impaired Home Maintenance Management related to low value ascribed to home safety and cleanliness
Including the medical diagnosis in the diagnostic statement	Impaired Home Maintenance Management related to arthritis	Do not include the medical diagnosis in the nursing diagnosis statement	Impaired Home Maintenance Management related to mobility, endurance, and comfort alterations

(Common errors adapted from Mundinger, M. O., & Jauron, G. D. [1975]. Developing a nursing diagnosis. *Nursing Outlook, 23*[2], 94–98. Guidelines for writing nursing diagnoses adapted from Iyer, P., Taptich, B., & Bernocchi-Losey, D. [1991]. *Nursing process and nursing diagnoses* [2nd ed.]. Philadelphia: Saunders)

Table 17-5
What a Nursing Diagnosis Is Not, and Why

What a Nursing Diagnosis is Not	Example	Rationale
Medical diagnosis	Diabetes mellitus	Although there is nursing care associated with medical illnesses, the illness is not primarily amenable to nursing intervention. Nursing's concern is the *person* who has the illness and the effect of the illness on human functioning.
Medical pathology	Hypoglycemia	Nurses need to understand the pathology underlying disease states to plan appropriate nursing care, but once again, nursing's focus is the person, not the pathology. The person's response to hypoglycemia, how hypoglycemia affects human functioning—these are the domain of *nursing* diagnoses.
Diagnostic tests, treatments, equipment	Fasting blood glucose Insulin therapy Insulin syringe Infusion pump	Nursing's concern is the person's response to the diagnostic study, treatment, or equipment. If the need for insulin therapy reveals a knowledge deficit or self-care deficit, this becomes the nursing diagnosis, not insulin therapy in and of itself.
Therapeutic client needs	Needs to learn the relation among diet, exercise, and insulin	The diagnosis should be written as a client health problem rather than a client need. *Example:* Altered Health Maintenance (Diabetic Care) related to lack of knowledge of relation among diet, exercise, and insulin.
Therapeutic nursing goals	To develop therapeutic diabetic self-care behaviors	The diagnosis should be written from the client perspective rather than the nursing perspective and phrased as a client health problem. *Example:* Self-Care Deficit: Diabetic Self-Care Behaviors, related to decreased value on life and decreased motivation to learn.
A single sign or symptom	After successfully administering own insulin for 3 days client tells nurse, "You give me my shot today."	A nursing diagnosis is not developed until a pattern or cluster of significant cues is detected. The signs and symptoms lead to the identification of the problem statement but are not the problem statement. In this situation, no nursing diagnosis is indicated until further data collection, interpretation, and analysis take place.
An *unvalidated* nursing inference	Above incident leads to the nursing inference: Noncompliance related to depression	This is a premature nursing diagnosis that may not accurately reflect a client problem. More data and the validation of the tentative nursing diagnosis (nursing inference) are needed before the diagnoses can be recorded.

noses were proposed and are now readily accepted. According to NANDA (1990), a "wellness diagnosis is a clinical judgment about an individual, family, or community in transition from a specific level of wellness to a higher level of wellness" (p. 117). The diagnostic statement for wellness diagnoses is a one-part statement that contains the label *Potential for Enhanced* followed by the desired higher-level wellness. Examples include Potential for Enhanced Family Coping, Potential for Enhanced Health Maintenance, Potential for Enhanced Parenting, Potential for Enhanced Self-Esteem.

Validating Nursing Diagnoses

Once a tentative nursing diagnosis is formulated, it should be validated. Price (1980, p. 670) indicates that an affirmative response to each of the following questions validates a tentative diagnosis:

- Is my data base sufficient, accurate, and derived from some concept of nursing?
- Does my synthesis of data (significant cues) demonstrate the existence of a pattern?
- Are the subjective and objective data I used to determine the existence of a pattern characteristic of the health problem I defined?
- Is my tentative nursing diagnosis based on scientific nursing knowledge and clinical expertise?
- Is my tentative nursing diagnosis able to be prevented, reduced, or resolved by independent nursing action?
- Is my degree of confidence above 50% that other qualified practitioners would formulate the same nursing diagnosis based on my data?

In addition, clients who are able to participate in decision making should be encouraged to validate the diagnosis. "It seems to me that bathing has become a problem now that you are afraid of falling in the tub. What's your sense of this?" Table 17-2 lists possible outcomes of validating tentative nursing diagnoses.

Prioritizing Nursing Diagnoses and Documentation

To develop a prioritized list of nursing diagnoses, the nurse needs guidelines for ranking diagnoses as high, medium, or low priority. High-priority diagnoses pose the greatest threat to the client's well-being. Non–life-threatening diagnoses are ranked as medium priorities, and diagnoses that are not specifically related to the current illness and prognosis are of low priority. In all levels, psychosocial needs must be considered as well as physiologic needs. Three helpful guides suggested by Atkinson and Murray (1990) for prioritizing client problems are Maslow's hierarchy of human needs, client preference, and anticipation of future problems.

Maslow's Hierarchy of Human Needs

Because lower needs must be met before a person can focus on higher ones, client needs may be prioritized according to the following hierarchy: physiologic needs—safety needs—love and belonging needs—self-esteem needs—self-actualization needs. *Example:* A geriatric client who is incontinent of urine and sitting in a wet disposable brief (physiologic need) will be unable to participate fully in a music therapy diversional activity (self-esteem need).

Client Preference

It is best to first meet the needs the client thinks are most important, if this order does not interfere with other vital therapies. *Example:* A woman is admitted to an orthopedic unit with a fractured pelvis and multiple lacerations after an automobile accident. The morning after the accident she complains of pain and needs assistance with bathing and attention to her lacerations, but she refuses to do anything until she calls home to find out who is caring for her 15-month-old twins.

Anticipation of Future Problems

The knowledge base of the nurse must be tapped to consider the potential effects of different courses of nursing action. Assigning low priority to a diagnosis the client wants to ignore when this can result in harmful future consequences for the client may be nursing negligence. *Example:* An obese client with multiple sclerosis and greatly decreased limb strength who spends most of her day in bed may see no value in diet modification and position changes. The nurse who is alert to the potential, serious problem of pressure ulcers would assign high priority to this diagnosis and incorporate weight management and position changes into the plan of care, despite the client's reluctance to do so.

Once the prioritized list of nursing diagnoses is developed, the nurse documents this on the nursing plan of care. Depending on the documentation system in use, nursing diagnoses also may be recorded on the multidisciplinary problem list at the front of the client record.

Critical Thinking Exercise 17-3

Interview several experienced nurses. Find at least one nurse who is strongly committed to using nursing diagnoses and another who believes they are a waste of time. Interview both until you can explain their different experiences with nursing diagnoses. List the benefits and limitations of using nursing diagnoses.

Nursing Diagnosis: A Critique

The current nursing diagnosis literature contains many examples of nurses writing about how using nursing diagnosis has improved their clinical practice; one also finds articles that detail the many benefits nursing diagnosis brings to the profession. Conversely, there are articles that point out the limitations of nursing diagnosis and that urge nurses to be cautious, so that an uncritical use of nursing diagnosis does not restrict their practices.

The primary benefit that nursing diagnosis offers the client is the individualization of client care. For example, nurses may be caring simultaneously for three women who have had a modified radical mastectomy because of breast cancer. Although the postoperative nursing management of these women will be similar, priorities of care may differ. A prioritized list of nursing diagnoses enables nurses to direct their energies toward these differing client priorities:

Client A: Body Image Disturbance
Ineffective Individual Coping
Client B: Pain
Self-Care Deficit
Client C: High Risk for Sexual Dysfunction
Powerlessness

The use of nursing diagnosis also allows clients to be informed and willing participants in their care as they validate their diagnoses and assist in prioritizing them.

Improved communication among nurses and other healthcare professionals is probably the most important benefit that accurate, up-to-date diagnoses—expressed in well-defined and standardized terminology—offer nurses. This communication aids in planning, charting, client data retrieval, health team conferences, change-of-shift reports, and healthcare follow-up. It also promotes nursing accountability for the problems that nurses diagnose.

Among the other benefits that nursing diagnoses offer the profession is help in defining the domain of nursing to healthcare administrators, legislators, and other healthcare providers; this is important when seeking funding for nursing and reimbursement for nursing services. Nursing diagnoses also are used to define curriculum content and to direct specialization and advancement in nursing and nursing research.

When the diagnostic process is used incorrectly, a client may be "misdiagnosed." Premature diagnoses based on an incomplete data base, erroneous diagnoses resulting from an inaccurate data base or a faulty data analysis, and routinized diagnoses resulting from the nurse's failure to tailor data collection and analysis to the unique needs of the client are common sources of error.

Failure to modify diagnoses and to identify new diagnoses as the client's status changes also may be problems. Failures in diagnosis lead to failures in nursing care. All of the above are not so much limitations of nursing diagnosis as they are limitations of the nurses who are diagnosing incorrectly.

Nurses who are inexperienced in working with diagnoses may become frustrated because attempts to standardize nursing diagnoses are still in the early stages; confusion exists about the need to standardize and the best way to do it. Individual nurses working together at any one time may have different exposures to nursing diagnoses and may differ widely in their commitment to the use of nursing diagnoses in practice. Once nurses master skills in developing nursing diagnoses and begin to use them to direct care, it is believed that these difficulties will be minimized.

More serious criticisms of nursing diagnosis are raised by nurses who claim that a classification of standardized nursing diagnoses limits nursing, curbing nurses' originality and ability to think things through.

Although some nurses believe that diagnosis offers a valued shortcut to practice, critics find this offensive, and respond that rather than invest nursing's energies in perfecting a shortcut, nurses need to change the working conditions that interfere with in-depth problem solving and thoughtful nursing care.

Critics of diagnostic labeling point out that instead of identifying what is unique and positive about nursing, nursing diagnoses make a clear statement that nurses are concerned about what is deviant, wrong, or pathologic (Hagey & McDonough, 1984). The ever-changing and dynamic human person with a need for nursing care becomes objectified (Gebbie, 1984).

Nurses who are sensitive to transcultural issues raise important concerns about the cultural limitations of the NANDA diagnoses. Foremost among these concerns is that NANDA diagnoses and behaviors assume that the client is "wrong" and the provider is "right," and deny the validity of cultural and healthcare beliefs and practices that are different from those of the nurse (Geissler, 1991). Examples of nursing diagnoses that often are misused in labeling such cultural deviations as abnormal include Impaired Verbal Communication, Impaired Social Interaction, and Noncompliance.

In conclusion, nursing diagnosis has become a valued and essential step in the nursing process. Used correctly, it is a powerful tool for individualizing client care, and ensures that nursing's energies are being used in the most efficient way to meet client needs. Nurses who are as concerned about the art and spirit of nursing as they are about its science are careful to avoid labeling clients in a way that objectifies them or limits the potential range of nurse–client interactions.

Key Points

- The purpose of diagnosing is the identification of (1) problems in the way the client is responding to health or illness, (2) factors that contribute to or cause these problems (etiologies), and (3) strengths the client can draw on to prevent or resolve the problems.
- Actual or potential health problems that independent nursing intervention can prevent or resolve are termed nursing diagnoses.
- Once significant client data are detected, the nurse looks for data clusters that signal a client strength or problem, and checks out these findings with the client.
- The interpretation and analysis of client data may lead to the identification of nursing diagnoses or collaborative problems (best treated by nurses working together with other healthcare professionals) or, when shared with a physician, may contribute to medical diagnoses.
- Most nursing diagnoses are written as either two-part statements that contain the client problem and its etiology connected by the words *related to*, or as three-part statements that include the problem's defining characteristics.
- A wellness diagnosis is a one-part statement that contains the label *Potential for Enhanced* followed by the desired higher-level wellness.
- The problem component of the nursing diagnosis identifies what is unhealthy about the client, indicating the need for change. It suggests the client goals. The etiology identifies the factors that are maintaining the unhealthy state or response and suggests the appropriate nursing intervention. The defining characteristics are the subjective and objective data that initially signaled the existence of the problem. They suggest evaluative criteria.
- Although nursing care may be related to the following, they are not nursing diagnoses and should not appear in the diagnostic statement: medical diagnosis, medical pathology, diagnostic tests, treatments, equipment, therapeutic client needs, therapeutic client goals, a single sign or symptom, and *unvalidated* nursing inferences.
- Other sources of error when writing nursing diagnoses include making legally inadvisable statements, reversing the clauses, identifying environmental factors rather than client factors as the problem, identifying as a client response what is not necessarily unhealthful, having both clauses say the same thing, and identifying as a client problem what cannot be changed.
- Three helpful guides for prioritizing client problems are Maslow's hierarchy of human needs, client preference, and anticipation of future problems.

Bibliography

Alfaro, R. (1994). *Applying the nursing process: A step-by-step guide* (3rd ed.). Philadelphia: Lippincott.

American Nurses Association. (1980). *Nursing: A social policy statement.* Washington, DC: ANA.

Anderson, B., & Hannah, K. J. (1993). A Canadian nursing data set: A major priority. *Canadian Journal of Nursing Administration, 6*(2), 7–13.

Aspinall, M. J. (1976). Nursing diagnosis: the weak link. *Nursing Outlook, 24*(7), 433–436.

Atkinson, J., & Murray, M. E. (1990). *Understanding the nursing process* (4th ed.). New York: Macmillan.

Brackstone, A., & Cooper-Page, L. (1993). Rekindling the nursing diagnosis flame. *The Canadian Nurse, 89*(4), 23–25.

Carnevali, D. L., Mitchell, P. H., Woods, N. F., & Tanner, C. A. (1984). *Diagnostic reasoning in nursing.* Philadelphia: Lippincott.

Carnevali, D. L., & Thomas, M. D. (1993). *Diagnostic reasoning and treatment decisionmaking in nursing.* Philadelphia: Lippincott.

Carpenito, L. J. (1985). Diagnostics: Actual, potential, or possible? *American Journal of Nursing, 85*(4), 485.

Carpenito, L. J. (1995). *Nursing diagnosis: Application to clinical practice* (6th ed.). Philadelphia: Lippincott.

Carroll-Johnson, R. M. (Ed.). (1991). *Classification in nursing diagnosis: Proceedings of the ninth conference.* Philadelphia: Lippincott.

Dobrzyn, J. (1995). Components of written nursing diagnostic statements. *Nursing Diagnosis, 6*(1), 29–35.

Dossey, B., & Guzzetta, C. E. (1981). Nursing diagnosis. *Nursing, 11*(6), 34–38.

Dougherty, C. M., Jankin, J. J., Lunney, M. R., & Whitley, G. G. (1993). Conceptual and research-based validation of nursing diagnoses: 1950–1993. *Nursing Diagnosis, 4*(4), 156–165.

Fitzpatrick, J. J., Kerr, M. E., Saba. V. K., Hoskins, L. M., Hurley, M. E., Milles, W. C., Rottkamp, B. C., Warren, J. J., & Carpenito, L. J. (1989). Translating nursing diagnosis into ICD code. *American Journal of Nursing, 89*(4), 493–495.

Gebbie, K. M. (Ed.). (1975). *Summary of the second national conference.* St. Louis: Clearinghouse for Nursing Diagnoses.

Gebbie, K. M. (1984). Nursing diagnosis: What is it and why does it exist? *Topics in Clinical Nursing, 5*(4), 1–9.

Gebbie, K. M., & Lavin, M. A. (1973). *Summary of the first national conference.* St. Louis: Mosby.

Geissler, E. M. (1991). Transcultural nursing and nursing diagnosis. *Nursing and Health Care, 12*(4), 190–192, 203.

Gordon, M. (1976). Nursing diagnosis and the diagnostic process. *American Journal of Nursing, 76*(8), 1298–1300.

Gordon, M. (1994). *Nursing diagnosis: Process and application* (3rd ed.). St Louis: Mosby.

Gordon, M. (1995). *Manual of nursing diagnosis: 1995–1996 edition.* St. Louis: Mosby–Year Book.

Hagey, R. S., & McDonough, P. (1984). The problem of professional labeling. *Nursing Outlook, 32*(3), 151–157.

Hammond, K. R. (1966). Clinical inference in nursing: A psychologist's view point. *Nursing Research, 15*(1), 27–38.

Hardy, E. (1983). The diagnostic wheel: Identifying care that is unique to nursing. *Canadian Nurse, 79*(3), 38–40.

Harvey, R. M. (1993). Nursing diagnosis by computers: An application of neural networks. *Nursing Diagnosis, 4*(1), 26–34.

Hurley, M. (Ed.). (1986). *Classification of nursing diagnoses: Proceedings of the sixth conference.* St. Louis: Mosby.

Iyer, P., Taptich, B., & Bernocchi-Losey, D. (1991). *Nursing process and nursing diagnosis* (2nd ed.). Philadelphia: Saunders.

Kerr, M., et al. (1993). Taxonomic validation: An overview. *Nursing Diagnosis, 4*(1), 6–14.

Kim, M. J., McFarland, G. K., & McLane, A. M. (Eds.). (1984). *Classification of nursing diagnosis: Proceedings of the fifth national conference.* St. Louis: Mosby.

Kim, M. J., & Moritz, D. A. (1982). *Classification of the third and fourth national conferences.* Highstown, NJ: McGraw-Hill.

Kritek, P. B. (1985). Nursing diagnosis in perspective: Response to a critique. *IMAGE: Journal of Nursing Scholarship, 17*(1), 3–8.

Lindsey, A. M. (1990). Identification and labeling of human responses. *Journal of Professional Nursing, 6*(3), 143–150.

Lunney, M. (1982). Nursing diagnosis: Refining the system. *American Journal of Nursing, 82*(3), 456–459.

Martens, K. (1986). Let's diagnose strengths, not just problems. *American Journal of Nursing, 86*(2), 192–193.

McLane, A. M. (Ed.). (1987). *Classification of nursing diagnoses: Proceedings of the seventh conference.* St. Louis: Mosby.

Mitchell, G. J. (1991). Nursing diagnosis: An ethical analysis. *IMAGE: Journal of Nursing Scholarship, 23*(2), 99–103.

Mundinger, M. O., & Jauron, G. D. (1975). Developing a nursing diagnosis. *Nursing Outlook, 23*, 94–98.

North American Nursing Diagnosis Association. (1990). *Taxonomy I revised with official diagnostic categories.* St. Louis: Author.

North American Nursing Diagnosis Association. (1994). *NANDA nursing diagnoses: Definitions and classification, 1995–1996.* Philadelphia: NANDA.

Nursing Diagnosis Newsletter. [Now a journal: *Nursing Diagnosis*]. North American Nursing Diagnosis Association.

Popkess, S. (1981). Diagnosing your patient's strengths. *Nursing, 11*(7), 34–37.

Popkess, S., & Vawter, S. (1991). Wellness nursing diagnosis: To be or not to be? *Nursing Diagnosis, 2*(1), 19–25.

Porter, E. J. (1986). Critical analysis of NANDA nursing diagnosis taxonomy I. *IMAGE: Journal of Nursing Scholarship, 18*(4), 136–139.

Price, M. R. (1980). Nursing diagnosis: Making a concept come alive. *American Journal of Nursing, 80*(4), 668–674.

Rasch, R. F. R. (1987). The nature of taxonomy. *IMAGE: Journal of Nursing Scholarship, 19*(3), 147–149.

Roberts, S. L. (1990). Achieving professional autonomy through nursing diagnosis and nursing DRGs. *Nursing Administration Quarterly, 14*(4), 54–60.

Rubenfeld, M. G., & Scheffer, B. K. (1995). *Critical thinking in nursing: An interactive approach.* Philadelphia: Lippincott.

Shamansky, S. L., & Yanni, C. R. (1983). In opposition to nursing diagnosis: A minority opinion. *IMAGE: Journal of Nursing Scholarship, 15*(2), 47–50.

Vincent, K. G., & Coler, M. S. (1990). A unified nursing diagnostic model. *IMAGE: Journal of Nursing Scholarship, 22*(2), 93–95.

Warren, J., & Hoskins, L. (1990). The development of NANDA's nursing diagnosis taxonomy. *Nursing Diagnosis, 1*(4), 162–168.

Weber, G. (1991). Making nursing diagnosis work for you and your client: A step-by-step approach. *Nursing and Health Care, 12*(8), 424–430.

Chapter 18

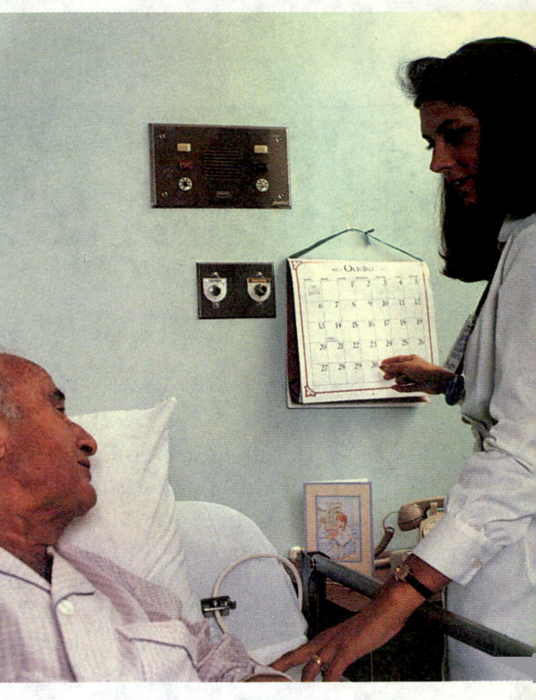

Planning

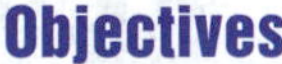

Objectives

After studying this chapter, the learner should be able to:

Define key terms used in the chapter.

Describe the purpose and benefits of planning.

Identify three elements of comprehensive planning.

Prioritize client health problems and nursing responses.

Describe how client goals/expected outcomes and nursing orders are derived from nursing diagnoses.

Develop a plan of nursing care with properly constructed goals/outcomes and related nursing orders.

Use criteria to evaluate planning skills.

Describe five common problems related to planning, their possible causes, and remedies.

Key Terms

client goal
clinical pathways/critical pathways
computerized nursing care plan
consultation
criteria
discharge planning
expected outcome
goal
Kardex care plan
nursing care plan
nursing order
planning
standardized care plan

After the nurse collects and interprets client data, identifies client strengths and health problems, and prioritizes nursing diagnoses, it is time to plan for nursing action. During the **planning** step of the nursing process, the nurse works with the client and family to (1) identify client goals/expected outcomes that, if achieved, prevent, reduce, or eliminate the problems specified in the nursing diagnoses, and (2) identify the nursing interventions that are most likely to assist the client in achieving these goals/outcomes.

A **goal** is an aim or an end. A **client goal** describes an expected client outcome, an expected conclusion to a client health problem. The words *goal, objective*, and outcome often are used interchangeably. In some practice settings, the term goal or objective is used to describe what is wanted and the term *outcome* is used to describe the results achieved. In nursing the term **expected outcomes** is used to refer to the more specific, measurable criteria used to evaluate whether the goal has been met. In this chapter we will use goal/outcome to refer to expected client outcomes.

Elements of planning (outlined in Fig. 18-1) include the following:

- Establishing priorities
- Writing goals/outcomes that determine the evaluative strategy
- Selecting appropriate nursing interventions
- Communicating the plan of nursing care

It is important that the nurse, client, and family work together as much as possible during planning. If the goals/outcomes specified in the plan of care are not valued by the client or do not contribute to the prevention, resolution, or reduction of the client's problems, then the plan of care may be meaningless. Goal/outcome determination is, therefore, a critical skill for the nurse who hopes to successfully intervene with clients.

In this chapter, planning is described as a formal process, a conscious, deliberate step in the nursing process. Informal planning is often observed by students in the practice setting. It is the link between the identification of a client strength or problem and the appropriate nursing response. When a nurse on a busy surgical unit learns that a postoperative client is complaining of incisional pain and quickly reshuffles priorities to allow time to assess the course and qualities of the pain and what nursing measures can be implemented to reduce discomfort, planning has occurred. When the postpartum nurse on the 3-to-11 shift realizes on the evening before discharge that he or she has not seen a particular father hold his new daughter and makes a mental note to observe the father–daughter interactions that evening and facilitate their bonding, planning has occurred. When a nurse in a geriatric daycare center hears a client choking and rushes to his side to perform the Heimlich maneuver if it becomes necessary, planning has occurred. Informal planning on a more conscious level is illustrated by a hospice nurse who ponders how best to support a client with terminal cancer who is gradually relinquishing her hold on life. When nurses find formal planning burdensome and are satisfied with this type of informal planning, they are depriving themselves and their clients of the benefits related to formal planning.

A formal plan of care allows the nurse to individualize care; set priorities; facilitate communication among nursing personnel; promote continuity of high quality, cost-effective care; coordinate care; evaluate the client's responses to nursing care; and promote the nurse's professional development. Core competencies needed to design effective plans of care are highlighted in the box on page 284.

Unique Focus of Nursing Planning

The primary purpose of the planning step of the nursing process is to design a plan of care for and with the client that, once implemented, results in the prevention, reduction, or resolution of client health problems. A comprehensive plan of care specifies any routine nursing assistance the client requires to meet basic human needs (eg, assistance with hygiene or nutrition) and describes appropriate nursing responsibilities for fulfilling the medical plan of care. For example, physicians may delegate to nurses caring for a surgical client the redressing of the surgical incision, the administration of

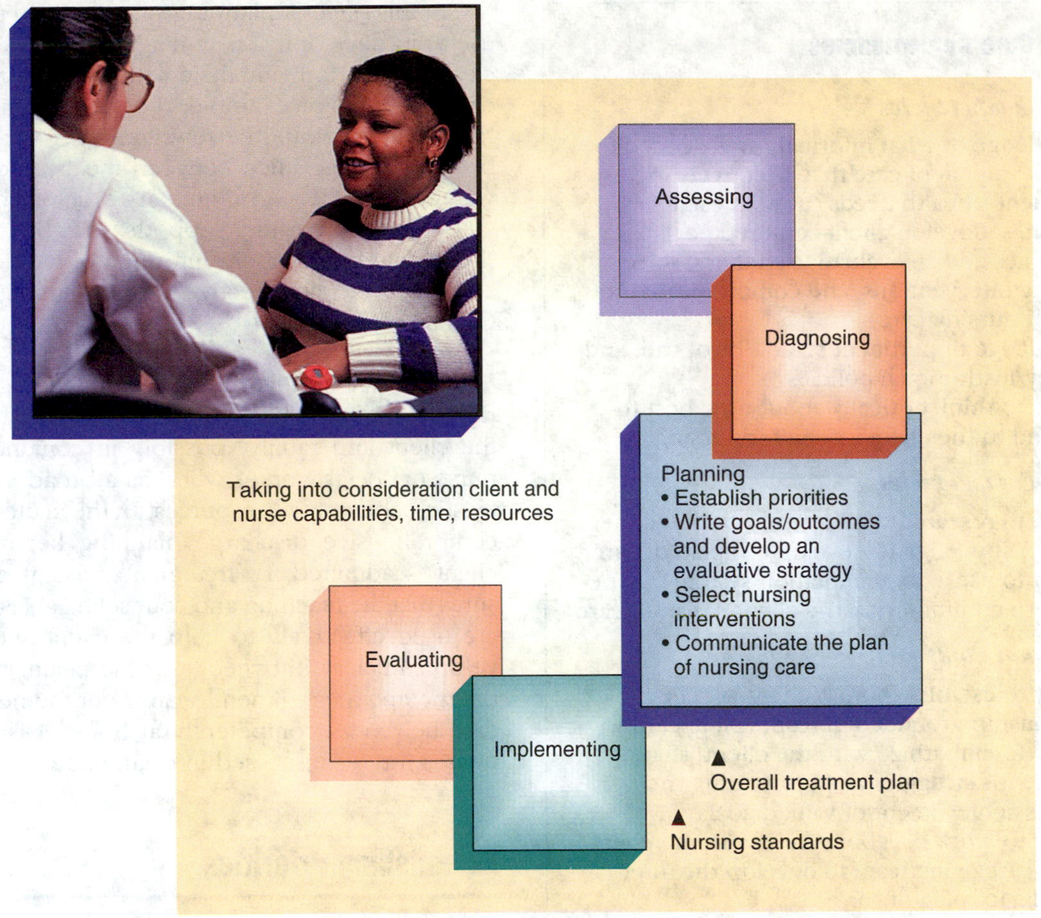

Figure 18-1
Planning. The nurse and client work together to develop client goals/outcomes and identify the nursing interventions most likely to assist the client to meet the goals. It is important for the plan of care to be consistent with nursing standards, congruent with other planned therapies, and realistic in terms of the client and nurses' abilities or resources. (Photo by Gates Rhodes, courtesy of School of Nursing, University of Pennsylvania.)

prescribed medications and intravenous therapy, and responsibility for scheduling laboratory studies. Nurses design plans of care that incorporate their independent and collaborative responsibilities. Because nursing is concerned with the client's responses to health and illness, the plan of care is supportive of nursing's broad aims—to promote wellness, prevent disease and illness, promote recovery, and facilitate coping with altered functioning.

Comprehensive Planning

In the acute care setting there are three basic stages of planning critical to comprehensive nursing care—initial, ongoing problem-oriented, and discharge. In other settings, initial and ongoing problem-oriented may be the primary stages used. The nurse who develops a comprehensive plan of care on the first meeting with the client and fails to update the plan will not have an effective or efficient plan. Failure to update the plan of care as needed is a common problem in all healthcare settings.

Initial Planning. The *initial plan* is developed by the nurse who performs the admission nursing history and the physical assessment. Comprehensive in nature, this plan addresses each problem listed in the prioritized nursing diagnoses and identifies appropriate client goals and the related nursing care. **Standardized plans of care** are prepared plans of care that identify the nursing diagnoses, goals/outcomes, and related nursing interventions common to a specific population or health problem. They can provide an excellent basis for the initial plan *if the nurse individualizes them.* Resources for standardized plans include computerized plans, textbooks with prepared care plans, and agency-developed plans/pathways. By using such standardized plans, the nurse is free to direct time and expertise to individualizing the plan.

Planning: Core Competencies

Cognitive Competencies

- Knowledge of what information is needed to develop a plan of care that effectively meets the client's health needs (how to establish priorities, develop client-centered goals/outcomes and an evaluative strategy, select nursing interventions, and communicate the plan of nursing care)
- Knowledge of pertinent standards of care and agency/institutional policies
- Ability to think critically about how best to respond to the client's need for nursing

Technical Competencies

- Ability to research the literature to obtain necessary knowledge to develop the plan of care
- Ability to use a documentation system competently to communicate the client's plan of care

Interpersonal Competencies

- Ability to establish a trusting nurse–client relationship grounded in responsible caring
- Ability to empathize with the client, sharing the client's struggles and celebrating the client's achievement of valued goals
- Ability to work collaboratively with members of the caregiving team to develop the interdisciplinary plan of care

Ethical/Legal Competencies

- Ability to communicate respect and to promote the client's sense of worth
- Commitment to do whatever is necessary to secure the client's well-being within the bounds of your professional responsibilities
- Ability to serve as a trusted and effective client advocate
- Consistent use of appropriate legal safeguards while developing and documenting the plan of care

Ongoing Planning. *Ongoing, problem-oriented planning* is carried out by any nurse who interacts with the client. Its chief purpose is to keep the plan up-to-date. As new data is collected and analyzed, the nurse caring for the client will use it to make the plan more specific and accurate and therefore more effective. The work of ongoing planning includes stating nursing diagnoses more clearly (both the problem statement and the cause); developing new diagnoses; making previously developed client goals/outcomes more realistic; developing new goals/outcomes as needed; and identifying those nursing interventions that will best accomplish the client goals.

At this stage of planning, standardized plans may be useful in developing new diagnoses, but the emphasis clearly is on individualizing the plan to meet unique client needs. For example, the standard nursing order "force fluids" would be rewritten as "offer 60 mL cranberry or orange juice between meals, and keep fresh water at bedside." A preliminary order such as "explore with the client existing supports" may be replaced with "keep daughter Barbara informed of mother's progress and coach her in effective support strategies (Barbara Clems, 448-3211)."

Discharge Planning. Discharge planning is best carried out by the nurse who has worked most closely with the client and family, possibly in conjunction with a nurse or social worker who has a broad knowledge of existing community resources. In the acute care setting, comprehensive discharge planning begins when the client is admitted for treatment. Careful planning ensures that the teaching and counseling skills of the nurse are used effectively to help the client and family develop sufficient knowledge of the health problem and the therapeutic regimen to carry out the necessary self-care behaviors competently at home. Discharge planning is further discussed in Chapter 12.

Establishing Priorities

Before developing or modifying the plan of care, it is helpful to review the prioritized list of nursing diagnoses to determine if they are correctly ranked as high priority (greatest threat to client's well-being), medium priority, and low priority (not specifically related to current illness and prognosis). Guidelines for establishing these priorities are presented in Chapter 17.

When planning nursing care for each day, it is helpful to consider the following:

- Have changes in the client's health status influenced what are considered the priority nursing diagnoses? For example, when a routine home visit of an older adult reveals evidence of possible elder abuse, a new set of priorities for care is needed.
- Have changes in the way the client is responding to health and illness or the plan of care affected those nursing diagnoses that can be realistically addressed? For example, the nurse may have identified ineffective individual coping as a high-priority diagnosis for the client who has learned of the medical diagnosis, and planned to initiate counseling. But if the client adamantly requests to be left alone for a day to think things through, the nurse has to modify priorities of care for that day.
- Are there relationships between diagnoses that require that one be worked on before another can be resolved?

- Can several client problems be dealt with together?

After answering these questions, the nurse ranks diagnoses in the order in which they will be addressed. Setting priorities enables the nurse to make sure that time and energy are being directed to the client's most important problems.

Critical Thinking Exercise 18-1

Write nursing diagnoses for three obese clients, making sure the etiologies for the problem statement (Altered Nutrition: More than body requirements) differ. Describe how these different etiologies result in different plans of care.

Writing Goals/Outcomes and Developing Evaluative Strategies

Deriving Goals/Outcomes from Nursing Diagnoses

Goals are derived from the problem statement of the nursing diagnosis. For each nursing diagnosis in the plan of care, at least one goal must be written that, if achieved, demonstrates a *direct resolution* of the problem statement (Table 18-1).

Other outcomes that contribute to the resolution of the problem may be written. For example, for the nursing diagnosis *Altered Nutrition: More than body requirements, related to excessive snacking and inactivity,* in addition to the goal, "within 12 weeks the client will lose 20 pounds and reach target weight: 122 lb," the following goals are appropriate:

- Within three days of teaching: the client will identify 10 low-calorie snack foods he is willing to try.
- The client will have 3-day diet recall consistent with nutritionally balanced 1500-calorie diet.
- The client will report incorporating three ½-hour periods of walking at 5 miles per hour into each week.

Table 18-1
Examples of Goals to Relieve Problems

Problem Statement of the Nursing Diagnosis	Related Client Goal/Outcome
Pain	By end of shift client will report pain is absent or diminished
Altered Nutrition: More than body requirements	By 12/6/98, client will reach target weight of 122 lb
Impaired Physical Mobility	Before discharge, client will ambulate length of hallway independently

The difference between these goals/outcomes and the goal/outcome that the client reach his target weight is that, whereas the achievement of the former may contribute to the resolution of the problem, they also may be achieved without the problem being resolved and the client's plan of care may mistakenly be terminated. Remember, *at least one goal per nursing diagnosis must directly resolve the problem statement in the nursing diagnosis.*

Long-Term Versus Short-Term Goals/Outcomes

Goals/outcomes may be either long-term or short-term. Simply defined, long-term goals/outcomes require a longer period (usually more than a week) to be achieved than do short-term goals. They also may be used as discharge goals, in which case they are more broadly written and communicate to the entire nursing team the desired end results of nursing care for a particular client. For example, two women, both aged 77, are on a nursing unit after undergoing similar operative procedures for fractured left hips. Whereas one woman has spent the past 2 years in bed in a nursing home, the other woman fractured her hip at the YMCA where she swims daily. Their nursing care should not be the same because it is directed to different long-term goals, although their short-term goals may be similar (see sample goals).

Cognitive, Psychomotor, and Affective Goals

Goals may be categorized according to the type of change they describe for the client. *Cognitive goals* describe increases in client knowledge or intellectual behaviors. *Example:* Within one day post-teaching, the client will list three benefits of continuing to apply moist compresses to leg ulcer after discharge. *Psychomotor goals* describe the client's achievement of new skills. *Example:* By 6/12/98, the client will correctly demonstrate application of wet-to-dry dressing on leg ulcer. *Affective goals* describe changes in client values, beliefs, and attitudes. Difficult both to write and to evaluate, affective goals may be critical to the resolution of a complex client problem. *Example:* By 6/12/98, the client will verbalize valuing health sufficiently to practice new health behaviors to prevent recurrence of leg ulcer. In this example, even if the client intellectually grasps the reasons for taking care of her leg and can competently redress her ulcer, unless she is motivated to take care of herself, her knowledge and skills will not result in healthy outcomes (Fig. 18-2).

Critical Thinking Exercise 18-2

Using one of the nursing diagnoses from Critical Thinking Exercise 18-1, write related cognitive, psychomotor, and affective goals. Explain the different purposes of each type of goal and why it may be necessary to include all three in order to resolve a client problem successfully.

Examples of Long- and Short-Term Goals

Client on Bed Rest From Nursing Home

Long-Term Goal

Mrs. Goldstein returns to the nursing home pain-free with her incision healed and her left leg in good alignment.

Short-Term Goals

- Whenever observed, client will be lying in bed with legs in correct alignment (abductor pillow in place if ordered).
- Before discharge, Mrs. Goldstein's hip incision will show signs of healing (skin surfaces approximate, free from signs of infection—redness, swelling, heat, purulent drainage).
- Whenever observed, client will report that comfort measures and medication are satisfactorily managing pain.

Active Client from Private Home

Long-Term Goal

Mrs. Silverstein returns home to her husband pain-free with incision healed, fully mobile (full weight-bearing on left leg), and capable of independent activities of daily living.

Short-Term Goals

- By 1/28/98, the client will verbalize willingness to participate in physical therapy program.
- By 2/4/98, the client will ambulate (with nursing assistance and walker) to bathroom (full weight-bearing).
- By 2/11/98, the client will ambulate with nursing assistance only (no walker) in her room.
- Goals for incision and pain relief same as for Mrs. Goldstein.

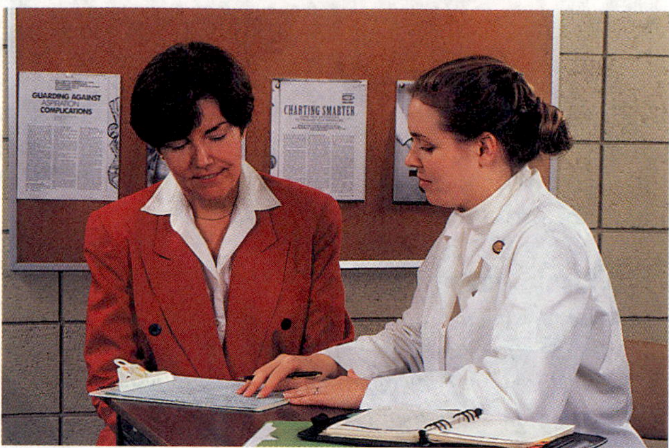

Figure 18-2
The nurse reviews short-term goals/outcomes with a family caregiver before the client's discharge from a healthcare facility. (Photo © B. Proud.)

Guidelines for Goal/Outcome Writing

One of the most important considerations in goal/outcome writing is to encourage the client and family to be as involved in goal development as their abilities and interest permit. The more involved they are, the greater the probability that the goals will be achieved. When developing client goals/outcomes, the nurse and client look at the problem statement of the nursing diagnosis and ask, "What client changes or outcomes will result in the prevention or resolution of this problem?" The answer, when carefully worded, becomes the client goal/outcomes (see the accompanying box.)

Each client goal/outcome must have a *subject*, which is the client; a *verb*, which indicates the action the client will perform; and **criteria**, which describe in *observable, measurable terms* the expected client behavior. The criteria must include a time criterion, which may be a realistic, actual date or other statement indicating time such as before discharge, after viewing film, whenever observed.

The following are examples of properly constructed client goals:

- By end of 3–11 shift, client's 24-hour fluid intake will total at least 2000 mL.
- At next visit, 12/23/98, the client will correctly demonstrate relaxation exercises.

It may be helpful to include special conditions when writing a goal if this information is important for other nurses (eg, "Before discharge, the client will ambulate independently the length of hallway and back, using Philadelphia collar to support cervical vertebrae").

Common Errors

Common errors when writing client goals/outcomes include the following:

- Expressing the *client* goal as a *nursing* intervention. *Incorrect:* Offer Mr. Myer 60 mL fluid every 2 hours while awake. *Correct:* Mr. Myer will drink 60 mL fluid every 2 hours while awake, beginning 2/24/98.
- Using verbs that are not *observable* and *measurable*. *Incorrect:* Mrs. Gaston will know how to bathe her newborn. *Correct:* After attending the infant care class, Mrs. Gaston will correctly demonstrate the procedure for bathing her newborn. Verbs to be avoided when writing goals include *know, understand, learn, become aware.* These verbs are considered too general and are unmeasurable. Verbs that are helpful when writing goals/outcomes that are observable and measurable are shown in the accompanying box.
- Including more than one client behavior in short-term goals/outcomes. *Incorrect:* Client will list

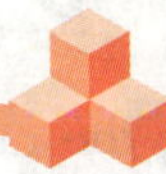

Guidelines for Nursing Care

Writing Goals/Outcomes

- Derive each set of goals/outcomes from only one nursing diagnosis.
- Make sure that at least one of the goals/outcomes clearly shows a direct resolution of the problem statement in the nursing diagnosis and that other goals/outcomes contribute to the prevention or resolution of the problem.
- Write goals/outcomes that are valued by the client and family.
- Check to make sure the goals/outcomes are supportive of the total treatment plan.
- Write goals/outcomes that are brief, specific (clearly describe an observable, measurable behavior), and phrased positively; specify timeline.
- Remember that each short-term goal/outcome can contain only one client behavior.

dangers of smoking and stop smoking. *Correct:* By next meeting, 3/11/98, the client will (1) identify three dangers of smoking and (2) describe a plan he is willing to try to stop smoking. By 6/20/98, the client will report that he no longer smokes.

- Writing goals/outcomes so vaguely that other nurses are unsure of the goal of nursing care. *Incorrect:* Client will cope better. *Correct:* After teaching, 10/20/98, the client will (1) describe two new coping strategies he is willing to try and (2) demonstrate decreased incidence of previously observed noneffective coping behaviors (chain smoking, withdrawal behavior, heavy alcohol consumption).

Developing Evaluative Strategy

Well-written goals define the evaluative strategy to be used by the nurse. Client goals/outcomes are meaningless unless nurses evaluate the client's progress toward their achievement. The nurse records the date the goal/outcome was written and the date it is achieved. Evaluative statements (see the accompanying box) include a statement about achievement of the desired goal/outcome (met, partially met, not met) and list actual client behavior as evidence supporting the statement. If the plan is not achieved, recommendations for revising the plan of care are included in the evaluative statement (Atkinson & Murray, 1990). Chapter 20 deals specifically with the evaluative component of the nursing process.

Verbs Helpful in Writing Goals

define
identify
list
describe
explain
apply
use
demonstrate
prepare
design
verbalize
choose
select
inject
perform

Selecting Nursing Interventions

Deriving Nursing Interventions From Nursing Diagnoses

Nursing interventions, like client goals, are derived from the nursing diagnosis. But whereas the problem statement of the diagnosis suggests the client goals, it is the cause of the problem that suggests the nursing interventions (Fig. 18-3). The effective nurse selects nursing interventions that specifically address factors that cause or contribute to the client's problems.

Evaluative Statement

Documents that client has met, partially met, or not met the goal/outcome.

Goal/Outcome Statement

Beginning 6/8/98, the client will ambulate half the length of hallway with assistance three times daily.

Evaluative Statement

6/8/98 Goal partially met; client refused to ambulate in the morning but did walk to the bathroom once in the afternoon with the assistance of one nurse.

Recommendation: Review reason for progressive ambulation with client; assess motivation to increase independence.

M. Stenulis, RN

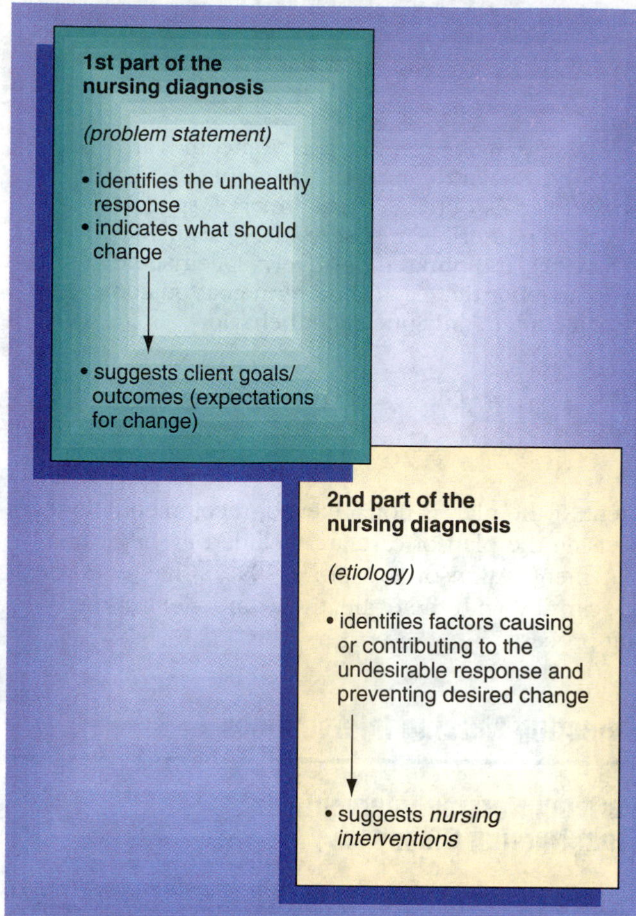

Figure 18-3
Deriving client goals and nursing orders from nursing diagnoses.

For example, many factors may contribute to obesity, such as deficient nutritional knowledge, convenience of high-calorie fast foods, lifetime snacking habits, limited food budget, little exercise, and low self-esteem. The nurse working with a client who wants to lose weight could attempt to deal with all these factors, but this approach would be inefficient. When a carefully developed nursing diagnosis identifies the specific factors that contribute to a particular client's weight problem, nursing interventions can be selected to deal directly with these factors.

For example, nursing interventions for the client with the diagnosis *Altered Nutrition: More than body requirements, related to lifetime snacking habits and heavy reliance on high-calorie fast foods* might include education about the fat content and calories in fast foods and an exploration of ways the client could change eating habits to eat more nutritionally balanced meals with fewer calories. Thus, not every client with a weight problem is nursed the same way. The art of nursing involves the careful identification of the specific nursing interventions which are needed by particular clients to meet their individual needs.

Identifying and Selecting Options

After the client goals/outcomes are written, the nurse identifies various nursing interventions to help the client achieve the goals/outcomes. The effectiveness of the nurse is directly proportional to his or her knowledge of varied nursing strategies. Consider these nursing care options identified by three nurses when they are asked to describe nursing care for a woman 2 days after caesarean delivery who is complaining of pain in her incisional area.

Nurse A

- Check to see what type of pain medication is ordered, and give it if the time interval is sufficient.

Nurse B

- Assess the quality of the pain, and use this time to communicate support by means of expression and squeeze of hand.
- Administer analgesic if indicated.
- Assess effectiveness of the analgesic ordered.

Nurse C

- Assess quality of the pain and explore the possibility of contributing factors such as the effects of increased gas in the abdominal area or concern about the newborn, herself, or other family members.
- Use empathic listening (possibly touch) to communicate support and to encourage the mother to share her concerns.
- Change the client's position in bed.
- Offer a back rub.
- If appropriate, suggest activity that will distract attention from the pain (eg, watching a film of newborn care or listening to music).
- Give the prescribed medication for pain and observe its effect.
- When administering the medication, use the power of positive suggestion to enhance its effectiveness: "This will start taking the pain away in about 10 minutes and will help you relax."

It is possible that the client simply needs her prescribed analgesic to achieve the goal/outcome: "Client will report minimal to no pain upon every 2-hour assessment." In that case, all three nurses would have been effective in meeting the client's need for nursing care. However, it is highly possible the prescribed medication is not working, or the pain is compounded by the mother's fears about caring for her new baby or by her worries that the baby will ruin her relationship with her husband. Therefore, Nurse C, whose knowledge level is more comprehensive, is most likely to be effective in resolving the client's problem.

The more varied the options available to the nurse, the more effective the nursing response will be. In different situations, a skilled nursing procedure, an appropriate use of silence, respectful listening, humor, teaching, counseling, and touch can all be effective nursing strategies. Nurses who are task oriented and satisfied to meet every client problem with a mechanical procedure are limiting their effectiveness.

When selecting nursing interventions for individual clients use the following guidelines. Nursing interventions should be:

- Consistent with standards of care, such as American Nurses Association/Canadian Nurses Association standards of practice, nurse practice acts, institutional standards, standards of accrediting agencies (eg, Joint Commission of Accreditation of Healthcare Organizations)
- Realistic in terms of the abilities, time, and resources available to the nurse and client
- Compatible with the client's values, beliefs, and psychosocial background
- Valued, whenever possible, by the client and family
- Compatible with other planned therapies

Use of these guidelines increases the chances that the client will successfully achieve the goal/outcome. Ongoing evaluation will enable the nurse to determine the effectiveness of the selected interventions. Nurse researchers are now attempting to establish a statistical pattern for predicting the probability of success of select nursing interventions. The competent nurse uses research findings (science of nursing) and knowledge of the client (art of nursing) to aid in the selection of effective nursing interventions. Consultation with nurse colleagues and continuing education enable the nurse to develop effective nursing approaches to client problems.

Consulting

The nurse designing the plan of care may discover that more information is needed about the nature of the problems underlying the need for nursing or about specific interventions. **Consultation**, a process in which two or more individuals with varying degrees of experience and expertise deliberate about a problem and its solution, often proves helpful at this point. Nurses may consult with nurse specialists and other members of the healthcare team, for example, physicians, nutritionists, social workers, pastoral caregivers, and ethicists. Consultations are a valuable means for nurses to expand their nursing knowledge and repertoire of effective strategies.

Nursing Orders

Nursing orders describe in writing, and thus communicate to the entire nursing staff and healthcare team, the specific nursing care to be implemented for the client (Fig. 18-4). Well-written nursing orders:

- Assist the client to meet specific goals/outcomes and are related directly to one goal/outcome

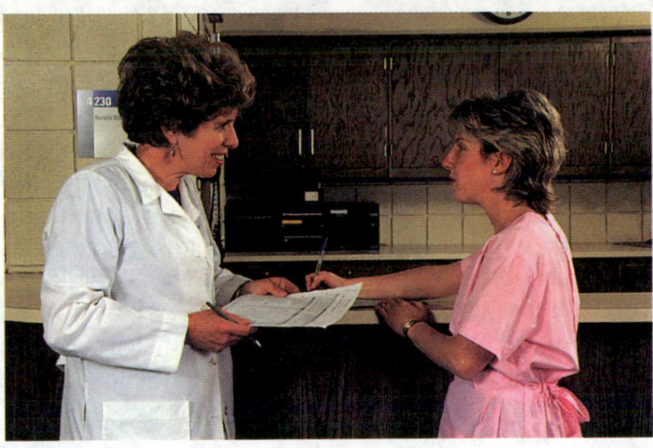

Figure 18-4
The nurse discusses client-centered nursing orders with another member of the staff. Nursing orders must be comprehensive. (Photo © B. Proud.)

- Clearly and concisely describe the nursing action to be performed (answer the questions who? what? where? when? and how?)
- Are dated when written and when the plan of care is reviewed
- Are signed by the nurse prescribing the order/intervention
- Use only those abbreviations accepted in the institution (these usually are found in the agency's policy manual; a list of commonly accepted abbreviations appears in Chapter 21)
- Refer the nurse to the agency's procedure manual or other literature for the steps of routine, lengthy procedures

The following are examples of well-stated nursing orders:

- Offer client 60 mL water or juice (prefers orange or cranberry juice) every 2 hours while awake for a total minimum P.O. intake of 500 mL.
- Teach client the necessity of carefully monitoring fluid intake and output; remind client each shift to mark off fluid intake on record at bedside.
- Walk with client to bathroom for toileting every 2 hours (on even hours) while client is awake.

The set of nursing interventions written to assist a client to meet a goal/outcome must be comprehensive. Comprehensive nursing orders specify what *observations* (assessments) need to be made and how often; what *nursing interventions* need to be done and when they must be done; and what *teaching, counseling, and advocacy needs* clients and families have.

Many sets of nursing orders are inadequate, in that they fail to indicate the ongoing assessment priority needs for a specific problem or goal. Clearly stating assessment priorities helps all nurses to be more sensitive to important client data. For example, when assisting a client who wants to lose weight to reach the target weight, appropriate nursing orders would include the following: 6/17/98—Continue to assess (1) client's motivation to participate in weight loss program, and (2) factors that positively or negatively influence weight loss.

Similarly, it often is assumed that all clients have the same teaching needs. Nothing is farther from the truth. In fact, many clients have an excellent knowledge base (which may be greater than that of the nurse for a particular disease). Their need for nursing may be a need for counseling, instead of teaching, as they learn to live with a chronic illness. Comprehensive nursing orders relate to individual client needs.

Writing the Plan of Nursing Care

The **plan of nursing care** (client care plan) is the written guide that directs the efforts of the nursing team in working with clients to meet health goals. It specifies nursing diagnoses, goals/outcomes, and associated nursing interventions. Well-written plans of care offer many benefits to the client, nurse, nursing unit, nursing administration, and nursing profession. Primarily, plans of nursing care ensure that the nursing team works efficiently to deliver holistic, goal-oriented, individualized care to clients. A well-written plan of nursing care:

- Represents an adequate philosophy of nursing and advances nursing's four aims: promotes wellness, prevents disease and illness, promotes recovery, facilitates coping with altered functioning
- Is responsive to the individual characteristics and needs of the client
- Clearly identifies the nursing assistance the client needs and nursing collaborative responsibilities for fulfilling the medical plan of care
- Directs the nurse's assessment priorities; caregiving behaviors; and teaching, counseling, and advocacy behaviors
- Is based on scientific principles and incorporates findings of nursing research
- Meets developmental, psychosocial, and spiritual needs of the client, as well as physiologic needs
- Addresses discharge needs of the client and family
- When appropriate, is compatible with the medical plan of care and that of the interdisciplinary team

Many suggestions for plans of care appear in the nursing literature. Each school of nursing and each healthcare institution and agency has its own format, which may reflect a particular nursing theory. Common to all formats is a minimum of three columns for documenting nursing diagnoses, client goals/outcomes, and nursing interventions. Formats differ in the way assessment data and nursing evaluation is addressed.

Institutional/Agency Plans of Care

The Joint Commission on the Accreditation of Healthcare Organizations (JCAHO) requires healthcare institutions and agencies to formulate, maintain, and support a client-specific plan for care, treatment, and rehabilitation (1994). There is great variety in the formats used to communicate the plan of care. In most institutions and agencies, the plans of care, regardless of their format, communicate directions for three different types of nursing care: nursing care related to basic human needs, nursing care related to nursing diagnoses, and nursing care related to the medical plan of care.

Nursing Care Related to Basic Human Needs. The plan should concisely communicate to caregivers data obtained during the nursing history about the client's usual health habits and patterns that are needed to direct daily

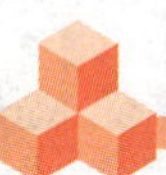

Guidelines for Nursing Care

Developing the Plan of Nursing Care

- Prepare and record the plan of nursing care on the day the nurse first meets the client, in a timely fashion—time is dictated by the client's condition.
- The nurse who best knows the client (the primary nurse or case manager) develops the initial plan, which is added to by other caregivers.
- Provide for as much client and family participation as possible.
- Sign and date the initial plan and subsequent additions and modifications.
- Write in ink according to agency policy as the plan of care becomes part of the client's permanent record (alternately, follow agency guidelines for computerized documentation).
- Clearly specify nursing diagnoses, client goals/outcomes, nursing interventions, and evaluation strategies.
- Use standardized symbols, abbreviations, and key phrases specified in the agency's policy manual, as opposed to lengthy descriptions.
- Refer to agency procedure manual for specific steps in new or complicated nursing procedures.
- Update the plan of care consistently to reflect changes in the client's status and related needs for nursing care.

care. For example, it is important to know if a toddler is toilet trained and what words he or she uses to indicate the need to void or defecate. Directives about the client's usual health habits and patterns may become modified by current treatment orders, such as an order to fast for a diagnostic procedure or to limit or increase activity. This information is useful to caregivers only if it is kept current as the client's condition changes. Any nurse should be able to find in the plan of care the instructions needed to provide care confidently and competently.

Nursing Care Related to Nursing Diagnoses. The plan contains goals/outcomes and nursing interventions for every nursing diagnosis, as well as a place to note client responses to the plan of care. This section is the heart of the plan of nursing care because it represents the independent component of nursing practice. If well developed, it demonstrates the clinical competence of the nurse (knowledge of the science of nursing), sensitivity to the individual needs of the client, and creativity.

Nursing Care Related to the Medical Plan of Care. The plan of care records current medical orders for diagnostic studies and treatment and specified related nursing care.

Kardex Plans of Care

Many healthcare institutions/agencies use a **Kardex care plan** in which the plan of nursing care for each client is concisely recorded on a 6 × 11–inch card and placed in a central Kardex file. Frequently the Kardex does not become part of the client's permanent record and is easily updated because most entries are written in pencil.

Computerized Plans of Care

In an increasing number of institutional settings, nurses are using computer software programs to generate **computerized plans of care**. Benefits of using computerized plans include ready access to an expanded knowledge base, improved record keeping with resultant improvement in audits and quality assurance, documentation by all members of the healthcare team with printouts for the client's record and for change-of-shift report, and reduction of time spent on paperwork. One nurse researcher is studying the negative impact computerized plans are having on the professionalization of staff nurses. Harris (1990) cautions that the computerized system for client care planning and the larger system in which it is embedded contribute to the loss of autonomy, loss of individualization of care, and loss of nursing expertise. Individual nurses as well as researchers must respond to Harris' challenge: "Does a lot of nursing time spent in procedural, rule-governed, step-by-step thinking processes destroy part of the nurse's ability to care, to empathize, to intuit, to gain insight, to function in the expert mode?" (p. 73).

Case Management Plans of Care

Case management is a healthcare delivery system with the objective of providing high-quality, cost-effective care for individuals, families, and groups. The emphasis is on clearly stating expected client outcomes and reasonable, specific times for achievement of these outcomes. **Clinical pathways (critical pathways)** are tools used to communicate the standardized, interdisciplinary plan of care for a particular group of clients. Chapter 21 provides examples of the use of critical pathways with select documentation tools in a computerized system. The accompanying boxes illustrate a standardized plan of care for a client with congestive heart failure. Care guidelines and outcomes are specified for each day of the client's stay. In this case, the client receives a version of the plan of care upon admission with the rationale that knowing what to expect will result in less stress, quicker recovery, and earlier discharge.

Student Plans of Care

The care plans that students are required to develop often are more detailed than those found in practice settings. The aim is to assist students to assimilate each of the five steps of the nursing process. Although care plan formats vary from one nursing program to another, most are designed so that the student will systematically proceed through each interrelated step in the nursing process, and many use a five-column format.

The sample student care plan on p. 294 demonstrates a plan developed for the client whose admission assessment form is in Chapter 16. This 72-year-old woman was admitted to the hospital after experiencing a ministroke (transient ischemic attack [TIA]) at home. Her condition is stable, and the three prioritized diagnoses developed on the plan address her inability to deal with this new medical diagnosis and to prevent a major stroke (high priority), ineffective coping (medium priority), and constipation (low priority). In the past year, her husband died and she sold her home and moved in with her daughter.

Assessing. In the assessment column, the student records the assessment data that led to the determination of each diagnosis. Recording these data helps to link specific defining characteristics with diagnostic problem statements. On some care plans, pertinent assessment data are recorded in the nursing diagnosis column.

Diagnosing. Priorities are assigned to each diagnosis, and these are recorded in the nursing diagnosis column. For each diagnosis, a clear and concise problem statement is followed by an etiology statement that identifies specific contributing factors.

(text continues on page 296)

Standardized Plan of Care

Chart 1
Sacred Heart–St. Mary's Hospitals, Inc.
PLAN OF CARE: CONGESTIVE HEART FAILURE
ESTIMATED LENGTH OF STAY: 4 Days
Supplies Given: Adm. Kit PN 2-1-94 **Urinal** PN 2-1-94 **Bedpan** PN 2-1-94 **Air Mattress** PN 2-1-94

FOCUS Date:	Day of Admission	Day 2	Day 3	Day 4
ACTIVITY	Activity intolerance related to dyspnea • Restrict activity 30 min before and 60 min after meals *Expected outcome* • Activity as tolerated PN 2-1	• Restrict activity 30 min before and 60 min after meals • Chair 30 min t.i.d. for meals • Ambulate 60 ft in hall w/assist • Bathroom privileges *Expected outcome* • Able to tolerate activity without distress PN 2-2	• Ambulate 100 ft t.i.d. *Expected outcome* • Able to perform ADLs and ambulation without the use of O_2 ____	• Prepare pt for discharge home *Expected outcome* • Able to tolerate activity without distress ____
NUTRITION Needs assist no Consult needed? no	NAS diet or ____ PN 2-1	NAS diet or ____	NAS diet or ____	NAS diet or ____
TREATMENTS Skin protocol PN 2-1 Fall protocol PN 2-1	Alteration in fluid balance related to compromised cardiac output • Vital signs q4h • I&O • Daily weight • Telemetry if ordered • Heparin lock • O_2 at 3 l/min • Assess lung and heart sounds q shift and p.r.n. • Assess pedal edema and pulses q shift	• Vital signs q4h • I&O • Daily weight • Telemetry if ordered • Heparin lock • O_2 at 3 l/min • Assess lung and heart sounds q shift and p.r.n. • Assess pedal edema and pulses q shift *Expected outcomes* • Pt's foot edema is decreased or pt has lost weight (min 1 lb) PN 2-2 • Pt has improved breath sounds PN 2-2	• Vital signs q shift • I&O • Daily weight • Discontinue telemetry if previously ordered ____ • Heparin lock • O_2 p.r.n. (If still needed, consult cardiopulmonary services for need for home O_2.) • Assess lung and heart sounds q shift • Assess pedal edema and pulses q shift	• Vital signs q shift • I&O • Daily weight • Discontinue heparin lock ____ • Discontinue O_2 ____ • Assess lung and heart sounds q shift • Assess pedal edema and pulses q shift *Expected outcomes* • Feet/ankle edema resolved ____ • Unlabored respirations ____
TEACHING	• Review Plan of Care with pt • Explain medications to pt. • Give copy of Plan of Care to pt • Give info sheet on congestive heart failure to pt • Home health referral needed yes PN 2-1-94 • Home O_2 needed possibly PN 2-1-94	*Expected outcome* • Pt can verbalize understanding of present medications PN 2-2	• Discharge medication sheets given ____ • Home health referral arranged if needed ____ • Home O_2 arranged if needed ____	*Expected outcomes* • Pt can verbalize understanding of present medications ____ • Discharge medication sheet reviewed and pt can verbalize understanding ____ • Discharge instructions reviewed and pt can verbalize understanding ____ • Pt can verbalize understanding for need of follow-up visit and when to call doctor ____

OTHER FOCAL AREAS
- Durable power of attorney yes PN 2-1
- Living will yes PN 2-1
- Code status full PN 2-1

Rasmussen, N., & Gengler, T. (1994). Clinical pathways of care: The route to better communication. *Nursing 94, 24*(2), 48–49. Used with permission.

Standard Plan of Care: Patient Copy

Chart 2
Sacred Heart–St. Mary's Hospitals, Inc.
PLAN OF CARE: CONGESTIVE HEART FAILURE **PATIENT COPY**
ESTIMATED LENGTH OF STAY: 4 Days

FOCUS Date:	Day of Admission	Day 2	Day 3	Day 4
ACTIVITY	You can move around as you are able. Avoid becoming overtired or short of breath. You should remain in bed 30 minutes before your meals and 60 minutes after your meals.	You should increase your activity slowly. Start by sitting up in the chair for meals and walking short distances with the help of the nurses twice a day.	You should be starting to feel better and should be able to do mild activities without your oxygen. If you can't tolerate this, your doctor may suggest using oxygen at home. A home care nurse would then come by to check on you for a few weeks.	You should be able to walk in the halls and take your own bath without trouble breathing. You'll go home today if your doctor feels you're ready.
NUTRITION	You'll be on a no-added-salt diet. The dietitian will come to talk to you about this if you don't understand. A salt substitute is available if you need it. (Salt causes your body to hold in extra fluids, making your swelling worse and causing your heart to work even harder.)	Low-salt diet	Low-salt diet	Low-salt diet. Ask your doctor or nurse if you should continue this diet at home.
TREATMENTS	The nurse will measure the amount of fluid you take in and put out. The nurse will listen to your heart and lungs to see if they are getting better. You may have to use oxygen for the first day or two to help you breathe easier. You'll be weighed daily. You'll have an intravenous needle placed in your hand or arm. This will be used to give you medication. You may have a telemetry heart monitor on. Nurses in the intensive care unit will monitor your heart's rhythm.	Treatments will remain the same.	Some treatments will remain the same. You'll use oxygen only when you feel you need it. The heart monitor will be discontinued if previously ordered.	Some treatments will remain the same. Your oxygen may be discontinued. Your needle will be removed if you're going home.
TEACHING	You'll need to understand what is going on with your body. Please ask questions if you don't understand something. You'll be given a sheet to explain what congestive heart failure is. Ask about your medications if you're unfamiliar with them.		You'll be given information sheets that explain the medication you'll take at home. You should know about the right foods to eat and what types of food you should avoid. Your doctor may order a follow-up by a home health nurse.	You'll need to follow up with your doctor. Make sure you know when your appointment is. Know what problems may require medical attention.

Rasmussen, N., & Gengler, T. (1994). Clinical pathways of care: The route to better communication. *Nursing 94, 24*(2), 48–49. Used with permission.

Student Care Plan

Assessment	Nursing Diagnosis	Goal/Outcome
Subjective data: "Will I get a stroke now? I don't think I could handle that." "How can I help myself prevent it?" *Objective data:* Admitting diagnosis: TIA BP: 184/120	High Risk for Alteration in Health Maintenance Response to TIA and Stroke Prevention related to knowledge deficit	Before discharge, the client will: • Describe the terms *TIA* and *stroke,* identifying the underlying disease process, causes, symptoms, and treatment
Strengths: Past pattern of adhering to prescribed health behaviors.		After discussion with the physician and nurse, the client will: • Correctly describe the treatment plan: • Medications (drugs, intended effect, dose, time, route) • Dietary modifications • Exercise prescription • Signs and symptoms to report • Follow-up appointment date
Subjective data: Husband died 8 months ago; moved in with daughter 6 months ago after selling family home Daughter reports mother has been a very independent, strong woman in the past—seemed to "crumple" after husband's death. History of headaches	Ineffective Individual Coping related to illness, recent death of husband, and relocation with daughter	Beginning 9/7/98, the client will: • Verbalize her feelings related to the loss of her husband, loss of family home, loss of health
Objective data: Clutches daughter's hand		• Identify coping patterns that have helped her in the past
Strengths: History of handling life stressors well		
Limitations: In the past, her husband was her primary support.		• Identify three personal strengths and three outside supports that will help her now
		Before discharge, the client will: • Verbalize that she feels "okay" (sufficiently in charge of her life) about returning home

Nursing Orders	Scientific Rationale	Evaluation
Assess what the client knows about TIA and stroke (correct any misinformation). Assess learning needs, readiness to learn, and factors that will influence learning.	Each person's learning needs are different; each person learns in own unique way; learning is dependent on readiness.	9/10/98 Goal not met. Client says her head is "too old" to learn all this stuff. Equates stroke with death. *Revision:* Reteach content in simpler terms. Reassess learning readiness. *C. Taylor, RN*
Plan teaching and learning sessions to involve family members designated by client.	The more support people knowledgeably committed to the plan of care, the greater the probability the client will achieve goals.	
Include in the teaching plan a description of TIA and stroke, the underlying disease process, causes, symptoms, and treatment plan.	New self-care behaviors are dependent on knowledge.	9/10/98 Too early to evaluate. *C. Taylor, RN*
Once the treatment plan has been developed, make sure the client and family can restate it (teaching) and *value* the prescribed lifestyle modification (counseling).	New self-care behaviors are dependent on motivation. Unless the client is committed to stroke prevention and values this outcome, she will not follow the treatment plan.	
Once a shift, primary nurse to sit at client's bedside for at least several minutes to communicate caring and to explore with the client her current stressors and the adequacy of her coping response. • Assess factors compounding her losses. • Reinforce her personal strengths and support systems; counsel her to tap into these now. • Suggest local support groups if indicated.	The nurse's unhurried, attentive, and caring presence communicates to the client that she is important to the nurse and that the nurse values her well-being. It is an invitation to the client to become actively involved in recovery. Also, it is logical to explore adequacy of past and current coping mechanisms before suggesting new approaches.	9/10/98 Goal partially met. Client speaks freely about how much she misses her husband and how fearful this hospitalization makes her. When asked about living with her daughter, she becomes uncharacteristically quiet. *C. Taylor, RN* 9/10/98 Goal met. Client talks about how everything seemed better in the past after she talked it over with her husband and God. *C. Taylor, RN* 9/10/98 Goal not met. Client couldn't think of anything about herself that is healthy or strong. Says "maybe" her family can help her now. *Revision:* Counsel regarding personal strengths. Help her to experience them. *C. Taylor, RN*
Primary nurse to explore with daughter, Lisa, how her mother's moving in with her has affected the family. Recommend support systems.	Adult children of aging parents are frequently experiencing overwhelming stress as they try to deal with own and their parents' problems. Supporting this family *is* supporting the client indirectly.	9/11/98 Too early to evaluate. *C. Taylor, RN*

(continued)

Student Care Plan *(continued)*

Assessment	Nursing Diagnosis	Goal/Outcome
Subjective data: "I move my bowels every 2 or 3 days; get constipated at least once a week. Often Metamucil helps." "I drink plenty of fluids and eat fruits and vegetables." History of hemorrhoids secondary to straining.	Colonic Constipation related to decreased physical activity and long-term laxative use (Metamucil)	Beginning 9/7/98, the client will: • Pass soft, formed stool every 1 to 3 days without use of laxatives

Objective data: No bowel movement in past 4 days
On bed rest since hospitalized
		By 9/10/98,the client will:
		• Verbalize the importance of the following natural aids to bowel elimination:
		  • Daily intake of foods high in bulk
		  • Daily fluid intake of 8 to 10 glasses
		  • Regular time for elimination
		  • Daily physical exercise: walking

Planning. The planning column contains the expected changes in client health status or in client behaviors (ie, the client goals/outcomes). If achieved, these resolve the problem statement in the nursing diagnosis.

Implementing. Sets of nursing orders which describe specific nursing interventions are written for each client goal/outcome. These specify *what* nursing interventions are to be performed, *how* they are to be performed, *when* they are to be performed, and by *whom* they are to be performed. In many nursing programs, students are asked to document the source of the nursing interventions they propose. Although students may be able to "pull from their head" some nursing strategies, developing the practice of consulting the nursing literature is a sure means to increase nursing knowledge. Some programs also require students to provide a scientific rationale for the interventions they propose. A succinct rationale statement demonstrates that the student is consciously choosing a nursing intervention because of its high probability to effect the desired change.

Critical Thinking Exercise 18-3

An alert, 82-year-old widow who has a history of unsafe behaviors has recently been discharged from the hospital to her home. Caregivers attempted to secure her consent to be transferred to a nursing home but she flatly refused. Being responsible for her home care, you list "Risk for Injury" as a priority nursing diagnosis. Independently with several students, list nursing measures that are most likely to achieve an outcome of injury prevention. Compare your lists of interventions and discuss how practicing nurses can be sure they select the best nursing interventions for each expected client outcome.

Evaluating. Incorporating evaluative statements on the plan of care clearly communicates the message that nursing care is never complete until client goal achievement is evaluated. Just as some say that teaching has not occurred if learning does not take place, so nursing care is incomplete if the desired client goals are not achieved.

Problems Related to Planning

Some of the common problems encountered while developing plans of nursing care are insufficient data collection, nursing diagnoses developed from inaccurate or insufficient data, stating goals/outcomes too broadly, developing goals/outcomes from poorly developed nursing diagnoses, failure to write nursing orders clearly, writing nursing orders that do not adequately resolve the problem, failure to involve the client in the planning process, and failure to update the plan of care.

Nursing Orders	Scientific Rationale	Evaluation
Monitor bowel elimination patterns; identify causative factors of constipation and successful corrective measures.	This client's elimination problems will not be resolved until all the specific causes of her constipation and successful corrective measures are identified. Needs to be an ongoing assessment priority.	9/10/98 Goal partially met. Soft, formed stool passed every 2 to 3 days with aid of colace. *C. Taylor, RN*
Explain the importance of adhering to a regular time for defecation (client suggests after breakfast)—adhere to this in the hospital.	This encourages positive use of circadian rhythms.	
When given medical clearance, assist client with progressive ambulation. Recommend that she include brisk walking into daily health habits (build strength to 20- to 30-minute brisk walk daily).	Peristalsis is stimulated by physical exercise.	9/10/98 Goal met. Client correctly related value of four natural aids to elimination. Questions whether or not she will be strong enough to walk. *Revision:* Encourage assisted ambulation. *C. Taylor, RN*
Explain the long-term effects of laxative abuse on the bowel and discourage their use.	Laxative abuse leads to decreased peristaltic response to food and loss of intestinal tone	
Reinforce the client's adequate fluid intake and ingestion of high-bulk foods such as fresh fruits and salad.	Commenting on these positive self-care behaviors reinforces them.	

Computer Applications in Nursing

Nursing Use of the Technology Assessment Framework

Nurses in all practice settings can use the technology assessment framework to evaluate technology for use in healthcare. The technology can be drugs, biomedical procedures, devices, organizational arrangements, or computer systems. The purpose of using the framework is to ensure that technologies with potential benefits and acceptable risks are made available, to constrain the diffusion and use of technologies that lack efficacy and safety, and to guide appropriate use of such technologies.

Whichever technology is being evaluated, the four areas addressed are safety, cost, efficacy/efficiency, and social impact. For example, if your nursing unit is considering the use of point-of-care computers for nursing documentation, you can use the technology assessment framework as a guideline to develop questions such as those listed below.

Safety

Safety questions refer to how secure, reliable, and safe from harm is the technology in question. It involves a judgment of the acceptability of risk in a specified situation.

- Has the point-of-care computer been tested by biomedical engineering to meet hospital standards? Has it been approved by Underwriters Laboratories for electrical safety?
- Can the device be cleaned?
- Is the device securely mounted in the room?
- Are there passwords and identification codes to protect the client from unauthorized use of the data?
- How does the nurse access the data if the system goes down?

Cost

Economic appraisal of a technology involves the cost of implementing the technology.

- Will the cost of using the system (hardware, software, training, etc.) outweigh the perceived benefits of using it?

(continued)

Computer Applications in Nursing *(continued)*

- Will the cost of using the system (hardware, software, training, etc.) outweigh the perceived benefits of using it?

Efficacy/Efficiency

Efficacy is the benefit of a technology under ideal conditions; effectiveness refers to the benefit of a technology under average conditions.

- Will the work of the nurse be harder or less time consuming with the use of this computer?
- Will the nurse have time to do more things for the client, such as client teaching?

Social Impact

Social impact involves the assessment of the ethical, legal, and political factors associated with the technology.

- Will the client perceive that I am nursing the computer or nursing him?
- Will client privacy and confidentiality be maintained with the use of the system? What laws or statues cover medical records?
- Can the computer be used for client teaching?
- What will be the impact on the nurses and the client of moving the activity from the nurses' station to the point where the care is administered?
- How will the use of the computer enhance the job of the nurse?

An example has been given using the technology assessment framework with a point-of-care system. It can be used with medications, procedures, other devices, and organizational arrangements as well (Happ, 1995; Pillar, Jacox & Redman, 1990).

Key Points

- During planning, the nurse works with the client and family to (1) develop client goals/outcomes that, if achieved, prevent, reduce, or eliminate the problems specified in the nursing diagnoses; and (2) identify the nursing interventions most likely to help the client achieve these goals.
- Conscious, deliberate planning individualizes care, helps communication among nurses, identifies priorities of care, promotes continuity of care, coordinates care, facilitates evaluation of the client's responses to care, and promotes the nurse's professional development.
- The three types of planning essential to comprehensive nursing care are initial, ongoing problem-oriented, and discharge.
- When planning care, the nurse reviews the prioritized list of nursing diagnoses to see that diagnoses are ranked according to the level of threat they present to client well-being. Any changes in the client's health status or in the way the client is responding to health and illness or the treatment plan may signal the need to reestablish client priorities.
- A client goal/outcome describes an expected client behavior. Client goals are derived from the problem statement of the nursing diagnosis, and once achieved, they contribute to the prevention or resolution of this problem.
- Each client goal/outcome must have a subject (the client), a verb (which clearly indicates the action the client is expected to perform), and criteria that describe in observable, measurable terms the expected client behavior.
- Client goals/outcomes should be valued by the client, be supportive of the total treatment plan, be brief, be specific, and be stated positively.
- Nursing interventions are derived from the etiology of the nursing diagnosis. The effective nurse chooses from various possible nursing interventions those that specifically address factors that cause or contribute to the client's problems.
- Effective nursing interventions are consistent with standards of care; realistic in terms of the abilities, time, and resources available to the nurse and client; compatible with the client's values, beliefs, and psychosocial background; valued by the client; and compatible with other planned therapies.
- Nursing orders clearly and concisely describe the nursing intervention to be performed; are signed by the nurse prescribing the order, and dated; use acceptable abbreviations, symbols, and key phrases; and refer nurses to procedure manuals for the steps of lengthy, routine procedures.
- Comprehensive nursing orders specify what observations need to be made and how often; what nursing interventions need to be done, how they are to be done, and when; and the teaching, counseling, and advocacy needs of clients and families.
- The plan of nursing care is the written guide that directs the efforts of the nursing team as they work with clients to meet health goals. Primarily, nursing care plans ensure that nursing care is goal-oriented, efficient, effective, and individualized.

- The nurse who best knows the client develops the plan of care within a reasonable time frame, dictated by the client's condition. The plan is written in ink (part of the client's permanent record) and signed and dated by the nurse who develops the plan. Alternately, the plan of care is entered into the computer as dictated by agency policy.
- Many institutions use a Kardex system of care planning, which specifies nursing care related to basic human needs, prioritized nursing diagnoses, and the medical plan of care. Each client's 6 × 11-inch Kardex care plan is placed in a central Kardex file.
- Standardized plans are prepared plans of care which specify care guidelines and outcomes for groups of clients with common care needs. These plans may be computerized. Interdisciplinary critical pathways are an example of one type of standardized plan.
- Most student care plans are designed to help students systematically proceed through each of the five steps of the nursing process. The assessment data establishing and validating nursing diagnoses often are recorded on the plan, scientific rationales and references may be requested for the nursing order chosen, and evaluative statements are documented.
- Some of the common problems encountered while developing plans of nursing care are insufficient data collection, nursing diagnoses developed from inaccurate or insufficient data, stating goals/outcomes too broadly, developing goals/outcomes from poorly developed nursing diagnoses, failure to write nursing orders clearly, writing nursing orders that do not adequately resolve the problem, failure to involve the client in the planning process, and failure to update the plan of care.

Bibliography

Ackley, B. J., & Ladwig, G. B. (1995). *Nursing diagnosis handbook: A guide to planning care* (2nd ed.). St. Louis: Mosby.

Alfaro-LeFevre, R. (1994). *Applying nursing process: A step-by-step guide* (3rd ed.). Philadelphia: Lippincott.

Atkinson, L. D., & Murray, M. E. (1990). *Understanding the nursing process* (4th ed.). New York: Pergamon.

Carpenito, L. J. (1995). *Nursing care plans and documentation* (2nd ed.). Philadelphia: Lippincott.

Carpenito, L. J. (1995). *Nursing diagnosis: Application to clinical practice* (6th ed.). Philadelphia: Lippincott.

Gage, M. (1994). The patient-driven interdisciplinary care plan. *JONA, 24*(4), 26–38.

Gulanick, M., Klopp, A., Galanes, S., Gradishar, D., & Puzas, M. K. (1994). *Nursing care plans: Nursing diagnosis and intervention.* St. Louis: Mosby.

Happ, B. (1995). Questions for success. *Nursing 95, 25*(9), 32X.

Harris, B. L. (1990). Becoming deprofessionalized: One aspect of the staff nurse's perspective on computer-mediated nursing care plans. *Advances in Nursing Science, 13*(2), 63–74.

Joint Commission on Accreditation of Healthcare Organizations. (1994). *1995 Accreditation manual for hospitals.* Oakbrook Terrace, IL: Author.

MacDonald, E. (1994). Start with the nursing care plan. *Canadian Nurse, 90*(11), 57, 59.

Marrelli, T. M., & Hilliard, L. S. (1996). *Home care and clinical paths.* St. Louis: Mosby.

Pillar, B., Jacox, A. K., & Redman, B. K. (1990). Technology, its assessment, and nursing. *Nursing Outlook, 38*(1), 16–19.

Rasmussen, N., & Gengler, T. (1994). Clinical pathways of care: The route to better communication. *Nursing, 24*(2), 47–49.

Rubenfeld, M. G., & Scheffer, B. K. (1995). *Critical thinking in nursing: An interactive approach.* Philadelphia: Lippincott.

Sparks, S. M. (1992). Computer consult: Exploring electronic support groups. *American Journal of Nursing, 92*(12), 62–65.

Tucker, S. M., Paquette, E. V., Canobbio, M. M., & Wells, M. F. (1996). *Patient care standards: Collaborative practice planning guide.* St. Louis: Mosby.

Ulrich, S. P., Canale, S. W., & Wendell, S. A. (1990). *Nursing care planning guides: A nursing diagnosis approach* (2nd ed.). Philadelphia: Saunders.

Vasey, E. K. (1979). Writing your patient's care plan . . . efficiently. *Nursing, 9*(4), 67–71.

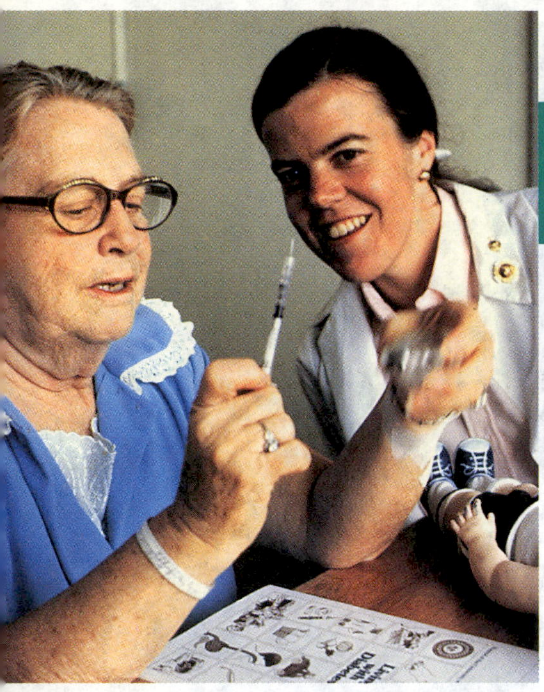

Chapter 19

Implementing

Objectives

After studying this chapter, the learner should be able to:

Define key terms used in the chapter.

Distinguish between independent, interdependent or collaborative, and dependent nursing interventions.

List advantages of having a standard classification of nursing interventions.

Use cognitive, interpersonal, technical, and ethical and legal competencies to implement a plan of nursing care.

Describe six variables that influence the way a plan of care is implemented.

Use seven guidelines for implementation.

Use ongoing data collection to direct revision of the plan of care.

Key Terms

delegation
dependent intervention
discharge summary
implementing
independent intervention
interdependent (collaborative) intervention
nursing interventions
protocol
report
standing order

During the **implementing** step of the nursing process, all the nursing actions developed during the planning step are carried out. The purpose of implementation is to assist the client in achieving desired health goals—promote wellness, prevent disease and illness, restore health, and facilitate coping with altered functioning. The plan of care is best implemented when clients who are able and willing to participate have maximum opportunities to provide self-care. Family members and other support people, as well as other healthcare professionals, also can become involved in the successful implementation of the plan of care (Table 19-1). During the implementation step, the nurse continues to collect data and to modify the plan of care as needed (Fig. 19-1). All activities are documented according to the form used in the nurse's institution.

Unique Focus of Nursing Implementation

In all nurse–client interactions, the nurse is concerned with both the client's response to health and illness and the client's ability to meet basic human needs. Whereas other healthcare professionals focus on selected aspects of the client's treatment regimen, the nurse is concerned with how the client is responding to the plan of care in general.

Types of Nursing Interventions

When implementing the plan of care, the nurse functions independently, dependently, and collaboratively.

Independent interventions or nursing actions involve carrying out nurse-prescribed orders written on the nursing plan of care, as well as any other actions that nurses initiate without the direction or supervision of another healthcare professional and that are the result of their assessment of client needs. Nurses are legally accountable for the assessments they make and for their nursing responses.

Dependent interventions or nursing actions involve carrying out physician-prescribed orders. Nurse practice acts make it clear from whom nurses can receive orders. Nurses are accountable for the dependent orders they implement and are thus responsible for the clarification of any questionable order.

Collaborative or **interdependent interventions** or nursing actions are those performed jointly by nurses and other members of the healthcare team. Because nurses are being increasingly respected as competent colleagues with a unique knowledge of the client, they are becoming more and more involved in collaborative ventures with the healthcare team.

To underscore the fact that nurses are always responsible for their actions, some nurses have moved away from the terminology independent and dependent nursing interventions, and replaced these terms with "nurse-initiated" or "nurse-prescribed" and "physician-initiated," or "physician-prescribed" interventions, respectively.

All these actions may be illustrated with reference to the care received by a depressed client with data indicative of a gastrointestinal blockage. If the physician orders a series of gastrointestinal studies, it is nursing's responsibility to prepare the client by executing the physician's orders for cleansing the bowel. These nursing actions are dependent interventions. If the nurse senses that the client seems unusually fearful of what the outcome of the studies will be, and plans to explore the client's fears and follow-up with appropriate teaching and counseling, then the nurse is involved in independent nursing actions. When a multidisciplinary team conference is held to discuss the client's failure to progress, the nurse works collaboratively with the psychiatrist, gastroenterologist, social worker, and pastoral counselor to develop a comprehensive plan of care; these are collaborative or interdependent nursing actions.

Practicing nurses as well as students beginning clinical experience may be surprised when they evaluate how much of their day is devoted to independent nursing practice (care organized by nursing diagnosis) and how much is spent carrying out dependent functions (medically delegated care—disease management, medical orders, and so forth). Using a circle, divide your day into segments that represent independent nursing practice, dependent nursing practice, collaborative nursing

Table 19-1
Professional Nursing Relationships: Role Responsibilities and Related Competencies

Relationship	Role Responsibilities	Related Competencies
Nurse–client	• Communicate to the client that someone is concerned about him or her (as well as the disease) and is interested in how this change in health state will affect his or her overall well-being. • Create an environment in which the client can commit his or her energies to health promotion or restoration or peaceful dying, confident that basic human needs are being addressed. • Challenge the client to maximally develop self-care abilities that promote holistic health.	• Repertoire of therapeutic interpersonal behaviors—attending, listening, interviewing, nonverbal communication, therapeutic communication, touching, facilitating, coaching • Ability to establish trusting nurse–client–family relationships • Demonstrated competence in the nursing roles of caregiver, teacher, counselor, advocate
Nurse–client–family	• Develop in the client and family the knowledge, attitude, and skills that will enable them to respond to the self-care challenge of their health or illness state. • Intervene as appropriate to promote healthy family functioning. • Educate the family to be wise and assertive health care consumers.	
Nurse–nurse	• Support one another's efforts to deliver quality nursing care; work collaboratively with nursing administration to improve quality care. • Provide creative leadership—formally or informally—to make the nursing unit a satisfying and challenging place to work. • Supervise the nursing care given by other nursing personnel; affirm the nursing strengths of others and constructively address the nursing deficiencies encountered. • Enhance the professional development of self and other nurses through active participation in professional organizations.	Communication Teaching/counseling/advocacy Assertiveness Collaboration Coordination Group process Organization Leadership Delegation Change strategies Problem solving Decision making Conflict resolution
Nurse–healthcare team	• Communicate clearly nursing's perspective regarding the client and family to the healthcare team. • Coordinate the inputs of the multidisciplinary team into a comprehensive plan of care. • Serve as a liaison between the client and family and the healthcare team, as necessary.	

practice, continuing education, and other activities. How your circle is divided illustrates your priorities, as well as the range of nursing interventions possible in your particular practice setting (Fig. 19-2).

The Nursing Interventions Taxonomy Structure

In 1992 McCloskey and Bulechek published *Nursing Interventions Classification* (*NIC*) (Iowa Intervention Project, 1992), a report of research to construct a taxonomy of nursing interventions. Each of the 336 interventions listed has a label, definition, set of activities that a nurse does to carry it out, and a short list of background readings. Advantages of having a standard classification of nursing interventions include:

- To standardize nomenclature
- To expand nursing knowledge
- To develop information systems
- To teach decision making
- To cost out nursing
- To allocate nursing resources
- To communicate nursing to non-nurses
- To link nursing content (Iowa Intervention Project, 1992, p. 14)

Table 19-2 illustrates the new taxonomy structure that helps clinicians to locate and select interventions most helpful for clients (McCloskey & Bulechek, 1996).

Protocols and Standing Orders

Protocols and standing orders may expand the scope of nursing practice in certain clearly defined situations. **Protocols** are written plans that detail the nursing activities to be executed in specific situations. Although some protocols specify routine aspects of nursing care (eg, protocols that describe nursing responsibilities when a client is admitted to or discharged from the institution), other protocols include **standing orders** that

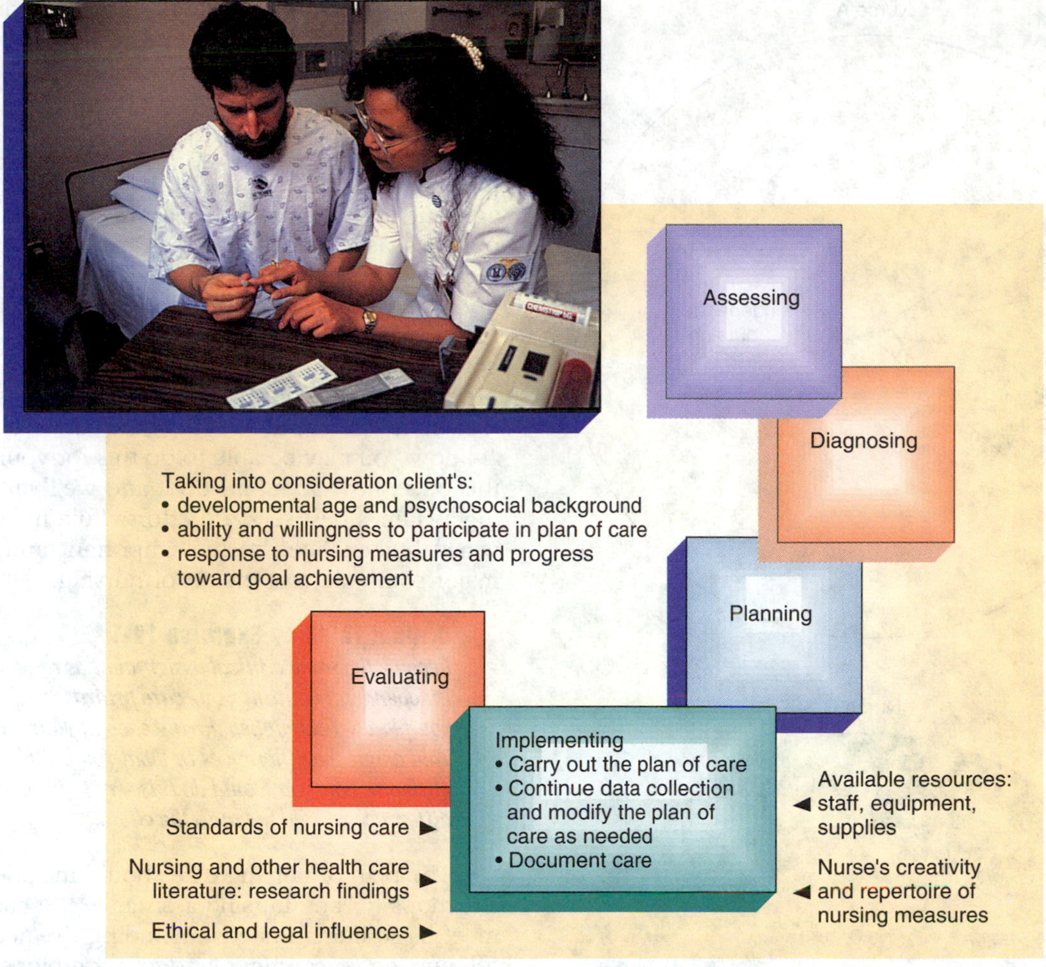

Figure 19-1
Implementing. Implementing involves the carrying out of the plan of care, which is modified in response to client changes. Numerous variables influence the way the plan of care is implemented (see arrows). (Photo © Kathy Sloane.)

empower the nurse to initiate actions that ordinarily require the order or supervision of a physician. Examples include admission protocols for obstetrics and gynecology clients, protocols for bowel programs that allow the nurse to select and administer necessary bowel interventions, standard orders for narcotic overdoses that specify the agents the nurse is to administer to reverse respiratory depression in an emergency, and standard orders for pain management that enable the nurse to select the strength of the medication to be given within preset ranges.

The Nurse as Coordinator

One of nursing's major contributions to the healthcare team is the role of coordinator. It is easy for care to become fragmented when clients are seen by numerous specialists—each interested in a different aspect of the client. At best, clients complain that no one person really knows them and can talk with them about what is going on and how it will affect them in the future. At worst, the orders of the different specialists may conflict with one another and be counterproductive. Therefore, it is important for nurses to make rounds with other healthcare professionals and to read the results of consultations that clients have had with various specialists. The nurse can then interpret the specialists' findings for clients and family members, prepare clients to participate maximally in the plan of care both before and after discharge, and serve as a liaison among the members of the healthcare team. Nurse case managers are specialists in the role of care coordinator.

Carrying Out the Plan of Care

When carrying out the plan of care, nurses use specialized abilities to (1) determine the client's need for nursing assistance, (2) promote self-care, and (3) assist the client to achieve health goals.

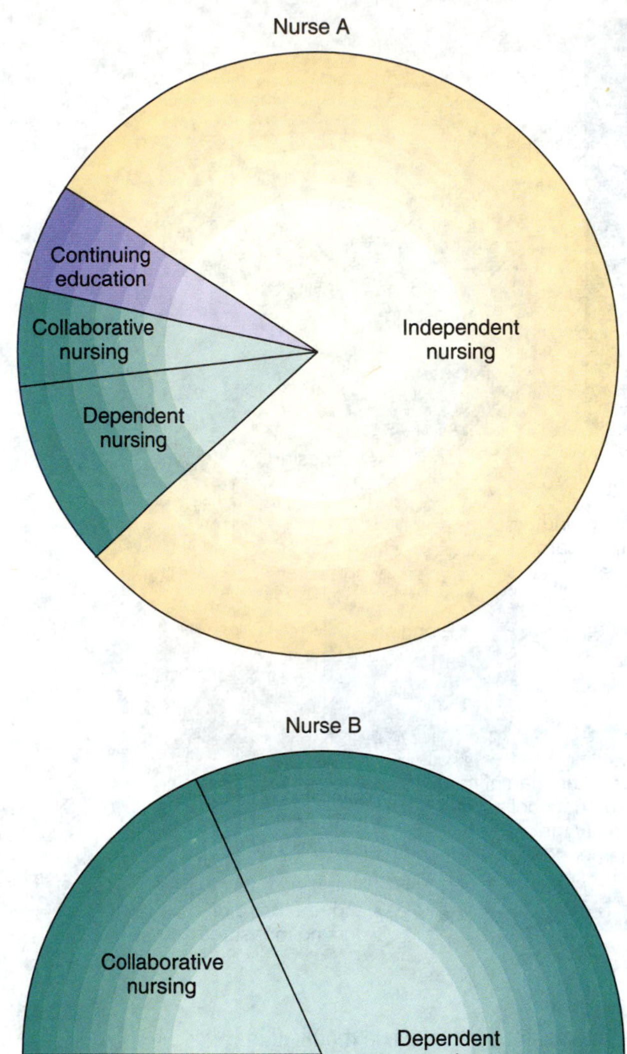

Figure 19-2
Division of nursing time. These circles illustrate the way two nurses in different practice settings spend their work day. This time division quickly indicates the emphasis on independent, dependent, and collaborative nursing.

Prerequisite Core Competencies

When implementing the plan of nursing care, nurses use cognitive, interpersonal, technical, and ethical and legal competencies. Each nurse possesses a unique blend of these competencies and is effective to the extent that his or her abilities are able to match the client's need for nursing care. These competencies are described in Chapter 15 and illustrated at the end of each clinical chapter.

Determining the Need for Assistance

Although most people are capable of independently meeting basic human needs, illness and the stress of diagnostic and therapeutic measures may interfere with a person's usual practice of self-care abilities. A careful nursing assessment of the client's abilities to independently meet human needs is indicated. Nursing often has failed clients by doing too much for them and by encouraging negative, sick role behaviors, such as inappropriate dependence. Conversely, there is a time and a place for the "tender loving care" that says to a client, "I know you may be able to do this for yourself, but just this once, how about if I do it and we'll talk!" Challenging a client's best self-care effort while meeting the universal human need to feel important and loved is an major component of the art of nursing.

Critical Thinking Exercise 19-1

Receive the same clinical assignment as another student. Independently outline your care priorities, specifying what you plan to accomplish during each of your clinical hours. Talk about the differences in what you both hope to accomplish and how you would do this. Try to imagine what these differences would mean to the client.

The plan of nursing care should include specific instructions for any nursing assistance the client needs to meet basic human needs, including the need for forceful nursing encouragement to promote greater independence in functioning. When routines of self-care are indicated (eg, colostomy management), instructions should include the time of the procedure, the equipment used, the process, and the level of client involvement. Continuity of nursing care is essential to the client's development of a comfortable routine.

Delegating Nursing Care

With the current pressure to reduce healthcare costs, many employers of nurses are increasing their utilization of unlicensed assistive personnel (UAP), or "nurse extenders." In some cases, the new mix of professional and nonprofessional staff is threatening client safety. Never has it been more important for nurses to critically identify which nursing interventions require professional nurses and which can be safely delegated. **Delegation** is the transfer of responsibility for the performance of an activity from one individual to another while retaining accountability for the outcome. Those new to nursing must understand that a nurse who delegates an intervention to a nursing assistant remains accountable for the delegated service.

Before delegating any nursing service, a number of factors should be considered: (1) the client's condition, (2) the complexity of the activity, (3) the capabilities of the UAP, and (4) the availability of professional staff to

Table 19-2
NIC Taxonomy

	Domain I	Domain II	Domain III	Domain IV	Domain V	Domain VI
Level 1 Domains	1. Physiological: Basic Care that supports physical functioning	2. Physiological: Complex Care that supports homeostatic regulation	3. Behavioral Care that supports psychosocial functioning and facilitates life style changes	4. Safety Care that supports protection against harm	5. Family Care that supports the family unit	6. Health System Care that supports effective use of the health care delivery system
Level 2 Classes	A Activity and Exercise Management: Interventions to organize or assist with physical activity and energy expenditure B Elimination Management: Interventions to establish and maintain regular bowel and urinary elimination patterns and manage complications due to altered patterns C Immobility Management: Interventions to manage restricted body movement and the sequelae D Nutrition Support: Interventions to modify or maintain nutritional status E Physical Comfort Promotion: Interventions to promote comfort using physical techniques F Self-Care Facilitation: Interventions to provide or assist with routine activities of daily living	G Electrolyte and Acid-Base Management: Interventions to regulate electrolyte/acid-base balance and prevent complications H Medication Management: Interventions to facilitate desired effects of pharmacologic agents I Neurologic Management: Interventions to optimize neurologic function J Perioperative Care: Interventions to provide care before, during, and immediately after surgery K Respiratory Management: Interventions to promote airway patency and gas exchange L Skin/Wound Management: Interventions to maintain or restore tissue integrity M Thermoregulation: Interventions to maintain body temperature within a normal range N Tissue Perfusion Management: Interventions to optimize circulation of blood and fluids to the tissue	O Behavior Therapy: Interventions to reinforce or promote desirable behaviors or alter undesirable behaviors P Cognitive Therapy: Interventions to reinforce or promote desirable cognitive functioning or alter undesirable cognitive functioning Q Communication Enhancement: Interventions to facilitate delivering and receiving verbal or non-verbal messages R Coping Assistance: Interventions to assist another to build on own strengths, to adapt to a change in function, or to achieve a higher level of function S Patient Education: Interventions to facilitate learning T Psychological Comfort Promotion: Interventions to promote comfort using psychological techniques	U Crisis Management: Interventions to provide immediate short term help in both psychological and physiological crises V Risk Management: Interventions to initiate risk reduction activities and continue monitoring risk over time	W Childbearing Care: Interventions to assist in understanding and coping with the psychological and physiological changes during the childbearing period X Lifespan Care: Interventions to facilitate family unit functioning and promote the health and welfare of family members throughout the lifespan	Y Health System Mediation: Interventions to facilitate the interface between patient/family and the health-care system a. Health System Management: Interventions to provide and enhance support services for the delivery of care b. Information Management: Interventions to facilitate communication among healthcare workers

McCloskey, J. C., & Bulechek, G. M. (Eds.) (1996). *Iowa Interventions Project: Nursing interventions classification* (2nd ed.). St. Louis: Mosby. Used with permission.

Implementing: Core Competencies

Cognitive Competencies

- Knowledge of what is needed to implement a plan of care that effectively meets the client's health needs
- Knowledge of pertinent standards of care and agency/institutional policies

Technical Competencies

- Ability to use equipment and techniques competently that are specified by the client's plan of care

Interpersonal Competencies

- Ability to establish a trusting nurse–client relationship grounded in responsible caring
- Ability to communicate to the client that you are more concerned about the client and his/her well-being than about rote implementation of the plan of care or accomplishment of discrete tasks
- Ability to work with members of the caregiving team collaboratively to implement the interdisciplinary plan of care

Ethical/Legal Competencies

- Commitment to do whatever is necessary to implement the plan of care successfully
- Ability to serve as a trusted and effective client advocate
- Consistent use of appropriate legal safeguards while implementing the plan of care

accomplish the unit workload. The American Nurses Association, which is committed to monitoring the regulation, education, and utilization of UAPs, recommends adherence to the following principles:

- It is the nursing profession that determines the scope of nursing practice.
- It is the nursing profession that defines and supervises the education, training, and utilization of any unlicensed assistant roles involved in providing direct nursing care.
- It is the RN who is responsible and accountable for nursing practice.

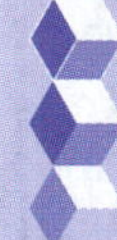

Through the Eyes of the Family Caregiver

The Nurses Never Told Me There'd Be Days Like This

I wasn't prepared for a roller coaster ride when my husband became ill. My husband was admitted to the hospital in an emergency condition, became confused when his electrolytes were off balance, went into cardiac arrest and had CPR, was placed on a ventilator, and was put to sleep because he was too apprehensive about the ventilator. I had reached the lowest point as I sat by his bedside for days, talking to him and wondering if he heard me.

My spirits soared the day they brought him out of his sleep state and he recognized me and was hungry for real food. The next day when I went to the hospital I plummeted to the low point again when he was crumpled in bed like a confused rag doll with his hospital gown up to his chest and the sheet to his ankles. I started to cry, and the nurse came and put her arm around me. She said, "Don't think he's taken a turn for the worse. There will be good days and bad days as he recovers." No one had prepared me for that—and her arm around me and her words were so consoling.

When I brought him home after 6 weeks in the hospital, I was not prepared for his anger at being confined to the house (in a heat wave) and not being allowed to drive. His reasoning that he had to get a haircut because he hadn't had one in 2 months made sense to him. My saying no one would care about the length of his hair did not soothe his anger.

He couldn't accept the fact that he was too weak to go up and down the steps more than once a day, so he insisted on going to the basement. Going down was simple; coming up wasn't. We forgot there was no railing (which he needed to haul himself up) on the last four steps. He solved the problem by sitting on the steps and lifting himself up a step at a time. Then he got to the floor at the top and couldn't stand up. I couldn't lift him. We were stuck. Again I took a nose dive.

I thought I understood how difficult it would be for him to readjust. I knew he would be depressed and expected him to lean on me. But I was not prepared for his frustration to come out as anger at me. It would have been helpful to have someone prepare me. Or it would be nice to have a nurse put her arm around me now when my roller coaster plummets.

—Eleanor Faven,
Philadelphia, Pennsylvania

- It is the RN who supervises any assistant involved in providing direct client care.
- It is the purpose of assistive personnel to work in a supportive role to the RN, carrying out tasks that will enable the professional nurse to concentrate on nursing care for the client (PNA, 1992).

Promoting Self-Care: Teaching, Counseling, and Advocacy

If clients and their families want to participate actively in seeking wellness, preventing disease and illness, recovering health, and learning to cope with altered functioning, it is important that they possess effective self-care behaviors. Nurses sensitive to the importance of clients learning to direct and manage their own care use nurse–client interactions for both planned and spontaneous teaching, counseling, and advocacy. These nursing roles are described in Chapters 23 and 24. For example, while caring for a child recently diagnosed as having cystic fibrosis, the nurses work continuously with the parents and siblings, helping them to develop the knowledge and skills that will enable them to care for the child on discharge. Referring families such as this to a community support group or other resources further enhances the self-care behaviors being developed.

Assisting Clients to Meet Health Goals

In this phase of the implementation process, the nursing team carries out the nursing orders detailed in the nursing plan of care. If the plan of care is well constructed, carrying out its orders is the nurse's most important task and should receive top priority. The nursing actions planned to promote client goal/outcome achievement and the resolution of health problems should be carefully executed (see implementation guidelines in the accompanying box).

Because understaffing continues to be a problem in many practice settings, it is important that nurses learn to use time wisely and to maximize each client encounter. A client bath can be simply that, or it can be an opportunity to gather additional focused data, to communicate concern for what the client is experiencing and to offer support, and to teach and counsel as appropriate. How the nurse uses the 30 minutes that he or she is in the client's room for the bath determines how effective the nurse is in helping the client to achieve his or her goals/outcomes.

Variables That Influence Goal/Outcome Achievement

When working with clients to achieve the goals/outcomes specified in the plan of care, remember that nothing about the plan of care is fixed. Some of the most important variables that influence the way the plan of care is implemented follow.

Client Variables. Ideally, the client is the primary determinant of how nursing interventions are implemented. Successful nurses modify their nursing actions according to the client's (1) changing ability and willingness to participate in the plan of care and (2) previous responses to nursing interventions and progress toward goal/outcome achievement. Other important client variables are developmental stage and psychosocial background.

Many nurses who have studied development believe that they have addressed the developmental needs of a

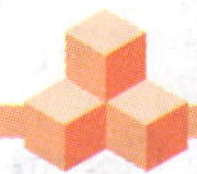

Guidelines for Nursing Care

Implementation

- Before implementing any nursing action, reassess the client to determine if the action is still needed.
- Approach the client competently. Know how to perform the nursing action, why the action is being performed, and potential adverse responses. Have all equipment and supplies ready.
- Approach the client caringly. Explain the nursing action using language the client understands. Communicate genuine concern for what the client is experiencing.
- Modify nursing interventions according to the client's (1) developmental and psychosocial background, (2) ability and willingness to participate in the plan of care, and (3) responses to previous nursing measures and progress toward goal/outcome achievement.
- Check to make sure that the nursing interventions selected are consistent with standards of care and within legal and ethical guides to practice.
- Always question that the nursing intervention selected is the best of all possible alternatives. Consult colleagues and the nursing and related literature to see if other approaches might be more successful. Evaluate the effectiveness of the intervention selected, noting any factors that positively or negatively influenced the outcome.
- Develop a repertoire of skilled nursing interventions. The more options one can choose from, the greater the likelihood of success.

client simply by identifying the client's developmental stage on the plan of care. What the developmental tasks related to this stage are and how these tasks are related to nursing care seldom are considered. Stereotypes about developmental stages and tasks also influence the care that clients receive. For example, the same student nurse who recommends that the parents of a premature infant make a tape of their voices to stimulate the infant in the neonatal intensive care unit may also work weekends in a nursing home where the developmental needs of older clients are routinely violated. This student has never thought to question the staff's selection of a radio station that plays rock music, or other staff actions—humorous comments about "romances" among some of the residents, infantilizing some residents by calling them cute names or putting bright, big bows in their hair, or planning childish group activities that many of the clients find demeaning. Perhaps the greatest violation is the belief that all older people have to do is wait to die, that there are no developmental challenges for this age group.

In implementing a comprehensive and holistic plan of care, nurses must find creative ways to meet developmental needs. This is of greatest importance when clients are separated from their families and home environments for long periods.

The same is true of the psychosocial needs of clients. Although few nurses would claim that people from all socioeconomic groups and cultures are the same, some practice nursing as if this were so. When choosing nursing interventions, it is important to consider and respect the client's background. Confronted with a malnourished client on a limited income who rents a single room in a boarding home, a nurse cannot simply teach the importance of including more protein in the diet. To be effective the nurse must explore the realistic possibility of the client being able to afford and obtain foods rich in protein. Moreover, the nurse needs to assess if the client values this intervention and is willing to make the necessary changes.

Nurse Variables. Nurse variables that influence the implementation of the plan of care include the nurses' levels of expertise, creativity (ability to match client needs with specific nursing strategies), willingness to provide care, and available time.

Critical Thinking Exercise 19-2

Team up with another student and take turns role playing a nurse visiting a homebound older male who needs assessment of his vital signs and nutritional status. Discuss with each other the truth or falsity of the claim: "Who the nurse is is as important as, and sometimes more important than, what the nurse does."

Resources. The most elaborately designed plan of care is doomed to failure on a chronically understaffed or undersupplied nursing unit. Adequate staff, equipment, and supplies are all important determinants of client care. The financial resources of the client and adequacy of community-based resources will also influence the plan of care.

Current Standards of Care. All nursing actions that are selected when implementing the plan of care must be consistent with standards for practice. Each nurse is responsible for learning the standards that dictate practice in his or her specialty. Failure to practice according to these standards may result in a charge of negligence.

Research Findings. Nurses concerned about improving the quality of nursing care use research findings to enhance their nursing practice. Reading professional nursing journals and attending continuing education workshops and conferences are excellent ways to learn about new nursing strategies that have proven effectiveness.

Ethical and Legal Guides to Practice. It is impossible to practice good nursing today and be ignorant of the laws and regulations that affect healthcare and the ethical dimensions of clinical practice. As the nurse implements the plan of care, sincere motivation to benefit the client and a conscientious attempt to implement nursing orders well are no longer sufficient. Each nurse is responsible for developing sensitivity to the ethical and legal dimensions of practice, and moral and legal accountability are inherent in the practice of professional nursing. Chapters 6 and 7 deal specifically with the ethical and legal dimensions of practice. Hospital risk managers and ethics committees are institutional resources that are increasingly available for nurses.

Responding to the Noncompliant Client

When a client fails to follow the plan of care in spite of the nurse's best efforts, it is time to reassess strategy. The first objective is to identify why the client is resisting therapy. One possibility is that the plan of care may not be right for this client. In this event, what is needed is not a change in the client, but rather a change in the plan of care. If the nurse determines, however, that the plan of care is adequate, she or he must identify and remedy the factors contributing to the client's noncompliance. Common reasons for noncompliance include (1) lack of family support, (2) lack of understanding about the benefits of compliance, (3) adverse physical or emotional effects of treatment (such as pain and fatigue), (4) inability to afford treatment, and (5) limited access to treatment. Wichowski and Kubsch (1995) recommend the following interventions if the client's negative outlook on illness and chance of recovery are contributing to noncompliance:

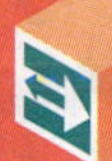

Developing Critical Thinking Skills

Situation

One of the nurses on your oncology unit wants to develop a "humor room" where clients, their families, and staff can "take a break" from the serious business of illness. Designed to lift the spirits, amuse, distract, and thus speed the healing process, humor rooms are gaining popularity as new therapeutic tools. Funny books, comic movies on a large-screen TV; games and puzzles; and ideally even clowns, magicians, musicians, and stand-up comedians are being envisaged (Buxman, 1991). Several nurses have vocally expressed their lack of support for the project and think the idea is "stupid" at best and potentially a great waste of money, time, and energy that could be devoted to "tried and true" methods of healing. You have been asked to support the project and must decide how to respond.

1. ***Identify Goal of Thinking***

   Clarify your thinking about humor as a therapeutic measure so that you can decide whether or not to support this project.

2. ***Assess Adequacy of Knowledge***

   Pertinent circumstances: The nurse who wants to develop the humor room is more popular with clients than she is with her colleagues. Her nurse friends are quick to point out that while it's true that she is "a bit flakey" and unorthodox, she is an efficient nurse who is well-loved by her clients and their families. The hospital is in the midst of cutting expenses and has laid off both professional and nonprofessional employees.

   Prerequisite knowledge: In order to decide how you should respond in this situation you need to research the healing benefits of humor. Are there clinical studies demonstrating its effectiveness as a therapeutic measure? Should studies point to humor's effectiveness you will need to determine (1) what priority it should have among other treatment modalities and (2) the feasibility of creating a humor room in the current climate of cutting expenses. Is there a creative way to finance this venture?

   Room for error: Since life and death do not hinge on how you elect to respond to this plea for support there is a relatively wide margin for error. However, since personal energy and finances are limited, you do not want to involve your unit in a futile project.

   Time constraints: There is no rush for an immediate decision on your part, which gives you adequate time to develop the knowledge base you need to make an informed decision.

3. ***Address Potential Problems***

   The most serious obstacle to critical thinking in this situation would be the lack of an open mind and refusal to weigh the merits of a new treatment modality. Complicating factors include divided loyalties among the nurses and the tendency to support or refuse support for the project on the basis of whether or not one likes the nurse advocating the project, rather than on the merits of the project. Finally, the lowered morale caused by lay-offs may squash all creativity and willingness to "dream new dreams."

4. ***Consult Helpful Resources***

   Your first challenge will be to learn more about humor as a healing measure. Ideally you may be able to consult a local expert and invite her or him to meet with the staff. Alternately, you can research the literature looking for clinical studies and reports of the first-person experiences of others.

5. ***Critique Judgment/Decision***

   After a search of the literature convinced you and some of the other nurses of the clinical benefits of humor, you decide to explore the feasibility of developing a humor room. Your options are to "play it safe" and not rock the boat during a difficult period in the hospital by trying something new, or to become an advocate for the project and commit your energies to making it happen. You decide that a creative project may be exactly what the staff needs to rediscover the "joy of nursing" and begin to explore means to fund the project. You plan to "start small" and to reassess the project every 6 months. Since your research educated you about the potential benefits *and harms* humor can create, you decide that your first objective must be to educate the staff.

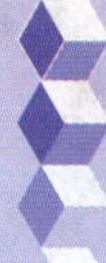

Through the Eyes of a Student

One of my first clients was a woman with a history of Alzheimer's disease. When I was assigned this client, I knew that I was not going to have a good day. I had been introduced to this client the week before, when I had orientation. She was sitting in a gerry chair in the hallway where she sang at the top of her lungs and threw tissues on the floor. Occasionally, she would curse at a person passing by.

I took a deep breath and entered her room. At her bedside I introduced myself. With a few choice words she told me to get out of her room. I tried to ignore her response and prepared her breakfast tray. She proceeded to throw her scrambled eggs around the room. After I took the tray away from her and finished cleaning up the mess, it was time for preconference. At preconference, my instructor told me we were going to "tub" my client. I had visions of a grand fiasco in the tub room, and I dreaded giving her the bath.

My instructor and I took her to the tub room by wheelchair. Once we convinced her to get in the tub, she did nothing but yell that it was cold. We started the water and she yelled even louder. I knew everyone could hear her in the hallway as she cursed and yelled, but as the bath proceeded she quieted down and stopped fighting me. We completed the bath and wheeled her back down the hall to her room. I bundled her up in blankets and put her in the gerry chair in the hallway. She was so relaxed from the bath that she let me brush her hair and put it in a ponytail. While I was brushing her hair, she fell asleep. I did my chart until her lunch arrived. When I set her up for her lunch and told her I would be leaving, she thanked me, and it made my day. All the struggling I went through all day with her and she thanked me. When I went home I felt really good about helping her. During all my worrying about the day being a fiasco and the embarrassment of having a client yell at me, I had lost sight of the client herself and what she needed me to do for her. By her thanking me at the end of the day, I realized that when my clinical instructor forced me to do something for my client that the regular staff of the hospital wouldn't do, I was meeting her basic needs, and my client recognized that.

—Jeanene C. Smith,
Delaware County Community College,
Media, Pennsylvania

1. Increase the client's expectations.
2. Offer a positive outlook; change the perception of illness from obstacle or setback to opportunity for growth.
3. Redirect negative behavior.
4. Develop a rapport.
5. Put a new spin on life.

Guide for Students

Student nurses trying in advance to organize their nursing care for a particular clinical day can use the guidelines for student clinical responsibilities in the accompanying box to help identify the nursing measures for which they will be responsible. Once these have been identified, working

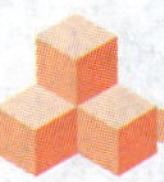

Guidelines for Nursing Care

Student Clinical Responsibilities

To organize clinical responsibilities, check:

1. Client profile
2. Name by which client wishes to be addressed
3. Client's current health status
   - Note any physical or emotional changes indicating the need to modify the plan of care
4. Routine assistance client needs to meet basic human needs
   - Note any special safety precautions needed
5. Priorities for nursing care
   - Prioritized nursing diagnoses, client goals/outcomes, and related nursing interventions
   - Medical orders that need to be implemented
   - Interdependent or collaborative nursing responsibilities
6. Special "events" of the day that may require special observation of the client, teaching, preparation, or aftercare
   - Diagnostic tests
   - Consultations with specialists
   - New therapies (physical therapy, medications, surgery, radiotherapy, and so forth)
7. Special teaching, counseling, or advocacy needs
8. Special needs of the family

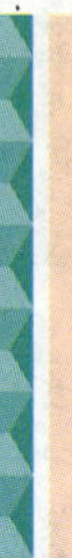

Computer Applications in Nursing

Computer Software to Enhance Clinical Skills

Mastering Clinical Skills by Marianne Yoder, Ph.D., RN, is a series of computer software programs designed for undergraduate and in-service programs. Topics include:

- Blood administration
- Oxygen administration
- Platelet administration
- Enteral feeding
- Managing chest tubes

It is available for IBM-compatible platforms from Lippincott-Raven Publishers, 227 East Washington Square, Philadelphia, PA 19106, 1-800-777-2295.

out a time schedule may provide clear direction for the clinical day and ensure that the client's needs are met.

Continuing Data Collection

An important nursing intervention is ongoing data collection. In every client encounter, the nurse needs to be sensitive to both subtle and dramatic changes in the client's condition or response to this condition. These assessment findings are used to update and revise the plan of care. Sensitivity to how the client is responding to nursing interventions and to the client's progress toward goal/outcome achievement allows the nurse to modify nursing interventions appropriately.

Critical Thinking Exercise 19-3

Describe how you probably would respond, and how you would like to respond (in case these are different), to hearing in the shift report that one of the clients you are assigned to was a real P.I.B. ["pain in the butt"] all day and "just impossible" to care for. Reflect on the importance of the language we use to report on a client to one another.

Nursing Oneself

It is difficult for nurses to be sincerely attentive to client needs when their own human needs are not being met. Because no one is perfectly healthy or "whole" all the time, it is important as nurses prepare for professional practice that they spend time getting to know themselves. In an excellent chapter on psychologic self-care written for nurses, Hill and Smith (1990) describe psychologic self-care as a constellation of activities practiced on a regular basis to promote psychologic health. These include self-awareness, communication, time management, preparation for crisis and loss, developing and maintaining support systems, and concurrent practice of self-care in all areas. The characteristics of emotional health include self-esteem, self-knowledge, satisfying interpersonal relationships, environmental mastery, stress management, a positive body image, a sense of humor, and the ability to provide oneself with pleasure.

Nurses who want to be competent practitioners learn early to nurse themselves and other nurses before attempting to nurse clients. Not only does improved personal health enable the nurse to practice more efficiently, but it also enables the nurse to be a health model for clients and their families. Nurses can help clients to imitate health behavior and eventually integrate it into daily life through the process of identification. Each clinical chapter contains a section titled "The Nurse as Role Model," which you may find helpful.

Key Points

- Implementing, the fourth step of the nursing process, is the carrying out of the plan of care. Its purpose is to assist clients to achieve desired health goals—to promote wellness, prevent disease and illness, restore health, and facilitate coping with altered functioning.
- The plan of care is best implemented when clients who are able and willing to participate have maximal opportunity to do so.
- Whereas other healthcare professionals focus on select aspects of the client's treatment regimen, nursing is concerned with how the *person* is responding in general to the plan of care.
- Nurses implement independent (nurse-prescribed), interdependent (collaborative), and dependent (physician-prescribed) nursing actions.
- A taxonomy of nursing interventions now exists which offers a means of standardizing nomenclature, expanding nursing knowledge, developing information systems, teaching decision making, costing out nursing, allocating nursing resources, communicating nursing to non-nurses, and linking nursing content.

- While carrying out the plan of care, nurses use cognitive, interpersonal, technical, and ethical and legal skills. Nursing's first challenge is the determination of how much nursing assistance the client needs to reach desired goals/outcomes.
- The nurse's teaching, counseling, and advocacy skills are used to assist clients to develop the self-care behaviors that enable them to direct and manage their own care.
- Nothing about the care plan or the way it is implemented is fixed. Client and nurse variables, as well as available resources, current standards of care, research findings, and ethical and legal guides to practice, may influence the plan's implementation.
- Ongoing data collection directs the revision of the plan of care.
- Improved personal health enables nurses to practice more effectively and to be a health model for clients and their families.

Bibliography

Alfaro-LeFevre, R. (1994). *Applying nursing process: A step-by-step guide* (3rd ed.). Philadelphia: Lippincott.

Benner, P. (1984). *From novice to expert: Excellence and power in clinical nursing practice.* Menlo Park, CA: Addison-Wesley.

Benner P., & Wrubel, J. (1989). *The primary of caring: Stress and coping in health and illness.* Menlo Park, CA: Addison-Wesley.

Blegen, M. A., Gardner, D. I., & McCloskey, J. C. (1992). Who helps you with your work? *American Journal of Nursing, 92*(1), 26–31.

Brider, P. (1992). The move to patient-focused care. *American Journal of Nursing, 92*(9), 26–33.

Bulechek, G. M., & McCloskey, J. C. (1987). Nursing interventions: What they are and how to choose them. *Holistic Nursing Practice, 1*(3), 36–44.

Buxman, K. (1991). Make room for laughter. *American Journal of Nursing, 91*(12), 46–51.

Cohen, E. L. (1995). *Nurse case management in the 21st century.* St. Louis: Mosby.

Dossey, B. (1991). Awakening the inner healer. *American Journal of Nursing, 91*(8), 31–34.

Eisenhauer, L. A. (1994). A typology of nursing therapeutics. *IMAGE: Journal of Nursing Scholarship, 26*(4), 261–264.

Ellis, J. R., & Hartley, C. L. (1995). *Managing and coordinating nursing care* (2nd ed.). Philadelphia: Lippincott.

Gibson, L. (1994). Healing with humor. *Nursing, 24*(9), 56–57.

Hansten, R., & Washburn, M. (1992). Delegation: How to deliver care through others. *American Journal of Nursing, 92*(3), 87–90.

Hansten, R., & Washburn, M. (1992). How to plan what to delegate. *American Journal of Nursing, 92*(4), 71–72.

Hill, L., & Smith, N. (1990). *Self-care nursing: Promotion of health* (2nd ed.). East Norwalk, CT: Appleton & Lange.

Iowa Intervention Project. (1993). The NIC taxonomy structure. *IMAGE: Journal of Nursing Scholarship, 25*(3), 187–192.

Iowa Intervention Project. McCloskey, J. C., & Bulechek, G. (Eds.). (1992). *Nursing intervention classification (NIC).* St. Louis: Mosby–Year Book.

Iowa Intervention Project. McCloskey, J. C., & Bulechek, G. (Eds.). (1995). Validating and coding of the NIC taxonomy structure. *IMAGE: Journal of Nursing Scholarship, 27*(1), 43–49.

Joint Commission on Accreditation of Healthcare Organizations. (1995). *Accreditation manual for hospitals.* Oakbrook Terrace, IL: JCAHO.

McCloskey, J. C., & Bulechek, G. M. (Eds.) (1996). *Iowa Interventions Project: Nursing interventions classification* (2nd ed.). St. Louis: Mosby.

Neighbors, M., Eldred, E., & Sullivan, M. (1991). Nursing skills necessary for competing in the high-tech health care system. *Nursing and Health Care, 12*(2), 92–97.

Paris, L. L. (1994). Improving the process of communication at the bedside. *Journal of Nursing Care Quality, 9*(1), 10–15.

Pennsylvania Nurses Association. (1992). Perspectives on practice: RNs working with unlicensed assistive personnel. *Pennsylvania Nurse,* January, 7–8.

Prescott, P. A., Phillips, C. Y., Ryan, J. W., & Thompson, K. O. (1991). Changing how nurses spend their time. *IMAGE: Journal of Nursing Scholarship, 23*(1), 23–28.

Rice, R. (1995). *Handbook of home health nursing procedures.* St. Louis: Mosby.

Rubenfeld, M. G., & Scheffer, B. K. (1995). *Critical thinking in nursing: An interactive approach.* Philadelphia: Lippincott.

Seeger Jablonski, R. A. (1992). Remember the person attached to the ventilator. *Nursing, 92*(4), 67–70.

Sundeen, S. J., Wiscarz, S., DeSalvo-Rankin, E. A., & Cohen, S. A. (1994). *Nurse–client interaction: Implementing the nursing process* (5th ed.). St. Louis: Mosby.

Valega, T. M. (1984). It's time for nurses to begin nursing. *Nursing and Health Care, 5*(6), 331–335.

Wichowski, H. C., & Kubsch, S. (1995). Improving your patient's compliance. *Nursing, 25*(1), 66–68.

Chapter 20

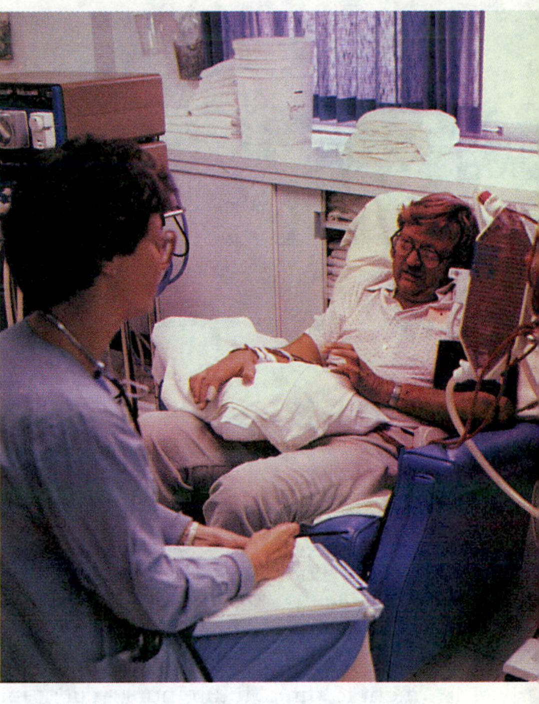

Evaluating

Objectives

After studying this chapter, the learner should be able to:

Define key terms used in the chapter.

Describe evaluation, its purpose, and its relation to other steps in the nursing process.

Evaluate the client's achievement of goals/outcomes specified in the plan of care.

Manipulate factors that contribute to the client's success or failure in goal/outcome achievement.

Use the client's responses to the plan of care to modify the plan as needed.

Explain the relation between quality assurance/quality improvement programs and excellence in healthcare.

Value self-evaluation as a critical element in developing the ability to deliver quality nursing care.

Key Terms

concurrent evaluation
criteria
evaluating
nursing audit
outcome evaluation
process evaluation
quality assurance
quality improvement
retrospective evaluation
standard
structure evaluation

During the fifth step of the nursing process, **evaluating**, the nurse and client together measure how well the client has achieved the goals/outcomes specified in the plan of care. While evaluating client goal/outcome achievement, the nurse identifies factors that contribute to the client's success or failure and, when necessary, modifies the plan of care. The purpose of evaluation is to allow client goal achievement to direct future nurse–client interactions. Based on the client's responses to the plan of care, the nurse decides to either (1) terminate the plan of care (each client goal/outcome is achieved), (2) modify the plan (client is having difficulty achieving goals/outcomes), or (3) continue the plan of care (client simply needs more time to achieve goals/outcomes). When evaluation points to the need to modify nursing care, each preceding step of the nursing process (assessing, diagnosing, planning, and implementing) is reviewed.

In summary, during the evaluation step of the nursing process, the nurse measures how well the client has achieved desired goals/outcomes; identifies factors that contribute to the client's success or failure; and terminates, continues, or modifies the plan of care as needed (Fig. 20-1). Core competencies for quality evaluation are highlighted in the box on page 316.

Unique Focus of Nursing Evaluation

As members of the healthcare team, nurses are involved in many types of evaluation. Nurses measure client goal/outcome achievement; how effectively nurses help targeted groups of clients to achieve their specific goals; the competence of individual nurses; and the degree to which external factors, such as different types of healthcare services, specialized equipment or procedures, or socioeconomic factors, influence health and wellness. The client, however, is always the nurse's primary concern. A nurse may perform a nursing procedure competently, caringly, and creatively, but if this nursing action does not help the client to reach desired goals, it is meaningless. Either directly or indirectly, the aim of all nursing evaluation is quality nursing care that aids client goal/outcome achievement. Therefore, the most important act of evaluation performed by the nurse is evaluating goal/outcome achievement with the client.

Critical Thinking Exercise 20-1

Interview experienced nurses from the same practice setting. Ask them what system variables (philosophy of care, client–nurse ratio, professional–nonprofessional staff mix, nursing management, adequacy of resources) most influence their ability to deliver quality care. Begin to identify variables you want to look for when you interview for a job.

Evaluation Criteria and Standards

The classic elements of evaluation are identifying evaluative criteria and standards (what you are looking for when you evaluate), collecting data to determine if these criteria and standards are met, interpreting and summarizing findings, and taking appropriate action. In the nursing process, evaluative criteria are the client goals/outcomes developed during the planning step. Because these reflect desired changes or outcomes in client behavior, and because nursing actions are directed toward these goals/outcomes, it is logical that they be at the core of evaluation. Determining whether these goals/outcomes have been met and then identifying the appropriate nursing response are the functions of evaluation.

Although the terms *criteria* and *standard* often are used interchangeably in the evaluation step, they have distinct definitions. **Criteria** are measurable qualities, attributes, or characteristics that specify skills, knowledge, or health states. They describe acceptable levels of performance by stating the expected behaviors of the nurse or the client.

Standards are acceptable, expected levels of performance by the nursing staff or other health team members. They are established by authority, custom, or consent.

Measuring Client Goal/Outcome Achievement

Collecting Evaluative Data

The nurse collects evaluative data to determine whether the client has met the desired goals/outcomes. Whereas the nurse collects data in the nursing assessment to identify client health problems, the data collected in

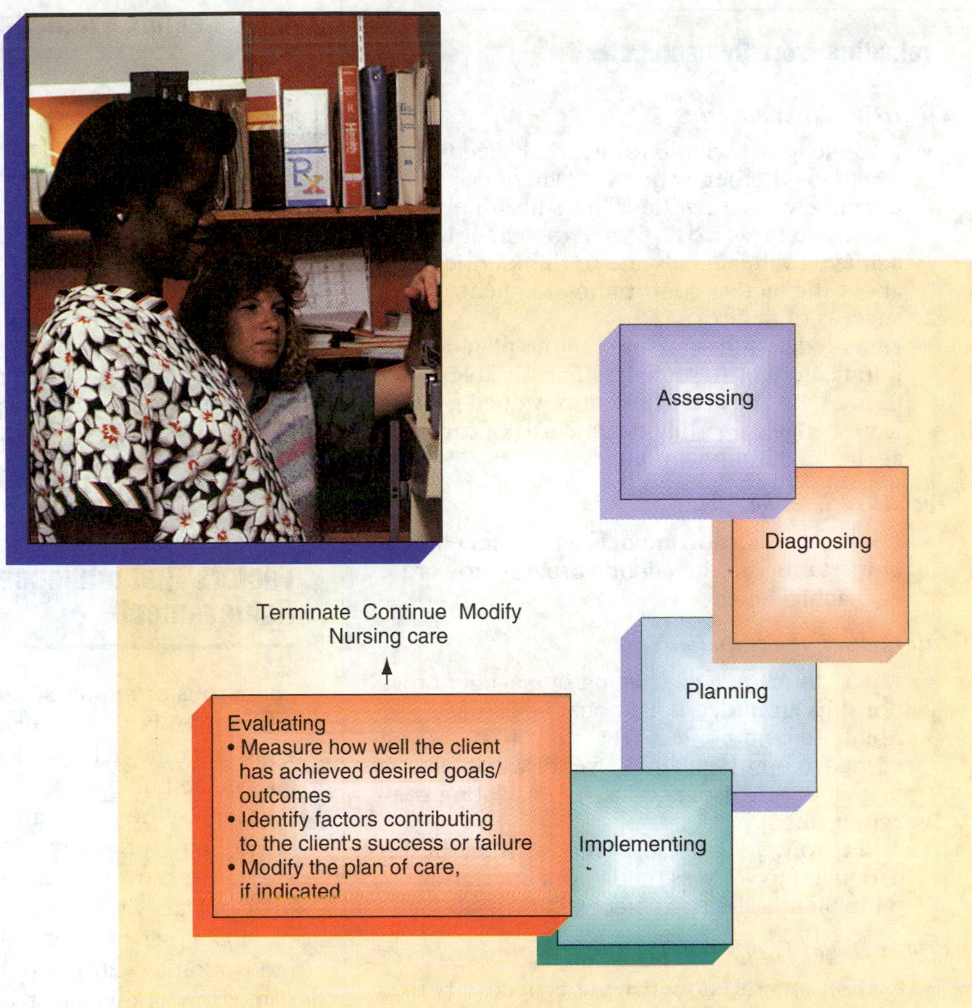

Figure 20-1
Evaluating. The nurse and client together measure how well the client has achieved the goals specified in the plan of care. Factors that contribute to the client's success or failure are identified, and the plan of care is modified if necessary. Client responses to the plan of care determine if nursing care is to be continued as is, modified, or terminated. (Photo by David Macklem, University of Wisconsin–Milwaukee Photo Services.)

the evaluation step is used to determine whether the identified health problems were resolved through goal achievement.

Types of Goals. The type of client data collected to support the evaluation of goal achievement is determined by the nature of the goal. *Cognitive goals* involve increases in client knowledge; these goals may be evaluated simply by having clients repeat information or, at a higher level of performance, by having clients apply the new knowledge to their everyday situations. For example, having clients describe new dietary restrictions is very different from having them plan a weekly menu compatible with these restrictions. *Psychomotor goals* describe the client's achievement of new skills; they are evaluated by having the client demonstrate the new skill. *Affective goals* pertain to changes in client values, beliefs, and attitudes; affective goals are more complex to evaluate. Observation of client behavior and conversation are used to determine whether these affective goals have been achieved.

In the final type of goal statement, *physical changes* in the client are the targeted outcome. To evaluate achievement of this type of goal, the nurse uses physical assessment skills to collect relevant data and compare these with previously acquired client data.

Samples of these goals are contained in the accompanying plan of care (p. 317). The data collected to determine the degree of goal achievement are recorded in the related evaluative statement.

Time Criteria. In addition to knowing what type of data to collect to determine goal/outcome achievement, it is important to know when to collect the data. In properly constructed client goals/outcomes, a time frame is established for determining whether the specified change in client behavior has been achieved. At the designated time, the nurse, in collaboration with the client, the family, and other members of the nursing team, evaluates the client's ability to demonstrate the desired behavior. If goals/outcomes are developed in observable and measurable terms, the task of collecting data for evaluation becomes clear-cut. Examples of three types of time criteria follow:

- By 7/8/98, the client will walk the length of hallway with support of walker.

Evaluating: Core Competencies

Cognitive Competencies

- Knowledge of what information is needed to evaluate whether or not the plan of care is effectively meeting the client's health needs (ability to measure how well the client has achieved valued goals and to think critically about the factors contributing to client success or failure)
- Knowledge of how to modify the plan of care, if indicated, or to remedy other variables interfering with the achievement of valued goals
- Knowledge of pertinent standards of care and agency/institutional policies

Technical Competencies

- Ability to use a documentation system competently to record the client's progress toward goal achievement

Interpersonal Competencies

- Ability to maintain a trusting nurse–client relationship grounded in responsible caring
- Ability to communicate that you are more concerned about the client's overall well-being than about the isolated task of evaluating goal achievement
- Ability to work collaboratively with the healthcare team to address the factors interfering with client's ability to meet valued goals

Ethical/Legal Competencies

- Commitment to do whatever is necessary to evaluate client achievement of goals in a timely fashion and to address whatever is interfering with goal achievement
- Ability to serve as a trusted and effective client advocate
- Ability to practice nursing accountable to self, client, the profession, and society

- Beginning 7/8/98, the client will demonstrate a weight loss of 3 lb per month until target weight (135 lb) is achieved (6/8/98, weight: 151 lb).
- Before discharge, parents will correctly demonstrate chest physiotherapy procedures for client.

It is important for nurses to evaluate client goal/outcome achievement as early as possible. Goal attainment, when celebrated with the client, usually results in the client's encouragement and leads to further goal achievement. When the client's failure to meet designated goals/outcomes is detected early, the plan of care can be modified to redress the failure. The most common mistake nurses make in evaluation in acute care settings is waiting until the day the client is to be discharged before evaluating goal/outcome achievement. At that point it is too late to do anything about the goals/outcomes the client has failed to achieve.

Documenting Evaluation

Once data have been collected to determine client goal/outcome achievement, the nurse writes an evaluative statement to summarize the findings. Atkinson and Murray (1990) have suggested using a two-part evaluative statement on the nursing plan of care to underscore the importance of evaluation. The evaluative statement includes a decision on how well the goal/outcome was achieved and all client data or behavior that support this decision. The nurse has three decision options—met, partially met, or not met. The nurse signs and dates the evaluative statement (see the box "Using Four Types of Goals in the Plan of Nursing Care").

Evaluative statement	=	Goal met Goal partially met Goal not met	+	Actual client behavior as evidence

Factors That Influence Goal/Outcome Achievement

Numerous client, nurse, and healthcare system variables contribute both positively and negatively to client goal/outcome achievement. Identifying these variables allows the nurse to reinforce positive factors by drawing on them in the future and to deal with those factors that are creating problems. The more sensitive and responsive nurses are to these variables, the more rewarding their practices will be.

Examples of positive factors include a client's strong motivation to learn new health behaviors, a nurse who comes to work well rested and with a new care idea read in a nursing journal, and a healthcare institution or agency that offers incentives for quality nursing and has an optimal nurse–client ratio.

Once the nurse understands what is helpful to the client who is trying to reach desired goals/outcomes, these factors often can be manipulated. For example, if a client is learning to ambulate independently after hip surgery and you notice that he seems to make his best effort when his wife is present, mention this observation to her and plan to ambulate the client at least once a day when she is present. Conversely, if the client seems more fearful when his wife is present, note in the plan of care that ambulation is best attempted when the client's wife is not on the unit. Ideally, this fear would be explored with the client before discharge so that he can continue to make progress when he is discharged home with his wife.

Table 20-1 presents common variables nurses encounter that can negatively influence client goal achievement. Tentative nursing approaches are suggested. What is important is that nurses become aware of the effects of these variables and respond creatively to them.

Critical Thinking Exercise 20-2

Interview five students who have personal fitness goals. Ask them to describe what personal factors have helped or hin-

Using Four Types of Goals

In the Plan of Nursing Care

Nursing Diagnosis: High Risk for Altered Parenting related to no previous experience in childrearing (fear)

Assessment Data: *Subjective:* "My husband and I are both afraid we won't know what to do when we get the baby home."

Objective: Both parents are single children, report no childrearing experience; healthy newborn son delivered 2/4/98; first born

Strengths: VIB (very important baby): parents are both 38; history of infertility with one miscarriage; strong motivation to learn and use good parenting skills; strong support network

Goals (Expected Outcomes)	Nursing Interventions	Evaluative Statement (Actual Outcomes)
Before discharge, parents will demonstrate confidence in: • Holding baby • Diapering, dressing baby • Bathing baby • Feeding baby (Psychomotor objectives)	Assess both parents' knowledge of childrearing practices; identify and reinforce motivation to learn; correct any misinformation. Develop and implement at a time convenient for both parents a teaching plan to include: • The primary nurse role-modeling techniques for comfortably and safely holding, talking to, and dressing baby • Parents independently viewing videocassettes on: Baby care Baby bath Breast-feeding Followed by one-on-one discussion • Class for new parents: nurse to demonstrate baby bath and discuss general principles of care • Primary nurse observing mother and infant during initial feeding sessions and offering teaching and support as necessary Answer parents' questions and address related concerns.	2/6/98 Goal partially met. Both parents have correctly demonstrated safe techniques for holding, dressing, and bathing the baby. Mother is still concerned baby is not getting enough milk. *Revision:* Continue to spend time with mother and infant during feeding—provide positive reinforcement. *F. Morales, RN*
By 2/6/98, parents will report appropriate action to be taken if questions or problems arise after discharge: • Name and number of primary nurse • Name and number of pediatrician • La Leche League contact and number (Cognitive objectives)	Assess parents' knowledge of infant problems frequently encountered by new parents. Inform parents of available community resources and describe appropriate action to take if questions or problems arise.	2/6/98 Goal met. Parents discussed some infant problems related to feeding, elimination, illness and reported appropriate community resource to contact. *F. Morales, RN*

(continued)

Using Four Types of Goals *(continued)*

In the Plan of Nursing Care

Goals (Expected Outcomes)	Nursing Interventions	Evaluative Statement (Actual Outcomes)
Before discharge, parents will verbalize decreased anxiety in regard to caring for son. (Affective objective)	Assess parents' level of anxiety and potential negative effects on childrearing. Discuss this with parents. Explore adequacy of parents' coping strategies—increased knowledge, practice in supportive environment, community resources. Counsel as necessary. Compliment parents on new parenting skills. Allow for ventilation of anxiety or specific fears. Respond with teaching or emotional support as necessary.	2/6/98 Goal partially met. Except for concern about breastfeeding, *both* parents expressed feeling comfortable and eager to care for their son at home. *F. Morales, RN*
At 1 month postpartal telephone interview, 3/4/98 (by parents' report), the baby will demonstrate adequate: • Weight gain (birth weight, 7 lb 6 oz) • Sleep-wakefulness patterns • Comfort level indicating adequate parenting. (Physical objectives)	Use a 1-month postdelivery telephone interview to assess the adequacy of parenting skills. With positive report of growth and development, compliment (reinforce) the parents. With negative report, teach or counsel and refer as appropriate.	3/4/98 Goal met. Parents' report of baby's weight gain and behavior indicates good parenting skills. *F. Morales, RN*

dered their achieving their goals. Note commonalities and differences. Reflect on how you can help clients tap personal strengths in order to better achieve their goals.

Modifying the Plan of Care

When evaluation reveals that the client has made little or no progress toward goal/outcome achievement, and attempts to identify the contributing factors point to problems with the plan of care, the nurse needs to reevaluate each preceding step of the nursing process for accuracy. After this study, new assessment data may need to be collected, diagnoses may be added or altered, goals/outcomes may need to be modified or rewritten, nursing orders may be changed, and evaluation may be targeted more frequently. See the checklist in this chapter for help in evaluating your use of the nursing process. Table 20-2 suggests appropriate nursing responses to common problems encountered during evaluation.

Once the nurse has identified the factors that contribute to the client's failure to achieve goals/outcomes, the evaluative statement can be used to suggest the necessary revision in the plan of care.

The following evaluative statement might be noted if the client fails to meet the behavior specified in the goal, "Client will participate in a minimum of two planned social activities per week beginning 9/20/98." "9/27/98 Goal not met. Resident refused to participate in any group activities this week."

Many courses of action are then available to the nurse. Possible revisions to follow the evaluative statement include the following:

Delete or modify the nursing diagnosis. This may not be a problem or concern for the resident. Evaluate and validate data pointing to the nursing diagnosis.

Make the goal statement more realistic. Carefully determine the resident's need for activities and ability or desire to participate in activities.

Adjust time criteria in goal statement. Reevaluate after 3 weeks; resident may need more time to adjust to being institutionalized and more encouragement.

Change nursing interventions. Make a special effort to familiarize yourself with the resident's interests, and match these with available programs and activities.

(text continues on page 322)

Table 20-1
Client, Nurse, and Healthcare System Variables That May Detract From Quality Nursing Care

Variables	Possible Solution
Client Variables	
Client who is physically and cognitively capable of self-care gives up—refuses to cooperate with therapeutic regimen or thwarts the regimen	Identify one nurse who is able to develop a trusting relationship with the client and determine the *reason* underlying the observed behavior: • No longer finds meaning and purpose in life • Overwhelming sense of powerlessness • Previous history of being "hurt," "exploited," "cheated" by the healthcare system • Inability to accept illness and related life-style changes Counsel appropriately. Use a team conference to develop a consistent plan of nursing care.
Client who quietly accepts whatever is done or not done for him or her; seldom communicates needs or dissatisfaction	Note on the plan of care the need to assess this client thoroughly because the client will probably not advocate for himself or herself. Educate the client to become a more assertive healthcare consumer.
Nurse Variables	
Nurse who sincerely desires to give 150% all the time and who becomes quickly frustrated when observing substandard care; may feel alienated from other staff; excellent candidate for burnout	Learn to give quality care during designated work period; leave on time; avoid the temptation to do the work of others; leave work concerns at work. After establishing a reputation for delivering quality nursing care, seek creative solutions for nursing problems (strategies to increase nursing resources, motivation, morale) and try them—hopefully with a support network. View concerns as challenges rather than overwhelming obstacles. Develop a realistic sense of how much nursing care and of what quality can be delivered with existing resources. If resources do not permit quality care, explore change strategies within the institution. If administration is not supportive, explore other practice settings.
Nurse with overwhelming outside concerns: • Preparation for marriage, childbirth, divorce • Illness (self or family members) • Role conflict (familial roles, school, work, and so forth) • New apartment, house	During periods of peak demand, may need to accept less than optimal performance at work. If this becomes the norm rather than the exception, carefully evaluate priorities. May need to cut work hours rather than "cheat" clients.
Nurse who is bored	After reflection, write down *personal* objectives related to work. Explore avenues within work setting for professional growth and development: Initiate changes in nursing unit to improve patient care and to stimulate peer development; join institutional committees; participate actively in staff development programs; develop patient and family support groups. Look for new position that offers new challenges within or outside the institution. Join professional organizations and participate actively. Evaluate educational goals and explore possibilities—continuing education programs and degree work.
Healthcare System Variables	
Inadequate staffing	Develop and use a client classification system that incorporates an identification of the kind and amount of nursing services required. Record staffing patterns and relate to needs for nursing care and client outcomes. Clearly demonstrate and *document* that adequate staffing makes a difference. Present these data to nursing administration with the request for additional staff. If necessary, use professional bargaining unit.
Nursing administration has sold out nursing; insensitivity to nursing demands within the institution	It may be impossible to practice quality, progressive nursing in this environment. If there seems to be no hope for change after appropriate channels have been explored, look for a new practice setting. Evaluate the new setting on the basis of what experience has taught you.

Table 20-2
Common Problems Noted During Evaluation of the Nursing Process

Problem	Effect on Nursing Process	Nursing Response
Assessing		
1. Data base is inaccurate.	1–3. Inaccurate nursing diagnoses. (Because the nursing diagnoses establish the client's *need* for *nursing,* inaccuracies here distort and may invalidate the entire plan of care.)	1. a. Identify the client or nurse variables responsible for inaccuracy. b. Revise the recorded data base.
2. Data base does not reflect changes in client condition.		2. Inservice the *entire* nursing staff on the importance of making assessment a priority in every client interaction as well as the *recording* of the new data obtained.
3. Data base is superficial: • Fails to communicate uniqueness of client. • Lacks sufficient detail on major problems or developments.		3. a. Rethink the critical relation between an adequate data base and quality care. b. Develop interviewing and physical assessment skills. c. Begin to identify the key data that need to be collected for specific nursing diagnosis and medical diagnosis and to assess client response to therapeutic regimen (use of a nursing diagnosis handbook may be helpful).
Diagnosing		
1. General sense that nursing diagnoses are "common sense" and therefore do not need to be put in writing.	1. "Common sense" nursing, which fails to address client's real problems, may ensue. Lack of continuity of care.	1. Carefully develop and record priority nursing diagnoses for several clients and fairly evaluate whether or not this makes a difference in terms of the continuity of quality care.
2. General sense that nurses are too busy doing treatments, "passing meds," and doing paperwork to develop nursing diagnoses carefully.	2. Independent dimension of nursing practice remains underdeveloped; clients experience nurses as busy "doers" who are insensitive to their concerns.	2. Examine practice and see if *independent* nursing has a place; what percentage of every day is devoted to independent nursing functions? If this percentage is nonexistent or small, there understandably may be *no felt need* for nursing diagnoses—but a desperate need to revise practice priorities.
3. Nursing diagnoses are too vague to be helpful.	3. Routinized client care results; individualized client problems are overlooked.	3. a. Revise the problem statement to describe more accurately what is *unhealthy* about the client (the behavior that needs to be changed). b. Revise the etiology to more accurately identify what is making the problem a problem—this should be a guide to nursing intervention. c. Check NANDA lists.
4. Nursing diagnoses are not up to date.	4. Nurses will not value or use the plan of care, assuming that it does not address the client's ongoing priorities.	4. Have a process for periodically reviewing the plan of care to delete nursing diagnoses when problems have been resolved and to add a new diagnosis as needed.

(continued)

Table 20-2 *(continued)*
Common Problems Noted During Evaluation of the Nursing Process

Problem	Effect on Nursing Process	Nursing Response
Planning		
1. The plan of care contains only the standard knowledge most nurses would know without a written plan.	1–2. Lack of personalized care; failure to address client's real problems; nursing staff works haphazardly on different priorities.	1. Make use of standardized (computerized) plans as a basis for care planning. Devote nursing energies to *individualizing* this plan.
2. The long-term goal is vague, standard; fails to make clear the discharge goal for this client.		2. Practice writing specific long-term goals that clarify for all nurses the aim toward which all nursing care is directed (eg, client returns home ambulatory with walker, right hip incision healing, able to manage activities of daily living with minimal assistance from spouse).
3. The nursing goals/outcomes, even if met, do not necessarily guarantee a resolution of the client problem.	3. Client problems are unresolved.	3. When writing goals, it often is helpful to develop outcomes related to etiologic factors. Because the stated etiology may be incomplete or inaccurate, it is essential that at least *one goal/outcome* be written so that if it is achieved, the problem in the nursing diagnosis is resolved.
4. The goals/outcomes are incorrectly developed.	4. Both the client and nurses may be unsure of the aims of care; progress toward goal/outcome achievement is difficult to evaluate.	4. After writing goals/outcomes, check them against the following criteria: • Subject is the client or some part of the client. • The client behavior is stated in observable, measurable terms. • Criteria of acceptable performance are specified. • Time criteria are included in notes.
5. Nursing orders are superficial.	5. Client receives routinized care; lack of continuity of care; client goals/outcomes may never be achieved. Each nurse must figure out a plan of nursing strategies.	5. Review nursing orders to ensure that they indicate the *specific* nursing strategies most likely to result in successful goal achievement *for this client* (eg, particular comfort measures that are successful adjuncts to analgesic administration for a particular client). In specifying the "who, what, when, where, how, and how much" of nursing actions, be sure to list the type of equipment and supplies needed in various treatments. As new client data are obtained, update nursing orders. Delete inappropriate or unnecessary orders.
6. The initial plan of care fails to be updated.	6. Plan of care will not be consulted by nurses—if used, it will be to client's detriment.	6. If personal accountability for updating plan fails, develop a process on the nursing unit to ensure care plan review and revision.

(continued)

Table 20-2 *(continued)*
Common Problems Noted During Evaluation of the Nursing Process

Problem	Effect on Nursing Process	Nursing Response
Planning *(continued)*		
7. The plan of care addresses the immediate needs of the client but fails to anticipate discharge needs.	7. Client returns home unable to manage self-care activities.	7. Work hard at developing the ability to project yourself into the client's home after discharge. Learn to anticipate problems and concerns and prepare the client and family for these. Use all discharge resources in the institution. Learn from clients what their needs were after previous discharge.
Implementing		
1. Nurses are not aware of client priorities and the plan of care; lack of continuity; inefficient use of nursing resources.	1. Client fails to achieve goals/outcomes.	1. a. Use shift report to update staff on status of priority nursing diagnosis and concomitant nursing care. b. Review plan of care and nursing notes before beginning care.
2. Nursing care becomes routinized and mechanized.	2. Client never has the sense that he or she is personally known by nurses.	2. Explore creative strategies to make quality nursing care on this particular unit a *challenge* rather than a *burden;* use ongoing education, problem-solving strategies by the nursing team, gaming, and other incentives.
3. Documentation is inadequate.	3. Because there is no complete written record of nursing care, *legally,* this care was never provided.	3. a. Develop the philosophy that quality nursing care *deserves* to be documented. Review legal reasons for careful documentation. b. Become familiar with the flow sheets and note format used within the work setting so that charting can be done quickly and comprehensively.
Evaluating		
1. It is not done.	1. Mastery of nursing process is stunted; severely limits accomplishment of nursing aims.	1. Develop the belief that quality nursing care does not happen automatically and that only ongoing evaluation will identify needed areas of revision. Devise an evaluative strategy and carry it out. Study its effect on quality of care after 6 months' implementation.

Evaluative Programs

In addition to each nurse's evaluation of client goal/outcome achievement and the subsequent modifications to the plan of care, many formal mechanisms exist to ensure quality nursing care. In the United States, regulatory agencies such as state boards of nursing, the Joint Commission on Accreditation of Healthcare Organizations (JCAHO), the Professional Standards Review Organization, and the National Health Planning and Resources Development Act of 1975 require nurses to document that nursing standards are being implemented and maintained. Each of these agencies is concerned with quality care and quality control. The availability of fewer resources to treat clients in hospitals and the unavailability of sufficient alternative treatment settings pose a strong challenge to the nursing profession to find ways to avoid a compromise in quality of care. Numerous professional nursing organizations are meeting this challenge.

Quality Assurance

Specially designed programs that have as their aim the promotion of excellence in nursing are called **quality-assurance programs**. These programs may be as small

Approaches to Quality Healthcare: Inspection or Opportunity?

There are two distinct approaches to ensuring quality. *Quality by inspection* focuses on "finding the bad apples (deficient workers) and removing them." Although client satisfaction is important, the focus of quality by inspection is on the technical delivery of care and the competence of clinicians. Clinicians subject to this type of quality assurance tend to be angry or afraid, and expend their energies proving that they are not deficient or incompetent—in negative ways.

In contrast, *quality as opportunity* focuses on finding opportunities for improvement and fosters an environment that thrives on teamwork, with people sharing the skills and lessons they have learned. Mistakes are not viewed as being caused by lack of motivation or lack of effort on the part of workers, but rather as a result of problems in the system. Workers are viewed as doing the best they can, and are respected as trying hard, acting in good faith, and not willfully failing to do what they know is correct. In this work environment, clinicians respond with openness and a desire to learn because their integrity and self-worth are not threatened.

Donna Ambler Peters suggests a different way of looking at the quality of healthcare and its measurement. She reminds us that how well quality is measured is based on the beliefs we hold about health, the nurse–client relationship, our coworkers, and the healthcare system.

> Without a personal commitment to quality and respect for oneself and others there is no means to achieve quality. There never will be sufficient financial resources, organizations artifice, or measurable standards to safeguard quality any other way. Each of us must care enough to make this happen—for ourselves, for our patients, and for our profession. (Peters, 1991, pp. 6–7)

Our goal should be to work in an environment in which quality measurements encourage our best efforts.

(Peters, D. [1991]. Measuring quality: Inspection or opportunity? *Holistic Nursing Practice, 5*[3], 1–7.)

as one conducted by the nurses on a small nursing unit or may have a scope as broad as that of an entire institution, state, province, or country.

Quality-assurance programs enable nursing to be accountable to society for the quality of care it provides. Such programs also are a response to the public mandate for professional accountability and the mandate of professional nursing law. They ensure professional survival, encourage nursing's fidelity to its moral and ethical responsibilities, and assist nursing to comply with other external pressures.

American Nurses Association Quality-Assurance Program

The American Nurses Association (ANA) in 1975 developed a model quality-assurance program consisting of seven steps: (1) identify values; (2) identify structure, process, and outcome standards and criteria; (3) measure the degree of attainment of criteria and standards; (4) make interpretations about strengths and weaknesses based on such measurements; (5) identify possible courses of action; (6) choose a course of action; and (7) take action. The ANA hoped that the model could be used at the local level to develop and implement quality-assurance programs.

The ANA model directs attention to three essential components of quality care—structure, process, and outcome. Different types of quality-assurance programs may focus exclusively on one component or on a mixture of components.

Structure. This type of **structure evaluation** or audit is focused on the environment in which care is provided. Standards describe physical facilities and equipment; organizational characteristics, policies, and procedures; fiscal resources; and personnel resources.

Process. The focus of the **process evaluation** is the nature and sequence of activities carried out by the nurse implementing the nursing process. Criteria make explicit acceptable levels of performance of nursing actions related to client assessment, diagnosis, planning, implementation, and evaluation.

Outcome. Outcome evaluations focus on measurable changes in the health status of the client or the end results of nursing care. Whereas the proper environment for care and the right nursing actions are important aspects of quality care, the critical element in evaluating care is demonstrable changes in client health status.

From Quality Assurance to Quality Improvement

Concern about the spiraling costs of healthcare, coupled with the success of industrial models for quality improvement, has led to a strong commitment to quality improvement in the 1990s. **Quality improvement** (also known as continuous quality improvement [CQI] or total quality management [TQM]) is "the commitment and approach used to continuously improve every process in every part of an organization, with the intent of meeting and exceeding customer expectations and outcomes"

(Schroeder 1994, p. 3). Unlike quality assurance, quality improvement is internally driven, follows client care rather than organizational structure, focuses on processes rather than individuals, and has no endpoints. Its focus is on *improving* quality rather than *assuring* quality. The major premises of quality improvement follow:

- Focus on organizational mission
- Continuous improvement
- Customer orientation
- Leadership commitment
- Empowerment
- Collaboration/crossing boundaries
- Focus on process
- Focus on data and statistical thinking (Schroeder, 1994, pp. 5–8)

From the client point of view, one of the most important outcomes of quality improvement is the recognition that client satisfaction is as important as customer service is in retail business. With increased competition for the healthcare dollar, providers are learning that it is important to offer the services that clients value and to offer them in a way that is valued by clients. More than one study has demonstrated that clients value care far more when it is delivered by a thoughtful, concerned, and respectful individual rather than by someone who is abrupt and concerned only with meeting narrowly defined professional standards of care (Coulter et al., 1994). By reemphasizing the critical nature of nursing's person- versus task-orientation, quality improvement underscores the need for nurses to successfully blend intellectual, technical, interpersonal, and ethical/legal competencies.

Nursing Audit

A **nursing audit** is a method of evaluating nursing care that involves a review of client records to assess the outcomes of nursing care or the process by which these outcomes were achieved. Successful nursing audits depend on careful nursing documentation.

Critical Thinking Exercise 20-3

Interview several clients and ask them what qualities in a nurse are most helpful as they try to achieve health goals. Similarly, ask what nurse qualities are most problematic. Reflect on how you measure up in terms of both positive and negative nurse qualities.

Concurrent Versus Retrospective. The evaluation of nursing care and client outcomes may be conducted while the client is receiving care (ie, a **concurrent evaluation**) or after the client has been discharged (ie, a retrospective evaluation). Concurrent evaluations are conducted by using direct observation of nursing care, client interviews, and chart review to determine whether the specified evaluative criteria are met.

Retrospective evaluations may use postdischarge questionnaires, client interviews (telephone or face to face), or chart review (nursing audit) to collect data. The type of retrospective audit most familiar to nurses working in hospitals is the JCAHO retrospective chart review. This accrediting body initially required hospitals to conduct a certain number of audits per year.

Self-Evaluation

Nurses who are sincerely committed to quality care learn early to make self-evaluation an integral part of their nursing practice. Self-evaluation skills promote professional development, enhance self-esteem, and develop self-awareness. The nurse who is just beginning to develop the caregiver role may find it helpful to conclude each caregiving experience with a brief moment of reflection that identifies and celebrates the nursing competencies that were skillfully used and targets competencies that need to be developed. This practice can keep one from becoming overwhelmed in the face of all that remains to be mastered and yet strongly motivated to learn new skills. The accompanying checklist will

Computer Applications in Nursing

"Point-of-Care" Computer Systems for Nursing Care

Nurses are now able to document care and access client records where the care is provided—at the "point of care." Locations for point-of-care systems include the bedside, the emergency room, ancillary departments, community clinics, the physician's office, and the client's home.

The devices used can be either stationary or portable terminals. In either case, data must be communicated to the main computer that stores the client data. This is done through either direct wiring or radio frequency waves. Data can be input directly from medical devices such as hemodynamic monitors, infusion pumps, or ventilators, or by the clinician. Some options for the nurse to input and retrieve data include the keyboard, function keys, light pen, touch screen, or voice.

Hardware for point-of-care systems is varied owing to the evolution of technology. The application software for point-of-care systems is divided into three main arenas: the medical–surgical inpatient units, home health, and the critical care environment.

The uses of point-of-care computer systems are relatively new in the healthcare arena. Watch for advances in this technology that help nurses improve their productivity, effectiveness, and the quality of care for the client (Hughes, 1995).

Checklist for Evaluating Your Use of the Nursing Process

Assessing

- ☐ The initial data base is obtained by means of a nursing history and nursing examination.
- ☐ Assessment data are documented:
  - ☐ Accurately—Questionable data are validated.
  - ☐ Completely—Use of a systematic guide ensures that recorded data describe (1) the client's functional ability to meet each basic human need and (2) responses to health and illness.
  - ☐ Concisely—Irrelevant data and meaningless generalizations are avoided.
  - ☐ Factually—Client behaviors are recorded rather than the nurse's interpretation of these behaviors.
- ☐ The initial data base communicates a "real sense" of the client that makes possible individualized care.
- ☐ Focused assessment data are recorded for each client problem.
- ☐ Data collection and documentation are ongoing and responsive to changes in the client's condition.

Diagnosing

- ☐ A prioritized list of nursing diagnoses is on the plan of care.
- ☐ Each nursing diagnosis describes an actual or potential client health problem that independent nursing intervention can prevent or resolve. Each nursing diagnosis:
  - ☐ Is derived from an accurate and validated interpretation of a cluster of significant client data or "cues"
  - ☐ Contains a precise problem statement describing what is unhealthy about the client and what needs to change—suggests client goals
  - ☐ Identifies factors that contribute to the problem (etiology)—these suggest nursing interventions
  - ☐ Uses nonjudgmental language and is written using legally advisable terms
- ☐ Old nursing diagnoses are deleted from the plan of care once resolved, and new diagnoses are added as soon as identified

Planning

- ☐ A comprehensive, individualized, and up-to-date plan of care that specifies client goals/outcomes and nursing orders for each nursing diagnosis is developed with the assistance of the client and family.
- ☐ Planning is comprehensive:
  - ☐ Initial
  - ☐ Ongoing
  - ☐ Discharge
- ☐ Long-term goals alert the entire nursing team to realistic client expectations after discharge.
- ☐ Short-term goals/outcomes:
  - ☐ When achieved, demonstrate a resolution of the problem specified in the nursing diagnosis
  - ☐ Describe a single, observable, and measurable client behavior
  - ☐ Are valued by the client and family
  - ☐ Are realistic in terms of the resources of the client and the nurse
- ☐ Nursing orders:
  - ☐ Clearly and concisely describe the nursing intervention to be performed (ongoing assessment; nursing treatments and procedures; teaching, counseling, advocacy)
  - ☐ Are individualized to the client
  - ☐ Are consistent with standards of care and supportive of other therapies
  - ☐ Are effective in accomplishing the desired client goals/outcomes
- ☐ The plan of care encourages client and family participation.

Implementing

- ☐ The client record contains daily documentation of the nursing measures used to (1) assist the client to meet basic human needs, (2) resolve health problems, and (3) implement select aspects of the medical plan of care.
- ☐ The plan of care is implemented:
  - ☐ Competently
  - ☐ Caringly
  - ☐ Creatively

Evaluating

- ☐ Evaluative statements are recorded on the plan of care to document the client's level of goal/outcome achievement at targeted times.
- ☐ Ongoing evaluation of the client's responses to the plan of care are used to make decisions about terminating, continuing, or modifying nursing care.

help you evaluate your personal skill in using the nursing process.

Identified in the client care studies that conclude each clinical chapter in this text are the specialized knowledge and skills the nurse needs to implement the plan of care. These include cognitive, technical, interpersonal, and ethical/legal skills. It is helpful when planning care to try to identify the nursing resources that are needed to ensure that you will be able to meet each encounter's challenge. Nurses sensitive to mastering both the art and the science of nursing care evaluate their possession of the prerequisite knowledge and skills for each nurse–client encounter as well as their ability to perceive, respond to, and appreciate the uniqueness of each client. Quality care is each nurse's responsibility.

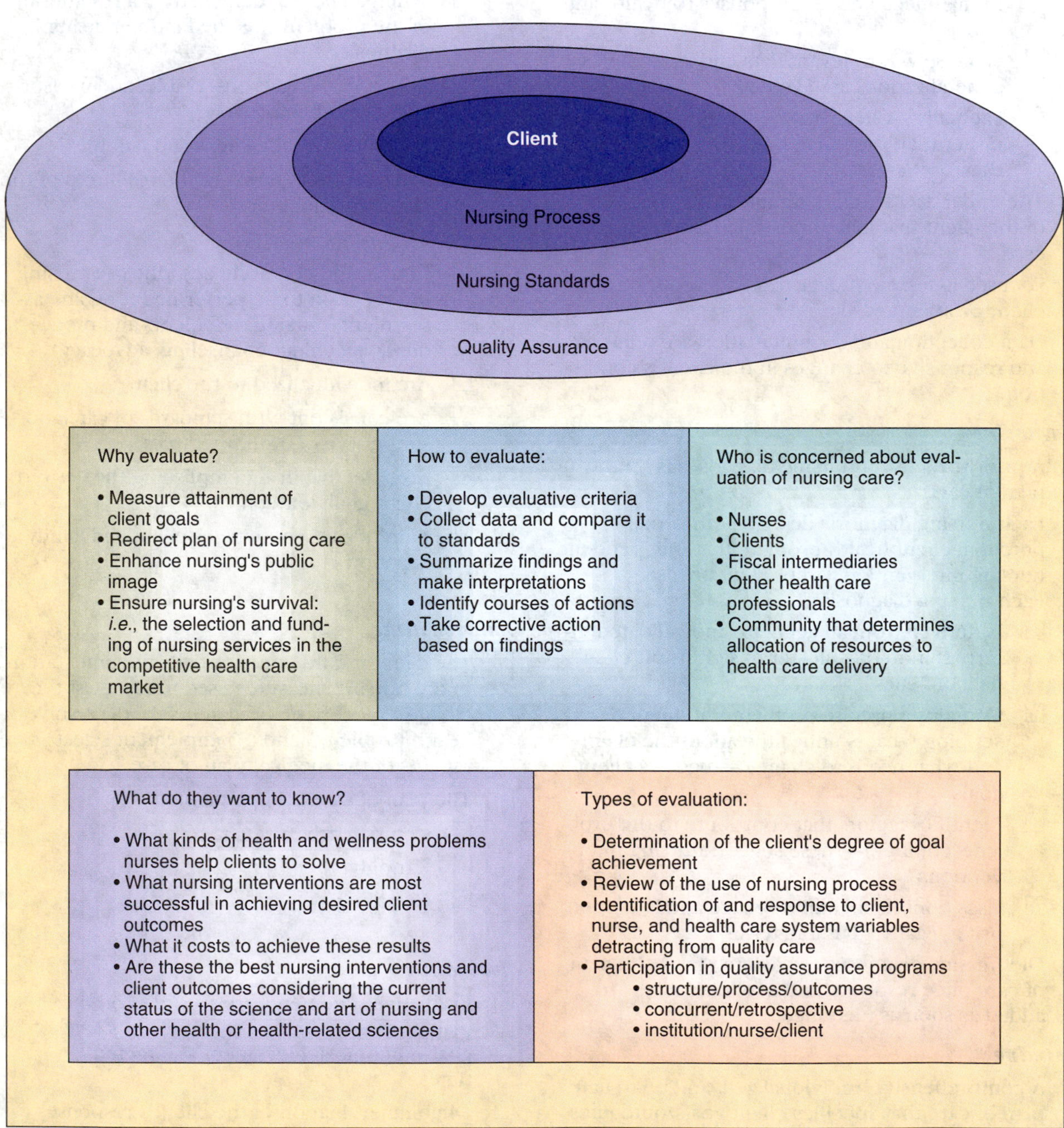

Figure 20-2
Overview and summary of the evaluative component of the nursing process.

Summary

The cultivation of evaluation as a critical component of the nursing process ensures nursing's continued success in achieving desired changes in client health status. Only a firm commitment to evaluation enables nurses to answer the following questions:

- What are nursing's values?
- How can these be formalized in standards and evaluative criteria?
- What data exist to determine whether the specified evaluative criteria are being met?
- How can these data best be collected, analyzed, and interpreted?
- To what courses of action do the findings lead?

Nursing actions are far too valuable and costly resources today to be haphazardly implemented. Evaluation, carefully planned and executed, can direct and redirect these actions to maximize client benefit. This is the goal and challenge of nursing evaluation. Criteria that may be helpful in determining the adequacy of the evaluative component of the nursing process include the following:

- Evaluation of the client's achievement of desired goals/outcomes
- Review of how the process is used and revision of the plan of care if necessary
- Participation in quality-assurance programs

Figure 20-2 provides a summary and overview of the evaluation step of the nursing process.

Key Points

- During evaluation, the nurse and client measure how well the client has achieved the goals/outcomes specified in the plan of care. Factors that have positively or negatively influenced goal/outcome achievement are identified, and a decision is made to terminate, continue, or modify care.
- When evaluation points to the need to modify nursing care, each preceding step in the nursing process is reviewed for accuracy.
- The type of evaluative data collected to support the decision regarding goal/outcome achievement (goal met, partially met, or not met) is determined by the nature of the goal/outcome. Goals/outcomes may be cognitive, psychomotor, or affective, or they may describe physical changes in the client.
- It is important for nurses to evaluate client goal/outcome achievement as early as possible. Achievement, when celebrated with the client, encourages further goal achievement. Failure directs necessary revisions in the plan of care. Waiting until a client is about to be discharged to evaluate goals/outcomes is the most common mistake nurses make in evaluation.
- Evaluative statements recorded on the plan of care alert the entire nursing staff to the client's level of goal/outcome achievement. Each evaluative statement includes a decision about how well the goal/outcome was achieved and the client data or behavior that supports the decision. The statement is dated and signed.
- Sensitivity to the client, nurse, and healthcare system variables that influence goal/outcome achievement enables the nurse to manipulate factors that will help the client reach desired goals.
- Common problems encountered during evaluation that may require a revision of the plan of care include inaccurate or incomplete data base, vague or missing nursing diagnoses, standardized plan of care, improperly developed nursing goals, superficial nursing orders, plan that is not kept up-to-date, failure to use evaluation to improve quality of nursing care, and insufficient communication among nurses.
- Historically, nursing has been a strong advocate for quality healthcare. The current availability of fewer resources to treat clients in hospitals and the unavailability of sufficient alternative treatment settings pose a serious challenge to nursing.
- Quality-assurance programs are evaluative programs designed to secure and implement excellence in nursing and healthcare. These programs may include process, structure, or outcome standards and have as their focus the client, the nurse, the institution, or the healthcare system.
- Quality-assurance/quality-improvement programs enable nursing to be accountable to society for the quality of its service. They also are a response to the public mandate for professional accountability and the mandate of professional nursing law. They ensure professional survival, encourage nursing's fidelity to its moral and ethical responsibilities, and assist nursing to comply with other external pressures.
- Self-evaluation skills promote professional development, enhance self-esteem, and develop self-awareness.

Bibliography

Alfaro-LeFevre, R. (1994). *Applying nursing process: A step-by-step guide* (3rd ed.). Philadelphia: Lippincott.

American Nurses Association. (1975). *A plan for implementation of the standards of nursing practice.* Kansas City, MO: ANA.

American Nurses Association. (1976). *ANA quality assurance workbook.* Kansas City, MO: ANA.

American Nurses Association. (1991). *Standards of clinical nursing practice.* Kansas City, MO: ANA.

Ardabell, T. R., Turjanica, M. A., Mastorovich, J., & Hirschman, V. (1995). Business process quality improvement: A step beyond continuous quality improvement. *MEDSURG Nursing, 4*(4), 279–288.

Atkinson, L. D., & Murray, M. E. (1990). *Understanding the nursing process* (4th ed.). New York: Pergamon.

Bloch, D. (1975). Evaluation of nursing care in terms of process and outcome: Issues in research and quality assurance. *Nursing Research, 24,* 256–263.

Christensen, P. J., & Griffith-Kenney, J. W. (1994). *Nursing process: Application of conceptual models* (4th ed.). St. Louis: Mosby.

Coulter, S. J., Atkins, P. M., Bailey, D., Blatt, M. E., Blashford, L., & Shumway, S. (1994). Patient satisfaction: A QI pilot project. In P. Schroeder, *Improving quality and performance.* St. Louis: Mosby.

Donabedian, A. (1980). *The definition of quality and its approaches.* Ann Arbor: Health Administration Press.

Donabedian, A. (1982). *The criteria and standards of quality: Explorations in quality assessment and monitoring.* Ann Arbor: Health Administration Press.

Hughes, S. J. (1995). Point-of-care information systems: State of the art. In M. J. Ball, K. J. Hannah, S. K. Newbold, & J. V. Douglas (Eds.). *Nursing informatics: Where caring and technology meet* (2nd ed.). New York: Springer-Verlag.

Joint Commission on Accreditation of Healthcare Organizations. (1994). *1995 accreditation manual for hospitals.* Oakbrook Terrace, IL: Author.

Katz, J. M., & Green, E. (1996). *Managing quality: A guide to improving performance in health care.* St. Louis: Mosby–Year Book.

Koch, M. W., & Fairly, T. M. (1993). *Integrated quality management: The key to improving nursing care quality.* St. Louis: Mosby–Year Book.

LaRochelle, D. R., & Shahinpour, N. (Eds.). (1995). Staff nurse initiated total quality management projects achieve quality nursing outcomes. *Nursing Clinics of North America, 30*(1), 1–162.

Ludwig-Beymer, P. (1993). Using patient perception to improve quality care. *Journal of Nursing Care Quality, 7*(2), 42–51.

Morin, G. D. (1995). A personal performance checklist. *Nursing Management, 26*(2), 325–326.

Peters, D. (1991). Measuring quality: Inspection or opportunity? *Holistic Nursing Practice, 5*(3), 1–7.

Phaneuf, M. (1976). *The nursing audit: Self regulation in nursing practice.* New York: Appleton-Century-Crofts.

Phaneuf, M. (1976). Quality assurance: A nursing view. *New Zealand Nursing Journal, 69*(2), 9–11.

Rubenfeld, M. G., & Scheffer, B. K. (1995). *Critical thinking in nursing: An interactive approach.* Philadelphia: Lippincott.

Schroeder, P. (1994). *Improving quality and performance: Concepts, programs, and techniques.* St. Louis: Mosby.

Western, P. (1994). QA/QI and nursing competence: A combined model. *Nursing Management, 25*(3), 44–46.

Wright, D. (1984). An introduction to the evaluation of nursing care: A review of the literature. *Journal of Advanced Nursing, 9*(5), 457–467.

Chapter 21

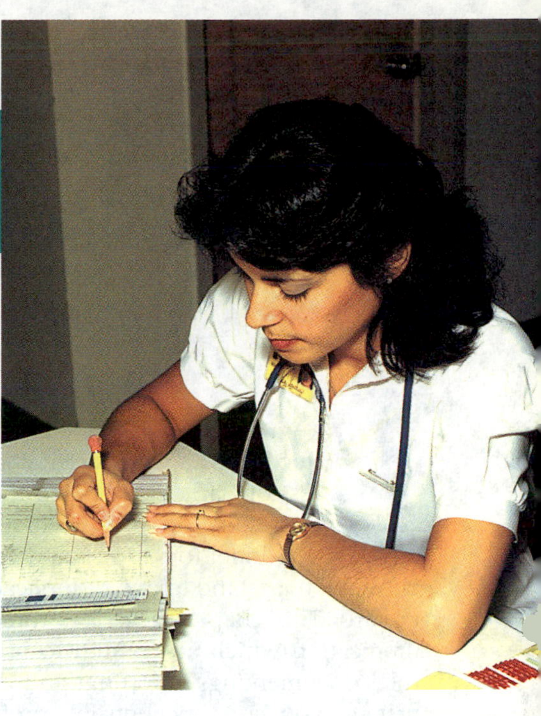

Documenting, Reporting, and Conferring

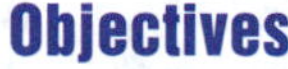

Objectives

After studying this chapter, the learner should be able to:

Define key terms used in the chapter.

List the guidelines for effective documentation.

Identify the abbreviations and symbols commonly used for charting.

Describe the purposes of client records.

Compare and contrast different methods of documentation: source-oriented record; problem-oriented record; PIE—problem, intervention, evaluation; focus charting; charting by exception; case management model; computerized records.

Describe the purpose and correct use of each of the following formats for nursing documentation: nursing assessment, nursing care plan, critical/collaborative pathways, progress notes, flow sheets, discharge summary, and home care documentation.

Document nursing interventions completely, accurately, concisely, and factually—avoiding legal problems.

Describe nursing's role in communicating with other healthcare professionals by reporting and conferring.

Key Terms

change-of-shift report
charting by exception
client record
critical/collaborative pathway
discharge summary
documentation
flow sheet
focus charting
graphic sheet
medication record
narrative notes
nursing care conference
nursing care round
PIE charting
problem-oriented record
progress notes
referral
report
SOAP format
source-oriented record
variance charting

Effective communication among healthcare professionals is essential to the coordination and continuity of care. Communicating effectively enables personnel to support and complement one another's services and to avoid duplications and omissions in care. This chapter describes three methods of communication which are central to nursing's professional role: documenting, reporting, and conferring. The very first day you care for clients in a professional setting you will find yourself needing to confer with colleagues, prepare a record of your interventions, and report on your client's progress toward valued goals/outcomes. A careful reading of this chapter will assist you to assume these responsibilities with greater confidence and skill. The communication process itself and specific communication techniques are discussed in Chapter 22.

Documenting Care

Documentation is the written, legal record of all pertinent interventions with the client—assessing, diagnosing, planning, implementing, and evaluating. Increasingly sophisticated management information systems are being designed to manage client-specific data and information. This data is used to facilitate client care, serve as a financial and legal record, help in clinical research, and support decision analysis. Information specialists aim to create an environment that supports timely, accurate, secure, and confidential recording and use of client-specific information (Joint Commission of Accreditation of Healthcare Organizations, 1995).

The **client record** is a compilation of a client's health information. Each healthcare institution/agency has policies that specify the nurse's documentation responsibilities. The Joint Commission for the Accreditation of Healthcare Organizations (JCAHO) specifies that nursing care data related to client assessments, nursing diagnoses or client needs, nursing interventions, and client outcomes are permanently integrated into the client record (1995). The accompanying box illustrates the JCAHO documentation standards. Each nurse is accountable to practice according to local policies and professional standards.

Guidelines for Effective Documentation

The client record is the only permanent legal document that details the nurse's interactions with the client and is the nurse's best defense if a client or client surrogate alleges nursing negligence. Unfortunately, it is not unusual to find critical omissions of nursing documentation, meaningless repetitious entries, and inaccurate entries. Although these errors may go undetected and have no effect on the client, they also may seriously affect the care the client receives, undermine nursing's credibility as a professional discipline, and cause legal problems for the nurse responsible. Adherence to the accompanying guidelines for documentation helps to prevent errors. In brief, documentation should be consistent with professional and agency standards; complete, accurate, relevant, factual, and timely; orderly and sequential; legally prudent; and confidential.

Agency Policies

Most agencies have specific policies concerning client records. All who have access to the record (direct caregivers) are expected to maintain its confidentiality. At no time may a nurse give a client's chart to any person other than an authorized caregiver. State laws differ as to whether the client has the legal right to review the chart. Most agencies grant student nurses access to client records for purposes of education. In this instance, the student assumes responsibility to hold the client information in confidence.

Agency policies also indicate which personnel are responsible for recording on each form in the record, and such policies also may describe the order in which the forms are to appear in the record. Additional policies may concern the frequency with which entries are to be made, whether routine care is recorded, the manner in which health personnel identify themselves after making an entry, which types of abbreviations are acceptable, and the manner in which an error in recording is handled. An issue of growing importance concerns documentation made by unlicensed personnel. Since professional nurses frequently supervise the care unlicensed personnel give, it is essential to clarify which assessments and interventions may be charted by unlicensed

Managing Patient-Specific Data and Information: Standards of the Joint Commission on Accreditation of Healthcare Organizations

The information-management function provides for the definition, capture, analysis, transformation, transmission, and reporting of individual patient-specific data and information related to the process(es) and/or outcome(s) of the patient's care.

1. **The organization initiates and maintains a medical record for every individual assessed or treated. The medical record incorporates information from subsequent contacts between the patient and the organization.**
   - Entries in medical records are made only by individuals authorized to do so as specified in the organization and medical staff policies.
2. **The medical record contains sufficient information to identify the patient, support the diagnosis, justify the treatment, document the course and results accurately, and facilitate continuity of care among health care providers. Each medical record contains at least the following:**
   - The patient's name, address, date of birth, and the name of any legally authorized representative;
   - The patient's legal status, for patients receiving mental health services;
   - Emergency care provided to the patient prior to arrival, if any;
   - The record and findings of the patient's assessment;
   - A statement of the conclusions or impressions drawn from the medical history and physical examination;
   - The diagnosis or diagnostic impression;
   - The reason(s) for admission or treatment;
   - The goals of treatment and the treatment plan;
   - Evidence of known advance directives;
   - Evidence of informed consent for medical procedures and treatments for which informed consent is required by organizational policy;
   - Diagnostic and therapeutic orders, if any;
   - All diagnostic and therapeutic procedures and tests performed and the results;
   - All operative and other invasive procedures performed, using acceptable disease and operative terminology that includes etiology, as appropriate;
   - Progress notes made by the medical staff and other authorized individuals;
   - All reassessments, when necessary;
   - Clinical observations;
   - The response to the care provided;
   - Consultation reports;
   - Every medication ordered or prescribed for an inpatient;
   - Every dose of medication administered and any adverse drug reaction;
   - Every medication dispensed to or prescribed for an ambulatory patient or an inpatient on discharge;
   - All relevant diagnoses established during the course of care; and
   - Any referrals and communications made to external or internal care providers and to community agencies.
3. **At discharge from inpatient care, a clinical resume concisely summarizes the reason for hospitalization, the significant findings, the procedures performed and treatment rendered, the patient's condition on discharge, and any specific instructions given to the patient and/or family, as pertinent.**
4. **Medical record data and information are managed in a timely manner.**
   - All significant clinical information pertaining to a patient is entered into the medical record as soon as possible after its occurrence.
   - Medical records of discharged patients are completed within the time period specified in medical staff rules and regulations, not to exceed 30 days.
5. **Verbal orders of authorized individuals are accepted and transcribed by qualified personnel who are identified by title or category in the medical staff rules and regulations.**
6. **All entries in medical records are dated and authenticated, and the organization establishes a method to identify the authors of entries.**
   - Authentication may be written signatures or initials, rubber-stamp signatures, or computer key.
   - When rubber-stamp signatures or computer key is authorized, the individual whose signature the stamp represents or whose computer key is authorized signs a statement that he or she alone will use the stamp or the code for the computer key. This statement is filed in the organization's administrative offices. Such a stamp or code for the computer key is not used by another individual.
   - The appropriate practitioner authenticates the parts of the medical record for which he or she is responsible.
7. **When a patient is admitted to the hospital or appears for a prescheduled ambulatory care appointment, the organization uses a patient information system to routinely assemble all divergently located record components. The system also ensures that all record components are assembled in a timely manner, as needed, for patients seen for unscheduled ambulatory and emergency services visits.**

From Joint Commission on Accreditation of Healthcare Organizations. (1995). *1995 accreditation manual for hospitals,* vol. 1. Oakbrook Terrace, IL: JCAHO. Used with permission of the publisher.

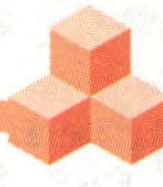

Guidelines for Nursing Care

Documentation

Content

- Enter information in a *complete, accurate, relevant* (concise), and *factual* manner.
- Record client findings (observations of behavior) rather than your interpretation of these findings.
- Avoid words such as "good," "average," "normal," or "sufficient," which may mean different things to different readers.
- Avoid generalizations such as "seems comfortable today." A better entry would be "on a scale of 1 to 10, client rates back pain 2 to 3 today as compared with 7 to 9 yesterday; vital signs returned to baseline."
- Note problems as they occur in an *orderly, sequential manner;* record the nursing intervention and the client's response; update problems or delete as appropriate.
- Document all medical visits and consultations of which other nurses should be aware, either because of their impact on the client or because of the nursing care the client now requires.
- Document in a *legally prudent manner.* Know and adhere to professional standards and agency/institutional policy for documentation.
- Document the nursing response to questionable medical orders or treatment (or failure to treat). Factually record the date and time the physician was notified of the concern and the exact physician response. If this occurs by phone, have a second nurse listen to the conversation and cosign the note. If a nurse administrator was contacted, document this. Documentation should give legal protection to the nurse, other caregivers, the healthcare agency or institution, and the client.
- Avoid the use of stereotypes or derogatory terms when charting.

Timing

- Chart in a *timely* manner. Follow agency policy regarding the frequency of documentation and modify this if changes in the client's status warrant more frequent documentation.
- Indicate in each entry the date and both the time the entry was written and the time of pertinent observations and interventions. This is crucial when a case is being reconstructed for legal purposes.
- Document nursing interventions as closely as possible to the time of their execution. The more seriously ill the client, the greater the need to keep documentation current. Never leave the unit for a break when caring for a seriously ill client until all significant data is recorded.
- Never document interventions before carrying them out.

Format

- Chart on the proper form as designated by agency policy.
- Print or write legibly. Use correct grammar and spelling. Use *standard terminology,* only commonly accepted terms and abbreviations and symbols (see Table 21-1 at end of chapter). Alternately, follow computer documentation guidelines.
- Date and time each entry.
- Chart nursing interventions chronologically on consecutive lines. Never skip lines. Draw a single line through blank spaces.

Accountability

- Sign your first initial, last name, and title to each entry. Do not sign notes describing interventions not performed by you which you have no way of verifying.
- Do not use dittos, erasures, or correcting fluids. A single line should be drawn through an incorrect entry and words "mistaken entry" or "error in charting" should be printed above or beside the entry and signed. The entry should then be rewritten correctly.
- Identify each page of the record with the client's name and identification number.
- Recognize that the client record is *permanent.* Follow agency policy pertaining to the color of ink and the type of pen or ink to be used. Ensure that the client record is complete before sending it to medical records.

Confidentiality

- Clients have a moral and legal right to expect that the information contained in their client health record will be kept private. Students should be familiar with agency policy and pertinent legislation about who has access to client records, other than the immediate caregiving team, and the process used to obtain access.
- Most agencies allow students access to client records for educational reasons. Students using client records are bound professionally and ethically to keep in strict confidence all the information they learn by reading client records. Actual client names and other identifiers should not be used in written or oral student reports.

personnel and which require documentation by a professional nurse.

The storage of client records is a function of the health agency's record department. Many client records are microfilmed for compact storage or are entered into a computer to expedite accessibility of information.

Purposes of Client Records

Client records serve many purposes.

Communication. The client record helps healthcare professionals from different disciplines who interact with the client at different times to communicate with one another. This is the primary purpose of the record.

Care Planning. Each professional working with the client has access to the client's baseline and ongoing data, and can see how the client is responding to the treatment plan from day to day. Modifications of the plan of care are based on this data.

Quality Review. Charts may be reviewed to evaluate the quality of care received and the competence of the nurses providing that care. For example, in a nursing audit, a committee decides in advance certain standards of care it wants to evaluate (eg, pertaining to nursing assessment, nursing documentation, or safety measures). A number of charts are then randomly selected and reviewed for evidence of the nurses' meeting the selected standards of care. If deficiencies are found, inservice can be used to remedy the problem and improve the quality of care. Accrediting agencies such as the JCAHO may also use chart review to determine if a particular agency or healthcare institution is meeting its standards.

Research. The record may be studied by researchers who are hoping to learn from study of similar cases how best to recognize or treat identified health problems.

Decision Analysis. Information from record review often provides the data needed by strategic planners to identify needs and the means and strategies most likely to address these needs. Record review may reveal both under- and over-utilized services, clients with prolonged stays who require special assistance, and financial information about which services generate revenue versus those that cost the institution/agency money.

Education. Healthcare professionals and students reading a client's chart can learn a great deal about the clinical manifestations of particular health problems, effective treatment modalities, and factors that affect client goal achievement.

Legal Documentation. Client records are legal documents that may be entered into court proceedings as evidence; as such, they play an important role in implicating or absolving health practitioners charged with improper care. The record also can be used in accident or injury claims made by the client.

Looking Into the Future

As healthcare reform initiatives evolve, outcomes will become the primary focus in evaluating the effectiveness of care. This focus will intensify as the Health Care Financing Administration and other reimbursement-management sources develop standard outcome measurements for all healthcare organizations. Outcome evaluations will be an important part of healthcare report cards for consumers buying health care in the managed-care environment. A key component to facilitate data and outcome comparisons will be *minimum data sets.* These specific categories of information will use uniform definitions to create a common language among multiple healthcare data users.

The *nursing minimum data set* is organized into three categories:

- nursing care elements (such as nursing diagnosis and intervention)
- patient demographic elements (such as sex, date of birth, and ethnicity)
- service elements (such as admission and discharge dates and expected payer for services)

Computerization will distribute this data among many caregivers in a standardized format allowing them to easily compare and uniformly evaluate patient progress.

Besides tracking the progress of individual patients, *outcome information* compares the progress of groups of patients with similar diagnoses. Results will contribute to research, education, and, ultimately, better and more efficient nursing practice.

Eggland, E. T. (1995). Charting smarter. *Nursing, 25*(9), 35–41. Used with permission.

Reimbursement. Client records are also used to demonstrate to payers that clients received the care for which reimbursement is being sought.

Historic Documentation. Because the dates of entries on records are specified, the record has value as an historic document. Years later, information may become pertinent concerning a client's past healthcare.

Methods of Documentation

Source-Oriented Records

A source-oriented record is one in which each healthcare group keeps data on its own separate form. Sections of the record are designated for nurses, physicians, laboratory and x-ray personnel, and so on. Notations are entered chronologically, with the most recent entry being nearest the front of the record. An advantage of the source-oriented record is that each discipline can easily find and chart pertinent data. The main disadvantage is that data are fragmented, and it is difficult to track problems chronologically with input from different groups of professionals.

Although the specifics vary among health agencies, general characteristics of the source-oriented record essentially have remained the same. Types of forms typically used in a source-oriented client record are presented in Table 21-2. Progress notes written by nurses in a source-oriented record are **narrative notes** which address both routine care, normal findings, and the client problems identified in the plan of care. They include a description of the status of the problem, related nursing interventions, client responses, and needed revisions to the plan of care. Sample traditional narrative nursing notes are given in Figure 21-1 (found at the end of the chapter). Traditional narrative nursing notes are also found in the nursing process client care studies that conclude each clinical chapter.

Problem-Oriented Medical Records

Another type of record used in some health agencies is the problem-oriented medical record (POMR) or problem-oriented record (POR), which was originated by Dr. Lawrence Weed in the 1960s. The **problem-oriented (medical) record** is organized around a client's problems, rather than around sources of information. An example is given in Figure 21-2 (found at the end of the chapter). All healthcare professionals record on the same forms. The advantages of this type of record are that the entire healthcare team works together in identifying a master list of client problems and contributes collaboratively to the plan of care. Progress notes are clearly focused on client problems. Table 21-3 and Figure 21-2 (found at the end of the chapter) describe and illustrate the major parts of the problem-oriented record—the defined data base, problem list, care plans, and progress notes.

The acronym SOAP (**SOAP** = **S**ubjective data, **O**bjective data, **A**ssessment [the caregiver's judgment about the situation], **P**lan) is used to organize data entries on the progress notes of the problem-oriented medical record. Caregivers select numbered problems from the master list on the front of the client record and then work-up the problem or "SOAP it" on the progress sheet. Some nurses believe that the SOAP method of charting focuses too narrowly on problems and are advocating a return to the traditional narrative format. Variants of the SOAP format include SOAPE, SOAPIE, and SOAPIER (**I**ntervention, **E**valuation, and **R**esponse). Figure 21-2*D* incorporates a SOAP note.

PIE—Problem, Intervention, Evaluation

The **PIE charting** system is unique in that it does not develop a separate plan of care. The plan of care is incorporated into the progress notes in which problems are identified by number. In this documentation system a complete client assessment is performed and documented at the beginning of each shift using preprinted fill-in-the-blank assessment forms. Client problems identified in these assessments are numbered, worked up using the problem (P), intervention (I), evaluation (E) format, and evaluated each shift. Figure 21-3 (found at the end of the chapter) is an example. Continuing problems are redocumented and numbered each day. One advantage of this system is that it promotes continuity of care. It also saves time since there is no separate plan of care. The disadvantage of not having a formal care plan, however, is that nurses need to read all the nursing notes to determine problems and planned interventions before initiating care.

Focus Charting

The purpose of **focus charting** is to bring the focus of care back to the client and client concerns. Instead of a problem list or list of nursing/medical diagnoses, a focus column is used that incorporates many aspects of a client and client care. The focus may be a client strength or a problem or need. Topics that may appear in the focus column include client concerns and behaviors; therapy and response; changes of condition; and significant events such as teaching, consultations, monitoring, management of activities of daily living, or assessment of functional health patterns. The narrative portion of focus charting uses the data (D), action (A), response (R) format (see Fig. 21-4 at the end of the chapter). The principal advantage of focus charting is the holistic emphasis on the client and the client's priorities. Ease of charting is also cited as an advantage of focus charting since there is no requirement that each note incorporate data, action, and response. Some nurses report that the DAR categories are artificial and not helpful when documenting care (Eggland, 1995).

Charting by Exception

Charting by exception is a shorthand documentation method that makes use of well-defined standards of practice; only significant findings or "exceptions" to these standards are documented in narrative notes. Benefits of this approach include decreased charting time (frees time for direct client care), greater emphasis on significant data, easy retrieval of significant data, timely bedside charting, standardized assessment, greater interdisciplinary communication, better tracking of important client responses, and lower costs. Widely billed as "a more efficient way to document," charting by exception is rapidly gaining advocates (Murphy & Burke, 1990; Comstock & Moff, 1991). Figure 21-5 (found at the end of the chapter) shows one example of this type of charting.

Case Management Model

Managed care's emphasis on quality, cost-effective care, delivered within a limited time frame, has led to the development of interdisciplinary documentation tools that clearly identify the outcomes select groups of clients are

Table 21-2
Examples of Forms and Information in Source-Oriented Client Records

Form	Typical Client Information Entered on the Form
Admission sheet	Legal name, identification number Age, birthdate, sex Marital status Occupation and employer Religious preference Next of kin and person to notify in case of emergency Date, time, reason for admission Name of the attending physician Insurance information Discharge data
Admission nursing assessment	Results of nursing history and physical assessment
Graphic sheet (see Fig. 21-9)	Daily temperatures, pulse and respiratory rates, blood pressure (vital signs) Daily weight Special measurements, such as the patient's fluid intake and output
Activity flowsheet (see Fig. 21-1)	Diet and how client has eaten Bathing and skin care Activity level, safety measures Respiratory interventions Elimination Diagnostic measures, treatments Isolation
Narrative nurse's notes (see Fig. 21-1)	Descriptions of pertinent observations of the client Statements that specify the nursing care, including teaching, received by the client and his or her responses to nursing care Statements that describe the client's condition and progress, or lack of progress, toward recovery and goal achievement Descriptions of the client's complaints and how the client is coping, or failing to cope, with them and nursing's response
Medication sheet (see Chapter 29)	Name of prescribed medications administered on a regular basis Dosage of the medication administered Route by which the medication was administered, unless given orally Time medication was administered Name or initials of the person administering the medication
Medical history and examination sheet	Results of the physical examination performed by the physician Current medical condition Health history, including previous illnesses Family medical history Confirmed or tentative diagnosis Plan of medical therapy
Physician's order sheet	Orders for medications Orders for treatments Other directives pertinent to a particular client's care
Physician's progress notes	Interpretations of the client's pathology Responses of the client to medical therapy
Miscellaneous forms	Laboratory reports X-ray film reports Consultation reports Dietary requirements Results of social service consultations Types and results of physical, respiratory, and x-ray therapy

expected to achieve on each day of care. A collaborative pathway for clients undergoing modified radical mastectomy is illustrated in Figures 21-6 to 21-8 (found at the end of the chapter). It is part of a computerized documentation system that integrates the collaborative pathway and documentation flowsheets designed to match each day's expected outcomes. Developed at Vanderbilt University, this system has reduced charting time by 40% and increased staff satisfaction with the amount of paperwork from 0% to 85%. These gains were accomplished with no decrease in audited charting quality. More importantly, a time study demonstrated a directly

Table 21-3
Organization of the Problem-Oriented Client Record

Part	Information
Data base (see Fig. 21-2A)	The data base is a compilation of all initial information about the client and includes the following: Health state profile prepared by the nurse Medical history and the physical examination, prepared by the physician Social history Initial diagnostic test results
Problem list (see Fig. 21-2B)	The multidisciplinary problem list itemizes major aspects of the client's life that require health attention and includes the following: Socioeconomic, demographic, psychologic, and physiologic problems Each problem is labeled, numbered, and categorized as active or inactive
Plan of care (see Fig. 21-2C)	An initial plan is formulated for each specifically numbered problem on the problem list. The nursing plan, whether *therapeutic, diagnostic,* or *educational,* is expressed through nursing orders.
Progress notes (see Fig. 21-2D) Narrative progress notes	Progress notes consist of narrative progress notes, flowsheets, and discharge notes, as follows: The narrative progress notes on the client follow the SOAP format, as follows: S–Subjective information reported by the client O–Objective observations made by health practitioners A–Assessments drawn from new data P–Plans or goals for action related to the client's problems
Flowsheets	Flowsheets are used for recording information that is monitored over time. This information provides data for making comparisons of a client's status at one time with his status later.
Discharge notes	Discharge notes are the entries made at the time an episode of the client's care is terminated and include the following information: The date of the resolution of each problem, as had been described while using the SOAP format Referrals made for the client Recommendations for unresolved or partially resolved problems

proportional increase in time spent with the client (Hatcher, 1995). Charting by exception is frequently used with critical pathway documentation systems.

The case management model promotes collaboration, communication, and teamwork among caregivers; makes efficient use of time; and increases quality by focusing care on carefully developed outcomes. The system works best for "typical" clients with few individualized needs. At present there is little consensus about which documentation tools will best record routine aspects of care and avoid repetition.

Variance Charting. When a client fails to meet an expected outcome or a planned intervention fails to be implemented, this variation or variance from the plan is documented. The usual format for **variance charting** is the unexpected event, the cause for the event, actions taken in response to the event, and discharge planning when appropriate. The variances most likely to be documented are those which affect quality, cost, or length of stay.

Computerized Records

In an increasing number of healthcare institutions, comprehensive computer systems have revolutionized nursing documentation in the client record. Computer capacities are in operation in which the nurse (1) calls up the admission assessment tool on the computer screen and keys in client data; (2) develops the plan of care using computerized care plans available for each North American Nursing Diagnosis Association–approved diagnosis; (3) adds to the client data base as new data are identified and modifies the plan of care accordingly; (4) receives a work list indicating the treatment, procedures, and medications necessary for the client throughout the shift; and (5) documents care immediately using the computer terminal at the client's bedside. The American Nurses Association has been instrumental in developing the Computer-Based Patient Record Institute (CPRI) in response to a recommendation by the Institute of Medicine that a computer-based client record be adopted by all healthcare providers and systems nationwide (Mulholland, 1992).

The increasing use of computerized client information systems to store client data has necessitated the development of policies and procedures to ensure the privacy and confidentiality of client information. Policies should specify what types of client information can be retrieved, by whom, and for what purpose. Client consent is necessary for the use and release of stored information.

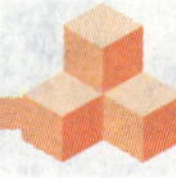

Guidelines for Nursing Care

Safe Computer Charting

The American Nurses Association, the American Medical Record Association, and the Canadian Nurses Association offer the following guidelines and strategies for safe computer charting.

- Never give your personal password or computer signature to anyone—including another nurse in the unit, a float nurse, or a doctor.
- Don't leave a computer terminal unattended after you have logged on.
- Follow the correct protocol for correcting errors. To correct an error after storage, mark the entry "mistaken entry," add the correct information, and date and initial the entry. If you record information in the wrong chart, write "mistaken entry—wrong chart" and sign off.
- Make sure that stored records have back-up files—an important safety check. If you inadvertently delete part of the permanent record, type an explanation into the computer file with the date, time, and your initials and submit an explanation in writing to your manager.
- Don't leave information about a client displayed on a monitor where others may see it. Keep a log that accounts for every copy of a computerized file that you've generated from the system.
- Follow the agency's confidentiality procedures for documenting sensitive material, such as a diagnosis of AIDS or HIV infection.

Charting tips. Computer charting: Minimizing legal risks. (1993). *Nursing, 23*(5), 86.

The accompanying box highlights guidelines for safe computer charting.

Formats for Nursing Documentation

When the nursing process is fully implemented, nursing documentation on the client's permanent record includes the following.

Initial Nursing Assessment

A typical form used to record the initial data base obtained from the nursing history and physical assessment is illustrated in Chapter 16. Accurate documentation of these data is important because they provide a baseline for later comparisons as a client's condition changes.

Plan of Nursing Care

The client record must utilize some means to communicate the client's problems or diagnoses, related goals/outcomes and interventions, and progress or resolution of the problems. The plan of nursing care may be written separately or incorporated into a multidisciplinary plan. In a traditional plan of nursing care, nursing diagnoses, goals/expected outcomes, and nursing interventions are written for each client (see the sample student plan in Chapter 18 and the plans of care at the end of each clinical chapter). Standardized plans of care may also be used that identify the common problems and related care for select client cohorts. These generally incorporate standards of high-quality care, but unless individualized, they may not sufficiently address individual client needs. Formats for plans of care vary greatly.

Critical/Collaborative Pathways

The case management plan is a detailed, standardized plan of care that is developed for a client population with a designated diagnosis. It includes expected outcomes, a list of interventions to be performed, and the sequence and timing of those interventions. The critical or collaborative pathway, illustrated in Figure 21-6 (found at the end of the chapter) and in Chapter 18, is an abbreviated summary of key information taken from the more detailed case management plan.

Progress Notes

The purpose of progress notes is to inform caregivers of the progress a client is making toward achieving expected outcomes. The method used to record client progress depends on the documentation system in place. Common examples include narrative nursing notes, SOAP notes, PIE notes, focus charting, charting by exception, and flow sheets. Advantages and disadvantages of each are listed in Table 21-4.

Flow Sheets

Flow sheet are documentation tools used to record routine aspects of nursing care.

Graphic (Clinical) Record. The graphic sheet is a form used to record specific client variables such as pulse, respiratory rate, blood pressure readings, body temperature, weight, bowel movements, and other client characteristics (see Fig. 21-9 at the end of the chapter).

24-Hour Fluid Balance Record. Forms are available to document the 24-hour intake and output of fluids for

Table 21-4
Advantages and Disadvantages of Different Documentation Formats

Format	Advantages	Disadvantages
Narrative Notes	Narrative notes allow nurses to describe a condition, situation, or response in their own terms, as they understand it.	It is time-consuming and difficult to read days and weeks of narrative notes to find a specific problem, its treatment, and client response.
SOAP Notes (Subjective Data, Objective Data, Assessment–Judgment, Plan)	The location of the problem list at the front of the chart alerts all caregivers to client priorities. Care and documentation of care is problem-focused. Easy retrieval of information facilitates quality review and research. Healthcare professionals from different disciplines chart on same progress notes. SOAP format is consistent with nursing process.	The level of ability and consistency of caregivers in organizing data into the SOAP format varies. Problem focus may reduce clients to "problems to be solved." Maintaining a neat, up-to-date problem list takes constant vigilance and routine review.
PIE (Problem, Intervention, Evaluation)	Without a formal, separate care plan the method saves time because a nurse does not have to create or update a plan. Consistent with nursing process.	Because there is no formal care plan, the nurse preparing to provide care will need to read all the nursing notes to determine problems, planned interventions, and evaluations to see if those interventions are effective.
Focus Charting	Ease of charting with DAR is an advantage because categories of data, action, and response are not required for each focus cited. Components of DAR can be cited alone or out of sequence.	Many nurses have difficulty in documenting information by separating the data into DAR categories. The "result" portion of the note seems to be a particularly difficult area since some nurses relate this portion to the resulting problems identified from the assessment data rather than to the client outcome of care following nursing intervention.
Charting by Exception	Abnormal status can be seen immediately with narrative easily retrieved. The flow sheet format shows overall trends in the client's condition. Guidelines provide specific but concise standard information regarding "normal" assessments and expected outcomes. Documentation time is decreased because standard care is not written in narrative and duplication of charting is eliminated. This results in charting being done in a more timely manner.	Preventive and wellness-promoting functions of nursing are not documented on this format because they do not address problems. The system requires predictable, defined client outcomes which are more difficult to predict for some clients and in some settings than others. More difficult to computerize.
Case Management Model	Makes efficient use of time because each day has planned interventions and client expected outcomes written on the plan. Increases the probability that a client will be discharged in a timely fashion. Care is goal-focused, which potentially increases quality. Promotes collaboration, communication, and teamwork among caregivers.	Effective for clients with one or two diagnoses and few complications; less helpful for clients with multiple variances. Space to document is limited on critical pathways and too much writing causes illegibility. Space for individualization is limited. Separate narrative notes must be used for documentation of care. The intervention flow sheet, nursing notes, and critical path must all be reviewed to get a picture of a client's condition.

Data for this chart was adapted in part from Eggland, E. T., and Heinemann, D. S. (1995). *Nursing documentation: Charting, recording and reporting*, Philadelphia: Lippincott.

clients with special needs. The forms include shift and daily fluid intake and output totals. A sample tool may be found in Chapter 46.

Medication Record. The client's record must include documentation of all the medications administered to the client (drug, dose, route, time), the nurse administering the drug, and, for some medications (eg, analgesics), the reason the drug was administered and its effectiveness. Sample medication records may be found in Chapter 29.

Daily Nursing Care Record. Flow sheets such as those illustrated in Figures 21-1 and 21-8 are often used to document routine aspects of nursing care. When well designed, they enable nurses to quickly document routine aspects of care that promote client goal achievement, safety, and well-being.

Discharge and Transfer Summary

At the time a client is discharged from care or transferred from one unit or institution/agency to another, a clinical resume should concisely summarize the reason for treatment, significant findings, the procedures performed and treatment rendered, the client's condition on discharge/transfer, and any specific instructions given to the client and/or family as pertinent. A copy of a discharge summary is given in Chapter 12.

Home Care Documentation

Documentation of home care visits that reports client progress serves two purposes. Sent to the attending physician with a request for signed medical orders to continue treatment, they ensure continuity of care. Sent to third-party payers, they establish the need for continuing home care that results in continued reimbursement for necessary services. Medicare, for example, reviews progress summaries written every 60 days to determine if a client meets one of these Medicare requirements:

- A client is homebound and still needs skilled nursing care.
- Rehabilitation potential is good (or client is dying).
- Client status is not stabilized.
- A client is making progress in expected outcomes of care. (Eggland, 1995, pp. 168, 172)

Chapter 13 contains a sample home health certification and skilled nursing note.

Potential Legal Problems in Documentation

One out of four malpractice suits is decided from the client's record. In the accompanying box, Eggland (1995) outlines documentation content and mechanics that increase a nurse's legal risk. No nurse can afford to be ignorant or careless with respect to agency policies and professional standards for documentation.

Potential Legal Problems in Documentation

Documentation Content That Increases Legal Risk

- The content is not in accordance with professional or healthcare organization standards.
- The content does not reflect client needs.
- The content does not include description(s) of situations that are out of the ordinary.
- The content overgeneralizes client assessment or nursing interventions.
- The content is incomplete or inconsistent.
- The content does not include appropriate medical orders.
- The content implies a potential or actual risk situation.
- The content implies attitudinal bias.

Documentation Mechanics That Increase Legal Risk

- Lines between entries
- Countersigning documentation
- Tampering
- Different handwriting or obliterations
- Illegibility
- Sloppiness (some lawyers infer sloppy care from sloppy charting)
- Dates and times of entries omitted or inconsistently documented
- Improper nurse signature or unidentifiable initials
- Transcription errors (notes are made at bedside and later transcribed into client record; problems include the amount of time that elapses between the event and when it is recorded and errors associated with recopying)

Eggland, E. T. & Heinemann, D. S. (1995). *Nursing documentation: Charting, recording and reporting.* Philadelphia: Lippincott. Used with permission.

Reporting Care

To report is to give an account of something that has been seen, heard, done, or considered. **Reporting** is the oral, written, or computer-based communication of client data with the purpose of informing others. A laboratory report, for example, may communicate to the healthcare team that a client's cardiac enzymes are normal or that a biopsy of breast tissue revealed malignant or atypical cells. A nurse's shift report or nursing note may communicate the progress a client is making toward goal achievement. Common methods for reporting among health practitioners, other than the client record, include face-to-face meetings, the telephone, a messenger, the written message, the audiotaped message, and

Table 21-5
Common Methods of Communication Among Healthcare Professionals

Method	Advantages	Disadvantages
Face-to-face meeting	• Message can be delivered immediately. • Nonverbal messages are readily conveyed. • Message can be clarified; receiver's questions can be raised and answered.	• Both the communicating and the receiving people must be available at the same time, in the same place. • Ordinarily there is no permanent record for later use.
Telephone conversation	• Message can be delivered immediately. • Message can be clarified; receiver's questions can be raised and answered. • Two parties need not be present in same place.	• Only the tone of voice and voice inflections can be communicated—no nonverbal messages. • Ordinarily there is no permanent record.
Written message	• Can be exchanged at times convenient for the people involved. • Record is available. • Time-efficient if message is understood.	• Message usually cannot be validated with the sender.
Audiotaped message	• Can be exchanged at times convenient for the people involved. • Record is available. • Time-efficient if information communicated is complete.	• Message usually cannot be validated with the sender.
Computer message	• Message can be delivered immediately—even to those at a great distance. • Parties need not be present in same place. • Two-way communication is possible via E-mail. • Record is available. • Many people can participate in exchange.	• No nonverbal messages can be communicated. • Privacy concerns remain an issue.

the computer message. Each of these methods has certain benefits and limitations, as detailed in Table 21-5.

Change-of-Shift Reports

A **change-of-shift report** is given by a primary nurse to the nurse replacing him or her or by the charge nurse to the nurse who assumes responsibility for continuing care of the client. The change-of-shift report may be given in written form or orally (Fig. 21-10) in a meeting, or it may be audiotaped. Many charge nurses find that using a tape decreases the amount of time spent reporting and allows more time for last-minute details.

Typical information shared among nurses during a change-of-shift report includes the following:

- Basic identifying information about each client—name, room number, bed designation, and current diagnosis
- Current appraisal of each client's health status:
  - Changes in medical condition (results of pertinent diagnostic studies) and client's response to medical therapy
  - Where the client stands in relation to identified nursing diagnoses and goal achievement
- Current orders (especially any newly changed orders):
  - Nurse-prescribed orders
  - Physician-prescribed orders (changes in medications, intravenous fluids, diet, activity level)
- Summary of each newly admitted client, including his or her diagnosis, age, plan of therapy, and general condition
- Report of clients who have been transferred or discharged

It is important to avoid unprofessional comments about clients that could predispose oncoming nurses to view and respond to clients negatively.

Telephone Reports

Telephones can link healthcare professionals immediately. Such linkage enables nurses to receive and give critical information about clients in a timely fashion. For example, hematology may call to report a dangerously low platelet count and the nurse may in turn notify the attending physician to obtain new medical orders. When reporting significant changes in a client's condition to physicians and other healthcare professionals, nurses should be prepared to:

- Identify themselves and the client, and state their relationship to the client. ("Dr. Gomez-Lobo, this is Ellen McLouglin, and I am calling about Mr. Clouser, a patient of yours who was just dis-

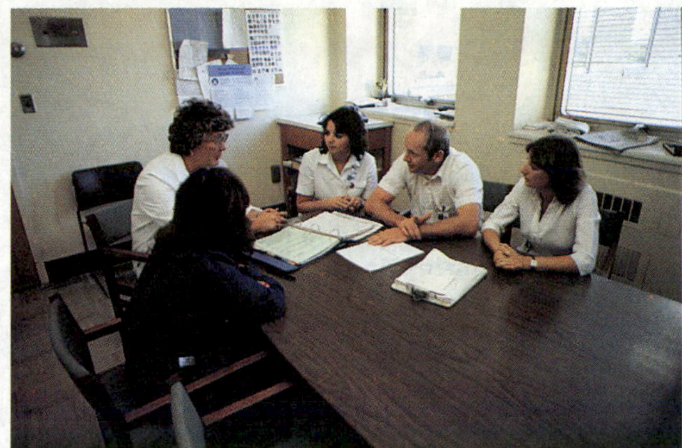

Figure 21-10
Oral change-of-shift report on a nursing unit.

charged home following a work-up for recurrent chest pain. I am his new nurse case manager.")

- Report concisely and accurately the change in the client's condition that is of concern and what has already been done in response to this condition. ("When I first arrived in his home he was complaining of feeling dizzy, and when I took his blood pressure it was 190/110. Yesterday morning in the hospital it was 150/90. His wife appears very flustered and says she doesn't know how she is going to take care of him. I had him rest for 30 minutes and when I checked his pressure at that time it was still 186/110.")
- Report the client's current vital signs and clinical manifestations.
- Have the client record at hand so that knowledgeable responses can be made to the physician's inquiries. In this situation the physician will probably want a complete set of vital signs and may ask questions about the treatment regimen both in the hospital and upon discharge.
- Concisely record the time and date of the call, what was communicated to the physician, and the physician's response.

Telephone Orders

Agency policy is followed regarding telephone orders. Every telephone order should be repeated back to the physician to ensure that the nurse correctly interpreted what was ordered. If the nurse is unsure of an order given by phone, he or she asks the physician to repeat what was said. Telephone orders must be transcribed on an order sheet; policy usually dictates that they be co-signed by the physician within a set time. If the nurse judges a telephone order to be inappropriate, another nurse should listen to the order also. Then agency guidelines for questioning inappropriate orders are followed.

Transfer and Discharge Reports

Nurses report a summary of a client's condition and care when transferring clients from one unit or institution/agency to another (eg, from the postanesthesia care unit to a surgical floor) and when discharging clients. It is critical for the nurse making the report to concisely summarize all the client data that caregivers need to provide immediate care. See Chapter 12 for transfer and discharge reporting guidelines.

Reports to Family Members and Significant Others

Nurses play a crucial role in keeping the client's family and significant others updated on the client's condition and progress toward goal achievement. It is essential for nurses to clarify with the client which visitors are entitled to progress reports. Similarly, nurses need to clarify what types of information they are able to communicate. The nurse is generally not the caregiver who initially informs the family that a client's biopsy revealed a malignancy. They do, however, often explain what this will mean for the client once the family has this information. Information should be shared in a manner that is honest, compassionate, and respectful of the person's ability to understand and apply medical concepts.

Conferring About Care

To confer is to consult with someone to exchange ideas or to seek information, advice, or instructions from another. A nurse may consult with another nurse, as when a primary care nurse consults with a nurse clinical specialist about a particular client's care. A school nurse may confer with a child's teacher or a psychologist about a behavior problem. A community health nurse and a physician may confer about a client's activity regimen. Health practitioners also confer to validate information. Healthcare professionals increasingly use electronic support groups to consult with clinicians who share similar interests or who have expertise in other specialty areas.

Consultations and Referrals

When nurses detect problems they are unable to solve because they lie outside the scope of independent nursing practice or their expertise, they make referrals to other professionals. The process of sending or guiding someone to another source for assistance is called a referral. A client may be referred by a hospital to a community health nursing service for assistance with home care. A school nurse may refer a student to a hospital emergency department. A community health nurse may refer a problem to the Department of Health.

Most health agencies have policies related to referrals. An agency may have a special form that personnel are to use when making referrals. The policies usually indicate who may initiate a referral, how it is to be done, and so on. Referrals are especially important in provid-

Computer Applications in Nursing

The Nursing Minimum Data Set

In order for a computer system to store, code, and retrieve data, information must be presented in a form that has uniform definitions and classification. The nursing minimum data set (NMDS) is a set of data elements necessary to document nursing care data in a paper or computer-based client record.

Many nations, including the United States and Canada, are working on a unified nursing language system for the nursing profession. The purposes of the NMDS are to:

- Establish comparability of nursing data across clinical populations, settings, geographic areas, and time
- Describe the nursing care of clients and their families in both inpatient and outpatient settings
- Show or project trends regarding nursing care needs and allocation of nursing resources according to nursing diagnosis
- Stimulate nursing research

Nursing elements of the NMDS are:

- Nursing diagnosis
- Nursing interventions
- Nursing outcomes
- Patient intensity

Since 1973 the North American Nursing Diagnoses Association (NANDA) has worked on a taxonomy of nursing diagnoses. Nursing diagnoses provide the basis for selection of nursing interventions to achieve outcomes for which the nurse is responsible. Based on nine "Human Response Patterns," the diagnoses use a numbering system that facilitates computerization of the taxonomy. NANDA continues to develop the taxonomy and the coding of nursing diagnoses for possible inclusion in the World Health Organization International Classification of Diseases.

A team of nurse researchers at the University of Iowa, Iowa City, is developing a *Nursing Intervention Classification* (NIC) in order to define the contributions nurses make to healthcare. An intervention consists of a label, a definition, a list of activities for implementing the intervention, and a set of readings related to the intervention. The interventions were developed from a review of the literature, expert opinion, and focus groups. Currently, the NIC defines 433 interventions within the realm of nursing practice. The classification is continuously being updated and upgraded.

Researchers at the University of Iowa have also embarked upon a project to define and classify *nursing-related outcomes.*

Patient intensity is an indicator of the acuity, intensity, or dependency used by each facility to classify its clients.

Although work is being done in the United States and many other countries to define a NMDS, much work remains (Bulechek, McCloskey, Titler, & Denehey, 1994; NANDA, 1994; Werley, Devine, & Zorn, 1988).

ing continuity of care for people who need a variety of services. It is essential that health practitioners to whom a client is referred are given information that is most useful to the continuity of care. The key question is, "What would I want to know about this client if I were the person who had to continue his or her care?" The client must know and approve of a referral to another agency or to other health personnel.

Before making a referral, it is important to determine which profession has the needed expertise and which of its practitioners are good referral sources. A great disservice is done clients when referrals are poorly made ("I guess if I just received this news I'd want to see an oncologist—too bad I don't know any to recommend."). Clients will also appreciate a phone number and practical tips about how to reach the referred practitioner most easily.

Nursing Care Conference

Nurses and other healthcare professionals frequently confer in groups to plan and coordinate client care. Such conferences are also used for instructing students and practitioners. A **nursing care conference** is a meeting of nurses to discuss some aspect of a client's care. For example, several nurses who have taken care of a generally uncooperative client may initiate a conference. This would allow each nurse an opportunity to offer his or her opinion about the client's problem and its cause, and then together they could discuss possible solutions to the problem.

Nurses may invite other healthcare practitioners to a nursing care conference to gain input concerning a particular client's care. For example, a clinical psychologist may be invited to the conference described above to address the possibility that a mental disorder is influencing this client's behavior.

Nursing Care Rounds

Nursing care rounds are procedures in which a group of nurses visit selected clients individually at each client's bedside. The primary purposes of nursing care rounds are to gather information that helps to plan nursing care, to evaluate the nursing care the client has received, and to provide the client with an opportunity to discuss his or her care with those administering it. As each client is visited, the nurse assigned provides a short summary of the client's nursing diagnoses and goals and the care being given. There are two principal advantages of nursing care rounds over a discussion in a meeting room: Nursing personnel can actually see the client as a report of care is given, and clients can participate in discussions of their care.

It is important that nursing personnel use language the client can understand when holding discussions at the bedside. Otherwise, the client is likely to feel excluded and cannot intelligently participate in the discussion. Nurses also may make rounds with physicians to inform them of nursing's input.

Key Points

- Nurses are responsible for documenting each step of the nursing process in the client record. Most healthcare institutions and professional and regulatory agencies have standards for documentation that detail the nurse's responsibilities.
- The client record is the only legal document that provides a comprehensive picture of the nursing care given to the client.
- Client-specific data and information are used to facilitate client care, serve as a financial and legal record, help in clinical research, and support decision analysis.
- Documentation should be consistent with professional and agency standards; complete, accurate, relevant, factual, and timely; orderly and sequential; legally prudent; and confidential.
- Each healthcare group keeps data on its own separate form in the source-oriented client record. In the problem-oriented record, recording is organized around the client's problems rather than around sources of information.
- The case management model of documentation uses a critical or collaborative pathway tool for groups of clients with the same diagnosis. The pathway includes expected outcomes and lists the interventions needed to secure these outcomes and the timing and sequence of these interventions.
- Computer records have simplified nursing documentation in many ways. Use of computer terminals at the client's bedside enables nurses to document care immediately.
- There are distinct advantages and disadvantages linked to common formats used by nurses to document client progress toward expected outcomes and related nursing care. Examples of these formats include narrative notes, SOAP notes, PIE charting, focus charting, charting by exception, and flow sheets.
- One out of four malpractice suits is decided from the client's record. No nurse can afford to be ignorant or careless with respect to agency policies and professional standards for documentation.
- Reporting is the oral, written, or computer-based communication of client data with the purpose of informing others. Common methods for reporting among health practitioners, other than the client record, include face-to-face meetings, the telephone, a messenger, the written message, the audiotaped message, and the computer message.
- To confer is to consult with someone to exchange ideas or to seek information, advice, or instructions. When nurses detect problems they are unable to solve because they lie outside the scope of independent nursing practice or outside the scope of their expertise, they make referrals to other professionals. The process of sending or guiding someone to another source for assistance is called a referral.

Bibliography

Barbera, M. L. (1994). Giving report: How to sidestep common pitfalls. *Nursing, 24*(9), 41.

Buckley-Womack, C., & Gidney, B. (1987). A new dimension in documentation: The PIE method. *Journal of Neuroscience Nursing, 19*(5), 256–260.

Bulechek, G. M., McCloskey, J. C., Titler, M. G., & Denehey, J. A. (1994). Nursing interventions' use in practice. *American Journal of Nursing, 94*(10), 59–62, 64.

Burke, L., & Murphy, J. (1988). *Charting by exception: A cost effective quality approach.* Albany, NY: Delmar.

Calfee, B. (1994). 7 things you should never chart. *Nursing, 24*(3), 43.

Capuano, T. A. (1995). Clinical pathways: Practical approaches, positive outcomes. *Nursing Management, 26*(1), 34–37.

Cohen, M. R. (1987). Play it safe: Don't use these abbreviations. *Nursing, 17*(7), 46–47.

Comstock, L. G., & Moff, T. E. (1991). Cost-effective, time-efficient charting. *Nursing Management, 22*(7), 44–48.

Cox, S. S. (1994). Taping report: Tips to record by. *Nursing, 24*(3), 64.

Eggland, E. T. (1995). Charting smarter. *Nursing, 25*(9), 35–41.

Eggland, E. T., & Heinemann, D. S. (1995). *Nursing documentation: Charting, recording and reporting.* Philadelphia: Lippincott.

Ferraro-McDuffie, A. (1993). Documenting the primary nurse's summary note. A leap toward professionalism. *Pediatric Nursing, 19*(2), 189–193.

Hatcher, I. (1995). Personal communication.

House, E. (1992). Resistance to documentation—A nursing research issue. *International Journal of Nursing Studies, 29*(4), 371–381.

Iyer, P. W., & Camp, N. (1995). *Nursing documentation: A nursing process approach* (2nd ed.). St. Louis: Mosby–Year Book.

Joint Commission on Accreditation of Healthcare Organizations. (1995). *Accreditation manual for hospitals.* Oakbrook Terrace, IL: Author.

Mandell, M. (1994). Not documented, not done. *Nursing, 24*(8), 62–63.

Marr, P. B. (1993). Bedside terminals and quality of nursing documentation. Part I. *Computers in Nursing, 11*(4), 176–182.

Marrelli, T. M. (1996). *Nursing documentation handbook* (2nd ed.). St. Louis: Mosby–Year Book.

Martin, F. (1994). Documentation tips to help you stay out of court. *Nursing, 24*(6), 63–64.

Meyer, C. (1992). Bedside computer charting: Inching toward tomorrow. *American Journal of Nursing, 92*(4), 38–44.

Murphy, J., & Burke, L. J. (1990). Charting by exception: A more efficient way to document. *Nursing, 20*(5), 65–69.

North American Nursing Diagnosis Association. (1994). *NANDA nursing diagnoses: Definitions and classification, 1995–1996.* Philadelphia: NANDA.

Rasmussen, N. (1994). Clinical pathways of care: The route to better communication. *Nursing, 24*(2), 47–49.

Rich, P. L. (1995). Protecting patient information. *Nursing, 25*(9), 32L.

Siegrist, L., Stocks, B., & Dettor, R. (1985). The PIE system: Complete planning and documentation of nursing care. *QRB, 11*(6), 186–189.

Simpson, R. L. (1994). Ensuring patient data privacy, confidentiality, and security. *Nursing Management, 25*(7), 18–20.

Werley, H. H., Devine, E. C., & Zorn, C. R. (1988). Nursing needs its own minimum data set. *American Journal of Nursing, 88,* 1652.

Windle, P. E. (1994). Critical pathways: An integrated documentation tool. *Nursing Management, 25*(9), 80 F–L, 80 P.

Wong, C. A., & Budgell, L. (1994). Documentation redesign. *Canadian Nurse, 90*(6), 38–41.

Table 21-1
Abbreviations and Symbols Commonly Used by Health Practitioners

Abbreviation	Meaning
Activities	
AMB	ambulatory
BRP	bathroom privileges
CBR	complete bed rest
OOB	out of bed
up ad lib	up as desired
Assessment Data	
abd	abdomen
BP	blood pressure
bx	biopsy
C	Celsius (centigrade)
cc	chief complaint
c/o	complains of
dx	diagnosis
F	Fahrenheit
GI	gastrointestinal
GU	genitourinary
h/o	history of
HPI	history of present illness
Imp	impressions
lt or Ⓛ	left
NAD	no apparent distress
neg	negative
P	pulse
PE	physical examination
PMH	past medical history
R	respirations
R/O	rule out
ROS	review of systems
rt or ®	right
RX	treatment
Sx	symptoms
T	temperature
WNL	within normal limits
⊕	positive
⊖	negative
Diseases	
ASHD	arteriosclerotic heart disease
ASCVD	arteriosclerotic cardiovascular disease
BPH	benign prostatic hypertrophy
CA	cancer
CAD	coronary artery disease
CHF	congestive heart failure
COPD	chronic obstructive pulmonary disease
CVA	cerebrovascular accident
DM	diabetes mellitus
HTN (↑ BP)	hypertension
MI	myocardial infarction
PVD	peripheral vascular disease
STD	sexually transmitted disease

(continued)

Table 21-1 *(continued)*
Abbreviations and Symbols Commonly Used by Health Practitioners

Abbreviation	Meaning
Diagnostic Studies	
ABG	arterial blood gases
BE	barium enema
CBC	complete blood count
CO_2	carbon dioxide
C&S	culture and sensitivity
CXR	chest x-ray
ECG (EKG)	cardiogram
lytes	electrolytes
RBC	red blood cells
UA	urinalysis
UGI	upper GI
WBC	white blood cells
Symbols	
>	greater than
<	less than
↑	increase
↗	increasing
↓	decrease
↙	decreasing
2°	secondary to
=	equal to
≠	unequal
♀	female
♂	male
°	degree
Orders	
$\bar{a}$	before
ad lib	as desired
AMA	against medical advice
BM	bowel movement
BP	blood pressure
$\bar{c}$ (C)	with
CPR	cardiopulmonary resuscitation
dc (disc)	discontinue
dx	diagnosis
DNR (no code)	do not resuscitate
hs	hour of sleep
I&O	intake and output
IV	intravenous
noc	night
NPO (npo)	nothing by mouth
NS (NlS) (N/S)	normal saline
O_2	oxygen
od	daily
$\bar{p}$	after
OT	occupational therapy
postop	postoperative
preop	preoperative
prep	preparation
PRN (prn)	as needed
PT	physical therapy
pt	patient
q	every
qs	quantity sufficient
ROM	range of motion
$\bar{s}$ (S)	without
STAT	immediately
TPR	temperature, pulse, respirations
VS	vital signs
×	times

Shift	11-7:30 AM	7-3:30 PM	3-11:30 PM
Diet or NPO	House = Soft	→	→
Nutrition		BR ☑ G ☐ F ☐ P LU ☐ G ☐ F ☐ P ☐ Feed ☑ Self	Di ☐ G ☑ F ☐ P HS Snack ☑ ☐ Feed ☑ Self
Bathing Skin Care	☑ Mouth Care ☐ Skin Care Keri lotion	☐ S ☑ P ☐ C ☑ Mouth Care ☑ AM Care	☑ PM Care ☑ Mouth Care
Activity	☑ CBR ☑ Pos. q2° ☐ BRP ☐ BRP c̄ Asst. ☐ OOB Chair c̄ Asst. ☐ OOB Chair s̄ Asst. ☐ AMB c̄ Asst. ☐ AMB s̄ Asst.	☑ CBR ☑ Pos. q2° ☐ BRP ☐ BRP c̄ Asst. ☐ OOB Chair c̄ Asst. ☐ OOB Chair s̄ Asst. ☐ AMB c̄ Asst. ☐ AMB s̄ Asst.	☑ CBR ☑ Pos. q2° ☐ BRP ☐ BRP c̄ Asst. ☐ OOB Chair c̄ Asst. ☐ OOB Chair s̄ Asst. ☐ AMB c̄ Asst. ☐ AMB s̄ Asst.
Resp. Assess-ment	☑ Cough/D. Breathe q2° ☐ Trach Care ☐ Suction Freq ____	☑ Cough/D. Breathe q2° ☐ Trach Care ☐ Suction Freq ____	☑ Cough/D. Breathe q2° ☐ Trach Care ☐ Suction Freq ____
Treat-ments	Assisted ROM	P.T. →	→
Protective Precau-tions	☐ Full ☑ Half	— ☐ Full ☐ Half	— ☐ Full ☐ Half
Restraints	☐ Posey ☐ Wrist ☐ Ankle ☐ None ☑ q2° Check ☐ Other	☐ Posey ☐ Wrist ☐ Ankle ☑ None ☐ q2° Check ☐ Other	☐ Posey ☐ Wrist ☐ Ankle ☑ None ☐ q2° Check ☐ Other
Elimina-tion Bowel Bladder ☐ Foley	bedpan voiding qs ☐ Commode	TBM Voiding qs bedpan ☐ Commode ☐ Foley Care	☐ Commode ☐ Foley Care
Diagnostic Studies +/or Specimens Obtained	—	CAT Scan	—
Isolation Type	—	—	—
Nursing Care Plan	☑ Reviewed ☐ Revised	☑ Reviewed ☐ Revised	☑ Reviewed ☐ Revised
Comments	awake @ 2am did not fall back to sleep	"when can I go home?" napped in pm	—
Signature	L. Gray RN	C Taylor RN	D. Kande RN

Nazareth Hospital
Activity Flowsheet/Patient Care Notes

Date / Time	
9/4/97 7 AM	Pt. awake and alert. Awoke at 2 AM to void — unable to fall back asleep. Refused sedative. Rested quietly. Speech clear, moving all extremities. — L. Gray RN
9/4/97 10 AM	Prune juice + cup of hot water with breakfast resulted in soft formed BM — about 1 hour p̄ breakfast (1st stool in 3 days). Keri lotion to dry skin on legs and arms. Strength seems to be increasing in left arm & leg. Performs lt. leg exercises independently. During bath talked about how much she misses her husband and her house. Explored feelings about participating in support group for widows — recommended by her friends. Feels good about babysitting her 2 grandchildren — C. Taylor, RN
2 pm	Spent 30 min. teaching client + daughter Lisa about T.I.A. and stroke. Strong family history of PVD, CVA and MI. Reviewed importance of dietary modifications, regular exercise and taking prescribed medication. Excellent motivation for self-care — S Taylor RN
9/4/97 8 pm	VS 98.8 – 7 – 18 136/92 Quiet this evening. – Napping – Not hungry at dinner: states "Busy day." Moving all extremities; alert. Daughter Barbara says her mother wants to do "too much." Still afraid TIA automatically means stroke & death! — D. Kande RN.

Figure 21-1
Sample of an activity flowsheet with narrative client care notes. (Courtesy of Nazareth Hospital, Philadelphia.)

Summary of data base for client (21-2A)

72 year old, white, recently widowed female

brought to hospital after sudden fall caused by temporary paralysis of left leg; admitting diagnosis: transient ischemic attack (TIA), R/O cerebrovascular accident

treated for hypertension since 1985, otherwise in good health; history of headaches—once or twice a week (increasing in severity)—for last six months

ht 5′2″ wt 63.6 kg 98.2 F-88-18 BP L—184/120, R—180/120
↓ strength ↓ movement left lower extremity (LLE)

Problem List (21-2B)

XXXX Medical Center 4629F

Date	No.	Problem	Identified	Resolved
9/2/97	#1	transient ischemic attack (TIA) R/O cerebrovascular accident	J. Gleer MD	
	#1A	impaired physical mobility related to weakness in left lower extremity	D. Kande RN	
9/4/97	#2	impaired adjustment related to major life stressors and decreased supports	D. Kande RN	

Plan of Care (21-2C)

Date	Problem
9/4/97	#2 Impaired adjustment related to major life stressors (including illness) and decreased supports Goal: Prior to discharge client reports feeling able to go home and take one day at a time Plan: *Diagnostic*: explore adequacy of client's usual patterns of coping and motivation to learn new strategies *Therapeutic*: 1) explain all tests/procedures to client who wants to know and understand what is happening to her 2) create a restful environment 3) talk with client's home minister (daughter will contact) *Educative*: Teach client new coping skills, e.g., relaxation exercises. Refer to community support group for widows. —D. Kande RN

Progress Notes (21-2D)

Date	Problem-Oriented Progress Notes
9/6/97	Impaired mobility related to weakness left lower extremity (LLE) **S** "My left leg still feels queer, pins and needles—but I can move it alright." **O** Able to lift left leg off bed, positive flexion, positive extension; muscle strength in LLE 3/5 (normal movement against gravity) **A** recovering mobility as strength returns **P** *therapeutic:* consult with physician about complete bed rest order; *diagnostic:* continue to monitor muscle strength and movement at least once/shift; be alert for any signs of recurrent TIA; *educative*: instruct not to try to get out of bed without assistance until diagnostic work-up is complete; reinforce need for safety precautions. —D. Kande RN

Figure 21-2
Sample of a problem-oriented client record.

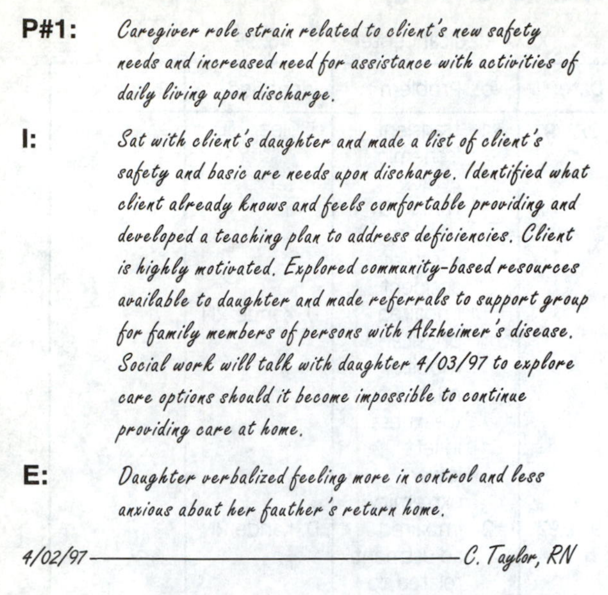

P#1: *Caregiver role strain related to client's new safety needs and increased need for assistance with activities of daily living upon discharge.*

I: *Sat with client's daughter and made a list of client's safety and basic are needs upon discharge. Identified what client already knows and feels comfortable providing and developed a teaching plan to address deficiencies. Client is highly motivated. Explored community-based resources available to daughter and made referrals to support group for family members of persons with Alzheimer's disease. Social work will talk with daughter 4/03/97 to explore care options should it become impossible to continue providing care at home.*

E: *Daughter verbalized feeling more in control and less anxious about her fauther's return home.*

4/02/97————————————————C. Taylor, RN

Figure 21-3
Sample PIE client care note.

Date/Time	Focus	Client Care Notes
7/11/97 9:15 am	*High risk for trauma*	**DATA:** *Client crying when I entered room; confided that she is afraid to go home because her injuries are the result of husband's battery*
		ACTION: *Attending notified and discharge cancelled; Abuse network called with client's permission and they are sending a counselor this afternoon to talk with her. ——————————————————C. Taylor, RN*
10:00 am	*Pain*	**DATA:** *Client complaining of pain in right rib area*
		ACTION: *Tylenol 3 administered as ordered.——————————————C. Taylor, RN*
10:30 am	*Pain*	**RESPONSE:** *Client reports relief from rib pain, still anxious about aftermath of discharge.————C. Taylor, RN*

Figure 21-4
Sample focus client care notes.

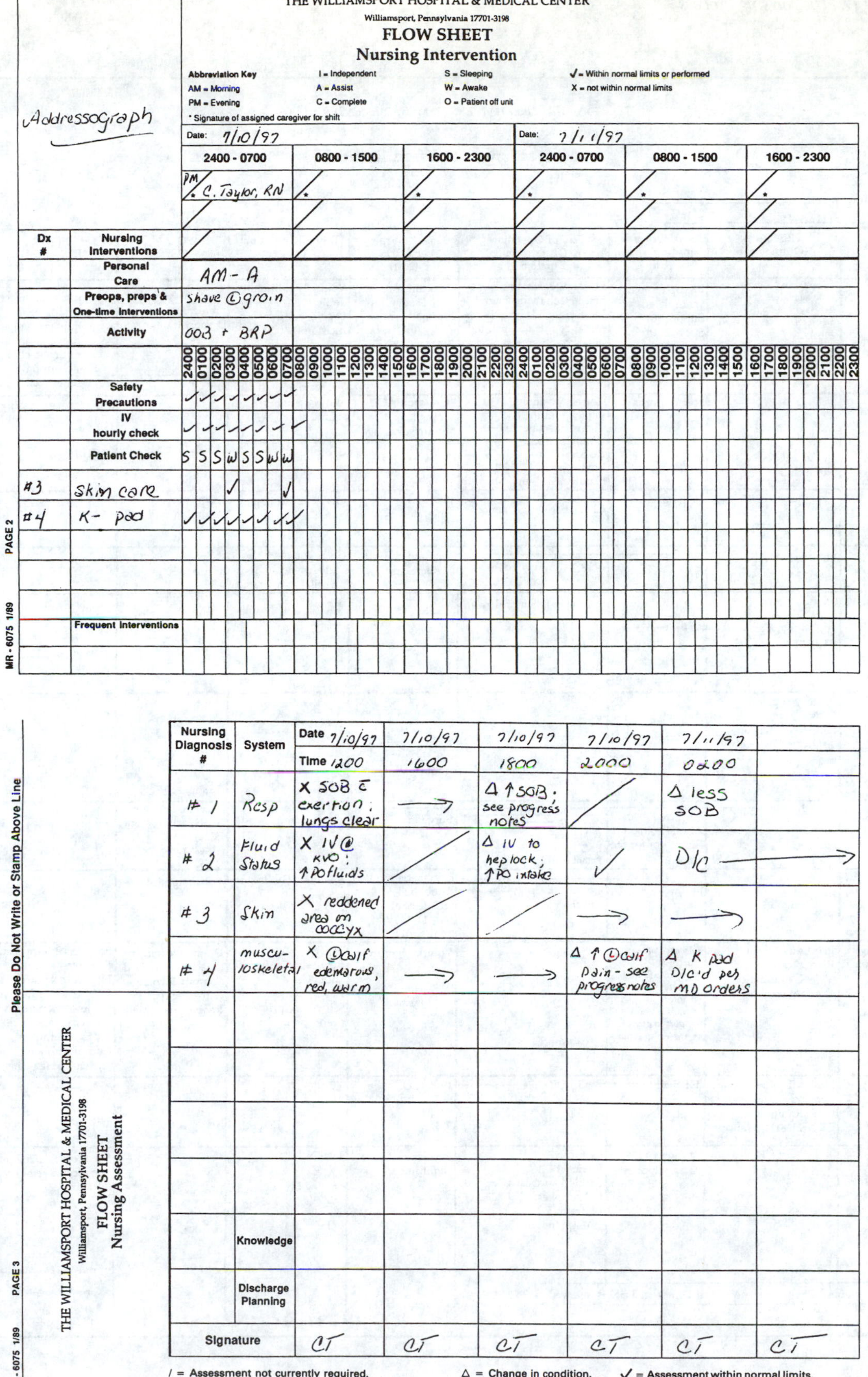

THE WILLIAMSPORT HOSPITAL & MEDICAL CENTER
Williamsport, Pennsylvania 17701-3198

FLOW SHEET
Nursing Intervention

Abbreviation Key
AM = Morning; PM = Evening
I = Independent; A = Assist; C = Complete
S = Sleeping; W = Awake; O = Patient off unit
✓ = Within normal limits or performed; X = not within normal limits
* Signature of assigned caregiver for shift

Addressograph

	Date: 7/10/97			Date: 7/11/97		
	2400 - 0700	0800 - 1500	1600 - 2300	2400 - 0700	0800 - 1500	1600 - 2300
	PM / * C. Taylor, RN	*	*	*	*	*
Dx # / Nursing Interventions						
Personal Care	AM - A					
Preops, preps & One-time Interventions	shave Ⓛ groin					
Activity	OOB c BRP					

Dx #	Nursing Interventions	2400	0100	0200	0300	0400	0500	0600	0700
	Safety Precautions	✓	✓	✓	✓	✓	✓	✓	✓
	IV hourly check	✓	✓	✓	✓	✓	✓	✓	✓
	Patient Check	S	S	S	W	S	S	W	W
#3	Skin care					✓			✓
#4	K- pad	✓	✓	✓	✓	✓	✓	✓	✓
	Frequent Interventions								

MR - 6075 1/89 PAGE 2

Please Do Not Write or Stamp Above Line

THE WILLIAMSPORT HOSPITAL & MEDICAL CENTER
Williamsport, Pennsylvania 17701-3198
FLOW SHEET
Nursing Assessment

Nursing Diagnosis #	System	Date 7/10/97 Time 1200	7/10/97 1600	7/10/97 1800	7/10/97 2000	7/11/97 0200	
#1	Resp	X SOB c exertion; lungs clear	→	Δ ↑ SOB; see progress notes	/	Δ less SOB	
#2	Fluid Status	X IV @ KVO; ↑ PO fluids	/	Δ IV to hep lock; ↑ PO intake	✓	D/C →	
#3	Skin	X reddened area on coccyx	/	/	→	→	
#4	musculoskeletal	X Ⓛ calf edematous, red, warm	→	→	Δ ↑ Ⓛ calf pain - see progress notes	Δ K pad D/C'd per MD orders	
	Knowledge						
	Discharge Planning						
	Signature	CT	CT	CT	CT	CT	CT

/ = Assessment not currently required.
D/C = System no longer requires assessment
Δ = Change in condition.
X = New problem.
✓ = Assessment within normal limits.
➡ = No change in condition since last assessment.

MR - 6075 1/89 PAGE 3

Figure 21-5
Sample documentation of nursing care using charting by exception. (Courtesy of the Department of Nursing, Williamsport Hospital and Medical Center, Williamsport, PA.)

VANDERBILT UNIVERSITY MEDICAL CENTER

Mastectomy: Modified Radical

DRG Number: ______________

ELOS: ______________

	Pre Op (Outpatient)	Day of Operation (Holding Room) 1 hr	Day of Operation (OR → close) 2 hr 15 min	Day of Surgery PACU (2 hr)	Day of Operation (9 S)	POD 1 (9S)	POD 2 (9S/Day of Discharge)
Goals	Pre-op testing complete and data available for review 1-4 days pre-op Pre-op testing results WNL for surgery Pt/family teaching complete Consent signed	Pre-op checklist completed Support to family Support to patient Permit signed	Pt. safety maintained → Sterile tech maintained → Pt. positioned correctly → Initial counts documented Final counts correct	Pain controlled VSS, Lung CTA Normothermia achieved $SaO_2 \geq 90\%$	Voids w/o difficulty Temp < 100° → Drsg dry & intact Incision w/o S/Sx infection → Drains patent & functioning → Tol reg diet w/o difficulty	Reach to Recovery referral made Demonstrates drain care	Home care teaching complete Drains patent and functioning till return to clinic F/U appointment scheduled
Treatments		Shave/prep	Correct position Pad extremities and bony prominence → Warm blanket → Pt. prep Bovie pad Counts x 3 if applicable	Standard PACU care Monitor drainage in hemovac Check dsg q 1 hr	No needle sticks, BP to ____ arm JP drains x 2 →		MD remove dressing Till RTC
Activity	Ad lib	Bedrest →	Check bony prominence	Progress as tolerated	OOB to chair in p.m.	OOB to chair Ambulate halls TID	
Diet	NPO at MN night before surg	NPO →		Sips and chips if tolerated	Clear liquids → advance to regular as tolerated		
Labs	SMA6 SMA12 CBC with plts PT, PTT UA } →	Pre-op value on charts	Specimen to Surgical Path.		PCV		
Tests	History & physical CXR EKG if > 50 yrs or indicated by history }	Test results on chart					
Consults	Anesthesia →	Surgical Resident → Anes. Resident → Circulator for the case	Core Staff → PCM (prn) PACU Notified Pathologist	Surgeon		Reach to Recovery (call early w/ bra size) Assess need for HIR	
Meds/IV		IV access → Pre-op meds	Anesthesia drugs → Ancef 1 gm	Pain meds prn IV Antibotic IV (if requested) May D/C IV (if ordered)	Analgesic (IV, IM on PO)	PO analgesic	
Teaching/ D/C Plan	Procedure Plan of care VUMC orientation Consent signed	Reinforce pre-op teaching Support to family • waiting room infor. • update phone call Support to pt. • answer questions • comfort		Volurex →	TCDB Request pain med if not PCA Assess home situation/primary care giver	Drain care (empty, reactivate, record output & change dressing q d) Request pain med	Post mastectomy teaching Exercises How to take care of arm F/U Reach to Recovery Review drain care, meds, activity, reportable S/Sx, precautions Complete "patient discharge list" sheet
Patient Flow	H&P MD office Labs: Pre adm testing CXR: Radiology EKG: Heart Station	HR →	To OR suite →	PACU	9S		
Equipment & Supplies		IV start kit Anes. supplies X-ray folder on bed	Case cart Bovie Padded armboard OR supplies JP drains x 2 PACU stretcher	Respirator equipment	IMED		Schedule F/U 5-7 days post op to remove drains

Mastectomy Modified Radical
6/3/94
General Surgery 1

Figure 21-6
Sample collaborative pathway.

VANDERBILT UNIVERSITY MEDICAL CENTER
COLLABORATIVE PATHWAY REPORT

PAGE: 1
DATE: 7/03/95
EST LOS: 3
Additional Dx:

Mastectomy - Modified Radical

PATIENT, TEST
ACCT# 111111111111 MR# 222222222
AGE: 55 YRS DOB: 1/01/1940
ADM DT: 7/03/1995 9228 GNS
DR: REYNOLDS, VERNON

NHO: T > 101.5°, SBP < 90 > 180, DBP < 50 > 110, P < 60 > 120 , R < > ,
UOP < 240 ml/shift

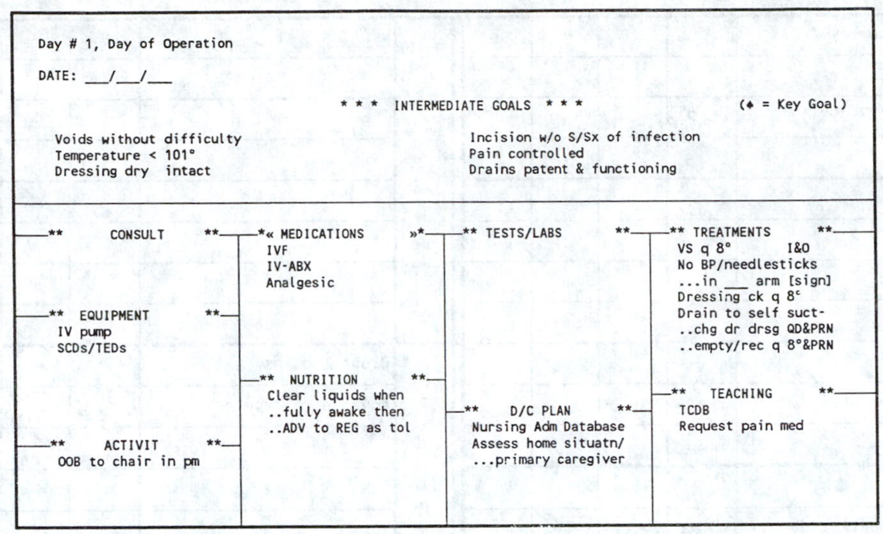

Day # 1, Day of Operation

DATE: __/__/__

* * * INTERMEDIATE GOALS * * * (♦ = Key Goal)

Voids without difficulty
Temperature < 101°
Dressing dry intact

Incision w/o S/Sx of infection
Pain controlled
Drains patent & functioning

** CONSULT **

** EQUIPMENT **
IV pump
SCDs/TEDs

** ACTIVIT **
OOB to chair in pm

« MEDICATIONS »
IVF
IV-ABX
Analgesic

** NUTRITION **
Clear liquids when
..fully awake then
..ADV to REG as tol

** TESTS/LABS **

** D/C PLAN **
Nursing Adm Database
Assess home situatn/
...primary caregiver

** TREATMENTS **
VS q 8° I&O
No BP/needlesticks
...in ___ arm [sign]
Dressing ck q 8°
Drain to self suct-
..chg dr drsg QD&PRN
..empty/rec q 8°&PRN

** TEACHING **
TCDB
Request pain med

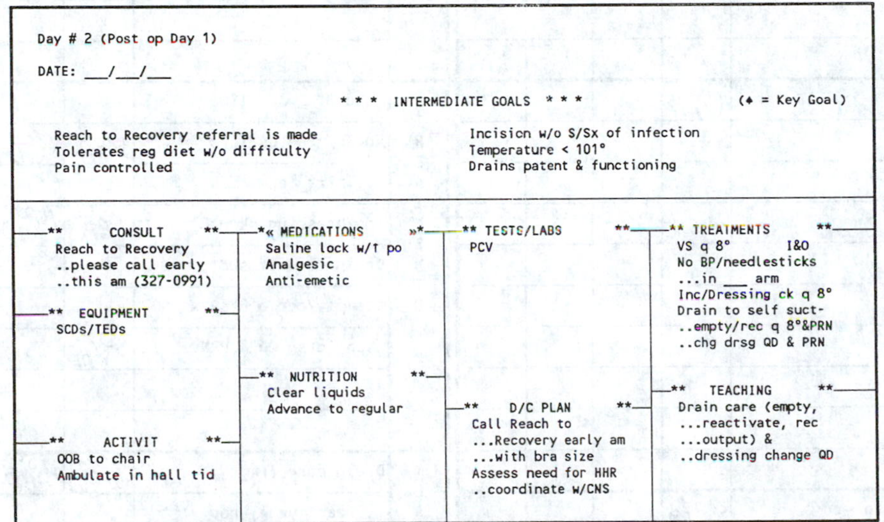

Day # 2 (Post op Day 1)

DATE: __/__/__

* * * INTERMEDIATE GOALS * * * (♦ = Key Goal)

Reach to Recovery referral is made
Tolerates reg diet w/o difficulty
Pain controlled

Incision w/o S/Sx of infection
Temperature < 101°
Drains patent & functioning

** CONSULT **
Reach to Recovery
..please call early
..this am (327-0991)

** EQUIPMENT **
SCDs/TEDs

** ACTIVIT **
OOB to chair
Ambulate in hall tid

« MEDICATIONS »
Saline lock w/T po
Analgesic
Anti-emetic

** NUTRITION **
Clear liquids
Advance to regular

** TESTS/LABS **
PCV

** D/C PLAN **
Call Reach to
...Recovery early am
...with bra size
Assess need for HHR
..coordinate w/CNS

** TREATMENTS **
VS q 8° I&O
No BP/needlesticks
...in ___ arm
Inc/Dressing ck q 8°
Drain to self suct-
..empty/rec q 8°&PRN
..chg drsg QD & PRN

** TEACHING **
Drain care (empty,
...reactivate, rec
...output) &
...dressing change QD

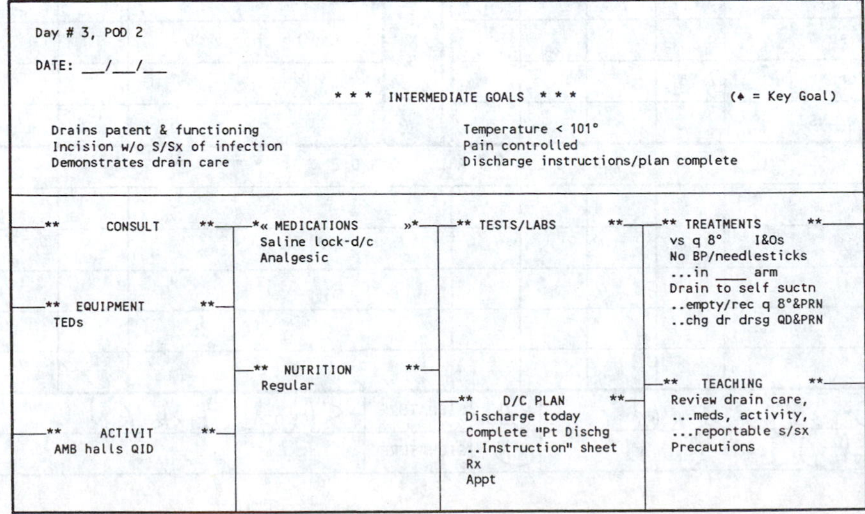

Day # 3, POD 2

DATE: __/__/__

* * * INTERMEDIATE GOALS * * * (♦ = Key Goal)

Drains patent & functioning
Incision w/o S/Sx of infection
Demonstrates drain care

Temperature < 101°
Pain controlled
Discharge instructions/plan complete

** CONSULT **

** EQUIPMENT **
TEDs

** ACTIVIT **
AMB halls QID

« MEDICATIONS »
Saline lock-d/c
Analgesic

** NUTRITION **
Regular

** TESTS/LABS **

** D/C PLAN **
Discharge today
Complete "Pt Dischg
..Instruction" sheet
Rx
Appt

** TREATMENTS **
vs q 8° I&Os
No BP/needlesticks
...in ____ arm
Drain to self suctn
..empty/rec q 8°&PRN
..chg dr drsg QD&PRN

** TEACHING **
Review drain care,
...meds, activity,
...reportable s/sx
Precautions

Figure 21-7
Sample collaborative pathway report. (Courtesy of Vanderbilt University Medical Center, Nashville, TN.)

VANDERBILT UNIVERSITY MEDICAL CENTER
DATE: 7 / 5 / 97

FLOWSHEET PAGE 2

PATIENT, TEST
ACCT# 111111111111 MR# 222222222
AGE: 55 YRS DOB: 1/01/1940 9228 GNS
DR: REYNOLDS, VERNON ADM DT: 7/03/1995

COLLABORATIVE PATHWAY: Mastectomy - Modified Radical
Day # 2 (Post op Day 1)

CONSULT	Reach to Recovery				
	..please call early				
	..this am (327-0991)	✓ 830 AB			
EQUIPMENT	SCDs/TEDs	✓ AB			
ACTIVITY	OOB to chair	830 AB			
	Ambulate in hall tid	845 AB	1600 CD	2300 EF	
TESTS/LABS	PCV	710 ✓ AB			
D/C PLAN	Call Reach to	830 AB			
	...Recovery early am				
	...with bra size				
	Assess need for HHR	850 AB			
	..coordinate w/CNS				

NUTRITION	Clear liquids	8 ✓ AB			
	Advance to regular	1230 ½ AB	1730 ½ CD		
TREATMENTS	VS q 8° I&O				
	No BP/needlesticks	✓ AB	✓ CD	✓ EF	
	...in rt_ arm				
	Inc/Dressing ck q 8°	8 AB	1620 CD	2200 EF	
	Drain to self suct-				
	..empty/rec q 8°&PRN				
	..chg drsg QD & PRN	850 ✓ AB			
TEACHING	Drain care (empty,	830 AB	1130 AB	2030 CD	
	...reactivate, rec				
	...output) &				
	..dressing change QD				

***** INCIDENTAL ORDERS *****

chemsticks BID					

SIGNATURE	Alice Boyd RN	AB	SIGNATURE	Ellen Fisk RN	EF
SIGNATURE	Carol David RN	CD	SIGNATURE		

Figure 21-8
Flowsheets that accompany the collaborative pathway on day 2, mastectomy—modified radical. (Courtesy of Vanderbilt University Medical Center, Nashville, TN.)

VANDERBILT UNIVERSITY MEDICAL CENTER
DATE: 7/5/97

FLOWSHEET PAGE 3

PATIENT, TEST
ACCT# 111111111111 MR# 222222222
AGE: 55 YRS DOB: 1/01/1940 9228 GNS
DR: REYNOLDS, VERNON ADM DT: 7/03/1995

COLLABORATIVE PATHWAY: Mastectomy - Modified Radical
Day # 2 (Post op Day 1)

ALLERGIES: penicillin

PREVIOUS DAY'S ACTIVE GOALS	Temperature < 101°	
TODAY'S PATHWAY GOALS (♦ = Key Goal)	Reach to Recovery referral is made ✓AB Tolerates reg diet w/o difficulty ✓EF Pain controlled ✓EF	Incision w/o S/Sx of infection ✓EF Temperature < 101° EF Drains patent & functioning ✓EK

Time		8	10	12	14	16	18	20	22	24	2	4	6
Activity		bed	ch	ch	amb	bed	amb	bed	→	→	→	→	→
Comfort	Scale												
Sal lock	flush q8												
Trach	Care												
Saline	lavage												
Suction	trach												
Tubefeed	residual												
NGT pH													
Neuro	Pupils												
	React												
	EyesOpen												
Verbal	Response												
Motor	Response												
Strength	RUE/LUE												
Strength	RLE/LLE												

Linen ∆	8³⁰ BB	Bath	A 8³⁰ BB	Mouth	✓BB	Skin	✓BB	Perineal	✓BB

****** SHIFT ASSESSMENTS ******

** TIME/INITIALS **	8¹⁵ AB	1510 CD	2030 EF	** TIME/INITIALS **	8¹⁵ AB	1510 CD	2030 EF
1. NEUROLOGICAL	✓	✓	✓	8. IV SITE	✓	✓	✓
2. CARDIOVASCULAR	✓	✓	✓	9. INCISION	✓	✓	✓
3. PULMONARY	✓	*	*	10. DRAINS	✓	✓	✓
4. MUSCULOSKELETAL	✓	✓	✓	11. PSYCHOSOCIAL	✓	*	→
5. GASTROINTESTINAL	✓	✓	✓	12. SAFETY	✓	✓	✓
6. GENITOURINARY	✓	✓	✓	13. COMFORT	✓	✓	✓
7. INTEGUMENT	✓	✓	✓				

IV SITE: LOC/TYPE	RFA/PIV	COLLABORATIVE PATH REVIEW	EF

SIGNATURE	Alice Boyd, RN	AB	SIGNATURE	Betty Brown CP	BB	✓ = No significant finding * = Significant finding see note -> = No change from last significant finding
SIGNATURE	Carol Dawn, RN	CD	SIGNATURE			
SIGNATURE	Ellen Fisk, RN	EF	SIGNATURE			

Figure 21-8 *(continued)*

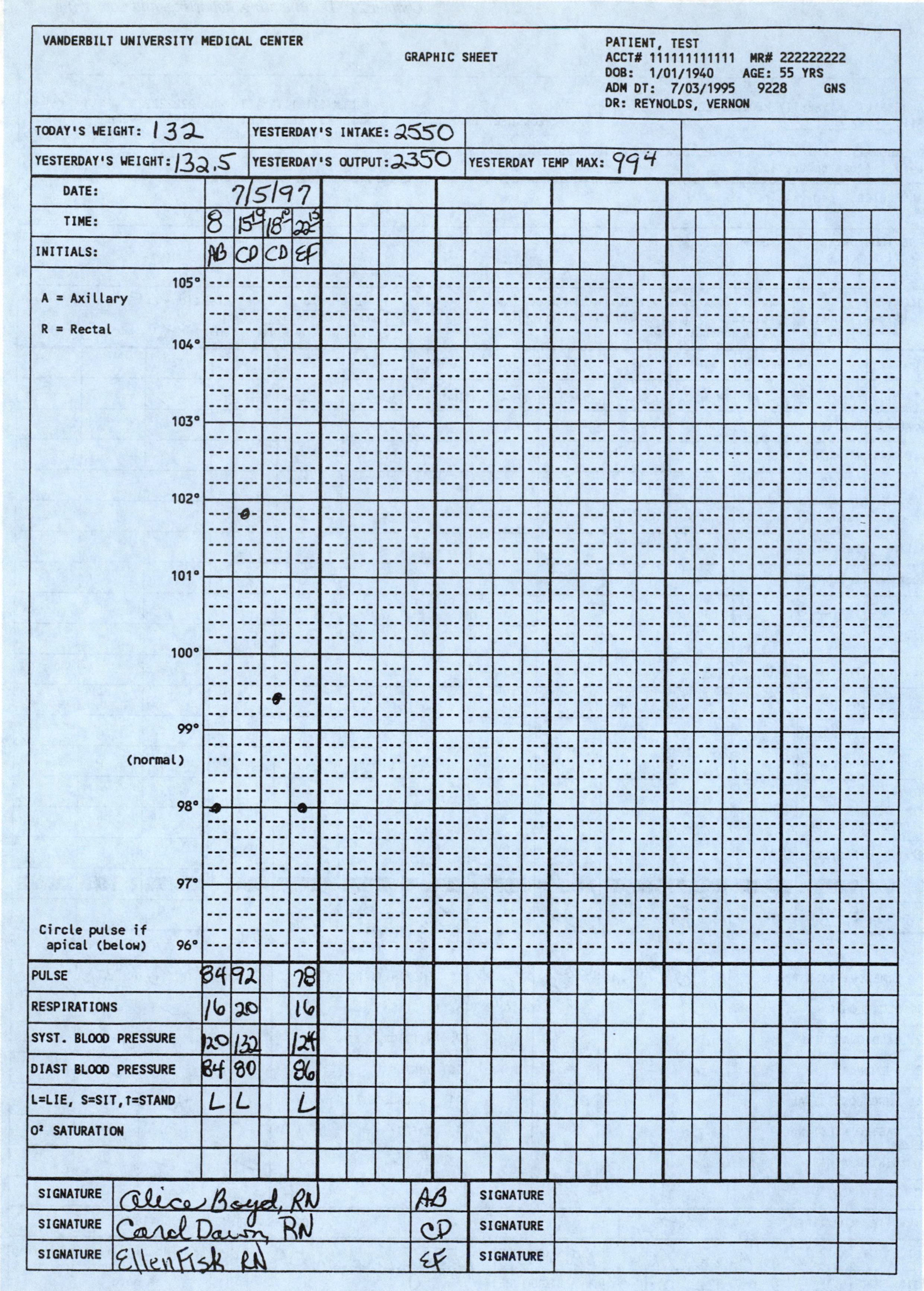

VANDERBILT UNIVERSITY MEDICAL CENTER

GRAPHIC SHEET

PATIENT, TEST
ACCT# 111111111111 MR# 222222222
DOB: 1/01/1940 AGE: 55 YRS
ADM DT: 7/03/1995 9228 GNS
DR: REYNOLDS, VERNON

TODAY'S WEIGHT: 132	YESTERDAY'S INTAKE: 2550		
YESTERDAY'S WEIGHT: 132.5	YESTERDAY'S OUTPUT: 2350	YESTERDAY TEMP MAX: 994	

DATE:	7/5/97			
TIME:	8	15^{19}	18^{10}	22^{15}
INITIALS:	AB	CD	CD	EF
A = Axillary R = Rectal 105° 104° 103° 102° 101° 100° 99° (normal) 98° 97° Circle pulse if apical (below) 96°				
PULSE	84	92		78
RESPIRATIONS	16	20		16
SYST. BLOOD PRESSURE	120	132		124
DIAST BLOOD PRESSURE	84	80		86
L=LIE, S=SIT, ↑=STAND	L	L		L
O² SATURATION				

SIGNATURE	Alice Boyd, RN	AB	SIGNATURE		
SIGNATURE	Carol Dawn, RN	CD	SIGNATURE		
SIGNATURE	Ellen Fisk RN	EF	SIGNATURE		

Figure 21-9
Graphic record that accompanies the collaborative pathway in Figure 21-6. (Courtesy of Vanderbilt University Medical Center, Nashville, TN.)

VANDERBILT UNIVERSITY MEDICAL CENTER
DATE: 7/5/97

I & O SHEET

PATIENT, TEST ADM: 7/03/1995
ACCT# 111111111111 MR# 222222222
DOB: 1/01/1940 AGE: 55 YRS
DR: REYNOLDS, VERNON 9228 GNS

T = Tubing Change
▲ = Dressing Change
D = Diuretic
+ = Positive Blood
- = Negative Blood

TIME	INIT	SITE✓	D5½NS c̄ 30K	meds	PO										urine	JP#1	JP#2		BM
			INTAKE								INTAKE OR OUTPUT				OUTPUT				
0700																			
0800	AB	✓	240/60		400										200				
0900																			T
1000	AB	✓	180/60	50	100														
1100																			
1200	AB	✓	120/60		400														
1300															400				
1400	AB	✓	60/60	50												15	25		
			240	100	900										600	15	25		
			Shift Cumulative Total						1240					Shift Cumulative Total				640	
1500																			
1600	CD	✓	T 1000/60												400				
1700																			
1800	CD	✓	930/70	T 100	240														
1900																			
2000	CD	✓	880/50		100														
2100															500				
2200	CD	✓	820/60	50												15	30		
			240	150	340										900	15	30		
			Shift Cumulative Total						730					Shift Cumulative Total				945	
2300															400				
2400	EF	✓	770/60	50															
0100																			
0200	EF	✓	705/65																
0300																			
0400	EF	✓	650/55																
0500																			
0600	EF	✓	580/60													10	25		
			240	50											400	10	25		
			Shift Cumulative Total						290					Shift Cumulative Total				440	
CUMULATIVE 24° TOTAL			INTAKE						2260					OUTPUT				2030	

SIGNATURE		SIGNATURE	
SIGNATURE		SIGNATURE	
SIGNATURE		SIGNATURE	

Figure 21-9 ***(continued)***

Unit V discusses the nurse's professional roles of communicator, teacher, counselor, leader, researcher, and advocate. These roles are interdependent, and each is an integral part of the broad nursing role of caregiver. The nurse uses these roles to help clients of all ages to meet needs along the health continuum.

To be effective as a caregiver, the nurse must be proficient in both the art and science of nursing roles. The role of the nurse as communicator is essential to each professional nursing role and is the heart of caring. Nursing is a person-centered service, based on relationships with clients, peers, and other members of the healthcare team. By developing effective interpersonal skills and using therapeutic communication skills, nurses are able to establish and maintain helping relationships with peers.

As teacher, the nurse uses communication skills to teach individuals and families. Teaching, implemented through the nursing process, is used to meet learning needs. As counselor, the nurse provides information, makes appropriate referrals, and assists the client in developing a systematic approach to problem solving and decision making. The nurse as leader practices assertive, self-directed nursing. Abilities for leadership and bringing about change begin with the student nurse and progress as the nurse develops self-confidence and skill in interpersonal relationships and experience in healthcare settings. As researcher, the nurse may conduct research, use research findings to improve client care, or participate in research done by others. As advocate, the nurse combines all these roles to promote the right of clients to make their own decisions about health and life and to protect human and legal rights.

The content of Unit V enables beginning nurse caregivers to enrich their professional practice by integrating the professional nursing roles of communicator, teacher, counselor, leader, researcher, and advocate. Nursing practice, as a specialized and unique service to others, is based on the application of knowledge and skill presented in this unit.

Roles Basic to Nursing Care

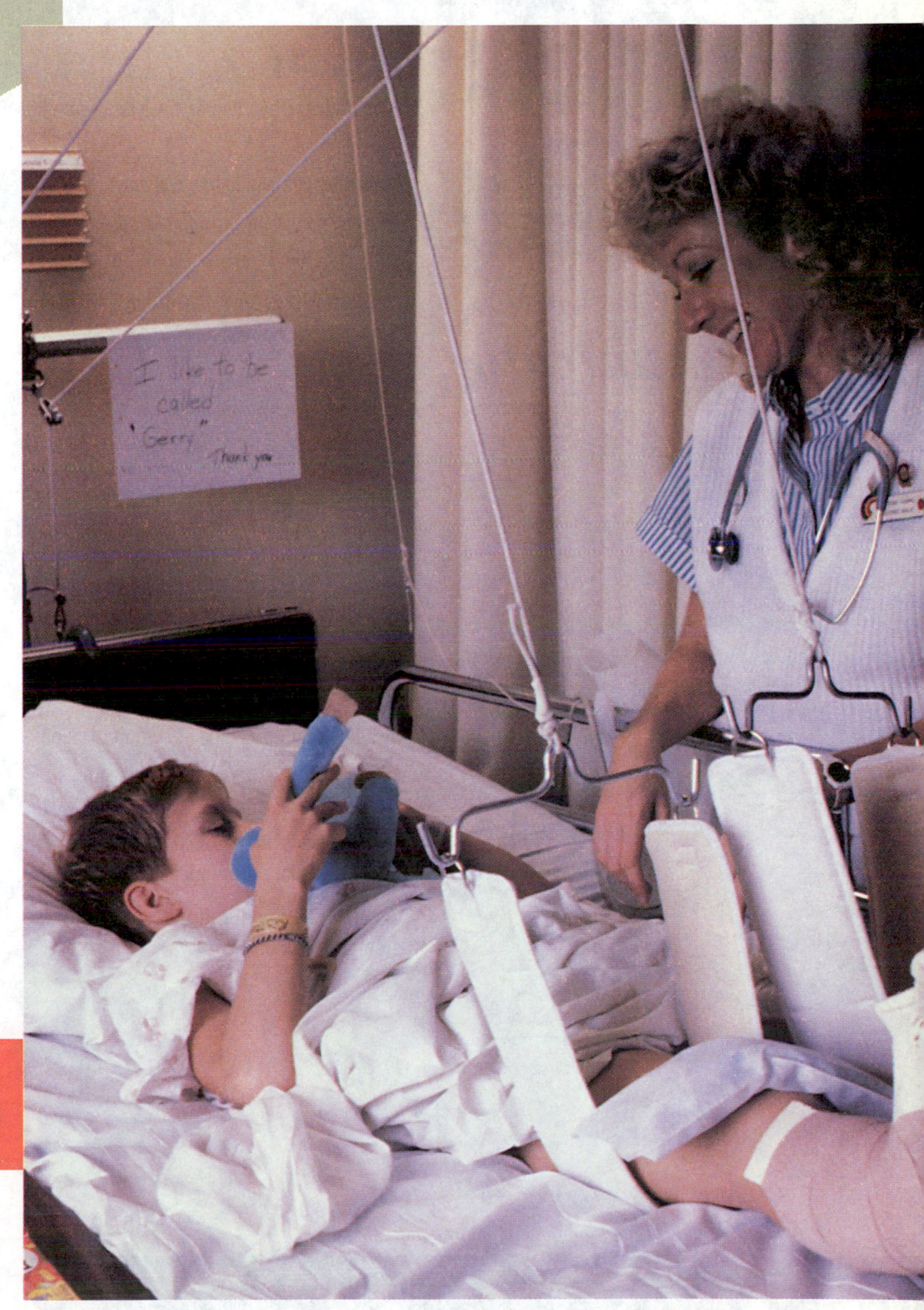

"Clinical competence . . . has three dimensions. . . . Care is the fundamental things we do to make a patient comfortable. . . . curative nursing, . . . the broader group of restorative and rehabilitative activities: to a sound knowledge of the principles on which they are based . . . counseling, . . . of emotional, intellectual, and psychological support . . ."

Frances Reiter (1904–1977)
the first chairperson of the ANA Committee on Education, she coined the term "nurse clinician" and advocated advanced preparation of nurse clinicians

Unit V

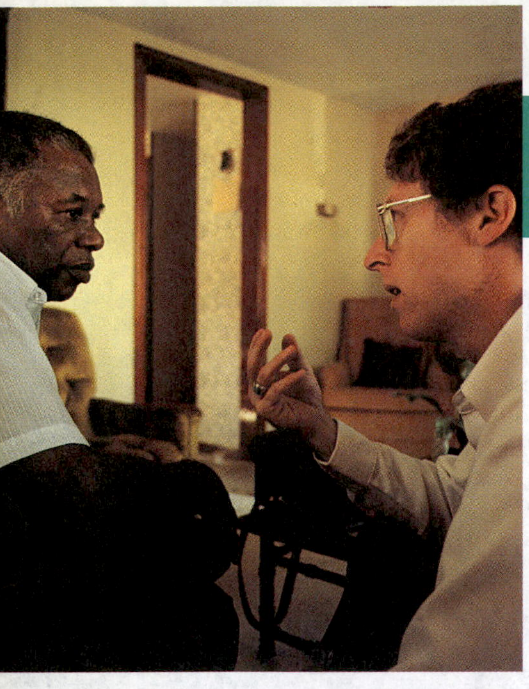

Chapter 22

Communicator

Objectives

After studying this chapter, the learner should be able to:

Define key terms used in the chapter.

Describe the communication process, identifying factors that influence communication.

List at least eight ways in which people communicate nonverbally.

Describe the interrelation between communication and the nursing process.

Identify client goals for each phase of the helping relationship.

Use effective communication techniques when interacting with clients from different cultures.

Evaluate self in terms of the interpersonal competencies needed in nursing.

Describe how each of the ineffective communication techniques hinders communication.

Establish therapeutic relationships with clients assigned to your care and describe effective interventions for clients with impaired verbal communication.

Compare and contrast effective and ineffective groups.

Key Terms

assertiveness
body language
channel
communication
empathy
feedback
group dynamics
helping relationship
interpersonal skills
interviewing techniques
language
message
nonverbal communication
rapport
receiver (decoder)
relationship
semantics
source (encoder)
therapeutic touch
verbal communication

Any nurse who wishes to be an effective caregiver must first learn to communicate. Good communication skills enable nurses to get to know their clients and, ultimately, to diagnose and meet their needs for nursing care. The student nurse who sits face to face with a client for the first time and is charged with the responsibility of obtaining a comprehensive nursing history intuitively grasps the importance of the communicator role of the nurse. Communication skills are the building blocks of professional relationships: nurse–client, nurse–nurse, and nurse–physician (and other health team members). Many experienced nurses identify the quality of their interpersonal relationships as the single most significant element in determining their helper effectiveness. Studies have shown that on nursing units where nurses freely exchange ideas and information, problem solve together when something goes wrong rather than assigning blame, compliment one another, and use humor creatively, staff morale is high and clients demonstrate enhanced well-being and increased compliance with treatments and procedures.

The Communication Process

Communication is the foundation of society. Without some form of communication it would be impossible to share family experiences, master an education, establish and maintain a government, and enjoy many current forms of entertainment. By nature humans are social and their needs are met in collaboration with other humans. Human relationships enable us to meet not only our physical and safety needs but also our psychosocial needs for love, belonging, and self-esteem. The ability to communicate is basic to human functioning and well-being.

Communication is the process of sharing information or the process of generating and transmitting meanings. The two definitions are not in conflict because information is produced and has meaning before it can be shared. David K. Berlo (1960) is credited with the classic description of the communication process, which involves a source (encoder), message, channel, and receiver (decoder). This process is illustrated in Figure 22-1. The function of the **source** or **encoder** is to prepare and send to the receiver a message that can be decoded with complete accuracy. The **message** is the actual product of the source or encoder. It might be a speech, interview, telephone conversation, chart, conversation, gesture, memorandum, or nursing note. The **channel** is the medium selected to convey the message and may target any of the receiver's senses. In a teaching session, a nurse may use auditory, visual, and tactile channels to communicate with a client. The **receiver (decoder)**, upon receiving the message, must translate it and make a decision about it. The nurse who is an effective communicator needs to consider the receiver at all times, seeking to select a message that appeals to the client's interests, is phrased in words the client understands, and requires minimal effort and time to decode. It is critical to look for verbal and nonverbal evidence—**feedback**—that the client has received and understood the message. Noise—factors that distort the quality of a message—may interfere with communication at any point in the process. Some examples of noise include a distracted source or receiver, a room that is uncomfortably warm, a noisy television program, and pain.

Communication is a reciprocal process in which both the sender and the receiver of messages participate simultaneously. The basic characteristics of communication are highlighted in the accompanying box.

Forms of Communication

People communicate in various environments involving a varying number of people. *One-to-one communication* occurs when only two people are involved in the communication process. A great deal of nursing situations involve the nurse and client in one-to-one communication.

Communication also occurs in *small groups* of 3 to 10 individuals. Nurses must learn to communicate effectively in small groups because they are often required to be members or leaders of such groups. *Large groups* comprise more than 10 people. Nursing instructors and students frequently experience the communication process in large groups. The nurse's role in teaching large groups is presented in Chapter 23. Attendance at

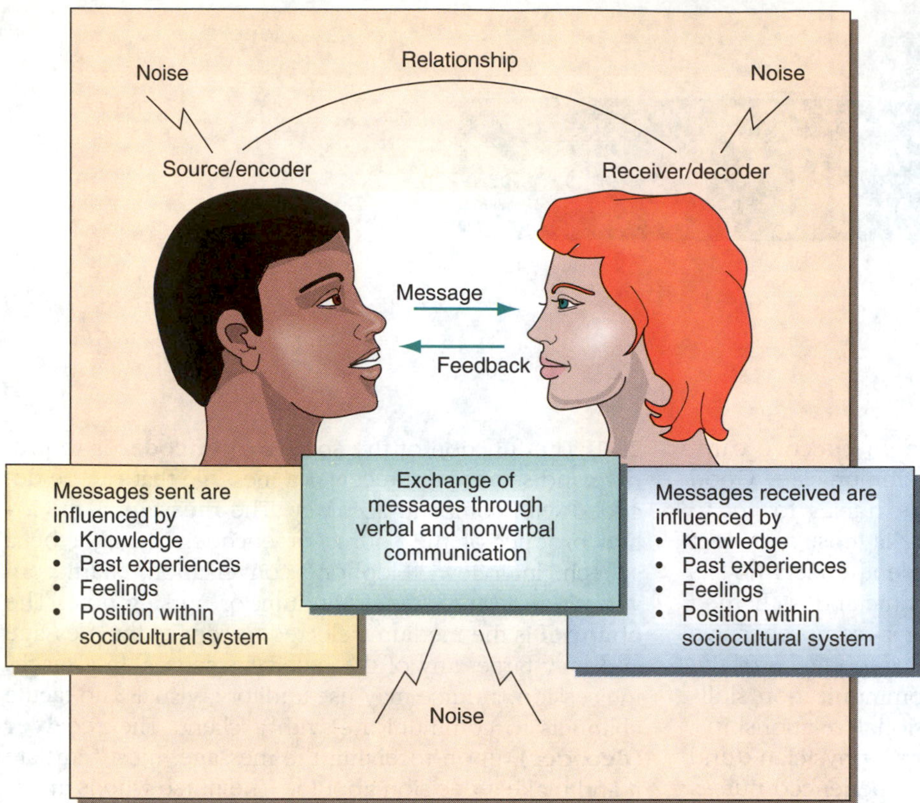

Figure 22-1
The various components in the process of communication.

social, religious, or political functions also involves large groups where communication may occur.

Communicating people receive and send messages through verbal and nonverbal means, which occur simultaneously. Learning about forms of communicating and developing skills in them are important parts of the nurse's education.

Verbal Communication

Verbal communication is an exchange of information using words and includes both the spoken and the written word. Verbal communication depends on language. **Language** is a prescribed way of using words so that people can share information effectively. Language includes a common definition of words as well as a method of arranging the words in a certain order.

Both written and spoken forms of communication reveal a great deal about a person. The way a person pronounces certain words or uses particular phrases gives clues to such things as geographic or ethnic origins. Vocabulary, sentence structure, and spelling give indications of a person's intellectual development or educational level and may also indicate that English is a second language. Language helps nurses assess what clients know and feel. In turn, nurses must develop their own language skills to aid in reciprocal responses in the communication process.

The verbal form of communication is used extensively by nurses when speaking with clients, giving oral reports to other nurses, writing care plans, and recording in nursing progress notes. Other examples of verbal communication include public speaking, writing for publication, and composing signs and posters. In each of these examples, words and language are communicated to others.

Nonverbal Communication

Nonverbal communication is the exchange of information without the use of words; it is what is not said. Sometimes referred to as **body language**, it often helps us to understand the subtle and hidden meanings in what is being said verbally. For instance, a person may respond to the question, "How are you?" by simply answering, "Fine." However, if this answer is accompanied by a rigid, tense facial expression, the true meaning of the response would need further investigation (Fig. 22-2).

Information is exchanged through nonverbal communication in various ways. It is generally accepted that nonverbal communication expresses more of the true meaning of a message than does verbal communication (Fig. 22-3). Therefore, nurses must be aware of both the nonverbal messages they send and the nonverbal messages they receive from clients. A great deal of variation exists in nonverbal communication, depending on one's individual or cultural patterns. Nurses working with clients from diverse cultural backgrounds should attempt to understand cultural variations to avoid misunderstanding nonverbal communication. The various forms of nonverbal communication follow.

Touch. Tactile sense has been studied seriously as a form of nonverbal communication only within the past

3 or 4 decades. Touch expresses personal behavior and means different things to different people. Investigations have shown that tactile experiences are largely shaped by familial, regional, class, and cultural influences. Such factors as age and sex also play a role in individualizing meanings associated with touch. Despite its individuality, touch is viewed as one of the most effective nonverbal ways to express feelings such as comfort, love, affection, security, anger, frustration, aggression, excitement, and many others.

Eye Contact. Communication often begins with eye contact. A glance, for example, is often an attention-getting method to open conversation. Eye contact also suggests respect and a willingness to listen and to keep communication open. Its absence often indicates anxiety or defenselessness or that a person is avoiding communication. However, young children and adolescents in some cultures are taught that it is disrespectful to look an adult in the eye. In other cultures, women are taught to avoid eye contact, or that out of respect eye contact should not be made with a superior. In addition, the eyes themselves carry nonverbal messages. For example, the eyes fix in a stare during anger, tend to narrow in disgust, and ordinarily open wide in fear. A blank stare can indicate daydreaming or inattentiveness.

Basic Characteristics of Communication

- Communication requires at least two people who, as a result of communicating, establish a relationship with each other.
- Communication is continuous and reciprocal.
- Communicating people receive and send messages through verbal and nonverbal means.
- Verbal and nonverbal communications occur simultaneously.
- Communicating people respond to messages they receive.
- The message cannot always be assumed to mean what the receiver believes it to mean or what the sender intended it to mean.
- Exchanging messages requires knowledge.
- Past experiences influence messages sent, and interpretation by the receiver is based on past experiences.
- Communication is influenced by the way people feel about themselves, the subject matter being communicated, and others.
- A person's position within a sociocultural system may influence the process of communication.

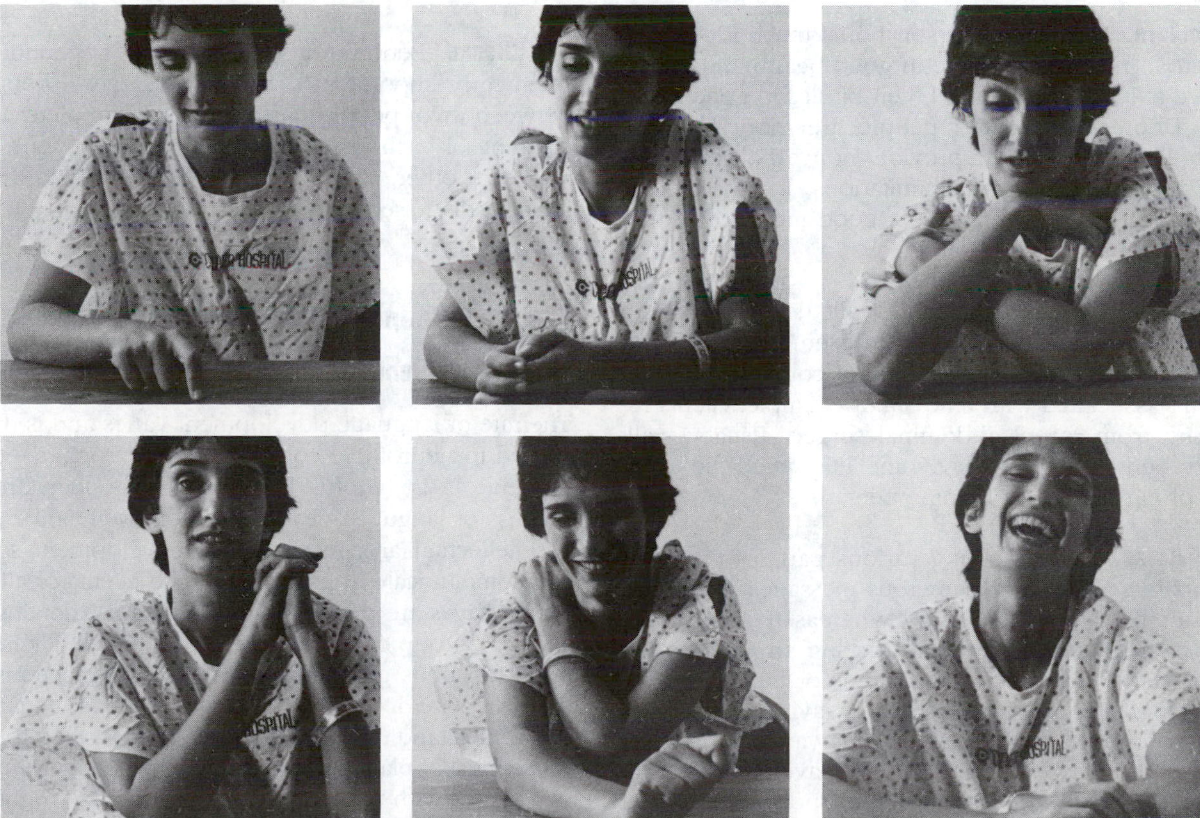

Figure 22-2
Eye contact, the lack of it, facial expression, posture, gesture, and silence send nonverbal messages to the receiver. What messages do you receive from each of these photographs? (Photos by Charles Field.)

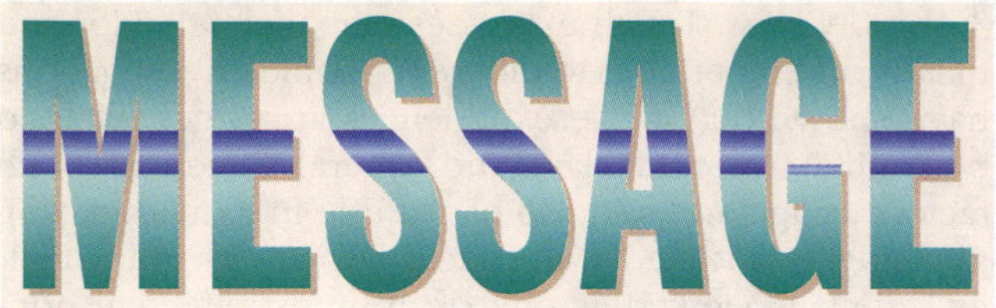

MESSAGE

Figure 22-3
Research in communication has shown that words contribute only a small percentage to the communication of a message (*the colored area*). Nonverbal expression, tone, timing, context, the other characteristics of an exchange complete the message communicated.

Facial Expressions. The face is the most expressive part of the body. Examples of the various messages facial expressions convey are anger, joy, suspicion, sadness, fear, and contempt. Some people have extremely expressive faces, whereas others mask their feelings, making it more difficult to determine what the person is really thinking. Nurses need to learn some control over their own facial expressions. For instance, a client with extensive burns may watch the nurse's reaction when burn dressings are changed for the first time. Any sign of repulsion or disgust could have grave implications for the client's self-image and recovery.

Posture. The way a person holds the body carries nonverbal messages. People in good health and with a positive attitude usually hold their bodies in good alignment. Depressed or tired people are more likely to slouch. Posture also often provides nonverbal clues concerning pain and physical limitations; for instance, a rigid, stiff appearance may be a good indicator of tension and pain.

Gait. A bouncy, purposeful walk usually carries a message of well-being. A less purposeful, shuffling gait often means the person is sad or discouraged. Certain gaits are associated with illness. For example, clients recovering from recent abdominal surgery usually walk slightly bent over and slowly and may need the assistance of handrails or a helping person.

Gestures. Gestures using various parts of the body are capable of carrying numerous messages; for example, thumbs up means victory whereas thumbs down carries a negative connotation; kicking an object often expresses anger; wringing the hands or tapping a foot usually indicates anxiety or anger; a waving hand serves to beckon someone to come, or, if waved in another way, signifies that someone should leave. Gestures are used extensively when two people speaking different languages attempt to communicate with each other.

General Physical Appearance. Most illnesses cause at least some alterations in general physical appearance. Observing for changes in appearance is an important nursing responsibility in detecting a particular illness or in evaluating effectiveness of care and therapy. For example, the person with an insufficient intake of fluids has dry skin that wrinkles easily, eyes that may be sunken and dull in appearance, and poor muscle tone. On the other hand, the person in good health tends to radiate his or her healthy status through general physical appearance.

Mode of Dress and Grooming. A person's clothing and grooming practices carry significant nonverbal messages. For example, healthy people with good self-esteem tend to pay attention to details of dress and grooming, whereas those with low self-esteem show much less interest in them. People feeling ill often demonstrate little interest in personal appearance, and it is often a sign of returning health when interest in mode of dress and appearance resumes.

Sounds. Crying, moaning, gasping, and sighing are oral but nonverbal forms of communication. Such sounds can be interpreted in numerous ways. For example, a person may cry because of sadness or joy. Gasping often indicates fear, pain, or surprise. A sigh may be a sign of reluctant agreement to do something or of relief.

Silence. Periods of silence during communication often carry important nonverbal messages. The silence between two people may indicate complete understanding of each other, or it may mean they are angry with each other. Silence and its possible uses and meanings are discussed later in this chapter.

Factors Influencing Communication

Developmental Considerations

The rate of language development varies and is directly related to neurologic competence and cognitive development. It is helpful for nurses to understand the process of language development as well as the stages of intellectual and psychosocial development so they can communicate appropriately with clients of all ages. These stages are presented in Chapter 8. Knowing how each age group commonly perceives health, illness, and body functions guides nurses in their interactions with their clients. For instance, a 10-year-old child has a limited understanding of what an infection is; therefore, the nurse must explain this in simple terms so that the child cooperates with the treatment without being frightened. Because adolescents are developing abstract thinking, more detailed and accurate explanations can be given to them. Being familiar with commonly used slang usually helps nurses when communicating with adolescents.

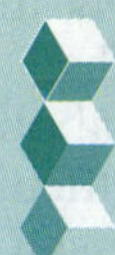

Research in Nursing: Making a Difference

Communicating Caring

To care for others and to experience caring are basic human needs. The following studies explore the significance of different types of nurse–client interactions in terms of their ability to communicate human caring.

Related Research

Bottorff, J. L., & Morse, J. M. (1994). Identifying types of attending: Patterns of nurses' work. *IMAGE: Journal of Nursing Scholarship, 26*(1), 53–60.
Verbal and nonverbal behaviors of nurses during interactions with cancer clients were examined by analyzing videotapes of caregiving. Five types of touch (comforting, connecting, working, orienting, and social) and four types of attending (doing more, doing for, doing with, and doing tasks) were identified. The findings provide support for an alternative method of classifying nurse–client interactions that captures patterns of caring.

Moore, J. R., & Gilbert, D. A. (1995). Elderly residents' perceptions of nurses' comforting touch. *Journal of Gerontological Nursing, 21*(1), 6–13.
Elderly nursing home residents often feel unwanted or unloved because of a lack of physical contact with others or their caregivers' inability to communicate love and belonging. A study of 25 elderly nursing home residents found that those who were subjected to comforting touch by their nurses perceived an increased feeling of affection and worth.

Allen, L. J., & Van Ess Coeling, H. (1995). Quality of life: Its meaning to long term care residents. *Journal of Gerontological Nursing, 21*(2), 20–25.
Although the physical and recreational environments have been shown to be important to the mental health of the long-term care resident, human relationships and social contact have been described as being far more important in determining quality of life. This study identifies two new findings as contributing to the quality of life—caring for oneself and the importance of helping others.

Summary

More research is needed to demonstrate the consequences of deficient human caring and to provide models that achieve excellence in communicating caring.

Communicating with adults can be affected by years of positive or negative health-related experiences and by inaccurate information. Nurses communicating with older clients must assess for any problems with hearing or sight (discussed later in this chapter), confusion, or depression, all of which could affect nurse–client interactions.

Gender

Men and women demonstrate different communication styles and may give different interpretations to the same conversation. Tannen (1990) believes that this is because girls and boys grow up communicating differently. Whereas girls generally play with "best friends" and use language to seek confirmation, minimize differences, and establish or reinforce intimacy, boys use language to establish their independence and to negotiate status activities in large groups. It is important for nurses to be sensitive to the fact that men and women may use communication differently as a result of these developmental experiences. Moreover, it may be necessary for nurses working with clients of the opposite gender to validate that both the nurse and client are accurately receiving the message trying to be communicated.

Sociocultural Differences

Nurses need to develop skills in recognizing the ways in which culture, economic condition, and overall lifestyle influence a client's preferred mode of communicating. For example, nurses working with pregnant women in an inner city ghetto will find it helpful to be familiar with the city's street language. This will enable the nurse to understand what the client is communicating and to use language the client understands. Women in some cultures may speak of personal things only to their spouses. For this reason maternal care nurses may have to talk with the client's partner about the woman's postdelivery care.

It is best to use lay terminology when speaking with clients unless a client is known to be a healthcare professional. Use of medical terminology (ie, myocardial infarction for heart attack, cerebrovascular accident for stroke, or cholecystectomy for gallbladder operation) usually alienates clients and can inhibit further communication.

Roles and Responsibilities

A person's occupation may give the nurse a general idea of his or her abilities, talents, interests, and economic status. Stereotyping a person according to occupation can be misleading, however, and should be avoided. This can be particularly dangerous when nurses assume that clients who are healthcare professionals know everything about their conditions and are in little need of nursing assistance, teaching, and counseling. The challenge for the nurse caregiver is to respect the roles and responsibilities of clients, especially as these influence their preferred manner of communicating, without denying the client needed care. A successful attorney may present a "take charge" demeanor and seem utterly self-sufficient; a skilled nurse will note this but provide an opening for the client to verbalize her or his needs: "You seem well prepared for this procedure and in control, but I know that clients often have questions that never get answered or fears that remain unvoiced. Is there anything I can help you with while I'm here?" Similarly, nurses should be careful not to ignore an uncomplaining indigent person who never asks for anything because the power differences in the healthcare professional–client relationship make communciation intimidating.

Space and Territoriality

People are generally most comfortable in areas they claim as their own. We are all familiar with the sense of relief we get when we come home, take our shoes and professional clothes off, and relax. This urge to mark and exercise an exclusive right to certain spaces is termed territoriality. You may have already noticed that clients behave differently when being interviewed in their homes, at a health fair in the mall, or in an institutional setting. Similarly, healthcare professionals may behave differently when they are "on their own turf" in a healthcare institution than when they enter a client's home as a guest caregiver. It is important to understand how this influences the nurse–client relationship.

The actual physical difference between the nurse and client during an interaction is also important. Each person has a sense of how much private space is needed and of what actual distance between persons is optimal; some of this is culturally dictated and some is idiosyncratic. Anywhere from 18 inches to 4 feet may be considered the optimal distance for a nurse to sit from a client during an intake interview. It is best to take cues from clients, noting if they are recoiling from nearness or leaning forward to draw the nurse closer. Since many nursing interventions place one in close proximity to clients and entail forced intimacy, it is critical to develop sensitivity to how offensive this may be to certain clients who are accustomed to large areas of private space.

Physical, Mental and Emotional State

The degree to which people are physically comfortable and mentally and emotionally free to engage in interactions will also influence communication. A full bladder, a dull headache or crushing chest pain, anxiety about a pending diagnosis or about what is happening back home or at work, and fear can all negatively influence communication. A client who thinks that a nurse wants to hurt him or who can think only about what it would be like to date the nurse will be difficult to interview. It is helpful for nurses to develop sensitivity to the physical, mental, and emotional barriers to effective communication.

Values

Communication is influenced by the way people value themselves, one another, and the purpose of any human interaction. The nurse who believes that teaching is an important aspect of nursing and who values empowering clients will communicate this to clients. Conversely, the nurse who believes teaching is an unimportant chore is unlikely to be an effective teacher. Similarly, the client's motivation (or lack of motivation) to develop new self-care behaviors cannot help but influence nurse–client communication.

Environment

Communication happens best when the environment facilitates an easy exchange of needed information. Depending upon the goals of interaction, this may require minimizing distractions, ensuring privacy, or using music, art, and decor to place a client at ease. A client newly diagnosed with HIV infection will find it difficult to provide the needed sexual history or to discuss genital warts if being interviewed in a crowded hallway because of the scarcity of private rooms in a clinic. A toddler may find it easier to communicate with a nurse if a parent, favorite stuffed animal, or blanket is nearby.

Using Communication in the Nursing Process

The nurse's ability to communicate with clients and with other nurses is essential to effective use of the nursing process. Knowledge of the communication process and of effective communication techniques is fundamental to all steps of the nursing process. At the same time, the nursing process provides the nurse with the guidance and direction needed to communicate with the client effectively.

Assessing. Because the major focus of the assessment step is information gathering, verbal and nonverbal communication are essential nursing tools. Nurses use the written word to obtain data concerning their clients. Nurses often read their clients' records or charts before meeting them. The spoken word is used to give and receive reports to and from other health personnel. This is a common practice when admitting a client to a hospital unit. Nurses use one-to-one communication to obtain thorough nursing histories and physical examinations. Effective communication techniques, as well as

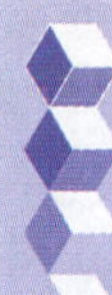

Through the Eyes of a Student

It was my first day of clinical rotation and I was assigned to Mr. Anderson, who was in his early nineties. He was in the hospital because he had had a second heart attack. Mr. Anderson had lived alone for 5 years after the death of his wife. He wanted to remain independent, but his daughter, who was herself in her late sixties, and his doctor believed that he would not be able to function well on his own any longer. Mr. Anderson was distressed about this belief.

Because it was my first day and, unlike some of my classmates, I had never worked in a hospital before, I felt insecure and nervous. There really wasn't a lot of work for us to do. We weren't allowed to give medication yet and my client was pretty self-sufficient. Because my skills were shaky, I took my time taking vital signs, assisted Mr. Anderson with his bath and toileting, and made his bed. After checking his chart, I began my nursing interview with him. I was overjoyed to discover that he was a real talker! His memory was tremendous—either that or he was a great improvisor! He recalled stories about his childhood and his wife with great detail and emotion. He smiled and laughed when he spoke of his daughter and grandchildren. He told me about his daughter's childhood illnesses as well as his own. We talked about the Depression and world wars and about music and art and education. He asked me about my family and I felt like I had made a friend.

The next day Mr. Anderson told me about his fears. He talked about losing his wife, about his health and body deteriorating, and about losing his independence and home. He despised having to be sent to a nursing home and having to depend on others. It hurt him a lot and made me sad. Mr. Anderson left on my second day, and as I said goodbye I wished I could do something for him.

I thought about him a lot since then and I've come to realize that in those 2 days that I knew Mr. Anderson, I did do something for him besides washing him and changing his sheets. I listened to him. Although his family had little time for him and the doctors quickly flew in and out of the room, I let him talk and heard all he said, both in words and in his eyes. He will always be a good memory for me—and I think I'll be a good memory for him.

—***Kristina Hofmeister, Holy Family College, Philadelphia, PA***

observational skills, are used extensively during this phase. The data collected verbally and nonverbally are analyzed and then passed on to the appropriate people through oral and written communications.

Diagnosing. Once a nurse formulates a nursing diagnosis, it must be communicated through the spoken and written word to other nurses as well as to the client. The written diagnosis becomes a permanent part of the client's record.

Planning. The planning step requires communication between the client, nurse, and other team members as goals and outcomes are developed and interventions selected. Because a nurse is rarely able to implement all parts of a plan alone, oral and written communication is relied on to inform others of what needs to be done to meet the set objectives or goals. Without communication, the nurse's plan would never proceed to the implementation phase.

Implementing. Nurses assume many roles when they implement the plan of care. Verbal and nonverbal communication allows nurses to enhance basic caregiving measures and to teach, counsel, and support clients and their families during the implementation phase. Even a simple nursing order such as "encourage to drink 100 mL of fluid every hour while awake" requires countless messages to be sent and received between the nurse and client. The nurse explains why fluids are important, what fluids are beneficial, and how often they are needed. The client, in turn, informs the nurse of his or her ability or inability to comply with the order. The client's verbal and nonverbal messages are assessed during each nurse–client interaction. The implementation of the order is then documented in the client's record.

Evaluating. Nurses often rely on the verbal and nonverbal cues they receive from their clients to verify whether client objectives or goals have been achieved. Communication also facilitates the revision of parts of the care plan through the exchange of positive and negative messages between the nurse and the client.

Documenting Communication. Any information required for the continual assessment of the client's needs and condition should be documented in the appropriate place, unless the information is confidential. This documentation serves to promote the continuity of care given by nurses and other healthcare providers. Because one nurse cannot provide 24-hour coverage for clients, significant information must be passed on to others through nursing progress notes and care plans. Documentation is discussed in Chapter 21.

Using Communication in the Helping Relationship

Most people enter the healthcare field because they want to help people. This is not accomplished randomly but rather through purposeful relationships. A **helping relationship** exists among people who provide and receive assistance in meeting human needs. In this book, the term is used to refer to the helping relationships between nurses and clients (Fig. 22-4). A helping relationship sets the climate for the participants to move toward common goals, which arise from human needs. Therefore, need gratification occurs as the result of a successful helping relationship.

When a nurse and client are involved in a helping relationship, the nurse assists the client to achieve goals that allow the client's human needs to be satisfied. The nurse is the helper and the client is the person being helped. The helping relationship between the nurse and client is sometimes called the nurse–client relationship.

The quality of one's relationship with another person is the most significant element in determining helping effectiveness. "Of all the problems that can arise in nursing care, perhaps the most common is failure to establish rapport and a helping–trust relationship with the other person" (Watson, 1985, p. 24).

A Helping Relationship Versus a Social Relationship

The difference between a helping relationship and a friendship must be emphasized. Helping relationships contain many of the qualities of a social relationship; they have in common the components of care, concern, trust, and growth. They also possess major differences:

- The helping relationship does not occur spontaneously, as do most social relationships. It occurs for a specific purpose with a specific person.

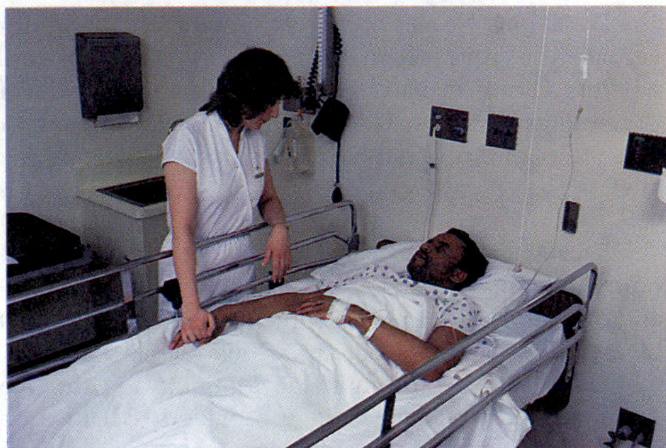

Figure 22-4
A helping relationship between the nurse and client sets the climate for participants to move toward common goals. (Photo © B. Proud.)

- The helping relationship is characterized by an unequal sharing of information. The client shares information related to personal health problems, whereas the nurse shares information in terms of a professional role. In a friendship, information sharing is more likely to be similar in quantity and type.
- The helping relationship is built on the client's needs, not on those of the helping person. In a friendship, needs of both participants are generally considered. A friendship may grow out of a helping relationship, but this is separate from the purposeful, time-limited interaction described as a helping relationship.

Characteristics of the Helping Relationship

The helping relationship is intangible and therefore difficult to describe. However, most authorities agree that it has at least the following three basic characteristics:

- It is dynamic. Both the person providing the assistance and the person being helped are active participants to the extent each is able.
- It is purposeful and time limited. This means there are specific goals that are intended to be met within a certain period.
- Although both parties in the helping relationship have responsibilities, the person providing the assistance is professionally accountable for the outcomes of the relationship and the means used to attain them. The helping person should present his or her helping abilities as honestly as possible and not promise to provide more assistance than he or she is capable of offering.

Goals of the Helping Relationship

The goals of a helping relationship between a nurse and a client are determined cooperatively and are defined in terms of the client's needs. Broadly speaking, common goals might include increased independence for the client, greater feelings of worth, and improved health and well-being. Depending on the goals/outcomes, the nurse selects nursing interventions that will move the person toward the goal. As the client's needs and goals change, so do the nursing care activities. The nurse may also have many needs to be met, but in the helping relationship between the nurse and the client, the nurse's needs are temporarily set aside and the focus is on the client's needs.

Phases of the Helping Relationship

The helping relationship is ordinarily described as having three phases: (1) the orientation phase, (2) the working phase, and (3) the termination phase. In the helping relationship, the communication process follows the sequence of the nursing process. Both processes are continuous and reciprocal. Table 22-1 summarizes goals for

Table 22-1
Summary of Client Goals for the Three Phases of the Helping Relationship

Orientation Phase	Working Phase	Termination
The client will call the nurse by name. The client will accurately describe the roles of the participants in the relationship. The client and nurse will establish an agreement about: • Goals of the relationship • Location, frequency, and length of the contacts • Duration of the relationship	The client will actively participate in the relationship. The client will cooperate in activities that work toward achieving mutually acceptable goals. The client will express feelings and concerns to the nurse.	The client will participate in identifying the goals accomplished or the progress made toward goals. The client will verbalize feelings about the termination of the relationship.

clients during the three phases of an effective helping relationship.

Orientation Phase

Ideally, the helping relationship between a nurse and a client is initiated when the nurse starts the data-gathering part of the nursing process. However, it can also be initiated at other times. In the orientation phase, the tone and guidelines for the relationship are established. The nurse and client meet and learn to identify each other by name. It is especially important that the nurse introduce himself or herself to the client; it may even be helpful for the nurse to write his or her name for the client. Failure to do so may result in the client becoming confused and mistrustful because of the number of caregivers with whom most clients come in contact.

The following activities generally occur during the orientation phase of the helping relationship:

- The roles of both people in the relationship are clarified. It has been observed that a successful relationship is more likely to occur when the responsibilities assigned to each participant are known and accepted and when there is leadership present. In the nurse–client relationship, the nurse, by virtue of role, generally assumes leadership. Leadership does not mean control in the restrictive or manipulative sense, but here implies taking the initiative to enlist the client's point of view. When cooperative planning occurs with consideration for the client's needs, the relationship between a nurse and a client is more likely to be mutually satisfactory.
- An agreement or contract about the relationship is established. The agreement is usually a simple verbal exchange or, occasionally, a written document, especially if the relationship extends over a long period. Elements in the agreement include the goals of the relationship; location, frequency, and length of the contacts; and the duration of the relationship. Depending on the purpose of the relationship, the agreement may also include the way in which personal information that the client may divulge will be handled.
- An orientation to the healthcare agency is provided. The nurse is responsible for seeing that the client is oriented to the health agency, its facilities/services, admission routines, and so on. The nurse identifies this orientation as one of the goals in the nurse–client helping relationship.

It is critical that trust begins to be established from the outset of the relationship. Some clients may engage in testing behavior, especially if they have had negative experiences in the past in their family or with other healthcare providers. The nurse's openness to and interest in the concerns of the client pave the way for trust to develop and communicate respect and care.

Working Phase

The working phase is usually the longest phase of the helping relationship. The nurse and the client work together to meet the client's needs. Interaction is the essence of the working phase. The nurse–client interactions that occur at this time are purposeful in that they have been designed to ensure achievement of mutually agreed upon health goals or objectives.

In the working phase, the nurse provides whatever assistance may be needed to achieve each goal. For example, an older client has a poor appetite and the goal is to increase food intake. The nurse discusses the idea of small, more frequent meals with the client. With the client's approval, the nurse makes the necessary arrangements. In another instance, a mother explains to a school nurse that she cannot afford dental care recommended for her child, although she would like to have the work done. The nurse asks if a referral to a social agency for financial assistance would be acceptable. With the mother's permission, the nurse contacts the agency.

When sentiments and feelings between people are unsatisfactory, they often cannot work cooperatively toward achieving a common goal. When sentiments and feelings are satisfactory, they can usually work together.

In the preceding examples, satisfactory sentiments and feelings between the nurse and clients might have been the key aspects. The older person's relationship with the nurse may have allowed a positive response to the small, more frequent meals. The mother's feelings about the nurse may have allowed her to accept financial assistance for dental care without feeling embarrassed.

In addition, the nurse as caregiver provides the client with whatever assistance may be needed to perform activities of daily living. For example, if a client with impaired mobility is unable to get out of bed except to use a bedside commode, the nurse needs to help with daily hygiene.

The nursing roles of teacher and counselor (see Chapter 23) are performed primarily during this phase. These roles involve motivating the client to learn and implement health-promotion activities, to comply with medical treatments such as medication regimens, and to express feelings about health problems, nursing care, any progress or setbacks, and any other areas of concern. This is where the nurse's interpersonal skills are used to their fullest (see the discussions of interpersonal skills and effective communication techniques later in this chapter). A breakdown of the helping relationship on one of these levels could result in serious consequences. For instance, a client begins to break clinic appointments, although he seemed to be interested in his health previously when he visited the clinic. When a community health nurse calls on the client at home, he says, "The nurse at the clinic seems too busy; she just doesn't seem to care if I come or go. I don't like to go to that clinic." The lack of satisfactory interaction between the nurse and the client discouraged him from continuing the relationship, even at the expense of his health. Had the nurse–client interaction been satisfactory, the problem most likely would not have occurred.

Satisfactory interaction preserves the integrity of people while promoting an atmosphere characterized by minimal fear, anxiety, distrust, and tension. People feel harmonious and contented with each other as they work cooperatively to reach common goals.

Termination Phase

The termination phase occurs when the conclusion of the initial agreement is acknowledged. This may happen at change-of-shift time, when the client is discharged, or when a nurse leaves on vacation or for employment elsewhere. The client and nurse examine the goals of the helping relationship for indications of their attainment or for evidence of progress toward them. If the goals/outcomes have been reached, this fact should be acknowledged. Such acknowledgment generally results in a feeling of satisfaction for both the client and nurse. If the goals/outcomes have not been reached, the progress can be acknowledged and either the client or the nurse may make suggestions for future efforts.

Ordinarily emotions are associated with the termination of a helping relationship. If the goals have been met, there is often regret about ending a satisfying relationship, even though a sense of accomplishment persists. If the goals have not been completely achieved, the client may experience anxiety and fear about the future. Whatever the feelings, the client should be encouraged to express his or her emotions about the termination.

The nurse can prepare for the termination of the helping relationship in various ways. The thoughtful nurse can set the stage for the client to establish a helping relationship with another nurse, if appropriate. The nurse can assist the client transferring from one agency to another or from one unit in an agency to another by offering explanations concerning the transfer. In some instances, the nurse may introduce the client to personnel who will be giving care.

Occasionally, termination of the helping relationship produces negative emotional reactions. The client may feel angry, rejected by the nurse, or depressed and helpless, or may deny that a relationship ever really existed. Should such reactions occur, the nurse should help and support the client rather than impose feelings of guilt or wrong for having these views. However, emotional reactions of this sort are less likely to occur if the client has been involved in establishing goals and has been helped to anticipate termination of the helping relationship.

Those wishing to explore the topic of interpersonal relations in nursing more fully are referred to the classic works of nursing theorists Orlando (1961), Paterson and Zderad (1976), Peplau (1952), Travelbee (1971), and Watson (1985).

Factors Promoting Effective Communication

Good **rapport**, a feeling of mutual trust experienced by people in a satisfactory relationship (Fig. 22-5), can be achieved by paying attention to the following variables.

Specific Objectives. Having a purpose for an interaction guides the nurse toward achieving a meaningful encounter with the client. One objective might be to do a quick head-to-toe physical assessment while greeting the client at the beginning of a shift. Another objective might be to discuss a client's feelings about newly diagnosed diabetes. The shortest encounter with a client can have an objective, even if it is as simple as conveying a feeling of friendliness. Flexibility is essential at all times. Cues from the client should be followed to work toward meeting all needs.

Comfortable Environment. A comfortable environment, in which both the client and the nurse are at ease, helps to promote interactions. Such items as suitable furniture, proper lighting, and a moderate temperature are important. Also, effective relationships are enhanced when the atmosphere is relaxed and unhurried. If the nurse seems preoccupied and on the run or if the client is ill at ease for fear of missing visitors or because of another commitment, communications are impaired.

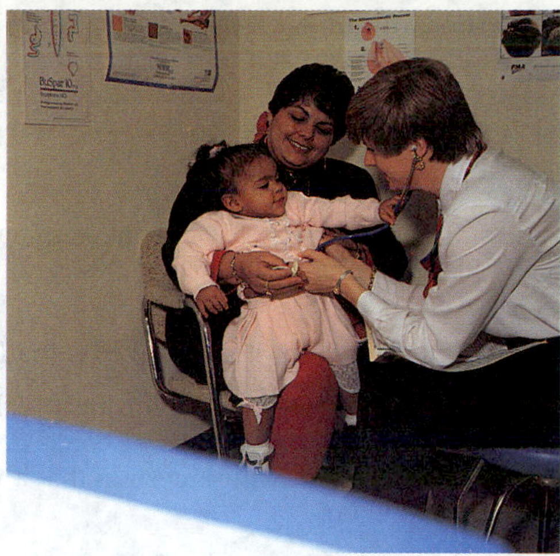

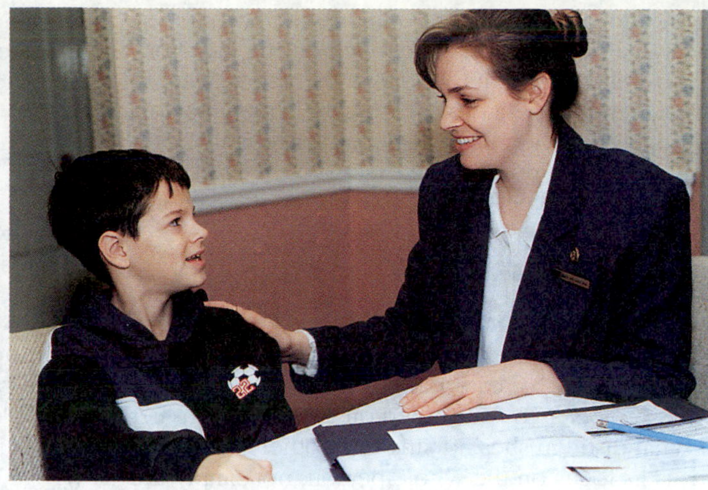

Figure 22-5
Rapport between the nurse and the client/family is a necessary first step in planning for care. (Left photo courtesy of Nursing Spectrum; right photo courtesy of Brett Ainsworth.)

Privacy. It may not always be possible to carry out conversations with only the client and the nurse in a room. However, every effort should be made to provide sufficient privacy so that conversations cannot be overheard by others. Sometimes merely drawing the curtains around the bed in a hospital or nursing home or sitting in a corner of a waiting room or lounge can provide the sense of privacy so necessary for most interactions. Home visits may need to be timed to ensure the privacy the client desires and needs.

Confidentiality. The confidentiality with which the information is to be treated should be established with the client. The nurse should indicate with whom the information the client gives will be shared. The client should know about the right to specify the people who may have access to the information. Failure to take this factor into account can be considered a breach of the client's right to privacy. See Chapter 21 for guidelines concerning client confidentiality.

Client Focus. Communication in the nurse–client relationship should focus on the client and the client's needs, not on the nurse or an activity in which the nurse is engaged. Consider the following example, in which the nurse's comment focuses on the client and the client's needs:

Client: I don't know why these injections scare me, but they do.
Nurse: You are afraid of these injections?

Now consider this example, in which the nurse's comment focuses on a nursing activity:

Client: I don't know why these injections scare me, but they do.
Nurse: Let's hurry and get this shot done. Then you won't have time to worry.

Use of Nursing Observations. *Observation,* which involves both seeing and interpreting, is especially useful for validating information. For example, a nurse suspects that a client is afraid to hear the results of certain blood tests, but the client insists that the tests are unimportant. However, the nurse observes the client pacing in the corridor while appearing to be in deep thought. Observing the client's behavior helps validate the nurse's suspicion that the client is fearful, and the client's assertion that he or she is unconcerned appears to be a coverup for truer feelings.

Observation serves several important purposes:

- It helps the nurse become aware of nonverbal messages the client is sending.
- It serves as the primary source of information when a client is unable or unwilling to communicate verbally.
- It demonstrates caring and an interest in the client. (Clients often recognize when a nurse is unobservant and, rightly or wrongly, usually conclude that the nurse does not care.)

Optimal Pacing. A nurse must consider the pace of any conversation or encounter with a client. For instance, it would be ineffective for the nurse to rush through a list of questions when obtaining a nursing history; it is more effective to let the client set the pace. The nurse can let the client know at the beginning of the interaction if time is limited. This way, the client will not feel that the nurse is rushing because of a lack of concern or personal interest.

Providing Personal Space. Perceptions of personal space vary. Nurses must try to determine each client's perception of personal space because invasion of this zone can evoke uncomfortable feelings. Nurses can assess a client's personal space through careful observations of nonverbal communication. For example, some people like to be close to the person with whom they are speaking. They may also use touch during their conversations and seem comfortable with others in close proximity. Others back away from close encounters or become nervous when their personal space is invaded. It is important for nurses to be sensitive to personal space so that clients feel comfortable during interactions.

Blocks to Communication

Failure to Perceive the Client as a Human Being. Clients report that nothing is more discomforting than to be treated as an object of care rather than as Ms. Jan Bennett who happens to be undergoing surgery on her colon. What distinguishes nursing from other health professions is its focus on the whole person, not simply the illness or dysfunction.

Failure to Listen. Clients may or may not feel able to speak freely to the nurse. Often the signals indicating their readiness to talk are subtle. Nurses may miss valuable opportunities for important communication if they approach clients with closed minds or focus on their own needs rather than on client needs.

Inappropriate Comments and Questions. Certain types of comments and questions should be avoided in most situations because they tend to impede effective communications. A description of each type follows.

Using Clichés. A *cliché* is a stereotyped, trite, or pat answer. Most clichés tend to indicate that there is no cause for anxiety or concern, or they offer false assurance. Their use tends to be interpreted as a lack of real interest in what has been said. For example, even though the common question, "How are you?" could start a conversation, it can cause a problem if the person has reason to suspect that the nurse is not sincerely interested in how the client feels. The following are some commonly used clichés that are usually best left unsaid because they tend to impede effective communications:

"Everything will be all right."

"Don't worry. You will be just fine in another day or two."

"Your doctor knows best."

"Cheer up. Tomorrow is another day."

Another type of cliché makes a sweeping generalization that does not necessarily apply to a specific client. It also tends to cut off communications and makes the person feel as though he or she is just another insignificant being. Consider the following examples:

"Men tolerate pain poorly. That must be why you are complaining of such severe pain."

"Everybody is afraid of surgery. Why should you be any different?"

"You teenagers are all alike. You aren't being cooperative because you want to defy authority."

Such comments rarely promote communication with clients to whom they are addressed.

Using Questions Requiring Only a Yes or No Answer. Questions that can be answered by simply saying yes or no tend to cut off discussion, even when the person might wish to continue. Consider the following question:

Nurse: Did you have a good day?

The question almost begs for a noncommittal answer, which tells the nurse little. A better way to comment is as follows:

Nurse: Tell me about the kind of day you have had.

Another pitfall is to pose a question to which the client can say no when his or her answer could present a problem. Consider the following question that a nurse asks a postoperative client:

Nurse: Are you ready to get out of bed?

By offering the client the chance to say no, the nurse may have created difficulties if the client is to be out of bed.

There are times when questions that can be answered with yes or no are legitimate. The following are examples:

Nurse: Did you take your insulin before breakfast this morning?

Nurse: Do you have pain when I move your arm this way?

The problem arises when the nurse is seeking more detailed information or when the question may create difficulty.

Using Questions Containing the Words *Why* and *How*. Questions using *why* and *how* tend to be intimidating. Consider the following questions:

Nurse: Why were you not tired enough to sleep?

Nurse: How did you ever decide to go on a crash diet?

These two questions would be better stated as follows:

Nurse: What were you doing while you were unable to sleep?

Nurse: What things prompted you to decide to go on a crash diet?

Using Questions That Probe for Information. Questions that appear to probe for information tend to cut off communication. Clients who are made to feel as though they are receiving the "third degree" become resentful and will usually stop talking and try to avoid further conversation. Although the nurse may feel more information is needed, it is better to follow the client's lead. Letting the client take the initiative allows the nurse to delve more deeply at a time when the client is ready. The person who says, "Let's get to the bottom of this" is likely to destroy conversation unless the client is ready to face the real cause of the problem.

Using Leading Questions. A leading question suggests a response that the speaker wishes to hear. Leading questions tend to produce answers that may please the nurse but are unlikely to encourage the client to respond without feeling intimidated. Consider the following examples:

Nurse: You aren't going to smoke that cigarette, are you?
Nurse: You have been well cared for by your nurses, haven't you?

These questions direct the client to give an answer that pleases the nurse rather than to express thoughts.

Using Comments That Give Advice. Giving advice often implies that the nurse knows what is best for the client and denies him or her the right to make decisions and have feelings. It also tends to increase the client's dependence on caregivers. However, advice does have a rightful place when it is requested, and the person giving the advice may have expert knowledge that the client does not.

Using Judgmental Comments. Using judgmental comments tends to impose the nurse's standards on the client. Consider the comment of a nurse who notes that a young woman is crying:

Nurse: You aren't acting very grown-up. How do you think your husband would feel if he saw you crying like this?

The nurse judges the client as being immature, and the apparent hostility could end effective communication. A better comment in this situation might be as follows:

Nurse: I would like to help. Tell me what causes you to cry.

Consider the following exchange between a nurse and a client about to have surgery:

Client: I think I have a right to be afraid of this operation.
Nurse: Tell me what has made you afraid.

This client is likely to feel safe when allowed to express feelings without being judged.

Changing the Subject. A quick way to stop conversation is by changing the subject. The client may be at a point of readiness to discuss something and can be expected to feel frustrated if put off by a change in the topic of conversation. The following example illustrates:

Client: When can I expect to be told about taking my own insulin?
Nurse: Let's discuss your diet now so that you will know what to eat when you get home. We can discuss your insulin some other time.

A nurse may also change the subject when feeling uncomfortable about the topic of conversation. For example, the client's needs are being met when the nurse allows the client to speak of impending death, thoughts of suicide, or a contemplated abortion. The nurse is ignoring the client when the subject is changed to meet the nurse's own needs.

Giving False Assurance. It is easier and more pleasant to deal with positive outcomes than with negative ones. Through comments, the nurse may sometimes try to convince the client that things are going to turn out well even when knowing the chances are not good. False assurance leaves many clients with the impression that the nurse is not interested in their problems. Clichés are frequently used when a nurse gives a client false assurance. Unintentionally impeding communication may sometimes occur. Being aware of it and explaining with an apology to the client will help promote a return to effective communication.

Gossip and Rumor. Gossip and rumor are common forms of communication in healthcare settings. Those new to nursing are invited to explore their beneficial and negative repercussions for clients, caregivers, and the healthcare agency or institution. Gossiping may be used to inform, influence others, entertain, or ventilate. Generally confined to small intimate groups, gossiping may be harmless but it may also damage the reputation of others. Rumors serve similar functions as gossip but tend to be more widespread. Among their negative consequences are damage to the reputation of authority figures, coworkers, or an organization; disharmony or divisiveness; and adversarial relations (Ribeiro & Blakeley, 1995).

Development of Therapeutic Communication Skills

Another basic characteristic of communication is that exchanging messages requires knowledge. The knowledge provided by a nursing education is useful in developing therapeutic communication skills. Although humans use communication in all of their waking moments, the therapeutic use of communication requires training and practice. As students realize the importance of communication in helping relationships, they may feel awkward at first and that the relationships are contrived; however, as the merits of effective communication become evident through practice, they will become more at ease with the process.

Effective Communication Techniques

Communication takes on many forms depending on the situation in which the communication occurs. If effective techniques are used appropriately, nurses can enhance the quality and purpose of any communication. At no time, however, should nurses put techniques of communication above the nurse–client relationship.

Conversational Skills

A good place to start is with conversation. *Conversation*, or the exchange of verbal communication, is a social in-

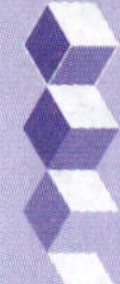

Through the Eyes of a Client

I know you come to clinical every day with your head full of all the important things you need to do for me. Probably you worry about whether or not you will remember the steps to both simple and complex procedures and fear that you will never get everything done in the time allotted. I'm sure that there are many things that your clinical instructor will use as a basis for your evaluation and perhaps other things that are important to you for your self-evaluation. But I thought you might like to know what's important to me. Most of what I've listed are simple things that you can communicate each time you walk into my home or room.*

- Really listen to me.
- Ask me what I think.
- Don't dismiss my concerns.
- Don't treat me like a disease, treat me like a person.
- Talk *to* me, not *at* me.
- Respect my privacy.
- Don't keep me waiting.
- Don't tell me what to do without telling me how to do it.
- Keep me informed.
- Remember who I used to be.
- Let me know you care.

Thanks for giving me this chance to share with you what matters to me.

* The list of nursing interventions that are valued highly by clients was compiled by Roberta Messner after a review of many patient satisfaction studies. These are cited in Messner, R. L. (1993). What patients really want from their nurses. *American Journal of Nursing, 93*(8), 38–41.

teraction. As social beings, humans learn as children how to converse with others. Therefore, a person coming into nursing has had years of experience in communicating verbally. However, nurses can improve their communications with clients and achieve a more effective helping relationship by considering the following points:

- Control the tone of your voice so you are conveying exactly what you mean to say and not a hidden message. The nurse's tone should indicate interest rather than boredom, patience rather than anger, acceptance rather than hostility, and so forth.
- Be knowledgeable about the topic of conversation and have accurate information. When possible, the nurse should be familiar with the subject of conversation before discussing it with the client. If the topic is an unfamiliar one, it is best to tell the client so. Convey confidence and honesty.
- Be flexible. The nurse may have selected a subject to discuss but learns the client wishes to discuss something else. It is better to follow the client's lead whenever possible; in due time, the nurse can return to the subject. For example, the nurse arrives at the client's bedside to administer a medication, but the client begins to talk about his or her diet. It is better to take a little time to allow the client to speak rather than to insist on carrying out a procedure when the time taken for the conversation is not contraindicated.
- Be clear and concise, and make statements as simple as possible. Clients are often anxious and fail to receive the nurse's message unless the conversation is geared to a level the client understands. Stay on one subject at a time.
- Avoid words that may be interpreted differently. The study of the meaning of words is called **semantics**. Even when two people speak the same language, some words—such as *love, hate, freedom*, and *liberty*—may have different meanings.
- Be truthful. The client will soon distrust the nurse if given false information. Admit not knowing and seek an answer rather than make a comment that is likely to be an error.
- Keep an open mind. An attitude of "I know better than the client" is quickly discerned by the client. Clients can make valuable contributions to their own health care.
- Take advantage of available opportunities. During most caregiving situations, the nurse can facilitate conversation that will make even the most routine task meaningful. For instance, when giving a bed bath to a client, a nurse can introduce the topic of the client's employment. This would allow the client to verbalize any positive or negative feelings about the job and the temporary absence from it, reducing the anxiety that often occurs with the loss of work. It is often comforting to know that someone understands and cares.

Listening Skills

Listening is a skill that involves both hearing and interpreting what is said. It requires attention and concentration to sort out, evaluate, and validate clues so that a person better understands the true meaning of what is being said (Fig. 22-6). The following recommended techniques may help improve listening skills:

- Whenever possible, sit when communicating with a client. Do not cross arms or legs; this type of body language conveys a message of being closed to the client's comments.
- Be alert but relaxed and take sufficient time so that the client feels at ease during the conversation.

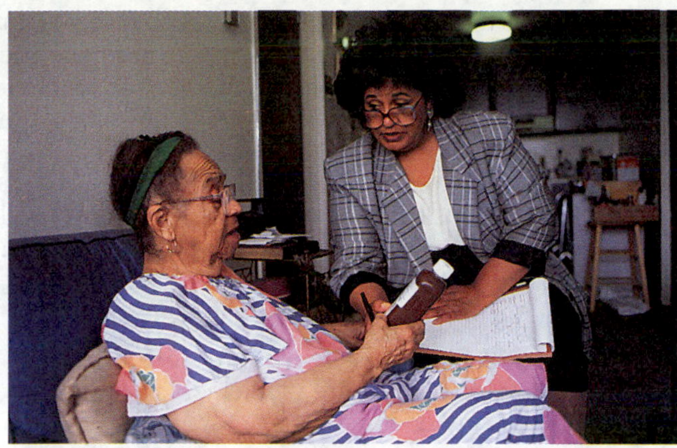

Figure 22-6
Listening attentively, with concentration and genuine concern, is key to productive communication. (Photo © Kathy Sloane.)

Keep the conversation as natural as possible, and avoid sounding overly eager.

- If culturally appropriate, maintain eye contact with the client, without staring, in a face-to-face pose. This technique conveys interest in the conversation and willingness to listen.
- Indicate that you are paying attention to what the client is saying by using appropriate facial expressions and body gestures. Be attentive to both your own and the client's verbal and nonverbal communication.
- Think before responding to the client. Responding impulsively tends to disrupt communication and listening.
- Do not pretend to listen. It is the rare client who is insensitive to an attitude of feigned attention or to boredom and apathy.
- Listen for themes in the client's comments. Consider the following questions to help detect them: What are the repeated themes in the person's speech and behavior? What topics does the client tend to avoid? What subjects tend to make the client shift the conversation to other subjects? What inconsistencies and gaps appear in the client's conversation?

Silence

The nurse can use silence appropriately by taking the time to wait for the client to initiate or continue speaking. During periods of silence, the nurse has the opportunity to observe the client without having to concentrate simultaneously on the spoken word. Periods of silence during communication can carry a variety of meanings, including the following:

- The client may be demonstrating comfort and contentment in the nurse–client relationship. Continuous talking is unnecessary.
- The client may be trying to demonstrate stoicism and the ability to cope without help.
- The client may be exploring inner feelings, and conversation would disrupt these thoughts. In this situation, the client is really saying, "I need some time to think."
- The client may be fearful and use silence as an escape from a threat.

In due time silence may be discussed with the client, especially if the nurse wishes to validate any speculation about its meaning. Fear of silence sometimes leads to too much talking by the nurse. Also, excessive talking tends to place the focus on the nurse rather than on the client.

Interviewing Techniques

The purpose of any interview is to obtain accurate and thorough information. In nursing, the interview is a major tool for collecting data during the assessment step of the nursing process (see Chapter 16). Consequently, every nurse needs to become proficient in the use of the communication techniques described previously, as well as in interviewing techniques, which are specifically designed to gather and validate information.

All interviews should begin with an explanation of the purpose of the interview. During the interview, the various interviewing techniques are used to obtain the information needed while remaining flexible in approach. The interview itself is a therapeutic interaction and may be an essential part of the orientation phase of the helping relationship. At the end of the interview, plans for further interactions can be made. The following interviewing techniques are useful in nearly all nurse–client interactions, especially the interview.

Open-Ended Question or Comment. When obtaining a nursing history, the nurse uses this technique to allow the client a wide range of possible responses. It encourages free verbalization. The greatest advantage of this technique is that it prevents the client from answering with a simple yes or no. Consider the following example of an open-ended question and the response:

Nurse: What did your physician tell you about your need for this hospitalization?
Client: He told me that my blood pressure is dangerously high and that I need some special tests done while I am here.

This open-ended question by the nurse allows the client to express what he or she understands to be true, yet is specific enough to prevent digressing from the issue at hand—the client's hospital admission. The nurse could continue with an open-ended comment such as

Nurse: Yes . . . and . . .
Client: Well, he thinks I could need a change in my blood pressure medicine too.

Now the nurse has even more information from the client and can continue to seek more information. This should be done in a way that does not make the client feel as though the nurse is prying or probing.

Closed Question or Comment. This technique allows limited choices in possible responses. It is used to gather specific information from a client and allows the nurse and client to focus on a particular area. The following is an example:

Nurse: What medicines have you been taking at home?
Client: Let me see, my doctor gave me a water pill and a blood pressure pill to take every day.

This technique gives the nurse the exact response that is being sought. Care should be taken to avoid overusing closed questions and comments because of the limiting effects they have on the client's responses.

Validating Question or Comment. This type of question or comment serves to validate what the nurse believes is heard or observed. To continue the example used in the previous technique, the nurse could validate what was said as follows:

Nurse: At home you have been taking both a water pill and a blood pressure pill every day. Did you take them today?
Client: Yes. I took one of each with my breakfast.

The nurse is able to ascertain that the client has been taking the medication regularly, as well as the correct dosage that day. However, overusing questions and comments to validate information may lead the client to suspect that the nurse is not listening.

Clarifying Question or Comment. By using this technique, a nurse can try to gain an understanding of a client's comment.

Client: I have never needed to take medicine before in my life.
Nurse: Is this the first health problem you have had?
Client: Yes, I've always been healthy.

The overuse of this technique can lead the client to believe that the nurse is not listening or is unknowledgeable. However, when used appropriately, it can avert possible misconceptions that could lead to an inappropriate nursing diagnosis. In the above example, by clarifying what the client's health has been previously, the nurse can assess his or her knowledge of the blood pressure problem and plan the necessary health teaching (see Chapter 23).

Reflective Question or Comment. This technique involves repeating what the person has said or describing feelings. It serves to encourage the client to elaborate on thoughts and feelings. An example of this technique follows:

Client: I've been really upset about my blood pressure and having to take these pills.
Nurse: You've been upset . . .
Client: I guess I'm worried about what could happen if my blood pressure gets too bad.

By saying this, the nurse has encouraged the client to expand on this topic by expressing a more specific concern. Again, overusing this technique or using it mechanically may lead the client to believe that the nurse is not listening or is uninterested.

Sequencing Question or Comment. Sequencing is used to place events in chronologic order or to investigate a possible cause-and-effect relationship between events. This technique is evident in the following example:

Client: I don't feel like myself anymore since I've been taking my blood pressure medicine. I'm tired and don't have any energy.
Nurse: Your tiredness began after you started taking your medicine?

This type of question could lead to a possible contributing factor to the client's problem. Nursing assessment is facilitated when events leading to a problem are placed in sequence.

Directing Question or Comment. It may become necessary at times to obtain more information about a certain subject brought up earlier in the interview or to introduce a new aspect of the current subject. In such an instance, the nurse can attempt to direct the client to the subject by using a technique similar to the following:

Client: Before I knew that I had high blood pressure, I was very active. I felt good at work and at home. I think the medicine is making me tired.
Nurse: When did your physician start you on your current medication?
Client: I've been on them for 6 weeks.
Nurse: Have you been told about eating foods high in potassium when on this medication?
Client: My doctor gave me some special diet to follow, but I haven't looked at it. I hate diets.

In this way, the nurse has gained valuable information to consider in assessing the client's health status and educational needs.

Touch

Touch is a powerful means of communication with multiple meanings. It can connect people, provide affirmation, be reassuring, decrease loneliness, share warmth, provide stimulation, and increase self-concept. It can also communicate frustration, anger, aggression, and punishment; invade personal space and privacy; and convey a negative (for example, subservient) type of relationship with another (Giger & Davidhizar, 1995, p. 28). Because of the personal nature of touching, a nurse needs to weigh the beneficial against the detrimental use of touch for each client. Touch can be a powerful therapeutic tool when used at the right time. However, anxiety or discomfort may result when a client does not understand the meaning of a tactile gesture or when the client simply dislikes being touched.

Touch is the most highly developed sense at birth. Tactile experiences of infants and young children appear essential for the normal development of self and awareness of others. It has also been found that many elderly people long for touch, especially when isolated from loved ones because of hospitalization or nursing home care. Many older people have no living family to provide them with the caring touch so necessary for the sense of well-being. In such an instance, a nurse can provide some special care by holding the client's hand (Fig. 22-7).

Many situations require the nurse to touch the client while implementing nursing care. Physical closeness between the client and the nurse is essential and inevitable. Therefore, every nurse needs to become comfortable with the judicious use of this nonverbal communication technique, so that security, rather than anxiety, will be promoted. Dexterity and sureness in the use of the hands help to assure the client of the nurse's expertise when measuring blood pressure or giving an injection.

Interest has been growing in the phenomenon known as **therapeutic touch**. Therapeutic touch involves "unruffling," or unblocking, congested areas of energy in the body and redirecting this energy. After assessing a client's "energy field," the nurse uses therapeutic touch to promote comfort, relaxation, healing, and a sense of well-being. Many nurses are studying therapeutic touch in nursing educational programs and through special courses or workshops. It is becoming a widely accepted form of therapy as well as a subject for nursing research.

Humor

Humor has come to be increasingly valued in recent years as both an interpersonal skill for the nurse and a healing strategy for clients. Nurses have a valuable tool when they are able to use humor effectively to maintain a balanced perspective in their work and to encourage clients to do the same. Nurses with a sense of humor are able to laugh at themselves and accept their failures, confront the absurdities in everyday practice without falling apart, and challenge clients to situate their current dilemma within the context of their larger life experiences. Laughter releases excess physical and psychologic energy and reduces stress, anxiety, worry, and frustration. Humor, like other interpersonal competencies, is a learned skill; when used inappropriately it can be destructive. Inexperienced nurses may find it helpful to identify nurses who use humor well and to "try on" behaviors they observe.

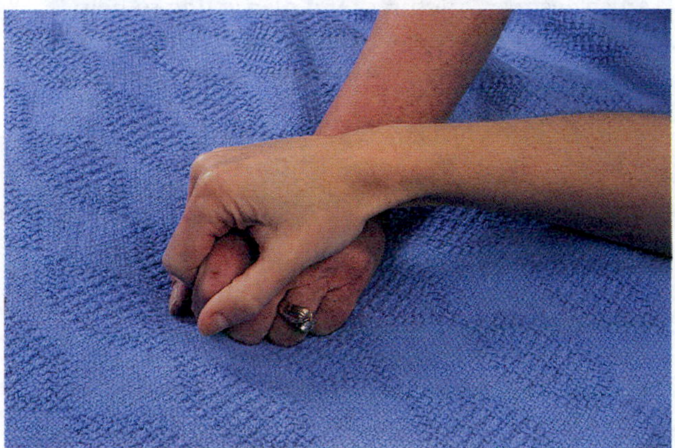

Figure 22-7
A reassuring handclasp uses touch to convey a message. Sometimes touch can be a more effective way of expressing concern and interest than verbal communication. (Photo © B. Proud.)

Interpersonal Competencies

The skills required for positive relationships between people are referred to as **interpersonal competencies**. In nursing, these competencies are essential to the promotion of a nurse–client relationship that will be therapeutic for the client.

Warmth and Friendliness. The helping relationship depends on the nurse's ability to begin the orientation phase successfully. A pleasant greeting accompanied by a smile can facilitate the initiation of this phase and allow the client to relax in the nurse's presence. By maintaining the qualities of warmth and friendliness throughout the helping relationship, the nurse conveys continuous acceptance of the client and interest in discussing the client's feelings and concerns.

Openness. A person who is open conveys an attitude of acceptance, frankness, and lack of prejudice. This is an important quality for a nurse, because a client who feels the nurse is judging could hold back significant information. The nurse must also be open to supporting the client's strengths and promoting the client's growth.

Empathy. Empathy is identifying with the way another person feels. An empathic nurse is sensitive to the client's feelings and problems but remains objective enough to help the client work toward positive outcomes. A nurse who retains this quality can establish successful helping relationships without becoming the cold, stern figure frequently portrayed in films and television.

Competence. Competent nurses are skilled in all aspects of basic nursing and are capable of meeting their client's healthcare needs through the use of technical, intellectual, interpersonal, and ethical/legal competencies. Nurses are responsible for evaluating their own strengths and for strengthening any weaknesses so that all clients will receive optimal care. Consequently, the clients develop trust in and respect for their nurses, facilitating helping relationships.

Respect and Commitment. Nurses need to develop sensitivity to the unique challenges presented by each client. Clients quickly sense if they are merely a "task to be performed" or a person of worth with a unique set of needs. Attention to the client variables that may influence the process of communicating (eg, gender, developmental level, culture, life experience) can make the difference between effective and ineffective interactions. The accompanying box highlights guidelines for relating to persons from different cultures.

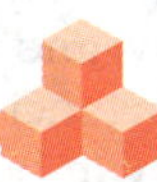

Guidelines for Nursing Care

Relating to Clients From Different Cultures

- Assess your personal beliefs surrounding persons from different cultures.
  - review your personal beliefs and past experiences
  - set aside any values, biases, ideas, and attitudes that are judgmental and may negatively affect care
- Assess communication variables from a cultural perspective.
  - determine the ethnic identity of the client, including generation in America
  - use the client as a source of information when possible
  - assess cultural factors that may affect your relationship with the client and respond appropriately
- Plan care based on the communicated needs and cultural background.
  - learn as much as possible about the client's cultural customs and beliefs
  - encourage the client to reveal cultural interpretation of health, illness, and health care
  - be sensitive to the uniqueness of the client
  - identify sources of discrepancy between the client's and your own concepts of health and illness
  - communicate at the client's personal level of functioning
  - evaluate effectiveness of nursing actions and modify nursing care plan when necessary
- Modify communication approaches to meet cultural needs.
  - be attentive to signs of fear, anxiety, and confusion in the client
  - respond in a reassuring manner in keeping with the client's cultural orientation
  - be aware that in some cultural groups discussion concerning the client with others may be offensive and may impede the nursing process
- Understand that respect for the client and communicated needs is central to the therapeutic relationship.
  - communicate respect by using a kind and attentive approach
  - learn how listening is communicated in the client's culture
  - use appropriate active listening techniques
  - adopt an attitude of flexibility, respect, and interest to help bridge barriers imposed by culture
- Communicate in a nonthreatening manner.
  - conduct the interview in an unhurried manner
  - follow acceptable social and cultural amenities
  - ask general questions during the information-gathering stage
  - be client with a respondent who gives information that may seem unrelated to the client's health problem
  - develop a trusting relationship by listening carefully, allowing time, and giving the client your full attention
- Use validating techniques in communication.
  - be alert for feedback that the client is not understanding
  - do not assume meaning is interpreted without distortion
- Be considerate of reluctance to talk when the subject involves sexual matters.
  - be aware that in some cultures sexual matters are not discussed freely with members of the opposite sex
- Adopt special approaches when the client speaks a different language.
  - use a caring tone of voice and facial expression to help alleviate the client's fears
  - speak slowly and distinctly, but not loudly
  - use gestures, pictures, and play acting to help the client understand
  - repeat the message in different ways if necessary
  - be alert to words the client seems to understand and use them frequently
  - keep messages simple and repeat them frequently
  - avoid using medical terms and abbreviations that the client may not understand
  - use an appropriate language dictionary
- Use interpreters to improve communication.
  - ask the interpreter to translate the message, not just the individual words
  - obtain feedback to confirm understanding
  - use an interpreter who is culturally sensitive

Used with permission from Giger, J.N., & Davidhizar, R.E. (1995). *Transcultural nursing: Assessment and intervention* (2nd ed.). St. Louis: Mosby, p. 38.

Assertive Skills

When interacting with clients, family members, nurses, physicians, and other members of the healthcare team, it is important for nurses to communicate in a way that demonstrates respect for all parties in the communication. Assertive behaviors, which are one hallmark of professional nursing relationships, need to be distinguished from aggressive (ie, harsh, injurious, or destructive) and avoidance or acquiescent behaviors—both of which are the opposite of true assertive behavior. Chenevert (1994) equated learning to be assertive with learning to stand up for yourself and your clients, to trust your feelings and respect your opinions, and to like yourself. The key to assertiveness is open, honest, and direct communication. "I" statements—"I feel . . ." and "I think . . ."—play an important role in assertive statements. Table 22-2 gives examples of assertive and nonassertive speech.

Four basic components of the assertive response or approach are as follows: (1) empathic component, (2) description of feelings or situation, (3) expectation, and (4) consequences (Angel & Petronko, 1983). For example, a student who is feeling overwhelmed by her weekly clinical assignments may communicate the following to her instructor:

Empathy: "I guess it must be hard for you to make our clinical assignments each week and to know what each one of us needs."

Description: "I have to share with you that right now I feel so overwhelmed that I go home from clinical in tears each week."

Expectation: "I am wondering if we could talk about this. I am willing to work hard but I seem to need some help pulling everything together."

Consequences: "I expect to do well in clinical but I am afraid that if things continue the way they are right now, I may not last the semester. I would appreciate any help you can give me."

Characteristics of the assertive nurse's self-presentation include a confident, open body posture; eye contact; use of clear, concise "I" statements; and the ability to honestly share thoughts, feelings, and emotions. The assertive nurse's attitude toward work is characterized by working to capacity with or without supervision, the ability to remain calm under supervision, freedom to ask for help when necessary, the ability to give and accept compliments, and honesty in admitting mistakes and taking responsibility for them. Table 22-3 highlights some of the advantages and disadvantages of nonassertive and assertive behavior.

Impaired Verbal Communication (NANDA)

Impaired verbal communication was accepted as a nursing diagnosis by the North American Nursing Diagnosis Association (NANDA) in 1973. Its definition, defining characteristics, and related factors are given here.

Definition: The state in which an individual experiences a decreased or absent ability to use or understand language in human interaction.

Defining Characteristics: Unable to speak dominant language; speaks or verbalizes with difficulty; does not or cannot speak; stuttering; slurring; difficulty forming words or sentences; difficulty expressing thought verbally; inappropriate verbalization; dyspnea; disorientation.

Related Factors: Decrease in circulation to the brain; brain tumor; physical barrier (tracheostomy, intubation); anatomic defect, cleft palate; psychologic barriers (psychosis, lack of stimuli); cultural differences; developmental or age related.

The accompanying displays describe communication disorders and identify where speech–language pathology and audiology services can be obtained; describe the speech, language, and hearing disorders that

Table 22-2
Examples of Assertive and Nonassertive Speech

	Assertive	Nonassertive
Nurse to Nurse	"I know we all lose track of time occasionally but I'm finding it harder and harder to cover for you when you take extra time for lunch. I don't think it's fair for your clients and I to have to wait an extra 30 minutes every day for you to come back from lunch. Can we talk about this?"	"Huh? No, I didn't really mind. Luckily I wasn't too busy today." Thought: "What a sucker I am. Now I'll have to grab a quick bite so that I can get back to the unit in time to do 2 PM treatments."
Nurse to Physician	"I know we talked about Mr. Esposito's pain medication before but I've collected some new data. Even with the change in dosage he is only getting 1 to 1½ hours of relief. I believe a different analgesic agent might work better for him."	"Um . . . yes I know you already changed the dosage. It's just that I thought it still wasn't working. Maybe I didn't give it enough time. Thanks for listening to me anyway. I'm sorry to bother you with this."
Student Nurse to Preceptor	"Miss Cheng has a new order to be straight cathed. I reviewed the procedure but I'd sure appreciate your talking me through this because I've never done it before and I'm terrified."	"Uh . . . I'm sorry to be such a pain again. I have to do this cath and don't know where to begin. I know you must be busy, but, uh, is there any way you might have time for me?"

Table 22-3
Advantages and Disadvantages of Assertive and Nonassertive Behavior

Assertive Behavior	Nonassertive (Passive) Behavior	
Advantages	*"Quasi" Advantages*	*Disadvantages*
Increased sense of personal integrity and self-worth	"Comfortable" maintenance of status quo	Decreased sense of personal integrity and self-worth
Resolution of conflict	Avoidance of conflict (and thereby hostility and rejection)	No resolution of problem causing inner turmoil
Personal growth: independence, honesty, decision making	Avoidance of responsibility	Increased anxiety and stress and decreased health
Increased leadership ability	Commendation for being a team player (not rocking the boat)	Decreased sense of control (increased dependence)
		Increased feelings of inadequacy and insecurity → aggressive behavior

Communication Disorders

What Are Communication Disorders?

Communication disorders can be grouped in two main categories:

1. People with *hearing disorders* do not hear sounds clearly. Such disorders may range from hearing speech sounds faintly, or in a distorted way, to profound deafness.
2. *Speech and language disorders* affect the way people talk and understand. These disorders may range from simple sound substitutions to not being able to use speech and language at all.

What Are The Signs Of A Communication Disorder?

Hearing: Hearing loss might be suspected when a person does not always hear sounds like a telephone or doorbell ringing, turns his or her ear towards the source of sound, frequently asks the speaker to repeat, turns the TV or radio up too loud, or shows obvious signs of confusion or misunderstanding of speech.

Speech and language disorders might be present when a person's speech or language is different from that of others of the same age, sex, or ethnic group; when a person's speech and/or language is hard to understand; when a person is overly concerned about his or her own speech; or when a person frequently avoids communicating with others.

Are Communication Disorders Serious Problems?

Yes. The ability to communicate is our most human characteristic. Human communication is essential to learning, working, and social interaction. Impaired communication can affect every aspect of a person's life.

Common Communication Disorders

Hearing

Conductive: sound is not conducted efficiently through the outer and/or middle ear, causing speech and other sounds to be heard less clearly or to sound muffled. This kind of hearing loss can often be medically or surgically corrected.

Sensorineural: caused by damage in the inner ear or nerve pathways to the brain. Certain sounds are heard less distinctly than others, causing distortion and reduced understanding of speech. While this kind of hearing loss is usually not medically correctable, people with sensorineural hearing loss can often be helped by using a hearing aid or other amplification device.

Mixed: a combination of conductive and sensorineural hearing loss.

Language

Delayed Language: a noticeable slowness in the development of the vocabulary and grammar necessary for expressing and understanding thoughts and ideas.

Aphasia: the loss of speech and language abilities resulting from stroke or head injury.

Speech Disorders

Stuttering: an interruption in the rhythm of speech characterized by hesitations, repetitions or prolongations of sounds, syllables, words, or phrases, for example, cow . . . boy, tuh-tuh-tuh-table, ssssun.

Articulation Disorders: difficulties with the way sounds are formed and strung together usually characterized by substituting one sound for another

(continued)

Communication Disorders *(continued)*

(wabbit for rabbit), omitting a sound (han for hand), or distorting a sound (shlip for sip).

Voice Disorders: inappropriate pitch (too high, too low, never changing or interrupted by breaks); loudness (too loud or not loud enough); or quality (harsh, hoarse, breathy, or nasal).

What Causes Communication Disorders?

Hearing: Some of the causes of hearing loss are chronic ear infections, heredity, birth defects, health problems at birth, certain drugs, head injury, viral or bacterial infection, exposure to loud noise, aging, and tumors.

Speech and Language: Some of the causes of speech and language disorders are related to hearing loss, cerebral palsy and other nerve/muscle disorders, severe head injury, stroke, viral diseases, mental retardation, certain drugs, physical impairments such as cleft lip or palate, vocal abuse or misuse, and inadequate speech and language models; frequently, however, the cause is unknown.

What Can You Do If You Suspect A Speech, Language, Or Hearing Problem?

A thorough evaluation by a speech–language pathologist or audiologist is needed to determine a person's communication strengths and weaknesses. After this evaluation, the speech–language pathologist or audiologist will be able to provide a plan for meeting individual needs.

What Is A Speech–Language Pathologist?

A speech–language pathologist is a professional educated in the study of human communication, its development, and its disorders. By evaluating the speech and language skills of children and adults, the speech–language pathologist determines if communication problems exist and decides the best way to treat these problems.

What Is An Audiologist?

An audiologist is a professional educated in the study of normal and impaired hearing. The audiologist determines if a person has a hearing impairment, what type of impairment it is, and how the individual can make the best use of remaining hearing. If a person will benefit from using a hearing aid or other listening device, the audiologist can assist with the selection, fitting, and purchase of the most appropriate aid and with training the individual to use the aid effectively.

Where Can You Find Speech–Language Pathology and Audiology Services?

Speech–language pathologists and audiologists provide professional services in many different types of facilities such as:

- public and private schools
- hospitals
- rehabilitation centers
- nursing care facilities
- community clinics
- colleges and universities
- private practice
- state and local health departments
- state and federal governmental agencies

A speech–language pathologist or audiologist will have a master's or doctoral degree and should hold a Certificate of Clinical Competence (CCC) from the American Speech-Language-Hearing Association and/or a license from the state.

(From *Recognizing communication disorders*. American Speech-Language-Hearing Association, Rockville, MD. Reprinted with permission.)

most frequently affect older people; and offer guidelines for communicating with clients with special needs.

Communicating in Groups

Nurses communicate in groups as well as one-on-one with clients and other caregivers. A *group* exists when two or more people are gathered together. To be functional, the members must communicate with one another for the purpose of achieving a goal or purpose.

When functional groups are observed or studied for their effectiveness or ineffectiveness, it is commonly referred to as *group dynamics.* Group dynamics involves the evaluation of whether a group is effective in making the changes that were planned. If the group is ineffective, the reason is investigated. Group dynamics also includes studying how the individual group members relate to one another during the process of working toward group goals. This observation can be done by the members themselves, the leader, or an outside observer. Much can be gained by the careful assessment of the dynamics or internal life of the group.

Types of Groups

Groups can be categorized by size—one-to-one, small, and large. Nurses, both professionally and personally, commonly belong to each of these types of groups. Many nursing situations involve the nurse and client in

(text continues on page 382)

Focus on the Older Adult

What Are the Disorders of Communication Which Most Frequently Affect Older People?

Our communication system, which involves speaking, hearing and understanding the speech of others, reading, and writing, is a unique human achievement. It plays a vital role in all aspects of everyday life—in our jobs, our families, and our recreation. When communication processes are damaged by disorders of speech, language or hearing, the effects are always serious.

Disorders of speech, language, and hearing are frequently found among older adults. These individuals often find themselves at a distinct disadvantage on social, economic, and personal levels. With the number of older adults growing rapidly, and with the increased numbers of survivors of illnesses and accidents which can result in speech, language, or hearing disorders, more and more older adults with communication problems will be encountered. They require the understanding of family and friends as well as services from professionals in communication disorders.

Disorders of communication which affect older people may result from hearing impairment, stroke, cancer or other disease of the larynx, parkinsonism, or other neurological disorders. The communication disorders vary widely and include difficulty with speaking and with understanding verbal messages. The effects of these disorders may be frustrating and bewildering and may lead to withdrawal and isolation. Participation on any social or economic level may become difficult or impossible either because of the disorder itself or the emotional consequences.

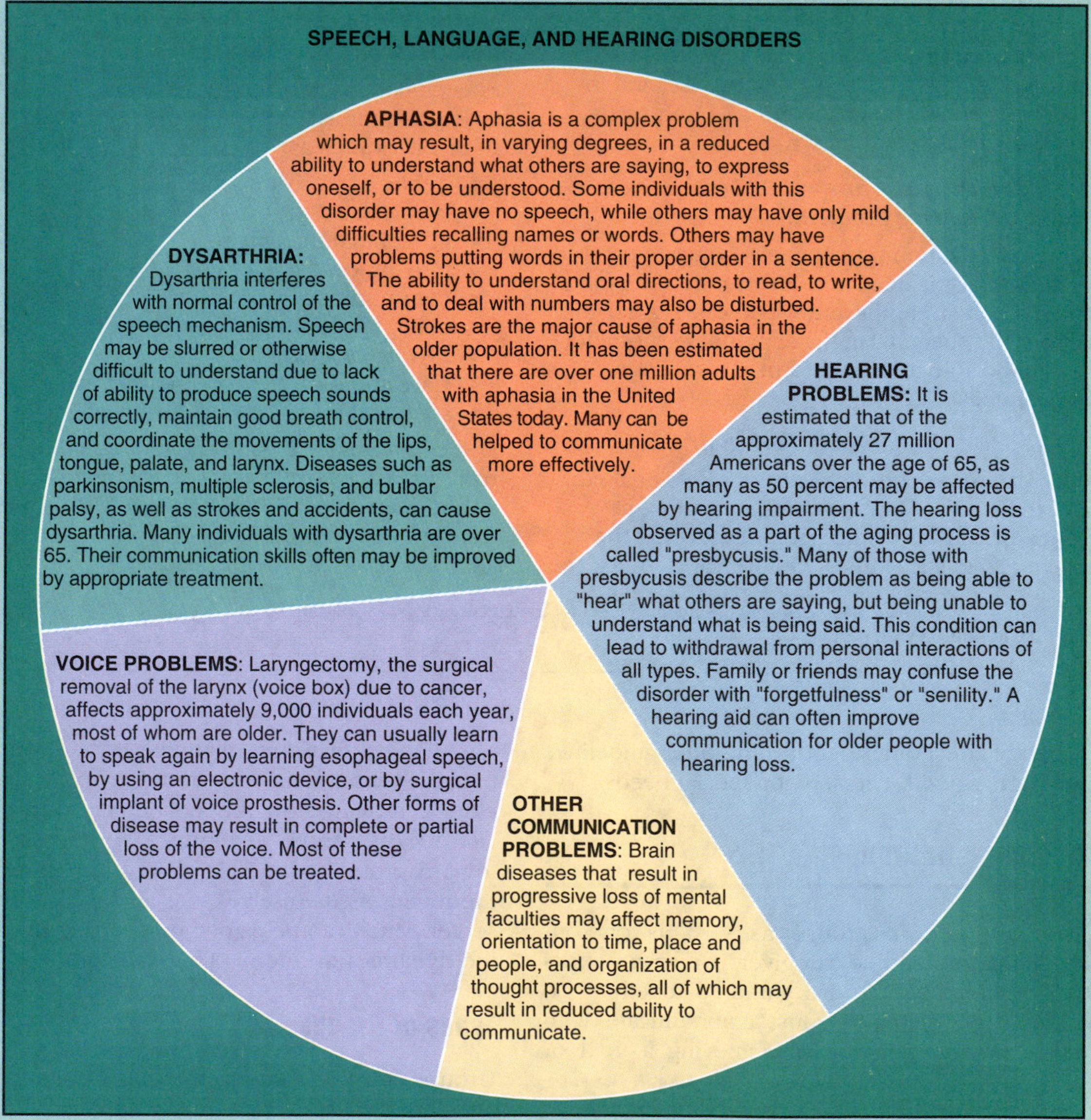

SPEECH, LANGUAGE, AND HEARING DISORDERS

APHASIA: Aphasia is a complex problem which may result, in varying degrees, in a reduced ability to understand what others are saying, to express oneself, or to be understood. Some individuals with this disorder may have no speech, while others may have only mild difficulties recalling names or words. Others may have problems putting words in their proper order in a sentence. The ability to understand oral directions, to read, to write, and to deal with numbers may also be disturbed. Strokes are the major cause of aphasia in the older population. It has been estimated that there are over one million adults with aphasia in the United States today. Many can be helped to communicate more effectively.

DYSARTHRIA: Dysarthria interferes with normal control of the speech mechanism. Speech may be slurred or otherwise difficult to understand due to lack of ability to produce speech sounds correctly, maintain good breath control, and coordinate the movements of the lips, tongue, palate, and larynx. Diseases such as parkinsonism, multiple sclerosis, and bulbar palsy, as well as strokes and accidents, can cause dysarthria. Many individuals with dysarthria are over 65. Their communication skills often may be improved by appropriate treatment.

HEARING PROBLEMS: It is estimated that of the approximately 27 million Americans over the age of 65, as many as 50 percent may be affected by hearing impairment. The hearing loss observed as a part of the aging process is called "presbycusis." Many of those with presbycusis describe the problem as being able to "hear" what others are saying, but being unable to understand what is being said. This condition can lead to withdrawal from personal interactions of all types. Family or friends may confuse the disorder with "forgetfulness" or "senility." A hearing aid can often improve communication for older people with hearing loss.

VOICE PROBLEMS: Laryngectomy, the surgical removal of the larynx (voice box) due to cancer, affects approximately 9,000 individuals each year, most of whom are older. They can usually learn to speak again by learning esophageal speech, by using an electronic device, or by surgical implant of voice prosthesis. Other forms of disease may result in complete or partial loss of the voice. Most of these problems can be treated.

OTHER COMMUNICATION PROBLEMS: Brain diseases that result in progressive loss of mental faculties may affect memory, orientation to time, place and people, and organization of thought processes, all of which may result in reduced ability to communicate.

(From *Communication Disorders and Aging*. American Speech-Language-Hearing Association, Rockville, Md. Reprinted with permission.)

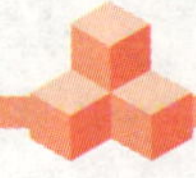

Guidelines for Nursing Care

Communicating in Special Circumstances

Clients Who Are Visually Impaired

- Acknowledge your presence in the client's room.
- Identify yourself by name.
- Remember that the visually impaired client will be unable to pick up most nonverbal cues during communication. Speak in a normal tone of voice.
- Explain the reason for touching the client before doing so.
- Indicate to the client when the conversation has ended and when you are leaving the room.
- Keep a call light or bell within easy reach of the client.
- Orient the client to the sounds in the environment and to the arrangement of the room and its furnishings.
- Be sure eyeglasses are clean and intact or that contacts are in place.

Clients Who Are Hearing Impaired

- Orient the client to your presence before initiating conversation. This may be done by gently touching the client or moving so you can be seen.
- Talk directly to the client while facing him or her. If the client is able to lip read, use simple sentences and speak in a quiet, natural manner and pace. Be aware of nonverbal communication.
- Do not chew gum or cover your mouth when talking with the client.
- Demonstrate or pantomime ideas you wish to express, as appropriate.
- Use sign language or finger spelling, as appropriate.
- Write any ideas that you cannot convey to the client in another manner.
- Be sure that hearing aids are clean, functioning, and inserted properly.

Clients With a Physical Barrier (Laryngectomy or Endotracheal Tube)

- Select one or more simple means of communication that the client is physically able to use. Options include eye blinks or hand squeezes to communicate yes or no; writing pads or magic slates; communication boards with words, letters, or pictures; flash cards; sign language.
- Be sure that everyone communicating with the client—family, friends, and caregivers—understands and is able to use the communication devices selected.
- Demonstrate patience with the time needed to communicate effectively, and reinforce the efforts made by the client.
- Ensure that the client has an effective means of signaling need for assistance, such as call bells or alarms.

Clients With Dementia

- Establish and maintain eye contact with the client to hold attention.
- Communicate important information in a quiet environment where there is little to distract the client's attention.
- Keep communication simple and concrete. Break down instructions into simple tasks and avoid lengthy explanations. Do not use pronouns or abstract terms. Use pictures or drawings when appropriate.
- Whenever possible, avoid open-ended questions. Ask "Would you like to wear the brown pants or the gray pants?" instead of "What would you like to wear?"
- Be patient and give the client time to respond. If the client does not respond after 2 minutes, repeat what you said. If there is still no response, take a break before continuing the conversation so that neither you nor the client becomes frustrated.

An Unconscious Client

- Be careful of what is said in the client's presence. Hearing is believed to be the last sense lost, and therefore the unconscious client is often likely to hear even though there is no apparent response.
- Assume the client can hear you. Talk in a normal tone of voice about things you would ordinarily discuss.
- Speak with the client before touching. Remember that touch can be an effective means of communication with the unconscious client.
- Keep environment noises at as low a level as possible. This helps the client focus on the communication.

Clients Who Speak a Foreign Language

- Use an interpreter whenever possible.
- Use a dictionary that translates words from one language to another so that you can speak at least some words in the client's language.
- Speak in simple sentences and in a normal tone of voice.
- Demonstrate or pantomime ideas you wish to convey, as appropriate.
- Be aware of nonverbal communication. Remember that many nonverbal communication cues are universal.

Computer Applications in Nursing

On-Line Resources for Nursing

More and more nurses are joining the information age. Student nurses use word processing to produce papers. Nurse administrators are communicating about management issues with colleagues around the world using electronic mail. Nurse researchers employ computers to collect and manage data. Nurse educators utilize teleconferencing to "attend" seminars simultaneously with nurses in other countries.

On-line means being connected to another computer separate from yours, either directly or through a telephone line. Now more hospitals and nursing schools are connecting to the Internet, a worldwide system of linked computers. If access to the Internet is not supplied by the workplace, nurses can purchase it through a commercial service and link to other nurses from home.

Electronic mail (e-mail) and mailing lists are the most widely used application. Nurses can communicate with others on a one-to-one basis or with a group of nurses using a mailing list. Over 15 mailing lists are geared to nursing specifically, with new ones emerging. Some of the more popular lists include from 800 to 1000 nurses in countries all over the world and focus on topics such as student nurses, general nursing, nursing education, nursing informatics, and nursing research.

Newsgroup is the term for an electronic bulletin board with access from the Internet. There are over 10,000 groups covering a multitude of topics. Many newsgroups focus on healthcare topics such as quitting smoking, supporting those with cancer, and nutrition and diet.

Available software allows the nurse to search for information stored on computers all over the world. Several sites contain nursing-specific information, and the number of nursing sites are expanding. This text-based software is affectionately known as "gopher," after the mascot of the developing university.

Another way to search for nursing-related information is on the World Wide Web (WWW). The Web, as it is commonly called, combines "hypertext" and "hypermedia" to access documents on computers all over the world. Hypertext refers to documents in which words or phrases are tagged as "links" to other documents. Hypermedia describes documents that can include text, graphics, sounds, and videos. Web browsers, just like the gopher software, allow the user to find documents. The WWW, a new phenomenon, is growing dramatically. There is great potential for nurses to explore and exploit the use of the WWW for nursing and patient education and research.

To get started on the information highway, you need a personal computer with a modem and a telephone line. You also need access to the Internet, either through your university or workplace or via a commercial service. Are you ready to join the information age?

a one-to-one group—a collaborative situation in which the nurse maintains a leadership advantage.

Nurses participate in groups both as members and as leaders. For example, a nurse may lead a group of family members in discussing how they can meet their mother's needs for supervision at home. The same nurse may also belong to the hospital safety committee and work toward achieving committee goals. In addition, many nurses choose to serve large groups of people through their involvement in community-based programs, such as community health–planning boards, health-promoting organizations (eg, American Red Cross, American Cancer Society, or American Heart Association), or even school board committees.

Groups can also be categorized as formal or informal. *Formal groups* usually stipulate membership requirements as well as group goals. The local chapter of the American Nurses Association (ANA) is an example of a formal group. *Informal groups* have fewer rules and regulations and sometimes none at all. A group of nurses gathered together during their lunch break is considered an informal group. A nurse who is discussing the hospital discharge policy with a group of clients in the lounge has formed an informal group.

Purpose of Groups

A group must have a purpose to bind its members together. The purpose may change and grow as the group develops or its membership changes. Most groups are formed for the purpose of effecting change, reflected in the group goals that are set. Some groups dissolve once the goals have been met; other groups may set new goals, thus continuing the group's existence.

The group's purpose may be clearly indicated by the group's name. Many formal groups have names that explain their purpose. Other groups may have more subtle or covert purposes, yet on inspection their mission becomes clear.

Roles of Group Members

Although effective leadership facilitates a group's achievement of its goals, the group's success or failure is largely a function of member behaviors. Ideally each

A Support Group for Families of Trauma Patients (Sample Outcomes, Problem Areas, and Solutions)

Family Outcomes

Sharing of experiences
Expression of emotions
Mutual support
Coping strategies (eg, instilling hope)
Education about hospital and community resources

Problem Areas and Solutions

Domination by one participant: leader channels discussion to include others and offers to meet individually

Late arrival of participants: no alteration of time frame; flexible format

Nursing Outcomes

Increased knowledge of family dynamics
Improved sensitivity among healthcare team
Holistic care planning

Adapted from Harvey, C., Dixon, M., & Padberg, N. (1995). Support group for families of trauma patients. *Critical Care Nurse, 15*(4), 59-63.

group member uses his or her talents and interpersonal strengths to help the group accomplish its goals while maintaining sensitivity to the needs of individual group members. Group members who attempt to dominate or thwart the group process are confronted. Effective and ineffective groups are contrasted in Table 22-4. Member roles have been categorized as task-oriented roles whose focus is the work to be done; group-building or maintenance roles whose focus is the well-being of people doing the work; and self-serving roles, which advance the needs of individual members at the group's expense. Examples of these roles follow:

Task roles—information giver, information seeker, clarifier, coordinator, delegator, energizer, evaluator

Maintenance roles—active listener, harmonizer, trust builder, tension reliever, supporter

Self-serving roles—attention seeker, dominator, blocker, special pleader, withdrawer, aggressor (Benne & Sheats, 1948)

One administrative team who recognized the critical value of staff participation in designing and implementing a hospital restructuring project used a team approach to secure needed change. The list of ground rules for team members is presented in the accompanying box.

Table 22-4
A Comparison of Effective and Ineffective Groups

Variable	Effective Group	Ineffective Group
Group identity	Members value and "own" the aims of the group; aims are clearly articulated	Group's aims are not of major importance to members
Cohesiveness	Members generally trust and like one another and are loyal to the group; high commitment; high degree of cooperation	Members often feel alienated from the group and from one another; low commitment; members tend to work better alone than with the group
Patterns of interaction	Honest, direct communication flows freely; members support, praise, and critique one another	Communication is sparing; little self-disclosure; self-serving roles (ie, dominator, blocker, or aggressor) may be unchecked
Decision making	Problems are identified, appropriate method of decision making is used (ie, individual, minority, majority, consensus, or unanimous); decision is implemented and followed through; group commitment to decision is high	Problems are allowed to build without resolution; little responsibility is shown for problem solving; group commitment to decision is low
Responsibility	Members feel strong sense of responsibility for group outcomes	Little responsibility for group felt by group members
Leadership	Effective style of leadership to meet desired aims	Ineffective leadership styles
Power	Sources of power are recognized and used appropriately; needs or interests of those with little power are considered	Power is used and abused to "fix" immediate problems; little attention to needs of powerless

Ground Rules for Team Members

- I know what I have to do and the team's goals are clear.
- Everyone takes some responsibility for leadership.
- There is active participation by everyone.
- I feel appreciated and supported by others.
- Team members listen when I speak.
- Different opinions are respected.
- We enjoy working together and have fun.
- We are aiming for excellence, not perfection.
- Everyone on the team has an equal voice.
- We are always open to more education and information.
- Ask anything, challenge anything.
- We have a clean slate.
- We color outside the lines.
- It is OK to take a risk and fail.

Scott, J., & Rantz, M. (1994). Change champions at the grass roots level: Practice innovation using team process. *Nursing Administration Quarterly, 18*(3), 13.

Key Points

- Nurses communicate thoughts, ideas, experiences, and facts to other nurses, clients, physicians, other healthcare workers, and families as part of their promotion of wellness and prevention of illness.
- The communication process can be defined in two ways: (1) the process of sharing information and (2) the process of generating and transmitting meanings. Communication, as a foundation of life, is a reciprocal process with simultaneous participation.
- People communicate one to one or in small or large groups by verbal and nonverbal means.
- Nonverbal communication includes touch, eye contact, facial expressions, posture, gait, gestures, physical appearance, sounds, and silence.
- Factors that can influence the process of communication include development, gender, sociocultural differences, roles and responsibilities, space and territoriality, physical and mental/emotional state, values, and environment.
- The ability of the nurse to communicate with others is essential to effective use of the nursing process.
- The three phases in the helping relationship are (1) orientation phase, (2) working phase, and (3) termination phase. A helping relationship is dynamic, purposeful, and time limited, and involves one person in a dominant role.
- Factors that benefit the helping relationship by promoting effective communication include having specific objectives, a comfortable environment, privacy, confidentiality, and client focus, as well as using nursing observations, allowing optimal pacing, and providing personal space.
- Effective communication techniques are conversational skills, listening skills, use of silence and touch, and interviewing techniques. The interview is a major tool for data collection in the assessment step of the nursing process.
- Interpersonal skills such as warmth and friendliness, openness, empathy, competence, and consideration of client variables are essential to a therapeutic nurse–client relationship.
- Assertive skills enable nurses to communicate with clients, nurses, and other members of the healthcare team in a direct, honest fashion that is respectful of the rights of all parties in the communication.
- The nurse must develop communication skills for special circumstances, especially when the client is visually impaired, hearing impaired, unconscious, has dementia, has a physical barrier such as a laryngectomy or endotracheal tube, or speaks a foreign language.
- In functional groups members communicate with one another for the purpose of achieving a goal. Group members may serve task, maintenance, or self-serving roles. When groups are studied to determine their effectiveness or ineffectiveness, the study is called group dynamics.

Bibliography

Allen, L.J. & Van Ess Coeling, H. (1995). Quality of life: Its meaning to the long term care resident. *Journal of Gerontological Nursing, 21*(2), 20–25.

Angel, G., & Petronko, D. K. (1983). *Developing the new assertive nurse: Essentials for advancement.* New York: Springer-Verlag.

Armstrong, J. (1996). Too close for comfort. *Nursing, 26*(4), 44–47.

Bergbom-Engberg, I. (1993). The communication process with ventilator patients in the ICU as perceived by the nursing staff. *Intensive Critical Care Nursing, 9*(1), 40–47.

Berlo, D. (1960). *The process of communication: An introduction to theory and practice.* New York: Holt, Rinehart, & Winston.

Bottorff, J.L. & Morse, J.M. (1994). Identifying patterns of attending: Patterns of nurse's work. *IMAGE: Journal of Nursing Scholarship, 26*(1), 53–60.

Chenevert, M. (1994). *STAT: Special techniques in assertiveness training for women in the health professions* (4th ed.). St. Louis: Mosby–Year Book.

Clark, C. C. (1978). *Assertive skills for nurses.* Wakefield, MA: Contemporary Publishing.

Deering, C.G. (1993). Working with people: Giving and taking criticism. *American Journal of Nursing, 93*(12), 56–60.

Fine, J.I. & Rouse-Bane, S. (1995). Using validation techniques to improve communication with cognitively impaired older adults. *Journal of Gerontological Nursing, 21*(6), 39–45.

Giger, J.N. & Davidhizar, R.E. (1995). *Transcultural nursing: Assessment and intervention* (2nd ed.). St. Louis: Mosby.

Grossman, D.& Taylor, R. (1995). Working with people: Cultural diversity on the unit. *American Journal of Nursing, 95*(2), 64–67.

Hagerty, B.M.K., Lynch-Sauer, J., Patusky, K.L. & Bouwsema, M. (1993). An emerging theory of human relatedness. *IMAGE: Journal of Nursing Scholarship, 25*(4), 291–296.

Harvey, C., Dixon, M. & Padberg, N. (1995). Support group for families of trauma patients. *Critical Care Nurse, 15*(4), 59–63.

Heidt, P. R. (1990). Openness: A qualitative analysis of nurses' and patients' experience of touch. *IMAGE: Journal of Nursing Research, 22*(3), 180–186.

Hermann, J. F., Cella, D. F., & Robinovitch, A. (1995). Guidelines for support group programs. *Cancer Practice, 3*(2), 111–113.

Laing, M. (1993). Gossip: Does it play a role in the socialization of nurses? *IMAGE: Journal of Nursing Scholarship, 25*(1), 37–43.

MacKay, M. (1990). *Empathy in helping relationship.* New York: Springer-Verlag.

Mackey, R.B. (1995). Discover the healing power of therapeutic touch. *American Journal of Nursing, 95*(4), 26–33.

Messner, R.L. (1993). What patients really want from their nurses. *American Journal of Nursing, 93*(8), 38–41.

Montagu, A. (1986). *Touching: The human significance of the skin* (3rd ed.). New York: Harper & Row.

Moore, J.R. & Gilbert, D.A. (1995). Elderly residents' perceptions of nurses' comforting touch. *Journal of Gerontological Nursing, 21*(1), 6–13.

Nance, T.A. (1995). Intercultural communication: Finding common ground. *JOGNN, 24*(3), 249–255.

Norris, R. M. (1989). Commonsense tips for working with blind patients. *American Journal of Nursing, 89*(3), 360–361.

North American Nursing Diagnosis Association. *NANDA Nursing Diagnoses: Definitions and Classification, 1995–1996.* Philadelphia: NANDA.

Orlando, I. J. (1990). *The dynamic nurse–patient relationship: Function, process and principles.* New York: National League for Nursing.

Paterson, J., & Zderad, L. (1976). *Humanistic nursing.* New York: Wiley.

Peplau, H. (1952). *Interpersonal relations in nursing.* New York: Putnam.

Quinn, J. F. (1988). Building a body of knowledge: Research on therapeutic touch. *Journal of Holistic Nursing, 6*(1), 37–45.

Ribeiro, V.F. & Blakeley, J.A. (1995). The proactive management of rumor and gossip. *JONA, 25*(6), 43–50.

Scott, J. & Rantz, M. (1994). Change champions at the grass roots level: Practice innovation using team process. *Nursing Administration Quarterly, 18*(3), 13.

Seldon, B. (1994). Communicating with Alzheimer's patients. *Journal of Gerontological Nursing, 20*(10), 51–53.

Sundeen, S. J., Stuart, G. W., Rankin, E. D., & Cohen, S. A. (1989). *Nurse–client interaction* (4th ed.). St. Louis: Mosby.

Tannen, D. (1990). *You just don't understand: Women and men in conversation.* New York: Morrow.

Tennant, K. F. (1990). Laugh it off: The effect of humor on the well-being of the older adult. *Journal of Gerontological Nursing, 16*(12), 11–17.

Travelbee, J. (1971). *Interpersonal aspects of nursing* (2nd ed.). Philadelphia: Davis.

Vanore-Black, N. (1990). Maintaining healthy relationships. *Holistic Nursing Practice, 4*(4), 39–45.

Watson, J. (1985). *Nursing: The philosophy and science of caring.* Boulder: Colorado Associated University Press.

White, C. & Howse, E. (1993). Managing humor: When is it funny–and when is it not? *Nursing Management, 24*(4), 80, 84, 86–96.

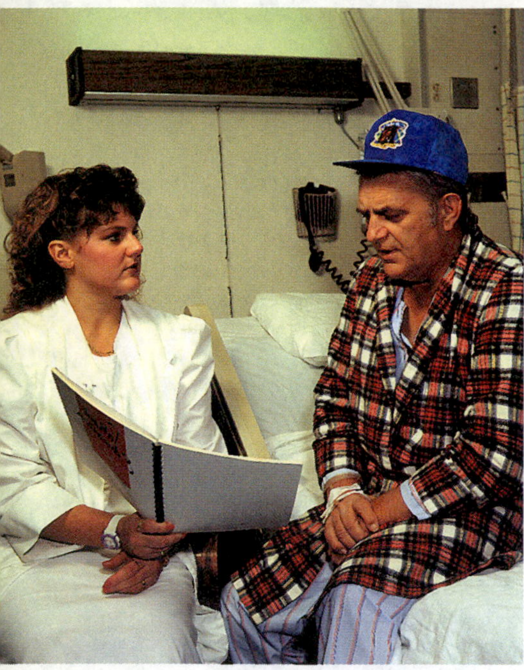

Chapter 23

Teacher and Counselor

Objectives

After studying this chapter, the learner should be able to:

Define key terms used in the chapter.

Describe the teaching–learning process, including domains, developmental concerns, and specific principles.

Describe what factors should be assessed for the learning process.

Formulate diagnoses for identified learning needs.

Explain how to create and implement a teaching plan for a client.

Name three methods for evaluating learning.

Explain what should be included in the documentation of the teaching–learning process.

Discuss the nurse's role as a counselor.

Summarize how the nursing process is used to assist clients in problem solving.

Describe how to use the counseling role to motivate a client toward health promotion.

Key Terms

affective learning
cognitive learning
contractual agreement
counseling
developmental crisis
formal teaching
informal teaching
learning
learning readiness
literacy
negative reinforcement
noncompliance
positive reinforcement
psychomotor learning
situational crisis
teaching

Many clients lack the knowledge and self-care abilities they need to achieve valued health goals. To work effectively with these clients nurses must be skilled teachers and counselors. Both roles require strong communication skills. The current trends toward shorter hospital stays and decreased time for healthcare professional–client interactions have increased the need for effective teaching and counseling. More acutely and chronically ill clients are at home in need of complex nursing assistance from their families, friends, and volunteers. Never has the demand for quality education and counseling been greater. Nurses who are skilled educators and counselors increase client health and well-being and reduce the demand for professional services.

Aims of Teaching and Counseling

The basic purpose of teaching and counseling is to help clients and families develop the self-care abilities (knowledge, attitude, and skills) that enable them to maximize their functioning and quality of life (or dignified death). When skillfully used by nurses, teaching and counseling are powerful tools for achieving nursing aims.

Promoting Wellness

A higher level of wellness is possible for all. Nurses can help clients to value health and develop specific health practices that promote wellness. Wellness teaching is varied and can range from teaching passive exercises to a client with left-sided paralysis to designing a safe exercise program for a young athlete.

Preventing Illness

Prevention, a major theme in health teaching and counseling, takes many forms. Nurses can counsel women of childbearing age about health practices that promote optimal fetal development, teach parents how to make their home safe for a toddler, or counsel individuals at high risk for heart disease, cancer, or communicable diseases.

Restoring Health

Once a client is ill, teaching and counseling focus on developing self-care practices that facilitate recovery. Preoperative and postoperative teaching, sexual counseling for a client recovering from a myocardial infarction, and lifestyle counseling for the client with an ostomy are all examples of teaching and counseling directed at restoring health.

Facilitating Coping

Developmental lifestyle changes and acute, chronic, and terminal illness all place demands on clients and families that may become overwhelming. Nurses work not only with clients but also with their families and friends to help them to come to terms with the illness and any lifestyle modifications it entails.

The nurse caregiver who is a skilled teacher and counselor can expect to effect the following outcomes:

- High-level wellness and related self-care practices
- Disease prevention or early detection
- Quick recovery from trauma or illness with minimal to no complications
- Enhanced ability to adjust to developmental life changes and acute, chronic, and terminal illness
- Family acceptance of the lifestyle changes necessitated by the illness or disability of a family member

General topics for health teaching are highlighted in the accompanying box.

The Nurse as Teacher

Nurses assume the role of teacher when clients have identifiable learning needs. This teacher–learner relationship is enhanced by the continuance of the helping relationship (see Chapter 22), in which mutual respect and trust have been established. The nurse builds on this trust by sharing information the nurse and client have mutually identified as important. The client may ask for this information or the nurse may initiate teaching as the result of assessment and diagnostic factors.

Topics for Health Teaching and Counseling

Promoting Wellness

- Developmental and maturational issues
- Normal childbearing
- Hygiene
- Nutrition
- Exercise
- Mental health
- Spiritual health

Preventing Illness

- First aid
- Safety
- Immunizations
- Screening
- Identification and management of risk factors

Restoring Health

- Orientation to treatment center and staff
- Client's and nurses' expectations of one another
- The illness and physical condition: anatomy and physiology, etiology of problem, significance of symptoms, prognosis
- The medical and nursing regimens and how the client can participate in care
- Self-care practices the client and family needs to manage the client's condition independently

Facilitating Coping

- How the client's physical and mental condition affects other areas of functioning; life-style counseling
- Measures that maximize independence and enhance self-concept
- Stress management
- Environmental alterations
- Community resources
- Appropriate referrals (eg, physical therapy, occupational therapy, self-help groups, psychiatric–mental health counselor)
- Grief and bereavement counseling

Teaching–Learning Process

How the human brain stores and retrieves information has not yet been fully determined. A person plays the role of learner throughout life, although what is learned and how learning occurs change according to developmental stages. Basic understanding of the teaching–learning process aids nurses in developing their own teaching and learning skills. The process is summarized in the accompanying box.

Teaching is a planned method or series of methods used to help someone learn. The person using these methods is the teacher. **Learning** is the process by which a person acquires or increases knowledge or changes behavior in a measurable way as a result of an experience.

Learning Domains

Learning can be divided into three domains—cognitive, affective, and psychomotor (Bloom, 1956). **Cognitive learning** involves the storing and recalling of new knowledge and information in the brain (eg, the client states how salt affects blood pressure). When a physical skill has been acquired, the change that has occurred is called **psychomotor learning** (eg, the client demonstrates how to change dressings using clean technique). **Affective learning** includes changes in attitudes, values, and feelings (eg, the client expresses renewed self-confidence following physical therapy). These three areas of learning give the nurse-teacher a way of categorizing the learning that is planned for the client (see the "Learner Objectives" column in the sample teaching plan, Table 23-1).

Developmental Considerations

One of the major learning theories is Piaget's theory of intellectual development (see Chapter 8). A nurse who understands how children and adolescents develop learning abilities can use this knowledge when teaching clients of any ages. For instance, if a 6-year-old girl must begin to take insulin every day, the nurses who are caring for her must recognize her limitations in understanding diabetes. Information should be simplified to provide only the most basic facts with accompanying concrete examples or demonstrations. At no time would a detailed discussion of the pathophysiology of diabetes be appropriate. The girl could be told that she needs a shot every day to keep her from getting sick or feeling funny. She could be allowed to play with the syringes and to give shots to a doll.

A nurse who is teaching a sexually active 16-year-old girl about contraceptive methods needs to assess whether the young client has reached the stage Piaget refers to as *formal operations* (the ability to use logical reasoning to solve hypothetical problems). If the client's intellectual development is delayed and is still in the period of *concrete operations* (use of logical reasoning to solve concrete problems), she may be unable to think abstractly. That is, she may not perceive pregnancy as a real possibility and therefore may be unable to understand the need for contraception. If so, the nurse can alter the teaching plan to include audiovisual (AV) teaching aids that explain the topic in concrete terms.

Some adults have not attained the formal operations stage. The nurse must be alert to this possibility and

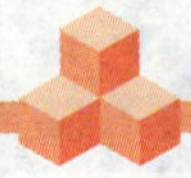

Guidelines for Nursing Care

Taking Steps in the Teaching–Learning Process

Assess the Client's Learning Needs

1. Use all appropriate sources of information.
2. Identify the knowledge, attitude, or skills needed by the client and family.
3. Assess emotional and experiential readiness to learn.
4. Assess the client's ability to learn.
5. Identify client strengths.
6. Use anticipatory guidance.

Diagnose the Learning Needs

1. Be realistic.
2. Validate with client or family, or both.

Develop a Teaching Plan

1. Formulate measurable learner objectives.
   - Identify short- and long-term objectives.
   - Prioritize.
   - Determine who should be included (ie, family members, significant others).
   - Include the client in planning.
2. Create a teaching plan.
   - Match content with appropriate teaching strategies and learner activities.
   - Directly relate teaching content to the client's interests, resources, and patterns of everyday living.
   - Schedule within limits of time constraints.
   - Decide on group versus individual teaching and formal versus informal.
   - Formulate a verbal or written contract with the client.

Implement the Teaching Plan

1. Prepare the physical environment.
2. Gather all audiovisual materials and equipment.
3. Deliver content in organized manner using teaching strategies.
4. Be flexible.

Evaluate the Teaching–Learning

1. Evaluate completion of learner objectives.
   - Client's comments
   - Direct questioning
   - Observational skills
   - Return demonstration
   - Postdischarge follow-ups
2. Reinforce and celebrate learning.
3. Evaluate teaching.
   - Self-evaluation
   - Client questionnaires
4. Revise plan of learner objectives not met.
   - Alter content and teaching strategies.
   - Use motivational counseling if needed.
   - Reschedule teaching sessions.
5. Document the teaching–learning process.

teach or re-teach material as needed. For example, an adult taking an antibiotic may be unable to grasp the importance of taking the capsules at the prescribed times to maintain the proper blood level for the best effect. If the nurse sees that the client is not complying with the schedule, the effectiveness of the teaching and learning should be evaluated. Showing a simple diagram of how erratic scheduling affects the body could give the concrete information the client needs to be motivated toward taking the antibiotic as ordered. In this way, the teaching is altered to meet the client's intellectual development.

Motor development is also a concern in the teaching–learning process. The 6-year-old girl diagnosed with diabetes may not be expected to learn to give her own insulin shots if she lacks the fine motor skills needed to manipulate the equipment for insulin injections. On the other hand, a 13-year-old client could probably master the technique quickly.

Other developmental concerns related to the teaching–learning process are emotional maturity and psychosocial development. Chronologic age does not guarantee maturity. It is possible that a 13-year-old client could respond more maturely to health teaching than a 30-year-old client. A great deal depends on how the client has learned to respond to changes and stressful events in the past.

Adult Learners. Many of the developmental concerns related to teaching and learning are exacerbated by age. As people age, their personalities as well as their learning abilities change. Most psychologists who have studied the teaching–learning process have based their work on children and adolescents, because a large amount of learning occurs early in life. The science of teaching—*pedagogy*—generally refers to the teaching of children and adolescents. In recent years, the study of teaching adults—*androgogy*—has become popular. This term emphasizes that adults need to be taught differently.

Knowles (1984) lists the following four assumptions concerning adult learners:

1. As a person matures, his or her self-concept is likely to move from dependence to independence.

Table 23-1
Sample Teaching Plan

Diagnosis: High Risk for Impaired Skin Integrity: Nipples, related to knowledge and skill deficit (nipple care)

Signs and symptoms: Complains of sore nipples; first baby; 1 day after delivery; fair skin with freckles; no redness or cracking yet; no prenatal preparation

Learner Objective	Met	Content	Teaching Strategy	Learner Activity
The Client		Prevention and care of sore nipples		
Morning Session				
Begins protective measures immediately (psychomotor)	√ 8/10/97 L.S.	Protective measures: • Avoid soap • Avoid exposure to air and sunlight • Apply lanolin or vegetable oil • Avoid plastic liners in bra or bra pads	Lecture with discussion Audiovisual: Flip chart on breastfeeding	Read handout: Nipple Care
Explains why feedings should be shorter and more frequent (cognitive)	√ 8/10/97 L.S.	Preparation for breast-feeding: • Feed baby more frequently —Every 2 hours during day —Arrange for rooming in • Nipple roll before the feeding	Discussion Audiovisual: Flip chart on breastfeeding	Read handout: Sore Nipples
Demonstrates nipple rolling (psychomotor)	√ 8/10/97 L.S.		Return demonstration	
10 AM Session				
Demonstrates correct feeding technique and after care (psychomotor)	√ 8/10/97 L.S.	Breastfeeding the baby: • Start baby on less sore side • Hold the breast properly • Get baby onto areolar area • Position properly • Change position for each feeding • Remove baby from breast	Discovery: Guide through each step; assist as necessary	Read handout: Positioning Baby for Breastfeeding
Describes a feeling of improved comfort with each feeding (affective)	√ 8/10/97 L.S.	After the feeding: • Air dry nipples • Inspect for open or cracked areas • Apply lanolin or vegetable oil	Discovery	Borrow books on breast-feeding from client's reference shelf
Afternoon Session				
Explains the importance of good nutrition and rest at home (affective) Lists the signs of thrush (cognitive)	√ 8/10/97 L.S.	Considerations for home: • Maintain "demand" feedings • Ensure good nutrition • Get adequate rest • Know the signs and symptoms of thrush	Lecture with discussion Audiovisual: Poster	Refer to handouts at home as needed; call the maternity department's information number for any questions

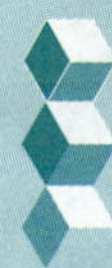

Research in Nursing: Making a Difference

Teaching Caregiving Behaviors

Nurses attempting to teach self-care skills to older adults or to prepare the family caregivers of older adults living at home confront unique challenges.

Related Research

Hussey, L.C. (1994). Minimizing effects of low literacy on medication knowledge and compliance among the elderly. *Clinical Nursing Research, 3*(2), 132–145.
Eighty-year-old adults were studied to determine their knowledge of and compliance with their medication regimen. The results suggest that nurses who work with the elderly must be aware of special learning needs. Barriers to compliance such as visual impairment and lack of dexterity may be routinely evaluated, but reading ability must also be included as part of the nursing assessment. A picture schedule for when medications are to be taken proved effective in increasing compliance—possibly because it was not necessary to be able to read to use it.

Archbold, P.G. et al. (1995). The PREP system of nursing intervention: A pilot test with families caring for older members. *Research in Nursing and Health, 18*(1), 3–16.
This study enrolled 22 families who were providing care to older adults. Those who received the PREP system of nursing intervention—designed to increase the **PR**eparedness and competence of family members providing long-term care for frail elderly people, to **E**nrich the caregiving process, and to make unpredictable caregiving situations more **P**redictable—scored higher on the care effectiveness scale.

Summary

Further research is needed to identify the barriers to learning needed care-giving measures and related nursing interventions.

2. The previous experience of the adult is a rich resource for learning.
3. The readiness to learn in an adult often is related to a developmental task or a social role.
4. The adult's orientation to learning is that material should be useful immediately, rather than at some time in the future.

Given these assumptions it is easy to see that androgogy has a problem-centered or need-centered focus with immediate application of new material.

It is generally accepted that adults must believe they need to learn before they are willing to learn. Nurses often use their counseling skills (discussed later in this chapter) to motivate clients to participate in the teaching–learning process. Adults may need to be shown the necessity of learning new information, health practices, or skills.

Many adults are afraid of the teaching–learning process. This may be the result of a fear of failure, because many adults have not participated in formal educational programs since their school days. As aging occurs, adults often express a concern over memory loss, and being required to learn new material can threaten their feelings of self-worth. Consequently, the sensitivity and concern of the nurse in the helping relationship are the foundation for a nonthreatening learning environment for the adult client.

Adults may resist learning because of preconceived ideas about the teaching–learning process and others' expectations. Honest and open communication provides the adult learner with a preview of what will be involved. Many adults willingly participate once they have received the reassurance that they are partners in the process. Retaining some control over what is taught and how it is taught gives adult learners the sense of control they are accustomed to in their daily lives.

Some older clients are especially fearful and threatened by the idea of having to learn new information. They may often refer to the old adage, "You can't teach an old dog new tricks," as a defensive attempt to avoid failure or change. Nurses find that a slower approach is needed when introducing new material so that older clients do not become discouraged or overwhelmed.

Literacy. About 20% of adults are functionally illiterate (unable to read and write). Many have learned to compensate for this disability and may fool even experienced nurses. Never presume **literacy** (the ability to read and write) in a client you are attempting to teach. By asking clients to read your name badge or a sheet of printed material you can assess their ability to understand printed material.

Principles of Teaching–Learning

Several basic principles of teaching–learning serve as guidelines for a nurse assuming the role of teacher (Fig. 23-1). They can be applied in situations in which the teaching–learning process is used to meet the needs of clients.

- The teaching–learning process is facilitated by the existence of a helping relationship (discussed in Chapter 22).

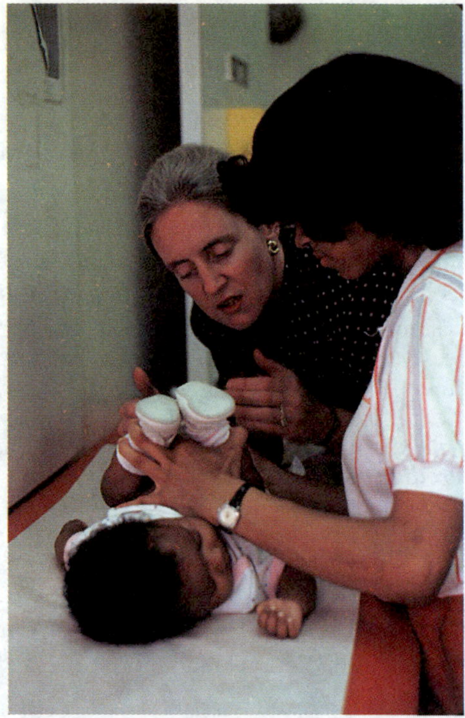

Figure 23-1
Principles of teaching–learning include such factors as a helping relationship; effective communication skills; assessment skills; planning that includes the client; use of a variety of strategies; expectation of realistic behavioral changes; attention to time, scheduling, and physical environment; and reassessment where necessary. (Photo by Gates Rhodes, courtesy of School of Nursing, University of Pennsylvania.)

- Nurse-teachers need to be able to communicate effectively with individuals, small groups, and, in some instances, large groups.
- Knowledge of the communication process is necessary for the assessment of verbal and nonverbal feedback.
- A thorough assessment of clients and the factors affecting learning helps to diagnose their learning needs accurately.
- The teaching–learning process is more effective when the client is included in the planning of learner objectives.
- Unless the client values these objectives, little learning is likely to occur.
- The implementation of a teaching plan should include varied strategies for sensory stimulation, which apparently promote learning.
- Relating new learning material to clients' past life experiences is effective in helping to assimilate new knowledge.
- Proposed behavioral changes must always be realistic and explored in the context of the client's resources and everyday lifestyle.
- Careful attention should be paid to time constraints, scheduling, and the physical environment.
- Learner objectives provide the basis for evaluating whether learning has occurred.
- When learning objectives have not been met, careful reassessment provides ideas for changing the teaching plan for subsequent implementation.

Client teaching is approached most effectively by following the steps of the nursing process. The teaching–learning process and the nursing process are interdependent.

Assessing the Client's Learning Needs

Sources of Information

Usually clients themselves are the best source of assessment information. By using effective interviewing techniques (see Chapter 22), the nurse can obtain the data needed to identify the client's learning needs. Relevant information can be obtained before actually meeting the client by reviewing the client's past and current medical records. These records provide a history of medical problems as well as documentation of the nursing assessments, nursing diagnoses, nursing physical examinations, and nursing interventions that have been performed.

The client's family and significant others are also valuable sources of assessment data. Sometimes the family or significant others are used for assessment data when the client is unable to communicate with the nurse because of health problems, language barriers, or impaired sensory functions. At other times, the family members or significant others may be the most appropriate source for certain information; for example, if seeking information pertaining to the use of salt in cooking, the nurse could speak with the person who prepares the meals in the client's home and then include that person in any teaching pertaining to food preparation. The client's permission should be secured before the nurse involves family members in the teaching–learning process.

Assessment Parameters

Four elements need to be considered in each assessment of client learning needs (Fig. 23-2). The nurse first identifies what new knowledge, attitudes, or skills are necessary for clients and families to independently manage their health care. The second focus of assessment is on **learning readiness**, a concept signifying the client's willingness to engage in the teaching–learning process (emotional readiness). The third focus is on experiential readiness to begin the challenge of learning. Readiness is distinguished from the client's physical ability to learn. The fourth focus of assessment is on client strengths, personal resources the nurse can assist clients to tap. Many factors influence each of these elements, and all should play a role in the assessment. These factors are highlighted in the accompanying box.

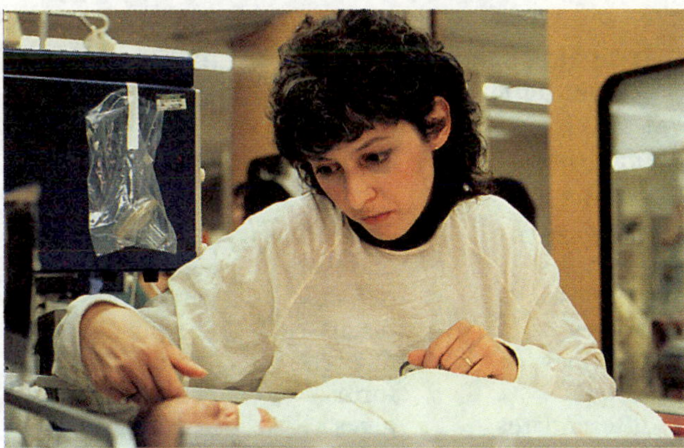

Figure 23-2
The nurse considers four elements in assessing this client's learning needs: knowledge, skills, and attitudes necessary for the client to independently manage health care; learning readiness; ability to learn; and learning strengths. (Photo by Gates Rhodes, courtesy of School of Nursing, University of Pennsylvania.)

Assessment Parameters: Factors That Affect Learning

Knowledge, attitudes, and skills needed for the client and family to manage health care independently

Readiness to Learn

- Emotional readiness
  - Emotional health
  - Motivation for learning
  - Self-concept and body image
  - Sense of responsibility for self
- Experiential readiness
  - Social and economic stability
  - Past experiences with learning
  - Attitude toward learning
  - Culture

Ability to Learn

- Physical condition
- Cognitive ability to learn
- Acuity of senses
- Developmental considerations
- Level of education
- Literacy
- Communication skills
- Primary language

Learning Strengths

- Successful learning in the past
- Above-average comprehension, reasoning, memory, or psychomotor skills
- High motivation
- Strong network
- Adequate financing

Diagnosing the Client's Learning Needs

When a lack of knowledge, attitude, or skill hinders a client's self-promotion of health, the nurse diagnoses the deficit. The nurse can use diagnoses or problem statements approved by the North American Nursing Diagnosis Association (NANDA) as a guide when diagnosing learning needs (see Chapter 17). If the nurse believes that a client's knowledge deficit is the primary problem, the nurse can write a diagnosis identifying a specific knowledge deficit as the problem followed by its etiology and the related signs and symptoms. For example:

Knowledge Deficit: Breastfeeding, related to inexperience as manifested by anxiety and multiple questions.

More often it is a knowledge deficit that results in an actual or potential problem; hence, the knowledge deficit is written as the etiology (second part of the diagnostic statement):

Infant at High Risk for Altered Nutrition: Less Than Body Requirements, related to mother's lack of knowledge about infant feeding and deficient learning readiness (as manifested by mother's quick frustration when breastfeeding, refusal to engage in learning process, and infant's weight loss).

Wellness diagnoses, such as Potential for Enhanced Parenting or Potential for Enhanced Self-Esteem, are written as one-part statements. Teaching and counseling are the primary nurse-prescribed interventions used to achieve related outcome criteria.

In addition to identifying the client's learning needs, nurses need to assess their own knowledge base and teaching skills. Nurses cannot teach information and skills to clients if they lack the information and skills to be taught. Often, knowing where to find information or an appropriate resource person is the first step in correcting one's own knowledge deficits.

Planning

Planning for learning involves the development of a teaching plan. Teaching plans are similar to nursing care plans—both follow the steps of the nursing process. One type of teaching plan is given in Table 23-1 as an example to follow during the remaining steps of the teaching–learning process. Standardized teaching plans (some computerized) are available for major topics of health teaching. When using these plans, it is imperative to individualize the plan to the client's unique learning needs and abilities. Examples of teaching plans that are incorporated into critical path documentation systems are featured in Chapters 18 and 21.

Thoughtful planning for a client's learning experiences maximizes the client's chances for learning while ensuring the most efficient use of the nurse's time and talents. Learner objectives are developed for each diagnosis of a learning need. The nursing orders become the content, teaching strategy, and learner activity columns of the written plan. This phase requires thought and creativity. The nurse's efforts are rewarded when the client successfully completes objectives at the end of the implementation phase.

When planning for learning, the nurse and client together must decide who should be included in the learning sessions. When the client is a young child, one or both parents may be the primary learners. When the client is an adult, a spouse or close friend who will be giving the care that is to be learned may be included. For instance, the person who does the household cooking is usually asked to be present for any nutritional teaching. If the client is ill and unable to participate in the teaching–learning process, people who will provide care at home must be taught procedures. Teaching plans are developed according to the needs of the person being taught.

One nurse or several nurses can prepare and use a teaching plan. When two or more nurses plan and coordinate the implementation of the plan, it is referred to as *team teaching.* An advantage of team teaching is that the talents of more than one nurse are used to promote learning for the client. Several factors should be considered during the formulation of any teaching plan.

Verbs That Can Be Used When Writing Learner Objectives

Cognitive Domain	*Affective Domain*	*Psychomotor Domain*
categorizes	answers	adapts
compares	chooses	arranges
composes	defends	assembles
defines	discusses	begins
describes	displays	changes
designs	forms	constructs
differentiates	gives	creates
explains	helps	demonstrates
gives examples	initiates	manipulates
identifies	joins	moves
labels	justifies	organizes
lists	relates	rearranges
names	revises	shows
prepares	selects	starts
plans	shares	works
solves	uses	
states		
summarizes		
writes		

Learner Objectives

Learner objectives are written in the same manner as the client goals of the nursing process (see Chapter 18). When planning for the client's learning, it is best to determine first which of the three learning domains (cognitive, psychomotor, or affective) will be used when teaching. The nurse can then write learner objectives that reflect what learning is to occur. A well-constructed learner objective serves as a guide for planning evaluation methods.

Choosing the verb for a learner objective is probably the most difficult part when writing objectives (see the accompanying box). Yet, if chosen carefully, it makes the planning of content, teaching strategies, learner activities, and evaluation methods easier.

The number of objectives needed for each diagnosis varies. It is better to have several specific objectives than to try to use only one or two broad objectives. Many nurses state one long-term objective for each diagnosis followed by several specific objectives. For example, a long-term objective for the sample teaching plan could be as follows: "The client will be able to breastfeed her infant as long as desired without sore nipples." This objective could be met in 2 weeks or 2 years. Long-term objectives are general statements. On the other hand, the objectives written in the "Learner Objective" column of the sample teaching plan (see Table 23-1) are specific behaviors to be accomplished within a short time.

Clients and appropriate family members or significant others should be included in the planning of learner objectives. Once clients value the learning objectives, learning readiness is enhanced and compliance is maximized.

Content

Once the learner objectives are completed, the nurse must decide what information the client needs to complete them successfully. This information is the content of the teaching plan. It is usually necessary to research the area to be taught to determine what information exists about the topic. Books, articles, and manuals are available in many nursing units for the nurse's research. It is becoming more common to have content that is already organized available for a variety of common health-teaching topics, thus shortening the required research time.

Nurses are concerned about what clients need to know about topics such as illness, procedures, medications, and surgeries. "How much should they know?" is a common topic for debate. It has been found that clients benefit from explanations of the physical sensations they will experience during a procedure. They appreciate advanced knowledge of what they will feel, taste, hear, see, and smell. See Table 23-1 for a sample teaching plan containing an example of content included for one client's learning needs.

Content explaining why certain treatments and medications are needed is included in a teaching plan. Information on the prevention of illness or its complications should also be covered. Compliance with the nursing and medical plans is a major objective for much of the health teaching done. People who have a basic understanding of their illness and its treatment usually comply with the treatment more readily than those who do not understand their illness.

Teaching Strategies

The techniques used by a teacher to promote learning are *teaching strategies.* Teaching strategies are planned before the actual teaching sessions so that every content area can be matched with an effective teaching technique. The strategies chosen depend on the teacher's familiarity with the method, the availability of computers and teaching aids such as audiovisual and printed materials, the facilities for using AV materials, and factors in the client's learning, such as educational level and cultural background. The nurse must also consider age-appropriate methods for her client; for example, a 10-year-old will be receptive to a comic book on personal safety, whereas an adult could learn similar material by discussing the safety measures with the nurse.

Experts in the field of education generally agree that the use of a variety of teaching strategies aids learning. In addition, some methods are better suited to certain learning objectives. The accompanying box gives suggested teaching strategies for the three learning domains. See Table 23-1 for the sample teaching plan, which shows how teaching strategies are varied for the learner objectives and content of that particular plan. Again, the nurse is free to use creativity in choosing the methods. However, the nurse should take care to stimulate as many of the client's senses as possible when teaching. Seeing, hearing, and touching are superior to hearing alone. Descriptions of common teaching strategies follow.

Role Modeling. The old saying "Actions speak louder than words" explains why role modeling is effective. Clients watch their nurses closely; the nurse can use this opportunity to affect a client's behavior positively. For example, nurses who were formerly smokers can be role models for clients who are trying to quit smoking for health reasons.

Suggested Teaching Strategies for the Three Learning Domains

Cognitive Domain

Lecture or discussion
Panel discussion
Discovery
AV materials
Printed materials
Programmed instruction
Computer-assisted instruction programs

Affective Domain

Role modeling
Discussion
Panel discussion
AV materials
Role playing
Printed materials

Psychmotor Domain

Demonstration
Discovery
AV materials
Printed materials

Lecture. In the purest sense, a *lecture* is a presentation of information by the teacher to the learners. However, to be more effective, lectures usually include question-and-answer periods to allow for clarification of material. This strategy is often used to deliver information to a large group of clients. It is rarely used for individual instruction, without the addition of other strategies.

Discussion. Discussion involves the two-way exchange of information, ideas, and feelings between the teacher and the learners. It is an effective method when used by a nurse who is comfortable with leading a group and knowledgeable in group process (see Chapter 22). It can also be an effective method for one-on-one instruction.

Panel Discussion. Panel discussion involves the presentation of information by two or more people. Panel discussions can be used to impart factual material but are also effective for sharing experiences and emotions. Debates are a form of panel discussion and allow for exposure of all aspects of a topic.

Demonstration. Demonstration of techniques, procedures, exercises, and the use of special equipment, combined with a lecture and discussion, is an effective strategy. Evaluation of the client's learning can be done by a return demonstration. Practice sessions are often included for the learner. Models of body parts or practice models such as a resuscitation model are frequently used. When teaching breast self-examinations, the use of a breast model allows the learner actually to feel different types of lumps commonly found in breast tissue. Childbirth educators usually demonstrate the birth of a baby by using a pelvic model, knitted uterus, and a baby doll.

Discovery. In discovery learning, the nurse presents a problem or situation to the client or group of clients and then guides the clients to discovering the solution or approach. Discussion of other possible approaches and solutions can follow the client's own solutions. This is a good method for teaching problem-solving techniques and independent thinking. For instance, a nurse could give a group of diabetic clients a short description of a situation that includes signs and symptoms. The group would decide if the signs and symptoms indicate *hypoglycemia* (low blood sugar) or *hyperglycemia* (high blood sugar) and would choose what measures to take. Next, the nurse could discuss the group decision as a further learning experience. Even if the clients chose a poor resolution, the nurse could turn it into an effective learning experience.

Role Playing. This strategy gives the learner a chance to experience, relive, or anticipate an event. The nurse explains the scenario and then allows the client to play out the scene with the teacher or with one or more clients. Role playing can be used to work through emotional traumas or to plan for possible traumas. For example, a nurse could help a teenage girl prepare herself to tell her mother about her pregnancy by letting the girl play her mother while the nurse plays the girl. This would help the client rehearse what she wanted to say and anticipate the emotional atmosphere that she will experience. Role playing is a good strategy for adults as well as children. Puppets and dolls can help young children express negative feelings that have resulted from hospitalization and traumatic procedures.

AV Materials. The use of AV materials can be an effective teaching and learning tool. AV materials include films, filmstrips with or without audiotapes, slides, television programs, videotapes, overhead transparencies, flip charts, posters, and diagrams. Their use is a popular and effective teaching strategy when combined with a lecture or discussion. Literacy should never be assumed in the client when using printed words. AV materials should never be the sole source of learning for the client. It is an accepted practice to allow the client to view AV material alone but to precede and follow it with a discussion of the material.

Printed Material. The use of printed material depends on its availability to the nurse. Many nurses have contributed to written materials for distribution to clients. Writing pamphlets, instruction sheets, books, and comic books for health teaching can be rewarding as well as useful. As with AV materials, the nurse usually uses printed materials in conjunction with other strategies. Use of specially prepared games, which are relatively easy to make, is a popular and fun way for clients to learn. For instance, cards with pictures of foods can be used to develop a nutritional instruction game.

Print materials should be selected carefully after evaluating how well they present needed content in a format that is attractive, understandable, and helpful. The Agency for Health Care Policy and Research has recently published excellent consumer guidelines for a number of common health problems. Three samples of client education materials appear in the accompanying boxes.

Programmed Instruction. Most programmed instruction books or booklets are prepared so that learners can

Sample Client Education Materials for Pain Control After Surgery: Pain Control Methods

Pain Control Methods You May Be Using

To get the best results, work with your doctors and nurses to choose the methods that will work best for you.

Your nurses and doctors want to make your surgery as pain free as they can. But you are the key to getting the best pain relief because pain is personal. The amount or type of pain you feel may not be the same as others feel—even those who have had the same operation.

Before Surgery

Drug treatment: Take pain medicine.

Non-drug treatment: Understand what operation the doctor is doing, why it is being done, and how it will be done. Learn how to do deep breathing and relaxation exercises (see example below).

During Surgery

Drug treatment: Receive general anesthesia, spinal anesthesia, or nerve blocks, or take a pain medicine through a small tube in your back (called an epidural).

After Surgery

Drug treatment: Take a pain medicine as a pill, shot, or suppository, or through a tube in your vein or back.

Non-drug treatment: Use massage, hot or cold packs, relaxation, music or other pastimes to distract you, positive thinking, or nerve stimulation (TENS).

What can you do to help keep your pain under control? These seven steps can help you help yourself.

Example—Slow Rhythmic Breathing for Relaxation*

1. Breathe in slowly and deeply.
2. As you breathe out slowly, feel yourself beginning to relax; feel the tension leaving your body.
3. Now breathe in and out slowly and regularly, at whatever rate is comfortable for you. You may wish to try abdominal breathing. If you do not know how to do abdominal breathing, ask your nurse for help.
4. To help you focus on your breathing and breathe slowly and rhythmically: Breathe in as you say silently to yourself, "in, two, three." Breathe out as you say silently to yourself, "out, two, three."
   or
   Each time you breathe out, say silently to yourself a word such as peace or relax.
5. You may imagine that you are doing this in a place that is very calming and relaxing for you, such as lying in the sun at the beach.
6. Do steps 1 through 4 only once or repeat steps 3 and 4 for up to 20 minutes.
7. End with a slow deep breath. As you breathe out say to yourself "I feel alert and relaxed."

Additional points: If you intend to do this for more than a few seconds, try to get in a comfortable position in a quiet place. You may close your eyes or focus on an object. This breathing exercise may be used for only a few seconds or for up to 20 minutes.

Before Surgery

1. Ask the doctor or nurse what to expect.
   - Will there be much pain after surgery?

(continued)

Sample Client Education Materials for Pain Control After Surgery: Pain Control Methods *(continued)*

- Where will it occur?
- How long is it likely to last?

Being prepared helps put you in control. You may want to write down your questions before you meet with your doctor or nurse.

2. Discuss the pain control options with your doctors and nurses. Be sure to:
   - Talk with your nurses and doctors about pain control methods that have worked well or not so well for you before.
   - Talk with your nurses and doctors about any concerns you may have about pain medicine.
   - Tell your doctors and nurses about any allergies to medicines you may have.
   - Ask about side effects that may occur with treatment.
   - Talk with your doctors and nurses about the medicines you take for other health problems. The doctors and nurses need to know, because mixing some drugs with some pain medicines can cause problems.
3. Talk about the schedule for pain medicines in the hospital.

   Some people get pain medicines in the hospital only when they call the nurse to ask for them. Sometimes there are delays, and the pain gets worse while they wait.

   Today, two other ways to schedule pain medicines seem to give better results.
   - Giving the pain pills or shots at set times. Instead of waiting until pain breaks through, you receive medicine at set times during the day to keep the pain under control.
   - Patient controlled analgesia (PCA) may be available in your hospital. With PCA, you control when you get pain medicine. When you begin to feel pain, you press a button to inject the medicine through the intravenous (IV) tube in your vein.

   For both ways, your nurses and doctors will ask you how the pain medicine is working and change the medicine, its dose, or its timing if you are still having pain.
4. Work with your doctors and nurses to make a pain control plan.

You can use a form to begin planning for pain control with your nurses and doctors. They need your help to design the best plan for you. When your pain control plan is complete, use the form to write down what will happen. Refer to it after your operation. Then keep it as a record if you need surgery in the future.

After Surgery

5. Take (or ask for) pain relief drugs when pain first begins.
   - Take action as soon as the pain starts.
   - If you know your pain will worsen when you start working or doing breathing exercises, take pain medicine first. It's harder to ease pain once it has taken hold.

   This is a key step in proper pain control.
6. Help the doctors and nurses "measure" your pain.
   - They may ask you to rate your pain on a scale of 0 to 10. Or you may choose a word from a list that best describes the pain.
   - You may also set a pain control goal (such as having no pain that's worse than 2 on the scale).
   - Reporting your pain as a number helps the doctors and nurses know how well your treatment is working and whether to make any changes.
   - They may ask you to use a "pain scale" (see Chapter 41, Fig. 41-5).
7. Tell the doctor or nurse about any pain that won't go away.
   - Don't worry about being a "bother."
   - Pain can be a sign of problems with your operation.
   - The nurses and doctors want and need to know about it.

   Stick with your pain control plan if it's working. Your doctors and nurses can change the plan if your pain is not under control. You need to tell the nurses and doctors about your pain and how the pain control plan is working.

* From McCaffery, M. and Beebe, A. (1989). *Pain: Clinical manual for nursing practice.* St. Louis: Mosby.

Acute Pain Management Guideline Panel. (1992). *Pain control after surgery. A patient's guide.* AHCPR Pub. 92-0021. Rockville, MD: Agency for Health Care Policy and Research. Public Health Service, U.S. Department of Health and Human Services.

use them independently of a teacher. However, educators generally agree that the teacher needs to spend time with the learner before and after the completion of the program to clarify information, answer questions, and provide the personal touch necessary for a learner's motivation. Because this is a self-paced strategy, it can be beneficial for many learners.

Computer-Assisted Instruction Programs. The use of computer programs for teaching is still in its infancy, but its possibilities are unlimited. Perhaps individual terminals will be made available in each client's room so that instruction will be available at any time. This method can even be personalized by programming the computer to address the learner by name and to give positive feedback

Sample Client Education Materials for Managing Cancer Pain: Pain Control Plan

Pain Control Plan

Pain control plan for ______________________

At home, I will take the following medicines for pain control:

Medicine	*How to take*	*How many*	*How often*	*Comments*

Medicines that you may take to help treat side effects:

Side Effect	*Medicine*	*How to take*	*How many*	*How often*	*Comments*

Constipation is a very common problem when taking opioid medications. When this happens, do the following:

- Increase fluid intake (8 to 10 glasses of fluid per day).
- Exercise regularly.
- Increase fiber in the diet (bran, fresh fruits, vegetables).
- Use a mild laxative, such as milk of magnesia, if no bowel movement in 3 days.
- Take ______________________ every day at ____________(time) with a full glass of water.
- Use a glycerin suppository every morning (this may help make a bowel movement less painful).

Nondrug pain control methods:

____

Additional instructions:

____

Important phone numbers:

Your doctor ______________________
Your nurse ______________________
Your pharmacy ______________________
Emergencies ______________________

Call your doctor or nurse immediately if your pain increases or if you have new pain. Also call your doctor early for a refill of pain medicines. Do not let your medicines get below 3 or 4 days' supply.

Cancer Pain Management Guidelines Panel. (1994). *Managing cancer pain: Patient guide.* AHCPR Pub. 94-0595. Rockville, MD: Agency for Health Care Policy and Research. Public Health Service, U.S. Department of Health and Human Services.

when appropriate. Currently, this method is not widely used because of limited access. This technique is only acceptable when personal, human attention is also available.

Contractual Agreements

A **contractual agreement** is a pact between two people made for the achievement of mutually set goals. The use of contracts between nurses and clients is becoming a common practice in many healthcare settings. Usually the contracts are rather informal and not legally binding. When teaching a client, such an agreement can serve to motivate both the client and the nurse to do what is necessary to attain the client's learning objectives. The agreement serves to point out the responsibilities of both the teacher and the learner, thus emphasizing the importance of the mutual commitment (see the accompanying box). Nurses can redirect "failures" to meet contracted objectives into new learning and decision-making situations and boost self-esteem by rewarding objectives that were achieved.

Sample Client Education Materials for Understanding HIV: Getting the Support You Need

Getting the Support You Need

A person or family living with HIV may need many kinds of support. Your health care provider and your local health and social services departments can help you find the support you need, including someone to:

- Answer your questions about HIV and AIDS.
- Help you find health care providers, get insurance, make health care decisions, and obtain food and housing.
- Provide transportation to and from health care appointments.
- Assist in planning ways to meet financial and daily needs.
- Refer you and your loved ones to support groups.
- Arrange for home nursing care or rehabilitation services.
- Represent you in legal matters.

Many people living with HIV feel better if they can talk with other people who also have HIV. Here are some ways to find others with HIV:

- Read HIV newsletters.
- Join support groups.
- Volunteer to help others
- Be an HIV educator or public speaker, or write a newsletter.
- Attend social events to meet other people who have HIV.

Additional Resources

There are many sources of information about living with HIV. Look in the telephone book for:

- Your local health department. They can tell you where to get tested for HIV and what services are available from public sources.
- Your local or state medical society to help you find a doctor.
- Your library. They may have many materials to help you learn about HIV and AIDS.

Some hospitals, churches, and the American Red Cross, as well as HIV and AIDS organizations, offer programs and sponsor support groups that may be listed in a special directory or your newspaper. Ask your librarian about newsletters and other printed materials.

Toll-free national hotlines and information clearinghouses can send you free publications and give you the latest news about drug-testing and clinical trials.

Here are some telephone numbers to help you get the information you need:

General Information

National AIDS Hotline
English . . . . (800) 342-AIDS (2437)
Spanish . . . . (800) 344-SIDA (7432)

TDD Service for the Deaf
(800) 243-7889

National AIDS Clearinghouse
(800) 458-5231

HIV/AIDS Treatment Information

American Foundation for AIDS Research
(800) 39AMFAR (392-6327)

AIDS Treatment Data Network
(212) 268-4196

Project Inform (800) 822-7422

Clinical Trials Conducted by the National Institutes of Health or Food and Drug Administration-Approved Trials:

AIDS Clinical Trials Information Service
800-TRIALS-A (874-2572)

Social Security Disability Benefits

For confidential assistance in applying for social security disability benefits, call the Social Security Administration at (800) 772-1213. You also may request a personal earnings and benefit estimate statement (PEBES) to help you estimate the retirement, disability, and survivor benefits payable on your social security record.

Start your own list of services, support groups, and where to get information now:

____
____
____
____
____
____
____
____
____
____
____
____
____
____
____
____
____
____
____
____

(continued)

Sample Client Education Materials for Understanding HIV: Getting the Support You Need *(continued)*

For Further Information

The information in this booklet was taken from the Clinical Practice Guideline on Evaluation and Management of Early HIV Infection. The guideline was written by a panel of private-sector experts sponsored by the Agency for Health Care Policy and Research. Other guidelines on common health problems also are being developed.

To order another copy of this booklet, call the National AIDS Hotline toll-free at (800) 342-AIDS, or write to:

AHCPR HIV Guideline
CDC National AIDS Clearinghouse
P.O.Box 6003
Rockville, MD 20849-6003

To order copies of AHCPR-sponsored guidelines on other topics, call (800) 358-9295 (for callers outside the U.S., only: (301) 495-3453 weekdays, 9 a.m. to 5 p.m., Eastern time, or write to:

Agency for Health Care Policy and Research
Publications Clearinghouse
P.O. Box 8547
Silver Spring, MD 20907

Evaluation and Management of Early HIV Guideline Panel. (1994). *Understanding HIV: Consumer guide.* AHCPR Pub. 94-0574. Rockville, MD: Agency for Health Care Policy and Research. Public Health Service, U.S. Department of Health and Human Services.

Learning Activities

While planning teaching strategies, the nurse also decides what learning activities the client is to do independently. There are many ways that the client can preview new material or reinforce what has already been taught. Use of printed material, AV materials, and programmed instruction materials is often assigned in the "Learning Activity" column of the teaching plan. This column is used to guide the client in learning activities that can be done before, between, and after planned learning sessions.

Practical Considerations

Time Constraints. Time constraints must be considered when planning for the client's learning. A problem for nurses is finding time to meet the client's learning needs. Priorities must be set so that essential content is taught thoroughly. Less important content is taught last so that the more important learner objectives are met within the time available. If time permits, the remaining content can be addressed. Note that in the sample teaching plan in Table 23-1, the client will be taught measures to use immediately.

To meet time constraints, nurses often plan together. Teamwork and cooperation allow nurses to meet deadlines. If teaching must continue beyond the hospitalization, home visit, or clinic visit, the nurse can schedule additional learning opportunities through outpatient programs or referrals to community-based programs. Home healthcare nurses often receive referrals from hospital nurses to continue teaching begun during a client's hospitalization. Discharge planning must be started early to ensure continuity of teaching.

Scheduling. It is better to plan for shorter, more frequent teaching sessions than for one or two longer sessions. Short sessions allow the client to digest the new material and prevent him or her from becoming too tired or uncomfortable because of the current health problem. Sessions of 15 to 30 minutes are generally well tolerated. Usually, more formal classroom programs last for more than 1 hour. In such cases, the nurse should provide breaks after every 50 minutes of class time. The client should be included in planning for the time and frequency of lessons.

Group Versus Individual Teaching. The nurse must consider several factors when choosing the type of setting for the client. Some learner objectives are met more readily in a one-to-one encounter, whereas others are achieved more easily in a group. For example, the objective "The client will change the dressing using sterile technique" would be evaluated during a private session with the nurse. The objective "The client will discuss feelings

Example of a Contractual Agreement Between a Nurse and a Client

I will participate in the learning activities needed to help me learn about my low-salt diet. During my hospital stay, I will attend the class on low-salt diets, read the materials given to me, and ask questions as I need to. I will work with S. Moore, RN, to plan my meals and food preparation at home. If I need help when I get home, I will contact S. Moore.

Jim Mall

I will provide Jim Mall with the experiences needed for him to follow his low salt-diet accurately.

S. Moore R.N.

Computer Applications in Nursing

Computer-Assisted Instruction

Nearly all nursing schools in the United States use computer technology for instructional purposes. Some computer-assisted instruction (CAI) programs are a required part of the student's coursework. Other CAI programs can supplement what is required.

The technology used varies depending upon when the CAI was written. Early programs still in use in many schools were written using monochrome monitors and do not take advantage of color or graphics. Programs are now available on microcomputers (either IBM compatible or Apple Macintosh formats), interactive videodiscs, and CD-ROM. Styles of CAI include simulations, drill and practice, authoring tools, games, tutorials, and tests.

CAI can be used to fill educational gaps, practice repetitive tasks, supplement classroom learning, refresh and enhance skills, and test mastery of skills. The student of nursing must be familiar with using a computer in order to take the National Council Licensure Examination (NCLEX) upon graduation.

There is a variety of content in the over 300 programs that are available to students and nurses for educational purposes. Some programs focus on learning or refreshing knowledge on basic nursing skills such as dosage calculation and EKG interpretation. Nursing practice programs teach subjects ranging from Lyme disease to physical assessment to anorexia. Nursing theory and research topics embrace nursing diagnosis, the nursing process, and an introduction to research. Nursing management CAI programs help to analyze a nursing salary budget and enhance discussion on nursing management issues.

Enormous possibilities exist for using computer-assisted instruction for the education of nurses, clients, and family members (Bolwell, 1993; Newbold, 1996).

about returning home after a heart attack" might be met more easily in a group discussion with other clients.

Formal Versus Informal Teaching. Most nurse–client interactions result in **informal teaching** being done by the nurse (Fig. 23-3). These unplanned teaching sessions are often effective because they deal with the client's immediate learning needs and concerns. Informal teaching often leads to additional planned, formal sessions. **Formal teaching** is the planned teaching done to fulfill learner objectives. Both forms are effective when the nurse uses them appropriately.

Implementing the Teaching Plan

Implementing the teaching plan requires use of interpersonal skills as well as effective communication techniques. Teaching the client can be a major part of the working phase of the helping relationship (see Chapter 22). The nurse must continually observe the client for additional assessment data that could alter the original teaching plan. This requires skill in adapting and reorganizing the teaching plan.

The nurse can facilitate client learning by continuing a warm and accepting approach. The nurse's attitude has more effect on the client than any other factor (Fig. 23-4). The nurse must avoid a condescending attitude. Moreover, it is always best to avoid technical and medical terms unless the client has a background in this area. A nonthreatening teaching–learning atmosphere allows learning to occur.

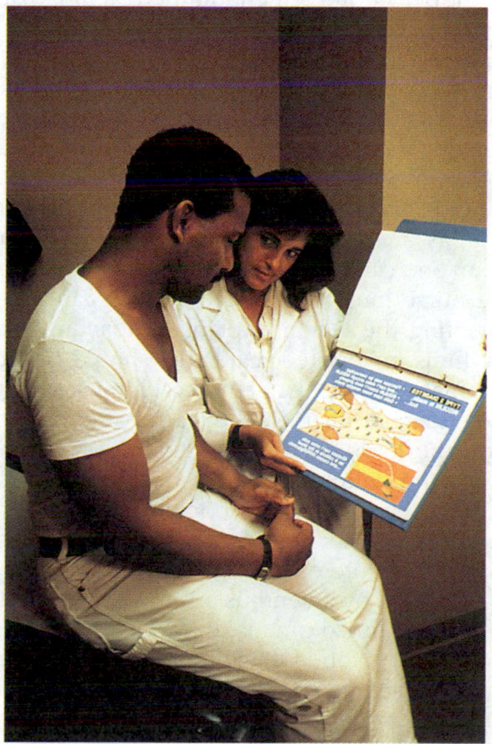

Figure 23-3
One-to-one teaching is used in many client–nurse situations. The nurse must be able to assess whether individual teaching is needed or whether learning can occur in a group. (Photo by Gates Rhodes, courtesy of School of Nursing, University of Pennsylvania.)

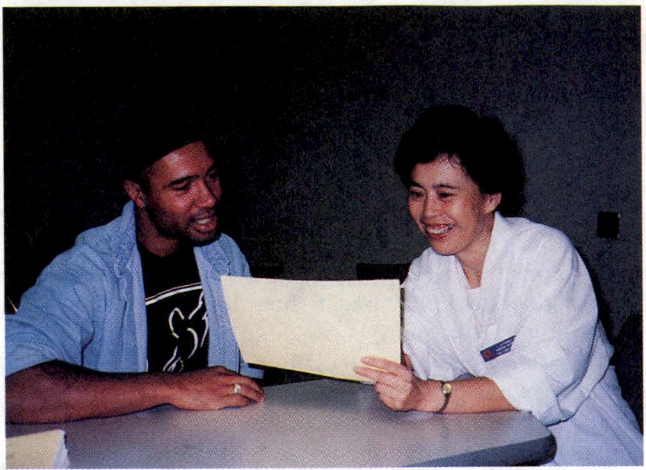

Figure 23-4
The nurse's warm approach is an important factor in interpersonal relationships.

The physical environment is another important consideration when implementing the teaching plan. Some preplanning may be needed to ensure adequate space and lighting, comfortable chairs, and good ventilation. Privacy is also important, as is freedom from distractions and interruptions.

During the implementation phase, the client as a learner must fulfill certain role functions. To avoid any misunderstandings, it is helpful to review the contractual agreement before implementing the teaching plan. The client is expected to listen, observe, and attempt to understand what is being taught.

Some people are uncomfortable in the role of learner; the nurse must assess this problem so that the client can be assisted to assume the role more easily. If special techniques or procedures must be learned (eg, colostomy care, self-injections, or eye medication instillation), the nurse can assure the client that it takes time and practice before anyone can perform new skills confidently.

The nurse must be prepared and organized before implementing the teaching plan. All teaching aids (eg, posters, films, or printed materials) should be gathered and organized before the actual teaching session. A disorganized teacher distracts the learner and has negative effect on the learning. If a procedure or skill is being taught, it is important to proceed in the correct sequence so that the client does not become confused.

An important nursing responsibility is to make each learning session interesting and enjoyable for the client. This is facilitated by an enthusiastic and positive attitude. In addition, the nurse can make learning fun through the creative use of planned teaching strategies. If the nurse approaches teaching positively, the client is more likely to approach learning in a similar way.

Evaluating Teaching–Learning

Evaluating Learning

It cannot be assumed that learning has occurred without some type of proof or feedback. The key to evaluation is the learner objectives written in the teaching plan (see Table 23-1), which describe what behaviors to measure. Methods for obtaining feedback of learning are discussed in the following section.

Methods of Evaluation. Methods of evaluation vary. For instance, cognitive domain learning may be evaluated through oral questioning; affective domain, through the client's response; and psychomotor domain, by return demonstration. Consider the following learner objective from the cognitive domain: "The client will be able to describe what a blood pressure reading represents." To evaluate this, the nurse could say to the client, "Tell me what this blood pressure reading means to you." The client then has a chance to talk about the current reading while the nurse evaluates the client's understanding of it.

Sometimes the nurse can use observational skills to determine if the client is using the material learned. For example, observing what the client has ordered for lunch tells the nurse if dietary lessons are being put into practice. The nurse depends on observation when evaluating the client's psychomotor skills. The nurse observes any new technique or skill that the client demonstrates to determine if it is performed satisfactorily.

The client's comments can be used to decide whether learner objectives have been met. Sometimes a client verbalizes understanding of information taught, yet avoids further discussion of the topic. In such instances, the use of effective communication techniques when reintroducing the topic at a later time might provide the evaluation data needed.

Using direct questions often provides an efficient method of evaluating learner objectives. The nurse simply asks the client a question to elicit a response that reflects the client's level of knowledge concerning a topic. This can also be used to evaluate the client's affective learning.

A return demonstration is an excellent evaluative method for the psychomotor domain (Fig. 23-5). Letting the client change his or her own dressing provides the nurse with concrete evidence of satisfactory or unsatisfactory performance of the procedure. Care must be taken to promote a nonstressful environment for the client's return demonstration.

Evaluation of learning may continue once the client has returned home. Home healthcare nurses may evaluate what was taught to the client in the hospital as well as what is being taught during home visits. Hospital nurses often check with family members or significant others after discharge to evaluate whether learner objectives have been met. Short-term objectives are usually evaluated while the client is still hospitalized.

Reinforcing and Celebrating Learning

Most people feel encouraged and supported when their efforts are acknowledged by another person, especially when the other person is trusted and valued. This is especially true in health care, where clients often feel overwhelmed by their illness. Nurses who recognize this

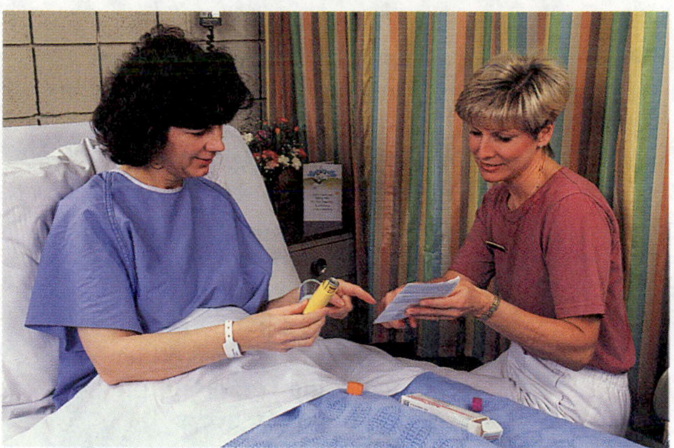

Figure 23-5
One type of evaluation is to ask the client questions concerning what he or she has been taught. (Photo © B. Proud.)

dynamic can use **positive reinforcement** to affirm the efforts of clients who have mastered new knowledge, attitudes, or skills. Reinforcement may be as simple as a few words of acknowledgment—"You've mastered this diet quickly"; as spontaneous as a warm hug; or as planned as the entire staff joining to celebrate a client's independent ambulation. **Negative reinforcement**—criticism or punishment—generally is ineffective; for the most part, undesirable behavior is best ignored. Behavior modification programs that reward desired behaviors and ignore undesired behaviors may be designed for some clients.

Evaluating Teaching

Nurses need to evaluate their teaching to capitalize on strengths and work on improving weaknesses. Like all nursing roles, teaching requires a great deal of practice and experience. Even nurse educators agree that they are always learning better ways to promote learning in students. It is important to avoid becoming discouraged when evaluations of teaching are less than perfect.

It is best to evaluate one's own teaching effectiveness immediately after each session. This involves a quick review of how the nurse-teacher feels the implementation of the plan went. Mentally noting both the strengths and weaknesses of the teaching session helps the nurse when planning for subsequent sessions.

Nurses can also seek feedback from clients. A simple questionnaire can be used at the end of each teaching session or after discharge to evoke the client's perception of the nurse's teaching effectiveness. The questionnaire may be a standardized form used throughout the hospital or agency or one prepared by the nurse-teacher. If it is an objective format, requiring only circles or checkmarks as answers, space should be provided for comments. The most honest and helpful evaluations are

Computer Applications in Nursing

Computer Use in Nursing Education

Nurses are using computers as a vehicle to obtain health-related education and as tools to help in practice. The benefits of using computers for education include increased effectiveness and efficiency, decreased cost, and the provision of essential knowledge and skills.

Computers are used in the school setting as well as in the work setting for educational purposes. Computer-assisted instruction serves as a teaching tool and as a way to refresh knowledge about nursing topics. Some nurses in rural areas use computer technology to take distance education classes by way of video conferencing. The instructor at one location and students at another are linked by cameras and microphones. In the future, nurses may use virtual reality to place the learner in a simulated role.

The nursing licensure examination is conducted only on the computer and not with pencil and paper as in the past. It uses the technique of computer adaptive testing in which each individual has a different test based on his or her response to a question.

Presentation graphics, word processing, spread sheets, and electronic mail may serve to disseminate information to the nurse. Nurses are also using on-line access to retrieve information from MEDLINE, other health-related databases, and expert systems. The Internet and the World Wide Web are emerging as educational tools for nurses and clients.

Currently most undergraduate nursing programs integrate computer technology into the curriculum. Some nurses seek to learn more about computer technology and the impact on nursing by obtaining degrees in information science or nursing informatics. "Nursing informatics is the specialty that integrates nursing science, computer science, and information science in identifying, collecting, processing, and managing data and information to support nursing practice, administration, education, research, and the expansion of nursing knowledge" (ANA, p. 3). There are two masters level and one doctoral programs in nursing informatics in the United States.

Computer technology is an important addition to the learning process of both the nursing student and the licensed nurse. The use of computers is limited only by our imagination (American Nurses Association, 1994; Hannah, Ball, & Edwards, 1994).

often those that are anonymous. Anonymity, however, is unnecessary and can sometimes bring forth harsh and nonproductive evaluations.

Revising the Plan

During evaluation, nurses and clients may establish that revisions are needed in the teaching plan. A reassessment may indicate that some client factors were not considered in the original plan. Adjustments may be made accordingly to meet the client's needs. Often, the selection of a different teaching strategy is all that is needed for a client to successfully achieve learner objectives. Revision is a natural part of the teaching–learning process and should not be viewed negatively.

Neither the nurse nor the client has failed when an objective is not met. Most objectives can be met with a change in approach; however, learner objectives are sometimes unrealistic. Further assessment by the nurse may reveal that the content may be too complex or the time too short for successful achievement.

Documenting

Because teaching is such an important nursing responsibility, it must be documented in the client's record. Documentation of the teaching–learning process includes a summary of the learning need, the plan, the implementation of the plan, and the evaluation results. The evaluative statement is crucial and must show whether the client has displayed concrete evidence that learning has occurred. If the desired learning has not occurred, the nurse's notes should indicate how the problem was resolved. It is insufficient to document only what was taught. The charting has to show evidence that the client or significant other has learned the material taught. See the accompanying box for an example of documentation.

Example of Documentation Using a Problem-Oriented Progress Note to Meet a Learning Need

8/10/98 #2 New Problem—High Risk for Impaired Skin Integrity: Nipples

S —Client stated that her nipples were sore during and after her newborn's first feeding

O—First day postpartum; client is fair skinned with freckles; no reddened areas, no cracking yet; no nipple preparation before delivery

A —At high risk to develop cracked, open areas; client lacks experience and knowledge of preventive measures

P —Develop teaching plan for nipple care

I —Teaching plan implemented

E —Client able to meet all of the objectives satisfactorily as recorded on the teaching plan; she currently is doing protective and preparatory care for her nipples; when breastfeeding, she uses the correct feeding technique with good aftercare; she states that her nipples are no longer sore, and she is able to explain what she should do when she goes home

R —None needed, but reinforcement of content will be continued

—L. Sweeney, RN

The Nurse as Counselor

Counseling is the interpersonal process of assisting clients to make decisions that promote their overall well-being. Often family members or significant others are included in the counseling sessions. Everyone participating must feel comfortable in the situation and surroundings.

The interpersonal skills of warmth, friendliness, openness, and empathy are necessary ingredients for successful counseling. The effective counselor needs to be a caring individual. Caring is based on humanistic philosophy (Watson, 1985), which is the core of nursing practice. A humanistic approach to counseling uses the caring process in helping the client strive toward the greatest health potential. Caring is important to all nursing roles but is fundamental in the counseling role.

Some nurses are advanced-practice psychiatric mental health nurses who specialize in counseling. The focus in this chapter is on the everyday counseling that is a basic component of each nurse's practice. This counseling involves listening carefully to the questions, concerns, demands, and complaints of the client or family and then responding in an effective and facilitative manner. Appropriate responses may be difficult for the nurse to give at first, but practice will help to develop this skill. Keep in mind that each nurse–client (or nurse–family) interaction is unique. A nursing response that works well with one client may intimidate or anger another. Sensitivity to the unique needs of each client and a willingness to get involved and make a difference are essential to effective counseling. Table 23-2 presents typical counseling situations that you might experience in your first year of nursing. Both effective and ineffective nursing responses are briefly analyzed. You may want to role-play these situations with a friend. It will quickly become apparent that the nurse who wishes to succeed as a caregiver and counselor needs to master the communication techniques described in Chapter 22.

Three Types of Counseling

The three types of counseling are short-term, long-term, and motivational. Following the descriptions of these three types is a discussion of strategies for dealing with

Table 23-2
An Analysis of Nursing Responses In Common Counseling Situations

Ineffective Response	Analysis	Effective Response	Analysis
Situation A: *You walk into the room of Ms. Goldstein, who learned earlier in the day that her tumor is malignant. She is crying.*			
"Oh cheer up! Tomorrow's got to be a brighter day."	Provides false reassurance; communicates insensitivity to client's feelings.	Touch forearm and sit next to her quietly. After several minutes, say, "I can't even begin to imagine how difficult this must be for you. Please let me know if there is anything I can do to help."	Uses touch, silence, and caring appropriately
Situation B: *You have been teaching 60-year-old Mr. Hyong diabetic self-care for 4 days and he is still asking the same questions and refusing to administer his own insulin or check his blood sugar.*			
"Well, I guess we are getting nowhere here. Is there anyone else who might be able to do this for you?"	Rejects client without first evaluating the teaching plan and exploring client variables that might be hindering learning.	"We may have a bit of a problem here. . . . I hear you asking the same questions every day. Let's see if together we can't figure out why this isn't making sense to you."	Enlists client in problem solving
Situation C: *The daughter of an elderly client with emphysema stops you at the nursing desk and starts screaming that none of the nurses is helping her mother.*			
"That's just not true! I was in your mother's room myself for a good part of the morning."	Gives a defensive response; may invite combat.	"I'm hearing a lot of concern from you about your mom and the care she is receiving. Tell me more about why you feel that the nurses aren't doing enough."	Affirms the daughter's concern and opens the door to communication that may reveal the daughter's true needs
Situation D: *One morning you walk into the room of an older resident who had withdrawn and become totally dependent on the nurses for basic care on her transfer into the nursing home. You are surprised to discover that she has washed and dressed herself—for the first time.*			
"Well, I'm happy to see that you have rejoined the ranks of the living. Did you wash off your glasses?"	Misses opportunity to celebrate the resident's achievement of an important goal.	Hugs resident warmly, looks her in the eye, and exclaims, "Don't you look wonderful today? What are you celebrating?" Defers an assessment of how thorough the morning care has been until later.	Rejoices spontaneously in the resident's achievement and reinforces this behavior. Gives the resident a reason to continue to make progress. Uses touch appropriately.
Situation E: *A 42-year-old male client who is in the step-down unit following a massive heart attack repeatedly tells you how pretty you are while you are assisting with his care. When you attempt to help him out of bed, he squeezes your breast.*			
Turn beet red, try to stammer a response, and flee the room.	Loses control of the situation. Is unable to meet the client's needs because own needs take precedence.	"Please stop. I am not comfortable with your remarks and I most certainly will not allow you to touch me like this. Often men feel like they need to test their virility and attractiveness after a serious illness. I am wondering if that might not be behind some of your behavior this morning?"	Retains control of the situation and keeps the focus on the client's needs. The nurse's second statement normalizes the client's behavior and gives him an opening to share his feelings. The nurse makes no judgment until all the data are in.

(continued)

Table 23-2 *(continued)*
An Analysis of Nursing Responses In Common Counseling Situations

Ineffective Response	Analysis	Effective Response	Analysis
Situation F: *You are helping Mr. Stein, who has been on bed rest for 2 weeks because of a painful and debilitating illness, out of bed. A fiercely independent man, he is embarrassed to need your support and looks disgusted with himself when he steps on your foot.*			
"What's the problem, Honey? Haven't been eating your Wheaties?"	Uses terms of endearment, which often denote disrespect and condescension to clients, no matter in what spirit they are uttered.	"No problem, Mr. Stein, my husband steps on my toes all the time when we go dancing!" After a few minutes . . . "It must be hard when you are used to doing everything for yourself to all of a sudden find yourself needing others for simple things . . . ?"	Uses humor and empathy appropriately; invites the client to share his feelings.
Situation G: *Ms. Berretta recently underwent surgery resulting in a urinary diversion. She should be able to change her own ostomy bag by this time but she is still unwilling to look at the stoma, and participate alone in her care. The nurses are getting impatient with her "childish" refusals to learn.*			
"Really Helen, I'll do it myself but you'll be the loser once you get home with this thing and there's no one around to help."	Uses a threat in an attempt to coerce learning (negative reinforcement). Displays unwillingness to explore what is blocking Ms. Berretta's readiness to learn.	Before beginning Ms. Beretta's care: "I think we need to talk before your treatment today. You will be discharged soon and I want you to feel confident about caring for your stoma. I understand that until you can accept it, you don't want to learn anything about it. Would you like to talk about this with me or would you prefer me to make a referral to someone else?"	Communicates respect for client and sensitivity to her needs, without ignoring what is a real problem. Offers the possibility of a referral to another health care professional if the client so wishes.
Situation H: *Ms. Congar is an alert 70-year-old woman who was admitted for a simple hypertension workup but has developed numerous complications and currently is in her fourth week of hospitalization. She has grown progressively more demanding and crotchety and now uses her call light several times each hour. She is a single woman without family or close friends.*			
Floor nurse to an agency nurse who does not know Ms. Congar: "Watch out for the witch in Room 52. Don't let her get to you . . . nothing pleases her."	Fails to see the client as a human with unique needs—the most effective block to communication.	Floor nurse to agency nurse: "We have really been having problems with Ms. Congar. She is so sick of being hospitalized right now that nothing pleases her. I try to make it a point to drop into her room frequently to see if she needs anything and then she doesn't use the light so often. Good luck."	Acknowledges a real problem but also offers a constructive solution; may be just enough information to help the agency nurse establish a meaningful relationship with the client, and thus be sympathetic to her needs.

uncooperative or noncompliant clients as well as a list of nursing diagnoses for which counseling is the primary intervention. Sometimes a client needs specialized counseling by nurses with advanced training or other healthcare professionals. In these cases, the best thing you can offer the client is a referral to the appropriate professional (eg, psychologist or psychiatrist, social worker, clergy, financial counselor, sex therapist, or occupational therapist). In other cases a simple referral to community-based resources, such as a neighborhood support group, may be all the client needs. In each of the clinical chapters in this text you will see a display entitled "HelpScan," which will begin to familiarize you with local resources. When making a referral you must be sure to address any barriers that may prevent the client from using the referral source. Clients may fail to follow up with a referral for financial reasons, because they do not understand the reason for or value the referral, because they lack transportation, or because the agency is not open during the times when they are free.

Short-Term Counseling

Short-term counseling focuses on the immediate problem or concern of the client or family. It can be a relatively minor concern or a major crisis, but whatever the situation it needs immediate attention (Fig. 23-6).

In counseling situations, the nurse does not tell the client what to do to solve the problem but instead assists and guides problem solving or decision making. Many people lack the knowledge and skills to approach a problem systematically. This is where the teaching and counseling roles can be combined to help the client solve the dilemma successfully.

The nursing process becomes an essential tool for the nurse in guiding and teaching the client. Nurses are educated to approach all nursing situations in a logical, systematic way. In a crisis situation, whether minor or major, the nurse can share problem-solving abilities with the client. The nursing process was used to organize the nurse–client counseling situation described in the accompanying box.

An example of when short-term counseling could be used is during a **situational crisis**, which occurs when a client faces an event or situation that causes a disruption in life. For example, a male client in the hospital finds out that his spouse has been involved in a car accident. His spouse received only a few scratches, but their only car was demolished. The nurse is in an excellent position to help the client decide what can be done to solve this situational crisis. The nurse can guide the client in solving the travel, financial, and emotional difficulties that arise as a result of the accident. This holistic approach is especially necessary because the crisis could adversely affect the client's recovery.

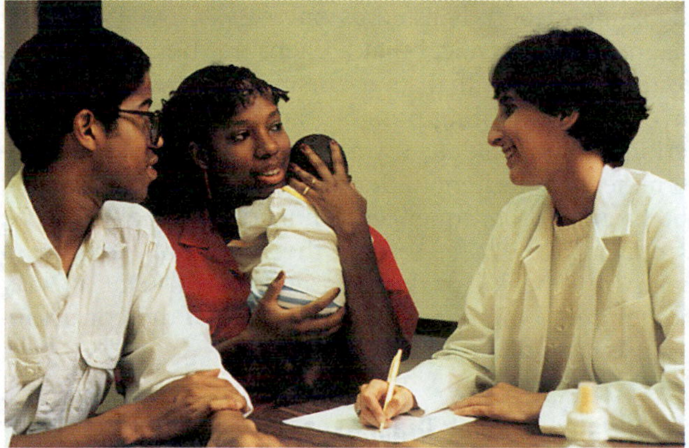

Figure 23-6
Counseling may involve a relatively minor concern that needs immediate attention. (Photo by Gates Rhodes, courtesy of School of Nursing, University of Pennsylvania.)

Long-Term Counseling

Counseling is considered *long-term* when it extends over a prolonged period. A client may need the counsel of the nurse at daily, weekly, or monthly intervals. A client experiencing a developmental crisis may need long-term counseling. A **developmental crisis** can occur when a person is going through a developmental stage or passage. For example, many women going through menopause need the assistance of a nurse when adjusting to the changes they experience. Nurses can lead support groups for the purpose of group counseling.

Another example of long-term counseling occurs when a nurse counsels a client who is breastfeeding. The nurse may give assistance and guidance until the baby is weaned, which could be over 2 to 3 years. This type of counseling is often done over the telephone, which saves the client the inconvenience of traveling to meet with the nurse.

Many hospital specialty units provide clients with a telephone number to call for counseling after discharge. Clients are often relieved to know they can call to talk to a nurse at any time of the day or night. After experiencing the close observation and supervision of hospitalization, this telephone connection has helped many clients make the transition from acute care to home care.

Motivational Counseling

Motivational counseling involves discussing feelings and incentives with the client. Nurses often become frustrated because their clients do not seem to want to get better or to learn how to care for themselves. Perhaps individual clients may not have the inner drive or motivation to cooperate in their own health care. Clients often express the thought, "I have nothing to live for." A nurse who has established a helping relationship with the client can help him or her work through these feelings of despair. The nurse may be able to get the client to talk about what is generating disinterest in recovery. If a problem is identified, the nurse and client can use the problem-solving technique to work toward an acceptable solution.

If a client shows an unwillingness to participate in learning activities, the nurse can assess any factors from the past or present that might be negatively influencing motivation for learning. Sometimes, if the nurse explains the need for certain knowledge and the consequences of not learning the material, the client will become more receptive to the teaching–learning process. A trial learning session can be suggested to allow the client to see what the sessions will be like. If the nurse uses the nurs-

An Example of Problem Solving That Follows the Nursing Process

Situation

Monday, 7:30 PM, Amy Purcell has been admitted to the children's unit with dehydration resulting from diarrhea. Amy is responding well to IV fluids. Her mother is visibly distraught.

Assessing

Amy is doing well but will need 24 hours of IV therapy.

Amy and her twin sister Susan have never been separated from their parents or each other. They are 2 years old.

Ms. Purcell has no idea of who will care for Susan when Mr. Purcell goes to work in the morning.

The Purcells have no regular child-care arrangements and have no family members in the area.

Ms. Purcell wants to stay with Amy during her hospitalization.

The Purcells' neighbor is home during the day. Sometimes Amy and Susan play at her house.

There is a day-care center near their home, but Susan might be upset about going there. It's also expensive.

Mr. Purcell cannot afford to take Tuesday off but will take Wednesday morning off.

Insurance does not cover a private room, which would allow Susan to come to stay in the hospital too.

Diagnosing

Anxiety related to stress of daughter's hospitalization, need for child care for Susan, and uncertain resources.

Planning Goal

Ms. Purcell will demonstrate decreased anxiety over the care of Susan during Amy's hospitalization.

Together, Ms. Purcell and the nurse have planned the following:

- The neighbor will come to the Purcell home to care for Susan when Mr. Purcell leaves for work on Tuesday morning.
- The neighbor will bring Susan to the hospital for the afternoon visiting hours to be with Ms. Purcell and Amy.
- Mr. Purcell will come to the hospital after work to have dinner with the family.
- Mr. Purcell will take Susan home for bedtime.
- On Wednesday morning, Mr. Purcell will take off work in the morning. He and Susan will go to the hospital to pick up Ms. Purcell and Amy.

Implementing

Plan implemented by the Purcells with support of the nursing staff.

Evaluating

Ms. Purcell told the nurse that she feels that both Amy and Susan did well with the care they received from their parents. The family's stress was minimized and she is relieved that everything went so well. The nurse decides that the goals were met.

ing process approach for counseling, a satisfactory change in the client's motivation may be achieved.

When a nurse assesses a motivational problem, considering the client's cultural values is important. Often the way a person feels about something is strongly influenced by cultural background. For instance, if a person has grown up in a family in which illness is perceived as an inevitable result of aging, it will be difficult to motivate that person to practice preventive measures for health. These problems seem insurmountable, yet a caring nurse can work toward helping the client become oriented toward promoting self-health. When discouraged, the nurse can confer with a colleague to help solve client-centered problems.

Noncompliant Client. When the nurse's best counseling efforts fail to produce motivation in the client to adhere to a treatment regimen, the client may be described as **noncompliant**. Noncompliance, defined as a person's informed decision not to adhere to a therapeutic recommendation, is listed as one of NANDA's accepted diagnoses. It is critical that a client not be labeled noncompliant until exhaustive nursing energies have been invested in exploring possible factors that may be interfering with the client's learning readiness. Once it is determined that a client understands his or her options and the probable consequences of noncompliance, the nurse is ethically bound to respect the treatment decisions a competent person makes. An ethical consultation may be helpful to the nurse who is unsure of the correct response in such a case.

Related Nursing Diagnoses

Nursing diagnoses for which counseling may be indicated are highlighted in the accompanying box.

Examples of Nursing Diagnoses

Counseling

Numerous NANDA-approved nursing diagnoses exist for which counseling is the appropriate nursing intervention. Some of these diagnoses follow:

- Altered Parenting
- Altered Role Performance
- Anxiety
- Body Image Disturbance
- Decisional Conflict (specify)
- Defensive Coping
- Dysfunctional Grieving
- Fear
- Health-Seeking Behaviors (specify)
- Hopelessness
- Impaired Adjustment
- Impaired Social Interaction
- Ineffective Denial
- Ineffective Family Coping
- Ineffective Individual Coping
- Personal Identity Disturbance
- Powerlessness
- Self-Esteem Disturbance
- Social Isolation
- Spiritual Distress (Distress of the Human Spirit)

Key Points

- Nurses use communication skills in their roles as teachers and counselors.
- The nursing roles of teacher and counselor require the use of the nursing process; the teaching–learning process follows the steps of the nursing process.
- With the trend toward shorter hospital stays, clients and families need more extensive instruction for home care. However, as the importance of teaching increases, the hospital time for teaching decreases. Consequently, the quality of teaching must improve.
- The outcomes of effective teaching and counseling include high-level wellness and related self-care practices; disease prevention or early detection; quick recovery from illness with minimal to no sequelae; enhanced ability to adjust to developmental life changes and acute, chronic, and terminal illness; and family acceptance of the lifestyle changes necessitated by the illness or disability of a family member.
- Learning can be divided into the following three domains: (1) cognitive learning, which involves the storing and recalling of new knowledge and information in the brain; (2) psychomotor learning, which indicates that a physical skill has been learned; and (3) affective learning, which involves changes in attitudes, values, and feelings.
- Assessment of learning needs focuses on the knowledge, attitude, and skills the client needs to independently manage health care; learning readiness; the physical ability to learn; and client strengths. Factors affecting each are explored, often in consultation with the family and significant others.
- Nursing diagnoses are developed that identify health problems related to client deficits in knowledge, attitudes, or skills.
- Teaching plans specify measurable learning objectives, related content, and specific teaching strategies and learning activities. A contractual agreement may facilitate learning.
- Implementing the teaching plan requires use of interpersonal skills as well as effective communication techniques. Teaching is part of the working phase of the helping relationship.
- The evaluation of learning provides the information needed for revisions and for documenting that learning has occurred. Positive reinforcement affirms and encourages learning.
- Counseling involves the nurse in teaching and assisting the client to learn problem-solving techniques.
- The three types of counseling are (1) short-term counseling, which focuses on an immediate problem; (2) long-term counseling, which extends over a prolonged period; and (3) motivational counseling, which involves discussing feelings and incentives with the client.
- Counseling may be needed for assisting the client through crises or for motivating the client to work toward health promotion.

Bibliography

American Nurses Association. (1994). *The scope of practice for nursing informatics.* Washington, DC: ANA.

Aquilera, D. C. (1994). *Crisis intervention: Theory and methodology* (7th ed.). St. Louis: Mosby–Year Book.

Archbold, P.G. et al. (1995). The PREP system of nursing intervention: A pilot test with families caring for older members. *Research in Nursing and Health, 18*(1), 3–16.

Babcock, D.E. & Miller, M.A. (1994). *Client education: Theory and practice.* St. Louis: Mosby.

Barnes, L.P. (1994). Useful tools in patient teaching—Interviewing skills. *MCN, 19*(5), 289.

Black, K. (1983). *Short-term counseling: A humanistic approach for the helping professions.* Menlo Park, CA: Addison-Wesley.

Bloom, B. S. (1956). *Taxonomy of educational objectives: The classification of educational goals.* New York: David McKay.

Bolwell, C. (1993). *Directory of education software for nursing* (5th ed.). New York: National League for Nursing; Athens, OH: Fuld Institute for Technology in Nursing Education.

Brazen, L. & Roth, R.A. (1995). Using learning style preferences for perioperative clinical education. *AORN Journal, 61*(1), 189, 191–195.

Canobbio, M. M. (1996). *Mosby's handbook of patient teaching.* St. Louis: Mosby.

Cordell, B. & Smith-Blair, N. (1994). Streamlined charting for patient education. *Nursing, 24*(1), 57–59.

Dellasega, C., Clark, D., McCreary, D., Schan, P. & Helmuth, A. (1994). Nursing process: Teaching elderly clients. *Journal of Gerontological Nursing, 20*(1), 31–41.

Doak, C.C., Doak, L.G. & Root, J.H. (1995). *Teaching patients with low literacy skills.* Philadelphia: Lippincott.

Elliot, L. & Kulwicki, G. (1993). Improving patient education documentation. *Nursing Management, 24*(10), 61–62.

Farthing, M. (1994). Health education needs of a Hutterite colony. *The Canadian Nurse, 90*(7), 20–26.

Griffiths, M. (1995). Patient education needs: Opinions of oncology nurses and their patients. *Oncology Nursing Forum, 22*(1), 139–144.

Hannah, K. J., Ball, M. J., & Edwards, M. J. A. (1994). *Introduction to nursing informatics.* New York: Springer-Verlag.

Harvey, C., Dixon, M. & Padberg, N. (1995). Support group for families of trauma patients: A unique approach. *Critical Care Nurse, 15*(4), 59–63.

Hussey, L.C. (1994). Minimizing effects of low literacy on medication knowledge and compliance among the elderly. *Clinical Nursing Research, 3*(2), 132–145.

Jabeck, M.E. (1994). Teaching the elderly: A commonsense approach. *Nursing, 24*(5), 70–71.

Jacono, B. & Jacono, J. (1995). The impact of teacher characteristics on teaching. *Journal of Nursing Staff Development, 11*(3), 146–149.

Jubeck, M. E. (1994). Teaching the elderly: A commonsense approach. *Nursing, 24*(5), 70–71.

Kelly, P. (1992). Counseling patients with HIV. *RN, 55*(2), 54–58.

Knowles, M. S. (1980). *The modern practice of adult education: From pedagogy to androgogy* (2nd ed.). Chicago: Follett.

Knowles, M. S. (1984). *The adult-learner: A neglected species* (3rd ed.). Houston: Gulf Publishing.

Lindberg, C.E. (1995). Perinatal transmission of HIV: How to counsel women. *MCN, 20*(4), 207–212.

Logan, J. & Boss, M. (1993). Nurses' learning patterns. *Canadian Nurse, 89*(3), 18–22.

Lorig, K. (1992). *Patient education: A practical approach.* St. Louis: Mosby–Year Book.

Melnyle, B.M. (1994). Coping with unplanned childhood hospitalization: Effects of informational intervention on mother and children. *Nursing Research, 43*(1), 50–55.

Miller, B. (1994). Determination of reading comprehension level for effective patient health education materials. *Nursing Research, 43*(2), 118–119.

Newbold, S. K. (1996). Maximizing technology for cost effective staff education and training. In B. R. Heller, M. E. Mills, & C. A. Romano (Eds.). *Information management in nursing and health care.* Springhouse, PA: Springhouse.

Price, J.L. & Cordell, B. (1994). Cultural diversity and patient teaching. *Journal of Continuing Education in Nursing, 25*(4), 163–166.

Rankin, S. H., & Stallings, K. D. (1990). *Patient education* (2nd ed.). Philadelphia: Lippincott.

Redman, B. K. (1992). *The process of patient education* (7th ed.). St. Louis: Mosby.

Reele, B.L. (1994). effect of counseling on quality of life for individuals with cancer and their families. *Cancer Nursing, 17*(2), 101–112.

Ruppert, R.A. (1996). Caring for the lay caregiver. *American Journal of Nursing, 96*(3), 40–45.

Schoenly, L. (1994). Teaching in the affective domain. *Journal of Continuing Education in Nursing, 25*(5), 209–212.

Sciartelli, C.H. (1995). Using a clinical pathway approach to document patient teaching for breast cancer surgical procedures. *Oncology Nursing Forum, 22*(1), 139–144.

Seley, J. (1994). Ten strategies for successful patient teaching. *AJN, 94*(11), 63–65.

Sitzer, C.R. (1995). A community-based breast cancer education and screening program for elderly women. *Geriatric Nursing, 16*(4), 151–154.

Wally, B. (1994). Reading, writing and health. *Canadian Nurse, 90*(2), 29–32.

Watson, J. (1985). *Nursing: The philosophy and science of caring.* Denver: Colorado University Press.

Weaver, J. (1995). Patient education: An innovative computer approach. *Nursing Management, 26*(7), 78–83.

Weinrich, S.P. & Boyd, M. (1992). Education in the elderly—Adapting and evaluating teaching tools. *Journal of Gerontological Nursing, 18*(1), 15–20.

Wong, M. (1992). Self-care instructions: Do patients understand educational materials? *Focus on Critical Care, 19*(2), 47–49.

Chapter 24

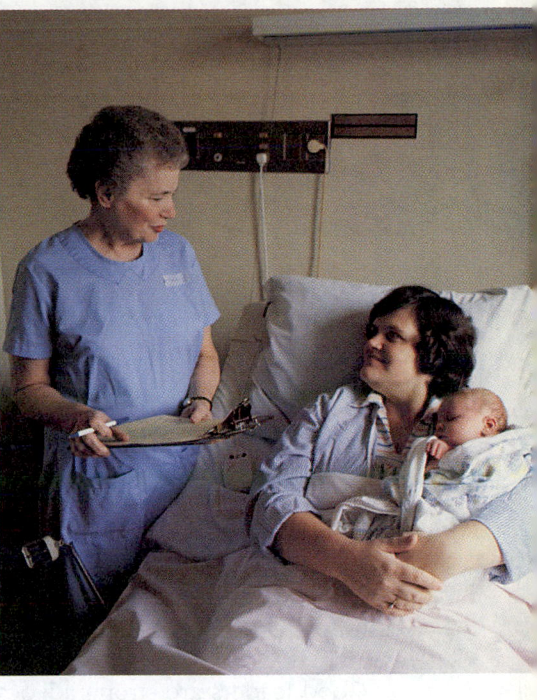

Leader, Researcher, and Advocate

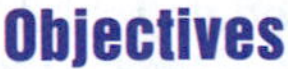

Objectives

After studying this chapter, the learner should be able to:

Define key terms used in the chapter.

Identify the qualities, four skills, and three styles of leaders.

List the four managerial functions.

Summarize the steps in the process of change.

Describe areas in which the beginning nurse can develop leadership skills that enhance the caregiver role.

Compare the strengths and limitations of three sources of nursing knowledge.

Describe three ways the beginning nurse can use research to enhance the caregiver role.

Explain different ways nurse caregivers can be advocates for clients.

Describe the nurse advocate's role in situations requiring ethical decision making.

Explain how two types of advance directives promote client dignity and well-being.

Key Terms

advocacy
assertiveness
autonomy
change
change agent
knowledge
authoritative knowledge
scientific knowledge
traditional knowledge
leadership
autocratic leadership
democratic leadership
laissez-faire leadership
transformational leadership
management
mentorship
power
preceptorship
professionalism
variables

Many changes in society and in the healthcare system are jeopardizing human health and well-being. Never before has there been such a need for nurses to work competently and collaboratively with other healthcare professionals to secure cost-effective quality health care for all. To do this successfully nurses must be skilled leaders, advocates, and researchers.

Good leaders are strong advocates of clients' rights because leadership and advocacy complement each other. Research provides a knowledge base on which the leader and advocate can build. Research adds the dignity of professionalism to teaching, counseling, and communication—all nursing skills applied to the leadership role.

Although some nurses function as full-time leaders, researchers, or advocates, this chapter explores how the roles of leader, researcher, and advocate enhance the basic caregiver role of the nurse. It takes time and experience to develop these skills; beginning nurses can monitor their progress by periodically reviewing the checklist provided to improve these skills.

The Nurse as Leader

Leadership Dynamics

Leadership is the ability to direct or motivate an individual or group toward the achievement of predetermined goals. Leaders have power, whether it is explicit or implied. Much of this power depends on the leadership style and how leadership responsibilities are fulfilled. The dynamics of leadership involve applying that power to growth or change. Nurses who use leadership skills can become proficient in effecting desired changes in many areas, including their clients' health patterns, the healthcare agency, the community, the nursing profession, and the healthcare system in general.

Leadership Qualities

Most people would agree that leaders should be dynamic, enthusiastic, and self-directed. They need to be comfortable with themselves (ie, have a positive self-image) and present themselves as role models to followers. Ideally they possess a vision that energizes the group and calls forth the best efforts of members. Critical thinkers and responsible decision makers, they commit high energy to goal achievement and are skilled in enlisting support and cooperation.

Leaders value learning and must be knowledgeable. Because it is impossible for nurse leaders to be knowledgeable about all aspects of the profession, they develop and use resources. They use one another and other healthcare workers as resources, respecting one another's expertise. Political awareness is also required of the nurse leader. Knowing how legislation at the local, state or province, and national levels affects health care allows the nurse to make informed decisions when voting for and supporting candidates.

Flexibility is a must for leaders. All nursing functions and roles require flexibility. The needs of clients, families, and the nursing team can change from minute to minute. A flexible, knowledgeable nurse is a welcomed team member.

Although aggression is rarely suited to the leadership role, leaders need assertiveness in nearly all leadership situations. It is used extensively when effecting change. Assertiveness is a learned quality all nurses can develop. (Assertiveness is discussed in Chapter 22.)

Leadership qualities exist in every nurse. With education and practice, these qualities can be developed to the point where a nurse is skilled in the many behaviors necessary for leadership. A discussion of each of these qualities and skills is beyond the scope of this text, but the checklist provides an overview of how one might approach the role of leader.

Leadership Skills

The four basic types of skills needed for nursing leadership are the following:

Communication skills—the ability to establish trusting interpersonal relationships with clients, peers, subordinates, and superiors that maximize goal achievement and enhance the personal growth of all participants

Checklist for the Beginning Nurse Who Wishes to Develop Leadership, Research, and Advocacy Skills

Basic Attitudes and Skills

Read the statements on the right and circle the appropriate response: (1) rarely characterizes me, (2) sometimes characterizes me, and (3) often characterizes me.

- ☐ 1 2 3 — 1. I am self-directed. I know what I want and take the necessary steps to get it.
- ☐ 1 2 3 — 2. I know my strengths and limitations and feel confident with who I am and who I am becoming.
- ☐ 1 2 3 — 3. I get an idea and energize others to help me "make it happen."
- ☐ 1 2 3 — 4. I coordinate or direct the activities of others, matching their abilities to the necessary task.
- ☐ 1 2 3 — 5. I reason objectively about a situation without letting my feelings or those of others bias my analysis.
- ☐ 1 2 3 — 6. Once I have identified a problem I work at it until I resolve it—to the extent that this is within my power.
- ☐ 1 2 3 — 7. When I need help, I know where to find it and ask for it.
- ☐ 1 2 3 — 8. I recognize the talents of others and offer sincere compliments.
- ☐ 1 2 3 — 9. I accept compliments and enjoy my success.
- ☐ 1 2 3 — 10. I confront individuals who are abusing my rights or those of others in my group.
- ☐ 1 2 3 — 11. I use assertiveness techniques when defending rights.
- ☐ 1 2 3 — 12. I am flexible and can change direction once I see the value of another course of action.
- ☐ 1 2 3 — 13. I follow an appropriate chain of command when problem solving.
- ☐ 1 2 3 — 14. I question how nursing interventions might be improved.

The higher your score the better. Reread the statements where you checked "1" and see how you might plan to improve in these areas.

Beginning Execution of Role Responsibilities: Leader, Researcher, Advocate

Read the list of behaviors on the right and check the appropriate box—met or not met.

MET	NOT MET	
____	____	1. Recognize some personal need you have been ignoring and take steps to ensure that it is met.
____	____	2. Think of some group you belong to (eg, school, work, church, or social) whose members' needs are not being met and plan with other members to tackle the problem.
____	____	3. Recognize the special advocacy needs of a client you believe is being underserved by the health care system. Become an advocate for this client.
____	____	4. Find a nursing research study that recommends a specific type of care for one of your clients. Implement the recommendation and compare your findings with those of the researchers.
____	____	5. Identify a researchable problem in your area of nursing practice. Describe what might make a good study.
____	____	6. Join a professional nursing organization and become an active member.
____	____	7. Analyze the media's portrayal of nurses in a specific television program, film, or book. Talk with a friend about how this portrayal of nursing influences your profession. Share your comments with the producer or author.
____	____	8. Contact your legislator to share your views about pending legislation.
____	____	9. Think about leaders you admire and respect; interview current nursing leaders; develop a plan for personal professional growth and development.
____	____	10. Develop a mentoring relationship with a nursing leader.

Problem-solving skills—the ability to analyze all sides of a problem, to explore multiple options, and to work to a creative solution; the ability to plan, implement, and stabilize change

Management skills—the ability to direct others toward goal achievement; this ability involves the recognition and fostering of unique talents and skills of others and the ability to match these with necessary tasks; organizational skills; financial skills; and the ability to generate and use resources wisely

Self-evaluation skills—the ability to honestly assess one's effectiveness and to accept both praise and blame; the ability to direct personal professional growth and development

Leadership Styles

Different styles of leadership are commonly identified in the nurse's work settings. Generally speaking, it is best for nurses to use the leadership style with which they are most comfortable if that style is effective for the task at hand and for the groups they are leading. The variables of the nurse's own personality, the group personality, and the tasks or objectives to be accomplished must be considered in each leadership situation (Fig. 24-1).

Autocratic Leadership. **Autocratic leadership**, also called directive leadership, occurs when the leader assumes complete control over the decisions and activities of the group. The nurse with an autocratic personality can be described as "firm, insistent, self-assured, and dominating with or without intent, and keeps at the center of attention" (Douglass, 1992). There can be extremes in autocratic leadership, such as a leader who makes all the decisions for the workers or followers without consideration of the followers' ideas or feelings.

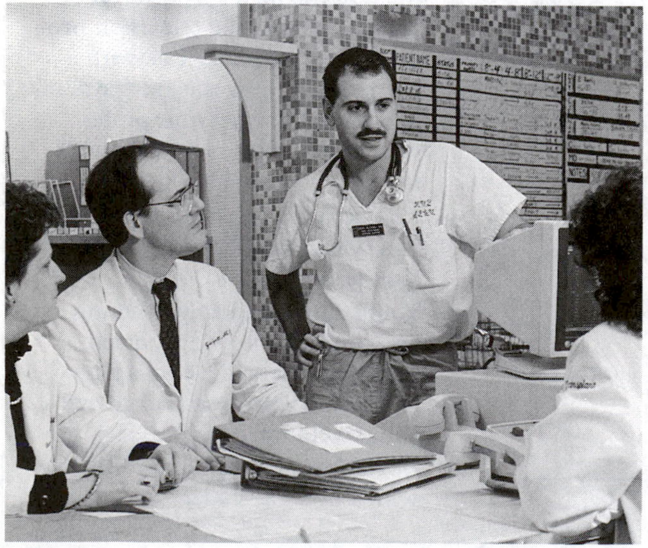

Figure 24-1
Leadership styles vary. The nurse should choose one that is comfortable and will be effective for the situation.

Many nurses are used to working under an autocratic leader. This approach has been used in most hospital settings until recently. It seems to have evolved from the military and religious images that nursing has developed historically. These images and this type of leadership are gradually being replaced by the democratic style of leadership, as nurses demand more participation in decision making.

Situation. Nurse A discovers that one of her clients is bleeding excessively from his surgical incision. She knows that he needs immediate attention, so she begins to give specific orders to another team member to attend to the needs of the other clients. She tells the registered nurse on her team to call the surgical resident to come as soon as possible. She implements a nursing plan of care to prevent further blood loss or complications.

Nurse A chose the autocratic style of leadership in this situation so that all of the necessary tasks would be accomplished immediately. Although she rarely uses this style, she implemented it effectively in this emergency situation.

Democratic Leadership. **Democratic leadership**, also called participative leadership, is characterized by a sense of equality among the leader and the followers. Decisions and activities are shared. The followers are encouraged to develop their skills and strengths within the group. The group and leader strive to work to accomplish mutually set goals and outcomes. The leader needs to develop skills in group dynamics to apply this type of leadership effectively.

More nurses currently are working toward the democratic style of leadership. Nurses, as professionals, tend to respond well to this type when they are the followers and feel more comfortable when they are the leaders of democratic groups. Group satisfaction and motivation can be excellent benefits of this style.

Situation. Nurse B, a head nurse, observes that staff members have not been documenting client teaching and learning in the nurse's progress notes. Nurse B is not sure why this has occurred but believes that this problem must be solved. He calls a staff meeting and leads a discussion to seek information on possible causes and planning strategies.

Nurse B has decided that staff members need to be included in the problem-solving approach. He thinks the staff will be more motivated to document their teaching and the clients' learning if they have a say in how the changes will be implemented. Nurse B has used the democratic style of leadership.

Laissez-Faire Leadership. In **laissez-faire leadership**, also called nondirective leadership, the leader relinquishes all power to the group. This encourages independent activity by the group members. An outsider would be unable to identify the leader in such a group.

This style depends on the strengths of the followers to direct the group activities.

This style is rarely seen in the hospital setting because task achievement is difficult when each nurse is working independently. However, it can be used effectively when the leader wants a problem to be solved completely by the group members. It has been successful in cases in which there is resistance to a certain policy or change and the leader allows the group to work to achieve an acceptable solution.

Situation. Nurse C, a clinical coordinator, has read an interesting research study that supports a change in the current instructions being given to new mothers who are breastfeeding. The article, with a summary of findings, is posted in all of the nurses' stations in the maternity unit.

Nurse C is using a laissez-faire leadership style and is confident that individual staff members are capable professionals who are concerned with keeping up with current research findings that they can use to improve their nursing care.

Transformational Leadership. A **transformational leader** creates revolutionary change and commits to the personal and professional growth of self and others. Qualities that describe transformational leaders and strategies for personal and professional transformation are highlighted in the accompanying box.

Situation. Nurse D, a transformational leader, is troubled by the plight of women and children in the inner city where she lives. She unites with other nurses and healthcare professionals to design and implement strategies to meet their needs; within 18 months a funded nursing center is up and running, improving maternal–child outcomes. The founding group of healthcare pro-

Transformational Leadership

Qualities of the Transformational Leader: Research Findings

- Individual consideration
  - Promotes others' growth
  - Recognizes and supports others' needs and feelings
  - Gives positive feedback and recognition
- Charisma
  - Inspires and motivates
  - Demonstrates enthusiasm
  - Communicates in a positive manner
- Intellectual stimulation
  - Creates a questioning environment
  - Acts as a mentor
  - Challenges others to grow and learn

Strategies for Personal Transformation

- Self-empowerment
  - Accept responsibility for own thoughts, feelings, and actions
  - Choose to think and behave in a positive, growth-promoting manner
  - Use affirmation and visualization to assist in changing limiting beliefs and attitudes
- Role modeling
  - Identify personal strengths and weaknesses in relationship to the qualities of the transformational leader
  - Practice qualities that need to be developed
- Positive attitude
  - Maintain a positive realistic approach
  - Focus on the vision
- Support
  - Seek support from others in implementing personal and professional changes
  - Network with like-minded friends and colleagues

Qualities That Describe the Transformational Leader

- Vulnerability
  - Communicates authentically and openly
  - Expresses emotions as well as ideas
  - Shares self with others
- Knowledge, concern, and courage
  - Seeks knowledge through study and experience
  - Shows concern and caring for others
  - Willing to take risks
- Feminine attributes
  - Maintains accessibility
  - Pays attention to process as well as outcomes
  - Practices balance in lifestyle

Strategies for Professional Transformation

- Vision crafting
  - Use a questioning approach to create a vision for practice
  - Ask what and how, not why
  - Communicate the vision in a context of finding common ground
  - Demonstrate passion for the vision
  - Create a specific action plan for implementation
  - Develop and commit to an evaluation and feedback process
- Empowerment of others
  - Discover what is empowering to staff and support them in it
  - Develop others' competence and expertise
  - Role model self-empowerment

Gurka, A.M. (1995). Transformational leadership: Qualities and strategies for the CNS. *Clinical Nurse Specialist, 9*(1), 170, 173. Used with permission.

fessionals continues to meet monthly to dream about future strategies and to support one another in the work that is being done. They are most proud of the new sense of esteem and independence demonstrated by many of the women they serve.

Leadership and Management

All nurses are leaders. Some nurses, because of their positions in the healthcare system, are also managers. The role of the nurse manager is to plan, organize, direct, and control available human, material, and financial resources to deliver quality care to clients and families.

Planning—identifying problems, developing goals, objectives, and related strategies
Organizing—mobilizing resources to meet objectives
Directing—leading others in goal achievement
Controlling—implementing mechanisms for ongoing evaluation

Hersey and Blanchard (1977) substituted motivating for directing as one of the four management functions. This substitution is compatible with the recent shift in emphasis in organizations from management (used to control enterprises) to leadership (used to bring out the best in people and to respond quickly to changes). Chief nurse executives have come to realize that nurse managers must be effective leaders to be successful. In all likelihood, nursing units with low morale, high turnover, and frequent physician and client complaints have unskilled leaders. Nursing managers who cannot create healthy group environments, who fail to define interpersonal issues that lower morale, and who are unable to develop a plan to resolve detrimental interpersonal issues lack leadership skills.

Models of Client Care Delivery

Models of nursing care delivery systems are highlighted in the accompanying box. Over time these have evolved from highly technical, industrial-based, assembly-line models to more professional, self-managed, cross-functional methods. According to Kerfoot, "As nurses have moved to accept more professional status and the responsibility of delegating and working through others, they have moved into advanced practice models in which there is less supervision, more opportunity for independent thought and creativity, and more accountability" (1995, p. 41). What is clear as one studies the evolving models of client care delivery is that professional nurses will be increasingly expected to possess significant managerial competence.

Effecting Change Through Leadership

Change is the process of transforming, altering, or modifying something. It may be planned, unplanned, or developmental. Nursing and the healthcare system are continually changing and evolving. Such factors as the increase in the number of chronically ill and older people, the increase in government and industry intervention in health care, the rising cost of health care, and the

Models of Client Care Delivery

Functional nursing	Nurses and other staff are assigned to specific tasks for a group of clients. Based on the assembly-line concept found in industry; specializing tasks increases efficiency but results in impersonal care
Team nursing	A team made up of a registered nurse and other caregivers provides care to a designated group of clients on a given shift. Modified the depersonalized approach of functional nursing and focused on individual client care
Total care or case nursing	A nurse as caregiver provides total care to a group of clients for a designated shift. A client-centered model; suffers from a lack of continuity between shifts and is expensive because highly paid nurses provide all aspects of care
Primary nursing	A nurse is accountable for planning, evaluating, and directing the care of clients 24 hours a day throughout the client's stay. A method of providing comprehensive, individualized, and consistent care; expensive
Case management	One nurse is responsible for overseeing the quality and financial outcomes of client care; the nurse works collegially with physicians and other caregivers as well as with payers to manage clients along an agreed-upon clinical pathway
Client-centered or client-focused care	Cross-functional teams consisting of groups of professionals and assistive personnel from nursing and other departments work together as a unit-based team to provide care to a given group of clients. Care is designed around the needs of the client and not the needs of the departments or professionals
Collaborative practice model	Nurses and physicians work together in collaborative practice models

changing patterns of healthcare delivery have helped provoke the need for innovation and change in health care.

Many theories of change exist, but most are modifications of the classic theory of change proposed by Kurt Lewin in 1951. Lewin posited the following three stages of change:

Unfreezing: The need for change is recognized.

Moving: Change is initiated after a careful process of planning.

Refreezing: Change becomes operational.

Planned change is a purposeful, systematic effort to alter or bring about change through the intervention of a change agent. Basic questions to consider before planning to make changes are highlighted in the accompanying box. The eight steps in the process of change loosely follow the steps of the nursing process:

1. Recognize symptoms that indicate a change is needed and collect data.
2. Identify a problem to be solved through change. Analyze the symptoms and reach a conclusion. Note resistance or barriers to change and factors that promote the desired change.
3. Determine and analyze alternative solutions to the problem. Consider the advantages, disadvantages, and consequences of each alternative. An analysis of various proposed solutions to a problem may result in using a combination of alternatives.
4. Select a course of action from possible alternatives. It is best to avoid initiating too many courses of action and thereby dissipating resources and energy.
5. Plan for making a change. This step is critical to effect change successfully. Start by stating specific objectives, designing a plan for change, developing timetables, selecting people to assist with making the change, and anticipating how to stabilize change and deal with resistance to change. Unless a plan is clearly designed, effecting change is likely to be a chaotic experience.
6. Implement the selected course of action to effect change. The plan for change is then put into effect. During this period, flexibility is important to adapt to unforeseen problems.
7. Evaluate the effects of change by comparing them with objectives stated in the plan for change. Adjustments can be made in the plan as necessary after evaluation. If the results of evaluation indicate that the course of action selected to solve a problem has been unsuccessful, an adjustment should be made or another course of action selected.
8. Stabilize the change. When a solution to a problem has been found, take measures to make the change permanent. Continue follow-up until the change is firmly established.

The same steps apply whether dealing with individuals or groups. Figure 24-2 illustrates the process of change.

Basic Questions to Consider Before Effecting Change

- ***What is amenable to change?*** The answer to this question may reveal behavior not amenable to change.
- ***How does the group function as a unit?*** A change agent can make certain deductions concerning forces within a group favoring change and forces likely to resist change.
- ***What resources are available to help make a change?*** If specific resources are unavailable, adjustments must be made in keeping with available resources.
- ***Is the person or group ready for change and, if so, at what rate can it be reasonably expected that change will be accepted?*** The pace of change must be consistent with the person's or group's readiness to assimilate change. *Readiness* is possessing the ability to change.
- ***Are the changes major or minor in nature?*** A series of small changes may be more easily accomplished than one large change. Also, stability in one area in which change has just occurred is necessary before change begins in another area.

Resistance to Change

People may resist change for various reasons. The leader must decide why there is resistance and what techniques will overcome the resistance.

Threat to Self. People tend to view change in terms of how they are affected personally. Personal threats may include a loss of self-esteem, a belief that more work will be required, and a belief that social relationships will be disrupted. For example, when unit management was instituted in health agencies, many nurses resisted because they felt the unit clerks would take away their responsibilities, for example, transcribing physicians' orders.

Lack of Understanding. The person who does not understand the nature of change is likely to resist. The involvement of people affected by change is important to overcome resistance. For example, nurses who do not realize the effectiveness of plans of care tend to resist preparing them because they believe they are not beneficial in providing client care.

Limited Tolerance for Change. Some people simply do not like to function in a state of flux or disequilibrium. A person may understand the need for change but may be unable to cope emotionally with the change itself. For

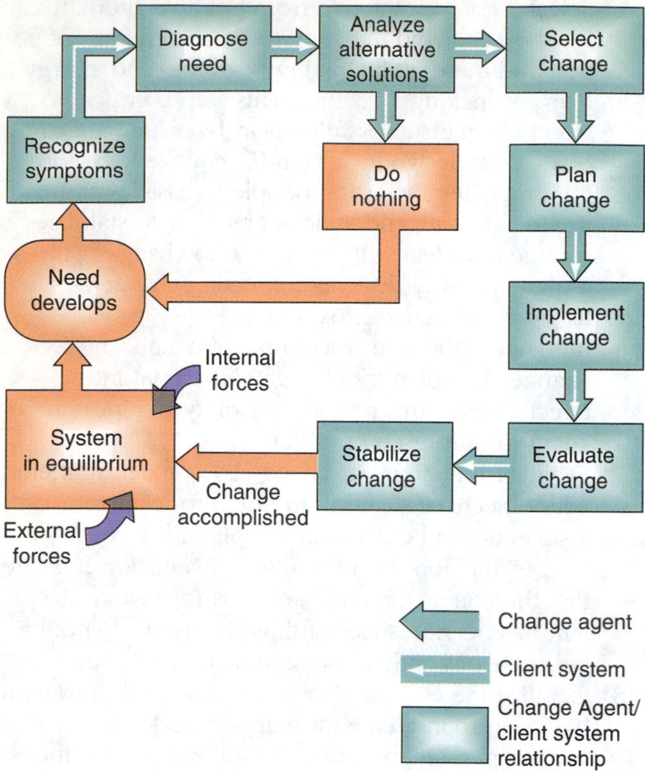

Figure 24-2
A planned change model demonstrating the logical process through which change is planned and implemented. The change agent and client system work together in the *green shaded* area. The *brown* area indicates when change is not taking place. Internal and external forces are at work on the system in equilibrium. (Spradley, B.W. [1980]. Managing change creatively. *Journal of Nursing Administration, 10*[5], 33.)

example, a nurse may resist change because of the confusion a change is likely to cause.

Disagreements About the Benefits of Change. Resistance may occur when the information available to the change agent and those resisting change is different. If the information provided by people resisting change is more accurate and relevant than information held by the change agent, the resistance may be beneficial. As an example, consider a plan that had been effective in implementing home health care in a middle-class section of a city. The supervisor of community-health services proposed that the plan be implemented in a low-income neighborhood. The nurse in charge of the health program in the low-income area resisted, believing that a plan suitable for a middle-class section of the community could not be used in a financially and educationally disadvantaged neighborhood.

Fear of Increased Responsibility. Many people are worried about having more complex responsibilities placed on them. This is especially true if they feel unprepared for the planned changes. The changes may seem overwhelming, so they respond by resisting.

Overcoming Resistance to Change

Nurses, in their leadership roles, find that they often must work to overcome resistance to change. Resistance can be subtle or distinct, gentle or aggressive. Responding to resistance is a leadership challenge in which a person's leadership qualities, leadership style, and knowledge of group dynamics are combined to influence individuals toward a desired outcome. The nurse acting as an agent of change will find the following guidelines helpful for overcoming resistance to change:

- Explain the proposed change to all affected people in simple, concise language.
- List the advantages of the proposed change, both for an individual and for members of a group.
- Relate the proposed change to the existing beliefs and values of the person or group.
- Help overcome resistance by providing opportunities for open communication and feedback.
- Indicate clearly how the change will be evaluated.
- Introduce change gradually. Involve everyone affected by the change in the design and implementation of the process.
- Provide incentives for commitment to change. Incentives may be money, status, time off, or a better working environment.

Power

Nurses who wish to be effective change agents are sensitive to both the uses and abuses of power. **Power**, the ability to influence others to achieve a desired effect, has many sources. Certain management positions within an institution (eg, director of nursing or nursing coordinator) have ascribed power associated with the role. Simultaneously, a group may attribute power to different individuals because of their expertise, leadership, or charisma. When introducing change, it is helpful to recognize and enlist the support of key power players who can then encourage others to become involved. Nursing leaders recognize the strengths and limitations of their own power and encourage the development and constructive use of power in others.

The Nurse Caregiver's Leadership Skills

No one is born a leader. People develop leadership qualities through observation, knowledge, and experience. Nurses develop their leadership qualities in the same way, although they may enter nursing with some background in leadership experiences.

Nursing students and beginning practicing nurses have some leadership responsibilities, but they are still working at developing skills and learning where and how to apply them. Fortunately, they have support systems for guidance.

Computer Applications in Nursing

Computer Use in Nursing Administration

Computers assist the nurse administrator in the planning, monitoring, and evaluation of nursing resources. Major benefits include:

- Better utilization of nursing staff resources
- Improved documentation, communication, and planning
- Standardized nursing practice
- Tracking of nursing services
- Measurement of outcomes
- Improved cost accountability
- Improved patient care (ANA, 1994)

Automated workload measurement systems help the nurse manager to plan staffing and scheduling based on client requirements. Computers help the executive to measure nursing care and resources consumed. The use of computers within the nursing service allows for the tracking of accreditation guidelines and maintenance of consistent standards of care and protocols, and facilitates the audit process.

Nursing administrators can benefit from the office automation functions of word processing, document storage and retrieval, and electronic mail. Personnel management systems are utilized to maintain data regarding degrees, licensure, in-services, continuing education, and performance appraisals.

Nurse executives are interested in using standard nursing terminology to track nursing diagnosis, interventions, and outcomes, to provide for a consistent and high standard of care regardless of the setting. Systems for documenting client care are now incorporating the capability to utilize the standard terminology.

Nurse executives can benefit from the use of computer technology to improve their role in managing resources and overseeing the quality of care that the client receives (Saba, Johnson, & Simpson, 1994).

Areas of Leadership

Leadership should be approached as any new role or skill is approached—slowly and carefully. The nursing student and beginning nurse should be prepared with all of the necessary tools or skills before attempting the new role. Initially, a nurse develops leadership skills in well-defined situations. With each experience, growth occurs and leadership is strengthened. It helps to remember that all nurse managers, nurse administrators, and nursing leaders also began as inexperienced nurses.

Client Care. Even new graduate nurses have leadership responsibilities when they begin working. Nursing leadership begins with nursing care of the individual client (Fig. 24-3). Nurses have to take the initiative in helping clients. Although clients are partners in their care planning, most do not have the knowledge base and skills to direct the plan. Through use of interpersonal skills and effective communication techniques, nurses lead their clients in acquiring new knowledge, solving problems, and changing behaviors.

Employee Responsibilities. Nurses have specific tasks or duties to perform. These tasks are determined by the plan and objective of the healthcare agency. It is important to read job descriptions carefully and to continue to evaluate how institutional factors influence an individual's practice of nursing. Factors that compromise quality care should be noted and addressed in consultation with experienced nurses.

Managerial Responsibilities. New graduate nurses use leadership techniques when they cover for nurse managers or direct the work of nonprofessional staff and volunteers. Gradually, new nurses assume increased leadership responsibilities as they become primary nurses, case managers, or unit coordinators.

Nursing Department. The nursing team can also be viewed in the broader sense of the entire nursing department of a healthcare institution or agency. Nurses should have an interest in the functioning of the depart-

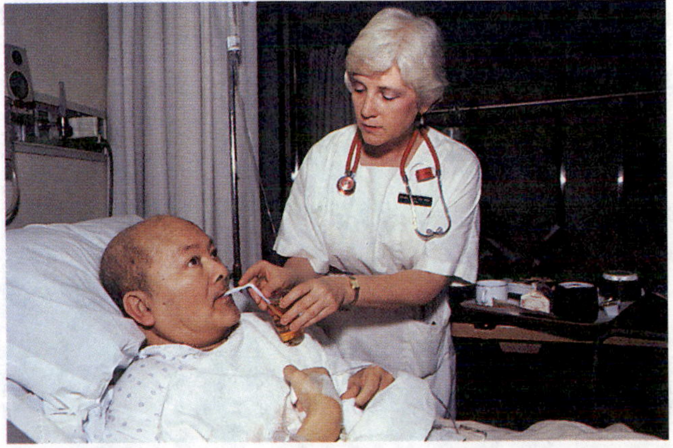

Figure 24-3
Nursing leadership begins with nursing care of the individual. (Photo © Kathy Sloane.)

ment. Using this knowledge, nurses can seek information or change through appropriate channels. The more nurses understand how the nursing department runs, the better able they are to constructively work toward the objectives of the department.

Employing Institution/Agency. Nurses at all levels need to be knowledgeable about the administrative structure and functions of the employing institution/agency. When problems arise concerning professional, unit, departmental, or institutional/agency objectives, nurses must be able to use the proper channels of communication. These channels are structured according to an organization chart. The organization chart shows the relationships among the various administrative positions, departments, and job titles. Sometimes the nurse is referred to committees that deal with specific problems or to other departments, such as public relations.

Research. Nurses need to be concerned with the advancement of nursing as a profession. Of the many ways to promote nursing's evolution toward greater autonomy and strength, an important facet is nursing research (Fig. 24-4). The nurse as researcher is more fully discussed later in this chapter. Nurses have given, and will continue to give, comprehensive and cost-efficient care by using the research findings of their colleagues. Nurse researchers can provide staff nurses with invaluable information to use in client care, but staff nurses also contribute to nursing research by doing the following:

- Observing all nursing care activities to look for any area that needs improvement
- Questioning one's own practice to see if the rationale behind caregiving activities is sound
- Participating in the client-care research done by colleagues or nurse researchers
- Making suggestions for specific topics to be researched

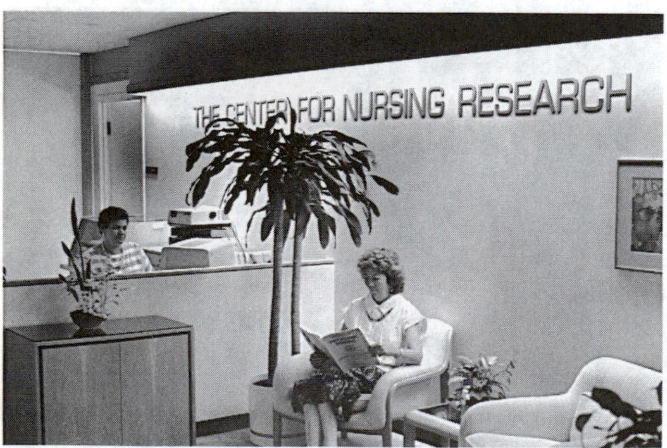

Figure 24-4
Research is an important way to promote nursing's evolution toward greater autonomy and strength by contributing to improvement of the quality of health care.

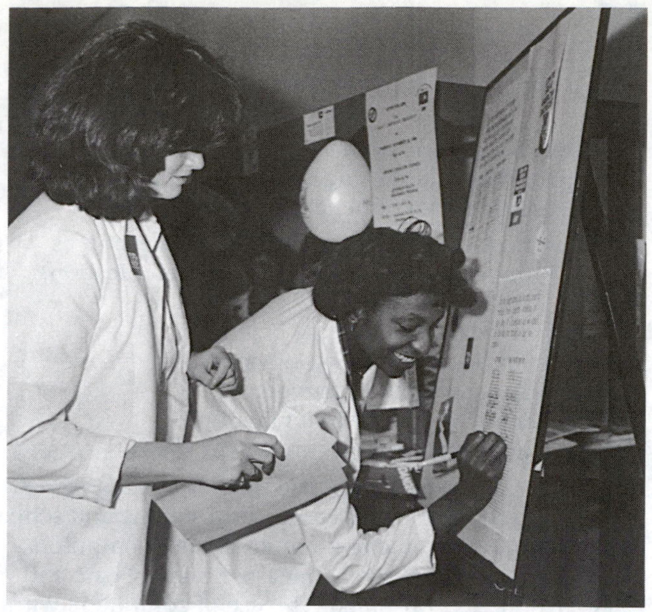

Figure 24-5
If all registered nurses (1.7 million in the United States alone) were active in movements for change and improvement in health care, they would command tremendous power and influence. (Photo by Robert Neroni, courtesy of Thomas Jefferson University.)

Legislation. Keeping informed about local, state or provincial, and national legislation allows nurses to write or call legislators before new laws are passed. Many nursing publications, newsletters, and papers have sections giving nurses specific information and guidelines on writing to elected officials concerning health-related legislation. The American Nurses Association (ANA) has lobbyists in Washington, DC, as well as in the state capitals. The potential influence of nurses in the continued improvement of health care is phenomenal (Fig. 24-5).

Public Image. Nurses create the public's image of nursing whenever they interact with others and are recognized as a nurse. It is critical for beginning practitioners of nursing to understand the power they have to positively or negatively affect nursing's image. Because nurses are often portrayed negatively by the media (eg, as sex objects or as uncaring females), it is important that the public encounter nurses who are intelligent, competent, and caring to reverse this image. Nurses can change negative portrayals of nursing by organizing, monitoring and reacting to the media, and fostering an improved image. Certainly not all nurses are interested in joining a media watch group, but all nurses can practice nursing care in a manner that promotes a positive image of nursing.

Support for Leadership Training

Mentorship. Mentorship is a relationship in which an experienced individual (the *mentor*) advises and assists a less experienced individual (*protégé* or *protégée*).

This is an effective way of easing a new nurse into the leadership responsibilities that will be expected in the future. Mentors link with protégés or protégées by common interest and provide support, information, and network links. The relationship does not include financial reward. Characteristics of effective mentors are highlighted in the accompanying box.

Mentorship is used in all types of nursing positions. As a nurse climbs the ladder of leadership responsibility, a mentor who is experienced in management and administrative functions may be chosen. A mentor can be a critical factor in helping the less experienced nurse successfully assume added responsibilities and position changes.

The role of mentor can be rewarding. Besides receiving the satisfaction of helping a newer nurse, the mentor is stimulated to further develop his or her own teaching, counseling, and leadership skills. Sometimes the mentor learns new knowledge and techniques when the newer nurse shares current information learned in school. Many mentorship relationships also become lasting friendships.

Preceptorship. An alternative model is **preceptorship**. The *preceptor* (experienced nurse) is selected (and generally paid) to facilitate the orientee's transition to new responsibilities by way of teaching and guidance. The relationship is limited by the orientee's needs.

Nursing Organizations. The many nursing organizations at the international, national, state or provincial, district, and local levels were discussed in Chapter 1. They are major forces for nursing leadership. These organizations have active groups in the United States and Canada. Membership and participation in professional organizations are important aspects of the nurse's leadership role (Fig. 24-6).

Continuing Education. Many programs that develop leadership, managerial, and administrative skills are available to nurses. Courses can even be taken by mail correspondence. Periodicals and current books also provide continuing education for the emerging leader. Many of the continuing education programs and methods serve to prepare nurses before they assume higher levels of leadership; some are geared to nurses already in such positions. Consequently, it is wise to choose a program carefully so that your learning needs are correctly met.

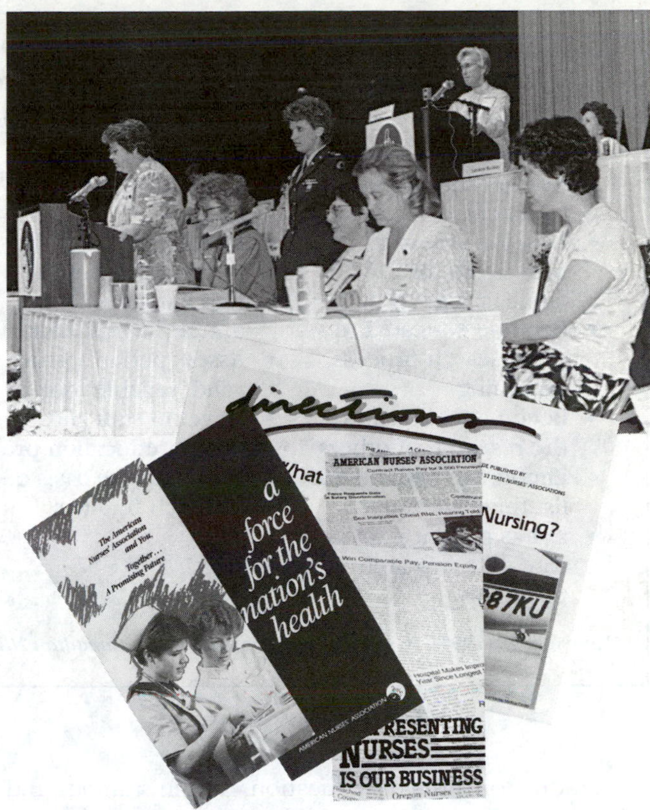

Figure 24-6
Membership and participation in professional nursing organizations help keep the individual nurse current on issues and recent developments, increase the strength of the group, and are important aspects of the nurse's leadership role. (Courtesy of the American Nurses' Association.)

Characteristics of Effective Mentor

- Gives upward mobility to your career
- Boosts self-esteem by believing in you
- Shares your dreams
- Provides advice, counsel, and support
- Teaches by example
- Introduces you to the corporate structure, players, and politics
- Imparts valuable information
- Gives feedback on your progress

Heidman, M. & Cobbold, D. (1995). Mentoring and career development revisited. *Registered Nurse,* 7(1), 29–30.

The Nurse as Researcher

While caring for victims of the Crimean War, Florence Nightingale kept careful and objective records. These records provided baseline data that she later used to determine which nursing interventions were most effective in treating her clients. Since that time, nursing research has taken many different pathways, which are highlighted in the accompanying box.

Nursing research was finally recognized by the public sector when the 1985 session of the U.S. Congress enacted legislation to establish a National Center for Nursing Research (NCNR) at the National Institutes of Health (NIH). Increasing numbers of healthcare institutions currently employ postgraduate nurses as researchers.

Research Options for Nurses

Utilization ←------ **Research** ------→ **Conduct**

Research approach	*Application of findings*	*Data collection and evaluation*	*Conduct of studies*
• Ask questions related to practice • Link the research process to the familiar, e.g. QI • Become educated re the research process, critiquing • Become involved in the research of others • Encourage patients to list their questions • Act as patient's advocate with research protocols.	• Critique research articles • Develop policies that are research-based • Join a research committee, journal club • Assess patients using valid, reliable tools • Develop staff and patient education programs on the basis of research findings.	• Use existing data bases to review demographics, practices • Conduct retrospective chart audits • Collect data prospectively • Replicate studies • Conduct pilot tests to introduce change.	• Participate as a research assistant • Become involved as a co-investigator on a research team • Assist with data collection, interpretation and communication • Conduct non-experimental research as a principal investigator • Conduct experimental research as a principal investigator.

Thurston, N. (1995). Hospital research comes of age. *Canadian Nurse, 91*(4), 35. Used with permission.

Studies on nursing education, administration, and practice all affect client care either directly or indirectly. Too often, practicing nurses mistakenly associate research with professions far removed from caring for clients at the bedside. This false impression has slowed the progress of practice-based nursing research. Yet much of what bedside nurses routinely do constitutes research. The nursing process (ie, assessing, diagnosing, planning, implementing, and evaluating) represents the basic framework of the research process. The top-ranked impediments to nursing research include access to resources, time to participate in research-related activities, and the educational preparation needed by nurses for research. Two major challenges face nursing research programs in the future:

- To continue to improve the link between research and practice
- To demonstrate nursing's unique contribution to health care delivery within the context of fiscal responsibility (Thurston, 1995)

Professionalism

Nursing research is fundamental to the recognition of nursing as a profession. As an occupation, nursing has existed since the beginning of human history. Many argue, however, that the profession of nursing is still in its infancy. One of the essential elements that differentiates an occupation from a profession is the existence of a unique and distinct knowledge base. The ultimate goal of expanding nursing's body of knowledge is to learn improved ways to promote and maintain health. As health care and illness patterns change, nursing interventions must change. Ongoing practice-based research reflects the nursing profession's commitment to meet the ever-changing demands of healthcare consumers.

Roots of Knowledge

How can nursing expand its knowledge base to meet the healthcare needs of clients? To answer this question, one must look to the roots of knowledge. Knowledge comes from a variety of sources. **Traditional knowledge** is that part of nursing practice passed down from generation to generation. When questioned about this aspect of nursing practice, nurses might reply, "We've always done it this way." Changing of bedclothes provides a practical illustration of how traditional knowledge has affected nursing practice. It is customary in acute-care settings to change a client's bedclothes daily, whether soiled or not. There are no data to support this, yet virtually millions of hospital beds are changed daily because this practice is accepted as a necessary component of quality client care. Until this practice is challenged scientifically, it will remain a traditional part of client care.

Authoritative knowledge comes from an expert and is accepted as truth based on a perceived level of expertise, for example, when a senior staff nurse teaches a new graduate nurse an easier way of doing a technical procedure such as inserting an intravenous catheter. The senior nurse has gained knowledge through experience, and the new graduate nurse accepts it as truth based on the perceived authority of the experienced nurse. Authoritative knowledge remains unchallenged as long as the presumed authority maintains his or her perceived expertise.

Scientific knowledge is that knowledge arrived at through the scientific method. The term *research* implies the scientific approach to acquiring new knowledge. New ideas are tested and measured systematically using objective criteria. Scientific study implies the presence of control over **variables**—factors that might interfere with results (outcomes). Different types of variables constitute a research study. **Independent variables** are the factors the researcher introduces into the study and can control. **Dependent variables** are those factors already in the situation that may respond to the independent variables. An example of scientific research that might be carried out at the bedside would be to measure the effects of two different skin emollients on opposite limbs of a client over the course of 2 days. The dependent variable in this example would be the client's limbs. The independent variable would be the skin emollients. With careful and objective data collection, the researcher might be able to determine which lotion elicited a better client result or outcome. By testing the results of the two emollients on the same client, the researcher would have maintained control within the study. Research as simple as this example could have vast implications on practice when results are shared among healthcare professionals. Scientific research relies on careful planning. If the emollients were tested on two clients, the results of the research might be affected by an unknown factor such as differing skin conditions in the two clients. These factors are called **extraneous variables**. Extraneous variables (ie, those that are not being studied) can sometimes result in inaccurate research findings.

Is one source of knowledge better than another? All sources of knowledge are useful to the collective body of knowledge that constitutes the nursing profession. Although these three methods provide nursing with important contributions, each has inherent strengths and limitations. Traditional and authoritative knowledge are practical to implement but are often based on subjective data, limiting their usefulness over a wide variety of practice settings. Scientific research, designed to achieve high levels of objectivity, is often costly and time-consuming and can be impractical given the complexities surrounding client care. However, because of its control and objectivity scientific knowledge can be generalized, making it highly useful in a variety of care settings. Acquiring new knowledge, then, is one reason why nurses must become more aware of and involved in the research process.

Consumerism

The social climate of consumerism surrounding health care has increased the importance of nursing research as well. The healthcare marketplace is characterized by rising concern over quality of care while assuring cost containment. Consumers have become dissatisfied with unproved, costly treatments; they demand effective methods of treatment at a reasonable cost. Nursing care, therefore, must focus on measurable results to assure the consumer of nursing's commitment to improve client care. Unless practice-based research is used to validate the effects of nursing interventions, consumers will not credit nursing for its important contribution.

The Nurse Caregiver's Research Skills

Relating Research to Practice. Unless the research findings of nurse researchers are used by practicing nurses to improve the quality of client care, clinical nursing research is useless. As students develop clinical skills, it is critical they understand the scientific rationale that makes one course of action preferable to another. Throughout this text, Research in Nursing boxes highlight current studies that have the potential to make a positive difference in nursing practice and client outcomes. Shown in the accompanying box are sources nurses can explore to find research studies pertinent to their concerns. Most librarians are willing to provide helpful introductions to these resources. As nurses develop their clinical and research skills, they will be better able to critique nursing research for validity, reliability, and applicability.

Identifying Researchable Problems. Because it is the nurse as caregiver who works most immediately with clients and families, it is critical for caregivers to continually approach their practice with the question, "Is this the best way to achieve the desired client outcomes?" The questions, insights, and recommendations of caring, practicing nurses have assisted many nurse researchers to refine their studies in significant ways.

Protecting the Rights of Subjects. Many nurses work in healthcare institutions in which clients are invited to participate in clinical research. With their focus on the overall well-being of the client, nurses play an important role in ensuring that client interests are not sacrificed to research interests. Nursing priorities on research units include determining that research studies have met appropriate scientific and ethical criteria before their implementation and protecting client rights. Specific rights of concern are **informed consent**, the client's right to knowledgeably consent to participate in the study without coercion (knowing that this consent may be withdrawn at any time) or to refuse to participate without jeopardizing the care that he or she will receive; the right to confidentiality; and the right to be protected from harm. Nurses caring for clients who are research subjects should be familiar with the ethical directives of the American Nurses Association (1985) or Canadian Nurses' Association (1983), Silva's *Ethical Guidelines in the Conduct, Dissemination, and Implementation of Nursing Research* (1995; see the accompanying box), and *The Belmont Report* (National Commission for the Protection of Human Subjects of Biomedical and Behavioral Research, 1978).

Computer Applications in Nursing

Computer Use in Nursing Research

Computer use in nursing research can provide tremendous benefits that include speed, accuracy, and flexibility. Quality of care is promoted by use of computers in all nursing settings. As a nurse you may be asked to take part in a research study conducted as a quality improvement effort.

In order to select computer programs for any stage of the project, the researcher must determine the function for which the program is to be used. Sample functions can be grouped into three major categories: management and analysis of research data, dissemination of research findings, and project management. After the functions are determined, the researcher selects software to meet these functions. The software selected dictates the hardware required. Some of the functions are highlighted here.

Data Collection, Tracking, and Transmission

Assembly of data in either a stand-alone or integrated information system can improve the quality of data. Reminders and edits are built into the computer software to check the quality of the data as they are entered. Data are easily retrieved using a computer system. Data can be transmitted to compare nursing interventions and client outcomes across patient care floors, hospitals, states, and countries.

Identification of Potential Problems

Risks can be identified and managed before they become problems. For instance, evaluation of incident reports can reveal problem areas to be rectified. Charted trends will reveal deficiencies or improvements.

Statistics

Statistics such as mathematical calculations, frequencies, percentages, means, medians, and standard deviations are frequently used in quality improvement research studies. Data manipulation is made significantly easier by use of a computer. Trended over time, statistics will reflect whether a specific criterion is improving or declining.

Case Identification

Automation can be used for fast and accurate case identification and retrieval. Criteria can be input with the computer instructed to retrieve all cases matching those criteria. Case identification can readily extract specific data—physical parameter readings, nursing diagnosis, treatment, room number, specific care provider, etc., for analysis purposes. Data for quality assurance studies may be easily extracted from a variety of sources provided they are on-line. Examples of sources are infection control and incident reports, medication error reports, client care plans, client classification data, nurse staffing and scheduling systems, client satisfaction surveys, diagnosis-related groups, census, and other client records.

Random Selection of Criteria for Evaluation

Some quality assurance studies require only a subset of the potential number of cases, and automation can select random cases in which to conduct studies without bias.

Presentation Mechanisms and Reports to Disseminate Findings

Graphically displayed statistical results enable the researcher to visualize improvements or departures from quality care. Various charts such as pie, bar, and graph are easily drawn and updated with the use of automation. Reporting, such as cardiac arrest critiques, operating room and emergency room audits, nosocomial disease reports, incident summary reports, and professional licensure reports, can be readily compiled, maintained, and trended with the aid of automation.

Project Management

Automated project management tools, word processing, spreadsheets, and data bases aid in management of research projects. Computers are used to gain access to on-line information from libraries and other sources. In short, computers can be used to help with all phases of the research process.

The Nurse as Advocate

Advocacy involves combining the three roles of teacher, counselor, and leader to form a new role through which the nurse protects and supports the client's rights. Nurses have always been advocates for clients' rights. This role is increasingly emphasized, perhaps because of clients' changing expectations and demands, as well as the importance placed on an individual's rights by the nursing profession.

Advocacy requires that nurses inform clients and then support them in their decisions. Nurses must recognize that clients have the right to make their own decisions. Through teaching and counseling, the nurse is able to give the client the information needed to make educated decisions about healthcare needs.

Nursing Research Resources

Major nursing journals with a science or research focus
- *Advances in Nursing Science*
- *Journal of Advanced Nursing*
- *Canadian Journal of Nursing Research*
- *Journal of Research in Nursing and Health*
- *Nursing Research*
- *International Journal of Nursing Studies*
- *Western Journal of Nursing Studies*

Indexes of journal articles
- *Cumulative Index to Nursing and Allied Health Literature* (CINAHL)
- *International Nursing Index*
- *Index Medicus*

Secondary resources
- *Annual Review of Nursing Research*
- *Review of Nursing Research in Nursing Education*

Computerized literature searches of research*
- *BIOETHICSLINE*
- Cumulative Index to Nursing and Allied Health Literature (CINAHL)
- *Educational Resources Information* (ERIC)
- Medical Literature Analysis and Retrieval System (MEDLARS)
- *Psychological Abstracts* (PsycINFO)

Individually subscribed computer bibliographic services
- *Knowledge Index* (available through *DIAGLOG Information Services*)
- *GRATEFUL MED* (available through the National Library of Medicine)
- *BRS Colleague* (available through W.B. Saunders)

* To access these arsenals of information, you need the following four items: (1) a telephone line, (2) a computer, (3) a modem, and (4) communications software. To access the desired data base, the user needs to obtain a password and an account number.

Many view advocacy as necessary only for those who cannot defend themselves. This is not true when considering the needs and rights of clients. Nearly all clients need a nurse advocate to provide the data needed for making informed decisions. Clients also need nurses to interpret what their rights are in given situations.

Client's Bill of Rights

As holism and holistic care became popular, clients began to demand their rights as healthcare consumers. In 1972, the American Hospital Association described *A Patient's Bill of Rights,* which includes the rights and responsibilities of the client who is receiving care in the hospital. The bill has been widely disseminated, and in some hospitals clients receive a copy on admission. (*A Patient's Bill of Rights* is discussed and reprinted in Chapter 6.)

In the United States, the Freedom of Information Act of 1967 and the Privacy Act of 1974 were enacted primarily to open personal government records to the people described in them. Medical records were included in this enactment. Clients in health agencies operated by the U.S. government (eg, the Department of Veterans' Affairs) and clients receiving Medicare currently are entitled to see their records. Although some specifics and interpretations of the laws have not been clarified, the trend is apparent: consumers are demanding their right to know about their health care and are seeking legislation to support this right. Nurses are responsible advocates of these client rights.

The Nurse Caregiver's Advocacy Skills

Representing Clients

Most nurses would agree that a great deal of nursing time is spent representing clients' interests or guiding clients in protecting their own rights. The nurse is often involved as an intermediary between the client and the family, especially when the client and family have conflicting ideas about the management of healthcare situations (Fig. 24-7).

For instance, a client with terminal cancer may want to go home to die. He has told this to his nurse. The client's family, however, has told the nurse that they cannot care for him at home. As an advocate, the nurse recognizes the rights of both the client and his family. The nurse then works to assist them in finding a solution that will benefit all concerned. By informing the family of the availability of home care and hospice care, the nurse has given them knowledge that may help satisfy the client's right to a dignified death. Most people on their own would have no way of getting the financial help needed for such care. The nurse has the resources available to help them and can arrange referrals from other healthcare workers, such as social workers, to achieve the desired outcomes.

Nurses may also serve as intermediaries between the client and the medical profession. Patricia Murphy (1990) documented a moving account of how nurses interceded for a 43-year-old woman with amyotrophic lateral sclerosis who was on a ventilator but wished to die. The client's primary physicians refused to help remove

Ethical Principles in the Conduct, Dissemination, and Implementation of Nursing Research

1. The investigator respects autonomous research participants' capacity to consent to participate in research and to determine the degree and duration of that participation without negative consequences.
2. The investigator prevents harm, minimizes harm, and/or promotes good to all research participants, including vulnerable groups and others affected by the research.
3. The investigator respects the personhood of research participants, their families, and significant others, valuing their diversity.
4. The investigator ensures that the benefits and burdens of research are equitably distributed in the selection of research participants.
5. The investigator protects the privacy of research participants to the maximum degree possible.
6. The investigator ensures the ethical integrity of the research process by use of appropriate checks and balances throughout the conduct, dissemination, and implementation of the research.
7. The investigator reports suspected, alleged, or known incidents of scientific misconduct in research to appropriate institutional officials for investigation.
8. The investigator maintains competency in the subject matter and methodologies of his or her research, as well as in other professional and societal issues that affect nursing research and the public good.
9. The investigator involved in animal research maximizes the benefits of the research with the least possible harm or suffering to the animals.

Silva, M. (1995). *Ethical guidelines in the conduct, dissemination, and implementation of nursing research.* Washington, DC: American Nurses Association. Used with permission.

her from the ventilator, and more than 20 other physicians declined to accept her as a client on learning what she wanted to do. After unsuccessful appeals for help to the county medical society and her own attorney, the client's visiting nurse, working with a supportive social worker, contacted her state nurses' association and finally secured the assistance she needed to help the client achieve her goal of a dignified death.

People with special advocacy needs include those who are uninformed concerning their rights and opportunities, those with sensory impairment, those who do not speak English, the very young and the elderly, those who are seriously ill, those who are mentally or emotionally impaired, and those with physical disabilities.

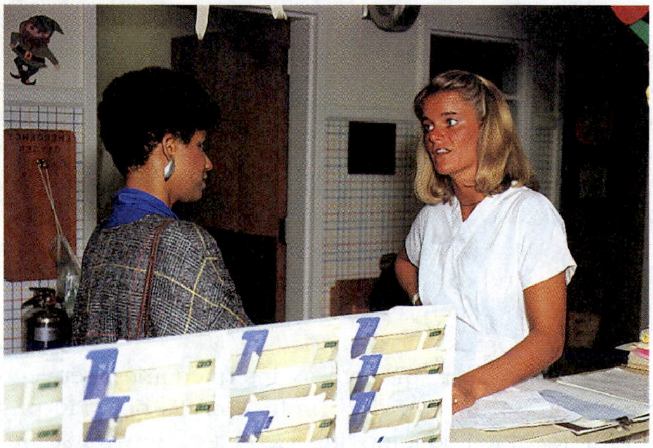

Figure 24-7
The nurse acts as a client advocate in discussing all aspects of the client's healthcare with the family members.

Being Assertive

To help clients attain their rights, nurses need to be assertive. Occasionally, they need to teach assertive techniques to their clients. Some individuals are intimidated in the healthcare environment; even when they disagree with a physician's treatment plan, they may feel unable to question or challenge the physician. Nurses can empower clients to claim and defend their right to knowledge, to respectful treatment, and to informed consent, by legitimizing these rights and by coaching clients in the assertiveness techniques that can help them secure these rights. Basic assertiveness techniques are described in Chapter 22.

Promoting Self-Determination

Advocacy is linked to the belief that making choices about health is a fundamental human right that promotes dignity and well-being. Ethical dilemmas may arise when people are unable or unwilling to make choices or when they are not given the opportunity to do so. Faulty communication between clients, family members, and caregivers frequently contributes to these dilemmas. Nurses play an important advocacy role in educating the public about the value of written **advance directives** (described in Chapter 33).

Nurses as advocates must realize that they do not make the ethical decisions for their clients. Instead, they facilitate the clients' decision making. Nurses interpret findings for their clients; inform them of the various aspects to be considered; let them verbalize and organize their feelings; call in those people who should be involved in the decision making (eg, family, primary nurse, physician, or clergy); and help clients assess all of their options in relation to their beliefs. In this way, nurses advocate for the right of clients to make their own decisions concerning health. It is important to recall that not all individuals want to make their own treatment decisions. The spirit of autonomy (self-determination) should not be violated by forcing it on anyone. Nurses sometimes advocate for clients by helping them to delegate a preferred decision maker whom they trust. In addition, in claiming to be a client advocate, nurses must be careful to clarify exactly what it is they mean by advocacy, because in most instances this is not simply supporting the client in all of his or her preferences. For example, if a client in the early stages of Alzheimer's disease, with the support of her husband, asked a nurse for help in terminating her life, the nurse would have excellent ethical grounds for refusing to advocate for this particular request. Advocacy is discussed in Chapter 6.

Being Politically Active

No discussion of nursing advocacy would be complete without noting nursing's continuing voice in the political arena on behalf of those least well served by the existing healthcare system. As the government becomes more involved in the delivery and funding of healthcare services and rationing plans speak seriously of age and other variables as criteria for limiting care, nurses must continue to advocate for the healthcare needs of those least empowered to do so for themselves, for example, homeless people, minorities, women, and children. Nurses represent a powerful block of voters whose potential for influencing healthcare legislation is just beginning to be tapped.

Key Points

- Nurses have the basic qualities and skills for leadership; they need to work toward developing these qualities and skills.
- Nurses choose leadership styles according to their own personality traits, the objectives to be achieved, and the characteristics of the followers.
- Nurse leaders are responsible for effecting positive changes, managing client and staff activities, and using administrative knowledge appropriately.
- Nursing leadership is involved in working for the benefit of the client, the nursing team, the nursing profession, and society.
- Research provides an important step toward expanding the professional role of nursing, acquiring new knowledge to improve client care, and remaining competitive in the healthcare marketplace.
- Beginning nurses can use research findings to improve their care; identify researchable problems; and protect the rights of research subjects to informed consent, confidentiality, and freedom from harm.
- Making choices about health is a fundamental human right that promotes client dignity and well-being.
- As an advocate, the nurse informs the client of rights and supports client decisions concerning rights and healthcare choices.
- Assertiveness is a necessary tool for the nurse to use in both advocacy and leadership roles. Nurses may also need to teach assertiveness techniques to clients and families.
- Educating the public about the benefits of advance directives is an important nursing advocacy role.

Bibliography

Leader

Benne, K. D., & Sheats, P. (1948). Functional roles of group members. *Journal of Social Issues, 4*(2), 41.

Bennis, W. G., Benne, K. D., Chin, R., & Corey, K. E. (1976). *The planning of change* (3rd ed.). New York: Holt, Rinehart & Winston.

Bernhard, L.A. & Walsh, M. (1994). *Leadership: The key to the professionalization of nursing* (3rd ed.). St. Louis: Mosby.

Brown, B.J. & Sample, S., Eds. (1994). Change: The challenge for nursing. *Nursing Administration Quarterly, 18*(3), entire issue.

Chenevert, M. (1993). *Pro-nurse handbook: Designed for the nurse who wants to thrive professionally* (2nd ed.). St. Louis: Mosby.

Douglas, L. M. (1992). *The effective nurse: Leader and manager* (4th ed.). St. Louis: Mosby–Year Book.

Grohar-Murray, M. E., & DiCroce, H. R. (1992). *Leadership and management in nursing.* Norwalk, CT: Appleton & Lange.

Gurka, A.M. (1995). Transformational leadership: Qualities and strategies for the CNS. *Journal for Advanced Nursing Practice, 9*(3), 169–174.

Hagenow, N.R. & McCrea, M.A. (1994). A mentoring relationship: Two viewpoints. *Nursing Management, 25*(12), 42–43.

Heidman, M. & Cobbold, D. (1995). Mentoring and career development revisited. *Registered Nurse, 7*(1), 29–30.

Hersey, P., & Blanchard, K. (1977). *Management of organizational behavior: Utilizing human resources* (3rd ed.). Englewood Cliffs, NJ: Prentice-Hall.

Kerfoot, K. (1995). Models of patient care delivery. In K.W. Vestal (Ed.). *Nursing management: Concepts and issues* (2nd ed.). Philadelphia: Lippincott, pp. 37–47.

Keenan, M. & Hurst, J.B. (1994). *A skills workbook for leading and managing in nursing.* St. Louis: Mosby.

Lewin, K. (1951). *Field theory in social science.* New York: Harper & Row.

Manfredi, C.M. & Valiga, T.M. (1994). Leadership in nursing. *Holistic Nursing Practice, 9*(1), entire issue.

Manion, J. (1995). Understanding the seven stages of change. *AJN, 95*(4), 41–43.

Marriner-Tomey, A. (1992a). *Guide to nursing management* (4th ed.). St. Louis: Mosby–Year Book.

Marriner-Tomey, A. (1992b). *Transformational leadership in nursing*. St. Louis: Mosby–Year Book.

Morrison, M. (1994). *Professional skills for leadership: Foundations of a successful career.* St. Louis: Mosby.

Nakata, J.A. & Saylor, C. (1994). Management style and staff nurse satisfaction in a changing environment. *Nursing Administration Quarterly, 18*(3), 51–57.

Pedersen, A. (1993). Qualities of the excellent head nurse. *Nursing Administration Quarterly, 18*(1), 40–50.

Porter-O'Grady, T. (1994). *The nurse manager's problem solver.* St. Louis: Mosby.

Tiffany, C.R., Cheatham, A.B., Doornbos, D., Loudermelt, l. & Momadi, G.G. (1994). Planned change theory: Survey of nursing periodical literature. *Nursing Management, 25*(7), 54–59.

Tiffany, C.R. (1994). Analysis of planned change theories. *Nursing Management, 25*(2), 60–62.

Trofino, J. (Ed.) (1992). Transformational leadership. *Nursing Administration Quarterly, 17*(1), entire issue.

Wolf, G.A., Boland, S. & Aukerman, M. (1994). A transformational model for the practice of professional nursing. Part I, The model. *JONA, 24*(4), 51–57.

Wolf, G.A., Boland, S. & Aukerman, M. (1994). A transformational model for the practice of professional nursing. Part II, Implementation of the model. *JONA, 24*(5), 38–46.

Researcher

American Nurses Association, Commission on Nursing Research. (1981). *Guidelines for the investigative function of nurses.* Kansas City, MO: ANA.

American Nurses Association. (1985). *Human rights guidelines for nurses in clinical and other research.* Kansas City, MO: ANA.

American Nurses Association. (1987). *Research in nursing: Toward a science of nursing.* Kansas City, MO: ANA.

Canadian Nurses Association. (1983). *Ethical guidelines for nursing research involving human subjects.* Ottawa: Author. (1994). Developing a strategic plan for nursing research. Nursing research in Alberta "by 2005." *AARN Newsletter, 50*(5), 8.

Larson, E., & McGuire, D. B. (1990). Patient experiences with research in a tertiary care setting. *Nursing Research, 39*(3), 168–171.

Lekander, B.J. (1994). Overcoming obstacles to research-based clinical practice. *AACN Clinical Issues in Critical Care Nursing, 5*(2), 115–123.

National Commission for the Protection of Human Subjects of Biomedical and Behavioral Research. (1978). *The Belmont report: Ethical principles and guidelines for the protection of human subjects of research* (DHEW Publication No. [OS]78-0012). Washington, DC: U.S. Government Printing Office.

Pettengill, M.M., Gillies, D.A. & Clark, C.C. (1994). Factors encouraging and discouraging the use of nursing research findings. *IMAGE: Journal of Nursing Scholarship, 26*(2), 143–147.

Phillips, J.R. (1994). A vision of nursing research priorities. *Nursing Science Quarterly, 7*(2), 52.

Polit, D.F. & Hungler, B.P. (1993). *Essentials of nursing research: Methods, appraisal, and utilization.* Philadelphia: Lippincott.

Price, C. (1994). Nursing research: Everybody's business . . . here are practical steps to develop any type of nursing research program. *MCN, 19*(1), 9–12, 14.

Roy, C.L. (1995). Developing nursing knowledge: Practice issues raised from four philosophical perspectives. *Nursing Science Quarterly, 8*(2), 79–85,

Sanchez-Sweatman, L. (1994). Research, patients and nurses. *Canadian Nurse, 90*(11), 53–54.

Silva, M. (1995). *Ethical guidelines in the conduct, dissemination, and implementation of nursing research.* Washington, DC: American Nurses Association.

Silva, M. (1995). *Annotated bibliography for ethical guidelines in the conduct, dissemination, and implementation of nursing research.* Washington, DC: American Nurses Association.

Thurston, N. (1995). Hospital research comes of age. *Canadian Nurse, 91*(4), 35.

Wuest, J. (1995). Breaking the barrier to nursing research. *Canadian Nurse, 91*(4), 29–33.

Advocate

American Hospital Association. (1992). *A patient's bill of rights.* Chicago: AHA.

Annas, G. J. (1992). *The rights of patients.* Totowa, NJ: Humana Press.

Copp, L.A. (1993). A response to, Patient advocacy—an important part of the daily work of the expert nurse. *Scholarship and Inquiry in Nursing Practice, 7*(2), 137–140.

Gadow, S. (1989). Clinical subjectivity: Advocacy with silent patients. *Nursing Clinics of North America, 24*(2), 535–541.

Kavanaugh, K.H. (1993). Transcultural nursing: Facing the challenge of advocacy and diversity/universality. *Journal of Transcultural Nursing, 5*(1), 4–13.

Kendrick, K. (1994). An advocate for whom—doctor or patient? How far can a nurse be a patient advocate? *Professional Nurse, 9*(12), 826–829.

Kenner, C. (1995). Use of professional associations for political action. The job of perinatal and neonatal nursing. *Journal of Perinatal and Neonatal Nursing, 9*(1), 78–88.

Kohnke, M. F. (1982). *Advocacy: Risk and reality.* St. Louis: Mosby.

Murphy, P. (1990). Helping Joanne die with dignity. *Nursing, 20*(9), 45–49.

Saba, V. K., Johnson, J. E., & Simpson, R. L. (1994). *Computers in nursing management.* Washington, DC: American Nurses Association.

Segesten, K. (1993). Patient advocacy—an important part of the daily work of the expert nurse. *Scholarship and Inquiry in Nursing Practice, 7*(2), 129–135.

Teasdale, K. (March 1994). Advocacy and the nurse manager. *Journal of Nursing Management, 2*(2), 93–97.

Unit VI focuses on the actions basic to nursing practice—those commonly planned and implemented to meet the healthcare needs of clients at any age, at any point along the health–illness continuum, and in both hospital and community-based settings. The nursing actions discussed in this unit include taking vital signs, conducting a health history and assessment, maintaining safety, administering medications, and providing perioperative care.

Chapter 25 describes nursing responsibilities related to the assessment of vital signs, and Chapter 26 discusses conducting a health history and assessment. Nursing assessment is both an art and a science. The art of performing a skill is integrated into the science of nursing so that variations from normal are identified and evaluated and necessary nursing actions are implemented. The findings from assessments provide a data base necessary to maintain or restore health and promote wellness.

Nurses are responsible for meeting basic human needs for physical safety and security. Chapter 27 discusses environmental safety and the nursing actions necessary to identify risk factors for clients at any age and to implement teaching and other nursing actions to prevent accidents. Chapter 28 explains medical and surgical aseptic techniques to prevent and control the spread of microorganisms.

Chapters 29 and 30 focus on collaborative and independent nursing actions necessary when administering medications and providing perioperative and wound care. In most instances, the physician prescribes the medications, performs the surgery, and writes orders for wound care, while the nurse orders and implements nursing interventions to promote client safety and knowledge and to facilitate optimal function or recovery in both hospital and home settings. Although procedures and protocols are often used in these situations, nursing actions are individualized to the unique needs of each person requiring care.

Unit VI introduces the learner to the knowledge and skills basic to nursing practice in any setting. Using the nursing process, nurses make accurate assessments, ensure safety, prevent and control the spread of microorganisms, administer medications knowledgeably and safely, and provide perioperative and wound care for clients in the hospital, home, and community.

Actions Basic to Nursing Care

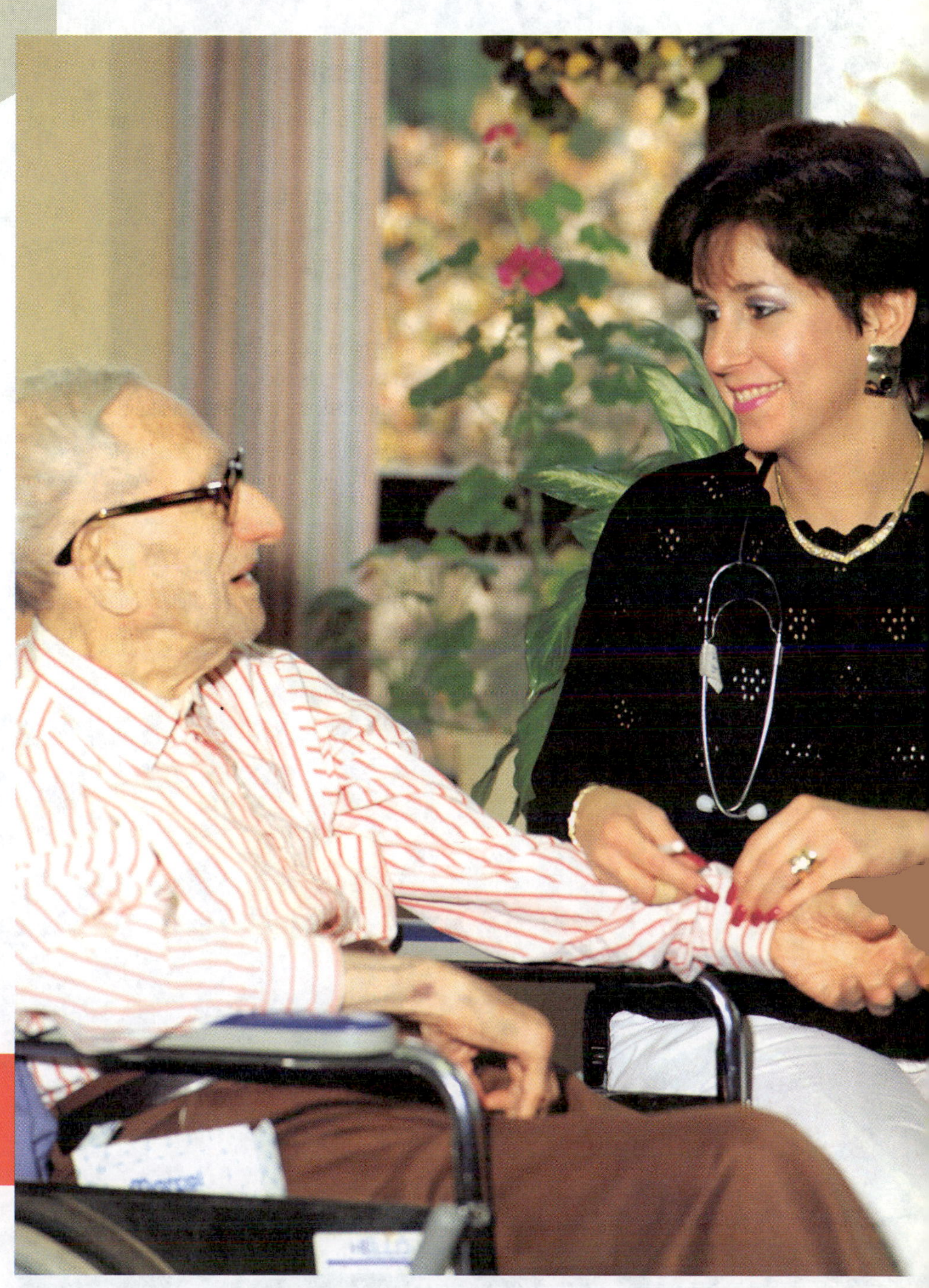

"Our intent when we lay hands on the patient in bodily care is to comfort."

Lydia Hall (1906–1969)
an innovator in nursing practice, she developed the theory that the direct nurse-to-patient relationship is itself therapeutic and that nursing care is the chief therapy for critically ill patients

Unit VI

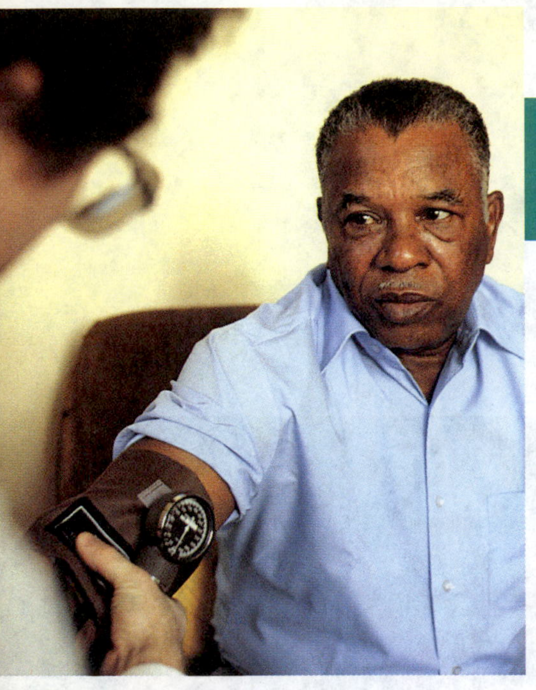

Chapter 25

Vital Signs

Objectives

After studying this chapter, the learner should be able to:

Define key terms used in the chapter.

Discuss nursing responsibilities in assessing temperature, pulse, respirations, and blood pressure.

Compare normal and abnormal vital sign assessments, including causes, effects, and implications of abnormal findings.

Describe the equipment necessary to assess vital signs.

Identify sites for assessing temperature, pulse, and blood pressure.

Provide information to clients about taking temperature, pulse, and blood pressure at home.

Key Terms

afebrile
apnea
blood pressure
bradycardia
bradypnea
crackles
diastolic pressure
dyspnea
dysrhythmia
eupnea
febrile
gurgles
hyperpyrexia
hypertension
hypotension
Korotkoff sounds
orthopnea
orthostatic hypotension
pulse
pulse deficit
pulse pressure
pyrexia
respiration
stertorous
stridor
systolic pressure
tachycardia
tachypnea
temperature
vital signs
wheezes

A basic nursing function in assessing the health status of an individual is taking vital signs. **Vital signs** are a person's temperature, pulse, respiration, and blood pressure. The physiologic status of the body is reflected by these indicators of body function, which are normally regulated by the body through homeostatic mechanisms and fall within certain normal ranges. A change from a person's normal pattern is considered indicative of a change in health.

Vital signs are taken and compared with accepted normal values and to the client's usual patterns in a wide variety of instances, including screenings at health fairs and clinics, in the home, upon admission to an institution or agency, when giving medications that affect readings, before and after diagnostic and surgical procedures, before and after certain nursing interventions, and in emergency situations. It is an independent nursing action to take and record vital signs as often as the condition of a client requires such intervention.

Although vital signs are taken frequently, careful attention to details of the procedures and accuracy of the interpretation of the findings is extremely important. It is the nurse's role to interpret vital sign findings. Each of the vital signs, with techniques and a discussion of normal and abnormal findings, is discussed in this chapter.

Frequency of Vital Sign Assessments

Assessing a person's vital signs is part of most home visits as well as agency admission procedures and ongoing care. These data provide part of the baseline and assessment information upon which a plan of care is developed, implemented, and evaluated. It is recommended that the nurse assess these signs whenever possible, rather than assigning the task to auxiliary nursing personnel who may have less knowledge about measuring and evaluating these important health-status indicators.

Institutional and agency policies govern when and how frequently vital signs are to be assessed. Vital signs are assessed at least every 4 hours in the hospital setting for clients with elevated temperatures, with either high or low blood pressures, with changes in pulse rate or rhythm, with respiratory difficulty, who are taking medications that affect cardiovascular or respiratory function, or who have had surgery. Severely ill clients may have vital signs taken more frequently. In the home setting and in some self-care and psychiatric units, assessments are often made on the basis of the nurse's judgment. When a client does not have abnormal blood pressure, temperature, pulse, or respirations, there seems to be little justification for taking these signs several times a day.

The use of technologically advanced monitoring devices has made it possible to keep clients' vital signs under constant surveillance in critical care settings. The lives of many clients have been saved because continuous assessment of vital signs provides an accurate means of observing the effects of pathology and therapy.

Auxiliary personnel may obtain vital signs in some situations, but the nurse responsible for the client is ultimately accountable for these assessments. If a client has untoward symptoms or demonstrates unexpected changes in vital signs, the nurse should double-check the measurements and further assess the client. The nurse should also be familiar with normal variations in vital signs that occur with age. These variations are described in the accompanying box.

Body Temperature

Body **temperature** is the heat of the body, measured in degrees. The degree of body temperature reflects the difference between heat production and heat loss. The core body temperature of a healthy person is maintained within a fairly constant range by the thermoregulatory center in the hypothalamus. This center receives messages from thermal receptors located throughout the body either to produce or conserve body heat or to increase heat loss. Under normal conditions, the thermoregulatory center's set point maintains body temperature within a range of 35.9°C (96.6°F) to 37.4°C (99.3°F). Core body temperatures reflect the temperature of the viscera and the muscles, which are insulated by the adipose tissue and skin to prevent heat loss. Heat is lost when heat from the body's inner core is transferred to the skin surface by circulating blood (Porth, 1994).

Focus on the Older Adult

Normal Variations in Vital Signs With Aging

Temperature

- Changes in temperature regulation may necessitate a longer time for body temperature to register, and the actual body temperature may normally be lower.

Pulse

- Although pulse rate may not differ from that of the middle-aged adult, there may be a change in rate, and dysrhythmias are more common.

Respirations

- As lung elasticity and gas exchange decrease with age, respirations are commonly more rapid and shallow.

Blood Pressure

- As age increases, the elasticity of arterial walls decreases, resulting in a higher systolic and diastolic blood pressure reading.
- Readings of 100 to 160 systolic and 60 to 95 diastolic are considered to be in the normal range.

Body temperatures differ in various parts of the body, with core body temperatures higher than surface body temperatures. Core temperatures are usually measured rectally, but they may also be measured in the esophagus, pulmonary artery, or bladder through invasive monitoring devices. Other sites for measuring body temperature are oral (sublingual), axillary, and the tympanic membrane.

Regulation of Temperature

Body temperature is regulated by balancing heat production and loss to maintain homeostasis. The regulation of body temperature is influenced by various factors, including circadian rhythms, age, gender, stress, and the temperature of the surrounding environment.

Heat Production

The primary source of heat in the human body is metabolism, with heat produced as a by-product of metabolic activities that generate energy for cellular functions. Various mechanisms increase body metabolism, including hormones, muscle movements, and exercise. When additional heat is required to maintain balance, epinephrine and norepinephrine (sympathetic neurotransmitters) are released and alter metabolism so that energy production decreases and heat production increases. Thyroid hormone, produced by the thyroid gland, also increases metabolism and heat production but does so over a much longer time period. Shivering, which is a response that increases the production of heat, is initiated by the hypothalamus and results in muscular tremors. Exercise increases heat production through muscular activity.

Heat Loss

The skin is the primary site of heat loss. The circulating blood brings heat to the skin's surface, where small connections between the arterioles to the venules lie directly below the surface. These connections, called arteriovenous shunts, may remain open to allow heat to dissipate to the skin and thus to the external environment, or they may close and retain heat in the body. Opening and closing of these shunts is controlled by the sympathetic nervous system in response to changes in core body temperature and in environmental temperature (Porth, 1994).

Other sources of heat loss include the contraction of pilomotor muscles of the skin. This reduces the size of the surface for heat loss and produces piloerection or "goose bumps." Other losses are through evaporation of sweat, through warming and humidifying of inspired air, and through urine and feces. Heat is transferred to the external environment through physical processes of radiation, convection, evaporation, and conduction. These processes are defined and illustrated in Table 25-1.

Factors Affecting Body Temperature

Many different factors affect body temperature. These factors include circadian rhythms, age, gender, stress, and environmental temperatures.

Circadian Rhythms. Many environmental and physiologic processes occur in repeated cycles of time. Some events in humans appear to recur at 24-hour intervals. This cycling pattern is referred to as **circadian** (meaning nearly every 24 hours) **rhythm**. Predictable fluctuations in measurements of body temperature and blood pressure are examples of functions that exhibit a circadian rhythm. For instance, body temperature is usually approximately 0.6°C (1° to 2°F) lower in the early morning than in the late afternoon and early evening. This variation tends to be somewhat greater in infants and children. Current research indicates that the peak elevation of a person's temperature occurs in late afternoon, between 4 and 7 PM.

Table 25-1
Mechanisms of Heat Transfer

	Radiation	Convection	Evaporation	Conduction
Definition	The diffusion or dissemination of heat by electromagnetic waves	The dissemination of heat by motion between areas of unequal density	The conversion of a liquid to a vapor	The transfer of heat to another object during direct contact
Example	The body gives off waves of heat from uncovered surfaces	An oscillating fan blows currents of cool air across the surface of a warm body	Body fluid in the form of perspiration and insensible loss is vaporized from the skin	The body transfers heat to an ice pack, causing the ice to melt
Illustration				

Age. Both the very young and the very old are more sensitive to changes in environmental temperature. The body temperature of infants and children responds more rapidly to both heat and cold air temperatures and requires careful attention so that harmful changes do not occur. With aging, the older adult loses some thermoregulatory control and is at risk for harm from extremes of temperature.

Gender. Women tend to have more fluctuations in body temperature than do men. This is most probably the result of changes in hormones; the increase in progesterone secretion at ovulation increases body temperature as much as 0.5° to 1°F.

Stress. The body responds to both physical and emotional stress as a threat, increasing the production of epinephrine and norepinephrine. As a result, the metabolic rate increases, raising the body temperature.

Environmental Temperature. Most of us respond to changes in the environmental temperature by wearing clothing that either allows increased heat loss when it is hot or retains heat when it is cold. However, when exposed to extreme cold without adequate protective clothing, heat loss may be increased to the point of *hypothermia* (low body temperature). Similarly, if exposed to extremes of heat for long periods of time, *hyperthermia* (high body temperature) may result. The causes, effects, and treatment of hypothermia and hyperthermia are outlined in Table 25-2.

Normal and Abnormal Body Temperature

Normal Body Temperature

Variations in normal body temperature occur in each person, with a range of 0.3° to 0.6°C (0.5° to 1.0°F) from the average normal temperature considered to be within normal limits. However, wider variations from the average temperature have been found to be normal for certain people.

A thermometer is placed under the tongue (sublingual area) of a person's mouth to obtain an oral temperature, in the anal canal to obtain a rectal temperature, in an axilla (armpit) to obtain an axillary temperature, and in the ear to obtain a tympanic temperature. Figure 25-1 and Table 25-3 show the average normal temperature standards for well adults at various body sites.

Elevated Body Temperature

Pyrexia is an increase in body temperature above normal. The lay term is *fever*. A person with an increased body temperature is said to be **febrile**. A person with a normal body temperature is referred to as **afebrile**. **Hyperpyrexia** is a high fever, usually above 41°C (105.8°F), and survival is rare when the temperature reaches 44°C (110°F). Death is probably due to damaging effects to the respiratory center but may be due also to inactivation of body enzymes and destruction of tissue proteins.

Pyrexia is a common symptom of illness, and there is sufficient evidence to indicate that an elevation in tem-

Table 25-2
Causes and Effects of Hypothermia and Hyperthermia

	Hypothermia	Hyperthermia
Temperature	Less than 35°C	More than normal (see below)

Causes	• Exposure to prolonged cold (atmosphere or submersion)
	• Older age
	• Contributing factors:
	  • Acute alcoholism
	  • Cardiovascular disease
	  • Cerebrovascular disease
	  • Malnutrition
	  • Homelessness
	  • Hypothyroidism
		• Exposure to prolonged heat
		• Prolonged muscular exertion
		• Older age
		• Cardiovascular disease
		• Drugs that increase muscle tone or reduce heat loss
		• Leaving infants or children in a closed car in hot weather
		• Damage to the spinal cord or brain

Effects	• Intense shivering • Increased heartbeat • Deep breathing • Rigid muscles • Decreasing blood pressure • Poor coordination • Slurred speech • Skin blue, puffy • Dilated pupils • Weak, irregular pulse • Loss of consciousness • Death	• Heat cramps (following vigorous activity) in heavily used muscles • Heat syncope: sudden onset of unconsciousness with a fall in blood pressure and cool damp skin • Heat exhaustion: thirst, fatigue, nausea, delirium, moist skin, rapid pulse, core temperature greater than 37.8°C (100°F) • Heatstroke: core temperature greater than 40°C (104°F), absence of sweating, nausea, dizziness, blurred vision, convulsions, coma, death
Treatment	• Rewarming (depending on degree, may involve applying blankets, giving warm fluids, immersing in warm water, applying heat pads or hot water bottles, instilling warmed fluids, supplying warmed oxygen, using extracorporeal blood warming) • Supporting vital functions • Preventing/treating complications	• Heat cramps: drink fluids containing salt and rest in a cool environment • Heat syncope: replace fluids (oral or intravenous) and rest in a cool place • Heat exhaustion: replace fluids and salt, rest in a cool place • Heatstroke: rapidly cool core temperature by submersing in cold water or applying icepacks

perature helps the body fight disease. In children, this response is often seen quickly. In the older adult, pyrexia may be one of the later signs of illness, and the temperature may be elevated only 1° or 2°F above normal, even when pathologic processes are extensive.

It is generally theorized that when a fever occurs, the set point regulated by the hypothalamus is readjusted to a higher level. As a result, heat loss is decreased or heat production is increased, or both occur through the following mechanisms—shivering, constriction of surface blood vessels, and absence of sweating. After the body temperature rises to the new set point, heat loss mechanisms are again used to control the body temperature from rising to dangerous levels. Most fevers are self-limiting; the body temperature returns to normal range after the disease process is in check. Relieving a moderately elevated body temperature may reduce the body's defenses against disease as well as alter the ability to assess the person's progress.

The client with a fever usually experiences loss of appetite; headache; hot, dry skin; flushed face; thirst; and general malaise. Young children or people with high fevers may experience periods of delirium or seizures. Observing for other potentially dangerous signs that accompany a fever, such as dehydration, decreased urinary output, and rapid heart rate, are important nursing assessments. The onset of an elevated body temperature may be sudden or gradual. Common terms used to describe the course of an elevated body temperature and its resolution are listed in Table 25-4.

Antipyretic, or fever-reducing, drugs, such as aspirin or acetaminophen, may be necessary in certain circum-

Axillary

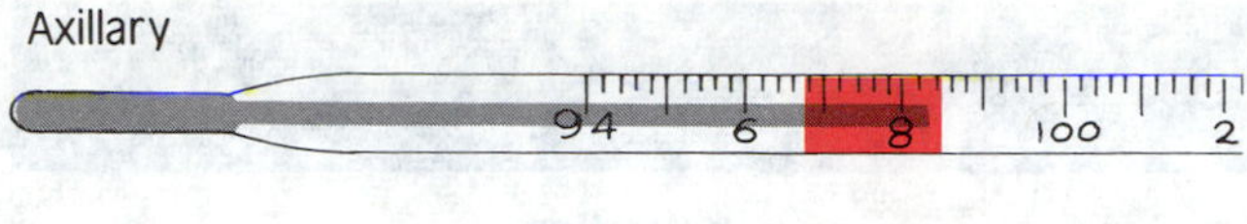

Oral

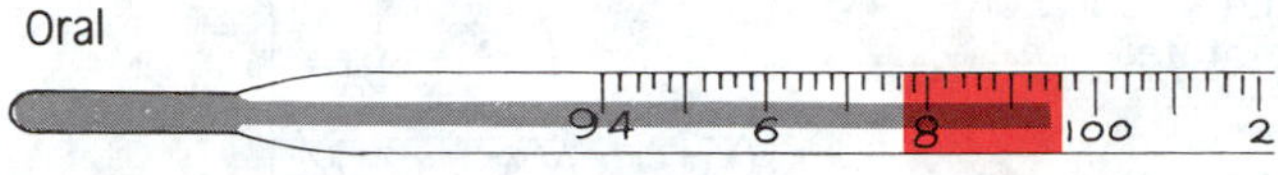

Rectal

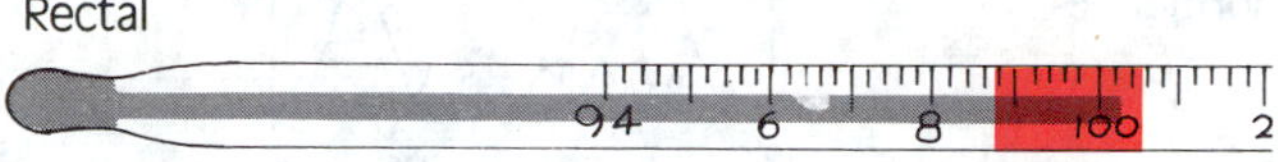

Figure 25-1
Comparison of normal adult axillary, oral, and rectal temperature ranges in Fahrenheit.

stances. These drugs are believed to lower the elevated set point regulated by the hypothalamus. They do not affect body temperature when it is within normal range. Body temperature may also be lowered through nonpharmacologic interventions. These interventions include cool sponge baths, cool packs, and cooling blankets.

Subnormal Body Temperature

A body temperature below the lower limit of normal is called **hypothermia** (see Table 25-2). Death may occur when the temperature falls below about 34°C (93.2°F), but survival has been reported in isolated cases when body temperatures have fallen in the range of severe hypothermia (28°C or 82.4°F). This may happen to a person drowning in cold water or buried by snow. Because body functions are almost imperceptible at this range, healthcare personnel should attempt to warm hypothermic clients and continue resuscitation efforts.

Just as an elevated body temperature is a protective device for the body, a lowered body temperature may be beneficial at times. Rates of chemical reactions in the body are slowed, thereby decreasing the metabolic demands for oxygen. Hypothermia as a form of therapy is discussed in clinical texts. Figure 25-2 illustrates the usual ranges of human body temperature.

Table 25-3
Average Normal Temperatures for Healthy Adults at Various Sites

Oral	Rectal	Axillary	Tympanic	Forehead
37.0°C 98.6°F	37.5°C 99.5°F	36.5°C 97.6°F	37.5°C* 99.5°F	34.4°C** 94.0°F

* The average normal tympanic temperature depends on the calibration and mode setting of the tympanic membrane thermometer.

** The manufacturer of Digitemp forehead thermometer (Hallcrest Products, 1820 Pickwick Lane, Glenview, IL 60025) says, "Most older children and adults have normal forehead temperatures between 93 and 95 degrees F."

Equipment

Body temperature may be assessed by using a variety of devices. These are glass thermometers, electronic thermometers, tympanic membrane thermometers, disposable thermometers, temperature-sensitive patches or tape, and automated monitoring devices.

Glass Thermometer. A glass thermometer with a mercury tip has traditionally been used to measure body temperature. This type of thermometer has two parts, as illustrated in Figure 25-1. The bulb contains liquid mercury, which expands when exposed to heat and rises within the stem. Most commonly, a long, thin bulb is found on glass thermometers used to take oral temperatures and a blunt bulb is found on glass thermometers used to take rectal temperatures.

Glass thermometers are generally calibrated in either degrees of centigrade (Celsius, C) or Fahrenheit (F). The range is about 34°C (94°F) to about 42.2°C (108°F). The degrees on a thermometer using the Celsius scale are subdivided into gradients of 0.1°; the subdivisions on a thermometer using the Fahrenheit scale are the equivalent of 0.2°. It is common practice to report the temperature to the nearest tenth of a degree when the mercury is a bit more or less from a line of calibration. Table 25-5 illustrates comparable centigrade and Fahrenheit temperatures and explains how temperatures are converted from one scale to the other. Assessing body temperature using a glass thermometer is discussed later in the chapter.

Electronic Thermometer. Electronic thermometers measure body temperature in 25 to 50 seconds. Most have two nonbreakable temperature probes, one for oral use and one for rectal use. They are equipped with disposable probe covers, a feature that minimizes chances for cross infection and decreases cleaning chores. A sound indicates when the peak temperature has been recorded. This helps the nurse avoid wasting time. Various models are available. Assessing body temperature using an electronic thermometer is discussed later in the chapter.

Tympanic Membrane Thermometer. Tympanic membrane thermometers use infrared sensors to detect heat given off by the tympanic membrane. The probe of the thermometer is covered with a probe cover, and the probe is inserted into the ear canal tightly enough to seal the opening. The reading is obtained in less than 2 seconds. However, there is some question about the accuracy of the reading obtained with these thermometers, especially in infants up to the age of 3 months. In one

Table 25-4
Common Courses of Pyrexia and Its Resolution

Term	Definition	Illustration
Intermittent fever	The body temperature alternates regularly between a period of fever and a period of normal or subnormal temperature	
Remittent fever	The body temperature fluctuates several degrees, more than 2°C (3.6°F), above normal but does not reach normal between fluctuations	
Constant fever	The body temperature remains consistently elevated and fluctuates little, less than 2°C (3.6°F)	
Relapsing fever	The body temperature returns to normal for at least a day, but then fever recurs	
Resolution of pyrexia by crisis	An elevated body temperature returns to normal suddenly	
Resolution of pyrexia by lysis	An elevated body temperature returns to normal gradually	

study (Selfridge & Shea, 1993) it was reported that the tympanic thermometer, although accurate in normal readings, sometimes indicated a fever when none was present.

Disposable Single-Use Thermometer. Disposable single-use thermometers register within seconds and are nonbreakable. Because they are used only once, they eliminate the danger of cross infection.

Temperature-Sensitive Patch or Tape. Temperature-sensitive patches or tape, commonly applied to the abdomen or forehead, change color at different temperature ranges. This type of equipment is often used with well infants born at term. Newborns usually are incapable of achieving a fever; assessment of temperature at this age is primarily to determine the infant's ability to regulate body heat. These devices may also be used when it is necessary to check the temperature of a toddler or young child who does not appear febrile. A thermometer should be used to check the temperature if the color on the tape or patch indicates that the temperature is either above or below normal average range.

Automated Monitoring Device. Automated monitoring devices are increasingly being used in a variety of healthcare settings to simultaneously measure a client's body temperature, pulse, and blood pressure. Their use

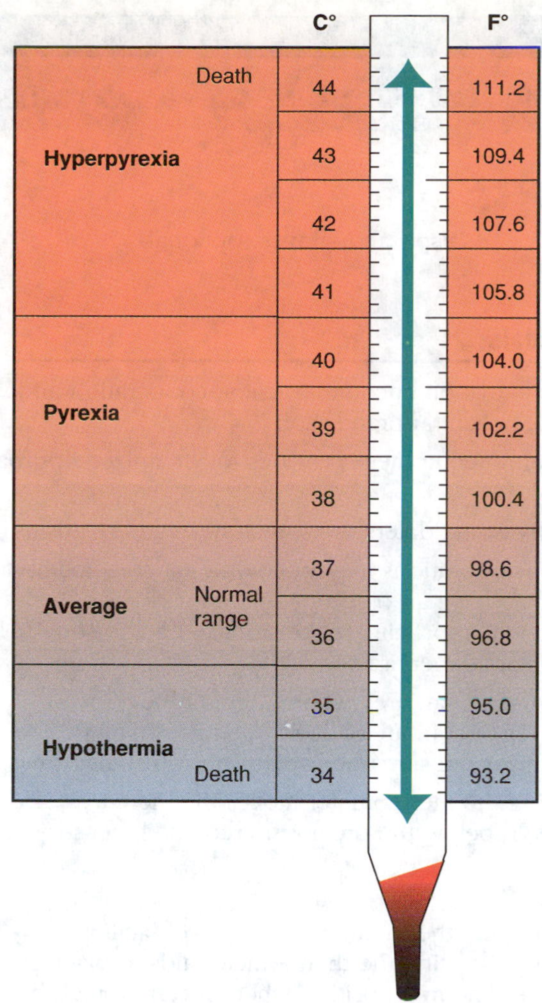

Figure 25-2
The range of human body temperature, as measured orally.

Table 25-5
Equivalent Centigrade and Fahrenheit Temperatures*

Centigrade	Fahrenheit	Centigrade	Fahrenheit
34.0	93.2	38.5	101.3
35.0	95.0	39.0	102.2
36.0	96.8	40.0	104.0
36.5	97.7	41.0	105.8
37.0	98.6	42.0	107.6
37.5	99.5	43.0	109.4
38.0	100.4	44.0	111.2

* To convert centigrade to Fahrenheit, multiply by 9/5 and add 32. To change Fahrenheit to centigrade, subtract 32 and multiply by 5/9.

requires less task-oriented nursing time, especially when these assessments are obtained frequently.

Assessment Sites and Methods

Health agencies specify the site to be used for obtaining clients' temperatures. Most agencies measure temperature by the oral route. However, the nurse is expected to select and use alternative sites in certain situations. Factors affecting the site selection include such things as age of client, state of consciousness, amount of pain, and other care being provided at the time. It is customary to indicate the site that was used to obtain the temperature when recording the measurement within the client's record.

Obtaining an Oral Temperature

Oral temperatures are most commonly assessed. One criterion for selecting an oral route is that the client must be able to close his or her mouth around the thermometer. Obtaining an oral temperature using a glass thermometer is contraindicated for unconscious, irrational, and seizure-prone clients, and for infants and young children because of the danger of breaking the glass thermometer in the mouth. Oral temperatures are also contraindicated for people with diseases of the oral cavity or who have had surgery of the nose or mouth. If a client has had either hot or cold food or fluids or has been smoking or chewing gum, it is generally recommended that a period of from 15 to 30 minutes elapse before an oral temperature is obtained to allow the oral tissues to return to normal temperature. Traditionally, oral temperatures have not been obtained on clients receiving nasal oxygen because it is believed that the oxygen causes a false low reading. Research is challenging this opinion. However, oral temperatures should not be obtained on clients receiving oxygen by mask, because the time it takes to obtain a reading using a glass thermometer is likely to result in a serious drop in the client's blood level of oxygen. Measures for obtaining an oral temperature are given in Procedures 25-1 and 25-2.

Obtaining a Rectal Temperature

The rectal temperature, a core temperature, is considered to be the most accurate of all measurements. Obtaining a rectal temperature is a possible alternative whenever obtaining an oral temperature is contraindicated (Procedure 25-3). It is also recommended practice to check the temperature rectally if the client's oral temperature changes considerably and unexpectedly. Some hospitals require rectal readings on all clients with an elevated temperature. However, the rectal site is not used in certain clients. Obtaining a rectal temperature is contraindicated for newborns and for clients having rectal surgery, diarrhea, and diseases of the rectum. Because the insertion of the thermometer can slow the heart rate by stimulating the vagus nerve, obtaining a rectal temperature may not be allowed in some institutions for people with certain heart diseases or following cardiac surgery.

(text continues on page 445)

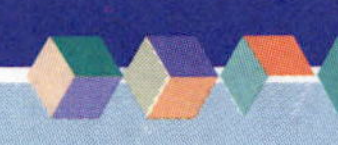

PROCEDURE 25-1

Assessing Body Temperature by Oral Method: Glass Clinical Thermometer

Equipment

Oral thermometer
Soft tissues
Pencil or pen
Paper or flow sheet
Disposable gloves (optional)

Action	Rationale
1. Explain the procedure to the client.	An explanation encourages client cooperation and reduces client apprehension.
2. Gather equipment.	Gathering equipment provides for organized approach to task.
3. Wash your hands.	Handwashing deters the spread of microorganisms.
4. If the thermometer has been stored in a chemical solution, wipe it dry with a firm, twisting motion, using clean, soft tissue.	Chemical solutions may irritate the mucous membrane and may have an objectionable odor or taste. Soft tissue will approximate the surface, and twisting helps to contact the entire surface.
5. Wipe once from the bulb toward the fingers with each tissue.	Wiping from an area where there are few or no organisms to an area where organisms may be present minimizes the spread of organisms to cleaner areas.
6. Grasp the thermometer firmly with the thumb and forefinger, and with strong wrist movements shake the thermometer until the mercury line reaches at least 36°C (95°F).	Shaking the thermometer moves the mercury back into the bulb below the previously recorded measurement.
7. Read the thermometer by holding it horizontally at eye level, and rotate it between the fingers until the mercury line can be seen clearly.	Holding the thermometer at eye level facilitates reading. Rotating the thermometer aids in placing the mercury line in a position where it can be read best.
8. Place the mercury bulb of the thermometer well within the back of the right or left pocket under the client's tongue, and instruct the client to close his or her lips around the thermometer.	When the bulb rests deeply in the posterior sublingual pocket, it is in contact with blood vessels lying close to surface and can accurately measure body temperature.

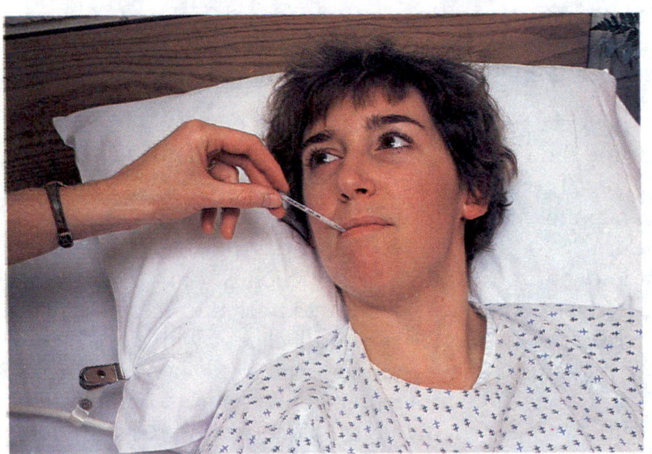

Action 8: Placing the thermometer.

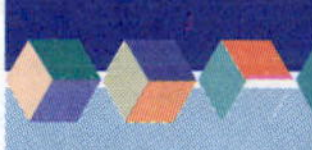

PROCEDURE 25-1 *(continued)*

Assessing Body Temperature by Oral Method: Glass Clinical Thermometer

Action	Rationale
9. Leave the thermometer in place for 3 minutes or according to time interval recommended by agency.	Allowing sufficient time for the mercury to expand ensures an accurate measurement.
10. Remove the thermometer, and wipe it once from the fingers down to the mercury bulb, using a firm, twisting motion.	Cleaning from an area where there are few organisms to an area where there are numerous organisms minimizes their spread to cleaner areas. Friction helps to loosen matter from the surface.
11. Read the thermometer to the nearest tenth.	Mercury may rise a bit above or below a calibration on a thermometer.

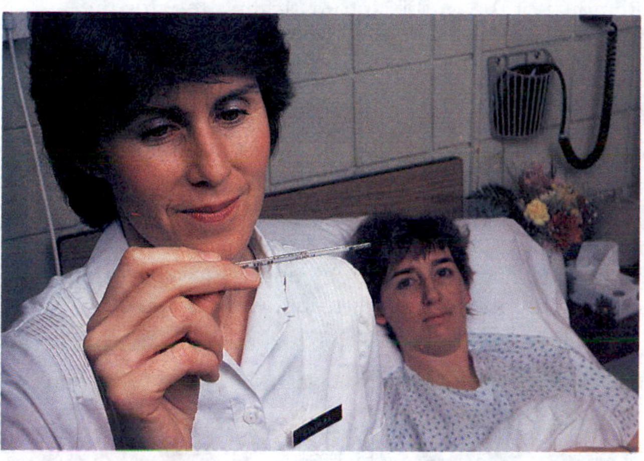

Action 11: Reading the thermometer. (Photos © Ken Kasper.)

Action	Rationale
12. Dispose of the tissue in a receptacle used for contaminated items.	Confining contaminated articles helps to reduce the spread of pathogens.
13. Wash thermometer in lukewarm soapy water. Rinse it in cool water. Dry and replace the thermometer in a container at the bedside.	Mechanical action of washing removes organic material and microorganisms.
14. Wash your hands.	Handwashing deters the spread of microorganisms.
15. Record temperature on flow sheet or paper. Report any abnormal findings to the appropriate person.	Recording the temperature provides accurate documentation.

Age Considerations

The axillary route, a temperature-sensitivity strip, or the tympanic membrane is the preferred method of evaluating the body temperature of a child younger than 6 years. These should also be the methods of choice for a confused or disoriented adult.

Home Care Considerations

Reinforce differences in temperature reading depending on route used. Axillary temperature is generally a degree less than an oral measurement; a rectal temperature is usually a degree higher.

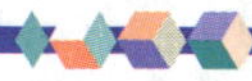

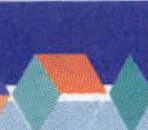

PROCEDURE 25-2

Assessing Body Temperature by Oral Method: Electronic Thermometer

Equipment

Thermometer with probe
Disposable probe cover
Soft tissues
Pencil or pen
Paper or flow sheet

Action	Rationale
1. Explain the procedure to the client. Gather equipment.	An explanation encourages client cooperation and reduces client apprehension.
2. Wash your hands.	Handwashing deters the spread of microorganisms.
3. Release the electronic unit from the charging area.	Charging sustains the power of the batteries when using the unit as a portable device.
4. Remove the temperature probe from within the recording unit.	Removal of the probe automatically prepares the machine to measure and record temperature.
5. Attach a disposable cover over the temperature probe. Make sure it is secure.	A disposable cover prevents the transmission of organisms.
6. Place the covered probe in the client's right or left sublingual pocket.	Thermometers placed in the middle area under the tongue have not registered as accurately as those placed in the areas to the sides.
7. Hold the probe in place while it is in the client's mouth.	If unsupported, the weight of the probe tends to fall away from the deepest areas under the tongue, causing the measurement to be less reliable.

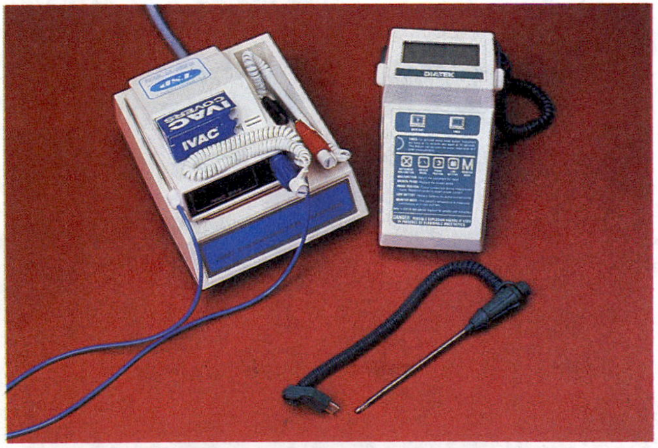

Two types of electronic thermometers and probes.

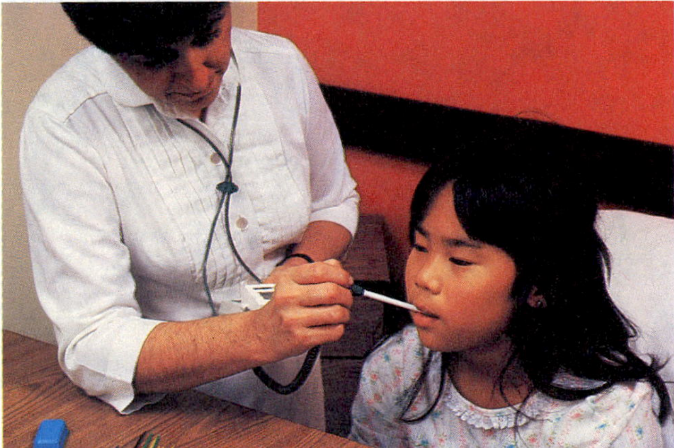

Actions 6 and 7: Placing and supporting the probe in place in the client's mouth.

Action	Rationale
8. Listen for a sound indicating that a maximum recording has been reached.	A sound indicates that the unit is not sensing any further change in the measurement.
9. Remove the probe from the client's mouth, and note the numbers displayed on the electronic unit.	An electronic thermometer is not calibrated with multiple numbers. It displays only the measured temperature.
10. Press the probe release button while holding it over a receptacle, such as a wastebasket.	The release button frees the disposable cover from the probe without being touched by the nurse's hands.
11. Return the probe to its storage location within the electronic unit.	The probe is protected from becoming broken if transported or stored within the recording unit.

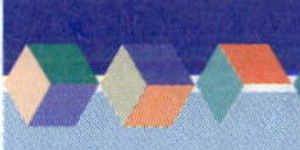

PROCEDURE 25-2 *(continued)*

Assessing Body Temperature by Oral Method: Electronic Thermometer

Action	Rationale
12. Wash your hands.	Handwashing deters the spread of microorganisms.
13. Record temperature on flow sheet or paper. Report any abnormal findings to the appropriate person.	Recording the temperature provides accurate documentation.
14. Return the electronic unit, and reconnect it to the source for charging the batteries.	Equipment needed by personnel for multiple client use should be readily available.

Age Considerations The axillary route, a temperature-sensitivity strip, or the tympanic membrane is the preferred method of evaluating the body temperature of a child younger than 6 years. These should also be the methods of choice for a confused or disoriented adult.

Home Care Considerations Reinforce differences in temperature reading depending on route used. Axillary temperature is generally a degree less than an oral measurement; a rectal temperature is usually a degree higher.

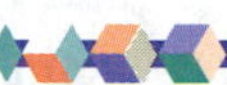

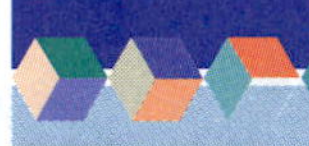

PROCEDURE 25-3

Assessing Body Temperature by Rectal Method: Glass Thermometer

Equipment

Rectal thermometer
Soft tissues
Pencil or pen
Paper or flow sheet
Storage container
Lubricant
Disposable gloves

Action	Rationale
1. Explain the procedure to the client.	An explanation encourages client cooperation and reduces client apprehension.
2. Gather equipment.	Gathering equipment provides for organized approach to task.

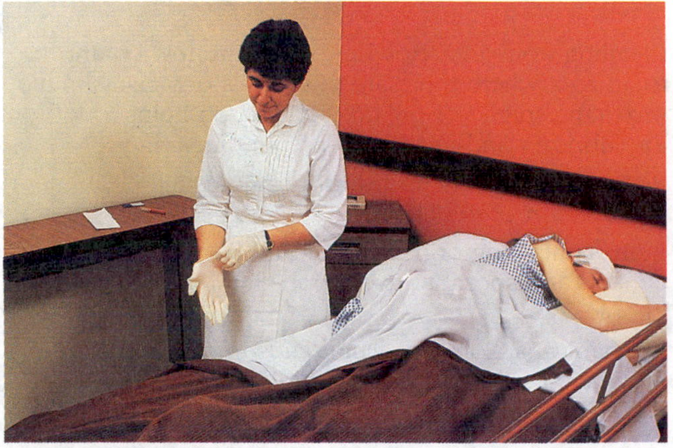

Action 3: Donning clean gloves.

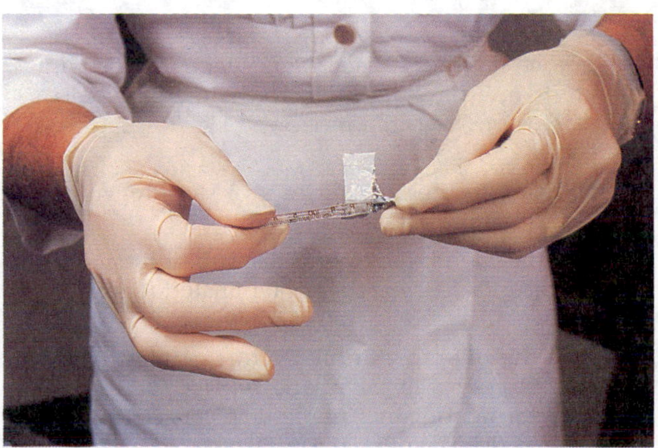

Action 5: Lubricating the mercury bulb.

(continued)

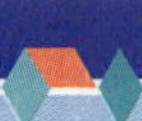

PROCEDURE 25-3 *(continued)*

Assessing Body Temperature by Rectal Method: Glass Thermometer

Action	Rationale
3. Wash your hands. Don a disposable glove on your dominant hand or on both hands.	Handwashing deters the spread of microorganisms. Disposable glove protects the nurse from microorganisms in the feces.
4. Wipe, shake, and read the rectal thermometer.	A rectal thermometer requires the same preparation as an oral thermometer.
5. Lubricate the mercury bulb and an area approximately 2.5 cm (1 inch) above the bulb.	Lubrication reduces friction and thereby facilitates insertion, minimizing irritation or injury to the mucous membrane of the anal canal.
6. Provide for privacy. With the client on his or her side, fold back the bed linen and separate the buttocks so that the anal sphincter is seen clearly.	If not placed directly through the anal opening, the bulb of the thermometer may injure the adjacent tissue or cause discomfort for the client.
7. Insert the thermometer for approximately 3.8 cm (1½ inches) in an adult, 2.5 cm (1 inch) in a child, and 1.25 cm (½ inch) in an infant.	Insertion length must be adjusted according to the anatomical size of the client's rectum.
8. Permit the client's buttocks to fall in place while holding the thermometer in place for 2 to 3 minutes.	The thermometer may become displaced internally or externally if it is not held in place.

Actions 6 and 7: Separating the buttocks and inserting the thermometer.

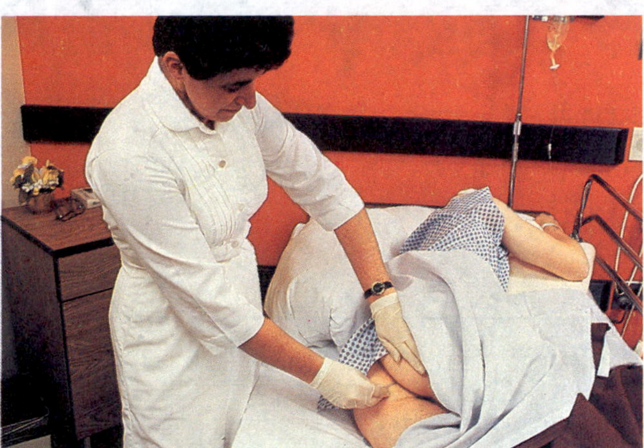

Action 8: Holding the thermometer in place.

Action	Rationale
9. Remove the thermometer, and wipe it once with soft tissue from the fingers to the mercury bulb, using a firm, twisting motion.	Cleaning from an area where there are few organisms to an area where there are numerous organisms minimizes the spread of organisms. Friction helps to loosen the lubricant and fecal matter from the surface.
10. Wipe any residue of lubricant or stool remaining about the anus.	Removing lubricant and stool promotes the cleanliness and comfort of the client.
11. Read the thermometer and dispose of the tissue in a receptacle used for contaminated items.	Items containing organisms should be placed in containers for disposal to avoid transmitting them to other people.
12. Wash thermometer in lukewarm soapy water. Rinse in cool water. Dry and replace the thermometer in container marked "rectal thermometer" at the bedside. Remove the disposable glove from the inside out and discard the glove.	Mechanical action of washing aids in removal of organic material and microorganisms.

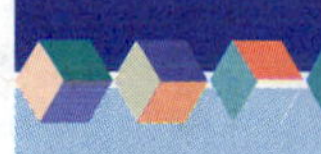

PROCEDURE 25-3 *(continued)*

Assessing Body Temperature by Rectal Method: Glass Thermometer

Action	Rationale
13. Wash your hands.	Handwashing deters the spread of microorganisms.
14. Record temperature on flow sheet or paper. Indicate that rectal route was used. Report any abnormal findings to the appropriate person.	Recording the temperature provides accurate documentation.

Age Considerations

The axillary route, a temperature-sensitivity strip, or the tympanic membrane is the preferred method of evaluating the body temperature of a child younger than 6 years. These should also be the methods of choice for a confused or disoriented adult.

Home Care Considerations

Reinforce differences in temperature reading depending on route used. Axillary temperature is generally a degree less than an oral measurement; a rectal temperature is usually a degree higher.

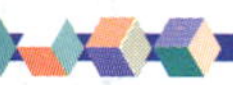

Obtaining a Tympanic Membrane Temperature

The tympanic membrane temperature is also considered a core body temperature. Infrared sensors in the thermometer sense heat from the body as it is given off by a heat source; in the ear canal, the primary heat source is the tympanic membrane. The thermometer does not touch the tympanic membrane.

The procedure for assessing a temperature using a tympanic membrane thermometer is as follows:

- Wash hands and attach tympanic probe cover to thermometer unit.
- Insert probe into ear canal with gentle but firm pressure (Fig. 25-3).
- Remove thermometer after reading is displayed on digital unit.
- Remove probe cover and dispose in proper container.
- Return thermometer to storage area.
- Wash hands and document temperature by TM (tympanic membrane).

Obtaining an Axillary Temperature

An axillary temperature is generally obtained when both oral and rectal temperatures are contraindicated or when the sites are inaccessible. Some hospitals obtain temperatures by the axillary method on healthy newborns to avoid the potential for perforating the wall of the rectum with the thermometer. If the axilla has just been washed, obtaining the temperature should be delayed because the temperature of the water and the friction created by drying the skin can influence the temperature. Most authorities believe that when proper procedure is used, axillary temperatures are as accurate as oral or rectal temperatures.

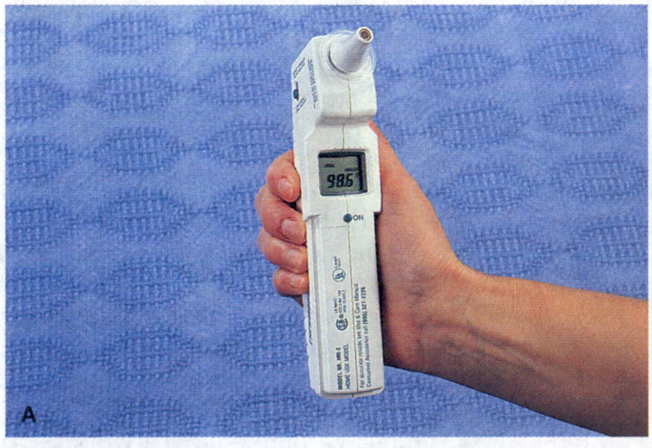

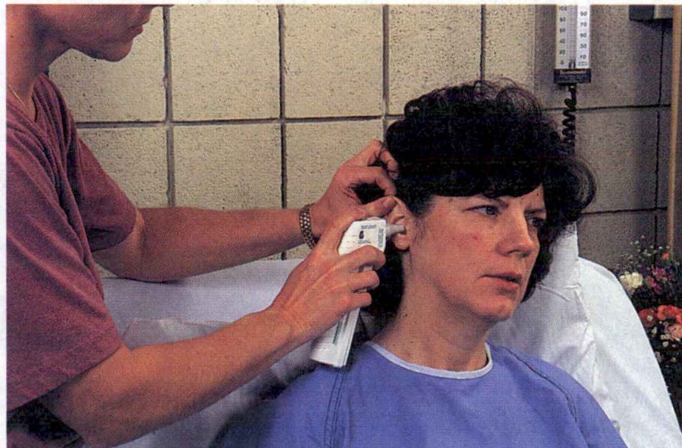

Figure 25-3
(A) Tympanic membrane thermometer. **(B)** Tympanic membrane thermometer with probe cover being placed in client's ear. (Photos © B. Proud.)

For most clinical purposes, it would appear equally satisfactory to obtain an oral, a rectal, a tympanic, or an axillary temperature provided proper technique is used and normal variations among the methods are considered. Figure 25-1 shows the differences in normal body temperature depending on the site selected. Comparing the recordings using two different sites may also be a method for double-checking the validity of an unusual measurement. The procedure for obtaining an axillary temperature is described in Procedure 25-4.

Care of Equipment

If glass thermometers are used within a healthcare institution, each client has his or her own thermometer for the length of in-client care. The thermometer is kept in the client's room, usually in a container of liquid disinfectant. It is recommended that glass thermometers used for clients with hepatitis (an infectious disease of the liver) and acquired immune deficiency syndrome be discarded when the client is discharged.

It is common practice in some agencies to have thermometers issued from a central supply unit. After being used one time for an individual client, they are returned for cleaning and disinfecting.

In the home, clean thermometers in lukewarm soapy water, rinse in cool water, and then store for reuse. If the thermometer is to be used by more than one person or if the person has a known or suspected infection transmitted by oral secretions, disinfect the thermometer with an appropriate solution after cleaning. The nurse should follow manufacturers' recommendations concerning the care and disposal of electronic and other types of thermometers and their sheaths.

Pulse

The **pulse** is a perceptible sensation as a wave of blood is pumped into the arteries by the contraction of the left ventricle. The pulse may be assessed at various sites of the body.

Regulation of Pulse

Each time the left ventricle of the heart contracts to eject blood into an already full aorta, the arterial walls in the blood system expand to compensate for the increase in pressure. This expansion of the aorta sends a wave through the walls of the arterial system that, on palpation, can be felt as a light tap. The pulse is regulated by the autonomic nervous system through the sinoatrial node (often called the pacemaker). Parasympathetic stimulation decreases the heart rate and sympathetic stimulation increases the heart rate.

The quantity of blood forced out of the left ventricle with each contraction is called the *stroke volume.* The average amount of blood per contraction is 70 mL for an adult. The *cardiac output* is the amount of blood pumped per minute. This volume is determined by using the following formula:

$$\text{cardiac output} = \text{stroke volume} \times \text{pulse rate}$$

Thus, the cardiac output of an adult with a stroke volume of 70 mL and a pulse rate of 72 beats per minute would be about 5000 mL. Many factors can affect both the heart rate (such as exercise), and the volume (such as a person's state of fluid balance). However, the body attempts to maintain a sufficient supply of blood to the cells at all times. For example, when the stroke volume decreases, such as when the blood volume is lowered because of hemorrhage, the contraction rate increases to try to maintain the same cardiac output. Conversely, in a physically fit athlete whose heart pumps a maximum volume of blood per stroke, the heart rate may be well at the low range or below the range of normal, yet the body cells remain adequately supplied.

Normal and Abnormal Pulses

The components of the pulse that are commonly assessed are the rate, rhythm, and pulse amplitude.

Pulse Rate

The *pulse rate* is the number of pulsations felt over a peripheral artery or heard over the apex of the heart in one minute. This rate normally corresponds to the same rate at which the heart is beating. There are wide ranges for normal pulse rates. Rates differ as individuals age, gradually diminishing from birth to adulthood as shown in Table 25-6.

Tachycardia. A rapid heart rate is called **tachycardia**. An adult has tachycardia when the pulse rate is 100 to 180 beats per minute. The following factors contribute to an increase in the pulse rate:

- Pain
- Strong emotions, such as fear, anger, anxiety, and surprise
- Exercise, when the heart's compensatory ability attempts to meet the need for increased blood circulation
- Prolonged application of heat
- A decrease in blood pressure, such as occurs with blood loss, when the heart's compensatory ability attempts to meet the need for increased output of blood from the heart
- An elevated temperature, which usually causes an increase of about 7 to 10 beats per minute for each 0.6°C (1°F) of elevation above normal
- Any condition resulting in poor oxygenation of blood, for example, chronic pulmonary disease or anemia
- Some medications (eg, Adrenalin)

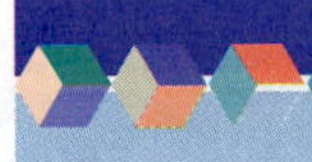

PROCEDURE 25-4

Assessing Body Temperature by Axillary Method: Glass Thermometer

Equipment

Thermometer
Soft tissues
Pencil or pen
Paper or flow sheet

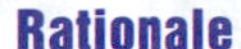

Action	Rationale
1. Explain the procedure to the client.	An explanation encourages client cooperation and reduces client apprehension.
2. Gather equipment.	Gathering equipment provides for organized approach to task.
3. Wash your hands.	Handwashing deters the spread of microorganisms.
4. Provide privacy and move gown to expose axilla.	Moving the gown to expose axilla ensures accurate placement of thermometer.
5. Wipe the thermometer with a clean tissue if it has been stored in a chemical solution. Use a firm, twisting motion to remove the moisture.	Chemical solutions may irritate the skin. The presence of solution may alter skin temperature. Soft tissue and friction help remove the solution.
6. Shake and read the thermometer as suggested in Procedure 25-1.	The mercury must be below the calibrations of the previous recording to assess the current temperature accurately.
7. Place the bulb of the thermometer into the center of the axilla.	The deepest area of the axilla provides the most accurate temperature measurement.
8. Bring the client's arm down close to his or her body, and place the client's forearm over his or her chest.	Surrounding the bulb with the skin surfaces of the axilla reduces the amount of surrounding air and ensures a reliable measurement.

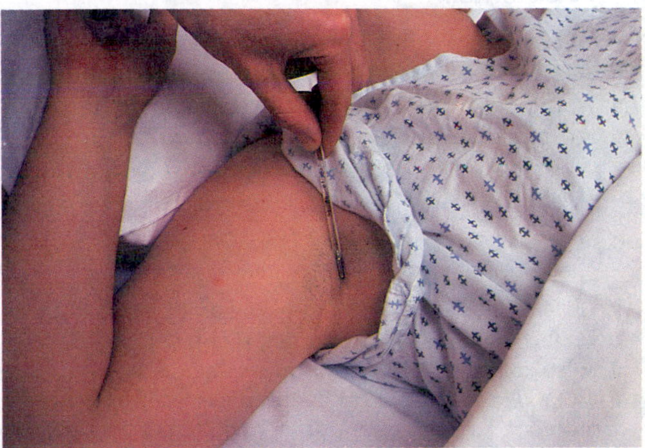

Action 7: Placing the bulb in the center of the axilla.

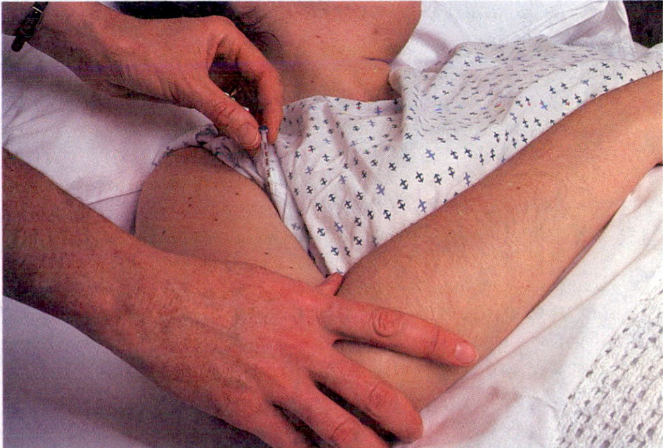

Action 8: Placing the client's arm close to the body. (Photos © Ken Kasper.)

Action	Rationale
9. Remain with the client and leave the thermometer in place for 10 minutes.	Additional time is required because the thermometer has not been placed in a body cavity and it takes longer for the mercury to rise to the maximum level of the client's temperature.

(continued)

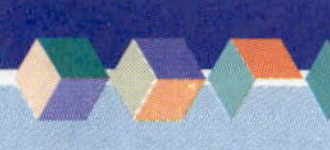

PROCEDURE 25-4 *(continued)*

Assessing Body Temperature by Axillary Method: Glass Thermometer

Action	Rationale
10. Remove and read the thermometer. Clean the thermometer and replace it in its location for reuse.	A thermometer that has been used for an axillary temperature should be cleaned before using it for another route and vice versa.
11. Wash your hands.	Handwashing deters the spread of microorganisms.
12. Record temperature on flow sheet or paper. Indicate axillary route. Report any abnormal findings to the appropriate person.	Recording the temperature provides accurate documentation.

Age Considerations

The axillary route, a temperature-sensitivity strip, or the tympanic membrane is the preferred method of evaluating the body temperature of a child younger than 6 years. These should also be the methods of choice for a confused or disoriented adult.

Home Care Considerations

Reinforce differences in temperature reading depending on route used. Axillary temperature is generally a degree less than an oral measurement; a rectal temperature is usually a degree higher.

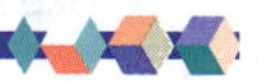

Bradycardia. The term used to describe the heart rate when it falls below 60 beats per minute in an adult is called **bradycardia**. A slow pulse rate during illness is less common than a rapid pulse rate but, when present, bradycardia should be reported promptly. The following are other factors that may slow the pulse:

- The pulse rate is generally slower at rest and on awakening.
- Males have a slower pulse rate than females.
- People with thin body size tend to have slower heart rates.
- Increasing age may be associated with a slower pulse.
- Medications, such as cardiotonic glycosides, slow the pulse rate.

Pulse Rhythm

The *pulse rhythm* is the pattern of the pulsations and the pauses between them. This rhythm is normally regular; that is, the beat and the pauses occur similarly throughout the time the pulse is being obtained. An irregular

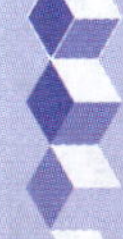

Through the Eyes of a Student

On the second week of my basic rotation, I went into my assigned client's room to take noon vital signs. I got a pulse only for a few seconds, and I kept losing it. I started getting nervous because I had no problem getting a.m. vital signs. Everyone in my group was getting ready to go to lunch. I went out of my client's room to tell my instructor that I couldn't get a good pulse—it kept fading in and out. My instructor and I entered my client's room. I went on the client's left side, and my instructor went on the right side. At this point, I was really nervous, because I kept thinking my instructor will get a pulse right away and I'll really feel stupid. She had a hard time getting a radial pulse, too. She told me to take an apical pulse. I was really nervous; I wasn't understanding what she was saying. In my mind, I was thinking axillary, so I put my hand near the client's axilla, feeling around for a pulse, and my instructor said, "Oh, you are trying for an axillary pulse. I think an apical would be easier to get." So then I am thinking, "She is going to fail me." She said, "Apical is near the heart." Then I thought, "I can't believe this is happening to me." So I put my hand near the heart for an apical pulse. My instructor said to use the stethoscope. "You can get an apical pulse that way." I was so embarrassed; I couldn't believe that happened to me. I knew where the apical pulse was! I was so nervous, I thought axilla. This was my most frightening clinical experience, and I will never forget it.

—***Elizabeth Ann McGrenra, Holy Family College, Philadelphia***

Table 25-6
Normal Pulse Rates per Minute at Various Ages

Age	Approximate Range	Approximate Average
Newborn to 1 mo	120–160	140
1 to 12 mo	80–140	120
12 mo to 2 yr	80–130	110
2 to 6 yr	75–120	100
6 to 12 yr	75–110	95
Adolescence to adult	60–100	80

pattern of heartbeats is called a **dysrhythmia**. Any irregularity in the heartbeat should be reported immediately. Common pulse rhythms are described and illustrated in Table 25-7.

Electrocardiograms (ECGs) are important for studying heart function and provide information about the rate and rhythm of the pulse. The record of the heart function may be displayed on an oscilloscope screen or on a paper graphic record, commonly called the ECG (Fig. 25-4). This figure also shows the association between the electrical system of the heart and the waves produced on the ECG. Note that the waves of each cardiac cycle are lettered as follows:

- The P waves occur when electrical changes, originating in the SA node, cause the atria to depolarize and contract.
- The QRS waves, as a whole, occur when the electrical charges result in ventricular depolarization and contraction; repolarization of the atria occur during this part of the cycle but are not normally visible on the ECG.
- The T wave represents relaxation of the ventricles and ventricular repolarization.

The ECG graph paper is ruled and calibrated to assist with interpretation of the timing and velocity of the waves of the cardiac cycle. When the heart is diseased or challenged by physical changes, the waves may be abnormal in size, form, and position. The time interval between waves also has diagnostic significance.

To take the recording, the client is placed in a supine position. Transmission gel is applied to the skin, and electrodes are placed at various sites over the anterior thorax and extremities. There is no discomfort involved. Clients who have never had the procedure will require an explanation of the purpose of the recording and how the electrodes are applied, and should be reassured that there is no transfer of electricity to the body during the procedure.

Pulse Amplitude

The *pulse amplitude* describes the quality of the pulse in terms of its fullness and reflects the strength of the left ventricular contraction. It is assessed by the feel of the blood flow through the vessel. Under normal conditions, the amplitude of each pulse beat is strong at all areas where an artery can be palpated. A strong pulse can be obliterated with relative ease by exerting pressure over the artery, but it remains perceptible with moderate pressure. Table 25-8 presents a scale commonly used to describe pulse amplitude.

Equipment

Stethoscope

Auscultation means listening for sounds within the body. The stethoscope is used to listen to and assess those sounds. The acoustical stethoscope, the most common type used, has an amplifying mechanism connected to ear pieces by tubing. Examples of amplifying devices include a *diaphragm*, which is a large, flat disc, or a *bell*, which has a hollowed, upright, curved appearance. Some acoustical stethoscopes have both.

The diaphragm is more useful for hearing high-frequency sounds because it is constructed to screen out low-frequency sounds. For example, the diaphragm is generally used for listening to respiratory sounds. The bell screens out high-frequency sounds and is more useful for hearing low-frequency sounds, such as those commonly made by the heart and the blood within the vessels. Figure 25-5 illustrates the bell and diaphragm of the acoustical stethoscope.

The ear tips of the stethoscope should be selected to fit the ear canals comfortably and snugly for the most effective auscultation. The tips should be sufficiently large to block out extraneous noises in the environment when the stethoscope is being used. The tips should be adjusted to be directed into the ear canal, not against the ear itself. The selection of an appropriate stethoscope for maximum efficiency during auscultation is an individual matter but should be considered carefully.

Assessment Sites and Methods

The rate, rhythm, and amplitude of the pulse may be assessed by compressing an artery against an underlying bone with the tips of the fingers. The thumb is not used to compress an artery because the nurse would tend to feel his or her own pulse rather than that of the client. The peripheral arteries located close to the skin surface are used most often. Most, but not all, are named for the bone to which each is adjacent. Common arteries used for assessment include the temporal, carotid, brachial, radial, femoral, popliteal, posterior tibial, and dorsalis pedis. Collectively, they are called *peripheral pulses* because they are distant from the heart. The location of these sites is illustrated in Figure 25-6.

The **apical pulse,** assessed by listening with the stethoscope over the apex of the heart on the thorax, is used when the peripheral pulse is irregular or nonpalpable and when giving medications that alter heart rate and rhythm.

Table 25-7
Various Pulse Rhythms

Term	Description	Illustration*
Regular	The pulsations and the pauses occur similarly throughout the entire minute	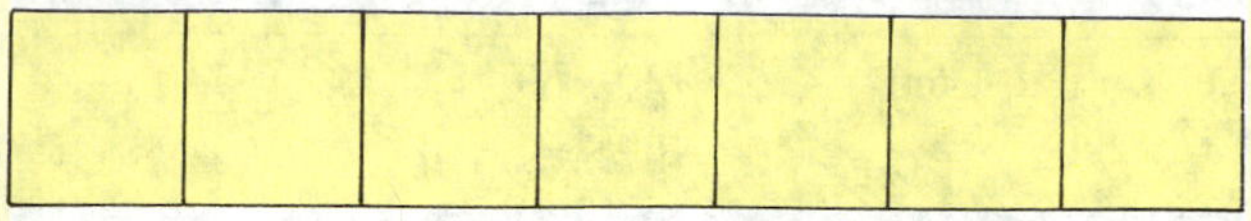 Normal
		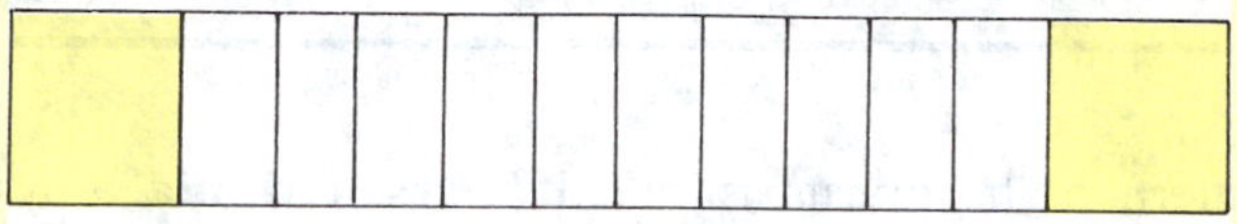 Tachycardia
		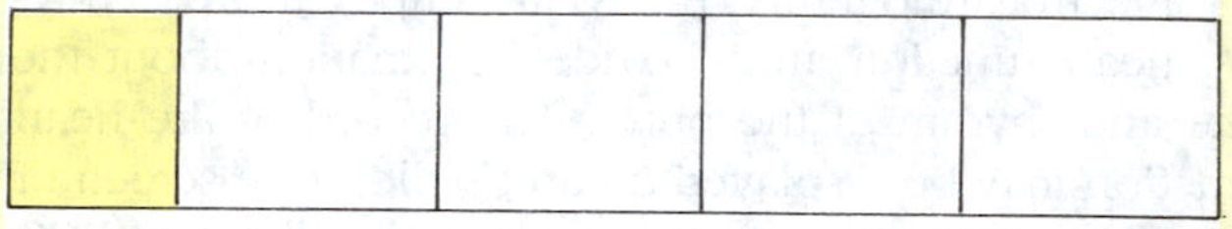 Bradycardia
Arrhythmia	The pulsations or length of pauses occur with no pattern or predictability	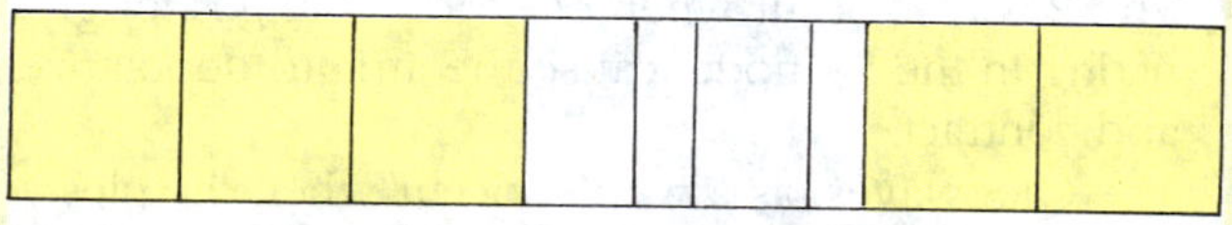 Intermittent — A normal pulse rhythm is broken by periods of irregularity.
		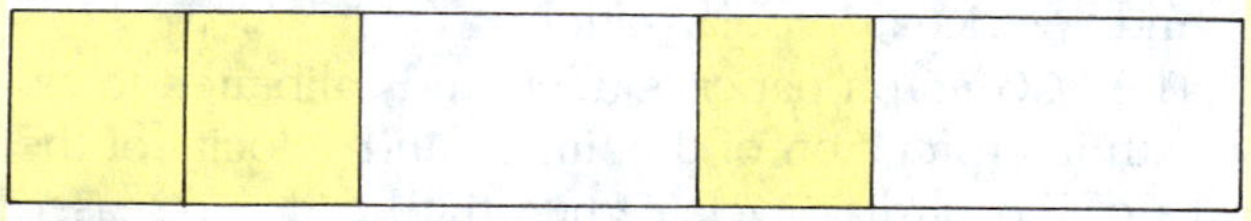 Bigeminal — A normal pulse rhythm of two beats is followed by a pause.
		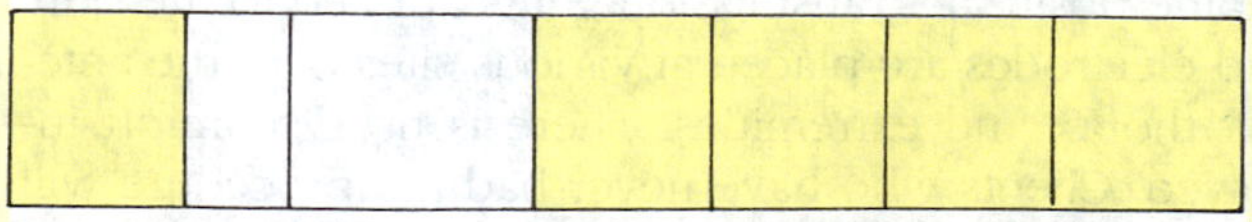 Premature beat — A heartbeat occurs before the normal one.

* Each vertical line represents one heartbeat.

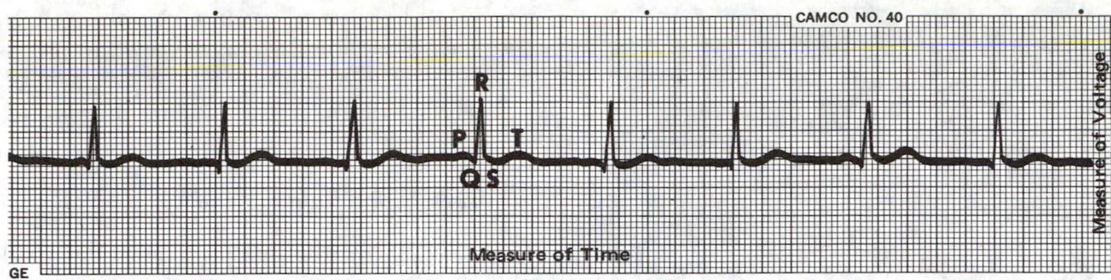

Figure 25-4
Calibrated paper used for the electrocardiogram shows time and voltage measures.

The pulse may be assessed by palpating (feeling) or auscultating (hearing). The following methods are used:

- The middle three fingers may be used to palpate all pulse sites except the apical pulse.
- A stethoscope may be used to auscultate the apical pulse (the procedure is discussed later).
- A Doppler ultrasound may be used to assess pulses that are difficult to palpate or auscultate. This device has an ultrasound transducer and an audio unit and transmits the sounds of red blood cells moving though the blood vessel. The procedure for assessing the pulse with this device is as follows:
  - Wash hands.
  - Collect the Doppler ultrasound stethoscope, the transducer in the Doppler probe (the probe looks like a small transistor radio), a stethoscope headset, and transmission gel.
  - Plug the headset into one of the two output jacks next to the volume control.

Table 25-8
Pulse Amplitude

Number	Definition	Description
0	Absent pulse	No pulsation is felt despite extreme pressure
1+	Thready pulse	Pulsation is not easily felt and slight pressure causes it to disappear
2+	Weak pulse	Stronger than a thready pulse; light pressure causes it to disappear
3+	Normal pulse	Pulsation is easily felt, takes moderate pressure to cause it to disappear
4+	Bounding pulse	The pulsation is strong and does not disappear with moderate pressure

(Timby, B.K., and Lewis, L.W. [1992]. *Fundamental skills and concepts in patient care* [5th ed.]. Philadelphia: Lippincott, p. 255.)

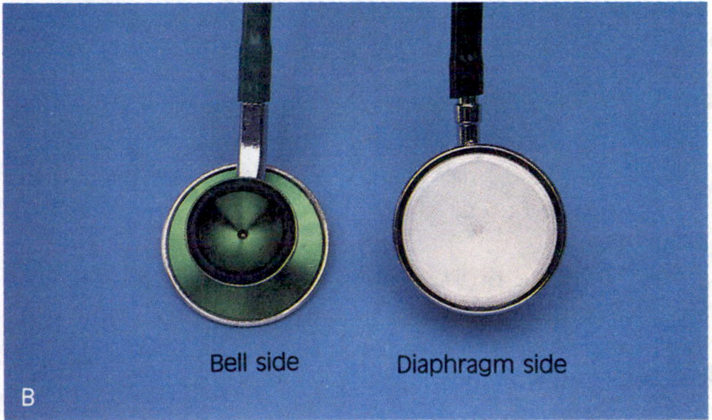

Figure 25-5
(A) Stethoscope. **(B)** Two sides of stethoscope amplifiers. (Photo © Ken Kasper.)

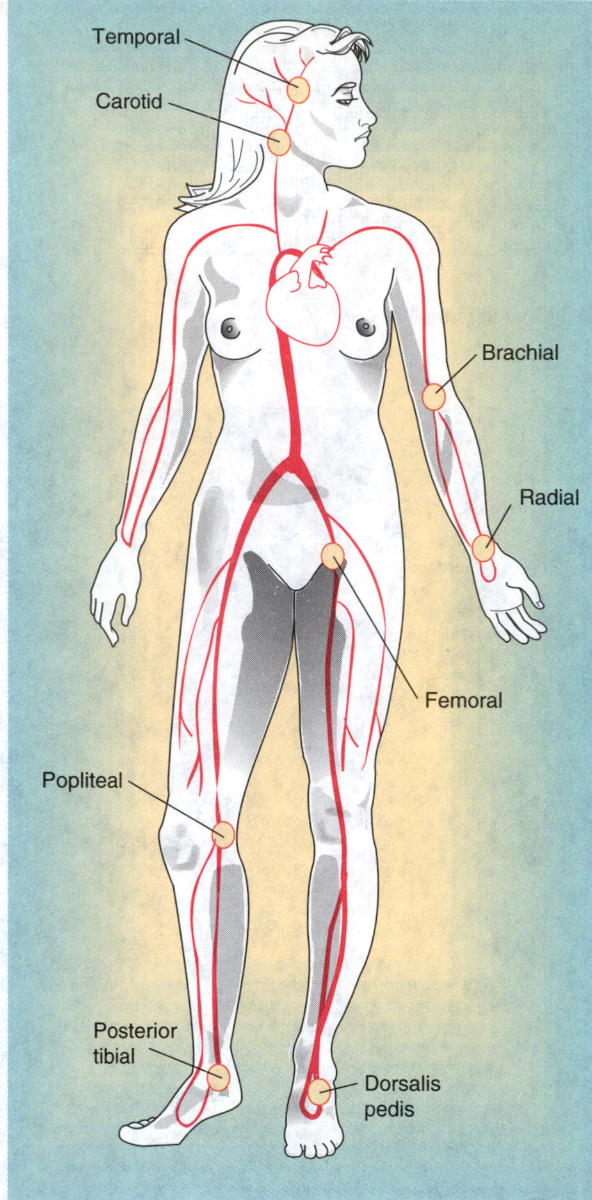

Figure 25-6
These arteries are located near the surface of the body. The pulse can be detected in any of these sites by light palpation.

- Apply a small amount of transmission gel to either the probe or to the client's skin over the selected area.
- Use the "on" button to activate the transducer.
- Hold the probe at a 45-degree angle to the skin over the pulse site while maintaining contact with the skin and the transmission gel.
- Listen for pumping sounds, indicating arterial pulse.
- Count the rate of the pulse for one minute.
- Remove gel from the probe and the client's skin; do not use alcohol to clean the transducer as it may damage the transducer covering.
- Wash hands and document pulse rate by Doppler.
- A cardiac monitor may be used to assess the apical pulse. The monitor produces a graph or digital reading of the pulse rate and amplitude.

Obtaining a Radial Pulse

Most commonly, the radial artery at the wrist is used for palpating the pulse because it is easily accessible. It is located on the inner, thumb side of the wrist. The location and the position of the fingertips during assessment are illustrated in Procedure 25-5. If this site is inaccessible, select an alternative artery that does not require exertion or cause discomfort for the person, which could alter the pulse rate. Procedure 25-5 describes how to obtain the pulse rate using the radial artery site.

Obtaining an Apical Pulse

If a peripheral pulse is difficult to assess accurately because it is irregular, feeble, or extremely rapid, the apical rate may be assessed. In the adult, the apical rate is counted for one full minute by listening with a stethoscope over the apex of the heart. The contraction of the heart can be heard in the space between the fifth and the sixth ribs, about 8 cm (3 inches) to the left of the median line and slightly below the nipple, as illustrated in Procedure 25-6. Nursing actions are given in Procedure 25-6. The apical rate of an infant is easily palpated with the fingertips.

Obtaining an Apical–Radial Pulse

When the radial pulse is irregular, the *apical–radial pulse rate* may be obtained by counting at the apex of the heart and at the radial artery simultaneously. The difference between the apical and radial pulse rates is called the **pulse deficit**. The following techniques are recommended to obtain an apical–radial pulse rate:

- Two nurses are needed; one listens with a stethoscope over the apex of the heart for the heartbeat, and the other counts the rate at the radial artery.
- The client's chest wall is exposed so that the stethoscope can be placed directly on the skin of the chest wall.
- One watch with a sweep second hand is placed so that both nurses can read it conveniently and simultaneously.
- The nurses determine where they can best hear and feel the pulse and decide on a time to start counting, such as when the second hand on the watch is at a specified place.
- Both nurses count for 1 full minute and record their counts.

(text continues on page 455)

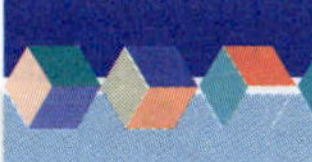

PROCEDURE 25-5

Assessing the Radial Pulse Rate

Equipment

Watch with second hand or digital readout
Pencil or pen
Paper or flow sheet

Action	Rationale
1. Explain the procedure to client.	An explanation encourages client cooperation and reduces client apprehension.
2. Gather equipment.	Gathering equipment provides for organized approach to task.
3. Wash your hands.	Handwashing deters the spread of microorganisms.
4. Have the client lie down and rest his or her arm alongside the body with the wrist extended and the palm of the hand downward. Or the client can sit with his or her forearm at a 90-degree angle to the body resting on a support and with the wrist extended and the palm of the hand downward.	These positions are ordinarily comfortable for the client and convenient for the nurse.
5. Place your first, second, and third fingers along the client's radial artery, and press gently against the radius; rest your thumb in apposition to fingers on the back of the client's wrist.	The fingertips, sensitive to touch, feel pulsation of the client's radial artery. If the thumb is used for palpating the client's pulse, the nurse's own pulse may be felt.
6. Apply only enough pressure so that the client's pulsating artery can be felt distinctly.	Moderate pressure allows the nurse to feel the superficial radial artery expand with each heartbeat. Too much pressure obliterates the pulse. If too little pressure is applied, the pulse is imperceptible.
7. Using a watch with a second hand, count the number of pulsations felt for 30 seconds. Multiply this number by two to obtain the rate for 1 minute.	Sufficient time is necessary to assess the rate, rhythm, and amplitude of the pulse.

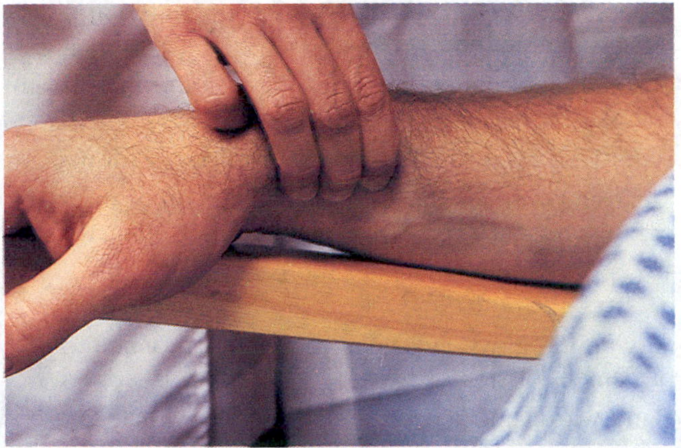

Action 5: Proper placement of the fingers along the radial artery.

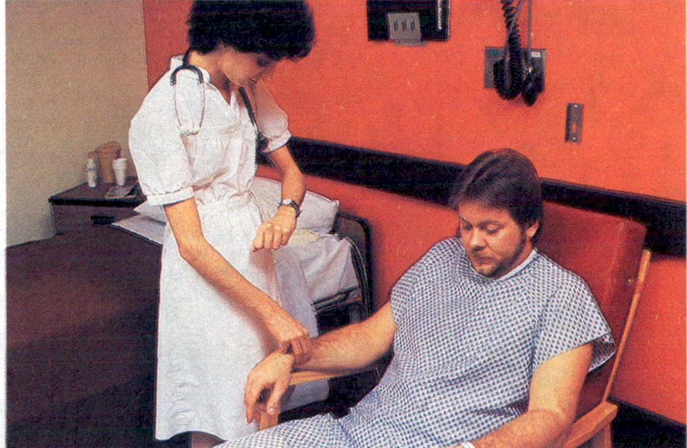

Action 7: Counting the pulsations felt for 30 seconds.

Action	Rationale
8. If the pulse rate is abnormal in any way, palpate the pulse for a full minute or longer.	When the pulse is abnormal, longer counting and palpation are necessary to identify most accurately the unusual characteristics of the pulse.

(continued)

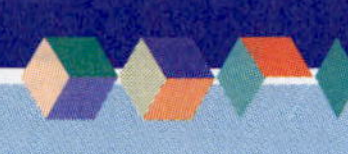

PROCEDURE 25-5 *(continued)*

Assessing the Radial Pulse Rate

Action	Rationale
9. Assess rhythm, amplitude, and elasticity of the vessel wall while counting rate.	Irregularity in heart rate may disrupt the cardiac output. Amplitude of pulse indicates the quality of the heart's contraction. Elasticity of blood vessel does not affect the pulse rate but does reflect status of the vascular system.
10. Record pulse rate on flow sheet or paper. Report any abnormal findings to the appropriate person.	Recording the pulse rate provides accurate documentation.
11. Wash your hands.	Handwashing deters the spread of microorganisms.

Home Care Considerations

Teach the client how to take own pulse.

Inform the client of availability of digital pulse monitoring devices.

Instruct family members about techniques used to locate and monitor other peripheral pulse sites.

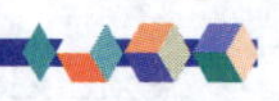

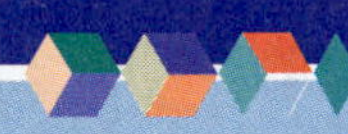

PROCEDURE 25-6

Assessing the Apical Pulse Rate

Equipment

Watch with second hand or digital readout	Stethoscope	Paper or flow sheet
	Pencil or pen	Alcohol swab

Action	Rationale
1. Explain the procedure to the client.	An explanation encourages client cooperation and reduces client apprehension.
2. Gather equipment.	Gathering equipment provides for organized approach to task.
3. Wash your hands.	Handwashing deters the spread of microorganisms.
4. Use alcohol swab to cleanse ear pieces and diaphragm of stethoscope, if necessary.	Cleansing with alcohol deters transmission of microorganisms.
5. Assist client to sitting position in bed or on a chair, if possible.	This position eases identification of site for nurse.
6. Provide privacy and move gown to expose upper chest area.	Moving the gown facilitates identification of site for placement of stethoscope.
7. Hold diaphragm of stethoscope against palm of hand for a few seconds.	Hand warms metal area of stethoscope, which may be cold and may startle client.
8. Palpate fifth intercostal space and move to left midclavicular line. Place diaphragm over apex of heart.	This is point of maximal impulse, where heartbeat is easier to hear.
9. Listen for normal heart sounds, identified as "lub dub" beat.	These sounds occur as blood flows through heart valves.

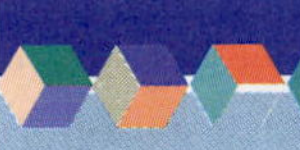

PROCEDURE 25-6 *(continued)*

Assessing the Apical Pulse Rate

Action	Rationale
10. Using a watch with a second hand, count the heartbeat for 30 seconds and multiply by two if rhythm is regular. Count for 60 seconds if irregular rhythm is present.	Longer time interval allows for more accurate assessment of heart rate.

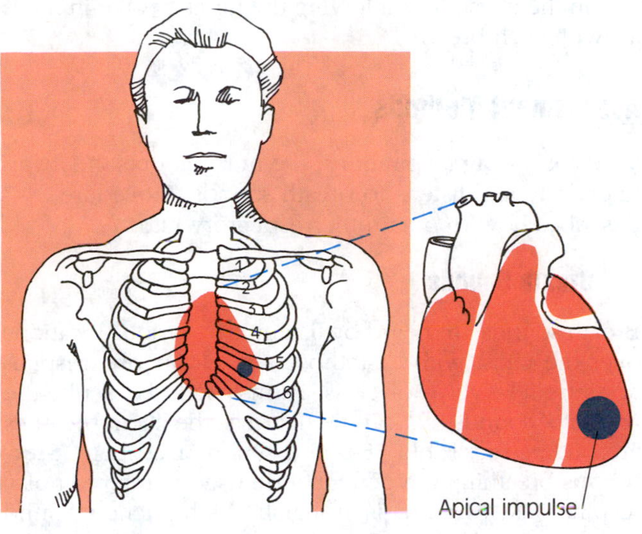

Schematic depiction of the thorax showing location of apical impulse.

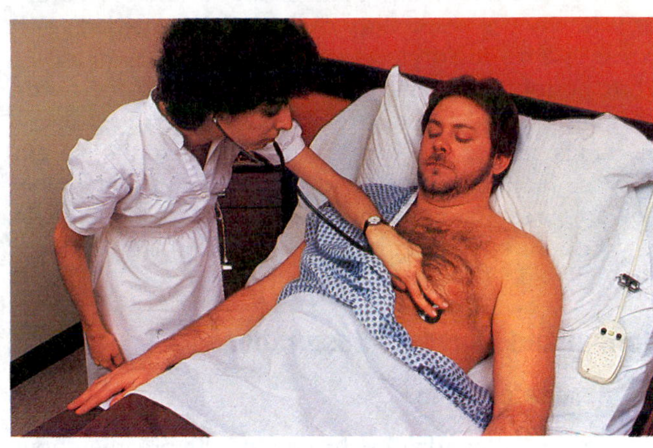

Action 10: Counting the heartbeat for 30 seconds.

Action	Rationale
11. Assess presence of any irregularity in heart rate and rhythm.	This assessment indicates adequacy of cardiac function.
12. Replace the client's gown and assist client to comfortable position.	Such action provides for privacy and comfort.
13. Record pulse rate on flow sheet or paper. Identify as apical rate. Report any abnormal findings to the appropriate person.	Recording the pulse rate provides accurate documentation.
14. Wash your hands.	Handwashing deters the spread of microorganisms.

Home Care Considerations

Inform client of availability of digital pulse monitoring devices.

Instruct family members about techniques used to locate and monitor other peripheral pulse sites.

Respiration

Respiration involves several physiologic events, including:

Pulmonary ventilation (or *breathing*)—movement of air in and out of the lungs; **inspiration** or inhalation is the act of breathing in, and **expiration** or exhalation is the act of breathing out.

External respiration—the exchange of oxygen and carbon dioxide between the alveoli of the lungs and the circulating blood

Internal respiration—the exchange of oxygen and carbon dioxide between the circulating blood and tissue cells

Although nurses assess the manifestations of changes in all of these respiratory events, the part that is measured as a vital sign is pulmonary ventilation, called respirations. The physiology and general principles of respiration are thoroughly discussed in Chapter 45; further information about respiratory system assessment is found in Chapter 26.

Regulation of Respiration

The cerebral cortex of the brain allows voluntary control of breathing, such as in singing or playing a musical instrument. The rate and depth of breathing can change in response to body demands. These changes are brought about by the inhibition or stimulation of the respiratory muscles by the respiratory centers in the medulla and pons. The respiratory centers are activated by impulses from peripheral chemoreceptors located in the aortic arch and carotids, from stretch and irritant receptors in the lungs, and from receptors in muscles and joints. An increase in carbon dioxide partial pressures is the most powerful respiratory stimulant, causing an increase in respiratory depth and rate.

Normal and Abnormal Respiration

Respiratory Rate

Under normal conditions, healthy adults breathe about 16 to 20 times each minute. Wider variations have also been observed in healthy people. The respiratory rate is more rapid in infants and young children. It has been noted that the relationship between the pulse rate and the respiratory rate is fairly consistent in well people, the ratio being one respiration to about four heartbeats.

During illness, the respiratory rate may vary from normal. When body temperature is elevated, the respiratory rate increases in response to the increased metabolic rate. Cells require more oxygen at this time and have a greater amount of carbon dioxide that must be removed. The rate increases as much as four breaths per minute with every 0.6°C (1°F) that the temperature rises above normal. Any condition causing an increase in carbon dioxide and a decrease in oxygen in the blood also tends to increase the rate and depth of respirations.

Some conditions characteristically predispose to slow breathing. An increase in intracranial pressure depresses the respiratory center, resulting in irregular or shallow breathing, slow breathing, or both. Certain drugs also depress the respiratory rate, especially narcotics.

Respiratory Depth

In a state of rest, the depth of each respiration is about the same. The depth of respirations is generally described as ranging from shallow to deep. Periodically, each person automatically inhales deeply, filling the lungs with more air than inhaled with the usual depth of respiration.

Certain terms are used to describe the nature and depth of respirations. **Apnea** refers to periods during which there is no breathing. This is a serious situation in which brain damage and death can occur if breathing is suppressed for more than 4 to 6 minutes. **Dyspnea** is difficult or labored breathing. A dyspneic client is likely to demonstrate rapid, shallow respirations, and to appear to be anxious. Dyspneic people can often breathe more easily in an upright position. The condition of being able to breathe easier in this manner is known as **orthopnea**. A sitting or standing position uses gravity to lower organs in the abdominal cavity away from the diaphragm. This gives more room for the lungs to expand within the chest, thus allowing the lungs to take in more air with each breath.

Assessment Methods

When assessing respirations, the nurse counts the respiratory rate and listens to breath sounds. Procedure 25-7 describes how to obtain the respiratory rate.

Breath Sounds

Breath sounds are heard by listening at various locations over the chest with a stethoscope. Ordinarily, respirations are relatively noiseless. Terms used to describe the nature of sounds that can be heard as the client breathes are outlined in Table 25-9 and summarized here. **Stertorous** breathing is a general term used to refer to noisy respirations. **Stridor** is a harsh, high-pitched sound heard on inspiration when there is a narrowing of the upper airway, such as the larynx or trachea. Infants or young children with croup often manifest stridor when breathing. A **wheeze** is a continuous, high-pitched squeak or musical sound made as air moves through a narrow or partially obstructed airway. **Crackles** (formerly called rales) are fine crackling sounds made as air moves through wet secretions; they are most often heard on inspiration. **Gurgles** (formally called rhonchi) are coarse wheezing or whistling sounds made as air moves through thick mucous or narrowed airways; they are best heard on expiration. Although stertorous respirations, stridor, and wheezes can be heard without amplification, crackles and gurgles are usually only heard by auscultation with a stethoscope.

Blood Pressure

Physiologic Factors

Blood pressure refers to the force of the blood against arterial walls. Maximum blood pressure is exerted on the walls of arteries when the left ventricle of the heart pushes blood through the aortic valve into the aorta during systole. The highest pressure thus is called **systolic pressure**. When the heart rests between beats (*diastole*), the pressure drops. The lowest pressure present on

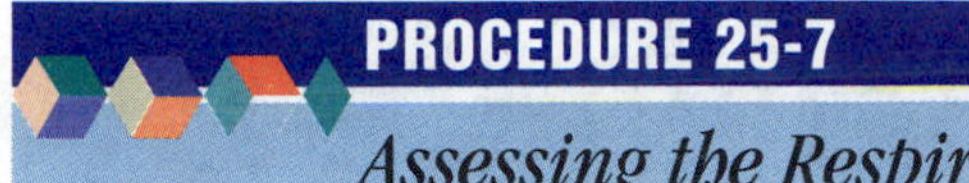

PROCEDURE 25-7

Assessing the Respiratory Rate

Equipment

- Watch with second hand or digital readout
- Pencil or pen
- Paper or flow sheet

Action	Rationale
1. While your fingertips are still in place after counting the pulse rate, observe the client's respirations.	Counting the respirations while presumably still counting the pulse helps to keep the client from becoming conscious of own breathing and possibly altering usual rate.
2. Note the rise and fall of the client's chest with each inspiration and expiration.	A complete cycle of inspiration and expiration constitutes one act of respiration.
3. Using a watch with a second hand, count the number of respirations for a minimum of 30 seconds. Multiply this number by two to obtain the client's respiratory rate per minute.	Sufficient time is necessary to observe rate, depth, and other characteristics.
4. If respirations are abnormal in any way, count the respiratory rate for a full minute. Repeat if necessary to determine the rate and characteristics of breathing.	Full-minute countings allow for the detection of unequal timing between respirations.
5. Record respiratory rate on flow sheet or paper. Report any abnormal findings to the appropriate person.	Recording the respiratory rate provides accurate documentation.
6. Wash your hands.	Handwashing deters the spread of microorganisms.

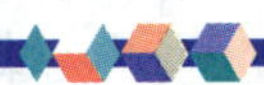

arterial walls at this time is called **diastolic pressure**. The difference between the two is called the **pulse pressure**. Blood pressure is measured in millimeters of mercury (mm Hg) and is recorded as a fraction. The numerator is the systolic pressure; the denominator is the diastolic pressure. For example, if the blood pressure is 120/80, 120 is the systolic pressure and 80 is the diastolic pressure. The pulse pressure, in this case, is 40.

Regulation of Blood Pressure

The following factors are responsible for maintaining blood pressure. Deviations from normal blood pressure may result from alterations in any of these factors, alone or in combination.

Peripheral Resistance. Once blood leaves the heart, it is circulated through a continuous loop of blood vessels consisting of arteries, arterioles, capillaries, and veins. *Arterioles* are fine, elastic tubes with the capacity to contract or dilate to regulate the distribution of blood to various organs, tissues, or cells, depending on their moment-by-moment requirements.

Normally, arterioles are in a state of partial contraction; they are neither totally constricted nor fully relaxed. This semicontracted state is *peripheral resistance*. It creates a relatively constant level of restraint to blood flow. Peripheral resistance is one of the main factors affecting blood pressure.

Pumping Action of the Heart. When increased amounts of blood are pumped into the arteries (ie, when cardiac output is increased), the arteries distend more, resulting in an increase in blood pressure. When less blood is pumped into the arteries (ie, when cardiac output is decreased), blood pressure falls. Hence, a weak pumping action results in a lower blood pressure than a strong pumping action.

Blood Volume. When blood volume is low, as may occur with hemorrhage or dehydration, blood pressure is low because there is decreased fluid within the arteries. Increasing the quantity of blood increases the pressure because there is more fluid volume creating pressure within the arteries.

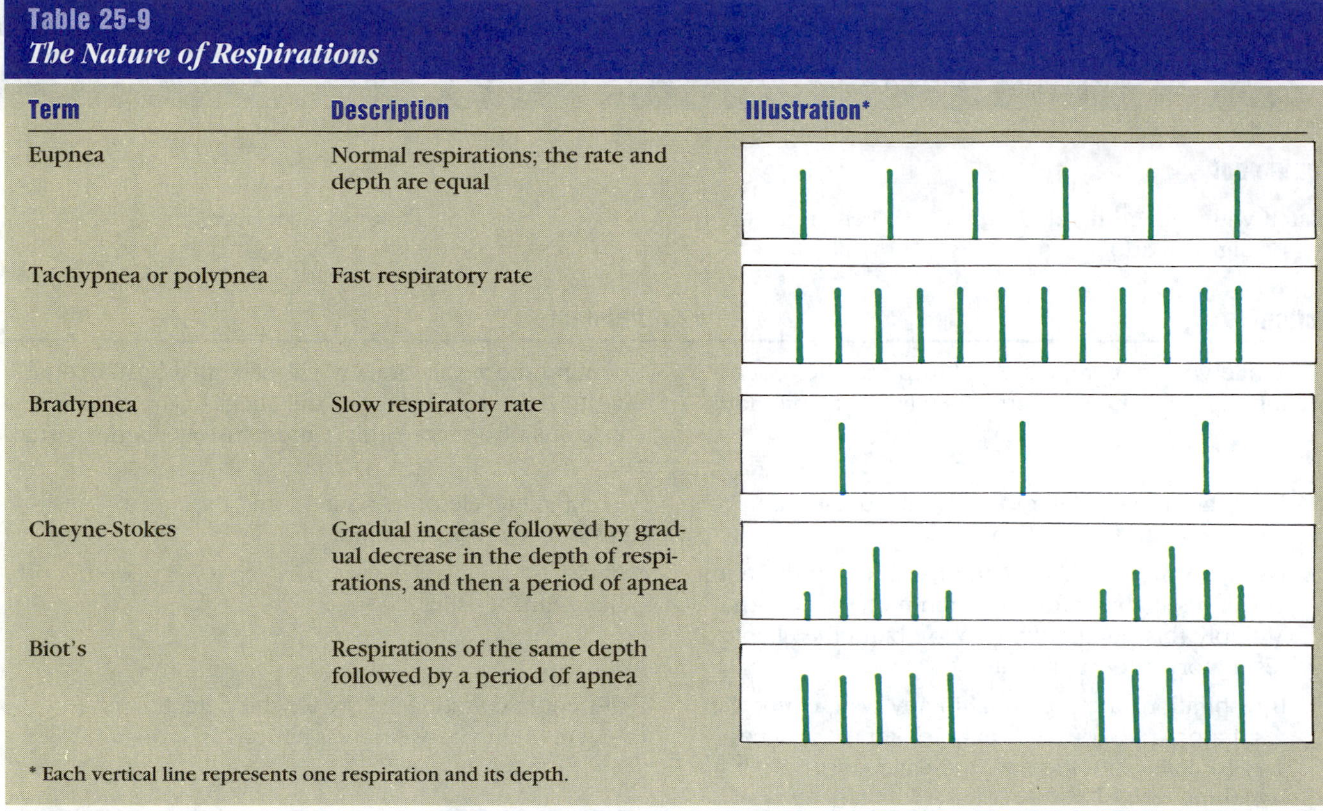

Table 25-9
The Nature of Respirations

Term	Description	Illustration*
Eupnea	Normal respirations; the rate and depth are equal	
Tachypnea or polypnea	Fast respiratory rate	
Bradypnea	Slow respiratory rate	
Cheyne-Stokes	Gradual increase followed by gradual decrease in the depth of respirations, and then a period of apnea	
Biot's	Respirations of the same depth followed by a period of apnea	

* Each vertical line represents one respiration and its depth.

Viscosity of Blood. **Viscosity** is the state of being sticky or gummy. The viscosity of the blood depends on the proportion of blood cells to plasma. The more viscous the blood, the higher the blood pressure. This occurs because the heart requires more force to move the concentrated fluid throughout the circulatory system.

Elasticity of Vessel Walls. Arteries have a considerable quantity of elastic tissue that allows them to stretch and distend (called *compliance*). When the heart rests between each beat, the walls of the arteries recoil, although pressure in them does not drop to zero. The state of pressure keeps the blood entering the capillaries and veins in a continuous flow, not in spurts. Simultaneously, the arterioles, normally in a moderate state of contraction, offer certain resistance. Therefore, the elasticity of the walls, in addition to the resistance of the arterioles, helps to maintain normal blood pressure.

With age, the walls of arterioles become less elastic, which interferes with their ability to stretch and dilate. This can subsequently limit adequate blood flow and contribute to rising pressure within the vascular system.

Normal and Abnormal Blood Pressure

Normal Blood Pressure

Studies of healthy people indicate that blood pressure can be within a wide range and still be normal. Because individual differences are considerable, it is important to know the normal blood pressure for a particular person. A rise or fall of 20 to 30 mm Hg in a person's blood pressure is significant, even if it is within the generally accepted normal range. Table 25-10 offers a guide for average normal and hypertensive levels of blood pressure measurements for people of various ages.

The following factors influence blood pressure in the average healthy adult:

- A person's age influences the blood pressure, with readings being lowest at birth, peaking at adolescence, and then slightly decreasing with aging. However, the older adult has decreased elasticity of the arteries, which increases peripheral resistance and therefore increases blood pressure.
- Normal fluctuations occur during the day. The blood pressure is usually lowest on arising in the morning. The blood pressure has been noted to rise as much as 5 to 10 mm Hg by late afternoon, and it gradually falls again during sleep.
- Women usually have a lower blood pressure than men of the same age.
- Blood pressure increases after eating food.
- Systolic blood pressure rises during periods of exercise and strenuous activity.
- Blood pressure is usually higher in people who are obese than in those who are thin.
- Emotions, such as anger, fear, excitement, and pain, generally cause the blood pressure to rise, but the pressure falls to normal when the situation passes.

Table 25-10
Average and Hypertensive Blood Pressures According to Age

Age	Average Blood Pressure	Hypertensive Level*
Newborn	40 mm Hg systolic	Undetermined
1 mo	85/54 mm Hg	Undetermined
1 yr	95/65 mm Hg	≥110/75 mm Hg
6 yr	105/65 mm Hg	≥120/80 mm Hg
10–13 yr	110/65 mm Hg	≥125/85 mm Hg
14–17 yr	120/80 mm Hg	≥135/90 mm Hg
18+ yr	120/80 mm Hg	≥140/90 mm Hg

* Levels determined by the 1984 Joint National Committee on Detection, Evaluation, and Treatment of High Blood Pressure.

- A person's blood pressure tends to be lower when in a prone or supine position than when sitting or standing.

Because of the many factors that influence blood pressure, a single blood pressure measurement is not necessarily significant. The American Heart Association recommends that blood pressure readings be averaged on two or more subsequent occasions before diagnosing a person with high blood pressure. Measurements should be taken after the client rests for at least 5 minutes and has not consumed caffeine or smoked for 30 minutes before the measurement. The U.S. Department of Health and Human Services, Public Health Service, has prepared recommended initial action and follow-up guidelines for subsequent blood pressure measurement. The Canadian Heart Fund (Ontario Division) advises that, in adults older than age 18 years who are not being treated for hypertension, a diastolic pressure below 95 mm Hg is considered normal, diastolic pressure between 95 and 104 mm Hg is considered borderline elevation, and diastolic pressure above 104 mm Hg is definitely elevated. People found to have a diastolic pressure above 104 mm Hg are referred for evaluation and care (Ontario Heart Fund Foundation, 1983). Blood pressure classifications and follow-up criteria are outlined in Table 25-11.

Hypertension

A person whose blood pressure is above normal for a sustained period is in a state of **hypertension**. When the cause of hypertension is due to known pathology, it is called *secondary hypertension*. *Primary* or *essential* hypertension is hypertension without a known cause.

Hypertension is a prevalent health problem. The public and health practitioners alike are becoming increasingly aware of the importance of having regular blood pressure measurements because of the many dangers associated with hypertension. Persistent diastolic hypertension is the most serious and most common blood pressure disturbance. It is a major cause of early death and serious disability in millions of people. Although the exact reason has not been determined, hypertension occurs almost twice as often in African Americans then in European Americans.

Hypotension

A blood pressure below normal is called **hypotension**. A consistently low blood pressure, for example, a systolic reading of 90 to 115 mm Hg in an adult, appears to cause no ill effects. Rather, this is usually associated with longevity.

Orthostatic (postural) **hypotension** is a low blood pressure associated with weakness or fainting when rising to an erect position. It is the result of peripheral vasodilation without a compensatory rise in cardiac output. This type of hypotension can usually be prevented by arising and moving about slowly, especially after a period of bed rest. Ordinarily it can be corrected by lowering the head, which restores blood flow to the brain.

Table 25-11
Blood Pressure Classification and Follow-Up Criteria

Category	Systolic BP (mm Hg)	Diastolic BP (mm Hg)	Follow-Up Recommended
Normal	<130	<85	Recheck in 2 years
High normal	130–139	85–89	Recheck in 1 year and discuss lifestyle modifications
Hypertension			
Stage 1 (mild)	140–159	90–99	Confirm within 2 months
Stage 2 (moderate)	160–179	100–109	Evaluate or refer within 1 month
Stage 3 (severe)	180–209	110–119	Evaluate or refer within 1 week
Stage 4 (very severe)	≥210	≥120	Evaluate or refer immediately

The recommendations for various blood pressure readings given are from the fifth report on the Joint National Committee on Detection, Education, and Treatment of High Blood Pressure. U.S. Department of Health and Human Services, Public Health Service, National Institutes of Health. (1993). (NIH Publication No. NIH 93-1088). Washington, DC: Author.

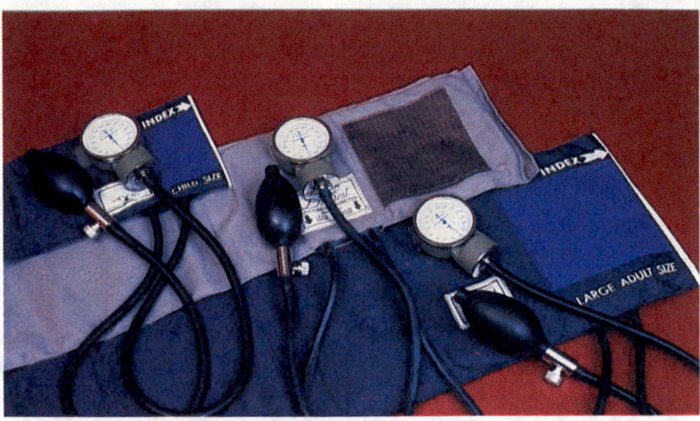

Figure 25-7
It is important to select a cuff of an appropriate size to obtain an accurate blood pressure reading. Shown hear are three cuff sizes: a small cuff for a child or a small or frail adult, a normal adult size cuff, and a large cuff, called a leg cuff, for measuring blood pressure on a leg or for use on an obese adult.

Clients with postural hypotension (most of whom are older adults) require special monitoring.

Some drugs, such as meperidine hydrochloride (Demerol) cause hypotension. There are also several illnesses associated with hypotension. For example, the blood pressure drops when a client is experiencing severe blood loss, burns, or severe vomiting and diarrhea, or when cardiac output is impaired after a heart attack.

Equipment

Sphygmomanometer

A **sphygmomanometer**, consisting of a cuff and a manometer, and a stethoscope are necessary for obtaining an indirect measurement of blood pressure.

Cuff. The sphygmomanometer has a cuff that contains an airtight, flat, rubber bladder covered with cloth. It is important to select a cuff of the proper width to obtain an accurate blood pressure reading (Fig. 25-7). If it is too narrow, the reading could be erroneously high because the pressure is not evenly transmitted to the artery. This occurs, for example, when an average size cuff is used on an obese person. If a cuff is too wide, the reading may be erroneously low because pressure is being directed toward a proportionately large surface area. For example, using an adult cuff on the thin arm of a child may cause this to occur. Recommendations for the selection of an appropriate size cuff are given in Table 25-12.

Cuffs are closed around the limb with contact closures, such as nylon fabric that can be fastened to itself (Velcro) or hooks. Some long cuffs are applied by encircling the arm several times.

Two tubes are attached to the bladder within the cuff. One is connected to a manometer; the other is attached to a bulb used to inflate the bladder. The bladder is inflated to the extent necessary to obstruct the flow of blood through the artery. A needle valve on the bulb allows the operator to deflate the cuff while the pressure is being read.

Manometer. A mercury *manometer* has a mercury-filled cylinder or tube calibrated in millimeters. When mercury rises in the tube, the upper or top surface of the mercury forms a convex curve called the *meniscus.* When determining blood pressure on the mercury manometer, the top of the curve of the meniscus within the calibrated cylinder correlates with the pressure. If the meniscus is observed above eye level, the pressure reading appears higher than it really is. If the meniscus is lower than eye level, it appears lower than it really is. The apparent change of position of an object when observed from two different angles is called *parallax.*

Table 25-12
Recommended Bladder Sizes for a Blood Pressure Cuff

Arm Circumference at Midpoint* (cm)	Cuff Name	Bladder Width (cm)	Bladder Length (cm)
5-7.5	Newborn	3	5
7.5-13	Infant	5	8
13-20	Child	8	13
24-32	Adult	13	24
32-42	Large adult	17	32
42-50†	Thigh	20	42

* Midpoint of arm is defined as half the distance from the acromion to the olecranon. Use nonstretchable metal tape.

† In persons with very large limbs, the indirect blood pressure should be measured in the leg or forearm.

(Reproduced with permission. "Recommendations for human blood pressure determination by sphygmomanometers," 1967, 1980, 1987. Copyright © American Heart Association.)

Figure 25-8 illustrates the meniscus and how pressure readings may be incorrect when the meniscus is above or below eye level.

Another type of manometer is called the *aneroid manometer*. It too has a cuff, but it is attached to a round, calibrated dial with a needle that indicates pressure. Figure 25-9 shows a mercury manometer and an aneroid manometer.

Stethoscope. The stethoscope is used to auscultate the sound heard directly over the artery as the pressure in the cuff is released and the blood is permitted to flow through the artery. The construction of the stethoscope magnifies the sounds in the artery as they are transmitted to the listener. The blood pressure reading is obtained by listening to the sounds and watching the manometer. The bell of the stethoscope amplifies low-frequency sounds, such as those commonly made by the heart and the blood within the vessels, and is most often used when assessing blood pressure.

Assessment Sites and Methods

The nurse assesses the blood pressure by listening for specific sounds, called Korotkoff sounds. Although various sites may be used to assess the blood pressure, the brachial artery and the popliteal artery are most commonly used. Alternate methods for assessing blood pressure include palpation and the use of mechanical devices.

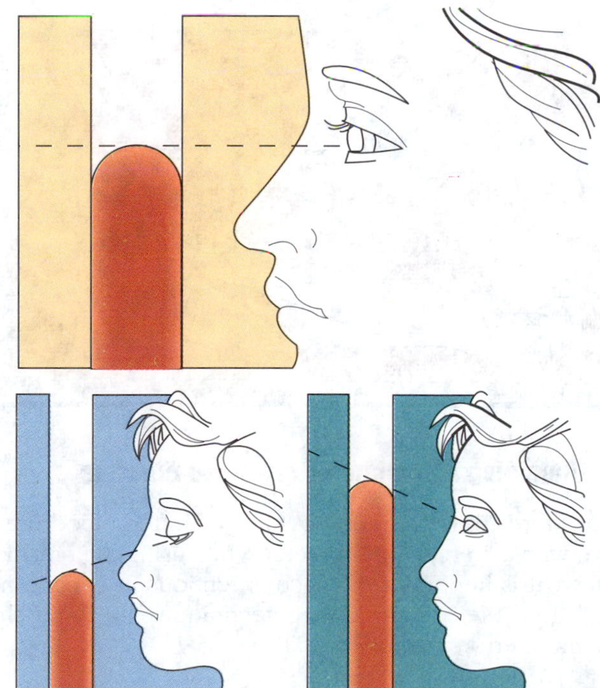

Figure 25-8
A blood pressure reading should be made with the eye at the level of the meniscus as shown in the top drawing. The two drawings at the bottom illustrate how parallax can affect the accuracy of a reading when the line of sight is not level with the meniscus.

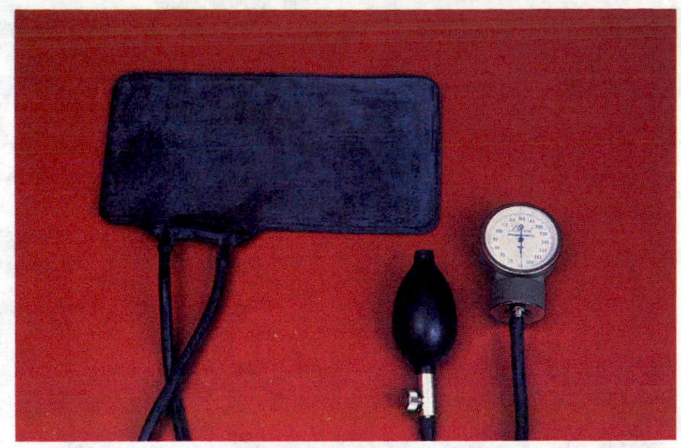

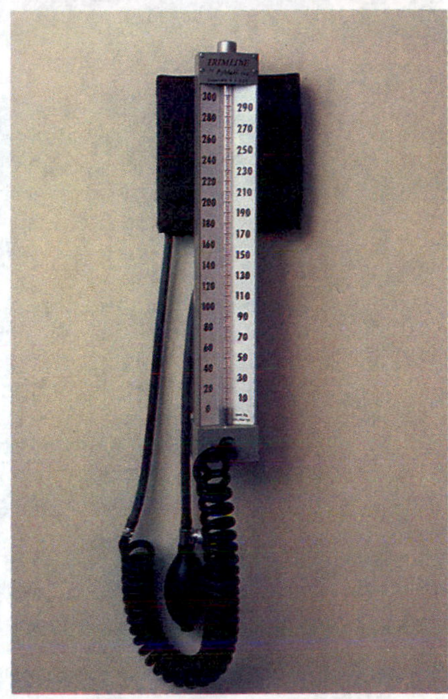

Figure 25-9
An aneroid manometer (*top*) and a mercury manometer (*bottom*).

Korotkoff Sounds

The series of sounds for which the nurse listens when measuring the blood pressure are called **Korotkoff sounds** and are described in Table 25-13. In some adults, each of these sounds is distinct, whereas in others, only the beginning and ending sounds are heard. It is important to determine institutional policy when recording blood pressure sounds, and to be consistent in taking and documenting the readings.

The first sound that is heard, which is the onset of phase I, represents the systolic pressure. It is recorded as the first number in the fraction; for example, if the blood pressure reading is 120/80, 120 is the systolic pressure. The second number, which represents the diastolic

Table 25-13
Korotkoff Sounds

Phase	Description	Illustration
Phase I	Characterized by the first appearance of faint but clear tapping sounds that gradually increase in intensity; the first tapping sound is the systolic pressure	
Phase II	Characterized by muffled or swishing sounds; these sounds may temporarily disappear, especially in hypertensive people; the disappearance of the sound during the latter part of phase I and during phase II is called the auscultatory gap and may cover a range of as much as 40 mm Hg; failing to recognize this gap may cause serious errors of underestimating systolic pressure or overestimating diastolic pressure	
Phase III	Characterized by distinct, loud sounds as the blood flows relatively freely through an increasingly open artery	
Phase IV	Characterized by a distinct, abrupt, muffling sound with a soft, blowing quality; in adults, the onset of this phase is considered to be the first diastolic figure	
Phase V	The last sound heard before a period of continuous silence; the pressure at which the last sound is heard is the second diastolic measurement	

pressure (in this case 80), notes the level at which either a change in or cessation of the loud, distinct sounds took place. This occurs in either phase IV or phase V.

The blood pressure is most commonly recorded with two numbers written as a fraction, with the bottom number indicating either the change of the sound or the last sound heard. However, the American Heart Association (1987) recommends that in instances when both a change in the sounds and a cessation of the sounds are heard, all numbers be recorded. In this case, the blood pressure would be recorded as 120/80/64. If the sounds are heard all the way down to zero, the blood pressure recording would be 120/80/0. It is important to determine the procedure for recording blood pressure at each agency or institution so that readings are consistent.

Obtaining a Brachial Artery Blood Pressure

Procedure 25-8 describes how to obtain the blood pressure with a mercury manometer while using the brachial artery. It is important to be conscientious in continuing to follow the recommended techniques to avoid the common errors identified in Table 25-14.

Obtaining a Popliteal Artery Blood Pressure

When the client's brachial artery is inaccessible, the nurse can obtain the blood pressure using the popliteal artery in the leg. It can be expected that the systolic pressure is likely to be 10 to 40 mm Hg higher using this site. A cuff of proportionately larger size should be used. The

(text continues on page 467)

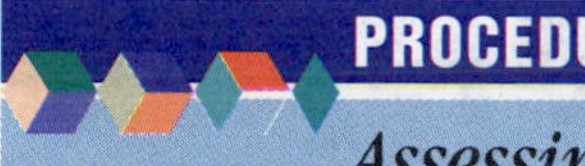

PROCEDURE 25-8

Assessing Blood Pressure

Equipment

Stethoscope
Sphygmomanometer
Blood pressure cuff of appropriate size
Pencil or pen
Paper or flow sheet
Alcohol swab

Action	Rationale
1. Explain the procedure to the client.	An explanation encourages client cooperation and reduces client apprehension.
2. Gather equipment.	Gathering equipment provides for organized approach to task.
3. Use alcohol swab to cleanse earpieces and diaphragm of stethoscope, if necessary.	Cleansing stethoscope deters the transmission of microorganisms.
4. Wash your hands.	Handwashing deters the spread of microorganisms.
5. Select a blood pressure cuff of an appropriate size for the client.	A cuff that is too large or too small produces a false reading.
6. Delay obtaining the blood pressure if the client is emotionally upset, is in pain, or has just exercised, unless it is urgent to obtain the blood pressure.	Factors such as emotional upset, exercise, and pain alter usual blood pressure measurements.
7. Select appropriate arm for application of cuff (no intravenous infusion, breast or axilla surgery on that side, cast, arteriovenous shunt, or injured or diseased limb).	Measurement of blood pressure may temporarily impede circulation to a diseased or compromised extremity.
8. Have the client assume a comfortable lying or sitting position with the forearm supported at the level of the heart and the palm of the hand upward.	This position places the brachial artery on the inner aspect of the elbow so that the bell of the stethoscope can rest on it easily.
9. Expose the area of the brachial artery by removing garments, or move a sleeve, if it is not too tight, above the area where the cuff will be placed.	Clothing over the artery interferes with the ability to hear sounds and may cause inaccurate blood pressure readings. Tight clothing on the arm causes congestion of blood and possibly inaccurate readings.
10. Center the bladder of the cuff over the brachial artery, approximately midway on the arm, so that the lower edge of the cuff is about 2.5 to 5 cm (1 to 2 inches) above the inner aspect of the elbow. The tubing should extend from the edge of the cuff nearer the client's elbow.	Pressure in the cuff applied directly to the artery provides the most accurate readings. If the cuff gets in the way of the stethoscope, readings are likely to be inaccurate. A cuff placed upside down with the tubing toward the client's head may give a false reading.
11. Wrap the cuff around the arm smoothly and snugly, and fasten it securely or tuck the end of the cuff well under the preceding wrapping. Do not allow any clothing to interfere with the proper placement of the cuff.	A smooth cuff and snug wrapping produce equal pressure and help promote an accurate measurement. A cuff too loosely wrapped results in an inaccurate reading.
12. Check that a mercury manometer is in a vertical position. The mercury must be within the zero area with the gauge at eye level. If an aneroid gauge is used, the needle should be within the zero mark.	Tilting a mercury manometer, inaccurate calibration, or improper height for reading the gauge can lead to errors in determining the pressure measurements.
13. Palpate the pulse at the brachial or radial artery by pressing gently with the fingertips.	Palpation allows for measurement of the approximate systolic reading.

(continued)

PROCEDURE 25-8 *(continued)*

Assessing Blood Pressure

Action | **Rationale**

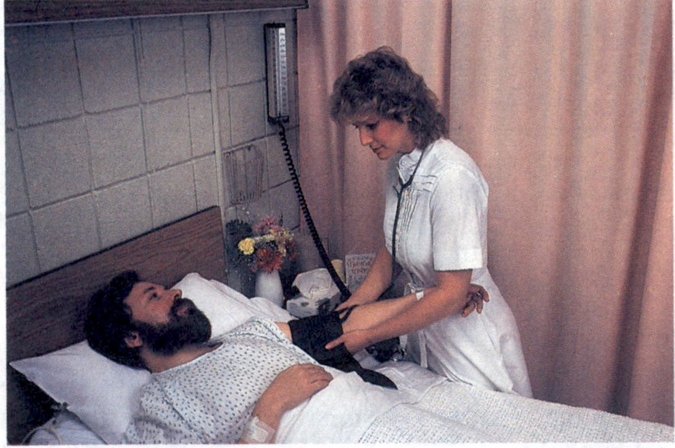

Actions 10 and 11: Centering the cuff over the brachial artery and wrapping smoothly and snugly.

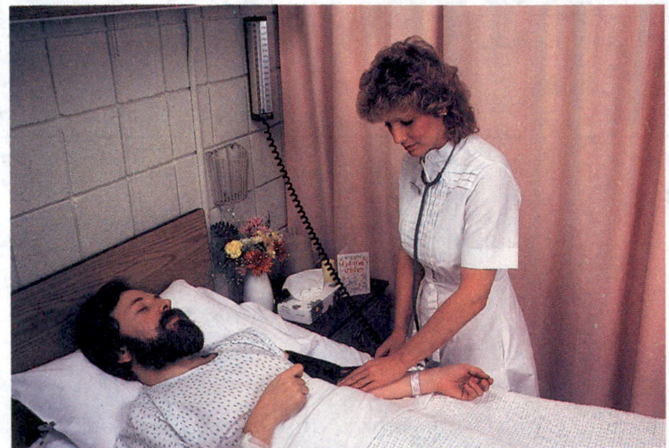

Action 13: Palpating the brachial artery.

14. Tighten the screw valve on the air pump.

The bladder within the cuff will not inflate with the valve open.

15. Inflate the cuff while continuing to palpate the artery. Note the point on the gauge where the pulse disappears.

The point where the pulse disappears provides an estimate of the systolic pressure. To identify the first Korotkoff sound accurately, the cuff must be inflated to a pressure above the point at which the pulse can no longer be felt.

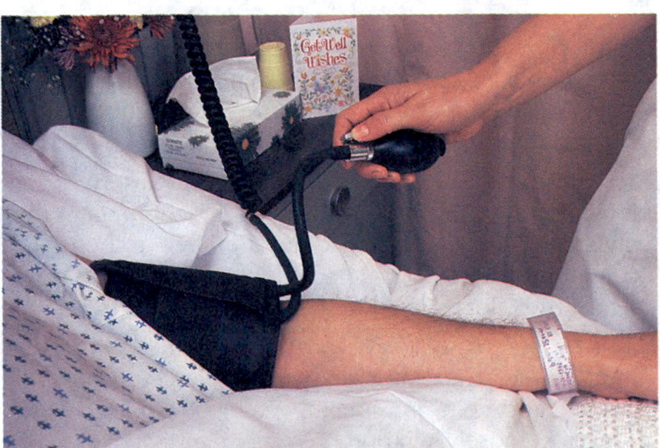

Action 14: Tightening the screw valve on air pump.

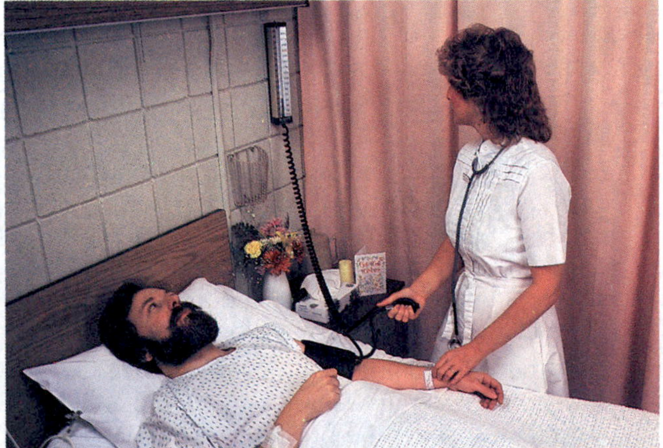

Action 15: Inflating cuff while palpating the radial artery.

16. Deflate the cuff and wait 15 seconds.

Allowing a brief pause before continuing permits the blood to refill and circulate through the arm.

17. Assume a position that is no more than 3 feet away from the gauge.

A distance of more than about 3 feet can interfere with accurate readings of the numbers on the gauge.

18. Place the stethoscope earpieces in the ears. Direct the eartips forward into the canal and not against the ear itself.

Proper placement blocks extraneous noise and allows sound to travel more clearly.

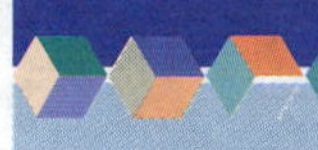

PROCEDURE 25-8 *(continued)*

Assessing Blood Pressure

Action	Rationale
19. Place the bell or diaphragm of the stethoscope firmly but with as little pressure as possible over the brachial artery. Do not allow the stethoscope to touch clothing or the cuff.	Having the bell or diaphragm directly over the artery makes more accurate readings possible. Heavy pressure on the brachial artery distorts the shape of the artery and the sound. Placing the bell or diaphragm away from clothing and the cuff prevents noise, which will distract from the sounds made by blood flowing through the artery.

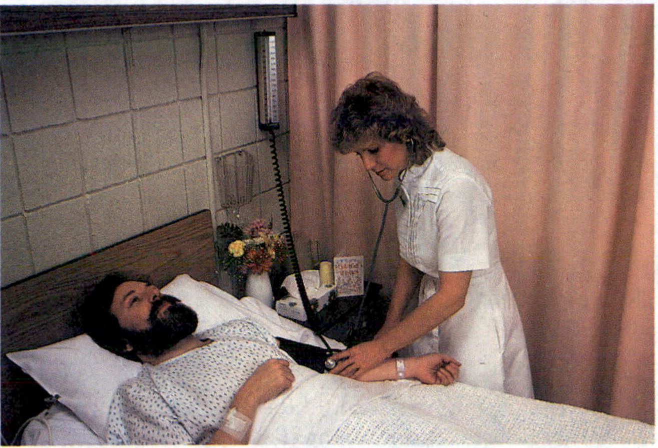

Actions 18 and 19: Placing amplifier of stethoscope over artery, reinflating cuff, and listening for disappearance of sound.

Action	Rationale
20. Pump the pressure 30 mm Hg above the point at which the systolic pressure was palpated and estimated. Open the valve on the manometer and allow air to escape slowly (allowing the gauge to drop 2 to 3 mm per heartbeat).	Increasing the pressure above where the pulse disappeared ensures a period before hearing the first sound that corresponds with the systolic pressure. It prevents misinterpreting phase II sounds as phase I.
21. Note the point on the gauge at which there is an appearance of the first faint, but clear, sound that slowly increases in intensity. Note this number as the systolic pressure.	Systolic pressure is the point at which the blood in the artery is first able to force its way through the vessel at a similar pressure exerted by the air bladder in the cuff. The first sound is phase I of Korotkoff sounds.
22. Read the pressure to the closest even number.	It is common practice to read blood pressure to the closest even number.
23. Do not reinflate the cuff once the air is being released to recheck the systolic pressure reading.	Reinflating the cuff while obtaining the blood pressure is uncomfortable for the client and may cause an inaccurate reading. Reinflating the cuff causes congestion of blood in the lower arm, which lessens the loudness of Korotkoff sounds.
24. Note the pressure at which the sound first becomes muffled. Also observe the point at which the sound completely disappears. These may occur separately or at the same point.	The point at which the sound changes corresponds to phase IV of Korotkoff sounds and is considered the first diastolic pressure reading. According to the American Heart Association, this is used as the diastolic pressure recording in children. The last sound heard is the beginning of phase V and is the second diastolic measurement.
25. Allow the remaining air to escape quickly. Repeat any suspicious reading, but wait 30 to 60 seconds between readings to allow normal circulation to return in the limb. Be sure to deflate the cuff completely between attempts to check the blood pressure.	False readings are likely to occur if there is congestion of blood in the limb while obtaining repeated readings.

(continued)

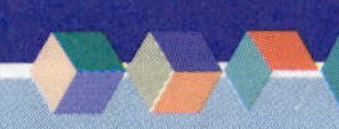

PROCEDURE 25-8 *(continued)*

Assessing Blood Pressure

Action	Rationale
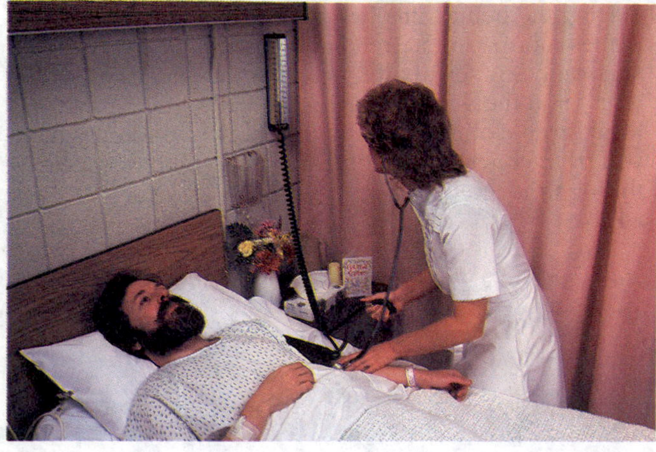	*Actions 20, 21, and 23: Listening for Korotkoff sounds and noting systolic and diastolic pressure readings. (Photos © Ken Kasper.)*
26. Remove the cuff, clean and store the equipment.	Equipment that must be shared among personnel should be left in a manner ready for use.
27. Wash your hands.	Handwashing deters the spread of microorganisms.
28. Record the client's position, the arm that was used to obtain the blood pressure, and the readings that correspond to the systolic and diastolic readings. Compare to previous readings and report any abnormalities to the appropriate person.	Circumstances for assessing the blood pressure should be consistent for future comparisons.

Special Considerations

If this is the initial nursing assessment of a client, take the blood pressure on both arms. It is normal to have a 5–10 mm Hg difference in the systolic reading between arms. Use the arm with the higher reading for subsequent pressures.

When having difficulty hearing the blood pressure sounds, the following technique is recommended:

- Raise the client's arm, with cuff in place, over his or her head for 15 seconds before rechecking the blood pressure.
- Inflate the cuff while the arm is elevated and then gently lower the arm while continuing to support it.
- Position the stethoscope and deflate the cuff at the usual rate while listening for Korotkoff sounds.

Raising the arm over the head helps relieve congestion of blood in the limb, increases pressure differences, and makes the sounds louder and more distinct when blood enters the lower arm.

Home Care Considerations

- Use cuff size appropriate for limb circumference. Inform client that cuff sizes range from a pediatric cuff to a large thigh cuff and that a poorly fitting cuff may result in an inaccurate measurement.
- Inform client about availability of digital blood pressure monitoring equipment. Though costly, most provide an easy-to-read recording of systolic and diastolic measurements.

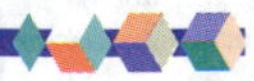

Table 25-14
Blood Pressure Assessment Errors and Contributing Causes

Error	Contributing Causes	Error	Contributing Causes
Falsely low assessments	• Hearing deficit • Noise in the environment • Viewing the meniscus from above eye level • Applying too wide a cuff • Inserting eartips of stethoscope incorrectly • Using cracked or kinked tubing • Releasing the valve rapidly • Misplacing the bell beyond the direct area of the artery • Failing to pump the cuff 20 to 30 mm Hg above the disappearance of the pulse	Falsely high assessments	• Using a manometer not calibrated at the zero mark • Assessing the blood pressure immediately after exercise • Viewing the meniscus from below eye level • Applying a cuff that is too narrow • Releasing the valve too slowly • Reinflating the bladder during auscultation

client should be positioned on the abdomen or with the knee flexed, if in a supine position. The technique for assessment is essentially the same as when using the arm.

Alternate Techniques

Palpating the Blood Pressure. Assessing the blood pressure through palpation is sometimes referred to as the *sensory detection method.* It requires only the use of the sphygmomanometer. The cuff is inflated 30 mm Hg above the point at which the pulsation in the artery disappears. As the air in the cuff is released, the nurse feels for the return of the pulse. Usually no diastolic pressure is recorded because the artery continues to pulsate as long as blood flows through it. Some home clients assess their blood pressure this way. Instead of palpating the artery, however, the person notes the pressure on the manometer when experiencing the onset and disappearance of the throbbing sensation. The measurements using this method have been fairly similar to those obtained using other, more sophisticated techniques for assessing blood pressure.

Using the Doppler Ultrasound. The blood pressure may also be taken with an ultrasound or Doppler apparatus, which amplifies sounds. This is especially useful if the sounds are indistinct or are inaudible with a regular stethoscope. Usually, the only measurement that can be obtained is the systolic reading. To use the Doppler, the nurse follows the same procedure as described for taking the pulse by this device.

Electronic Indirect Blood Pressure Meters. Electronic blood pressure meters sense vibrations within the artery wall, record the pressure readings, and display them in digital numbers (Fig. 25-10). These devices are helpful for people who wish to obtain their own blood pressure measurements, and are used by clients in their own homes. They are also advantageous for those people who have a hearing impairment because listening for Korotkoff sounds is unnecessary. No stethoscope is required. However, because of their delicate instrumentation, electronic machines should be recalibrated when readings are more than a few points different from the person's normal pattern. Clients using these devices at home should also have their blood pressure checked periodically by health personnel.

Direct Electronic Measurement. It is possible to measure blood pressure directly through the insertion of a thin catheter into an artery (an **arterial line**). The tip of the catheter has the ability to sense pressures and transmit the information to a machine that displays the systolic and diastolic pressure in a waveform. This technique is used primarily in intensive care areas.

Care of Equipment

It is important that equipment used for measuring blood pressure be in good repair and function accurately. Improperly functioning equipment is a major cause of

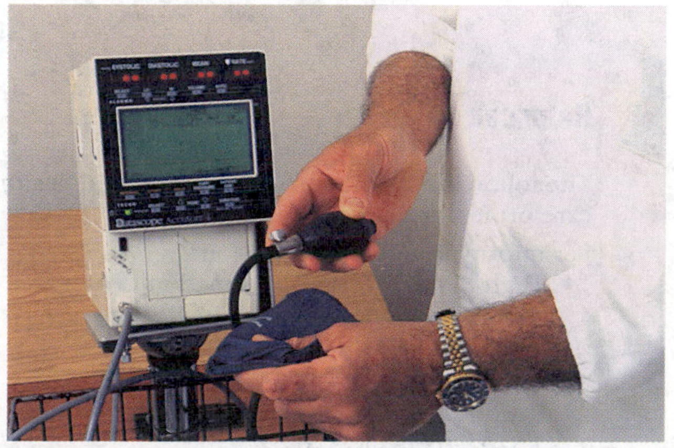

Figure 25-10
The automatic blood pressure monitor reports systolic, diastolic, and mean blood pressure. (Photo © B. Proud.)

inaccurate measurements. The nurse should check routinely to see that there are no air leaks in the rubber bladder, sphygmomanometer connectors, tubing, or valve. For pressure to be measured accurately, the mercury meniscus and the needle on the aneroid manometer should be checked to see that they are exactly on zero when the cuff is deflated. The mercury manometer should be cleaned and checked at least annually to see that the mercury is free of foreign matter and air. The aneroid manometer must be checked for accurate calibration frequently against an accurate mercury manometer. Some authorities recommend weekly calibration for the aneroid manometer, whereas others suggest checking it every 6 months. Any time the accuracy of the equipment is questioned, it should be checked and repaired or replaced, as indicated.

Teaching About Vital Signs for Home Care

Clients at home often need to check their own temperature, pulse, or blood pressure. Guidelines for teaching self-assessment and care of equipment follow.

Taking the Temperature

- The temperature may be taken with a glass thermometer, a single-use disposable thermometer, or a temperature-sensitive tape.
- Adults who use a glass thermometer usually take an oral temperature. It is important that the temperature be taken at least 30 minutes after eating or drinking hot or cold foods or fluids or after smoking, to be sure an accurate temperature is obtained.
- Infants and small children should have their temperature taken either with a temperature-sensitive tape on the forehead or a single-use thermometer in the axilla (armpit). Infants and small children should not have rectal temperatures taken because of the risk of damage to the rectal area.
- Shake the mercury down into the bulb of the thermometer until the level of the mercury is below 98°F (36.5°C). To see the mercury level, hold the thermometer sideways at eye level and rotate it until the mercury can be seen. If the thermometer uses a Fahrenheit scale, each long mark is one degree and each short mark is two tenths of a degree; a centigrade scale uses long marks for one half of a degree and short marks for one tenth of a degree.
- Place the glass thermometer as far back as possible under the side of the tongue and close the lips. Do not talk while the thermometer is in the mouth.
- Leave the thermometer in place for 2 to 3 minutes.
- Remove the thermometer and determine the point at which the mercury is level. This is the body temperature. Call your healthcare provider if the temperature is greater than 100°F (37.7°C), or if you are concerned.
- Wash the thermometer with soap and warm water, rinse it with cold water, dry it well, and store it in a clean, dry area. Do not use the thermometer to take another person's temperature unless it has been cleaned. If several members of the household have an infection or illness, the thermometer should soak in 70% isopropyl alcohol between uses; be sure to rinse off the alcohol with cold water before using it again.

Taking the Pulse

- The pulse is often taken before taking certain medications, such as those to make the heartbeat stronger. It is also taken by people who exercise and use it as an indicator of the effectiveness of the exercise on heart function.
- It is necessary to be able to see a watch or a clock with a second hand when taking the pulse.
- Place one arm on a firm surface so the palm is upward. Using the middle three fingers of the other hand, gently feel the outside of the arm just below the wrist with the fingertips. Do not press hard. When pulsations are felt, watch the second hand of the watch or clock and begin to count when the second hand reaches 12 (any number is fine, but it is often easier to remember to always begin count-

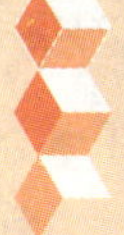

Helpscan

The following are resources for clients and health care professionals:

For information on hypertension:

- High Blood Pressure Information Center
  120 '80 National Institutes of Health
  Bethesda, MD 20205

For information on heart disease:

- American Heart Association
  7320 Greenville Ave.
  Dallas, TX 75231
  (214) 373-6300

For information on lung diseases:

- American Lung Association
  740 Broadway
  New York, NY 10019
  (212) 315-8700

ing when the second hand is on 12). Count each pulsation (beat) for one minute (when the second hand again reaches 12) and write the number down.

- If the speed of the pulse is very fast, very slow, or irregular, or if you have any concerns, contact your healthcare provider.

Taking the Blood Pressure

- The blood pressure is often taken to determine how well medications are working to control high blood pressure. The blood pressure is usually checked once a week. A record of blood pressure readings over time is more important than one reading.
- The blood pressure can be measured at home with a blood pressure monitoring device or by using the mechanical devices found in many grocery or discount stores that have a pharmacy. It is important to use the same device or machine each time, and to write down the numbers.
- If a home device is used, be sure the cuff is the proper size and that all parts of the device are working properly. The measurement should be taken while sitting comfortably, and the arm should be supported on a firm surface.
- If the blood pressure numbers increase or decrease by more than 10, or if you have any concerns, contact your healthcare provider.

Key Points

- Assessing vital signs, a traditional nursing responsibility, involves obtaining temperature, pulse, respiration, and blood pressure as part of the baseline data from which a plan of care is developed.
- The frequency of assessing vital signs is governed by the healthcare agency's policies and the client's health status.
- Humans are warm blooded and maintain body temperature independently of their environment. The hypothalamus in the central nervous system maintains body temperature of the well human within a fairly constant range, called a set point.
- Pyrexia, or fever, an elevation of normal body temperature, is a common symptom of disease. Most fevers are self-limiting. On the other hand, hypothermia is a temperature below the lower limit of normal. Both may be means by which the body fights disease.
- Temperature may be assessed by glass clinical thermometer, electronic thermometer, disposable single-use thermometer, temperature-sensitive patch or tape, or automated monitoring device. Although most agencies measure temperature by the oral route, rectal and axillary routes are alternative sites.
- When the left ventricle of the heart contracts to eject blood into the filled aorta, arterial walls expand or distend; this expansion can be felt as a wave and is called the pulse. Pulse rate is the number of pulsations felt in a minute; pulse rhythm is the pattern of the pulsations and the pauses between them; and pulse amplitude describes the quality of the pulse.
- Arteries most commonly used for assessment are peripheral pulses or those close to the skin surface (ie, temporal, carotid, brachial, radial, femoral, popliteal, posterior tibial, and dorsalis pedis). The radial pulse at the wrist is most commonly used.
- Respiration is the act of breathing and includes the body's use of oxygen and elimination of carbon dioxide. Inspiration or inhalation is the act of breathing in. Expiration or exhalation is the act of breathing out.
- Healthy adults breathe about 16 to 20 times per minute with a fairly consistent relationship of pulse rate to respiratory rate of one respiration to about four heartbeats.
- Apnea refers to periods in which there is no breathing; dyspnea is difficult or labored breathing, demonstrated by rapid and shallow breathing. Dyspneic clients frequently are able to breathe easier in an upright position. Being able to breathe easier in this manner is known as orthopnea.
- Blood pressure refers to the force of blood against arterial walls. The highest pressure, exerted when the left ventricle of the heart pushes blood through the aortic valve into the aorta during systole, is called systolic pressure. When the heart rests between beats (diastole), the pressure drops; the lowest pressure is called diastolic pressure. Blood pressure, measured in millimeters of mercury (mm Hg), is recorded as a fraction. The numerator is the systolic pressure; the denominator is the diastolic pressure (eg, 120/80).
- Deviations from normal blood pressure are likely due to alterations in any one or more of these functions: peripheral resistance, heart's pumping action, blood volume, blood viscosity, and elasticity of vessel walls.
- Blood pressure can be within a wide range and still be normal. Many factors influence a normal, healthy adult's blood pressure.
- Hypertension is a state in which a person's blood pressure is above normal. Primary or essential hypertension has an unknown cause, whereas secondary hypertension is due to known pathologic factors. Blood pressure below normal is called hypotension. Orthostatic or postural hypotension is associated with weakness or fainting when rising to an erect position.

- A sphygmomanometer, consisting of a cuff and manometer, and a stethoscope are necessary for obtaining an indirect measurement of blood pressure. The series of sounds heard in this measurement are called Korotkoff sounds. They are written as fractions (eg, 120/80).
- Blood pressure also can be assessed using palpitation, electronic indirect blood pressure meters, or direct electronic measurements.
- Clients providing self-care at home need to know how to take their own temperature, pulse, and blood pressure.

Study Questions

1. An elevation of the body temperature above normal is labeled
   a. pyrexia
   b. hypothermia
   c. hypertension
   d. afebrile
2. For which of the following clients would you use an oral thermometer?
   a. a 6-month-old infant
   b. a client receiving oxygen therapy
   c. a 42-year-old healthy female
   d. an unconscious client
3. Insertion of a rectal thermometer may cause a potentially harmful condition. This condition is
   a. an increase in heart rate
   b. a decrease in heart rate
   c. an involuntary loss of stool
   d. an increase in respirations
4. While taking an adult client's pulse, the nurse finds the rate to be 140. The nurse would report and document this finding as
   a. hyperthermia
   b. bradycardia
   c. palpitations
   d. tachycardia
5. A client complains of severe abdominal pain. When assessing the vital signs, the nurse would not be surprised to find
   a. an increase in the pulse rate
   b. a decrease in body temperature
   c. a decrease in blood pressure
   d. an increase in body temperature
6. The apical pulse is obtained by using
   a. a sphygmomanometer
   b. an electronic thermometer
   c. a stethoscope
   d. a Doppler apparatus
7. The difference between the apical and radial pulse rates is called the
   a. pulse deficit
   b. pulse amplitude
   c. ventricular rhythm
   d. heart arrhythmia
8. The normal respiratory rate in adults is considered to be
   a. 1 to 6 breaths per minute
   b. 16 to 20 breaths per minute
   c. 60 to 80 breaths per minute
   d. 100 to 120 breaths per minute
9. A client is having dyspnea. To facilitate respirations, the nurse would
   a. remove pillows from under the head
   b. elevate the head of the bed
   c. elevate the foot of the bed
   d. take the blood pressure
10. Blood pressure is the measurement of
    a. the flow of blood through the circulation
    b. the force of blood against arterial walls
    c. the force of blood against venous walls
    d. the flow of blood through the heart
11. With aging, blood pressure is often higher due to
    a. loss of muscle mass
    b. changes in exercise and diet
    c. decreased peripheral resistance
    d. decreased elasticity in arterial walls
12. A client has a blood pressure reading of 130/90 when visiting a clinic. The nurse would recommend
    a. follow-up measurements of blood pressure
    b. immediate treatment by a physician
    c. nothing, because the nurse considers this reading is due to anxiety
    d. a change in diet and exercise
13. In recording a blood pressure of 120/80, the 120 represents
    a. the pulse rate
    b. the diastolic pressure
    c. the systolic pressure
    d. the pulse deficit
14. It is important to have the appropriate cuff size when taking the blood pressure. A cuff that is too large or too small may result in
    a. an incorrect reading
    b. injury to the client
    c. prolonged pressure on the arm
    d. loss of Korotkoff sounds
15. A client has intravenous fluids infusing in the right arm. When taking a blood pressure on this client, the nurse would
    a. take the blood pressure in the right arm
    b. take the blood pressure in the left arm
    c. use the smallest possible cuff
    d. report inability to take the blood pressure

Answers With Rationale

1. The correct response is *a.* Pyrexia is an elevation of body temperature. Hypothermia is low body temperature. Hypertension is elevated blood pressure. Afebrile means that there is not an elevation of body temperature.
2. The correct response is *c.* Use of oral thermometers is contraindicated in infants, clients receiving oxygen therapy, and unconscious clients.
3. The correct response is *b.* Insertion of a rectal thermometer may stimulate the vagus nerve, which, in turn, would decrease heart rate. This may potentially be harmful for clients with cardiac problems.
4. The correct response is *d.* A pulse rate of 100 to 180 beats per minute in an adult is tachycardia. Hyperthermia is high body temperature. Bradycardia is an adult pulse rate of below 60 beats per minute. The sensation one feels in being aware of the heartbeat is called palpitations.
5. The correct response is *a.* The pulse often increases when an individual is experiencing pain. Pain does not affect body temperature, and may increase (not decrease) blood pressure.
6. The correct response is *c.* The apical pulse can only be obtained by listening with a stethoscope.
7. The correct response is *a.* The difference between the apical and radial pulse rate is called the pulse deficit. The other responses are names given to volume and rhythm of the pulse.
8. The correct response is *b.* The normal respiratory rate for adults is 16 to 20 breaths per minute.
9. The correct response is *b.* Dyspnea is difficult respirations. Elevating the head of the bed allows the abdominal organs to descend, giving the diaphragm greater room for expansion and facilitating lung expansion. Any other intervention would not facilitate respirations.
10. The correct response is *b.* Blood pressure is the measurement of the force of blood against arterial walls. Other responses are incorrect in describing blood pressure.
11. The correct response is *d.* With aging, elasticity in arterial walls is decreased, contributing to an elevated blood pressure reading. The other responses may contribute to changes in readings, but they are not the physiologic basis for blood pressure findings in the older adult.
12. The correct response is *a.* A single blood pressure reading that is mildly elevated is not significant, but the measurement should be taken again over time to determine if hypertension is a problem. The nurse would recommend a return visit to the clinic for a recheck.
13. The correct response is *c*—120 is the systolic pressure. The diastolic pressure is 80. The other responses relate to pulse rather than blood pressure.
14. The correct response is *a.* A blood pressure cuff that is not the right size may cause an incorrect reading. It will not cause injury or loss of sounds.
15. The correct response is *b.* The blood pressure should be taken in the arm opposite the one with the infusion. Blood pressure should not be taken in the arm with an intravenous infusion because the pressure of inflating the cuff may allow the artery to clot.

Bibliography

American Heart Association. (1987). *Recommendations for human blood pressure determination by sphygmomanometers* (Publication No. 701005). Kansas City, MO: AHA.

Anderson, F., Cunningham, S., & Maloney, J. (1993). Indirect blood pressure measurement: A need to reassess. *American Journal of Critical Care, 2*(4), 272–274.

Anderson, F., & Maloney, J. (1994). Taking blood pressure correctly—it's no off-the-cuff matter. *Nursing 94, 24*(11), 34–39.

Braun, L., Potempa, K., Holm, K., Fogg, L., & Szidon, J. (1994). The role of catecholamines, age, and fitness on blood pressure reactivity to dynamic exercise in patients with essential hypertension. *Heart and Lung: Journal of Critical Care, 23*(5), 404–412.

Devine, E., & Reifschneider, E. (1995). A meta-analysis of the effects of psychoeducational care in adults with hypertension. *Nursing Research, 44*(4), 237–245.

Grossman, D., Jorda, M., & Farr, L. (1994). Blood pressure rhythms in early school-age children of normotensive and hypertensive parents: A replication study. *Nursing Research, 43*(4), 232–237.

Grossman, D., Keen, M., Singer, M., & Asher, M. (1995). Current nursing practices in fever management. *MEDSURG Nursing, 4*(3), 193–198.

Hill, M., & Grim, C. (1991). How to take a precise blood pressure. *American Journal of Nursing, 91*(2), 38–42.

Hogstel, M. (1994). Vital signs are really *vital* in the old-old. *Geriatric Nursing, 15*(5), 252–255.

Iyriboz, Y., & Hearon, C. (1992). Blood pressure measurement at rest and during exercise. *Journal of Cardiopulmonary Rehabilitation, 12*(4), 277–287.

Johannsen, J. (1993). Update: Guidelines for treating hypertension. *American Journal of Nursing, 93*(3), 42–49.

McCaffrey, M., & Ferrell, B. R. (1992). How vital are vital signs? *Nursing, 22*(1), 42–46.

Melby, C., Toohey, M., & Cebrick, J. (1994). Blood pressure and blood lipids among vegetarian, semivegetarian, and nonvegetarian African Americans. *American Journal of Clinical Nutrition, 59*(1), 103–109.

Nash, C., & Jensen, P. (1994). When your surgical patient has hypertension. *American Journal of Nursing, 94*(12), 38–45.

Ontario Heart Fund Foundation. (1983). *Proposed guidelines for hypertension screening.* Ontario: OHFF.

Porth, C. (1994). *Pathophysiology: Concepts of altered health states* (4th ed.). Philadelphia: Lippincott.

Selfridge, J., & Shea, S. (1993). The accuracy of the tympanic membrane thermometer in detecting fever in infants 3 months and younger in the emergency department setting. *Journal of Emergency Nursing, 19*(2), 127.

Thomas, D. (1995). Fever in children: Friend or foe? *RN, 58*(4), 42–48.

Trottier, D., & Kochar, M. (1992). Around-the-clock blood pressure monitoring: How to get good results. *Nursing 92, 22*(11), 66–68.

U.S. Department of Health and Human Services, Public Health Service, National Institutes of Health. (1993). *The fifth report of the Joint National Committee on Detection, Evaluation, and Treatment of High Blood Pressure* (NIH Publication No. 93-1088). Washington, DC: Author.

Winslow, E. (1994). What's so normal about 98.6°F? *American Journal of Nursing, 94*(6), 57.

Chapter 26

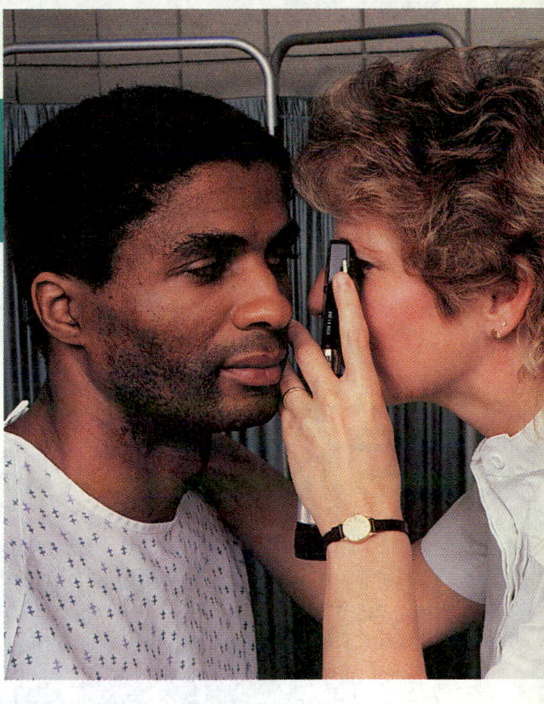

Health Assessment

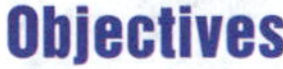

Objectives

After studying this chapter, the learner should be able to:

Define key terms used in the chapter.

Identify the purposes of the health assessment.

Describe the techniques used during a health assessment.

Discuss client preparation for a health assessment.

Identify equipment used in performing a health assessment.

Describe positioning used for each body system assessment.

Conduct a health assessment in a systematic manner, identifying normal and abnormal findings.

Document significant health assessment findings in a concise, descriptive manner.

Describe nursing responsibilities before, during, and after diagnostic procedures.

Key Terms

adventitious breath sounds
auscultation
bronchial sounds
bronchovesicular sounds
bruits
cyanosis
ecchymosis
edema
flushing
inspection
jaundice
pallor
palpation
percussion
petechiae
precordium
tremor
turgor
vesicular breath sounds

Health assessment is an integral component of holistic nursing care and is the basis of the nursing process. Assessments are used to initiate, implement, and evaluate care provided to promote an optimal level of wellness through interventions focused on prevention of illness, restoration of health, and facilitation of coping with disabilities or death.

Health assessments may be conducted in any setting. The two components of health assessment are a health history and a physical assessment. The nurse uses communication skills and interviewing techniques during the health history to gather data to determine the client's health status. The physical assessment may focus on one specific body system or may be a head-to-toe, system-by-system physical assessment of the client. Both subjective and objective data are collected during the health history and the physical assessment. The purposes of the health assessment are to:

- Establish a nurse–client relationship
- Gather data about the client's general health status, integrating physiologic, psychologic, cognitive, sociocultural, developmental, and spiritual dimensions
- Identify client strengths
- Identify actual and potential health problems
- Establish a base for the nursing process

Health History

A health history is a collection of subjective and objective data that provides a detailed profile of the client's health status. A nurse collects the information through an interview with the client. The components of the health history and specific interviewing skills are found in Chapters 16 and 22.

Physical Assessment

The physical assessment is usually conducted in a head-to-toe sequence, but can be adapted to meet the needs of the client being examined. This section discusses commonly used positions and techniques for the healthy adult. It is often necessary to modify the sequence, positions, and specific assessments to the client's age, energy level, and physical state and to time constraints. Even when modified, the physical assessment should be conducted in an organized and knowledgeable manner. Conducting an accurate physical assessment takes time and practice.

General Guidelines

This section discusses the general guidelines for the physical assessment, including instrumentation, positioning, draping, preparation of the environment, client preparation, and techniques of physical assessment.

Instrumentation

The instruments (or equipment) used during a physical assessment should be readily accessible, clean or sterile, in proper working order, and organized in the sequence of use (Fig. 26-1). Any equipment that will touch the client should be warmed (either with the examiner's hands or with warm water) before use. Although all of the instruments described may not be needed in an assessment, they are commonly used in the total assessment of clients. Additional equipment and supplies are listed in the accompanying box.

Ophthalmoscope. An *ophthalmoscope* is a lighted instrument used to visualize the interior structures of the eye. It consists of two parts—a body, containing the light source, and a detachable head, containing the magnifying lens used to bring the internal eye structures into focus. The magnification of the lens can be adjusted using a rotating dial. The head is placed into the body and secured. The dial located on the head, when depressed and turned, provides illumination. At the beginning of the assessment, the lens should be positioned at 0 diopters (the 0 magnification power of the lens). The numbers on the rotating dial range from −20 to +40, corresponding to the magnification power of the lens,

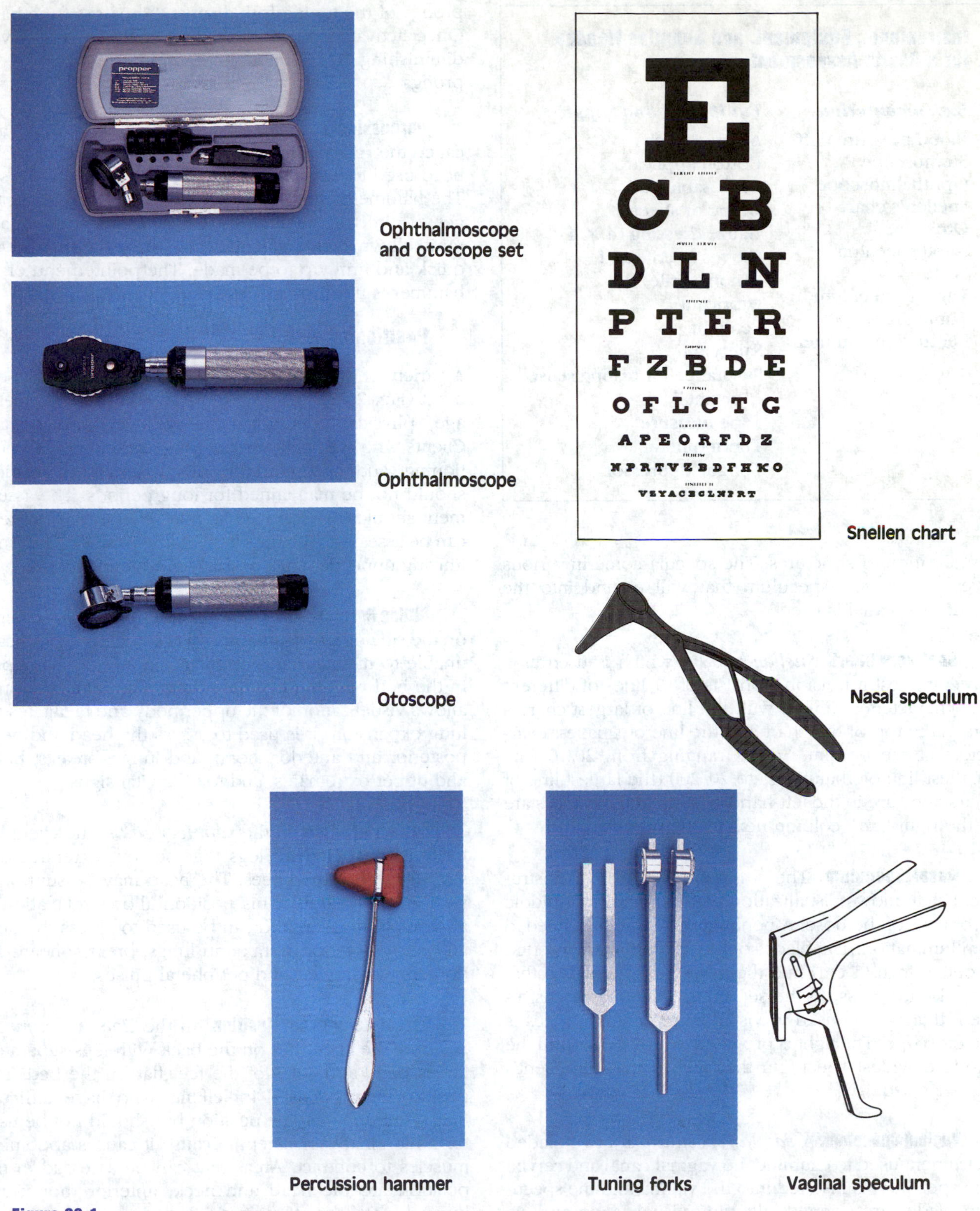

Figure 26-1
Instruments used in the physical examination. (Photos © Ken Kasper.)

with the negative numbers in red and the positive numbers in black. The system of negative and positive numbers compensates for nearsightedness and farsightedness and allows the examiner to visualize structures more clearly.

Otoscope. The *otoscope* is a lighted instrument used for examining the external ear canal and the tympanic membrane. The ophthalmoscope and otoscope heads are interchangeable on the same body. An attached speculum directs the light in a narrow beam to improve

Instruments, Equipment, and Supplies Needed for a Health Assessment

Instrumentation	*Equipment and Supplies*
Blood pressure cuff	Alcohol swabs
Stethoscope	Cotton applicators
Ophthalmoscope	Disposable pad
Snellen's chart	Drape or sheet
Otoscope	Gauze dressing (4 × 4)
Nasal speculum	Gloves (sterile and non-sterile)
Scale	Lubricant
Vaginal speculum	Penlight
Tuning fork	Safety pin
Percussion hammer	Substance for testing sense of smell
	Tape measure
	Thermometer
	Tongue depressor

visualization of structures. The specula come in various sizes; the largest speculum that will extend into the client's ear canal is used.

Snellen's Chart. *Snellen's chart,* which is used as a screening test for vision, consists of 11 lines of different size characters arranged with the line of largest characters at the top of the chart and the line of smallest characters at the bottom. Scores ranging from 20/10 (the smallest line of characters) to 20/200 (the largest line of characters) are in the left-hand column and distances are in the right-hand column next to the numbers.

Nasal Speculum. The *nasal speculum* is an instrument that allows visualization of the lower and middle turbinates of the nose. A penlight or flashlight is needed for illumination. The blades of the speculum are inserted about ½ inch (1 cm) into the nares and opened so that they do not press on the septum. An alternative instrument that can be used to visualize the internal nares is the otoscope. The light is provided by the scope, and the shortest, widest speculum that will fit into the client's nares is used.

Vaginal Speculum. A *vaginal speculum* is a two-bladed instrument used to examine the vaginal canal and cervix. The speculum is inserted into the vagina and the speculum blades are opened, allowing visualization and assessment of the vagina and cervix. Warming and lubrication of the speculum (either with warm water or with a water-soluble agent) are essential before insertion.

Tuning Fork. A *tuning fork* is a two-pronged metal instrument used for testing auditory function and vibratory perception. The fork is activated by gently tapping the prongs of the tuning fork against the palm of the hand. Once activated, the fork is held at the base to avoid diminishing the sound or vibration produced by the prongs.

Percussion Hammer. The *percussion hammer,* also called the *reflex hammer,* is an instrument with a rubber head used to test reflexes and determine tissue density. The hammer is held between the thumb and index finger to direct a brisk tap on the selected body area. A rapid downward and backward wrist action allows a quick and firm tap to be made. The pointed end of the hammer is used for smaller areas.

Positioning

A variety of positions are used during a physical assessment (Fig. 26-2). It is important to consider the client's age, physical condition, energy level, and privacy. Clients who are weak may require assistance with positioning, and uncomfortable or embarrassing positions should not be maintained for long periods. The assessment should be organized so that several body systems can be assessed with the client in one position, thus minimizing unneeded and possibly tiring movements.

Sitting Position. The client may sit upright in a chair or on the side of an examining table or bed or, if physically unable to maintain an upright position, may lie supine in the bed with the head elevated. This *sitting* position allows visualization of the upper body and facilitates full lung expansion. It is used to assess the head and neck, posterior and anterior thorax and lungs, breasts, heart, and upper extremities, and to take vital signs.

Supine Position. In the *supine position,* the client lies flat on the back with legs together but extended and slightly bent at the knees. The head may be supported with a small pillow. This position allows relaxation of abdominal muscles and can be used to assess the head and neck, anterior thorax and lungs, breasts, heart, abdomen, extremities, and peripheral pulses.

Dorsal Recumbent Position. In the *dorsal recumbent position,* the client lies on the back with legs separated, knees bent, and soles of the feet flat on the bed. This position may be used for clients who have difficulty maintaining the supine position but should not be used for abdominal assessment because it causes abdominal muscles to contract. Areas that can be assessed in this position are the head and neck, anterior thorax and lungs, breasts, heart, extremities, and peripheral pulse.

Sims' Position. In the *Sims' position,* the client lies on either the right or left side. The lower arm is behind the body and the upper arm is bent at the shoulder and elbow. The knees are both bent, with the uppermost leg more acutely bent. The Sims' position is used to assess the rectum or vagina.

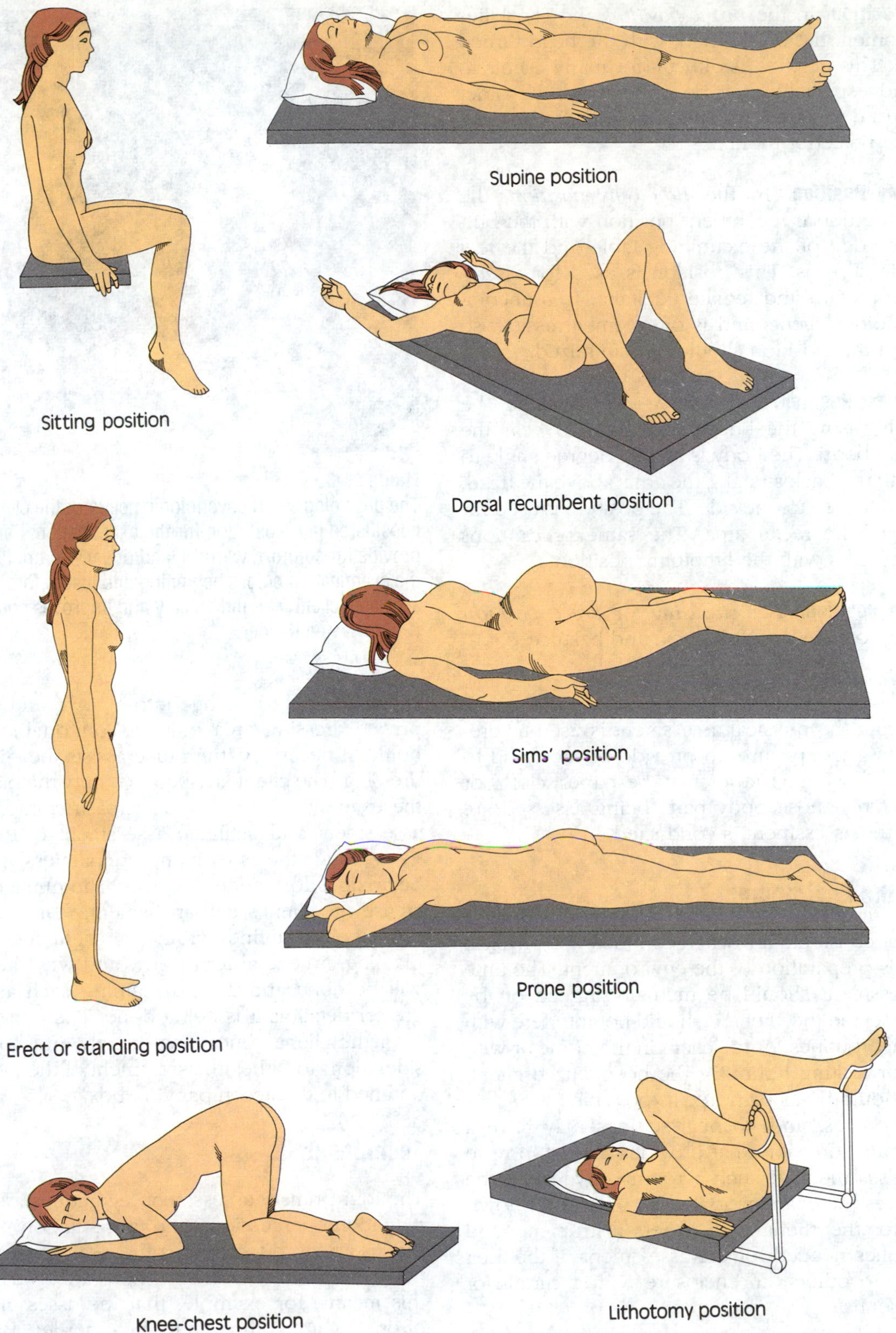

Figure 26-2
Various client positions used during the nursing examination.

Prone Position. In the *prone position,* the client lies on the abdomen, flat on the bed, with the head turned to one side. This position is difficult for many clients to assume, and especially may be difficult for the older adult. It is used to assess the hip joint and can be used to assess the posterior thorax.

Lithotomy Position. In the *lithotomy position,* the client is in the dorsal recumbent position with the buttocks at the edge of the examining table and the feet supported in stirrups. This position is used for assessment of the rectum and female genitalia. It is uncomfortable for older clients and is often embarrassing, so time spent in this position should be minimized.

Knee–Chest Position. In the *knee–chest position,* the client kneels, using the knees and chest to bear the weight of the body. The body is at a 90-degree angle to the hips, with the back straight, the arms above the head, and the head turned to one side. The position is used for assessment of the rectal area. The same precautions should be used as with the lithotomy position.

Standing Position. The *standing,* or *erect, position* may be used to assess posture, gait, and balance.

Draping

Draping during the physical assessment is used to prevent unnecessary exposure, to provide privacy, and to keep the client warm. Drapes may be paper, cloth, or bed linens. Only those body parts being assessed are exposed as the assessment is conducted.

Preparing the Environment

An important consideration when conducting a physical assessment is preparation of the environment. The time for the assessment should be mutually agreed on by both the nurse and the client. It should not interfere with meals or daily routines for the client in the home or with treatments or visiting hours for the hospitalized client. The client should be as pain free as possible.

Clinics, offices, and hospital settings may have a special examination room that provides a quiet, private space for assessment. If such a room is available, the nurse prepares the examination table, provides a gown and drape for the client, and gathers instruments and special supplies needed for the assessment. If the area is accessible to others, an enclosure with a curtain or screen is essential.

Preparing the Client

Both physiologic and psychologic needs of the client should be considered before and during the physical assessment (Fig. 26-3). Explain that a physical assessment will be done by the nurse, that body structures will be examined, and that the assessments are painless. The client is asked to change into a gown and directed to a private dressing area or to a comfortable area in the home. If necessary, the nurse assists the client with undressing. The client is asked to empty the bladder before the examination begins to increase comfort during the assessment and facilitate assessment of the abdomen. Even though the assessments are painless, the client may be anxious for various reasons. The nurse can help decrease the client's embarrassment, fear of possible abnormal physical findings, or fear of "failing" a test by explaining in general terms how and why the assessment will be done and then explaining each assessment in greater detail as it is being done. The nurse should answer the client's questions directly and honestly. Considerations for a health assessment of the older adult are outlined in the accompanying box.

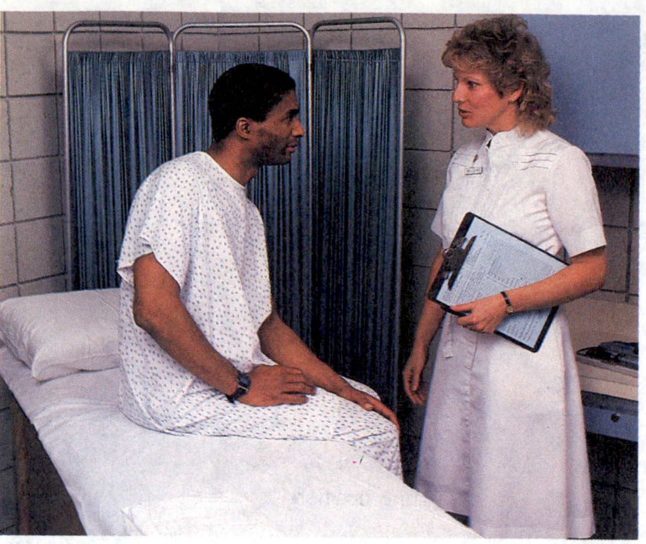

Figure 26-3
The physiologic and psychologic needs of the client must be considered in preparation for the examination. Care is taken to provide for comfort, warmth, and privacy. A brief explanation of the examination before beginning and just before each stage alleviates client fear and anxiety and improves cooperation. (Photo © Ken Kasper.)

Techniques

The four primary assessment techniques are inspection, palpation, percussion, and auscultation. These techniques are used to conduct the health assessment of all body systems. Bilateral body parts are always compared; this means, for example, that the assessment findings of one leg are compared to the other leg. Bilateral body parts should be symmetric; that is, they should have the same size and shape as well as the same characteristics, such as movement or pulses.

Inspection

Inspection is the process of deliberate, purposeful observations performed in a systematic manner. Observa-

Focus on the Older Adult

Health Assessment

Considerations when assessing the older adult include:

- Know the normal physiologic changes that occur with aging.
- Remove only clothing necessary to assess specific body parts, and ensure the client does not become chilled.
- Organize the assessment so that like body systems are assessed together to minimize fatigue. If the client tires easily, conduct focused assessments only.
- Ask if the client would prefer to have a family member present during the assessment.
- Respect cultural differences in disrobing and exposing body parts (especially if the nurse is not the same gender as the client).
- Ask clients what name they prefer to be called.
- Adapt questions and assessment techniques to any identified changes in vision and hearing. If the client wears glasses or a hearing aid, be sure they are available, clean, and in good repair.
- Collect information about past illnesses and surgeries, as well as about traditional and nontraditional treatments, while conducting the physical assessment.
- Allow time for the client to respond to questions.

tions are made by using visual, auditory, and olfactory senses to gather data throughout the assessment. Inspection begins at the time of initial contact with the client and continues throughout the entire assessment. Adequate lighting, either natural or artificial, is essential for distinguishing color, texture, and moisture of body surfaces. A quiet environment eliminates extraneous noises and allows sounds to be heard without interference.

The nurse inspects each area of the body for size, color, shape, position, and symmetry (equal size, shape, and position of bilateral parts), making observations of normal findings and any deviations from normal. Inspection may be combined with the palpation phase of the assessment.

Palpation

Palpation is a technique that uses the sense of touch. The hands and fingers are sensitive tools and are used to assess temperature, turgor, texture, moisture, vibrations, and shape. The dorsum, or back, of the hand and fingers is used for gross measure of temperature. When a discriminatory sense is needed for differentiating between texture, shape, fluid, size, consistency, and pulsation, the palmar surface of the fingers and finger pads is used. Vibration is palpated best with the palm of the hand (Fig. 26-4).

General guidelines to follow during palpation include the following:

- The client should be provided with a warm, comfortable, and relaxed environment.
- The nurse's hands should be warm and fingernails short.
- Any area of tenderness is palpated last.

Light or deep palpation may be used and is controlled by the amount of pressure applied. For light palpation, apply light pressure by placing the fingers together and depressing the skin and underlying structures about ½ inch (1 cm; Fig. 26-5, *top*). For deep palpation, press inward about 1 inch (2 cm; see Fig. 26-5, *bottom*). Deep palpation, with the risk of possible internal injury, should be used with caution and only after considerable practice. Applying intermittent pressure to a specific area allows assessment of surface characteristics and under-

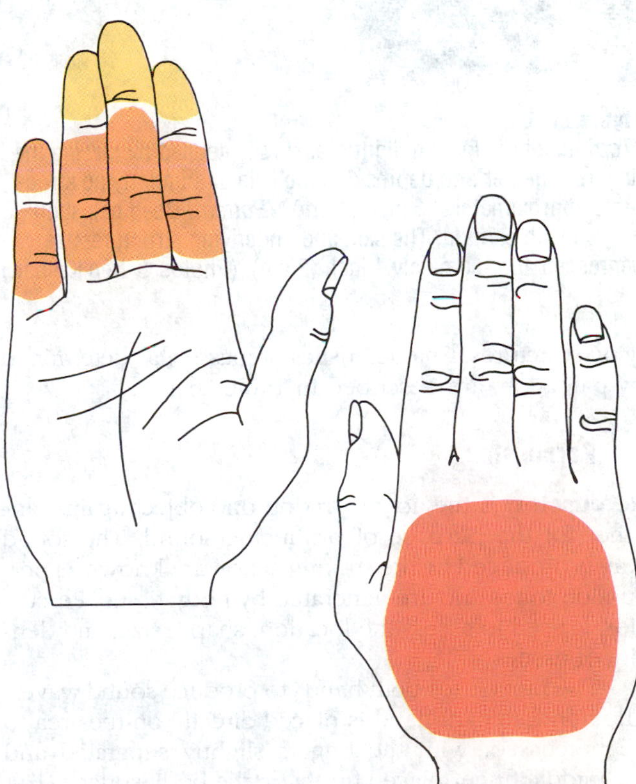

Figure 26-4
(Top) Palmar surfaces of the examiner's fingertips and finger pads are used for discriminatory sensation, such as texture, presence of fluid, or size and consistency of a mass. *(Bottom)* The dorsum, or back of hand, is used to assess surface temperature.

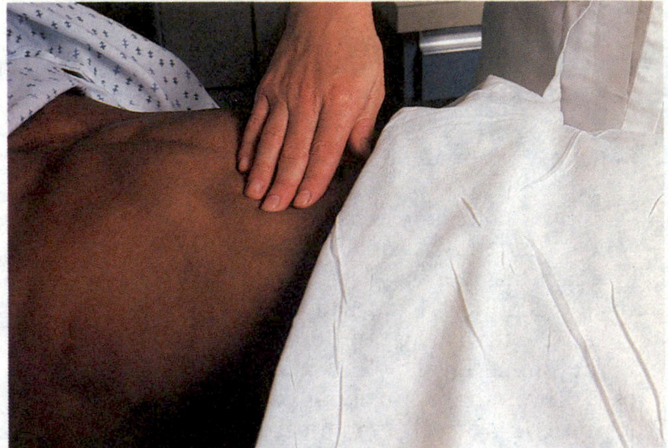

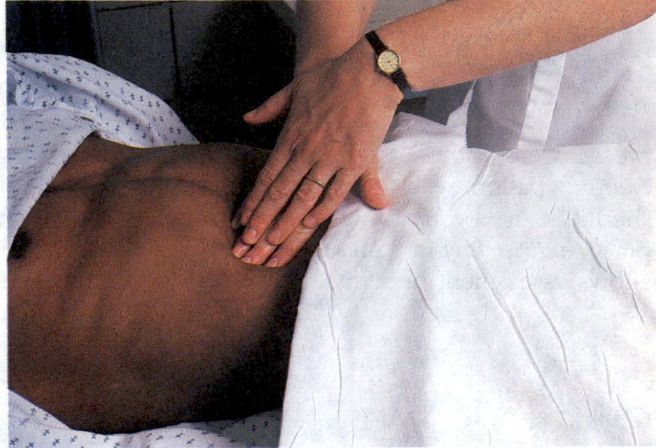

Figure 26-5
(Top) In light palpation, light pressure is applied by placing the fingers together and depressing the skin and underlying structures approximately ½ inch (1 cm). *(Bottom)* Deep palpation is used with caution. The skin and underlying structures are depressed approximately 1 inch (2 cm). (Photos © Ken Kasper.)

lying structures. Characteristics of masses, as determined by palpation, are described in Table 26-1.

Table 26-1
Characteristics of Masses Determined by Palpation

Quality	Characteristics to Determine
Shape	Round Ovoid Tubular Irregular
Size	Measured in centimeters
Consistency	Firm Edematous Spongy Cystic
Surface	Smooth Nodular Granular
Mobility	Fixed or nonmobile Mobile
Tenderness	Amount of tenderness to touch
Pulsatile	Pulsation can or cannot be felt in the mass

Percussion

Percussion is the act of striking one object against another for the purpose of producing sound. The sound waves produced by the striking action are known as percussion tones and are generated by body tissue. Percussion is used to assess the location, shape, size, and density of tissues.

The nurse uses both hands to produce sound waves. The nondominant hand is placed directly on the area to be percussed, with the fingers slightly separated and the middle finger placed firmly on the body surface (Fig. 26-6, *left*). The opposite hand (or dominant hand) is the striking force, which is initiated by sharp downward wrist movement with the forearm stationary and the wrist relaxed. The tip of the middle finger of the dominant hand strikes the joint of the middle finger of the opposing hand (see Fig. 26-6, *right*). This action produces a vibration that allows the nurse to discriminate among five different tones. The five percussion tones are as follows:

Tympany—loud, drumlike sound that is illustrated by the sound produced by percussing a puffed-out cheek; heard when percussing the stomach, an air-filled organ

Resonance—moderate to loud, lower-pitched, hollow sound percussed over lung tissue

Hyperresonance—very loud, low-pitched sound with a booming quality; most often percussed over the emphysematous lung

Dullness—soft to moderate, high-pitched sound with a thud-like quality; percussed over the liver

Flatness—soft, high-pitched sound that is flat; usually percussed over muscle tissue

Table 26-2 summarizes percussion tones and their characteristics.

Auscultation

Auscultation is the act of listening to sound produced within the body by using a stethoscope. Chapter 25 discusses types of stethoscopes, their uses, and specific characteristics.

Auscultation is performed by firmly placing the stethoscope diaphragm or bell against the body part being assessed. The diaphragm of the stethoscope is used to detect high-pitched sounds, such as normal lung and bowel sounds. The bell of the stethoscope is used to detect low-pitched sounds, such as those produced by the heart and vascular system.

Four characteristics of sound should be assessed by auscultation. They are (1) *pitch* (ranging from high to low); (2) *loudness* (ranging from soft to loud); (3) *qual-*

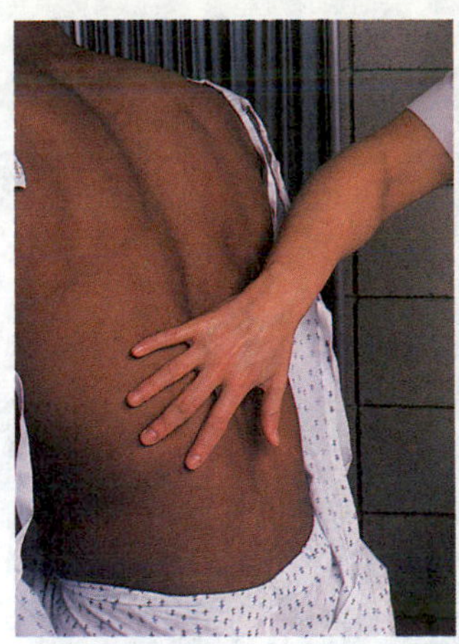
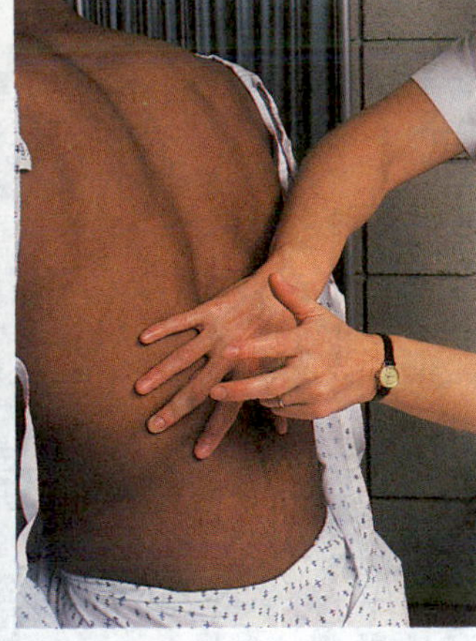

Figure 26-6
Percussion is used to access the location, shape, size, and density of tissues. *(Left)* The nondominant hand is placed directly on the area to be percussed, and the middle finger placed firmly on the body surface. *(Right)* The tip of the middle finger of the dominant hand strikes the joint of the middle finger of the opposite hand. (Photos © Ken Kasper.)

ity (eg, gurgling or swishing); and (4) *duration* (described as short, medium, or long).

General Survey

The general survey is the first phase of the health assessment. Some information, such as the client's appearance and behavior, is assessed during the health history. Measuring the vital signs, height, and weight are also a part of the general survey.

General Appearance

Assessment of general appearance includes the following:

- Gender and race
- Body build, posture, and gait (note proportion of height to weight, erect or slumped posture, coordination of movements, pattern of gait)
- Hygiene, grooming (note cleanliness, body odors, appropriate dress for age and environment)
- Signs of illness (note posture, skin color, respirations, nonverbal communications of pain or distress)
- Affect, attitude, mood (note speech, facial expressions, ability to relax, eye contact, behavior)
- Cognitive processes (note speech content and patterns, orientation, appropriate verbal responses)

Vital Signs

Vital signs are measured to establish a data base and to detect actual or potential health problems. Vital signs are discussed in Chapter 25.

Height and Weight

In adult clients, the correlation (or ratio) of height and weight is an assessment of overall health and nutrition. Both height and weight should be measured using accurate scales and measuring devices, and the client should remove shoes and heavy clothing if the measurements are taken before undressing. If the client is unable to stand erect, weight can be obtained by using a chair or bed scales. The client's actual height and weight can be compared with recommended average weights on a standardized chart as a general guideline for assessing nutritional status and health (see Chapter 12).

Assessment of Body Systems

This section discusses the physical assessment of each body system. Accompanying the discussion of each system are factors for consideration during assessment, positions, assessment techniques, and common normal and abnormal findings. Normal alterations in physical assessments with aging are outlined in the accompanying box.

Table 26-2
Percussion Tones and Their Characteristics

Tone	Relative Intensity	Relative Pitch	Relative Duration	Sample Location
Flatness	Soft	High	Short	Thigh
Dullness	Medium	Medium	Medium	Liver
Resonance	Loud	Low	Long	Normal lung
Hyperresonance	Very loud	Lower	Longer	Emphysematous lung
Tympany	Loud	* High	*	Gastric air bubble or puffed-out cheek

* Distinguished mainly by its musical timbre.

(Bates, B. [1995]. *A guide to physical examination and history taking* [6th ed.]. Philadelphia: Lippincott, p. 243.)

Focus on the Older Adult

Normal Alterations in Physical Assessments With Aging

Integument

- Wrinkles, dryness, scaling
- Decreased turgor
- Raised dark areas (senile keratosis)
- Flat brown age spots (senile lentigines)
- Small, round, red spots (cherry angioma)
- Fine, brittle, gray or white hair
- Loss of hair (alopecia)
- Coarse facial hair in women, decreased body hair in both men and women
- Thick, yellow toenails; may be ingrown

Head and Neck

- Dry mucous membranes of mouth
- Unable to taste or smell as acutely
- White ring around iris (arcus senilis)
- Decreased tear production
- Clouding of lens (cataracts)
- Decrease in near vision (presbyopia), in peripheral vision, and in accommodation
- Decreased hearing acuity (presbycusis)

Thorax and Lungs

- Increase in dorsal spinal curve (kyphosis)
- Decreased breath sounds
- Hyperresonance on percussion
- Systolic murmurs are common

Breasts

- Less firm, pendulous, more nodular

Peripheral Vascular

- Rigid, tortuous veins and arteries
- Increased systolic and diastolic blood pressure
- Increased systolic pressure, widening pulse pressure

Abdomen

- Decreased bowel sounds
- Decreased abdominal tone
- Liver span shorter and liver border more easily palpated

Genitalia

- Decrease in size of labia
- Decreased vaginal secretions
- Shortened vaginal vault
- Decrease in size of penis

Musculoskeletal

- Loss of muscle mass and strength
- Decrease in range of motion
- Decrease in height

Neurologic

- Slower thought processes and verbal responses
- Decreased sensory ability
- Slower coordination and voluntary movements
- Decreased or slower reflex responses

Integument

The structures of the integumentary system that are assessed are the skin, the nails, and the hair and scalp.

Skin

The skin is a general indicator of a client's health status and provides information that may signify an underlying disease. Before assessing the skin, ask about exposure to harmful environmental materials or increased sun exposure, recent changes in skin condition, or current medications.

The skin is assessed by inspection and palpation. The assessment begins with an overall inspection of the skin condition; specific areas of the skin can be assessed while performing other body system assessments. Adequate lighting is essential for accurate assessments.

Inspection

The skin is inspected for color, vascularity, and lesions. Body odors are also included in inspection (Fig. 26-7).

Color. The skin color varies among races and among individuals. Normally, skin color ranges from a pinkish white to various shades of brown, depending on the person's race. The skin areas that are normally exposed, such as the face and hands, may have a somewhat different color than areas that are usually covered by clothing, but generally the color is relatively constant. Special care must be taken to detect color changes in dark-skinned people, such as African Americans, Hispanics, Native Americans, people of Mediterranean descent, and Caucasians who are deeply suntanned. Some body areas of dark-skinned people, such as the palms of the hands and the soles of the feet, normally have less pigmentation than other areas of the body. Various terms used to

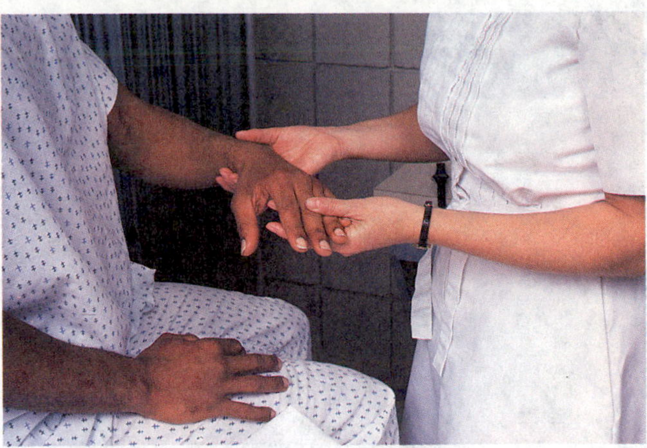

Figure 26-7
The skin is inspected for color, vascularity, and lesions.

describe abnormal appearance of the skin are summarized in Table 26-3.

The changes in skin color that may be assessed include flushing, cyanosis, jaundice, and pallor. These color changes are much easier to assess in light-skinned people. **Flushing** is redness of the skin, as in sunburn. It is often associated with an elevated body temperature, and is more often seen in the face and the neck. **Cyanosis** is a dusky, bluish color in people with light skin color. In dark-skinned people, cyanosis may be detected in the conjunctiva and inside the mouth. **Jaundice** is a yellow color of the skin, usually first observed in the sclera of the eyes and then in the skin and mucous membranes. Jaundice in dark-skinned people is more difficult to observe because the sclera often has a normal yellowish color. **Pallor** is paleness of the skin, often resulting from an inadequate amount of circulating blood or hemoglobin, both of which cause inadequate oxygenation of the body tissues. Depending on severity, pallor may be visible over the entire skin surface or only in the lips, nailbeds, mucous membranes, and conjunctiva. Pallor is more difficult to assess in dark-skinned people.

Vascularity. The skin is inspected for vascularity, bleeding, or bruising, because these signs may be related to cardiovascular, hematologic, or liver dysfunctions. **Ecchymosis** is a collection of blood in the subcutaneous tissues, causing purplish discoloration. **Petechiae** are small, hemorrhagic spots caused by capillary bleeding. If present, assess location, color, and size.

Lesions. The skin is assessed by inspection for the presence of lesions, which are areas of diseased or injured tissue (Table 26-4). Normally, the skin is smooth and intact. Evidence of bruises, scratches, cuts, insect bites, and wounds are noted. A *wound* is a break in the continuity of the skin and is assessed for size, shape, depth, location, and presence of drainage or odor. *Scars* are healed wounds. (Wounds are discussed in Chapter 30.) A *rash* is a skin eruption. The descriptive details of a rash include the type, size, elevation, coloring, and presence or absence of drainage or itching. Document the exact body surface areas involved.

Palpation

The temperature, moisture, turgor, and texture of the skin are determined by palpation.

Temperature and Moisture. The skin is normally warm and dry. An increase in skin temperature and moisture can indicate an elevation of body temperature. An excessive amount of perspiration, such as when the entire skin is moist, is called *diaphoresis.* When the body is *dehydrated* the skin is dry.

Table 26-3
Skin Color Assessment

Color Variations	Assessment Areas	Causes
Redness (erythema; flushing)	Facial area, localized area of skin on the body	Blushing, alcohol intake, fever, injury trauma, infection
Bluish (cyanosis)	Exposed areas, particularly the ears, lips, inside of the mouth, hands and feet, nailbeds	Cold environment, cardiac or respiratory disease (decreased oxygenation)
Yellowish (jaundice)	Overall skin areas, mucous membranes, and sclera	Liver disease (increase in bilirubin levels)
Paleness (pallor)	Exposed areas, particularly the face and lips, conjunctivae, and mucous membranes	Anemia (decreased hemoglobin)
	Overall skin areas, lips, nailbeds, conjunctivae	Shock (decreased blood volume)
Vitiligo	Whitish patchy areas on the skin	Depigmentation (congenital or autoimmune conditions)
Tanned or brown	Sun-exposed areas	Overexposure (increased melanin production), pregnancy (brown spots?)

Table 26-4
Basic Types of Skin Lesions

Lesion Name	Description	Example
Primary Lesions*		
Circumscribed, Flat, Nonpalpable Change in Skin Color		
Macule	Lesion ≤1 cm	Petechiae, freckle
Patch	Lesion >1 cm	Vitiligo
Palpable, Elevated Solid Masses		
Papule	Mass ≤0.5 cm	Mole
Plaque	Mass >0.5 cm	Coalesced papules
Nodule	Mass 0.5–2 cm; firmer than a papule	Nevus (wart)
Tumor	Mass >2 cm	Lipoma
Wheal	Irregular, superficial area of localized skin edema	Hives, mosquito bite
Circumscribed, Superficial Skin Elevations Formed by Free Fluid in a Cavity Within the Skin Layers		
Vesicle	Filled with serous fluid, ≤0.5 cm	Herpes simplex
Bulla	Filled with serous fluid, >0.5 cm	2nd-degree burn
Pustule	Filled with pus	Acne, impetigo
Secondary Lesions†		
Loss of Skin Surface		
Erosion	Loss of superficial epidermis, moist, nonbleeding surface	Moist area after rupture of a vesicle, as in chickenpox
Ulcer	Loss of epidermis and dermis, may bleed and scar	Stasis ulcer
Fissure	Deep linear crack, extends into dermis	Athlete's foot
Material on the Skin Surface		
Crust	Dried residue of serum, pus, or blood	Impetigo
Scale	Thin flake of exfoliated dermis	Dandruff, dry skin
Miscellaneous Lesions		
Lichenification	Thickened and roughened epidermis, with increased visibility of skin furrows	Atrophic dermatitis
Atrophy	Thinning of the skin, loss of skin furrows, shiny appearance	Peripheral vascular disease
Excoriation	Scratch of the epidermis	
Scar	Fibrous tissue replaces tissue in the dermis or subcutaneous layer	
Keloid	Hypertrophied scar	
Other Common Skin Lesions, Not Technically Primary or Secondary		
Comedo	Plugged opening of a sebaceous gland, a hallmark of acne	Common blackhead
Telangiectasia	Small, dilated, red or bluish surface vessels; may be part of a basal cell carcinoma or skin injury from radiation	
Nevus	Flat to slightly elevated, round, evenly pigmented	Common mole

* May arise from previously normal skin.
† Result from changes in primary lesions.

Turgor. **Turgor** (Fig. 26-8) is the fullness or elasticity of the skin. Normal turgor results in elasticity of the skin, allowing it to be picked up in a fold and to return to its shape when released. When the client is dehydrated, normal skin elasticity and fullness are decreased and the skin fold returns to normal slowly. This, however, may be a normal finding in the older client. Difficulty in lifting a skin fold may indicate excess fluid in the tissues, or **edema**. Edema is characterized by swelling, with taut and shiny skin over the edematous area. If the area of edema is palpated with the fingers, an indentation may remain after the pressure is released. Edema may be described on a scale, as follows:

0 = none
+1 = trace
+2 = moderate
+3 = deep
+4 = very deep

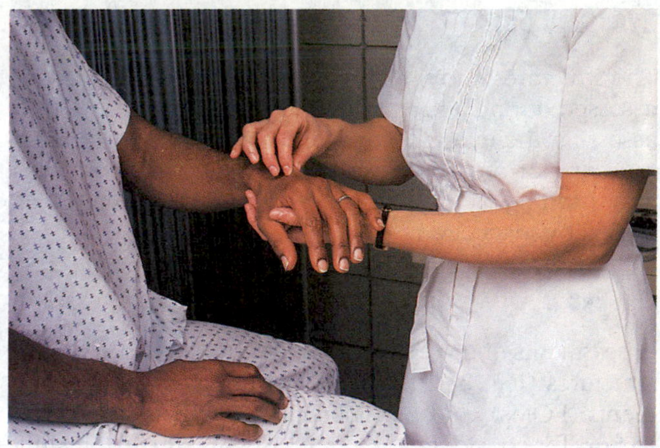

Figure 26-8
To assess skin turgor, a small fold of skin is picked up and then released to return to its normal shape. Difficulty in lifting a skin fold may indicate presence of edema. (Photo © Ken Kasper.)

Texture. The texture of the skin may vary from smooth and soft to rough and dry. In the dehydrated client, the texture is loose and wrinkled and the mucous membranes are cracked and dry.

Nails

The nails are inspected for shape, texture, and color. The shape of the nails should be somewhat convex and follow the natural curve of the finger. The angle between the nail and its base in the finger should be about 160 degrees. The texture of the nails should be smooth, and the nail base, when palpated, should be firm and nontender. Abnormal findings include indentations, called *Beau's lines*; infection (*paronychia*); painless separation of the nail plate from the nail bed (called *onycholysis*); increased brittleness and angulation; changes in the thickness or texture; and clubbing. Figure 26-9 illustrates nail abnormalities.

Hair and Scalp

The hair is normally resilient, evenly distributed, and neither excessively dry or oily. Hair is found on all body surfaces except the palms of the hands, the soles of the feet, and parts of the genitalia. The hair is examined for color, texture, and distribution. Abnormal findings include unusual balding (*alopecia*) and excessive amounts of hair on the body (*hirsutism*). Decreased oxygenation of peripheral tissues, especially of the lower extremities, may cause loss of hair.

Separate the hair to inspect the scalp for color, dryness, scaliness, lumps, lesions, or lice. If any lumps or masses are palpated, note location, size, tenderness, and mobility.

Head and Neck

Assessment of the head and neck includes the skull, face, eyes, ears, nose and sinuses, mouth and pharynx, trachea, thyroid gland, and lymph nodes. Structures of the head and neck are assessed by inspection and palpation, with the client in the sitting position. Factors for

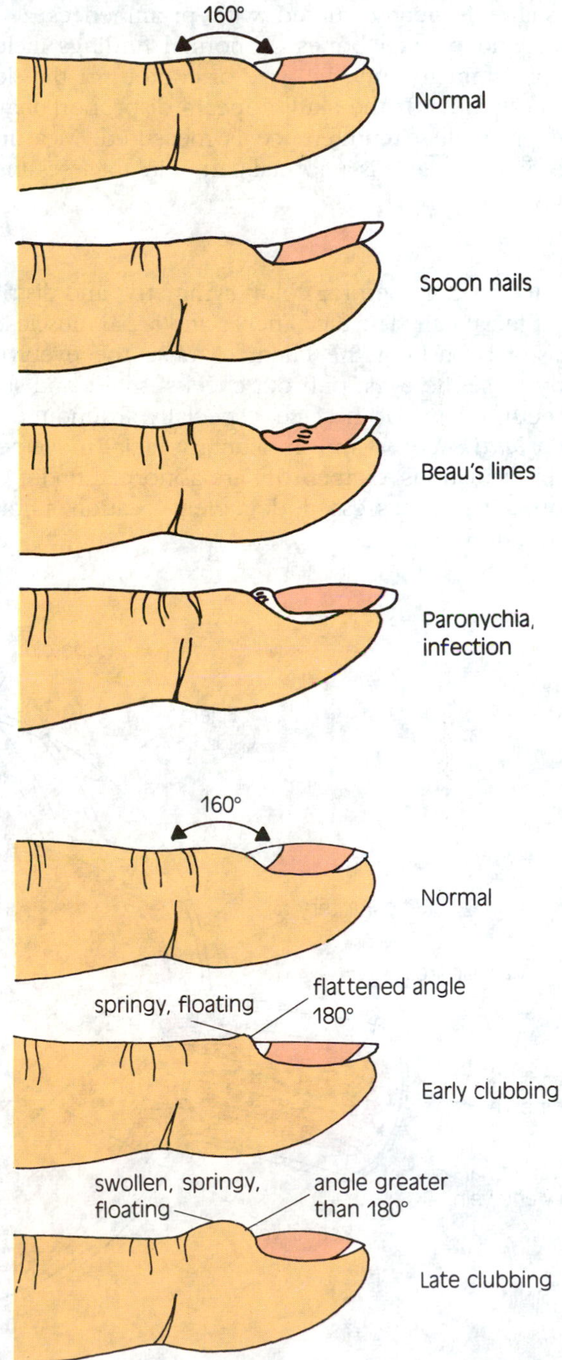

Figure 26-9
Examples of nail abnormalities.

consideration while assessing the head and neck include allergies, smoking history, head injury, increased levels of stress, and thyroid dysfunction.

Skull

The skull is assessed for size and shape by inspection and palpation. The parts of the head and face should be in proportion to each other and symmetric. Although the shape of the normal skull varies considerably, generally the shape is gently curved with prominences at the frontal and parietal bones. Abnormal findings include lack of symmetry, unusual size or contour of the skull, and tenderness. If the skull appears disproportionately large or small, circumference is measured. Measuring head circumference is a normal part of infant assessment.

Face

The face is examined for color, symmetry, and distribution of facial hair. The facial nerve and facial muscles are assessed by asking the client to raise the eyebrows, tightly close the eyes, puff out cheeks, smile, and show the teeth. Edema of the face, especially around the eye (*periorbital edema*), and involuntary facial movements (tic, fasciculations, or **tremor**) are abnormal findings. If abnormalities are assessed, document location, amount, and timing.

Eyes and Ears

The structures and the function of the eyes and ears are assessed during a health history. The equipment used in assessing the eyes and ears are a penlight, an ophthalmoscope or otoscope, an eye chart, a watch that ticks, and a tuning fork. The eyes and ears are primarily assessed by inspection.

Eye

Assessments of the eye include external and internal eye structures (Fig. 26-10). Visual acuity, extraocular movements (EOMs), and peripheral vision are also assessed. Factors for consideration while assessing the eye include age, use of corrective lens, artificial eye, allergies, pain, visual disturbances, and health-related factors such as high blood pressure or diabetes.

External Eye Structures. The eyes, eyebrows, eyelids, eyelashes, lacrimal gland, and the pupils and iris are inspected for position and alignment (Fig. 26-11). The eyes are inspected for symmetry and parallel alignment. The eyebrows should have equal distribution, and the eyelashes should curl outward. The eyelids are examined for color, edema, and equal coverage of the eyeball. The lacrimal glands are inspected and palpated for edema and pain.

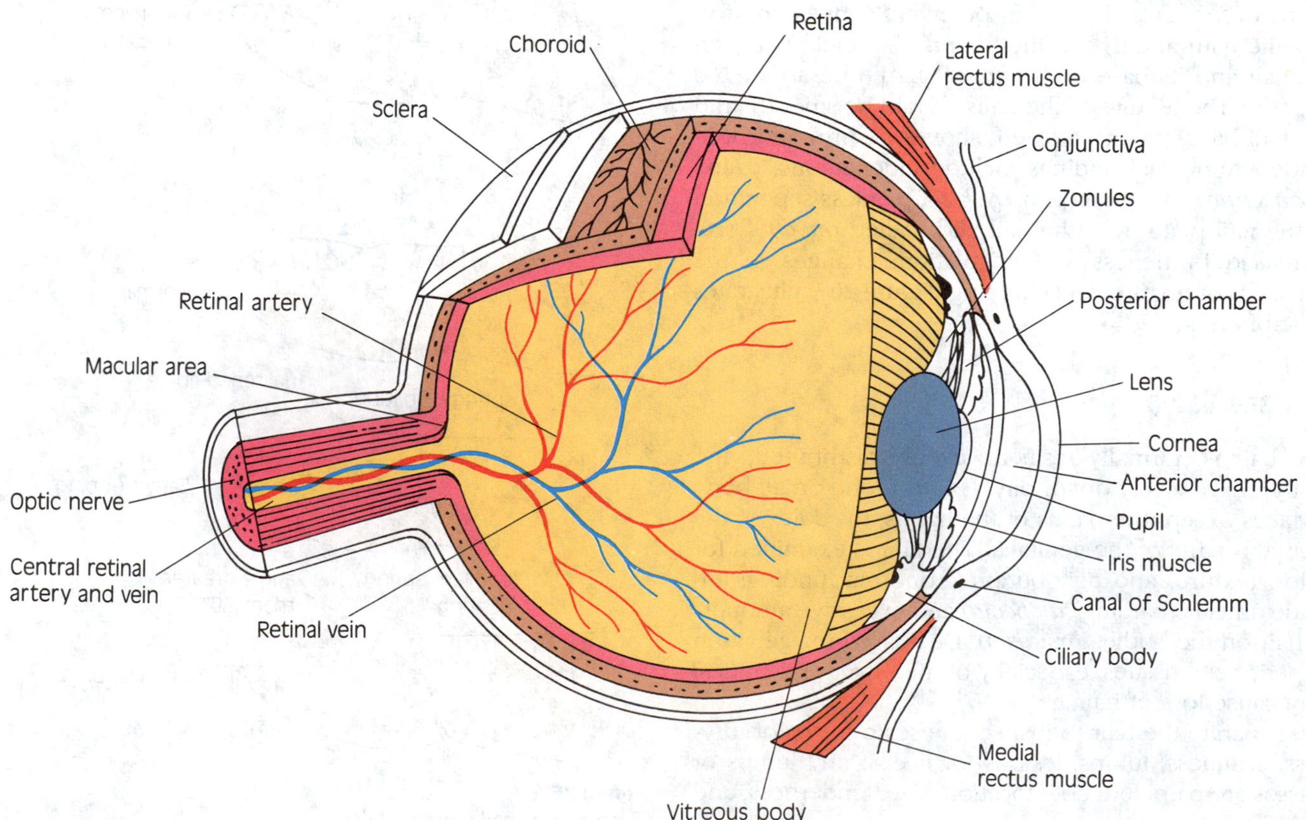

Figure 26-10
A cross section of the eye.

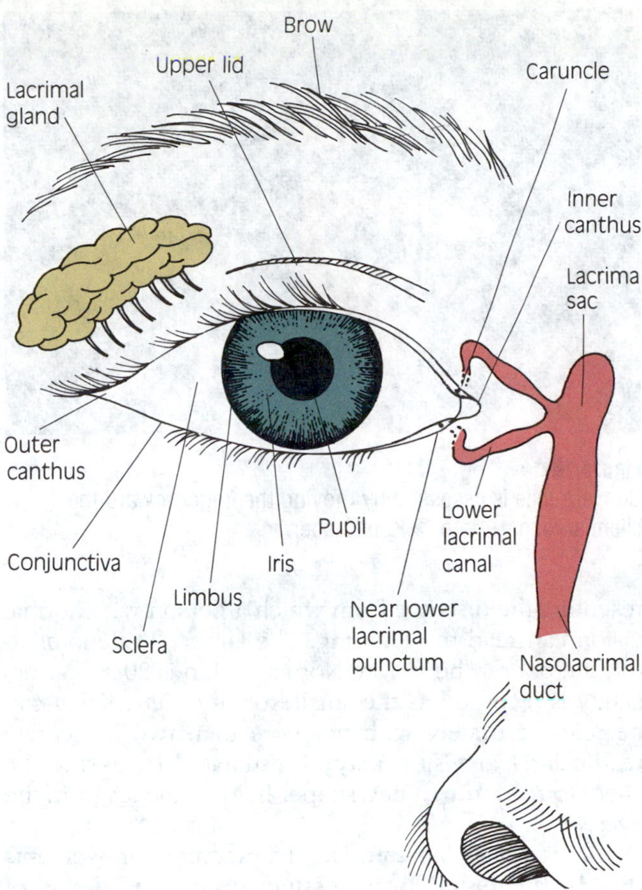

Figure 26-11
The eye and surrounding structures.

Pupil and Iris. The pupils are normally black, equal in size, round, and smooth. The pupils may be pale and cloudy if the client has cataracts. Injury to the eye, glaucoma, and certain medications may cause the pupil to dilate (*mydriasis*); certain drugs can cause constriction (*miosis*); and unequal pupils may result from central nervous system injury or illness. The pupils are assessed for reaction to light and accommodation, and for convergence.

Assess *reaction to light* by following these five steps (Fig. 26-12):

- Ask the client to look straight ahead.
- Bring the penlight from the side of the client's face and shine the light on the pupil.
- Observe the pupil's reaction; normally it will constrict (*direct response*).
- Repeat the procedure and observe the other eye; normally it too will constrict (*consensual reflex*).
- Repeat the procedure with the other eye.

Accommodation is assessed by following these steps (Fig. 26-13):

- Hold the forefinger, a pencil, or other straight object about 10 to 15 cm (4 to 6 inches) from the bridge of the client's nose.
- Ask the client to first look at the object, then at a distant object, then back to the object being held.

Normally the pupil should constrict when looking at a near object and dilate when looking at a distant object.

Convergence is assessed by moving the examiner's finger toward the client's nose; the client's eyes should normally converge (assume a cross-eyed appearance; Fig. 26-14).

Internal Eye Structures. The internal eye (Fig. 26-15) is examined with the ophthalmoscope to assess the fundus, including the retina, optic nerve disc, macula, fovea centralis, and retinal vessels. Using the ophthalmoscope takes practice. Normal findings are a uniform red reflex; clear, yellow optic nerve disc; reddish retina; and light red arteries and dark red veins, the veins being about

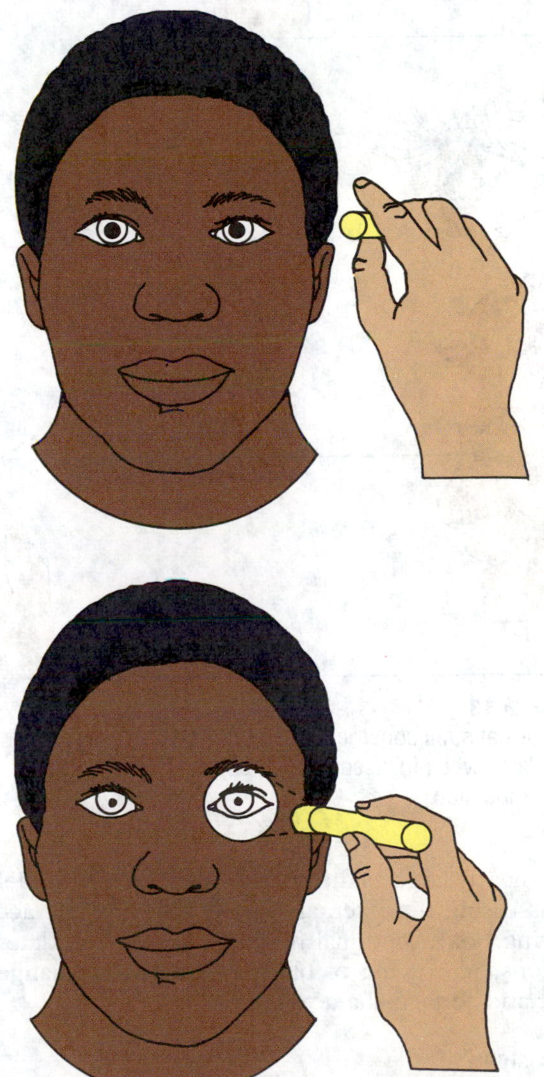

Figure 26-12
To test pupillary reaction to light, a penlight is moved from the side of the client's face *(top)* to in front of the eye *(bottom)*. The pupil should constrict when the light is present. The dilation or constriction shown is exaggerated for clarity.

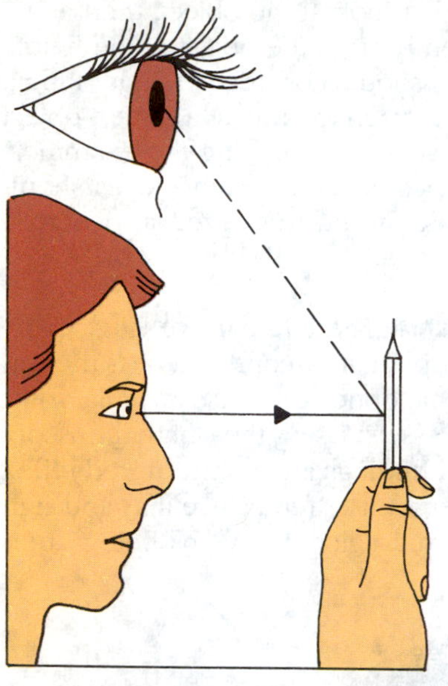

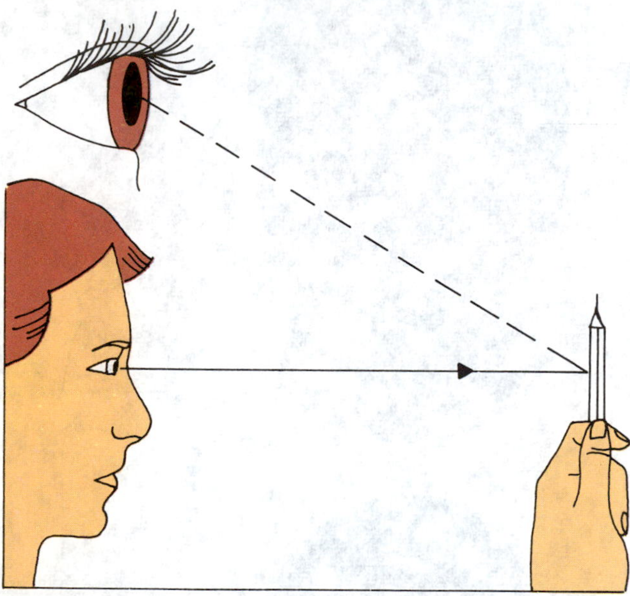

Figure 26-13
The normal pupil constricts when focused on a near object and dilates when focused on a far object. This is called accommodation.

1½ times as large as the arteries (Fig. 26-16). Guidelines for assessing the internal eye are listed in the accompanying box. Abnormal findings include cloudiness of the lens, narrowing of blood vessels, and changes in color and surface characteristics.

Vision

Visual Acuity. Visual acuity is assessed by placing the client 20 feet from Snellen's chart and testing each eye. The client is asked to read the smallest possible line of letters, first with both eyes and then with one eye at a time. Visual acuity is measured by standardized numbers listed on the side of the chart. The numerator is 20, representing the distance from which a person with normal vision can read the lettering. The larger the denominator, the poorer the vision. Normal vision is 20/20. Visual acuity is recorded as the smallest line of letters that can be read accurately with no more than two inaccurate readings. Near vision may be estimated by asking the client to read from a newspaper held 14 inches from the eyes.

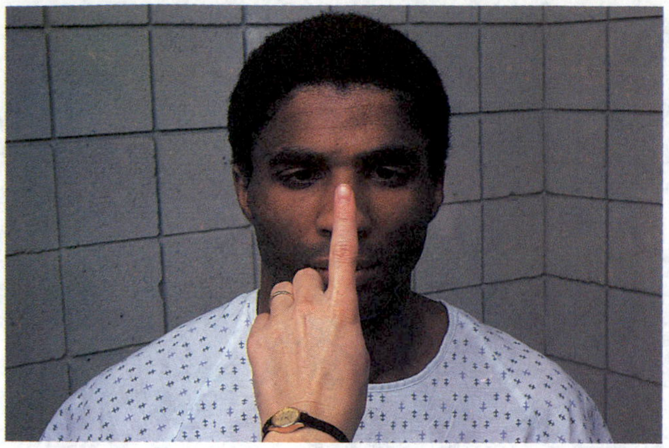

Figure 26-14
Convergence is assessed by moving the finger toward the client's nose. (Photo © Ken Kasper.)

Extraocular Movements. Extraocular movements (EOMs) are tested by assessing the cardinal fields of vision for coordination and alignment (Fig. 26-17). Normally both eyes move together, are coordinated, and are parallel. To assess EOMs, follow these three steps:

- Ask the client to sit or stand about 2 feet away, facing the examiner, who is also sitting or standing on eye level with the client.
- Ask the client to hold the head still and follow the movement of the examiner's forefinger or a penlight with the eyes.

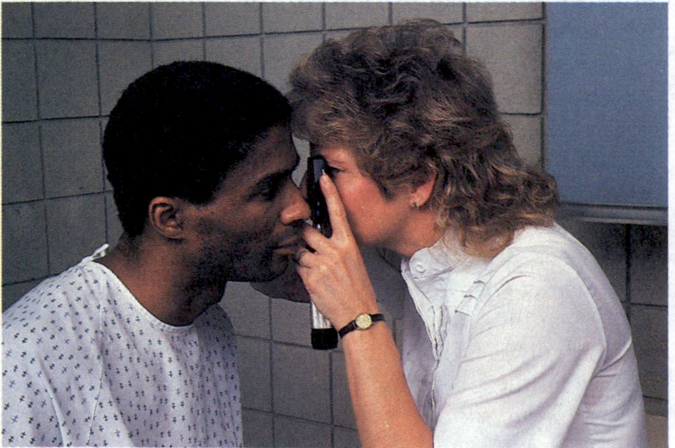

Figure 26-15
Examination of the internal structures of the eye using an ophthalmoscope. (Photo © Ken Kasper.)

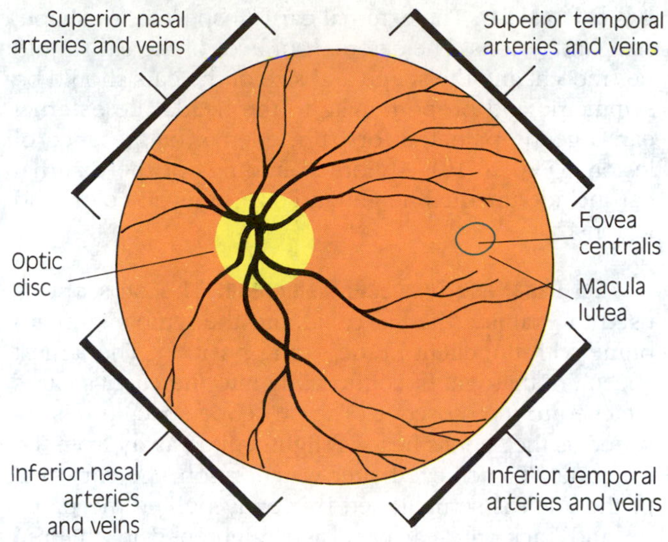

Figure 26-16
The normal fundus as seen through an ophthalmoscope.

- Keeping the finger or light about 1 foot from the client's face, move it slowly through the cardinal positions—up and down, left and right, diagonally up and down to the left, diagonally up and down to the right.

Peripheral Vision. Tests for peripheral vision (or visual fields) assess retinal function and optic nerve function. Normally, the client will have full peripheral vision. Assess visual fields by following these seven steps:

- Have the client stand or sit about 2 feet away, facing the examiner at eye level.
- Ask the client to cover one eye with a hand or an index card.
- Ask the client to look directly at the examiner's nose, and fix the eyes on that spot.
- The examiner covers his or her own eye opposite the client's closed eye.
- The examiner holds one arm outstretched to one side (right or left) and moves his or her fingers into the visual fields from various peripheral points.
- The client is asked to indicate verbally when the fingers are first seen (both the examiner and the client should see the fingers at the same time).
- Repeat the procedure for the other eye.

Abnormalities of the external eye, pupil and iris, and visual assessment include asymmetry of position and alignment, inability to open and close the upper lids, scanty eyebrows and eyelashes, edema, redness or drainage, decreased or absent pupillary response, inability of the eyes to accommodate or converge, and alterations in the visual fields.

Ear

Each ear comprises the external ear, the middle ear, and the inner ear (Fig. 26-18). Risk factors for consideration when assessing the ears are environmental hazards, such as exposure to chemicals or uncontrolled loud noises. The use of corrective hearing devices should be included in the assessment documentation.

The client remains sitting while the nurse assesses the ears and hearing ability by inspection and palpation. An otoscope with a suitably sized ear speculum may be used to inspect the ear canal; a tuning fork is used in hearing acuity assessment.

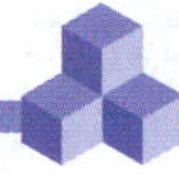

Focused Assessment Guide

Internal Eye

General guidelines for assessment of the internal eye are as follows:

- Assemble the ophthalmoscope, beginning with the light setting at the large white light and the lens wheel at 0 setting.
- Darken the room and have the client remove glasses. Allow time for the client's pupils to dilate. The client should be sitting.
- Sit facing the client and ask him or her to look straight ahead during the examination.
- Keep both eyes open while looking through the ophthalmoscope viewer.
- Use your right hand and eye to examine the client's right eye, and your left hand and eye for the client's left eye.
- Shine the light on the pupil and observe the round red or orange glow (the red reflex).
- Focusing on the red reflex, slowly move the ophthalmoscope toward the client's eye.
- Rotate the lens wheel until internal eye structures are sharp and clear.
- Follow blood vessels toward the midline to locate the optic disc; note color, size, shape, margins, and central area (physiologic cup).
- Follow blood vessels outward to each of the four quadrants, assessing color, size, and pattern.
- Ask the client to look up, down, and from side to side, assessing the characteristics of the retina.
- Locate the macula by first locating the optic disc and then looking toward the client's temple for a small circular structure near the disc; note color, characteristics, and area of reflected light (fovea centralis).

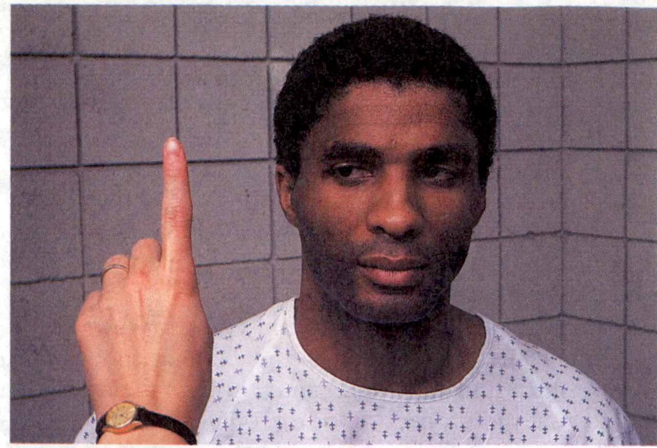

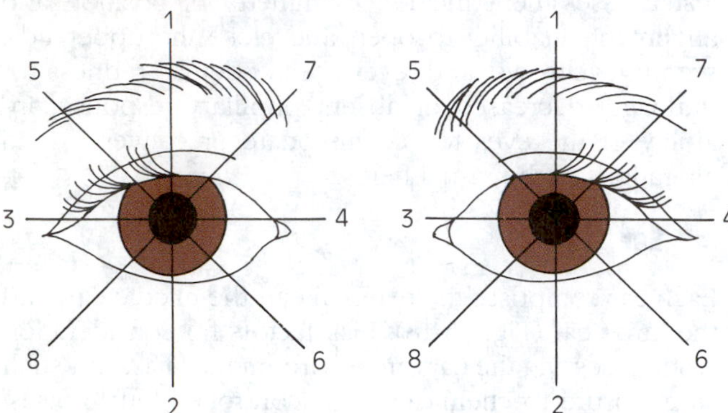

Figure 26-17
Test extraocular movement of the eye by asking the client to hold his head still and follow the movement of your forefinger *(top)* through the cardinal positions of the eye *(bottom)* (Photo © Ken Kasper.)

External Ear. The external ear is inspected for shape, size, and lesions. The external surfaces of the ear should be smooth, and the shape and size of the ears should be symmetric and proportionate to the head. The external ear is gently palpated for pain, edema, or presence of lesions (Fig. 26-19). Abnormal findings of the external ear include unequal height and size, uneven color, and lesions.

Ear Canal and Tympanic Membrane. The otoscope is used to examine the ear canal and the tympanic membrane with the client in the sitting position. The largest speculum that will fit comfortably into the client's ear is attached to the otoscope. The otoscope speculum is inserted as the client's head is slightly tilted away from the examiner. To achieve better visualization, the ear canal of the adult is straightened by gently pulling the pinna up and back (the ear canal is straightened in children younger than age 3 years by pulling the pinna down and back). The ear canal should be smooth and pinkish in color. It is examined for wax, discharge, and foreign bodies. The tympanic membrane should be intact and without redness or discharge. The membrane is translucent, shiny, and gray (Fig. 26-20). Typical abnormal findings include pain when manipulating the pinna, redness of the canal, nodules on the auricle, mastoid tenderness, a red and swollen eardrum, a perforated eardrum, wax plugs in the ear canal, and drainage.

Hearing. Hearing is assessed, one ear at a time, by determining if the client can hear the nurse's whispered voice or a ticking watch from a distance of 1 to 2 feet. The nurse must be certain the client is not lip-reading

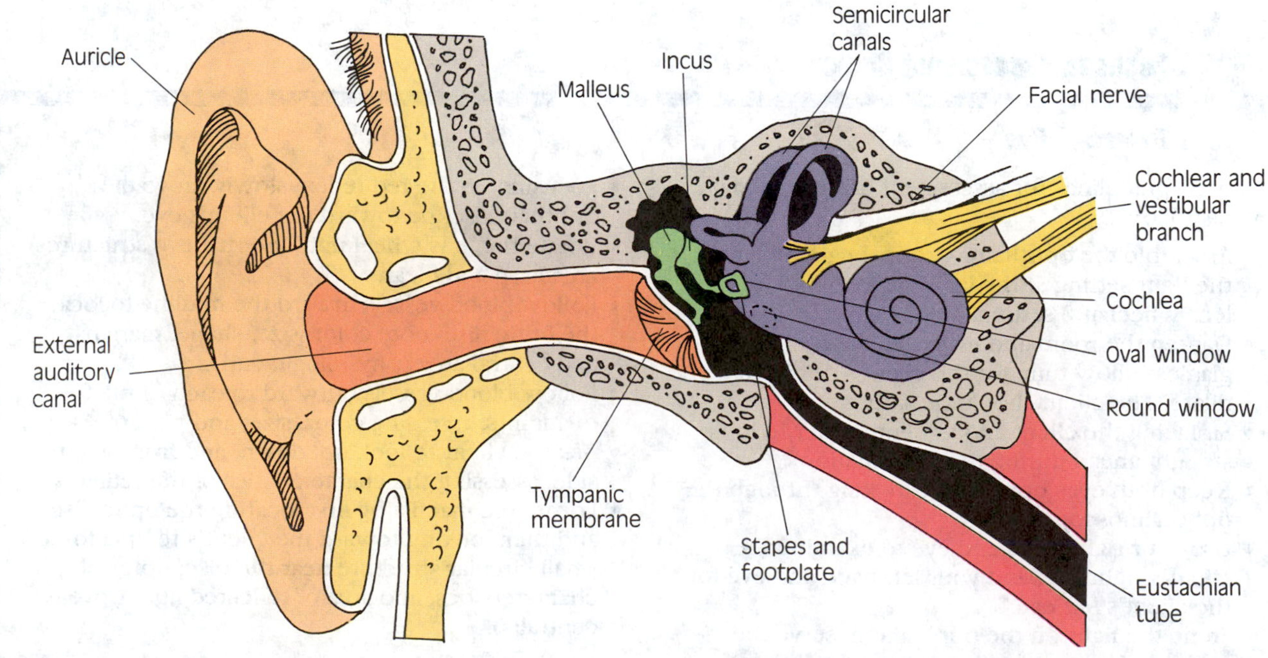

Figure 26-18
Internal structures of the ear.

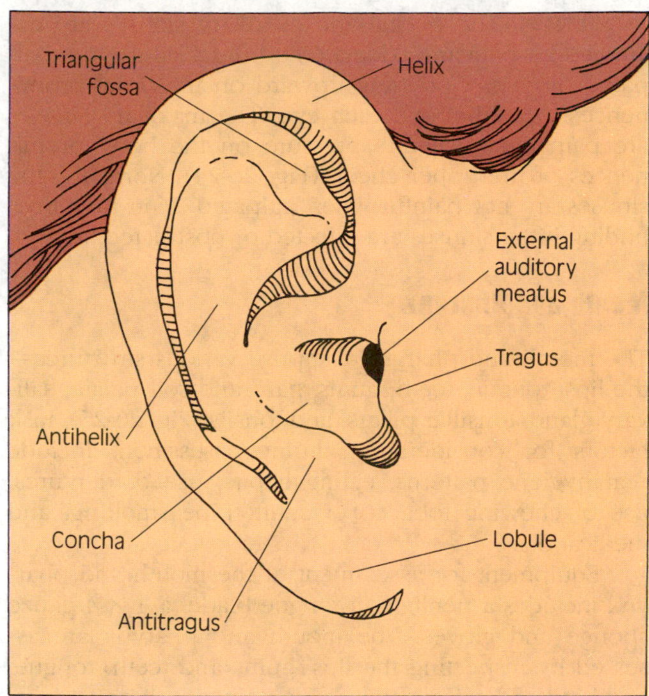

Figure 26-19
External structures of the ear.

and assesses hearing acuity out of the line of vision, with the opposite ear plugged. When hearing loss is found, a tuning fork or audiometer may be used for more precise assessments of hearing; audiometry is not generally used in routine physical assessment. Tuning fork tests are used to assess the type of hearing loss. Hearing loss may be *conductive*, that is, the result of a problem with the transmission of sound waves through the outer and middle ear; *sensorineural*, resulting from inner ear damage; or *mixed*, a combination of both. Weber's and Rinne's tests are used.

Weber's test is used to assess bone conduction. The three-step procedure is as follows:

- Hold the tuning fork at its base and strike it against the palm of the opposite hand so the fork vibrates.
- Place the base of the tuning fork on the center of the top of the client's head.
- Ask the client where the sound is heard best.

Clients with conductive hearing loss hear the sound better in the affected ear because bone transmits the sound directly to the ear. Normal findings would be sound heard in both ears or in the midline.

Rinne's test compares air conduction (AC) with bone conduction (BC). The four-step test is as follows:

- Activate the tuning fork.
- Hold the base of the tuning fork against the mastoid process of the client and ask the client to tell you when the sound can no longer be heard.
- Immediately place the still-vibrating tuning fork close to the external ear canal and ask if the client can hear the sound; the normal ear will do so.
- Repeat the test with the other ear.

Normally, air conduction is better than bone conduction (positive Rinne's test with AC exceeding BC). If the hearing loss is conductive, bone conduction will be the same or greater than air conduction.

Nose and Sinuses

Assessment of the nose and sinuses is conducted by examining the external nose, the *nares*, and the *turbinates* (Fig. 26-21). The maxillary sinuses are located in the maxillary bone; the frontal sinuses are located in the frontal bone (Fig. 26-22).

Factors to consider when assessing the nose and sinuses include allergies; frequent respiratory infections; use of cocaine; and use of nasal drops, sprays, and medications. The nose is assessed by inspection, and the sinuses by inspection and palpation. The client is in a sitting position with the head slightly tilted back.

Nose. The nose is tested for nasal patency by occluding one nostril at a time and asking the client to inhale and exhale through the nose. Each nostril is inspected, using an otoscope with a short, wide tip or with a nasal speculum and penlight (Fig. 26-23). The mucous membranes are examined for color and the presence of exudate or growths. The nasal septum is inspected for intactness and deviation. Normally, the nasal mucosa is moist and redder than the oral mucosa. Abnormal findings that should be noted when assessing the nose are swelling of the mucosa, bleeding, discharge, perforation or deviation of the nasal septum, and polyps.

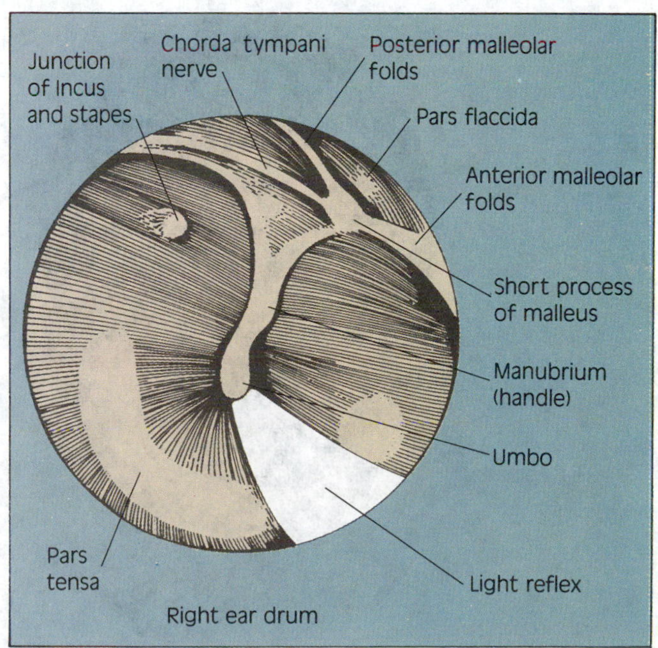

Figure 26-20
Normal tympanic membrane, as seen through an otoscope.

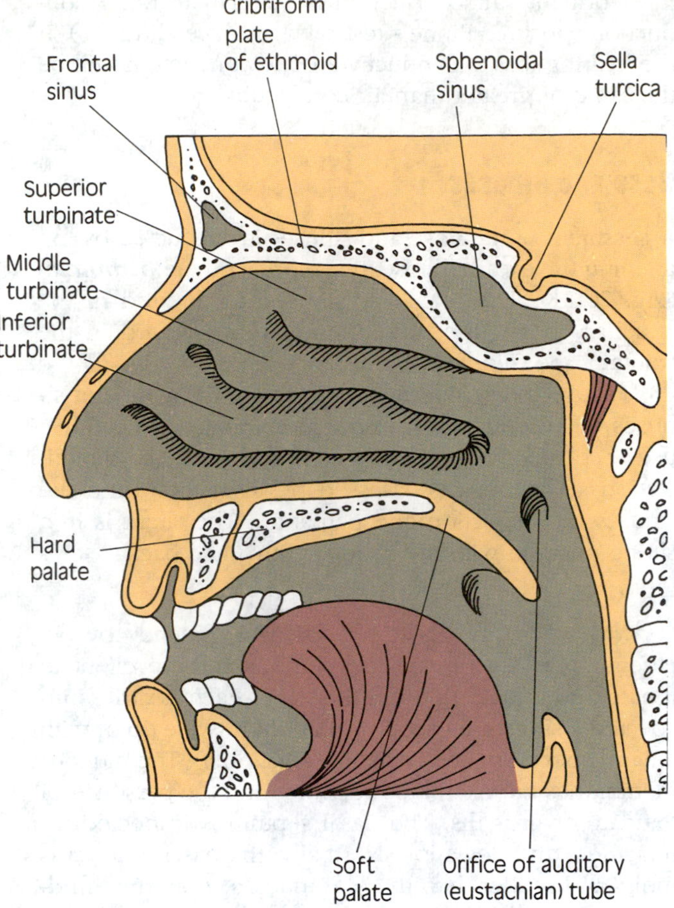

Figure 26-21
Cross section of the nasal cavity.

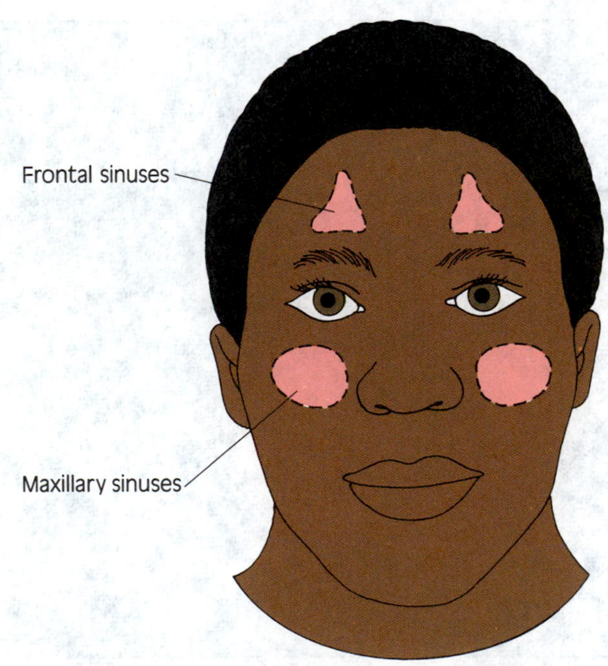

Figure 26-22
Location of the frontal and maxillary sinuses.

Sinuses. The frontal and maxillary sinuses are examined for pain and edema. The frontal sinuses are palpated by gently pressing upward on the bony prominences located above each eye. The maxillary sinuses are palpated by gentle pressure on the bony prominences of the upper cheek (Fig. 26-24). Normally, the sinuses are not painful when palpated. Pain may be a finding if the sinuses are infected or obstructed.

Mouth and Pharynx

The mouth and pharynx comprise various structures—the lips, tongue, teeth, gums, hard and soft palate, salivary gland, tonsillar pillars, and tonsils (Fig. 26-25). Risk factors for consideration during assessment include oral hygiene patterns, eating habits, use of dentures, use of chewing tobacco or snuff, pipe smoking, and medications.

Equipment for assessment of the mouth and pharynx includes a penlight, a tongue blade, a 4 × 4 gauze sponge and gloves. The mouth and pharynx are assessed by inspecting the lips, gums and teeth, tongue, and hard and soft palates, using palpation if any abnormalities are noted during inspection. The client is in the sitting position with the head tilted backward and is instructed to open the mouth wide. The nurse wears gloves when assessing a client's mouth and may use the gauze 4 × 4 to hold the tongue for palpation.

The lips should be pink, moist, and smooth. The tongue and mucous membranes are normally pink in color, moist, and free of swelling or lesions. If the client wears dentures, they are removed for inspection of the gums and roof of the mouth. The gums should be pink and smooth. With the tongue relaxed on the floor of the mouth, the mucous membrane of the oropharynx is examined as the base of the tongue is depressed with a tongue depressor. The uvula normally is centered and freely movable. The tonsils, if present, are small, pink, and symmetric in size. The teeth should be regular and

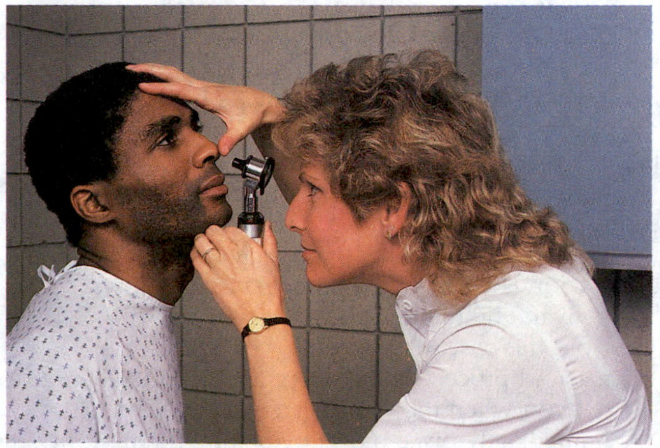

Figure 26-23
Examination of the nasal passages using an otoscope with a wide speculum. (Photo © Ken Kasper.)

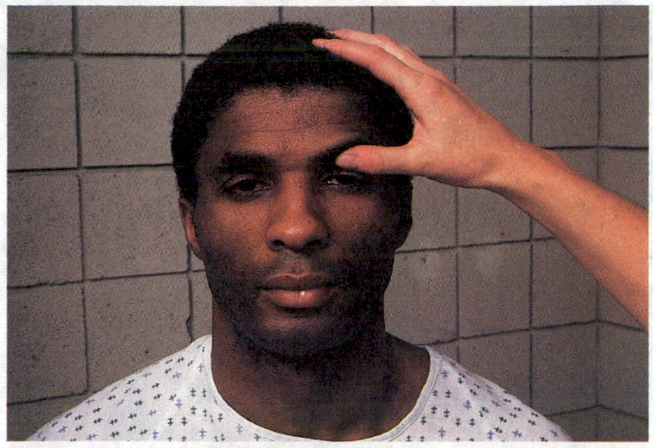

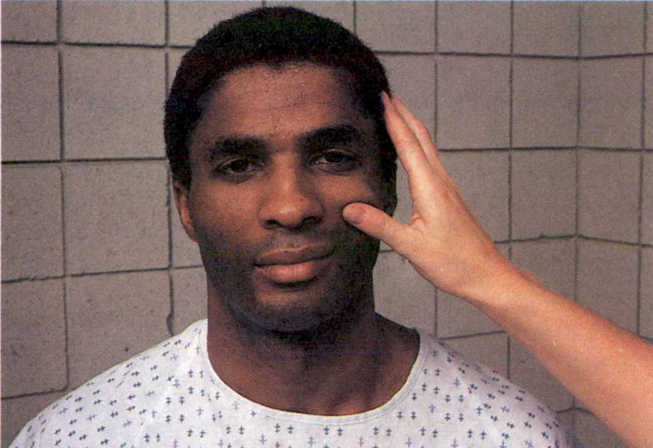

Figure 26-24
(Top) The frontal sinuses are palpated by gently pressing upward on the bony prominences above each eye. *(Bottom)* The maxillary sinuses are palpated by applying gentle pressure on the bony prominences of the upper cheek. (Photos © Ken Kasper.)

free of cavities or have dental restoration. Abnormal findings of the mouth and pharynx are pallor, cyanosis, redness and swelling of the mucous membranes; lesions of the mucosa and lips; swollen, red tonsils; swollen, red, and bleeding gums; poorly aligned, missing, or carious teeth; a hairy, fissured, or bright red tongue; and paralysis of the tongue.

Neck

With the client in the sitting position, the neck (Fig. 26-26) is assessed by inspection and palpation. The neck should be slightly hyperextended. Risk factors to consider when assessing the neck include past injury, infections, and evidence or history of thyroid problems.

The neck is assessed for size and position of the trachea and thyroid (Fig. 26-27), range of motion, lymph nodes, and venous distention. Range of motion is assessed by asking the client to tilt the head backward, forward, and side to side. The neck should be symmetric with full range of motion. No neck vein distention should be visible.

Trachea. The trachea, normally midline at the supersternal notch, is palpated for alignment and position. An unequal space between the trachea and the sternocleidomastoid muscle on each side is an abnormal finding indicating tracheal displacement.

Thyroid. The thyroid gland is assessed by palpation, but in many individuals is normally not palpable. The client is sitting, with the examiner using the posterior approach (Fig. 26-28). Palpate for size, shape, symmetry, tenderness, and presence of any nodules. Follow these five steps to palpate the thyroid gland:

- Standing behind the client, the examiner's hands are placed around the client's neck, with the fingertips over the lower half of the neck and trachea.
- Ask the client to swallow, and feel for enlargement of the gland as it rises.
- Palpate each lobe of the thyroid by having the client turn the head slightly toward the side to be examined; then gently displace the trachea with one hand.
- Ask the client to swallow, and palpate the thyroid with the other hand.
- Repeat for the other side.

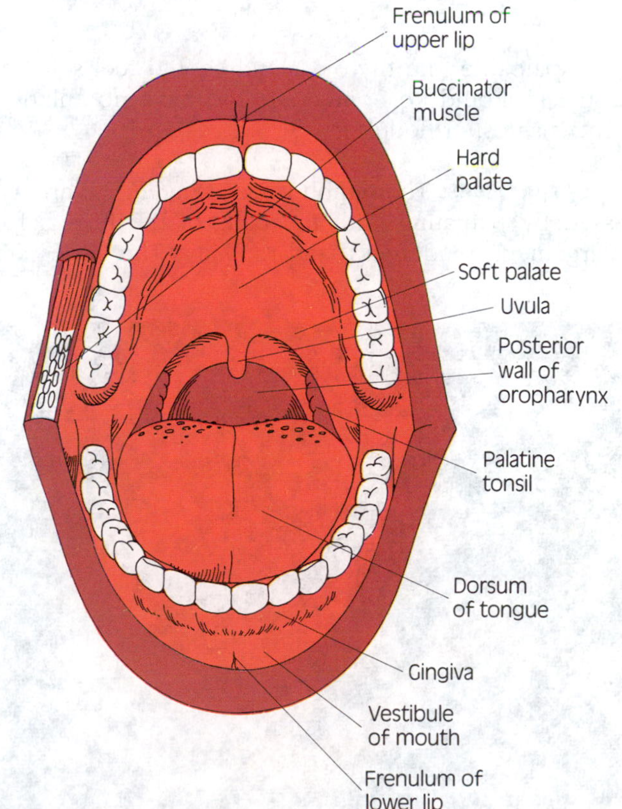

Figure 26-25
Structures of the mouth.

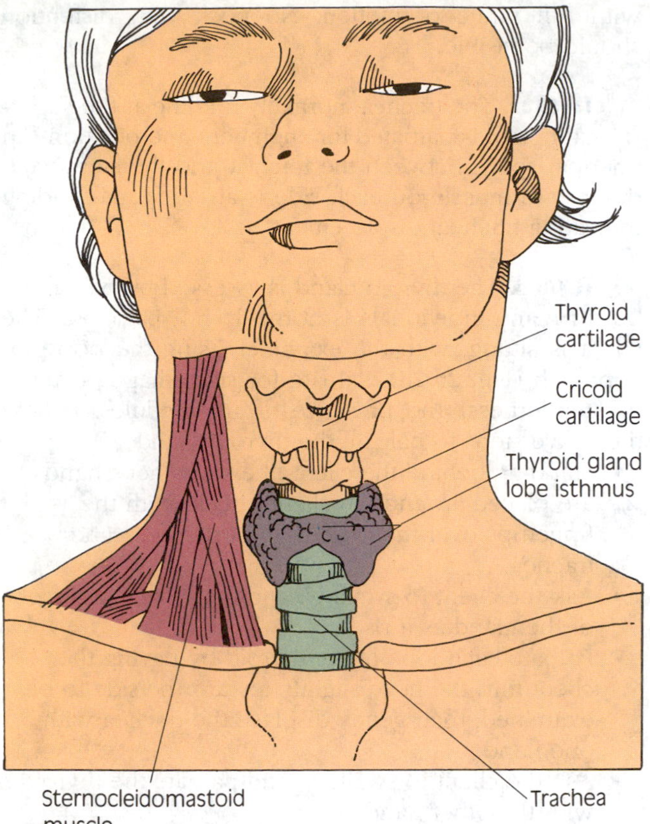

Figure 26-26
Structures of the neck.

If palpable, the thyroid gland should feel soft but elastic. It should be nontender, and have no enlargement, masses, or nodules.

Lymph Nodes. The lymph nodes (Fig. 26-29) are assessed by palpating with the pads of the fingers for enlargement, tenderness, and mobility. The nodes are

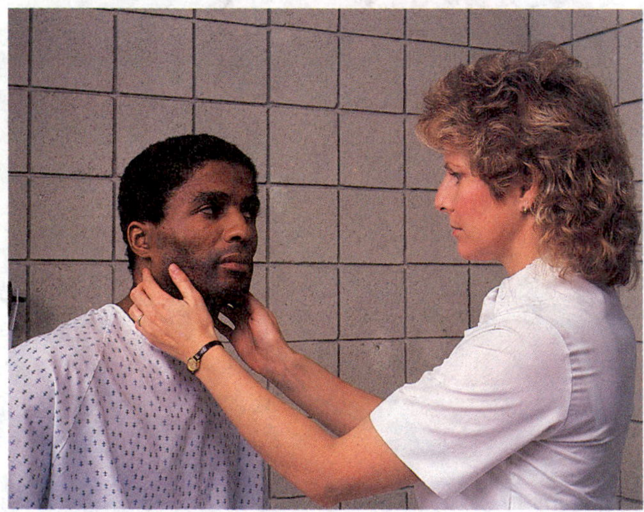

Figure 26-27
Palpation of the neck. (Photo © Ken Kasper.)

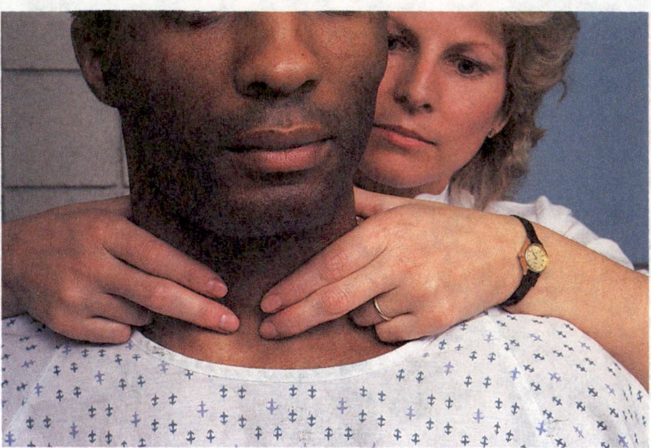

Figure 26-28
Examination of the thyroid. (Photo © Ken Kasper.)

generally not palpable; if palpable, they should be small, mobile, smooth, and nontender. If palpable, assess location, size, consistency, mobility, and tenderness. Abnormal findings of the neck include limited neck movement, enlargement of veins, tracheal deviation, thyroid enlargement, and palpable lymph nodes. Consistent hoarseness should also be documented.

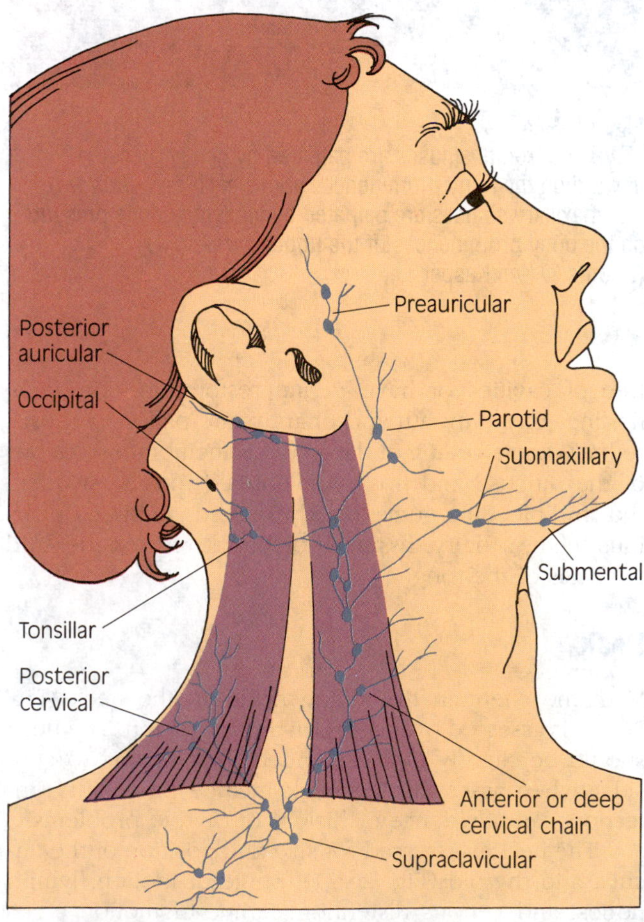

Figure 26-29
Location of the lymph nodes of the neck.

Thorax and Lungs

The thorax (Fig. 26-30) comprises the lungs, rib cage, cartilage, and intercostal muscles. Risk factors for consideration when assessing the thorax and lungs include environmental pollutants, smoking, nutritional status, heart disease, allergies, respiratory disease, and frequent or chronic respiratory infections.

The equipment needed for this assessment includes a stethoscope (warmed) and a tape measure. The environment should be warm and have adequate lighting. The techniques for this assessment include inspection,

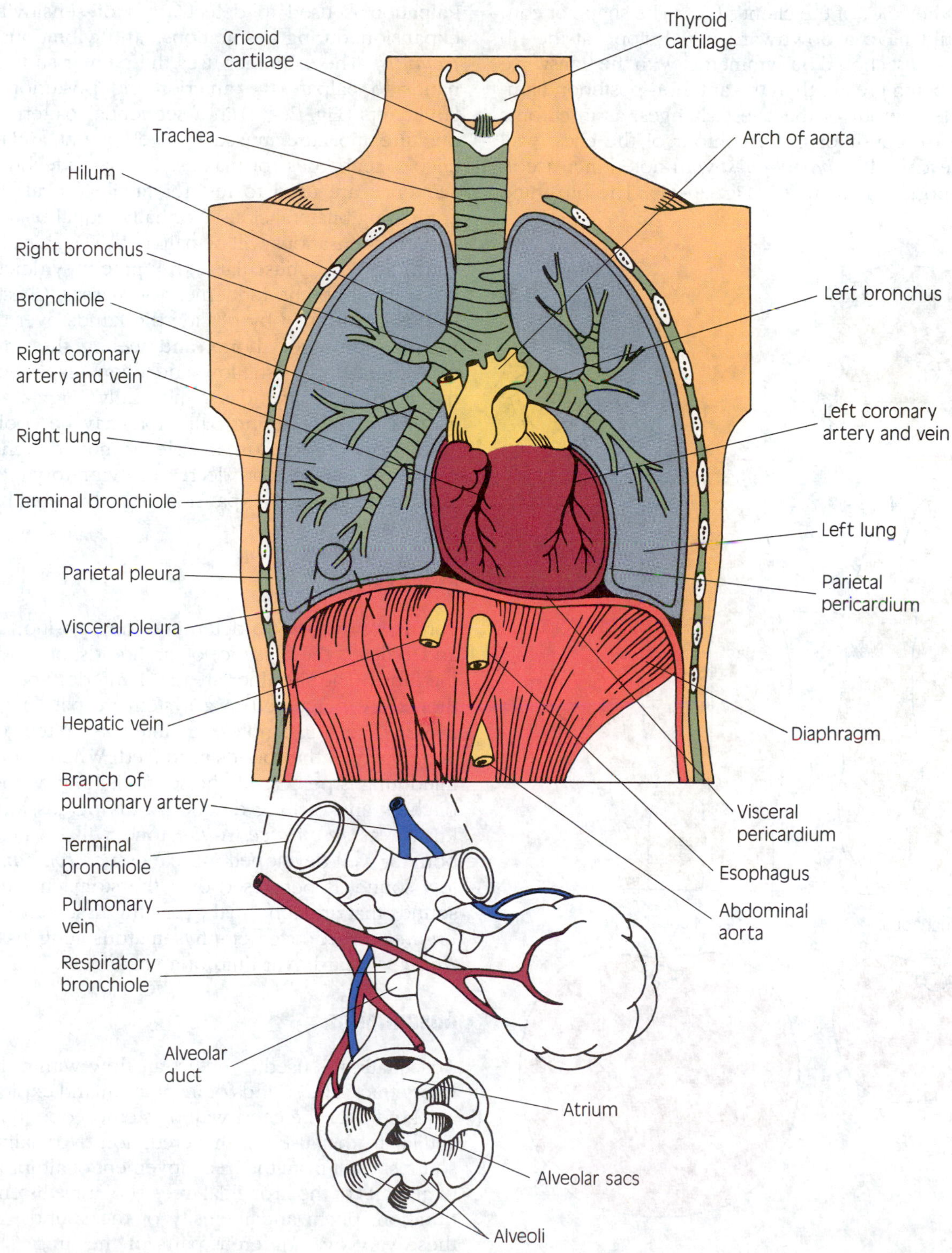

Figure 26-30
Structures of the thorax, with inset of alveoli.

palpation, percussion, and auscultation. The client is in a sitting position during the assessment.

Inspection

Inspection begins with observation of the client's chest for color, shape or contour, breathing patterns, and muscle development. The color should be even and consistent with the color of the client's face. The shape or contour should have a downward equal slope at the rib cage. The chest should be symmetric, with the transverse diameter being greater than the anterior–posterior diameter. If the contour of the chest changes, as in chronic lung disease conditions, the contour of the chest wall can be described as *barrel-chest* with noted increase in anterior–posterior diameter (Fig. 26-31). The breathing patterns should be smooth and even, ranging from 12 to 20 breaths per minute. Abnormal findings during inspection include an increase in chest size and contour, abnormal breathing patterns with use of accessory muscles, and changes in skin color.

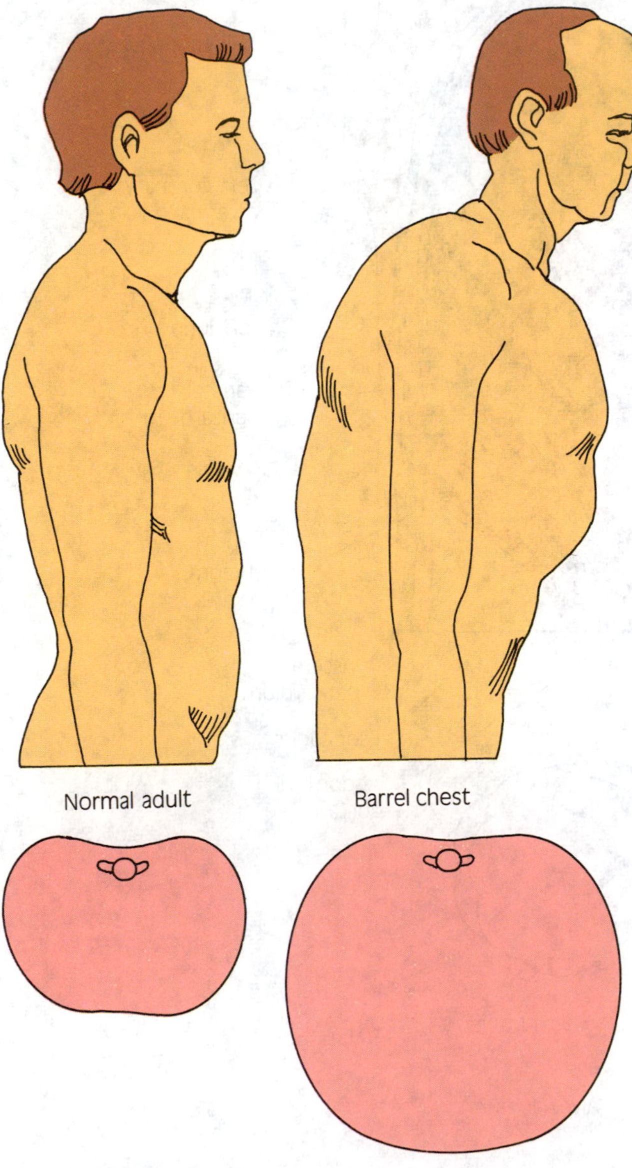

Figure 26-31
Profile and anteroposterior diameter of normal adult chest and barrel chest.

Palpation

Palpation is used to detect areas of sensitivity, chest expansion during respirations, and vibrations (called *fremitus*). The examiner uses the palmar surface of the hands to palpate the anterior and posterior thoracic landmarks (Fig. 26-32) in a sequential pattern for temperature, moisture, muscular development, and the presence of tenderness or masses. The same technique and sequence are used to test for tactile (vocal) fremitus, comparing bilateral sides. Normally, equal bilateral mild vibratory sensations will be palpated. The skin should be warm and dry, muscular development symmetric, and there should be no tenderness or masses. Chest expansion is determined by placing the hands over the anterior and posterior thorax and feeling the amount of movement during shallow and deep respirations. The thorax should expand symmetrically (Fig. 26-33). Abnormal findings during palpation may be cool, excessively dry or moist skin; muscle asymmetry; tenderness; masses; increased or decreased vibratory sensation; asymmetric thoracic expansion; and abnormal breathing patterns (Fig. 26-34).

Percussion

Percussion is used to determine lung position and size and to detect the presence of air, liquids, or solids within the lungs. The shoulder area and anterior and posterior thorax are percussed in a systematic pattern (see Fig. 26-32). The nurse notes the intensity, pitch, duration, and quality of the sounds produced. When a normal air-filled lung is percussed, the sound is hollow, loud, low-pitched, and of long duration. This percussion tone is known as *resonance*. A *flat* tone will be heard over bony or well-developed muscle tissue. *Tympany*, a hollow sound, is percussed over the stomach. Percussion sounds that are abnormal over lung tissue are *hyperresonance*, heard over emphysematous lung tissue, and *dullness*, heard over fluid or a solid mass.

Auscultation

Auscultation is used to detect air flow within the respiratory tract. The sounds of inspiration and expiration are assessed over the chest wall by stethoscope in a pattern similar to that used with percussion. Normally, breath sounds result from the free movement of air into and out of all parts of the bronchial tree. The nurse listens for the duration, pitch, and intensity of the sounds; normally these vary over different parts of the lung. The client should be placed in a sitting position and asked to breathe slowly and deeply through the mouth. The

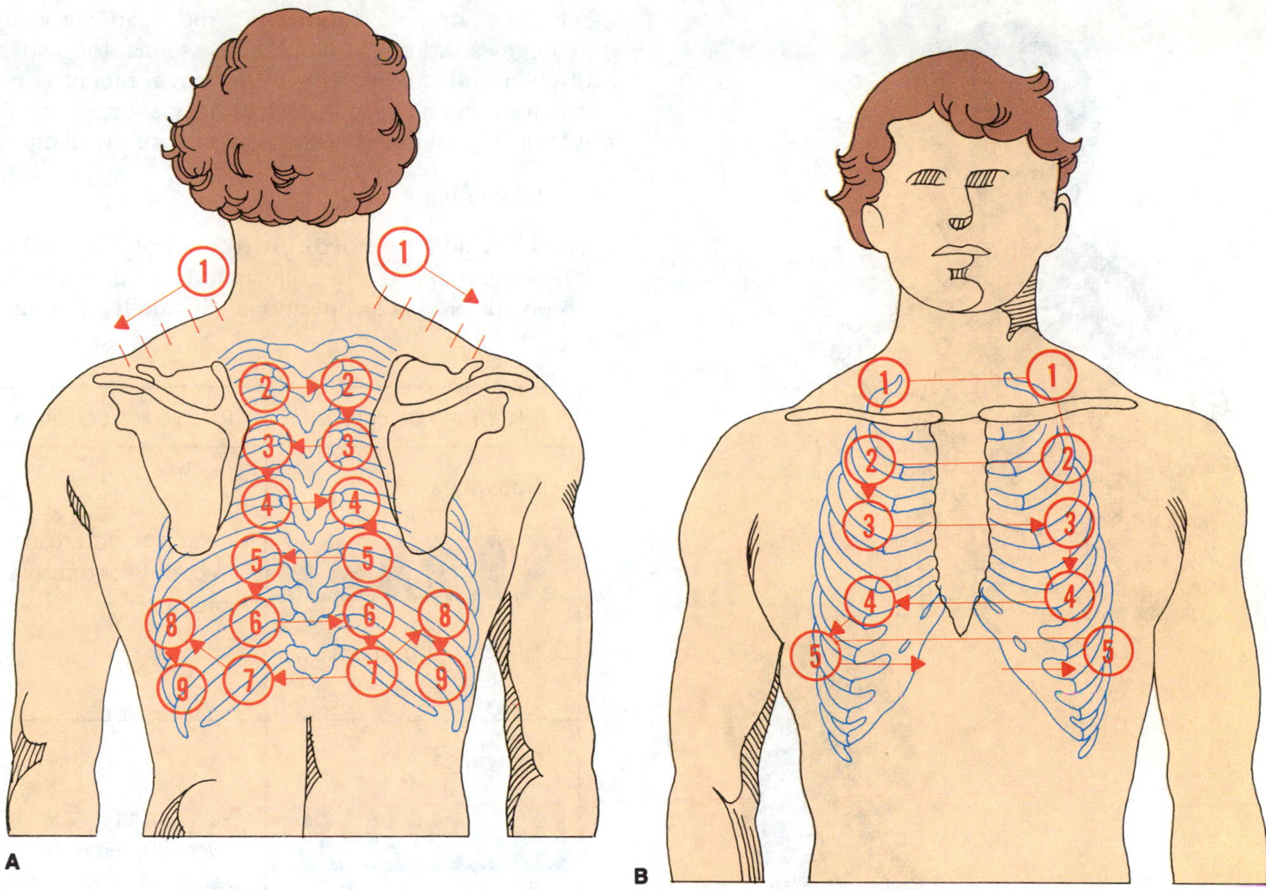

Figure 26-32
Posterior **(A)** and anterior **(B)** chest—landmarks and systematic sequence of examination. The pattern is used for palpation, percussion, and auscultation of the chest.

warmed diaphragm of the stethoscope is placed over the thoracic landmarks, and breath sounds are auscultated in the same sequential pattern as used for palpation and percussion (see Fig. 26-32).

Normally, **bronchial sounds** are heard over the trachea and are high-pitched, harsh sounds, with expiration being longer than inspiration. **Bronchovesicular sounds** are heard over the mainstem bronchus, and are moderate "blowing" sounds, with inspiration equal to expiration. **Vesicular breath sounds** are soft, low-pitched sounds, heard best over the base of the lungs during inspiration, which is longer than expiration (Fig. 26-35).

Adventitious breath sounds are sounds not normally heard in the lungs, but if present, they may be auscultated along with normal breath sounds. Crackles are discrete, discontinuous sounds that have a dry or wet crackling quality. They are most often heard on inspiration. Crackles are described as fine when they are made by air passing through moisture in small air passages and alveoli, and as coarse when they are made by air passing through moisture in the bronchioles, bronchi, and trachea. These sounds may also be labeled *rales.* Wheezes are continuous sounds that originate in small air passages that are narrowed by secretions, swelling, or tumors. They may be inspiratory or expiratory and are high-pitched sounds. Gurgles, formerly called *rhonchi,* are also continuous sounds, originating in large air passages that are narrowed or contain mucus. Gurgles are best heard on expiration, are low-pitched, and may be altered by coughing. A *pleural friction rub* is a grating sound, caused by an inflamed pleura rubbing against the chest wall (Fig. 26-36).

If a productive cough occurs during assessment of the thorax and lungs, the sputum should be assessed for color, consistency, and amount.

Cardiovascular and Peripheral Vascular Systems

Cardiovascular and peripheral vascular assessment is conducted through physical assessment of the heart and the extremities.

Risk factors for consideration during this assessment include nutritional status, cholesterol levels, triglyceride levels, hypertension, chronic respiratory illnesses, congenital disorders, stress, use of tobacco, alcohol consumption, and use of medications.

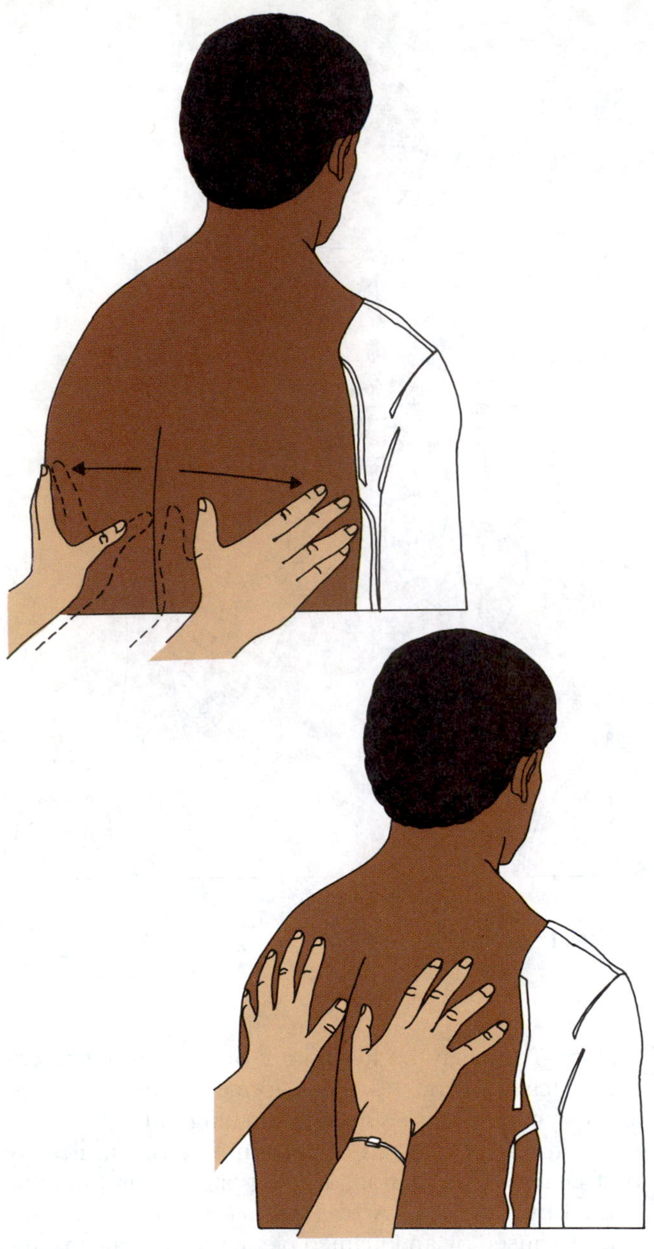

Figure 26-33
(Top) Palpation of the posterior thorax excursion. The examiner's hands are placed symmetrically on the client's back. As the client inhales, the examiner's hands should move apart symmetrically. *(Bottom)* Palpation of the posterior thorax for vocal or tactile fremitus. The examiner uses the palms of the hands to detect vibrations transmitted through the lung to the chest wall.

Heart

The techniques used for assessment of the heart (Fig. 26-37) include inspection, palpation, and auscultation. (Inspection and palpation, although discussed separately here, are usually combined.) Equipment used in this assessment are a stethoscope with a bell and diaphragm and a sphygmomanometer. The client is in a sitting or supine position with the head raised about 30 degrees. Adequate lighting is essential for inspection of color and pulsations. A quiet environment is necessary for accurate auscultation of heart sounds. The nurse is usually positioned at the right side of the client.

Inspection

The neck and **precordium** (the aortic, pulmonic, tricuspid, and apical areas, illustrated in Figure 26-38) are observed for visible pulsations. Generally, there are no

Pattern and Description	Pathological Conditions
Bradypnea 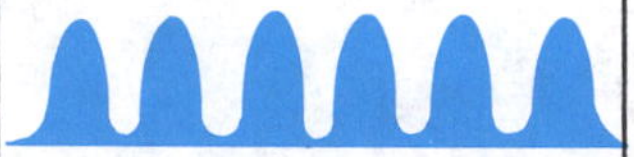 Rate < 12 respirations per minute	Neurologic disturbance Electrolyte disturbance Infection
Tachypnea 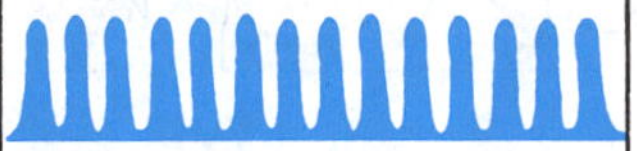 Persistent rate > 20 respirations per minute	Pain or injury Liver enlargement Ascites
Cheyne-Stokes 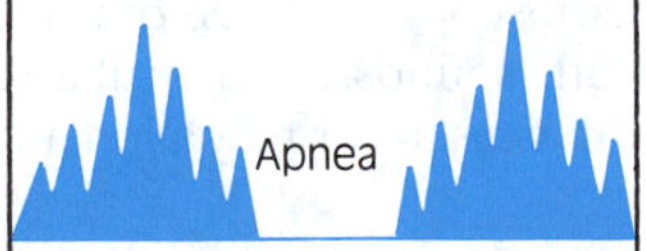 Apnea Cyclic pattern of respirations which progress from slow and shallow to rapid and deep respirations with a gradual return to slow and shallow respirations followed by a period of apnea	Congestive heart failure Renal failure Increased intracranial pressure
Kussmal 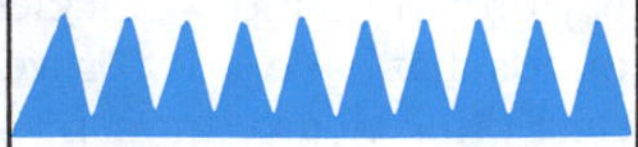 Faster and deeper respirations than normal without pauses	Diabetic ketoacidosis Metabolic acidosis Renal failure

Figure 26-34
Abnormal breathing patterns.

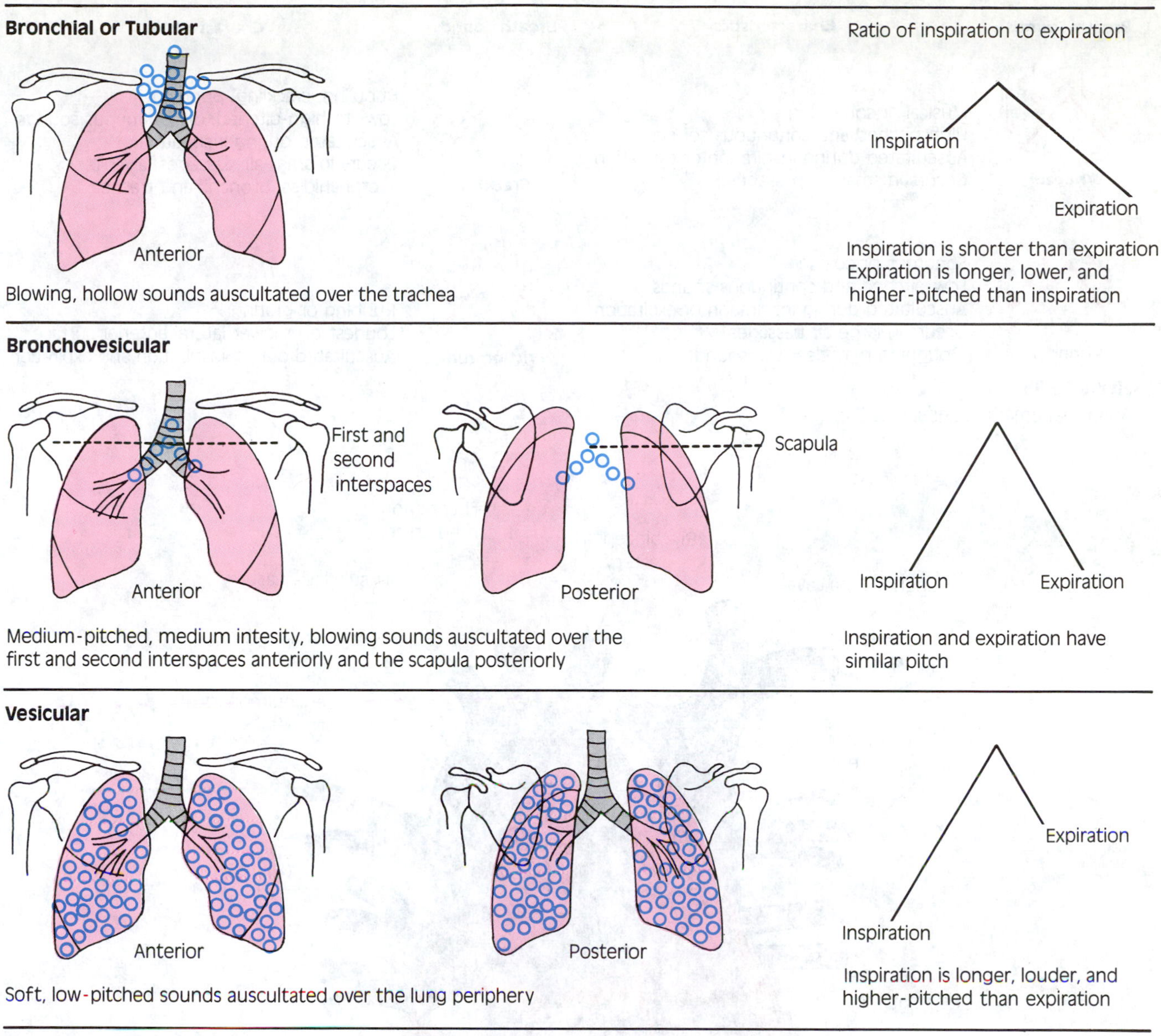

Bronchial or Tubular

Anterior

Blowing, hollow sounds auscultated over the trachea

Ratio of inspiration to expiration

Inspiration

Expiration

Inspiration is shorter than expiration
Expiration is longer, lower, and higher-pitched than inspiration

Bronchovesicular

First and second interspaces

Scapula

Anterior

Posterior

Inspiration

Expiration

Medium-pitched, medium intesity, blowing sounds auscultated over the first and second interspaces anteriorly and the scapula posteriorly

Inspiration and expiration have similar pitch

Vesicular

Anterior

Posterior

Expiration

Inspiration

Soft, low-pitched sounds auscultated over the lung periphery

Inspiration is longer, louder, and higher-pitched than expiration

Figure 26-35
Normal breath sounds.

visible pulsations, except the apical impulse (or the point of maximal impulse [PMI]), located approximately at the fourth or fifth intercostal space at the left mid-clavicular line. Inspect the epigastric area at the tip of the sternum for pulsation of the abdominal aorta. Findings of neck vein distention or visible pulsations in precordial areas other than the PMI are considered abnormal.

Palpation

The precordium is palpated for the presence of pulsations. The nurse's hands, which should be warm, are used to palpate gently using the palmar surface with the four fingers held together. Palpation proceeds in a systematic manner, with assessment of specific cardiac landmarks—the aortic, pulmonic, tricuspid, and mitral areas (Fig. 26-39).

Each area is palpated to determine if a pulsation is felt. Identify the PMI and record the apical impulse by interspace and relationship to the midsternal line or mid-clavicular line. Identify any precordial *thrills*, which are fine, palpable, rushing vibrations over the right or left second intercostal space; and *lifts* or *heaves*, which involve a rise along the border of the sternum with each heartbeat.

Normal findings include no pulsation palpable over the aortic and pulmonic areas, with a palpable pulsation at the PMI. Abnormal findings include visible pulsations; palpable thrill at the aortic, pulmonic, tricuspid, or mitral areas; and lifts or heaves.

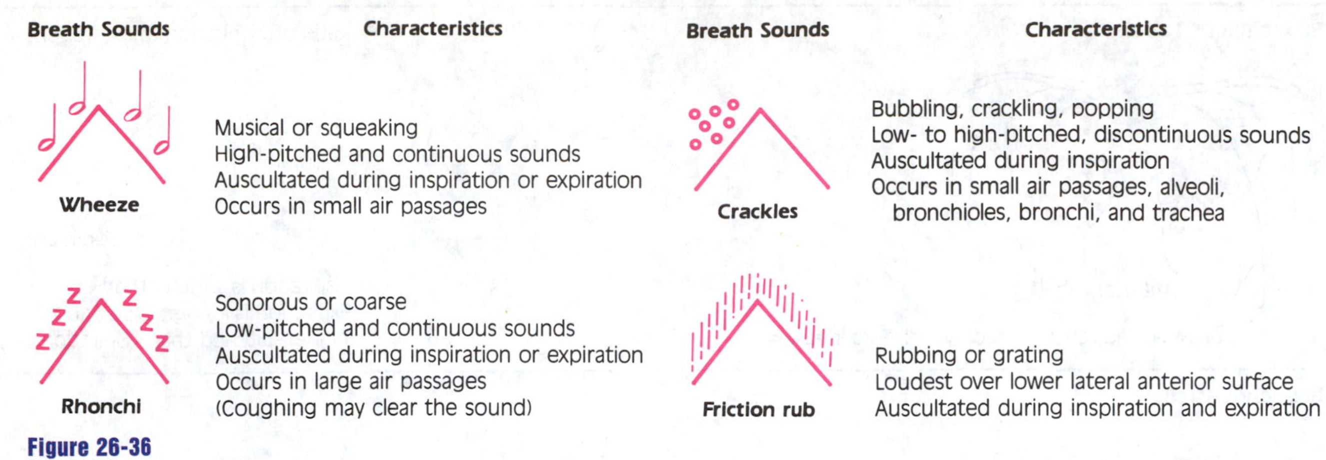

Figure 26-36
Abnormal breath sounds.

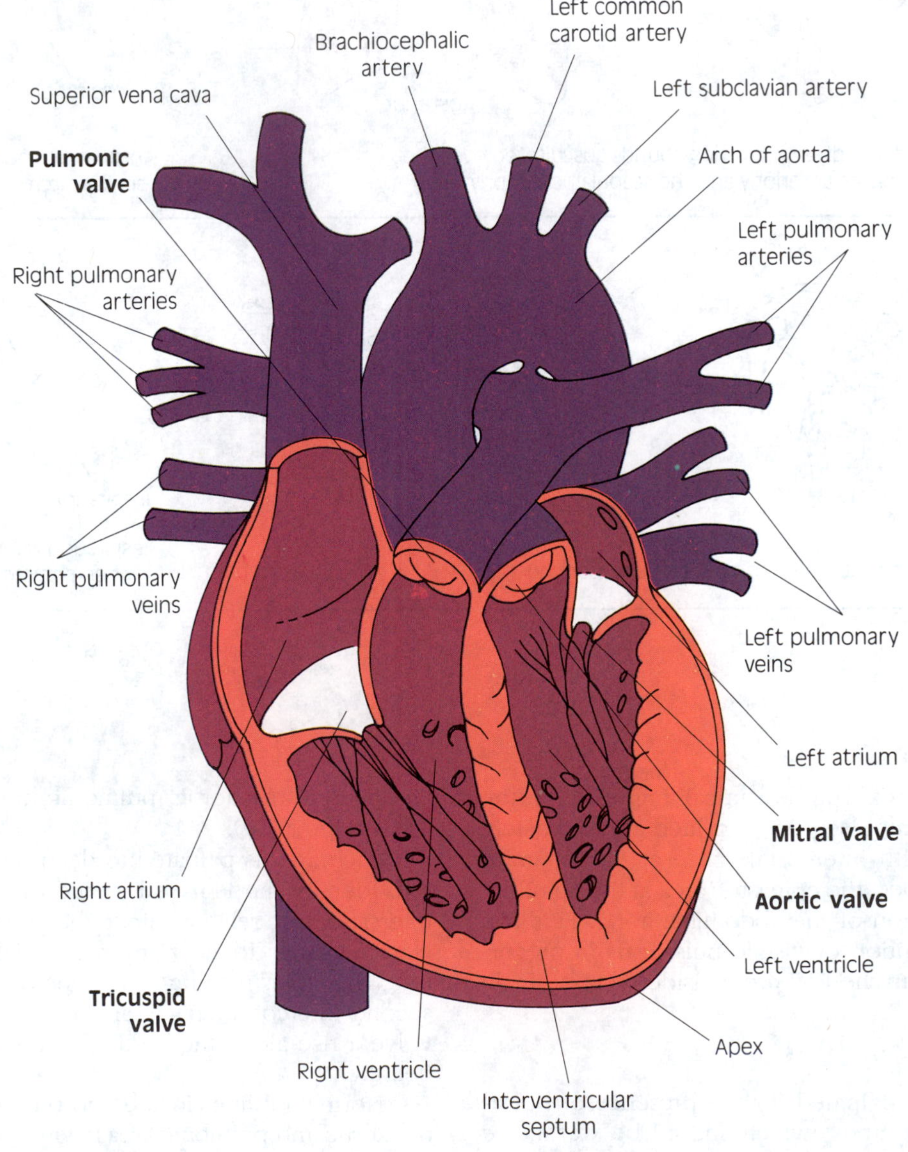

Figure 26-37
View of the interior of the heart showing the atrioventricular and semilunar valves responsible for normal heart sounds.

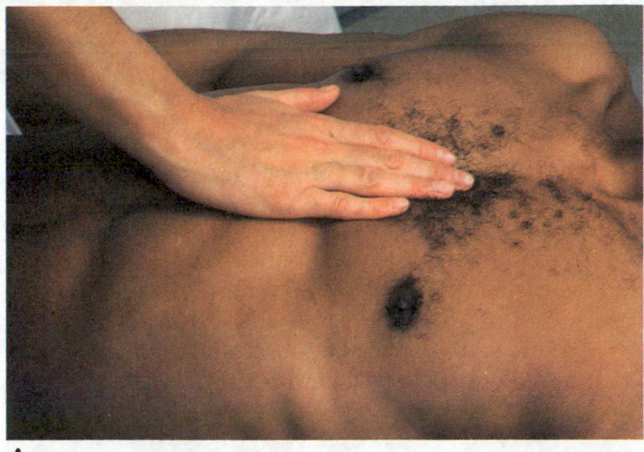

A

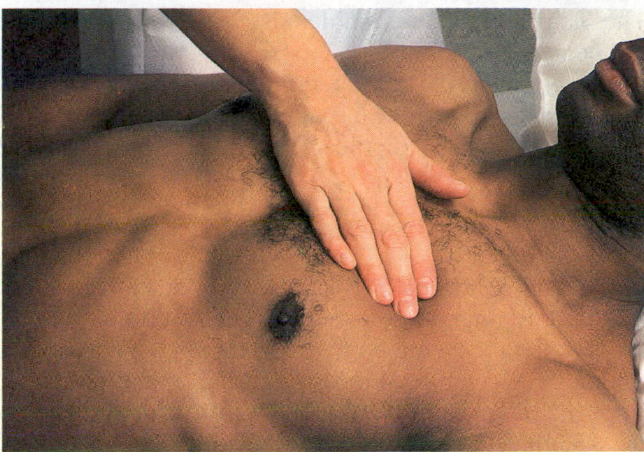

B

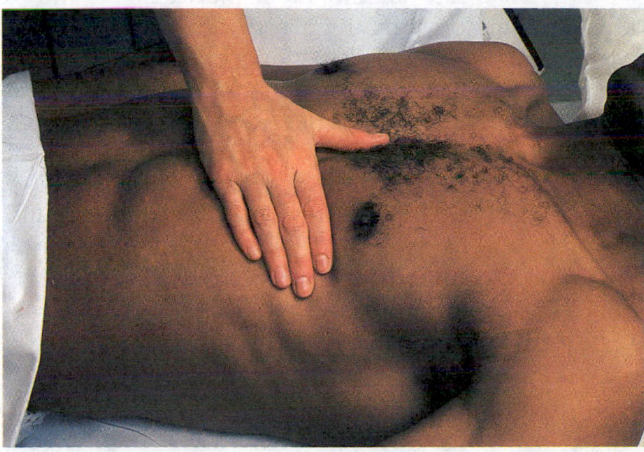

C

Figure 26-38
Palpation of areas of the precordium: **(A)** aortic area, **(B)** pulmonic area, and **(C)** apical and tricuspic area. (Photo © Ken Kasper.)

Auscultation

Auscultation is used to determine the heart sounds caused by closure of the heart valves. A systematic approach is used as the nurse listens at all cardiac landmarks (see Fig. 26-39). Auscultation is done systematically, beginning at the aortic area, moving to the pulmonic, then to the tricuspid, and last to the apical areas. The client should breathe normally. The stethoscope diaphragm is first used to listen to high-pitched sounds, followed by use of the stethoscope bell to listen to low-pitched sounds. The closure of the four valves is responsible for normal heart sounds. The nurse focuses on the overall rate and rhythm of the heart and the normal heart sounds (S_1 and S_2).

During auscultation, the first heart sound is heard as the "lub" of "lub-dub." This sound occurs when the mitral and tricuspid valves close and corresponds with the onset of ventricular contraction (Fig. 26-40). The sound, low-pitched and dull, is called S_1, and is heard best at the apical area. The second heart sound, S_2, occurs at the termination of systole and corresponds with the onset of ventricular diastole. It is the "dub" of "lub-dub" and represents the closure of the aortic and pulmonic valves. The sound of S_2 is higher pitched and shorter than S_1. The two sounds occur within 1 second or less, depending on the heart rate.

Normal findings include S_1 to be louder at the tricuspid and apical areas, with S_2 louder at the aortic and pulmonic areas. Abnormal findings include extra heart sounds at any of the cardiac landmarks, and abnormal rate or rhythm.

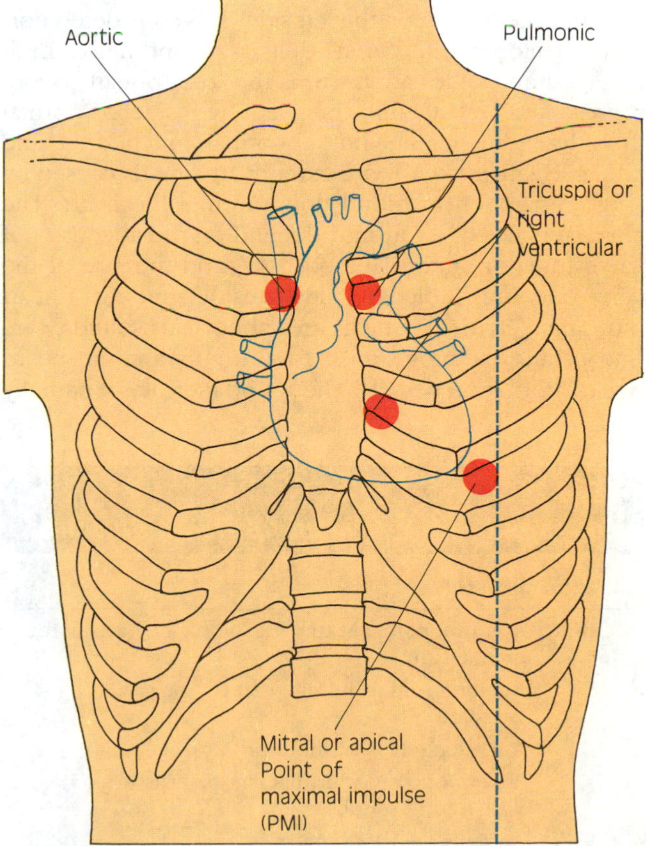

Figure 26-39
Cardiac landmarks and sequence of examination using auscultation.

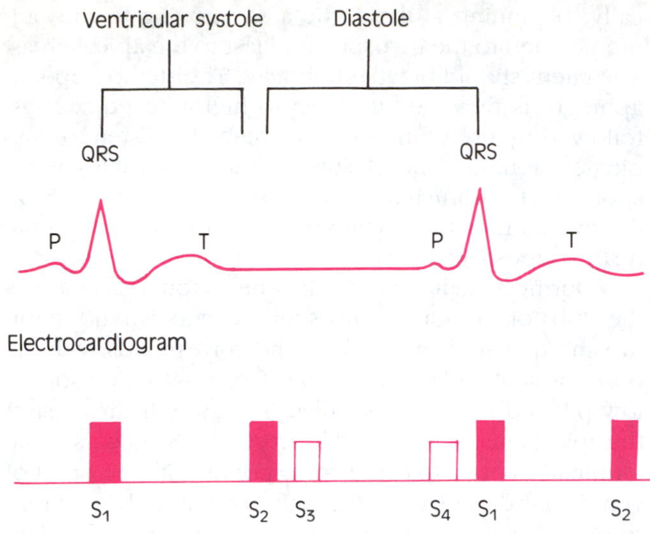

Figure 26-40
Heart sounds in relation to the cardiac cycle and an electrocardiogram.

Extra heart sounds may be S_3, S_4, murmurs, or bruits. S_3, known as the *third heart sound,* often is represented by a "lub-dub-dee" pattern ("dee" being S_3); this sound is best heard with the stethoscope bell at the mitral area, with the client lying on the left side. S_3 is considered normal in children and young adults and abnormal in middle-aged and older adults. S_4 is the fourth heart sound, represented by "dee-lub-dub." S_4 is considered normal in older adult clients but abnormal in children and adults. Heart *murmurs* are extra heart sounds caused by some disruption of blood flow through the heart. The characteristics of a murmur depend on the adequacy of valve function, rate of blood flow, and the size of the valve opening. Table 26-5 illustrates the grading of heart murmurs. **Bruits**, which are abnormal sounds, are "swooshing" sounds similar to murmurs and are heard over major blood vessels. The sound indicates a partially blocked or overextended artery, causing blood to swirl rather than flow normally. Bruits are most commonly heard over the carotid arteries, over the abdominal aorta, and over the femoral arteries.

Table 26-5
Common Grading System for Heart Murmurs

Grade	Description
I	A murmur so faint that it can only be heard with great effort
II	A faint murmur but one that can be easily detected
III	A moderately loud murmur
IV	A very loud murmur that is usually associated with a thrill sound
V	An extremely loud murmur
VI	An exceptionally loud murmur that can be heard while the stethoscope is lifted off the skin

Peripheral Vascular System

The peripheral vascular assessment includes measuring the blood pressure, assessing peripheral vascular pulses, and assessing peripheral vascular perfusion. Assessments are done by inspection and palpation, with the client in the sitting or supine position. Peripheral vascular assessments may be combined with assessment of other body areas.

Inspection

The skin of the extremities is inspected for color, temperature, continuity, lesions (as described previously for assessment of the integument), venous patterns, and edema. There are normally no venous patterns (eg, varicosities, rashes, or ulcers) or edema on the lower extremities.

Palpation

To palpate peripheral pulses, use the pads of the index and middle fingers; palpate the pulse for rate, rhythm, amplitude, and symmetry. Palpate the carotid (one at a time and with caution); brachial, radial, femoral, popliteal, dorsalis pedis, and posterior tibial pulses. Figure 25-6 illustrates the location for palpation of each of these peripheral pulses.

The pulse rate should range between 60 and 90 beats per minute, with a regular rhythm and strong and equal pulses bilaterally. It is unnecessary to determine rate on all peripheral pulses (eg, a strong palpable dorsalis pedis pulse is significant of good peripheral circulation). Abnormal findings include an increased or decreased rate, irregular rate, regularity with pauses or skipped beats, weak or thready pulse, forceful or bounding pulse, and asymmetry of pulses. Related abnormal assessments include cold, pale, cyanotic skin; dark red skin; edema; and varicosities. The blood pressure may be taken at this time or during the general survey.

Breasts and Axillae

The breasts and axilla are assessed in both men and women. Each breast comprises a lymphatic network that drains into the underlying axilla (Fig. 26-41). Although assessments and disorders focus on the female breast, both male and female clients should have breast assessments. Men as well as women may have diseases of the breast.

Risk factors for consideration when assessing the breasts include age, changes in breast tissue, pain, discharge from the nipple, and knowledge and practice of breast self-examination (discussed in Chapter 35). In-

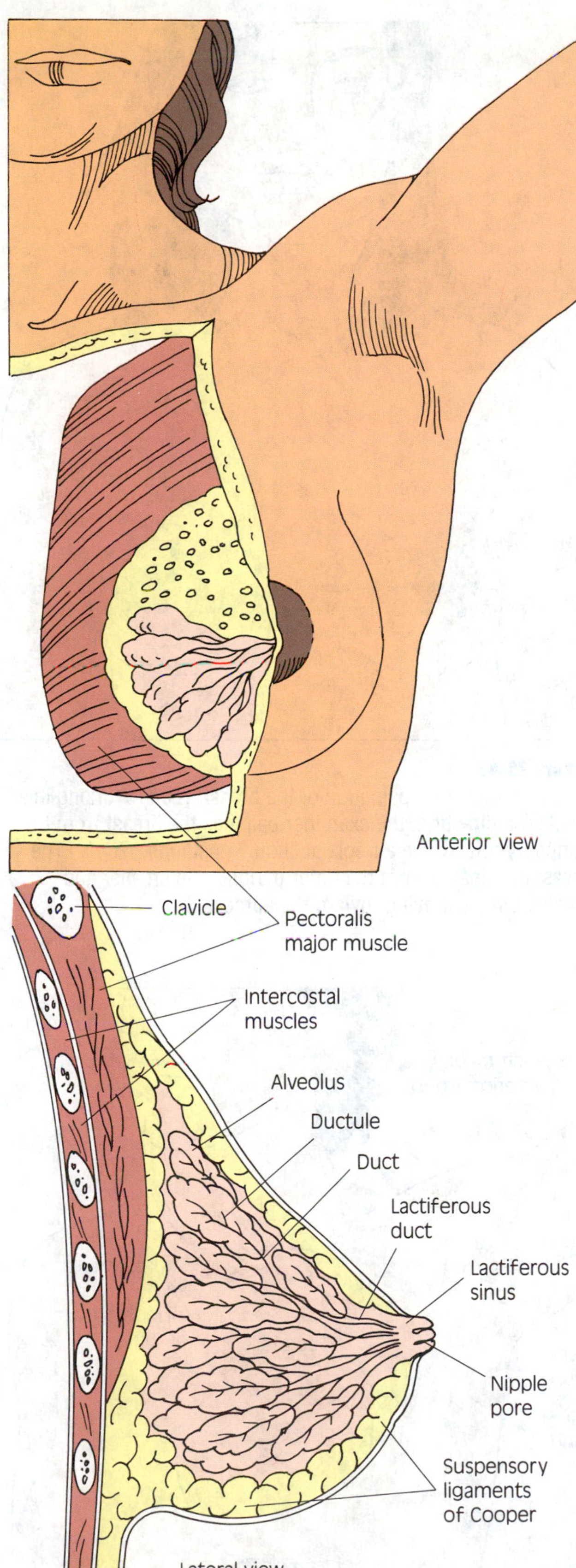

Figure 26-41
Anterior and lateral views of the female breast.

spection and palpation are used in the assessment. The client is in a sitting and supine position. When sitting, the client should sit erect, arms at sides or raised overhead. When supine, the client's hand on the side being examined is under the head.

Inspection

The breasts and axilla are inspected for size, shape, symmetry, color, texture, and skin lesions. The breasts should be relatively symmetric, although variations are normal. The size varies among individuals. The shape of the breasts is round and smooth, and there should be no skin depressions (*retraction*) or puckering (*dimpling*). The color should be consistent with the rest of the skin, and the texture of the skin should be soft.

The areola and nipples are inspected for size and shape; the nipples are inspected for discharge, crusting, and inversion. The areolar and nipple areas should be equal in size, round or oval, with a smooth surface. Montgomery's tubercles are a normal component of the areola. The nipples are normally everted. Lesions and discharge from the nipples are abnormal findings.

Palpation

The primary purpose of palpation is to detect any abnormal masses or lumps. The nipple and areola are palpated, and the nipple is gently compressed between the thumb and forefinger to assess for discharge. The breast is divided into four quadrants: the outer upper quadrant, the outer lower quadrant, the inner upper quadrant, and the inner lower quadrant (Fig. 26-42). Using the pads of the first three fingers, the examiner palpates each quadrant of each breast in a systematic method as the breast tissue is gently compressed against the chest wall (Fig. 26-43). The breast tissue should be smooth and firm with a granular consistency. If a mass is detected, the location, size, shape, consistency, and tenderness should be carefully assessed. The breasts are normally tender the week before menstruation.

The axillary areas are palpated for lymph nodes (Fig. 26-44), which normally are nonpalpable and nontender. If any nodes are palpable, assess location, size, shape, consistency, tenderness, and mobility. Abnormal findings include the presence of a lump, dimpling, nipple discharge, lesions, asymmetry, and palpable lymph nodes.

Abdomen

The abdominal cavity (Fig. 26-45) contains several vital organs: the stomach, the small intestine, the large intestine, the liver, the gallbladder, the pancreas, the spleen, the kidneys, and the urinary bladder. Not all of these organs can be assessed. The abdominal cavity also contains the female reproductive organs, discussed in the following section.

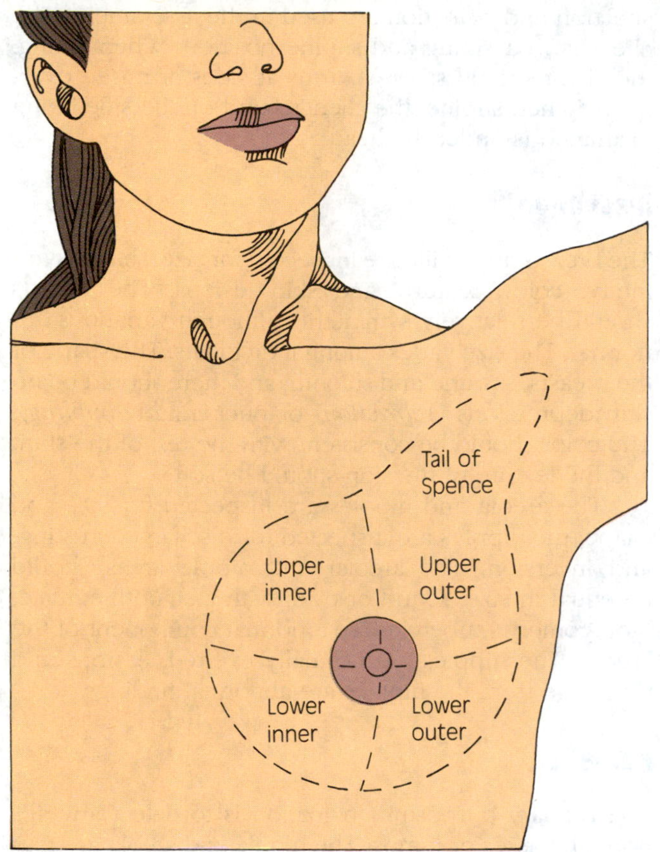

Figure 26-42
Location of assessment findings of the breast are identified by quadrant.

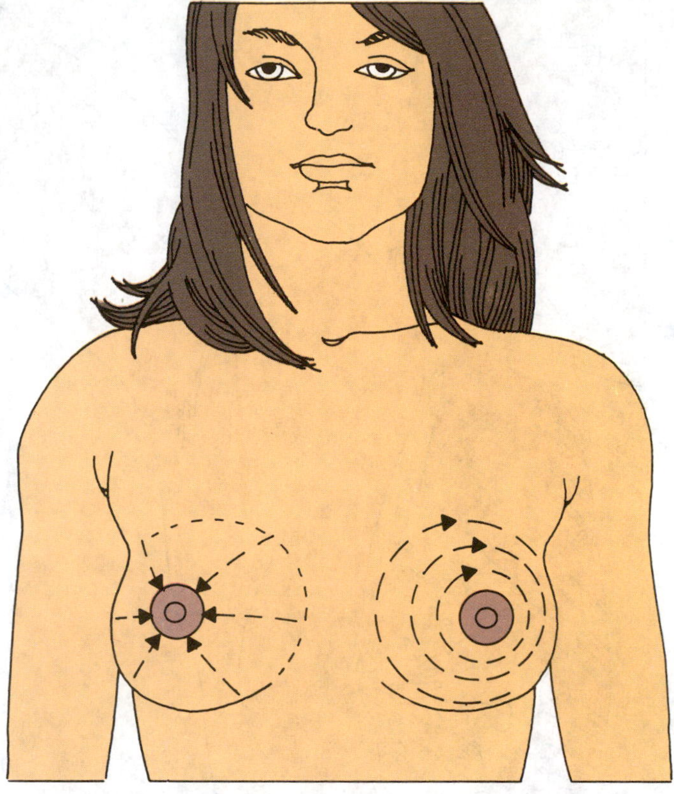

Figure 26-43
Two techniques for palpation of the breast. *(Left)* Working in a clockwise direction, the examiner palpates the breast from the periphery toward the aureola at "hour" positions. *(Right)* The breast is palpated from the outer periphery in smaller and smaller circles moving toward the aureola.

Factors to consider during assessment of the abdomen include nutrition, use of alcohol, stress, urine and stool characteristics, frequency of bladder and bowel elimination, infectious diseases, trauma, and medications. A warm stethoscope, adequate lighting, and warm hands with short fingernails are needed for abdominal assessment. The client is placed in the supine position with the head slightly elevated and arms at sides. Small pillows may be placed under the head and knees. The client should have an empty bladder and be warm. These measures, as well as the position, help prevent contraction of the abdominal muscles, which makes palpation difficult.

To better locate organs and to make documentation more specific, the abdomen can be divided into four quadrants: right upper, right lower, left upper, and left lower (Fig. 26-46). The sequence of techniques used to assess the abdomen is inspection, auscultation, percussion, and palpation. Percussion and palpation stimulate bowel sounds and thus are done after auscultation of the abdomen.

Inspection

The nurse inspects the abdomen while sitting at the side of the client, allowing a tangential view that enhances shadows and contours. Inspection is made of skin color

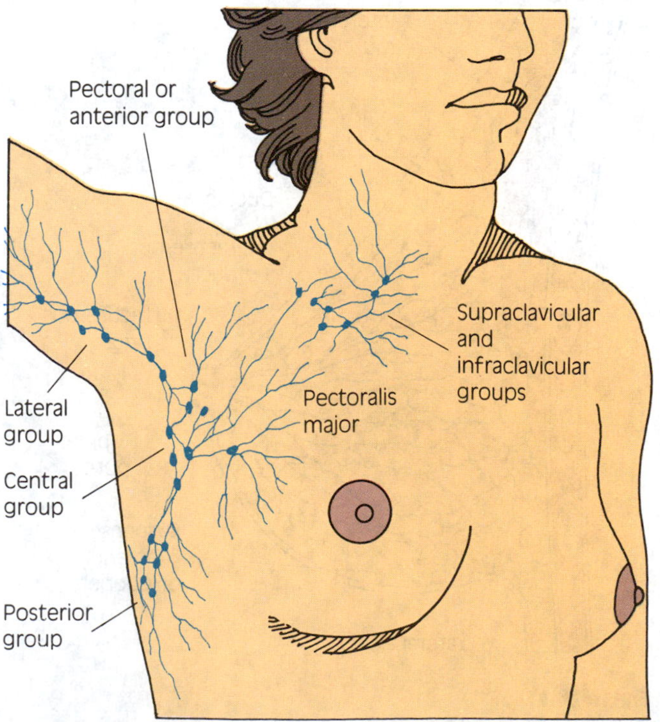

Figure 26-44
Location of the cervical, axillary, and mammary lymph nodes.

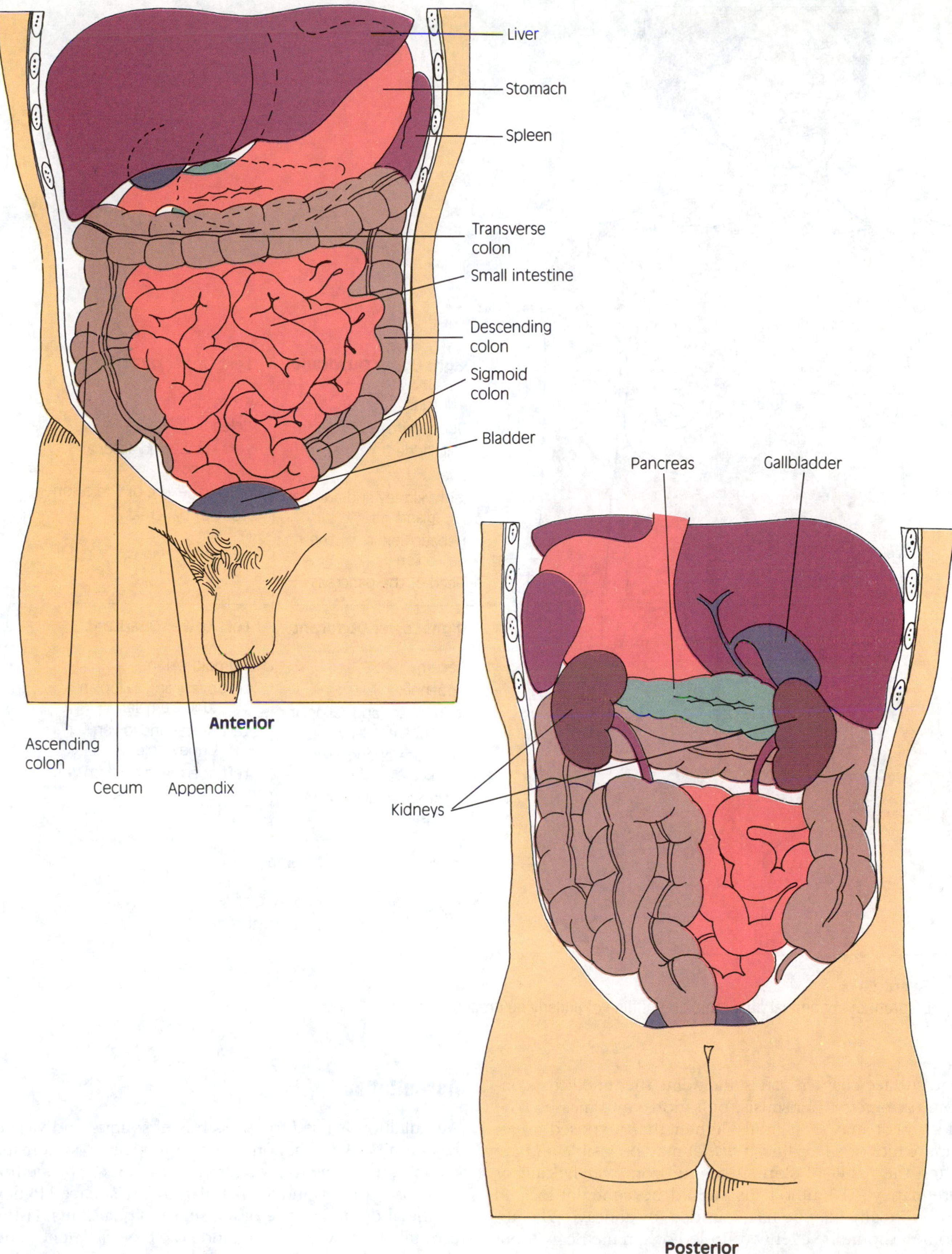

Figure 26-45
Organs of the abdominal cavity.

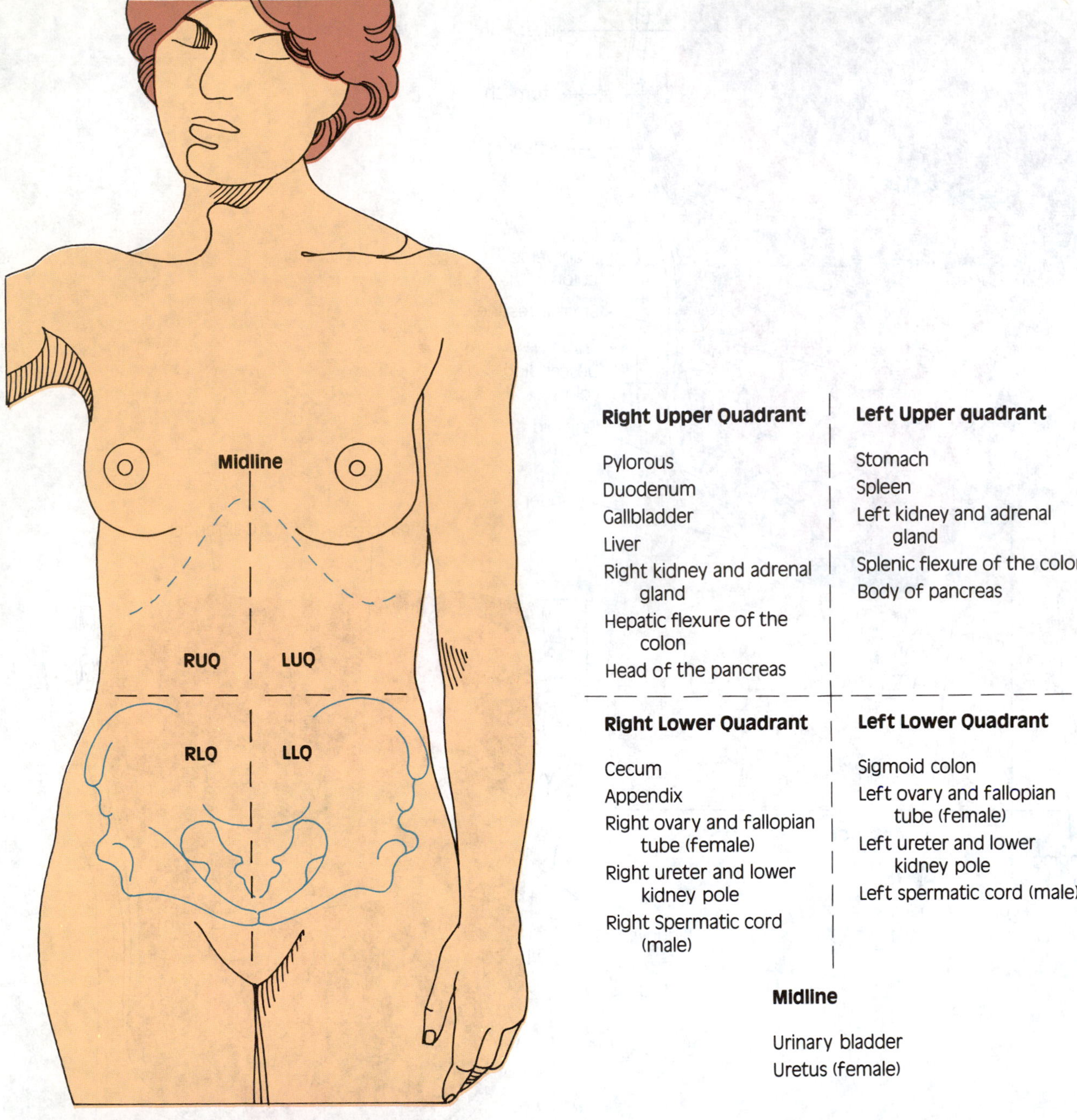

Figure 26-46
Diagram of abdominal quadrants and outline of underlying organs.

and surface characteristics, including the umbilicus, contour, symmetry, peristalsis, pulsations, and masses. The skin color may be slightly lighter than exposed areas. Fine white or silver lines (*striae*) may be visible and are often the result of skin stretching from weight gain or pregnancy. The umbilicus should be centrally located and normally may be flat, rounded, or concave. The abdomen should be evenly rounded or symmetric, without visible peristalsis. In thin people, an upper midline pulsation may normally be visible.

Auscultation

Auscultation is used to assess bowel sounds and vascular sounds. Auscultation is performed in a systematic manner, using the four quadrants as a guide. The stethoscope is warmed, and the flat diaphragm is placed lightly on the abdomen in one of the selected quadrants. Listen carefully for bowel sounds, and note their frequency and character; they are heard as clicks and gurgles and usually occur every 5 to 20 seconds. Move the stethoscope in a clockwise manner, assessing all four quadrants systematically. Using the bell of the stethoscope, auscultate over the aorta, renal arteries, and iliac arteries for bruits. Abnormal findings include increased, decreased, or absent bowel sounds (established after auscultating each quadrant for 5 minutes) and bruits.

Percussion

All four quadrants are percussed in a systematic, clockwise manner to identify fluid, masses, or air. The nurse should note the distribution of sounds. Normal sounds are tympany over the abdomen, dullness over the liver, and dullness over a full bladder. The predominate percussion note in abdominal assessment is tympany. Abnormal findings include decreased tympany and increased dullness, possibly caused by fluid or a mass.

Palpation

The pads of the fingers are used to palpate with a light, gentle, dipping motion. Watch the client's face for nonverbal signs of pain during palpation. Palpate each quadrant in a systematic manner, noting muscular resistance, tenderness, enlargement of the organs, or masses. If the client verbalizes abdominal pain, palpate the area of pain last. The abdomen should normally be soft, relaxed, and free of tenderness. Abnormal findings include involuntary rigidity, spasm, and pain.

Male and Female Genitalia

This section discusses inspection and palpation of the genitalia. A description of an internal pelvic assessment is also included in this chapter, although individual health agency policies vary on whether this is included as part of the health assessment. However, nurses often assist in performing vaginal examinations and need to be familiar with the procedure. Equipment required includes a vaginal speculum (for the female examination), a good light source, and disposable gloves.

Female Genitalia

The external female genitalia consist of the mons pubis, labia majora and minora, clitoris, vestibular glands, vaginal vestibule, vaginal orifice, and urethral opening (Fig. 26-47). Factors in assessing the female genitalia include menstrual history, sexual history, sexually transmitted diseases, use of contraceptives, and frequency of pelvic assessments. The client should empty the bladder before the examination. The woman is placed in the lithotomy position on the examination table, legs in stirrups, and draped so that only the genitalia are exposed. She should be told about the procedure and helped to relax as it is carried out. The nurse wears gloves during this assessment.

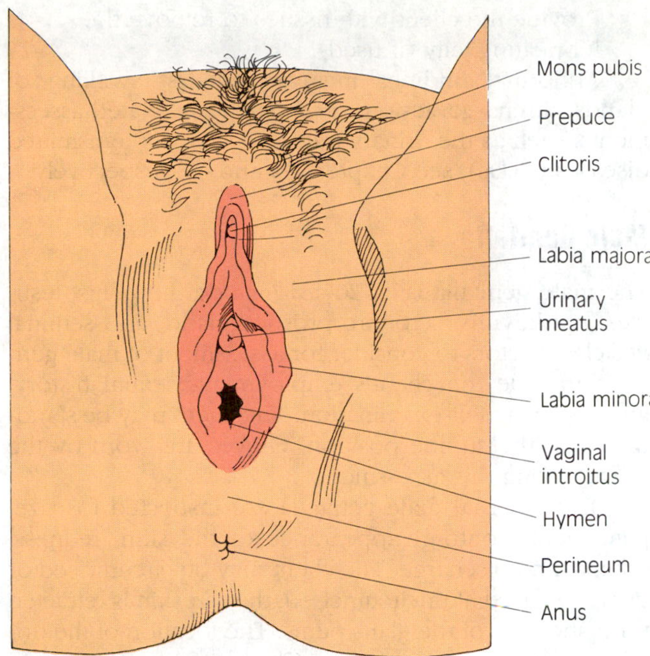

Figure 26-47
External female genitalia.

The external genitalia are inspected first. The pubic area is inspected for color, size, lesions, and discharge. The vulva normally has more pigmentation than other skin areas, and the mucous membranes will be dark pink and moist. The skin and mucosa should be smooth, without lesions or swelling. There may normally be a small amount of clear or whitish vaginal discharge.

A speculum is used to inspect the cervix and vagina. The procedure is as follows:

- Explain the procedure to the client.
- Warm the speculum under warm, running water; if cytologic specimens are to be taken, the water serves as the lubricant; if no specimens are needed, a water-soluble lubricant may be used.
- Don gloves.
- Using two fingers placed just inside the vagina, press down gently on the posterior vaginal wall.
- Insert the speculum blades vertically into the vagina, the posterior portion pointed at a 45-degree angle. Ensure that no pubic hair is caught in the speculum.
- Turn the speculum so that the handle is down and the blades are in a horizontal position.
- Open the blades and close the screw that locks the blades open.
- Inspect the cervix and os for size, color, shape, lesions, and discharge.
- Obtain specimens if needed.
- Withdraw the blades slowly, observing the vaginal walls.
- When the speculum blades are clear of the cervix, release the screw so that the blades close, and withdraw the speculum from the vagina.

- Provide the client with tissues to remove the lubricating jelly (if used).

Abnormal findings include redness, swelling of glands, discharge, lesions, and pain. For related assessments, such as the urinary tract and sexually transmitted diseases (STDs), see Chapters 35 and 43, respectively.

Male Genitalia

The male genitalia (Fig. 26-48) include the penis, testicles, epididymis, scrotum, prostate gland, and seminal vesicles. Factors to consider for assessment of male genitalia include the client's employment, sexual history, and testicular self-examination. The client may be standing or in the supine position. Gloves are worn by the nurse during this assessment.

The external male genitalia are inspected for size, placement, contour, appearance of the skin, redness, edema, and discharge. The client may be circumcised or uncircumcised; if uncircumcised, the foreskin is retracted for inspection of the glans penis. The location of the urinary meatus is also assessed. The scrotum is inspected for symmetry; it is not unusual for the left testicle to lie lower in the scrotal sac than the right testicle. The size, shape, and consistency of the scrotal contents should be similar. Abnormal findings are the presence of lesions, redness, edema, pain, discharge, fluid-filled masses in the scrotum, and displacement of the urinary meatus or difficulties with voiding. (See Chapters 35 and 43 for further discussion of the male urinary tract and STDs.)

Rectum and Anus

The rectum and anus are not assessed in all clients, but this is a part of a total health assessment. Techniques used to assess the rectum and anus are inspection and palpation. Necessary equipment includes lubricant and good lighting. The nurse wears gloves during this assessment. The client may be in the Sims', knee–chest, or lithotomy position or may be standing while leaning over the examination table.

Inspection is used to assess the anal area. The area normally has increased pigmentation and some hair growth. Palpation is used to assess the rectum, using a well-lubricated, gloved index finger. Sphincter tone at the anus should be firm and the mucosal lining smooth. (Fecal specimens may be taken at this time, if necessary.) Abnormal findings include relaxed sphincter tone; skin cracks, nodules, or hemorrhoids at the anal sphincter; bleeding; discharge; and hard or abnormally colored stools.

The prostate gland in men can be assessed for size, shape, and consistency by palpation through the anterior rectal wall; the gland is normally smooth, firm, and about 13/4 inches (4 cm) in size. Abnormal findings include enlargement or changes in consistency. In women, the cervix may be felt as a small, round mass when palpating the anterior rectal wall. Abnormal findings include changes in consistency.

Musculoskeletal System

The primary structures of the musculoskeletal system are the bones, muscles, cartilage, ligaments, tendons, and joints. Assessments are made of muscles, bones, and joints. During the assessment, the client assumes a variety of positions, including standing, sitting, and supine. Assessments of the musculoskeletal system can be integrated into the assessment of other body systems. Factors to consider during this assessment include a history of arthritis, trauma, or neurologic disorders; pain; and changes in function.

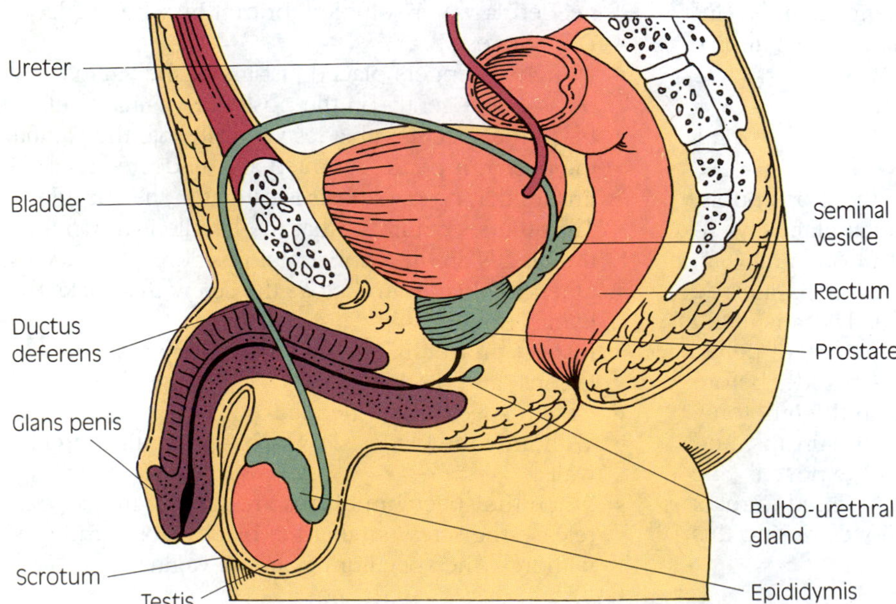

Figure 26-48
Organs of the male urogenital system.

Muscles

The muscles are examined by inspection and palpation of muscle groups and by testing muscle tone and strength. Muscle groups are observed for bilateral symmetry and palpated for tenderness; normally they are symmetric and are nontender. Muscle *tone* (the normal condition of a muscle at rest) is evaluated by putting each joint and extremity through passive range of motion. Bilateral equal resistance should be present. Muscle strength is assessed by asking the client to move against resistance. Observe muscle contraction and determine muscle strength exerted. An individual's dominant side is normally stronger than the nondominant side. Techniques for testing muscle strength are illustrated in Figure 26-49. Muscle strength should be bilaterally equal with slight increase on the dominant side.

Muscles are normally firm, with good strength and tone. Abnormal findings include *atrophy*, a decrease in size; tremors, involuntary movements; and *flaccidity*, weakness of muscles. Other abnormal findings are loss of strength and tone, decreased range of motion, uncoordinated movements, swelling, and pain.

Bones and Joints

Bones are palpated for normal contour and prominences, as well as for bilateral symmetry. Abnormal findings include pain, enlargement, asymmetry, and changes in contour.

Joints are assessed by inspection and palpation. Normally, each joint has full range of motion (ROM), is nontender, and moves smoothly. Each joint is put through full ROM, and the degree is assessed. Joint movements include flexion, extension, hyperextension, abduction, adduction, supination, and pronation. Joints are palpated for the abnormal findings of pain, swelling, nodules, and *crepitation* (a grating sound heard or felt on movement). See Chapter 39 for further discussion and illustration of joint mobility.

Neurologic System

The neurologic assessment is conducted to detect normal and abnormal findings for cerebral function, cranial nerve function, cerebellar function, motor and sensory function, and reflexes. Cerebral function is assessed by observing the client's behavior throughout the interview and assessment, and includes mental status, memory, emotional status, cognitive abilities, and behavior. Cerebellar function is evaluated by assessing fine motor skills, coordination, and balance. The sensory system is assessed by having the client identify various sensory stimuli, and the reflexes are evaluated by contraction of specific muscles.

Factors for consideration in the neurologic assessment include environmental hazards (eg, exposure to lead, insecticides, or chemicals); emotional and intellectual status; use of alcohol or other chemicals; medication; and history of seizures, dizziness, weakness, or numbness.

Equipment for this assessment includes vials of aromatic substances (eg, peppermint and vanilla); visual acuity chart; penlight; sharp object (such as a large safety pin); cotton balls; vials of solution to test taste (eg, salt or sugar); tuning fork; tongue depressor; reflex hammer; and familiar objects (eg, a key or coin). The client should be in a sitting position, and the environment should be quiet.

Mental Status

Components of the mental status assessment include assessment of orientation, level of consciousness, behavior and appearance, memory, abstract reasoning, and language. The following discussion of each of these components includes sample questions or specific assessments to use during the assessment.

Orientation

Orientation to time, place, and person are evaluated to assess a person's level of awareness. The following questions may be used:

Time

- What is today's date?
- What day of the week is it?
- What season of the year is this?
- What was the last holiday?

Place

- Where are you now?
- What is the name of this city?
- What state are we in?

Person

- What is your name?
- How old are you?
- Who came to visit you this morning?

Although exceptions may occur, individuals who have impaired awareness first lose time orientation, followed by place orientation, and then person orientation. Remember that it is often difficult to know the exact date when one is ill, in pain, or in unfamiliar surroundings.

Level of Consciousness

Consciousness is the degree of wakefulness or the ability of a person to be aroused. This is not the same as orientation; a client may be conscious but not oriented. Two methods to assess consciousness are (1) level of consciousness and (2) the Glasgow Coma Scale.

Level of consciousness is described as follows:

Awake and alert—fully awake; oriented to person, place and time; responds to all stimuli, including verbal commands

Lethargic—appears drowsy or asleep most of the time but makes spontaneous movements; can be

(*text continues on page 512*)

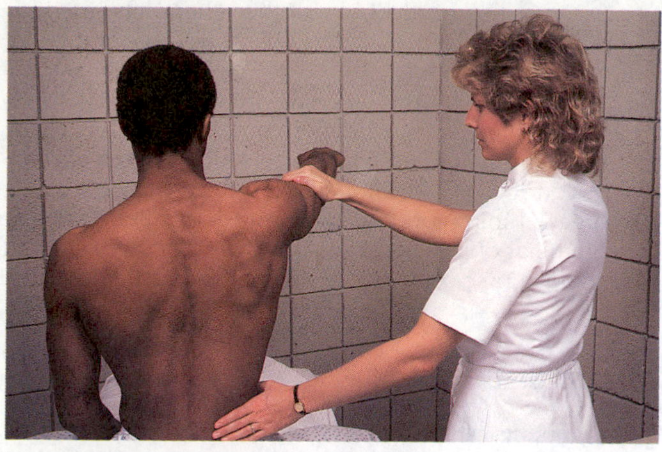

The client flexes shoulder muscle against resistance of examiner's hand.

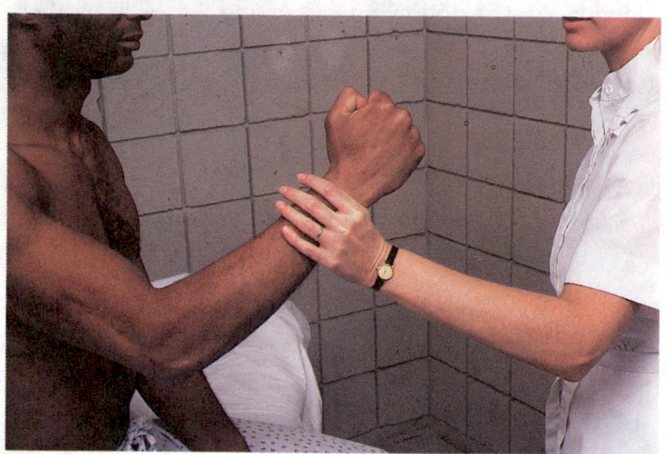

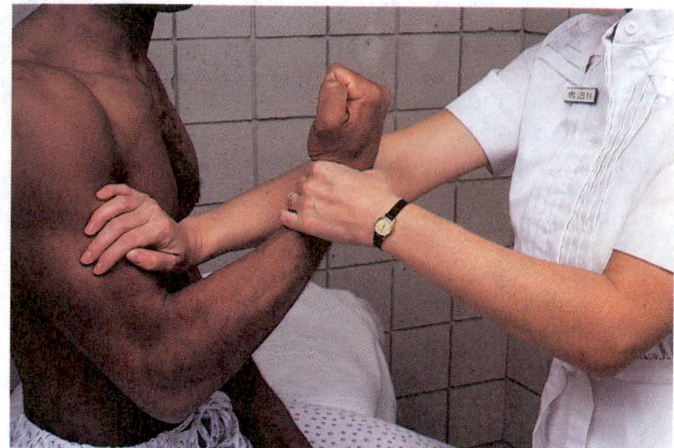

Elbow extension and flexion. The client first extends elbow against resistance by the examiner, then flexes elbow against resistance.

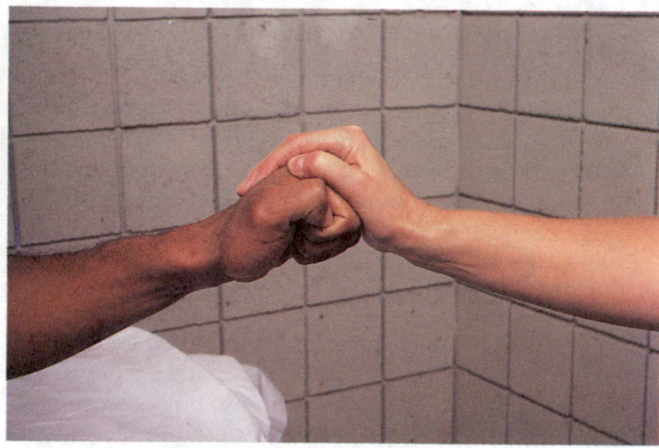

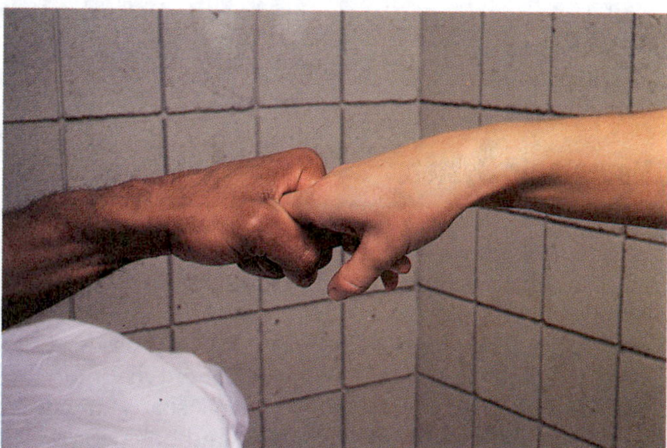

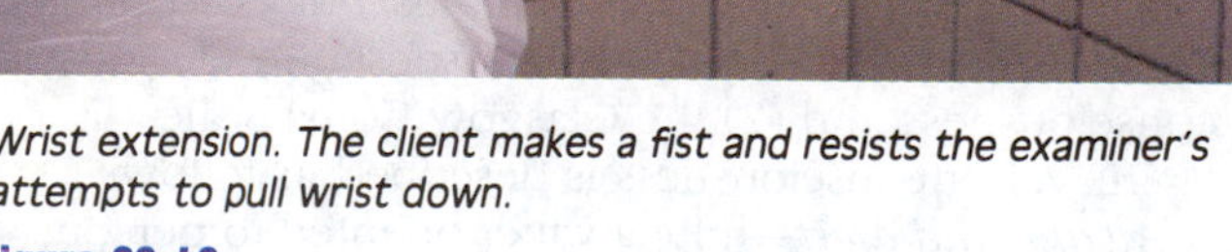

Wrist extension. The client makes a fist and resists the examiner's attempts to pull wrist down.

Testing grip. Client squeezes examiner's index and middle fingers.

Figure 26-49
Techniques for testing muscle strength. (Photos © Ken Kasper.)

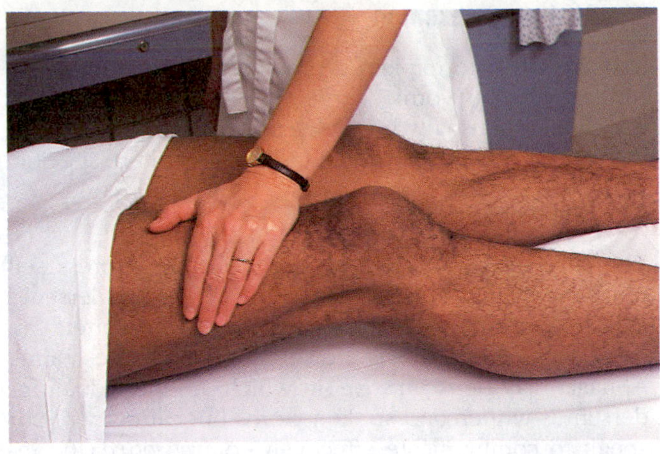

Hip flexion. Client attempts to raise his thigh against examiner's resistance.

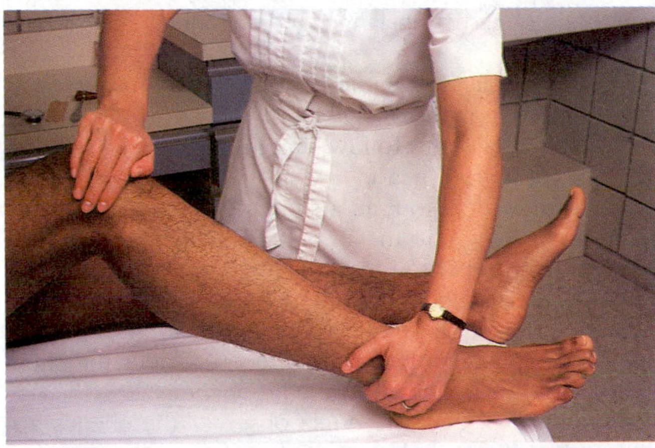

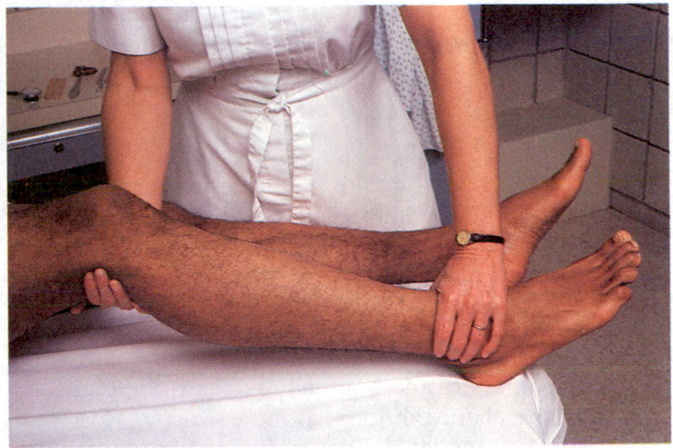

Knee flexion and extension. With the client's knee bent and foot on the examining table, the client attempts to keep foot down while examiner attempts to straighten the client's leg to test flexion. To test extension, the examiner supports client's knee, and the client attempts to straighten his leg against examiner resistance at the ankle.

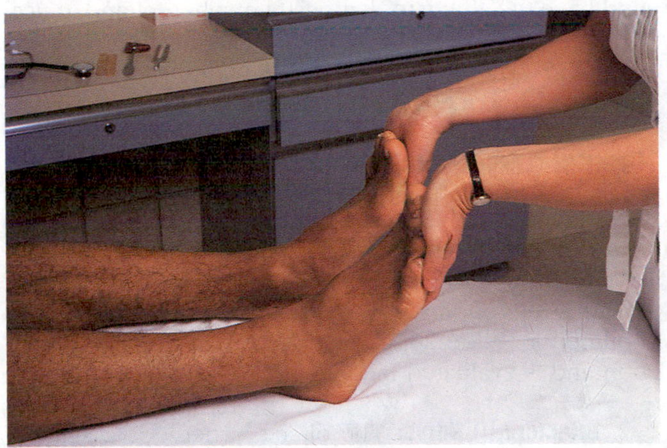

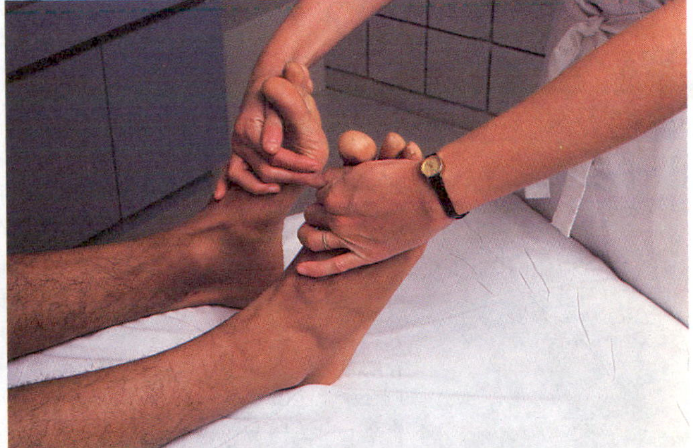

Ankle plantar flexion and dorsiflexion. The client first pushes the balls of the feet against resistance of examiner's hands, then attempts to pull against examiner's resistance.

Figure 26-49 (continued)

aroused by gentle shaking and saying client's name

Stuporous—unconscious most of the time; no spontaneous movement; must shake or shout to arouse; can make verbal responses, but these are less likely to be appropriate; responds to painful stimuli with purposeful movements

Comatose—cannot be aroused, even with use of painful stimuli; may have some reflex activity (as gag reflex); if no reflexes present, is in a deep coma

The Glasgow Coma Scale is a standardized assessment tool that assesses level of consciousness. Three parameters are evaluated—eye opening, motor response, and verbal response. Scores are given in each category and a total score is recorded, with higher scores indicating a more normal level of functioning. A score of 7 or less defines coma. This is a more accurate evaluation of mental status over time. The scale is illustrated in Table 26-6.

Memory

Memory is assessed by asking questions that call for answers demonstrating immediate recall and recall for past events. The following may be used:

Immediate

- Ask the client to repeat a series of numbers forward or backward (eg, three, six, nine). Start with three numbers and gradually increase the digits until the client cannot respond correctly. Most adults can repeat a series of five to eight numbers forward and four to six digits backward.
- Ask: What did you eat for breakfast this morning?

Past

- Ask: When is your birthday? or When is your wedding anniversary?

Table 26-6
Glasgow Coma Scale

Component	Response	Score
Eye opening	Spontaneous	4
	To verbal command	3
	To pain	2
	No response	1
Motor response	To verbal command	6
	To localized pain	5
	Flexes/withdraws	4
	Flexes abnormally	3
	Extends abnormally	2
	No response	1
Verbal response	Oriented/talks	5
	Disoriented/talks	4
	Inappropriate words	3
	Incomprehensible sounds	2
	No response	1

Abstract Reasoning

Ask the client to explain a proverb such as "The early bird catches the worm." If intellectual ability is impaired, the client will usually give a literal explanation or repeat the phrase. Be sure that the phrase is not culture specific.

Language

The cerebral cortex controls the ability to express self through writing, words, or gestures and to understand the spoken and written word. Injury to the cortex can cause *aphasia*, which is a disorder of language ability. Aphasia may be *expressive* (in which the individual understands written and spoken words but cannot write or speak to communicate effectively) or *receptive* (the individual cannot understand written or spoken words). These aphasias also may be combined. Some simple methods of assessing language capabilities include the following:

- Ask the client to name items in the room (eg, bed, flowers, gown, pajamas).
- Ask the client to follow simple commands, such as "Point to your head."
- Ask the client to read a short sentence aloud.
- Ask the client to match printed and spoken words with appropriate pictures.

On initial contact, the nurse begins to evaluate the client's orientation level to person, place, and time, as well as cognitive abilities and affect (eg, does the client know who he or she is, where he or she is, and the day or month or year). The nurse observes the client's appearance, general behavior, and responses to questions. Any variation in responses should be noted. The nurse also assesses the client's ability to speak clearly. The client should have a clean, neat appearance with erect posture; be oriented to person, place, and time; have memory recall (both short-term and long-term memory); and have the ability to demonstrate coherent and logical thought processes. Abnormal findings include poor hygiene, inappropriate dress, disorientation, absent memory recall, and incoherent or illogical thought processes.

Cranial Nerve Function

The function of the twelve cranial nerves is assessed primarily during the neurologic assessment, although parts of cranial nerve function are assessed with other body systems (eg, pupillary response). The cranial nerves are outlined in Table 26-7. Each nerve has a specific function and is evaluated individually.

Olfactory (I) Nerve. The olfactory nerve is a sensory nerve and its function is the sense of smell. Two or three substances with aromatic odors, such as coffee, vanilla, or peppermint, are used to assess this sense. The client is asked to close the eyes and occlude one nostril (by pressing a finger against the side of the nose). The client is then asked to take a breath as the vial is placed under the open nostril, and to identify the odor; the process is

Table 26-7
Cranial Nerves

Nerve (Number)	Type	Functions	Methods for Examining Nerve
Olfactory (I)	Sensory	Sense of smell	Test each nostril for smell reception and interpretation
Optic (II)	Sensory	Sense of vision	Test vision for acuity and visual fields
Oculomotor (III)	Motor	Pupil constriction Raise eyelids	Test pupillary reaction to light and ability to open and close eyelids
Trochlear (IV)	Motor	Downward inward eye movement	Test for downward and inward movement of the eye
Trigeminal (V)	Motor	Jaw movements—chewing and mastication	Ask client to open and clench jaws while palpating the jaw muscles
	Sensory	Sensation on the face and neck	Test face and neck for pain sensations, light touch, temperature
Abducens (VI)	Motor	Lateral movement of the eyes	Test ocular movement in all directions
Facial (VII)	Motor	Muscles of the face	Ask the client to raise eyebrows, smile, show teeth, puff out cheeks
	Sensory	Sense of taste on the anterior two thirds of the tongue	Test for the taste sensation with various agents
Acoustic (VIII)	Sensory	Sense of hearing	Test hearing ability
Glossopharyngeal (IX)	Motor	Pharyngeal movement and swallowing	Ask the client to say "ah," and have client yawn to observe upward movement of the soft palate; elicit gag response; note ability to swallow
	Sensory	Sense of taste on the posterior one third of the tongue	Test for taste with various agents
Vagus (X)	Motor	Swallowing and speaking	Ask the client to swallow and speak; note hoarseness
Accessory (XI)	Motor	Movement of shoulder muscles	Ask the client to shrug shoulders against your resistance
Hypoglossal (XII)	Motor	Movement of the tongue; strength of the tongue	Ask the client to protrude tongue; ask client to push tongue against cheek

then repeated for the opposite nostril. Normal findings are equal and bilateral sense of smell; abnormal findings are the inability to identify the odor or absence of smell.

Optic (II) Nerve. The optic nerve is a sensory nerve whose function is vision. Vision is tested for acuity and visual fields, as described earlier in the chapter in the discussion on assessment of the eye. Abnormal findings include changes in vision; blurring of vision; or inability to identify letters, numbers, or pictures.

Oculomotor (III), Trochlear (IV), and Abducens (VI) Nerves. The oculomotor, trochlear, and abducens nerves are motor nerves that control movement of the eyes through the cardinal fields of gaze; pupil size, shape, response to light, and accommodation; and opening of the upper eyelids. These assessments are discussed earlier in the chapter in the assessment of the eye. Normal findings include round pupils that are equal in size, direct and consensual pupillary response, lid margin flush with the surface of the eyeball, equal and complete bilateral lid closure, and parallel movements of the eyes. Abnormal findings include asymmetric eye position, a portion of the eye not covered by the eyelid, lesions, edema, abnormal eye movements, and inability for one or both eyes to follow the cardinal fields.

Trigeminal (V) Nerve. The trigeminal nerve is a sensory and motor (sensorimotor) nerve. Motor function is assessed by observing the facial muscles for deviation of the jaw to one side and by instructing the client to clench the jaw and palpating the tone of the muscles. Sensory status of the nerve is assessed by testing the ability to discriminate between sharp, dull, and light touch. The client is asked to close the eyes, and as the nurse touches each side of the client's face with a sharp object or paper clip, to report whether the sensation is sharp or dull. The same procedure is used for light touch, using a wisp of cotton and asking the client to tell you when and where on the face the sensation is felt. Normally, the client will correctly identify sharp, dull, and soft sensation of the face and neck bilaterally. Abnormal findings are decreased or absent sensations unilaterally or bilaterally.

Facial (VII) Nerve. The facial nerve is a sensorimotor nerve that innervates the muscles of the face and functions also to provide the taste sensation of the anterior two thirds of the tongue. Motor function is evaluated by observing a series of expressions the client is asked to make, such as raising the eyebrows, smiling and showing the teeth, and puffing out the cheeks. Facial expressions should be symmetric. Abnormal findings are asymmetry and lack of expression. The taste sensation of the tongue is tested by placing a small amount of different substances (eg, sugar, salt, or lemon) on the anterior two thirds of the tongue as the client, with eyes closed, protrudes the tongue. Various substances should be correctly identified. Abnormal findings include incorrect identification of substances or the inability to taste.

Acoustic (VIII) Nerve. The acoustic nerve is a sensory nerve that is tested by assessing hearing ability, as described previously in assessment of the ear. The client should be able to hear bilaterally; abnormal findings are the inability to hear unilaterally or bilaterally.

Glossopharyngeal (IX) Nerve. The glossopharyngeal nerve is a sensorimotor nerve that allows tongue movement and swallowing, as well as taste sensations of the posterior one third of the tongue. The motor function of this nerve is assessed with the vagus (X) nerve, and the taste function is assessed with the facial (VII) nerve. The client should be able to identity various taste substances correctly, have a gag reflex, and be able to move the tongue symmetrically.

Vagus (X) Nerve. The vagus nerve is a motor nerve that is assessed by asking the client to open the mouth and say “Ah” as the upward movement of the soft palate is observed. The uvula should remain midline and rise symmetrically. The swallowing reflex can be assessed by having the client sip and swallow water.

Accessory (XI) Nerve. The accessory nerve is a motor nerve that controls the movement of the head and shoulders. Ask the client to shrug the shoulders upward and turn the head against the resistance of your hands (Fig. 26-50). There should be equal movement and strength of the muscles of the shoulder and head bilaterally.

Hypoglossal (XII) Nerve. The hypoglossal nerve is a motor nerve that affects the movement and strength of the tongue. Ask the client to protrude the tongue forward and to push out the cheek with the tongue. The protrusion should be symmetric, and the cheek should have a puffed-out appearance. Abnormal findings include asymmetry of movements, drooping, weakness, tremors, and loss of strength.

Motor, Sensory, and Reflex Function

This part of the neurologic assessment includes the motor, sensory, and reflex abilities of the client. Motor ability is evaluated by assessing balance, gait, and coordination; sensory function is assessed by testing sensory discrimination of pain, light touch, and vibrations; and deep tendon reflexes are evaluated to determine the functioning ability of specific spinal segment levels.

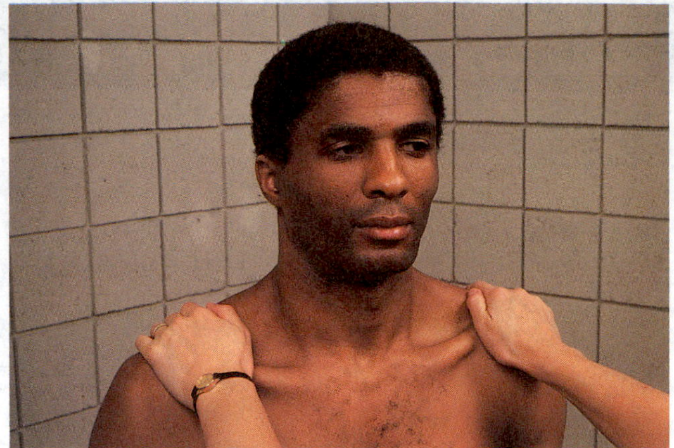

Figure 26-50
Test of the spinal accessory nerve. The client shrugs his shoulders against the resistance of the examiner's hands. (Photo © Ken Kasper.)

Motor Function

Balance and Gait. Balance and gait are evaluated by having the client walk across the room on the toes, on the heels, and heel-to-toe. The nurse observes posture, balance, and arm and leg movements. The posture should be erect, with slight swaying in the standing position, and the gait even with simultaneous arm movements. Abnormal findings include loss of balance, shuffling, wide-based gait, and abnormal patterns of gait.

Motor Function and Coordination. Motor function and coordination are evaluated by having the client rapidly touch each finger with the thumb, rapidly pat the hand on the thigh, and tap the foot against the floor (or against your hand, if the client is supine). Normally, the movements are coordinated.

Sensory Function. Sensory perception is tested by evaluating the client's response to pain, light touch, and vibration. With the client's eyes closed, a sharp object and a soft object are used randomly to touch upper and lower extremities to test sensation. This assessment proceeds from distal (ie, hands, arms, feet, or legs) to proximal (ie, trunk). The client should be able to distinguish between sharp (pain) and soft or dull touch. The same process is repeated by using the tuning fork to test for vibratory sensation and placing the fork on bony prominences. Abnormal findings include inability to perceive pain or light touch, inability to identify the location of touch, and absence of vibratory sensation.

Reflex Function. The reflexes are assessed to evaluate the function of specific spinal segment levels. The reflex hammer is used to elicit muscle contraction and reflexes.

The client may be either sitting or supine. The reflexes are illustrated in Table 26-8. Usually they are graded on a scale of 0 to 4+, as listed in Table 26-9.

Biceps Reflex. The client's arms should be partially flexed at the elbow, with the palms down. The examiner places a thumb or finger firmly on the client's biceps muscle, and strikes with the reflex hammer, aimed directly toward the finger. Observe for flexion at the elbow, and feel for contraction of the biceps muscle.

Table 26-8
Normal Responses of Commonly Tested Reflexes

Reflex	How to Test Reflex	Normal Response
Biceps	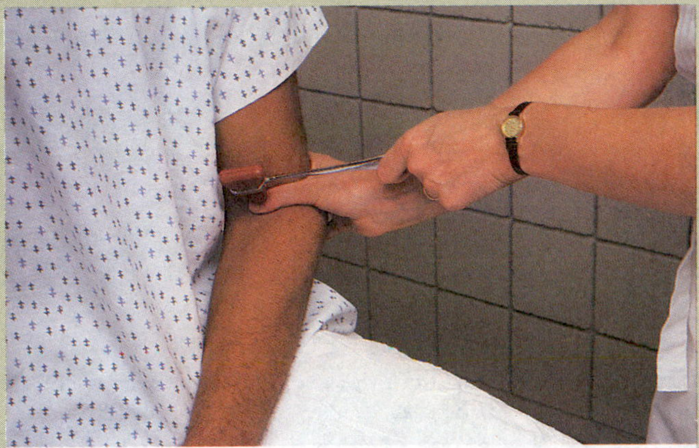	The contraction of the biceps can be seen and felt. To test the biceps reflex, the elbow is slightly bent, and the palm faces downward. The examiner's thumb is placed on the biceps tendon at the bend in the elbow. The percussion hammer strikes the examiner's thumb.
Triceps	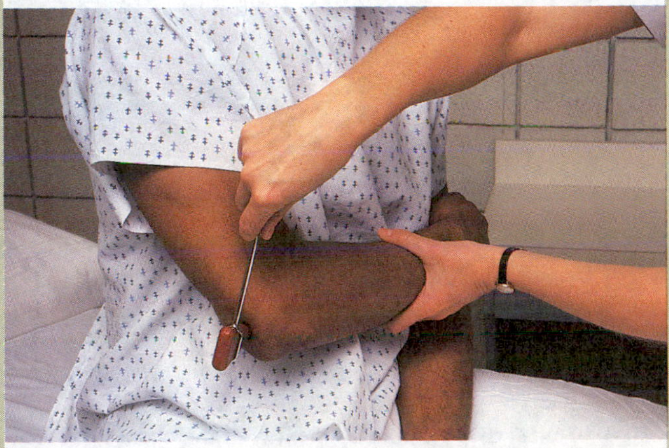	The contraction of the triceps can be seen as the elbow extends. To test the triceps reflex, the client's elbow is sharply bent; the forearm is placed across the chest wall with the palm turned toward the body. The triceps muscle is struck with the percussion hammer just above the elbow.
Knee	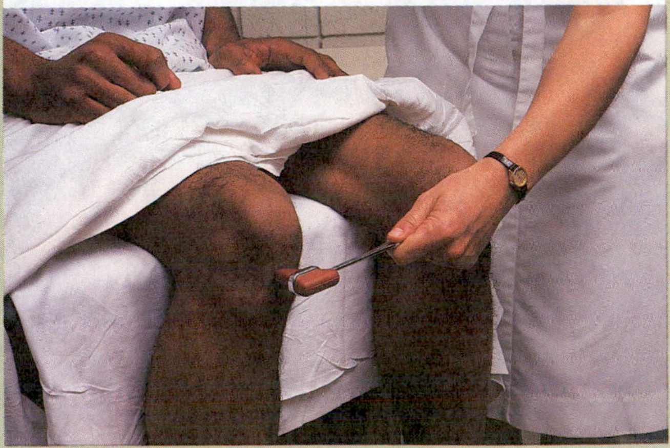	The contraction of the quadriceps causes the knee to extend. To test the knee reflex, the client is in the sitting position. The patellar tendon just below the patella is struck with the percussion hammer. If the client is lying down, the reflex is tested while the examiner's hands are placed under the knees to bend them.

(continued)

Table 26-8 *(continued)*
Normal Responses of Commonly Tested Reflexes

Reflex	How to Test Reflex	Normal Response
Ankle	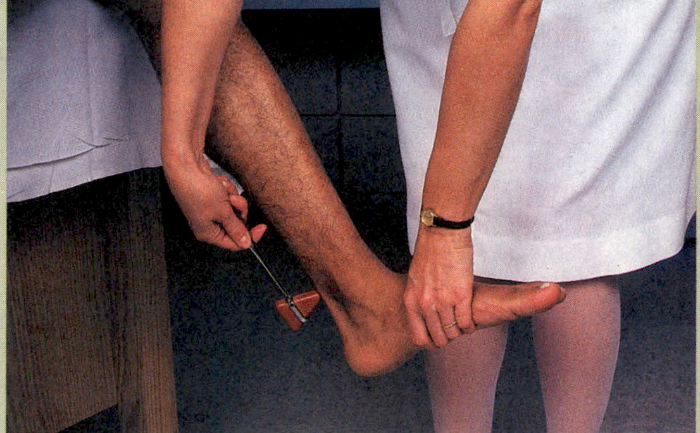	The foot jerks and moves downward. To test the ankle reflex, the leg is bent at the knee and the foot is supported in a walking position. The Achilles tendon is struck with the percussion hammer.
Babinski	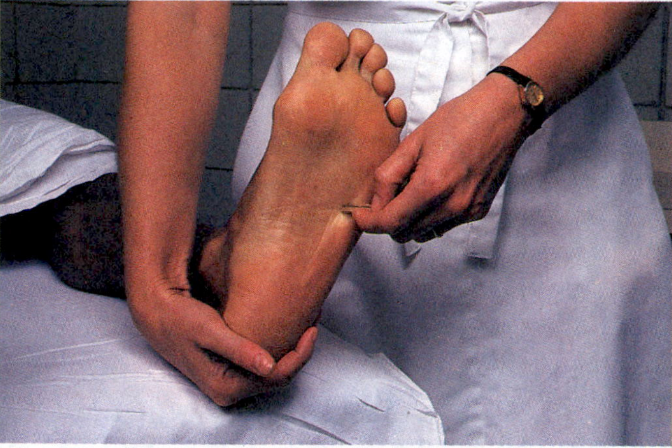	The toes bend or curl. The lateral aspect of the sole of the foot is stroked with an object, such as a key or a thumbnail, from the heel to the ball of the foot.
Abdominal	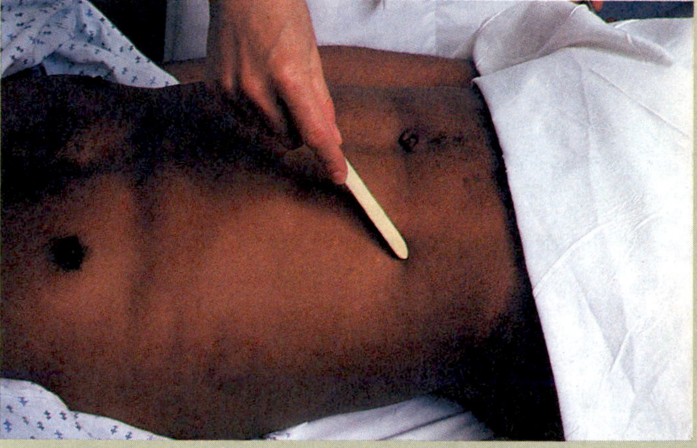	The contraction of abdominal musculature can be seen. To test the abdominal reflex, with the client lying on the back, each side of the abdomen is stroked from the sides toward the center with a tongue blade or key.

(Photos © Ken Kasper.)

Table 26-9
Grading of Reflexes on a 0 to 4+ Scale

Grade	Description
4+	Very brisk, hyperactive; often indicative of disease; often associated with clonus (rhythmic oscillations between flexion and extension)
3+	Brisker than average; possibly but not necessarily indicative of disease
2+	Average; normal
1+	Somewhat diminished; low normal
0	No response

Triceps Reflex. Flex the client's arm at the elbow, with the client's palm facing the body, and position it across the client's chest. Strike the triceps tendon above the elbow. Observe for contraction of the triceps muscle and extension at the elbow.

Brachioradialis or Supinator Reflex. Rest the client's forearm on the abdomen or in the lap, with the palm facing downward. Strike the tendon on the client's radius 1 to 2 inches above the wrist. Observe for flexion and supination of the forearm.

Patellar or Knee Reflex. The client is placed in a sitting or supine position with the knees in a flexed position. Briskly tap the patellar tendon just below the patella and observe for contraction of the quadriceps with knee extension.

Achilles Tendon Reflex or Ankle Reflex. The client's leg should be slightly flexed at the knee, with dorsiflexion of the foot at the ankle joint. Strike the Achilles tendon and observe for plantar flexion at the ankle. Reflexes are graded according to their response, with a 2+ considered a normal or active response.

Documenting the Data

After completing the nursing history and assessment, the nurse organizes all assessment data to identify actual and potential health problems, make nursing diagnoses, plan appropriate care, and evaluate the client's responses to treatment. Often a pattern is established that begins during the history and is confirmed during the physical assessment. The data are documented, with each system recorded individually.

The Nurse's Role in Diagnostic Procedures

The results of diagnostic procedures are also used by nurses in assessment of health status, and nurses participate in diagnostic tests performed for clients. The basic responsibilities of nurses, who assist before, during, and after tests, are listed in the accompanying box. The nurse

(*text continues on page 520*)

Application of Nursing Process Model to Pre-, Intra-, and Post-test Care

Assessment Parameters

Assess Indications for Testing

- Screen for risk factors or occult diseases
- Evaluate signs and symptoms requiring medical diagnosis
- Rule out presence of disease
- Differentiate one pathologic condition from another
- Monitor response to therapy and evaluate prognosis
- Determine disease severity

Assess Factors That Interfere With Test Outcomes

- Certain medications, over-the-counter drugs, vitamins, iron preparations, pretest diet, or fluid intake
- Undisclosed drug, smoking, and alcohol use
- Stress, high anxiety levels, fear, and confusion
- Improper specimen collection
- Strenuous exercise, age, and gender
- Communication errors (improper labeling and incomplete identification of specimen)
- Nondisease factors (pregnancy)
- Past illness and present health status

Assess for Contraindications to Testing

- Pre-existing conditions (ex: diabetes, pregnancy)
- Inability to comprehend and follow directions, to physically cooperate with testing; disorientation
- Allergies to contrast substances (iodine), drugs, and latex
- Influence of previous testing procedures
- Presence of bleeding disorders

Focus Data Collection Upon These Points

- Age and developmental stage
- Pertinent health history data: allergies, medication history, vision, hearing, and mobility deficits; social history and habits (drugs, smoking, and alcohol)
- Ability to follow instructions and cooperate in procedural protocols (ex: anxiety, mental confusion, physical weakness, casts, immobilization, and diseases)
- Cultural differences and language barriers
- Nutritional status (ex: special nutritive requirements—tube feeding, gastrostomy tubes, IV lines)

(continued)

Application of Nursing Process Model to Pre-, Intra-, and Post-test Care *(continued)*

Nursing Diagnoses

Formulate Appropriate Nursing Diagnoses Based Upon Nurse-Identified Need for Care

These diagnoses are also nurse-treated. Suggested examples vary; others are possible.

- Knowledge Deficit related to lack of or misinterpretation of information, purpose, preparation, equipment, and need for patient cooperation.
- Anxiety and/or Fear related to lack of knowing (not wanting to know) test outcome results, possible need for further treatment, perception of diagnostic procedures as frightening and environment as uncaring and hostile, fear of equipment.
- Ineffective Individual Coping related to test outcome results and inability to accept diagnosis of serious disease.
- Powerlessness related to unfamiliar procedures, strange environment, cultural differences.
- Impaired Social Interactions related to language barrier and lack of an interpreter.
- Anxiety of child related to separation from parents; anxiety of parents related to separation from child.
- Risk for Injury related to venipuncture; special preparation (for example, prolonged bowel preparation for a patient who is elderly, frail, chronically ill); risks of the procedure as in cardiac catheterization, radiopharmaceuticals, contrasts, and complications.
- Risk for Injury related to limited mobility or decline in physical skills.
- Potential for Noncompliance to test protocols related to anxiety, confusion, denial, refusal, or inability to follow instructions.
- Altered Family Processes related to lengthy and complicated diagnostic test regimens.
- Risk for Infection related to arterial, venous, or other invasive lines.
- Impaired Adjustment related to denial or nonacceptance of test results/need for lifestyle changes.
- Knowledge Deficit related to significance of test outcome deviation and related lifestyle change requirements.
- Decisional Conflict related to test outcome and need for surgery versus medical treatment and lifestyle changes.
- Pain related to diagnostic procedure.

Planning Parameters

Include Pre-, Intra-, and Post-test Nursing Orders in the Care Plan

- Take into account age, language, cultural diversity, compliance, understanding, and care setting.
- *Pretest care focus* is on proper patient preparation and individualized patient education.
- *Intratest care focus* is on collection of specimens, comfort and reassurance, administration of ordered analgesics and sedatives, assisting physician during procedure, and monitoring during testing. Express confidence in patient's ability to tolerate procedure to completion. Reassure patient.
- *Post-test care focus* is on follow-up activities, observation, surveillance to prevent complications, and appropriate actions if complications occur. Identification of patient and test outcomes and plans for discharge are part of this nursing process step.
- Incorporate patient's need for information as well as pre- and post-test care (self- or nurse-administered) into plan. Include modalities to help patient cope with the actual diagnostic procedure and test outcomes. Be alert to patients with special needs such as hearing- or sight-impaired patients, ostomy patients, diabetics, the comatose, the confused, children, and the elderly. Develop a plan that allows the patient to maintain dignity and some control over scheduling and participation in the process.

Implementation Parameters

Prepare Patient Properly

- Know certain facts: what type of sample is needed and method of collection—invasive or noninvasive; contrast substance injected or instilled; is the patient required to swallow any contrast substance; need to fast; fluid restrictions; force fluids; medications instilled; length of procedure; is a consent form needed; sedation required?
- Review current and previous test results. The plan of care is developed or changed on the basis of these test results. Know how to sequentially gather diagnostic information from records (review the most recent data first to determine the current patient status; then work backwards to note trends and changes).

Place Special Emphasis Upon Patient Education Activities

- Give accurate and precise instructions according to the patient's level of understanding and condition. Avoid medical jargon. Ascertain communication barriers (cognitive, language).
- Provide both sensory and objective information about the test. Talk about sensations, equipment used, length of procedure, people present.
- Reinforce information about the diagnostic process, time frames, and the patient's role. Use resource people if necessary.

(continued)

Application of Nursing Process Model to Pre-, Intra-, and Post-test Care *(continued)*

Collect Samples for Testing, Assist With and Carry Out Diagnostic Procedures

- Obtain properly signed, witnessed, informed consents for specific diagnostic procedures such as HIV, genetic testing, use of injected pharmaceuticals, and all invasive procedures such as cardiac catheterization and certain x-ray and endoscopic procedures in select settings.
- Follow universal precautions, infection control measures, and sterile techniques as appropriate.
- Provide support. Be a caring, listening presence.
- Alleviate psychologic concerns. These can affect reliable test outcomes and the patient's physiologic state during testing.
- Recognize anxiety, fear, and other patient responses to undesirable test outcomes. Help patients work through anxiety and depression. Assist patient and family to make lifestyle and self-concept adjustments.

Prevent Complications, Provide Patient Safety, and Manage Risk

- Be aware that the most common complications after invasive procedures are bleeding, infection, respiratory difficulties, and perforation of organs.
- Use special cautions when iodine contrast is to be used or barium has been infused.

Evaluation Parameters	*Expected Outcomes*	*Unexpected Outcomes*
	Anticipated outcomes will be achieved.	Some anticipated outcomes may not be achieved. Reasons may be related to specific patient behaviors.
Evaluate the Effectiveness of Care During Diagnostic Treatment • Evaluate progress toward goal achievement. A goal may simply be that the patient can tolerate the diagnostic procedure to its completion.	Patients and family should be able to describe the testing process and purpose and patient should be able to properly perform expected activities.	Inability to fully participate in teaching/learning process as evidenced by verbal and nonverbal cues. Inability to properly perform expected activities.
Interpret Test Outcomes Correctly • Reassess interfering factors and patient compliance that may influence test results if test outcomes significantly deviate from normal. • Report critical values to the physician immediately and take appropriate nursing actions. • No test is perfect. However, the greater the degree of abnormal test result, the more likely that this outcome deviation is significant or represents a real disorder.	If test outcomes are abnormal, the patient will make appropriate lifestyle changes.	Noncompliance with test preparation guidelines and post-test recommended lifestyle changes.
Initiate Posttesting Modalities • Monitor for complications and incorporate safety precautions.	Should complications occur, they will be optimally resolved.	Complications not fully resolved; health state compromised.
Reassess, Review, and Revise Care Plans • When tests are completed, test reports become available, new tests are ordered, patient's condition changes, expected outcomes are met, or unexpected outcomes occur: reassess, review, and revise care plans. • Emphasize importance of follow-up visits for repeat testing and treatment problems identified through diagnostic evaluation.	Anxiety and fears will be alleviated and will not interfere with testing process.	Unable to collect specimens properly or accurately perform procedure steps because of anxiety or fear. Unable to calm and reassure patient.

(continued)

Application of Nursing Process Model to Pre-, Intra-, and Post-test Care *(continued)*

• Provide psychosocial support. If patients get "bad news," they may not be good, effective listeners.	Does not develop complications; remains free from injury.	Exhibition of untoward signs and symptoms (for example, allergic response, shock, bleeding, nausea, vomiting, and retention of barium).
Evaluate Patient Outcomes and Counsel Appropriately • Compare actual outcomes with expected outcomes.	With support and comfort, able to cope with test outcomes revealing chronic or life-threatening disease.	Lack of appropriate problem-solving behaviors; uncertainty and/or denial about test outcomes; extreme depression and abnormal patterns of responses; refusal to take control of the situation.

Documentation Parameters

Record All Pre-, Intra-, and Post-test Care

- Enter appropriate assessment data and note patient concerns and questions that help to define nursing diagnosis and direction for care planning.
- Document specific preparation of patient before procedure.
- Indicate that the preparation, side effects, expected results, and interfering factors have been explained.
- Record medications, treatments, food and fluids, intake status, beginning and end of specimen collection and procedure times, outcomes, and patient condition during all phases of diagnostic care.
- Completely and clearly describe any adverse reactions or complications along with follow-up care and instructions for post-test care and monitoring.
- Record patient's refusal to undergo diagnostic tests. Note the reason for refusal using the patient's own words if possible.
- Record all nursing interventions, specific surveillance measures, and nursing evaluations made during diagnostic testing.

F. T. Fischbach. [1995]. *Quick reference to common laboratory and diagnostic tests.* Philadelphia: Lippincott. Used with permission.

is also responsible for other activities associated with diagnostic tests, such as witnessing the client's consent, scheduling the test, preparing the client physically and emotionally for the test, providing care after the test, disposing of used equipment, and transporting specimens.

Diagnostic tests provide critical information about a client's state of health. Most clients undergo some type of diagnostic evaluation during their lifetime. Decisions concerning which diagnostic tests to schedule are made by clinicians when problems are noted during the health history or physical assessment or because of a problem stated by the client. Table 26-10 presents an overview of different types of diagnostic procedures. Nurses consider the scheduling or results of these evaluations when making their assessments and during the rest of the nursing process.

Table 26-10
A Guide to Common Laboratory and Diagnostic Procedures

Procedure	Description	Examples
Aspiration procedures	Studies in which a needle or similar instrument is inserted into a body organ or cavity. Fluid or tissue is aspirated, prepared, labeled, and sent to the laboratory for examination.	Liver biopsy Lumbar puncture Paracentesis Thoracentesis
Electrical impulse procedures	Studies that use a machine with electrodes attached to the body to monitor electric activity. Electric impulses are recorded on a graph and displayed on paper or an oscilloscope screen.	Electrocardiography (EKG) Electroencephalogram (EEG)

(continued)

Table 26-10 *(continued)*
A Guide to Common Laboratory and Diagnostic Procedures

Procedure	Description	Examples
Endoscopic procedures	Studies that allow for direct visual examination of various body cavities and organs by means of a hollow, lighted tube, called an endoscope. The tube may be flexible or rigid. May be used to obtain tissue specimens for biopsy or microscopic examination.	Bronchoscopy Colonoscopy Gastroscopy Sigmoidoscopy Laparoscopy
Laboratory procedures	Studies in which body fluids, secretions, or tissues are sent to the laboratory for analysis.	Blood studies Urine studies Sputum studies Fecal studies Biopsies
Radiography procedures	Because of the ability of x-rays to penetrate human tissues, x-ray studies provide a picture of body structures that looks like a negative of a photograph.	Chest x-ray Dye-enhanced cardiac catheterization
Magnetic resonance imaging (MRI)	The computer-based procedure provides physiologic information and detailed views of fluid-filled soft tissues.	MRI of the brain, spine, extremities, joints, heart, pelvis, abdomen
Nuclear scanning	Studies that use the administration of a radionuclide and subsequent measurement of radiation from an organ to detect functional abnormalities.	Brain scan Heart scan Lung scan Bone scan
Ultrasonography	Studies in which a harmless, high-frequency sound wave is emitted that penetrates the organ being studied. The sound waves bounce back to the sensor and are electronically converted into a picture of the organ or the contents of the organ.	Ultrasound of the pelvis, abdomen, heart, uterus

Key Points

- Data collection during a health assessment includes a health history and a physical assessment. Data from nursing assessments are used to formulate nursing diagnoses.
- Four techniques are used in performing a health assessment—inspection, palpation, percussion, and auscultation.
- The nurse should plan the health assessment at a time that is appropriate for both the client and the nurse. The nurse should prepare the room, gather instruments and equipment, ensure privacy, and meet the client's physical and psychologic needs.
- Various positions are used during the health assessment. The client's privacy and comfort should be considered in each position.
- Each body system is assessed for normal and abnormal findings; included are the integument, the head and neck, the thorax and lungs, the breasts and axilla, the abdomen, the male and female genitalia, the rectum and anus, the musculoskeletal system, and the neurologic system. The techniques of assessment are used to assess the health status of the client systematically.
- The nurse carefully documents normal and abnormal findings.
- Diagnostic tests provide valuable information about a client's health status. Nursing responsibilities associated with diagnostic tests may include witnessing a client's consent, scheduling the test, physical and emotional preparation of the client, nursing care after the test, disposal of equipment, and proper care of any specimen.

Study Questions

1. The internal structures of the eye can be visualized by using which of the following instruments?
   a. an otoscope
   b. an ophthalmoscope
   c. a stethoscope
   d. a tuning fork
2. To make accurate assessments during inspection, the nurse must
   a. compare bilateral body parts
   b. have 20/20 vision
   c. focus on selected body systems
   d. use touch judiciously

3. Palpation is a physical assessment technique that uses the sense of
   a. intuition
   b. vision
   c. hearing
   d. touch
4. When percussing over the stomach, the nurse notes the finding of a loud, drumlike sound. The term to document this percussion tone is
   a. dullness
   b. flatness
   c. tympany
   d. resonance
5. The bell of the stethoscope is used to hear
   a. tympanic sounds
   b. bowel sounds
   c. lung sounds
   d. heart sounds
6. Skin turgor may be assessed by which of the following techniques?
   a. indenting with the fingertips
   b. using special lighting
   c. touching to detect moisture
   d. lightly pinching a skin fold
7. Visual acuity may be assessed by using Snellen's chart. If a client has acuity of 20/40 in both eyes, this means
   a. the client can see twice as well as normal
   b. the client has double vision
   c. the client has less than normal vision
   d. the client has normal vision
8. When using an otoscope to assess the tympanic membrane of an adult, the ear canal is straightened by gently pulling the pinna
   a. up and back
   b. down and forward
   c. away from the examiner
   d. in any direction
9. When percussing the thorax and lungs, a dull sound indicates
   a. an air-filled structure
   b. a bony structure
   c. emphysematous tissue
   d. fluid or a solid mass
10. When auscultating the thorax and lungs, coarse gurgling sounds are heard on expiration. These sounds can be broadly labeled as
    a. adventitious breath sounds
    b. bronchovesicular breath sounds
    c. vesicular breath sounds
    d. bronchial sounds
11. Heart sounds are the result of
    a. blood flow through the heart
    b. movement of blood into the heart from the aorta
    c. closure of the heart valves
    d. contraction of the cardiac muscle
12. When palpating the breast, the assessment should be conducted by which division of areas?
    a. quadrants
    b. halves
    c. entire breast tissue
    d. bilateral comparison
13. When assessing the abdomen, which assessment technique should be conducted after inspection?
    a. percussion
    b. palpation
    c. auscultation
    d. sequence does not matter
14. Which of the following assessments of mental status is *not* an assessment of orientation?
    a. time
    b. place
    c. person
    d. consciousness
15. As part of the assessment of cranial nerves, the nurse asks the client to raise the eyebrows, smile, and show the teeth. These actions provide information about which cranial nerve?
    a. olfactory
    b. optic
    c. facial
    d. vagus

Answers With Rationale

1. The correct response is *b.* None of the other instruments can be used to visualize the internal eye.
2. The correct response is *a.* A comparison of bilateral body parts is necessary for recognizing abnormal findings. Perfect vision is unnecessary; the nurse examines all body systems and uses touch during palpation.
3. The correct response is *d.* Palpation is the technique that uses the sense of touch. The other responses are incorrect.
4. The correct response is *c.* Tympany is a loud, drumlike sound, heard over an air-filled organ. Dullness has a thud-like quality. Flatness is a flat, high-pitched sound. Resonance is a hollow sound heard over lung tissue.
5. The correct response is *d.* The bell of the stethoscope is used to hear low-pitched sounds, such as those produced by the heart and vascular system. The diaphragm of the stethoscope is used to hear high-pitched sounds, such as normal lung and bowel sounds.
6. The correct response is *d.* Skin turgor is assessed by lightly pinching a fold of skin and allowing it to return to its shape when released. None of the other techniques would determine skin turgor.

7. The correct response is *c*. Normal vision is 20/20. A finding of 20/40 would mean that a client has less than normal vision.
8. The correct response is *a*. The ear canal of an adult is straightened by gently pulling the pinna of the ear up and back. In children younger than age 3 years, the ear canal is straightened by pulling the pinna gently down and back.
9. The correct response is *d*. A dull sound is heard when percussing over fluid or a solid mass. A flat tone is heard over a bony structure. Tympany is heard over an air-filled structure. Hyperresonance is heard over emphysematous lung tissue and is an abnormal finding.
10. The correct response is *a*. Adventitious breath sounds are sounds not normally heard in the lungs (such as rales or rhonchi). The other responses are normal breath sounds.
11. The correct response is *c*. Heart sounds are the result of closure of the heart valves. The other responses do not result in heart sounds.
12. The correct response is *a*. The breast is divided into four quadrants—outer upper quadrant, outer lower quadrant, inner upper quadrant, and inner lower quadrant. Each quadrant is systematically palpated in a clockwise direction. Any abnormal findings are recorded by location of the involved quadrant.
13. The correct response is *c*. When assessing the abdomen, the sequence is inspection, auscultation, percussion, and palpation. Auscultation follows inspection because percussion and palpation stimulate bowel sounds.
14. The correct response is *d; a, b,* and *c* are assessments of orientation. Consciousness is the degree of wakefulness or the ability of a person to be aroused, which is not the same as orientation.
15. The correct response is *c*. Motor function of the facial nerve (cranial nerve VII) is assessed by asking the client to raise the eyebrow, smile, and show the teeth. The other responses are also cranial nerves, but have different techniques of assessment.

Bibliography

Andresen, G. (1992). How to assess the older mind. *RN, 55*(7), 34–41.

Barker, E., & Moore, K. (1992). Neurological assessment. *RN, 55*(4), 28–35.

Barker, E., & Moore, K. (1992). Perfecting the art: Cranial nerve assessment. *RN, 55*(5), 62–69.

Bates, B. (1995). *Guide to physical examination and history taking* (6th ed.). Philadelphia: Lippincott.

Cook, M. (1994). Nursing assessment for the older woman. *RN, 57*(9), 40–44.

Dettenmeier, P. (1995). *Radiographic assessment for nurses.* St. Louis: Mosby.

Dykes, P. (1993). Minding the 5 Ps of neurovascular assessment. *American Journal of Nursing, 93*(6), 38–39.

Finesilver, C. (1992). Respiratory assessment. *RN, 55*(2), 22–30.

Fischbach, F. (1995). *Quick reference to common laboratory and diagnostic tests.* Philadelphia: Lippincott.

Flory, C. (1992). Perfecting the art: Skin assessment. *RN, 55*(6), 22–27.

Fuller, J., & Schaller-Ayers, J. (1994). *Health assessment: A nursing approach* (2nd ed.). Philadelphia: Lippincott.

Holgren, C. (1992). Abdominal assessment. *RN, 55*(3), 28–34.

Hunt, L. (1992). Ophthalmic nursing assessment. *Insight, 17*(3), 9–11.

Irwin, M. (1991). Assessing color changes for dark skinned patients. *Advancing Critical Care, 6*(6), 8–11.

Kuhn, J., & McGovern, M. (1992). Peripheral vascular assessment of the elderly client. *Journal of Gerontological Nursing, 18*(12), 35–38.

Lower, J. (1992). Rapid neuro assessment. *American Journal of Nursing, 92*(6), 38–45, 47–48.

McConnell, E. A. (1988). Getting the feel of lymph node assessment. *Nursing, 18*(8), 54–57.

McGovern, M., & Kuhn, J. (1992). Skin assessment of the elderly client. *Journal of Gerontological Nursing, 18*(4), 39–43.

Morton, L. (1991). Cardiac assessment. *RN, 54*(12), 28–35.

Pagana, K., & Pagana, T. (1994). *Diagnostic testing and nursing implications: A case study approach.* St. Louis: Mosby.

Pagana, K., & Pagana, T. (1994). *Mosby's diagnostic and laboratory test reference.* St. Louis: Mosby.

Poncar, P. (1995). Who has time for a head-to-toe assessment? *Nursing 95, 25*(3), 59.

Rhoads, M., & Jepson, T. (1994). A quick screening assessment tool for students. *Nurse Educator, 19*(1), 6.

Smeltzer, S., & Bare, B. (1996). *Brunner and Suddarth's textbook of medical–surgical nursing* (8th ed.). Philadelphia: Lippincott-Raven.

Stiesmeyer, J. (1993). A four-step approach to pulmonary assessment. *American Journal of Nursing, 93*(8), 22–31.

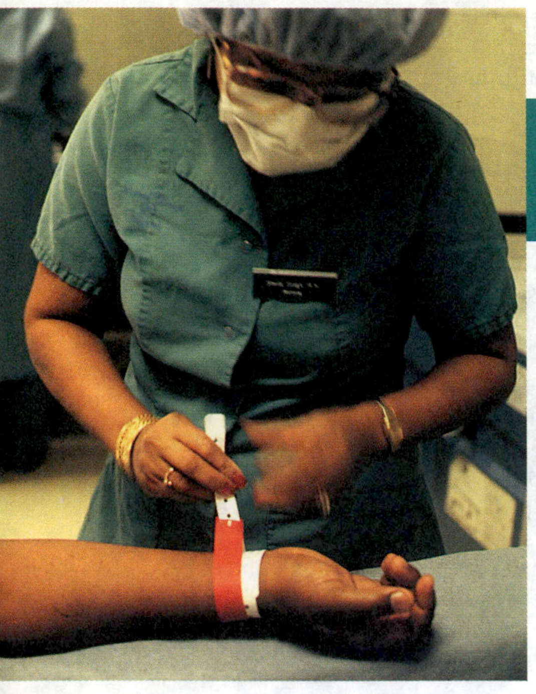

Chapter 27

Safety

Objectives

After studying this chapter, the learner should be able to:

Define key terms used in the chapter.

Identify factors that may be safety hazards in the client's environment.

Describe ways in which the client's safety can be promoted in the home and healthcare setting.

Identify clients at risk of falling.

Describe preventive strategies to decrease the incidence of client falls.

Identify alternatives to using restraints.

Identify nursing diagnoses associated with a client in an unsafe situation.

Describe nursing responsibilities for fire safety.

Identify teaching strategies that should be included in a safety program to prevent poisoning and suffocation.

Key Terms

asphyxiation

ground

incident report

macroshock

microshock

restraint

Safety and security are basic human needs. Safety is a paramount concern that underlies all nursing care, and it is the responsibility of *all* healthcare providers. The focus on safety encompasses all healthcare facilities as well as the home, workplace, and community. There are universal safety concerns common to all age groups as well as unique safety considerations for each.

Injuries and deaths from motor vehicle accidents, falls, fire, and poisoning occur with alarming regularity across the life span. Violent behavior and its aftermath have also become a significant public safety concern. Statistics verify the incidence and particular groups at risk:

- Motor vehicle accidents are the leading cause of death in the United States for ages 1 to 34; frequently, alcohol is cited as a major contributor to these accidents (Hingson, 1993).
- Falls are the major safety problem in healthcare facilities, and each year, approximately 30% of older adults in the community will fall (Stanley & Beare, 1995). Although falls can occur at any age, older people and young children are particularly at risk.
- A house fire occurs every 66 seconds in the United States. Despite the fact that smoke detectors are now present in 82% of all homes, usually one third of those detectors do not function because the batteries are dead (Milford & Manser, 1995). Often a fire in a home results in injury or death to family members and frequently the victims are young children or older residents.
- Children are most vulnerable to poisoning between the ages of 1 and 3, but accidental deaths by poisoning across the life span increased by 12% in 1993 (Accident Facts, 1994). Drug use is on the rise again among high school students; particularly alarming is a sharp increase in marijuana use in eighth graders (Famighetti, 1995).
- In the United States, gunshot injuries and deaths among children and adolescents have increased sharply since 1990. Gun-related homicides, suicides, and accidents are now responsible for 14 deaths every day in this vulnerable population (Fingerhut, 1993).

Providing a safe, secure environment requires an awareness of potential hazards for each developmental level. Studies have confirmed that pregnant women who use drugs, consume alcohol, and smoke expose their unborn children to substances that may adversely affect normal growth and development. The nurse frequently is the initial healthcare provider who has contact with an abused child or a battered woman. Prompt recognition is crucial, and nursing assessment may play a vital role in identifying a harmful environment. Adolescents face great dangers when they choose a pattern of drug or alcohol abuse or high-risk sexual activity. The increasing number of adolescents who become pregnant or are victims of alcohol-related motor vehicle accidents, sexually transmitted diseases, and suicide is a devastating outcome of these unsafe behaviors. Nurses have become more aware of the growing crisis of elder abuse, which according to the House Select Committee on Aging may affect between 1 and 2 million older Americans (Lachs & Pillemer, 1995). Nurses have firsthand experience with the specific hazards confronting each age group and situation.

Study of this chapter provides the student with the problem-solving tools needed to address these safety issues. Use of the nursing process facilitates the nurse's ability to recognize, assess, diagnose, and plan the nursing interventions that will effectively ensure safety for all ages in all environments.

Factors Affecting Safety

Nursing strategies that identify potential hazards and promote wellness evolve from an awareness of the various factors that affect safety in the environment. Table 27-1 lists statistics for the principal causes of accidental death in the United States.

Developmental Considerations

Each developmental level has its own particular risks. Promoting safety and preventing injury are a nurse's dual responsibilities. The nurse and client or family cooperate and together strive to eliminate or reduce accident risks in the home, community, or healthcare setting. Education to promote awareness of potentially dangerous situations must begin as early as possible and continue throughout the life span.

Table 27-1
Deaths Due to Unintentional* Injuries in the United States for 1993

Type	Death Total	Death Rate per 100,000 Population
Motor-vehicle accidents	42,000	16.3
Falls	13,500	5.2
Poisoning by solids and liquids	6,500	2.5
Drowning	4,800	1.9
Fires, burns, and deaths associated with fires	4,000	1.6
Suffocation by ingested object	2,900	1.1
Firearms	1,600	0.6
Poisoning by gases and vapors (eg, carbon monoxide)	700	0.3
All other types (eg, medical complications, machinery, air and water transport)	14,000	5.4
Total	90,000	34.9

* The term "unintentional" covers most deaths from injury and poisoning. Homicides, suicides, deaths for which none of these categories can be determined, and war deaths are excluded from these totals.

(Adapted from National Safety Council [1994]. *Accident Facts.* Itasca, IL: NSC.)

Identification of prenatal high-risk factors allows for appropriate intervention to prevent a developing fetus from being harmed. Newborns of mothers who smoke have a lower birth weight. Excessive alcohol consumption and use of addictive drugs may cause adverse effects that are readily apparent at birth. Pregnant women also should avoid exposure to x-rays in the first trimester, certain pesticides, and anything that is a potential risk for the general population.

The infant or young child has a limited awareness of danger. Parents should be encouraged to teach their children about potential dangers at as early an age as possible. Many childhood accidents are preventable. As motor skills develop, the child's environment expands and potential hazards multiply. Protecting an infant or young child may involve childproofing activities in the home, simple instruction about potentially dangerous situations such as crossing a street, and careful observation during routine activities. Protecting a child also includes a heightened awareness by caregivers of manifestations that indicate child abuse. In 1992, more than 2.9 million cases of suspected physical and sexual child abuse were reported in the United States and countless more went unreported (Devlin & Reynolds, 1994). Any suspicion of child abuse deserves immediate investigation and swift intervention, once verified, so that the child can be removed from the dangerous environment and receive treatment. All 50 states now have laws that require reporting of suspected child abuse.

Adolescents are particularly at risk for becoming involved in motor vehicle accidents. Conflicts with parental values coupled with peer pressure may lead to experimentation with drugs and alcohol, creating an even higher potential for accidents. Young and middle-aged adults are more susceptible to accidents when alcohol is used in response to stressful situations. Many motor vehicle accident fatalities that occur in this age group are alcohol related. The National Highway Traffic Safety Administration (NHTSA) estimates that in 1993, 38% of adolescent motor vehicle fatalities resulted from alcohol-related accidents (American Academy of Pediatrics, 1994). NHTSA also reports that adolescent drivers, unlike adults, are less likely to drive after drinking but more likely to have an accident when alcohol and driving are combined.

Domestic violence is widespread in the United States. Every 15 seconds an act of adult domestic violence occurs, and women are usually the victims; it is the most common cause of injury to women. Three quarters of men who abuse their spouse also batter their children (Chez, 1994). Counseling and education are interventions that promote safety and well-being and interrupt the cycle of violence.

Although older adults have more experience with their environment, illness or some degree of motor or sensory impairment may increase their risk for accidents. They are vulnerable to falls, exposure to unfavorable environmental conditions, and fire hazards, in addition to elder abuse. Realistic concerns exist for older clients who have slowed reflexes and continue to operate motor vehicles in an overly cautious or inadvertently careless manner. Failing sight, hearing difficulties, memory lapses, or inadequate communication from the healthcare providers may be responsible for noncompliance with medication regimens. Elder abuse frequently goes unreported because the older adult fears that his or her home care situation may be jeopardized. The typical victim is a white female, over 75 years of age, who has a physical and/or mental impairment; the abuser is most often a family member who is caring for the older adult (All, 1994). Elder abuse is more likely to occur when stress and conflict exist in a family situation. It is difficult to identify, and is a sensitive safety issue.

Older adults admitted to healthcare facilities are more likely to experience a fall, and the mortality rate associated with falls increases with age (Brady et al., 1993). More older women fall than men, which may reflect the fact that there are more women than men in this age group and osteoporosis is more common in women. More than one third of falls in the older population are associated with the need to urinate. Checklists that can be used to assess the potential for a fall occurring in the home or healthcare setting are included in the discussion of nursing assessment later in this chapter.

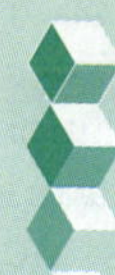

Research in Nursing: Making a Difference

Safety

The growing number of older individuals in the population has prompted nurses to investigate methods of preventing falls and to explore the effectiveness of alternative measures instead of restraints. Falls are the second leading cause of accidental death and until recently, restraints have traditionally been one solution nurses used to protect the client and prevent falls. Recent research has focused on the effectiveness of alternative strategies, implementations of these measures in healthcare facilities, and the benefits of gait training for clients at risk of falling.

Related Research

Werner, P., Cohen-Mansfield, J., Koroknav, V., & Braun, J. (1994). Reducing restraints: Impact on staff attitudes. *Journal of Gerontological Nursing, 20*(12), 19–24.
When asked why they used restraints on older clients, nursing staff members consistently cited the need to ensure client safety and make their work less worrisome. After an inservice on restraints and nursing care alternatives, a majority of staff indicated a change in their perception of the need for applying restraints. Slow implementation of a restraint-reduction policy coupled with ongoing continuing education and administrative support decreased staff feelings of frustration and stress with the restraint policy.

Galindo-Ciocon, D., Ciocon, J., & Galindo, D. (1995). Gait training and falls in the elderly. *Journal of Gerontological Nursing, 21*(6), 10–17.
A mobility scale was administered to a group of older clients who had a history of gait disorders accompanied by a recent fall. Part of this group participated in a balance and gait training program, which resulted in improved scores on the mobility scale and a decrease in the number of falls. The nurse can promote safety and facilitate increased independence in this population by reinforcing gait training and instructing the client and caregivers on the importance of making the home environment safe and manageable for the client.

Mahoney, D. (1995). Analysis of restraint-free nursing homes. *IMAGE: Journal of Nursing Scholarship, 27*(2), 155–160.
A systematic plan for change is recommended rather than a trial-and-error approach. Once restraint-free care is implemented, positive feedback and daily monitoring further support this policy. Administrators should also explore alternative strategies for restraints to determine clinical and cost effectiveness.

Summary

The nurse is responsible for ongoing assessment of both the client at risk of falling and the safety of his or her surroundings. Implementations that promote safety and meet the client's individualized needs can minimize the potential for falls. Responsible care of all clients, particularly the older individual, must focus on safety.

Lifestyle

Certain occupations, recreational activities, and environments place people in more hazardous situations. A worker who operates heavy industrial machinery, functions in perilous settings, or is involved with chemical agents on a consistent basis is at greater risk of accidental injury. Certain agents are being investigated that may place healthcare workers at risk. Reproductive hazards may exist for women with long-term exposure to certain anesthetic agents, and an antiviral preparation (Ribavirin) used for respiratory infections in infants and children may be harmful to a developing fetus (Worthington, 1994). Exposure to excessive noise levels, such as those experienced at a construction site or from extremely loud music, may eventually lead to hearing loss.

Some people, by nature, are more inclined to take risks and place themselves at jeopardy. Failure to wear seat belts or abide by safety precautions is common behavior for some people. Stress may precipitate unhealthful lifestyles that involve drug or alcohol abuse. Although much has been done to identify and control environments affected by pollutants, certain areas may statistically prove more hazardous and may expose residents to potentially unhealthy circumstances.

Living in an area where crime is prevalent may pose an additional threat to physical and emotional well-being. Security measures, such as locks and adequate exterior lighting, provide additional safety reassurances.

Mobility

Any limitation in mobility is potentially unsafe. An older client with an unsteady gait is prone to falling, and an unfamiliar setting may further aggravate the situation. Someone with paralysis or a spinal cord injury may require assistance with even the simplest movement. Supportive devices, such as canes, walkers, and wheelchairs, may facilitate movement, but they require careful instruction and preparation for safe use. Recent surgery or a prolonged illness can temporarily affect mobility and necessitate special precautions to prevent falls or injuries. Nurses must assess a client's risk for injury with a view toward maintaining independence and fostering self-esteem while providing a safe, predictable environment.

Sensory Perception

Alterations in sensory perception can have a devastating effect on safety. Any impairment in sight, hearing, smell, taste, or sense of touch can reduce sensitivity to the environment. Visual changes may cause a person to stumble, lose his or her balance, and fall. A hearing deficit interferes with normal communication and may result in a client who is insensitive to safety alarms, automobile horns, and sirens and unable to understand instructions relating to healthcare. A reduction in one's ability to distinguish odors may mean failure to detect leaking gas or smoke. Loss of taste bud receptors can foster unsafe eating habits or result in ingestion of tainted food. A client whose tactile sense is impaired may be unable to perceive extremes in temperature as a threat to safety.

Knowledge

An awareness of safety precautions is crucial in promoting and maintaining wellness. A client needs instruction to adhere accurately to a medical regimen or to follow safety precautions when oxygen is in use. He or she requires a certain amount of knowledge to manage new equipment and unfamiliar procedures. Nursing assessment includes identification and recognition of potentially threatening circumstances. Recommendations for specific safety precautions are included throughout this chapter.

Ability to Communicate

Communication between the environment and the senses is basic to safety. The nurse must be sensitive to any factor that influences the client's ability to receive and send messages. Fatigue, stress, medication, aphasia, and language barriers are examples of factors that can affect any personal interchange and interfere with an accurate perception of events. A valid assessment by the nurse not only identifies the client's level of understanding, but also facilitates a positive communication experience.

Health State

Anything that affects the health state of the client potentially has the ability to affect the safety of the environment. When a person is chronically ill or in a weakened health state, the focus of healthcare includes preventing accidents as well as promoting wellness and restoring the client to a healthy state. The nurse caring for a client who is recovering from a stroke identifies the client's neuromuscular impairment, pays particular attention to health teaching concerning the client's maintaining a sense of balance, and carefully assists with ambulation to prevent falls. Many of the clients who fall have a primary or secondary diagnosis of cardiovascular disease. Prevention of complications and return to the optimal level of functioning require attention to safety and become primary concerns during the stroke rehabilitation program. The nurse strives to maximize the client's potential by considering safety factors in all phases of the illness and recovery experience.

Psychosocial State

Stressful situations tend to narrow a person's attention span and make him or her more prone to accidents. Stress may be sustained over long periods, but the effects tend to be more devastating in the later years, when there is less adaptive and coping capacity. Depression, when it develops, may result in confusion and disorientation, accompanied by reduced awareness or concern about environmental hazards. Social isolation or lack of social contact may be responsible for a reduced level of concentration, errors in judgment, and a diminished awareness of external stimuli.

Assessing Safety

Environmental safety hazards result in falls, fires, poisoning, suffocation, and accidents involving motor vehicles, equipment, and procedures. Nursing assessment includes identifying clients at risk and unsafe situations. This requires a knowledge of the various factors mentioned above that influence safety and predispose people to accidents. Recognition of these considerations facilitates development of an individualized plan of care and has implications for nursing interventions aimed at protecting the client. Assessment includes an awareness of risk factors in the home and the healthcare agency.

As student nurses become increasingly involved in community and home care settings, it is also appropriate to assess personal environmental safety when visiting an unfamiliar area. Use the self-assessment checklist in the accompanying box to evaluate your attention to maintenance of personal safety.

The Client

Nursing History. In an effort to provide a safe environment, the nurse must be alert for any history of falls or accidents because a person with a history of falling is likely to fall again. Any assistive devices that the client uses (eg, cane, walker) should be noted. The nurse also should attempt to confirm if there is a history of drug or alcohol abuse. Family members or significant others often are valuable resources. Knowledge of family support systems and the home environment is vital as the nurse prepares to plan protective health measures.

Promoting Wellness

Safety in the Community

Use the following assessment checklist to determine how well you are meeting your need for maintaining personal safety as you assist with healthcare delivery in the community. Then develop a prescription for self-care by choosing appropriate behaviors from the list of suggestions.

Assessment Checklist

almost always	sometimes	almost never	
☐	☐	☐	1. I wear a badge or clothing that identifies me as a healthcare worker.
☐	☐	☐	2. I dress in an unobtrusive, professional manner.
☐	☐	☐	3. I keep my car in good working order.
☐	☐	☐	4. I am aware of neighborhoods where personal safety and security may be a problem.
☐	☐	☐	5. I use appropriate precautions to maintain optimum personal safety.
☐	☐	☐	6. I only enter clients' homes when invited in by responsible adult.

Self-Care Behaviors

1. Call clients to schedule visits for an agreeable time.
2. Carry a map of the communities you plan to visit.
3. Avoid isolated areas.
4. Request that pets be secured prior to your visit.
5. Do not carry money, credit cards, or handbag on your person. If necessary, lock them in your trunk.
6. Avoid wearing expensive jewelry.
7. Consider the advantages of a mobile car phone.
8. Request escort services as appropriate or make joint visits.
9. Keep your car locked when driving and when parked.
10. Make sure agency is aware of time/location of scheduled visits.

Physical Examination. The nurse needs to assess the client's mobility status, ability to communicate, level of awareness or orientation, and sensory perception as a nursing examination is completed. Early detection and identification of any potential safety hazards are essential. The nurse's concern for personal safety includes recognition of any manifestations that suggest domestic violence or neglect. Chapters 4 and 9 discuss families who are experiencing violence, neglect, or abuse.

Accident-Prone Behavior. Some people seem to be more likely than others to have accidents. Once an older adult has suffered one fall, it is likely that he or she will fall again. It is not uncommon for some children to be involved in multiple mishaps resulting in fractured bones. Some adolescent drivers repeatedly have motor vehicle accidents. They appear unable to predict situations that may prove hazardous. Opinion varies as to the probable cause of this accident-prone behavior, but the consensus is that a client with a history of accidents is likely to have another one.

The Environment

Assessment of the environment requires the same attention to safety risks. The home, community, and healthcare agency are all settings that have the potential to cause injury. Each must be reviewed on an individual basis with the focus on the client's developmental level and health status. Potential safety hazards in the client's environment that need assessment and appropriate intervention are reviewed in detail later in this chapter in the Implementing section.

Specific Risk Factors

The nurse needs to be aware of those clients who are most at risk for injury as well as specific factors that have consistently been implicated as hazards.

Falls. Assessment for risk of falling includes use of the nursing history and nursing examination. The nursing examination includes inspecting for faulty vision and hearing, mobility problems such as alterations in gait or posture, and postural hypotension. A recent study indicated that a hospitalized older adult is most likely to fall when satisfying elimination needs, seeking rest or change of position, or obtaining food or fluids (Brady et al., 1993). Ryan, Dinkel, and Petrucci (1993) suggest that when assessing risk of falls, it may be relevant to question older adults about "near fall" incidents. They define a "near fall" as a situation where loss of balance occurs and a fall appears imminent but the individual is able to catch him or herself before landing on the ground. Fear of falling or "fallaphobia" may cause anxiety and panic in an individual with a balance or gait problem and make an older adult more vulnerable for a fall (Stanley & Beare, 1995).

Falls can occur at any age but are the leading cause of accidental death in persons 79 years and older (Accident Facts, 1994). A client is considered a high-risk candidate for a fall if he or she has any of the following characteristics:

- Age greater than 65 years
- Documented history of falls
- Impaired vision or sense of balance
- Altered gait or posture
- A medication regimen that includes diuretics, tranquilizers, sedatives, hypnotics, or analgesics
- Postural hypotension
- Slowed reaction time
- Confusion or disorientation
- Impaired mobility
- Weakness and physical frailty
- Unfamiliar environment

Surveillance of environmental hazards in the healthcare facility and the home environment and of clients who are at risk for falls must be continuous. Most healthcare agencies have fall prevention programs. Nurses have the responsibility to identify those clients who are at high risk for falls, document pertinent assessments on the chart, and plan appropriate interventions to ensure their safety. A checklist for preventing falls in a healthcare facility appears in the accompanying box.

Home Healthcare Alert

Instruct family members/caregivers to notify the nurse or physician if the client has any unusual episodes of unsteadiness or confusion.

Fires. Many home fires are started by someone smoking in bed or falling asleep on a sofa or chair while smoking. The majority of all fatal home fires occur while people are sleeping and most people who die in house fires die not from burns but from smoke inhalation. Kitchen stoves, candles, and electric heaters are other causes of home fires. Faulty wiring and unsafe electrical equipment cause fires in homes and healthcare facilities. Risk factors for home fires can be determined by assessing the knowledge of clients and families.

For clients of limited financial resources, questioning as to how a client heats the house is important, since the electricity or gas may have been turned off and space or kerosene heaters, wood stoves, or a fireplace may be the sole source of heat. A sample of a fire prevention checklist that may be used in the home is given in the accompanying box.

Fire prevention and emergency response programs in healthcare facilities often are viewed by staff as time-consuming and unnecessary exercises, but the nurse must be prepared at all times to protect clients from injury. Hospitals are required by law to establish safety boards and to inspect the facilities regularly for possible hazards. Equipment must be checked periodically, and escape routes must be kept open. Nurses, as part of their daily care procedures, must be aware of their agency's smoking policy, review equipment and its proper functioning, and assess when and how often drills are performed.

Poisoning. Although the incidence of childhood poisoning has been reduced dramatically in the past 10 years, accidental poisoning remains a concern in the 25-to-44-year age group, which had the greatest increase in death rate, up to 4.5 per 100,000 people in 1991 (Accident Facts, 1994). Causes of fatalities from unintentional poisoning are listed in Table 27-2. Not all poisons, however, cause death.

Developmental considerations must be taken into account when making assessments. Younger children are more apt to ingest household chemicals, whereas older children may swallow medicines in a suicide attempt. Preschool children also are at risk for ingestion of lead-containing substances. Experimentation with drugs by adolescents and young adults may result in accidental poisoning and death. An older person may inadvertently consume an overdose of a medication because of confusion or forgetfulness. Poor vision also is a factor in accidental poisoning in the older population.

Most exposures to toxic fumes occur in the home. Poisoning may result from improper mixing of household substances, prolonged use of strong cleaning products, or malfunctioning household appliances (gas, oil, and kerosene heaters) that can release carbon monoxide gas. Carbon monoxide (CO) gas is colorless, odorless, tasteless, and nonirritating, which makes it especially dangerous because it requires a special device to test its presence. Exposure can result in mild symptoms or progress to serious and long-term effects, and may be life threatening. Young children and older adults appear to be most vulnerable to the fumes.

Many poison control centers provide checklists for poison-proofing a home and lists of toxic household items as displayed in the adjacent box. Reviewing these items will help in assessing and teaching the family about poisonous materials.

Suffocation and Choking. Suffocation, or **asphyxiation**, may occur in any age group, but the incidence is greater in children. It results in a lack of air reaching the lungs and a stoppage of breathing.

Common causes of suffocation include drowning, choking on a foreign substance inhaled into the trachea, and gas or smoke poisoning. An infant may suffocate when a pillow or a piece of plastic inadvertently covers the nose and mouth. A young child may be accidentally strangled by the shoulder harness of a seat belt or become trapped while playing in a discarded refrigerator and suffocate.

Drowning is a form of suffocation. Nearly half of all drowning victims are children under age 5. Most drowning deaths in young children occur because of inadequate supervision in the bathtub and in pools—even

Checklist: Prevention of Falls in the Healthcare Facility

Client's name ______________________________ Age __________

Diagnosis ______________________________

Nursing unit/station ______________________________

A *no* answer to any of these questions indicates the need to take additional measures to guarantee the client's safety.

	Yes	*No*	*Comments*
1. Has risk assessment for the client been completed?	☐	☐	____________
2. If client is at risk, have room and chart been clearly identified to alert all caregivers?	☐	☐	____________
3. Are side rails up?	☐	☐	____________
4. Is bed in low position?	☐	☐	____________
5. Are bed wheels locked?	☐	☐	____________
Wheelchair brakes on?	☐	☐	____________
6. Is call bell within the client's reach?	☐	☐	____________
7. Does the client understand how to use the call bell?	☐	☐	____________
8. Is the night light on?	☐	☐	____________
9. Have physical hazards in the room been eliminated (eg, wet area on floor, clutter in pathway to bathroom)?	☐	☐	____________
10. Does the client wear nonskid footwear?	☐	☐	____________
11. Are the client's water, tissues, bedpan/urinal within reach?	☐	☐	____________
12. Is the client aware of activity restrictions?	☐	☐	____________
13. Have any changes in the client's cognitive or sensory status been reported at change of shift?	☐	☐	____________
14. Are alternative measures to restraints being implemented?	☐	☐	____________
What are they?			____________
15. If necessary, are restraints being used? What type?	☐	☐	____________
16. Is client checked every hour and call bell answered promptly?	☐	☐	____________
17. Are visitors aware of safety protocols?	☐	☐	____________

small wading pools. Older children are more likely to drown while swimming or boating.

Educating the public about the various causes of suffocation is the strongest factor in promoting wellness in this category. Assessing the knowledge level of clients—especially parents—is vitally important. The following questions might be included in an assessment for hazards that might cause a child to asphyxiate or choke:

Are plastic bags within reach of young children or infants?

Do you have soft pillows or thick blankets in your infant's crib?

Do you ever place your baby on a water bed to sleep?

Do you cut food into small pieces before giving it to young children?

Do you give peanuts, hard candy, or other small treats to your preschooler?

Are your children playing with toys appropriate for their age?

Do their toys have small or loose parts?

Have you ever left your infant or young child alone in a bathtub—even for a moment?

Does your child have access to a swimming pool?

Checklist: Fire Safety in the Home

How safe is your home from fire? Take a few minutes to walk through your home, looking for these common fire hazards.

Yes	No	*Electricity*
☐	☐	Are electrical cords in good condition—not frayed or worn?
☐	☐	Do you avoid threading electric cords, including extension cords, under carpeting or pinching them behind furniture?
☐	☐	When a fuse blows, do you replace it with a proper fuse—and not a penny?

Yes	No	*Alternative Heating Measures*
☐	☐	Do you use an electric space heater? Does it have an automatic shut-off in case it's tipped over? Do you keep the electric heater out of damp or wet areas?
☐	☐	Do you turn off a kerosene heater when no one is in the room and at bedtime?
☐	☐	Is the flue open when a fire is burning in the fireplace?
☐	☐	Does a firescreen cover the entire opening of the fireplace?
☐	☐	Do you start the fire properly—not with charcoal starter or gasoline?
☐	☐	Is a metal pail available to carry out the ashes and are the ashes cold?
☐	☐	Is the chimney cleaned annually?
☐	☐	Is the fuel for the fireplace—kindling, newspapers, firewood—stacked at least 3 feet from the hearth?
☐	☐	Are Christmas tree branches or needles properly discarded and not used to start or maintain a fire?
☐	☐	Are draperies and furniture more than 3 feet away from the fireplace?

Yes	No	*Smoking Habits*
☐	☐	If there are smokers in the house, are ashtrays readily available?
☐	☐	Do you enforce a strict "no smoking in bed" policy?
☐	☐	Do you also avoid smoking in a comfortable chair where you might fall asleep while smoking?
☐	☐	After a party, do you check waste baskets, ashtrays, furniture, and carpets for carelessly discarded cigarettes?

Yes	No	*Smoke Detectors*
☐	☐	Are smoke detectors installed outside every sleeping area?
☐	☐	Are smoke detectors operable?
☐	☐	Do you replace smoke alarm batteries twice a year with long-lasting, 9-volt lithium batteries?
☐	☐	Do you resist disconnecting the detectors if they sound because the batteries are weak or because the toast is burning in the kitchen?
☐	☐	Do you forbid anyone to "borrow" the batteries from the detectors?

Yes	No	*Children's Play (Matches/Lighters/Candles)*
☐	☐	Are matches and lighters stored out of children's reach?
☐	☐	Are all lighted candles kept out of the reach of children?
☐	☐	Are all candles extinguished?

Yes	No	*Escape Route and Drills*
☐	☐	Have you determined two escape routes out of the bedroom in case there is a fire?
☐	☐	Have you had a home fire drill?
☐	☐	Have you reviewed with the babysitter what to do if a fire occurs?
☐	☐	If your house has rooms above the ground floor or if you live in an upper story, have you installed rope or chain ladders or discussed how to escape from the upper floors quickly?

Yes	No	*Appliances*
☐	☐	Are all appliances turned off before you go to bed or leave the house?
☐	☐	When working over the stove, do you wear garments with short or snug sleeves?
☐	☐	Is baking soda (not baking powder or flour) handy to snuff out a grease fire?
☐	☐	Do you have a fire extinguisher handy?

(continued)

Checklist: Fire Safety in the Home *(continued)*

Yes	No	*Storage of Flammable Substances*
☐	☐	Is trash—particularly oily or paint-saturated rags—kept from accumulating in your garage?
☐	☐	Do you store oily rags, gasoline, or other flammables away from heating sources or open flames, such as the pilot light of the water heater?
☐	☐	Do you use gasoline or paintbrush cleaner in an open area, where fumes can be dissipated and won't drift toward a source of ignition?

Yes	No	*Storage of Flammable Substances (continued)*
☐	☐	Do you refuse to allow anyone in your home to use gasoline as a cleaner for clothing or furniture?

Scoring

A *no* answer to any of these questions indicates that you are not doing all you can to minimize the risk of fires in your home. Although no house is fireproof, fires can be prevented. You should take all the fire-prevention steps suggested in the questions.

(Adapted from: *Aide Magazine.* [October 1991]. USAA, San Antonio; *USAA Magazine.* [August 1995]. USAA, San Antonio.)

Is pool rescue equipment nearby?
Is your child closely supervised when near water?
Do you know how to perform cardiopulmonary resuscitation and an abdominal thrust (Heimlich maneuver)?

Firearm Injuries. Firearm injury prevention has become a major concern of the health community. Many people feel that keeping a gun in the home provides protection for family and property. According to Kellerman et al. (1993), keeping a gun in the home has dangerous consequences. It increases the risk of domestic homicide threefold and may be responsible for unintentional injury and death. Young children are curious and like to explore their surroundings. If they encounter a loaded gun, the outcome may be tragic.

Gun ownership is a sensitive issue and nurses need to approach this topic in a nonjudgmental manner with the focus on injury prevention. The intent is to inform families about risks from firearm injury and discuss appropriate safety measures. The following questions address these concerns:

If you own a gun, do you keep it unloaded and locked up?
Do you lock and store bullets in a separate location?
Do you make certain that children do not have access to the keys?
Have you discussed the risk of injury from guns with your children?
Have you told your children that they should never touch a gun or remain in a friend's house where a gun is accessible?

Diagnosing

Once the nurse has identified an unsafe situation or a client at risk, the nursing diagnosis and plan of care should reflect this. The actual or potential statement of the client's health status must be followed by the appropriate contributing or risk factors to individualize the nursing plan of care.

Samples of nursing diagnoses pertaining to safety risks include the following:

Risk for Injury related to lack of awareness of environmental hazards; visual or auditory sensory deficits; history of falling; unsteady gait; substance abuse; refusal to use seat belt or child safety seat;

Table 27-2
Unintentional Poisoning Deaths for 1991

	Age						
Type of Poisoning	*All Ages*	*<5 years*	*5–14*	*15–24*	*25–44*	*45–64*	*≥65*
Drugs, medicines and biologicals	5,215	48	16	357	3,501	725	568
Other solids and liquids (including alcohol)	483	14	11	57	193	147	61
Gases and vapors (all types)	736	14	29	147	254	134	158

(Adapted from National Safety Council. [1994]. *Accident Facts.* Itasca, IL: NSC.)

Checklist: Prevention of Poisoning in the Home

Complete the following checklist to see if your home is safe from potential poisons. Check this list to see if all poisons are safely stored out of reach of small children and pets.

Kitchen

- ☐ Cleaners—carpet or upholstery cleaners, furniture polish, soaps or detergents
- ☐ Corrosives—automatic dishwashing detergents, drain cleaners, ammonia, metal cleaners, oven cleaners
- ☐ Medicines—pain relievers such as aspirin and acetaminophen, diet aids, vitamins or iron pills, pet medications
- ☐ Insecticides

Bedroom

- ☐ Cosmetics—nail polish or remover, baby powder
- ☐ Perfumes
- ☐ House plants
- ☐ Jewelry cleaners
- ☐ Medicines

Laundry Room

- ☐ Bleaches
- ☐ Laundry detergents
- ☐ Disinfectants

Bathroom

- ☐ Medicines
- ☐ Aftershave
- ☐ Mouthwashes
- ☐ Cleaners
- ☐ Deodorizers or sanitizers
- ☐ Drain openers
- ☐ Shampoo or hair products
- ☐ Hair removers
- ☐ Fluoride rinses

Garage, Basement, Storage Areas

- ☐ Antifreeze
- ☐ Pesticides
- ☐ Gasoline or kerosene
- ☐ Lighter fluid
- ☐ Paint remover or thinner
- ☐ Paint stripper
- ☐ Weed killer
- ☐ Mothballs

Living Room

- ☐ Cigarette butts, cigarettes
- ☐ Chocolate (hazardous to pets)
- ☐ Plants (check with the poison center to see if they are poisonous)
- ☐ Lamp oil

Miscellaneous

- ☐ Alcoholic beverages
- ☐ Outdoor plants—azalea, rhododendron, poke berry, holly berry

In the event of poisoning, contact the local poison control center.

(Poison Control Center, 1 Children's Center, Philadelphia, PA 19104)

effects of medication; age greater than 65; generalized weakness

Risk for Poisoning related to impaired vision; medications stored in unlocked medicine cabinet that is accessible to a child; presence of poisonous plants; excess alcohol intake; use of illicit drugs; knowledge deficit

Risk for Suffocation related to plastic bag that is accessible to a young child; child left unattended in bathtub; smoking in bed; placing an infant prone in a water bed; lack of safety precautions (door left on discarded refrigerator); unfamiliarity with fire prevention guidelines

Risk for Trauma related to history of previous falls; unsteady gait; presence of unsecured scatter rugs; smoking in bed; inoperable smoke detector; history of substance abuse; lack of experience operating an automobile; presence of unsecured loaded gun in the home

Impaired Home Maintenance Management related to insufficient finances; substance abuse; physical disability

Risk for Disuse Syndrome related to use of physical restraints

Planning: Expected Outcomes

Many accidental injuries and deaths are preventable. The nurse considers the varied factors and environment that affect the client's safety and formulates expected outcomes uniquely suited to each situation and circumstance. Nursing interventions focus on meeting these safety needs.

Expected outcomes for clients that promote safety and prevent injury include the following. The client will:

- Identify unsafe situations in his or her environment
- Identify potential hazards in his or her environment

- Demonstrate safety measures to prevent falls and other accidents
- Establish safety priorities with family members or significant others
- Demonstrate familiarity with his or her environment
- Identify resources for safety information
- Remain free of injury during hospitalization

Implementing

Integral to the nursing plan of care is the client's safety. The nurse intervenes to control or modify the client's environment. Safety recommendations throughout this section apply to health agency settings, the home, and the community. Nursing implementations are discussed for each developmental level as well as for specific hazards in the environment.

Teaching to Prevent Accidents

Teaching is an important factor in accident prevention and health promotion (Fig. 27-1). Resources the nurse or family can use are given in the accompanying box. Many teaching opportunities concerning safety measures arise while the nurse performs regular client care. Careful assessment, diagnosis, and planning prepare the nurse to use these opportunities wisely.

Assessment data and statistical information often prove helpful to healthcare personnel who are developing a safety program for clients at risk. Safety education classes, in addition to situational health teaching, can be worthwhile for the hospitalized client and his or her family. Recent studies have demonstrated that early assessment of vulnerable clients and preventive education programs can decrease the incidence of falls (Algase, 1992; Croft & Foraker, 1993; Roberts & Wykle, 1993).

All-purpose fire extinguishers for the home

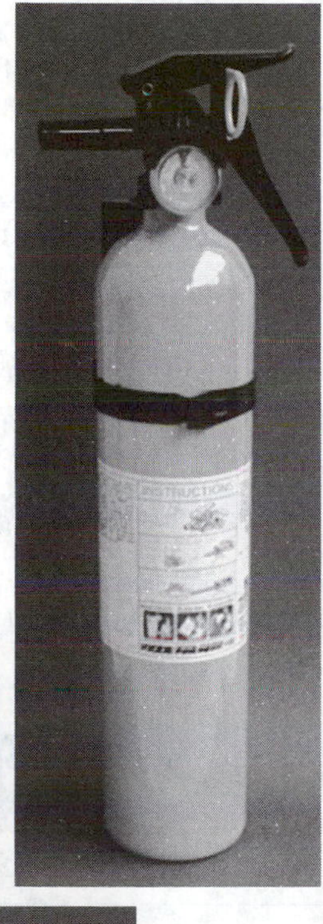

3-prong plug adapters with grounding wire

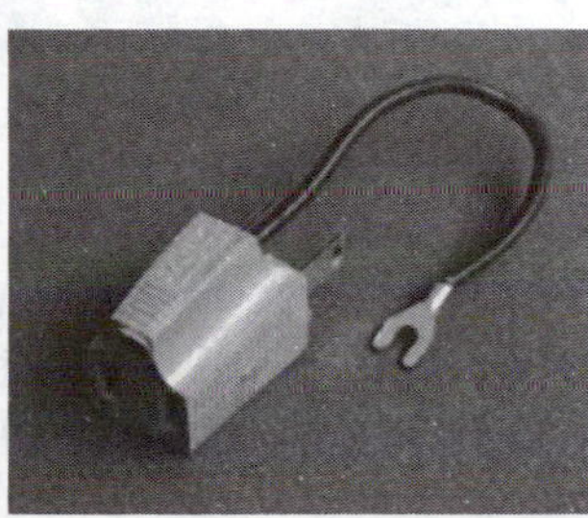

Smoke detectors for the home

Outlet covers protect curious tots from electrical shock

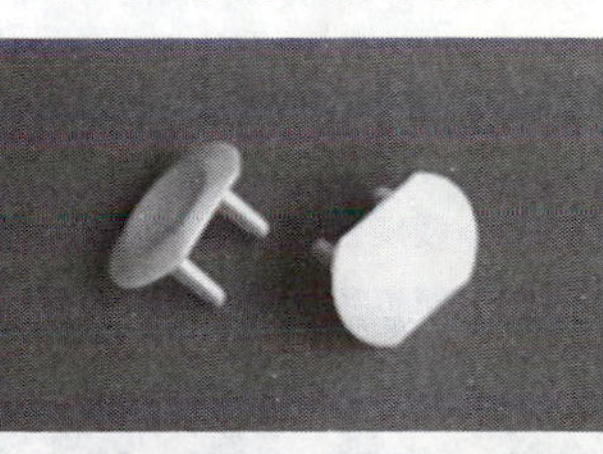

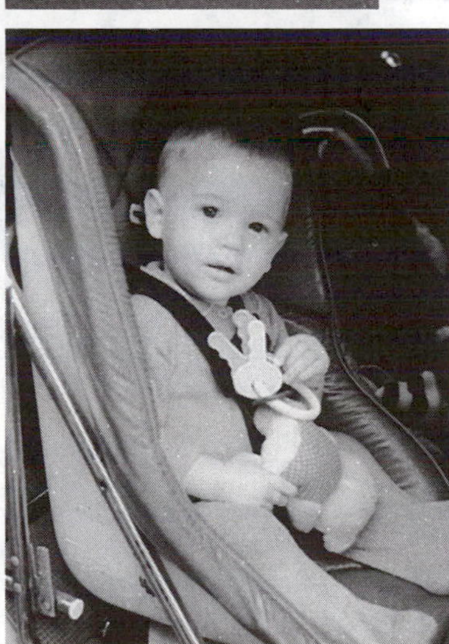

Car seats for infants and small children

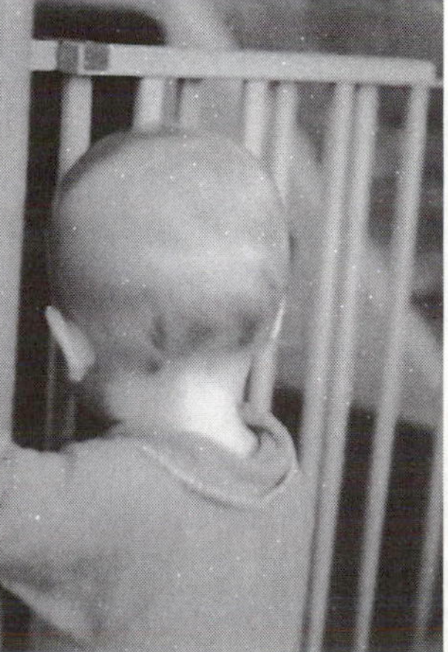

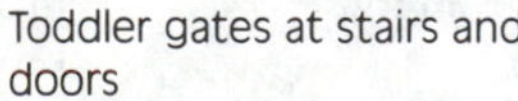

Toddler gates at stairs and doors

Figure 27-1
The nurse's responsibility in home safety is primarily that of education and counseling, including providing information about home safety devices and sources for additional information.

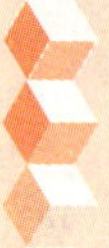

Helpscan

The following are resources for clients and health-care professionals:

For pamphlets on safety for older adults:

- National Safety Council
  444 N. Michigan Avenue
  Chicago, IL 60611
  (800) 621-7619 (ext. 6900)
- Canada Safety Council
  2750 Stevenage Dr., Unit 6
  Ottawa, ON KIG 3N2
  (613) 739-1535

Hotline numbers for victims of abuse:

- National Organization for Victim Assistance (NOVA)
  (800) TRY-NOVA
- National Child Abuse Hotline
  (800) 422-4453

For health care professionals with concerns/questions about restraints:

- Mary Weick Brady
  FDA, Center for Devices and Radiological Health
  1350 Piccard Drive (HFZ-520)
  Rockville, MD 20850
  (301) 594-1144

Hotline for health professionals to voluntarily report problems or serious adverse effects with healthcare-related products (drugs, medical devices, food, cosmetics, etc.):

- MEDWATCH
  The FDA Medical Products Reporting Program
  Food and Drug Administration
  5600 Fishers Lane
  Rockville, MD 20852-9787
  (800) FDA-1088

A school nurse has multiple opportunities and a ready audience for health teaching about safety, including screening programs (eg, vision and hearing), fire prevention sessions, drug and alcohol prevention programs, firearm safety, and classes covering various accident prevention techniques. Management of minor accidents that involve children at school provides a forum for teaching additional preventive strategies.

Considering Developmental Levels

Table 27-3 lists types of accidents according to developmental age, and safety topics that should be discussed with parents and in the school. The material in the remainder of this section on environmental safety is adaptable to teaching.

Fetus. Consideration for safety begins with an awareness of behaviors that may harm the developing fetus. A pregnant woman's knowledge of the risks associated with excess alcohol consumption, smoking, drug use, and exposure to other dangers in the environment, as listed in Table 27-3, should be reinforced.

Infant. The nurse has many opportunities to educate parents about safety and accident prevention for infants

Table 27-3
Developmental Considerations and Safety Topics to Be Taught

Developmental Age	Accidents	Safety Topics
Fetus	Abnormal growth and development	Alcohol consumption Smoking Use of drugs (addicting, prescription, and over the counter) X-ray exposure Pesticides
Neonate	Falls	Neonatal supervision Proper method of caring for neonate Environment—crib, bath, and changing area Infant car seats Use of vitamins, iron medications Feeding
Infant (first 6 mo)	Falls Injuries from toys Burns	Many of above topics Infant supervision Development—rolling over and falls Toy safety—size, construction, lead-free paint

(continued)

Table 27-3 *(continued)*
Developmental Considerations and Safety Topics to Be Taught

Developmental Age	Accidents	Safety Topics
		Flame-retardant clothes and inflammable toys Smoke alarms Sunburns, bathwater temperature, smoking, hot beverages Kitchen safety Electrical cords and outlets Using medications
Infant (second 6 mo)	Falls Injuries from toys Burns Suffocation or drowning Inhalation or ingestion Foreign bodies	Many of above topics Close supervision for active child Development—crawling, pulling up to stand, and pulling down objects (curiosity) Safety on stairs (gates) Teaching siblings about infant safety Plastic bags Tub and pool safety Childproofing entire house and any houses the infant visits Poisonous plants Child-resistant packaging of medications and all poisonous substances
Toddler	Falls Cuts from sharp objects Burns Suffocation or drowning Inhalation or ingestion Foreign bodies	Poison Control Center and instructions for emergencies Many of above topics Toddler supervision Development—inquisitive nature Outdoor safety—cars, driveways, parking lots Safety glass on doors, lock doors and windows, screens Animal safety—pets and strange animals Child car seats Storage of hazardous substances (indoors and outdoors) Poisonous plants (indoors and outdoors) Car safety (car seats, unattended children, cars parked in sun) Storage of matches, use of hot liquids Water safety—tubs, jacuzzis, and wading and swimming pools, swimming lessons
Preschooler	Falls Cuts Burns Drowning Inhalation or ingestion Guns and weapons	Many of above topics, plus use of safety equipment when riding bicycles or skateboards Safe play areas (equipment and supervision, streets) Tricycles, scissors, other toys Guns or rifles in the house Begin to teach safety measures to child Fire safety—prevention, emergency measures, fire drills
School-age child	Burns Drowning Broken bones Inhalation or ingestion Guns and weapons Substance abuse	Many of above topics Safety on way to school (traffic, child abuse) Play equipment—bicycles, skateboards, roller skates Competitive sports Use of machinery (farm, lawn, cooking) Teaching safety measures (bicycle, use of phone in emergencies, policeman as helper, substance abuse) Parental role modeling Drug and alcohol abuse education Sexuality education
Adolescent	Drowning Vehicle accidents Guns and weapons Inhalation or ingestion	Many of above topics Responsibilities of new freedoms of being a teenager Driving (driver education, traffic safety, drinking and driving, motorcycles and snowmobiles) Competitive sports (proper equipment, physical examination before beginning sports or going to camp) Safety around water and water sports Emergency procedures, first-aid training Gun safety Substance abuse and role modeling for siblings Stress and coping Sexuality education and discussion of sexually transmitted diseases (including AIDS)

and young children. Lack of mobility in early infancy limits opportunities for hazardous activity, but minimal safeguards are vital if accidents are to be prevented.

Safe care entails never leaving the infant unattended, using crib rails, and monitoring objects that the infant could place in the mouth and swallow. As the infant becomes more active, parents and caregivers must be alert to hazards that a curious, mobile infant may encounter. All items within reach must be carefully inspected and, if dangerous, secured in a safe place. Household products, medicines, electric outlets, and sharp instruments may cause injury and death. Because an infant frequently climbs or pulls up on objects, scalding hot liquids must be placed out of reach. Lead-free paint on all furniture and toys ensures that the infant will not be exposed to lead poisoning. All 50 states mandate the need for safe infant car seats and carriers when transporting a child in a motor vehicle. A rear-facing safety seat is recommended for infants who weigh less than 20 lb (9.1 kg); a forward-facing car seat may be used for larger infants and toddlers. The American Academy of Pediatrics (1992) released a revised statement from NHTSA reinforcing their admonition that rear-facing safety seats not be placed in the front seat of a vehicle with passenger-side air bags, but indicated that a forward-facing child restraint may be used in the front seat if the child's age and weight meet the restraint manufacturer's requirements and the vehicle seat is moved as far back as possible. The high force of sudden air bag inflation has the potential to cause injury to an infant in the safety seat. Additional safety counseling measures that focus on tasks and behavior typical for this developmental level are included in Table 27-3.

Toddler and Preschooler. To prevent accidental injury and death during the toddler and preschool years, the focus of parental responsibility is on childproofing the environment. Play areas must allow for exploration but must provide for safety. Vigilant supervision by parents and guardians should anticipate hazardous elements and protect with precautionary devices such as safety locks, guard rails, and electric outlet covers. Childproofing products are available that help children recognize dangerous items in the home.

Ingestion of poisons or medications is a major threat for preschoolers. Their overconfidence and initiative make them more likely to dart into the street while chasing a ball, climb into a discarded refrigerator, or play with matches. When riding in a motor vehicle, children who have outgrown their safety seats should use a booster seat with a shield or harness; older children can use lap and shoulder belts. Nursing measures that safeguard toddlers and preschoolers are included in Table 27-3.

School-Age Child. As a child becomes more independent during the school years, accidents continue to be a leading cause of death. Although increasingly independent behavior is typical of this age group, children need assistance to evaluate activities that are potentially dangerous. The nurse needs to counsel parents of school-age children about specific interventions that provide for safety at home, at school, and in the neighborhood.

Adolescent. Nurses and parents must collaborate to reinforce safety behaviors in the adolescent. Much of the adolescent's time is spent away from home, with his or her peer group, or in automobiles. Education must focus on safe driving skills, including wearing a seat belt, discussions about drug and alcohol use as well as ways to solve arguments without guns and violence, and formulation of a healthful lifestyle in response to the stress of daily living. Providing safety information is crucial in helping the adolescent to make mature decisions about health hazards peculiar to this age group.

Adult. Young and middle-aged adults need to be reminded about the effects of stress on their lifestyle. Coping with the demands of raising a family and establishing and promoting a career may lead to the development of unsafe health practices and reliance on drugs or alcohol. Unsafe behaviors can be modified and changed, but this requires considerable effort and commitment on the part of the adult client. The nurse may be directly involved in health education and counseling measures or may suggest resources to contact for additional support.

Older Adult. Most accidents that involve older adults are preventable. Falls, fires, and motor vehicle accidents are significant hazards for this age group. Many risk factors for falls (listed earlier in this chapter) apply to the older person.

Visual changes and slowed reaction time are realistic concerns that affect the older driver. Some become overly cautious, whereas others are prone to careless responses. Interventions aimed at helping the older client drive safely include maintaining the automobile in optimum driving condition, scheduling regular eye examinations, wearing corrective lenses when necessary, and keeping noise from radio and other equipment to a minimum. Some states require additional testing for the older person to renew a driving license.

The older person is at greater risk for suffering burn injuries. Confusion, forgetfulness, and diminished visual and olfactory senses are factors. More fires occur in the home than in healthcare facilities, and smoke inhalation frequently is the cause of death. Nursing interventions directed at helping to promote a fire-safe environment for the older client at home include admonitions not to smoke in bed, recommendations for installing a smoke-detecting device, and encouragement to wear nonflammable clothing.

Accidental overdosing on medications also is a safety risk. Poor eyesight or confusion may result in dosage errors. Special devices, such as medication trays, can be prefilled, and serve as a reminder to prevent the older person from taking additional doses.

Orienting the Person to Surroundings

A person who is familiar with his or her surroundings is less likely to suffer an accidental injury. As part of the admission routine, the nurse orients the client to all the safety features and equipment in the room. An explanation and demonstration of the adjustable bed and side rails, call system, telephone, television, and bathroom area facilitate adjustment to the new environment. Application of an identification bracelet and discussion of agency routine further ensure safety and assist the client to adapt to an unfamiliar setting. Similarly, the nurse addresses the importance of orienting an older person to new surroundings when taking up residence with a son, daughter, or other caregiver.

Preventing Falls

Major causes of falls in the home include slippery surfaces, poor lighting, clutter, and improperly fitting clothing or slippers. The living room, hall, bedroom, bathroom, and stairs are the areas in the home where most falls occur. Measures as simple as hand rails in bathrooms and on stairs, good lighting, and discarding or repairing broken equipment about the home help prevent accidents.

The following safety measures are recommended to reduce the number of falls in acute and extended care facilities:

- Thorough orientation to surroundings
- Careful survey of physical surroundings for hazards
- Bed wheels locked and bed in low position
- Call bell and personal articles within client's reach
- Examination of client's footwear
- Appropriate use of restraints only when alternative measures have failed and their use has been prescribed

Some examples are shown in Figure 27-2.

Using Side Rails

Side rails provide support and aid equilibrium but are especially important for the safety of clients who are likely to be disoriented, restless, confused, or unconscious (see Fig. 27-2). When in doubt about the client's mental status, it is better to err in the overuse of side rails than to contribute to a situation that results in a person's falling out of bed. A confused client may attempt to climb over side rails or out the foot of the bed. The client may fall out of bed or disturb tubes, equipment, dressings, or wounds. In such cases, it may be necessary to use restraints with raised side rails as a temporary solution to protect the client. An explanation frequently facilitates cooperation with their use.

Recent guidelines for long-term care facilities indicate that side rails can be viewed as restraints in certain situations. If the client chooses to have side rails raised, then side rails are not considered to be a restraining device. As part of the assessment process, the nurse assigns one of the following risk levels to a client:

Level 1—Low Risk: Side rails are not necessary but client may choose to have them raised.

Level 2—Moderate Risk: Client desires to get out of bed unassisted but is unable to do this safely. For this client, side rails are considered restraints and require a physician's order.

Level 3—High Risk: Client requires side rails because alternative measures have failed and there are no other options. Side rails in this instance are restraints, should be used on a short-term basis, and require a physician's order (Donius & Rader, 1994).

Using Restraints and Alternatives

Restraints are physical or chemical devices used to limit a client's movement. Side rails, geriatric chairs with attached trays, and appliances tied at the wrist, ankle, or waist are types of physical restraints. Chemical or pharmacologic agents, such as sleeping pills, sedatives, and tranquilizers, also may either intentionally or inadvertently restrain activity and behavior. Older clients are more likely to be restrained than younger clients. During hospitalization, Mion et al. (1994) reported that one fifth of older adults on medical and surgical units were restrained. Frequently, more than one type of restraint is used but the vest device is the most common one. Figure 27-3 shows types of physical restraints used for adults and children.

In the last decade, the federal government and accrediting agencies have actively supported the reduction or elimination of the practice of using restraints. This focus on strengthening the rights of clients is not without precedent. In Europe, restraint use is practically nonexistent; in Canada, restraints have been available only by prescription since 1981 (Weick, 1992). Guidelines formulated by the Health Care Financing Administration as part of the 1987 Omnibus Budget Reconciliation Act (OBRA) emphasized the limited use of restraints in long-term settings. After several years of collecting data about injuries and deaths attributed to restraint use, the Food and Drug Administration (FDA), in 1991, issued a warning about restraints with recommendations for their limited use. Reports to the FDA indicated that there were more than 100 deaths per year directly related to the use of restraints (Weick, 1992). The FDA also required that manufacturers label restraints as available by prescription only rather than over the counter. An additional FDA safety alert, in 1992, stated that clients or their representatives need information about the risks and benefits of restraint use (see adjacent box) and recommended an informed consent be obtained (U.S. Food and Drug Administration, 1992). More recently the Commission on Accreditation of Rehabilitation Facilities (CARF) and the Joint Commission on Accreditation of Healthcare Organizations (JCAHO) have targeted the need for specific standards and policies including physician's orders, time

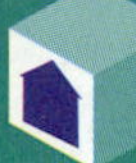

Home Care: Bridging the Gap

Preventing Falls

Exterior	Suggested Improvements
Lighting	Replace burnt-out or dim bulbs. Arrange for lighting along all walking areas.
Walking areas	Surfaces should be even and in good repair.
Steps	Secure hand rails should be available with adequate lighting provided.
General environment	Keep uncluttered and free of debris.
Interior	
Bathroom	
Floor surface	Apply nonslip adhesive strips on floor in front of toilet, at sink, and in front of and inside shower area.
Toilet	Install raised toilet seat with support arms.
Grab bars	Position secure grab bars next to toilet and in tub or shower area.
Scatter rugs	Eliminate or attach double-faced, nonslip adhesive strips to underneath surface of rug.
Thresholds	Replace with threshold even with floor or plane down existing one.
Lighting	Provide adequate lighting for all areas (toilet, washing areas, medicine cabinet).
Accessories	Use contrasting colors for easier visibility. Use liquid soap in dispenser or bar soap on a rope.
Limited space	Provide grab bars in appropriate locations and modify bathroom fixtures with nonslip adhesive strips to provide nonslippery support area.
Kitchen	
Cabinets and shelves	Have secure, sturdy stool with nonslip treads available. Reposition shelves to allow for easier reach.
Lighting	Provide adequate lighting, particularly in working areas.
Accessibility of objects	Use hand-held reaching device for inaccessible objects.
Floor area	Install nonslip adhesive strips on floor in front of sink and stove. Remove any scatter rugs.
Chairs	Use sturdy chairs with armrests. Height should be appropriate to allow for easy rising. Avoid chairs with crossbar between front legs because it interferes with placing feet firmly under chair when rising.
Bedrooms and Other Living Areas	
Lighting	Provide adequate lighting. Use night lights where appropriate.
Floor area	Avoid scatter rugs. Use nonslip adhesive strips where surface is slippery. Secure raised edges of carpet with tape to prevent catching heel or toe of shoe.
Chairs	Use sturdy chairs with armrests.
Accessory tables	Replace wobbly tables that may be used for support while walking. Keep table surfaces uncluttered. Place colored nonslip adhesive strips on edges of glass tables.
Stairs	
Lighting	Provide adequate lighting. Install light switch at top and bottom of stairs.
Steps	Paint or carpet in contrasting color for improved visibility. Install nonslip rubber strips to accentuate stair edges. Keep stairs free of clutter.
Support	Provide secure hand rails on both sides of steps.

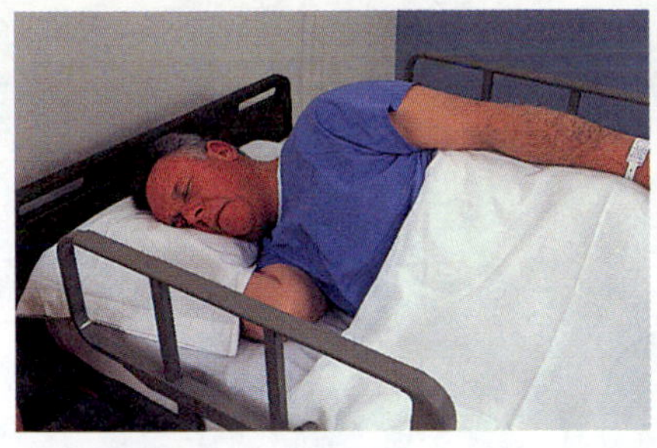
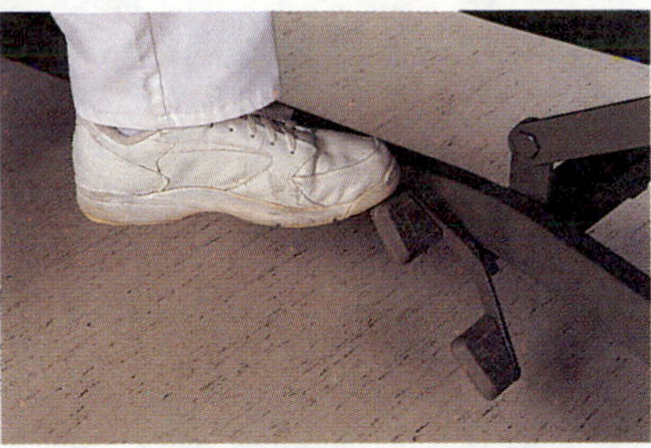
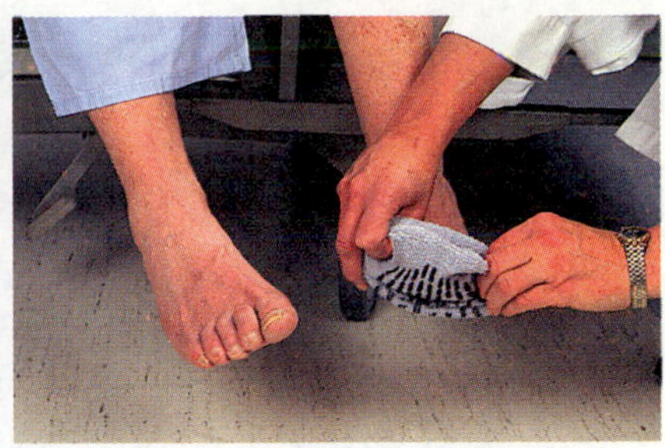

Figure 27-2
Side rails on beds, locking devices on wheeled equipment, and non-skid slippers are some of the safety devices used in healthcare agencies and the home to prevent falls. (Photos © B. Proud.)

limitations for application, and observation intervals in rehabilitative and acute care facilities (Stolley, 1995). The JCAHO guidelines clearly state that restraints should only be applied when less-restrictive or alternative measures have proved ineffective in protecting the client (Corr & Corr, 1994).

Nurses consistently cite the risk of injury from falls as the primary reason for applying restraints (Varone et al., 1992; Werner et al., 1994; Hardin et al., 1994). Other justifications include protection of the healthcare facility from a lawsuit, compensation for inadequate staffing, and prevention of any interference with medical treatment such as attempting to remove tubes and catheters (Haddad, 1994). Research has demonstrated that restraints do not guarantee safety and, in fact, can cause harm to clients. The following are physiologic hazards associated with the use of restraints:

- Danger of suffocation from improperly applied vests
- Impaired circulation
- Altered skin integrity (eg, abrasions, skin tears, bruises)
- Pressure ulcers and contractures
- Diminished muscle and bone mass
- Fractures
- Altered nutrition and hydration
- Aspiration and breathing difficulties
- Incontinence

Tappen & Beckerman (1993) reported that older clients who were restrained for more than 4 days also had an increased risk of developing hospital-acquired infections. Another recent study questioned the effectiveness of restraints in preventing falls and observed that restrained older people were three times as likely to sustain fall-related injuries (Tinetti, Liu, & Ginter, 1992). In addition, it is not uncommon for the restrained person to become more confused, agitated, angry, depressed, and embarrassed.

Nurses frequently have ambivalent feelings about using restraints or protective devices. Their dilemma results when concern about the client's potential risk of injury conflicts with the nurse's awareness of the indignity, as well as the regression an older person may suffer when placed in restraints. Although safety is a priority concern, Varone et al. (1992) report that there are more successful fall-related lawsuits involving use of restraints than nonuse of restraints. Also, litigation in cases of nonrestraint is uncommon because U.S. courts are reluctant to uphold the duty to restrain an individual because of the belief that they may violate the quality of an individual's life (Stolley, 1995).

An awareness of the potential harm restraints can cause has prompted nurses to look for alternative methods of ensuring client safety and preventing serious falls (see Fig. 27-4 for restraint alternatives). Careful nursing assessment is the key. Identifying the cause of the problem—although it may require more time and effort than simply applying a restraint or giving a medication—is the critical ingredient in finding a solution. A Canadian staff nurse reported that the time required to monitor a client in restraints (her agency policy specifies 15-minute checks) would be more effectively utilized attempting alternative measures (Janelli, Kanski, & Neary, 1994). Individualized nursing interventions may effectively reduce confusion or agitation and provide a safe environment (see the accompanying box).

Despite all efforts, restraints may be the only solution in some situations. It is important to explain to the client and his or her family that the restraints are being applied as a protective device, not as a punishment measure. Documentation should include alternative strategies that were ineffective, the reason for restraining the client, the type of restraint and the time it was applied, pertinent nursing assessments, and the regular intervals when restraints were removed. Procedure 27-1 demonstrates the proper method for applying restraints.

A physician's order ordinarily is required to apply restraints, but some agencies allow nurses to apply them in certain emergencies provided a verbal or written time-limited physician's order is obtained. A clearly stated agency policy assists the nurse in determining when to apply restraints as well as which type to use, and reflects the institution's concern for client safety as well as its respect for the quality of human life. Constant re-evaluation of the need for the restraint is vital. Student nurses, from their earliest clinical experiences, need help to identify and assess the cause of a client's behavior and not just the behavior itself (Schott-Baer, Lusis, & Beauregard, 1995). Careful client assessment provides the bridge to developing creative alternative strategies.

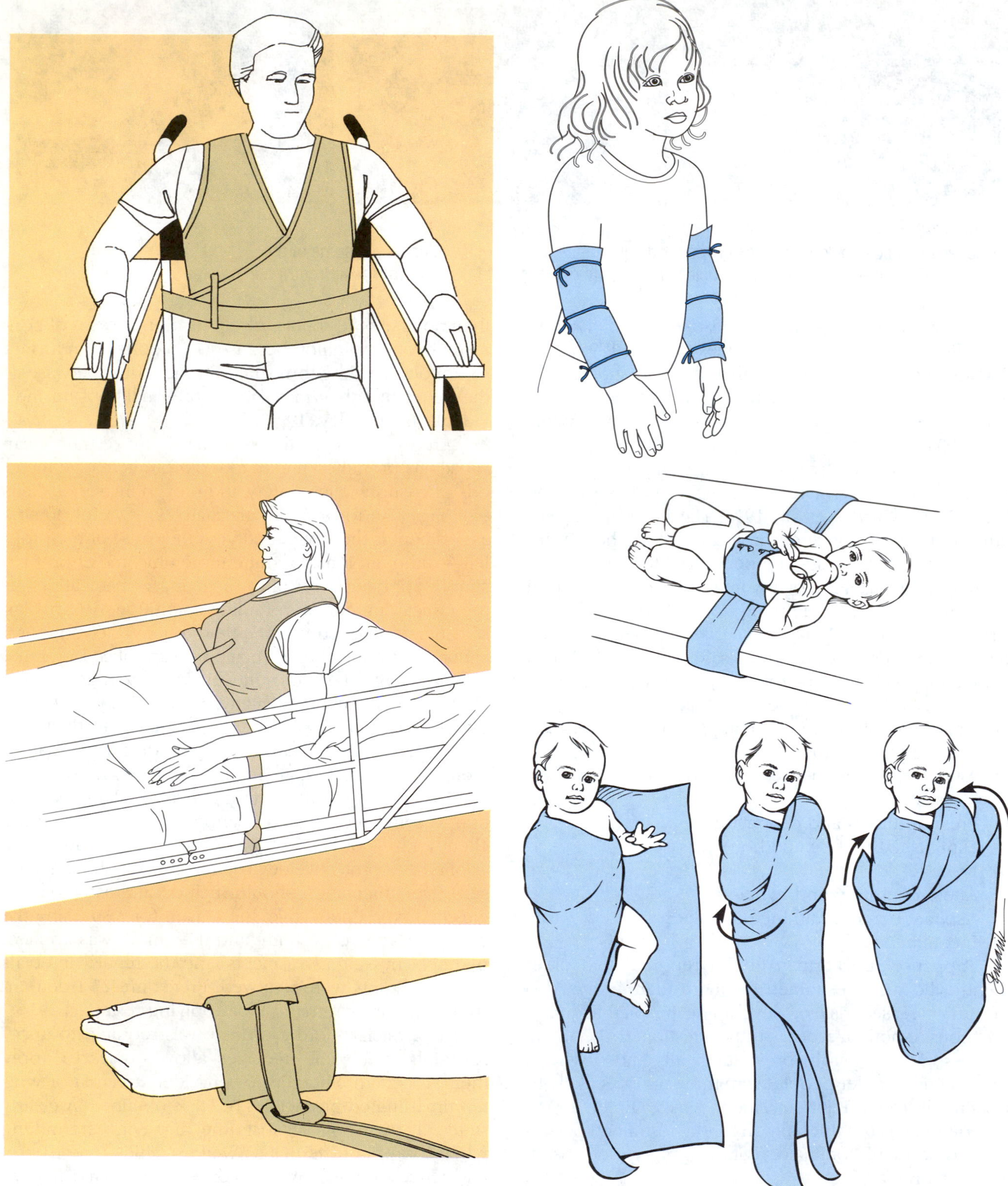

Figure 27-3
A variety of restraints used for adults and children. The purpose of restraints is to help prevent the client from being harmed. Restraints should not interfere with physiologic functioning, such as impairing circulation, limiting muscular activity to the point of immobilization, or interfering with respiration. Restraints that can be adjusted to the desired activity limitation are most likely to be accepted by the client and family.

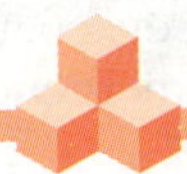

Guidelines for Nursing Care

Using Patient Restraints Correctly

Physical patient restraints can be useful in protecting the patients/residents from falls and from wandering or straying. However, restraints are not the only solution to these difficulties, and in some cases may be more dangerous. The following are important tips that can make you more aware of when and how restraints should be used. It will also help you identify problems that could have serious consequences if not responded to.

Patient Rights: Patients/residents have the right to be free from restraints. Restraint use should not be a first-choice solution. Before allowing yourself or a loved one to be restrained, be sure to understand the reason for the restraint use, request a limited time frame for restraint use, and be sure that all other solutions to the problem have been exhausted.

Facility Policy: All healthcare facilities must have a written policy on use of patient restraints. Ask to see this document and be sure that you understand and are comfortable with the policy set forth by your facility.

Prescription Device: Restraints are prescription devices and may only be used if a physician, or other healthcare professional licensed to prescribe in your state, has specifically ordered a restraint for an individual. The need for the restraint must be well documented in the patient chart and assessment of the need should continue even after the device has been ordered.

Patient Criteria: Not all patients/residents are appropriate for restraint use. For example, an agitated or seriously confused patient may not be a good candidate for restraints. The use of restraints may only add to this agitation or confusion and place the patient in jeopardy as he or she may try to escape from the device. These medical symptoms combined with the use of a restraint may lead to a serious injury or death.

Appropriate Size: It is very important to be sure that the appropriate size of restraint is selected. A restraint that is too small will be uncomfortable for the patient and may cause agitation or constriction of bodily parts. A restraint that is too large or loose, where the patient can slide down or forward, may result in asphyxiation.

Good Labeling: Manufacturers of patient restraints are being required to develop better labeling. They are also being encouraged to use graphics in improved labels, sewn directly on the device, to help ensure proper application. Look for these labels and alert a healthcare provider if it appears a device is on incorrectly or a patient is uncomfortable in a restraint.

Proper Use: For wheelchair use, be sure that the patient is upright and securely seated in the chair before applying the restraint. See device directions for correct application. Incorrect application is more likely to result in the patient sliding forward which may result in asphyxiation. For use in a bed, be sure the restraint is *never* tied to the bed rails or mattress. The restraint should only be tied to the bed springs. Also, most restraints are not indicated for use with regular beds or regular chairs, including geri-chairs. Consult the manufacturer labeling for correct application of the restraint to any bed or chair.

Length of Wear: Any patient/resident in a restraint must be free of that restraint at frequent intervals to ensure good patient health. Long-term immobilization can contribute to various health problems including decubitus ulcers, nerve damage, incontinence, and sensory deprivation. Consult with the facility policy for the maximum length of each period of restraint use. During the time when the patient is free of the restraint, be sure that exercise, such as walking, is available and encouraged.

Patient Monitoring: Patients/residents must be monitored frequently while wearing a restraint device. As with any other medical device, supervision and monitoring are critical to ensure the safety of the patient.

Ask your facility what alternatives exist or are being developed to reduce the use of restraints. Restraints should never be used as a substitute for nursing care. They are an adjunct to proper care. In many cases, volunteers may be all a facility needs to help keep patients free from restraints. However, if you are aware of the potential dangers of restraint use and know what to look for and what to do if you see a restraint being used incorrectly, it could save a patient from a serious injury or even death.

(U.S. Department of Health and Human Services, Food and Drug Administration, Rockville, MD 20857.)

Preventing Fires and Maintaining Fire Safety

Careless smoking, faulty electrical equipment, or combustion of anesthetic agents are most frequently implicated as causes of hospital fires; cigarettes, grease, and electrical problems are most often responsible for fires in the home.

Healthcare Agency. Orientations to healthcare agencies stress fire prevention information and the agency's smoking policy. The nurse is responsible for the client's safety and needs to be familiar with the agency's fire safety plan, exits, location and operation of fire extinguishers, and any special directions to report the fire.

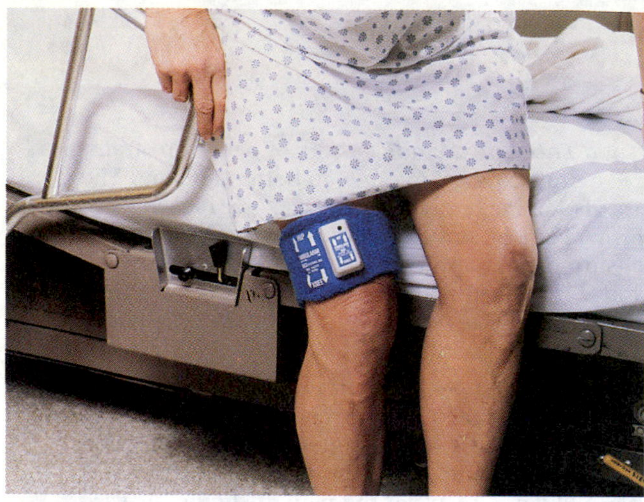

Figure 27-4
The use of a position-sensitive electronic alarm is an alternative to restraints. (Photo of AMBULARM courtesy of AlertCare, Inc.)

Most hospital procedures emphasize the following priorities:

- Move anyone in immediate danger out of the area first.
- Call for help and activate the fire code system.
- Use the appropriate type of fire extinguisher to confine the fire (Fig. 27-5).

Home. The focus of nursing education for home fire safety includes a plan of action similar to that used in a healthcare setting. Priorities and practical suggestions include the following:

- Keep emergency numbers near the telephone.
- Rehearse response to fire alarm and fire evacuation routes with family members before an emergency occurs.
- Evacuate family members as soon as smoke or fire is detected.
- Use the stairs to exit; do not use the elevator.
- Use a fire extinguisher if one is available and the fire is small.
- Close the doors to rooms. Open or break a window only if this is necessary to obtain fresh air.
- Remain close to the floor because smoke rises.
- Cover your nose and mouth with a wet washcloth to prevent smoke inhalation.
- Do not run if your clothing catches fire. Lie down and roll on the floor to extinguish the flames. Another person may smother the flames with a blanket or coat. Remember: *Stop, drop, and roll.*
- Install approved smoke detectors with working batteries in recommended locations.
- Do not let children play near space heaters, wood-burning stoves, or fireplaces.

Home Healthcare Alert

Encourage family members to replace smoke detector batteries once a year or when the detector chirps to signal that the battery is dead. Instruct them not to borrow smoke detector batteries for other uses.

Preventing Poisoning

Concerted efforts by individuals, communities, state governments, and the federal government have reduced the number of accidental deaths by poisoning. Child-

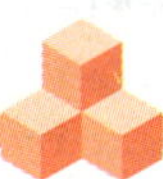

Guidelines for Nursing Care

Choosing Alternatives to Restraints

- Determine if behavior pattern exists.
- Provide pain relief.
- Involve the family in client's care.
- Reduce noise.
- Check environment for hazards.
- Use night light.
- Identify door of room (eg, use of balloon, sign, client's picture, ribbon).
- Use an alarm system (eg, bed or position-sensitive alarms).
- Allow restless client to walk after ensuring that environment is safe.
- Use half rails or keep side rails in down position.
- Use a large plant or piece of furniture as a barrier to limit wandering from designated area.
- Maintain low bed position.
- Use therapeutic touch.
- Play music or video selections of the client's choice.
- Use pillows wedged against the side of the chair to keep client positioned safely.
- Assist with toileting at frequent intervals.
- Arrange for a bedside commode.
- Make the environment as homelike as possible.
- Provide a warm beverage.
- Provide comfortable rocking chairs.
- Allow the client to assist the staff with simple tasks.
- Encourage daily exercise.
- Investigate possibility of discontinuing bothersome treatment devices (eg, IV, catheter, feeding tube).

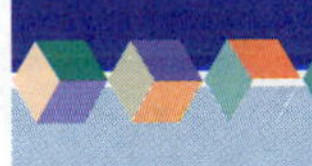

PROCEDURE 27-1

Applying Restraints

Equipment

- Restraint
- Padding, if necessary, for bony prominences

Action	Rationale
1. Determine the need for restraints.	Restraints (physical or chemical) should be used only as a last resort when alternative measures have failed.
2. Confirm agency policy for application of restraints. Secure a physician's order.	Policy protects the client and the nurse and specifies guidelines for application as well as type of restraint to be used.
3. Explain reason for use to client and family. Clarify how care will be given and needs will be met and that use of restraint is a temporary measure.	Explanation to client and family may lessen confusion and anger and provide reassurance. A clearly stated agency policy on application of restraints should be available for client and family to read.
4. Obtain informed consent from the client or family before applying the restraint.	FDA advises informed consent. If client and/or family refuse the use of restraints, document the refusal along with the reasons you believe restraints are indicated.
5. Wash your hands.	Handwashing deters the spread of microorganisms.
6. Apply restraints according to manufacturer's direction:	Proper application ensures that there is no interference with client's respiration and circulation. FDA advises manufacturers place "front" and "back" labels on vest restraints and that correct size be used.
a. Choose the least restrictive type of device that allows the greatest possible degree of mobility.	This provides minimal restriction.
b. Pad bony prominences	Padding prevents skin breakdown.
c. For restraint applied to extremity, ensure that two fingers can be inserted between the restraint and client's wrist or ankle.	This prevents impaired circulation to extremity.

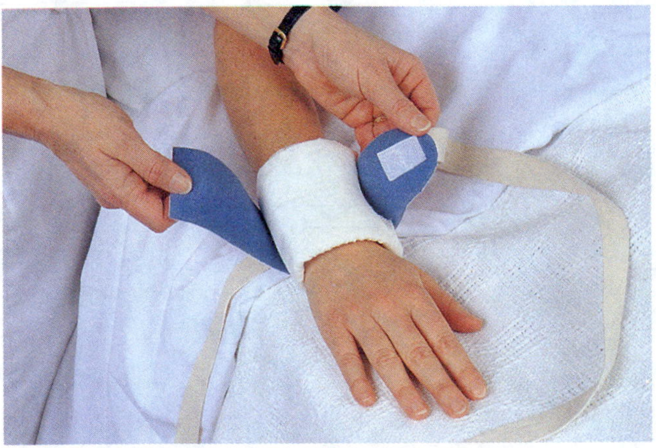

Action 6b: Applying restraint over padded bony prominences.

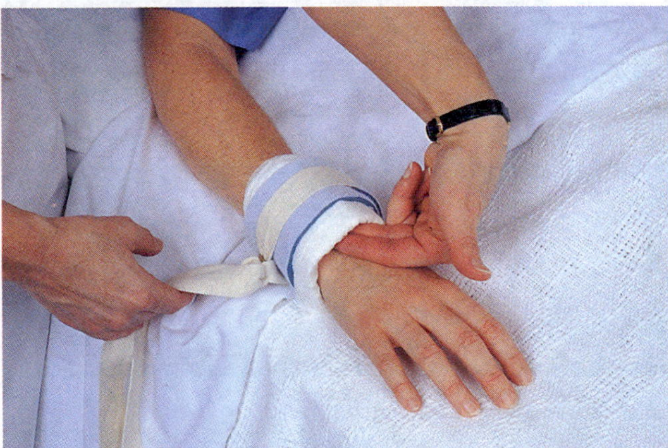

Action 6c: Ensuring that two fingers can be inserted between the restraint and the wrist.

(continued)

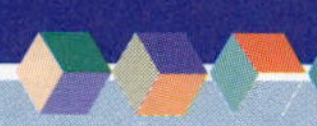

PROCEDURE 27-1 *(continued)*

Applying Restraints

Action	Rationale
d. Maintain restrained extremity in normal anatomic position.	This lessens possibility for development of contracture or musculoskeletal injury.
e. Use appropriate tie for all restraints.	A quick-release knot ensures that restraint will not tighten when pulled and can be removed quickly in an emergency.
f. Fasten restraint to the bed frame and not the side rail. Site should not be readily accessible to the client.	Restraint secured to a side rail may injure the client when side rail is lowered. Tying restraint out of client's reach promotes security.

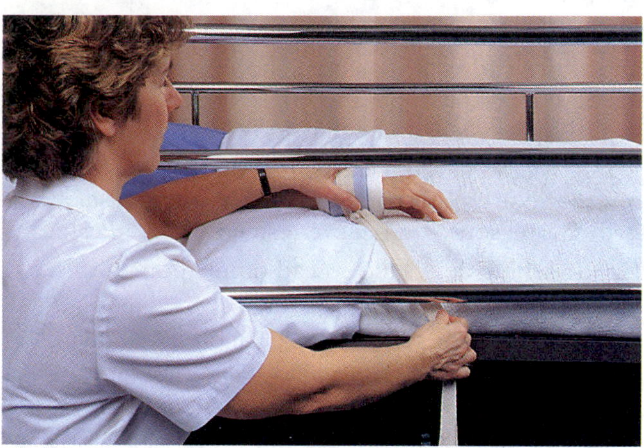

Action 6d: Keeping extremity in normal anatomic position.

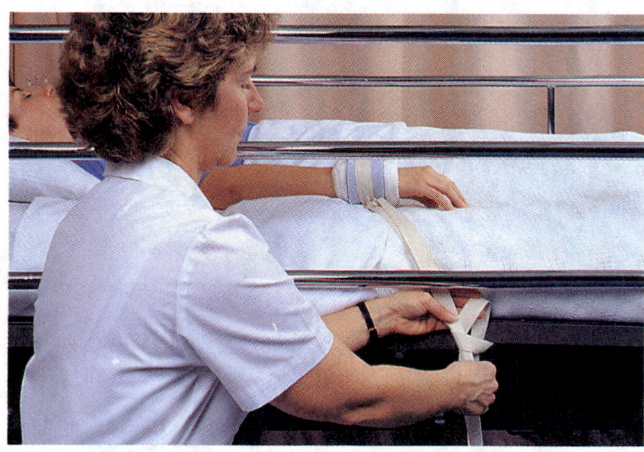

Action 6f: Fastening restraint to bed frame.

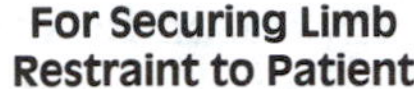

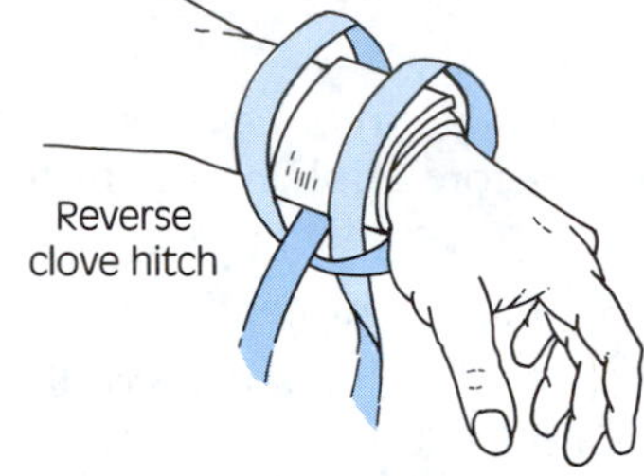

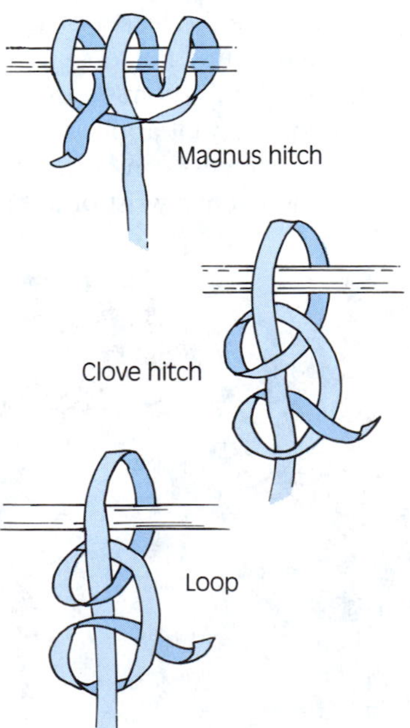

Action 6e: Knots for restraints.

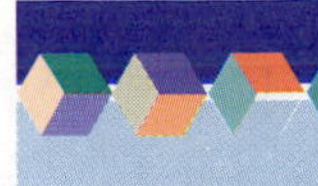

PROCEDURE 27-1 *(continued)*

Applying Restraints

Action	Rationale
7. Remove restraint at least every 2 hours or according to agency policy and client need.	Removal allows for assessment of client and reevaluation of need for restraint.
a. Check for signs of decreased circulation or impaired skin integrity.	Improperly applied restraints may cause skin tears, abrasions, or bruises. Decreased circulation may result in paleness, coolness, decreased sensation, tingling, numbness, or pain in an extremity.
b. Perform range-of-motion exercises before reapplying.	Exercise increases circulation in the restrained extremity.
8. Reassure client at regular intervals.	Reassurance demonstrates caring and provides opportunity for sensory stimulation as well as ongoing assessment and evaluation.
9. Assess for signs of sensory deprivation, such as increased sleeping, day-dreaming, anxiety, panic, and hallucinations.	Use of restraints may decrease environmental stimulation and result in sensory deprivation.
10. Wash your hands.	Handwashing deters the spread of microorganisms.
11. Document reason for restraining client, alternative measures attempted before applying the restraint, time of application, type of restraint, times when removed, and result and frequency of nursing assessment for every shift.	Careful documentation supports use of restraints, alternative measures to ensure safety, and assessment data.

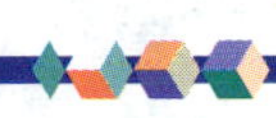

proof containers are primarily responsible for this reduction. Nursing education efforts can also impact on behaviors that place older adults at risk for poisoning. Suggestions for a safe medical regimen are included in the accompanying box.

Nursing intervention involves health education aimed at preventing accidental poisoning in the home. Parents need to be aware of hazardous substances that could result in poisoning if ingested. Plants frequently are implicated as a dangerous poison that is available in or near the home. Toxic household substances should be removed or stored safely out of a child's reach. Local poison control centers can provide information about poisonous substances found in or near the home. Additional suggestions for childproofing homes are listed in the box.

It is vital that every household have the telephone number of the nearest poison control center readily available. The nurse should emphasize to parents that they should call the poison control center immediately, before they attempt any home remedy. Parents should be instructed to keep syrup of ipecac on hand but not to administer it unless directed to do so by medical authorities to induce vomiting. They may be instructed to bring the child immediately to an emergency facility for treatment. The focus of emergency treatment of poisoning is to stabilize vital body functions, prevent the absorption of the poison, and encourage excretion of the toxic substance.

The nurse should recommend that a carbon monoxide (CO) detector be installed to alert family members to toxic levels of the gas. The gas company, oil company, or local health authority can provide help with identifying and removing sources of CO contamination. The U.S. Consumer Product Safety Commission (CPSC) has proposed national mandatory installation of CO detectors in all new residential construction beginning in 1995 and has also recommended installation of these monitors in all existing homes (Centers for Disease Control, 1994).

Home Healthcare Alert

To prevent food poisoning, caution family members never to taste or feed the client any fresh or prepared foods that look or smell spoiled. Even a small taste can introduce dangerous bacteria into the body and cause a serious illness to develop.

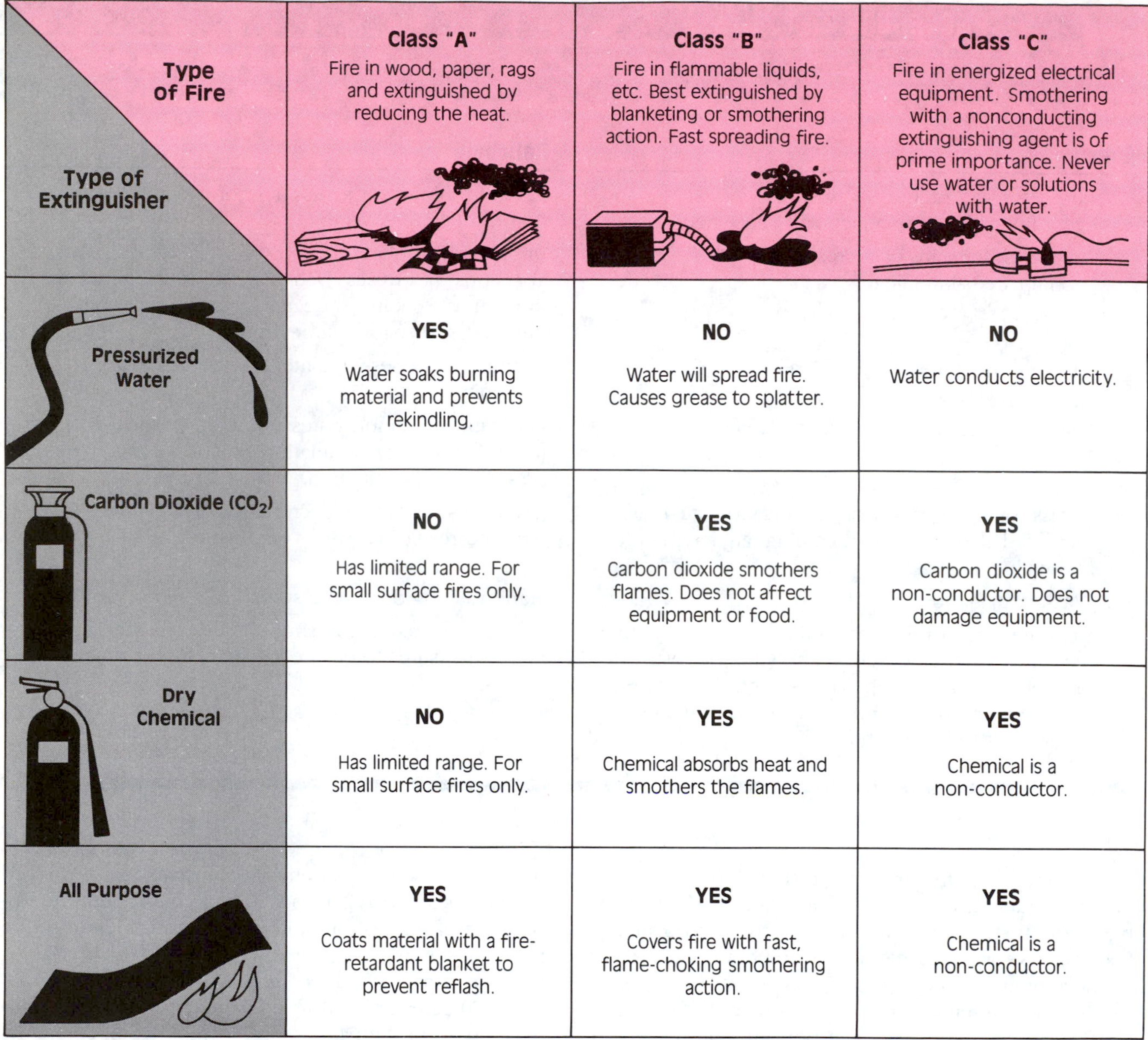

Type of Extinguisher / Type of Fire	Class "A" Fire in wood, paper, rags and extinguished by reducing the heat.	Class "B" Fire in flammable liquids, etc. Best extinguished by blanketing or smothering action. Fast spreading fire.	Class "C" Fire in energized electrical equipment. Smothering with a nonconducting extinguishing agent is of prime importance. Never use water or solutions with water.
Pressurized Water	**YES** Water soaks burning material and prevents rekindling.	**NO** Water will spread fire. Causes grease to splatter.	**NO** Water conducts electricity.
Carbon Dioxide (CO_2)	**NO** Has limited range. For small surface fires only.	**YES** Carbon dioxide smothers flames. Does not affect equipment or food.	**YES** Carbon dioxide is a non-conductor. Does not damage equipment.
Dry Chemical	**NO** Has limited range. For small surface fires only.	**YES** Chemical absorbs heat and smothers the flames.	**YES** Chemical is a non-conductor.
All Purpose	**YES** Coats material with a fire-retardant blanket to prevent reflash.	**YES** Covers fire with fast, flame-choking smothering action.	**YES** Chemical is a non-conductor.

Figure 27-5
Appropriate fire extinguisher usage for specific types of fires.

Preventing Suffocation

Suffocation results almost immediately in unconsciousness, followed by respiratory and cardiac arrest. Emergency measures must be undertaken without delay and involve removing any obstruction and initiating cardiopulmonary resuscitation.

The educated and alert parent can reduce the risk of suffocation in the home. The nurse may be involved in child care instruction that emphasizes careful supervision of children when they are drinking from a bottle, eating, bathing, or playing near a swimming pool. When riding in a motor vehicle, a child less than 55 inches (1.4 m) tall needs to be restrained using an appropriate car seat rather than an adult seat belt and shoulder harness, which can slip with impact and cause neck injury. Other potential hazards include plastic bags, balloons, soft pillows or thick blankets in a crib, and allowing an infant to sleep on a water bed. Health education is a valuable preventive force.

Preventing Injury From Firearms

Nurses are in a unique position to raise awareness and reduce high-risk behavior that may lead to injury or death from firearms. In homes, schools, and other health-care settings, nurses have the opportunity to provide the information that may persuade parents to keep guns away from children. Parents may be unaware of the magnitude of gunshot injuries or misinformed about the dan-

Focus on the Older Adult

Preventing Poisoning in the Elderly

Although poisonings happen more frequently in children, poison control centers receive many calls from adults, particularly older adults, regarding accidental poisonings. The older population uses more medications than any other age group and may also be more susceptible to the effects of various drugs. The following information includes suggestions for preventing poisonings in the older individual, as well as adults of any age:

- Do not hesitate to call the physician, nurse, or pharmacist with any questions.
- Keep the telephone numbers for your health-care providers and the Poison Control Center in a readily accessible place.
- Develop good communication with your physician, nurse, and pharmacist.
- Report side effects from medications to health-care provider.
- Do not stop taking any prescription drug or change the dose without first consulting with the physician or nurse.
- Request large-print labels from your pharmacist.
- Use a medication calendar or diary to keep track of your dosing schedule.
- Use a pill dispenser as a medication reminder tool.
- Avoid doubling a dose if you forget a medication. Check with the physician or nurse first.
- Avoid mixing alcohol with medicines without first checking with the pharmacist.
- Do not share medications with others or take their pills.
- When a drug is discontinued, throw away any remaining medication.

ger and implications for injury when a gun is accessible for children and young adults. As a prevention partner, the nurse can begin to have an impact on controlling this epidemic of gun injuries and death.

Preventing Equipment-Related Accidents

Healthcare Agency. With the marked increase in the use of highly sophisticated equipment, it is especially important for health practitioners to learn to use equipment properly and to recognize the signs that indicate that the equipment is not functioning correctly. For example, failure to use protective belts or side rails on carts and to lock wheelchair wheels can result in client injury. Using suction devices with inadequate vacuum and rate regulators or infusion equipment that delivers erratic amounts of solution also has resulted in equipment-related accidents.

Electrical equipment can present a particular safety hazard to both client and health practitioner when safety

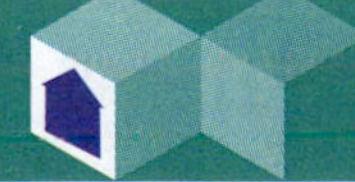

Home Care: Bridging the Gap

Preventing Childhood Poisoning

- Keep all medications and toxic products in original containers.
- Keep childproof caps on toxic products if children live in the home or are frequent visitors.
- Keep all medications, including vitamins, out of the reach of children, in a locked chest.
- Keep household chemical products out of the reach of children.
- Do not treat medicines as candy.
- Do not take or give medicine in the dark.
- Read labels carefully before using drugs or toxic products.
- Keep emergency poison control telephone numbers handy.
- Have emergency drugs in the home—syrup of ipecac and epsom salts.
- Use toxic chemical products in a well-ventilated area.
- Do not mix common household cleaning products.
- Destroy all old medications.
- Destroy unused medications by flushing down toilet or washing down sink rather than by throwing in trash.
- Use childproof containers when available.
- Identify any poisonous houseplants, and keep seeds, bulbs, leaves, and fruits of such plants away from children.

(Spencer, R.T., Nichols, L., Lipkin, G., Henderson, H., & West, F. [1993]. *Clinical pharmacology and nursing management* [4th ed.]. Philadelphia: Lippincott.)

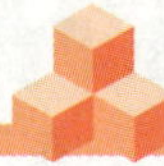

Guidelines for Nursing Care

Decreasing Equipment-Related Accidents

- Use equipment only for the use for which it was intended.
- Do not operate equipment with which you are unfamiliar.
- Handle equipment with care to prevent damaging it.
- Use three-prong electric plugs whenever possible.
- Do not twist or bend electric cords. The wires inside the cord may break.
- Be alert to signs that indicate equipment is faulty, such as breaks in electric cords, sparks, smoke, electric shocks, loose or missing parts, and unusual noises or odors. Report signs of trouble immediately.
- Make certain that electric cords are not in a position to be trapped as beds are raised or lowered. This can strip insulation covering the electric wires.
- Be alert for wet surfaces on areas where electric cords or connections are present.

measures are ignored. Most electrical equipment used in hospitals is equipped with three-prong plugs. The third prong, when inserted into a properly wired wall outlet, provides a ground for the piece of equipment. A **ground** is a connection from an electricity source to the earth through which electric current leakage can be harmlessly conducted. Current leakage is not uncommon in electrical equipment, but a grounding system renders the equipment safe.

Most people have experienced a tingling sensation in the extremities and trunk resulting from an electric current passing through a relatively large area of the body. This is known as **macroshock**, and although it is unpleasant, it usually is not harmful. Macroshock often results from an ungrounded appliance or one in which the electric wiring has been damaged.

Microshock is the transmission of an electric current through a relatively small area of the body, usually directly into the heart. Because of the sensitivity of the myocardium to electric impulses, microshock can cause serious or even fatal heart irregularities. People with tubes, wires, or electrodes implanted in their chests or hearts are susceptible to microshock because the tubing or wire can conduct leakage electricity directly to the heart muscle. Particularly because of microshock dangers, only equipment with three-prong plugs is recommended for use in healthcare agencies. Suspicion of ungrounded current leakage, including even a slight tingling sensation when touching a piece of equipment, or any other malfunction of electrical equipment should be reported immediately. The accompanying box lists guidelines to help reduce the number of equipment-related accidents.

Home. Accidents in the home frequently result from the careless use of equipment or from using malfunctioning or poorly maintained equipment. Many injuries and deaths from electric shock can be avoided. Overload of electric circuits, faulty appliances, frayed wires, careless use of electrical equipment, and handling of electrical devices and cords when shoes and hands are wet often result in injury and death.

Preventing Procedure-Related Accidents

The nurse must always be cautious and alert to prevent a procedure-related accident. The potential for error exists when the nurse is administering medications or intravenous solutions, transferring a client, changing a dressing, or applying external heat to a client's extremity. It is vital that the nurse follow correct procedures when administering care. Safeguards to prevent errors include making sure that the client is correctly identified (Fig. 27-6). A system of checking and rechecking further ensures the client's safety. The availability and use of resources further corroborate any question about correct procedure and prevent procedure-related accidents.

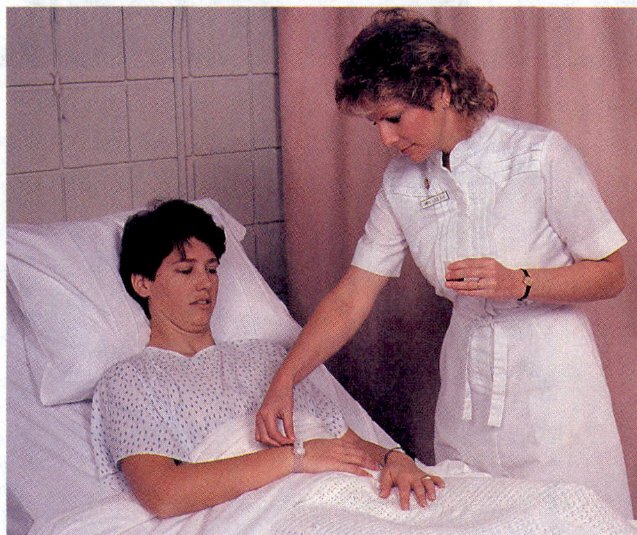

Figure 27-6
An essential nursing responsibility is checking the client's identification bracelet before any procedure. Here the nurse checks the client's identification before administering medications.

Filing an Incident Report

An accident in a healthcare agency requires the completion of an incident report, a confidential document that objectively describes the circumstances of the accident. The report also provides details concerning the client's response and the examination and treatment of the client after the incident. The nurse completes the incident report immediately after an accident and is responsible for recording the occurrence of the accident and its effect on the client in the medical record. The incident report itself is not a part of the medical record and should not be mentioned in the documentation. Laws may differ in each state and the nurse has a responsibility to be aware of the appropriate state law.

All incident reports are carefully reviewed to detect any potentially threatening situation or pattern. The focus of a conference after the incident report has been filed is prevention of a similar occurrence and continuation of efforts to deliver quality nursing care. Incident reports are discussed in greater detail in Chapter 7.

Evaluating

The nurse must evaluate the effectiveness of interventions to promote environmental safety and prevent injury. If expected client outcomes have been met and evaluative criteria have been satisfied, the client will:

- Correctly identify real and potential unsafe environmental situations
- Implement safety measures in the environment
- Use available resources for safety information
- Incorporate accident prevention practices into the activities of daily living
- Remain free of injury

Key Points

- Safety is the responsibility of all healthcare providers in every environment.
- Falls are the major safety problem in healthcare facilities as well as the leading cause of accidental death for older people.
- Clients at high risk of falling include older people and those who have previously fallen.
- Careless smoking and faulty electrical equipment are frequently implicated as causes in hospital fires.
- Hazards associated with the use of restraints include suffocation from improperly applied vests, impaired circulation, sensory deprivation, and emotional distress.
- Careful nursing assessment is the critical element in finding creative, resourceful alternatives to using restraints.
- The focus of emergency treatment of poisoning is to stabilize vital body functions, prevent the absorption of the poison, and encourage excretion of the toxic substance.
- Orientation to new surroundings, introduction to staff members, and explanations about equipment and procedures facilitate the client's transfer to a new healthcare setting.
- An incident report must be filed when an accident occurs in a healthcare agency. The report should objectively document the circumstances of the accident.

Study Questions

1. The most common cause of injury to women is
   a. motor vehicle accidents
   b. domestic violence
   c. occupational hazards
   d. accidental falls
2. When transporting a toddler in a motor vehicle, car seats are mandatory
   a. in all 50 states
   b. in 36 of the 50 states
   c. if a seat belt is not available
   d. on interstate highways
3. Which child has the greatest risk for choking and suffocating?
   a. a toddler playing with his 9-year-old brother's construction set
   b. a 4-year-old eating yogurt for lunch
   c. an infant covered with a small blanket and asleep in the crib
   d. a 3-year-old drinking a glass of juice
4. A class C electrical fire is appropriately extinguished by
   a. using an all-purpose extinguisher
   b. spraying it with water
   c. smothering it with a blanket
   d. taking the burning item outside
5. The leading cause of accidental death for people 79 years and older is
   a. fires
   b. exposure to temperature extremes
   c. drug overdose
   d. falls

6. Nursing education efforts that focus on prevention of firearm injuries are important because
   a. the elder population is particularly at risk
   b. deaths among adolescents and children have increased sharply
   c. the National Safety Council recommends that every household have a gun to protect family members
   d. since 1990, they have successfully contributed to a decrease in injuries and deaths from guns
7. Nurses most frequently restrain an older client because
   a. administration requires it
   b. the family has requested it
   c. they are short-staffed
   d. they fear the client may fall
8. Mr. Kennedy is a disoriented, older resident who likes to wander the halls in a long-term care facility. As an alternative to using restraints, the nurse might
   a. seat him in a geriatric chair
   b. use the sheets to secure him snugly in his bed
   c. keep the bed in the high position
   d. identify his door with his picture and a balloon
9. While discussing home safety with the nurse, Mrs. Fuller admits that she always smokes a cigarette in bed before falling asleep at night. An appropriate nursing diagnosis would be
   a. Impaired Gas Exchange related to cigarette smoking
   b. Anxiety related to inability to stop smoking
   c. Risk for Suffocation related to unfamiliarity with fire prevention guidelines
   d. Knowledge Deficit related to lack of follow-through of recommendation to stop smoking
10. Mr. D'Ambro has weakened knees due to arthritis. The home healthcare nurse is aware that he understands the need for safety modifications at home because he
    a. uses the towel bar for support to stand up from the commode
    b. leans on the pedestal table in his bedroom when he dresses
    c. sits only in chairs with armrests
    d. uses a small stepladder to reach an item on an upper shelf
11. When a fire occurs in a client's room, the nurse's priority should be to
    a. rescue the client
    b. extinguish the fire
    c. sound the alarm
    d. run for help
12. The nurse is planning health teaching for a young mother about responding to a poisoning emergency. She should instruct the mother to first
    a. use salt water to induce vomiting
    b. rush the child to the emergency department
    c. call the poison control center
    d. administer syrup of ipecac
13. After reviewing Mr. Sennett's past history of injuries and completing the assessment, the nurse suspects elder abuse. The nurse is aware that
    a. the client is probably the best source of information about the injuries
    b. the typical victim is a black male
    c. the abuser usually is a paid healthcare employee
    d. a family in which conflict and stress exist is frequently implicated
14. The nurse orients an older client to the safety features in her hospital room. A vital component of this admission routine is to
    a. explain how to use the telephone
    b. introduce the client to her roommate
    c. review the hospital policy on visiting hours
    d. explain how to operate the call bell
15. When completing an incident report, the nurse should
    a. include suggestions to prevent the accident from recurring
    b. provide minimal information about the incident
    c. discuss the details with the client before documenting them
    d. objectively describe the incident in detail

Answers With Rationale

1. The correct response is *b.* Domestic violence is widespread and represents the most common cause of injury to women. Older people and young children are particularly at risk of injury from falls; adolescents are injured in motor vehicle accidents more than any other group. The incidence of injury from occupational hazards is relatively low for all groups.
2. The correct response is *a.* All 50 of the states require safety car seats for infants and toddlers at all times.
3. The correct response is *a.* A young child may place small or loose parts in his or her mouth; thus, a toy that is safe for a 9-year-old could kill a toddler. An infant sleeping in a crib without a pillow or large blanket and a 3- and 4-year-old drinking juice and eating yogurt are not particular safety risks.
4. The correct response is *a.* An all-purpose extinguisher will put out an electrical fire because the chemical used is a nonconductor. Water conducts electricity, and smothering with a blanket or moving a burning item outside is ineffective and dangerous.
5. The correct response is *d.* Falls are the leading cause of accidental death in the population 79

years and older. Fires, exposure to temperature extremes, and drug overdose are significant causes of accidental death, but not in this age group.

6. The correct response is *b.* Deaths among adolescents and children have increased sharply since 1990. Keeping a gun in the home can have dangerous consequences and increases the risk for domestic violence. Young children may also be unintentionally injured or killed. Recently, efforts to prevent injuries from guns have become more serious as violent behavior has increased.
7. The correct response is *d.* Nurses most commonly apply restraints to a client because they fear he or she will fall and sustain an injury. Administrators usually say that they do not want clients restrained unless necessary, but may not support the nurse if the client falls. The family also may have ambivalent feelings, but neither their request nor short-staffing is the primary reason that nurses apply restraints.
8. The correct response is *d.* Identifying his door with his picture and the balloon may work as an alternative to restraints. Using the geriatric chair and sheets are forms of physical restraint. Leaving the bed in the high position is a safety risk and will probably result in a fall.
9. The correct answer is *c.* Because Mrs. Fuller is not aware that smoking in bed is extremely dangerous, she is at risk of suffocation from fire. The other three nursing diagnoses are correctly stated but not a priority for this situation.
10. The correct response is *c.* Chairs with armrests increase the client's leverage as he attempts to rise. Towel bars are not designed to provide support, the pedestal table is unsteady and unsafe, and standing on a stool and reaching places the client at risk of falling.
11. The correct response is *a.* The client's safety is always the priority. Sounding the alarm and extinguishing the fire are important once the client is safe. Calling for help, rather than running for assistance, allows you to remain with your clients and is more appropriate, if possible.
12. The correct response is *c.* Always call the poison control center before attempting any home remedies or administering syrup of ipecac. These responses may be dangerous for the victim. The poison control center can supply the doctor or emergency department with specific information to assist in the victim's care.
13. The correct response is *d.* One out of 20 (5%) older Americans is abused, and most often the abuse involves family members rather than a paid employee. The family situation frequently is a stressful one, with some kind of conflict. For a variety of reasons—fear or shame—the abused older person is reluctant to report a family member for abuse.
14. The correct response is *d.* Knowing how to use the call bell is a safety priority, whereas knowing how to use the phone, meeting one's roommate, and an awareness of visiting hours will not necessarily prevent an accidental injury.
15. The correct response is *d.* An incident report is a legal document and must be stated as objectively and completely as possible. It is not a collaborative effort with the client, and any suggestions to prevent this from happening again should be discussed at a postincident conference.

Bibliography

Accident Facts. (1994). Itasca, IL: National Safety Council.

Algase, D. (1992). A century of progress: Today's strategies for responding to wandering behavior. *Journal of Gerontological Nursing, 18*(11), 28–34.

All, A. (1994). A literature review: Assessment and intervention in elder abuse. *Journal of Gerontological Nursing, 20*(7), 25–32.

American Academy of Pediatrics. (1992). Update on air bags. *Safe Ride News, 11*(3), 3.

American Academy of Pediatrics. (1994). AA = alcohol and adolescents. *Safe Ride News, 13*(4), 2–4.

American Academy of Pediatrics/Center to Prevent Handgun Violence. (1994). *Stop: Steps to prevent firearm injury.* Elk Grove Village, IL: AAP.

Brady, R., et al. (1993). Preventing falls in the hospital. *Nursing, 23*(10), 32X.

Carpenito, L. (1995). *Nursing diagnosis: Application to clinical practice* (6th ed.). Philadelphia: Lippincott.

Centers for Disease Control. (1994). Carbon monoxide poisoning—Weld County, Colorado, 1993. *Journal of the American Medical Association, 272*(19), 1489–1490.

Chez, N. (1994). Helping the victim of domestic violence. *American Journal of Nursing, 94*(7), 33–37.

Cohen, C., Neufeld, R., Dunbar, J., Plug, L., & Brever, B. (1996). Old problem, different approach: Alternatives to physical restraints. *Journal of Gerontological Nursing, 22*(2), 23–29.

Corr, K., & Corr, D. (1994). Taking the gloves off: Caring for confused patients without using restraints. *Nursing, 24*(9), 70–72.

Croft, W., & Foraker, S. (1993). Preventing falls in the hospital. *Nursing, 23*(10), 32X.

Devlin, B., & Reynolds, K. (1994). Child abuse: How to recognize it, how to intervene. *American Journal of Nursing, 94*(3), 26–31.

Donius, M., & Rader, J. (1994). Use of siderails: Rethinking a standard of practice. *Journal of Gerontological Nursing, 20*(11), 23–26.

Famighetti, R. (Ed.). (1995). *World almanac and book of facts.* Mahwah, NJ: Funk & Wagnalls.

Fingerhut, L. (1993). Firearm mortality among children and youth. *Advance data from vital and health statistics of the National Center for Health Statistics.* Washington, DC: U.S. Department of Health and Human Services.

Haddad, A. (1994). Acute care decisions: Ethics in action. *RN, 57*(3), 18–20.

Hardin, S., Magee, R., Stratmann, D., Vinson, M., Owen, M., & Hyatt, E. (1994). Extended care and nursing home staff attitudes towards restraints. *Journal of Gerontological Nursing, 20*(3), 23–31.

Hingson, R. (1993). Prevention of alcohol-impaired driving. *Alcohol Health & Research World, 17*(1), 28–33.

Janelli, L., Kanski, G., & Neary, M. (1994). Physical restraints: Has OBRA made a difference? *Journal of Gerontological Nursing, 20*(6), 17–21.

Joint Commission 1994 accreditation manual for hospitals. Volume I: Standards. (1993). Oakbrook Terrace, IL: JCAHO.

Kellermann, A., et. al. (1993). Gun ownership as a risk factor for homicide in the home. *New England Journal of Medicine, 329*(15), 1084–1091.

Lachs, M., & Pillemer, K. (1995). Abuse and neglect of elderly persons. *New England Journal of Medicine, 332*(7), 437–443.

Leger-Krall, S. (1994). When restraints become abusive. *Nursing, 24*(3), 54–56.

Markiewicz, T. (1993). Recognizing, treating, and preventing lead poisoning. *American Journal of Nursing, 93*(10), 59–64.

McConnell, E. (1996). Applying wrist restraints. *Nursing, 26*(1), 28.

Milford, P., & Manser, A. (1995, February 8). Smoke detectors best defense against fires. *News Journal* (Wilmington, DE), B1.

Mion, L., et al. (1994). Use of physical restraints in the hospital setting: Implications for the nurse. *Geriatric Nursing, 15*(3), 127–131.

Mondov, E., & Wray, M. (1994). What's the matter with Johnny? *Canadian Nurse, 90*(4), 35–38.

Myers, Y. (1994, Summer). Poisonings in the elderly. *Poison Pen Notes.* Philadelphia: Poison Control Center.

Rice, R. (1994). Safety in the community. *Home Healthcare Nurse, 12*(3), 70.

Roberts, B., & Wykle, M. (1993). Pilot study results: Falls among institutionalized elderly. *Journal of Gerontological Nursing, 19*(5), 13–20.

Ryan, J., Dinkel, J., & Petrucci, K. (1993). Near falls incidence: A study of older adults in the community. *Journal of Gerontological Nursing, 19*(12), 23–28.

Schott-Baer, D., Lusis, S., & Beauregard, K. (1995). Use of restraints: Changes in nurses' attitudes. *Journal of Gerontological Nursing, 21*(2), 39–44.

Stanley, M., & Beare, P. (1995). *Gerontological nursing.* Philadelphia: F.A. Davis.

Stolley, J. (1995). Freeing your patients from restraints. *American Journal of Nursing, 95*(2), 27–30.

Tappen, R., & Beckerman, A. (1993). A vulnerable population: Multiproblem older adults in acute care. *Journal of Gerontological Nursing, 19*(11), 38–42.

Tinetti, M., Liu, W., & Ginter, S. (1992). Mechanical restraint use and fall-related injuries among residents of skilled nursing facilities. *Annals of Internal Medicine, 116*(5), 369–374.

U.S. Food and Drug Administration. (1992, July 15). *FDA safety alert: Potential hazards with restraint devices.* Rockville, MD: U.S. Department of Health and Human Services.

Varone, L., Tappen, R., Dixon-Antonio, E., Gonzales, I., & Glussman, B. (1992). To restrain or not to restrain? The decision-making dilemma for nursing staff. *Geriatric Nursing, 13*(5), 269–272.

Weick, M. (1992). Physical restraints: An FDA update. *American Journal of Nursing, 92*(11), 74–80.

Werner, P., Cohen-Mansfield, J., Koroknay, V., & Braun, J. (1994). Reducing restraints: Impact on staff attitudes. *Journal of Gerontological Nursing, 20*(12), 19–24.

Wojner, A. (1993). Seconds count when a child is poisoned. *RN, 56*(10), 46–52.

Worthington, K. (1994). Workplace hazards: The effect on nurses as women. *American Nurse, 26*(2), 15.

Chapter 28

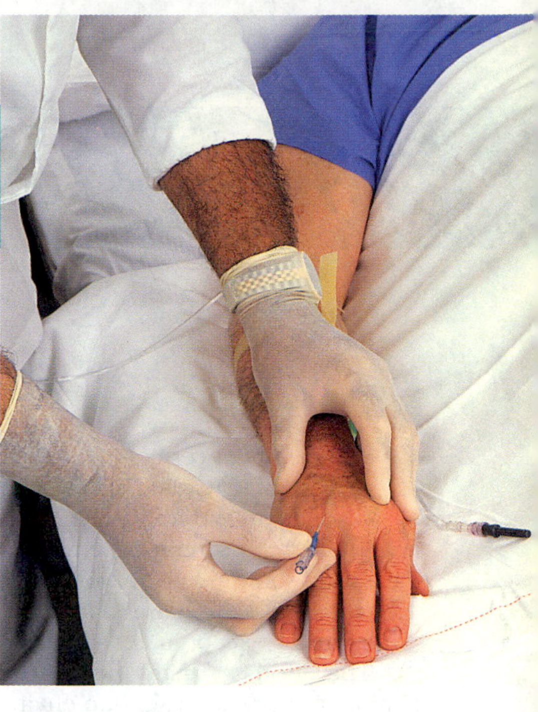

Asepsis

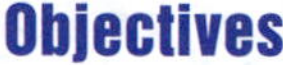

Objectives

After studying this chapter, the learner should be able to:

- Define key terms used in the chapter.
- Explain the infection cycle.
- Describe nursing interventions used to break the chain of infection.
- List the stages of an infection.
- Identify clients at risk for developing an infection.
- Identify factors that reduce the incidence of nosocomial infection.
- Identify situations in which handwashing is indicated.
- Identify nursing diagnoses associated with a client who has an infection or is at risk of developing an infection.
- Compare CDC guidelines for standard and transmission-based precautions with category-specific, disease-specific, universal, and the body substance isolation systems.
- Describe recommended techniques for medical and surgical asepsis.

Key Terms

aerobic
anaerobic
asepsis
bacteria
Centers for Disease Control
endogenous
exogenous
fungi
host
iatrogenic infection
infection
isolation
medical asepsis
nosocomial infection
pathogen
reservoir
surgical asepsis
virus

A major concern of health practitioners is the danger of spreading microorganisms from person to person and from place to place. Microorganisms are naturally present in the environment. Some are beneficial and some are not. Some are harmless to most people, and others are harmful to many people. Still others are harmless except in certain circumstances.

The efforts of many people are involved in maintaining a microorganism-safe environment: government agencies at the international, national, state, and local levels; health personnel; and individuals. Such efforts include mass immunization programs, laws concerning safe sewage disposal, regulations for the control of communicable diseases, and hospital infection-surveillance programs. Medical science continues to grapple with increasingly virulent organisms that may be drug resistant and with immunologically compromised hosts, and prevention of infection becomes a major focus for the nurse. As the primary caregiver the nurse needs to be involved in identifying, preventing, controlling, and teaching the client about infection. Consistent application of the nursing process can prove critical in breaking the chain of infection.

Infection Prevention and Control

Infection Cycle

An **infection** is a disease state that results from the presence of pathogens in or on the body. A **pathogen** is a disease-producing microorganism. An infection occurs as a result of a cyclic process, as shown in Figure 28-1. The six components in the infection cycle are as follows:

- Infectious agent
- Reservoir
- Portal of exit
- Means of transmission
- Portal of entry
- Susceptible host

Infectious Agent. Some of the more prevalent agents that are capable of causing infection include bacteria, viruses, and fungi. **Bacteria** are the most significant and most commonly observed infection-causing agents in healthcare institutions. Bacteria can be categorized in various ways. According to shape, they are classified as spherical (cocci), rod-shaped (bacilli), or corkscrew (spirochetes). Based on their reaction to the Gram stain, bacteria may be either gram-positive or gram-negative. *Gram-positive bacteria* have a thick cell wall that resists decolorization (loss of color) and are stained violet. *Gram-negative bacteria* have chemically more complex cell walls and can be decolorized by alcohol. This difference is vital information when the physician is selecting an antibiotic to prevent or treat an infection. Antibiotics may be either specifically effective against only gram-positive organisms or classified as broad-spectrum and be effective against several groups of microorganisms.

Another distinguishing characteristic of bacteria is their need for oxygen. Most bacteria require oxygen to live and grow and are referred to as **aerobic**. Those that can live without oxygen are **anaerobic** bacteria.

A **virus** is the smallest of all microorganisms and can be seen only by using an electron microscope. Many infections are caused by viruses, including the common cold and the deadly disease acquired immunodeficiency syndrome (AIDS).

Fungi are plantlike organisms (molds and yeasts) that also can cause infection. They are present in the air, soil, and water, and many are resistant to treatment.

An organism's potential to produce disease depends on a variety of factors, including the following:

- Number of organisms
- *Virulence* of the organism, or its ability to cause disease
- Competence of a person's immune system
- Length and intimacy of the contact between a person and the microorganism

Under normal conditions, an organism may not produce disease. Microorganisms that commonly inhabit various body sites and are part of the body's natural defense system are referred to as *normal flora.* Other factors may intervene and cause this relatively harmless organism to become the source of an infection. Bacteria that may potentially be harmful are referred to as *opportunists.* For example, *Escherichia coli,* which normally resides in the intestinal tract, may produce infection when it migrates into the urinary tract.

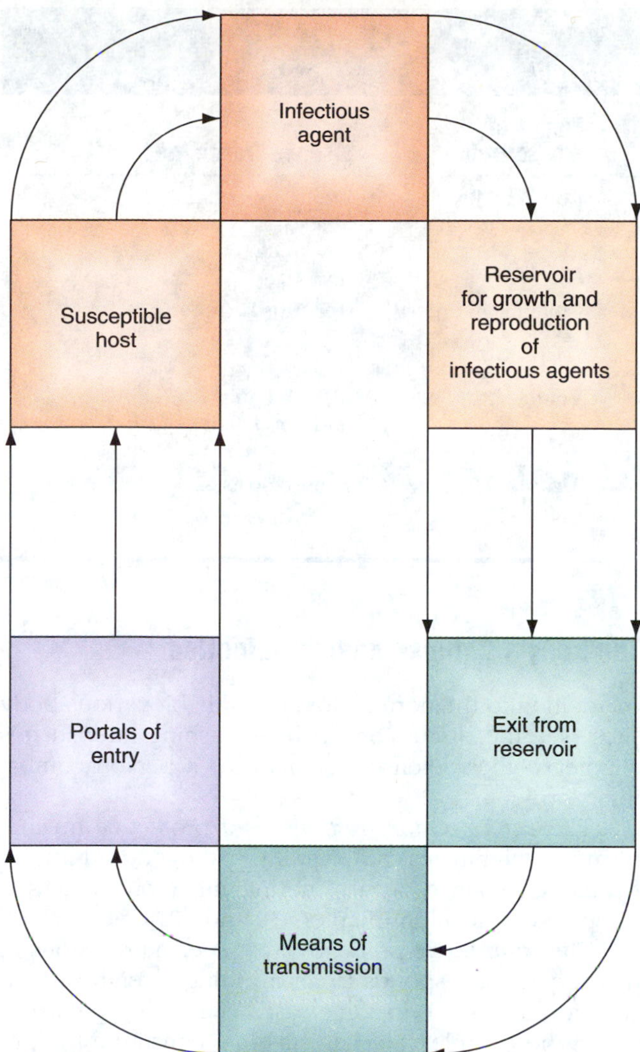

Figure 28-1
Infection process cycle. An infection occurs as a result of interrelated factors. An infection will not develop if the sequence is interrupted. Hence efforts to control infections are directed toward interrupting the sequence.

Reservoir. The **reservoir** for growth and multiplication of microorganisms is the natural habitat of the organism. Possible reservoirs that support organisms pathogenic to humans include other humans, animals, food, water, milk, and inanimate objects.

Other Humans. The tubercle bacillus and the spirochete that causes syphilis are examples of pathogens whose reservoirs are inhabited by the infectious agent and exhibit symptoms of disease, whereas others are *carriers* of the disease but do not show any symptoms of illness. For example, a person who has tested positive after a human immunodeficiency virus (HIV) antibody test probably has been infected with HIV. Even though symptoms of AIDS may not be present, the virus may be transmitted by intimate sexual contact, sharing a contaminated needle and syringe, and transfusion with contaminated blood or blood products and from an infected mother to her child during pregnancy or birth. A person's own normal flora can serve as a reservoir of pathogens.

Animals. The rabies virus is an example of a pathogen whose reservoir is various animals, notably dogs, squirrels, and raccoons.

Soil. Organisms that cause gas gangrene and tetanus are examples of pathogens whose reservoir is soil.

Portal of Exit. The *exit from the reservoir* is the point of escape for the organism. The organism cannot extend its influence unless it moves away from its original source. There usually is a primary exit route for each type of microorganism. In humans, common escape routes are the respiratory, gastrointestinal, and genitourinary tracts, as well as breaks in the skin. Blood and tissue also can serve as an exit for pathogens.

Means of Transmission. An organism may be transmitted from its reservoir by various means or routes. Some organisms can be transmitted by more than one route. Organisms can enter the body by way of the *contact* route, either directly or indirectly. Direct contact involves proximity between the susceptible host and an infected person or a carrier, such as occurs in touching, kissing, and sexual intercourse. The indirect contact route requires personal contact with an inanimate object such as a contaminated instrument. Contaminated blood, food, water, or inanimate objects (fomites) are *vehicle* routes of transmission. *Vectors,* such as mosquitoes, ticks, and lice, are nonhuman carriers that transmit organisms from one host to another. Microorganisms also can be spread by means of the *airborne* route by droplet nuclei when coughing, sneezing, and talking or by becoming attached to dust particles. Table 28-1 presents a summary of the means of transmission for several organisms, their reservoirs, and examples of diseases they transmit.

Portal of Entry. The organism must find a portal of entry on a host. The *portal of entry* is the point at which organisms enter a host. The entry route often is the same as the exit route. The urinary, respiratory, and gastrointestinal tracts and the skin are common entry points.

Susceptible Host. For microorganisms to continue to exist, they must find a source that is acceptable (a **host**) and overcome any resistance mounted by the host's defenses. *Susceptibility* is the degree of resistance the potential host has to the pathogen. It is not uncommon for a person admitted to a hospital to be in a weakened state of health due to illness. Many factors influence a host's susceptibility and are discussed later in the chapter.

Stages of Infection

An understanding of the stages in the development of an infection is necessary if the nurse is to intervene and disrupt the infection cycle. An infection progresses through the following phases:

Table 28-1
Reservoir, Mode of Transmission, and Disease Transmitted

Organism	Reservoir	Means of Transmission	Disease Transmitted
Staphylococcus aureus	Skin surface Mouth Nose Throat	Contact (direct)	Wound infection Abscess Carbuncle Boil
Hepatitis B virus	Blood Feces Body fluids/excretions	Contact (indirect)	Hepatitis B
Human immunodeficiency virus (HIV)	Blood Semen Vaginal secretions	Vehicle	AIDS (Acquired Immunodeficiency Syndrome)
Mycobacterium tuberculosis	Sputum (respiratory tract)	Airborne	Tuberculosis
Borrelia burgdorferi	Ticks (sheep, cattle, deer, mice)	Vectors	Lyme disease

- Incubation period
- Prodromal stage
- Full stage of illness
- Convalescent period

The course and severity of the infection as well as the client's response influence the extent and type of nursing care provided.

Incubation Period. The *incubation period* is the interval between the invasion of the body by the pathogen and the appearance of symptoms of infection. During this stage the organisms are growing and multiplying, and the length of incubation may vary. For example, the common cold develops in 1 to 2 days, whereas tetanus has an incubation period ranging from 2 to 21 days.

Prodromal Stage. A person is most infectious during the *prodromal stage.* Early signs and symptoms of disease are present but are vague and nonspecific, ranging from fatigue and malaise to a low-grade fever. This period lasts from several hours to several days.

Full Stage of Illness. The presence of specific signs and symptoms indicates the *full stage of illness.* The type of infection determines the length of the illness and the severity of the manifestations. Symptoms that are limited or restricted to a discrete area are referred to as *localized symptoms,* whereas *systemic symptoms* are manifested throughout the entire body.

Convalescent Period. The *convalescent period* represents recovery from the infection. The signs and symptoms disappear, and the person returns to a healthy state. Convalescence may vary according to the severity of the infection and the client's general condition.

The Body's Defense Against Infection

In addition to the normal flora that inhabit various body sites (see the discussion on handwashing later in this chapter), other defense systems help a person combat infection.

The *inflammatory response* is a protective mechanism that eliminates the invading pathogen and allows for tissue repair to occur. The inflammation process is discussed in detail in Chapters 30 and 32.

The *immune response* involves specific reactions in the body as it responds to an invading foreign protein such as bacteria or, in some cases, the body's own proteins. The complex mechanisms that constitute the immune response occur as the body attempts to protect and defend itself. The foreign material is called an *antigen,* and the body commonly responds to the antigen by producing an *antibody.* This antigen–antibody reaction is one component of the overall immune response; it also is known as *humoral immunity.* The cell-mediated defense, or cellular immunity, involves an increase in the number of lymphocytes (white blood cells) for the purpose of destroying or reacting specifically with cells the body recognizes as harmful. Although these complicated chemical and mechanical responses are not completely understood, it is known that they help to defend the body specifically against bacterial, viral, and fungal infections as well as malignant cells.

Factors Affecting the Risk of Infection

The susceptibility of the host is influenced by various factors, including the following:

- Intact skin and mucous membranes protect the body against microbial invasion.
- The normal *p*H levels of gastric secretions and of the genitourinary tract help to ward off microbial invasion.

- The body's white blood cells influence resistance to certain pathogens.
- Age, sex, race, and hereditary factors influence susceptibility, although the reasons are not always clear. Neonates and elderly people appear to be more vulnerable to infection than the general population. The accompanying box discusses older adults' predisposition to infection.
- Immunization, natural or acquired, acts to resist infection.
- Fatigue, climate, nutritional and general health status, the presence of preexisting illnesses, previous or current treatments, and some kinds of medications may play a part in the susceptibility of a potential host.
- Stress may adversely affect the body's normal defense mechanisms.
- The increasing use of invasive or indwelling medical devices provides more potential sources of disease-producing organisms, particularly in a client whose defenses are already weakened by disease.

Lifestyle also places a person at risk for developing an infection. Health habits that promote wellness positively influence the susceptibility of a host. Sensible nutrition, adequate rest and exercise, stress reduction techniques, and good personal hygiene habits are examples of activities that can help to maintain optimum bodily function and immune response. Unsafe sex practices and sharing intravenous needles are potentially dangerous and can introduce pathogens that cause infection.

ASSESSING

The nurse's critical role in controlling infection begins with early detection and surveillance techniques. The extent of the nursing interventions is determined by the susceptibility of the host, the virulence of the organism, and the client's signs and symptoms.

Home Healthcare Alert

Remind family members and caregivers that older adults may exhibit unusual manifestations of an infection. Lethargy, confusion, anorexia, immobility, and falls may indicate the presence of an infection and should be reported to the nurse or physician.

To formulate an individualized nursing plan of care, the nurse inquires about the client's immunization status and previous or recurring infections, observes nonverbal cues, and elicits information regarding the history of the current disease process. A review of laboratory data provides further insight into the presence of an infectious process. Any of the laboratory test results outlined in the accompanying box may indicate the presence of an infection.

This compilation of assessment data constitutes a unique nursing data base that suggests nursing interventions for clients at risk for infection or those in whom an infection is already present.

Focus on the Older Adult

Predisposition for Infection

There are specific *physiologic alterations* that predispose an older adult to infection. Common infections seen in the elderly are pneumonia, tuberculosis, and urinary tract and skin infections. Morbidity and mortality are increased in this age group, and the signs and symptoms may be atypical. In addition to a *reduced inflammatory response* and a *decrease in immune function,* specific physiologic alterations in each body system that are associated with the development of these common infections include:

Pulmonary Infections (Pneumonia and Tuberculosis)

Decreased cough reflex

Decreased elastic recoil of the lungs

Decreased activity of the cilia

Abnormal swallowing reflexes

Urinary Tract Infections

Incomplete emptying of the bladder

Decreased sphincter control

Bladder outlet obstruction due to an enlarged prostate gland

Skin Infections

Loss of elasticity

Increased dryness

Thinning of epidermis

Slowing of cell replacement

Decreased vascular supply

Atypical clinical manifestations of infection in an older adult include confusion, disorientation, lethargy, anorexia, delayed fever response, and failure to thrive.

Laboratory Data Indicating an Infection

- Elevated white blood cell (leukocyte) count—normal value is 5000 to 10,000/mm^3
- Increase in specific types of white blood cells (differential count or % of each cell type)

Neutrophils	Normal = 60 to 70%	Increased in acute infections that produce pus; may be decreased in acute bacterial infection
Lymphocytes	Normal = 20 to 40%	Increased in chronic bacterial and viral infections
Monocytes	Normal = 2 to 8%	Increased in severe infections and function as a scavenger or phagocyte
Eosinophil	Normal = 1 to 4%	May be increased in allergic reaction and parasitic infection
Basophil	Normal = 0.5 to 1%	Usually unaffected by infections

- Elevated erythrocyte sedimentation rate (ESR)—red blood cells (RBCs) settle more rapidly to the bottom of a tube of whole blood when an inflammation is present
- Presence of pathogen in urine, blood, sputum, or other draining cultures

DIAGNOSING

The potential for infection or the presence of an infection in a client suggests possible nursing diagnoses. The direction or focus of nursing care depends on a nursing diagnosis that accurately reflects the client's condition. The following are examples of nursing diagnoses that relate to an infectious process:

Risk for Infection related to presence of chronic disease; altered immune response; effects of medication; altered skin integrity; malnutrition; presence of invasive or indwelling medical device; lack of proper immunization

Social Isolation related to presence of communicable disease (AIDS)

Altered Oral Mucous Membrane related to ineffective dental hygiene; trauma

Diversional Activity Deficit related to lack of visitors; restrictions imposed by airborne isolation precautions

Risk for Altered Body Temperature related to obstructed urine outflow

Anxiety related to high risk for infection

PLANNING: EXPECTED OUTCOMES

Effective nursing interventions can control or prevent infection. The nurse reviews the assessment data, considers the cycle of events that results in the development of an infection, and incorporates principles of infection control as client outcomes are formulated. Planning outcomes that prevent infection or interfere with the infection cycle provides an exciting challenge for the nurse and an opportunity to see positive results because of these efforts. The following expected client outcomes are appropriate to prevent infection. The client will:

- Demonstrate effective handwashing
- Identify the signs of an infection
- Maintain adequate nutritional intake
- Demonstrate proper disposal of soiled articles
- Use appropriate cleansing and disinfecting techniques
- Demonstrate an awareness of the necessity of proper immunizations
- Demonstrate stress reduction techniques

IMPLEMENTING

The nurse uses principles of aseptic technique to halt the spread of microorganisms and minimize the threat of infection. To control the number of organisms, medical and surgical asepsis are vital. The practice of **asepsis** includes any activities that prevent infection or break the chain of infection. It is divided into two types—medical asepsis and surgical asepsis. **Medical asepsis**, or clean technique, involves procedures and practices that reduce the number and transfer of pathogens. **Surgical asepsis**, or sterile technique, includes practices used to render and keep objects and areas free from microorganisms.

Teaching About Infection Control

Teaching about medical asepsis and infection control is a challenging nursing responsibility. Clients need to be aware of techniques that prevent the spread of infection. Consistent application of the nursing process protects both the client and the nurse.

In the home, medical asepsis techniques are appropriate for most procedures with the exception of self-injection technique. The client frequently must make adjustments and improvise with the resources and supplies available for his or her use. The nurse emphasizes effective handwashing and hygiene practices that interrupt the infection chain. In order to satisfy OSHA requirements, many home care agencies have either a full-time or part-time infection control practitioner (ICP).

Clients should be taught to use basic principles of asepsis at home and in public facilities. These involve activities of daily living (refer to Chapter 37 for a discussion of personal hygiene). The following are examples of medical asepsis practices recommended in the home:

- Wash hands before preparing food and before eating.
- Prepare foods at temperatures sufficiently high to ensure that they are safe to eat, the most common example being the preparation of fresh pork.
- Use care with cutting boards and utensils, and wash hands before and after handling raw meat.
- Keep foods refrigerated, especially those containing mayonnaise.
- Wash raw fruits and vegetables before serving them.
- Use pasteurized milk.
- Wash hands after using the bathroom.
- Use individual personal care items, such as washcloths, towels, and toothbrushes.

Observe infection prevention in public facilities by following these guidelines:

- Wash hands after using any public bathroom.
- Use paper towels or hot-air dryers in restrooms.
- Use individually wrapped drinking straws.
- Use tongs to lift food from common service trays in cafeterias, food stores, and salad bars.

The community reinforces medical asepsis practices in various ways, including the following:

- Use of sterilized combs and brushes in barber and beauty shops
- Examination of food handlers for evidence of disease
- Enforcement of frequent handwashing by food handlers

Using Medical Asepsis

Medical asepsis is used continuously both within and outside health agencies because it is always assumed that pathogens are likely to be present. For example, public drinking cups are unsanitary because pathogens may be present on the cup after being used by someone who may be harboring them. In a healthcare facility, if a specific pathogen is known to be present, special methods of medical asepsis are used to prevent further spread of the organism. Nearly every nursing activity includes practices of medical asepsis. Breaking the chain of infection is the nurse's responsibility. It involves giving safe client care and protecting the client as well as oneself from microorganisms that have at least the potential to cause disease. See the accompanying box for basic practices of medical asepsis that nurses should use when giving care to clients.

Preventing Nosocomial Infections

For various reasons and sometimes despite best efforts, certain clients in health agencies develop infections that were not noted to be present on admission. The term **nosocomial** is used to describe a hospital-acquired infection. In its broad meaning, nosocomial means that the infection results while the client is receiving health care, and the source may be either exogenous or endogenous. An **exogenous** infection means that the causative organism is acquired from other people; an **endogenous** infection means that the causative organism comes from microbial life the person himself harbors. An infection is referred to as **iatrogenic** when it occurs as a result of a treatment or diagnostic procedure. Not all nosocomial infections have an iatrogenic component.

Prevention of nosocomial infections poses a major challenge for healthcare providers. At least 5 to 10% of all people admitted to a hospital contract a nosocomial infection, and these hospital-acquired infections are a direct cause of death for approximately 80,000 people a year in the United States (Turner, 1993). The cost of the additional hospital care days necessary to treat a nosocomial infection is staggering, particularly in light of the concerted efforts to control spiraling expenses associated with healthcare.

Most hospital-acquired infections are caused by bacteria. *Escherichia coli, Staphylococcus aureus, Streptococcus faecalis, Pseudomonas aeruginosa,* and *Klebsiella* species have been implicated as common causative organisms. Urinary tract infections account for 39% of all nosocomial infections, and indwelling urinary catheters have been implicated in 80% of these (Hoeprich et al., 1994). Surgical wounds are a common site for infections to develop, but nosocomial pneumonia is the most difficult infection to prevent and has the highest mortality rate (Mylotte et al., 1993; Calianno, 1996). The increasing use of biomedical equipment frequently is cited as a causative agent. In addition to indwelling urinary catheters, devices most frequently implicated include hemodynamic monitoring lines, hemodialysis equipment, and respiratory equipment. Often the hands of the healthcare worker using the instruments are the most significant means for the transmission of the hospital-acquired pathogens.

A significant and disturbing trend in the last decade continues to be the development of hospital-acquired pathogens that are often resistant to antibiotics. The increasingly common use of broad-spectrum antibiotics has been a factor in the emergence of these resistant organisms. *S. aureus,* frequently cited as the cause of nosocomial wound and skin infections that occur postoperatively, in recent years has developed resistance to the antibiotic methicillin, which has been the drug of choice to treat this infection. Vancomycin-resistant enterococcus (VRE) has now emerged as a serious pathogen in hospitals. Enterococci, a species of streptococcus often found in the normal intestinal and female genital tracts, can cause nosocomial infections that have a mortality rate of 40 to 50% if the organism is vancomycin resistant (Hospital Infection Control, 1994). VRE is particularly alarming because no alternative to vancomycin, which is the drug of choice to treat most serious infections, is

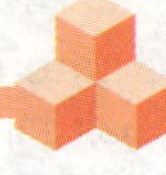

Guidelines for Nursing Care

Practicing Basic Principles of Medical Asepsis in Client Care

- Wash hands frequently but especially before handling foods, before eating, after using a handkerchief, after going to the toilet, before and after each client contact, and after removing gloves.
- Keep soiled items and equipment from touching the clothing. Carry soiled linens or other used articles so that they do not touch the uniform.
- Do not place soiled bed linen or any other items on the floor, which is grossly contaminated. It increases contamination of both surfaces.
- Avoid having clients cough, sneeze, or breathe directly on others. Provide them with disposable tissues, and instruct them, as indicated, to cover their mouth and nose to prevent spread by airborne droplets.
- Move equipment away from you when brushing, dusting, or scrubbing articles. This helps prevent contaminated particles from settling on the hair, face, and uniform.
- Avoid raising dust. Use a specially treated cloth or a dampened cloth. Do not shake linens. Dust and lint particles constitute a vehicle by which organisms may be transported from one area to another.
- Clean the least soiled areas first and then the more soiled ones. This helps prevent having the cleaner areas soiled by the dirtier areas.
- Dispose of soiled or used items directly into appropriate containers. Wrap items that are moist from body discharge or drainage in waterproof containers, such as plastic bags, before discarding into the refuse holder so that handlers will not come in contact with them.
- Pour liquids that are to be discarded, such as bath water, mouth rinse, and the like, directly into the drain so as to avoid splatterings in the sink and onto you.
- Sterilize items that are suspected of containing pathogens. After sterilization, they can be managed as clean items, if appropriate.
- Use practices of personal grooming that help prevent spreading microorganisms. Examples include shampooing the hair regularly, keeping it short or pinned up to limit the possibility of carrying microorganisms on hair shafts, keeping the fingernails short and free of broken cuticles and ragged nail edges, and avoiding wearing rings with grooves and stones that may harbor microorganisms.
- Follow guidelines conscientiously for isolation or barrier techniques as prescribed by agency.

available at present; in addition, this organism has the potential ability to transfer its resistance to other species.

Nurses, by nature of their role, are in a unique position to prevent the transmission of nosocomial infections. VRE, for example, is most often transmitted by the hands of the healthcare provider. Careful assessment and evaluation of high-risk clients and situations, coupled with strict observance of medical and surgical asepsis techniques, will minimize infection and reduce the unnecessary suffering imposed on clients. Using nursing diagnoses to generate appropriate nursing interventions makes a significant difference and improves the quality of nursing care.

Health agencies have found the following measures to be successful in reducing the incidence of nosocomial infections:

- Instituting constant surveillance by infection-control committees and nurse epidemiologists. Their work has been noted to reduce infections significantly when aggressive control measures resulting from their findings are initiated.
- Having written infection prevention practices for all agency personnel. The Omnibus Budget Reconciliation Act (OBRA '87), which became effective in October 1990, mandates that all long-term care facilities have formal infection-control programs with emphasis on policies and procedures to prevent the spread of infection (Stolley & Buckwalter, 1991). Adherence to thorough handwashing and barrier precautions or isolation techniques can prevent many nosocomial infections. Typical guidelines are described later in this chapter.
- Using practices to help promote and keep clients in the best possible physical condition. Measures include meeting the client's needs for nutrition, fluids, rest, oxygen, and physical and psychologic comfort and security.

Outbreaks of nosocomial infection in either acute-care hospitals or long-term care facilities are costly, frequently difficult to control, and debilitating for clients. Infection-control measures save lives and reduce the risk of transmission of pathogens to clients as well as personnel.

Handwashing

Handwashing is the most effective way to help prevent the spread of organisms. Differences of opinion persist about proper cleaning agents, length of time for washing, and ideal frequency of adequate handwashing, but everyone agrees that handwashing is the most important procedure in preventing nosocomial infections. Attention needs to be refocused on this simple procedure that can interrupt the chain of infection.

Bacterial Flora on Hands. Two types of bacterial flora normally are found on the hands—transient bacteria and resident bacteria. *Transient bacteria,* normally picked up by the hands in the usual activities of daily living, are relatively few on clean and exposed areas of the skin. They are attached loosely to the skin, usually in grease, fats, and dirt, and are found in greater numbers under the fingernails. Transient bacteria, pathogenic as well as nonpathogenic, can be removed with relative ease by washing the hands thoroughly and frequently. *Resident bacteria,* normally found in creases in the skin, are relatively stable in number and type. They cling tenaciously to the skin by adhesion and adsorption, and considerable friction with a brush is required to remove them. Also, they are less susceptible than transient bacteria to the action of antiseptics. It is not considered possible to clean the skin of all bacteria.

Transient bacteria may adjust to the environment of the skin if the flora are present in large numbers over a long enough time. They then become resident bacteria. If pathogenic organisms become resident bacteria on the skin, the hands are then carriers of the particular organism. Therefore, it is important that the hands be cleaned promptly when visibly soiled, after each contact with contaminated materials, and after removing gloves to help prevent transient bacteria from becoming resident bacteria on the hands.

Cleansing Agents. Various products are available for handwashing. Soaps and detergents, also referred to as *nonantimicrobial* agents, are considered adequate for routine mechanical cleansing of the hands and removal of most transient microorganisms. They help remove soil because they lower surface tension and act as emulsifying agents. Bar, liquid, leaflet, or powder are all effective, but the factor that determines selection may be the preference of personnel or agency choice.

Using handwashing products that contain an *antimicrobial* or antibacterial ingredient is recommended for any setting in which there is a high risk for infection. When present in certain concentrations, these agents can kill bacteria or suppress their growth. Antimicrobial soaps are suggested for intensive care units, emergency departments, and any client-care setting in which exposure to blood and body fluids is likely or clients are immunosuppressed. Some soaps containing antimicrobial agents have reportedly caused skin dryness and cracking. Usually this irritation can be traced to the detergent base of the soap rather than to any antiseptic that is present. These irritations defeat the purpose of decreasing the number of surface organisms because damaged skin harbors organisms and is difficult to clean adequately. Some products are available that contain an emollient or softening agent, but lotions may also be used to comfort damaged skin. They are best applied after client care is completed. Small containers, nonrefillable and for personal use, are recommended.

Recommended Techniques. Recommended handwashing techniques for medical asepsis are listed in Procedure 28-1. Handwashing that incorporates surgical asepsis is described in texts that deal with operating and delivery room procedures. Effective handwashing requires at least a 10 to 15-second scrub with plain soap or disinfectant and water. Hands that are visibly soiled need a longer scrub. Studies abound in the literature about the merits of handwashing, and several agencies have published directions and recommendations. The Association for Professionals in Infection Control and Epidemiology (APIC) has recently published guidelines for handwashing in various settings and reviewed the variety of products available for handwashing.

Most guidelines recommend removal of all jewelry except wedding bands and advise particular attention to the area beneath the fingernails, where bacteria tend to accumulate. Rings also have the added disadvantage of increasing the likelihood that gloves may tear when donned over the jewelry. Nails should be kept short since a majority of organisms are found under and around the nails. Nail polish does not appear to increase the number of microorganisms, but a clear color is preferable because the area under the nails is more visible. Artificial nails are not recommended because they harbor more bacteria than natural nails, and a person with artificial nails is less likely to vigorously scrub that area (Sheldon, 1994).

Even though healthcare personnel are aware of the importance of handwashing, most studies report that compliance with this simple preventive measure is difficult to achieve. Despite intensive educational efforts, handwashing is infrequently practiced. Wearing gloves does not substitute for proper handwashing. In reality, the warmth and moisture inside gloves create an ideal environment for bacteria to multiply, making it even more important to wash hands before and after gloves are applied. Research also indicates that gloving does not guarantee complete protection from infectious organisms. Olsen et al. (1993) reported that gloves provide a barrier but are not impenetrable. According to their study, a leak in a glove occurred after 13% of exposures to clients' mucous membranes, and many of the healthcare workers failed to identify that a leak had occurred. Routine handwashing should be done after each client contact, whether or not gloves were worn.

Controlling Infectious Agents by Sterilization and Disinfection

Cleansing, disinfection, and sterilization help to break the chain of infection and prevent nosocomial disease. Most health agencies provide items for client care that are sterile when purchased and disposed of after use. Some items, such as pitchers, water glasses, and ther-

(text continues on page 566)

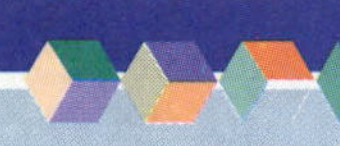

PROCEDURE 28-1

Handwashing

Equipment

Liquid, bar soap, granules, or leaflet
Paper towels
Lotion (optional)

Action	Rationale
1. Stand in front of the sink. Do not allow your uniform to touch the sink during the washing procedure.	The sink is considered contaminated. Uniforms may carry organisms from place to place.
2. Remove jewelry, if possible, and secure in a safe place or allow plain wedding band to remain in place.	Removal of jewelry facilitates proper cleansing. Microorganisms may accumulate in settings of jewelry. If jewelry was worn during care, it should be left on during hand washing.
3. Turn on water and adjust force. Regulate the temperature until the water is warm.	Water splashed from the contaminated sink will contaminate your uniform. Warm water is more comfortable and has less tendency to open pores and remove oils from the skin. Organisms can lodge in roughened and broken areas of chapped skin.
4. Wet the hands and wrist area. Keep hands lower than elbows to allow water to flow toward fingertips.	Water should flow from the cleaner toward the more contaminated area. Hands are more contaminated than forearms.
5. Use about 1 teaspoon liquid soap (3–5 ml) from dispenser or rinse bar of soap and lather thoroughly. Cover all areas of hands with the soap product. Rinse soap bar again and return to soap dish.	Rinsing the soap before and after use removes the lather that may contain microorganisms.
6. With firm rubbing and circular motions, wash the palms and backs of the hands, each finger, the areas between the fingers, the knuckles, wrists, and forearms. Wash at least one inch above area of contamination. If hands are not visibly soiled, wash to one inch above the wrists.	Friction caused by firm rubbing and circular motions helps to loosen dirt and organisms that can lodge between the fingers, in skin crevices of knuckles, on palms and backs of the hands, as well as the wrists and forearms. Cleaning less contaminated areas (forearms and wrists) after hands are clean prevents spreading organisms from the hands to the forearms and wrists.

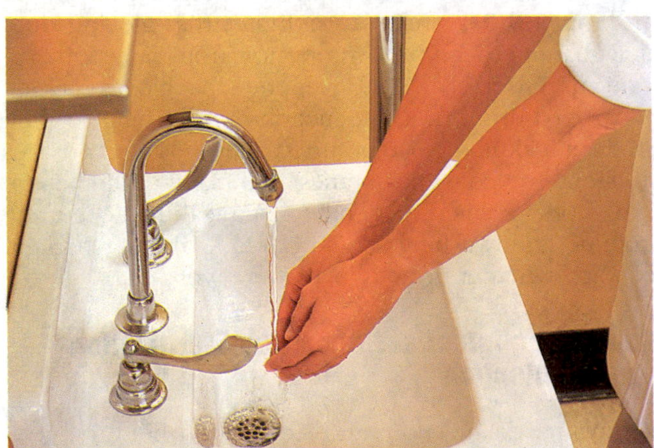

Action 4: Wetting hands and wrists.

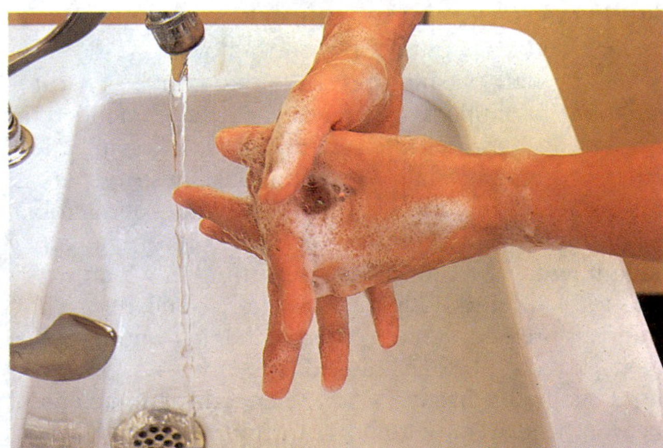

Action 6: Washing hands and forearms with firm rubbing and circular motions.

(continued)

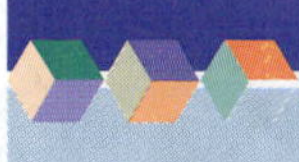

PROCEDURE 28-1 *(continued)*

Handwashing

Action	Rationale
7. Continue this friction motion for 10 to 15 seconds.	Length of handwashing is determined by degree of contamination.
8. Use fingernails of the other hand or a clean orangewood stick to clean under fingernails.	Area under nails has a high microorganism count and organisms may remain under the nails where they can grow and be spread to others.
9. Rinse thoroughly.	Running water rinses organisms and dirt into the sink.
10. Dry hands, beginning with the fingers and moving upward toward forearms, with a paper towel and discard it immediately. Use another clean towel to turn off the faucet. Discard towel immediately without touching other clean hand.	Drying the skin well prevents chapping. Dry hands first because they are the cleanest and least contaminated area. Turning the faucet off with a clean paper towel protects the clean hands from contact with a soiled surface.
11. Use lotion on hands if desired.	Lotion helps to keep the skin soft and prevents chapping. It is best applied after client care is complete and from small, personal containers.

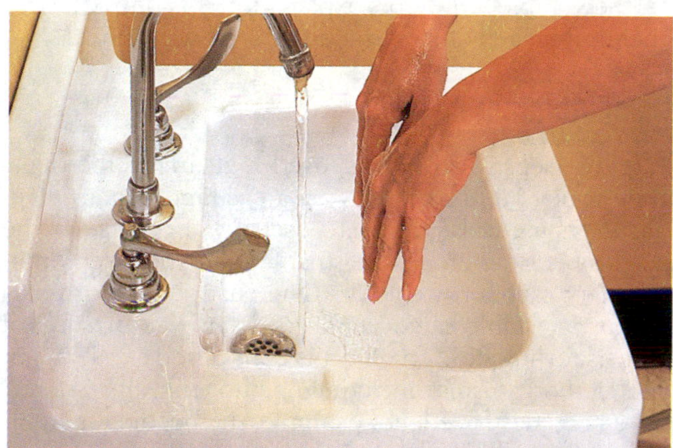

Action 9: Rinsing thoroughly.

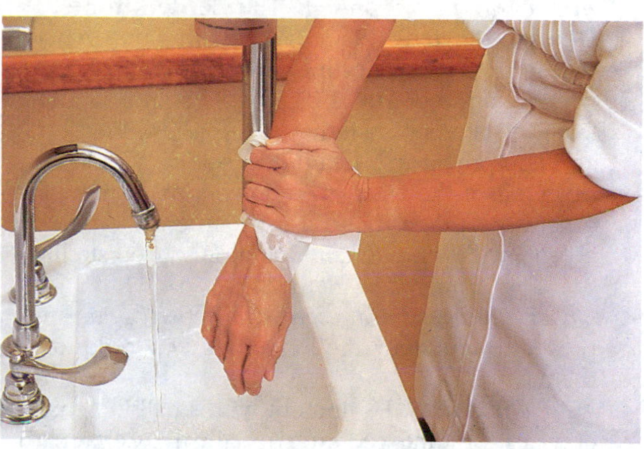

Action 10: Finishing drying with a paper towel.

Age Considerations

Instruct children at early age in proper handwashing techniques.

Special Considerations

An antimicrobial soap product is recommended prior to an invasive procedure and after exposure to blood or body fluids. The length of the scrub will vary based on need.

Special scrubbing techniques can reduce the risk for nurses who do not remove their rings. Research by Jacobsen and colleagues demonstrated that a 1-minute scrub using liquid soap and a scrub brush, followed by a 1-minute rinse can remove any additional surface bacteria (Jacobsen et al., 1985).

Sinks with various faucet controls are available. In addition to the more common hand faucets, knee- and foot-operated controls may be used. Sinks with elbow controls are generally used in a surgical setting.

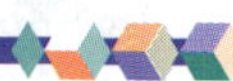

mometers, may be used repeatedly but by one client only; they are then discarded or sent home with the client on discharge.

Health agencies usually maintain a central supply unit where most reusable equipment is cleaned, kept in good working order, and sterilized as indicated. There are times, especially in homes and in some small health agencies, when the nurse is required to make decisions about how to prepare equipment and supplies so that they are safe for client use. Although nurses may not be directly involved in the actual process, they must be aware of the critical role they play in preventing infection.

Several processes are used to destroy microorganisms. *Disinfection* destroys all pathogenic organisms except spores; *sterilization* is the process by which all microorganisms, including spores, are destroyed. Disinfection and sterilization of contaminated or infected objects and good handwashing diminish and often eliminate microorganisms as potential sources of infection.

Factors in Selecting Method. Various factors must be considered when selecting sterilization and disinfection methods. They include the following:

Nature of organisms present: The **Centers for Disease Control** (CDC) is a government agency whose responsibilities include investigation, prevention, and control of disease. Recommendations from this agency state that all supplies, linens, and equipment in a healthcare setting should be treated as if the client were infectious. Some organisms are easily destroyed, whereas others are able to withstand certain commonly used sterilization and disinfection methods.

Number of organisms present: The more organisms present on an item, the longer it takes to destroy them.

Type of equipment: Equipment with small lumens, crevices, or joints require special care. Certain articles may be damaged by various sterilization and disinfection methods and require special handling.

Intended use of equipment: The need for medical or surgical asepsis influences the preparation and cleaning of equipment. In the home setting it may be safe to use equipment and supplies that are clean, but most health agencies prefer to use sterilized articles for client care.

Available means for sterilization and disinfection: The choice of chemical or physical means of sterilization and disinfection is made on the basis of the nature and number of organisms, the type and intended use of the equipment, and the availability and practicality of the means.

Time: Time is a key factor when sterilizing or disinfecting articles. Failure to observe recommended time periods is grossly negligent.

Cleaning Supplies and Equipment. Proper cleaning of items used in health care before they are sterilized or disinfected is essential to reduce the number of organisms and to dislodge them from crevices and from under layers of contaminating substances. The following techniques are recommended for cleaning equipment:

- Wear waterproof gloves at all times.
- Rinse the articles first with cold running water to remove organic material. Heat coagulates certain organic material, which makes removal more difficult.
- Wash the articles, after rinsing them, in warm water that contains detergent or soap. The combination of warm water and soap facilitates emulsification and removal of dirt and debris.
- Use a brush with stiff bristles as indicated to clean the articles thoroughly. Friction aids in the removal of organisms and debris from difficult-to-reach areas.
- Rinse and dry the article thoroughly.
- Prepare the cleaned equipment for sterilization or disinfection.
- Consider the brush, gloves, and the sink or basin in which the articles were cleaned as highly contaminated, and treat or discard them accordingly.

See Table 28-2 for explanation of physical and chemical means of sterilization and disinfection.

Using Surgical Asepsis

Surgical asepsis techniques, used regularly in the operating room, labor and delivery areas, and certain diagnostic testing areas, also are used by the nurse at the client's bedside. Procedures that involve the insertion of a urinary catheter, sterile dressing changes, and preparing an injectable medication are examples of surgical asepsis techniques. An object is considered sterile when all microorganisms, including pathogens and spores, have been destroyed. For example, the needle for an injection is handled so that it is sterile when inserted into a client. A sterile forceps or sterile gloves are used to handle sterile dressings to protect from contamination. The basic principles of surgical asepsis are listed in the accompanying box.

In observing medical asepsis, areas are considered contaminated if they bear or are suspected of bearing pathogens. In observing surgical asepsis, areas are considered contaminated if they are touched by any object that is not also sterile. One of the most important aspects of surgical and medical asepsis is that the effectiveness of both depends on the faithfulness and the conscientiousness of those carrying them out. It is far better to err on the side of safety when using surgical asepsis than to take the slightest chance of possible contamination.

Explanation of the surgical asepsis procedure facilitates cooperation of the client. An awareness of which objects and areas may not be touched, as well as directions to avoid sudden movements that may contaminate the equipment and the area, are vital for the client to assist the nurse in maintaining the sterility of the procedure.

Table 28-2
Methods of Sterilization and Disinfection

Method	Discussion	Caution
Physical		
Steam	Higher temperature caused by higher pressure destroys organisms (eg, autoclaving)	Most plastic and rubber devices are damaged by autoclaving
Boiling water	Frequently used in the home—simple and inexpensive; boil item for at least 15 minutes	Spores and some viruses are not destroyed by boiling
Dry heat	Alternative sterilization method for home. Used for metal items. Heat oven to 350°F for 2 or more hours	Insufficient to destroy all microorganisms. Not used in health care agencies
Radiation	Used for pharmaceuticals, foods, plastics, and other heat-sensitive items	Object must be directly exposed to ultraviolet radiation on all surfaces. Poses risk to personnel
Chemical		
Ethylene oxide gas	Destroys microorganisms and spores by interfering with metabolic processes in cells. Gas is released while items (oxygen and suction gauges, blood pressure equipment) are contained in autoclave	Precautions necessary because gas is toxic to humans
Chemical solutions	Generally used for instrument and equipment disinfection and for housekeeping disinfection. Chlorines are useful for disinfecting water and for housekeeping purposes. A solution of sodium hypochlorite (household bleach) in a 1:100 dilution effectively inactivates human immunodeficiency virus. Betadine or alcohol are also used as disinfectants	Method does not destroy all spores and may cause corrosion on metal surfaces

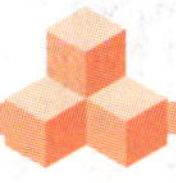

Guidelines for Nursing Care

Practicing Basic Principles of Surgical Asepsis

- Only a sterile object can touch another sterile object. Unsterile touching sterile means contamination has occurred.
- Open sterile packages so that the first edge of the wrapper is directed away from the worker to avoid the possibility of a sterile surface touching unsterile clothing. The outside of the sterile package is considered contaminated. Opening a sterile package is shown and described in Figure 28-2.
- Avoid spilling any solution on a cloth or paper used as a field for a sterile setup. The moisture penetrates through the sterile cloth or paper and carries organisms by capillary action to contaminate the field. A wet field is considered contaminated if the surface immediately below it is not sterile.
- Hold sterile objects above the level of the waist. This will help ensure keeping the object within sight and preventing accidental contamination.
- Avoid talking, coughing, sneezing, or reaching over a sterile field or object. This helps to prevent contamination by droplets from the nose and the mouth or by particles dropping from the worker's arm.
- Never walk away from or turn your back on a sterile field. This prevents possible contamination while the field is out of the worker's view.
- All items brought into contact with broken skin, or used to penetrate the skin in order to inject substances into the body, or to enter normally sterile body cavities, should be sterile. These items include dressings used to cover wounds and incisions, needles for injection, and tubes (catheters) used to drain urine from the bladder.
- Use dry, sterile forceps when necessary. Forceps soaked in disinfectant are not considered sterile.
- Consider the edge (outer 1 inch) of a sterile field to be contaminated.
- Consider an object contaminated if you have any doubt as to its sterility.

Handling Sterile Objects

Sterile gloves or sterile forceps are used for handling items when maintaining sterility is necessary.

Opening a Sterile Package and Preparing a Sterile Field

Handwashing is a necessity before opening any sterile item. Sterile packages may be opened after being placed on a flat surface or while hand-held. Opening the flaps in the appropriate sequence eliminates reaching over the sterile field and maintains the sterility of the contents (Fig. 28-2). A sterile item may need to be covered if it is not being used immediately. Reapply the cover by touching only the outside of the wrapper and reversing the opening order. Procedure 28-2 demonstrates the correct method for preparing a sterile field.

Using Sterile Forceps

Various forceps are available for use in sterile procedures (Fig. 28-3). They may be used during a dressing change procedure or to transfer a sterile item from one place to another. They are usually prepared in a package and discarded or resterilized after use. Forceps that were stored in a germicidal solution and then reused are not sterile and are unsafe. As with other sterile objects, forceps should be kept above waist level. If handled with the bare hand, only the tips can be considered sterile. Sterile forceps should not touch the edge of a container or sterile wrapper because this outer area is considered unsterile. The forceps' tips need to be held downward, particularly if they become wet, so that fluid will not flow from a contaminated area to a sterile one.

Pouring Sterile Solutions

Care is necessary when pouring sterile liquids onto a sterile dressing or into a sterile basin (Fig. 28-4). The outer surfaces of the bottle and cap are unsterile. Remove the cap carefully, and do not allow the inner surface of the lid to touch an unsterile area. Pour a small amount of the solution into a sink or waste container to clean the lip of the bottle. Be sure the label side of the container is uppermost when pouring so that the label does not become wet and soiled. Hold the bottle outside the edge of the sterile field and pour carefully so as not to splash the solution. The tip of the bottle should never touch the sterile container or dressing. Touch only the outside of the cap when recapping.

Once a solution has been opened, the outer bottle should be labeled and dated if it is to be reused. Most solutions are considered sterile for 24 hours after they are opened.

Adding Sterile Supplies to a Sterile Field

After establishing a sterile field, it may be necessary to add items to the sterile field (see Procedure 28-2, actions 8 through 10). The nurse should open the sterile item and drop it onto the sterile field from a safe distance, being careful that the outside wrapper does not touch the sterile field. If the item is wrapped in a sterile cloth, the nondominant hand should be used to secure the loose ends away from the item and protect them from contaminating the sterile field.

Putting on Sterile Gloves

Sterile gloves are donned so that only the inside of the gloves comes in contact with the hands. Procedure 28-3 explains the proper technique for putting on sterile gloves. After the gloves are on, sterile items may be handled with the sterile-gloved hands. Careful removal of the gloves reduces any hand contact with contaminated materials. Good handwashing technique before and after putting on sterile gloves is imperative.

Positioning a Sterile Drape

The sterile drape, which ideally is waterproof, may be applied to extend the sterile working area. Using sterile gloves to apply the drape allows the nurse to handle the entire surface. For protection when positioning, the

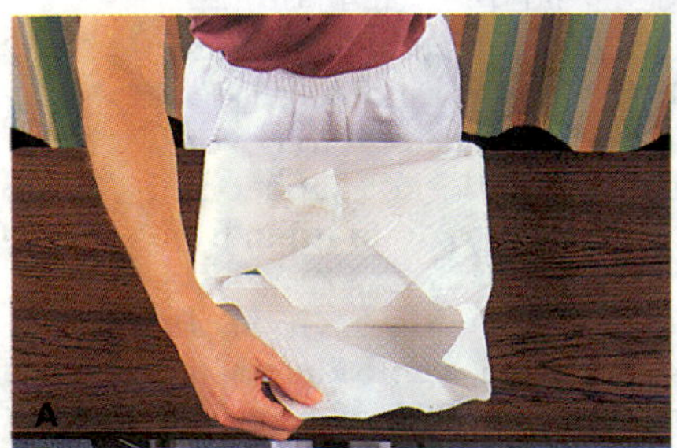

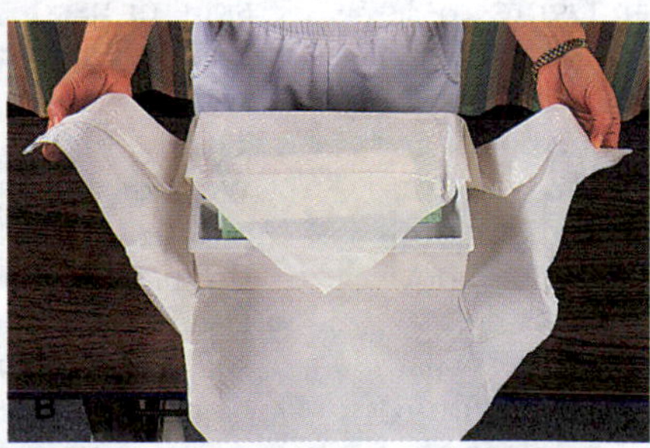

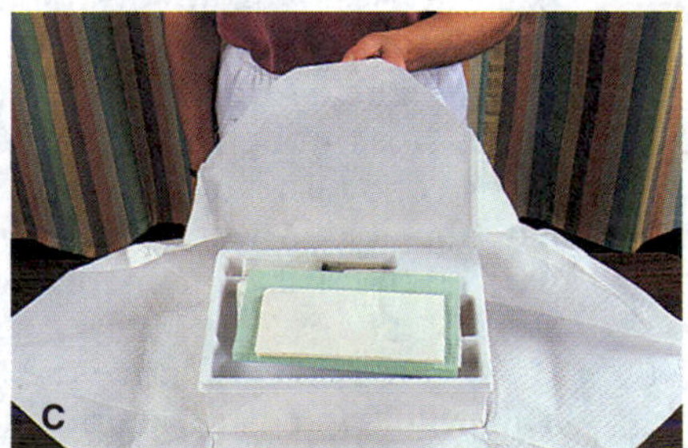

Figure 28-2
Opening a sterile tray. **(A)** The nurse folds the topmost part of the covering wrapper away from the nurse. **(B)** Then he or she opens the next layer of the wrapper to the sides. **(C)** The last layer of the wrapper is opened toward the nurse to prevent any reaching over the sterile field. (Photos © B. Proud.)

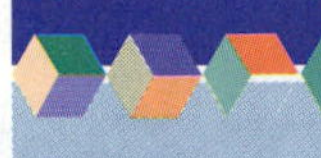

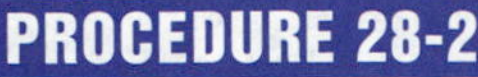

PROCEDURE 28-2

Preparing a Sterile Field

Equipment

Sterile wrapped drape or commercially prepared sterile package

Additional sterile supplies as needed (dressings, container, solution)

Action	Rationale
Initially Preparing the Field	
1. Explain procedure to client.	An explanation encourages client cooperation and reduces apprehension.
2. Gather equipment.	Preparation provides for an organized approach to task.
3. Wash your hands.	Handwashing deters the spread of microorganisms.
4. Check that sterile wrapped drape or package is dry and unopened. Also note expiration date.	Moisture contaminates a sterile package. Expiration date indicates period that package remains sterile.
5. Select a work area that is waist level or higher.	Work area is within sight. Bacteria tend to settle, so there is less contamination above waist level.
6. Open sterile wrapped drape or commercially prepared sterile package.	
a. For *sterile wrapped drape,* open outer covering. Remove sterile drape lifting it carefully by its corners. Shake open, hold away from your body, and lay drape on selected work area.	Outer 1 inch (2.5 cm) of drape is considered contaminated. Any item touching this area is also considered contaminated.
b. Place *commercially prepared package* in center of work area. Touching outer surface only, carefully reach around item and fold topmost flap of wrapper away from you. Open right and left flap before grasping the nearest flap and opening toward you.	Proper placement prevents contamination by reaching across sterile field. Touching outer side of wrapper maintains sterile field.
7. Place additional sterile items on field as needed.	Sterile field is maintained.

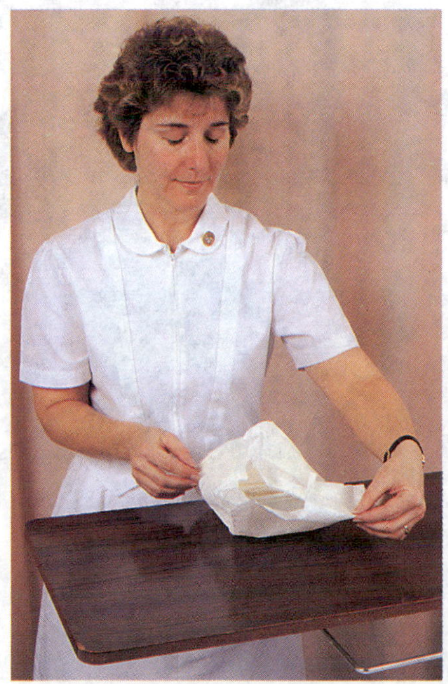

Action 6b: Folding topmost flap of wrapper away from body.

(continued)

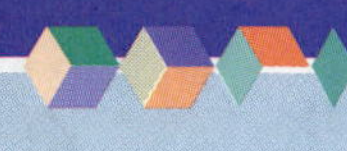

PROCEDURE 28-2 *(continued)*

Preparing a Sterile Field

Action	Rationale
Adding a Sterile Item to a Sterile Field	
8. Open agency-prepared item or commercially packaged item:	
a. Hold *agency-wrapped item* in one hand with top flap opening away from you. With other hand, unfold top flap and both sides. Keeping a secure hold on item, grasp the corners of the wrapper and pull back toward wrist, covering hand and wrist.	Only sterile surface and item are exposed before dropping onto sterile field.
b. If *commercially packaged item* has an unsealed corner, hold package in one hand and pull back on top cover with the other hand. If edge is partially sealed, use both hands to carefully peel apart.	Contents remain uncontaminated by hands.
9. Drop sterile item onto sterile field from a 6-inch (15 cm) height or add item to field from the side. Be careful to avoid 1-inch border.	Wrapper does not contaminate sterile field. Any items landing on 1-inch border are considered contaminated.
10. Discard wrapper.	A neat work area promotes proper technique.

Action 8b: Using both hands to peel apart edges of sterile item packaging.

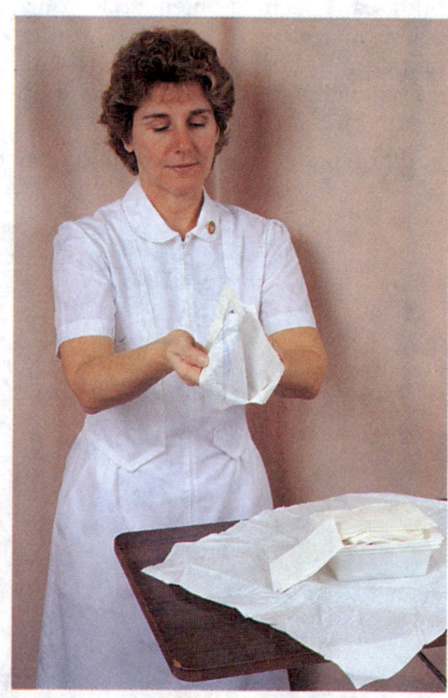

Action 9: Dropping sterile item into sterile field, avoiding 1-inch border.

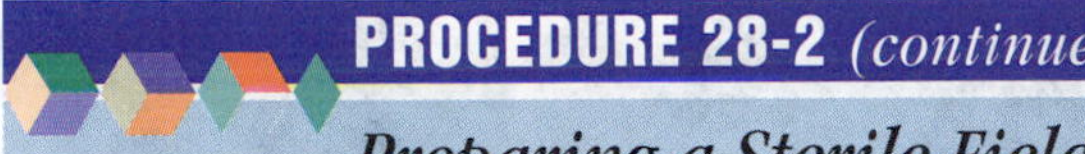

PROCEDURE 28-2 *(continued)*

Preparing a Sterile Field

Action	Rationale
Pouring a Sterile Solution	
11. Obtain appropriate solution and check expiration date.	Once opened, a bottle should be labeled with date and time. Solution remains sterile for 24 hours.
12. Open solution container according to directions and place cap on table with edges up.	Sterility of inside cap is maintained.
13. If bottle has previously been opened, "lip" it by pouring a small amount of solution into waste container.	This cleanses the lip of the bottle.
14. Hold bottle outside the edge of the sterile field with the label side uppermost and prepare to pour from a height of 4 to 6 inches (10 to 15 cm).	Label remains dry and solution may be poured without reaching across sterile field. Minimal splashing occurs from that height.
15. Pour required amount of solution steadily into sterile container positioned at side of sterile field. Avoid splashing any liquid.	Moisture contaminates sterile field.
16. Touch only the outside of the lid when recapping.	Solution remains uncontaminated.

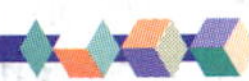

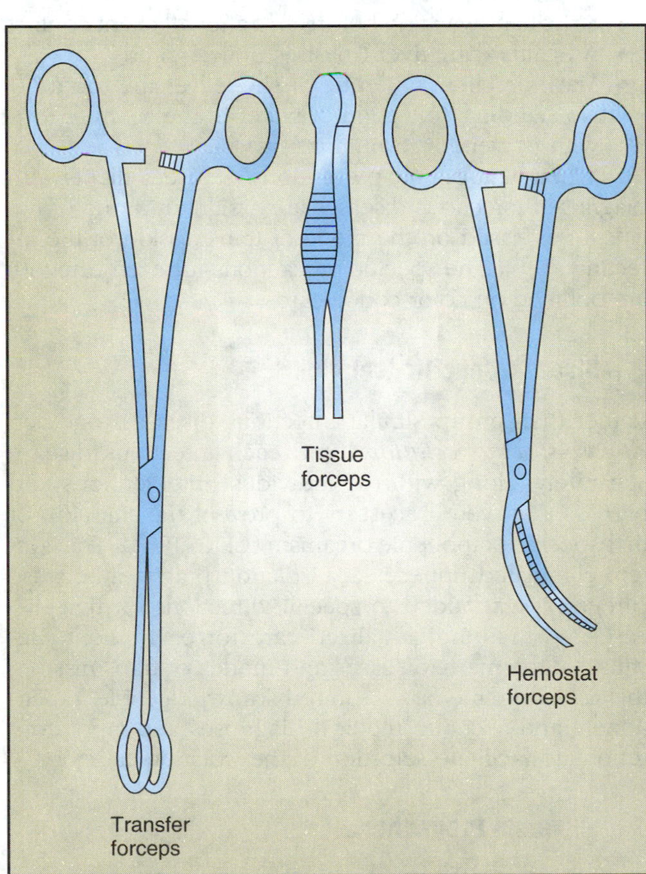

Figure 28-3
Examples of forceps used for sterile procedures.

upper edges of the drape should be folded over the sterile-gloved hands (Fig. 28-5). When sterile gloves are not worn, the nurse is allowed to touch only the outer 1 in (2.5 cm) of the drape. Caution must be used when shaking the drape open so as not to touch the uniform or an unsterile object. Holding the drape by the 1-in upper edge, the nurse positions the drape over the desired area. The nurse must not reach over the drape because this would contaminate a sterile area.

Using Isolation and Barrier Techniques for Infection Prevention and Control

Isolation is a protective procedure that limits the spread of infectious diseases among hospitalized clients, hospital personnel, and visitors. The transfer of pathogens from person to person can be decreased when dissemination of pathogens is limited. The most practical means of accomplishing this is to develop barriers that prevent common vehicles from transmitting them. Figure 28-6 demonstrates the ability of barriers to break the infection cycle. The following discussion gives the historical background to current CDC isolation precautions, including category-specific isolation, disease-specific isolation, universal precautions, and body substance isolation.

Early isolation practices involved quarantining infected persons together in a separate facility where few, if any, aseptic techniques were employed. At the beginning of the 20th century, efforts at isolation moved toward placing infected individuals together in one hospital or a hospital ward where caregivers used gowns

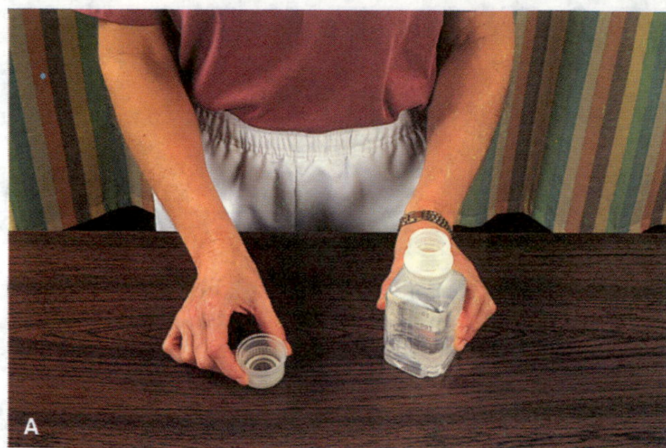

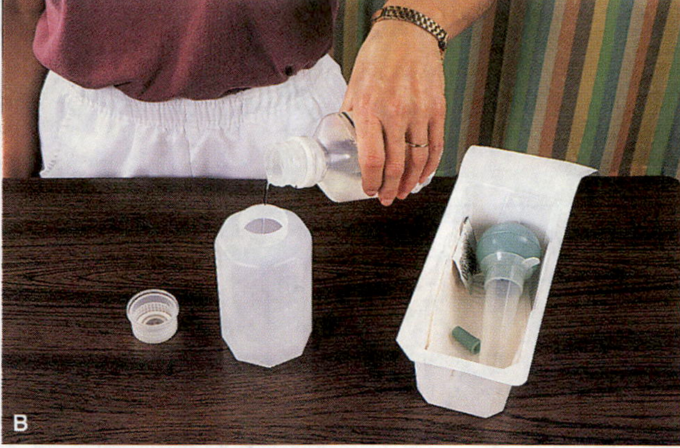

Figure 28-4
Pouring sterile liquids. **(A)** The nurse opens the sterile liquid container while touching only the outside of the cap. The cap is then placed aside with the open side up. **(B)** The nurse pours the sterile liquid into a sterile container without reaching over a sterile field. (Photos © B. Proud.)

and antiseptic solutions for handwashing as barriers to transmitting a disease. Eventually infectious disease hospitals began closing, including those set aside for people with tuberculosis, and infected clients were routinely placed on general hospital units in separate rooms or in multiple-client rooms.

By 1970, the CDC was actively involved in developing and recommending infection-control practices and procedures for hospitals. Guidelines from the CDC included procedures for category-specific and disease-specific isolation categories. Concern about the transmission of blood-borne diseases (eg, AIDS, hepatitis B) and the increasing incidence of nosocomial infections caused a shift in the focus of infection-control programs. Universal precautions or body substance isolation systems were adopted in healthcare institutions.

In an effort to simplify isolation practices and ensure that a consistent approach is utilized to prevent the many infections that are transmitted through varied modes, the CDC recently consolidated and synthesized isolation practices; these practices are reviewed later in the chapter. Nurses need an understanding of the various isolation or barrier techniques if they are to use them correctly and minimize infection risks to clients as well as themselves. One thing is certain: *handwashing before and after the care of a client with a communicable illness is mandatory for all health personnel in every situation*.

Category-Specific Isolation

In 1970 the CDC recommended *category-specific isolation* in which all infectious diseases that require similar infection-control techniques were grouped together in categories. In 1983 the list of CDC categories was expanded and the protective isolation category was eliminated (CDC, 1983). Table 28-3 summarizes these categories. Studies revealed that clients who were immunosuppressed more often than not became infected from organisms harbored in their own bodies rather than from pathogens present in the environment or transmitted from other people. Some hospitals and nursing homes still use protective isolation (now referred to as neutropenic precautions) on occasion for an immunosuppressed client (eg, one recovering from transplantation surgery). Recommendations for this particular type of isolation include:

- Single room for client
- Strict handwashing before and after all client contact
- A healthy caregiver (mask is not required)
- Mask on client when he or she leaves the room
- No standing collection of water in the room (eg, with flowers or in humidifiers)

When neutropenic precautions are used, clients with diagnosed infectious diseases are assigned to one of the categories based on the mode of transmission of the infecting agent. The specific precautions for each category are outlined on color-coded cards.

Disease-Specific Isolation

Rather than group similar infectious diseases together, *disease-specific isolation* listed each infectious disease separately, along with the individual interventions and barriers that were necessary to prevent transmission of that specific pathogenic organism (CDC, 1983). This system eliminated unnecessary isolation practices because caregivers responded to specific directions for that disease and thus individualized care for each client. Because of the many diseases and modes of transmission, this isolation method required knowledgeable practitioners and accurate medical diagnoses and laboratory reports to facilitate selection of the isolation category.

Universal Precautions

In 1987, in an effort to protect healthcare workers from exposure to HIV, hepatitis B virus, and other blood-borne pathogens, the CDC issued recommendations for

(text continues on page 576)

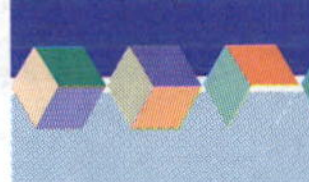

PROCEDURE 28-3

Donning and Removing Sterile Gloves

Equipment

Sterile gloves (size of gloves is indicated on outer wrapping; select appropriate size)

Action	Rationale
To Apply Gloves	
1. Wash and dry hands carefully.	Handwashing deters the spread of microorganisms. Gloves are easier to don when hands are dry.
2. Place sterile glove package on clean, dry surface above your waist.	Moisture could contaminate the sterile gloves. Any sterile object held below the waist is considered contaminated.
3. Open the outside wrapper by carefully peeling the top layer back. Remove inner package, handling only the outside of it.	This maintains sterility of gloves in inner packet.
4. Carefully open the inner package and expose the sterile gloves with the cuff end closest to you.	The inner surface of the package is considered sterile.

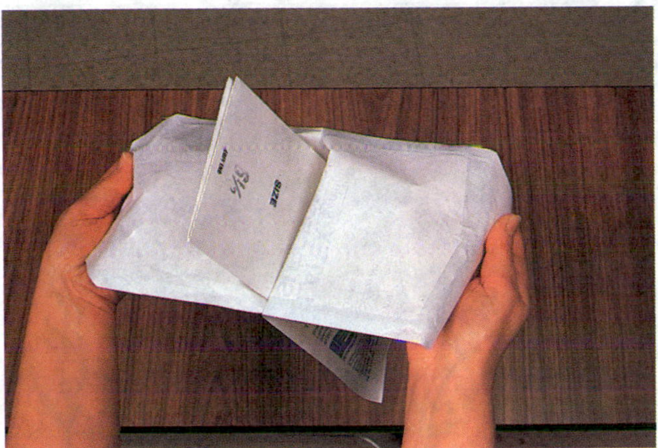

Action 3: Peeling back top layer of outer package.

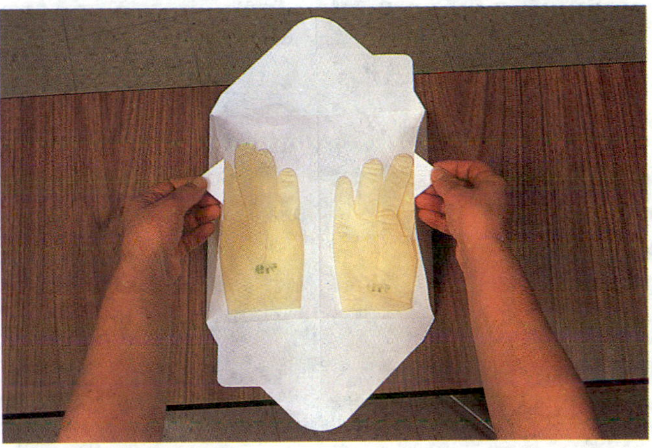

Action 4: Opening inner package.

Action	Rationale
5. With the thumb and forefinger of nondominant hand, grasp the top edge of the folded cuff of the sterile glove for dominant hand.	Unsterile hand only touches inside of glove. Outside remains sterile.
6. Lift and hold glove with fingers down. Be careful it does not touch any unsterile object.	Glove is contaminated if it touches unsterile objects.
7. Carefully insert the dominant hand into glove and pull glove on. Leave cuff folded down until other hand is gloved.	Attempts to turn upward with unsterile hand may result in contamination of sterile glove.
8. Holding thumb outward, slide fingers of gloved hand under cuff of remaining glove and lift glove upward.	Thumb is less likely to become contaminated if held outward.
9. Carefully insert nondominant hand into glove. Adjust gloves on both hands touching only sterile areas.	Sterile surface touching sterile surface prevents contamination.

(continued)

PROCEDURE 28-3 *(continued)*

Donning and Removing Sterile Gloves

Action | **Rationale**

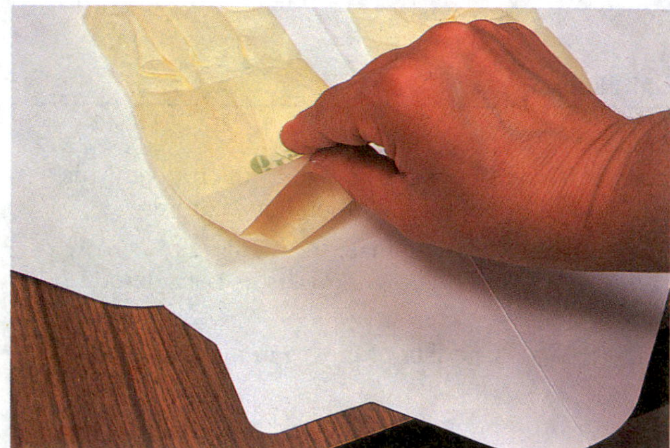

Action 5: Grasping edge of folded cuff.

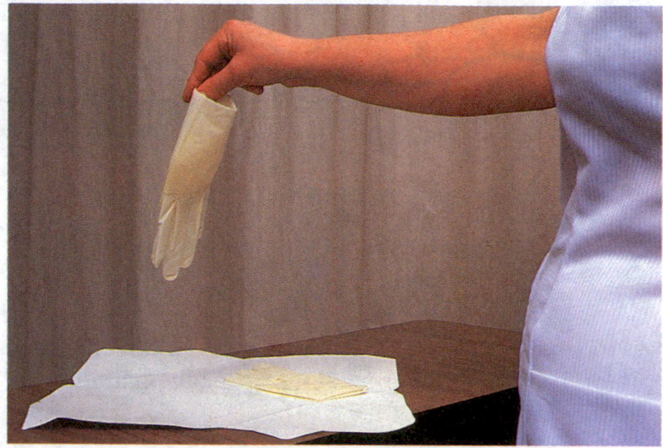

Action 6: Lifting and holding glove with fingers down.

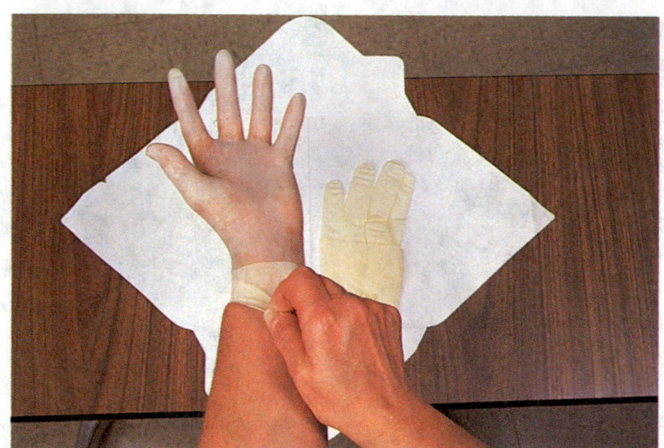

Action 7: Pulling first glove on with cuff folded.

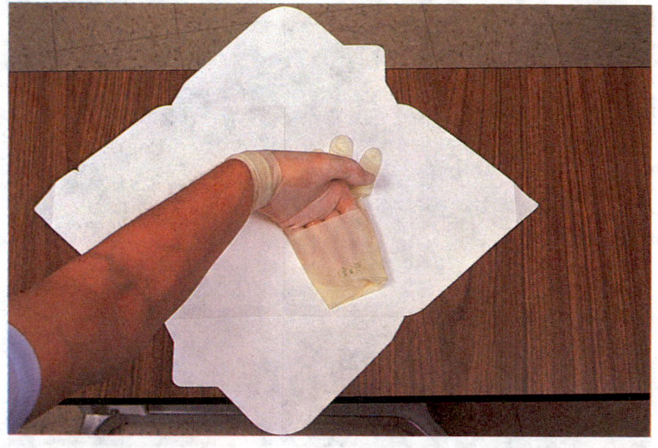

Action 8: Sliding fingers of gloved hand under cuff of second glove.

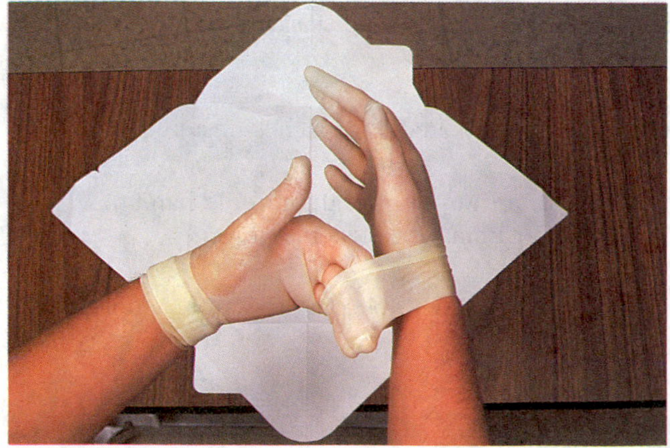

Action 9: Inserting hand with cuff folded.

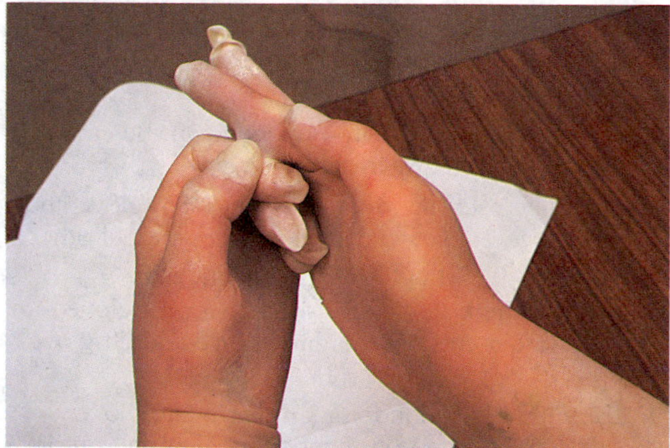

Action 9: Adjusting gloves on both hands.

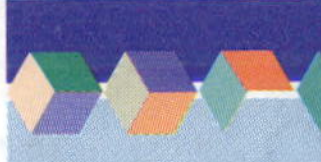

PROCEDURE 28-3 *(continued)*

Donning and Removing Sterile Gloves

Action	**Rationale**
To Remove Gloves	
1. Using dominant gloved hand, grasp other glove near cuff end and remove by inverting it, keeping the contaminated area on the inside. Continue to hold on to glove.	Contaminated area does not come in contact with hands or wrists.

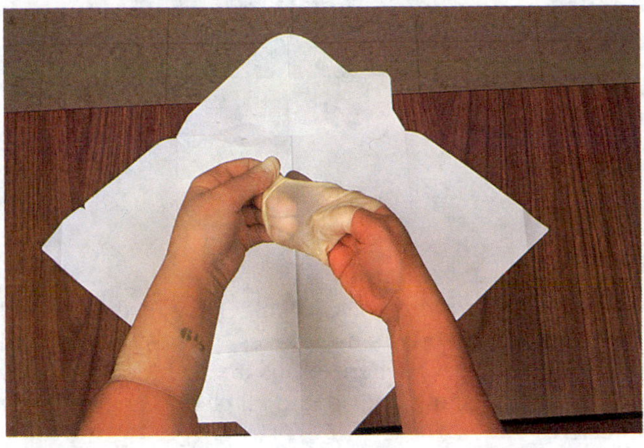

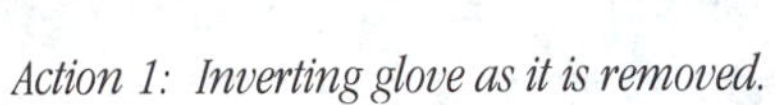

Action 1: Inverting glove as it is removed.

2. Slide fingers of ungloved hand inside the remaining glove. Grasp glove on inside and remove by turning inside out over hand *and other* glove.	Contaminated area does not come in contact with hands or wrists.

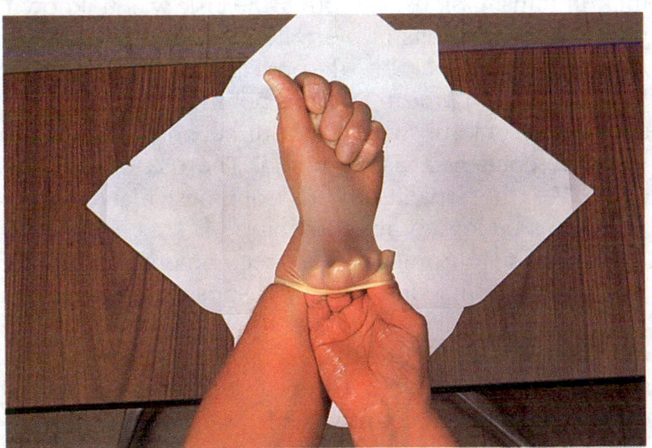

Action 2: Sliding ungloved fingers inside second glove.

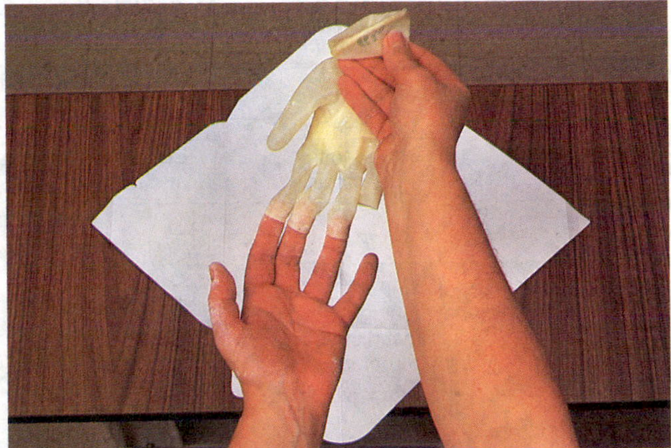

Action 2: Removing second glove inside out.

3. Discard gloves in appropriate container and wash hands.	Handwashing reduces the spread of microorganisms.

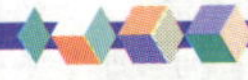

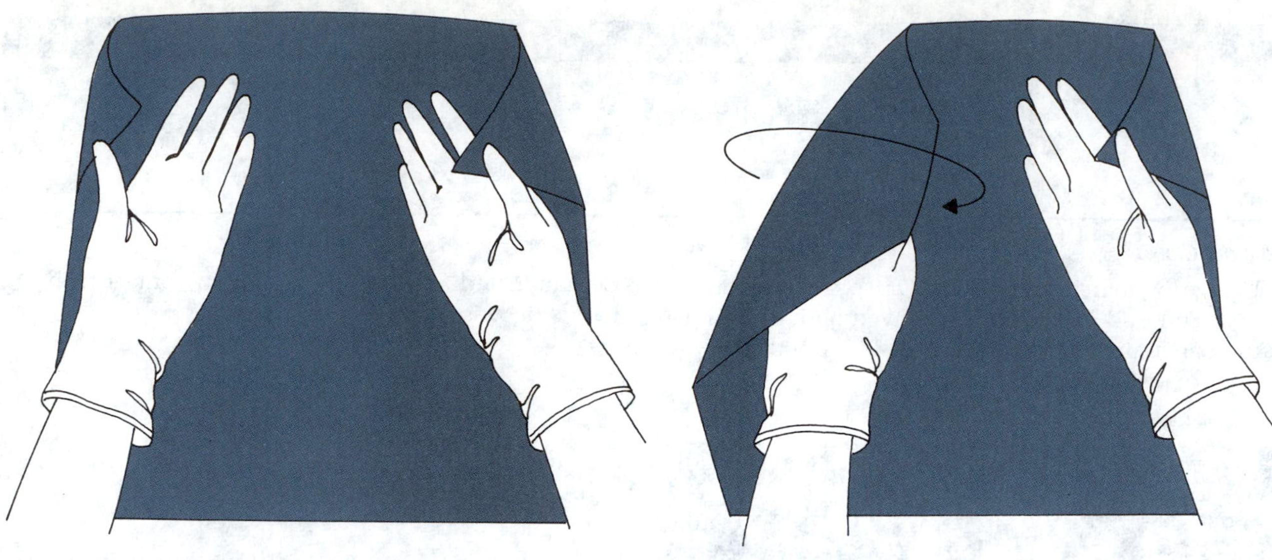

Figure 28-5
Techniques of cuffing a sterile drape over gloved hands.

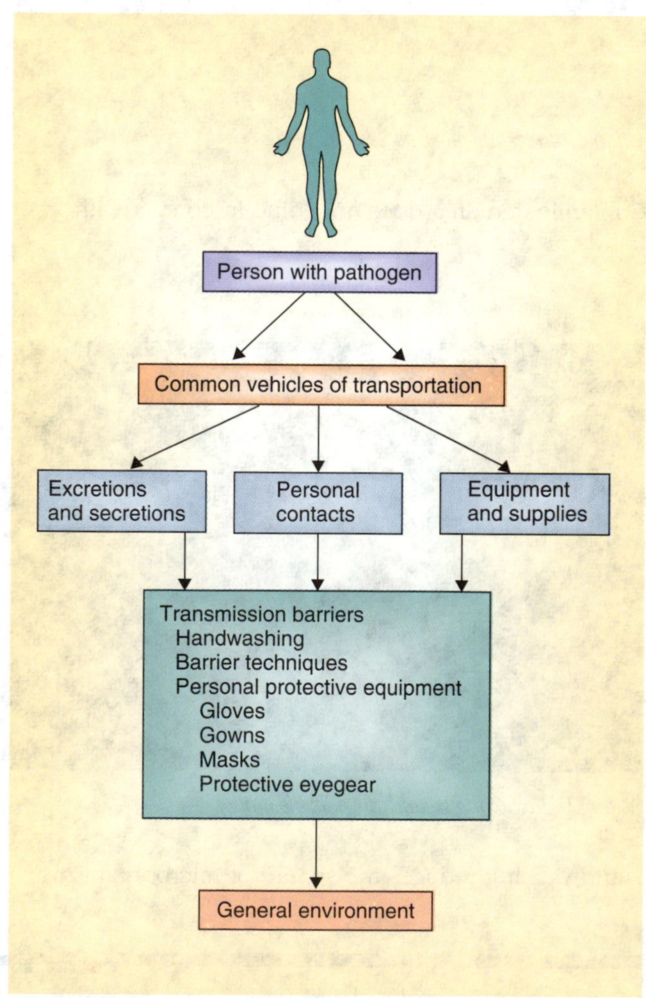

Figure 28-6
Transmission barriers prevent common vehicles from transporting pathogens from the infected person to the general environment.

universal precautions (CDC, 1988). They recommended that healthcare workers use gloves, gowns, masks, and protective eyewear when exposure to blood or body fluids was likely and considered all clients as potentially infected.

A 1988 update from the CDC clarified the specific body fluids affected by universal precautions (see the summary of these universal precautions in the accompanying box). Epidemiologic evidence implicated only blood, semen, vaginal secretions, and possibly breast milk in transmissions. Although the risk was unknown, universal precautions also applied to cerebrospinal, synovial, pleural, peritoneal, pericardial, and amniotic fluids. Universal precautions did not include feces, nasal secretions, sputum, sweat, tears, urine, and vomitus, unless they contained visible blood. The risk of transmitting HIV or the hepatitis B virus from these materials was thought to be low to nonexistent.

Universal precautions also recommend the use of puncture-resistant containers for disposing of all needles and sharps. Needles were not to be recapped, since most needlestick injuries occur at this time. Approximately 800,000 needlesticks occur each year to healthcare workers in this country (Gurevich, 1994). Some experts believe that as many as two out of every three of these needlesticks injuries are never reported (Doan-Johnson, 1992). The movement toward using protected needles or needleless systems significantly reduces the risk of accidental needlesticks, but cost has deterred many employers from adopting these systems. Studies in several healthcare facilities, however, determined that higher costs for the newer equipment may be almost totally offset when compared with the cost of treatment and follow-up for a needlestick injury to an employee (Cornman & Inglott, 1994; Doan-Johnson, 1992). Even

Table 28-3
Summary of Category-Specific Isolation System

Type	Purpose	Sample Diseases Requiring Isolation
Strict	Prevent transmission of highly contagious infections spread by air and contact	Varicella
Contact	Prevent transmission of highly transmissible infections not requiring strict isolation	Acute respiratory tract infections in infants and young children Multiple resistant bacterial infections
Respiratory	Prevent transmission of infectious disease, primarily over short distances by air droplets	Measles Meningitis
Tuberculosis	For client with active TB (positive sputum or x-ray)	Tuberculosis
Enteric Precautions	Prevent infections transmitted by direct or indirect contact with feces	Hepatitis (Type A) Acute diarrhea with infectious cause
Drainage-Secretion Precautions	Prevent infections transmitted by direct or indirect contact with purulent material or drainage from infected site	Abscess Skin or wound infection
Blood–Body Fluid Precautions	Prevent infections transmitted by direct or indirect contact with blood or body fluid	AIDS Hepatitis (Type B)

though alternative equipment is available, nurses must still be accountable for their own safe work practices (see the accompanying box for recommendations to prevent needlestick injuries).

Home Healthcare Alert

Remind clients at home to place sharps containers in a safe place that is out of the reach of small children.

The use of universal precaution strategies was not meant to replace other isolation system safeguards. The CDC recommended using universal precautions in conjunction with category-specific or disease-specific isolation systems. They also continued to emphasize that wearing gloves does not eliminate the need for good handwashing technique. Hands should be thoroughly washed before and after care and after any contact with blood or blood-tinged fluids. Because of frequent and extensive involvement in client care, nurses in particular need to conscientiously practice these risk-reduction behaviors.

Summary of Universal Precautions in Use Before 1996

General precautions to prevent transmission of HIV, Hepatitis B virus, and other blood-borne pathogens in health care settings:

- Consider *all* clients as potentially infected.
- Wear gloves when touching blood, body fluids containing blood, and body fluids to which universal precautions apply. Change gloves after each contact with a client.
- Use protective barriers (ie, wear masks, protective eyewear or face shields and gowns or aprons) when performing procedures likely to produce blood or body fluid droplets or splashes.
- Wash hands and skin surfaces immediately and thoroughly with warm soap and water if contaminated with blood or other body fluids to which universal precautions apply. Wash hands between clients and after removal of gloves even when they are intact.
- Take precautions to prevent injuries from needles, scalpels, and other sharp instruments during procedures, when cleaning instruments, during disposal, or when handling. Needles should not be recapped, purposely bent or broken by hand, removed from disposable syringes, or otherwise manipulated. After use, disposable syringes and needles, scalpel blades, and other sharp items should be placed in puncture-resistant containers for disposal.
- Use mouthpieces, resuscitation bags, or other ventilation devices when mouth-to-mouth resuscitation is likely to be performed in emergency situations.

VRE Guidelines. In addition to universal precautions, some healthcare facilities recently implemented CDC recommendations to help check the spread of vancomycin-resistant enterococci (VRE) (Hospital Infection Control, 1994). The following aggressive infection control measures are included in the advisory from CDC to control this resistant organism:

- Put VRE-infected clients in single rooms or in the same room as other clients with VRE.
- Wear clean gloves and a gown (if substantial contact with the client is expected) when entering the room. Remove the protective items before leaving the room.
- Wash hands immediately with an antiseptic or antimicrobial soap.
- Keep equipment that will be reused (blood pressure cuff, stethoscope, glass thermometer, etc.) in the client's room.
- Keep client in VRE isolation until at least three cultures—taken 1 week apart—are negative.

OSHA Regulations. The *Occupational Safety and Health Administration* (OSHA) is a government agency that administers the Occupational Safety and Health Act of 1970 and establishes minimum health and safety standards for workers. In December 1991 it issued regulations for use of universal precautions in all situations and settings in which occupational exposures to blood and other potentially infectious materials were possible. This ruling reinforced CDC guidelines for universal precautions and made violations punishable with severe fines. Recognizing that the hepatitis B virus poses the greatest blood-borne risk to healthcare workers, OSHA also required that employers offer HBV vaccine free of charge to employees to prevent transmission of hepatitis B. As many as 300 U.S. healthcare workers die each year from hepatitis B (Richardson, 1992). The American Nurses Association is urging OSHA to consider extending this directive to provide immunization and mandate protection against blood-borne diseases for nursing students who practice in these healthcare facilities.

OSHA has also fined hospitals that have failed to evaluate and adopt equipment or devices that reduce the risk of needlestick injuries for employees (Gurevich, 1994).

Body Substance Isolation

Body substance isolation (or body substance precautions) was an extension of universal precautions. First implemented by Lynch and colleagues (1990) at Harborview Medical Center in Seattle in 1985, it was designed to reduce the risk for cross-transmission of organisms between clients and minimize the risk for infection in healthcare personnel. Body substance isolation considered *all* body substances potentially infective, regardless of a person's diagnosis, and advocated consistent use of barriers whenever healthcare personnel had contact with moist body substances, mucous membranes, and nonintact skin. The more inclusive term body substance extended precautions to include not only blood and blood-tinged fluids but also feces, urine, wound drainage, oral secretions, vomitus, and any other body sub-

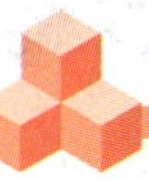

Guidelines for Nursing Care

Preventing Needlestick Injuries

- Dispose of syringes and needles in designated sharps containers *immediately* after use.
- Never lay used syringes and needles on bedding or bedside table or place in dressings at the bedside.
- If necessary to recap a needle, use a "one-handed scoop" technique (see photograph) or a needle recapping device.
- Use needleless systems or protected needle devices if available in healthcare facility.

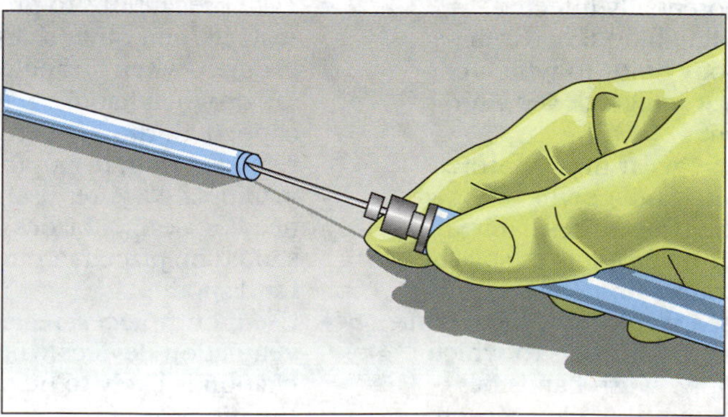

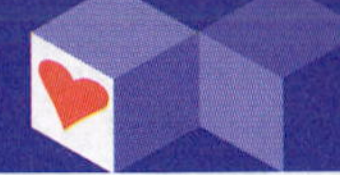

Promoting Wellness

Isolation/Barrier Techniques

Use the assessment checklist to determine how well you are observing isolation or barrier precautions as you care for clients in a healthcare facility or in a community setting. Then develop a prescription for self-care by choosing appropriate behaviors from the list of suggestions.

Assessment Checklist

almost always	sometimes	almost never	
☐	☐	☐	1. I wash my hands before and after contact with a client.
☐	☐	☐	2. I wear gloves if contact with blood or body fluids is a possibility.
☐	☐	☐	3. I use additional protective equipment (gowns, masks, goggles) to protect my clothing, skin, and mucous membranes from contamination with blood or other body substances.
☐	☐	☐	4. I avoid recapping any needles.
☐	☐	☐	5. I place needles or other sharp objects in a puncture-proof disposable container.
☐	☐	☐	6. I dispose of used or contaminated objects/equipment in a leak-resistant plastic trash bag.

Self-Care Behaviors

1. Read infection control standards published by OSHA and CDC.
2. Attend programs that provide updates on current CDC/OSHA policies.
3. Maintain strict personal hygiene habits.
4. Obtain immunizations when available.
5. Assess for any signs and symptoms of an infection.
6. Wash hands frequently with soap and water or use available antiseptic cleanser or hand wipes.
7. Wash hands immediately after removing gloves.
8. Protect myself with the barriers necessary to prevent exposure to blood/body fluids or secretions.
9. Follow agency policy if any exposure to blood or body substance occurs.
10. Never eat, drink, smoke, apply cosmetics or lip moistener, or handle contact lenses in an area where occupational exposure is possible.

stance. The accompanying box lists the elements of body substance isolation. Advocates of body substance isolation considered it a simple, straightforward approach to infection control.

Using body substance isolation eliminated the need for category-specific or disease-specific systems except for certain airborne diseases that required special precautions. Varicella (chickenpox) and pulmonary tuberculosis are examples of airborne diseases that necessitated a private room with the door closed and a "Stop Sign Alert" on the door. This requested visitors to check with the nurse before entering the room. Mask use depended on the organism and the visitor's immune status.

Reminder signs for body substance isolation were strategically placed throughout the unit and near client care areas. Some nurses expressed concern that not having a sign outside a client's room designating the particular disease and prevention strategy decreased their awareness. By its design, body substance isolation reduced risks for clients and personnel by treating all people in a similar manner, thus minimizing potential infection from unknown, undiagnosed diseases.

Body Substance Isolation

The following precautions should be observed by everyone at all times, regardless of the client's diagnosis:

- Wear gloves when contact with moist body substances, mucous membranes, or nonintact skin is likely.
- Wear a gown or plastic apron to prevent soiling of clothing from body substances.
- Wear masks or eyegear to protect mucous membranes of eyes, nose, and mouth from splattering of body substances.
- Use good handwashing technique before and after each client contact and when gloves are removed if hands are visibly soiled.
- Place uncapped needles and sharp instruments in puncture-proof containers.
- Bag soiled linen securely before transporting to laundry area. Dispose of trash in plastic bags according to agency policy.

Disposable gloves and needle disposal containers were placed in every room. Each client interaction required good handwashing technique before and after care. Clean gloves were required for each client, and high-stress care situations often required that gloves be changed several times while caring for one client. When gloves were removed, body substance isolation recommended handwashing only if hands were visibly soiled. Some healthcare experts cited this lack of emphasis on handwashing after glove removal as a disadvantage of this system.

Body substance isolation also provided a consistent approach to soiled linen, trash disposal, and laboratory specimens. Laundry bags were secured and transported in the usual manner. Visible soiling on the outside required double-bagging. Laundry workers were educated to wear heavy gloves when handling soiled linen and to follow good handwashing technique. Trash was disposed of in securely tied plastic bags according to hospital policy or local and state requirements. All laboratory specimens were placed in plastic bags and sealed to prevent leakage during transportation. No special labels were applied to specimen containers or bags.

Current CDC Recommendations for Isolation Precautions in Hospitals

The latest guideline from the CDC replaces all previous recommendations (CDC, 1996). It includes the major features of universal and body substance precautions but uses new terminology so as not to be confused with the previous systems. It recognizes the importance of body fluids, secretions, and excretions in the transmission of nosocomial pathogens. The revised guideline designates two tiers of precautions:

Standard Precautions: Precautions used in the care of all hospitalized persons regardless of their diagnosis or possible infection status. They apply to blood, all body fluids, secretions, and excretions *except sweat* (whether or not blood is present or visible), nonintact skin, and mucous membranes.

Transmission-Based Precautions: Precautions used in addition to Standard Precautions for clients in hospitals with suspected infection with pathogens that can be transmitted by *airborne, droplet,* or *contact* routes. These precautions encompass all the diseases or conditions previously listed in the disease-specific or category-specific classifications. These categories recognize that a disease may have multiple routes of transmission.

The three types of transmission-based precautions (airborne, droplet, or contact) may be used alone or in combination but always in addition to Standard Precautions. The accompanying boxes list a summary of these CDC guidelines and specific recommendations that are strongly supported and viewed as effective for each of the two tiers of precautions. Hospitals are encouraged to modify these recommendations as needed for implementation of their infection-control strategy.

CDC Isolation Guideline: Types of Procedures and Patients Requiring Them

Standard Precautions

Use Standard Precautions for the care of all patients

Airborne Precautions

In addition to Standard Precautions, use Airborne Precautions for patients known or suspected to have serious illnesses transmitted by airborne droplet nuclei. Examples of such illnesses include:

1. Measles
2. Varicella (including disseminated zoster)*
3. Tuberculosis (see CDC Guidelines for Preventing the Transmission of Tuberculosis in Health-Care Facilities)

Droplet Precautions

In addition to Standard Precautions, use Droplet Precautions for patients known or suspected to have serious illnesses transmitted by large particle droplets. Examples of such illnesses include:

1. Invasive *Haemophilus influenzae* type b disease, including meningitis, pneumonia, epiglottitis, and sepsis
2. Invasive *Neisseria meningitidis* disease, including meningitis, pneumonia, and sepsis
3. Other serious bacterial respiratory infections spread by droplet transmission, including:
   a. Diphtheria (pharyngeal)
   b. Mycoplasma pneumonia
   c. Pertussis
   d. Pneumonic plague
   e. Streptococcal pharyngitis, pneumonia, or scarlet fever in infants and young children
4. Serious viral infections spread by droplet transmission, including:
   a. Adenovirus*
   b. Influenza
   c. Mumps
   d. Parvovirus B19
   e. Rubella

(continued)

CDC Isolation Guideline: Types of Procedures and Patients Requiring Them *(continued)*

Contact Precautions

In addition to Standard Precautions, use Contact Precautions for patients known or suspected to have serious illnesses easily transmitted by direct patient contact or by contact with items in the patient's environment.

Examples of such illnesses include:

1. Gastrointestinal, respiratory, skin, or wound infections or colonization with multidrug-resistant bacteria judged by the infection control program, based on current state, regional, or national recommendations, to be of special clinical and epidemiologic significance
2. Enteric infections with a low infectious dose or prolonged environmental survival, including:
   a. *Clostridium difficile*
   b. For diapered or incontinent patients: enterohemorrhagic *Escherichia coli* O157:H7, *Shigella,* hepatitis A, or rotavirus
3. Respiratory syncytial virus, parainfluenza virus, or enteroviral infections in infants and young children
4. Skin infections that are highly contagious or that may occur on dry skin, including:
   a. Diphtheria (cutaneous)
   b. Herpes simplex virus (neonatal or mucocutaneous)
   c. Impetigo
   d. Major (noncontained) abscesses, cellulitis, or decubiti
   e. Pediculosis
   f. Scabies
   g. Staphylococcal furunculosis in infants and young children
   h. Staphylococcal scaled skin syndrome
   i. Zoster (disseminated or in the immunocompromised host)*
5. Viral/hemorrhagic conjunctivitis
6. Viral hemorrhagic fevers (Lassa fever or Marburg virus)

* Certain infections require more than one type of precaution.

(Centers for Disease Control. [1996]. Guideline for isolation precautions in hospitals. Part II: Recommnendations for isolation precautions in hospitals. *American Journal of Infection Control, 24*[1], 32–52).

Summary of Recommended Practices for Standard and Transmission-Based Precautions

Standard Precautions

* Wash hands after touching blood, body fluids, secretions, excretions, and contaminated items, regardless of whether gloves are worn. Wash hands immediately after gloves are removed, between patient contacts, and whenever indicated to prevent transfer of microorganisms to other patients or environments. Use plain soap for routine handwashing and an antimicrobial or waterless antiseptic agent for specific circumstances.
- Wear clean non-sterile gloves when touching blood, body fluids, excretions of secretions, contaminated items, mucous membranes, and nonintact skin. Change gloves between tasks on the same patient as necessary and remove gloves promptly after use.
- Wear mask, eye protection, or face shield during procedures and care activities that are likely to generate splashes or sprays of blood or body fluids. Use gown to protect skin and prevent soiling of clothing.
- Ensure that used patient-care equipment that is soiled with blood or identified body fluids, secretions, and excretions is handled carefully to prevent transfer of microorganisms, or cleaned, and appropriately reprocessed if used for another patient.
- Use adequate environmental controls to ensure that routine care, cleaning, and disinfection procedures are followed.
- Handle, transport, and process linen soiled with blood and body fluids, excretions, and secretions in a manner that prevents skin and mucous membrane exposures, contamination of clothing, and transfer of microorganisms.
- Use previously identified techniques and equipment to prevent injuries when using needles, sharps, and scalpels, and place these items in appropriate puncture-resistant containers after use.

(continued)

Summary of Recommended Practices for Standard and Transmission-Based Precautions *(continued)*

Transmission-Based Precautions

The following precautions are recommended in addition to Standard Precautions:

Airborne Precautions

- Place patient in private room that has monitored negative air pressure in relation to surrounding areas, 6 to 12 air changes per hour, and appropriate discharge of air outside or monitored filtration if air is recirculated. Keep door closed and patient in room.
- Use respiratory protection when entering room of patient with known or suspected tuberculosis. If patient has known or suspected rubeoloa (measles) or varicella (chicken pox), respiratory protection should be worn unless person entering room is immune to these diseases.
- Transport patient out of room only when necessary and place a surgical mask on the patient if possible.
- Consult CDC Guidelines for additional prevention strategies for tuberculosis.

Droplet Precautions

- Use a private room, if available. Door may remain open.
- Wear a mask when working within 3 feet of patient.
- Transport patient out of room only when necessary and place a surgical mask on the patient if possible.

Contact Precautions

- Place the patient in a private room if available.
- Change gloves after having contact with infective material. Remove gloves before leaving the patient environment, and wash hands with an antimicrobial or waterless antiseptic agent.
- Wear a gown if contact with infectious agent is likely or patient has diarrhea, an ileostomy, colostomy, or wound drainage not contained by a dressing.
- Limit movement of the patient out of the room.
- When possible, dedicate the use of non-critical patient-care equipment to a single patient to avoid sharing equipment.

(Centers for Disease Control. [1996]. Guideline for isolation precautions in hospitals. Part II: Recommendations for isolation precautions in hospitals. *American Journal of Infection Control, 24*[1], 32–52.)

Personal Protective Equipment and Supplies

According to the 1992 OSHA ruling, healthcare agencies must provide employees with the equipment and supplies necessary to minimize or prevent exposure to infectious material. This personal protective equipment (PPE) includes gloves, gowns, masks, and protective eye gear. Procedure 28-4 summarizes proper use of this equipment.

Gloves. Wearing gloves is not a substitute for good handwashing. Gloves are worn only once, discarded appropriately according to agency policy, and then hands should be thoroughly washed. Each client interaction requires a clean pair of gloves, and some care activities for an individual client may necessitate changing gloves more than once.

Concern has been expressed about the integrity of the various types of gloves. Korniewicz and Garzon (1994) reported that both latex and vinyl gloves provided some barrier protection, but that latex gloves seemed to be more useful in stressful care situations because they are more flexible and durable; also, by nature of the latex composition tiny glove punctures reseal automatically. Of concern, however, are reports from the Food and Drug Administration (FDA) that from 1988 to 1992 there were more than 1000 allergic reactions, including 16 fatal responses, to latex products (Gold, 1994). Reactions have ranged from urticaria (hives) to systemic anaphylaxis, an exaggerated allergic reaction that resulted in death for several clients undergoing a barium enema procedure with a latex-cuffed tip on an enema tube. The FDA recommends that client questioning about drug and food allergies should be expanded to include queries about sensitivity to latex products. A client is at risk if he has ever experienced any redness, wheezing, itching, swelling, or other abnormal reaction to any latex product (eg, when blowing up a balloon, using condoms, or wearing rubber gloves). If a latex allergy is confirmed or suspected, the client should wear a nonlatex ID wrist band that indicates this allergy. Latex-free equipment should be used during care; if he or she is scheduled for any surgery, the OR personnel must be notifed of this sensitivity. Screening tests are available to determine latex sensitivity but are not used routinely because of the risk of an adverse reaction. The skin prick test (SPT) is easy to administer and causes minimal discomfort; results are easily interpreted.

Healthcare workers must be aware of any sensitivity on their part to latex products and should consider wearing a Medic-Alert bracelet stating this allergy. The healthcare facility should have a written policy dealing with latex-sensitive employees and clients. It may also be necessary to use powderless latex surgical gloves since the latex antigen in the powder may become air-

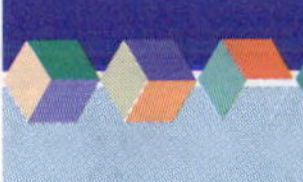

PROCEDURE 28-4

Using Personal Protective Equipment

Equipment (may vary)

Gloves
Gown
Mask (surgical or particulate respirator)
Protective eyewash

Action	Rationale
1. Check physician's order for type of isolation and review precautions in Infection Control Manual.	Mode of transmission or organism determines type and degree of precautions.
2. Plan nursing activities and gather necessary equipment prior to entering client's room.	Organization facilitates performance of task and adherence to isolation precautions.
3. Provide instruction about isolation precautions to client, family members, and visitors.	An explanation encourages cooperation of client and family and reduces apprehension about isolation procedures.
4. Wash your hands.	Handwashing deters the spread of microorganisms.
5. Put on gown, gloves, mask and protective eyewear, if recommended as isolation precaution:	Interrupts chain of infection. Protects client and nurse.
a. Tie gown securely at neck and waist.	Gown should protect entire uniform.
b. Use clean disposable gloves. If worn with gown draw glove cuffs over gown sleeves.	Protect hands and wrists from microorganisms.
c. Mask must be securely tied and fitted to face.	Protects nurse from droplet nuclei and large particle aerosols.
d. Eyewear must have protection on side of face or side shields.	Protects mucous membranes in the eye from splashes.
6. When client care is completed, remove gloves first.	Gloves have been involved in client care and are most soiled.
a. Untie waist strings of gown first. Grasp outside of one glove and turn inside out to remove. Continue to hold on to glove.	Ungloved hand is clean and should not touch contaminated areas. Waist strings of gown are considered contaminated.

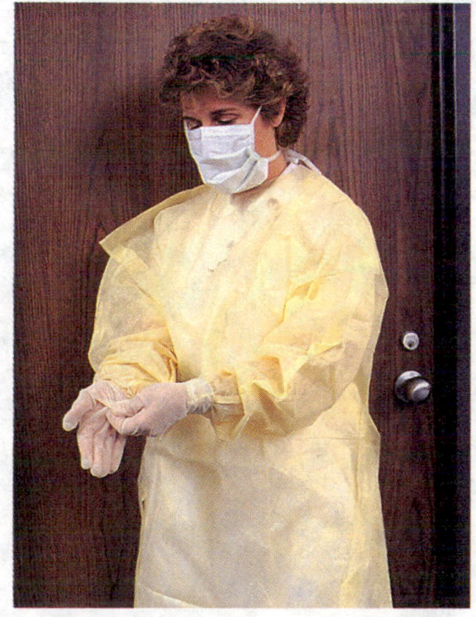

Action 6a: Grasping outside of first glove and pulling it off inside out.

(continued)

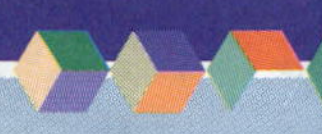

PROCEDURE 28-4 *(continued)*

Using Personal Protective Equipment

Action	Rationale
b. Insert fingers of ungloved hand inside the cuff of the remaining glove. Grasp glove on inside and remove by turning inside out. Drop in appropriate container.	

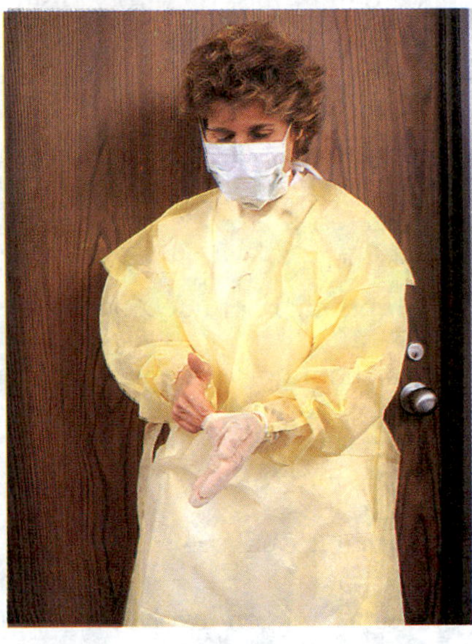

Action 6b: Placing fingers of ungloved hand inside cuff of the remaining glove.

Action	Rationale
7. After gloves are removed, remove mask:	
Surgical mask	
a. Untie mask and drop by strings into waste container.	Center of mask is contaminated. Strings are considered clean.
Particulate Respirator	
b. Use hand to hold respirator in place.	Prevents respirator from falling off face onto floor.
c. Pull bottom strap up and over head.	
d. Pull top strap over head.	
e. Remove respirator from face and save for future use or discard according to manufacturer's directions.	
8. Remove gown:	
a. Gown that is not visibly soiled requires no particular technique for removal	
For gown that is visibly soiled:	
b. Untie neck strings of gown. Remove gown without touching outside of gown by keeping one hand up and under the gown cuff and using this protected hand to pull the opposite sleeve down and off.	Neck strings are considered clean. Outside of gown is contaminated.

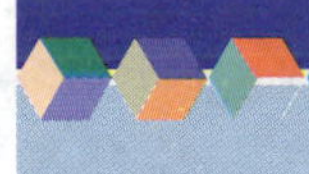

PROCEDURE 28-4 *(continued)*

Using Personal Protective Equipment

Action	Rationale
c. Use ungowned arm and hand to grasp the gown from the inside and remove from the remaining arm. Remove gown and turn inside out and drop in appropriate container.	

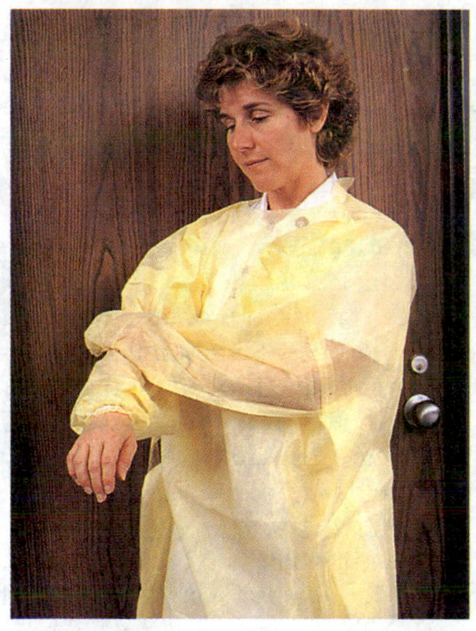

Action 8b: Using protected hand to pull the opposite sleeve down and off.

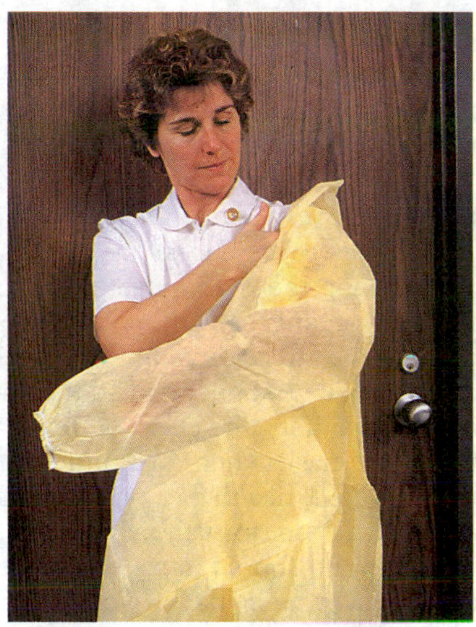

Action 8c: Using ungowned hand to grasp gown from the inside.

Action	Rationale
9. Remove eyewear last and clean according to agency policy.	Eyewear is reusable.
10. Wash hands thoroughly.	Prevents spread of microorganisms.

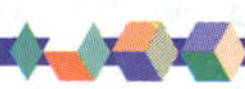

borne and be inhaled by others in the area who are sensitive. Nonlatex gloves may be worn over or under a latex pair, depending on who is sensitive.

In high-risk settings such as the operating room, double-gloving may be recommended. A recent study, however, demonstrated that wearing a single pair of latex gloves was as effective in preventing exposure to blood and body fluids as wearing two sets of latex gloves (Korniewicz et al., 1994). A stronger latex surgical glove is being developed that offers more protection and is an alternative to double-gloving.

Home Healthcare Alert

Awareness of a latex allergy is vital to provide safe home care. Ask clients if they have experienced any unusual signs or symptoms when blowing up balloons, using latex condoms, or wearing rubber gloves for dishwashing or cleaning.

Gowns. In most instances, gowns are worn to prevent soiling of the healthcare worker's clothing from the client's blood and body fluids. They provide barrier protection and should be donned immediately before entering the client's room. Individual gown technique is recommended. This means that gowns are worn only once and then discarded appropriately according to agency policy. If a gown becomes heavily soiled or moistened with blood or body fluids when caring for a client, it should be removed, hands should be thoroughly washed, and a clean gown should be donned. There is no special technique for applying a gown, but recommended practices for removing a soiled gown are included in Procedure 28-4.

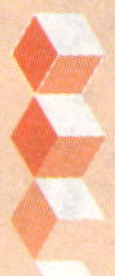

Helpscan

The following are resources for clients and health-care professionals:

- For guidelines to help health-care workers prevent and manage latex allergy:
  American College of Allergy and Immunology (ACAI)
  800 E. Northwest Highway, Suite 1080
  Palatine, IL 60067
- For information related to OSHA regulations:
  Occupational Safety and Health Administration (OSHA)
  Office of Public and Consumer Affairs
  US Department of Labor, Room N3637
  200 Constitution Ave. NW
  Washington, DC 20210
  (202) 523-8148

Masks. Masks are intended to prevent the wearer from inhaling large-particle aerosols, which usually travel short distances (about 3 ft), and small-particle droplet nuclei, which can remain suspended in the air and travel longer distances. Masks also discourage the wearer from touching the eyes, nose, and mouth, thus limiting contact of organisms with mucous membranes.

Various practices are observed in the use of masks. In some instances, all personnel and all the client's visitors wear masks; in others, the client on respiratory precautions wears the mask when transported outside his or her room to protect healthcare personnel and other clients from any exposure to pathogens. A mask should be worn only once and should *never* be lowered around the neck and then brought back over the mouth and nose for reuse. The length of time to wear one mask while caring for one client is debatable. It should certainly be changed before it becomes damp from the wearer's exhalations. Recommended practices when wearing a mask are summarized in Procedure 28-4.

The serious increase in the number of multidrug-resistant (MDR) tuberculosis cases prompted new guidelines to prevent the transmission of this disease. In 1990 the CDC recommended a more tightly fitting mask, called a *particulate respirator*, to better protect healthcare personnel from this particularly virulent, drug-resistant form of tuberculosis. Updated guidelines from the CDC (1994) focused on early detection and treatment of tuberculosis, careful examination and protection of healthcare workers who might unknowingly transmit the disease, and the use of a High-Efficiency Particulate Air filter mask (HEPA) when exposed to this pathogen. NIOSH (the National Institute of Occupational Safety and Health) has recently tested and certified a Type N95 respirator designed for use in healthcare settings that meets CDC and OSHA guidelines for TB exposure control (National Institute of Occupational Safety and Health, 1995). Caregivers expressed difficulty wearing the HEPA-style respirator for extended periods of time, but the more recent Type N95 respirator is designed to filter out particles as small as 1 micron with 95% efficiency and fit more comfortably against the face (Fig. 28-8). It costs considerably less than the HEPA filter respirators. The elastic straps on these respirators also provide more protection and better fit than the ties on regular surgical masks.

Protective Eyewear. Protective eyewear, such as goggles or a face shield, should be available on the unit whenever there is a risk of contaminating the mucous membranes of the eyes. Suctioning a tracheostomy or assisting with an invasive procedure may result in splattering of blood or other body fluids and require protection for the caregiver. Plain glasses are unacceptable because side shields are required.

Other Isolation Supplies and Procedures. Used equipment may either be disposed of after use or, if reusable,

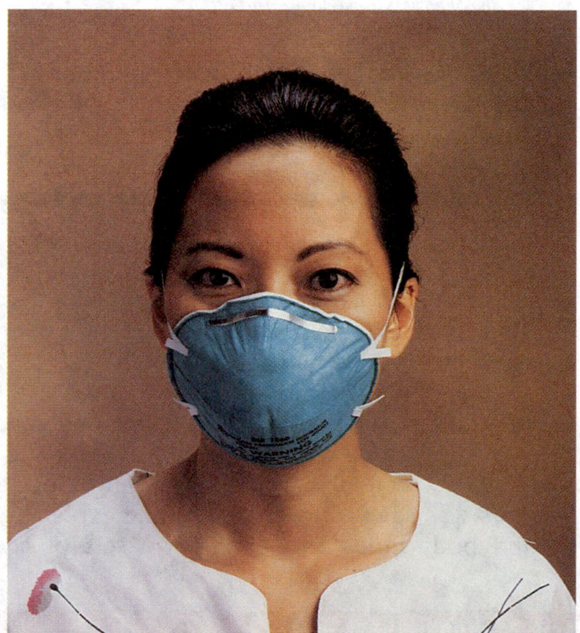

Figure 28-8
The new Type N95 healthcare particulate respirator is NIOSH approved. It meets CDC guidelines for tuberculosis exposure control and is designed specifically for use in a healthcare setting. (Courtesy of 3M Health Care.)

bagged according to agency policy, sent to a central cleaning area, and sterilized or disinfected to reduce risk of transmission of pathogenic organisms. Double-bagging may be required if the single bag is not secure or is soiled on the outside. A contaminated item should never be used for another client.

Double-bagging of trash and linen is advisable only if the outside of the bag is visibly soiled. Some linen bags are water-soluble and dissolve in hot water, making it unnecessary for workers to handle the contaminated linen. Paper trays and plastic eating utensils do not prevent transmission of organisms and are no longer recommended. The combination of hot water and detergent that is used in commercial dishwashers sufficiently decontaminates dishes, glasses, and utensils. Special cleaning techniques are no longer considered necessary for a person with a communicable disease. It is recommended that all spills of body fluids or substances be immediately cleaned with the appropriate chemical germicide or disinfectant.

Meeting Psychologic Needs of Clients in Isolation

The psychologic implications of isolation precautions usually are great, whether the client is strictly separated from others or needs only to observe relatively simple precautions. Isolation methods that treat all people in a similar manner greatly minimize the psychologic trauma of feeling unclean and undesirable. This feeling is intense for most clients; they feel frightened, lonely, unclean, guilty, and rejected. The likelihood of suffering sensory deprivation and loss of self-esteem is a troublesome accompaniment. Friends and relatives as well as healthcare personnel may be inclined to spend less time with the client because they are afraid that they will contract the disease or because of the inconvenience of coping with isolation procedures. Nursing measures to help prevent sensory deprivation and loss of self-esteem are discussed in Chapters 31 and 34.

Teaching and supportive measures are probably the two biggest contributions the nurse can make during this period of a client's illness. The client and family must have an accurate understanding of the pertinent epidemiologic facts of the situation and of how to carry out the specific precautions. The idea that it is the pathogenic organism that is unwanted, not the person, must be emphasized. The client who resents and ignores precautions also needs help in being accepted as a person and in constructively expressing his or her feelings.

Studies have shown that extensive separation of people from others can be traumatic. Isolation precautions should be discontinued as soon as it is deemed safe. The problem of striking a balance between what is best for both the client and others is a delicate one that often requires the nurse's utmost skill and ingenuity.

A well-informed nurse who understands how to protect self and clients and a well-informed client who is cooperating in his or her care are superior communicable disease precautions.

Raising Ethical Concerns About Infection Risks

Isolation and barrier techniques minimize infection risks for clients as well as healthcare workers. The increasing numbers of people infected with HIV and hepatitis B and C virus also has resulted in serious ethical concerns

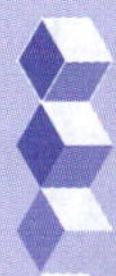

Through the Eyes of a Student

She was the cutest little girl I have ever known. She was infected with the HIV from birth. Her mother was an IV drug user and engaged in unprotected sex with multiple partners. This little girl, who came into the world with an innocent, fresh, new face full of unconditional love, could not walk, could not talk, could not chew, could not control her urine or bowel movements—but boy could she smile! In the beginning I was so terrified of contracting AIDS that I couldn't walk into her room without a mask, gown, gloves, protective eyewear, and basically a full protective body spacesuit. At the end I wanted to take her into my home and give her all the love, support, and care she needed. I am not saying that I didn't wear gloves when I changed her diapers or when I flushed her heparin lock because I did . . . I was very careful. But I realized that she is a person, a person full of feelings, a person who needed me and from whom I could learn. People with the AIDS virus are just that—people. We need to learn to treat them as such.

I also learned not to fear the person who is diagnosed with HIV infection or AIDS. I know that I will take the proper safety precautions with this person. The person I need to fear is the cute little old man who would never have AIDS because "he's not the type." If I don't use universal precautions, it is possible that one day I'll become infected through contact with someone who is "not the type." If that should ever happen, I hope everyone who cares for me will treat me as a real person and not be afraid.

—Karmi N. Soder, Georgetown University Washington, DC

Nursing Today: Challenges and Solutions

AIDS

Challenges

- The World Health Organization estimates that by the year 2000, 30 to 40 million persons will be HIV-infected and 12 to 18 million will have AIDS (Early HIV Infection Guideline Panel, 1994).
- By 2000, AIDS will be the third most common cause of death in the United States (Early HIV Infection Guideline Panel, 1994).
- More than 15,000 13- to 24-year olds have been diagnosed with AIDS (Veroneau & Campbell, 1995).
- AIDS is the number-one killer of Americans aged 25 to 44 (Veroneau & Campbell, 1995).
- Women are the fastest-growing population of people with HIV disease (Walker & Frank, 1995).
- By 2000, as many as 126,000 children in the United States may be motherless because of AIDS (Collins, 1994).

Nursing Solutions

- A school nurse incorporated age-appropriate HIV information into a 4-year comprehensive family planning curriculum she established at a school in Londonderry, Vermont. Her efforts related to AIDS education also include community meetings, newspaper articles, letters to parents, and teacher in-services (Campbell, 1995).
- Nurses are involved in hosting town meetings on HIV issues in various parts of the country. Discussion at these town forums has resulted in the establishment of HIV/AIDS task forces to deal with issues of concern (Campbell, 1995).
- A nurse-managed outpatient center in Denver, Colorado, provides education to HIV-positive clients and their friends, families, and other support personnel, in addition to fostering professional healthcare practices based on research findings (*American Nurse,* 1993).
- Nurses interested in getting involved in community efforts can contact Nurses Unite Against AIDS Hotline at (800) 807-6276.

and controversy related to the risk for transmitting these diseases. At issue are the rights of the client versus the rights of the healthcare worker and the healthcare agency. The following questions are being discussed and debated:

- Should all hospital clients be routinely tested for HIV infections?
- Should HIV testing be mandatory for all healthcare workers?
- Should healthcare workers infected with HIV be permitted to perform exposure-prone invasive procedures?
- Should AZT prophylaxis be routine for all exposed healthcare workers?
- What procedures should be considered exposure prone?
- Will healthcare facilities be liable if they allow HIV-positive staff to care for clients?
- Should pregnant healthcare providers be expected to care for clients with infectious diseases?

The CDC and various medical and nursing groups are attempting to reach agreement and consensus on these issues based on scientific information and valid statistical evidence. All are in agreement, however, that healthcare workers who conscientiously adhere to isolation or barrier technique recommendations seriously reduce the risk for infection for clients and themselves.

Reporting an Accidental Exposure

The nurse is accountable for his or her own safety. Any needlestick injury or accidental exposure to blood or body fluids must be reported immediately so that appropriate interventions can be initiated. Failure to notify an employer of an exposure may result in personal jeopardy as well as loss of compensation should an infection develop. An agency's plan for this type of exposure should include the following:

- Wash the exposed area immediately with warm water and soap.
- Report the incident to the appropriate person and complete an incident or injury report if required by the agency.
- Inform agency of the source (client's name) and nature of the exposure.
- Consent to initial baseline blood test, if agreeable, to determine personal HIV/hepatitis B (HBV) status. Repeat blood test 6 weeks after exposure and at 3-month, 6-month, and 1-year intervals.
- Await blood test results of the involved client (with his or her consent) to determine HIV/HBV status. State laws may vary concerning this practice.
- Begin post-exposure treatment, if recommended, at the appropriate time.
- Attend counseling session regarding safe practices to protect self and others (Bowles & Lynch, 1992).

Using the Infection-Control Nurse

In the hospital, the infection-control nurse is responsible for educating clients and staff about effective infection-control techniques and for collecting statistics about infections. Many hospitals rely on this specialized practitioner to survey laboratory reports and review records for clients at risk as well as suggest approaches to potentially dangerous situations. Intensive investigative strategies create a positive environment to significantly reduce the incidence of nosocomial infections in healthcare facilities. The infection-control nurse is aware of the devastating effects of infection and is intent on promoting health and fostering a systematic approach to infection control.

In the home care setting, the infection control nurse's duties include surveillance for agency-associated infections, education, consultation, epidemiologic investigation, quality-improvement activities, and policy and procedure development (Bennett, 1994). Comprehensive infection-control programs for home care agencies that include nationally accepted criteria for infections that develop in the home setting are currently being developed.

EVALUATING

Nurses, by nature of their role as the primary caregiver, can intervene in and positively affect a client's outcome. By assessing the person at risk, selecting appropriate nursing diagnoses, planning, and intervening to maintain a safe environment, the nurse can reduce a client's potential for developing an infection. Evaluation of the plan of care determines whether the individual's need for safety is being effectively met. Ongoing systematic evaluation is critical for the nurse who is striving to maintain a secure environment for her clients as well as a safe workplace for herself. If client goals have been met and evaluative criteria have been satisfied, the client will:

- Correctly use techniques of medical asepsis
- Identify health habits and lifestyle patterns that promote health
- State the signs and symptoms of an infection
- Identify unsafe situations in the home environment

Key Points

- The infection chain consists of six components and can be interrupted by measures that halt the spread of disease.
- The stage of an infection and the client's response influence the extent and type of nursing care provided.
- Sterilization and disinfection may be accomplished by physical or chemical means, based on the nature and number of organisms, the type and intended use of equipment, and the availability and practicality of the means.
- Handwashing is the single most effective way to prevent the spread of infection and decrease the incidence of nosocomial infection.
- The most common nosocomial infections are urinary tract infections, surgical wound infections, and pneumonia.
- Medical asepsis, or clean technique, is concerned with reducing the number of pathogens.
- Surgical asepsis, or sterile technique, includes practices that keep objects and areas free of microorganisms.
- Isolation procedures develop barriers that prevent the transmission of pathogens and break the infection cycle.
- The category-specific and disease-specific isolation systems require that an infectious disease be diagnosed before initiating the appropriate infection-control techniques.
- CDC recommendations for universal precautions state that healthcare workers use gloves, gowns, masks, and protective eyewear when exposure to blood, semen, vaginal secretions, or body fluids is likely. All clients should be considered potentially infected.
- The body substance isolation system considers all body substances potentially infective and advocates consistent use of barriers whenever healthcare personnel have contact with moist body substances, mucous membranes, and nonintact skin.
- The recently revised CDC guideline recognizes the importance of all body fluid secretions and excretions in transmitting nosocomial infections and consists of Standard Precautions and Transmission-Based Precautions.
- Multidrug-resistant tuberculosis requires the use of a Type N95 particulate respirator to protect the caregiver from droplet infection.

Study Questions

1. The smallest infectious agents capable of causing an infection are
   a. bacteria
   b. viruses
   c. molds
   d. yeasts
2. Your client has developed a low-grade fever and states that she has felt very tired lately. This phase of an infection is known as the
   a. incubation period
   b. prodromal stage
   c. full stage of illness
   d. convalescent period
3. The highest mortality rate is associated with nosocomial infections that involve the
   a. respiratory tract
   b. integumentary system
   c. urinary tract
   d. intestines
4. A client develops a urinary tract infection after an indwelling urinary catheter has been inserted. This would most accurately be termed
   a. a viral infection
   b. a chronic infection
   c. an iatrogenic infection
   d. an opportunistic infection
5. The nurse has opened his sterile supplies and donned two sterile gloves to complete a sterile dressing change. Maintaining surgical asepsis requires that he
   a. keep splashes on his sterile field to a minimum
   b. cover his nose and mouth as he sneezes with his gloved hands
   c. use the dominant hand to cleanse the incision with a moist saline sponge and then apply the dry dressing
   d. consider the outer 1 in of the sterile field as contaminated
6. The CDC's Standard Precaution recommendations apply to:
   a. only clients with diagnosed infections
   b. only blood and body fluids with visible blood
   c. all body fluids including sweat
   d. all clients receiving care in hospitals
7. In addition to Standard Precautions, the nurse caring for a client with rubella would plan to implement:
   a. Droplet Precautions
   b. Airborne Precautions
   c. Contact Precautions
   d. Universal Precautions
8. The nurse in a healthcare agency that uses body substance isolation wears gloves when caring for an incontinent client. She is aware that
   a. gloves can be used between clients if they are intact
   b. long fingernails and rings compromise the safety of gloves
   c. glove use is optional in this situation
   d. gloves protect her when frequent handwashing is not possible
9. The guidelines for minimum protection standards for infection prevention and control were initially developed by
   a. OSHA
   b. individual healthcare facilities
   c. the state governing body
   d. the CDC
10. The recommended sequence when the nurse removes soiled personal protective equipment as she prepares to leave the client's room is
    a. remove gown, goggles, mask, gloves, and exit the room
    b. remove gloves, wash hands, remove gown, mask, and goggles
    c. remove gloves, mask, gown, goggles, and wash hands
    d. remove goggles, mask, gloves, gown, and wash hands
11. For the nurse, under normal conditions with unsoiled hands, effective handwashing between clients requires
    a. at least a 10–15 second scrub
    b. at least a 2–3 minute scrub
    c. use of an antimicrobial product
    d. that a mask be worn when scrubbing
12. Which hospitalized client is most at risk for developing a nosocomial infection?
    a. Mr. Y, a 60-year-old who smokes two packs of cigarettes daily
    b. Mrs. J, a 40-year-old who has a white blood cell count of 6000/μL
    c. Mr. L, a 65-year-old who has an indwelling urinary catheter in place
    d. Mrs. M, a 60-year-old who is a vegetarian and slightly underweight
13. A client develops food poisoning from contaminated potato salad. The means of transmission for the infecting organism is
    a. direct contact
    b. vectors
    c. vehicle
    d. airborne
14. A nurse is caring for an obese 62-year-old client with arthritis who has developed an open reddened area over his sacrum. A priority nursing diagnosis is
    a. Altered Nutrition: More Than Body Requirements, related to immobility
    b. Impaired Physical Mobility related to pain and discomfort
    c. Chronic Pain related to immobility
    d. Risk for Infection related to altered skin integrity
15. The nurse teaches a client at home to use clean technique when changing a wound dressing. This is
    a. the nurse's preference
    b. safe for the home setting
    c. unethical behavior
    d. grossly negligent

Answers With Rationale

1. The correct response is *b.* A virus is the smallest of all microorganisms and can only be seen with a microscope. Molds and yeasts, which are fungi, and bacteria are larger infectious agents.
2. The correct response is *b.* During the prodromal stage, the person has vague signs and symptoms, such as fatigue and a low-grade fever. There are no obvious symptoms of infection during the incubation period, and they are more specific during the full stage of illness before disappearing by the convalescent period.
3. The correct response is *a.* Urinary tract infections and surgical wounds are common sites for nosocomial infections to develop, but the highest mortality rate is associated with those infections that involve the respiratory tract. The intestine is not particularly prone to nosocomial infections.
4. The correct response is *c.* An infection that develops as a result of the insertion of an indwelling catheter is termed iatrogenic. Because this infection just developed, it is not chronic, nor did it occur because of any altered physiology that may give an opportunistic organism a chance to cause infection. These infections are bacterial, not viral.
5. The correct response is *d.* Considering the outer inch of a sterile field as contaminated is a principle of surgical asepsis. Moisture contaminates the sterile field, and sneezing contaminates the sterile gloves. The sterile hand that cleaned a wound should not be used or should be regloved before applying a sterile dressing.
6. The correct response is *d.* Standard Precautions apply to all clients receiving care in hospitals regardless of their diagnosis or possible infection status. These recommendations include blood, all body fluids, secretions, and excretions except sweat, nonintact skin, and mucous membranes.
7. The correct response is *a.* Rubella is an illness transmitted by large particle droplets and requires Droplet Precautions in addition to Standard Precautions. Universal Precautions and Body Substance Isolation are incorporated into the new CDC Standard Precautions recommendations.
8. The correct response is *b.* Long fingernails and rings may cause tears in the gloves, allowing contamination of the nurse's hands. Gloves should never be used for more than one client, and body substance isolation precautions necessitate use of gloves as a barrier for any contact with body substances. Wearing gloves is not a substitute for handwashing.
9. The correct response is *d.* The CDC established the initial minimum requirements for infection prevention and control. OSHA has issued and monitors regulations for use of universal precautions in situations and settings in which exposure to blood and other infectious materials is possible.
10. The correct response is *c.* Gloves are always removed first because they are most likely to be contaminated and hands should be washed thoroughly after the equipment has been removed and before leaving the room.
11. The correct response is *a.* Hands that are not visibly soiled can be effectively cleaned with a 10–15 second scrub. Neither a mask nor an antimicrobial product is required in this situation or setting. Hands that are visibly soiled require a longer scrub.
12. The correct response is *c.* Indwelling urinary catheters have been implicated in a majority of nosocomial infections. Cigarette smoking, a normal white blood cell count, and a vegetarian diet have not been implicated as risk factors for developing an infection.
13. The correct response is *c.* Contaminated food is a vehicle for transmitting an infection. Direct contact requires proximity between the susceptible host and an infected person. A vector is a nonhuman carrier, such as an insect, and the airborne means of transmission carries the organism in droplet nuclei or with dust.
14. The correct response is *d.* The priority diagnosis in this situation is the possibility of an infection developing in the open skin area. The others may be potential or probable diagnoses for this client and also may require nursing interventions once the first one is addressed.
15. The correct response is *b.* In the home setting, where the client's environment is more controlled, medical asepsis usually is recommended with the exception of self-injection. This is the appropriate procedure for the home and is neither unethical nor grossly negligent.

Bibliography

Bennett, G. (1994). Developing an effective infection control program for home care. *Caring, 13*(11), 50–53.

Boutotte, J. (1993). Protecting yourself against T.B. *Nursing, 23*(10), 64–66.

Bowles, K. & Lynch, M. (1992). These products and procedures prevent needlesticks. *RN, 55*(7), 42–45.

Campbell, K. (1995). Nurses combat HIV/AIDS in adolescent community. *American Nurse,* 27(8), 16.

Carpenito, L. (1995). *Nursing diagnosis: Application to clinical practice* (6th ed.). Philadelphia: Lippincott.

Casey, K. (1993). Fighting MDR-TB. *RN, 56*(9), 26–30.

Centers for Disease Control. (1983). *Guidelines for prevention and control of nosocomial infections.* Atlanta: U.S. Department of Health, Education, and Welfare, Public Health Service.

Centers for Disease Control. (1988). Update: Universal precautions for prevention of transmission of human immunodeficiency virus, hepatitis B virus, and other blood-borne pathogens in health-care settings. *Morbidity and Mortality Weekly Report, 37*(24), 377–388.

Centers for Disease Control. (1990). Guidelines for preventing the transmission of tuberculosis in health-care settings with special focus on HIV-related issues. *Morbidity and Mortality Weekly Report, 39*(RR-17), 1–29.

Centers for Disease Control. (1994). Draft guidelines for isolation precautions in hospitals; Notice. *Federal Register, 59*(214), 55552–55570.

Centers for Disease Control. (1994). Guidelines for preventing the transmission of tuberculosis in health care facilities. *Federal Register, 59*(208), 54242–54303.

Centers for Disease Control. (1996). Guideline for isolation precautions in hospitals, Part I: Evolution of isolation practices. *American Journal of Infection Control, 24*(1), 24–31.

Centers for Disease Control. (1996). Guideline for isolation precautions in hospitals, Part II: Recommendations for isolation precautions in hospitals. *American Journal of Infection Control, 24*(1), 32–52.

Collins, H. (1994, March 29). AIDS orphans in U.S. may total 175,000 by end of decade. *Philadelphia Inquirer,* A1, 13.

Cornman, L. & Inglot, D. (1994). One hospital's solution. *RN, 57*(11), 50–51.

Doan-Johnson, S. (1992). Taking a closer look at needle sticks. *Nursing, 22*(8), 24–27.

Early HIV Infection Guideline Panel. (1994). *Evaluation and management of early HIV infection: Clinical practice guideline.* (AHCPR Pub. No. 94-0572). Rockville, MD: AHCPR Public Health Service, U.S. Department of Health and Human Services.

Eggleston, B. (1994). Infection control update. *Nursing, 24*(3), 70–72.

Fraser, D. (1993). Patient assessment: Infection in the elderly. *Journal of Gerontological Nursing, 19*(7), 5–11.

Fritsch, D. & Pilat, D. (1993). Exposing latex allergies. *Nursing, 23*(8), 46–48.

Gold, J. (1994). Ask about latex. *RN, 57*(6), 32–34.

Gurevich, I. (1994). Preventing needlesticks. *RN, 57*(11), 44–51.

Hoeprich, P. & Jordan, M. (1994). *Infectious diseases* (5th ed.). Philadelphia: Lippincott.

Hofland, S. & Mort, J. (1994). Infections in long-term care facilities: Issues for practice. *Geriatric Nursing, 15*(5), 260–264.

Korniewicz, D. & Garzon, L. (1994). How to choose and use gloves. *Nursing, 24*(9), 18.

Korniewicz, D. et al. (1994). Barrier protection with examination gloves: Double versus single. *American Journal of Infection Control, 22*(1), 12.

Larson, E. (1995). APIC guideline for handwashing and hand antisepsis in health care settings. *American Journal of Infection Control, 23*(4), 251–269.

Lynch, P., Cummings, M. Roberts, T., Herriott, M., Yates, B., & Stamm, W. (1990). Implementing and evaluating a system of generic infection precautions: Body substance isolation. *American Journal of Infection Control, 18*(1), 1–12.

Marwick, C. (1994). New guidelines to avoid TB transmission issued. *Journal of the American Medical Association, 272*(19), 1484.

Mylotte, J., Niederman, M. & Summer, W. (1993). Staying on top of hospital infections. *Patient Care, 27*(3), 116–145.

National Institute of Occupational Safety and Health (1995). Respiratory protective devices. *Federal Register, 60*(110), 30336–30402.

Olsen, R., Lynch, P., Coyle, M., Cummings, J., Bokete, T. & Stamm, W. (1993). Examination gloves as barriers to hand contamination in clinical practice. *Journal of the American Medical Association, 270*(3), 350–353.

Reiss, P. (1996). Battling the super bugs. *RN, 59*(3), 36–40.

Rice, R. (1993). Principles of Universal precautions/body substance isolation. *Home Healthcare Nurse, 11*(4), 55–59.

Richardson, D. (1992). OSHA releases final standard on HIV/hepatitis B exposures. *American Nurse,* 24(1), 1.

Sheldon, J. (1994). 25 tips on handwashing. *Nursing, 24*(1), 20.

Spechko, P. (1993). Blood borne pathogens: Can you become infected from your older patient? *Journal of Gerontological Nursing, 19*(7), 13–15.

Staff. (1993). States work to combat HIV/AIDS crisis. *American Nurse, 25*(3), 21–22.

Staff. (1994). VRE and other resistant pathogens threaten return to pre-antibiotic area. *Hospital Infection Control, 21*(7), 89–93.

Stolley, J. & Buckwalter, K. (1991). Iatrogenesis in the elderly: Nosocomial infections. *Journal of Gerontological Nursing, 17*(9), 30–34.

Turner, J. (1993). Handwashing behavior versus handwashing guielines in the ICU. *Heart and Lung, 22*(3), 275–277.

Veroneau, P. & Campbell, K. (1995). Grants are foundation of ANA's work on HIV/AIDS issues. *American Nurse,* 27(3), 30, 38.

Walker, M. & Frank, L. (1995). HIV/AIDS: An imperative for a new paradigm for caring. *Nursing and Health Care Perspectives on Community, 16*(6), 311–315.

Chapter 29

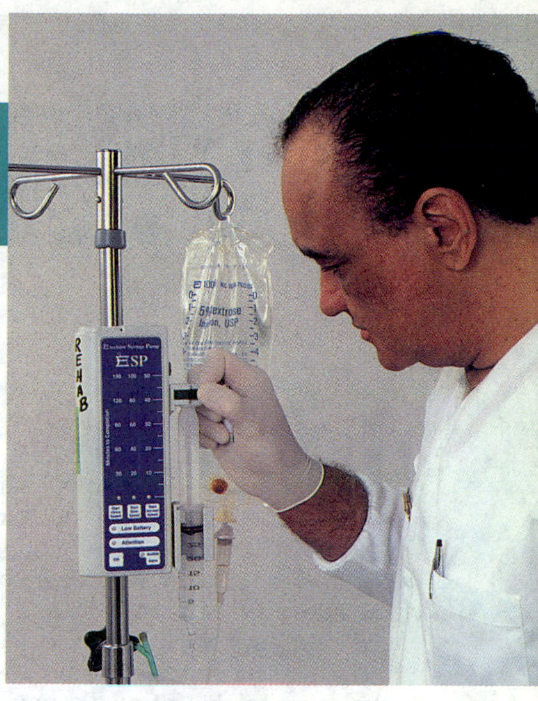

Medications

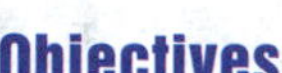

Objectives

After studying this chapter, the learner should be able to:

Define key terms used in the chapter.

Discuss drug legislation in the United States and Canada.

Describe drug names, types of preparations, and types of drug orders.

Identify drug classifications and actions.

Discuss adverse effects of drugs, including allergy, tolerance, cumulative effect, idiosyncratic effect, and interactions.

Obtain client information necessary to establish a medication history.

Calculate drug dosages, using the various systems of equivalents.

Describe principles used to safely prepare and administer medications orally, parenterally, topically, and by inhalation.

Develop teaching plans to meet client needs specific to medication administration.

Key Terms

absorption
ampule
anaphylactic reaction
antagonist effect
chemical name
cumulative effect
distribution
excretion
generic name
idiosyncratic effect
inhalation
intradermal injection
intramuscular injection
intravenous route
metabolism
official name
parenteral
subcutaneous injection
synergistic effect
topical application
trade name
vial
Z-track

Medication administration is a basic nursing function that involves skillful technique and consideration of the client's development and safety. The nurse administering medications is expected to have a knowledge base concerning drugs, including drug names, preparations, classifications, adverse effects, and physiologic factors that affect drug action.

The nursing process can be applied to the fundamental nursing skill of medication administration. Assessment entails a comprehensive medication history as well as ongoing assessments of the client's response during and after drug therapy. Nursing diagnoses are developed from the assessment data. Client-centered outcomes are evaluated after implementation of the plan of care, tailored to the client's needs.

A *drug* or *medication* is any substance that modifies body functions when taken into the living organism. The study that deals with chemicals that affect the body's functioning is called *pharmacology*. A *pharmacist* is a person licensed to prepare and dispense drugs. The physician is legally responsible for prescribing medications. Legislation in some states grants nurse practitioners this privilege also. The physician or nurse practitioner conveys the medication plans to others by an order called a *prescription*. After the medication is prepared by the pharmacist, the nurse administers the medication to the client.

Some medications are given frequently, and the nurse becomes familiar with the facts concerning these drugs. Other medications may not be given by the nurse often, and the nurse needs to seek information before administering the drugs. Information about specific drugs is more appropriately discussed in pharmacology texts. Many references are available to nurses to help them develop a personal medication data base.

Drug Legislation

United States

In 1906 the Pure Food and Drug Act designated the United States Pharmacopeia (USP) and the National Formulary (NF) as official standards of drugs and empowered the federal government to enforce these standards. This legislation was updated in 1938 by the Federal Food, Drug and Cosmetic Act. The Food and Drug Administration is responsible for enforcing this law. Extensive testing of new drugs is required before they may be marketed for use. An amendment to the Federal Food, Drug and Cosmetic Act in 1952 distinguished prescription (legend) drugs from nonprescription (over-the-counter) drugs and provided directions for dispensing prescription drugs.

The Comprehensive Drug Abuse Prevention and Control Act, also known as the Controlled Substances Act, was passed in 1970. This law regulates the distribution of narcotics and other drugs of abuse. Such drugs have been categorized according to their therapeutic usefulness and potential for abuse. Government programs for the prevention and treatment of drug abuse were established.

Canada

Drug legislation in Canada includes the Canadian Food and Drug Act, passed in 1953, which addresses regulations for the manufacture and sale of drug substances. This law has been amended often. According to the act, drugs must comply with standards outlined in specific pharmacopeias and formularies (British Pharmacopeia, Canadian Formulary). The regulations of the Canadian Narcotic Control Act, enacted in 1961, restrict the sale, possession, and use of opiates, coca, and marijuana. Amendments made since 1961 include restrictions on methadone. Only authorized people can possess narcotics. Enforcement of this law has been the charge of the Royal Canadian Mounted Police.

Introduction to Pharmacology

Drug Preparations

Nomenclature

One drug can have several names. The **chemical name** is a precise description of the drug's chemical composition; it identifies the drug's atomic and molecular structure. This name is of significance to the pharmacist. The

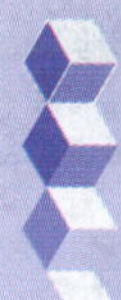

Through the Eyes of a Student

I entered my client's room, knowing that she had had surgery less than 12 hours before my arrival, and introduced myself. I asked how she was feeling, to which she immediately responded, "I need pain medication—*now!*" I told her that I would check the medication orders and be back as soon as possible. I walked quickly to the medication Kardex, and there it was glaring at me in neatly printed black and white: "Demerol 100 mg IM q 3–4 hr prn." My mind raced as I thought, "I have never given an IM injection. There has to be something else ordered for pain." I knew there wasn't. I found my clinical instructor and announced, "My client needs an IM injection." Given the anxiety I was feeling, everything went surprisingly well as we prepared the medication. I went over the procedure one last time before entering the client's room.

We approached the client just in time for her to look at us in sheer terror and cry, "I hope that shot isn't for me; I hate them," which did nothing for my already shaking hands. I explained that she couldn't take a pill because she could not have anything by mouth because of the nature of her surgery. My instructor and I positioned the client on her side—a feat in itself—so that I could give her the shot in the dorsogluteal area. I marked the landmarks at least half a dozen times, wiped the area with alcohol, and asked her if she was ready for the injection. *Big mistake!* She swiftly replied, "No, but get it over with."

A little voice in my head repeated the words my technologies professor had said a million times, "Darting action is the key to a successful injection." So I aimed at the bull's-eye that appeared in front of my eyes. My hand, which seemed to be moving in slow motion, propelled downward at a 90-degree angle. Secretly I prayed that I would not hit my own hand. I must have closed my eyes because the next thing I remember was the loudest scream I had ever heard! I looked down and it was a bull's-eye, thank God, but the needle had not penetrated the muscle! The client successfully tensed her muscle tight enough to intercept the needle midflight. At that moment she relaxed, probably because she thought the worst was over, and I pushed the needle into place. I slowly drew back the plunger to make sure no blood appeared in the syringe. I began injecting the Demerol slowly, watching my hands shake. Then I withdrew the needle and gently applied pressure over the site. It was over and I wanted to scream, "I did it!" but I kept my composure to feign the experience I lacked. Giving my first IM injection was not as bad as I thought it would be!

—Alison L. Moriarty, Georgetown University, Washington, DC

generic name is the name assigned by the manufacturer that first develops the drug. Often the generic name is derived from the chemical name. The **official name** is the name by which the drug is identified in the official publication, *United States Pharmacopeia and National Formulary* (USP and NF). The **trade name**, also referred to as the *brand name* or *proprietary name*, is selected by the drug company that sells the drug and is copyrighted. A drug can have several trade names when produced by different manufacturers.

Nurses should be familiar with a drug's generic and trade names. For example, acetaminophen (generic name) is known by such trade names as Tylenol, Tempra, and Liquiprin.

Types of Preparations

Drugs are available in many forms, or preparations. The form in which the drug is prepared may determine the route of administration. Some drugs may be prepared in only one form to be administered by a certain route. Others may be supplied in several preparations, which allow them to be given through various routes. One type of preparation may be desirable in a given situation. For example, a liquid preparation of a medication would be indicated for young children who are not able to swallow solid preparations such as tablets. Drug preparations are available for oral, topical, and injectable administration. Table 29-1 describes drug preparations commonly used by the nurse.

Classifications

How does the nurse organize the vast amount of information about medications? Where does the nurse begin the study of medications? It is recommended that the nurse focus on drug classifications.

Drugs can be classified from different perspectives. For example, drugs may be classified by body systems (eg, drugs that affect the respiratory system, drugs that affect the cardiovascular system), by the symptom relieved by the drug, or by the clinical indication for the drug (eg, analgesic, antibiotic).

Mechanisms of Drug Action

Pharmacodynamics

Drugs act at the cellular level to achieve their desired effects. The process by which drugs alter cell physiology is called *pharmacodynamics* (Abrams, 1995). One

Table 29-1
Common Types of Drug Preparations

Preparation	Description
Capsule	Powder or gel form of an active drug enclosed in a gelatinous container
Elixir	Medication in a clear liquid containing water, alcohol, sweeteners, and flavor
Extended release	Preparation of a medication that allows for slow and continuous release over a predetermined period; may also be referred to as CR or CRT (controlled release), SR (sustained or slow release), SA (sustained action), LA (long acting), or TR (timed release)
Liniment	Medication mixed with alcohol, oil, or soap, which is rubbed on the skin
Lotion	Drug particles in a solution for topical use
Lozenge	Small oval, round, or oblong preparation containing a drug in a flavored or sweetened base, which dissolves in the mouth and releases the medication; also called *troche*
Ointment	Semisolid preparation containing a drug to be applied externally; also called an *unction*
Pill	Mixture of a powdered drug with a cohesive material; may be round or oval
Powder	Single or mixture of finely ground drugs
Solution	A drug dissolved in another substance (eg, in an aqueous solution the drug has been dissolved in water)
Suppository	An easily melted medication preparation in a firm base such as gelatin that is inserted into the body (rectum, vagina, urethra)
Suspension	Finely divided, undissolved particles in a liquid medium; should be shaken before use
Syrup	Medication combined in a water and sugar solution
Tablet	Small, solid dose of medication, compressed or molded; may be any color, size, or shape; *enteric-coated tablets* are coated with a substance that is insoluble in gastric acids to reduce gastric irritation by the drug
Transdermal patch	Unit dose of medication applied directly to skin for diffusion through skin and absorption into the bloodstream

mechanism of drug action is a drug–receptor interaction in which the drug interacts with one or more cellular structures to alter cell function. These specialized structures are called *receptor sites.* The drug fits the receptor as a key fits a lock. Drugs may also combine with enzymes to achieve the desired effect, which is referred to as a *drug–enzyme interaction.* Some drugs act on the cell membrane or alter the cellular environment.

Pharmacokinetics

Pharmacokinetics is the study of the movement of drug molecules in the body in relation to the drug's absorption, distribution, metabolism, and excretion.

Absorption. Absorption is the process by which a drug is transferred from its site of entry into the body to the bloodstream. Absorption of a drug is influenced by several factors:

Route of administration: Injected medications usually are absorbed more rapidly than oral medications.

Drug solubility: Liquid medications are absorbed more rapidly than solid preparations. Liquid preparations do not have to be dissolved in the gastrointestinal fluids. Most drugs are weak acids and bases. When in solution, drugs are a mixture of ionized and un-ionized forms. The un-ionized form is more readily absorbed.

pH: The form in which the drug is found depends on the pH of the environment. Acidic drugs are well absorbed in the stomach. Drugs that are basic remain ionized or insoluble in an acid environment. These drugs are not absorbed before reaching the small intestine. The concept of acid–base balance is further discussed in Chapter 46.

Local conditions at the site of administration: The more extensive the absorbing surface, the greater the absorption of the drug and the more rapid the effect. A client with burns would have poor absorption from an intramuscular injection. Food in the stomach can delay the absorption of some medications or enhance the rate of absorption of other drugs. Drug absorption can be manipulated with sustained-release preparations or enteric-coated preparations. Enteric-coated preparations are resistant to the digestive action of the stomach.

Drug dosage: A loading dose is higher than body capacity. A maintenance dose is a lower dosage that becomes the usual or daily dosage. Clients who receive digoxin or phenobarbital may receive loading does when therapy is initiated.

Distribution. After a drug has been absorbed into the bloodstream, it is distributed throughout the body. The drug accumulates in specific tissues for its action. **Dis-**

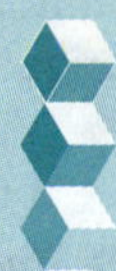

Research in Nursing: Making a Difference

Medications

Nursing competence with drug administration involves far more than just passing medications to clients. It requires that the nurse have knowledge of a drug's action and purpose, possible side effects, contraindications to use, and the range for safe dosage. Nursing responsibility also includes correctly calculating medication doses and teaching clients about potential drug interactions and adverse effects. Various authors have conducted research on nursing strategies that facilitate safe administration of medication and focus on decreasing the risk for adverse effects and drug interactions in older adults.

Related Research

Rice, P., Jensen, M., Lyons, M., & Murphy M. (1994). Medications in well and institutionalized elders. *Geriatric Nursing, 15*(4), 216–218.
Well older people in the community use fewer drugs than those who are in healthcare facilities. Nurses who work with older adults need to monitor their use of over-the-counter drugs and prescription drugs because of the potential for polypharmacy and drug interactions. Client education is vital and nurses can promote optimal independence and quality of life in this population by improving their knowledge of their medications. A thorough drug history that includes prescribed and OTC medications and encouragement to carry a medication profile card appear to support this goal.

Pollow, R., Stoller, E., Forster, L., & Duniho, S. (1994). Drug combinations and potential for risk of adverse drug reactions among community-dwelling elderly. *Nursing Research, 43*(1), 44–48.
Older adults living in the community take drug combinations that have the potential to cause adverse effects. Every year, 10 to 30% of older clients are admitted to the hospital because of drug interactions. Nurses who work with this population in the community need to take a detailed medication history to identify those clients who may be at risk for drug–drug or drug–alcohol interactions and prevent common adverse effects of hypotension and cognitive impairment.

Calliari, D. (1995). The relationship between a calculation test given in nursing orientation and medication errors. *Journal of Continuing Education, 26*(1), 11–14.
Medication errors can adversely affect the client and the institution. In order to prevent these errors, a medication test was given to nurses during their hospital orientation. In reviewing data, it was found that nurses who failed this test were more prone to make a medication error. Providing additional supervision during orientation and periodic observation when administering medications may improve attention to detail for this group of nurses and prevent errors.

Summary

Medication regimens for older adults are complex. Concern about the potential for nurses to make medication errors has prompted researchers to investigate the value of drug calculation tests during orientation activities. Early identification provides opportunity for additional support for these professionals. Older clients who overmedicate benefit from education regarding hazardous drug combinations that have the potential to impact negatively on their independence and quality of life.

tribution depends on the rate of perfusion and capillary permeability to the drug. Certain other factors may also influence distribution. The drug may bind to plasma proteins, which causes unequal distribution and may prevent the drug from reaching its intended site of action. The blood–brain barrier is poorly permeable to water-soluble drugs. Some drugs fail to penetrate the tissues of the central nervous system as readily as others. The placenta, on the other hand, is not a selective barrier to the distribution of drugs. Drugs move across the placenta readily, and many produce harmful effects in the fetus.

Metabolism. Metabolism, or biotransformation, is the breakdown of the drug to an inactive form. The liver is the primary site for drug metabolism. Various processes and enzymes are involved in metabolism. Physiologic changes associated with aging or the presence of liver disease may complicate the process. The reader is referred to a pharmacology text for a further explanation of metabolism.

Excretion. After the drug is broken down to an inactive form, **excretion** of the drug from the body occurs. Most drugs are excreted by the kidneys. The lungs are the primary route for the excretion of gaseous substances, such as inhalation anesthetics. Many drugs are excreted through the intestines. The sweat, salivary, and mammary glands also are routes of drug excretion.

Some medications may be contraindicated or dosages may need to be adjusted downward if renal excretion is affected by age or disease.

Factors Affecting Drug Action

Certain variables influence the action or effect of a medication.

Developmental Considerations

During pregnancy, most drugs are contraindicated because of their possible adverse effects on the fetus. A child's dose for medication is smaller than an adult's dose. Infants especially are responsive to medications because of the immaturity of their organs. Older people are responsive to medications because their bodies have experienced physiologic changes associated with the aging process, including decreased gastric motility, acid production, and blood flow, which affect drug absorption. Small body size, reduced weight, and reduced body water also alter distribution, as do decreases in cardiac output and organ perfusion. Decreased plasma binding increases the possibility of drug toxicity. Liver function declines with advancing age and changes in hepatic enzymes involved in drug metabolism. Blood flow to the liver decreases secondary to a decrease in cardiac output. Drugs are excreted more slowly from the body as a result of changes in kidney function. Receptor sensitivity is altered in older people and their sensitivity to certain drugs increases. The physiologic changes in older people that increase drug susceptibility are summarized in the accompanying box.

Home Healthcare Alert

The nurse should investigate OTC drugs that the client may be taking along with their prescription drugs. Older clients particularly are at risk for drug-drug interactions related to physiologic changes associated with aging.

Weight

Expected responses to drugs are based largely on those reactions that occur when the drugs are given to healthy adults (ages 18 to 65, 150 lb [68 kg]). The nurse should be aware of the usual dose for a particular medication. Drug doses for children are calculated by weight or body surface area.

Sex

This variable refers to the difference in the distribution of body fat and fluids in men and women and is usually thought to be a minor factor affecting drug action. To

Focus on the Older Adult

Altered Drug Response in Older People

Physiologic Basis	Adverse Reaction	Nursing Action
• Decreased gastric emptying time and increased pH of gastric juices	Stomach irritation and ulceration	Assess for symptoms of stomach discomfort. Test stools for blood.
• Increased adipose tissue and decreased total body fluid in proportion to the total body mass Decreased number of protein-binding sites Decline in liver function and enzyme production needed for drug metabolism Decreased kidney function, resulting in diminished filtration and excretion	Increased possibility of drug toxicity	Assess for early signs of drug interactions or toxicity. Monitor blood levels of drugs. Monitor laboratory values.
• Altered peripheral venous tone	More pronounced hypotensive effects from medications (particularly antihypertensives and diuretics)	Monitor vital signs. Caution client to change position slowly.
• Changes in blood–brain barrier allowing for easier penetration of fat-soluble drugs	Increased risk of dizziness and confusion, particularly with beta blockers	Assess for dizziness and lightheadedness. Be aware of safety precautions.

date, most research on drugs and their actions and effects has been conducted on males. Future clinical drug trials are expected to include more women so that the effect of hormonal fluctuations can also be studied and documented.

Genetic and Cultural Factors

Differences in the responses of clients receiving the same medication may be attributed to genetic and cultural differences. *Pharmaco-anthropology*, a relatively new field of study, investigates differences in drug response in various ethnic or racial groups (Kudzma, 1992). Enzyme deficiencies or metabolic disturbances can alter the way the body handles medication or metabolizes a drug. For example, Asian clients may require smaller doses of a drug because they metabolize it at a slower rate. A drug dose that is normal for a Caucasian may cause unexpected side effects in an Asian; body heights and weights do not appear to be a factor in this response. African Americans appear to require larger doses of some medications that are used to lower blood pressure. Culturally related health beliefs can also affect compliance and response to a medication regimen. Herbal treatments that are popular in some cultures may interfere with or counteract the action of prescribed medication. Nurses who are aware of the specific needs and beliefs of culturally diverse clients are better able to communicate effectively with them. The accompanying box gives guidelines for effective communication about medication with culturally diverse clients.

Psychologic Factors

The client's expectations of the medication affect the response to the medication, as, for instance, in studies of drug effects where some clients receive a placebo. A *placebo* is a pharmacologically inactive substance. In clinical drug trials, one group of clients receives the active drug, while another group receives a placebo to study the drug's effects. Some clients appear to have the same response with the placebo as with the active drug.

Pathology

The presence of disease can affect drug action. The liver is the primary organ for drug breakdown. Pathologic conditions that involve the liver may slow down metabolism.

Environment

The client's environment may influence the response to medications. Sensory deprivation and overload may affect drug responses. The relative oxygen deprivation at high altitudes may increase sensitivity to some drugs. The client who receives pain medication or a sedative in an active environment may not be able to benefit fully from the medication's effects. Nutritional state can also affect the body's reaction to certain drugs.

Time of Administration

The presence of food in the stomach delays the absorption of orally administered medications. Some medications should be given with food to prevent gastric irritation, and the nurse should consider this when establishing a client's medication schedule. Human rhythms and cycles may also influence drug action.

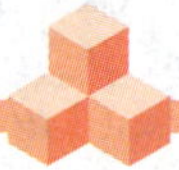

Guidelines for Nursing Care

Communicating Effectively About Medication With Culturally Diverse Clients

- Acquire basic information about health beliefs and practices of various cultural groups in your healthcare setting.
- Be alert to atypical drug responses or unexpected side effects that may occur in certain ethnic groups.
- Ask specifically about the use of folk or home remedies prescribed by a nontraditional healer.
- Utilize printed or audiovisual information that is in the language spoken by your clients.
- Encourage cultural sensitivity in healthcare workers in your particular setting.
- Recognize that diversity exists within cultural groups. For example, the Hispanic population includes Mexicans, Cubans, Puerto Ricans, and other Latino groups.
- Emphasize threads or messages in health teaching that are common to all cultures (eg, concern about family, faith, and home).
- Include culturally sensitive information in all basic health teaching.
- Help culturally diverse clients to value and understand the importance of communicating concerns and asking questions about prescribed medications.

(Adapted from National Council on Patient Information and Education. [1994]. *Talk about prescriptions,* p. 8.)

Adverse Drug Effects

Although therapeutic effect is the desired effect in medication administration, sometimes adverse effects may occur. Drug reactions may be unpredictable and harmful. Adverse effects are effects that are not intended or desired. Thirty percent of adverse drug reactions result in serious injury or death with as many as 140,000 fatalities each year related to adverse drug reactions (O'Donnell, 1992).

Home Healthcare Alert

Written instructions encourage compliance with a medication regimen at home. Emphasize special instructions and adverse effects that need to be reported promptly to the physician or nurse.

An *iatrogenic disease* is caused unintentionally by drug therapy. *Drug allergy* occurs in a person who has been previously exposed to the drug and has developed antibodies. Drug allergies can be manifested in a variety of symptoms ranging from minor to serious. The reaction can occur immediately after the client receives the medication or be delayed for hours to days. Some of the signs and symptoms of a drug allergy are rash, urticaria, fever, diarrhea, nausea, and vomiting. A life-threatening immediate reaction is called an **anaphylactic reaction** and results in respiratory distress, sudden severe bronchospasm, and cardiovascular collapse. This reaction is treated with epinephrine, bronchodilators, and antihistamines. Serious adverse drug reactions must be documented according to agency policy and reported to the FDA's MEDWATCH program. According to their criteria, a serious drug event is defined as an action that is life threatening, requires intervention to prevent death or permanent impairment, and leads to death, hospitalization, disability, or congenital anomaly (Cantrell, 1994).

Drug tolerance exists when the body becomes accustomed to a particular drug over a period of time. Larger doses of the drug must be given to the client to produce the same effects. A **cumulative effect** occurs when the body cannot metabolize one dose of a drug before another dose is administered. The drug is taken in more frequently than it is excreted, and each new dose increases the total quantity in the body. An **idiosyncratic effect** is any abnormal or peculiar response to a drug that may manifest itself by overresponse, underresponse, or response different from the expected outcome. Older clients often have unpredictable or erratic responses to medications. Idiosyncratic effects are thought to be the result of genetic enzyme deficiencies that lead to an abnormal mechanism for drug breakdown.

In a *drug interaction*, the combined effect of two or more drugs acting simultaneously produces either an effect less than that of each drug alone (**antagonist effect**) or greater than that of each drug alone (**synergistic effect**). Alcohol and barbiturates, when taken together, create a synergistic effect. Nurses must be knowledgeable and alert for drug interactions and effects of drug therapy.

ASSESSING THE MEDICATION HISTORY

Assessment of the client receiving medications begins during a nursing history, one component of which is the medication history. During the interview, the nurse's questions can be adapted or elaborated to meet the client's needs and level of understanding. The nurse should avoid using medical jargon that the client may not understand. Familiar terms the client or family recognizes should be chosen. For instance, the client may refer to a diuretic as the "water pill" or to an anticoagulant as a "blood thinner."

Areas to be included in the medication history are listed in the accompanying box.

Assessment is an ongoing process. The nurse not only assesses the client with regard to medications during the nursing history but also continues the assessment during and after medication administration. A discussion of how the nurse would measure the client's response to medications is included in the evaluation section later in this chapter. Refer to the accompanying box for medication self-care behaviors for healthcare workers.

DIAGNOSING

Data that the nurse collects may lead to the development of several nursing diagnoses related to the medication administration experience. The following are examples of appropriate nursing diagnoses:

- Altered Health Maintenance related to lack of knowledge about anticoagulant medication regimen
- Altered Sexuality Patterns related to adverse effects of antihypertensive drug
- Anxiety related to daily self-injection of insulin
- Body Image Disturbance related to effects of chemotherapy
- Risk for Aspiration related to impaired swallowing of oral medications
- Risk for Poisoning related to confusion about medication dosages
- Knowledge Deficit related to lack of interest in learning about medication regimen
- Noncompliance With Medication Regimen related to adverse drug effects, cost of medications, confusion, lack of motivation, visual impairment, complexity of regimen
- Sleep Pattern Disturbance related to consistent use of sedative–hypnotics

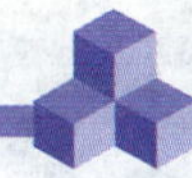

Focused Assessment Guide

Medications

Factors to Assess	Questions and Approaches
Previous and current drug use	What medications are you taking that the doctor prescribed for you?
	What over-the-counter medications are you taking on a regular basis?
	Do you use nonmedicinal drugs on a regular basis (eg, alcohol, caffeine, home remedies)?
	What is the reason for taking the medication?
	What medications have you taken during the past year and for what reasons?
Medication schedule	At what times do you take your medications?
	Is there any special way your medication has to be prepared (eg, crushing and mixing with applesauce)?
	Do you have any special method for remembering to take your medications?
Response to medications	Have the medications had the expected effects?
	Have you ever experienced any adverse or unexpected reactions to the medications?
	Is there a family history of this type of reaction to medication?
	Do you have any allergies to medications?
	What happens when you take this medication?
Attitude toward drugs and use of drugs	How do you feel about taking medications?
	Why do you take the medications?
Compliance with regimen	Do you understand the reason for taking the medications?
	Do you adhere to the medication schedule?
	Are there any problems that prevent you from adhering to the medication regimen?
Storage	Where are your medications stored at home?
	How long do you keep medications in the home?
	Can you show me any medications you have on hand?

EXPECTED OUTCOMES FOR MEDICATION ADMINISTRATION

Medication Orders

No medication may be given to a client without a *medication order* from a physician. Each health agency has a policy specifying the manner in which a physician writes an order. In most instances, orders are written on a form specifically designed for a physician's order. This becomes part of a client's permanent record. Some healthcare facilities utilize a computer-generated pharmacy order system while others have the capability to receive a medication order by fax from the physician.

Safe practice dictates that a nurse follow only a written order. A written order by a physician is least likely to result in error or misunderstanding. Under certain circumstances, such as in an emergency, a verbal order from the physician may be given to a registered nurse or a pharmacist. In most settings, a student nurse is not permitted to accept a verbal order from a physician. The legal implications for dispensing and administering an agent without a written order vary, and the nurse is cautioned to be familiar with the exact agency policy whenever called on to administer therapeutic agents. The legal implications of verbal orders are discussed in Chapter 7.

Usual hospital policy dictates that when a client is admitted, unless specific orders to the contrary are written, all drugs that the physician may have ordered while the client was at home are discontinued. This may prove to be a problem when a client brings medications from home to the hospital. To avoid the possibility of having the client continue taking the home medications while receiving the same ones or others under new orders, all medications should be sent home with the family or removed from the client's unit and placed in safekeeping.

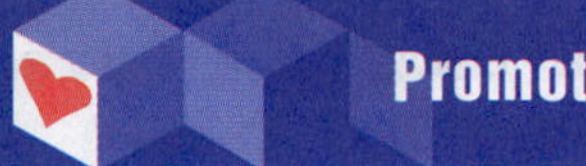

Promoting Wellness

Medications

Use the following assessment checklist to determine how well you are meeting your own need for safe medication practices. Then develop a prescription for self-care by choosing appropriate behaviors from the list of suggestions.

Assessment Checklist

almost always	sometimes	almost never	
☐	☐	☐	1. I store medications in a safe place (eg, a cool, dry place, away from direct sunlight, out of the reach of children).
☐	☐	☐	2. I discard medications that have passed their expiration date.
☐	☐	☐	3. I wear a Medic-Alert tag or carry information that identifies a drug allergy or required medication.
☐	☐	☐	4. I am cautious about combining prescribed medication with OTC drugs, alcohol, or foods that can interact with the drug.

Self-Care Behaviors

1. Finish all prescriptions as ordered by physician or nurse practitioner.
2. Avoid foods, alcohol, or OTC drugs that may interact with a prescribed drug.
3. Use available resources (textbooks, pharmacist, physician) to verify the potential for drug interactions or possible side effects of a medication.
4. Use a reminder system to maintain medication schedule.
5. Avoid sharing medications or taking someone else's prescribed pills.
6. Complete any laboratory tests necessary for maintenance or adjustment of a medication regimen.
7. Practice safe behaviors when storing medications.
8. Purchase drugs from the same pharmacy as an additional safeguard with multiple medication regimens.

This requires an explanation to the client and the family of how the client's drug plan is to be implemented.

In some inpatient facilities, clients keep their medications at their bedside and learn or continue to administer them as they would at home. It is believed that this approach helps to promote the clients' independence. The nurse should be aware when clients are allowed to take their own medications while hospitalized and should know each agent's purpose and possible adverse effects. Also, a notation should be made on the client's plan of care, so that everyone knows the client has medications at the bedside.

When a client has had surgery or is transferred to another clinical service or another health agency, it is general practice that all orders related to drugs are discontinued, and new orders are written. To keep physicians aware of orders in effect, some hospitals specify a day of the week when orders are to be rewritten or they automatically are discontinued.

Types of Orders

There are several types of orders that a physician may write.

A *standing order* is carried out as specified until it is canceled by another order. Many physicians whose practices are limited to a particular clinical area have a specified set of written orders for all their hospitalized clients. These are also referred to as standing orders. Occasionally, a physician writes a standing order and its cancellation simultaneously; that is, the physician specifies that a certain order is to be carried out for a stated number of days or times. After the stated period has passed, the order is canceled automatically.

The physician may write an *"as needed" (prn) order* for medication. The client receives medication when it is requested or needed. A prn order commonly is written for postoperative pain medication.

Another type of order is called a *single order*; that is, the directive is carried out only once, at a time specified by the physician. Medication to be administered immediately before surgery is an example of a single order.

A *stat order* also is a single order but one that is carried out at once. A stat order for epinephrine or an antihistamine would be carried out immediately for a client who is experiencing an anaphylactic drug reaction.

Parts of the Medication Order

The medication order consists of seven parts:

- Client's name
- Date and time the order is written
- Name of drug to be administered
- Dosage of the drug
- Route by which the drug is to be administered
- Frequency of administration of the drug
- Signature of person writing the order

Client's Name. The client's full name is used. The middle name or initial should be included to avoid confusion with other clients. In most agencies, the client's full name and identification number and the physician's name are mechanically imprinted on all sheets on the client's chart, including the physician's order sheet.

Date and Time the Order Is Written. The date the order is written is given. In some situations, the time the order is written is included. Because the nursing staffs in inpatient agencies change several times during each 24-hour period, the date and time help to prevent errors of oversight as different nurses take charge of a unit. When an order is to be followed for a specified number of days, the date and time are important, so that the discontinuation date and time can be determined accurately. The length of time an order for a narcotic remains valid is determined by law. Therefore, the date and time the order is written are essential for determining when the order for a narcotic becomes invalid.

Name of Drug to Be Administered. The name of the drug is stated in the order, either by the brand name or by the generic name. Certain brand names are well known, but the practice of using the generic name is considered safest and is required by some healthcare agencies.

If the nurse is unfamiliar with a drug, there are several sources for obtaining information. The USP and NF is the official source in the United States. In Canada, the *Compendium of Pharmaceutical Specialties* (CPS) is published with information written by the pharmaceutical companies. Most other countries have similar references that describe official therapeutic agents. Many agencies also provide their own book listing the official drugs commonly used by the agency. The *Physician's Desk Reference* (PDR) is another source of information. It is published by Medical Economics, Inc., from information supplied by pharmaceutical companies. In addition, the nurse may obtain information about drugs from the hospital pharmacist, the physician, and any of several texts written specifically for the nursing role in the management of drug therapy.

Dosage of the Drug. The dosage of a drug can be stated in either the apothecary or the metric system. The metric system has been adopted internationally. A similar system (le Système international d'unités), abbreviated as SI, is used in Canada. It includes familiar metric units with some differences (eg, the base unit of weight is the kilogram, not the gram, and temperature is measured in Celsius). In SI, the spelling of liter is litre.

Apothecary measurements are being used less frequently. Forty-two percent (42%) of the nurses in one survey reported that the apothecary system is rarely used for medication orders, while another 19% of the respondents stated they never see a drug ordered in this format (Cohen et al., 1993). A medication error may occur if nurses are unfamiliar with the apothecary system, the doctor's handwriting is illegible, or administration equipment, such as syringes, cups, or reference sources use only metric measurement. Manufacturers are considering making some syringes without the minim scale because of the potential for error. Self-administered drugs commonly are labeled in household measurements to facilitate administration. Most agencies post a table of common equivalent dosages for people who have learned to use one system and find that the agency for which they work uses the other system. Although these tables are convenient and useful, the nurse should be prepared to convert from one system to the other, since such tables are not available in every situation. The nurse should also be familiar with common equivalent measurements when using household equipment, such as teaspoons and tablespoons, since usually the home is not equipped with special measuring devices. The most common equivalents can be found in Appendix A.

Certain standard abbreviations are used to indicate drug amounts, and the nurse should know the common abbreviations before administering drugs. Table 29-2 lists some of the most commonly used abbreviations.

Route by Which the Drug Is to Be Administered. The route to be used when administering a medication is stated clearly because some drugs can be given in more than one way and some may be used safely only through one route. Table 29-3 describes common routes by which medications are administered.

Frequency of Administration of the Drug. The time and frequency with which a drug is to be administered usually are stated in standard abbreviations in the medication order. Common abbreviations used in writing prescriptions, including time and frequency, are listed in Table 29-4.

The nursing service department of inpatient facilities usually determines the hours at which routine drugs are

Table 29-2
Common Abbreviations for Measures

Abbreviation	Unabbreviated Form
ʒ	Dram
gt	Drop
gtt	Drops
gr	Grain
g	Gram
μg or mcg	Microgram
mg or mgm	Milligram
mL or ml	Milliliter
m or min	Minim
℥ or oz	Ounce
tbsp	Tablespoon
tsp	Teaspoon

Table 29-3
Routes for Administering Drugs

Route	How Drug Is Administered	Term Used to Describe Route
Given by mouth	Having patient swallow drug	Oral administration
Given by way of respiratory tract	Having patient inhale drug	Inhalation
Given by injection	Injecting drug into	Administration by injection
	Subcutaneous tissue	Subcutaneous injection
	Muscle tissue	Intramuscular injection
	Corium (under epidermis)	Intradermal injection
	Vein	Intravenous injection
	Artery	Intraarterial injection
	Heart tissue	Intracardial injection
	Peritoneal cavity	Intraperitoneal injection
	Spinal canal	Intraspinal injection
	Bone	Intraosseous injection
Given by placing on skin or mucous membrane	Inserting drug into	
	Vagina	Vaginal administration
	Rectum	Rectal administration
	Placing drug under tongue	Sublingual administration
	Placing drug between cheek and gum	Buccal administration
	Rubbing drug into skin	Inunction
	Placing drug into direct contact with mucous membrane	Instillation
	Flushing mucous membrane with drug in solution	Irrigation
	Applying medicated patch to skin	Topical application

given. For example, if certain drugs are to be given every 4 hours, the nursing service policy indicates the times. Every 4-hour administration may be at the times of 12 noon, 4 PM, 8 PM, 12 midnight, 4 AM, and 8 AM. Another agency may use the hours 1 PM, 5 PM, 9 PM, 1 AM, 5 AM, and 9 AM. To lessen the risk of error, some healthcare facilities use the 24-hour clock (or military time) which designates midnight as 0000 hours and runs until 2400 hours. If a drug is ordered to be given before or after meals, time of administration depends on the hours at which meals are served.

If a drug is to be given only once or twice a day, the decision as to which hours to use depends on the nature of the drug and the client's plan of care. Whenever possible, the client's choice of time should be considered.

Drugs should be administered punctually as ordered. A nurse administering drugs to several clients, however, cannot give all of the drugs exactly on the hour indicated. Agency policies vary, but a common one is that drugs should be administered within a half hour before or after the indicated hour. Thus a drug to be administered at 9 AM can be administered any time between 8:30 AM and 9:30 AM, using this policy. This policy does not apply to all drugs. A preoperative medication ordered to be given at 7:30 AM should be administered at that hour, since the time was planned in relation to the time surgery is to begin. This also holds true when clients are given drugs before certain diagnostic procedures and stat orders.

Signature of Person Writing the Order. The signature of the person writing the order follows the order. The signature is of importance for legal reasons because the authority to prescribe drugs is defined by state laws. Also, if there is a question about the order, the signature indicates who should be contacted.

Checking the Medication Order

Agency policy specifies the manner in which the medication order is checked. Various systems are used. Nurses should be familiar with the system used in the agency where they care for clients and should implement it correctly to minimize errors in administering therapeutic agents.

In many institutions, the order is copied onto the client's medication record, often called a *Kardex*. Increasing numbers of healthcare facilities are computerizing client records, including medication records. An example of a computerized record appears in Figure 29-1. The nurse is responsible for checking that the transcription of the medication order is correct by comparing it with the original order.

Questioning the Medication Order

The nurse is legally responsible for drugs administered. Any drug order suspected to be in error should be questioned. The suspected error may be in any part of the order. The legal implications are serious in a situation in

Table 29-4
Common Abbreviations Used in Prescribing Medications

Abbreviation	Meaning
ac	Before meals
ad lib	As desired
aq	Water
bid	Twice a day
c̄	With
cap	Capsule
DC	Discontinue
elix	Elixir
hs	At bedtime; hour of sleep
IM	Intramuscular
IV	Intravenous
IVPB	IV piggyback
KVO	Keep vein open
OD	Right eye
OS	Left eye
OU	Both eyes
pc	After meals
PO	By mouth
prn	As needed; when necessary
q	Every
qd	Every day
qh	Every hour
q2h	Every 2 hours
qid	Four times a day
qod	Every other day
qs	Quantity sufficient
Rx	Take
s̄	Without
SC	Subcutaneous
stat	Immediately
supp	Suppository
susp	Suspension
tid	Three times a day
tinct	Tincture

which there is an error in a drug order and in which the nurse could be expected, based on knowledge and experience, to have noted and reported the error.

On occasion, the nurse may not think that there is an error in the order but may not understand why the medication has been prescribed. In such instances, the nurse should ask how the order relates to the client's plan of care.

Confusion over the placement of a decimal point can lead to a medication error. A zero should always precede a decimal point (eg. 0.1 mg) for clarity but there is no need to use a zero after a decimal point (eg. 1.0 mg) since this can cause confusion if the decimal point is unclear or missed completely (Davis, 1994a).

A drug to which the client is allergic may be inadvertently prescribed. The client may describe past adverse reactions with the drug. It is general practice to indicate any drug allergies clearly on the client's chart. The drug should not be given, and the order should be questioned when, in the nurse's judgment, the client is allergic to a drug. An allergic reaction can be life threatening to the client.

A nurse may have difficulty reading an order. Guessing is gross carelessness. Rechecking with the person who wrote the order is the only safe procedure.

The nurse has the right to refuse to administer any medication that, based on knowledge and experience, may be harmful to the client. Although this situation seldom occurs, the nurse needs to understand that the client's safety is a primary objective in the administration of medications.

Medication Supply Systems

Medications are supplied in a number of ways. With a *stock supply* system, large quantities of medications are kept on the nursing unit. With an *individual supply* system, each client is supplied with the medication needed for a period of time. The nurse is responsible for accurately measuring the dosage from the medication containers. In the *unit dose* system, the pharmacist simplifies medication preparation by packaging and labeling each dosage for a 24-hour period. In some inpatient facilities, clients self-administer medications.

Most nursing units use a medication cart for the administration of medications. The cart contains individual drawers into which the medications for each client are placed. The drawer is labeled with the client's name. The nurse moves the cart from room to room when dispensing medications. A medication cart is shown in Figure 29-2.

Dosage Calculations

Systems of Measurement

Nurses need to be proficient in the use of weights and measures as well as systems of measurement to calculate drug dosages and prepare medications for administration. There are three systems of measurement in use for administering medications—the metric system, the apothecary system, and the household system.

Metric System. The metric system is the most widely accepted and convenient system. The official system used in Canada is the SI, which is similar to the metric system. The basic units of measurement are the meter (linear), the liter (volume), and the gram (weight). The metric system is a decimal system, in which each unit can be divided into multiples of 10 (10, 100, 1000). To do calculations in the metric system, the decimal point

ADMIT DATE 10/15/98	WATERFORD COMMUNITY HOSPITAL MEDICATION ADMINISTRATION RECORD FIVE DAY MEDICATION SUMMARY FROM 10/15/98 00:01 TO 10/19/98 24:00				PAGE: ** PERMANENT COPY *
ORDER INFORMATION	10/15	10/16	10/17	10/18	10/19
FERROUS SULFATE 325mg PO TID DAILY ROUTINE 325mg 325mg/1 TAB TAB EC 10/15 20:00 TO / :	2000 KMM	0800 AMD 1400 AMD 2000 AMD	0800 MAK 1400 MAK 2000 JBM	0800 CLG 1400 CLG 2000 MJM	0800 CLG 1400 CLG 2000 MJM
COUMADIN THERAPY QD (COU) DAILY ROUTINE TAB FOR 10-19-98 DOSE=2.5mg 10/15 22:00 TO / :	2200 KMM D=10mg	2200	2200 JBM D=3mg	2200 MJM D=7.5mg	2200 MJM D=2.5mg
PAROXETINE PAXIL 10mg PO QD DAILY ROUTINE 20 MG 10 MG/0.5 TAB TAB 10/19 10:00 TO / :					1000 CLG-
		PRN ORDERS			
ACETAMINOPHEN TAB TYLENOL 650mg PO Q6HRSPRN DAILY PRN 325MG/TAB 650 MG/2 TAB 2TAB-PK 10/15 13:06 TO / :	2400 APK D=2 TABS			1700 MJM D=2 TABS	
DEMEROL 50/VISTARIL 50 MEPERIDINE 50mg HYDROXYZINE HCL 50mg IM Q4HRSPRN DAILY PRN 10/15 22:07 / : Renewed 10/17 20:00		0045 APK SITE=LVG	0200 BLB SITE=RVG	0600 BLB SITE=LVG	
INJECTION SITE: A-ARM					*CANC* - CANCELLED
NAME JONATHAN MORGAN PT NO: 463 AGE: 78 SEX: M UNIT: 3B ROOM: 302301					
10/20/98 01:43 OCMARDF1					

Figure 29-1
Example of a medication administration record.

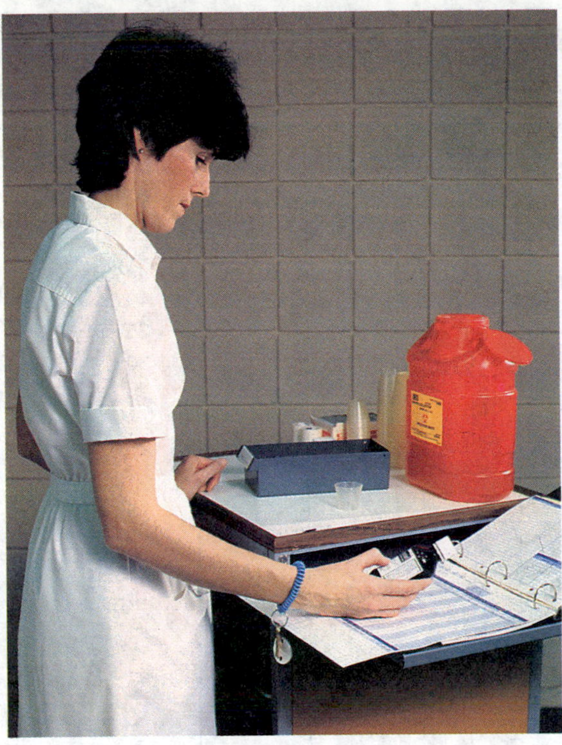

Figure 29-2
The mobile medication cart and the Kardex are taken to the client's room when medications are given. Each client's medications are stored in a separate drawer. The nurse carefully checks the medication he or she will give with the Kardex to avoid errors. The cart is stored between uses in a locked room near the nurses' station.

is moved to the right or left. In the preparation of medications, the nurse usually uses the following metric units:

Weight
1 kilogram = 1000 grams
1 gram = 1000 milligrams
1 milligram = 1000 micrograms

Volume
1 liter = 1000 milliliters or cubic centimeters

Converting Dosages. It may be necessary to convert drug dosages to a different unit in the metric system. To convert a larger unit into a smaller unit, move the decimal point to the right (the new number is larger than the original). To convert a smaller unit into a larger unit, move the decimal point to the left (the new number is smaller than the original).

Example
0.5 g = ? mg
Move decimal point three places to right.
Answer = 500 mg
900 mg = ? g
Move decimal point three places to the left.
Answer = 0.9 g

Apothecary System. The apothecary system is less convenient and precise than the metric system and infrequently used. The basic unit of weight is the grain. The minim, dram, ounce, pint, and quart are used for volume. In the apothecary system, Roman numerals are used to express numbers (grains X) and quantities less than 1 are written in fraction form (grains ¼).

Household System. The household system is the least accurate system of measurement. It is not widely used except in home settings. Teaspoon, tablespoon, teacup, and glass are commonly used household measures.

Equivalents of Measurement. All three systems of measurement are in use in the United States. The nurse may be called on to convert dosages from one system to another. It is then extremely important that the nurse know and be able to calculate commonly used equivalents as listed in Appendix A.

Formulas for Computing Drug Dosages

Sometimes drugs are prepared and supplied in the amount ordered by the physician and the nurse can see that no calculation is necessary when checking the medication label. At other times, drugs are not prepared and supplied in the exact quantities called for in the medication order, and the nurse must do a dosage calculation to determine what quantity of medication the client is to receive.

Several formulas can be used to calculate drug dosages. One such formula consists of ratios to set up a proportion and can be used to calculate dosages for both solid and liquid preparations. A ratio shows the relation between numbers. A proportion contains two ratios. The nurse usually is seeking the quantity of on-hand medication that is equal to the desired dosage (the dosage ordered). The formula is as follows:

$$\frac{\text{dose on hand}}{\text{quantity on hand}} = \frac{\text{dose desired}}{\text{X (quantity desired)}}$$

The dosage must be in the same unit of measurement. This applies to the quantity as well. Dosages are on the top line of the proportion and quantities on the bottom line. After the numbers are placed in the proportion, the nurse cross-multiplies to find the desired quantity.

Example: Amoxicillin 625 mg PO is ordered. It is supplied as a liquid preparation containing 250 mg in 5 mL. How much would the nurse administer?

$$\frac{250\text{ mg}}{5\text{ mL}} = \frac{625\text{ mg}}{\text{X mL}}$$

cross-multiply:

$$3125 = 250\text{X}$$
$$\text{X} = 12.5\text{ mL}$$

Example: Phenobarbital gr i PO is ordered. It is available in 30-mg tablets. How many tablets would the nurse administer?

There are two systems of measurement in this problem. The nurse checks the list of equivalents to learn that 60 mg is equivalent to grains i.

$$\frac{30\text{ mg}}{1\text{ tablet}} = \frac{60\text{ mg}}{X\text{ tablets}}$$

$$60 = 30X$$

$$X = 2\text{ tablets}$$

Another formula that can be used to calculate drug dosages is:

$$\frac{\text{dose desired}}{\text{dose on hand}} \times \text{quantity on hand} = \text{desired quantity}$$

This formula can be used for both liquid dosages and fractions of tablets.

Pediatric Calculations

Pediatric dosages are calculated according to the child's weight or *body surface area* (BSA).

The *BSA formula* provides the most accuracy in calculating pediatric dosages because it considers weight and height. To find a child's BSA, the West nomogram is used (Fig. 29-3). The child's height is located by a point in the left-hand column and the weight is located by a point in the right-hand column. The two points are connected with a straight line. The point at which the line crosses the surface area column is the child's BSA. The formula for calculating the child's dosage is:

$$\frac{\text{BSA (child)}}{\text{BSA (adult)}} \times \text{adult dose} = \text{child's dose}$$

The average adult BSA is 1.7 square meters.

A less commonly used formula is *Clark's rule* for children age 2 years or younger. This formula assumes that the average adult weighs 150 lb (68 kg) and is calculated as follows:

$$\text{usual adult dose} \times \frac{\text{weight of child in pounds}}{150} = \text{child's dose}$$

Accepted pediatric dosages according to milligram per kilogram weight per 24 hours for many drugs are listed in medication references.

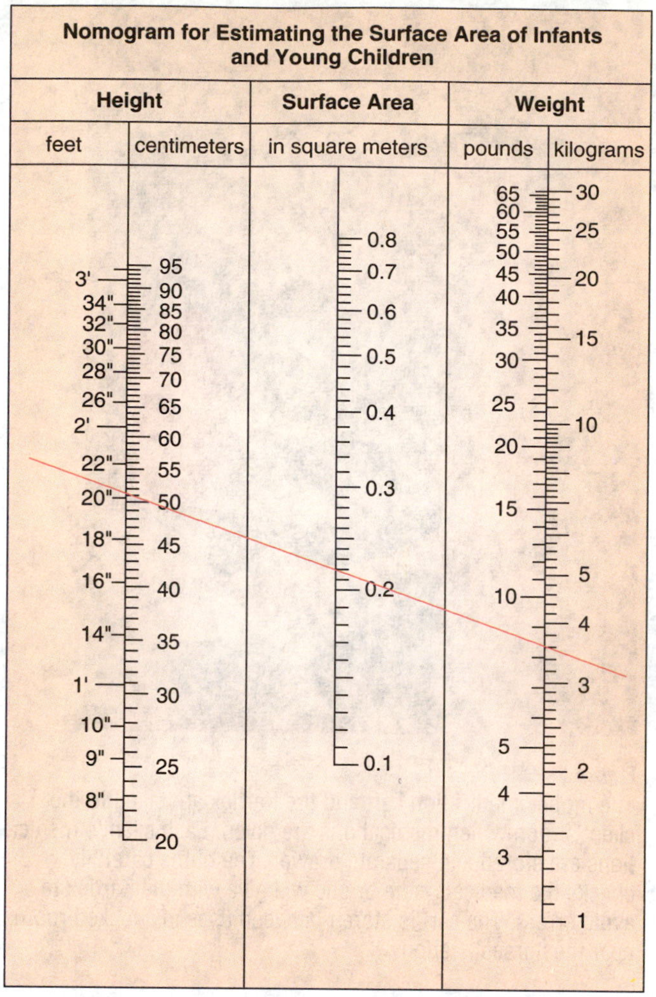

Nomogram for Estimating the Surface Area of Infants and Young Children

Height (feet, centimeters) | Surface Area (in square meters) | Weight (pounds, kilograms)

Figure 29-3

Body-surface nomogram. To determine the surface area of the child, draw a straight line between the point representing his or her height on the left vertical scale to the point representing weight on the right vertical scale. The point at which this line intersects the middle vertical scale represents the child's surface area in square meters. (Courtesy of Abbott Laboratories)

Using Safety Measures While Preparing Drugs

Safety is of the utmost importance in preparing and implementing drug administration. The nurse observes the *three checks* and the *five rights* when administering medications.

Three Checks. The label on the medication container should be checked three times during medication preparation. The label may be read (1) when the nurse reaches for the container or unit dose package, (2) immediately before pouring or opening the medication, and (3) when replacing the container to the drawer or shelf or prior to giving the unit dose medication to the client.

Five Rights. The *five rights* help to ensure accuracy when administering medications. The nurse gives the (1) *right medication* to the (2) *right client* in the (3) *right dosage* through the (4) *right route* at the (5) *right time.*

The importance of the three checks and the five rights cannot be overemphasized. The safe nurse does not allow automatic habits of preparing medications to replace constant thinking, purposeful action, and repeated checking for accuracy.

Maintaining a Safe Environment

An environment that promotes safety and good working habits contributes to accuracy in the preparation of drugs for administration. It is important that good lighting be available when preparing drugs. Also, the nurse who is preparing drugs should work alone. This practice helps to avoid distractions and interruptions, which may lead to errors.

After the nurse begins to prepare drugs for administration, they should not be left unattended. If it is imperative to leave for a short time, the drugs that have been prepared should be placed in a locked area. The nurse who prepares the medication also administers the drug and records the drug administration. When the nurse is not working at the medication cart, it should be locked.

Caring for Controlled Substances Safely

Controlled substances are kept in a double-locked drawer, box, or room. This precaution is observed as a safety measure. Narcotics or controlled substances may be ordered only by physicians who are registered with the Department of Justice, Bureau of Narcotics and Dangerous Drugs, or as specified by the Narcotic Control Act and Regulations (Canada). According to federal law, a record must be kept for each narcotic that is administered. Healthcare agencies provide forms for keeping such records, and these forms are kept with the narcotics. Although the forms differ, the following information usually is required: the name of the client receiving the narcotic, the amount of the narcotic used, the hour the narcotic was given, the name of the physician who prescribed the narcotic, and the name of the nurse who administered the narcotic. It is common practice to check narcotics daily at specified intervals. In hospitals, checking usually is performed at each shift change. The amount of narcotics on hand is counted, and each used narcotic must be accounted for on the narcotic record. Some agencies use a computerized system for dispensing narcotics. The nurse has a secure identification code that provides access into the system, identifies the client via name or identification number, and verifies the count for each drug as it is removed. Unless the number is incorrect, this eliminates the need to check the narcotic count at specific intervals each day. Figure 29-4 is an example of a computerized narcotic withdrawal form. A narcotic count that does not check must be reported immediately. The law requires these special precautions in the use of narcotics, to aid in the control of drug abuse. The nurse administering narcotics has an important responsibility to see that the federal law is observed. If for any reason a narcotic prepared for administration has to be discarded, a second person should act as a witness and that person should also sign the narcotic sheet.

Pyxis MEDSTATION 2SOUTH
Version 1.3h
Tues Apr 18 18:26:08 1998

REMOVED MED

MED : ALPRAZOLAM 0.25mg TAB

Qty : 2

For : Aiken, Paul
ID : 78593035

Patient
Notes : Dr. : Dr. : 390260

By : BUNK

2SOUTH drawer 5, pocket E. 18 Meds remain.

Figure 29-4
A sample computerized narcotic withdrawal form that includes client's name and ID number, physician's ID number, nurse's entry code, and number of medications remaining in drawer.

Identifying the Client

The nurse prepares medications, considering safety at all times, as discussed in the previous sections. Positive identification of the client is essential to safe drug administration. Before administering the drug, the nurse must check carefully to see that the right drug is given to the right client. Clients in inpatient healthcare agencies usually wear identification bracelets. The nurse identifies the client by checking the identification bracelet, as shown in Figure 27-6. Also, the client should be asked to state his or her name if possible. It is considered unsafe to call the client by name because the client may respond even when the nurse has used an improper name.

IMPLEMENTING: ADMINISTERING A MEDICATION

The nurse should remain with the client and see that the medication is taken. If the client receives several drugs, offer them separately so that if one is refused or dropped, positive identification can be made and the drug recorded or replaced. Never leave medications at the bedside for the client to take later. This is unsafe practice because the client may forget to take the medication or someone else may take the medication. The nurse records medication administration as soon as possible after the client takes the medication. Some agencies allow clients to self-administer certain drugs to promote the client's independence. The nurse should be familiar with agency policy on this matter. Nursing responsibilities for administering drugs are listed in the accompanying box.

Nursing Responsibilities for Administering Drugs

- Assessment of the client and clear understanding of why the client is receiving a particular medication
- Preparing the medication to be administered (ie, checking labels, preparing injections, observing proper asepsis techniques with needles and syringes)
- Accurate dosage calculations
- Administration of the medication (proper injection techniques, aids to help swallowing, topical methods)
- Documentation of medications given
- Monitoring the client's reaction and evaluating the client's response
- Educating the client regarding his or her medications and medication regimen

Administering Oral Medications

Drugs given orally are intended for absorption in the stomach and small intestine. The oral route is the most commonly used route of administration. It usually is the most convenient and comfortable and the safest for the client. After oral administration, drug action has a slower onset and a more prolonged but less potent effect.

There are certain situations in which oral medications would not be administered, such as when the client has difficulty swallowing, is unconscious, is to receive nothing by mouth, or is vomiting.

Oral medications are available in solid and liquid form. Solid preparations include tablets, capsules, and pills. Some tablets are scored for easy breaking if a partial quantity is needed. Enteric-coated tablets are covered with a hard surface that impedes absorption until the tablet has left the stomach. Absorption takes place in the small intestine because the active ingredient of the drug is irritating to the stomach mucosa. Enteric-coated tablets should not be chewed or crushed.

Liquid preparations include elixirs, spirits, suspensions, and syrups. Some are water-based solutions and others are alcohol-based solutions. Disposable, calibrated cups are available for the preparation of liquid medications. For clients who find it difficult to take liquids from a cup, the medication can be placed in the mouth directly from a plastic syringe without a needle. The syringe should be placed between the gum and cheek, and the liquid given to the client slowly. These techniques, in addition to an upright or side-lying position, help to prevent the client from choking and aspirating the medication.

Certain narcotics and insulin that were previously administered parenterally can now also be administered in a lollipop or oral-transmucosal form (O'Donnell, 1994).

If a label becomes difficult to read or accidentally comes off the container, the container should be returned to the pharmacy. A medication should never be given from a bottle without a label or with a label that cannot be read with accuracy. Because of the danger of error, unused medications should not be returned to their bottles. Care should be exercised in pouring, to prevent unnecessary loss. Medications should not be transferred from one pharmacy container to another. Many medication bottles now have an identification code number on them. If similar medications were mixed and a client had a reaction, it would be difficult to identify which drug was responsible. A medication with an unexpected precipitate should not be used, nor should one that has changed color.

Procedure 29-1 describes the techniques for preparing and administering oral medications.

Special Techniques

Certain drugs that are given orally discolor the teeth or damage the enamel. Such medications are mixed well with water or some other liquid vehicle; the client takes it through a drinking straw, and water is taken after administration. This practice reduces the strength of the drug that comes in contact with the teeth.

Some clients object to the taste of certain medications. The following techniques are suggested to disguise or mask the objectionable taste.

- Sometimes it is necessary to crush a medication or add it to food so the client can swallow it. Some drugs cannot be crushed (eg, enteric-coated and sustained-release capsules). Check with the pharmacist or a pharmacology reference when uncertain about crushing a medication.
- Allow the client to suck on a small piece of ice for a few minutes before taking the medication. The ice numbs the taste buds, and the objectionable taste is less discernible.
- Store oily medications in the refrigerator. Cold oil is less aromatic than oil at room temperature.
- Place the medication in a syringe, and place the syringe well back on the tongue, being careful not to trigger the client's gag reflex. This places the medication on the part of the tongue where there are few taste buds.
- Offer oral hygiene immediately after giving the medication.
- Give the medication with generous amounts of water or other liquids, if permitted, to dilute the taste.

Children. Nurses find administration of medications to infants and children challenging as well as frustrating at times. Children under age 5 years have difficulty swallowing tablets and capsules. Most medications are avail-

(text continues on page 614)

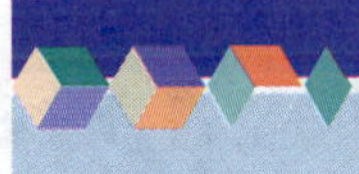

PROCEDURE 29-1

Administering Oral Medications

Equipment

Medication Kardex, cards, or computer-generated MAR
Medication cart or tray
Medication cups (disposable)
Straws
Water or juice

Action	Rationale
1. Gather equipment. Check each medication order against the original physician's order according to agency policy. Clarify any inconsistencies. Check the client's chart for allergies.	This comparison helps to identify errors that may have occurred when orders were transcribed. The physician's order is the legal record of medication orders for each agency.
2. Know the actions, special nursing considerations, safe-dose ranges, purpose of administration, and adverse effects of medications to be administered.	This knowledge aids the nurse in evaluating the therapeutic effect of the medication in relation to the client's diagnosis.
3. Wash your hands.	Handwashing prevents the spread of microorganisms.
4. Move the medication cart to the outside of the client's room or prepare for administration in the medication area.	Organization facilitates error-free administration and saves time.
5. Unlock the medication cart or drawer.	Locking of the cart or drawer safeguards each client's medication supply.
6. Prepare medications for one client at a time.	This prevents errors in medication administration.
7. Select the proper medication from the drawer or stock and compare with the Kardex or order. Check expiration dates and perform calculations if necessary:	Comparison of medication to physician's order reduces errors in medication administration. Verify calculations with another nurse if necessary. This is the *first* safety check.
a. Place unit dose–packaged medications in a disposable cup. *Do not open wrapper* until at bedside. Keep narcotics and medications that require special nursing assessments in a separate container.	The label is needed for an additional safety check. Prerequisites to giving certain medications may include monitoring of certain vital signs.
b. When removing tablets or capsules from a bottle, pour the necessary number into the bottle cap and then place the tablets in a medication cup. Break only scored tablets, if necessary, to obtain the proper dose.	Pouring medication into the cap allows for easy return of excess medication to bottle. Pouring tablets or capsules into the nurse's hand is unsanitary.
c. Hold liquid medication bottles with the label against the palm. Use the appropriate measuring device when pouring liquids, and read the amount of medication at the bottom of the meniscus at eye level. Wipe the lip of the bottle with a paper towel.	Accuracy is possible when the appropriate measuring device is used and then read accurately. Liquid that may drip onto the label makes the label difficult to read.
8. Recheck each medication package, card, or preparation with the order as it is poured.	This is a *second* check to guard against a medication error.
9. When all medications for one client have been prepared, recheck once again with the medication order before taking them to the client.	This is a *third* check to ensure accuracy and to prevent errors.

(continued)

PROCEDURE 29-1 *(continued)*

Administering Oral Medications

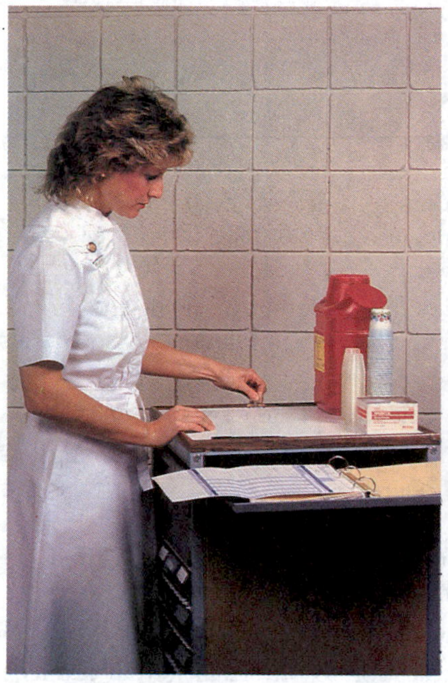
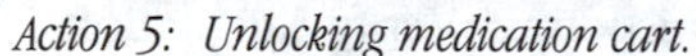

Action 5: Unlocking medication cart.

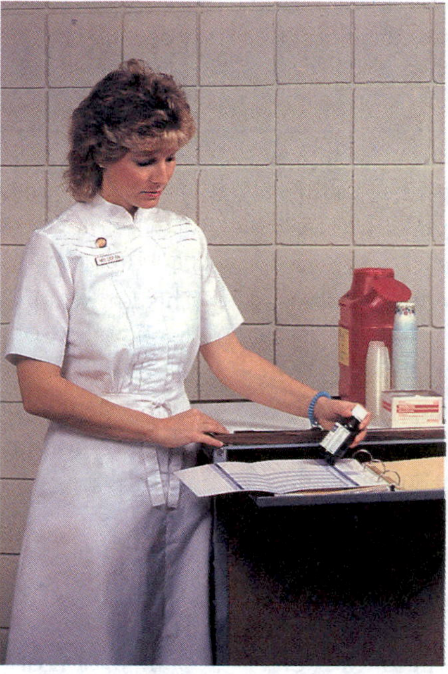

Action 7: Comparing medication with Kardex or order.

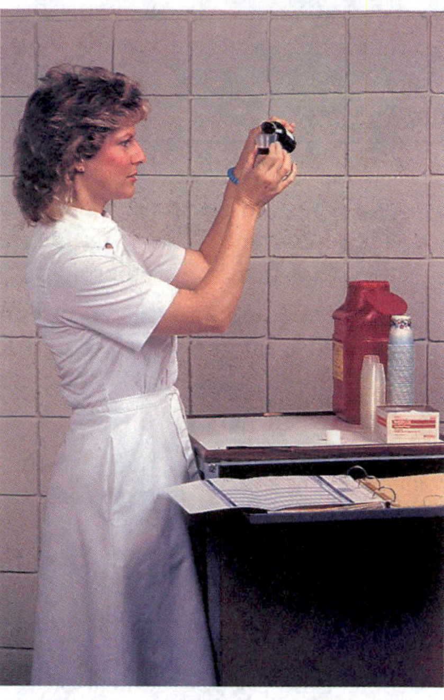

Action 7c: Measuring at eye level.

Action	**Rationale**
10. Transport medications to the client's bedside carefully, and keep the medications in sight at all times.	Careful handling and close observation prevent accidental or deliberate disarrangement of medications.
11. See that the client receives medications at the correct time.	Check agency policy, which may allow for administration within a period of 30 minutes before or 30 minutes after designated time.
12. Identify the client carefully. There are three correct ways to do this:	Identifying the client is the nurse's responsibility to guard against error.
a. Check the name on the client's identification band.	This is the most reliable method. Replace the identification band if it is missing or inaccurate in any way.
b. Ask the client his or her name.	This requires a response from the client, but illness and strange surroundings often cause clients to be confused.
c. Verify the client's identification with a staff member who knows the client.	This is another way to double-check identity. Do not use the name on the door or over the bed because these may be inaccurate.
13. Complete necessary assessments before administration of medications. Check allergy bracelet or ask client about allergies. Explain the purpose and action of each medication to the client.	Assessment is a prerequisite to administration of medications.
14. Assist the client to an upright or lateral position.	Swallowing is facilitated by proper positioning. An upright or side-lying position protects the client from aspiration.

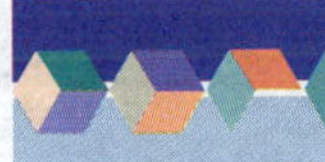

PROCEDURE 29-1 *(continued)*

Administering Oral Medications

Action	Rationale
15. Administer medications:	
a. Offer water or other permitted fluids with pills, capsules, tablets, and some liquid medications.	Liquids facilitate swallowing of solid drugs. Some liquid drugs are intended to adhere to the pharyngeal area, in which case liquid is not offered with the medication.
b. Ask the client's preference regarding medications to be taken by hand or in a cup and one at a time or all at once.	This encourages the client's participation in taking the medications.
c. If the capsule or tablet falls to the floor, it must be discarded and a new one administered.	This prevents contamination.
d. Record any fluid intake if intake and output measurement is ordered.	This provides for accurate documentation.
16. Remain with the client until each medication is swallowed. Unless the nurse has seen the client swallow the drug, it cannot be recorded that the drug was administered.	The client's chart is a legal record. Only with a physician's order can medications be left at the bedside.

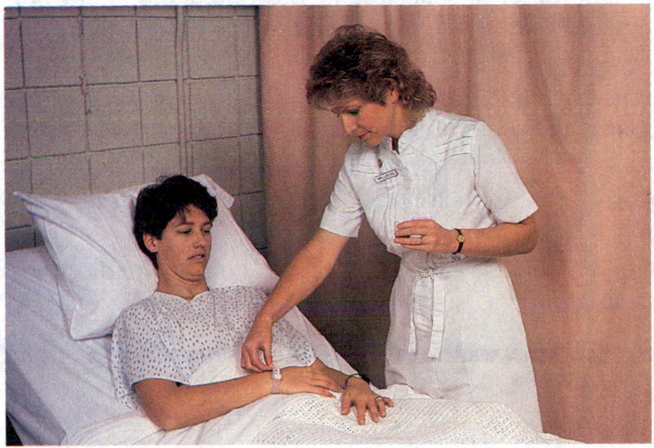

Action 12a: Checking client identity.

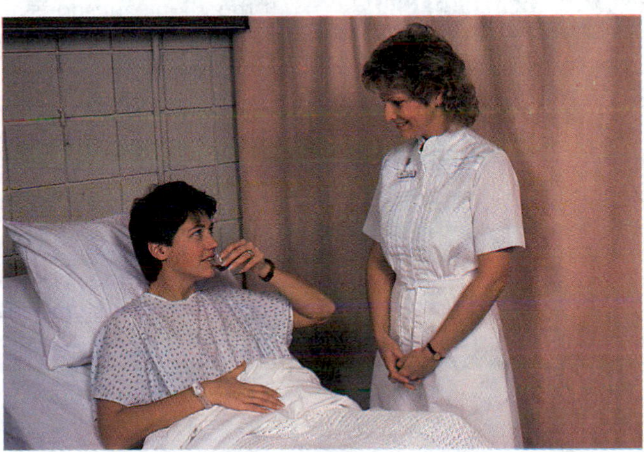

Action 16: Observing client swallowing medication. (Photos © Ken Kasper.)

Action	Rationale
17. Wash your hands.	Handwashing prevents the spread of microorganisms.
18. Record each medication given on the medication chart or record using the required format.	Prompt recording avoids the possibility of accidentally repeating the administration of the drug.
a. If the drug was refused or omitted, record this in the appropriate area on the medication record.	This verifies the reason medication was omitted.
b. Recording of administration of a narcotic requires additional documentation on a narcotic record stating drug count and other specific information.	Controlled substance laws necessitate careful recording of narcotic use.
19. Check on the client within 30 minutes to verify response to medication.	This provides opportunity for further documentation and additional assessment.

(continued)

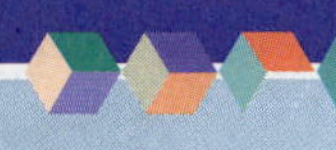

PROCEDURE 29-1 *(continued)*

Administering Oral Medications

Age Considerations

Special devices are available in a pharmacy to ensure accurate dose calculations for young children and infants.

Elderly clients with arthritis may have difficulty opening child-proof caps. On request, the pharmacist can substitute a cap that is easier to open. A rubber band twisted around the cap may provide a more secure grip for older clients.

The FDA has received reports of infants choking on the plastic caps that fit on the end of syringes used to administer oral medication. They recommend: removal and disposal of caps before giving syringes to clients or families, caution family caregivers to dispose of caps on syringes they buy over the counter, and report any problems with syringe caps to the FDA.

Home Care Considerations

Encourage the client to discard outdated prescription medications.

Discuss safe storage of medications when there are children and pets in the environment.

Devices are available to help the client remember to take medications as scheduled. These may be simple charts or appliances that can be made in the home, or more elaborate devices that can be purchased in a pharmacy or from the manufacturer.

Special Considerations

If the client questions a medication order or states the medication is different from the usual dose, *always* recheck and clarify with the original order before giving medication.

If the client's level of consciousness is altered or his or her swallowing is impaired, check with the physician to clarify the route of administration or alternative forms of medication.

Provide a straw for the client who has to swallow a liquid medication that may have a harmful effect on the teeth or mucous membranes.

Clients with poor vision can request labels printed with larger type on medication containers. A magnifying lens also may prove helpful.

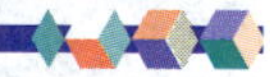

able in liquid form. Nursing responsibility also includes teaching and preparing family members to administer medications to a child at home. In addition to understanding the medication order and the reason for the medication, the caregiver should be able to demonstrate any special techniques involved in administering the prescribed drugs. Helpful strategies for administering medications to children are included in the accompanying box.

Older Clients. Techniques for administering medications to older people include the following:

- Allow extra time to administer medications to older clients because their reflexes may be slowed and their understanding of the treatment decreased.
- Older clients may experience some difficulty swallowing medications and may find it easier to take their medications when crushed or given in liquid form. Swallowing can be initiated by massaging the laryngeal prominence or the area just below the chin prominence. The pressure from the gentle massage creates the desire to swallow.
- Reevaluation of the drug dosage is necessary with the older client. Weight and age should be used as criteria for determining the dosage.
- The nurse should assist the older client to set up a home medication schedule. Some form of a weekly medication dispenser tray may be helpful.
- Monitor carefully for adverse effects associated with the drug regimen. These may be magnified in older individuals.
- Teach clients the names of drugs rather than distinguishing them by color. Manufacturers may vary the colors of generic drugs, and the visual changes associated with aging may make it more difficult to identify medications by their color.

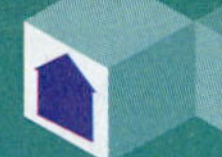

Home Care: Bridging the Gap

Administering Medications to Children

The following are helpful techniques when administering medications to children:

- Use a dropper to give infants or very young children liquid medications while holding them in a sitting or semisitting position. Place the medication between the gum and cheek to prevent possible aspiration.
- Crush uncoated tablets or empty a soft capsule and mix the medication with soft foods, such as potatoes or cereal, for clients who are likely to aspirate liquids. Proper absorption may not occur if coated tablets or hard capsules are added to food.
- Explain to the child when a medication has an objectionable taste if the child is old enough to understand. Failing to warn the child is likely to decrease the child's trust in the nurse.
- Care should be taken when selecting the food to be mixed with the medication. The item should not be an essential part of the child's diet such as formula or the child's favorite food. The child may refuse a food associated with medications.
- Offer the child a flavored ice pop or frozen fruit bar immediately before taking the medication. It numbs the tongue, making the taste of the medication less evident.
- Praise the child for a job well done after he or she swallows the medication.

Administering Medications Through a Gastrointestinal Tube

It is not uncommon for clients with a gastrointestinal tube (nasogastric, nasointestinal, J-tube, or G-tube) to receive medication through the tube. The insertion of the tube and care of the client with a tube are described in Chapter 42. The following are suggestions for giving medications through the tube:

- Use liquid medications or medications that can be crushed and combined with liquid.
- Bring the liquid medication to room temperature. Cold liquids may cause client discomfort.
- Remove the clamp from the tube and use the recommended procedure for checking tube placement in the stomach or intestine *before* administering the drug.
- Flush the tube with 15 to 30 mL of water (5–10 mL for children) before giving the medication and immediately after giving the medication. Flushing before may warn you if the tube is clogged and helps to maintain tube patency.
- It is best to give medications separately and flush with water in between each drug. Some medications may interact with each other or become less effective if mixed with other drugs.
- If the tube is connected to suction, keep it disconnected from the suction and clamped for 20 to 30 minutes after administration of the medication to allow for absorption.
- Disconnect a continuous tube feeding before giving medications and leave tube clamped for a short period of time after medication has been given according to agency protocol.
- Document water intake via tube on I&O record. Adjust amount of water used if client is on restricted fluid intake.

Administering Medications Sublingually

Certain drugs, sublingual nitroglycerin being typical, are administered *sublingually*; that is, a tablet is placed under the client's tongue. This area is rich in superficial blood vessels, which allows the drug to be absorbed relatively rapidly into the bloodstream for quick systemic effects. This type of medication should not be swallowed but held under the tongue so that complete absorption can occur.

Administering Parenteral Medications

The term *enteral* means within the intestines; **parenteral** means outside the intestines or alimentary canal. Many people use the term parenteral to refer to injection routes only, although technically the term includes routes for administering agents given by inhalation, those placed on the skin, and most of those placed on the mucous membrane.

Table 29-3 defines terms used to describe various types of *injections*. Medications may be injected into an artery, the peritoneum, heart tissues, the spinal canal, and bones. Techniques for injecting medications into these areas are discussed in clinical texts. In most instances, physicians are responsible for these procedures, and the nurse acts as an assistant.

Absorption occurs more rapidly with injection than when other routes are used. It is also more nearly complete; therefore, the results are more predictable, and the desired dosage can be determined with greater accuracy.

Giving drugs by injection is necessary if the drug is available in no other form. Injections are particularly desirable for clients who are irrational, unconscious, or having gastrointestinal disturbances. The injection of drugs is also used in emergencies because absorption and desired results occur rapidly.

Needles and Syringes. Needles are available in various lengths and gauges with different size bevels. Figure 29-5 shows the parts of a needle. Needle lengths vary from ½ to 2 inches (1.3 to 5.1 cm). The length of the needle is determined by the route of administration. The gauge is determined by the width of the needle. Needle gauges are numbered 18 through 27. As the diameter of the needle increases, the gauge number decreases. An 18-gauge needle is larger than a 27-gauge needle. The bevel of the needle is its sloped edge, designed to make a narrow, slit-like opening that closes quickly.

Syringes are supplied in various sizes. Most syringes are plastic and disposable. Some syringes are supplied with the needle attached, whereas others are not, in which case the nurse selects an appropriate needle. The parts of a syringe are shown in Figure 29-5.

The nurse chooses the equipment needed for an injection based on the following criteria:

Route of administration: A longer needle is required for an intramuscular injection than for an intradermal or a subcutaneous injection.

Viscosity of the solution: Some medications are more viscous than others and require a large-lumen needle to inject the drug.

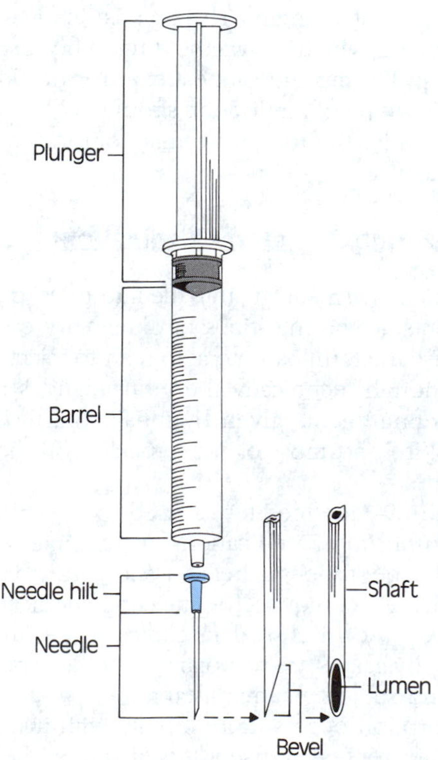

Figure 29-5
Parts of a needle and syringe.

Quantity to be administered: The larger the amount of medication to be injected, the greater the capacity of the syringe.

Body size: An obese person requires a longer needle to reach muscle tissue than a thin person.

Type of medication: There are special syringes for certain uses. An example is the insulin syringe used to inject insulin. Some medications, such as iron dextran injection (Imferon), are irritating to subcutaneous tissue. Therefore, a longer needle should be used to ensure proper placement of the medication in the muscle tissue.

After use, the needles and syringes are placed in puncture-resistant containers without being recapped. Most needlestick injuries occur during recapping. The one-handed technique for use if a needle must be recapped and additional measures to protect healthcare workers from accidental transmission of infectious diseases are discussed in Chapter 28.

Techniques of surgical asepsis must be strictly followed for parenteral injections to help avoid introducing organisms into the body. The parts of the syringe and needle that must be kept sterile during the procedure of preparing and administering an injection are the inside of the barrel, the part of the plunger that enters the barrel, the tip of the barrel, and the needle, except for the needle's hub.

Surgical asepsis applies to cleaning the skin for an injection. The skin is cleaned with alcohol or povidone-iodine (Betadine) in a circular motion, working from the center of the designated site outward. The skin is then considered clean enough to pierce with a sterile needle.

Needleless Systems. The risk of an accidental needlestick and possible exposure to blood-borne pathogens is reduced significantly with the use of needleless devices or protected needles. Chapter 28 summarizes the rationale for movement toward these systems of protection for healthcare workers. These devices prevent needlestick injuries in a variety of ways. Examples include needles that can be sheathed in a plastic guard once the needle is withdrawn from the skin or syringes that have a retractable needle that locks and seals inside the syringe barrel. Needleless systems are also available for intravenous use and include recessed and shielded IV needle connectors as well as blunt cannulas that are inserted into special receptor sites on tubing or lock setups. All needleless devices or blunt cannulas are discarded in special containers that are puncture-proof, leak-proof, clearly labeled, and available at various locations on each healthcare unit. Figure 29-6 displays one type of needleless device.

Preparing Medications for Administration by Injection

Drugs for administration by injection are packaged in several ways. Those that deteriorate in solution usually are dispensed as powders and are reconstituted imme-

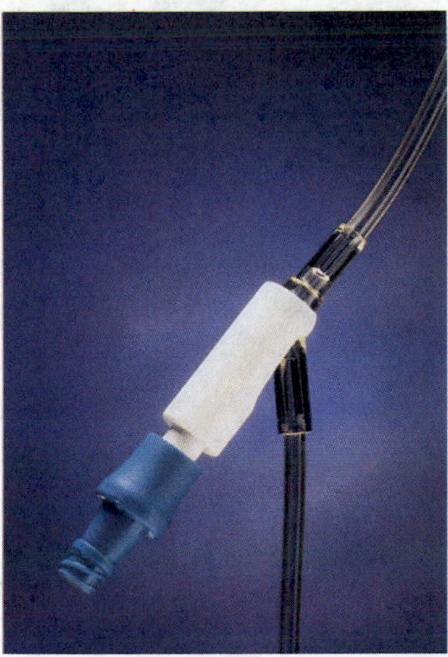

Figure 29-6
Example of a needleless system. (Courtesy of ICU Medical, Inc., San Clemente, CA.)

diately before injection. If drugs remain stable in solution, they usually are dispensed in ampules, bottles, or vials in an aqueous or oily solution or suspension.

Drugs may be dispensed in single-dose glass ampules, single-dose rubber-capped vials, multidose rubber-capped vials, and prefilled cartridges. Figure 29-7 shows several types of ampules and vials as well as a prefilled cartridge.

Ampules. An **ampule** is a glass flask that contains a single dose of medication for parenteral administration. There is no way to prevent airborne contamination of any unused portion of medication once the ampule is opened. If all the medication is not used, the remainder must be discarded. Medication can be removed from an ampule by breaking its thin neck. The ampule can be inverted or placed on a flat surface to draw the solution into the syringe. Care must be taken not to contaminate the needle by touching the rim of the ampule. Procedure 29-2 shows how to remove medication from an ampule.

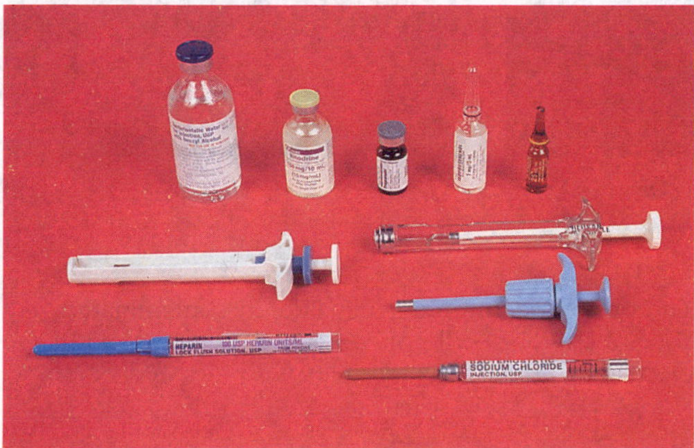

Figure 29-7
Ampules, vials, prefilled cartridges, and holders.

Vials. As Figure 29-7 shows, a **vial** is a glass bottle with a self-sealing stopper through which medication is removed. For safety in transporting and storing, the single-dose rubber-capped vial usually is covered with a soft metal cap that can be easily removed. The rubber stopper that is then exposed is the means of entrance into the vial.

Some drugs are dispensed in vials that contain several doses. This means that the nurse can remove several doses from the same container. To facilitate removal of medication, the nurse injects air into the vial. The amount of air is the same as the desired quantity of solution. Procedure 29-3 shows how to remove medication from a vial.

Prefilled Cartridges. Prefilled cartridges provide a single dose of medication. The nurse inserts the cartridge into a reusable holder. Before giving the injection, the nurse checks the dosage in the cartridge and clears the cartridge of excess air. Most prefilled cartridges are overfilled, and the nurse should eject any excess medication to give an exact dose and avoid a medication error. Tubex and Carpuject are two types of prefilled cartridges.

Mixing Medications in One Syringe

Preparation of medications in one syringe depends on how the medication is supplied. When using a single-dose vial and a multidose vial, air is injected into both vials and the medication in the multidose vial is drawn into the syringe first. This prevents the contents of the multidose vial from being contaminated with the medication in the single-dose vial. The nurse must ensure that the two drugs are compatible.

The steps to follow when preparing medications from two multidose vials in one syringe are illustrated in Figure 29-8 and are as follows:

1. Inject air into vial A, keeping the needle from touching the medication.
2. Inject air into vial B and withdraw the quantity of medication needed.
3. Change the needle if possible. This prevents the contents of vial A from being contaminated with the contents of vial B.
4. Carefully withdraw the needed quantity of medication from vial A. The two medications are now combined in the syringe. Excess medication must not be reinjected into vial A because this may cause an imbalance in the two dosages.

When preparing medications from an ampule and a vial, the medication in the vial is prepared first. The medication in the ampule is drawn up after the medication in the vial.

It is important for the nurse to be aware of drug incompatibilities when preparing medications in one syringe. Certain medications, such as diazepam (Valium),

(text continues on page 622)

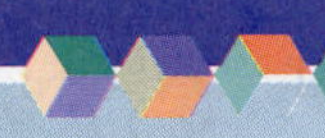

PROCEDURE 29-2

Removing Medication From an Ampule

Equipment

Sterile syringe and needle (size depends on medication being administered and client)
Ampule of medication
Medication card, Kardex, or computer-generated MAR
Alcohol swab or gauze pad
Filter needle (optional)

Action	Rationale
1. Gather equipment. Check the medication order against the original physician's order according to agency policy.	This comparison helps to identify errors that may have occurred when orders were transcribed.
2. Wash your hands.	Handwashing deters the spread of microorganisms.
3. Tap the stem of the ampule or twist your wrist quickly while holding the ampule vertically.	This facilitates movement of medication in the stem to the body of the ampule.
4. Wrap a small gauze pad or dry alcohol swab around the neck of the ampule.	This protects the nurse's fingers from the glass as the ampule is broken.
5. Use a snapping motion to break off the top of the ampule along the prescored line at its neck. Always break away from your body.	This protects the nurse's face and fingers from any shattered glass fragments.

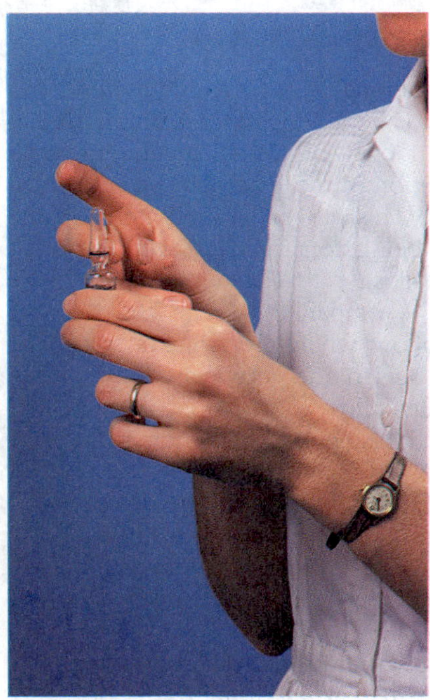

Action 3: Tapping stem of ampule.

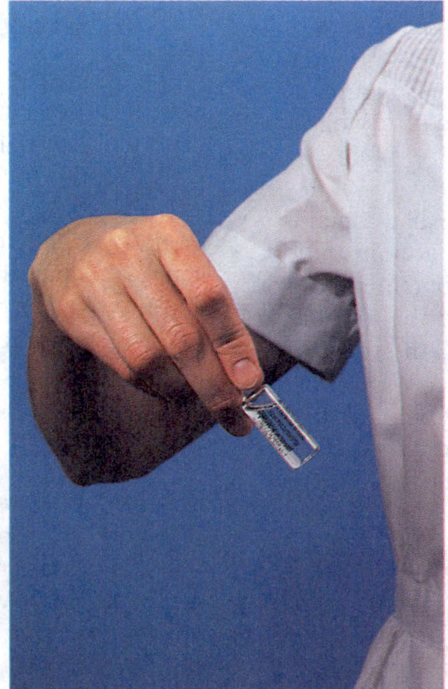

Action 3: Twisting motion of wrist while holding ampule.

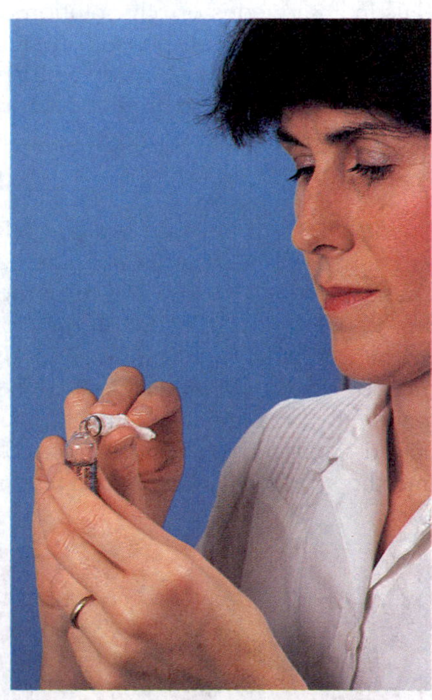

Action 5: Snapping off top of ampule.

Action	Rationale
6. Remove the cap from the needle by pulling it straight off. Insert the needle into the ampule, being careful not to touch the rim. (Some agencies recommend use of a filter needle when withdrawing solution from an ampule.)	The rim of the ampule is considered contaminated. (Use of a filter needle prevents the accidental withdrawing of small glass particles with the medication.)

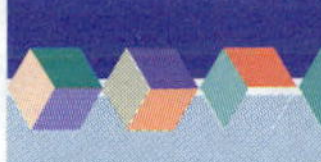

PROCEDURE 29-2 *(continued)*

Removing Medication From an Ampule

Action	Rationale
7. Withdraw medication in the amount ordered. Do not inject air into solutions. Use either of the following methods:	
a. Insert the tip of the needle into the ampule, which is *upright* on a flat surface, and withdraw fluid into the syringe. Touch plunger at knob only.	The contents of the ampule are not under pressure; therefore, air is unnecessary and will cause the contents to overflow. Handling plunger at knob only will keep shaft of plunger sterile.
b. Insert the tip of the needle into the ampule and *invert* the ampule. Keep the needle centered and not touching the sides of the ampule. Remove the prescribed amount of medication. Touch plunger at knob only.	Surface tension holds the fluid in the ampule when inverted. If the needle touches the sides or is removed and then reinserted into the ampule, surface tension is broken and fluid runs out. Handling plunger at knob only will keep shaft of plunger sterile.

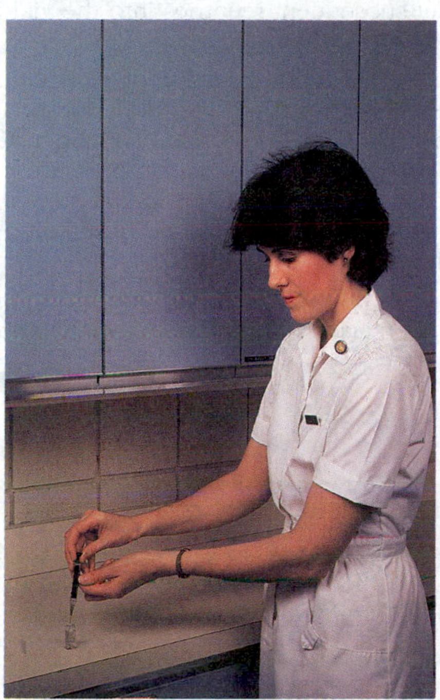

Action 7a: Withdrawing medication from upright ampule.

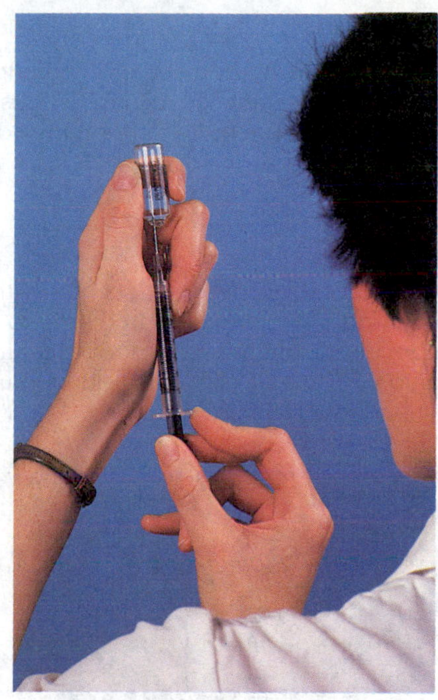

Action 7b: Withdrawing medication from inverted ampule. (Photos © Ken Kasper.)

Action	Rationale
8. Do not expel any air bubbles that may form in the solution. Wait until the needle has been withdrawn to tap the syringe and expel the air carefully. Check the amount of medication in the syringe and discard any surplus.	Ejecting air into the solution increases pressure in the ampule and can force the medication to spill out over the ampule.
9. Discard the ampule in a suitable container after comparing with the medication card or Kardex.	If all of the medication has been removed from the ampule, it must be discarded because there is no way to maintain sterility of contents in an opened ampule.
10. Cap the needle on the syringe.	This prevents contamination of the needle and protects the nurse against inadvertent needlesticks.
11. Wash your hands.	Handwashing deters the spread of microorganisms.

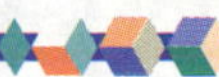

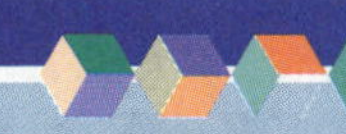

PROCEDURE 29-3

Removing Medication From a Vial

Equipment

Sterile syringe and needle (size depends on medication being administered and client)
Vial of medication
Medication card, Kardex, or computer-generated MAR
Alcohol swab
Filter needle (optional)

Action	Rationale
1. Gather equipment. Check medication order against the original physician's order according to agency policy.	This comparison helps to identify errors that may have occurred when orders were transcribed.
2. Wash your hands.	Handwashing deters the spread of microorganisms.
3. Remove the metal or plastic cap on the vial that protects the rubber stopper.	The metal cap prevents contamination of the rubber top.
4. Swab the rubber top with the alcohol swab.	Alcohol removes surface bacteria contamination. This is not necessary the first time the rubber stopper is entered but subsequent reentries into the vial require the use of alcohol cleansing.
5. Remove the cap from the needle by pulling it straight off. (Some agencies recommend use of a filter needle when withdrawing premixed medication from multidose vials.)	Before fluid is removed, injection of an equal amount of air is required to prevent the formation of a partial vacuum because a vial is a sealed container. If not enough air is injected, the negative pressure makes it difficult to withdraw the medication. (Use of a filter needle prevents any solid material from being withdrawn through the needle.)
6. Pierce the rubber stopper in the center with the needle tip and inject the measured air into the space above the solution. (Do not inject air into the solution.) The vial may be positioned upright on a flat surface or inverted.	Air bubbled through the solution could result in withdrawal of an inaccurate amount of medication.

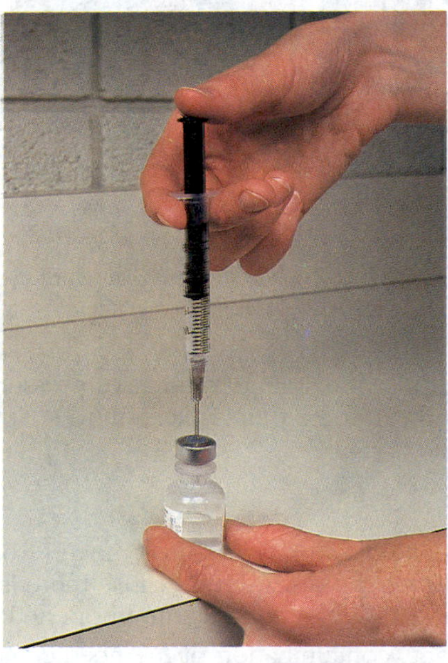

Action 6: Injecting air with vial upright.

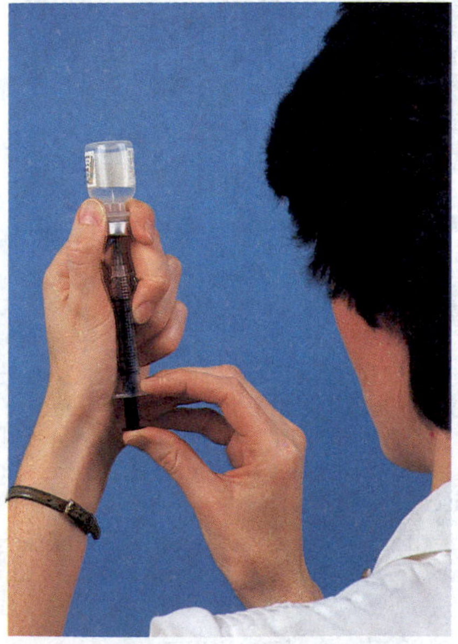

Action 6: Injecting air with vial inverted and needle above solution.

Removing Medication From a Vial

Action	Rationale
7. Invert the vial and withdraw the needle tip slightly so that it is below the fluid level.	This prevents air from being aspirated into the syringe.
8. Draw up the prescribed amount of medication while holding the syringe at eye level and vertically. Be careful to touch the plunger at knob only.	Holding the syringe at eye level facilitates accurate reading, and the vertical position makes removal of air bubbles from the syringe easy. Handling plunger at knob only will keep shaft of plunger sterile.
9. If any air bubbles accumulate in the syringe, tap the barrel of the syringe sharply and move the needle past the fluid into the air space to reinject the air bubble into the vial. Return the needle tip to the solution and continue withdrawal of the medication.	Removal of air bubbles is necessary to ensure accurate dose of medication.

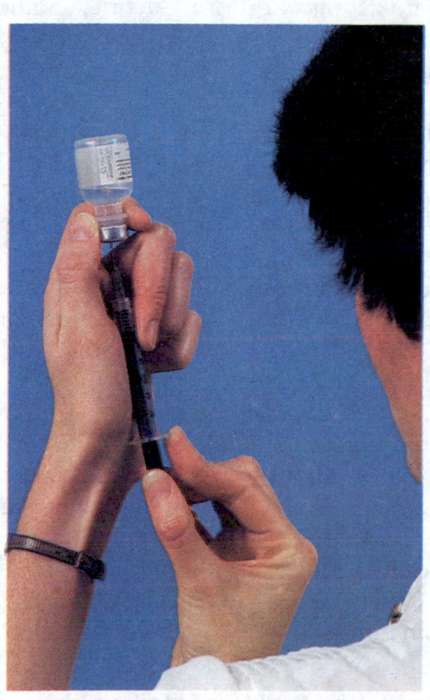

Action 8: Withdrawing medication at eye level.

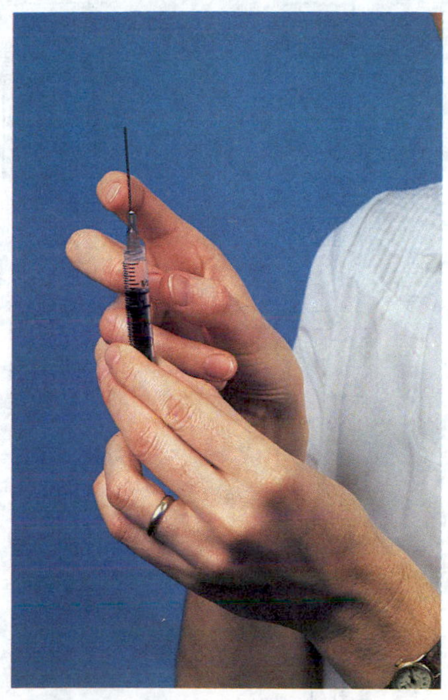

Action 9: Tapping to remove air bubbles. (Photos © Ken Kasper.)

Action	Rationale
10. Once the correct dose is withdrawn, remove the needle from the vial and cap it.	This prevents contamination of the needle and protects the nurse against accidental needlesticks.
11. If a multidose vial is being used, store the vial containing the remaining medication according to agency policy.	Because the vial is sealed, the medication inside remains sterile and can be used for future injections.
12. Wash your hands.	Handwashing deters the spread of microorganisms.

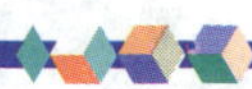

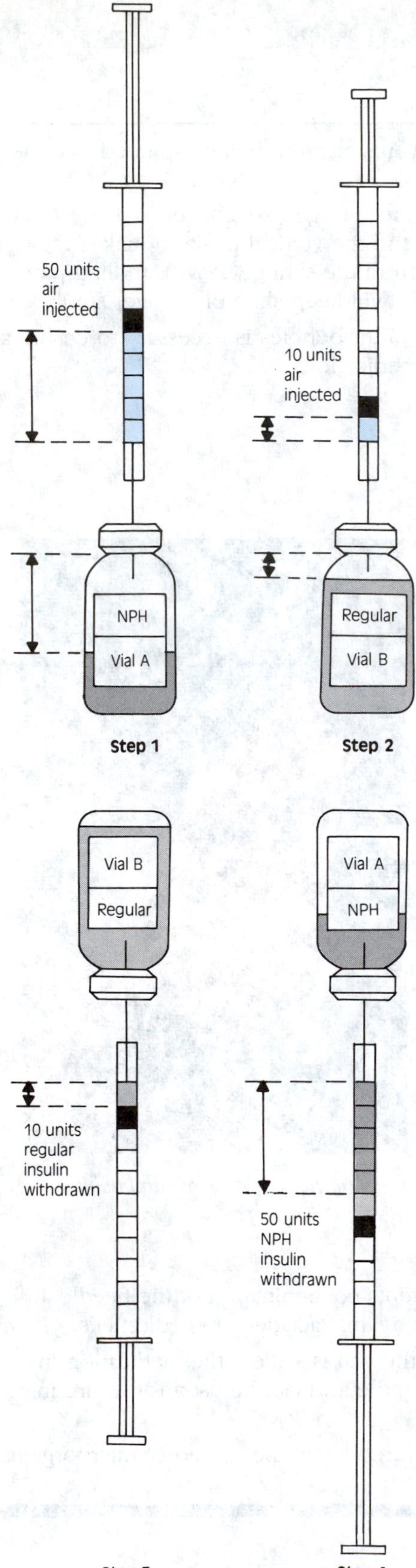

Figure 29-8
Mixing medications in one syringe.

are incompatible with other drugs when combined in the same syringe. Other drugs have limited compatibility and should be administered within 15 minutes of preparation. Incompatible drugs may become cloudy or form a precipitate in the syringe. Such medications are discarded and reprepared in separate syringes. A drug compatibility table should be available to nurses who are preparing medications.

Mixing Insulins in One Syringe

Insulin, a naturally occurring hormone produced by the islets of Langerhans in the pancreas, enables cells to use carbohydrates. Clients with diabetes mellitus produce no insulin or produce insulin in insufficient amounts. Several types of insulin are available for use by clients with diabetes mellitus. Insulins vary in their onset and duration of action and are classified as short-acting, intermediate-acting, and long-acting. Some insulins have a modifying protein that slows absorption. The modifying proteins are globin and protamine (NPH, globin zinc, protamine zinc).

Insulin dosages are calculated in units. The scale commonly used is U-100, which is based on 100 units of insulin contained in 1 mL of solution. An insulin syringe is calibrated in units also. Before administering insulin, the nurse should check the dosage with the physician's orders. Many clients with diabetes mellitus are regulated with a combination of two insulins (eg, regular and NPH insulins).

Procedure 29-4 gives the steps for mixing two types of insulins in the same syringe.

The importance of rotating injection sites for insulin administration cannot be overemphasized. A discussion of injection sites is included under Administering Medications Subcutaneously. Insulin should be stored in a cool place. It can be warmed before administration by rolling the vial between the palms. Some insulins are stable at room temperature.

Reconstituting Powdered Medications

Several drugs, including many antibiotics, are supplied as powders in vials. A liquid, or *diluent*, must be added to the powder before it is administered as a solution. The technique of adding a diluent to a powdered drug is called *reconstitution*. Information needed for reconstitution and dosage calculation usually is located on the vial label. The nurse must know the amount and type of diluent to be added to the powder. Common diluents are sterile water for injection and 0.9% sodium chloride injection. After the diluent is added to the solution, the nurse reads the label further to determine the concentration of drug per milliliter of solution. This is essential to the dosage computation. If all the medication is not used at the time of reconstitution, the nurse refers to the vial label for storage instructions. Additional sources of information about reconstitution of medications are package inserts and the pharmacist.

PROCEDURE 29-4

Mixing Insulins in One Syringe

Equipment

Two vials of insulin
Medication card, Kardex, or computer-generated MAR
Sterile insulin syringe with 25-gauge or 27-gauge needle
Alcohol swabs

Action	Rationale
1. Gather equipment. Check medication order against the original physician's order according to agency policy.	This comparison helps to identify errors that may have occurred when orders were transcribed.
2. Wash your hands.	Handwashing deters the spread of microorganisms.
3. If necessary, remove the metal cap that protects the rubber stopper on each vial.	The metal cap prevents contamination of the rubber top.
4. If insulin is a suspension, rotate the vial between your palms to mix before withdrawal.	Shaking vials creates froth that may interfere with withdrawal of accurate dose. Regular insulin is clear because it does not contain any modifying agents to slow its absorption.
5. Cleanse the rubber tops with alcohol swabs.	Alcohol removes surface bacteria contamination. This is not necessary the first time a metal cap is removed, but subsequent reentries into the vial require use of alcohol cleansing.
6. Remove cap from needle. Inject air into the modified insulin preparation (eg, NPH insulin). Touch plunger at knob only. Use an amount of air equal to the amount of medication to be withdrawn. Do not allow the needle to touch the medication in the vial. Remove the needle.	Regular, or short-acting, insulin should never be contaminated with NPH or any insulin modified with added protein. Placing air in the NPH insulin first without allowing the needle to contact the insulin ensures that regular insulin is not contaminated with the additional protein in the NPH. Handling the plunger by the knob only assures sterility of shaft of plunger.
7. Inject air into the clear insulin without additional protein (eg, regular insulin). Use an amount of air equal to the amount of medication to be withdrawn. Do not bubble the air through the medication.	An equal amount of air must be injected into the vacuum to allow easy withdrawal of medication.

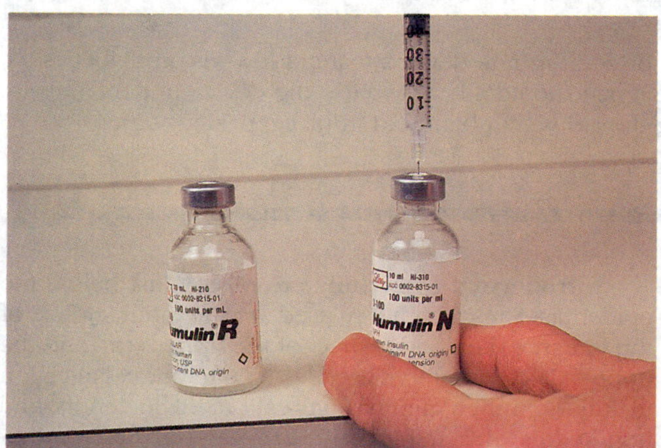

Action 6: Injecting air into modified insulin preparation.

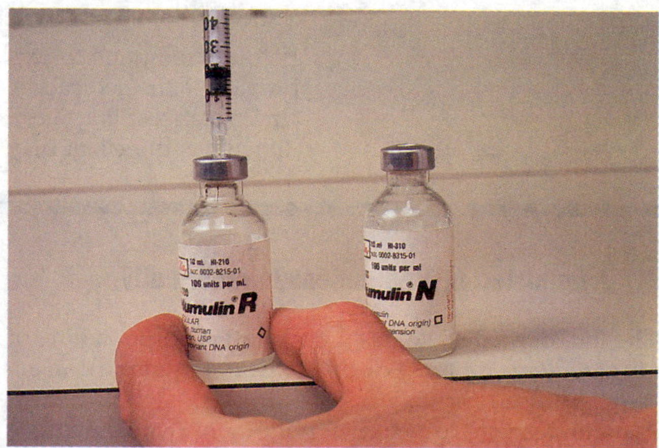

Action 7: Injecting air into clear insulin.

(continued)

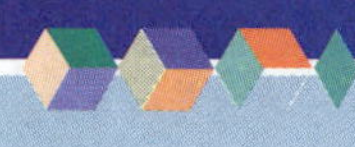

PROCEDURE 29-4 *(continued)*

Mixing Insulins in One Syringe

Action	Rationale
8. Invert the vial of clear insulin and aspirate the amount prescribed. Remove the needle from the vial.	Regular insulin that contains no additional protein is not contaminated by insulin that contains globulin or protamine.
9. Cleanse the rubber top of the modified insulin vial. Insert the needle into this vial, invert it, and withdraw the medication. Cap the needle.	Previous addition of air eliminates need to create positive pressure. Capping the needle prevents contamination and protects the nurse against accidental needlesticks.

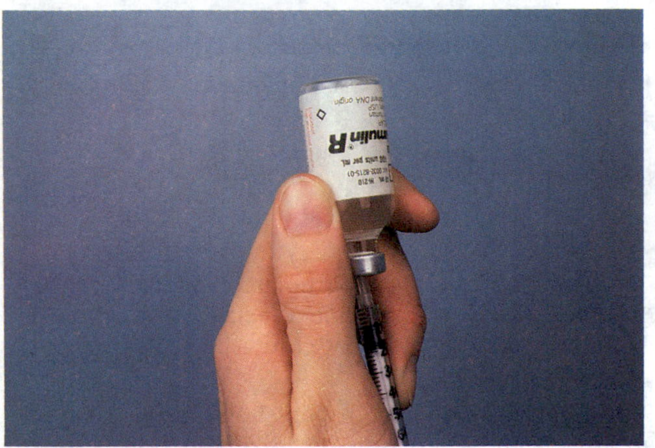

Action 8: Withdrawing clear insulin.

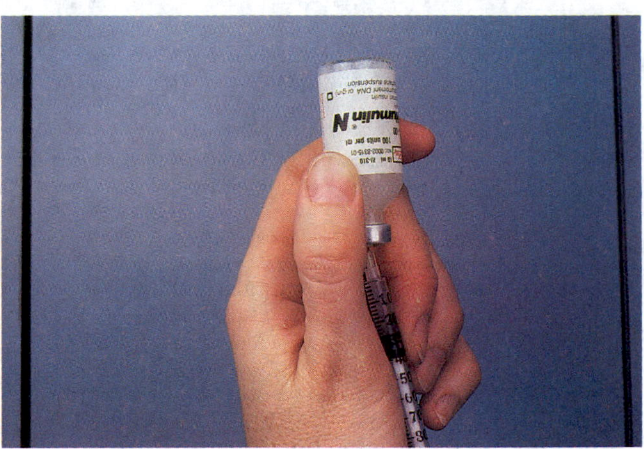

Action 9: Withdrawing modified insulin. (Photos © Ken Kasper.)

Action	Rationale
10. Store the vials according to agency recommendations.	Insulin need not be refrigerated but must be protected from temperature extremes.
11. Wash your hands.	Handwashing deters the spread of microorganisms.

Special Considerations

An insulin-dependent diabetic who is visually impaired may find it helpful to use a magnifying apparatus that fits around the syringe.

An insulin-cartridge pen (the Novalin Pen) is available that allows the client to dial the correct dose of insulin and press a button to quickly release the dose through a short, fine, 27-gauge needle.

Before attempting to explain or demonstrate devices that aid low-vision diabetics to prepare their medication, the nurse should attempt to use the device under similar circumstances. Practice using the aid with a blindfold in place, to detect any difficulties the client may experience.

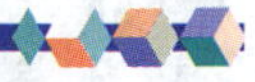

Administering Medications Intradermally

The intradermal route has the longest absorption time of all parenteral routes. For this reason, intradermal injections are used for diagnostic purposes, such as the tuberculin test and tests to determine sensitivity to various substances. The advantage of the intradermal route for these tests is that the body's reaction to substances is easily visible, and degrees of reaction are discernible by comparative study.

Intradermal injections are placed just below the epidermis. Sites commonly used are the inner surface of the forearm, the dorsal aspect of the upper arm, and the upper back. Equipment used for an intradermal injection includes a tuberculin syringe calibrated in tenths and hundredths of a milliliter. The dosage given intradermally is small, usually less than 0.5 mL. A 1/4- to 1/2-inch (0.6 to 1.3 cm), 26- or 27-gauge needle is used. Procedure 29-5 shows the procedure for administering an intradermal injection.

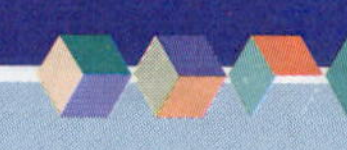

PROCEDURE 29-5

Administering an Intradermal Injection

Equipment

Medication
Medication card, Kardex, or computer-generated MAR
Sterile syringe and needle (size depends on medication being administered and client)
Alcohol swab
Acetone and 2 × 2 sterile gauze square (optional)
Disposable gloves

Action	Rationale
1. Assemble equipment and check the physician's order.	This ensures that the client receives the right medication at the right time by the proper route. Many intradermal drugs are potent allergens and may cause a significant reaction if given in an incorrect dose.
2. Explain the procedure to the client.	Explanation encourages cooperation and reduces apprehension.
3. Wash your hands. Don disposable gloves.	Handwashing deters the spread of microorganisms. Gloves act as a barrier and protect the nurse's hands from accidental exposure to blood during the injection procedure. They are recommended by the CDC's recent Standard Precautions guideline.
4. If necessary, withdraw medication from an ampule or vial as described in Procedures 29-2 and 29-3.	
5. Select an area on the inner aspect of the forearm that is not heavily pigmented or covered with hair. The upper chest or upper back beneath the scapulae also are sites for intradermal injections.	The forearm is a convenient and easy location for introducing an agent intradermally. Hair or lesions at the injection site may interfere with assessments of skin changes at the site.
6. Cleanse the area with an alcohol swab while wiping with a firm, circular motion and moving outward from the injection site. Allow the skin to dry. If the skin is oily, clean the area with a pledget moistened with acetone.	Pathogens on the skin can be forced into the tissues by the needle. Introducing alcohol into tissues irritates the tissues and is uncomfortable for the client. Acetone is effective for removing oily substances from the skin.
7. Use the nondominant hand to spread the skin taut over the injection site.	Taut skin provides an easy entrance into intradermal tissue.
8. Remove the needle cap with the nondominant hand by pulling it straight off.	The cap protects the needle from contact with microorganisms. This technique lessens the risk of an accidental needlestick.
9. Place the needle almost flat against the client's skin, bevel side up, and insert the needle into the skin so that the point of the needle can be seen through the skin. Insert the needle only about 1/8 inch.	Intradermal tissue is entered when the needle is held as nearly parallel to the skin as possible and is inserted about 1/8 inch.
10. Slowly inject the agent while watching for a small wheal or blister to appear. If none appears, withdraw the needle slightly.	If a small wheal or blister appears, the agent is in intradermal tissue.
11. Withdraw the needle quickly at the same angle that it was inserted.	Withdrawing the needle quickly and at the angle at which it entered the skin minimizes tissue damage and discomfort for the client.

(continued)

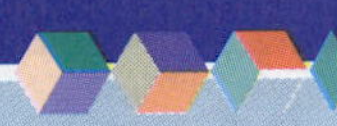

PROCEDURE 29-5 *(continued)*

Administering an Intradermal Injection

Action	Rationale
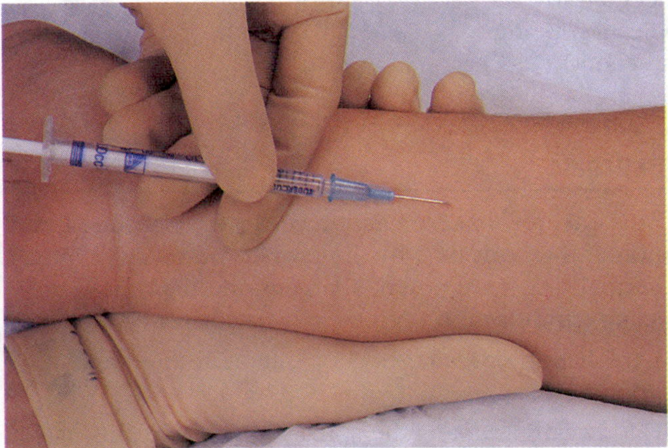 *Action 9: Inserting the needle almost level with the skin.*	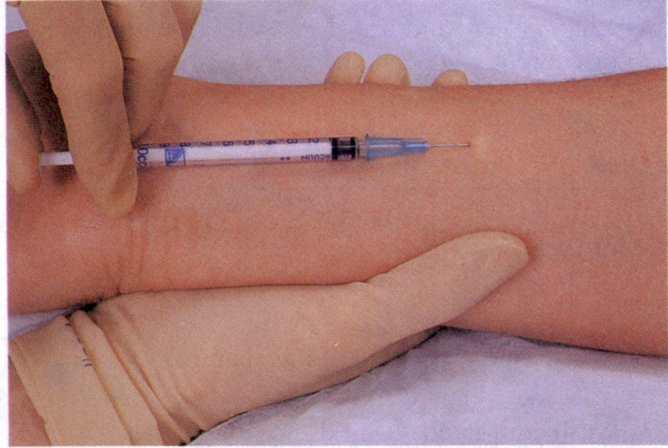 *Action 10: Observing for wheal while injecting medication.*
12. Do not massage the area after removing the needle.	Massaging the area where an intradermal injection is given may interfere with test results by spreading medication to underlying subcutaneous tissue.
13. Do not recap the used needle. Discard the needle and syringe in the appropriate receptacle.	Proper disposal of the needle protects the nurse from accidental injection. Most accidental puncture wounds occur when recapping needles.
14. Assist the client to a position of comfort.	This provides for the well-being of the client.
15. Remove gloves and dispose of them properly. Wash your hands.	Handwashing deters the spread of microorganisms.
16. Chart the administration of the medication.	Accurate documentation is necessary to prevent medication error.
17. Observe the area for signs of a reaction at ordered intervals, usually at 24- to 72-hour periods. Inform the client of this inspection. In some agencies, a circle may be drawn on the skin around the injection site.	This easily identifies the site of the intradermal injection and allows for careful observation of the exact area.

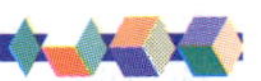

Administering Medications Subcutaneously

Subcutaneous tissue lies between the epidermis and the muscle. Because there is subcutaneous tissue all over the body, various sites are used for **subcutaneous injections**. These sites are the outer aspect of the upper arm, anterior aspects of the thigh, lower abdominal wall, and upper back. Figure 29-9 includes the sites on the body where subcutaneous injections can be given. This route is used to administer insulin, heparin, and certain immunizations.

Equipment used for a subcutaneous injection depends on the medication to be given. For instance, insulin is prepared with an insulin syringe. Heparin is prepared with a tuberculin syringe or supplied in a prefilled cartridge. A ½- to 1-inch, 25-gauge needle is used for this route. Ordinarily, no more than 1 mL of solution is given subcutaneously. Giving larger amounts adds to the client's discomfort and may predispose to poor absorption.

The skin is cleaned for a subcutaneous injection in the same manner as for an intradermal injection. The nurse chooses the angle of needle insertion based on the amount of subcutaneous tissue present and the length of the needle. In most cases, a ⅝-inch (1.6 cm) needle is inserted at a 45-degree angle and a ½-inch needle is inserted at a 90-degree angle. The client's size also may determine the angle of needle insertion. The amount of tissue that can be bunched or grasped is an indication.

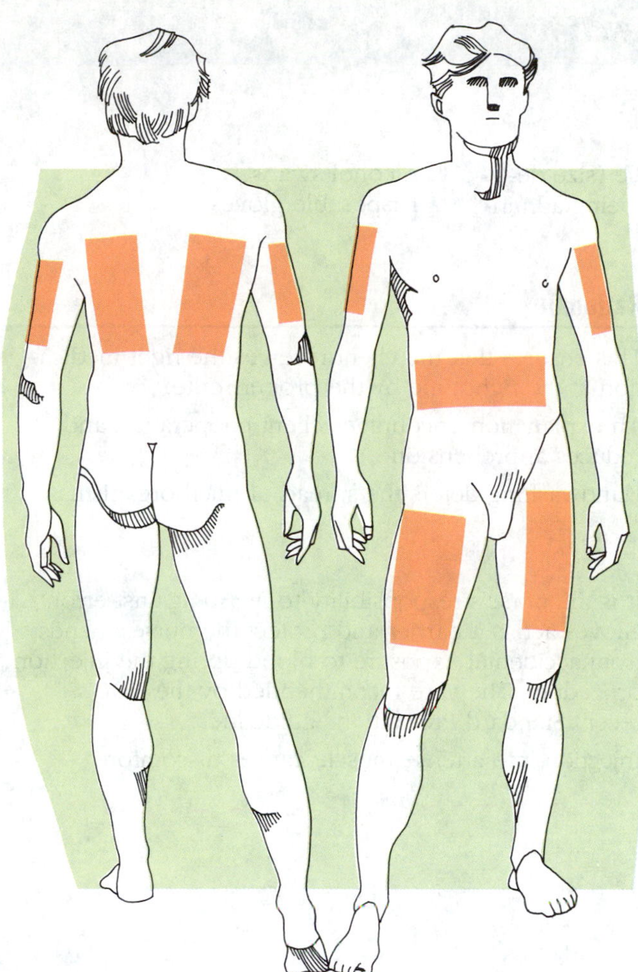

Figure 29-9
Sites on the body where subcutaneous injections can be given.

A 90-degree angle is used if 2 inches (5.1 cm) of tissue can be grasped at the site, and a 45-degree angle is recommended when 1 inch of tissue is grasped. Stretching or spreading the skin taut allows for easier insertion of the needle.

After the needle is in place, the nurse gently pulls back on the plunger to determine that the needle has not entered a blood vessel. When clients are taught to administer their own injections, this step is frequently omitted since there is not agreement on whether it is necessary. Recent information reported by Drass (1992) suggests that aspiration prior to an insulin injection is recommended for children or those with superficial blood vessels at the injection site (eg, thin adults or athletes with well-developed muscle underlying the skin). If blood enters the barrel of the syringe, the needle is removed and the medication, syringe, and needle should be discarded appropriately and a new dose prepared for administration at another site.

If no blood enters the barrel of the syringe, the medication is injected into the client. Aspiration of the plunger is not recommended with administration of subcutaneous heparin because this action can result in hematoma formation. The site is gently massaged, except in the case of heparin and insulin because massaging the site can increase the rate of absorption of these agents. The site of administration is recorded in the client's record. Procedure 29-6 shows the procedure for administering medications subcutaneously.

It is necessary to rotate sites or areas for injection if the client is to receive frequent injections. This helps to prevent irritation and permits complete absorption of the medication. Clients who receive injections repeatedly in one site are likely to develop hardened and tender tissue. It is recommended that clients administering their own insulin use the same area of the body at the same time every day (intrasite injection) to ensure more consistent absorption (Drass, 1992). For instance, every morning the client uses the anterior aspect of her right thigh for her insulin injection and every evening before dinner she injects the insulin into her abdomen. In each case, the injections should be given an inch away from the previous injection site so that the same area will not be used again in the same month. A small spot bandage or piece of tape can be used to mark the first injection site, with subsequent injections rotated in a circle around that site. Once this area has been used, an adjacent site, an inch away, can be selected, using the same rotation format. A marked diagram incorporated into the client's plan of care is also helpful for noting alternative sites. It is futile to rely on memory. Not even the client can always recall the site of the previous injection. Techniques for reducing discomfort in subcutaneous administrations are listed after the discussion Administering Medications Intramuscularly.

Administering Medications Intramuscularly

The intramuscular route often is used for drugs that are irritating because there are few nerve endings in deep muscle tissue. If a sore or inflamed muscle is entered, the muscle may act as a trigger area, and severe referred pain often results. It is best to palpate a muscle before injection. A site should be selected that does not feel tender to the client and where the tissue does not contract and become firm and tense.

Absorption occurs as in subcutaneous administration but more rapidly because of the greater vascularity of muscle tissue. The amount of 4 mL is considered the maximum to be given in one site for an adult with well-developed muscles (Beyea & Nicoll, 1995).

Intramuscular Injection Sites. An important point in the administration of an **intramuscular injection** is the selection of a safe site, one that is away from large nerves, bones, and blood vessels (Fig. 29-10). When care is not taken, common complications include abscesses, necrosis and skin slough, nerve injuries, lingering pain, and periostitis (inflammation of the membrane covering a bone).

The sites for injecting intramuscular medications should be rotated when therapy requires repeated in-

(text continues on page 631)

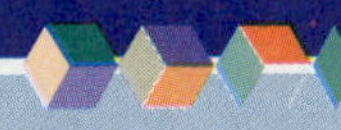

PROCEDURE 29-6

Administering a Subcutaneous Injection

Equipment

- Medication
- Medication card, Kardex, or computer-generated MAR
- A sterile syringe and needle (size depends on medication being administered and client)
- Alcohol swabs
- Disposable gloves

Action	Rationale
1. Assemble equipment and check the physician's order.	This ensures that the client receives the right medication at the right time by the proper route.
2. Explain the procedure to the client.	An explanation encourages client cooperation and reduces apprehension.
3. Wash your hands.	Handwashing deters the spread of microorganisms.
4. If necessary, withdraw medication from an ampule or vial as described in Procedures 29-2 and 29-3.	
5. Identify the client carefully. See Procedure 29-1, action 12. Close the curtain to provide privacy. Don disposable gloves.	It is the nurse's responsibility to guard against error. Gloves act as a barrier and protect the nurse's hands from accidental exposure to blood during the injection procedure. They are recommended by the CDC's recent Standard Precautions guideline.
6. Have the client assume a position appropriate for the site selected: a. Outer aspect of upper arm—the client's arm should be relaxed and at the side of the body. b. Anterior thighs—the client may sit or lie with the leg relaxed. c. Abdomen—the client may lie in a semirecumbent position. d. Scapular area—the client may be prone, on side, or in a sitting position.	Injection into a tense muscle causes discomfort.
7. Locate the site of choice according to directions given in this chapter. Ensure that the area is not tender and is free of lumps or nodules.	Good visualization is necessary to establish the correct location of the site and avoid damage to tissues. Nodules or lumps may indicate a previous injection site where absorption was inadequate.
8. Clean the area around the injection site with an alcohol swab. Use a firm, circular motion while moving outward from the injection site. Allow the antiseptic to dry. Leave the alcohol swab in a clean area for reuse when withdrawing the needle.	Friction helps to clean the skin. A clean area is contaminated when a soiled object is rubbed over its surface.
9. Remove the needle cap with the nondominant hand, pulling it straight off.	The cap protects the needle from contact with microorganisms. This technique lessens the risk of an accidental needlestick.
10. Grasp and bunch the area surrounding the injection site or spread the skin at the site.	This provides for easy, less painful entry into the subcutaneous tissue. The decision to pinch or spread tissue at the injection site depends on the size of the client. If the client is obese, skin needs to be bunched to allow the needle to penetrate below the fatty layer in the subcutaneous tissue.
11. Hold the syringe in the dominant hand between the thumb and forefinger. Inject the needle quickly at an angle at 45 to 90 degrees, depending on the amount and turgor of the tissue and the length of the needle, as shown.	Subcutaneous tissue is abundant in well-nourished, well-hydrated persons and spare in emaciated, dehydrated, or very thin persons.

Administering a Subcutaneous Injection

Action	Rationale
12. After the needle is in place, release the tissue and immediately move your nondominant hand to steady the lower end of the syringe. Slide your dominant hand to the tip of the barrel.	Injecting the solution into compressed tissues results in pressure against nerve fibers and creates discomfort. The nondominant hand secures the syringe and allows for smooth aspiration.

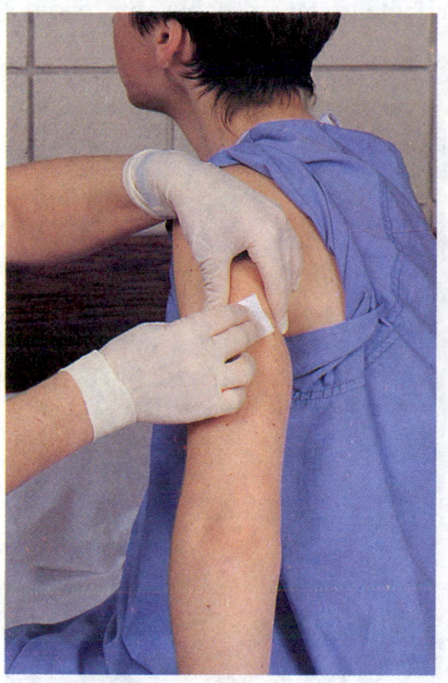
Action 9: Cleaning injection site.

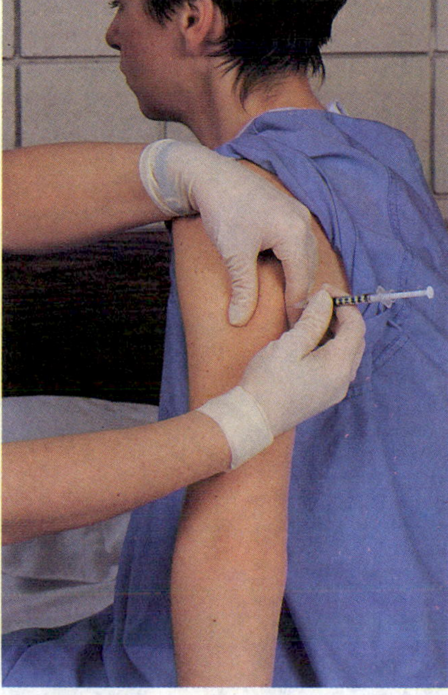
Action 11: Bunching tissue around injection site.

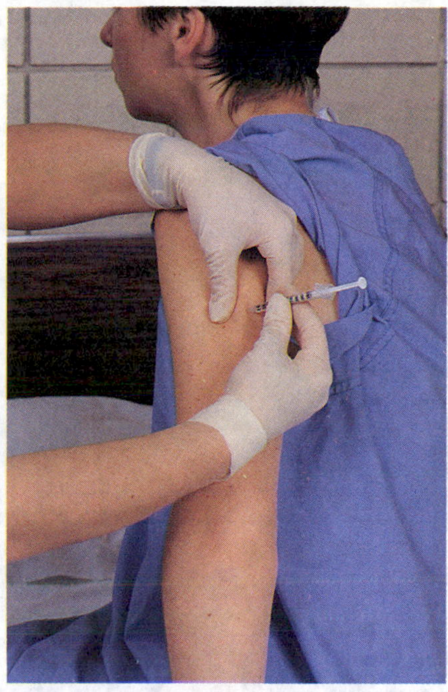
Action 12: Inserting needle.

Action	Rationale
13. Aspirate by pulling back gently on the plunger of the syringe to determine whether the needle is in a blood vessel (optional). If blood appears, the needle should be withdrawn and the medication, syringe, and needle are discarded, and a new syringe with new medication prepared. (Most agencies recommend that a subcutaneous anticoagulant injection should not be aspirated.)	Discomfort and possibly a serious reaction may occur if a drug intended for subcutaneous use is injected into a vein. Heparin is an anticoagulant and may cause bruising if aspirated. Aspiration is recommended for children, thin adults, and athletic individuals who may have more superficial blood vessels.
14. If no blood appears, inject the solution slowly.	Rapid injection of the solution creates pressure in the tissues, resulting in discomfort.
15. Withdraw the needle quickly at the same angle at which it was inserted, as shown.	Slow withdrawal of the needle pulls the tissues and causes discomfort. Applying countertraction around the injection site helps to prevent pulling on the tissue as the needle is withdrawn. Removing the needle at the same angle at which it was inserted minimizes tissue damage and discomfort for the client.

(continued)

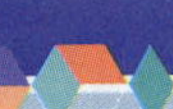

PROCEDURE 29-6 *(continued)*

Administering a Subcutaneous Injection

Action	Rationale
16. Massage the area gently with the alcohol swab. (Do not massage a subcutaneous heparin or insulin injection site.)	Massaging helps to distribute the solution and hastens its absorption. Massaging the site of a heparin injection causes additional bruising. Massaging after an insulin injection may contribute to unpredictable absorption of the medication.

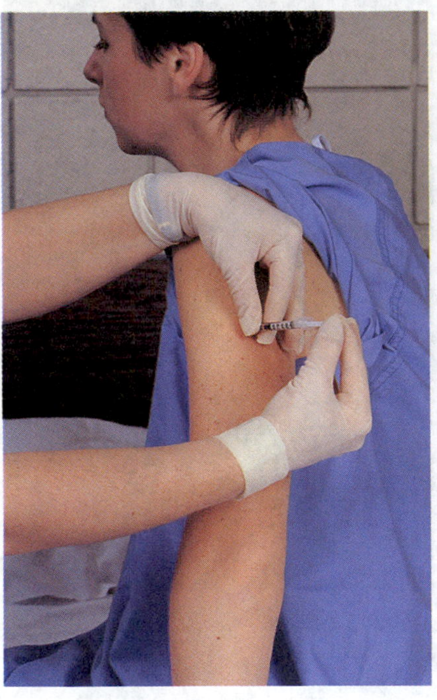

Action 14: Aspirating.

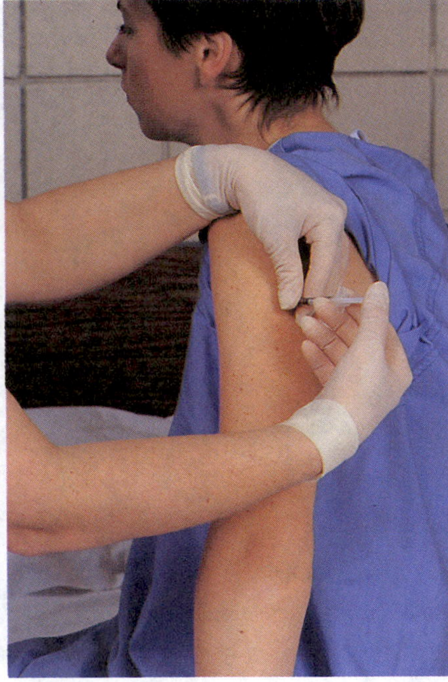

Action 15: Injecting medication.

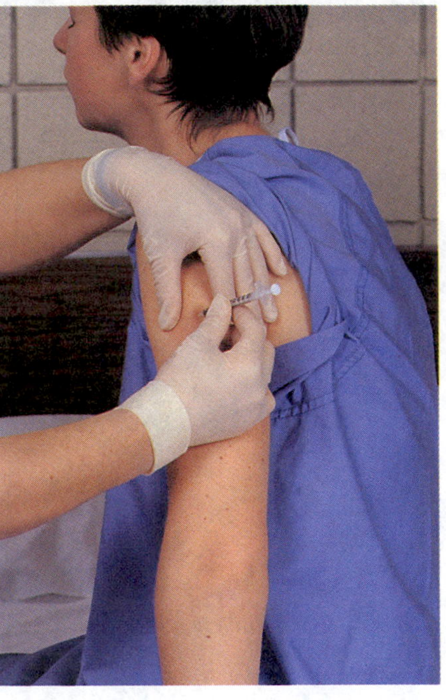

Action 16: Withdrawing needle. (Photos © B. Proud.)

Action	Rationale
17. Do not recap the used needle. Discard the needle and syringe in the appropriate receptacle.	Proper disposal of the needle protects the nurse from accidental injection. Most accidental puncture wounds occur when recapping needles.
18. Assist the client to a position of comfort.	This provides for the well-being of the client.
19. Remove gloves and dispose of them properly. Wash your hands.	Handwashing deters the spread of microorganisms.
20. Chart the administration of the medication.	Accurate documentation is necessary to prevent medication error.
21. Evaluate the response of the client to medication within an appropriate time frame.	Reaction to medication given by the parenteral route may occur within 15 to 30 minutes after injection.

Home Care Considerations

If a diabetic client is visually impaired, several insulin syringes may be preloaded and stored in the refrigerator for future use.

A poster or body log may be used to indicate sites for systematic rotation of insulin injections as well as to record the location of injections.

Refer the diabetic client to the American Diabetic Association for additional information and assistance.

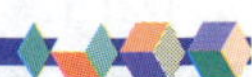

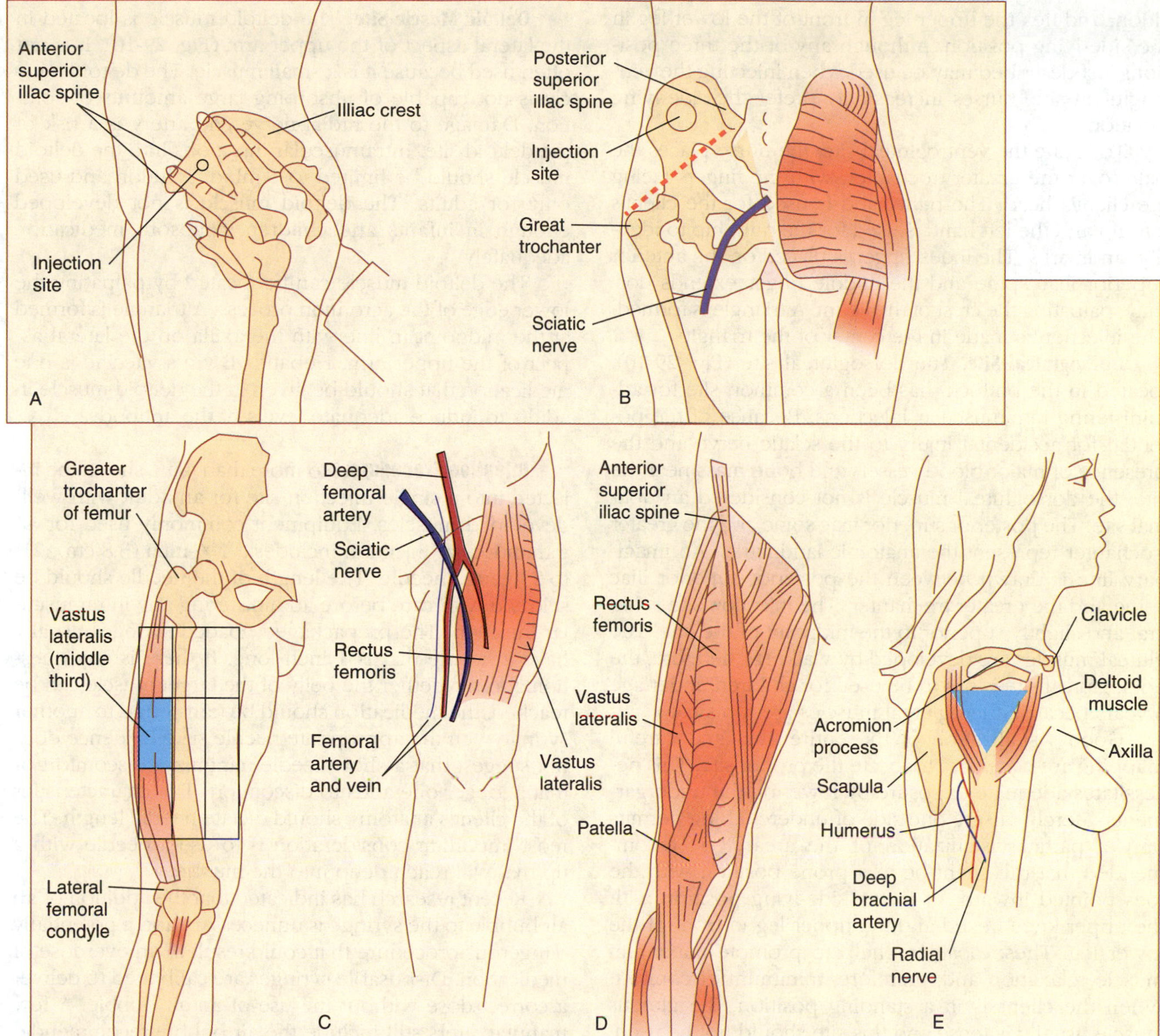

Figure 29-10
Sites for intramuscular injections. Descriptions for locating the sites are given in the text. **(A)** The *ventrogluteal site* is located by placing the palm on the greater trochanter and the index finger toward the anterior superior iliac spine. **(B)** The *dorsogluteal site* is lateral and slightly superior to the midpoint of a line drawn from the trochanter to the posterior superior iliac spine. **(C)** The *vastus lateralis site* is identified by dividing the thigh into thirds horizontally and vertically. **(D)** The *rectus femoris site* is located on the anterior part of the thigh. It is used only when others are contraindicated. **(E)** The *deltoid muscle site* is located by palpating the lower edge of the acromion process.

jections. The sites described in this chapter may all be used on a rotating basis. Whatever pattern of rotating sites is used, a description of it should appear in the client's plan of nursing care.

Ventrogluteal Site. The ventrogluteal site (Fig. 29-10) involves the gluteus medius and gluteus minimus muscles in the hip area. The ventrogluteal site is recommended for both adults and children over 7 months of age as a safe site for the majority of intramuscular injections (Beyea & Nicoll, 1995). There are no large nerves or blood vessels in the injection area, it is removed from bone tissue, the area is clean because fecal contamination is rare at this site, and the client can be on the back, abdomen, or side for the injection. To relax the gluteal muscle, the client may flex the knees while lying on the back, point the toes inward while lying in the prone position, and flex the upper leg in front of the lower leg in the side-lying position. Although any of the three positions just described may be used when injecting the ventrogluteal site, nurses increasingly prefer the side-lying position.

To locate the ventrogluteal site, the nurse places the palm over the greater trochanter, with the fingers facing the client's head. The right hand is used for the client's left hip and the left hand is used for the right hip to identify landmarks. The index finger is placed on the anterior superior iliac spine and the middle finger extends dorsally, palpating the crest of the ileum. A triangle is formed. The injection is made in the center of the triangle.

Dorsogluteal Site. The dorsogluteal site (Fig. 29-10), located in the buttock, has been a common site for administering intramuscular injections. Because of the potential for accidental injury to the sciatic nerve and the presence of major blood vessels and bone mass near the site, the dorsogluteal muscle is not considered an optimal site. The posterior superior iliac spine and the greater trochanter represent the anatomic landmarks. An imaginary line is drawn between the posterior superior iliac spine and the greater trochanter. The injection site is lateral and slightly superior to the midpoint of the line. The gluteal muscles are developed by walking; therefore, the dorsogluteal site is not to be used for children under age 3 years because their gluteal muscles are too small.

Good visualization of the entire area and careful mapping are necessary to locate the proper site. This necessitates adequate exposure by lowering the undergarments. Merely raising one side of underclothing permits only a partial visualization of the area. It is recommended that the client be in a prone position with the toes pointed inward, or in the side-lying position with the upper knee flexed and the upper leg in front of the lower leg. These positions help to promote maximum muscle relaxation and, therefore, minimum discomfort. When the client is in a standing position, the gluteus muscle usually is tense and this site should not be used.

Vastus Lateralis Site. The vastus lateralis muscle is being recommended more frequently for the injection of medications (Fig. 29-10). It is a thick muscle, and there is little or no danger of serious injury. There are no large nerves or vessels in proximity, and it does not cover a joint. The muscle covers the anterolateral aspect of the thigh. It is bounded by the midanterior thigh on the front of the leg and the midlateral thigh on the side. The thigh is divided into thirds horizontally and vertically. The injection is given in the *outer middle* third. This space provides a large number of injection sites. The syringe is held parallel to the surface of the bed. The vastus lateralis site is particularly desirable for infants and children, whose gluteal muscles are poorly developed.

Rectus Femoris Site. The rectus femoris muscle is on the anterior part of the thigh. The site (Fig. 29-10) is used only when others are contraindicated, since many clients find it uncomfortable. Some clients who must inject themselves at home use this site because of its convenience.

Deltoid Muscle Site. The deltoid muscle is located in the lateral aspect of the upper arm (Fig. 29-10). It is not often used because it is a small muscle. The deltoid muscle is not capable of absorbing large amounts of solution. Damage to the radial nerve and artery is a risk of the deltoid site. Intramuscular injections into the deltoid muscle should be limited to 1 mL of solution and used only for adults. The deltoid muscle is not developed enough in infants and children to absorb medication adequately.

The deltoid muscle can be located by palpating the lower edge of the acromion process. A triangle is formed at the midpoint in line with the axilla on the lateral aspect of the upper arm. Hepatitis B virus vaccine is one medication that should be given in the deltoid muscle in adults to induce adequate levels of the antibody.

Injection Procedure. No more than 4 mL should be injected into a single injection site for an adult with well-developed muscles. Equipment commonly used for an intramuscular injection includes a 1½-inch (3.8 cm), 21- to 23-gauge needle. The length of the needle should be selected with care before administering any intramuscular injection. The prepackaged, loaded syringes usually have a needle that is 1 inch long. If there is any question about whether the belly of the target muscle can be reached, the medication should be transferred to another syringe with the appropriate needle size. Evidence does not suggest that a short needle minimizes discomfort or that a longer one adds to discomfort. The characteristics of the client's anatomy should dictate needle length. The most important consideration is to use a needle with a tip that will reach deep into the muscle.

Recent research has indicated that the addition of an air bubble to the syringe is unnecessary and a potentially dangerous procedure that could result in an overdose of medication. Disposable syringes are calibrated to deliver a correct dose without the use of an air bubble. A few manufacturers still include the air bubble recommendation for specific medications but research is not available that validates this technique (Beyea & Nicoll, 1995). *An air bubble is no longer recommended for use with an intramuscular injection.*

To administer an intramuscular injection, the nurse cleans the site, prepares to use the Z-track technique or spreads the skin taut with the nondominant hand, and inserts the needle in a dartlike manner at a 90-degree angle into the skin. The nurse aspirates the plunger and injects the medication if the needle is not in a blood vessel. Gentle pressure is applied after the injection and the site is recorded in the client's record. The procedure for administering an intramuscular injection is outlined in Procedure 29-7. Figure 29-11 compares the angles for needle insertion for all the injections.

Z-Track Technique. Any intramuscular injection may be given using the Z-track technique. Taylor (1992) states that Z-track is the safest and most comfortable technique for giving any IM injection. This prevents

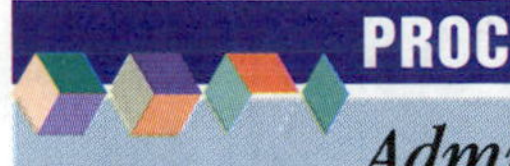

PROCEDURE 29-7

Administering an Intramuscular Injection

Equipment

Medication
Medication card, Kardex, or computer-generated MAR
Sterile syringe and needle (size depends on medication being administered and client)
Alcohol swab
Dry sponge
Disposable gloves

Action	Rationale
1. Assemble equipment and check the physician's order.	This ensures that the client receives the right medication at the right time by the proper route.
2. Explain the procedure to the client.	Explanation encourages cooperation and alleviates apprehension.
3. Wash your hands.	Handwashing deters the spread of microorganisms.
4. If necessary, withdraw medication from an ampule or vial as described in Procedures 29-2 and 29-3.	
5. Do not add air to the syringe.	The addition of air to the syringe is potentially dangerous and may result in an overdose of medication.
6. Provide for privacy. Have the client assume a position appropriate for the site selected. a. Ventrogluteal—the client may lie on the back or side with the hip and knee flexed. b. Dorsogluteal—the client may lie prone with toes pointing inward or on the side with the upper leg flexed and placed in front of the lower leg. c. Vastus lateralis—the client may lie on the back or may assume a sitting position. d. Deltoid—the client may sit or lie with arm relaxed.	Injection into a tense muscle causes discomfort.
7. Locate the site of choice according to directions given in this chapter and ensure that the area is nontender and free of lumps or nodules. Don disposable gloves.	Good visualization is necessary to establish the correct location of the site and avoid damage to tissues. Nodules or lumps may indicate a previous injection site where absorption was inadequate. Gloves act as a barrier and protect the nurse's hands from accidental exposure to blood during the injection procedure. They are recommended by the CDC's recent Standard Precautions guideline.
8. Clean the area thoroughly with an alcohol swab, using friction. Allow alcohol to dry.	Pathogens present on the skin and alcohol can be forced into the tissues by the needle.
9. Remove the needle cap by pulling it straight off.	The cap protects the needle from contact with microorganisms. This technique lessens the risk of an accidental needlestick.
10. Displace the skin in a Z-track manner or spread the skin at the site using your nondominant hand.	This makes the tissue taut and minimizes discomfort. Z-track prevents seepage of the medication into the needle track and is less painful.
11. Hold the syringe in your dominant hand between the thumb and forefinger. Quickly dart the needle into the tissue at a 90-degree angle.	A quick injection is less painful. Inserting the needle at a 90-degree angle facilitates entry into muscle tissue.

(continued)

PROCEDURE 29-7 *(continued)*

Administering an Intramuscular Injection

Action	Rationale

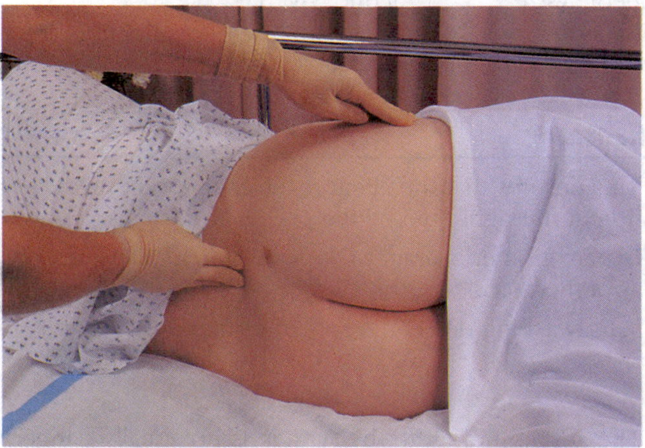

Action 7: Identifying landmarks for dorsogluteal injection site.

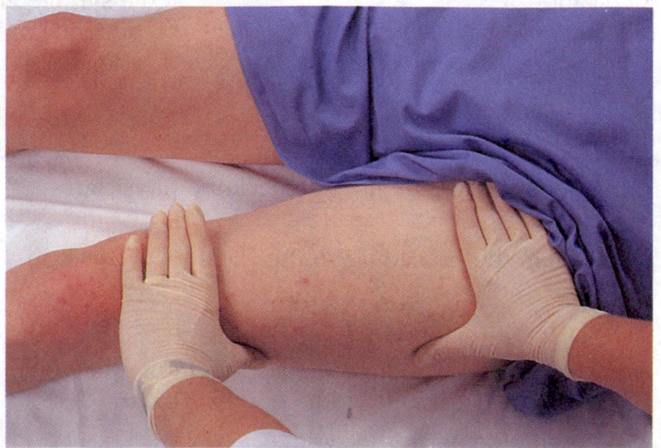

Action 7: Identifying vastus lateralis injection site.

Action	Rationale
12. As soon as the needle is in place, use your nondominant hand to hold the lower end of the syringe. Slide your dominant hand to the tip of the barrel.	This acts to steady the syringe and allows for smooth aspiration.
13. Aspirate by slowly (for at least 5 seconds) pulling back on the plunger to determine whether the needle is in a blood vessel. If blood is aspirated, discard the needle, syringe, and medication, prepare a new sterile setup, and inject another site.	Discomfort and possibly a serious reaction may occur if a drug intended for intramuscular use is injected into a vein. Allowing at least 5 seconds for aspiration facilitates back-flow of blood even if needle is in a small, low-flow blood vessel.
14. If no blood is aspirated, inject the solution slowly (10 seconds per mL of medication).	Injecting slowly helps to reduce discomfort by allowing time for the solution to disperse in the tissues.

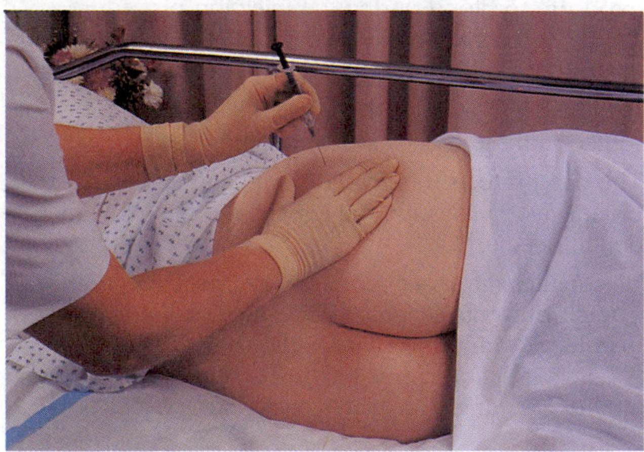

Action 10 and 11: Pulling the skin to one side at the site and darting in at 90-degree angle.

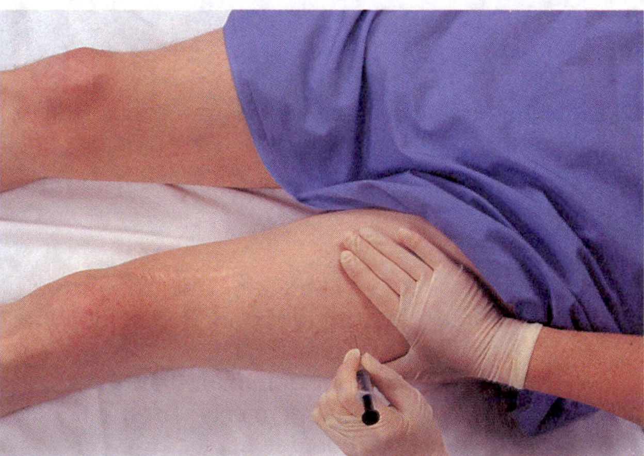

Action 10 and 11: Spreading the skin at vastus lateralis site and darting needle into the tissue. (Photos © B. Proud.)

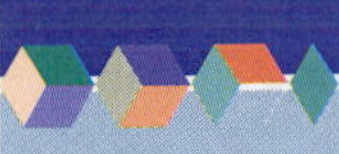

PROCEDURE 29-7 *(continued)*

Administering an Intramuscular Injection

Action	Rationale
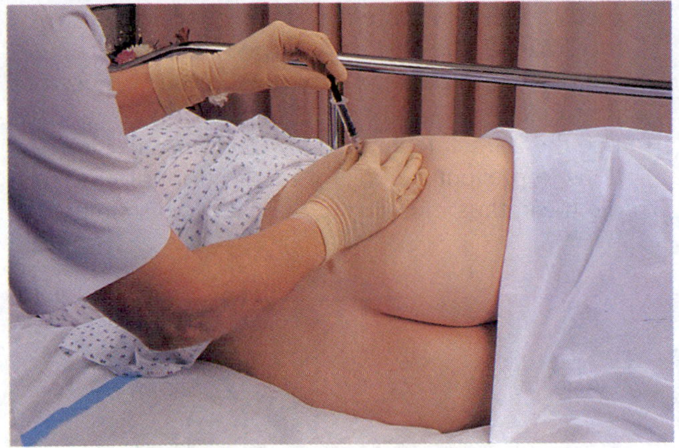 *Action 13: Aspirating.*	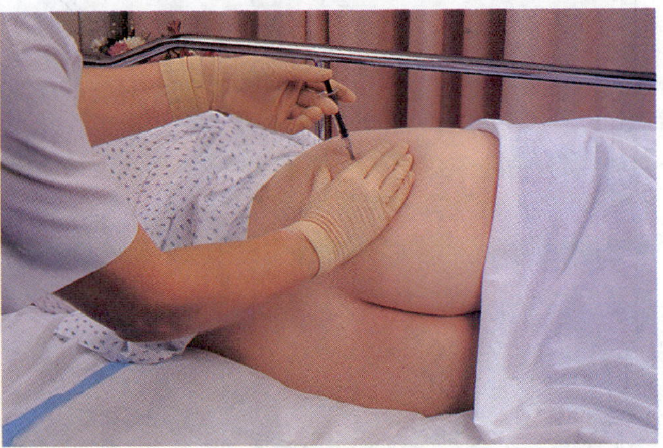 *Action 14: Injecting.*
15. Wait 10 seconds and remove the needle quickly. Release displaced tissue if Z-track technique was used.	A 10-second delay allows the medication to begin to be diffused through the muscle. Removing the needle quickly is less painful.
16. Apply gentle pressure at the site with a small, dry sponge.	Light pressure causes less trauma and irritation to the tissues.
17. Do not recap the used needle. Discard the needle and syringe in the appropriate receptacle.	Proper disposal of the needle protects the nurse from accidental injection. Most accidental puncture wounds occur when recapping needles.
18. Assist the client to a position of comfort. Encourage client to exercise leg if possible.	Exercise promotes absorption of the medication.
19. Remove gloves and dispose of them properly. Wash your hands.	Handwashing deters the spread of microorganisms.
20. Chart the administration of the medication.	Accurate documentation is necessary to prevent medication error.
21. Evaluate the response of the client to the medication within an appropriate time frame. Assess site, if possible, within 2–4 hours after administration.	Reaction to medication given by the parenteral route is a possibility. Assessment also allows for visualization of the site for any untoward effects.

Age Considerations

Safe administration of an intramuscular injection into an infant's vastus lateralis muscle may require use of a 1-inch needle rather than the commonly used 5/8-inch needle. A 1-inch needle consistently allows penetration into the muscle and safe administration of the medication.

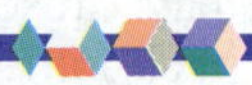

seepage of the medication into the needle track and reduces the pain and discomfort, particularly for clients receiving injections over an extended period. In the past the Z-track, or zig-zag, technique was recommended only to administer medications that were highly irritating to subcutaneous tissues—for example, iron dextran injection (Imferon)—and included the addition of 0.2 to 0.3 mL of air to the syringe. Although some manufacturer's directions still recommend adding air, available research does not validate the addition of air.

In the Z-track technique, a clean needle is attached to the syringe to prevent the injection of medication on the needle into superficial tissues. The needle should be a minimum of 1½ inches (3.8 cm) long. The ventro-

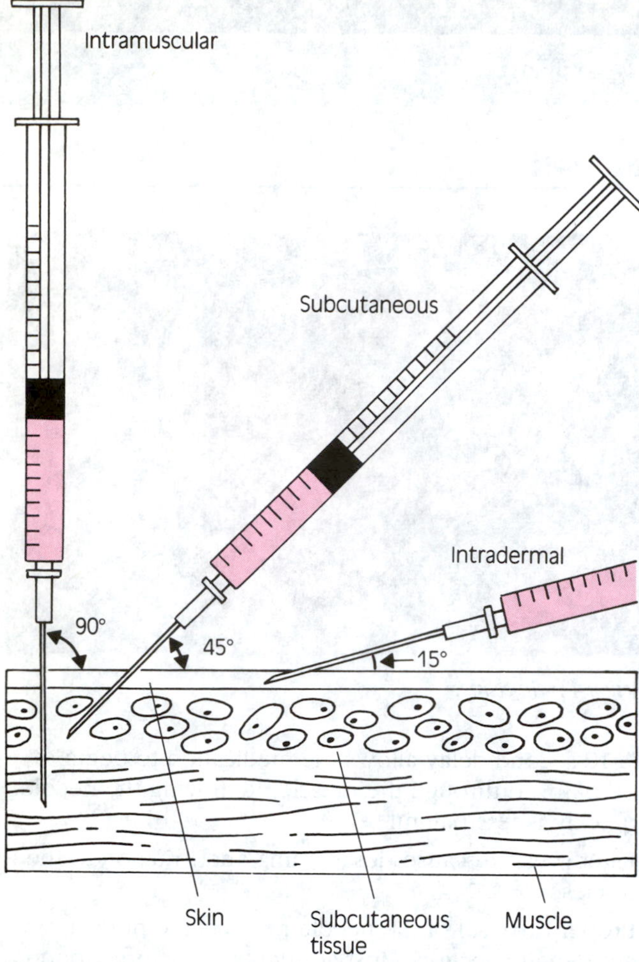

Figure 29-11
Comparison of the angles of insertion for intramuscular, subcutaneous, and intradermal injections.

gluteal, dorsogluteal, or vastus lateralis sites can be used for this procedure. The skin is pulled down or to one side, about 1 inch (2.5 cm), and held in this position with the left hand for a right-handed person. The needle is inserted and aspirated for at least 5 to 10 seconds for blood. The solution is injected slowly and the needle is allowed to remain in place for 10 seconds after injecting the medication. The needle is then withdrawn and the displaced tissue is released and allowed to return to its normal position.

Massage of the site is not recommended because it may cause irritation by forcing the medication to leak back into the needle track, but gentle pressure may be applied with a dry sponge. The procedure for administering a Z-track injection is outlined in Figure 29-12.

Reducing Discomfort in Subcutaneous and Intramuscular Administrations

The following are recommended techniques to help reduce discomfort when injecting medications subcutaneously or intramuscularly:

- Select a needle of the smallest gauge that is appropriate for the site and solution to be injected and select the correct needle length.
- Be sure the needle is free of medication that may irritate superficial tissues as the needle is inserted. Recommended procedure is to use two needles—one to remove the medication from the vial or ampule and a second one to inject the medication. If medication is in a prefilled syringe with a nonremovable needle and has dripped back on the needle during preparation, dry the needle with a sterile gauze.
- Use the Z-track technique for intramuscular injections to prevent leakage of medication into the needle track, thus minimizing the client's discomfort.

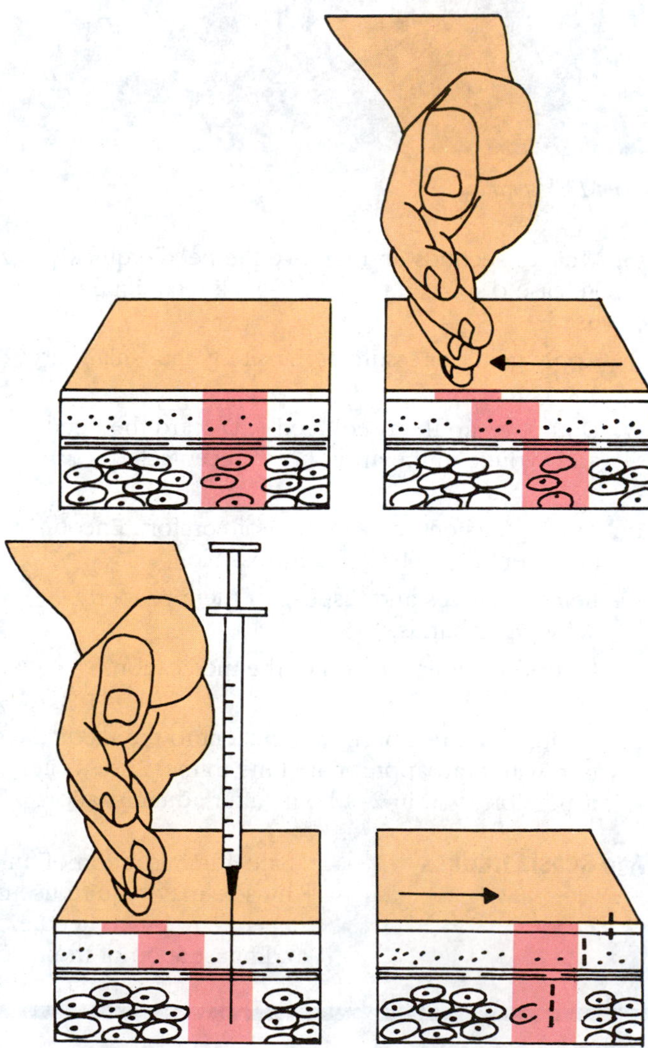

Figure 29-12
The Z-track or zigzag technique is used to administer medications that are irritating to subcutaneous tissue. The skin is pulled to one side. The needle is aspirated for blood by pulling back on the plunger, and the solution is injected. When the needle is withdrawn and the displaced tissue is allowed to return to its normal position, the solution is prevented from escaping from the muscle tissue.

- Inject the medication into relaxed musculature. There is more pressure and discomfort when the medication is injected into a contracted muscle.
- Do not inject areas that feel hard on palpation or tender to the client.
- Insert the needle with a dartlike motion without hesitation, and remove it quickly at the same angle at which it was inserted. These techniques help to reduce discomfort and tissue irritation.
- Do not administer more solution in one injection than is recommended for the site. Injecting more solution creates excess pressure in the area and increases discomfort.
- Inject the solution slowly so that it may be dispersed more easily into the surrounding tissue (10 seconds/1 mL).
- Apply gentle pressure after injection, unless this technique is contraindicated.
- Allow the client who is fearful of injections to talk about the fears. Answer the client's questions truthfully, and explain the nature and purpose of the injection. Taking the time to offer support often allays fears that ordinarily add to the discomfort of the procedure for the client.
- Rotate the sites when the client is to receive repeated injections. Injections in the same site may cause undue discomfort, irritation, or abscesses in tissues.

Administering Medications Intravenously

Medications administered intravenously have an immediate effect. The **intravenous route** is the most dangerous route of administration. Because the drug is placed directly into the bloodstream, it cannot be recalled nor can its actions be slowed. Intravenous administration would be the route chosen in an emergency situation when immediate absorption is required. There also are many clinical situations in which drugs are administered intravenously when an emergency does not exist. Patient-controlled analgesia allows the client to control administration of an intravenous analgesic for pain management and is discussed in Chapter 41. Procedure 46-1 describes the basic technique for administering an intravenous infusion.

There are several ways to administer medications intravenously. Medications may be added to the client's infusion solution. The recommended procedure is for the pharmacist to add the prescribed drug to a large volume of intravenous solution, but sometimes the drug is added in the nursing unit, in which case sterile technique must be maintained. Steps for adding medications to intravenous solutions are given in Procedure 29-8.

When medication is administered by *continuous infusion*, the client receives it slowly and over a long period. Although sometimes this can be an advantage when it is desirable to give the medication slowly, it is a disadvantage when it is necessary for the client to receive the drug more quickly. Also, if for some reason all of the solution cannot be infused, the client will not receive the prescribed amount of the medication. The client receiving medication by a continuous intravenous infusion should be checked for possible adverse effects at least every hour.

A medication can be administered as an intravenous *bolus* or push (IVP). This involves a single injection of a concentrated solution administered directly into an intravenous line (Procedure 29-9).

Medications can be administered by *intermittent intravenous infusion*. The drug is mixed with a small amount of the intravenous solution, such as 50 to 100 mL, and administered over a short period at the prescribed interval—for example, every 4 hours. As mentioned earlier, needleless devices effectively prevent needlesticks and provide access to the primary venous line. The client with an intravenous line in place receives the solution containing the medication by way of a piggyback setup or a tandem setup. The intravenous *piggyback* delivery system (Fig. 29-13) requires the intermittent or additive solution to be placed higher than the primary solution container. An extension hook provided by the manufacturer provides for easy lowering of the main intravenous container. The port on the primary intravenous line has a backcheck valve that automatically stops the flow of the primary solution, allowing the secondary or piggyback solution to flow when connected. A *tandem* delivery setup is similar, except that both solutions remain at the same height and there is no backcheck valve at the secondary port on the primary line. If the two solutions are incompatible, the primary infusion may be temporarily clamped and the nurse must flush the primary intravenous tubing below the secondary port with a sterile solution (usually 0.9% sodium chloride solution) before and after the tandem intravenous administration. Since manufacturer's designs vary, the nurse is advised to check the directions carefully for agency systems. The nurse is responsible for calculating and manually adjusting the flow rate of the intravenous intermittent infusion or regulating the infusion with an infusion pump or controller. The intravenous piggyback setup is explained in Procedure 29-10.

Medications also can be placed in a controlled-volume administration set (Soluset, Buretrol) for intermittent intravenous infusion. The medication is diluted with a small amount of solution and administered through the client's intravenous line (Procedure 29-11). This type of equipment is also used for infusing solutions into children and older clients when the volume of fluid infused must be carefully monitored.

The minisyringe pump for intermittent infusion allows medication mixed in a syringe to be connected to the primary line and delivered by mechanical pressure applied to the syringe plunger (see Fig. 29-14).

A *heparin lock*, or intermittent venous access device, is used for a client who requires intermittent intravenous medication but not a continuous intravenous infusion. This device consists of a needle or catheter connected to

(text continues on page 641)

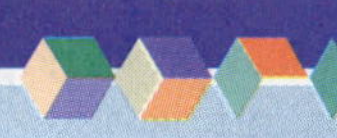

PROCEDURE 29-8

Adding Medications to an IV Solution Container

Equipment

Medication prepared in a syringe with a 19- to 21-gauge needle (or needleless device)
Alcohol swab
IV fluid container (bag or bottle)
Label to be attached to the IV container

Action	Rationale
1. Gather all equipment and bring to the client's bedside. Check the medication order with the physician's order.	Having equipment available saves time and facilitates performance of the task. Checking the orders ensures that the client receives the correct medication at the correct time and in the right manner.
2. Explain the procedure to the client.	Explanation allays the client's anxiety.
3. Wash your hands.	Handwashing deters the spread of microorganisms.
4. Identify the client by checking the band on the client's wrist and asking the client his or her name.	This ensures that medication is given to the right person.
5. Add the medication to the IV solution that is infusing:	
a. Check that the volume in the bag or bottle is adequate.	The volume should be sufficient to dilute the drug.
b. Close the IV clamp.	This prevents backflow directly to the client of improperly diluted medication.
c. Clean the medication port with an alcohol swab.	This deters entry of microorganisms when the needle punctures the port.
d. Steady the container, uncap the needle, and insert the needle into the port. Inject the medication.	This ensures that the needle enters the container and medication can be dispersed into the solution.
e. Remove the container from the IV pole and gently rotate the solution.	This mixes the medication with the solution.

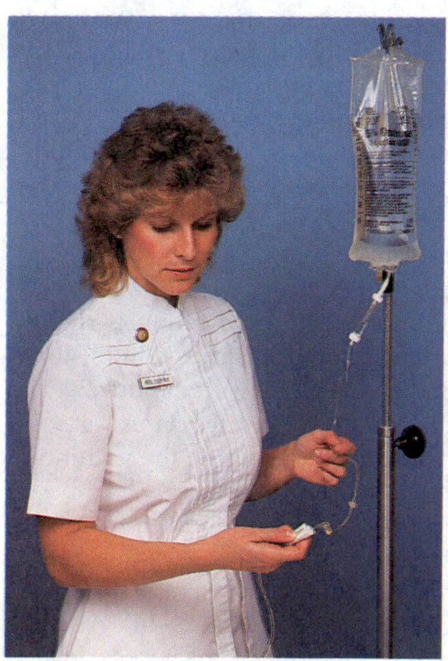

Action 5b: Closing the IV clamp.

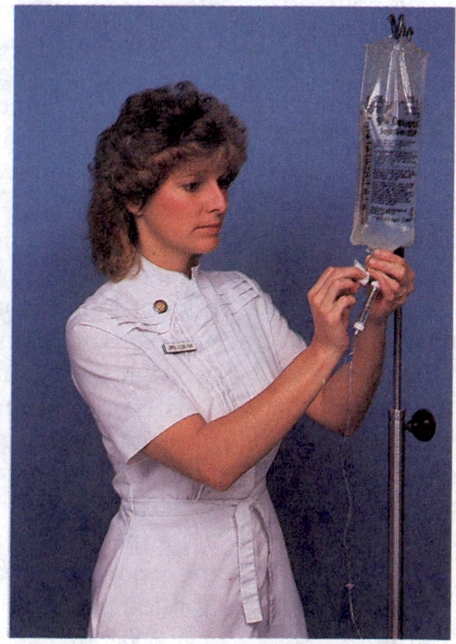

Action 5c: Cleaning the medication port.

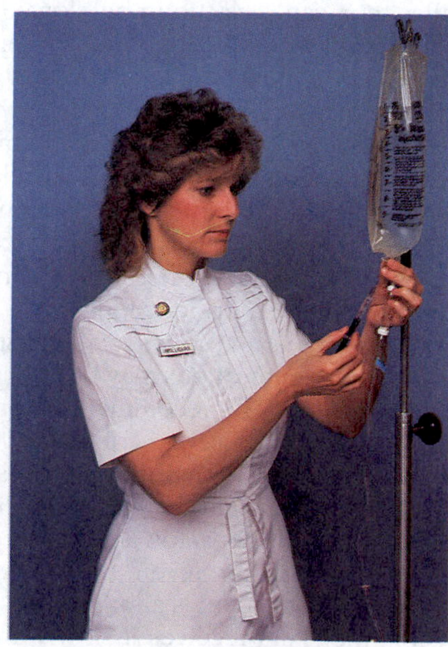

Action 5d: Inserting the needle into the port.

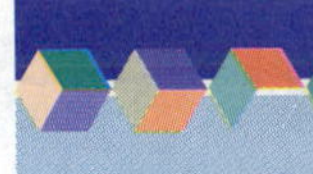

PROCEDURE 29-8 *(continued)*

Adding Medications to an IV Solution Container

Action	Rationale
f. Rehang the container, open the clamp, and readjust the flow rate.	This ensures the infusion of the IV with medication at the prescribed rate.
g. Attach the label to the container so that the dose of medication that has been added is apparent.	This confirms that the prescribed dose of medication has been added to the IV solution.

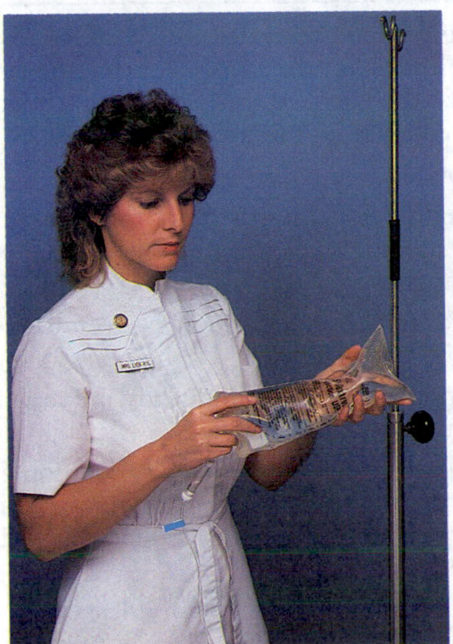

Action 5e: Rotating solution to distribute medication.

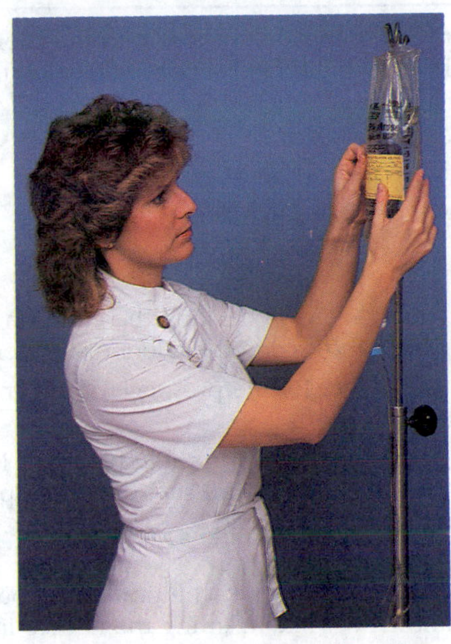

Action 5g: Labeling container to show medication. (Photos © Ken Kasper.)

Action	Rationale
6. Add the medication to the IV solution before infusion:	
a. Carefully remove any protective cover and locate the injection port. Clean with an alcohol swab.	This deters entry of microorganisms when the needle punctures the port.
b. Uncap the needle and insert into the port. Inject the medication.	This ensures that the needle enters the container and that medication can be dispersed into the solution.
c. Withdraw the needle and insert the spike into the proper entry site on the bag or bottle.	This punctures the seal in the IV bag or bottle.
d. With tubing clamped, gently rotate the IV solution in the bag or bottle. Hang the IV.	This mixes medication with the solution.
e. Attach the label to the container so that the dose of medication that has been added is apparent.	This confirms that the prescribed dose of medication has been added to the IV solution.
7. Dispose of equipment according to agency policy.	This prevents inadvertent injury from the equipment.
8. Wash your hands.	Handwashing deters the spread of microorganisms.
9. Chart the addition of medication to the IV solution.	Accurate documentation is necessary to prevent medication errors.
10. Evaluate the client's response to medication within the appropriate time frame.	Clients require careful observation because medications given by the IV route may have a rapid effect.

Special Consideration If a needleless device is used, the medication port (and IV setup) must be compatible and able to accept this system.

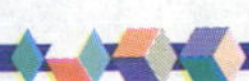

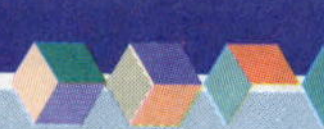

PROCEDURE 29-9

Adding a Bolus IV Medication to an Existing IV

Equipment

Medication prepared in a syringe with 23- to 25-gauge, 1-inch needle (or needleless device)
Alcohol swab
Watch with second hand
Disposable gloves

Action	Rationale
1. Gather the equipment and bring to the client's bedside. Check the medication order with the physician's order.	Having the equipment available saves time and facilitates performance of the task. Checking the orders ensures that the client receives the correct medication at the correct time and in the right manner.
2. Explain the procedure to the client.	Explanation allays the client's anxiety.
3. Wash your hands. Don clean gloves.	Handwashing deters the spread of microorganisms. Gloves protect the nurse from exposure to bloodborne pathogens.
4. Identify the client by checking the band on the client's wrist and asking the client his or her name.	This ensures that the medication is given to the right person.
5. Assess the IV site for the presence of inflammation or infiltration.	IV medication must be given directly into a vein for safe administration.
6. Select the injection port on the tubing that is closest to the venipuncture site. Clean the port with an alcohol swab.	Using the port closest to the needle insertion site minimizes dilution of the medication. Cleaning with alcohol deters entry of microorganisms when the needle punctures the port.
7. Uncap the syringe. Steady the port with your nondominant hand while inserting the needle into the center of the port.	This supports the injection port and lessens the risk of accidentally dislodging the IV or entering the port incorrectly.
8. Move your nondominant hand to the section of IV tubing just beyond the injection port. Fold the tubing between your fingers to temporarily stop the flow of the IV solution.	This minimizes the dilution of the IV medication with IV solution.
9. Pull back slightly on the plunger just until blood appears in the tubing.	This ensures injection of medication into a vein.

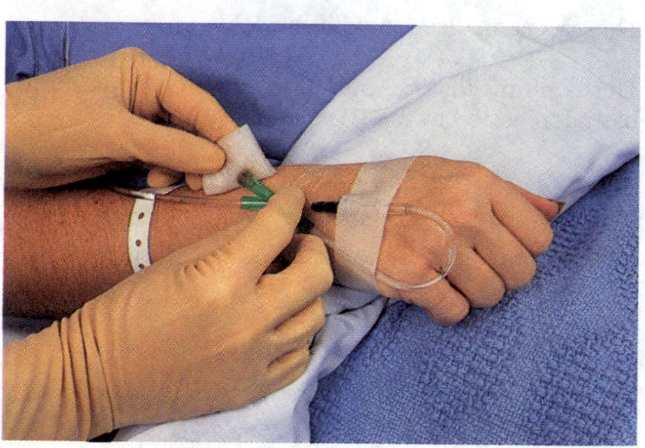

Action 6: Cleaning injection port.

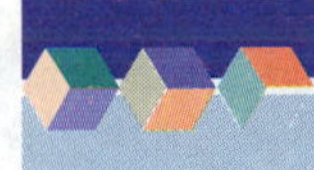

PROCEDURE 29-9 *(continued)*

Adding a Bolus IV Medication to an Existing IV

Action	Rationale
10. Inject the medication at the prescribed rate.	This delivers the correct amount of medication at the proper interval.

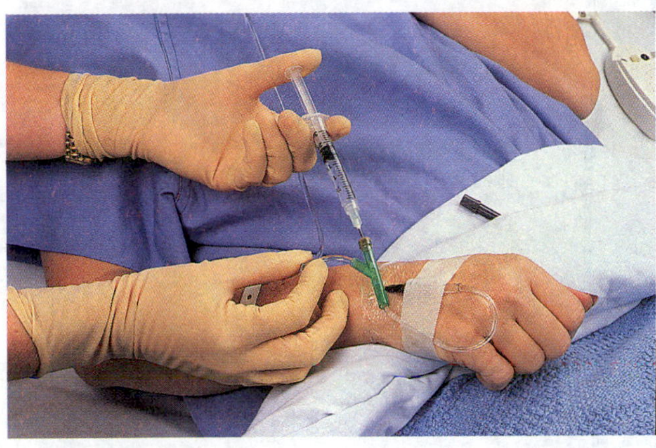

Action 10: Injecting medication while interrupting IV flow. (Photos © B. Proud.)

Action	Rationale
11. Remove the needle. Do not cap it. Release the tubing and allow the IV to flow at the proper rate.	This prevents accidental needlestick.
12. Dispose of the needle and syringe in the proper receptacle.	Proper disposal of the needle prevents accidental injury and spread of microorganisms.
13. Remove gloves and wash your hands.	Handwashing deters the spread of microorganisms.
14. Chart the administration of the medication.	Accurate documentation is necessary to prevent medication errors.
15. Evaluate the client's response to the medication within the appropriate time frame.	The client requires careful observation because medications given by an IV bolus injection may have a rapid effect.

Special Consideration If needleless device is used, the medication port (and IV setup) must be compatible and able to accept this system.

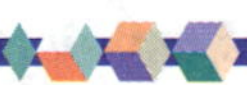

a short length of tubing capped with a sealed injection port. A heparin lock is shown in Procedure 29-12. After the needle is in place in the client's vein, the needle and tubing are anchored to the client's arm so that the needle remains in place until the client no longer requires the repeated medication intravenously.

A heparin lock allows the client more freedom than a continuous intravenous infusion. The client is connected to the intravenous line when it is time to receive the medication and disconnected when the medication is completed. A saline flush rather than a heparin flush is used by many institutions to maintain patency of the heparin lock. Using saline eliminates any possible systemic effects on coagulation or drug incompatibility that may occur when a heparin solution is used. The intermittent infusion is not started until the nurse confirms intravenous placement. The heparin lock is flushed after the infusion is completed to clear the vein of any medication and to prevent clot formation in the needle. The procedure for flushing an intravenous or heparin lock with saline is discussed in Procedure 29-12. The intravenous site is assessed for complications discussed in Chapter 46. If infiltration or phlebitis occurs, the heparin lock is removed and replaced in a new site.

Intermittent intravenous medication may be administered through a centrally placed line into the subclavian or internal jugular veins or via peripherally inserted central catheters (PICCS). These venous access devices are discussed in more detail in Chapter 46. Medications are prepared under laminar flow in a sterile environment if they are to be administered through a central intravenous line, such as a Hickman catheter. Aseptic tech-

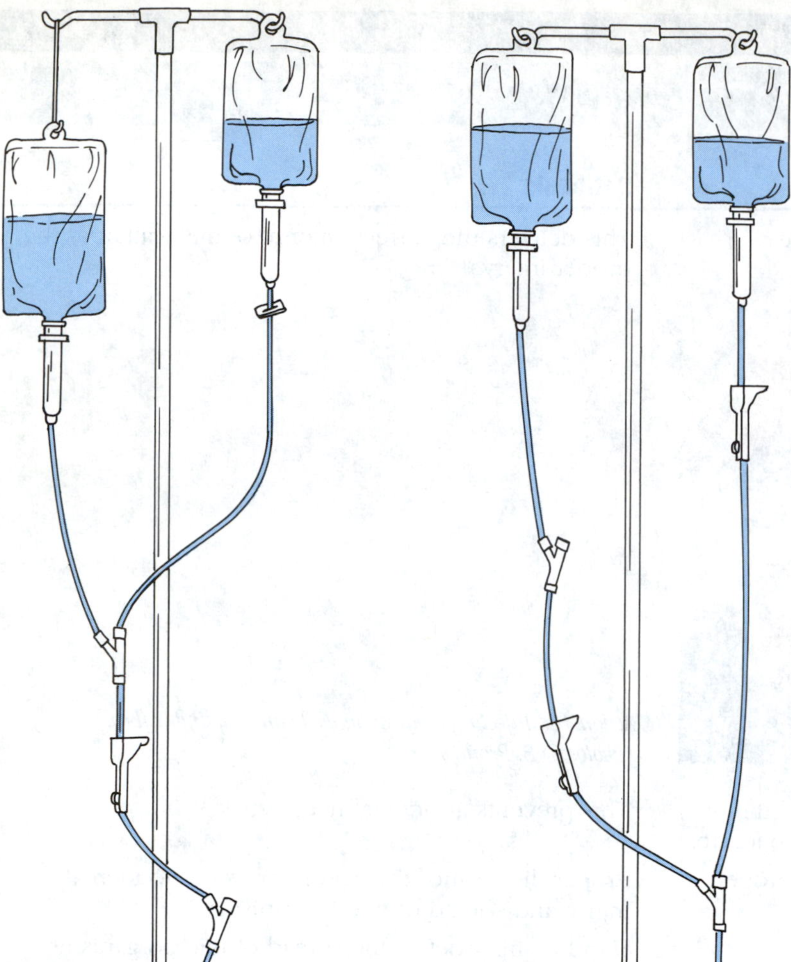

Figure 29-13
Piggyback and tandem setup for intermittent delivery of IV medications.

nique is observed when the nurse administers medications through a central intravenous line. All connections are cleaned with povidone–iodine or an antiseptic agent.

Administering Topical Medications

When a drug is applied directly to a body site, it is called a **topical application**. Other terms used include the *dermal* and *mucosal route.*

Topical applications usually are intended for direct action on a particular site, although some systemic effect may also occur. The action depends on the type of tissue and the nature of the agent.

If the site of application is readily accessible, such as the skin, an agent can easily be placed on it. If it is a cavity, such as the nose, or is enclosed, such as the eye, it is necessary to use a mechanical applicator for introducing the drug.

Skin Applications

The skin is a mechanical and chemical barrier that protects the underlying tissues. It is a sense organ, having receptors that respond to touch, pain, pressure, and temperature. The skin helps in excretion, in regulating body temperature, and in storing essentials to the body, such as water, salts, and glucose.

When a drug is incorporated in an agent, such as an ointment, and rubbed into the skin for absorption, the procedure is referred to as an *inunction.* On normal skin, drugs are absorbed into the lining of the sebaceous glands. Absorption is hindered because of the protective outer layer of the skin, which makes penetration difficult, and because of the fatty substances that protect the lining of the glands. Absorption can be enhanced by cleaning the skin well with soap or detergent and water before administration and then rubbing the medicated preparation into the skin. Absorption can also be improved by using a drug mixed in an ointment or added to a liniment that will mix with the fat in the gland lining. When indicated, local heat applied to the application area can improve blood circulation and promote absorption. The following are typical preparations applied to skin areas, their primary purposes, and specific nursing interventions:

(text continues on page 646)

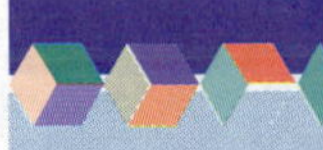

PROCEDURE 29-10

Administering Medications by IV Piggyback

Equipment

Medication preparation in labeled piggyback set (50 to 100 mL)
Secondary infusion tubing (microdrip or macrodrip)
Date label for tubing
Sterile needle (21 to 23 gauge) or needleless device
Alcohol swab
Tape
Metal or plastic hook (optional)
Infusion controller or IV pump (optional)

Action	Rationale
1. Gather all equipment and bring to the client's bedside. Check the medication order against the original physician's order according to agency policy.	Having equipment available saves time and facilitates performance of the task. Checking the orders ensures that the client receives the correct medication at the correct time and in the right manner.
2. Explain the procedure to the client.	Explanation allays the client's anxiety.
3. Wash your hands.	Handwashing deters the spread of microorganisms.
4. Assess the IV site for the presence of inflammation or infiltration.	IV medications must be given directly into a vein for safe administration.
5. Attach the infusion tubing to the piggyback set containing diluted medication. Open the clamp and prime the tubing (see action 5, Procedure 29-8). Close the clamp. Connect the capped sterile needle to the sterile end of the tubing. Place label on tubing with appropriate date.	This removes air from the tubing and preserves the sterility of the setup. Tubing for piggyback setup may be used for 48 to 72 hours depending on agency policy.

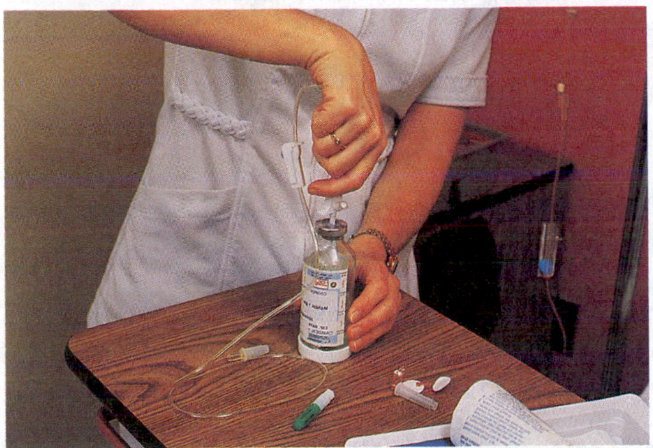

Action 5: Attaching infusion tubing to piggyback set containing medication.

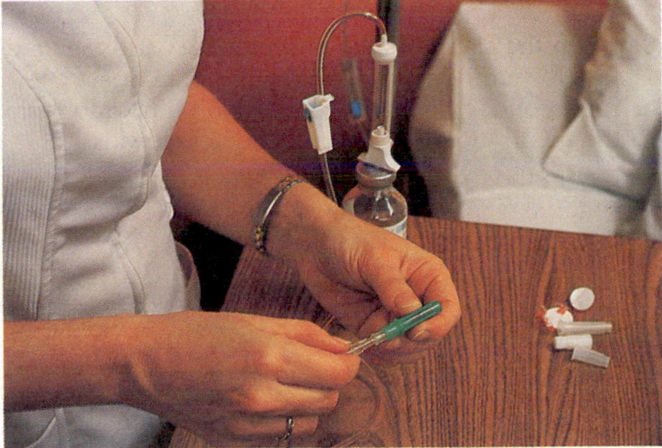

Action 5: Connecting capped sterile needle to tubing.

Action	Rationale
6. Hang the piggyback container on the IV pole, positioning it higher than the primary IV according to the manufacturer's recommendations. Use metal or plastic hook to lower primary IV.	The position of the container influences the flow of the IV fluid into the primary setup.
7. Identify the client by checking the identification band on the client's wrist and asking the client his or her name.	This ensures that the medication is given to the right person.
8. Use an alcohol swab to clean the secondary IV port closest to the top of the primary tubing.	This deters entry of microorganisms when the needle punctures the port.

(continued)

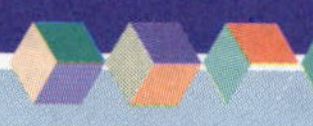

PROCEDURE 29-10 *(continued)*

Administering Medications by IV Piggyback

Action	Rationale
9. Remove the cap and insert the needle into the secondary port. Use a strip of tape to secure the secondary set tubing to the primary infusion tubing. Primary line is left unclamped if port has a back-flow valve.	The tape stabilizes the needle in the infusion port and prevents it from slipping out. Backflow valve in primary line secondary port stops flow of primary infusion while piggyback solution is infusing. Once completed, the backflow valve opens and flow of primary solution resumes.

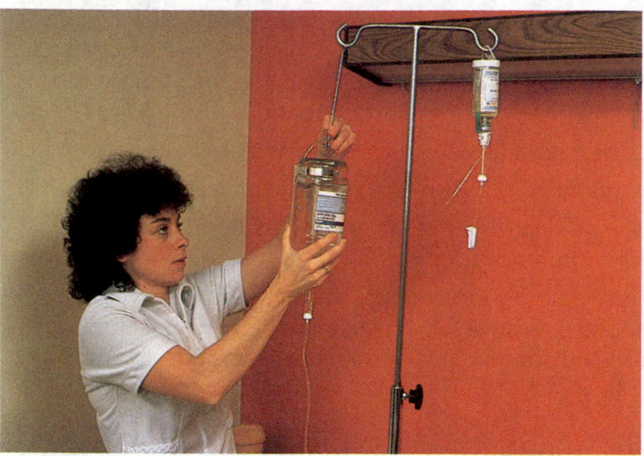

Action 6: Hanging on IV pole.

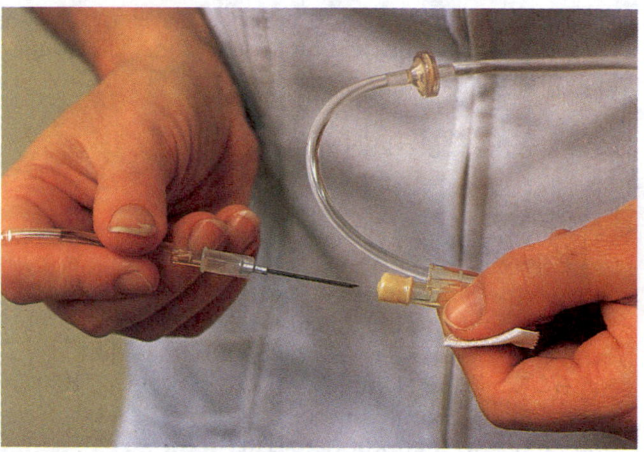

Action 9: Inserting needle into secondary port.

Action	Rationale
10. Open the clamp on the piggyback set and regulate the flow at the prescribed delivery rate or set rate for secondary infusion on infusion pump. Monitor the medication infusion at periodic intervals.	Delivery over a 30- to 60-minute interval is a safe method of administering IV medication.
11. Clamp the tubing on the piggyback set when the solution is infused. Follow agency policy regarding disposal of equipment.	This reduces the risk of contaminating the primary IV setup.
12. Readjust the flow rate of the primary IV.	Piggyback medication administration may interrupt the normal flow rate of the primary IV. Readjustment of the rate may be necessary.
13. Wash your hands.	Handwashing deters the spread of microorganisms.
14. Chart the administration of medication after it has been infused.	Accurate documentation is necessary to prevent medication errors.
15. Evaluate the client's response to medication within the appropriate time frame.	The client requires careful observation because medications given by the IV route may have a rapid effect.

Special Considerations

If needleless device is used, the medication port (and IV setup) must be compatible and able to accept this system.

Alternate method to prime IV line of "continued" piggyback set is to lower the piggyback bag below the main bag, open the clamp, and allow the primary solution to move up the tubing and into the secondary set drip chamber. This requires that piggyback set be connected to primary line below the backflow valve. If medication in secondary set is incompatible with primary solution, flush the primary line with saline solution before attaching the secondary set.

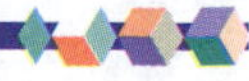

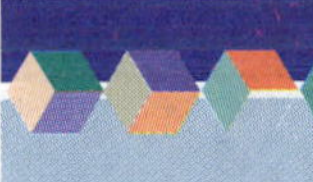

PROCEDURE 29-11

Administering IV Medications by Volume-Control Administration Set

Equipment

Volume-control administration set (50 to 100 mL)
Medication (in vial or ampule)
Syringe with 20- or 21-gauge needle or needleless device attached
Alcohol swab
Medication label

Action	Rationale
1. Gather all equipment and bring to the client's bedside. Check the medication order against the original physician's order according to agency policy.	Having equipment available saves time and facilitates performance of the task. Checking of the orders ensures that the client receives the correct medication at the correct time and in the right manner.
2. Explain the procedure to the client.	Explanation allays the client's anxiety.
3. Wash your hands.	Handwashing deters the spread of microorganisms.
4. Assess the IV site for the presence of inflammation or infiltration.	IV medications must be given directly into a vein for safe administration.
5. Withdraw medication from the vial or ampule into the prepared syringe. See Procedure 29-2 or 29-3.	The correct dose is prepared for dilution in the IV solution.
6. Identify the client by checking the identification band on the client's wrist and asking the client his or her name.	This ensures that medication is given to the right person.
7. Open the clamp between the IV solution and the volume-control administration set or secondary setup. Follow the manufacturer's instructions and fill with the desired amount of IV solution. Close the clamp.	This dilutes the medication in the minimal amount of solution. Reclamping prevents the continued addition of fluid to the volume to be mixed with the medication.
8. Use an alcohol swab to clean the injection port on the secondary setup.	This deters entry of microorganisms when the needle punctures the port.
9. Remove the cap and insert the needle into the port while holding the syringe steady. Inject the medication. Mix gently with IV solution.	This ensures that the medication is evenly mixed with solution.

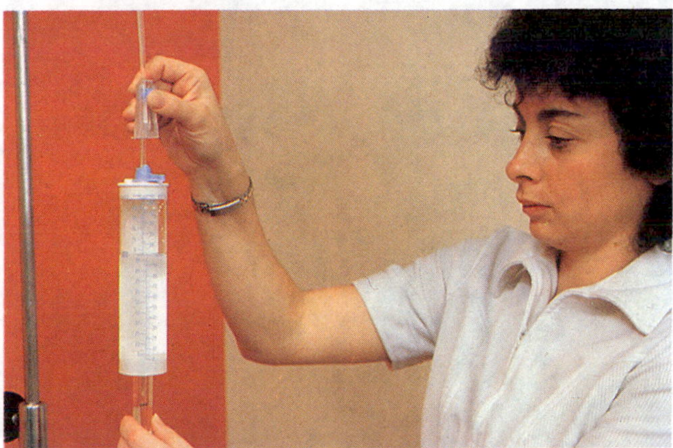

Action 7: Filling volume-control set.

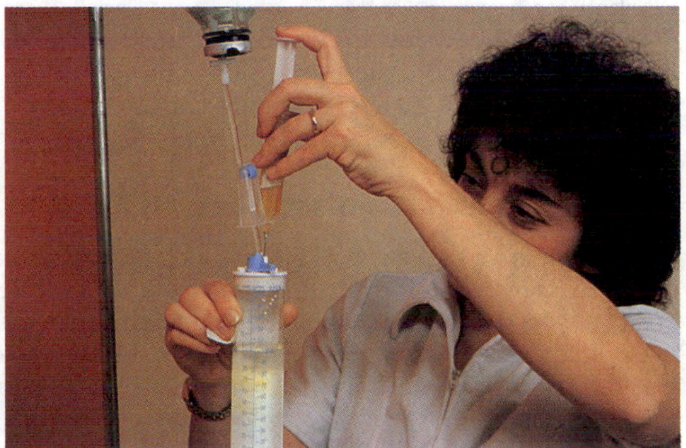

Action 9: Injecting medication.

(continued)

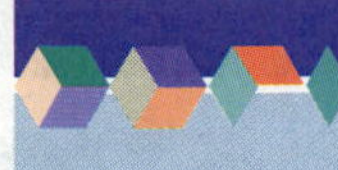

PROCEDURE 29-11 *(continued)*

Administering IV Medications by Volume-Control Administration Set

Action	Rationale
10. Open the clamp below the secondary setup and regulate at the prescribed delivery rate. Monitor the medication infusion at periodic intervals.	Delivery over a 30- to 60-minute interval is a safe method of administering IV medication.
11. Attach the label to the volume-control device.	This prevents medication error.
12. Place the syringe with the uncapped needle in the designated container.	Proper disposal of the needle prevents inadvertent needlestick.
13. Wash your hands.	Handwashing deters the spread of microorganisms.
14. Chart the administration of the medication after it has been infused.	Accurate documentation is necessary to prevent medication errors.
15. Evaluate the client's response to the medication within the appropriate time frame.	The client requires careful observation because medications given by the IV route may have a rapid effect.

Special Consideration If needleless device is used, the medication port on the volume-control administration set must be compatible with this system.

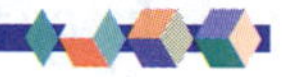

Powders are used to promote drying of the skin and prevent friction on the skin. Use caution when applying to prevent inhalation of the medicated powder.

Ointments provide prolonged contact of a medication on the skin and soften the skin. They are usually thoroughly massaged into intact skin.

Creams and oils lubricate and soften the skin and prevent drying of the skin. The preparation should be warmed in the hands or fingers if a large part of the body is to be covered, to prevent chilling.

Lotions protect and soothe the skin. Shake lotions thoroughly before using and apply with cotton balls or gauze.

The transdermal route is being used more frequently to deliver medication. Despite a slow onset of action, transdermal drug patches maintain consistent serum drug levels (see the accompanying box).

Eye Instillations and Irrigations

The receptors for the sense of sight are located in the eye. The outer layer of the eyeball is called the *sclera.* The cornea is the transparent part of the sclera in front of the eyeball. The sclera is fibrous and tough, but the cornea is easily injured by trauma. For this reason, applications to the eye seldom are placed directly onto the eyeball.

Because direct application cannot be made onto the sensitive cornea, applications intended to act on the eye or the lids are placed onto, or instilled or irrigated into, the lower conjunctival sac.

The eye is a delicate organ, highly susceptible to infection and injury. Although the eye is never free of microorganisms, the secretions of the conjunctiva have a protective action against many pathogens. For maximum safety for the client, equipment, solutions, and ointments introduced into the conjunctival sac should be sterile. If this is not possible, the most careful measures of medical asepsis should be followed.

Eyedrops. Instillation of eyedrops is performed for their local effects, such as for pupil dilatation or constriction when examining the eye or for treating an infection. The type and amount of solution depend on the purpose of the instillation. See the accompanying box

(text continues on page 650)

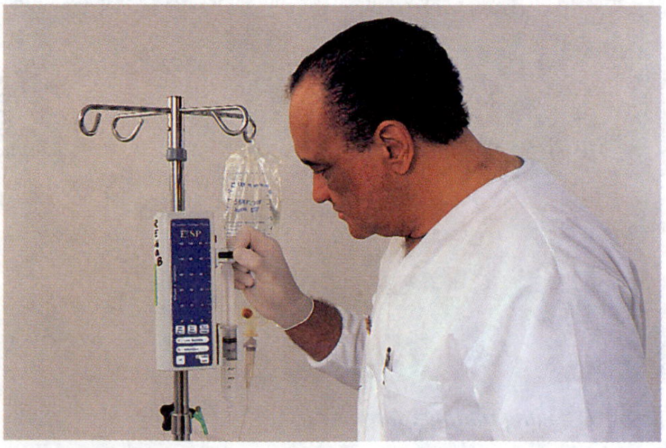

Figure 29-14
The nurse prepares the mini-pump to deliver IV antibiotics. (Photo © B. Proud.)

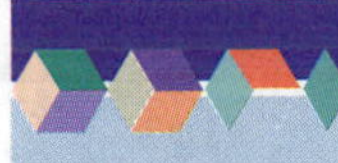

PROCEDURE 29-12

Introducing Drugs Through a Heparin or Intravenous Lock Using the Saline Flush

Equipment

Medication
Medication card, Kardex, or computer-generated MAR
Saline vial
Sterile syringe with 25-gauge needle or needleless device
Alcohol swabs
Watch with second hand or digital readout
Disposable gloves
For bolus injection
Sterile syringe with medication and 25-gauge needle or needleless device
For intermittent IV delivery
IV setup with 25-gauge needle or needleless device attached to tubing
Additional sterile 25-gauge needle or needleless device
Adhesive tape
IV pump or infusion controller (optional)

Action	Rationale
1. Assemble the equipment and check the physician's order.	This ensures that the client receives the right medication at the right time by the proper route.
2. Explain the procedure to the client.	Explanation alleviates the client's apprehension about IV drug administration.
3. Wash your hands.	Handwashing deters the spread of microorganisms.
4. Withdraw 1 to 2 mL of sterile saline from the vial into the syringe as described in Procedure 29-3.	Using saline eliminates concern about drug incompatibilities and effect on systemic circulation that exists with heparin flush.
5. Don the clean gloves.	Gloves protect the nurse's hands from contact with the client's blood.
6. Administer the medication. *For bolus IV injection:*	
a. Check the drug package for the correct injection rate for the IV push route.	Using the correct injection rate prevents speed shock from occurring.
b. Clean the port of the lock with an alcohol swab.	Cleaning removes surface bacteria at the heparin lock entry site.
c. Stabilize the port with your nondominant hand and insert the needle on the syringe into the port.	This allows for careful insertion of the needle into the center circle of the lock.

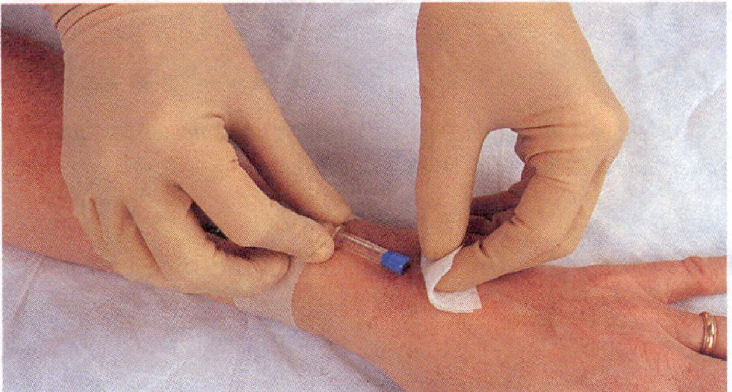

Action 6b: Cleaning the port (bolus injection).

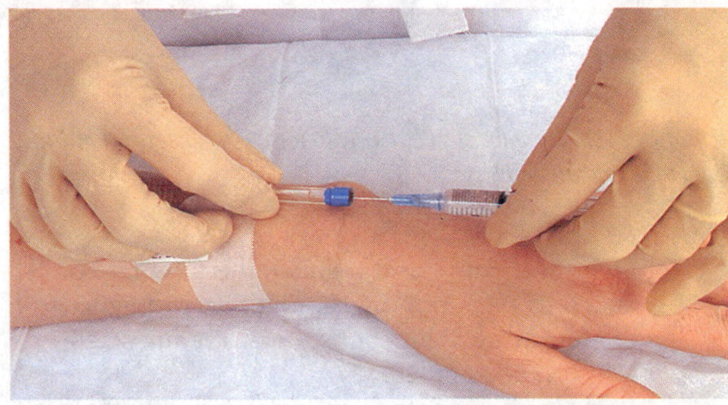

Action 6c: Stabilizing the port while inserting the needle (bolus injection).

(continued)

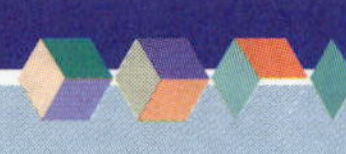

PROCEDURE 29-12 *(continued)*

Introducing Drugs Through a Heparin or Intravenous Lock Using the Saline Flush

Action	Rationale
d. Gently inject the medication, using a watch to verify correct injection rate. Do not force the injection if resistance is felt. If the lock is clogged, it has to be changed. Remove the medication syringe and needle when administration is completed.	Easy instillation of the medication usually indicates that the lock is still patent and in the vein.
For administration of a drug by way of an intermittent delivery system:	
a. Use a drug resource book to check for the correct flow rate of the medication. (The usual rate is 30 to 60 minutes.)	Using the correct injection rate prevents speed shock from occurring.
b. Connect the infusion tubing to the medication setup according to the manufacturer's directions. Hang the IV setup on a pole. Open clamp and allow solution to clear IV tubing of air. Reclamp tubing.	This removes air from the tubing and preserves the sterility of the setup.
c. Attach sterile 25-gauge needle to the end of the infusion tubing.	A small-gauge needle prevents damage to the lock.
d. Clean the port of the lock with an alcohol swab. Stabilize the port with your nondominant hand and insert the needle on the tubing into the port. Secure with tape.	Cleaning removes surface bacteria at the lock entry site. Tape secures the needle in the lock port.

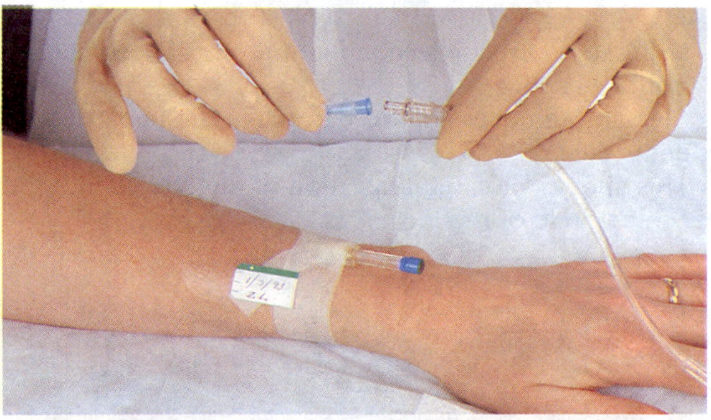

Action 6c: Attaching the sterile needle to the end of the infusion tubing (intermittent delivery).

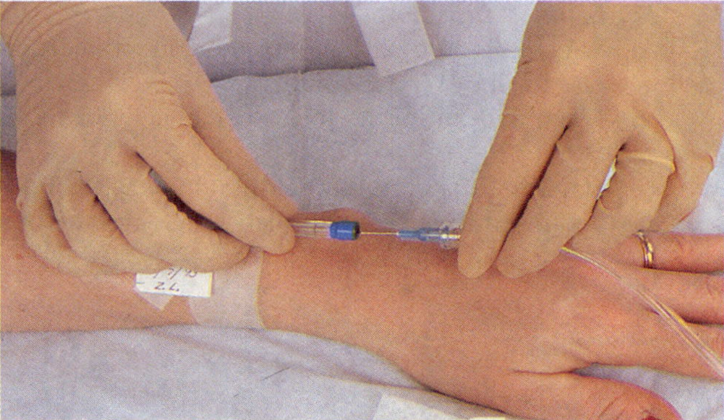

Action 6d: Stabilizing the port while inserting the needle into the port (intermittent delivery). (Photos © B. Proud.)

Action	Rationale
e. Open the clamp and regulate the flow rate or attach to IV pump or controller according to manufacturer's directions. Close clamp when infusion is complete.	This ensures that the client receives the medication at the correct rate.
f. Remove the needle from lock. Carefully replace the uncapped used needle on the tubing with a sterile covered needle. Allow the medication setup to hang on the pole for future use according to agency policy.	This prevents possible needlestick with contaminated needle. Agency policy specifies length of time for safe use of IV infusion tubing.
g. Dispose of uncapped used needle appropriately.	This prevents possible needlestick injury.

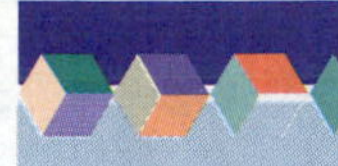

PROCEDURE 29-12 *(continued)*

Introducing Drugs Through a Heparin or Intravenous Lock Using the Saline Flush

Action	Rationale
7. Insert the needle of the syringe containing saline and flush the reservoir with 1 to 2 mL of sterile saline. Remove the syringe and needle and discard in the appropriate receptacle. Remove gloves and discard appropriately.	Saline clears the line of medication with less of the systemic effects of the heparin flush.
8. Wash your hands.	Handwashing deters the spread of microorganisms.
9. The injection site and IV lock should be checked at least every 8 hours and a small amount of saline administered if medication is not given at least that often.	This ensures the patency of the system for continuing injections.
10. The heparin lock should be changed at least every 48 hours or according to agency policy. A clogged lock should be changed immediately.	Changing a heparin lock regularly and having it free of clotted blood reduces dangers of infection and emboli in the circulating blood.
11. Chart the administration of the medication or saline flush.	Accurate documentation is necessary to prevent medication error.

Safety Considerations Some agencies recommend the use of single-dose saline vials without preservatives in the solution. Preservatives may be linked to an increased incidence of phlebitis with heparin locks.

Special Consideration If needleless device is used, the heparin or intravenous lock setup must be compatible with this system.

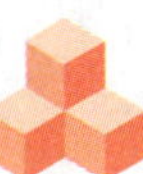

Guidelines for Nursing Care

Managing Transdermal Patches

- Wear gloves when applying or removing patches. Handwashing is also a necessity.
- Monitor the client's response carefully. Be alert for adverse effects specific to the medication applied.
- Apply the patch at the same time of the day and write the date and time on the patch. Document application on the MAR.
- Rotate application sites.
- Remove the old patch before applying the new one.
- Check for dislodgement of the patch if the client is active. Read information about the patch or consult with the pharmacist to determine reapplication schedule and procedure.
- Follow directions and use the patch as prescribed.
- Aluminum backing on a patch necessitates precautions if defibrillation is required. Burns and smoke may result.
- Assess for any skin irritation. If necessary, remove the patch, wash the area carefully with soap and water, and allow skin to air dry.
- Dispose of old patches carefully. Keep out of the reach of children and away from pets.

(Buttaro, M. [1994]. Staying on top of transdermal drug patches. *Nursing, 24*[11], 41–44.)

for a description of techniques to expose the lower conjunctival sac and instill eyedrops.

Ointments. Various types of medication in an ointment form may be prescribed for the eye. These ointments usually are used in the presence of a local infection or irritation. Eye ointments are dispensed in a tube. A small amount of ointment is distributed along the exposed lower conjunctival sac after the eyelids and eyelashes have been cleansed. About ½ inch of ointment is squeezed from the tube along the exposed sac. After the application, the eyes should be closed. The warmth helps to liquefy the ointment. Also, the client should be instructed to move the eye because this helps to spread ointment under the lids and over the surface of the eyeball.

Eye Irrigation. An eye *irrigation* is performed to remove secretions from the eye. In an emergency, eye irrigation can be used to remove chemicals that may burn the eye. Copious amounts of tap water should be used to remove chemicals such as acid. The irrigation should continue for at least 15 minutes, and then professional help should be sought.

The techniques for administering a conjunctival irrigation are described in Procedure 29-13.

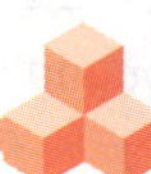

Guidelines for Nursing Care

Instilling Eyedrops

- Offer the client paper tissues to remove solution and tears that may spill from the eye during the procedure.
- Wash hands before putting on gloves.
- Clean the eyelids and eyelashes of any drainage with cotton balls or gauze pledgets moistened with normal saline solution because debris can be carried into the eye when the conjunctival sac is exposed. Use each cotton ball for only one stroke, moving from the inner toward the outer canthus to prevent carrying debris to the lacrimal ducts.
- Tilt the client's head back slightly if sitting, or place the client's head over a pillow if lying down. The head may be turned slightly to the affected side to prevent solution or tears from flowing toward the opposite eye.
- Invert the monodrip plastic container that is commonly used to instill eyedrops.
- Have the client look up while focusing on something on the ceiling.
- Place the thumb or two fingers near the margin of the lower eyelid immediately below the eyelashes, and exert pressure downward over the bony prominence of the cheek. The lower conjunctival sac is exposed as the lower lid is pulled down.
- Hold the dropper close to the eye, but avoid touching the eyelids or lashes, which may startle the client and cause blinking. Also, avoid touching the eyeball with the dropper because this could easily injure the eye.
- Squeeze the container and allow the prescribed number of drops to fall in the lower conjunctival sac. Do not allow drops to fall onto the cornea because of the danger of injuring it and the unpleasant sensation it causes the client.
- Release the lower lid after the eyedrops are instilled. Ask the client to gently close the eyes.
- Apply gentle pressure over the inner canthus to prevent the eyedrops from flowing into the tear duct. This minimizes the risk of systemic effects from the medication.

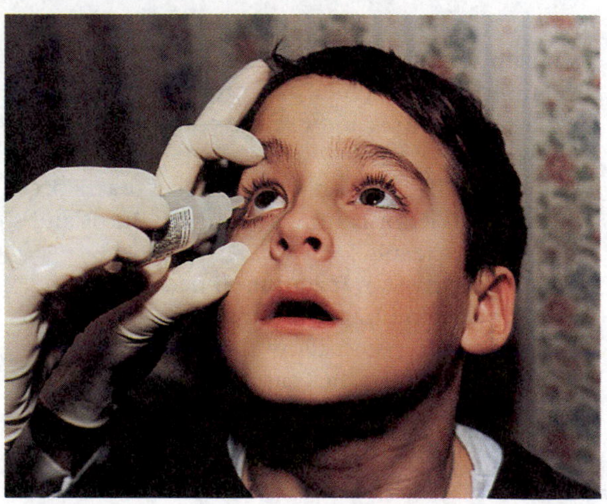

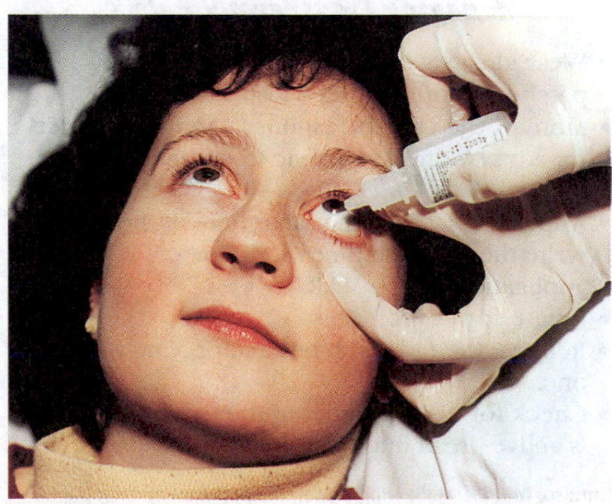

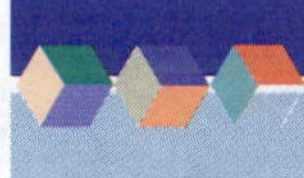

PROCEDURE 29-13

Administering an Eye Irrigation

Equipment

Sterile irrigating solution (warmed to 37°C [98.6°F])
Sterile irrigation set (sterile container and irrigating or bulb syringe)
Cotton balls
Emesis basin or irrigation basin
Disposable gloves
Waterproof pad
Towel

Action	Rationale
1. Explain procedure to client.	Explanation facilitates cooperation and reassures the client.
2. Assemble equipment.	This provides for an organized approach to the task.
3. Wash your hands.	Handwashing deters the spread of microorganisms.
4. Have the client sit or lie with the head tilted toward the side of the affected eye. Protect the client and the bed with a waterproof pad.	Gravity aids the flow of solution away from the unaffected eye and from the inner canthus of the affected eye toward the outer canthus.
5. Don disposable gloves. Clean the lids and the lashes with a cotton ball moistened with normal saline or the solution ordered for the irrigation. Wipe from the inner to the outer canthus. Discard the cotton ball after each wipe.	Materials lodged on the lids or in the lashes may be washed into the eye. This cleaning motion protects the nasolacrimal duct and the other eye.
6. Place the curved basin at the cheek on the side of the affected eye to receive the irrigating solution. If the client is sitting up, ask him or her to support the basin.	Gravity aids the flow of solution.
7. Expose the lower conjunctival sac and hold the upper lid open with your nondominant hand.	The solution is directed onto the lower conjunctival sac because the cornea is sensitive and easily injured. This also prevents reflex blinking.

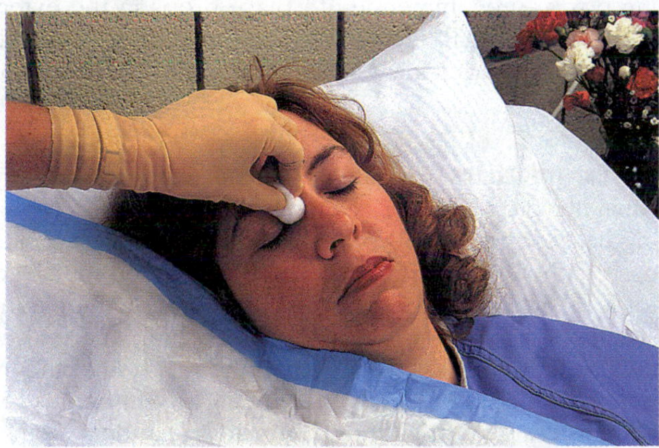

Action 5: Cleaning lids and lashes from inside of eye to outside.

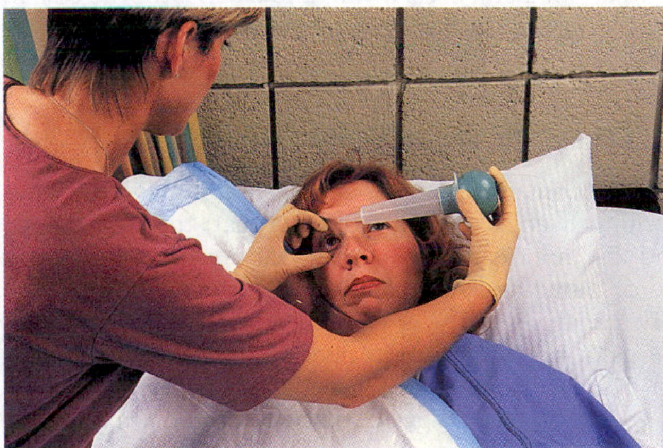

Action 7: Preparing to irrigate the eye. (Photos © B. Proud.)

(continued)

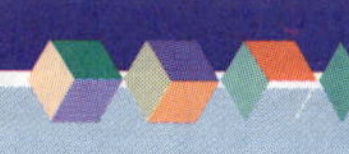

PROCEDURE 29-13 *(continued)*

Administering an Eye Irrigation

Action	Rationale
8. Hold the irrigator about 2.5 cm (1 inch) from the eye. Direct the flow of the solution from the inner to the outer canthus along the conjunctival sac.	This minimizes the risk of injury to the cornea. Solution directed toward the outer canthus helps to prevent the spread of contamination from the eye to the lacrimal sac, the lacrimal duct, and the nose.
9. Irrigate until the solution is clear or all of the solution has been used. Use only sufficient force gently to remove secretions from the conjunctiva. Avoid touching any part of the eye with the irrigating tip.	Directing solutions with force may cause injury to the tissues of the eye, as well as to the conjunctiva. Touching the eye is uncomfortable for the client.
10. Have the client close the eye periodically during the procedure.	Movement of the eye when the lids are closed helps to move secretions from the upper to the lower conjunctival sac.
11. Dry the area after the irrigation with cotton balls or a gauze sponge. Offer a towel to the client if the face and neck are wet.	Leaving the skin moist after an irrigation is uncomfortable for the client.
12. Remove gloves and wash your hands.	Handwashing deters the spread of microorganisms.
13. Chart the irrigation, appearance of the eye, drainage, and the client's response.	This provides accurate documentation.

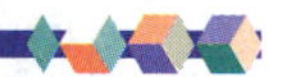

Eye Medication Discs. An eye medication disc is flexible, resembles a contact lens, and contains medication that is gradually released into the conjunctival sac. It can remain in place for up to a week before being removed and discarded. When properly placed, the disc is completely covered by the lower eyelid, allowing the client to wear contact lenses, swim, and sleep with the disc in place. Gloves should be worn when applying and removing the disc.

Ear Instillations and Irrigations

The ear contains the receptors for hearing and for equilibrium. It consists of the external ear, the middle ear, and the inner ear. The external ear consists of the auricle or pinna and the exterior auditory canal. The auditory canal serves as a passageway for sound waves. Drugs or irrigations are instilled into the auditory canal.

Drugs in solution are placed in the auditory canal for their local effect. They are used to soften wax, relieve pain, apply local anesthesia, destroy organisms, or destroy an insect lodged in the canal, which can cause almost intolerable discomfort.

The tympanic membrane separates the external ear from the middle ear. Normally, it is intact and closes the entrance to the middle ear completely. If it is ruptured or has been opened by surgical intervention, the middle ear and the inner ear have a direct passage to the external ear. When this occurs, instillations and irrigations should be performed with the greatest of care to prevent forcing materials from the outer ear into the middle ear and the inner ear. Sterile technique is used to prevent infection.

Ear Drops. The techniques listed in the accompanying box are recommended to place drops in the external auditory canal. Photos show a nurse about to instill drops into an adult's ear and instillation of ear drops for a child.

Ear Irrigations. Irrigations of the external auditory canal are ordinarily for cleaning purposes or for applying heat to the area. Typically, normal saline solution is used, although an antiseptic solution may be indicated for local action. An irrigation syringe is used in most instances. An irrigating container with tubing and an ear tip also may be used, especially if the purpose of the irrigation is to apply heat to the area. The techniques for administering an irrigation of the external auditory canal are described in Procedure 29-14.

Nasal Instillations

Besides serving as the olfactory organ, the nose functions as an airway to the lower respiratory tract and protects the tract by cleaning and warming the air taken in by inspiration. Cilia project on most of the surfaces of the nasal mucous membrane and are important in help-

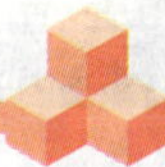

Guidelines for Nursing Care

Instilling Ear Drops

- Warm the solution to be instilled to body temperature to minimize discomfort for the client.
- Clean the external ear of drainage with cotton balls moistened with normal saline solution, as necessary. (Disposable gloves should be worn if drainage is present.)
- Place the client on the unaffected side in bed, or if ambulatory, have the client sit with the head well tilted to the side so that the affected ear is uppermost. This positioning prevents the drops from escaping from the ear.
- Draw up the amount of solution needed in the dropper. Excess medication should not be returned to a stock bottle. A monodrip plastic container may also be used.
- Straighten the auditory canal by pulling the cartilaginous portion of the pinna up and back in an adult and down and back in an infant or a child under age 3 years, and straight back for a school-age child. Pulling on the pinna as described helps to straighten the canal properly for ear instillation.
- Hold the dropper in the ear with its tip above the auditory canal. For an infant or an irrational or restless client, protect the dropper with a piece of soft tubing to help prevent injury to the ear.
- Allow the drops to fall on the side of the canal. It is uncomfortable for the client if drops fall directly onto the tympanic membrane.
- Release the pinna after instilling the drops, and have the client maintain the position to prevent the escape of the medication.
- Gently press on the tragus a few times to help move the medication from the canal toward the tympanic membrane.
- If ordered, loosely insert a cotton ball to prevent medication from leaking out.
- Wait 5 minutes before instilling drops in the second ear, if ordered.

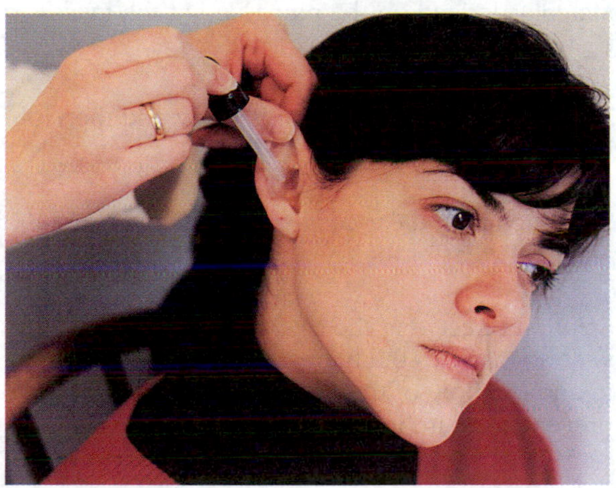

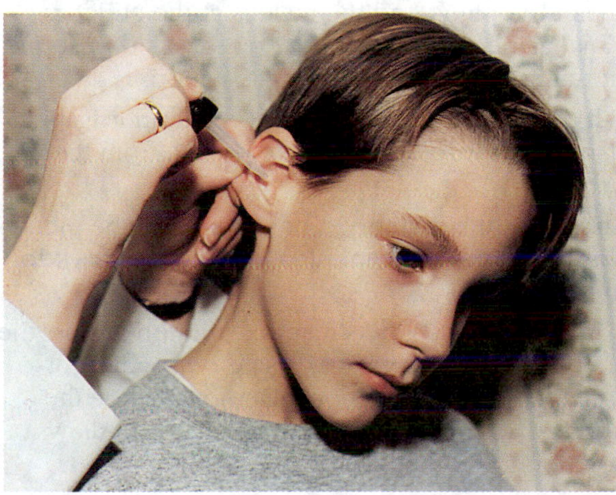

ing to remove particles of dirt and dust from the inspired air. The nose also serves as a resonator when speaking and singing.

Nasal instillations are used to treat sinus infections and nasal congestion. Medications that have a systemic effect, such as vasopressin, may also be prepared as a nasal instillation. The nose normally is not a sterile cavity, but because of its connection with the sinuses, medical asepsis should be carefully observed when using nasal instillations. See the accompanying box for recommended techniques to instill nose drops.

Solutions that are instilled by drops may also be applied to the nasal mucous membrane by using a spray. A small atomizer is used. The end of the nose is held up, and the tip of the nozzle is placed just inside the nares and directed backward. Only sufficient force to bring the spray into contact with the membrane is used. Too much force may drive the solution and contamination into the sinuses and eustachian tubes.

Vaginal Applications

A healthy vagina contains few pathogens but many nonpathogenic organisms. The nonpathogens are important because they protect the vagina from the invasion of pathogens. The normal secretions in the vagina are acidic and further serve to protect the vagina from microbial invasion. Therefore, the normal mucous membrane is its own best protection.

Creams can be applied intravaginally, using a narrow, tubular applicator with an attached plunger. Suppositories that melt when exposed to body heat are also

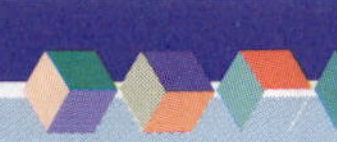

PROCEDURE 29-14

Administering an Ear Irrigation

Equipment

Prescribed irrigating solution (warmed to 37°C [98.6°F])
Irrigation set (container and irrigating or bulb syringe)
Emesis basin
Cotton-tipped applicators
Disposable gloves (optional)
Cotton balls
Waterproof pad

Action	Rationale
1. Explain the procedure to the client.	Explanation facilitates cooperation and provides reassurance for the client.
2. Assemble the equipment. Protect the client and bed linens with a moisture-proof pad.	This provides for an organized approach to the task.
3. Wash your hands.	Handwashing deters the spread of microorganisms.
4. Have the client sit up or lie with the head tilted toward the side of the affected ear. Have the client support a basin under the ear to receive the irrigating solution.	Gravity causes the irrigating solution to flow from the ear to the basin.
5. Clean the pinna and the meatus at the auditory canal as necessary with the applicators dipped in normal saline or the irrigating solution.	Materials lodged on the pinna and at the meatus may be washed into the ear.
6. Fill the bulb syringe with solution. If an irrigating container is used, allow air to escape from the tubing.	Air forced into the ear canal is noisy and therefore unpleasant for the client.
7. Straighten the auditory canal by pulling the pinna down and back for an infant and up and back for an adult.	Straightening the ear canal aids in allowing solution to reach all areas of the canal easily.
8. Direct a steady, slow stream of solution against the roof of the auditory canal, using only sufficient force to remove secretions. Do not occlude the auditory canal with the irrigating nozzle. Allow solution to flow out unimpeded.	Solution directed at the roof of the canal aids in preventing injury to the tympanic membrane. Continuous in-and-out flow of the irrigating solution helps to prevent pressure in the canal.

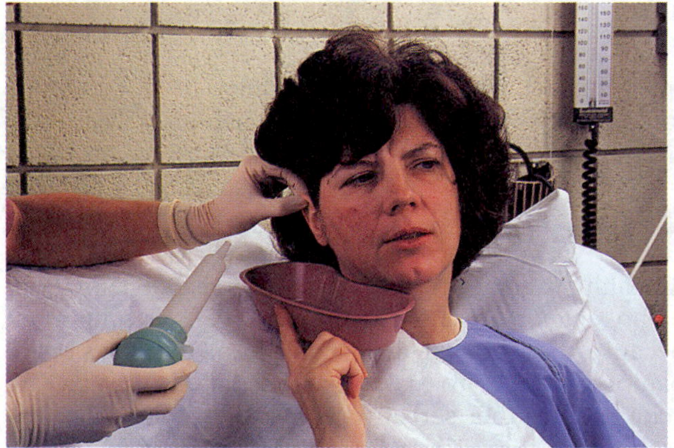

Action 7: Straightening the auditory canal.

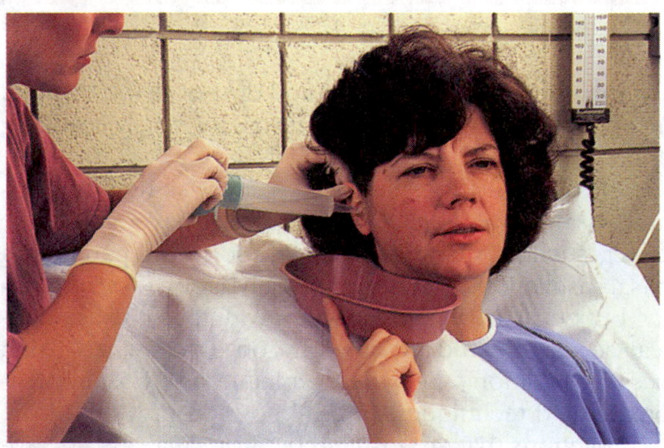

Action 8: Instilling irrigation fluid. (Photos © Ken Kasper.)

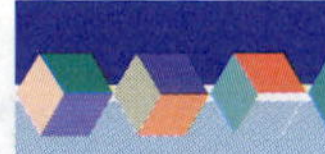

PROCEDURE 29-14

Administering an Ear Irrigation

Action	Rationale
9. When the irrigation is completed, place a cotton ball loosely in the auditory meatus and have the client lie on the side of the affected ear on a towel or an absorbent pad.	The cotton ball absorbs excess fluid and gravity allows the remaining solution in the canal to escape from the ear.
10. Wash your hands.	Handwashing deters the spread of microorganisms.
11. Chart the irrigation, the appearance of the drainage, and the client's response.	This provides accurate documentation.
12. Return in 10 to 15 minutes and remove the cotton ball and assess drainage.	Drainage or pain may indicate injury to the tympanic membrane.

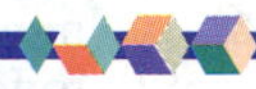

prepared for vaginal insertion. Suppositories should be refrigerated for storage.

The client should be asked to void before inserting the medication. The client is positioned lying on her back with the knees flexed. Privacy should be maintained with draping. Adequate light should be available to visualize the vaginal opening (see the accompanying box).

Rectal Instillations

Rectal suppositories are used primarily for their local action, such as a laxative and a fecal softener. Systemic effects are also achieved with rectal suppositories. Acetaminophen suppositories are used for an antipyretic effect, and many antiemetics are available in suppository form to relieve nausea and vomiting.

Be sure to use a clean disposable glove to protect your hand and prevent contamination with feces and microorganisms. See Nursing Guidelines for Inserting a Rectal Suppository and the accompanying figure in Chapter 44. Once the suppository is inserted, the client should remain in that position for 5 minutes, unless the suppository is for laxative purposes, in which case it must remain in position for 35 to 45 minutes or until the client feels the urge to defecate.

Administering Medications by Inhalation

The lungs are richly supplied with blood and have a large surface area. These characteristics allow drugs to be absorbed from the lower respiratory tract. The smaller the particles of inhaled medication, the lower in the respiratory tract the medication tends to travel. A disadvantage of using this route is that the drug dosage is difficult to establish.

Drugs classified as bronchodilators and decongestants commonly are administered by inhalation. They act to decrease resistance to air flow by enlarging the passageway. Decongestants are local vasoconstrictors. Bron-

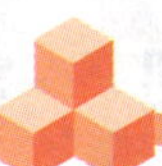

Guidelines for Nursing Care

Instilling Nose Drops

- **Provide the client with paper tissues and ask that the client blow his or her nose prior to instilling the nose drops.**
- **Have the client sit up with head tilted well back. Or, if the client is lying down, tilt the head back over a pillow. These positions allow the solution to flow well back into the nares.**
- **Draw sufficient solution into the dropper for both nares. Excess solution should not be returned to a stock bottle.**
- **Hold up the tip of the nose and place the dropper just inside the nares, about one third of an inch. Instill the prescribed number of drops in one naris and then into the other. Protect the dropper with a piece of soft tubing when the client is an infant or young child.**
- **Avoid touching the nares with the dropper because it may cause the client to sneeze.**
- **Have the client remain in position with the head tilted back for a few minutes to prevent the escape of the solution.**

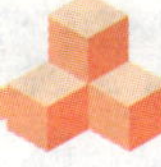

Guidelines for Nursing Care

Inserting Vaginal Suppository or Cream

- Fill a vaginal applicator with the prescribed amount of cream, or have a suppository ready.
- Lubricate the applicator with water, as necessary. A suppository may be lubricated with a water-soluble gel. Ordinarily, lubrication is unnecessary but may be used to reduce friction while inserting the applicator or suppository.
- Wear disposable gloves.
- Use clean aseptic technique to administer the medication.
- Spread the labia well with the fingers, and clean the area at the vaginal orifice with cotton balls and warm water to remove discharge, as necessary. With each cotton ball, use a single stroke moving from above the orifice downward toward the sacrum. These techniques prevent contamination of the vaginal orifice with debris surrounding the anus.
- Introduce the applicator gently in a rolling manner while directing it downward and backward to follow the normal contour of the vagina for its full length. Push the plunger to its full length, and then gently remove the applicator with the plunger depressed. After the applicator is properly positioned, the labia may be allowed to fall in place to free the nurse's hand for manipulating the plunger. Insert a suppository with gloved fingers well into the vagina.
- Ask the client to remain in the supine position for 5 to 10 minutes after insertion.
- Offer the client a perineal pad to collect excess drainage.
- Teach proper techniques to the client who wants to administer vaginal suppositories and creams herself.

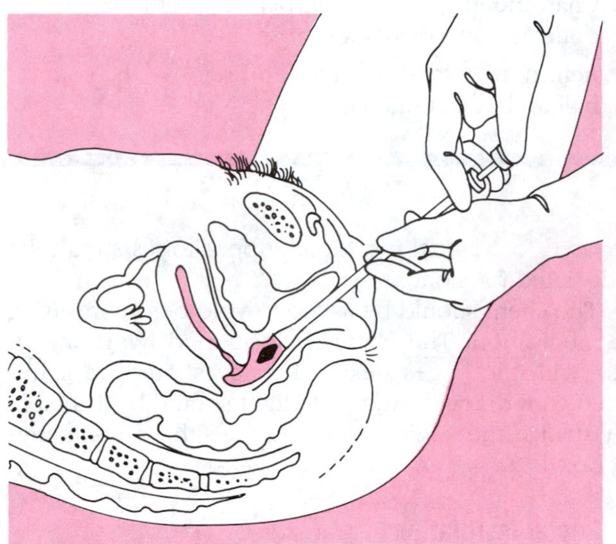

chodilators promote relaxation of musculature in the tracheobronchial tree. The relaxed passages produce less resistance to air flow and provide an opened respiratory passageway. Bronchodilators are further discussed in Chapter 45.

Drugs for inhalation may be administered by a hand atomizer or a nebulizer. These devices work to cause increased pressure in the unit, which forces solution into a specially constructed strictured chamber. The force with which the solution is made to move through the stricture and to leave the container is sufficient to break the large droplets of medication into a mist.

The hand-held, metered-dose inhaler (MDI) is often misused and the correct dose of medication is not delivered. After surveying a group of clients and healthcare workers, Interiano and Guntupalli (1993) concluded that 65% of the clients, 82% of the nurses, and 39% of the physicians tested were able to perform only two of six steps identified as necessary for correct operation of a metered-dose inhaler. See Nursing Guidelines for using an inhaler in Chapter 45.

Nebulization can also be accomplished by using the force of an oxygen stream or compressed air passed through the fluid in a nebulizer or an atomizer. This method is valuable for clients who require inhalation of a drug several times a day when the hand atomizer or nebulizer is fatiguing. The oxygen stream is also useful in the production of vapors when high humidity is needed continuously for long periods. One of the most common means of administering a nebulized drug using air pressure is the intermittent positive-pressure breathing machine also discussed in Chapter 45.

Documenting Medication Administration

The medication record is a legal document. Recording each dose of medication as soon as possible after it is given provides a documented record that can be consulted if there are any questions as to whether the client received the medication. The nurse should not record medications before they are given: if the medication is then not given, the medication record would show that the client received the medication when in fact that was not true. Different forms are used for recording medications. An example is given in Figure 29-15. The name of the medication, dosage, route of administration, time given, and nurse's initials are noted on the form. The site used for an injection should be recorded. The nurse's full signature must appear on the form for initial identification. Other specific client information may be required.

CROZER-CHESTER MEDICAL CENTER
MEDICATION ADMINISTRATION + PARENTERAL THERAPY RECORD

FORM NS-MAR-1

Legend for Injection Sites

RA- Right Arm | RT- Right Thigh
LA- Left Arm | LT- Left Thigh
RB- Right Buttock | R.Abd.- Right Abdomen
LB- Left Buttock | L.Abd.- Left Abdomen

Allergies: Penicillin

Operative Date:
Procedure:

STANDING ORDERS (MEDICATION ORDERED PER ROUTINE SCHEDULE OR WITH SPECIFIC NUMBER OF DOSES)

ORDER DATE & RN INIT.	EXP. DATE & TIME	MEDICATION, DOSAGE, FREQUENCY, ROUTE	HOURS	11/29		11/30		12/1		12/2		12/3		12/4		12/5		12/6		12/7		12/8	
				INJ. SITE	INIT.	INJ. SITE	INIT.	INJ. SITE	INIT.	INJ. SITE	INIT.	INJ. SITE	INIT.	INJ. SITE	INIT.	INJ. SITE	INIT.	INJ. SITE	INIT.	INJ. SITE	INIT.	INJ. SITE	INIT.
11/29/97 SM		Digoxin 0.25 mg po QD	10A		AC		AC		CL														
					AR = 88		AR = 92		AR = 86														
11/29/97 SM		Lasix 20 mg QD po	10A		AC		AC		CL														
11/29/97 SM		Trental 400 mg TID po	10A		AC		AC		CL														
			2P		AC		AC		CL														
			6P		PR		PR		PR														
11/29/97 SM		Slow K+ po QD	10A		AC		AC		(CL)														
11/29/97 SM		Serax 15 mg po q. 8°	6A		SP		SP		MS														
			2P		AC		AC		CL														
			10P		PR		PR		PR														
11/29/97 SM		Procardia 20 mg po TID	10A		AC		AC		CL														
			2P		AC		AC		CL														
			6P		PR		PR		PR														

SINGLE ORDERS (STAT, PRE-OP, ONE TIME DOSE, ON CALL, DIAGNOSTIC PREP)

ORDER DATE & RN INIT.	MEDICATION, DOSAGE, ROUTE	TO BE GIVEN DATE	TO BE GIVEN TIME	INJ. SITE	RN INIT.	ORDER DATE & RN INIT.	MEDICATION, DOSAGE, ROUTE	TO BE GIVEN DATE	TO BE GIVEN TIME	INJ. SITE	RN INIT.
11/29 PR	Dalmane 15 mg po now	11/29	11P	–	PR						
11/30	Dulcolax tab. iii po at 6 pm	11/30	6P		PR						

Figure 29-15
Example of a medication record.

PRN MEDICATIONS (ENTER DATE, TIME GIVEN, INJECTION SITE AND RN INITIALS)

ORDER DATE & RN INIT.	EXP. DATE & TIME	MEDICATION, DOSES, FREQUENCY, ROUTE		DOSES GIVEN													
11/29/97 sm		Tylox tab ii po q 3° prn	DATE	11/29	11/30												
			TIME	1p	3A												
			INJ. SITE														
			RN INIT.	AC	SP												
11/29/97 sm		Maalox 30cc po q 6° prn	DATE														
			TIME														
			INJ. SITE														
			RN INIT.														
			DATE														
			TIME														
			INJ. SITE														
			RN INIT.														
			DATE														
			TIME														
			INJ. SITE														
			RN INIT.														
			DATE														
			TIME														
			INJ. SITE														
			RN INIT.														
			DATE														
			TIME														
			INJ. SITE														
			RN INIT.														
			DATE														
			TIME														
			INJ. SITE														
			RN INIT.														

PATIENT NAME:

PARENTERAL THERAPY

ORDER DATE & RN INIT.	I.V. SOLUTIONS	SCHEDULE
11/29/97 sm	1000 cc D_5W	q 8°

DOCUMENTATION FOR MEDICATION WITHHELD

DATE	TIME	MEDICATION	REASON FOR WITHHOLDING
12/1	10A	Slow K tab ii	patient refused

RN IDENTIFICATION

INIT.	SIGNATURE	INIT.	SIGNATURE	INIT.	SIGNATURE
AC	A. Christopher RN				
PR	P Rogers RN				
SP	S. Pointer RN				
CL	C. Lewis RN				

Figure 29-15 *(continued)*

For instance, the pulse rate may be recorded when administering some cardiac drugs, or a description of the effects on the client's pain when administering analgesics.

Omitted Drugs

Drugs may be omitted intentionally or inadvertently. The omission and the reason for it are documented on the client's record. Drugs may be omitted intentionally for the following reasons:

- The client is to have a diagnostic test and is to fast before the test. Oral drugs usually are omitted or their administration is delayed, depending on the physician's orders.
- The problem for which the medication is intended no longer exists. For example, a laxative has been ordered for a client. The client has had a bowel movement and no longer needs the laxative. The laxative is then omitted.
- The client is suspected of having an allergy to the medication. Any suspected allergy should be reported to the physician.

In an effort to reduce the incidence of medication errors, many healthcare facilities are using computerized medication administration record systems. These automated records give the pharmacy the capability to track statistical information, maintain inventory control of drugs, and integrate this information with the central billing system. See Figure 29-1 for an example of a computer-generated medication administration record.

Refused Drugs

If the client refuses a drug that is considered essential to the therapeutic regimen, the nurse should report this promptly. The nurse often can play an important role in determining the reason for the refusal and can help the client accept needed drugs. If reasonable efforts fail to accomplish this, it is unwise to continue urging the client who adamantly refuses a medication. Clients have the right to refuse therapy, and the nurse should recognize and respect that right. Refusals to take prescribed drugs and the manner in which the situation was managed should be described on the client's record and reported according to agency policy.

Medication Errors

The conscientious nurse takes every precaution to avoid errors when administering therapeutic agents. Lilley and

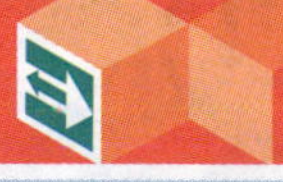

Developing Critical Thinking Skills

Situation

You are caring for two residents in a long-term care facility. One of your residents is scheduled to receive a B_{12} injection, and since it will be your first intramuscular injection it has you more than a little apprehensive. You are eagerly awaiting the moment when your instructor will be free to supervise your injection. Meanwhile she has cleared you to administer the 10:00 AM meds, and you bring a multivitamin, a diuretic, and an antiinflammatory agent to one of your assigned residents. When you go to record the medications you administered you suddenly realize to your horror that you brought them to the wrong resident. When you grab your buddy and confide your error, she says, "Whatever you do, don't tell Miss McMullen [the clinical instructor]. She gets spastic about med errors and has a reputation for gleefully failing students!" You remember that the resident who received the wrong medications has no known drug allergies and think that she probably wouldn't suffer any adverse effects from the meds she received. What should you do?

1. ***Identify Goal of Thinking***
   Determine how you ought to respond to the realization that you administered medications to the wrong resident.
2. ***Assess Adequacy of Knowledge***
   Pertinent circumstances: A resident has received three medications which were not ordered for her. You are a nursing student in your first clinical rotation and fear your clinical instructor's response should you inform her about your error. You are unsure of the harm that might result from the resident receiving the wrong medication.

   Prerequisite knowledge: In order to decide how you should respond in this situation you need to understand your professional obligations, which include your moral and legal accountability for having committed a medication error. You will need knowledge of the pharmacologic action of each of the medications you administered and their potential adverse effects for the resident who received them (possible interactions with other medications she is receiving, contraindications with related adverse effects, etc.). You recognize that there is no way for you to get the knowledge you need to make a morally and legally defensible response unless you admit your error to a responsible party.

(continued)

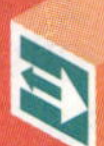

Developing Critical Thinking Skills *(continued)*

Room for error/Time constraints: Since you do not know the effects of these medications you are not in a position to judge how much room there is for error, nor are you able to make a prudent decision about how much time you have to act. The only defensible response is to seek help to clarify your position immediately since a resident's well-being is potentially at stake. No imagined personal costs would justify a delay in your admission of your error.

3. ***Address Potential Problems***
   The most serious obstacle to critical thinking in this situation would be an inability to think rationally about your obligation to report the error because of your fear of being censured by your clinical instructor. You will want to critically examine your friend's claim that your instructor will respond harshly, since this may, in fact, not be the case. You will also want to test your friend's unstated assumption that your primary obligation in this sort of situation is to take care of yourself—even if this course of action results in harm to a client. It would be helpful to think through the consequences of every healthcare professional behaving in this manner.

4. ***Consult Helpful Resources***
   Given that you are new to medication administration and are unable to assess the potential harm caused to the resident who received the wrong medications, you will find that your most helpful resource is your instructor and you will need to enlist her/his assistance immediately. She or he will probably want to contact the resident's physician to determine if there are any contraindications to this resident's receiving the medications you administered or possible interactions with other medications. A pharmacist may also need to be consulted. You will want to be familiar with the institution's policy on medication errors and will need to know how to complete an incident report. If the nursing home has a risk manager you may want to consult with him or her.

5. ***Critique Judgment/Decision***
   You have two options here: admit your error and initiate appropriate follow-up, or attempt to cover-up your error and "hope for the best." Your decision will basically be decided on the strength of your moral conviction that your primary obligation is to safeguard client well-being, even should this involve some self-sacrifice. Once you recognize the potential disastrous consequences of clients not being able to trust healthcare professionals to act in their best interests, you decide that there really is only one professionally acceptable response in this situation and you inform your instructor. It turns out that the resident who received the wrong medications suffered no adverse reactions. You, on the other hand, spend an awful morning following up on your error, and even have to delegate your B_{12} injection to another student while you are admitting your error to the resident, her attending, and the charge nurse and completing the incident report. At the end of the day your instructor compliments you for your honesty and sense of responsibility and cautions you not to repeat the mistake. You are grateful that your worst fears (*failing*) weren't confirmed and leave the unit having learned a powerful lesson about the costs of being accountable.

Guanci (1994a) list the common types of medication errors:

- Inappropriate prescribing of the drug (eg, incorrect dose, quantity, or route, or inadequate instruction)
- Extra, omitted, or wrong doses
- Administration of a medication to a client that was not ordered for him or her
- Administration of a drug via an incorrect route or rate
- Giving the drug in a dose that is different from that prescribed
- Failure to give a medication within the prescribed time interval
- Incorrect preparation of a drug before giving it
- Improper technique when administering a drug
- Giving a drug that has deteriorated

Prompt acknowledgement of errors may minimize their possible detrimental effect. The immediate priority is the safety of the client. The following steps are recommended when a medication error occurs.

1. Check the client's condition immediately when the error is noted. Observe for the development of adverse effects related to the error.
2. Notify the nurse manager and the physician to discuss possible courses of action depending on the client's condition.
3. Write a description of the error on the client's medical record, including remedial steps that were taken.
4. Complete a special form for reporting errors, as dictated by agency policy. These forms, called *accident, incident,* or *unusual occurrence reports*, re-

quire an objective, complete account of the medication errors. Include the steps that were taken after the error was recognized. For legal reasons, it is essential that an error be described fully and accurately. Medication errors are a common allegation in nursing liability cases (Lippman, 1993).

Though incident reports have a negative connotation for many nurses, they can provide vital information that can be used to prevent the error from being repeated in the future. With a continuous quality focus, the emphasis should be on the collaborative efforts necessary to provide safe client care and decrease the incidence of errors. The accompanying box discusses continuous quality improvement as a management tool to prevent medication errors.

Peer review committees have proved effective in some healthcare settings. According to Long (1992), after an error has occurred, the nurse completes a Medication Error Tool and receives varying types of counseling based on a score tallied from the forms. Recommendations and suggestions for improvements from the committee concerning delivery protocols have also proved helpful.

Teaching About Medications and Abuse

In many cases, clients continue a prescribed medication regimen at home after discharge from the hospital. A factor that affects the client's compliance to the medication regimen at home is education about the prescribed medications. Teaching should be tailored to the client's level of understanding. Written instructions can be used as a reference for the client and should include:

- The drug name and what it is supposed to do
- Special instructions about taking the medication
- What to do when adverse effects occur
- Foods, beverages, and other medications that should be avoided while taking a medication
- Proper storage of the drug
- What to do if a dose is missed (Hasegawa, 1993)

Techniques of medication administration should be explained to the client and family. Before discharge from a healthcare facility, the client should practice the necessary techniques under the supervision of a nurse to acquire sufficient skill for safe administration. Many clients have learned to give themselves injections, as well as many other medications, when the teaching has been well planned and the client is able and willing to learn.

The nurse must stress the importance of taking medications as prescribed and for as long as prescribed. A common error made by clients is simply omitting a drug, either through carelessness or because they believe that missing a dose is not important. Various aids are available to help nurses identify clients who are noncompliant and remind the client to take his or her medication on schedule. Medication containers that beep when a dose is due to be taken, scratch-off dots on a medication

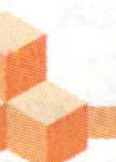

Guidelines for Nursing Care

Eliminating Potential Medication Error Situations: Continuous Quality Improvement

Nurses, as human beings, will occasionally make mistakes. Human error when administering medications can have potentially devastating effects. FMEA (Failure Mode and Effects Analysis) is a continuous quality improvement process that can effectively identify possible error situations, predict effects of this error on the client, and recommend opportunities for improvement. A continuous quality improvement (CQI) approach recognizes that it's not people who are the problem—it's processes that don't work. Physicians who order medications, pharmacists who dispense them, and nurses who administer medications are all valuable resources who can analyze error-prone products and procedures and suggest preventive strategies. Cohen and Senders (1994) and Davis (1994) recommend the following techniques to help prevent medication errors:

- Maintain a system of repetitive checks.
- Use fail-safe setups or systems.
- Remove unnecessary or dangerous items from the nursing unit.
- Limit access to dangerous drugs.
- Avoid confirmation bias (selecting an item because it's what you expect to see).
- Adapt equipment that is designed so it can only be used for the purpose intended.
- Choose products with unique packaging or distinctive shapes or use tactile cues to help identify drugs.
- Use warning labels on hazardous drugs.
- Rely on computer-generated medication records, bar codes, and other technological advances to prevent errors.
- Develop protocols and procedures and adhere to their standards.
- Use documentation to verify therapy and confirm the client's response to a medication.
- Refer to available resources to check on a medication or questionable drug order (eg, drug reference book, procedure and policy manual).

label, and an electronic cap that signals dosage time and records each time the cap is removed are compliance aids that are now available.

Home Healthcare Alert

Nurses should advise clients to keep their medications with them when they travel. If luggage is lost or misplaced, refilling the prescription may be difficult.

The client should be instructed not to alter the dosage without consulting the physician. Medications should not be discontinued when symptoms disappear. Drugs used to maintain health, such as those to control high blood pressure, need to be continued as ordered to avoid recurrence of symptoms.

Caution the client not to share prescribed medications with other family members or with friends and neighbors. Inappropriate use of another person's drugs can have serious consequences.

Nurses have a teaching responsibility in relation to the abuse of any drug. Teaching may take place on an individual basis or on a family or community level. Drug abuse is a major public health concern worldwide, according to authorities on the subject, especially among teenagers and young adults. Not only is continued public and individual education indicated, nurses are also expected to teach by setting high standards for their own behavior and the use of drugs. The increasing incidence of impaired providers makes it imperative that nurses observe, document, and intervene, for the client's safety, if drug abuse by a professional caregiver is suspected.

EVALUATING THE CLIENT'S RESPONSE TO MEDICATIONS

Drug effectiveness can be assessed in several ways. Clinical observation is the first method. Subjective data from the client (eg, "My pain has disappeared") can be collected. Objective data (eg, the client's vital signs) help the nurse evaluate medication effectiveness. The alert nurse assesses the client for adverse drug effects.

Measurement of drug levels in body fluids provides data about the client's response to a particular medication. For many drugs, including digoxin, theophylline, anticonvulsants, and aminoglycoside antibiotics, monitoring blood levels is an important component of therapy. The client is tested to determine if the drug level in the blood is within the therapeutic range. Drug dosages may be adjusted as a result of the serum drug level.

Monitoring systems can also assist the nurse in evaluating drug effectiveness. For the client with an arrhythmia, a cardiac monitor would show a change in heart rhythm.

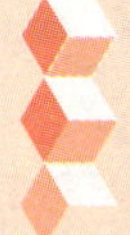

Helpscan

The following are resources for clients and healthcare professionals:

- Hotline for health professionals to voluntarily report serious adverse effects with drugs, devices, or biologicals:
  MEDWATCH
  The FDA Medical Products Reporting Program
  Food and Drug Administration
  5600 Fishers Lane
  Rockville, MD 20852-9787
  (800) FDA-1088
- For healthcare professionals who have made a medication error and want to help prevent a similar error elsewhere, call:
  United States Pharmacopeial Convention
  (800) 23-ERROR
  Your name and the name of your facility will be kept confidential.
- For Medication Fact Sheets available in English, Spanish, and Chinese, contact:
  Srx Medication Education for Seniors
  1095 Market Street, Room 602
  San Francisco, CA 94103
  (415) 626-1650

Key Points

- Medications have several names. The nurse should be aware of a drug's generic and trade names. Drugs can be classified by body system and by the symptom they relieve (clinical indication).
- Drugs are available in many forms. Some drugs are supplied in a number of preparations; others are available in only one form.
- Factors that influence drug absorption include route of administration, local conditions at the site of administration, drug solubility, pH, and drug dosage.
- Variables that influence the action of medications are age, weight, sex, genetic factors, psychologic factors, illness, environment, and time of administration.

- Known adverse drug effects include iatrogenic disease, drug allergy, drug tolerance, cumulative effect, idiosyncratic reaction, and drug interactions.
- Assessment of clients receiving medications includes obtaining a comprehensive medication history.
- Components of a medication order are client's name, date and time order is written, name of the drug, dosage, route, frequency, and signature of the prescriber. The nurse questions any unclear medication order before the order is implemented.
- Pediatric dosages are calculated by the child's weight or body surface area.
- The nurse observes the *five rights* and *three checks* in medication preparation and administration. The nurse who prepares a medication administers the medication. The medication area is locked when not in use.
- The nurse identifies the client correctly before administering a medication and remains with the client until the medication is taken. The nurse records the medication on the client's record as soon as possible after administration.
- Selection of equipment for a parenteral injection is based on the route of administration, viscosity of the drug, quantity to be administered, type of medication, and client's body size.
- After use, needles should never be recapped and are placed in a puncture-resistant container. Most needlestick injuries occur during recapping. Needleless equipment effectively prevents needlestick injuries.
- Sterile equipment is used to prepare a drug for injection.
- A vial of unmodified insulin should never be contaminated with modified insulin when preparing two insulins to be mixed in the same syringe.
- Proper site selection for an intramuscular injection should include palpation of anatomic landmarks. The Z-track method for an intramuscular injection is safer and less painful for most adults.
- Intravenous medications can be administered as a continuous infusion, as a bolus, or intermittently. A bolus dose and an intermittent infusion may be administered through the primary intravenous line or through a heparin lock. The nurse checks the placement of a heparin lock before administering any medication.
- Topical medications are applied to the skin and mucous membranes primarily for their local effects, although some systemic effects may occur.

Study Questions

1. The official name of a drug that is selected by the pharmaceutical company selling the drug and copyrighted by it is the drug's
   a. chemical name
   b. generic name
   c. official name
   d. trade name
2. The process by which a drug is transferred from its site of entry into the body to the bloodstream is known as
   a. absorption
   b. distribution
   c. metabolism
   d. excretion
3. A client has an abnormal, unexpected response to a drug. This is defined as
   a. drug tolerance
   b. a cumulative effect
   c. an idiosyncratic effect
   d. an anaphylactic reaction
4. A medication order reads: "Digoxin, 0.125 mg PO qod." The nurse correctly gives this drug
   a. daily before bedtime
   b. by mouth every other day
   c. twice a day by way of the oral route
   d. once a week after recording an apical rate
5. In addition to checking a client's identification bracelet, the nurse can correctly verify his identity by
   a. asking Mr. Brown his name
   b. reading his name on the sign over the bed
   c. asking his roommate to verify his name
   d. asking, "Are you Mr. Brown?"
6. Medication needs to be administered by way of a nasogastric tube. Before giving the medication, it is important for the nurse to
   a. crush the enteric-coated pill for mixing in a liquid
   b. flush open the tube with 60 mL of very warm water
   c. check for proper placement of the nasogastric tube
   d. take the client's vital signs
7. The medication order reads: "Meperidine, 50 mg IM stat." The prefilled cartridge is available with a label reading 50 mg/1 mL. The cartridge contains 1.2 mL of meperidine. The nurse should
   a. give all the medication in the cartridge because it expanded when it was mixed
   b. call the pharmacy and request the proper dose
   c. refuse to give the medication
   d. dispose of 0.2 mL correctly before administering the drug
8. A client requires 40 units of NPH insulin and 10 units of regular insulin daily subcutaneously. The correct sequence when mixing insulins is
   a. inject air into the regular insulin vial and withdraw 10 units; then, using the same syringe, in-

ject air into the NPH vial and withdraw 40 units of NPH insulin
   b. inject air into the NPH insulin vial, being careful not to allow the solution to touch the needle; next, inject air into the regular insulin vial and withdraw 10 units; then, withdraw 40 units of NLH insulin
   c. inject air into the regular insulin vial, being careful not to allow the solution to touch the needle; next, inject air into the NPH insulin vial and withdraw 40 units; then, withdraw 10 units of regular insulin
   d. inject air into the NPH insulin vial and withdraw 40 units; then, using the same syringe, inject air into the regular insulin vial and withdraw 10 units of regular insulin

9. Ms. Hall has an order for meperidine, 100 mg q 4 h prn. The nurse notes that according to Ms. Hall's chart, Ms. Hall is allergic to Demerol. The order for medication was signed by Dr. Long. Which of the following would be the correct procedure for this situation?
   a. Administer the medication; the doctor knows best.
   b. Call Dr. Long and ask that she change the medication.
   c. Ask the supervisor to administer the medication.
   d. Ask the pharmacist to provide a medication to take the place of Demerol.
10. The nurse manager on your unit prepared medications for Mr. Giles. She is called to the phone and asks you to give the client his medications. Which is the best response to this request?
   a. Give Mr. Giles the medication and record it in his chart.
   b. Tell the nurse manager that you do not have time and ask her to get someone else.
   c. Tell the nurse manager that because you did not pour the medication, you cannot administer it.
   d. Give the medication to Mr. Giles but have the nurse manager chart it.
11. Which of the following is the reason the intravenous method of medication administration is called the most dangerous route of administration?
   a. The vein can take only a small amount of fluid at a time.
   b. The vein may harden and become nonfunctional.
   c. Blood clots may become a serious problem.
   d. The drug is placed directly into the bloodstream and its action is immediate.
12. Mr. King is receiving heparin subcutaneously. Which of the following demonstrates correct technique for this procedure?
   a. Aspirate before giving and gently massage after the injection.
   b. Do not aspirate; massage the site for 1 minute.
   c. Do not aspirate before or massage after the injection.
   d. Massage the site of the injection; aspiration is not necessary but will do no harm.
13. A client refuses to take her noon medication, saying that she does not need it. Which of the following would be the best response?
   a. Tell her that she must take the medication because the doctor ordered it.
   b. Tell her that you went through a lot of preparation to get her medications ready and it's the least she can do.
   c. Tell her that you don't care whether she takes the medications or not.
   d. Tell her that you will return the medications to the cart but would like to discuss her reasons for refusing the medications.
14. The nurse discovers that she has made a medication error. Which of the following would be the first response?
   a. Record the error on the medication sheet.
   b. Notify the physician regarding course of action.
   c. Check the client's condition to note any possible effect of the error.
   d. Complete an incident report, explaining how the mistake was made.
15. The nurse takes an 8 AM medication to the client and properly identifies her. The client asks the nurse to leave the medication on the bedside table and states that she will take it with breakfast when it comes. What is the best response to this request?
   a. Leave the medication and return later to make sure that it was taken.
   b. Tell her that it is against the rules and take the medication with you.
   c. Tell her that you cannot leave the medication but will return with it when breakfast arrives.
   d. Take the drug from the room and record it as refused.

Answers With Rationale

1. The correct response is *d.* The chemical name identifies the drug's chemical composition and molecular structure. The generic name is assigned by the manufacturer who develops the drug, and the official name is the name that identifies the drug in the official publication.
2. The correct response is *a.* Distribution, metabolism, and excretion occur after the drug has been absorbed.
3. The correct response is *c.* Drug tolerance results when the body becomes accustomed to the drug over time. A cumulative effect occurs when the

body cannot metabolize one dose of a drug before another one is given. An anaphylactic reaction is a life-threatening, immediate response to a drug that can result in respiratory distress and cardiovascular response.

4. The correct response is *b.* The abbreviation qod refers to every-other-day administration.
5. The correct response is *a.* A sign over the client's bed may not always be current and updated. The roommate is an unsafe source of information, and the client may not even hear his name and reply in the affirmative (eg, a person with a hearing deficit).
6. The correct response is *c.* Tube placement should always be checked before administering any medication to prevent the possibility of aspiration if the tube is not in the stomach. Enteric-coated pills should never be crushed, and very warm water may injure stomach mucosa. Taking the vital signs is not necessary unless a particular medication requires it before administration.
7. The correct response is *d.* Many cartridges are overfilled, and some of the medication needs to be discarded. Giving the excess medication in the cartridge may result in adverse effects for the client. For this dose, it is not necessary to call the pharmacy or refuse to give the medication, provided the order is written correctly.
8. The correct response is *b.* Regular or short-acting insulin should never be contaminated with NPH or any insulin modified with added protein. Placing air in the NPH vial first without allowing the needle to contact the solution ensures that the regular insulin will not be contaminated.
9. The correct response is *b.* The nurse is responsible for any medications he or she gives and must contact the doctor to inform her of the client's allergy to the drug. The nurse should not give the medication and might speak with the supervisor only if he or she is uncomfortable with the physician's response once she is notified. The nurse is legally unable to order a replacement medication, as is the pharmacist.
10. The correct response is *c.* The nurse should never give medications prepared by someone else, since she is responsible for what she administers.
11. The correct response is *d.* The intravenous route is a direct access to the bloodstream, and medications act quickly when given intravenously. The condition of the veins is not as important as the rapid effect of the medication administered by way of the intravenous route.
12. The correct response is *c.* Heparin that is given subcutaneously should not be aspirated or massaged, so as not to cause trauma or bleeding in the tissues.
13. The correct response is *d.* The client has the right to refuse medications, but the nurse should assess the client's reasons for refusal, document them, and report them to the physician.
14. The correct response is *c.* The nurse's first responsibility is the client, and careful observation is necessary to assess for any effect of the medication error. The other nursing actions are pertinent but only after checking the client's welfare.
15. The correct response is *c.* Safe nursing practice requires that a medication never be left at the client's bedside. It is not correct to say that the client has refused medication in this situation.

Medication Calculation Problems

1. Metoprolol (Lopressor), 25 mg PO, is ordered. Metoprolol is available as 50-mg tablets. How many tablets would the nurse administer?
2. Phenytoin (Dilantin), 100 mg PO, is ordered to be given through a nasogastric tube. Phenytoin is available as 30 mg/5 mL. How much would the nurse administer?
3. Captopril (Capoten), 12.5 mg PO, is ordered. Captopril is available as 25-mg tablets. How many tablets would the nurse administer?
4. Potassium chloride (Micro-K), 20 mEq, is ordered. Potassium chloride is available as 10 mEq per tablet. How many tablets would the nurse administer?
5. Digoxin (Lanoxin), 0.0625 mg PO, is ordered. Digoxin is available as 0.125-mg tablets. How many tablets would the nurse administer?
6. Propantheline bromide (Pro-Banthine), 15 mg, is ordered. Propantheline bromide is available as 7.5-mg tablets. How many tablets would the nurse administer?
7. Ciprofloxacin (Cipro), 500 mg PO, is ordered. Ciprofloxacin is available as 250-mg tablets. How many tablets would the nurse administer?
8. Furosemide (Lasix), 20 mg PO, is ordered. Furosemide is available as 40-mg tablets. How many tablets would the nurse administer?
9. Theophylline elixir, 100 mg PO, is ordered by way of a percutaneous endoscopic gastrostomy tube. Theophylline elixir is available as 8 mg/15 mL. How much would the nurse administer?
10. Clinidine (Catapres), 0.1 mg PO, is ordered. Clinidine is available as 0.2-mg tablets. How many tablets would the nurse administer?
11. Vitamin K, 10 mg IM, is ordered. Vitamin K is available as 5 mg/mL. How much would the nurse administer?
12. Meperidine (Demerol), 35 mg IM, is ordered. Meperidine is available as 50 mg/mL. How much would the nurse administer?

13. Midazolam (Versed), 3 mg IM, is ordered. Midazolam is available as 5 mg/mL. How much would the nurse administer?
14. Hydroxyzine (Vistaril), 50 mg IM, is ordered. Hydroxyzine is available as 25 mg/mL. How much would the nurse administer?
15. Epoetin alfa (Epogen), 2000 units SC, is ordered. Epoetin alfa is available as 4000 units/mL. How much would the nurse administer?
16. Nalbuphine (Nubain), 1.5 mg IM, is ordered. Nalbuphine is available as 1 mg/mL. How much would the nurse administer?
17. Ocreotide acetate (Sandostatin), 50 µg SC, is ordered. Ocreotide is available as 100 µg/mL. How much would the nurse administer?
18. Morphine sulfate, 4 mg SC, is ordered. Morphine sulfate is available as 8 mg/mL. How much would the nurse administer?
19. Prochlorperazine (Compazine), 7.5 mg IM, is ordered. Prochlorperazine is available as 5 mg/mL. How much would the nurse administer?
20. Glycopyrrolate (Robinul), 0.4 mg IM, is ordered. Glycopyrrolate is available as 0.2 mg/mL. How much would the nurse administer?

Answers to Medication Calculation Problems

1. $$\frac{\text{dose on hand}}{\text{quantity on hand}} = \frac{\text{dose required}}{\text{X (quantity desired)}}$$

$$\frac{50\text{ mg}}{1\text{ tablet}} = \frac{25\text{ mg}}{\text{X}}$$

cross-multiply:

$$50\text{X} = 25$$
$$\text{X} = 0.5 \text{ or } 1/2 \text{ tablet}$$

2. $$\frac{\text{dose on hand}}{\text{quantity on hand}} = \frac{\text{dose desired}}{\text{X (quantity desired)}}$$

$$\frac{30\text{ mg}}{5\text{ ml}} = \frac{100\text{ mg}}{\text{X}}$$

cross-multiply:

$$30\text{X} = 500$$
$$\text{X} = 16.66 \text{ or } 17\text{ mL}$$

3. $$\frac{\text{dose on hand}}{\text{quantity on hand}} = \frac{\text{dose desired}}{\text{X (quantity desired)}}$$

$$\frac{25\text{ mg}}{1\text{ tablet}} = \frac{12.5\text{ mg}}{\text{X}}$$

cross-multiply:

$$25\text{X} = 12.5$$
$$\text{X} = 0.5 \text{ or } 1/2 \text{ tablet}$$

4. $$\frac{\text{dose on hand}}{\text{quantity on hand}} = \frac{\text{dose desired}}{\text{X (quantity desired)}}$$

$$\frac{10\text{ mEq}}{1\text{ tablet}} = \frac{20\text{ mEq}}{\text{X}}$$

cross-multiply:

$$10\text{X} = 20$$
$$\text{X} = 2 \text{ tablets}$$

5. $$\frac{\text{dose on hand}}{\text{quantity on hand}} = \frac{\text{dose desired}}{\text{X (quantity desired)}}$$

$$\frac{0.125\text{ mg}}{1\text{ tablet}} = \frac{0.0625\text{ mg}}{\text{X}}$$

cross-multiply:

$$0.125\text{X} = 0.0625$$
$$\text{X} = 0.5 \text{ or } 1/2 \text{ tablet}$$

6. $$\frac{\text{dose desired}}{\text{dose on hand}} \times \frac{\text{quantity}}{\text{on hand}} = \text{X (desired quantity)}$$

$$\frac{15\text{ mg}}{7.5\text{ mg}} \times 1\text{ tablet} = \text{X}$$

$$2 \times 1 = 2 \text{ tablets}$$

7. $$\frac{\text{dose desired}}{\text{dose on hand}} \times \frac{\text{quantity}}{\text{on hand}} = \text{X (desired quantity)}$$

$$\frac{500\text{ mg}}{250\text{ mg}} \times 1\text{ tablet} = \text{X}$$

$$2 \times 1 = 2 \text{ tablets}$$

8. $$\frac{\text{dose desired}}{\text{dose on hand}} \times \frac{\text{quantity}}{\text{on hand}} = \text{X (desired quantity)}$$

$$\frac{20\text{ mg}}{40\text{ mg}} \times 1\text{ tablet} = \text{X}$$

$$1/2 \times 1 = \text{X}$$
$$\text{X} = 1/2 \text{ tablet}$$

9. $$\frac{\text{dose desired}}{\text{dose on hand}} \times \frac{\text{quantity}}{\text{on hand}} = \text{X (desired quantity)}$$

$$\frac{100\text{ mg}}{80\text{ mg}} \times 15\text{ ml} = \text{X}$$

$$\frac{1500}{80} = \text{X}$$

$$\text{X} = 18.75 = 19\text{ mL}$$

10. $\frac{\text{dose desired}}{\text{dose on hand}} \times \frac{\text{quantity}}{\text{on hand}} = \text{X (desired quantity)}$

$$\frac{0.1\text{ mg}}{0.2\text{ mg}} \times 1\text{ tablet} = X$$

$$\tfrac{1}{2} \times 1 = X$$
$$X = \tfrac{1}{2}\text{ tablet}$$

11. $\frac{\text{dose on hand}}{\text{quantity on hand}} = \frac{\text{dose desired}}{\text{X (quantity desired)}}$

$$\frac{5\text{ mg}}{1\text{ mL}} = \frac{10\text{ mg}}{X}$$

cross-multiply:

$$5X = 10$$
$$X = 2\text{ mL}$$

12. $\frac{\text{dose on hand}}{\text{quantity on hand}} = \frac{\text{dose desired}}{\text{X (quantity desired)}}$

$$\frac{50\text{ mg}}{1\text{ mL}} = \frac{35\text{ mg}}{X}$$

cross-multiply:

$$50X = 35$$
$$X = 0.7\text{ mL}$$

13. $\frac{\text{dose on hand}}{\text{quantity on hand}} = \frac{\text{dose desired}}{\text{X (quantity desired)}}$

$$\frac{5\text{ mg}}{1\text{ mL}} = \frac{3\text{ mg}}{X}$$

cross-multiply:

$$5X = 3$$
$$X = 0.6\text{ mL}$$

14. $\frac{\text{dose on hand}}{\text{quantity on hand}} = \frac{\text{dose desired}}{\text{X (quantity desired)}}$

$$\frac{25\text{ mg}}{1\text{ mL}} = \frac{50\text{ mg}}{X}$$

cross-multiply:

$$25X = 50$$
$$X = 2\text{ mL}$$

15. $\frac{\text{dose on hand}}{\text{quantity on hand}} = \frac{\text{dose desired}}{\text{X (quantity desired)}}$

$$\frac{4000\text{ U}}{1\text{ mL}} = \frac{2000\text{ U}}{X}$$

cross-multiply:

$$4000X = 2000$$
$$X = \tfrac{1}{2}\text{ mL}$$

16. $\frac{\text{dose desired}}{\text{dose on hand}} \times \frac{\text{quantity}}{\text{on hand}} = \text{X (desired quantity)}$

$$\frac{1.5\text{ mg}}{1\text{ mg}} \times 1\text{ mL} = X$$

$$1.5 \times 1 = X$$
$$X = 1.5\text{ mL}$$

17. $\frac{\text{dose desired}}{\text{dose on hand}} \times \frac{\text{quantity}}{\text{on hand}} = \text{X (desired quantity)}$

$$\frac{50\ \mu\text{g}}{100\ \mu\text{g}} \times 1\text{ mL} = X$$

$$\tfrac{1}{2} \times 1 = X$$
$$X = \tfrac{1}{2}\text{ mL}$$

18. $\frac{\text{dose desired}}{\text{dose on hand}} \times \frac{\text{quantity}}{\text{on hand}} = \text{X (desired quantity)}$

$$\frac{4\text{ mg}}{8\text{ mg}} \times 1\text{ ml} = X$$

$$\tfrac{1}{2} \times 1 = X$$
$$X = \tfrac{1}{2}\text{ mL}$$

19. $\frac{\text{dose desired}}{\text{dose on hand}} \times \frac{\text{quantity}}{\text{on hand}} = \text{X (desired quantity)}$

$$\frac{7.5\text{ mg}}{5\text{ mg}} \times 1\text{ ml} = X$$

$$1.5 \times 1 = X$$
$$X = 1.5\text{ mL}$$

20. $\frac{\text{dose desired}}{\text{dose on hand}} \times \frac{\text{quantity}}{\text{on hand}} = \text{X (desired quantity)}$

$$\frac{0.4\text{ mg}}{0.2\text{ mg}} \times 1\text{ ml} = X$$

$$2 \times 1 = X$$
$$X = 2\text{ mL}$$

Bibliography

Abrams, A. (1995). *Clinical drug therapy* (4th ed.). Philadelphia: Lippincott.

Bailey, A., Ferguson, E., & Voss, S. (1995). Factors affecting an individual's ability to administer medication. *Home Healthcare Nurse, 13*(5), 57–63.

Beyea, S., & Nicoll, L. (1995). Administration of medications via the intramuscular route: An integrative review of the literature and research-based protocol for the procedure. *Applied Nursing Research, 8*(1), 23–33.

Beyea, S., & Nicoll, L. (1996). Back to basics: Administering IM injections the right way. *American Journal of Nursing, 96*(1), 34–35.

Buttaro, M. (1994). Staying on top of transdermal drug patches. *Nursing, 24*(11), 41–44.

Cantrell, S. (1994). How to respond to adverse drug reactions. *Nursing, 24*(11), 82–84.

Carpenito, L. (1995). *Nursing diagnosis: Application to clinical practice* (6th ed.). Philadelphia: Lippincott.

Cohen, M. (1993). What you said about the apothecary system. *Nursing, 23*(7), 56–58.

Cohen, M., & Senders, J. (1994). 12 ways to prevent medication errors. *Nursing, 24*(2), 34–41.

Davis, N. (1994a). Decimal point dangers. *American Journal of Nursing, 94*(1), 9.

Davis, N. (1994b). Teaching patients to prevent errors. *American Journal of Nursing, 94*(5), 17.

Davis, N. (1995). Preventing omission errors. *American Journal of Nursing, 95*(4), 17.

Dickerson, R. (1992). 10 Tips for easing the pain of intramuscular injections. *Nursing, 22*(8), 55.

Drass, J. (1992). Insulin injections. *Nursing, 22*(11), 40–43.

Gillespie, J. (1995). Five things you should know about medicine cabinets. *Nursing, 25*(1), 29.

Hasegawa, G. (1993). Ensuring patient compliance. *Nursing, 23*(1), 17.

Hussar, D. (1993). Reviewing drug interactions. *Nursing, 23*(9), 50–57.

Interiano, B., & Guntupalli, K. (1993). Metered-dose inhalers: Do health care providers know what to teach? *Archives of Internal Medicine, 153*(1), 81.

Jaffe, M. (1993). *Nursing procedures for home care.* Albany, NY: Delmar Publishers, Inc.

Kelly, M. (1996). Medications and the visually impaired elderly. *Geriatric Nursing, 17*(2), 60–62.

Kudzma, E. (1992). Drug response: All bodies are not created equal. *American Journal of Nursing, 92*(12), 48–50.

Lilley, L., & Guanci, R. (1994a). Getting back to basics. *American Journal of Nursing, 94*(9), 15.

Lilley, L., & Guanci, R. (1994b). Now what? After an error. *American Journal of Nursing, 94*(11), 18.

Lippman, H. (1993). Rx: Error-free meds. *RN, 56*(6), 65–69.

Long, T. (1992). Pointing out medication errors. *American Journal of Nursing, 92*(2), 76–78.

McConnell, E. (1992). Using a metered-dose nebulizer correctly. *Nursing, 22*(2), 18.

McGovern, K. (1992). 10 Golden rules for administering drugs safely. *Nursing, 22*(3), 49–56.

Messner, R., & Gardner, S. (1993). Start with the medicine cabinet. *RN, 56*(1), 51–53.

Miller, D., & Miller, H. (1995). Giving meds through the tube. *RN, 58*(1), 44–48.

Newton, M., Newton, D., & Fudin, J. (1992). Reviewing the big three injection routes. *Nursing, 22*(2), 34–41.

O'Donnell, J. (1992). Understanding adverse drug reactions. *Nursing, 22*(8), 34–39.

O'Donnell, J. (1994). Drug therapy: 20 ways your role will change. *Nursing, 24*(3), 46–48.

Osbourne, E. (1993). Administering aerosol therapy. *Nursing, 23*(12), 24C–24H.

Parisi, S. (1994). What to do after a med error. *Nursing, 24*(6), 59.

Powers, M. J., et al. (1995). Medication administration: How safe is your patient? *American Journal of Nursing, 95*(10), 44–59.

Rice, P., Jensen, M., Lyons, M., & Murphy, M. (1994). Medications in well and institutionalized elders. *Geriatric Nursing, 15*(4), 216–218.

Rice, R. (1995). *Handbook of home health nursing procedures.* St. Louis: Mosby.

Taylor, H. (1992). Patients deserve painless injections. *RN, 55*(3), 25–26.

Chapter 30

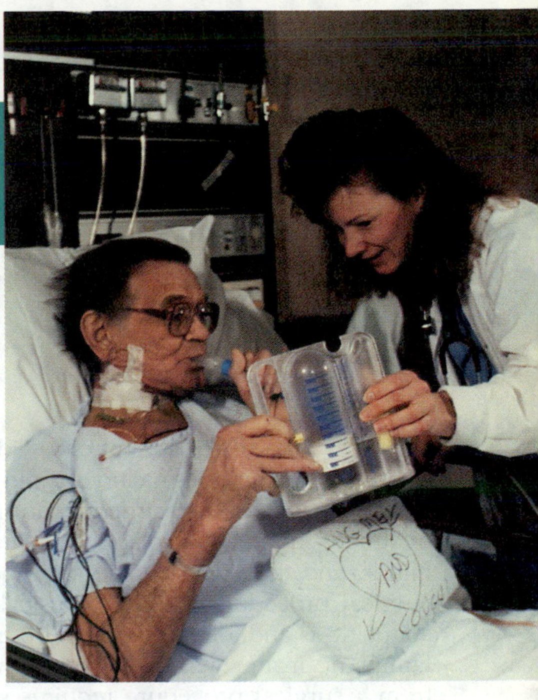

Perioperative Nursing

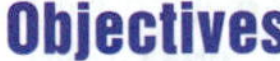

Objectives

After studying this chapter, the learner should be able to:

Describe the surgical experience, including perioperative phases, categories of surgery, types of anesthesia, and informed consent.

Conduct a preoperative nursing history and physical assessment to identify client strengths as well as factors that increase surgical and postoperative complication risk.

Teach preoperative exercises: deep breathing, coughing, and leg exercises.

Prepare a client physically and psychologically for surgery.

Identify assessments specific to the prevention of complications in the immediate postoperative phase.

Use the nursing process to knowledgeably develop an individualized plan of care for the surgical client during each phase of the perioperative period.

Discuss the processes involved in wound healing.

Describe wound care, including emergency treatment and factors that affect wound healing.

Implement dressing changes for different kinds of wounds.

Provide information to clients and caregivers for self-care at home.

Key Terms

bandage
binder
dehiscence
dressing
elective surgery
emergency surgery
evisceration
general anesthesia
granulation tissue
informed consent
intraoperative phase
perioperative nursing
perioperative period
postoperative phase
preoperative phase
regional anesthesia
scar
wound

Often the treatment of a wide variety of illness and injuries includes some type of surgical intervention. Surgery is an invasive method of treatment that may be planned or unplanned, major or minor, and that may involve any body part or system. Surgical procedures require physical and psychosocial adaptations and are stressors for both the client and the family, no matter what the extent. The client's recovery from a surgical procedure requires skillful and knowledgeable nursing care whether the surgery is done on an outpatient basis or in the hospital setting. All phases of the nursing process are used perioperatively to make assessments and provide interventions necessary to promote the recovery of health, prevent further injury or illness, and facilitate coping with alterations in physical structure and function.

This chapter discusses nursing care appropriate to preparing the client for surgery, supporting the client during surgery, and assisting with recovery after surgery. The nurse's role during each stage is described, using the phases of the nursing process. The care of wounds is described, and includes wound healing, factors affecting wound healing, wound complications, and the applications of dressings. Selected nursing diagnoses and expected outcomes are included for each phase of care of the surgical client.

The Surgical Experience

Regardless of the surgical intervention required or the setting in which the surgery is performed, all clients progress through specific perioperative phases, have a defined surgical procedure, require some type of anesthesia, and give their consent for surgery. This part of the chapter describes those components of the surgical experience to serve as a knowledge base for the application of the nursing process when giving nursing care to the client who is undergoing surgery.

Phases of the Perioperative Period

The client who is having surgery progresses through several distinct phases, with the entire time frame labeled the **perioperative period**. **Perioperative nursing** is the name given to the wide variety of nursing activities carried out before, during, and after surgery. The three phases of the perioperative period are the **preoperative phase**, beginning with the decision that surgical intervention is necessary and lasting until the client is transferred to the operating room table; the **intraoperative phase**, extending from admission to the surgical department (or operating room) to transfer to the recovery area; and the **postoperative phase**, lasting from admission to the recovery area to the complete recovery from surgery. With an increasing trend toward short-stay or same-day surgical treatment, the nursing interventions in each phase may be somewhat altered, but still remain basically the same. The nursing process is used during each phase to meet physical and psychosocial needs and facilitate the client's return to health. Each of these phases, with related client needs and nursing activities, are described in the remainder of the chapter.

Classification of Surgical Procedures

Surgical procedures usually are categorized by the major classifications of urgency, risk, and purpose. Table 30-1 lists each classification, with purposes and selected examples for each. The classifications are described below.

Based on Urgency. Surgery may be classified as **elective surgery**, meaning that it is preplanned and based on the client's choice; *urgent surgery*, in which the surgery is necessary for the client's health but not an emergency; and **emergency surgery**, when surgery must be done immediately to preserve the client's life, body part, or body function.

Based on Degree of Risk. Surgery is classified as *minor* or *major* based on the degree of risk for the client. Minor surgery is almost always performed in settings such as a physician's office, an outpatient clinic, or in same-day surgery settings. This classification means that the surgical procedure usually is brief, carries a low risk, and results in few complications. In contrast, major surgery always requires hospitalization, usually is prolonged, has a higher degree of risk, involves major body organs or life-threatening situations, and has the potential of post-

Table 30-1
Classification of Surgical Procedures

Classification	Purpose	Examples
Based on Urgency		
Elective: Delay of surgery has no ill effects; can be scheduled in advance based on client's choice	• To remove or repair a body part • To restore function • To improve health • To improve self-concept	Tonsillectomy, hernia repair, cataract extraction and lens implant, hemorrhoidectomy, hip prosthesis, scar revision, facelift, mammoplasty
Urgent: Usually done within 24–48 hours	• To remove or repair a body part • To preserve or restore health • To restore function • To prevent further tissue damage	Removal of gallbladder, coronary artery bypass, surgical removal of a malignant tumor, colon resection, amputation
Emergency: Done immediately	• To preserve life (plus purposes as listed above)	Control of hemorrhage, repair of trauma, perforated ulcer, intestinal obstruction, tracheostomy
Based on Degree of Risk		
Major: may be elective, urgent, or emergency	• To preserve life • To remove or repair a body part • To restore function • To improve or maintain health	Carotid endarterectomy, cholecystectomy, nephrectomy, colostomy, hysterectomy, radical mastectomy, amputation, trauma repair
Minor: Primarily elective	• To restore function • To remove skin lesions • To correct deformities	Teeth extraction, removal of warts, skin biopsy, dilatation and curettage, laparoscopy, cataract extraction, arthroscopy
Based on Purpose		
Diagnostic	• To make or confirm a diagnosis	Breast biopsy, laparoscopy, bronchoscopy, exploratory laparotomy
Ablative	• To remove a diseased body part	Appendectomy, subtotal thyroidectomy, partial gastrectomy, colon resection, amputation
Palliative	• To relieve or reduce intensity of an illness; is not curative	Colostomy, nerve root resection, debridement of necrotic tissue, balloon angioplasties, arthroscopy
Reconstructive	• To restore function to traumatized or malfunctioning tissue • To improve self-concept	Scar revision, plastic surgery, skin graft, internal fixation of a fracture, breast reconstruction
Transplant	• To replace organs or structures that are diseased or malfunctioning	Kidney, liver, cornea, heart, joints
Constructive	• To restore function in congenital anomalies	Cleft palate repair, closure of atrial-septal defect

operative complications. However, advances in the use of laser techniques and microscopic techniques involving very small incisions have made even major surgery less traumatic and therefore require shortened hospital stays.

Based on Purpose. Descriptors used to classify surgical procedures based on purpose include *diagnostic, ablative, palliative, reconstructive, transplant*, and *constructive* (see Table 30-1).

Combinations. Surgical procedures may combine several classifications and labels (eg, a client who has been in an automobile accident and has severe trauma and bleeding may require major, reconstructive, emergency surgery). It is important to remember that no matter the defined degree of risk, any surgical procedure imposes physical and psychologic stress and seldom is considered minor by the client.

Anesthesia

Anesthesia, depending on its classification as *general* or *regional*, produces such states as narcosis (loss of consciousness), analgesia, relaxation, and loss of reflexes. General anesthesia produces all of these responses, whereas regional anesthesia does not cause narcosis, but does result in analgesia and reflex loss. Anesthetic agents are administered by a physician, an anesthesiologist (medical doctor), or a nurse anesthetist.

General Anesthesia. When a client is given drugs by inhalation, intravenous, rectal, or oral route to produce central nervous system depression, it is termed **general anesthesia**. The desired action of general anesthesia is loss of consciousness, relaxation of skeletal muscles, and reduction of reflex action. The choice of route and type of anesthesia is primarily made by the anesthesiologist after discussion with the client. Many factors influence the choice, including the type and length of surgery and the physical and psychologic status of the client (Meeker & Rothrock, 1991). Inhalation anesthesia often is used because it has the advantage of rapid excretion and reversal of effects.

There are three phases of general anesthesia—induction, maintenance, and emergence. Induction begins with administration of the anesthetic agent and continues until the client is ready for the incision. Maintenance continues from this point until near the completion of the procedure. Emergence starts as the client begins to "emerge" from the anesthesia and usually ends when the client is ready to leave the operating room; the length of time depends on the depth and length of anesthesia (Meeker & Rothrock, 1991).

General anesthesia has both advantages and disadvantages. The advantages are that it can be used for clients of any age and for any surgical procedure, leaving the client unaware of physical trauma. There are, however, major risks of circulatory and respiratory depression.

Regional Anesthesia. Regional anesthesia occurs when an anesthetic agent is injected or applied topically near a nerve or nerve pathway, inhibiting the transmission of sensory stimuli to central nervous system receptors. The client receiving the regional anesthesia remains awake but loses sensation in a specific part of the body. In some instances, reflexes also may be lost. Regional anesthesia may be accomplished by surface anesthesia, local infiltration, nerve blocks, or subdural or epidural blocks. These are defined as follows:

- Surface (topical) anesthesia is used on mucous membranes, open skin surfaces, wounds, and burns. Cocaine, 4% to 10% solution, is the most commonly used agent; others are lidocaine (Xylocaine) and benzocaine.
- Local infiltration with an agent such as lidocaine or tetracaine 0.1% is used in minor surgical procedures such as skin biopsy and suturing small wounds.
- Nerve blocks are accomplished by injecting a local anesthetic around a nerve trunk supplying the area of surgery, such as the jaw, face, and extremities.
- Subdural blocks are used to provide spinal anesthesia. The injection of a local anesthetic into the subarachnoid space (through a lumbar puncture) causes sensory, motor, and autonomic blockage and is used for surgery of the lower abdomen, perineum, and legs. Adverse effects of spinal anesthesia may include hypotension, headache, and urine retention.

Informed Consent

Informed consent is when a client voluntarily agrees to undergo a particular procedure or treatment (such as surgery) after having received the following information, which should be given to the client in understandable words:

- Description of the procedure or treatment
- Name and qualifications of the person performing the procedure or treatment
- Explanation of the risks involved, including potential for damage, disfigurement, or death
- Explanation that the client has the right to refuse treatment and that consent can be withdrawn

Informed consent protects the client, the physician, and the healthcare institution. The form that is signed is a legal document as well as an ethical imperative. The responsibility for securing informed consent from the client lies with the person who will perform the procedure; this usually is the physician. The nurse, signing as witness, signifies that the client signed the consent form and was alert and aware of the act. The client always has the right to refuse treatment.

Consent forms are not legal if the client is confused, unconscious, sedated, mentally incompetent, or considered a minor (specific guidelines for minors are written in states in the United States and in provinces in Canada). Consent may be given in those instances by a parent, spouse, next of kin, or legal guardian. In emergency situations, the physician may obtain consent over the telephone or by court order. More detailed information about informed consent is included in Chapter 7.

Ambulatory Surgery

Surgical procedures performed in ambulatory (also referred to as outpatient or same-day) surgical settings are becoming more common as hospitals respond to government regulations formulated to reduce length of hospital stay as well as costs to third-party insurance companies. These surgical settings may be found as freestanding units, in hospitals, and in physicians' offices.

Many procedures that formerly required hospitalization are done routinely in ambulatory surgery and are in fact mandated by the federal government and the Health Care Financing Administration. Included are such procedures as cataract extraction, arthroscopy, hemorrhoidectomy, crushing of kidney stones and gallstones with sound waves, and gynecologic procedures.

By allowing the client to spend the night before surgery at home and to return to his or her own home to convalesce, much of the stress associated with surgery is eliminated. Clients who are older or chronically ill or who do not have support systems to provide the care needed after surgery may require additional teaching and home care.

Preoperative nursing assessments and teaching are key elements in providing care for the ambulatory surgical client (Fig. 30-1). Preoperative teaching often can be combined with preoperative screening tests, which usually are done 2 to 5 days before the scheduled surgery. Preoperative teaching for ambulatory surgery includes the following instructions to the client:

- List medications routinely taken and ask the physician which should be taken or omitted the morning of surgery.
- Notify the surgeon's office if a cold or infection develops before surgery.
- List allergies and be sure the operating staff is aware of these.
- Remove nail polish and do not wear makeup for the procedure.
- Leave all jewelry and valuables at home.
- Wear clothing that buttons in front; short-sleeved garments are better for surgery on the hands.
- Have someone available for transportation home after recovery from anesthesia.

Teaching should also include written instructions covering the following:

- Limitations on eating or drinking before surgery, with a specific time to begin the limitations
- When and where to arrive for the procedure as well as the estimated time when the procedure will be performed

Preoperative Nursing Care

Clients who require surgical intervention and nursing care enter the healthcare setting in a wide variety of situations, ranging from essentially healthy people who have planned elective procedures to emergency admissions for treatment of trauma. Surgical clients may be any age and at any point on the health–illness continuum. It is the nurse's responsibility to identify factors that affect risk from a surgical procedure; assess physical and psychosocial needs of the client and family; and establish a plan of care, based on appropriate nursing diagnoses, that includes interventions to meet needs and facilitate recovery as the client progresses through the perioperative period. The desired outcomes of the plan of care for the surgical client, outlined by the Association of Operating Room Nurses (1993), are that the client will:

- Be free from injury related to positioning; retained foreign objects; or chemical, physical, or electrical hazards
- Be free from infection
- Maintain fluid and electrolyte balance
- Maintain skin integrity
- Demonstrate an understanding of the physiologic and psychologic responses to the planned surgery
- Participate in a rehabilitation process following surgery

ASSESSING

The importance of preoperative assessment cannot be overemphasized. Surgery is a major trauma to the body, and preoperative assessments identify factors that may place the client at greater risk for complications during and after surgery. Assessment of the surgical client includes a nursing history and physical assessment to establish baseline data, identify risk factors, and determine teaching and psychosocial needs of the client and the client's family. The assessment is often conducted several days before surgery as part of preoperative laboratory screening and teaching. It may be conducted in the hospital or, as is more likely in today's healthcare system, in a surgical clinic, office, or even in the client's own home.

Nursing History

The nursing history identifies risk factors and strengths in the client's physical and psychosocial status. Information significant to the surgical experience includes a health history, lifestyle habits, and coping patterns and support systems, including client perceptions of self and surgery.

Health History

Health history data that identify risk factors and individualize assessments are developmental level, medical history, medications, previous surgeries, and perceptions and knowledge of the surgery to be done.

Developmental Considerations. Infants and older adults are at a greater risk from surgery than are children and young and middle-aged adults. The infant has a lower total blood volume, making even a small loss of blood a serious consideration because of the risk of dehydration and the inability to respond to the need for increased oxygen during surgery. The infant also has difficulty maintaining stable body temperature during surgery because the shivering reflex is not well developed, making potential hypothermia or hyperthermia more likely.

Physiologic changes associated with aging (described in Chapter 10) increase the surgical risk for the older client (Fromm & Metzler, 1993). These changes, summarized in the accompanying box, decrease the older adult's ability to respond to the stress of surgery, alter the response to preoperative and postoperative medications and anesthesia, and prolong or alter wound healing processes. With an increasingly older adult population, assessment of physiologic changes is critical in providing knowledgeable, safe, holistic nursing care to the older surgical client. Other chronic illnesses, more

PRE-ADMISSION TEACHING/TESTING PERI-OPERATIVE ASSESSMENT

DATE OF VISIT:

SURGICAL HISTORY:

ANESTHESIA HISTORY:

SYSTEMS REVIEW: **Allergy:**

Dental:

CONTACT LENS/IOL:

HEARING AID:

CARDIOVASCULAR

Rheumatic Fever: Murmur:

Hypertension: Infarction:

Date Last EKG:

RESPIRATORY

Pneumonia: TBC:

Asthma: Recent URI:

Date Last CXR:

HEMATOLOGY

Bleeding Tendency:

GI

Recent Vomiting: Diarrhea:

Jaundice: Hepatitis:

GYN

L.M.P.: Para:

Gravida:

GU

UTI/Problems:

NEUROPSYCH

Syncope: Epilepsy:

MUSCULOSKELETAL

Arthritis: Neck or Back Inj.:

R.O.M.: Prothesis:

Skin Integrity:

METABOLIC

Diabetes:

Thyroid:

MEDICATIONS:

B/P ____ T. ____ P. ____ R. ____ WT. ____ HT. ____

PLANNED SURGERY & DATE:

Lab Ordered:

Abnormal Lab work called to

Dr. ____ on ____ Initials ____

X-ray

Abnormal X-ray called to

Dr. ____ on ____ Initials ____

EKG

Abnormal EKG work called to

Dr. ____ on ____ Initials ____

PRE-OP TEACHING GUIDELINES

___ Pre-Op Injection	___ Shave Prep
___ Transported to Holding Room	___ Awake in Recovery Room
___ Visitors To Waiting Room	___ Oxygen Face Tent
___ I.V. Fluids	___ Deep Breaths & Cough
___ Pneumatic Boots (Appr. Surg.)	___ Frequent Check BP & P
___ Leggins (Cysto or GYN)	___ NPO after MN or Liq. Breakfast
___ Taken to O.R.	___ Cannot Drive Self Home
___ Strap	___ Jewelry, Make-up Left Home
___ BP Cuff, Monitor Pads	___ Wear Loose Clothing
___ Bovie Pad	___ Video ____
	___ Hand-out/Packet ____

NOTES:

RECOVERY ROOM FOLLOW UP:

POST-OP FOLLOW-UP:

PHONE:

Figure 30-1
Example of a same-day surgery assessment record.

Focus on the Older Adult

Physiologic Changes With Aging That Increase Surgical Risk

System	Change	Preoperative Nursing Interventions
Cardiovascular	• Decreased cardiac output, heart rate, and cardiac reserve • Decreased peripheral circulation • Increased vascular rigidity	• Establish baseline data of vital signs. • Assess peripheral pulses. • Teach leg exercises, turning, and ambulating. • Document normal activity levels and tolerance of fatigue.
Respiratory	• Reduced vital capacity • Diminished cough reflex • Decreased oxygenation of blood	• Establish baseline data of respiratory depth and rate. • Teach coughing and deep-breathing exercises. • Assess color of skin.
Neurologic	• Sensory deficit • Decreased reaction time	• Orient to surroundings. • Institute safety measures (eg, elevate side rails, use night light). • Allow additional time for questions and teaching.
Renal	• Decreased renal blood flow • Reduced bladder capacity	• Assess amount and times of voiding. • Monitor fluid and electrolyte status. • Institute intake and output.
Integument	• Decreased vascularity • Dry, inelastic	• Assess skin status. • Monitor fluid status. • Monitor nutritional status.

common in the older population, also increase surgical risk and may require adaptations of usual perioperative procedures. For example, the client with congestive heart failure may be more easily fatigued and so unable to be up and about as rapidly after surgery, or the client with chronic obstructive pulmonary disease may have increased respiratory difficulty and require more frequent postoperative respiratory assessments and interventions.

Medical History. The medical history provides information about past and current illnesses; pathologic changes associated with past and current illnesses increase surgical risk as well as the potential for postoperative complications. Preoperative assessments and documentation are necessary to provide a data base for individualized assessments and interventions in the intraoperative and postoperative phases of care. The following are selected examples and associated risks:

Cardiovascular diseases such as thrombocytopenia, hemophilia, recent myocardial infarction or cardiac surgery, congestive heart failure, or dysrhythmias increase the potential for hemorrhage and hypovolemic shock, hypotension, venous stasis, thrombophlebitis, and overhydration with intravenous fluids.

Pulmonary disorders such as pneumonia, bronchitis, asthma, or chronic obstructive pulmonary diseases increase the possibility of respiratory depression from anesthesia as well as postoperative pneumonia, atelectasis, and alterations in acid–base balance.

Kidney and liver function alterations influence the client's response to anesthesia, affect fluid and electrolyte as well as acid–base balance, alter the metabolism and excretion of drugs, and impair wound healing.

Metabolic disorders, especially diabetes mellitus, increase the potential for hypoglycemia or acidosis and slow wound healing.

Medications. Use of drugs, whether prescribed or over-the-counter, can affect the client's reaction to and increase the risk from the stress of surgery and the effects of the anesthetic agent. Many medications are cancelled when a client goes to surgery, but it is important for the nurse to know the purposes and specific actions of drugs as well as physician's orders; specific medications may be given even when the client is going to surgery (eg, clients with heart or cardiovascular problems and those with diabetes mellitus).

Surgical risk is increased by drugs in the following categories:

Anticoagulants—may precipitate hemorrhage

Diuretics—may cause electrolyte imbalances, with resulting respiratory depression from anesthesia

Tranquilizers—may increase the hypotensive effect of anesthetic agents

Adrenal steroids—abrupt withdrawal may cause cardiovascular collapse in long-term users

Antibiotics—those in the mycin group, when combined with certain muscle relaxants used during surgery, can cause respiratory paralysis

Previous Surgery. Data about previous surgeries provide a knowledge base for meeting physical and psychologic needs throughout the perioperative period. Physical implications of previous surgeries are important to the intraoperative and postoperative phases (eg, previous heart or lung surgery may necessitate adaptations in anesthesia and in positioning during surgery). Complications after prior surgery, such as pneumonia, thrombophlebitis, or wound infection, provide data to support careful postoperative monitoring.

The client's past experiences with surgery also affect the plan of care established in the preoperative phase, especially if those experiences were negative. When the interview elicits negative feelings about the surgical experience, pain control, or nursing interventions carried out to prevent complications during previous surgeries, teaching and mutual goal setting are even more important.

Perceptions and Knowledge of Surgery. Included in the medical history review are the client's perceptions and knowledge of the surgical procedure to be performed. Questions asked or statements made by the client provide a base for meeting psychologic and family needs when preparing the client for surgery.

Lifestyle

The nursing history data about the client's lifestyle provide valuable information about surgical risk and postoperative recovery and rehabilitation. Areas especially important for the surgical client are nutrition, use of alcohol or nicotine, activities of daily living, and occupation.

Nutrition. Both malnutrition and obesity increase surgical risk. Surgery increases the body's need for nutrients, necessary for normal tissue healing and resistance to infection. The client who is malnourished is at higher risk for alterations in fluid and electrolyte balance, delay in wound healing, and wound infection. The obese client is at increased risk for pulmonary, cardiovascular, and gastrointestinal problems. Fatty tissue is more difficult to suture and has less resistance to infection; postoperative complications of delayed wound healing, wound infection, and disruption in the integrity of the wound are more common (Smeltzer & Bare, 1996).

Use of Alcohol or Nicotine. Clients whose alcohol intake habitually is large require larger doses of anesthetic agents and postoperative analgesics, increasing the risk of drug-related complications. Clients who smoke are at higher risk for respiratory complications after surgery. Pulmonary secretions are retained by all clients during anesthesia, but the smoker, who already has increased mucous secretions and decreased ciliary action in the tracheobronchial tree, has more difficulty clearing the respiratory passages after surgery. In addition, the tracheobronchial mucosa is chronically irritated in people who smoke; anesthesia further increases this irritation.

Activities of Daily Living. Exercise and rest and sleep habits are important considerations in preventing postoperative complications and facilitating recovery. A client with a well-established exercise program has improved cardiovascular, respiratory, metabolic, and musculoskeletal function, thereby lowering the risks of surgery. Rest and sleep are essential to physical and emotional adaptation and recovery from the stress of surgery. Information from the nursing history allows the nurse to individualize interventions to promote rest and sleep.

Occupation. Many surgical procedures require a delay in returning to a career or occupation or may necessitate a change in the way the client supports self and family. Knowledge of a client's usual work and concerns about returning to work prepare the nurse for necessary teaching and referrals.

Coping Patterns and Support Systems

Assessment of the client's psychologic, sociocultural, and spiritual dimensions is as important as the physical history and examination. Surgery is a major psychologic stressor and affects coping patterns, support systems, and sociocultural needs.

Coping Patterns. A surgical procedure, no matter whether planned or unexpected, major or minor, causes anxiety and fear. The nursing history interview often is a time when the nurse can use cues from verbal and nonverbal communication of the client and family to identify fears and concerns and to plan nursing interventions to provide information and emotional support necessary to the successful recovery from surgery.

Surgery is an unknown experience over which a person has no control; the resulting anxiety may be expressed in many ways, such as anger, withdrawal, apathy, confrontation, or questioning. Therapeutic communication skills are essential in establishing the trusting nurse–client relationship necessary to identify and resolve fear. The causes of fear in the preoperative phase include the following:

Fear of the unknown: The client has fears about the surgery itself, the anesthesia, the diagnosis, the future, financial and family responsibilities, response to pain, or possible disfigurement or disability.

Fear of pain or death: Common fears are that the anesthesia will not "put me to sleep," that death

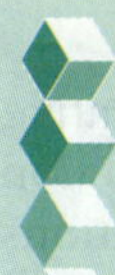

Research in Nursing: Making a Difference

Postoperative Nursing Care

Nursing care of the client in the postoperative period must be individualized to meet the complex needs of the client and facilitate a return to health. The studies discussed here illustrate the wide variety of problems that may occur and interventions that may be implemented during the care of clients after surgery.

Related Research

Kane, A., & Kurlowica, L. (1994). Improving the postoperative care of acutely-confused older adults. *MEDSURG Nursing, 3*(6), 453–458.
Acute confusion is often the first indication of an acute medical problem in the older surgical client. If untreated, it can lead to negative postoperative outcomes, including injury, risk of increased illness or death, increased costs, and longer hospital stays. Nursing management includes early management through recognition of confusion behaviors and contributing factors; ongoing assessment of the effects of other illnesses and the side effects of medications; and interventions to maintain environmental safety, provide orientation, promote normal sleep patterns, and enhance client awareness. Clinical practice guidelines for this at-risk population were developed based on actual client situations.

Hawthorne, M. (1994). Gender differences in recovery after coronary artery surgery. *IMAGE: Journal of Nursing Scholarship, 26*(1), 75–80.
Coronary artery bypass surgery is one of the most commonly performed surgical procedures for coronary artery disease. This study explored how perceptions of cardiac surgery differ by gender and role expectations, and how such differences can influence recovery. Data from interviews of men and women in two studies were analyzed for themes. The researchers found that coronary artery surgery in men constitutes a major life crisis, precipitating a realization of their own mortality and vulnerability. They were more likely to follow specific discharge guidelines, and to feel a special intimacy with the surgeon and other caregivers. Women regarded the surgery as less threatening, and as having a lesser impact on perception of self and lifestyle than did men. Women were more likely to use role responsibilities and fatigue as guides for activities and rehabilitation than they were to follow specific instructions. The goal of this research was to stimulate thinking about clients in new ways and to increase caregiver awareness of gender bias.

Good, M. (1995). A comparison of the effects of jaw relaxation and music on postoperative pain. *Nursing Research, 44*(1), 52–57.
The purpose of this study was to compare the effects of jaw relaxation and music, individually and combined, on postoperative pain. Subjects were 84 clients who had elective abdominal surgery in four hospitals during a 7-month period. The subjects were assigned to four groups: relaxation, music, combination, and control (no relaxation or music). Contrary to expectations, none of the clients reported effective pain reduction with these interventions. The researchers suggest that other methods of relaxation may be more effective as alternate methods of pain control, and that further studies should investigate appropriate interventions in relation to contextual and personal variables. These interventions may include jaw relaxation and music in clients who are interested, capable, and adequately medicated for pain.

Summary

These studies illustrate the ways in which nurses identify client needs and solve problems in client care during the postoperative period. As the population continues to age, consideration of the special needs of the older adult will become increasingly important. Gender differences in responses to illness and treatment are an emerging focus of individualized care. Nursing interventions to provide alternate methods of pain self-management are a significant part of holistic care. Nursing research in these areas will continue to provide the knowledge base for interventions to improve client outcomes following surgery.

will occur during surgery, or that the client will not be able to handle postoperative pain.

Fear of changes in body image and self-concept: Surgical procedures often leave the client with permanent changes in body structure, function, or appearance. Clients commonly fear alterations in physical attractiveness, social relationships, lifestyle, and sexuality.

The nurse should encourage the client to identify and verbalize fears; often simply talking about fears helps to diminish the magnitude that has built up. At the same time, incorrect knowledge can be identified and corrected, strengths can be identified, and teaching can be done. The reduction of fear is of major importance in preoperative preparation; emotional stress added to the physical stress of surgery increases surgical risk.

Support Systems. Coping with stress can be facilitated through various support systems identified during the assessment phase of preoperative nursing care. As much as possible, family members or significant others should be part of the initial interview and should be included in discussions of fears and concerns. Family members should be encouraged to be part of the surgical experience, providing support before and after surgery.

By identifying spiritual beliefs in the nursing history, the nurse can support the client's spiritual needs through acceptance, participation in prayer, or referral to clergy or chaplain. Faith in a higher being provides support and helps to reduce fears.

The need for other support systems also can be identified in the initial interview (eg, the client having a colostomy or mastectomy may have many questions answered and anxieties reduced by a preoperative visit from a person who has had the same operation and adapted successfully).

The nursing history should elicit those ways in which a client provides self-support to reduce stress. These are discussed in Chapter 32 and range from listening to music to actively practicing relaxation techniques.

Sociocultural Needs. A person's perceptions of and reactions to the surgical experience are influenced by sociocultural factors, including family health beliefs and practices, economic factors, and cultural background.

As discussed in Chapter 4, each person is influenced by family health beliefs and practices. A client who requires surgery but has grown up in a family that believes that surgical intervention is the last possible option in treating illness may refuse to have surgery or may be convinced that death will result. The resulting anxiety may make this particular client even more susceptible to surgical risk. Reactions to teaching, physical care, and pain also are influenced by family values and cultural/ethnic identity (eg, the male client reared with the belief that it is unmanly to acknowledge pain presents a stoic acceptance of pain and refuses needed medications postoperatively).

Cultural influences also affect the client's responses to and perceptions of the surgical experience. Cultural backgrounds may require that nursing interventions be individualized to meet needs in such areas as language, food preferences, family interactions and participation, personal space, and health beliefs and practices (eg, a client from a culture that believes that bed rest is the most important treatment for illness or injury may have difficulty accepting the need for postoperative exercises and ambulation).

Physical Assessment

Assessing the client's current physical status provides data for interventions to decrease surgical risk and potential postoperative complications. Depending on the situation, the physical assessment is conducted as described in Chapter 26. Table 30-2 summarizes assessments specific to the surgical client.

Screening Tests

Various screening tests conducted in the preoperative phase provide objective data of normal body function or, if abnormal, provide data for medical interventions to improve physical status and thus decrease potential surgical complications. The nurse's role is to ensure that the tests are ordered and done, that the results are recorded in the client's record before surgery, and that abnormal findings are reported. Additionally, abnormal results provide data to support nursing diagnoses and collaborative problems. Usual screening tests include chest x-ray, electrocardiography, complete blood count, measurement of electrolyte levels, and urinalysis. Normal findings for laboratory tests are found in Appendix B. Significant abnormal findings include an elevated white blood cell count (presence of infection), decreased hematocrit and hemoglobin level (presence of bleeding, anemia), hyperkalemia or hypokalemia (increased risk of cardiac problems), elevated blood urea nitrogen or creatinine levels (possible renal failure), and abnormal urine constituents (indicating infection, fluid imbalances, renal failure).

DIAGNOSING

Nursing diagnoses for the client in the preoperative phase may be identified for various actual or potential problems, based on the analysis of subjective and objective data obtained from the nursing history and physical examination as well as information from other health team members and screening tests. Many diagnoses reflect assessment of potential risk and are made to provide interventions to meet client needs during the intraoperative and postoperative phases. Nursing care throughout the perioperative period must be consistent and documented; the preoperative nursing diagnoses are the bases for consistent, holistic care from admission through recovery.

Examples of nursing diagnoses appropriate to the preoperative period are as follows:

- Anticipatory Grieving related to perceived loss of normal body image resulting from scheduled amputation of left leg
- Anxiety related to the effects of surgical procedure on ability to function as primary wage earner and head of the family
- Fear related to surgery for treatment of cancer of the breast and unknown future
- Risk for Infection related to age (77), obesity, and abdominal incision to remove intestinal tumor
- Ineffective Airway Clearance related to 25-year history of smoking and administration of anesthesia during surgery
- Ineffective Individual Coping related to conflict between need for surgery and religious belief (member of Christian Scientist faith)

Table 30-2
Preoperative Physical Assessments

Component	Assessment	Purpose
General survey	• Height • Weight • Vital signs	• Indicates nutritional status, especially obesity and malnutrition • Provides baseline data for intraoperative and postoperative phases • May indicate fluid and electrolyte imbalances or underlying infection
	• General appearance	• Reflects energy levels, physical and emotional status
Status of skin	• Oral cavity • Skin turgor • All skin surfaces, especially over bony prominences	• Indicates hydration levels • Significant in hydration status • Indicates potential for injury or pressure ulcers during and after surgery
Respiratory status	• Respiratory depth, rate • Adventitious sounds on auscultation • Diameter and shape of thorax	• Any abnormalities found would indicate potential respiratory difficulties during surgery, or postoperative atelectasis or infection
Cardiovascular status	• Apical pulse: character, rate, rhythm • Peripheral pulses • Presence of edema	• Provides baseline data for intraoperative and postoperative phases • Abnormal findings indicate potential complications intraoperatively and postoperatively, such as thrombophlebitis, emboli, congestive heart failure, arrhythmias
Abdominal status	• Size, shape, symmetry • Bowel sounds • Last bowel movement	• Provides baseline data for postoperative assessments
Neurologic status	• Level of consciousness • Mood • Motor and sensory function	• Provides baseline data for postoperative assessments • Especially important to postoperative assessment after spinal anesthesia

PLANNING: EXPECTED OUTCOMES

Preoperative nursing care is affected by the length of the preoperative phase. Clients who enter the hospital through the emergency department with the need for immediate surgery and those who have ambulatory surgery may not have time for comprehensive assessments and teaching. There has been a tremendous increase in the number of same-day and short-stay surgeries, in which clients are admitted early the morning of surgery. In such cases, it is imperative for the nurse to use standardized preoperative plans and individualize the plans for the particular client and family. Outcome criteria are standard for all clients having surgery, but nursing interventions must be designed to meet priority needs of specific clients and situations.

Planning for the entire perioperative period is done in the preoperative phase and includes expected outcomes that are mutually discussed and agreed on by the nurse, the client, and the family. Specific outcomes that would be appropriate are as follows. The client will:

- Be physically and emotionally prepared for surgery
- Demonstrate turning, coughing, and deep-breathing exercises
- Verbalize understanding of postoperative pain control
- Maintain fluid intake and nutritional balance to meet needs

To help the client meet these goals during the preoperative phase, the nurse must accomplish the following:

- Establish a data base and plan of care to meet client needs throughout the perioperative period
- Identify and meet client and family learning needs
- Identify physical and psychosocial risk factors
- Provide interventions to maximize physical and emotional safety and security

IMPLEMENTING

Preoperative nursing interventions provide the client with the necessary physical and psychologic preparation for surgery and the postoperative phase. This section of the chapter discusses implementing the plan of care to meet established client goals; Procedure 30-1 outlines the actions and rationales for preoperative client care.

Preparing the Client Psychologically

Surgery is almost always viewed as a life crisis and evokes anxiety and fear. Anxiety can be reduced and recovery can be facilitated by nursing actions that focus

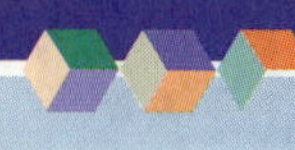

PROCEDURE 30-1

Preoperative Client Care: Hospitalized Client

Action	**Rationale**
General	
1. Identify clients for whom surgery is a greater risk: a. Very young and elderly clients b. Obese or malnourished clients c. Clients with fluid and electrolyte imbalances d. Clients in poor general health from chronic diseases and infectious processes e. Clients taking certain medications (ie, anticoagulants, antibiotics, diuretics, depressants, steroids) f. Clients who are extremely anxious	This allows for recognition of clients who may be prone to complications after surgery.
2. Reviewing nursing data base, history, and physical examination. Check that baseline data are recorded.	Review identifies clients who are surgical risks.
3. Check that diagnostic testing has been completed and results are available.	This check may influence type of surgery and anesthetic as well as timing of surgery or need for additional consultation.
4. Promote optimal nutrition and hydration status.	This promotes wound healing.
5. Identify learning needs of client. Conduct preoperative teaching regarding the following: a. Coughing and deep-breathing exercises b. Management of pain after surgery c. Leg exercises and ambulation d. Postoperative equipment and monitoring devices	This minimizes surgical risk and allays anxiety by preparing clients for postoperative period.

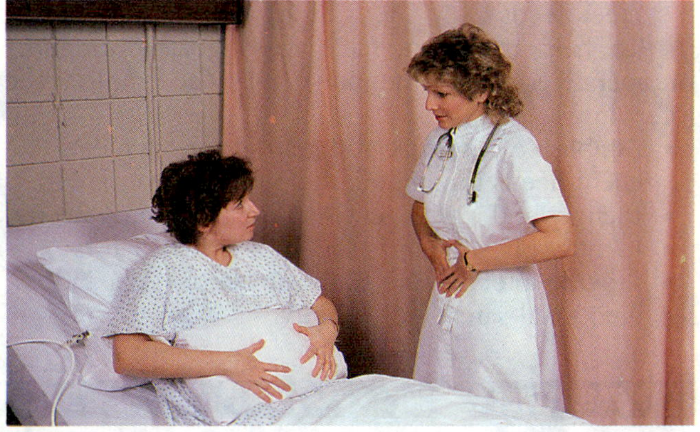

Action 5a: Teaching client to splint incision before coughing. (Photo © Ken Kasper.)

Action 5a: Teaching client to cough. (Photo © Ken Kasper.)

Action	**Rationale**
Day Before Surgery	
6. Provide emotional support. Answer questions realistically. Provide spiritual assistance if requested.	This allays client's misconceptions and fears.

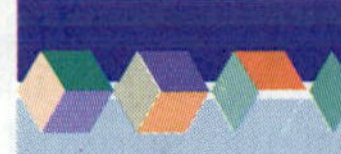

PROCEDURE 30-1 *(continued)*

Preoperative Client Care: Hospitalized Client

Action	Rationale
7. Follow preoperative dietary restrictions.	This reduces risk of vomiting and aspiration during surgery. Anesthetic agents temporarily depress gastrointestinal function and processes.
8. Prepare for elimination needs during and after surgery.	Anesthetic agents and abdominal surgery interfere with normal elimination function. A urinary catheter inserted preoperatively minimizes risk of inadvertent trauma to bladder during surgery.
9. Attend to client's special hygiene needs (ie, use of antiseptic cleaning agents).	This decreases potential for infection.
10. Provide for adequate rest.	Rest minimizes stress before surgery.
Day of Surgery	
11. Check that proper identification band is on client.	Double-checking ensures identity of client.
12. Check that preoperative consent forms are signed and medical record is in order.	This fulfills legal requirement related to informed consent.
13. Check vital signs. Notify physician of any pertinent changes (ie, rise or drop in blood pressure, elevated temperature, cough, symptoms of infection).	This provides baseline data for comparison.
14. Provide hygiene and oral care. Remind client not to swallow water if NPO for surgery.	This promotes comfort.
15. Continue nutritional and hydration preparation.	This prepares client for operative procedure.
16. Remove cosmetics and prostheses (eg, contact lenses, false eyelashes, dentures, and so forth). Assess for loose teeth.	These interfere with assessment during surgery.
17. Have client empty bladder and bowel prior to surgery.	An empty bladder and bowel minimize risk of injury or complications during and after surgery.
18. Place valuables in appropriate area. Hospital safe is most appropriate place for valuables. They should not be placed in narcotics drawer.	This ensures safety of valuables and personal possessions.
19. Attend to any special preoperative orders.	This prepares client for operative procedure.
20. Complete preoperative checklist and record of client's preoperative preparation.	This ensures accurate documentation.
21. Administer preoperative medication as ordered by physician.	Medication reduces anxiety, provides sedation, and diminishes salivary and bronchial secretions.

on therapeutic communications and client and family teaching.

Communicating

The nurse uses therapeutic communication skills and techniques, as described in Chapter 22, to establish a supportive and trusting nurse–client relationship and to facilitate psychologic safety and security. Guidelines for the nurse in meeting psychologic needs of the surgical client are as follows:

- Establish and maintain a therapeutic relationship, allowing the client to verbalize fears and concerns.
- Use active listening skills to identify and validate verbal and nonverbal responses indicative of anxiety and fear.
- Use touch, as appropriate, to demonstrate genuine empathy and caring.

- Be prepared to respond to common client questions about surgery:
  - Will I lose control of body functions while I'm having surgery?
  - How long will I be in the operating and recovery rooms?
  - Where will my family be?
  - Will I have pain when I wake up?
  - Will the anesthetic make me sick?
  - Will I need a blood transfusion?
  - How long will it be before I can eat?
  - What kind of scar will I have?
  - When will I be able to be sexually active?
  - When can I go back to work?

Remember that each client is a unique individual and will respond to the surgical experience in a unique way. One note of caution: The nontherapeutic use of false reassurance must be avoided. In an attempt to allay anxiety and fear, the nurse may be tempted to reassure the client that he or she will be fine. These responses deny the client's emotional needs, shut off therapeutic communications, and may not be true.

Teaching

Teaching about postoperative activities is implemented in the preoperative phase and is the nurse's responsibility. Clients and families need to know about surgical events and sensations, how to manage pain, and how to perform the physical activities necessary to decrease postoperative complications and facilitate recovery. The teaching–learning process (see Chapter 23) is individualized to meet both specific and common client needs.

The timing of teaching is a significant consideration; teaching that is done too far in advance of surgery or when the client is anxious will be less effective. In today's healthcare delivery system, clients often enter the hospital the day before or the day of surgery, and teaching must be adapted to this schedule. Many institutions provide teaching sessions before admission so that the client is prepared for surgery. Whether done before or after admission, a preoperative teaching checklist gives nurses organized and comprehensive guidelines for instruction (see the accompanying box).

Nursing research has indicated that the success of preoperative teaching varies with the timing of the teaching, the individual client and his or her support systems, the type of surgery, and group versus individual sessions. Preoperative teaching has proved to be beneficial in decreasing postoperative complications and in positively influencing recovery.

Surgical Events and Sensations. Clients and their families need to know when surgery is scheduled; about how long surgery and recovery room care will last; and what will be done before, during, and after surgery (procedures, medications, equipment). If the surgery is elective, a tour of the operating room suite is helpful in reducing anxiety and fear of the unknown (although especially helpful for children, this also is useful in teaching adult clients). An explanation of the surgical events includes a description of the various members of the healthcare team. An outline of surgical events is found in the preoperative teaching checklist box.

Sample Preoperative Teaching: Activities and Events for In-Hospital Surgery

Preoperative phase

- ☐ Exercises and physical activities
  - ☐ Deep-breathing exercises
  - ☐ Coughing
  - ☐ Incentive spirometry
  - ☐ Turning
  - ☐ Leg exercises
- ☐ Pain management
  - ☐ Meaning of prn orders
  - ☐ Timing for best effect
  - ☐ Splinting incision
- ☐ Visit by anesthesiologist
- ☐ Physical preparation
  - ☐ NPO
  - ☐ Sleeping medication the night before
  - ☐ Preoperative checklist (review items)
- ☐ Visitors and waiting room
- ☐ Transported to operating room by stretcher

Intraoperative phase

- ☐ Holding area
  - ☐ Skin preparation
  - ☐ Intravenous fluids
  - ☐ Medications
- ☐ Operating room
  - ☐ Operating room table
  - ☐ Lights
  - ☐ Restraints
  - ☐ Sensations
  - ☐ Staff

Postoperative phase

- ☐ Postanesthesia recovery area
  - ☐ Frequent vital signs
  - ☐ Dressings
  - ☐ Intravenous lines
  - ☐ Pain medications
  - ☐ Family notification
  - ☐ Sensations
  - ☐ Staff
- ☐ Transfer to unit (on stretcher)
  - ☐ Frequent vital signs
  - ☐ Sensations
  - ☐ Pain medications
  - ☐ NPO, diet
  - ☐ Exercises
  - ☐ Ambulation
  - ☐ Family visits

Clients also need to know what sensations they will be experiencing during the perioperative period. Although the sensations will differ depending on the type of surgery, teaching should include the following:

- Feelings experienced from preoperative medications, such as a dry mouth and drowsiness
- Sensations that normally occur after surgery and anesthesia, such as a sore throat from an endotracheal tube, a gradual return of feeling and movement after spinal anesthesia, and a lower tolerance of activity with increased fatigue
- Sensations experienced after surgery, such as incisional pain, intravenous catheters and fluids, tight dressings, dry mouth, and drowsiness

Pain Management. Pain is a normal part of the surgical experience and an area of major concern for the client and family. Guidelines for the management of acute surgical pain have been established by the Agency for Health Care Policy and Research (1992). These guidelines are based on a philosophy that (1) the pain reported by the client is the determining factor of pain control, (2) pain must be assessed as often as every two hours after major surgery, and (3) the older client is a risk for both under- and overtreatment of pain. The following are guidelines for teaching the client about pain control:

- Medications to relieve pain will be ordered by the physician and administered by the nurse.
- Pain medications may be ordered to be given on a regular basis or on an as-needed (PRN) basis. If medication is ordered PRN, there is a time restriction between doses (eg, every 2 to 4 hours). The client needs to ask for the medication and should do so before the pain is severe. If the medication does not control the pain, a different one can be ordered.
- Medications for pain usually are given by injection for the first few days (and as long as the client is NPO). With food intake and decreasing pain levels, oral medications can be used.
- There is little danger of addiction to pain medications when they are used in the postoperative management of pain.
- The use of relaxation techniques (such as deep breathing and guided imagery) facilitates the effects of pain medications.
- Pain medications facilitate the management of pain and increase the ability to carry out activities and exercises necessary for recovery.

Alternative methods of pain control, including transcutaneous electrical nerve stimulation (TENS) and patient-controlled analgesia (PCA), may be used after surgery. TENS is a nonpharmacologic technique that increases nerve fiber activity to close the gate to small nerve fibers; it also is believed to stimulate the release of endorphins, which are chemicals produced in the body that mediate pain perception. A TENS unit has electrodes that are placed on the skin along each side of the surgical incision. The client controls the electric current by pushing a button when feeling pain. A PCA pump allows the client to administer his or her own analgesic. When the client pushes the control button on the pump, a preset dose of analgesic medication is administered automatically. The time intervals between doses and the amount of medication that can be used within a given period are programmed into the device. The client must be taught before surgery how to use both of these methods of pain control, and the nurse is responsible for assessing the effectiveness of the pain relief. Further discussion of pain management is found in Chapter 41.

Physical Activities. The most common causes of postoperative complications are cardiovascular and pulmonary alterations, including atelectasis, pneumonia, thrombophlebitis, and emboli. Physical activities to reduce the potential of these complications are taught in the preoperative period. The following sections describe deep (diaphragmatic) breathing, coughing, incentive spirometry, leg exercises, and turning in bed. The client should be able to verbalize the purpose and demonstrate the activities before going to surgery. (This section gives the rationale for the activities; postoperative complications are discussed later in the chapter.)

Deep Breathing. During surgery, the cough reflex is suppressed, mucus accumulates in the tracheobronchial passageways, and the lungs do not fully ventilate. After surgery, respirations often are less effective as a result of the anesthesia, pain medications, and pain from the incision (eg, clients who have thoracic or high abdominal incisions are especially prone to shallow breathing because of incisional pain with deeper respirations). As a result, alveoli do not inflate and may collapse and secretions are retained, increasing the potential for atelectasis and pulmonary infection. Deep-breathing exercises hyperventilate the alveoli and prevent their recollapse, improve lung expansion and volume, help to expel anesthetic gases and mucus, and facilitate oxygenation of tissues.

The following are guidelines for teaching effective deep-breathing exercises:

- Place the client in semi-Fowler's position, with support for the neck and shoulders.
- Ask the client to place the hands over the rib cage, so he or she can feel the chest rise as the lungs expand.
- Ask the client to:
  - Exhale gently and completely.
  - Inhale through the nose gently and completely.
  - Hold his or her breath and mentally count to three.
  - Exhale as completely as possible through the mouth with lips pursed (as if whistling).
  - Repeat three times.
- This exercise should be done every 1 to 2 hours while the client is awake for the first 24 to 48 hours after surgery and as necessary thereafter, depending on risk factors and pulmonary status.

Coughing. Coughing facilitates the removal of retained mucus from the respiratory tract and usually is taught in conjunction with deep breathing. Coughing is painful; the client should be taught how to splint the incision (ie, to support the incision with a pillow or folded bath blanket, as shown in Procedure 30-1) and to use the period after pain medication has been administered to best advantage. The following are guidelines for teaching effective coughing:

- Place the client in a semi-Fowler's position, leaning forward.
- Provide a pillow or folded bath blanket to use in splinting the incision.
- Ask the client to:
  - Inhale and exhale deeply and slowly through the nose three times.
  - Take a deep breath and hold it for 3 seconds.
  - "Hack" out for three short breaths.
  - With mouth open, take a quick breath.
  - Cough deeply once or twice.
  - Take another deep breath.
- Repeat the exercise every 2 hours while awake.

Incentive Spirometry. An incentive spirometer often is ordered for clients having surgery, and the proper technique for using it should be practiced preoperatively. This device helps to increase lung volume and inflation of alveoli and facilitates venous return. The following points should be included in client teaching:

- Sit upright or elevate the head of the bed 45 degrees.
- Take two or three normal breaths and then insert the spirometer's mouthpiece into the mouth.
- Inhale through the mouth and hold the breath for 3 to 5 seconds.
- Exhale slowly and fully.
- Repeat the sequence 10 times during each waking hour for the first 5 days after surgery (except immediately before or after meals).

Leg Exercises. During surgery, venous blood return from the legs slows; some surgical positions also may decrease venous return. With circulatory stasis of the legs, thrombophlebitis and resultant emboli are potential complications. Leg exercises increase venous return through flexion and contraction of the quadriceps and gastrocnemius muscles. The following are guidelines for teaching the client leg exercises (Fig. 30-2):

- Alternately point toes toward the chin (dorsiflex) and toward the foot of the bed (plantar flex); then, make a circle with the toes.
- Flex and extend the knees, pressing them down toward the mattress on extension.
- Raise and lower each leg, keeping the leg straight.
- Repeat the exercises every 1 to 2 hours.

Leg exercises must be individualized to client needs, physical condition, physician preference, and agency protocol.

Turning in Bed. Turning in bed improves venous return, respiratory function, and gastrointestinal peristalsis.

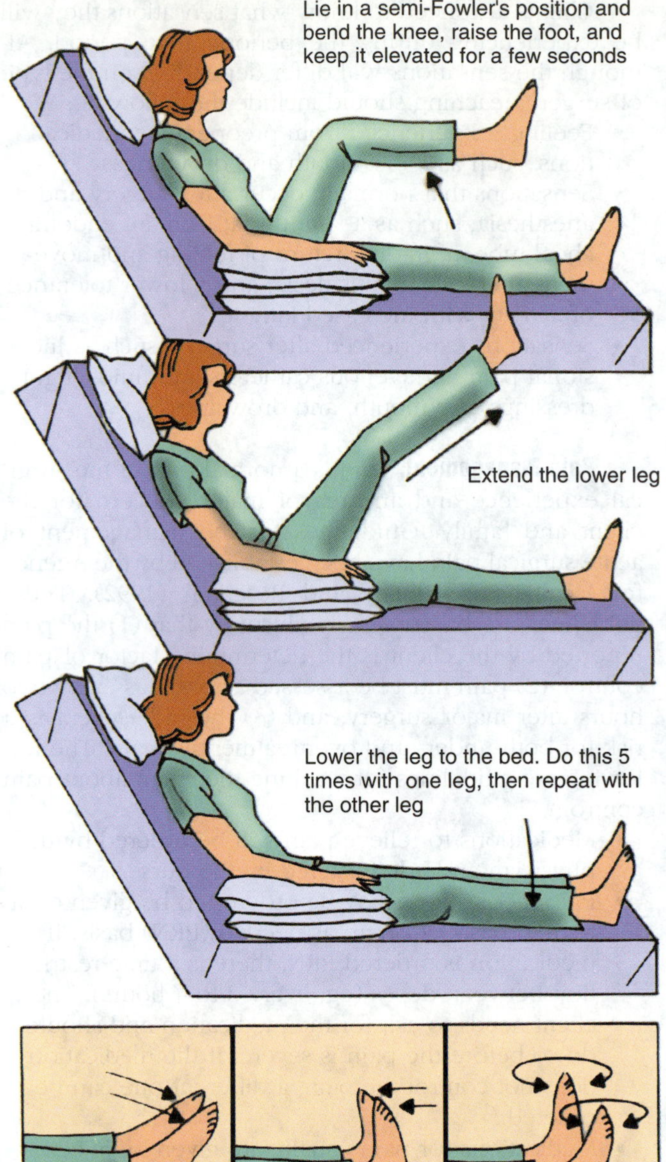

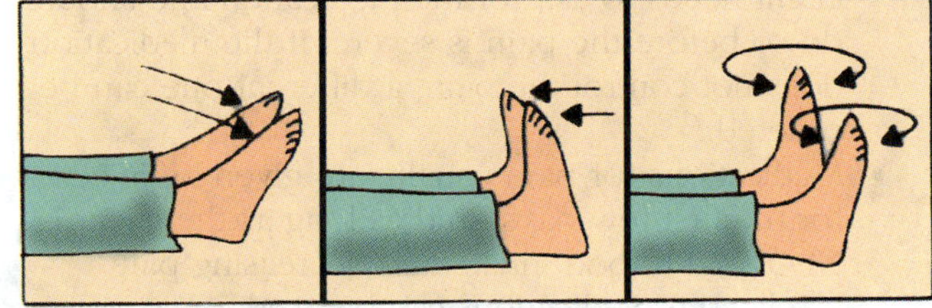

A. Point the toes of both feet toward the foot of the bed. Relax both feet
B. Pull toes toward the chin. Relax both feet
C. Make circles with both ankles. First circle to the right, then to the left. Repeat 3 times, relax feet

Figure 30-2
Leg exercises to increase venous return.

Although turning in bed sounds like a simple procedure, incisional pain makes it more difficult, and it should be practiced before surgery. To turn in bed, the client should raise one knee, reach across to grasp the side rail (on the side toward which he or she is turning), and roll over while pushing with the bent leg and pulling on the side rail. A small pillow is useful in splinting the incision while turning. The client should turn from side to side every 2 hours.

Preparing the Client Physically

The physical preparation of the client for surgery may vary, depending on the client's physical status and special needs, type of surgery to be done, and physician's orders. Certain nursing interventions are appropriate for all surgical clients in the areas of hygiene and skin preparation, elimination, nutrition and fluids, and rest and sleep. The nurse also is responsible for the preparation and safety of the client on the day of surgery.

Hygiene and Skin Preparation

Intact skin is the body's first line of defense against microorganisms, and an alteration in skin integrity (such as the surgical incision) provides a potential source of infection. Therefore, the skin is prepared to minimize skin contamination and decrease the risk of postoperative wound infection.

The skin is cleaned by scrubbing the operative site one or more times with an antibacterial soap or solution to remove bacteria. This can be done by the client while taking a bath or shower. Ideally, a shower is taken the evening before or the morning of surgery. Shampooing the hair and cleaning the fingernails also help to reduce the number of organisms present.

The incisional area usually is shaved before surgery because hair serves as a reservoir for bacteria. This may be done on the unit or in surgery. Although shaving the skin was once done routinely the evening before surgery, it is now most often done immediately before the operation, usually in the surgical holding area, based on findings that small cuts made by the razor serve as sites for bacterial growth. Increased time for growth of bacteria increases the risk of infection. Depilatory creams or hair clippers may be used to remove hair and are recommended by the Centers for Disease Control. Agency protocol should be followed for timing, people responsible, and method.

Elimination

Emptying the bowel of feces is no longer a routine procedure before surgery, but the nurse should use preoperative assessments to determine the need for an order for bowel elimination. If the client has not had a bowel movement for several days or has had preoperative barium diagnostic tests, an enema helps to prevent postoperative constipation.

If the client is scheduled for surgery of the gastrointestinal tract, cleansing enemas usually are ordered. Peristalsis does not return for 24 to 48 hours after the bowel is handled, so preoperative cleansing helps to decrease postoperative constipation. An empty bowel also prevents contamination of the surgical area during surgery.

Insertion of an indwelling urinary catheter may be ordered before surgery, especially in clients having pelvic surgery, to prevent bladder distention or accidental injury. If an indwelling catheter is not in place, the client should void immediately before receiving preoperative medications to ensure an empty bladder during surgery.

Nutrition and Fluids

The diet order for the client having surgery depends on the type of surgery and type of anesthesia to be used. Clients having general anesthesia or major regional anesthesia are made NPO 8 to 12 hours before the surgery (often at midnight before next-morning surgery) to prevent aspiration of gastric contents if the client should vomit while anesthetized. However, more current practice is to allow clients to have clear liquids until 2 to 4 hours before surgery. The nurse explains the reason for being NPO to the client, removes all food and fluids from the bedside, and places a sign over the bed so that all health team members and visitors know about the restriction. If the client eats or drinks, the physician should be notified at once.

Clients need to be well nourished and hydrated before surgery to counterbalance fluid, blood, and electrolyte loss during surgery and to facilitate tissue healing after surgery. Preoperative assessments provide a base for physical preparation for surgery, including the need for supplemental nutrition, fluids, or electrolytes. The client who is undernourished may require parenteral nutrition (see Chapter 42) and intravenous electrolyte replacements. If the client's screening tests show a hemoglobin level of less than 10 g/dL and a hematocrit less than 33%, blood may be given preoperatively to maintain volume and increase oxygenation of tissue during surgery.

Rest and Sleep

Rest and sleep are important components in reducing stress before surgery and in healing and recovery after surgery. The nurse can facilitate rest and sleep in the immediate preoperative period by meeting psychologic needs, carrying out teaching, providing a quiet environment, and administering the prescribed bedtime sedative medication.

Preparing the Client on the Day of Surgery

The preoperative checklist in the accompanying box outlines the nurse's responsibilities on the day of surgery; these activities must be completed before the client is transported to surgery. Some of these activities have already been described (NPO, preoperative teaching, informed consent, skin preparation, screening tests, bladder elimination); other nursing responsibilities include the following:

- Take and record vital signs to serve as baseline data for the intraoperative phase, and assess for and report any abnormal findings (such as an elevated temperature).
- Prepare the client physically for the intraoperative phase.

Checklist for Preoperative Surgery

- ☐ Pre-op hypo ordered
- ☐ NPO after midnight or as ordered
- ☐ ID band on patient
- ☐ Pre-op teaching done
- ☐ Surgical permit signed
- ☐ Informed consent signed
- ☐ Operative area shave prepped
- ☐ History and physical dictated
- ☐ CBC report on chart
- ☐ Urinalysis report on chart
- ☐ Profile report on chart if ordered
- ☐ Blood screened (typed and matched)
- ☐ PT and PTT
- ☐ Chest x-ray report on chart
- ☐ EKG
- ☐ T ______ P ______ R ______ BP ______
- ☐ Dentures or partial plate removed
- ☐ Contact lenses or glasses removed
- ☐ Jewelry removed or secured
- ☐ Hairpins, makeup, and nail polish removed
- ☐ Hearing aid to OR with patient
- ☐ Bathed
- ☐ OR gown on patient
- ☐ Voided or catheterized and Foley emptied
- ☐ Pre-op antibiotic given if ordered
- ☐ Pre-op medication given
- ☐ Allergies
- ☐ Family OR waiting room
- ☐ Old chart to OR
- ☐ X-ray films from floor to OR

Comments: ______________________________

____

- Have the client remove all personal clothing and put on an operating room gown.
- Remove all hairpins or hairpieces. This prevents injury to the client during surgery as well as possible loss of hairpieces or wigs.
- Remove makeup and fingernail polish to allow intraoperative and postoperative assessment of skin and nailbeds for circulation and oxygenation of tissues.
- Remove all prostheses, such as dentures or partial plates, eyeglasses, contact lenses, and artificial limbs. Dentures may cause respiratory obstruction during anesthesia; other prostheses may be damaged or lost. Be sure items are stored safely while the client is in surgery.
- Remove jewelry to prevent loss or injury from swelling during or after surgery; if the client prefers not to remove a wedding band, it can be securely taped to the finger (in some types of surgery, leaving jewelry on is not allowed). When jewelry is removed, it should be given to a family member or locked in a safe place.
- Leave on a hearing aid, and be certain that operating and recovery room nurses know the client has one.
- Be sure that the client's identification bracelet is in place to ensure accurate identity.
- Note allergies according to institutional policy (eg, on the front of the client's record or on an allergy bracelet).

- Carry out any special procedures that are ordered, such as securing previous records, inserting a nasogastric tube, starting an intravenous line, applying antiembolic stockings or compression devices, or giving medications.
- Give the preoperative medications that are prescribed, either at a scheduled time or "on call" (the operating room will call and tell the nurse to give the medication). Commonly ordered medications are as follows:
  - *Sedatives and tranquilizers*, such as pentobarbital (Nembutal), chlorpromazine (Thyroxin), or diazepam (Valium), to alleviate anxiety and facilitate anesthesia induction
  - *Anticholinergics*, such as atropine and glycopyrrolate (Robinul), to decrease pulmonary and oral secretions and to prevent laryngospasm
  - *Narcotic analgesics*, such as morphine and meperidine hydrochloride (Demerol), to facilitate client sedation and relaxation and to decrease the amount of anesthetic agent needed
  - *Neuroleptanalgesic agents* (Innovar) to cause a general state of calmness and sleepiness
  - *Histamine-receptor antihistaminics*, such as cimetidine (Tagamet) and ranitidine (Zantac), to decrease gastric acidity and volume
- Maintain client safety by elevating side rails, lowering the bed (if possible), and instructing the client to stay in bed or on the stretcher.
- Meet the family (or other support person's) needs. The family of the hospitalized surgical client is told where the client will be taken after surgery (if a different location, such as the intensive care unit). The waiting area for the family is described, and the family is taken there after the client leaves for the operating room. The ambulatory surgery client usually waits in the waiting area with family members until it is time for surgery. The family is told that the surgeon will come to the waiting room to tell them what happened in surgery.
- Document, through checklists and narrative charting, the nursing interventions carried out.
- Assist in moving the client from the bed to the operating room stretcher when it is time to transport the client to surgery, ensuring accurate identification.

- Prepare the hospitalized client's bed (make a surgical bed) and room for postoperative care.
    - Have necessary equipment and supplies in the room for postoperative care (equipment to measure vital signs, intravenous standard, and so forth).

EVALUATING

Evaluating the plan of care for the preoperative phase is based on the expected outcomes. The plan is effective if the client is physically and emotionally prepared for surgery, can verbalize events and sensations of the perioperative period, and can demonstrate postoperative exercises and activities.

Intraoperative Nursing Care

The intraoperative phase of surgery begins with admission of the client to the surgical area and lasts until the client is transferred to the recovery area. Although the surgeon has the dominant role during this phase, the nurse has specific responsibilities and roles in collaboratively meeting client needs. The nursing process uses the preoperative data and plan as a base.

The type of surgery scheduled influences the assessments and interventions carried out by the nurse. For example, the nurse's role when caring for the client having ambulatory surgery may be that of providing client care from admission through dismissal, whereas the nurse's role for hospital-based surgery usually is specific to the phases (ie, one group of nurses provides care on the hospital unit preoperatively and postoperatively, another group practices operating room nursing, and still another group provides specific postanesthesia recovery room care). This section of the chapter discusses the role of the nurse specific to intraoperative care.

ASSESSING

The first room the client enters when transferred to the surgical area usually is the holding area. Nurses in surgical scrub dress identify the surgical client, assess the client's emotional and physical status, and verify the information on the preoperative checklist. They also may carry out ordered immediate preoperative care, including performing skin preparation, starting intravenous fluids (using a large-gauge intercatheter), and giving preoperative medications. The client's response to procedures is assessed and events of surgery are explained. When the operating room is prepared, a nurse from the operating room arrives to transport the client to the operating room.

In the operating room, the client is positioned on the operating table, anesthetized, and draped. The operating room nurse assesses the client and reviews preoperative data, paying particular attention to factors that increase surgical risk. The nurse also assesses the client during positioning and monitors supplies used to maintain safety for the client.

DIAGNOSING

Client problems in the intraoperative period are primarily related to the position of the client during the procedure, the effects of the anesthesia, and the incision. Appropriate nursing diagnoses include the following:

Impaired Skin Integrity related to 4-inch midline abdominal incision

Fluid Volume Deficit related to loss of blood during surgery

Risk for Injury related to positioning, anesthesia, and environmental hazards

Collaborative problems might include the following (Carpenito, 1995):

Potential complication: Hemorrhage

Potential complication: Infection

Potential complication: Neuromuscular damage

PLANNING: EXPECTED OUTCOMES

The planning phase of the nursing process focuses on preventing potential complications and client problems and on ensuring client safety. The expected outcomes are that the client will:

- Remain free of neuromuscular damage
- Maintain intact skin surfaces
- Have symmetric breathing patterns
- Be free of injury from burns, inaccurate count of supplies, and wound contamination

During the intraoperative phase, the nurse performs the following activities:

- Assesses and monitors the client's physiologic response
- Positions the client to prevent injury or alterations in skin, respiratory, or neuromuscular function
- Maintains the client's physical safety
- Maintains aseptic technique

IMPLEMENTING

During surgery, nurses function either as scrub nurses or as circulating nurses. *Scrub nurses* assist the surgeon during the surgery and maintain surgical asepsis while draping and handling instruments and supplies. The *circulating nurse* assesses the client on admission to the operating room, helps to position the client on the operating table, helps with monitoring devices, gets additional supplies, and (at the end of the surgical procedure) counts the number of instruments, needles, and gauze sponges used during the surgery to prevent the accidental loss of an item in the wound.

Positioning

The client is placed in a specific operative position after anesthesia has produced loss of consciousness and reflexes. The nurse must ensure client safety and comfort in positioning to prevent alterations in respiratory, vascular, and neuromuscular function (Walsh, 1993). The potential for skin injury is avoided by lifting, rather than rolling or pulling, the client to a position. Rolling or pulling can cause a shearing force, in which two or more tissue layers slide on each other, stretching subcutaneous blood vessels, obstructing blood flow, and contributing to pressure ulcers.

Although the various operative positions are not included here, the nurse needs to know which position was used and significant nursing considerations for that position. Two examples are as follows:

Trendelenburg's position: The downward displacement of the abdominal viscera decreases diaphragm movement and respiratory exchange; blood pools in the upper torso and blood pressure increases; hypotension can result with return to the supine position.

Lithotomy position: The placement of legs in stirrups causes pooling of blood in the legs, increasing the potential of thrombophlebitis. Pressure also can damage the peroneal nerve, with resultant footdrop.

Draping

Drapes are used to establish a sterile field around the operative site, preventing the passage of microorganisms between sterile and nonsterile areas. The only area left exposed is the incision site. Plastic adhesive drapes may be used to form a complete seal over the skin; with these drapes, skin color is visible and the incision is made through the drape.

Documenting

Throughout surgery, the nurse documents item counts, monitored data, positioning, medications, dressings, and so forth on the intraoperative record.

Transferring to the Postanesthesia Recovery Room

After the surgery, the client is carefully moved from the operating table to a stretcher. This is an especially critical time; sudden or rough handling can cause severe hypotension or potentially lethal cardiac or respiratory arrest. The client is then moved to the postanesthesia recovery (PAR) room, and relevant preoperative and postoperative assessments and interventions are communicated to the PAR nurses.

EVALUATING

Evaluation of the effectiveness of the plan of care for the intraoperative phase is based on the expected outcomes. If met, the plan was effective.

Postoperative Nursing Care

The postoperative phase can be divided into two stages—immediate care (usually provided in the postanesthesia recovery [PAR] room in both in-hospital and ambulatory surgery centers) and ongoing postoperative care, lasting from return to the unit through convalescence. Nursing assessments and interventions are consistent with those in the preoperative and intraoperative phases and are carried out to maintain function, promote recovery, and facilitate coping with alterations in structure or function.

In this section, assessments and nursing interventions are combined in discussing immediate postoperative care; the phases of the nursing process are used to describe ongoing postoperative care.

Immediate Postoperative Care

Nurses in the PAR assess postoperative clients, with emphasis on preventing complications from anesthesia or the surgery. Assessments are continuous and ongoing, using preoperative and intraoperative data as the bases for comparison. The assessments made in the PAR include respiratory status, cardiovascular status, central nervous system status, fluid status, wound status, and general condition. These assessments are made every 10 to 15 minutes initially. The average PAR stay is about 2 hours but depends on the type of surgery, length of anesthesia, and client response.

Respiratory Status

Assessments of respiratory function are made by monitoring respiratory rate, rhythm, and depth; by auscultating breath sounds; and by observing skin color. During the surgical procedure with general anesthesia, an artificial airway is inserted to maintain patent air passages. The airway is not removed until the laryngeal and pharyngeal reflexes return, allowing the client to control the tongue, cough, and swallow. Cardiovascular and mental status assessments provide data about oxygenation. The following assessments indicate ineffective ventilation:

- Restlessness, apprehension
- Unequal chest expansion with use of accessory muscles
- Shallow, noisy respirations
- Cyanosis
- Rapid pulse rate

Respiratory obstruction is the most common PAR emergency. It may be due to secretion accumulation, ob-

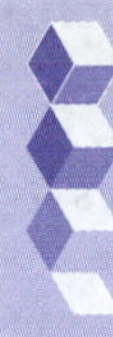

Through the Eyes of a Student

The first time I took care of a patient with "multiple tubes," I was horrified at the thought of actually touching the patient. I hadn't really been exposed to that many critically ill patients until my last semester as a student nurse. I remember being assigned a patient in the cardiothoracic intensive care unit in the hospital where I trained. The patient was a "fresh heart," commonly known as a cardiopulmonary bypass graft patient who had just been operated on that morning.

I remember walking into the room and thinking, "What do I do with all of these tubes?" and then with horror thinking "What if one of them falls out?" Needless to say, I was overwhelmed and frightened but at the same time excited at the challenge that faced me. I asked my preceptor what each tube was for and where it was hooked up and whether or not it would fall out if I touched it. She answered all my questions with patience and understanding and asked me if I wanted to actually handle the lines. I looked at her as if she were insane, but went ahead and did it. Would you believe that nothing fell out! I must admit that the experience taught me a lot, but also got me over the fear of tubes.

I now chuckle every time I see a nursing student's face with that same look of horror as I had and I try to answer every question with the same degree of patience and understanding that my preceptor had for me.

—Lynda L. Ullmer, R.N.
Gaithersburg, MD

struction by the tongue, laryngospasm (a sudden, violent contraction of the vocal cords), or laryngeal edema. Assessments of respiratory obstruction include those previously outlined plus wheezing or crowing sounds with respiratory effort.

Positioning, administering oxygen, and suctioning may be used to maintain a patent airway and tissue oxygenation.

Cardiovascular Status

Evaluation of cardiovascular function includes assessing blood pressure and pulses, skin color, respirations, and the wound.

Blood pressure findings are compared with baseline data from the preoperative period; hypotension may be the result of varied factors, including anesthetic agents, preoperative medications, position changes, blood loss, respiratory alterations, and peripheral blood pooling. Transient hypertension also can occur as a result of anesthetic effects, respiratory insufficiency, the surgical procedure, or the excitement phase of recovery from anesthesia. Low blood pressure can be increased by oxygen administration, deep breathing, leg exercises, verbal stimulation (to help expel anesthetic gases and facilitate increasing level of consciousness), and maintaining accurate intravenous flow rates.

All pulses are assessed for bilateral equality, rhythm, rate, and character. Of special significance are assessments of abnormal function—irregular rhythm, absence of pulses, and tachycardia. Tachycardia, an early symptom of shock, must be carefully evaluated. Other related assessments are cyanosis, edema, a cool skin temperature, and a decrease in urine output.

Central Nervous System Status

Anesthetics cause loss of consciousness and reflexes; the return of central nervous system function is assessed through response to stimuli and orientation. Reflexes return in reverse order, with the usual pattern being (1) unconsciousness, (2) response to touch and sounds, (3) drowsiness, (4) awake but not oriented, and (5) awake and oriented. Nurses in the PAR verbally reorient the client by touching and calling him or her by name.

Fluid Status

Fluid imbalance may be the result of such factors as preoperative fluid restriction, fluid loss during surgery, wound drainage, or stress (with retention of sodium and water). Fluid volume deficit or excess is a risk for all surgical clients but is especially so in children and older adults. Assessments of fluid status include skin turgor, vital signs, urine output, wound drainage, and intravenous fluid intake. Assessments of intravenous fluids include the type of fluid ordered, the rate, the needle insertion site, and the tubing.

Wound Status

The nurse in the PAR assesses the wound dressing for amount, consistency, and color of drainage as well as for any tubes or drains and drainage by that route. It also is important to assess underneath the client for drainage.

Large amounts of bright red drainage combined with other abnormal physical status assessments (restlessness, pallor, cold moist skin, decreasing blood pressure, increasing pulse and respiratory rates) may indicate hemorrhage and hypovolemic shock. These symptoms should be reported immediately.

General Condition

Other assessments and interventions are made to ensure physical and emotional comfort and safety. If the client is having pain and his or her condition has stabilized, pain medications are given (usually by the intravenous route). Most clients are cold and should be covered with blankets to keep them warm. Psychologic comfort is provided by constant reorientation and reassurance that the surgery is over. Physical safety is maintained by careful assessments, proper positioning, and use of side rails and restraints.

The client is dismissed from the PAR when physical status and level of consciousness are considered stable. The family is notified that the client is being transferred back to his or her room, and the PAR nurse gives a verbal report to the unit nurse about the assessments and interventions during the intraoperative and immediate postoperative phases.

Ongoing Postoperative Care

Nurses use the nursing process during all phases of perioperative care, with the focus being the special and unique needs of each client in each phase. Ongoing postoperative care is planned to facilitate recovery from surgery and coping with alterations. The plan of care is based on individualized nursing diagnoses and includes promoting physical and psychologic health, preventing complications, and teaching self-care when the client returns home. Procedure 30-2 outlines postoperative client care.

ASSESSING

The nurse on the unit assists PAR personnel in transferring the client to the bed in the unit room and, using data from the preoperative and intraoperative phases, makes an initial assessment. A postoperative checklist or flow sheet (Fig. 30-3) may be used. The initial assessment often is combined with the implementation of postoperative physician orders and includes the following:

Vital signs: Assess temperature, blood pressure, and pulse and respiratory rates. Note alterations from postoperative and PAR data as well as symptoms of complications (as discussed under Immediate Postoperative Care).

Color and temperature of skin: Assess for warmth, pallor, cyanosis, diaphoresis.

Level of consciousness: Assess orientation to time, place, and person as well as reaction to stimuli and ability to move extremities.

Intravenous fluids: Assess type and amount of solution, flow rate, tubing, and infusion site.

Wound: Assess dressing and dependent areas for drainage (color, amount, consistency). Assess drains and tubes and be sure they are intact, patent, and properly connected to drainage systems.

Other tubes: Assess indwelling urinary catheter, gastrointestinal suction, and so forth, for drainage, patency, and amount of output. Be sure dependent drainage bags are hanging properly and suction drainage is attached and functioning. If oxygen is ordered, ensure placement of ordered application and flow rate.

Comfort level: Assess for pain (location, duration, intensity) and, if present, determine if analgesics were given in the PAR room. Assess for nausea and vomiting.

Position and safety: Place the client in an ordered position (eg, after spinal anesthesia, client may have to remain flat for a specified period), or if the client is not fully conscious, place him or her in the side-lying position. Elevate the side rails and place the bed in low position.

Comfort: Cover the client with a blanket, reorient him or her to the room as necessary, and allow family members to remain with the client after initial assessment is completed.

After assessment, document time of arrival and all assessments. Follow agency protocol for assessment routines: common time frames are every 15 minutes until stable, changing to every 1 to 2 hours for the first 24 hours, and every 4 hours thereafter. Although agency protocols are used for guidelines in the immediate postoperative period, the nurse is responsible for adjusting the frequency and priorities of assessment to the specific needs of each client.

DIAGNOSING

Nursing diagnoses in the postoperative phase may be made for actual or potential altered responses or for collaborative problems to implement nursing actions necessary for monitoring and preventing postoperative complications. When making nursing diagnoses, the nurse uses assessment data and plans of care established before and during surgery and includes the family. Examples of postoperative nursing diagnoses include the following:

Risk for Infection related to traumatic wound of right arm in farm vehicle accident

Pain related to right flank incision

Altered Family Processes related to loss of economic stability following surgical treatment for bone malignancy

Impaired Verbal Communication related to repair and wiring of fractured jaw

Impaired Skin Integrity related to incision on left anterior thorax

Impaired Physical Mobility related to inability to be independent in movement secondary to surgical repair of fractured right hip

Appropriate collaborative problems for the client in the postoperative period include the following (Carpenito, 1995):

Potential complication: Hemorrhage
Potential complication: Evisceration
Potential complication: Dehiscence
Potential complication: Urinary retention
Potential complication: Thrombophlebitis
Potential complication: Paralytic ileus

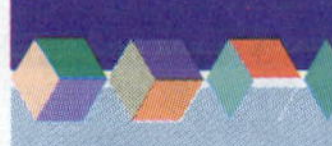

PROCEDURE 30-2

Postoperative Care When Client Returns to Room

Action	**Rationale**
Immediate	
1. Place client in safe position on side with face down and neck slightly extended. Note level of consciousness.	This prevents aspiration of vomitus and airway obstruction.
2. Monitor and record vital signs frequently. Assessment order may vary, but usual frequency includes taking vital signs every 15 minutes the first hour, every 30 minutes the next 2 hours, every hour for 4 hours, and, finally, every 4 hours.	Comparison with baseline preoperative vital signs may indicate impending shock or hemorrhage.
3. Provide for warmth. Assess skin color and condition.	Depressed level of functioning results in fall in body temperature.
4. Check dressings for color, odor, and amount of drainage, and feel under client for bleeding.	Hemorrhage and shock are life-threatening complications of surgery.

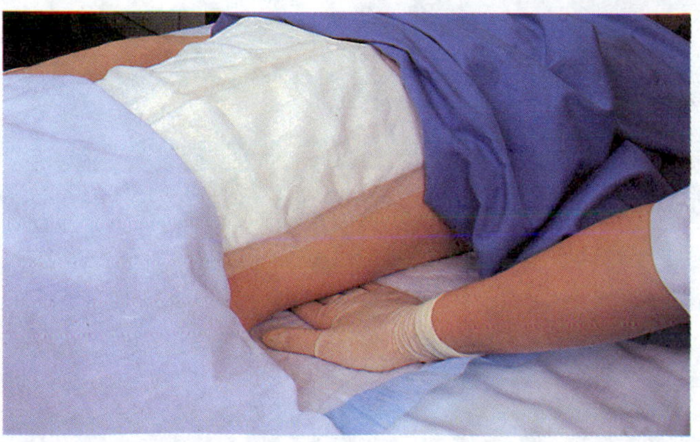

Action 4: Feeling under client for bleeding. (Photo © B. Proud.)

Action	**Rationale**
5. Verify that all tubes are patent and equipment is operative.	This ensures maintenance of vital functions.
6. Maintain intravenous infusion at correct rate.	This provides nutrition and prevents dehydration and electrolyte imbalances.
7. Provide for a safe environment. Keep bed in low position with side rails up. Have call bell within client's reach. Have NO SMOKING sign posted if client is receiving oxygen.	This prevents accidental injury.
8. Relieve pain by administering medications ordered by physician. Check record to verify if analgesic medication was administered in recovery room.	Analgesics are used for relief of postoperative pain.
9. Record assessments and interventions on chart.	This provides for accurate documentation.
General	
10. Promote optimal respiratory function: a. Coughing and deep breathing b. Incentive spirometry c. Early ambulation d. Frequent position change e. Administration of oxygen as ordered	Anesthetic agents may depress respiratory function: clients who have existing respiratory or cardiovascular disease or abdominal or chest incisions or who are obese or elderly or in a poor state of nutrition are at greater risk of developing respiratory complications.

(continued)

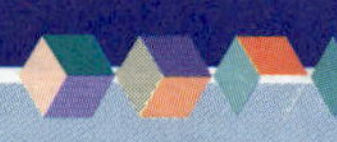

PROCEDURE 1-1 *(continued)*

Postoperative Care When Client Returns to Room

Action	Rationale
11. Maintain adequate circulation: a. Maintenance of intravenous therapy b. Early ambulation c. Application of antiembolic stockings if ordered by physician d. Leg and range-of-motion exercises if not contraindicated	Preventive measures can improve venous return and circulatory status.
12. Assess urinary elimination status: a. Promote voiding by offering bedpan at regular intervals b. Monitor catheter drainage if present c. Measure intake and output	Anesthetic agents may temporarily depress bladder tone and response.
13. Promote optimal nutrition status and return of gastrointestinal function: a. Assess for return of peristalsis b. Assist with diet progression c. Encourage fluid intake d. Monitor intake e. Medicate for nausea and vomiting as ordered by physician	Anesthetic agents depress peristalsis and normal functioning of gastrointestinal tract.

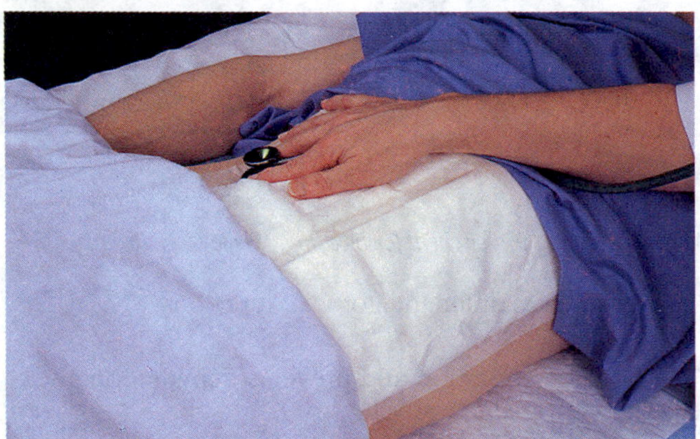

Action 13a: Assessing for return of peristalsis. (Photo © B. Proud.)

Action	Rationale
14. Promote wound healing: a. Use surgical asepsis b. Assess condition of wound c. Assess any drainage	Alterations in nutrition, circulatory, and metabolic status may predispose clients to infection and delayed healing.
15. Provide for rest and comfort.	This shortens recovery period and facilitates return to normal function.
16. Provide emotional and spiritual support.	This facilitates individualized care and client's return to normal health.

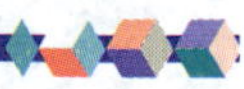

PLANNING: EXPECTED OUTCOMES

The plan of care in the postoperative phase begins in the preoperative phase, when nursing activities to reduce stress and teach postoperative activities are carried out. From admission, the client and family are prepared for uneventful recovery and self-care on dismissal. Specific expected outcomes are individualized, based on risk factors, surgical procedure, and unique needs. Examples of postoperative outcomes for a clients following major surgery are as follows. The client will:

- Carry out leg exercises every 2 to 4 hours

Name ____________

M.R. # ____________

POST-OP PROGRESS FLOW RECORD

DATE										
TIME										
BP										
PULSE										
RESPIRATIONS										
TEMPERATURE										
I.V.										
WOUND										
DRAIN (S)										
LOC										
PAIN										
NAUSEA										
FOLEY/ OTHER CATH OR VOIDING										
TURN, COUGH DEEP BREATHE										
MOVES ALL EXTREMITIES										
Initials										

Key

640-044-830/0800751

Figure 30-3
Example of a postoperative progress record.

- Deep breathe and cough effectively every 2 hours
- Verbalize decreasing levels of pain
- Have a balanced intake and output
- Regain normal bowel and bladder elimination
- Have a well-healed surgical incision
- Remain free of infection
- Verbalize any concerns about appearance of wound
- Verbalize and demonstrate self wound care

The aims of nursing are as follows:

- Assess and monitor client's physical and emotional status
- Promote physical and psychologic comfort and safety
- Prevent complications
- Facilitate coping with alterations in structure or function
- Promote a return to health and maximize wellness

IMPLEMENTING

Many nursing activities implemented in the postoperative phase have been discussed in this chapter or are fully discussed in other chapters; therefore, this section focuses on the nursing interventions implemented to meet the expected outcomes of the plan of care. Nursing care to prevent complications, promote a return to health, and facilitate coping with alterations are discussed.

Preventing Postoperative Complications

A wide variety of factors increase the risk of postoperative complications. These have been described in the preoperative and intraoperative sections of this chapter and include age, health habits, physical condition, medical history, psychologic status, and surgical intervention (anesthesia, positioning, wound). Preoperative assessments and teaching are implemented to decrease the risk of postoperative complications; this section describes the implementation of those activities, focusing on preventing respiratory, cardiovascular, and wound complications.

Preventing Cardiovascular Complications

Nursing interventions to prevent or monitor for cardiovascular complications are as follows:

- Assess and document vital signs as ordered and as the client's status dictates using preoperative assessments as a baseline.
- Provide covers as necessary to prevent chilling.
- Maintain fluid balance:
  - Maintain accurate intake and output.
  - Monitor rate and type of intravenous fluids.
  - Assess skin turgor and hydration of mucous membranes.
- Monitor amount, color, and consistency of wound drainage.
- Implement leg exercises and turning in bed every 2 hours.
- Assist with ambulation. Ambulation usually begins the evening of surgery and increases as tolerated; blood pressure and pulse and respiratory rates monitor tolerance.
- Apply and follow protocols for antiembolic stockings or compression devices, if ordered.
- Administer prescribed anticoagulant medications.
- Measure bilateral calf and thigh circumference daily. This is a more accurate assessment of thrombophlebitis than Homan's sign (pain in the calf when the foot is dorsiflexed).
- Avoid positioning that impedes venous return (eg, do not raise the knee gatch or place pillows under the knees).

Specific cardiovascular complications include shock, hemorrhage, thrombophlebitis, and pulmonary embolus.

Shock. Shock is the body's reaction to acute peripheral circulatory failure as the result of an alteration in circulatory control or to a loss of circulating fluid. The type of shock most commonly seen in the postoperative client is *hypovolemic shock*, which occurs from a decrease in blood volume. Common assessments of shock are hypotension; cold, clammy skin; a weak, thready, and rapid pulse; deep, rapid respirations; decreased urine output; thirst; apprehension; and restlessness. The primary purpose of care for the client in shock is to improve and maintain tissue perfusion by eliminating the cause of the shock. The following are recommended interventions in caring for the client in shock:

- Maintain airway.
- Place the client in a flat position with the legs elevated 45 degrees. (The Trendelenburg or "shock" position is no longer recommended because it causes the diaphragm to ascend, reducing total lung volume and ventilation.)
- Be prepared to assist with fluid administration as well as administration of whole blood or its components.
- Administer oxygen therapy as indicated.
- Place extra covering on the client to maintain warmth.
- Administer medications as ordered.
- Monitor vital signs and general condition continuously.
- Provide psychologic support to the client and family.

Hemorrhage. *Hemorrhage* is an excessive blood loss, either internally or externally. Hemorrhage may lead to hypovolemic shock. It may occur from a slipped suture, a dislodged clot in the wound, or stress on the operative site; it also may be the result of pathophysiologic conditions or certain medications. Common assessments of hemorrhage are restlessness, anxiety, and frank bleeding, as well as the symptoms listed above for shock. The primary purposes of care for the client having a hemorrhage include stopping the bleeding and replacing blood volume. The following interventions are recommended when caring for the client who is hemorrhaging:

- Apply a pressure dressing to the bleeding site.
- Be prepared to have the client return to the operating room if bleeding cannot be stopped or is massive.
- Provide nursing care as outlined for the client in shock.

Thrombophlebitis. *Thrombophlebitis* is an inflammation of a vein associated with thrombus (blood clot) formation. Thrombophlebitis is most commonly seen in the legs of the postoperative client (Bright & Georgi, 1994). Common assessments of thrombophlebitis are pain and cramping in the calf or thigh of the involved extremity, redness and swelling in the affected area, elevated temperature, and an increase in the diameter of the involved extremity. Care for the client with thrombophlebitis includes preventing a clot from breaking loose and becoming an embolus that travels to the lungs, heart, or brain and preventing further clot formation. Interventions in caring for the client with thrombophlebitis are as follows:

- Administer anticoagulant medications as ordered.
- Maintain bed rest as ordered.
- Use high antiembolic stockings or sequential pneumatic compression devices (see the accompanying box), and follow protocols for care.
- Elevate the affected leg to heart level.

Pneumatic Compression Devices

Pneumatic compression devices are composed of an air pump, connecting tubes, and an extremity sleeve. The sleeve may cover the entire leg or may extend from the foot to the knee. A variety of types are available; the accompanying figure provides one example. The devices apply brief pressure to the legs to enhance blood flow and venous return, thereby decreasing the risk of thrombophlebitis after surgery. The devices may apply either intermittent or sequential pressure. Intermittent pneumatic compression devices fit over the entire leg, with inflation and deflation of the sleeve covering the leg alternating from one leg to the other via a preset timer. Sequential pneumatic compression devices are designed so that pressure moves up the leg in increments. They may inflate and deflate alternating from one leg to the other or may do so for both legs at once.

Nursing Care

- Explain the purpose of the device to the client.
- Apply the device so that two fingers fit between the leg and the sleeve.
- Position the tubing so the client can move about without interrupting the air flow.
- Remove the sleeves at least once a day for skin care and assessment.
- Assess the extremities for peripheral pulses, edema, changes in sensation, and movement on a regular schedule.

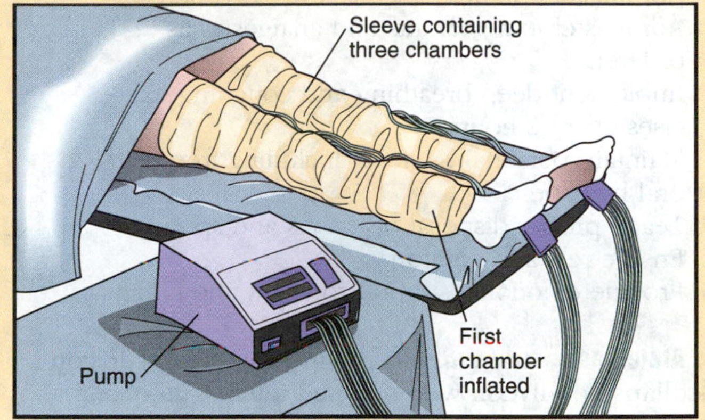

- Do *not* massage or rub the legs.
- Give analgesics and use external heat applications as ordered.
- Measure bilateral calf or thigh circumference every shift.
- Provide emotional support to the client and family.

Pulmonary Embolus. An *embolus* is a blood clot or other foreign substance that is dislodged and travels through the bloodstream until it lodges in another smaller vessel. In postoperative clients, the embolus often is part of a thrombus that breaks free from a vein wall. If the embolus lodges in the pulmonary vessels, it is called a *pulmonary embolus.* Common assessments of a pulmonary embolus include dyspnea, chest pain, cough, cyanosis, rapid respirations, tachycardia, and anxiety. The primary purposes of care are to stabilize cardiovascular and respiratory function and to prevent further emboli. The following are recommended interventions for the client with a pulmonary embolus:

- Contact the physician immediately if symptoms occur; pulmonary embolus is a life-threatening complication and immediate treatment is necessary.
- Maintain bed rest with the client in semi-Fowler's position.
- Maintain fluid balance; avoid overhydration with intravenous fluids.
- Administer oxygen therapy as appropriate.
- Administer anticoagulant medications as ordered.
- Administer prescribed analgesic medications for pain; use caution with narcotic analgesics, which depress respirations.
- Assess vital signs and general status frequently.
- Instruct client to avoid Valsalva's maneuver (forced exhalation against a closed glottis, such as straining to have a bowel movement) to prevent increased intrathoracic pressure and, possibly, increased emboli.
- Provide emotional support for client and family.

Preventing Respiratory Complications

Nursing interventions to prevent or monitor for respiratory complications are as follows:

- Assess and monitor vital signs, using preoperative assessments as a baseline.
- Implement deep breathing, coughing, incentive spirometry, and turning in bed every 2 hours.
- Ambulate as ordered.
- Maintain hydration.
- Avoid positioning that decreases ventilation.
- Carefully monitor responses to narcotic analgesics.

Specific respiratory complications include pneumonia and atelectasis.

Pneumonia. *Pneumonia* is an inflammation of the alveoli as the result of an infectious process or presence of foreign material. Pneumonia may occur postoperatively as a result of aspiration; infection; depressed cough reflex; and increased secretions from anesthesia, dehydration, and immobilization. Assessments common to pneumonia are an elevated temperature, chills, cough productive of purulent or rusty sputum, crackles and wheezes, dyspnea, and chest pain. The purposes of care are to treat the underlying infection, maintain respiratory status, and prevent the spread of microorganisms. The following are recommended interventions in caring for the client with pneumonia:

- Promote full aeration of the lungs by positioning the client in semi-Fowler's or Fowler's position.
- Administer oxygen therapy as indicated.
- Maintain nutritional and fluid status.
- Administer antibiotic medications as ordered.
- Administer expectorants and analgesics as ordered.
- Implement deep-breathing and coughing exercises every 2 hours.
- Maintain personal hygiene, including frequent oral hygiene.
- Teach proper disposal of tissues and sputum.
- Ensure rest and comfort.
- Provide emotional support to client and family.

Atelectasis. *Atelectasis* is the incomplete expansion or collapse of alveoli with retained mucus, involving a portion of the lung and resulting in poor gas exchange. Assessments of atelectasis are decreased lung sounds over affected areas, dyspnea, cyanosis, crackles, restlessness, and apprehension. The primary purposes of care for the client with atelectasis are to ensure oxygenation of tissues, prevent further atelectasis, and expand involved lung tissues. The following are recommended interventions in caring for the client with atelectasis:

- Position the client in semi-Fowler's position.
- Administer oxygen therapy as indicated.
- Implement deep breathing, coughing, and incentive spirometry every 2 hours.
- Implement leg exercises every 2 hours and ambulate as ordered.
- Maintain hydration.
- Administer analgesics for pain as ordered.
- Provide emotional support to client and family.

Preventing Wound Complications

The nurse provides care for wounds to restore health and prevent complications. Nursing care of wounds is discussed in the second half of this chapter. Nursing interventions to prevent or monitor for wound complications are as follows:

- Assess vital signs, especially monitoring for elevated temperature.
- Maintain hydration.
- Maintain nutritional status; encourage diet selection high in carbohydrates, proteins, calories, and vitamins.
- Use medical asepsis (handwashing) protocols.
- Maintain aseptic technique in dressing changes and care of tubes or drains.

Promoting a Return to Health

Nurses provide interventions in ongoing postoperative care to promote the return of clients' physical and psychologic functioning to as near a normal state as possible. The plan of care includes activities to meet elimination, fluid and electrolyte, nutrition, and rest and comfort needs.

Meeting Elimination Needs

Both urinary and bowel elimination can be altered by anesthesia, manipulation of organs during the surgical procedure, inactivity, and altered fluid and food intake during the perioperative period.

The return of normal *bowel elimination* is promoted by the following nursing assessments and interventions:

- Assess for the return of peristalsis by auscultating bowel sounds every 4 hours when client is awake.
  - Assess abdominal distention, especially if bowel sounds are not audible or are high-pitched (indicative of possible *paralytic ileus*, which is an absence of intestinal peristalsis).
  - Assess client's ability to pass flatus or stool.
- Assist with movement in bed and ambulation (to help relieve gas pains, a common postoperative discomfort).
- Encourage food and fluid intake when ordered, especially fruit juices and high-fiber foods.
- Maintain privacy when client is using the bedpan, commode, or bathroom.
- Administer colon tubes, suppositories, or enemas if ordered.

The return of normal *urinary elimination* is promoted by the following nursing assessments and interventions:

- Monitor intake and output balance.
- Assist with assumption of normal position to void.
  - Place client in upright sitting position when using bedpan.
  - Use bedside commode or assist client to bathroom, when able.
  - Help male clients stand upright to void.
- Assess for distention of the bladder (palpate above the symphysis pubis) if the client does not void within 8 hours after surgery or if the client voids frequently with amounts of less than 50 mL.
- Maintain ordered rate of intravenous fluids.
- Encourage PO fluids, when ordered.
- Provide privacy when the client is using the bedpan, commode, or bathroom.
- Carry out catheterization procedure, if ordered.

Meeting Fluid and Nutrition Needs

Fluid and nutrition needs can be met by the following nursing assessments and interventions:

- Monitor intake and output.
- Maintain intravenous fluids as ordered.

- Assess for dehydration and weight loss, if appropriate.
- Provide oral hygiene before meals and as needed.
- Monitor tolerance of ordered diet. (After surgery, diets usually progress from clear liquids to full liquids to soft to regular.)
- Maintain an environment conducive to good appetite (keep bedside articles clean and neat, eliminate odors).
- Encourage the client to sit up in bed or in a chair for meals.
- Encourage family participation in meals.
- Remember that the presence of drains, gastric suction, fever, and intravenous therapy increases the risk of fluid and electrolyte imbalances in the surgical client.

Meeting Comfort and Rest Needs

After surgery, comfort needs often are a priority for the client. Alterations in comfort are the result of many factors, including nausea, vomiting, hiccups, thirst, and surgical pain. The following are nursing interventions to meet comfort and rest needs by providing relief for various disturbances.

Nausea and Vomiting

- Maintain a clean environment.
- Provide oral hygiene as needed.
- Avoid a large intake of food or fluids at one time, especially after being NPO.
- Maintain bowel elimination.
- Assess allergic response to antibiotics or analgesics.
- Administer ordered medications.

Thirst

- Provide oral hygiene as needed.
- Offer sips of water or ice chips when NPO (if allowed).

Hiccups

- Have the client do the following:
- Take several swallows of water while holding his or her breath (if not NPO).
- Rebreathe into a paper bag.
- Eat a teaspoon of granulated sugar.
- Administer ordered medications.

Surgical Pain

- Assess for pain, and offer prescribed analgesics every 2 to 4 hours on a regular schedule during the first 24 to 36 hours after surgery.
- Reinforce preoperative teaching about pain management.
- Offer other comfort measures: position changes, back rubs, relaxation techniques.

Comfort and rest also are facilitated by providing personal hygiene, keeping the bed linens and environment clean, providing quiet during rest periods and at night, and allowing family members to remain with the client.

Helping the Client Cope

Surgical incisions often alter physical appearance and normal physiologic function, leading to actual or potential alterations in self-concept and body image and threatening psychologic security. Changes in a person's self-perception can influence all of the human dimensions and areas of human functioning—self-esteem, relationships with others, sexual identity, spiritual beliefs, sociocultural values, and independent conduct of activities of daily living and work.

Many surgical clients have the same reaction to loss of a body part as to a death (crisis is discussed in Chapter 32; loss and grief are discussed in Chapter 33). The response and the adaptation made by the client are influenced by multiple factors, including age, cultural values and beliefs, sociocultural background, significance of the body part, visibility of the body part, time to prepare for the change, and support people available. The nurse must be aware and accepting of the client's needs and must establish interventions to meet needs in coping with change. The nursing process is used to implement interventions, beginning with the client's decision to have surgery and continuing through convalescence. Nursing activities to facilitate coping are as follows:

- Accept each client as a unique individual.
- Identify through verbal and nonverbal cues clients who are at risk for alterations in self-concept (risk is increased if the client has little support from others, a visible alteration, or an alteration that will seriously affect functional ability).
- Allow time for clients and families to verbalize feelings about the alteration, and do not assume that all clients will have problems.
- Support strengths and effective coping mechanisms.
- Allow the client to be part of goal-setting and decision-making throughout the surgical experience.
- Provide teaching and honest information to the client and family about all aspects of care.
- Work collaboratively with other members of the health team and provide referrals as necessary to meet physical, psychologic, and spiritual needs.

Providing Ambulatory Surgery Postoperative Care

Evaluating the client's postoperative status after ambulatory surgery focuses on ensuring that the client can safely be cared for at home. After surgery and recovery from the anesthetic, the client is asked to sit up and drink liquids. The client who is no longer drowsy or dizzy, has stable vital signs, and has voided is allowed to go home accompanied by a responsible adult. The client is not allowed to drive a car to go home. The usual length of time from completion of surgery to dismissal from the facility is 1 to 3 hours, providing established criteria have been met. Written and verbal instructions for home care are given to the client and family.

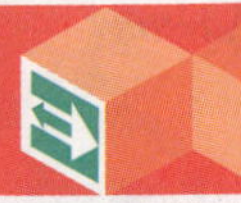

Developing Critical Thinking Skills

Situation

During both clinical days in one week you (a female student) have been assigned to care for a middle-aged woman who has had a breast removed because of cancer. The client, Mrs. Nola, is an attractive woman who usually is cheerful and eager to get better and return home. However, on both days she turned her head away and would not look at the incision when her dressing was changed. She tells you that she "just can't stand to look at herself." Her husband has left the room during the dressing changes after telling you that "it makes me sick to see what happened to my wife." Mrs. Nola is to be discharged to her home the next day and needs to learn how to provide self-care for her wound. What do you do?

1. ***Identify Goal of Thinking***

   Determine the most effective way of ensuring wound care and at the same time assisting Mrs. Nola in accepting her altered self-image.

2. ***Assess Adequacy of Knowledge***

   Pertinent Circumstances: The diagnosis of cancer was made only one day prior to the surgical removal of the breast. The client is to be discharged to her home the next day. The wound from her mastectomy has not completely healed and will require dressing changes for another 3 or 4 days. Mrs. Nola has had a disfiguring surgery and is coping with not only a change in body image but also the diagnosis of cancer. She has never before been seriously ill nor had surgery. She has a strong, loving relationship with her husband, but he is unable to deal with the physical disfigurement at this time.

   Prerequisite Knowledge: Before you decide what to do in this situation, you need to know at what level Mrs. Nola is in coping with the diagnosis of cancer. If she is still in denial about the disease, it is likely that she is also denying the surgical procedure and the changes in her body. You will need to review responses to the diagnosis of cancer as well as the stages of grief and loss. You will have to learn what her sources of support are, and how she can best access and use them. You will need to assess how best to help her achieve wound care in the face of her continued refusal even to look at the wound.

   Room for Error: If she is forced to look at the wound or made to feel inadequate because of her inability to do so, she will feel threatened and most likely will become angry in response to the perceived threat.

   Time Constraints: Some decision about wound care must be made prior to her discharge the next day.

3. ***Address Potential Problems***

   There are several potential obstacles to critical thinking in this situation. As a student you want to exhibit safe, knowledgeable care, and the importance of teaching for home care has been an emphasis in this course. As a woman, you have a sense of what the loss of a breast must mean. Having had a family member die of cancer, you find yourself wanting to do everything for Mrs. Nola. As a novice in nursing, you find it difficult to handle these emotional components of client care and find yourself wanting to scold both the client and her husband for being so silly about something as simple as a dressing.

4. ***Consult Helpful Resources***

   You must first understand the loss and grief Mrs. Nola is experiencing, and you must then relate that to her response to self-care of the wound. Your best source of information about her coping methods and sources of personal strength is Mrs. Nola herself. You also discuss the most effective way of providing wound care at home with your instructor and the case manager for Mrs. Nola.

5. ***Critique Judgment/Decision***

   After talking to Mrs. Nola, your instructor, and the case manager, you mutually agree that Mrs. Nola cannot be hurried into acceptance of her medical diagnosis or her body changes. The case manager consults with Mrs. Nola's physician, who writes an order for a home health nurse to visit for the next 4 days and complete the dressing change. After talking with Mrs. Nola, you identify that she is still very much in denial. You discuss with her the possibility of having a visitor from "Reach to Recovery," a support group for women with breast cancer who have had a mastectomy. Mrs. Nola tells you that she thinks she would like to talk to someone with the same problem, and you call a referral for her. When you tell Mrs. Nola that a home health nurse will be visiting her for the first few days at home to change her dressing, tears come into her eyes. She says "I am so scared, I just don't know what to do." You realize that insisting that Mrs. Nola do her own dressing would have been extremely stressful for her, and that you would have considered the wound as more important than the client. When you share the situation in postconference, your clinical group supports your decision.

Wounds and Wound Care

A **wound** is a disruption in the normal continuity of the skin. The nurse cares for wounds, but only as one aspect of the nursing care given to the *client* with the wound. In other words, it is the *client* to whom care is given. Using the nursing process, an individualized plan of care is developed to assess, to identify and prevent complications, to implement and evaluate skills essential to wound care, and to provide the necessary physical and emotional support so that healing, adaptation, and self-care are facilitated. Wound care may be required in both emergency situations and as a part of hospital or home-based client care. Nurses need to know how to assess and implement care for clients and their wounds, and to do so with knowledge and skill.

Types of Wounds

Wounds may be intentional or unintentional, open or closed. These broad classifications are discussed here; more specific descriptors are found in Table 30-3.

An *intentional wound* is the result of planned therapy or treatment that requires invasive measures. Examples of intentional wounds are those that result from surgical incisions, intravenous therapy, lumbar puncture, thoracentesis, and paracentesis. The wound edges are clean, and bleeding usually is controlled. Because the wound is made under sterile, aseptic conditions with sterile supplies and skin preparation, the risk of infection is decreased and healing is facilitated.

Unintentional wounds occur from unexpected trauma, such as from accidents, forcible injury (such as stabbing, gun shots), and burns. Because the wounds occur in an unsterile environment, contamination is likely. Wound edges usually are jagged, multiple trauma is common, and bleeding is uncontrolled. These factors create a high risk for infection and a longer healing time.

An *open wound* occurs from intentional or unintentional trauma. The skin surface is broken, providing a portal of entry for microorganisms. Open wounds may be accompanied by bleeding, tissue damage, and increased risk for infection. A *closed wound* is the result of a blow, force, or strain sustained in traumatic situations such as a fall, an assault, or a motor vehicle accident. The skin surface is not broken, but soft tissue is damaged and internal injury and hemorrhage may occur.

Wounds may also be clean or contaminated and superficial or deep. Table 30-3 lists the types, causes, de-

Table 30-3
Types of Wounds and Risk of Infection

Type	Cause	Description and Implications
Contusion (bruise)	Blow from a hard object	A closed wound, results in soft-tissue damage and ruptured blood vessels; causes swelling and pain. If internal organs are contused, serious effects may result.
Incision	Made with a sharp instrument or needle	See intentional (open) wound.
Abrasion	An accidental injury or fall that scrapes or rubs off the skin surface; or an intentional dermatologic procedure	A painful open wound; involves only the skin
Laceration	Accidental trauma	Tissues are torn, and wound edges are ragged. Depth of wound varies, and affects risk of complications. Often caused by an unclean object, increasing risk of infection.
Puncture	Made by a sharp instrument or object that penetrates the skin and underlying tissue	May be intentional, or unintentional (see above)
Possibility and Degree of Contamination		
Clean	Surgical incision or closed wound	Contains no pathogenic organisms. Surgery did not enter the respiratory, gastrointestinal, or genitourinary systems.
Clean-contaminated	A specific surgery	Surgery enters the respiratory, gastrointestinal, or genitourinary system; risk of infection is increased.
Contaminated	Open accidental wounds, surgery with a major break in asepsis, or surgery with major contamination from the gastrointestinal system	Tissue becomes inflamed; risk of infection is high.
Infected	A wound with demonstrated pathogens; an old, traumatic wound; or a surgical incision into an infected area	Wound demonstrates inflammation, heat, purulent drainage, skin separation.

scriptions, and implications of different types of wounds. Many wounds combine several descriptors; for example, an intentional wound to remove the appendix usually is a clean, open wound. In comparison, after an automobile accident, a person may have an unintentional, open laceration considered to be contaminated.

Wound Healing

The healthy body has an innate capacity to protect and restore itself. Increasing the blood supply to the damaged area, walling off and removing cellular and foreign debris, and initiating cellular development are parts of the body's healing process. The healing process occurs normally, without assistance, although some care measures can help to support the process. For example, keeping the injured area free of debris by proper cleaning helps to promote tissue healing, as does positioning the wounded area to promote circulation to that part.

General Principles of Tissue Healing

The following principles and rationale are significant in wound healing.

The body's ability to handle tissue trauma is influenced by the extent of the damage and by the person's general state of health. The capacity to deal adequately with an injury is limited when a healthy person sustains a massive injury, when the client has a chronic illness, or when the client is very young or very old. The promotion of wellness to improve resistance to an insult to the body is partially directed toward maintaining adequate body reserves to deal with traumatic experiences.

The body's response to injury is more effective if proper nutrition has been maintained. Undernourished clients have difficulty mounting their cell-mediated defense system associated with T-lymphocyte activity. These clients may demonstrate diminished immune response to an antigen. Some leukocytic functions are diminished in the presence of protein deficiency. Undernourished clients, then, are at higher risk for developing a wound infection. Although the role of fatty acids in wound healing is not understood, it is known that certain quantities of glucose are necessary to meet the energy requirements of wound healing.

Various vitamins, minerals, and trace elements are needed for efficient wound healing. Vitamin A is necessary for collagen synthesis and epithelialization. Vitamin B complex serves as a cofactor of enzyme reactions needed for wound healing. Vitamin C is needed for collagen synthesis, capillary formation, and resistance to infection. Vitamin K is needed for the synthesis of prothrombin. Zinc, copper, and iron assist in collagen synthesis. Manganese serves as an enzyme activator.

The body responds systematically to trauma in any of its parts. Local physical responses to an injury cannot be separated from an overall body reaction. For example, an injured foot or hand or an abdominal incision can cause a variety of systematic reactions, which include increased body temperature, increased heart and respiratory rates, anorexia or nausea and vomiting, musculoskeletal tension throughout the body, and harmful hormonal changes. Adequate rest, relief of emotional stress, and sufficient nutrients and fluids are particularly important for the person undergoing a response to trauma.

The blood transports substances to and from injured tissue. An adequate blood supply is essential for the body's normal response to any injury. The blood brings increased amounts of leukocytes, erythrocytes, and platelets to the site of injury. Antibodies also are carried by the plasma. Increased circulation to the injured part provides for the removal of toxins and debris and allows for nutrients, oxygen, and other cell-building materials to be supplied. Areas of the body that have a good blood supply, such as the head and the neck, heal faster than areas in which the blood supply is not as great, such as the distal part of an extremity.

Intact skin and mucous membranes serve as first lines of defense against microorganisms. A break in the continuity of the skin or mucous membranes increases the likelihood of a wound infection. Surgical asepsis is used in caring for an open wound to minimize the possibility of pathogens entering the site. Precautions also are taken for people with closed wounds because the resistance of the damaged tissue is lowered and pathogenic organisms may be present. Careful handwashing before caring for a wound is probably the single most effective method for preventing wound infections.

Normal healing is promoted when the wound is free of foreign bodies, including bacteria. Healing does not start until foreign bodies are removed from the wound. Excessive exudate, dead or damaged tissue cells, pathogenic organisms, or embedded fragments of bone, metal, glass, or other substances can all act as foreign bodies. The body's rejection mechanisms are sufficient to remove many foreign substances. Sometimes mechanical means may be used to assist the process. In some situations, the body walls off a collection of pus or another foreign body, and healing occurs around it. This localized collection of pus is called an *abscess.* The person can be expected to develop symptoms at the unhealed site, although they may be delayed in their appearance.

Phases of Wound Healing

An injury to tissues results in two major responses—the stress response and the inflammatory response. All wounds follow the same phases in healing, although differences occur in the length of time required for each phase of the healing process and in the extent of granulation tissue formed. The phases of wound healing are described as they occur in the surgical wound.

Inflammatory Phase. The inflammatory phase begins with the incision for surgery and lasts through the third or fourth postoperative day. The two major physiologic activities are hemostasis and phagocytosis. The inflammatory response is immediate and prepares the tissues for healing.

As a major stressor, injury initiates the local adaptation syndrome (described in Chapter 32). As a result, there is first an immediate and brief constriction of blood vessels, allowing clotting of blood to seal the wound. This is followed by vasodilation, allowing increased blood flow to the area, which permits white blood cells (leukocytes) to invade the area of injury and engulf bacteria and debris. About 24 hours after injury, a large phagocytic cell (a microphage) enters the area and secretes an angiogenesis factor that stimulates the formation of epithelial buds at the end of injured vessels so that reanastomosis can occur.

During the inflammatory phase, the client has a generalized body response, including a mildly elevated temperature, leukocytosis, and generalized malaise.

Proliferation Phase. The proliferation phase begins about day 3 or 4 and lasts to about day 21. Fibroblasts rapidly synthesize collagens and ground substance. These two substances form the scaffold for the final repair of the wound. A thin layer of epithelial cells was formed across the wound during the inflammatory phase; now capillaries grow across the wound. This revascularization brings oxygen and nutrients required for continued healing. Fibroblasts also migrate from the bloodstream into the wound, depositing fibrin that stretches through the clot. A thin layer of epithelial cells forms across the wound, and blood flow across the wound is reinstituted. The new tissue, called **granulation tissue**, is highly vascular and reddish and bleeds easily.

The systemic symptoms should disappear, and the client looks and feels better. During this phase, adequate nutrition and oxygenation as well as prevention of strain on the suture line are important client care considerations.

Maturation Phase. This final stage of healing begins about day 21 and can continue for as long as 1 to 2 years after injury. Collagen that has been haphazardly deposited in the wound is remodeled, making the healed wound stronger and more like adjacent tissue. New collagen continues to be deposited, which compresses the blood vessels in the healing wound, so that the scar eventually becomes a flat, thin, white line. The **scar** is avascular collagen tissue that does not sweat, grow hair, or tan in sunlight.

Processes of Wound Healing

Wounds heal by one of three processes—primary, secondary, or tertiary intention (Fig. 30-4). Most surgical incisions and small sutured lacerations heal by *primary intention.* The wound is a clean, straight line with little loss of tissue. All wound edges are well approximated with sutures. These wounds normally heal rapidly with minimal scarring. *Secondary intention* healing takes place in large wounds that have considerable tissue loss, so that the edges cannot be approximated. Healing occurs by formation of granulation tissue. Because the wounds are more open, there is a greater chance of infection, healing time is longer, and scars are larger. *Tertiary intention* healing occurs when the interval between the wound's occurrence and its suturing is extended. This delay allows access for pathogens, so that there is an increased risk for infection. There also is a greater inflammatory reaction and more granulation tissue in comparison to healing by primary intention, so scars are large and less likely to shrink to a flat line.

Wound Drainage

During the first two phases of wound healing, the inflammatory response results in exudate that escapes from the wound. The exudate is composed of fluid and cells that escape from blood vessels and are deposited in or on tissue surfaces. This exudate is called *wound drainage* and is described as *serous, sanguineous,* or, if infected, *purulent.* These types of exudate can be further described as follows:

Serous—composed primarily of the clear, serous portion of the blood and from serous membranes. Serous drainage is clear and watery.

Sanguineous—consists of large numbers of red blood cells and looks like blood. Bright red sanguineous drainage is indicative of fresh bleeding, whereas darker drainage indicates older bleeding.

Purulent—made up of white blood cells, liquefied dead tissue debris, and both dead and live bacteria. Purulent drainage is thick, often has a musty or foul odor, and varies in color, depending on the causative organism.

Drainage may be a mixture of these three types. Surgical wounds most commonly have a mixture of serum and red blood cells, called *serosanguineous* drainage.

Factors Affecting Wound Healing

Wound healing is affected by a variety of factors. These factors include age, circulation to and oxygenation of tissues, condition of the wound, and overall client wellness.

Developmental Considerations. Children and healthy adults heal more rapidly than do older adults, in whom physiologic changes caused by aging have resulted in diminished fibroblastic activity and circulation. The older adult is more likely to have one or more chronic illnesses, with pathologic changes that impede the healing process (see the accompanying box).

Circulation and Oxygenation. A number of physical conditions can affect wound healing. The presence of large amounts of subcutaneous and tissue fat (which has fewer blood vessels) in obese people may slow wound healing because fatty tissue is more difficult to suture, more prone to infection, and takes longer to heal. Circulation may be impaired in older adults and in people

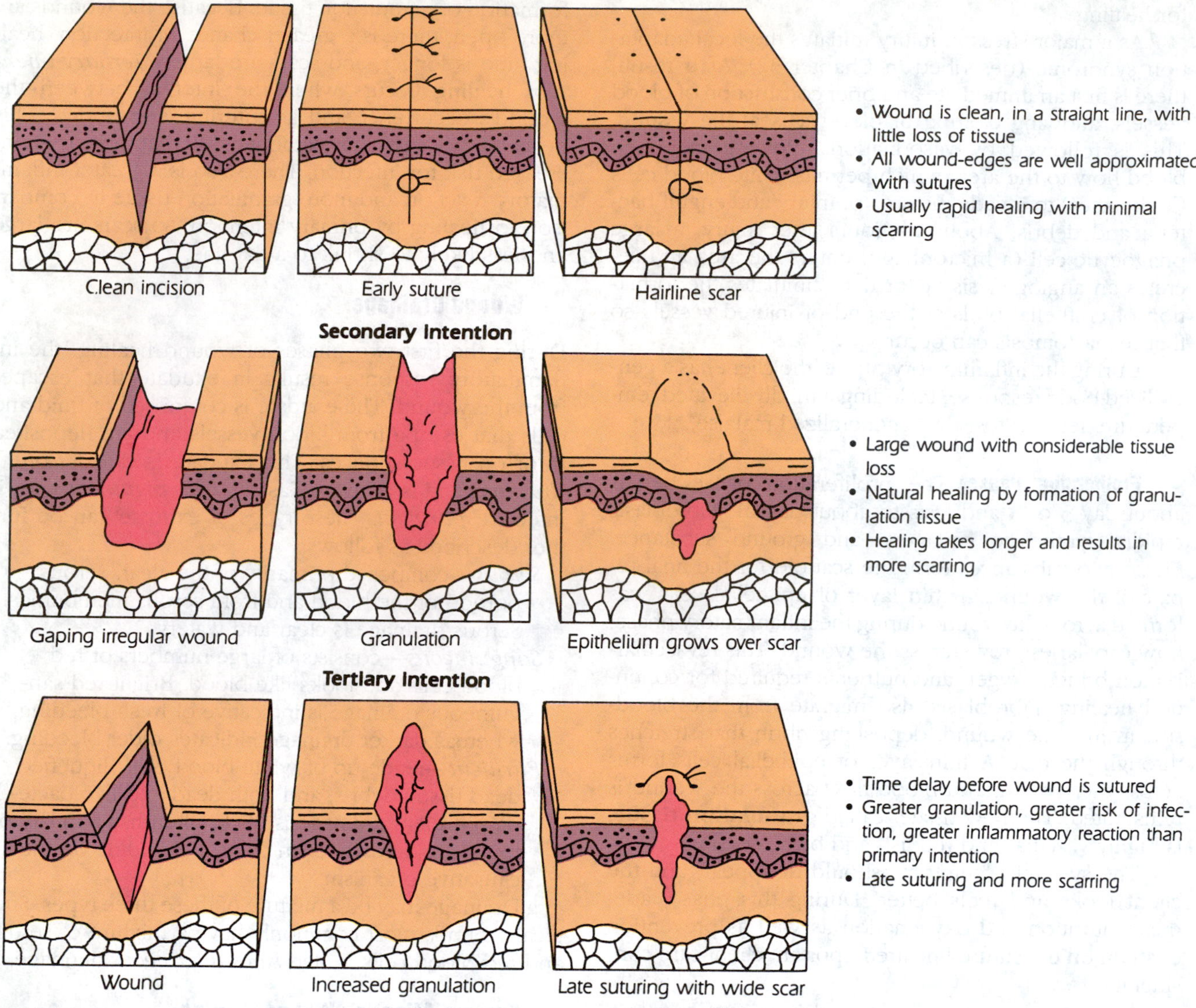

Figure 30-4
Types of wound healing.

with peripheral vascular disorders, cardiovascular disorders, hypertension, or diabetes mellitus. Oxygenation of tissues is decreased in people with anemia or chronic respiratory disorders and in those who smoke.

Wound Condition. The specific condition of the wound affects how quickly and effectively the wound heals. For example, large, contaminated, infected wounds or wounds that retain foreign bodies heal slowly. Some wounds may fail to heal. Table 30-3 describes types of wounds that are prone to complications.

Overall Client Wellness. Clients who have inadequate nutrition, are taking steroid drugs, or require postoperative radiation therapy have a high risk of delayed healing and wound complications. Additionally, the presence of a chronic physical illness or severe emotional stress can negatively affect wound healing. In some instances, it is necessary to improve nutritional status or treat underlying conditions before surgery is done.

Wound Complications

Wound complications increase the risk of generalized illness and death, lengthen the client's hospital stay, and add to healthcare costs. Wound complications include infection, hemorrhage, dehiscence, and evisceration.

Infection

Invasion of the wound by bacteria can occur at the time of trauma, during surgery, or at any time after the initial wound. A contaminated wound is more likely to become infected, as is a surgical wound resulting from a procedure that involves the intestines, in which the risk of

Focus on the Older Adult

Factors That Affect Wound Healing in Older Adults

Changes in Skin

- Skin loses turgor and is more fragile.
- There is increased risk of further injury from cleaning agents and tape.

Nutrition

- Decreased secretion of enzymes and absorption of nutrients and minerals may have potential risk for altered nutrition, which would delay wound healing.

Potential for Infection

- Age reduces antibody production and functioning of the endocrine system, both of which increase susceptibility to infection.
- The incidence of chronic illnesses that compromise circulation and oxygenation of tissues (such as diabetes mellitus and cardiovascular problems) further decreases resistance to infection.

contamination with fecal material is high. Symptoms of wound infection usually become apparent within 2 to 7 days after the injury or surgery. This means that with the trend toward decreased hospital stay, infection may appear after the client has left the hospital. Symptoms of infection include purulent drainage, increased drainage, pain, redness and swelling in and around the wound, increased body temperature, and increased white blood cell count. Nursing care of infected wounds is discussed later.

Hemorrhage

Hemorrhage may indicate a slipped suture, a dislodged clot from stress at the suture line or operative site, infection, or the erosion of a blood vessel by a foreign body (such as a drain). Postoperative wounds require careful nursing assessment so that hemorrhage is detected early. Hypovolemia may not be immediately evident. Therefore, the dressing (and the wound under the dressing if possible) should be checked frequently during the first 48 hours after surgery and no less than every 8 hours thereafter. If excessive bleeding does occur, additional sterile pressure dressings or packing may be necessary, fluid replacement will probably be necessary, and surgical intervention may be required.

Dehiscence and Evisceration

Dehiscence and evisceration (Fig. 30-5) are the most serious postoperative wound complications. **Dehiscence** is the partial or total disruption of wound layers. **Evisceration** is the protrusion of viscera through the incisional area. These are frightening occurrences for both the client and the nurse. Careful nursing assessment can help to identify the predisposing signs of these events. An appreciable increase in the flow of serosanguineous fluid into the wound dressings between the 5th and 12th postoperative days is a clue to impending dehiscence. Wound disruption often is preceded by a sudden straining, such as coughing, sneezing, or vomiting. It is not uncommon for the client to comment that "something has suddenly given way." If dehiscence or evisceration occurs, the wound area should be covered with sterile towels soaked in saline solution, and the physician should be notified immediately. Both these situations are emergencies that require prompt preparation for surgical repair.

Psychologic Effects of Wounds

Trauma, with resultant wounds, causes psychologic stress as well as physical injury. Because the skin functions as a sensory organ and plays a major role in the way we communicate with others and feel about ourselves, wounds require adaptation in the emotional as well as the physical dimensions of the traumatized per-

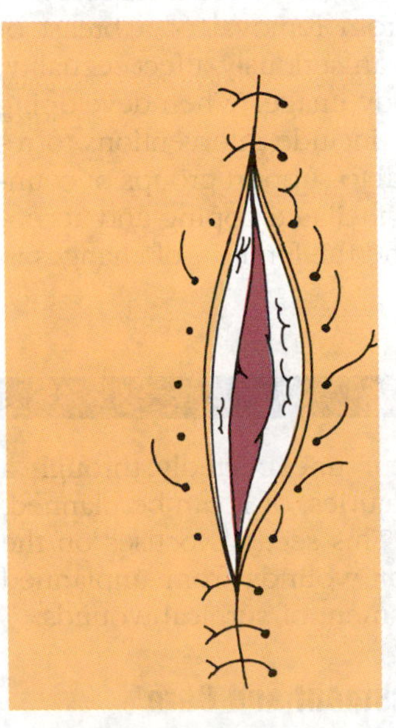

Figure 30-5
Wound complications.

son. Although stress and adaptation are highly individualized, actual and potential emotional stressors are common to all clients with wounds. These stressors include pain, anxiety, fear, and alterations in self-concept.

Pain. Pain is part of almost any trauma, from a small cut on the finger to a large abdominal incision made during bowel surgery. Although pain can be considered to be a physical complication, there is a large psychologic component as well. Pain from wounds often is increased by activities such as ambulating, coughing, moving in bed, and dressing changes. The actual pain may be worsened for the client by anticipatory apprehension of such activities. Nursing interventions to reduce pain through skill and explanations can greatly reduce emotional stress.

Anxiety and Fear. Anxiety and fear are common responses to a wound. Clients are apprehensive about the wound strength, how much privacy will be lost as the wound is cared for, and how they and others will react to the sights and smells of the wound. They may actually fear the sight of blood or the sight of what they consider mutilation of their bodies. As nurses care for clients with wounds, it is important that they be accepting and empathic, encourage ventilation of feelings, answer questions accurately and honestly, and avoid excessive exposure of body parts when giving wound care.

Alterations in Self-Concept. The self-concept of each person is that of a whole entity. When the skin and tissues are traumatized, that concept is changed, and the person must adapt and reformulate the concept of self. Wounds and scars that are visible to others, especially on the face, can leave the client with feelings of being conspicuous and ugly and of less worth. Large scars, such as those remaining from removal of a breast or from colostomy openings, can seriously affect sexuality, social relationships, and body image. When developing a plan of care, nurses must include interventions to resolve these concerns; referral to support groups or counselors may be necessary to facilitate coping and acceptance—by both the client and the family—of changes in body structure or function.

ASSESSING THE WOUND

Trauma to tissues can occur unexpectedly through a wide variety of accidental injuries, or it can be planned, as in surgical intervention. This section focuses on the assessment and first aid for wounds from unplanned trauma as well as the assessment of surgical wounds.

Emergency Wound Assessment and Care

The following are general guidelines for emergency wound assessment and client care.

- The priority is assessment of the general condition of the wounded person. If the injury is serious, assess for an open and intact airway, spontaneous respirations, and a strong pulse. A helpful way to remember these important areas of assessment is by using the mnemonic *ABC*:
  - A = airway
  - B = breathing
  - C = circulation

  (This pattern of assessments should be the priority in any emergency situation.)
- Assess the severity of the wound. In the case of major trauma or serious bleeding, either call for emergency care or have someone else call while you remain with the injured person.
- Control bleeding that is severe by applying direct pressure over the wound. If possible, cover the wound with a clean dressing.
- Assess for any other traumatic injuries—fractures, internal bleeding, spinal cord injuries, head injuries.
- For anything other than a minor wound, be sure the injured person goes to an emergency department or emergency care facility. Immediate treatment reduces the risk of infection and decreases scar formation. Tetanus immunization is usually recommended if the person has not had one within the past 5 years. The emergency assessment and care of specific wounds are discussed in the accompanying box.

Assessing the Surgical Wound

Surgical wounds are defined here as wounds that result from intentional surgical therapy or wounds that were unintentional but have been treated (cleaned and sutured). Wounds are assessed by inspection (sight and smell) and palpation for appearance, drainage, and pain. Included in the assessment are sutures, drains or tubes, and signs of possible complications.

Appearance. A wound is assessed for the approximation of wound edges, color of the wound and surrounding area, drains or tubes, sutures, and signs of dehiscence or evisceration. The wound edges should be clean and well approximated, with a crust along the wound edges. The wound's edges initially are reddened and slightly swollen, but by the end of about a week, the skin should be closer to normal in appearance and the wound edges should be healed together. Skin surrounding the wound may at first be bruised, but this, too, returns to normal as blood is reabsorbed. If an infection is present, the wound is swollen, has increased redness, and feels hot. If dehiscence is impending or present, the wound edges are separated.

Drainage. The amount, color, odor, and consistency of wound drainage is assessed. The amount and color

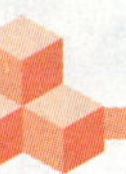

Guidelines for Nursing Care

Providing Emergency Assessment and Care of Specific Wounds

Abrasion

- Assess extent and depth of wound.
- Flush with running water and wash with soap and water.
- If small, leave open; if large, cover with light dressing.

Laceration

- Assess length, depth, and location of wound.
- Clean with soap and water.
- Hold wound edges together with tape or a dressing.
- Refer for further treatment, as necessary.

Puncture

- Assess cause (animal bite, outdoors) and last tetanus shot.
- Allow bleeding to flush out saliva or dirt.
- Clean with soap and water.
- Refer for further treatment, as necessary.

Impaled Object

- Assess cardiopulmonary status.
- *Do not* remove the object.
- Control the bleeding by putting pressure around the object.
- Secure immediate emergency care.

Amputations

- Assess blood loss and cardiopulmonary status.
- Control bleeding by direct pressure to wound or over pressure points.
- Elevate the affected extremity.
- Place amputated digits or extremity in a sealed plastic bag and immerse bag in ice-filled container.
- Secure immediate emergency care; transport amputated part with client.

depend on the wound location and size, with larger wounds having more drainage. Wound drainage, as previously described, may be serous, serosanguineous, sanguineous, or, if infected, purulent. Purulent drainage usually has a musty or foul odor; it is thick and either yellow, green, or brown. Frankly sanguineous drainage is indicative of hemorrhage. Drainage can be assessed on the wound, on the dressings, in drainage bottles or reservoirs, or, depending on the location of the wound and the amount of drainage, under the client.

Pain. If the client complains of increased or constant pain from the wound, or if wound edges are swollen with purulent or increased drainage, further assessments should be made and symptoms should be documented and reported. Pain, especially when accompanied by an increased or purulent flow of drainage, indicates delayed healing or the presence of an infection. Incisional pain usually is most severe for the first 2 to 3 days and then progressively diminishes.

Sutures and Staples. Skin sutures, which may be black silk, synthetic material, metal staples, fine wire, or metal skin clips, are used to hold tissue and skin together. Retention sutures are used to provide extra support for obese clients and for wounds with increased risk of dehiscence (Fig. 30-6).

Sutures are removed when enough tensile strength has developed to hold the wound edges together during healing. This stage varies from client to client, depending on age, nutritional status, and wound location. Silk sutures should be removed within 6 to 8 days to prevent suture marks, even though collagen formation and remodeling takes at least 21 days altogether. That means the scar may still stretch and widen after the silk sutures have been removed. Special subcutaneous techniques have now been developed to minimize this problem. Small wound closure strips of adhesive (Steri-Strips) may now be applied directly to the wound to help hold it together. Unless otherwise directed, Steri-Strips are not removed during wound care.

Sutures are removed with a suture removal set; staples are removed with a special staple remover. The steps in removing sutures and staples are summarized in the accompanying box. After the removal of skin sutures, Steri-Strips are sometimes applied across the healed wound to give additional support as the wound continues to heal. The status of skin sutures is included in wound assessment.

Drains and Tubes. Drains and tubes are inserted into or near a wound when it is anticipated that a collection of fluid in a closed area will delay healing. After a surgical procedure, the physician places one end of the tube or drain in or near the area to be drained and passes the other end through the skin, either directly through the incision or through a separate opening called a stab wound. Drains and tubes may or may not be sutured in

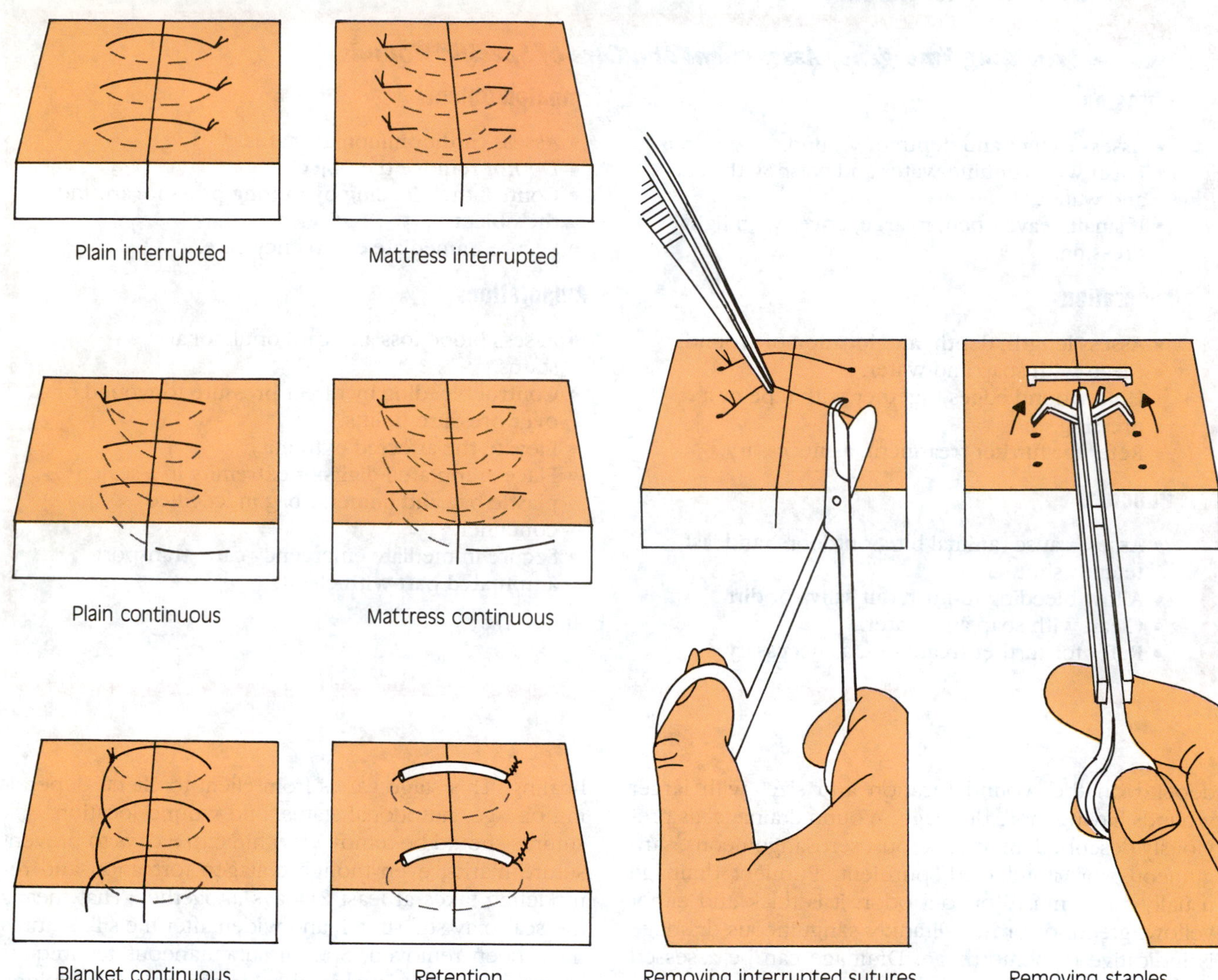

Figure 30-6
Types of sutures and techniques for removal.

place; drains placed directly through the wound (for example, a Penrose drain) usually have a large safety pin in the part outside the wound to prevent them from slipping back into the incised area and are not sutured (Fig. 30-7). Tubes that are connected to suction or that have a built-in reservoir to maintain constant low suction usually are sutured to the skin (for example, a Jackson-Pratt drainage tube or a Hemovac). It is important to know which type of drain or tube was inserted during surgery, so that accurate assessment can be made. The patency and placement of tubes or drains are included in wound assessment. Table 30-4 describes the purpose and common use of selected drains and tubes.

Related Assessments. In addition to assessments of the wound, the nurse evaluates the client's general condition and laboratory test results. *Infection* may cause generalized malaise, increased pain, anorexia, and an elevated body temperature and pulse rate; laboratory data include an elevated white blood cell count and, if a wound culture is done, a causative organism. *Hemorrhage* is further identified by restlessness, anxiety, a drop in systolic blood pressure, increased pulse and respiratory rates, decreased urinary output, and decreased hemoglobin levels and hematocrit.

IMPLEMENTING WOUND CARE

In caring for the client with a wound, the nurse carries out interventions to promote wound healing, prevent further injury or alteration in skin integrity, prevent infection, promote physical and emotional comfort, and facilitate coping.

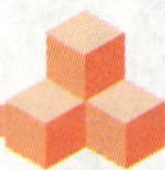

Guidelines for Nursing Care

Removing Staples and Sutures

The removal of staples or sutures may be done by the physician or by the nurse with a physician's order. Agency protocol should be followed, but general guidelines are as follows:

- Use sterile techniques, following recommended CDC guidelines for care of wounds.
- Wash hands before and after the procedure.
- Explain the procedure to the client. Describe the sensation that will be experienced as a pulling or slightly uncomfortable experience.
- Use proper technique to remove and dispose of old dressings.
- Clean the incision from the center of the wound outward, using hospital policy and procedure for type of agent.
- Remove every other suture or staple to be sure wound edges are healed; if they are, remove remaining sutures or staples as ordered.
- Remove or reapply dressing, depending on physician preference and agency policy.
- Some physicians order Steri-Strip application to the healed wound after removal of staples or sutures to give additional support to the wound as it continues to heal. Follow agency protocol and physician preference for placement of these tapes.

Specifics for Suture Removal

- Use a sterile suture removal kit.
- Using the sterile forceps, grasp the knot of the first suture and gently lift the knot.
- Using the sterile scissors, cut one side of the suture below the knot close to the skin.
- Grasp the knot with the forceps and pull the cut suture through the skin (be sure to pull through the healed wound only the portion of the suture that has been inside the tissue).

Specifics for Staple Removal

- As directed on the package, gently position the sterile staple remover under the staple to be removed.
- Firmly close the staple remover to straighten the staple ends (do not lift upward while disengaging staple ends).
- Carefully lift upward with the closed staple remover to remove the staple from the incision line. It may be necessary to remove one end of the staple and then the other if it does not easily lift out.

Using Dressings

The goal of wound care is to promote tissue repair and regeneration so that skin integrity is restored. There are two methods of caring for wounds—the closed method, in which a **dressing** is used as a protective cover over the wound, and the open method, in which no dressing is used.

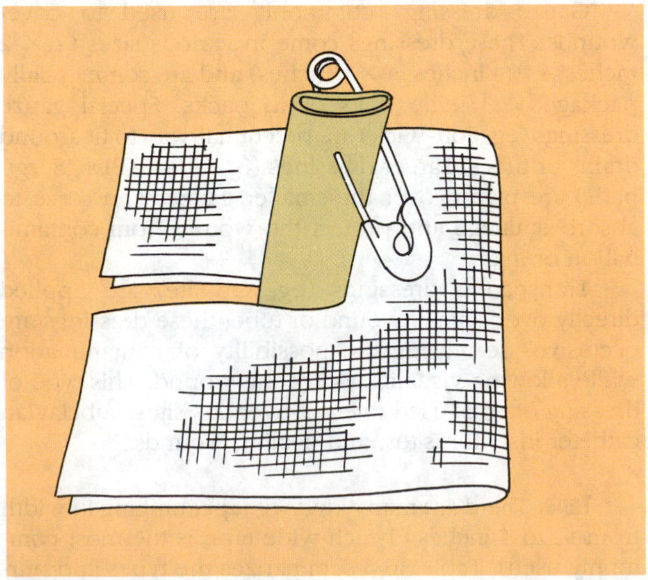

Figure 30-7
Penrose drain.

Most dressings, especially for the surgical wound, consist of three layers. The dressing applied directly over the wound, called the contact layer, allows drainage to pass into the middle layer. This layer should be able to be removed without causing further tissue damage. The middle layer dressings absorbs the drainage, and the outer layer keeps the two inner layers in place. There are many different types of dressings, but all have essentially the same purposes (Erwin-Toth & Hocevar, 1995, p. 46):

- Remove necrotic tissue
- Prevent, eliminate, or control infection
- Absorb drainage
- Maintain a moist wound environment
- Protect the wound from further injury
- Protect the skin surrounding the wound

Dressings have advantages and disadvantages. The advantages are listed in the box; the disadvantages are that dressings can rub or stick to the wound, causing further superficial injury. Dressings also can create a warm, damp, and dark environment—all components conducive to the growth of organisms, with resultant infection. Most wounds are covered with a dressing, and nurses are responsible for most dressing changes. This section deals with the supplies needed for dressing changes, guidelines for prevention of infection, and procedures for changing selected types of dressings.

Table 30-4
Common Types of Drains

Type	Purpose	Example
Penrose	Provides sinus tract	After incision and drainage of abscess, in abdominal surgery
T-tube	For bile drainage	After gallbladder surgery
Jackson-Pratt	Decrease dead space by collecting drainage	After breast removal, abdominal surgery
Hemovac	Decrease dead space by collecting drainage	After abdominal, orthopedic surgery
Gauze, iodoform gauze, NuGauze	Allow healing from base of wound	Infected wounds, after removal of hemorrhoids

Gathering Supplies for Dressings

Before changing a dressing, the nurse gathers needed supplies. The items may be gathered individually or they may be packaged in a sterile dressing tray. The setting in which wound care is provided determines how supplies are collected. Some hospital units have special dressing carts, with all dressing supplies located in one area. Wound care in the home is based on the availability of supplies provided by the client or family.

The supplies needed vary with the type, location, and amount of wound drainage; the nursing plan of care should include specifics about each client's dressing procedure and supplies. Materials and supplies include cleaning agents, materials to cover the wound (the dressing), and materials used to secure the dressing and support the wound.

Cleaning Agents. Many possible antiseptic cleaning agents can be used to clean the wound. Some commonly used agents are Betadine, 70% alcohol, 3% hydrogen peroxide, and sterile normal saline solution. Some authorities question the use of any agent other than saline solution because of the caustic effect on skin, tissues, and granulating tissue of the other agents. The choice of cleaning agent largely depends on agency protocol and physician preference.

Advantages of Wound Dressings

- Dressings absorb drainage to help promote wound healing.
- Dressings protect the wound from mechanical injury.
- Dressings, when used as a pressure dressing or with elastic bandages, promote hemostasis, help prevent hemorrhage, and aid in wound edge approximation.
- Dressings splint or immobilize the wound, facilitating healing and preventing further trauma.
- Dressings prevent contamination from the external environment.
- Dressings provide physical, psychologic, and aesthetic comfort.

Dressing Supplies. The number and types of dressings used depend on the location and size of the wound as well as on the amount and type of drainage. In discussing dressings, supplies are defined as they are used from the incision outward. An incision line often is covered with sterile petrolatum gauze or a special gauze called Telfa. Telfa's shiny outer surface is applied to the wound and allows drainage to pass through and be absorbed by the center (or outer) absorbent layer. Both these protective dressings prevent outer dressings from adhering to the wound and causing further injury when removed.

Gauze dressings commonly are used to cover wounds. These dressings come in various sizes (2 × 2 inches, 4 × 4 inches, 4 × 8 inches) and are commercially packaged as single units or in packs. Special gauze dressings (eg, Soft-Wick) are precut halfway to fit around drains or tubes. Larger dressings (8 × 10s, ABDs, Surgipads) are placed over the smaller gauzes and serve to absorb drainage and protect the wound from contamination or injury.

Transparent dressings (eg, Op-Site) are applied directly over a small wound or tube; these dressings are occlusive, decreasing the possibility of contamination while allowing visualization of the wound. This type of dressing often is used over intravenous sites, subclavian catheter insertion sites, and healing wounds.

Tape. There are many kinds of tape, ranging in width from ½ to 4 inches (1-inch-wide tape is the most commonly used). Table 30-5 summarizes the types and purposes of different tapes.

Table 30-5
Types of Tape

Type	Purpose
Adhesive (can cause occlusion, allergy, skin maceration, shearing)	Used for strength, support, and economy • To secure dressings and splints • To strap joints to prevent athletic injuries • To immobilize or stabilize body parts • To provide pressure • To approximate wound edges
Paper, plastic, acetate	Increased comfort, decreased allergic and skin problems • To close small wounds • To secure dressings
Microfoam	Used for compression or pressure dressings

Cleaning a Wound and Applying a Clean Dressing

The nurse prepares the client for the dressing change by explaining what will be done before starting the procedure. Proper screening is used to provide privacy. The client is assisted to a position that is comfortable and also convenient for the person changing the dressing. The area is exposed while maintaining proper draping.

It is important to use appropriate aseptic techniques when changing the dressing. It is especially important to wash hands thoroughly before and after changing dressings and to follow universal precautions. Among the most common causes of nosocomial infections is carelessness in observing medical and surgical asepsis when changing dressings.

The wound is cleaned and the dressing changed as described in Procedure 30-3. The nurse often is afforded an excellent opportunity for teaching while changing the client's dressing. Teaching becomes especially important when the client will be changing his or her own dressings at home. The client should be encouraged to help as much as possible, beginning with such assistance as preparing adhesive strips.

A client may be disturbed by the sight of the wound. The nurse should listen carefully to what the client is saying and observe for nonverbal communication as well. In some instances, the client may not want to look at the wound. This is apt to occur when a client has a wound that involves a change in normal body functions or appearance, such as a wound resulting from the removal of a breast, the amputation of an extremity, or the placement of a tube in a draining wound. Patience and emotional support help the client become accustomed to the sight of the wound in time.

The frequency with which dressings should be changed cannot be stated categorically. It depends on the amount of drainage, the physician's preference, and the nature of the wound. It is customary for the physician to perform the first dressing change, usually within 24 to 48 hours after surgery. Thereafter, nurses change the dressings on an as-needed basis or daily. Frequency for dressing changes should be noted on the client's nursing care plan.

Applying Bandages and Binders

Bandages and binders are used to secure dressings, apply pressure, and support the wound; they are especially useful in injuries of the extremities. **Bandages** are strips of cloth, gauze (eg, roller gauze, Kerlix, Kling), or elasticized material (eg, Ace bandages) used to wrap a body part. They come packaged in rolls and vary in width from 1 to 6 inches. **Binders** are designed for a specific body part and include slings, abdominal binders, chest binders, and T-binders. They may be made of cloth (flannel, muslin) or of an elasticized material that fastens together with Velcro.

A well-applied bandage or binder is comfortable, durable, neat, and clean. This is important for the client's emotional security as well as for promoting the best possible physiologic functioning of the body. The following principles guide action for applying bandages and binders.

Unclean bandages and binders may cause infection if applied over a wound or skin abrasion. This fact guides what may be a rather obvious action: bandages and binders should be kept clean and free of contamination. Medical asepsis is observed when applying bandages and binders. Skin abrasions and wounds are first covered with sterile dressings before clean bandages and binders are applied to protect the wound from trauma and contamination. Certain bandages and binders may be reused, but they should be changed if they become soiled or wet.

Prolonged heat and moisture on the skin may cause skin breakdown. This principle indicates that the area to be covered should be cleaned and dried thoroughly before applying a bandage or binder. An unnecessarily thick or extensive bandage should be avoided, so that the part being covered does not become excessively warm. Porous materials are preferable to nonporous ma-

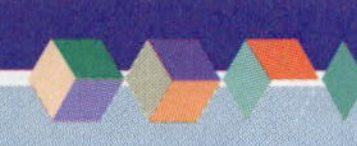

PROCEDURE 30-3

Cleaning a Wound and Applying a Clean Dressing

Equipment

Sterile gloves
Gauze dressings or squares
Sterile dressing set or suture set (contains scissors and forceps)
Cleaning solution
Clean disposable gloves
Sterile basin (optional)
Sterile drape (optional)
Plastic bag for soiled dressings
Waterproof pad
Bath blanket
Tape or ties
Surgi-pads or ABDs
Additional dressing supplies as needed or ordered (antiseptic ointments, extra dressings)
Acetone or adhesive remover (optional)
Sterile normal saline (optional)

Action	Rationale
1. Explain procedure to client.	An explanation encourages client cooperation and reduces apprehension.
2. Gather equipment.	This provides for organized approach to task.
3. Wash your hands.	Handwashing deters spread of microorganisms.
4. Check physician's order for dressing change. Note if drain is present.	This clarifies type of dressing.
5. Close door or curtain. Use bath blanket as needed when exposing area to be redressed. Position waterproof pad under client if desired.	This provides for privacy and warmth.
6. Assist client to comfortable position that provides easy access to wound area.	This provides for comfort.
7. Place opened, cuffed plastic bag near working area.	Soiled dressings may be placed in disposal bag without contaminating outside surfaces of bag.
8. Loosen tape on dressing. Use adhesive remover if necessary. If tape is soiled, don gloves.	It is easier to loosen tape before putting on gloves.
9. Don clean disposable gloves, and remove soiled dressings carefully in a clean to less clean direction. Do not reach over wound. Check position of drains before removing dressing. If dressing is not wet-to-dry application and is adhering to skin surface, it may be moistened by pouring a small amount of sterile saline onto it. Keep soiled side of dressing away from client's view.	This protects the nurse from handling contaminated dressings. Cautious removal of dressing is more comfortable for client and ensures that drain is not removed if one is present. Sterile saline provides for easier removal of dressing.
10. Assess amount, type, and odor of drainage.	Wound healing process or presence of infection should be documented.
11. Discard dressings in plastic disposal bag. Pull off glove inside out and drop it in bag.	This prevents spread of microorganisms by contaminated dressings.
12. Using aseptic technique, open sterile dressings and supplies on work area.	Supplies are within easy reach, and sterility is maintained.
13. Open sterile cleaning solution, and pour over gauze sponges in plastic container or over sponges placed in sterile basin.	Sterility of dressings and solution is maintained.
14. Don sterile gloves.	Maintains surgical asepsis.

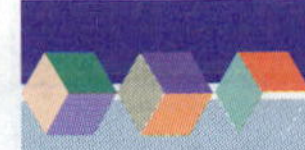

PROCEDURE 30-3 *(continued)*

Cleaning a Wound and Applying a Clean Dressing

Action	Rationale
15. Clean wound or surgical incision. Use sterile forceps if desired.	
a. Clean from top to bottom or from center outward.	Clean from least to most contaminated area.
b. Use one gauze square for each wipe, discarding each square by dropping into plastic bag. Do not touch bag with forceps.	Previously cleaned area is not recontaminated.
c. Clean around drain, if present, moving from center outward in a circular motion. Use one gauze square for each circular motion.	Move from least to most contaminated area.
d. Dry wound using gauze sponge and same motion.	Moisture provides medium for growth of microorganisms.
e. Apply antiseptic ointment if ordered.	Growth of microorganisms may be retarded and healing process improved.
16. Apply a layer of dry, sterile dressings over wound. Use sterile forceps if desired.	Primary dressing serves as a wick for drainage.
17. Use sterile scissors to cut sterile 4 × 4 gauze square to place under and around drain if one is present or use precut sterile gauze (see Fig. 30-7).	Drainage is absorbed and surrounding skin area is protected.
18. Apply second gauze layer to wound site.	This provides for increased absorption of drainage.
19. Place Surgi-pad or ABD dressing over wound as outermost layer.	Wound is protected from microorganisms in environment.

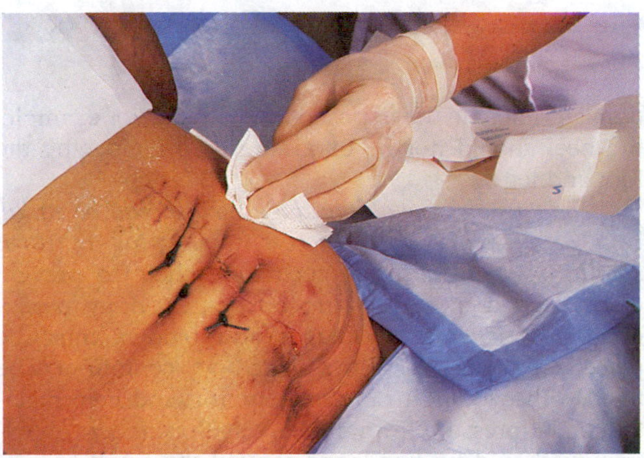

Action 15: Cleaning a surgical incision.

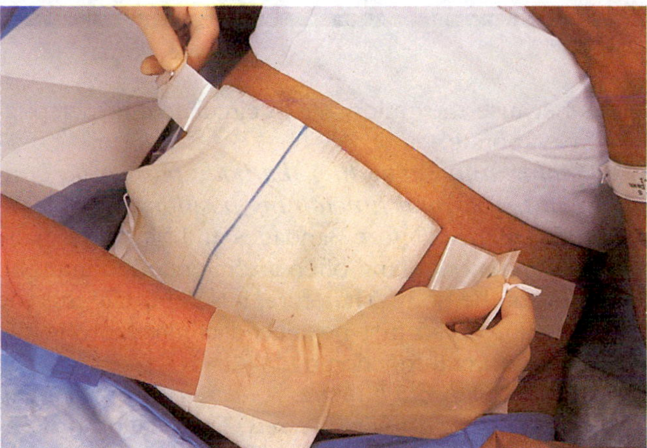

Action 19: Applying Montgomery straps over outer layer of dressing.

Action	Rationale
20. Remove gloves from inside out, and discard them in plastic waste bag. Apply tape or tie existing tapes to secure dressings.	Tape is easier to apply after gloves have been removed.
21. Wash hands. Remove all equipment, and make client comfortable.	This prevents spread of microorganisms.

(continued)

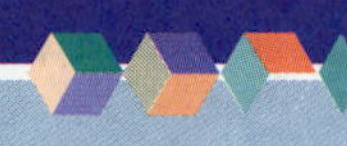

PROCEDURE 30-3 *(continued)*

Cleaning a Wound and Applying a Clean Dressing

Action	Rationale
22. Check dressing and wound site every shift. Record dressing change and appearance of wound, and describe any drainage in chart.	This provides accurate documentation of procedure.

Age Considerations

To keep a dressing intact or to prevent contamination of wound and supplies on an infant or young child, it may be necessary to restrain the child's hand. An old stocking or piece of stockinette may be used to encircle child's hand and then may be secured to the bed or crib with a tie or safety pin. Care must be taken not to compromise circulation to that extremity.

Home Care Considerations

Reinforce need for thorough handwashing before and after dressing change.

Have plastic bag available for safe disposal of soiled dressings and equipment.

Boil any nondisposable equipment (eg, forceps) for 10 minutes to ensure sterility after washing carefully in warm soapy water.

Inform client about availability of disposable wound care supplies.

Special Considerations

Client must be instructed that any break or interruption in the suture line may require immediate intervention and the surgeon should be notified immediately. Instruct client and family about significant changes that need to be reported to the nurse or physician.

Encourage splinting of wound during activity (coughing, sneezing, sudden movement, or change in position).

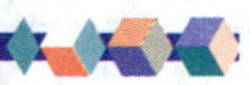

terials because they allow air to circulate and perspiration to evaporate.

Placing and supporting the body part to be bandaged in the normal functioning position prevents deformities and discomfort. Bandages and binders usually restrict some motion and often are intended to immobilize a part of the body. Therefore, it is important that the body part involved first be placed comfortably in the position of normal functioning.

Blood flow through tissues is decreased by applying excessive pressure on blood vessels. The healing process is impaired and tissue cells may die if the blood supply is inadequate to remove wastes and bring nourishment to the body part involved. The bandage or binder is applied with sufficient pressure to provide the amount of immobilization or support desired, to remain in place, and to secure a dressing if one is present. Pressure should not be so great, however, that circulation in the body part involved is impeded. Leaving a small portion of an extremity exposed, such as the fingers or toes, allows the nurse to assess for proper circulation in the bandaged area. Leaving a considerable portion of the end of an extremity exposed is likely to impede circulation if swelling in the exposed area occurs. For example, the heel should not be exposed when bandaging the foot and leg.

The tension of each bandage turn should be equal, and unnecessary and uneven overlapping of turns should be avoided. These techniques help to prevent undue and uneven pressure on tissues. Bony prominences over which bandages and binders must be placed are padded. Hollows in the body contour may be filled with padding to provide comfort and help maintain equal pressure from the bandage or binder. An extremity should be bandaged toward the trunk to promote venous return and impaired circulation in the distal part. After a bandage or binder has been applied, the body part is assessed frequently for signs of impaired circulation. In addition to being dangerous, a bandage applied too tightly is uncomfortable for the client.

Pins and knots, if used to secure a bandage or binder, are placed well away from the wound, a pressure point, or a tender and inflamed area. Pins and knots as well as seams in a bandage or binder cause undue and uneven pressure. They also cause discomfort for the client if located incorrectly.

Applying Roller Bandages

A roller bandage is a continuous strip of material wound on itself to form a cylinder or roll (Fig. 30-8). Plain gauze, elastic webbing, and stretchable roller bandages are made in various widths and lengths. When the bandaging is begun, the free end is held in place with one hand while the other hand passes the roll around the body part. After the bandage is anchored, the roll is passed or rolled around the body part, taking care that equal tension is exerted with each turn. It is easier to keep tension equal by unwinding the bandage gradually and only as it is required. The basic turns for roller bandages are:

Circular Turn. When using the circular turn, the bandage is wrapped around the body part with complete overlapping of the previous bandage turn. It is used primarily for anchoring a bandage where it is begun and where it is terminated.

Spiral Turn. When using the spiral turn, the bandage ascends in a spiral manner so that each turn overlaps the preceding one by one half or two thirds the width of the bandage. The spiral turn is useful when the body part being bandaged is cylindrical, such as the area around the wrist, the fingers, and the trunk.

Spiral-Reverse Turn. A spiral-reverse turn is a spiral turn in which reverses are made halfway through each turn. Spiral-reverse turns are particularly effective for bandaging a cone-shaped body part, such as the thigh, the leg, or the forearm.

Figure-of-Eight Turn. The figure-of-eight turn consists of making oblique overlapping turns that ascend and descend alternately. Each turn crosses the one preceding it so that it appears like a figure eight. It is effective for use around joints, such as the knee, the elbow, the ankle, and the wrist. Because it provides a snug bandage, it often is used for immobilization.

Spica Turn. The spica turn consists of ascending and descending turns that overlap and cross one another to form an angle. It is particularly useful for bandaging the thumb, the breast, the shoulder, the groin, and the hip.

Recurrent-Stump Bandage. Sometimes a recurrent type, or stump bandage, is applied. It is used for fingers and for the stump of an amputated limb. After a few circular turns to anchor the bandage, the initial end of the bandage is placed in the center of the body part being bandaged, well back from the tip to be covered. The bandage is passed back and forth over the tip, first on the one side and then on the other side of the center piece of bandage. Figure 30-9 shows how to apply a recurrent bandage to a stump, using the figure-of-eight turn to finish the bandage. Recurrent bandages also are used effectively for head bandages.

Whichever turn is being used, care should be taken to provide even overlapping of one half to two thirds the width of each bandage, except for the circular turn. All skin surfaces should be covered by the finished bandage to prevent pinching the skin between turns of the bandage. The bandage is completed well away from the wound or inflamed and tender areas. The terminal end of the bandage may be secured with adhesive, special clamps, or a safety pin, being careful to avoid undue pressure.

When removing a roller bandage, it is best to cut the bandage with a bandage scissors to prevent excessive manipulation of the part. Cutting should be done on the side opposite the injury or the wound, from one end to the other, so that the bandage can be folded open for its entire length. If the bandage is to be reused, it may be unwound by keeping the loose end together and passing it as a ball from one hand to the other while unwinding it.

Applying Binders

T-Binders. A T-binder is so named because it looks like the letter *T.* T-binders are particularly effective for securing dressings on the rectum and perineum and in the groin. The single T-binder is used for female clients, and the double T-binder is used for male clients. The belt is passed around the waist and secured with safety pins. The single or double tails are passed between the legs and pinned to the belt.

Many-Tailed Binders. A many-tailed binder, or scultetus binder, consists of a rectangular piece of fabric, with tails that are each about 5 cm (2 inches) wide attached to its sides. The binder supports the abdomen or holds dressings on it or on the chest. When a scultetus binder is applied to the abdomen, the client lies on his or her back on the center of the binder. The lower end of the binder is placed well down on the hips, but not so low that it interferes with the use of a bedpan or with walking. The tails are brought out to the sides of the client's body, with the bottom tail in position to wrap around the lower part of the abdomen first. A tail from each side is brought up and placed obliquely over the abdomen until all tails are in place. The last tails are fastened with safety pins.

Sling. A sling is used to support an arm. Most health-care agencies use commercial strap slings or sleeve slings. In the home setting, a large piece of cloth folded into a triangle can be used as a sling.

Straight Binders. A straight binder is a straight piece of material, usually about 15 to 20 cm (6 to 8 inches) wide and long enough to more than circle the torso. It is used for the chest and the abdomen. Straight binders may be pinned, or as is more common, fastened with Velcro. A straight binder for the chest often is provided

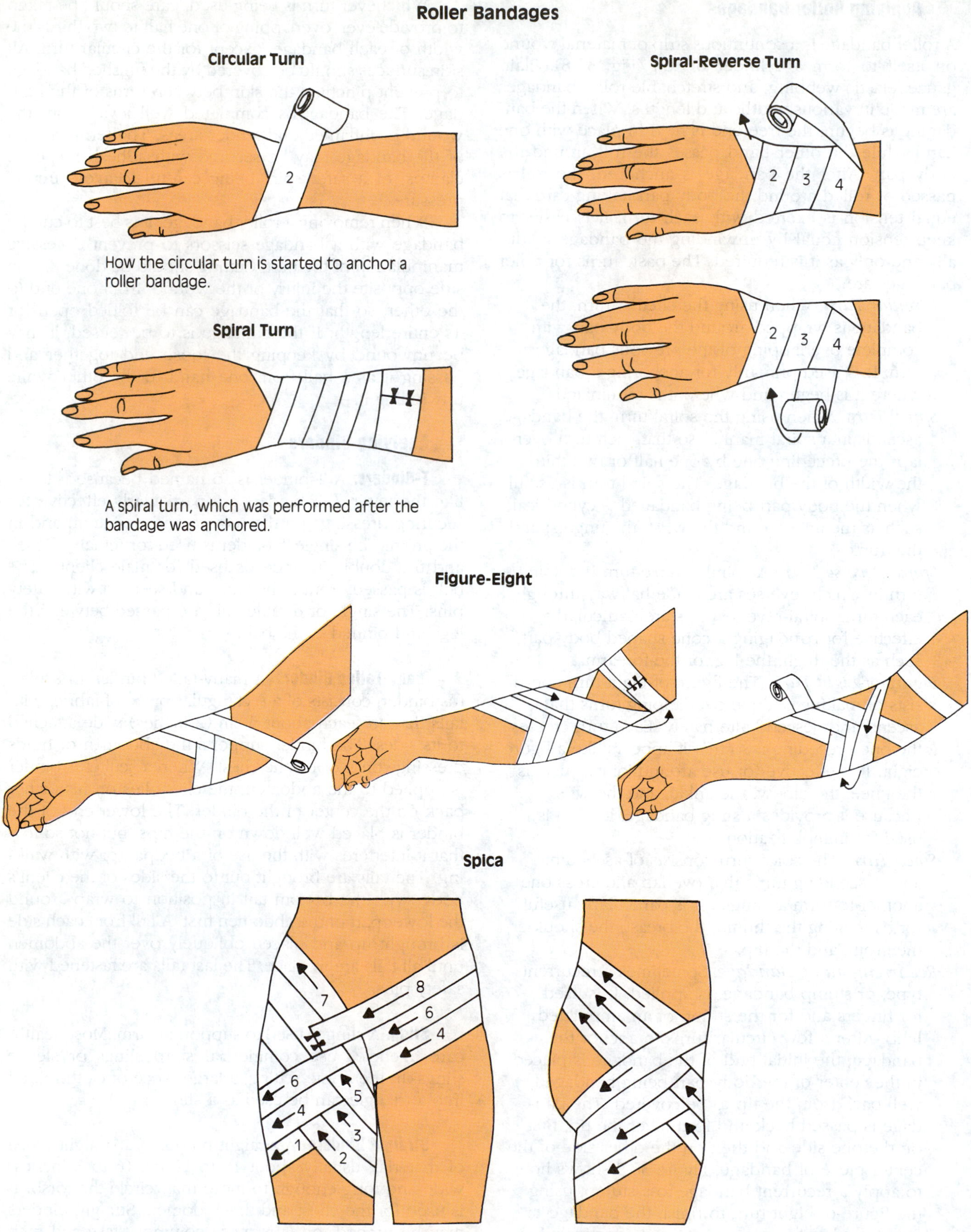

Roller Bandages

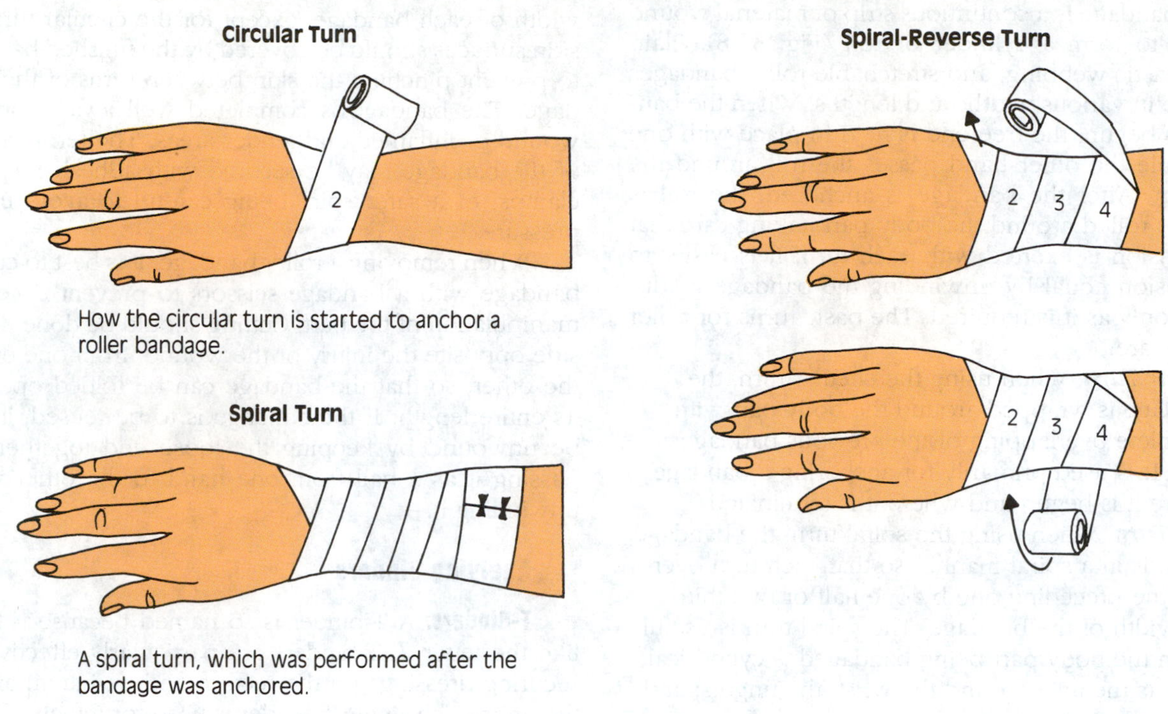

Figure-Eight

Spica

8
7
6
4
6
5
4
3
1
2

Figure 30-8
Techniques for applying various types of bandages.

Recurrent—Stump Bandage

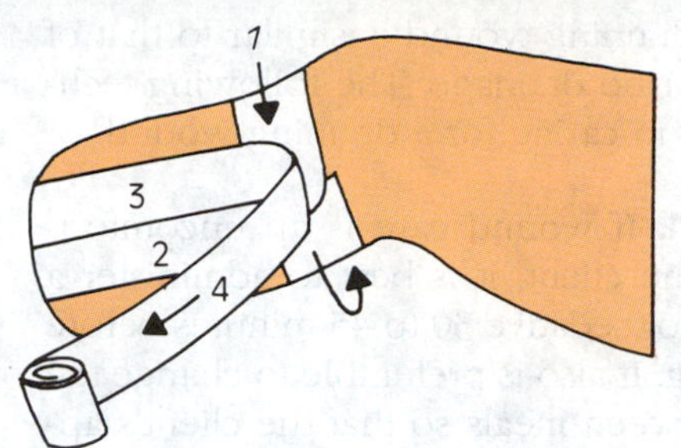

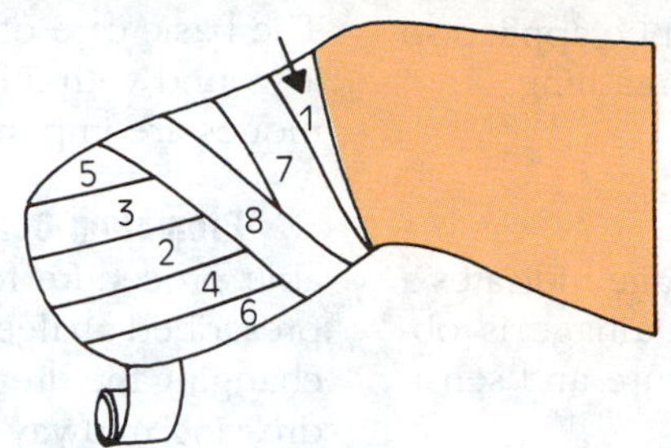

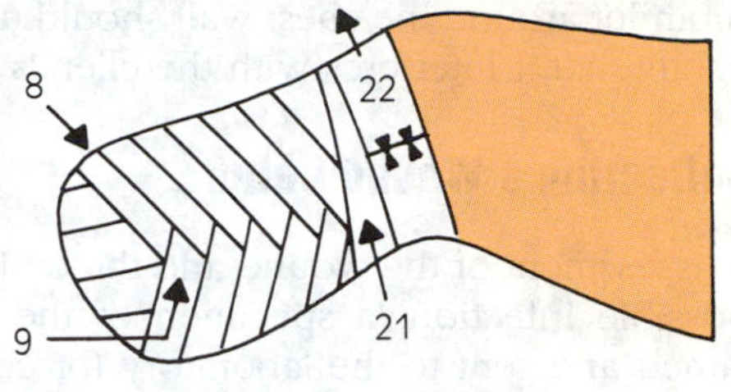

Binders

T-binders

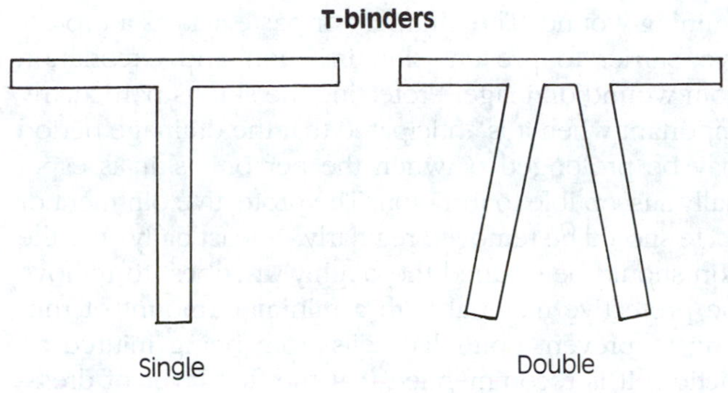

Many-Tailed Binders

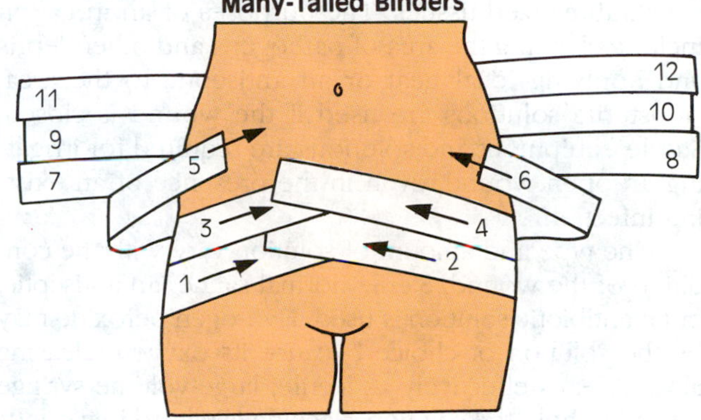

Slings

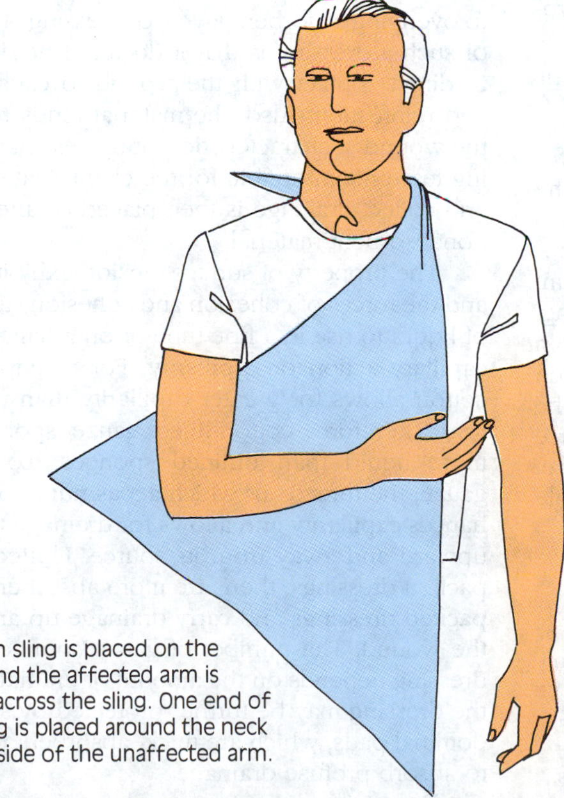

An open sling is placed on the chest and the affected arm is placed across the sling. One end of the sling is placed around the neck on the side of the unaffected arm.

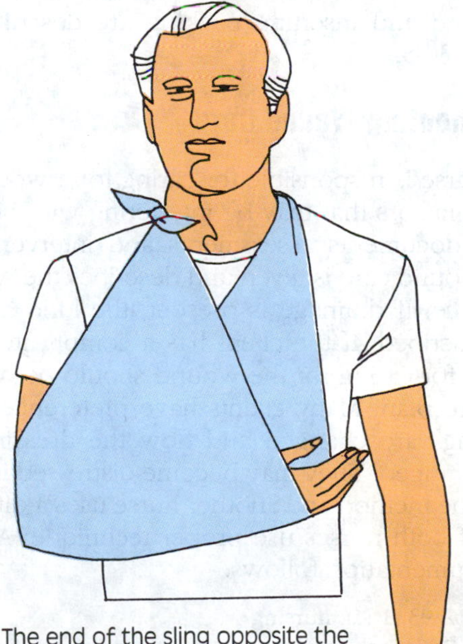

The end of the sling opposite the shoulder is placed over the affected arm, and the ends are tied at the side of the neck so that the knot does not rub over the cervical vertebra. The material at the elbow is folded neatly and may be secured with a pin placed behind the sling so that it is out of sight.

Figure 30-8 *(continued)*

with shoulder straps, so that it does not slip down on the trunk, and may require tucks to fit the body's contours. A binder around the chest wall should not be applied so tightly that it interferes with the client's breathing.

Collecting a Wound Culture

If assessment of the wound and the drainage indicates a possible infection, a specimen of the drainage is obtained and sent to the laboratory for culture and sensitivity, as outlined in Procedure 30-4.

Irrigating and Packing a Wound

An irrigation consists of directing a flow of solution over traumatized tissues. The purposes of an irrigation include cleaning the area of pathogens and other debris and applying local heat or an antiseptic to the area. Nonsterile solutions are used if the wound is closed. Sterile equipment and solutions are required for irrigating an open wound, even in the presence of an existing infection.

The type and amount of solution vary with the condition of the wound. Sterile normal saline, an antiseptic, or an antibiotic solution is used. Hydrogen peroxide may be the solution of choice because its oxygen-releasing ability cleans effectively. A sterile, large-volume syringe is used to hold the solution. Packing is placed in wounds to allow granulation tissue and healing by secondary intention to take place. The techniques for irrigating a wound and inserting packing are described in Procedure 30-5.

Documenting Wound Care

The nurse is responsible for caring for a wound and for noting factors that may be interfering with healing. The nurse documents assessments and interventions each time wound care is given and describes the wound's appearance. If drainage is present, the kind and amount are described. If the client has a complicated dressing, details for caring for the wound should be described in the care plan. Many clients have preferences for when dressings are changed and how the dressings can be best arranged. They may become distressed if one nurse uses one method and another nurse uses a different one, even if both nurses use proper technique. An example of documentation follows:

> 1/12/93, 1 PM, nursing
>
> Four-inch midline abdominal incision cleaned with sterile NS. Wound edges well approximated, skin sutures intact. Crust along suture line, edges of incision slightly edematous and dark pink. Penrose drain present in lower 1/4 of incision. Old dressing moderately saturated with serosanguineous drainage. New dressing applied with sterile technique, using Telfa, four 4 × 4s, and two ABDs applied with nonallergenic tape.
>
> A. Bowman, RN, CNS

Changing a Dressing for a Draining Wound

The basic care of a draining wound is similar to that of a wound with little or no drainage. The following techniques are important in caring for a draining wound.

Promoting Comfort. If wound care is an uncomfortable procedure for the client, it is best to administer a prescribed analgesic or sedative 30 to 45 minutes before changing the dressing. It also is preferable to change the dressing midway between meals so that the client's appetite and mealtimes are not disturbed.

Maintaining Skin Integrity. A protective ointment or paste may be applied to cleaned skin surrounding the draining wound. The ointment or paste acts as a protective barrier to prevent skin irritation and excoriation from wound drainage. Protecting the skin is particularly important when it is anticipated that the drainage period may be prolonged or when the person's skin is especially susceptible to irritation. The protective ointment or paste should be removed regularly, at least daily, and the skin should be cleaned thoroughly. It is best to remove the protective material with a minimal amount of rubbing to prevent epithelial cells from being injured by friction. It is recommended that the first layer of dressing material applied directly to a draining wound be nonabsorbent but hydrophilic (ie, capable of carrying moisture). This type of material allows drainage from the wound to pass from the first dressing without absorption to overlying absorbent layers of dressing. The advantage of such a dressing is that it does not hold the drainage in direct contact with the wound to cause maceration and reinfection. Also, the material tends not to stick to the wound, a characteristic that makes changing a dressing less uncomfortable for the client. Material to absorb and collect drainage is then placed on the first layer of nonabsorbent material.

The property of surface tension exhibited by liquids and the forces of cohesion and adhesion cause a column of liquid to rise in a fine tube or on a hair. This is called capillary action or capillarity. For example, absorbent cotton allows for greater capillarity than untreated cotton. Therefore, cotton-lined gauze sponges soak up more liquid than unlined sponges. Loosely packed gauze, the threads of which act as numerous wicks, enhances capillarity and allows for drainage to be directed upward and away from its source. Fluffed and loosely packed dressings, then, are more absorbent than tightly packed dressings and carry drainage up and away from the wound. The number of gauze sponges used in the dressing depends on the amount of drainage. The top of the dressing may be further protected by surgical or abdominal pads, which are thick, absorbent pads that help to absorb profuse drainage.

Because a draining wound requires more frequent changes of dressing than a wound without drainage, it

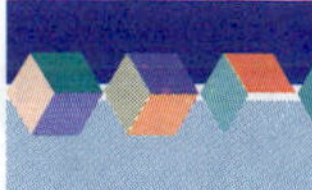

PROCEDURE 30-4

Collecting a Wound Culture

Equipment

Sterile Culturette tube with enclosed swab (or culture tube with individual swabs)
Sterile gloves
Clean disposable gloves
Plastic bag for soiled dressing
Label for Culturette tube
Laboratory requisition with rubber band or plastic bag

Action	Rationale
1. Explain procedure to client.	An explanation encourages client cooperation and reduces apprehension.
2. Gather equipment.	This provides for organized approach to task.
3. Wash your hands.	Handwashing deters the spread of microorganisms.
4. Don clean disposable gloves. Remove dressing and assess wound and drainage (see Procedure 30-3, actions 5 to 11).	This protects nurse from handling contaminated dressings.
5. Using aseptic technique, don sterile gloves and clean wound (see Procedure 30-3, action 15). Remove sterile gloves.	Previous drainage and skin flora are removed.
6. Twist cap to loosen swab in Culturette tube, or open separate swab and remove cap from culture tube, keeping inside uncontaminated.	Supplies are within easy reach, and sterility is maintained.
7. Don clean glove or new sterile glove, if necessary.	Use of Culturette does not require immediate contact with skin or wound. If contact with wound is necessary to collect specimen, wear sterile glove on that hand.
8. Carefully insert swab into drainage and roll gently. Use another swab if collecting specimen from another site.	Cotton tip absorbs wound drainage. This prevents cross-contamination of wound.
9. Place swab in Culturette tube, being careful not to touch outside of container. Twist cap to secure.	Outside of container is protected from contamination with microorganisms.
10. If using Culturette tube, crush ampule of medium at bottom of tube.	Swab with drainage can be surrounded by culture medium.

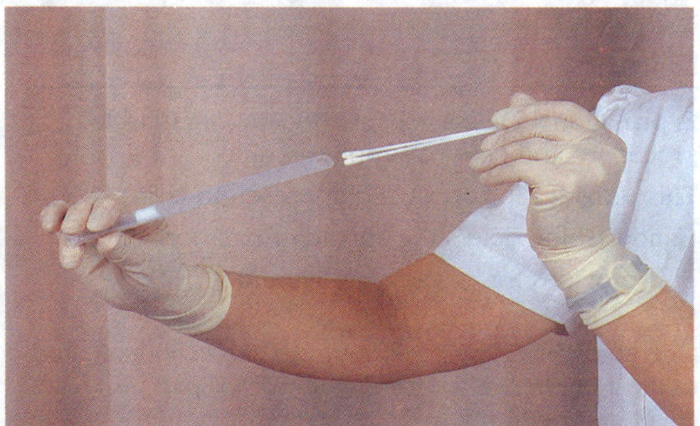

Action 9: Placing swab in a Culturette tube.

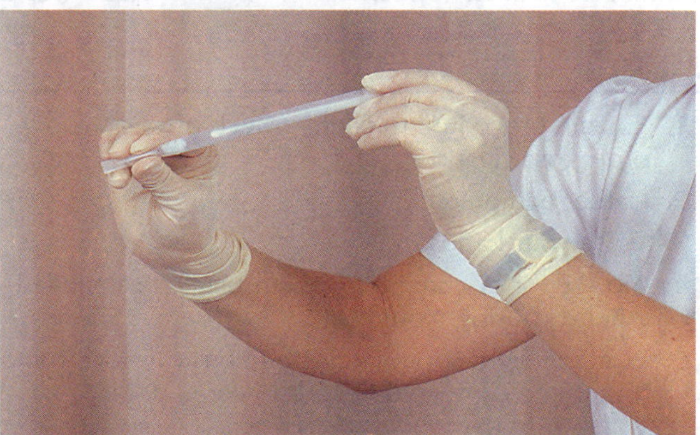

Action 10: Crushing ampule of medium at bottom of tube. (Photos © B. Proud.)

(continued)

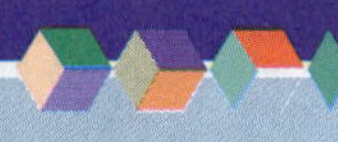

PROCEDURE 30-4 *(continued)*

Collecting a Wound Culture

Action	Rationale
11. Remove gloves from inside out, and discard them in plastic waste bag.	This prevents spread of microorganisms.
12. Wash your hands.	Handwashing deters the spread of microorganisms.
13. Apply clean dressing to wound (see Procedure 30-1, actions 16 to 20).	Drainage from wound is absorbed.
14. Wash your hands. Remove all equipment, and make client comfortable.	Handwashing deters the spread of microorganisms.
15. Label specimen container appropriately (client's name, date, time, nature of specimen). Attach laboratory requisition to tube with rubber band or place tube in plastic bag with requisition attached. Send to laboratory within 20 minutes.	This ensures proper identification of specimen. Overgrowth of other organisms can interfere with test results if specimen remains at room temperature for extended period.
16. Record collection of specimen, appearance of wound, and description of drainage in chart.	This provides for accurate documentation of procedure.

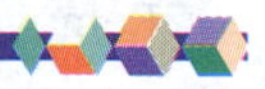

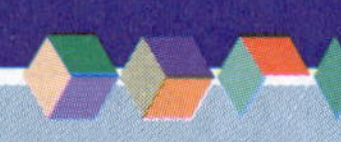

PROCEDURE 30-5

Irrigating a Sterile Wound

Equipment

Sterile irrigation set (basin, container for irrigant, irrigating syringe)
Prescribed irrigating solution (warmed to body temperature or 34°–37°C [93.2°–98.6°F])
Sterile soft catheter (optional)
Sterile gloves
Clean disposable gloves
Sterile dressing set or suture set (contains scissors and forceps)
Waterproof pad
Sterile gauze and surgipads or ABDs (for dressing change)
Plastic bag for soiled dressings
Packing gauze (as specified by physician)
Gown (optional)
Goggles (optional)
Bath blanket
Tape

Action	Rationale
1. Explain procedure to client. Check physician's order for irrigation.	Explanation facilitates client cooperation. Clarifies procedure and type of supplies required.
2. Gather equipment.	This provides for organized approach to task.
3. Wash your hands.	Handwashing deters the spread of microorganisms.
4. Close door or curtain. Use bath blanket as needed when exposing wound site.	This provides for privacy and warmth.
5. Position client so irrigating solution will flow from upper end of wound toward lower end. Place waterproof pad under client.	Gravity directs flow of liquid from least contaminated to most contaminated area. Waterproof pad protects client and bed linens.
6. Warm sterile irrigating solution to body temperature.	Warmed solution is more comfortable for client and promotes vasodilation.

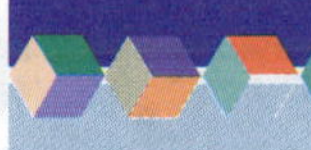

PROCEDURE 30-5 *(continued)*

Irrigating a Sterile Wound

Action	Rationale
7. Place opened, cuffed plastic bag near working area. Don gown and goggles if recommended.	Soiled dressings and packing may be placed in disposal bag without contaminating outside surfaces of bag. Gown protects uniform from contamination if splashing should occur. Goggles protect mucous membranes of eyes from contact with irrigant fluid.
8. Loosen tape on dressing, and put on clean gloves to remove soiled dressings.	Nurse is protected from handling contaminated dressings.
9. Assess amount, type, and odor of drainage. Observe condition of wound.	This provides information about wound healing process or presence of infection.
10. Discard dressings in plastic disposal bag. Remove gloves inside out and drop in bag.	Spread of microorganisms by way of contaminated dressings is prevented.
11. Using aseptic technique, open sterile dressings and supplies on work area.	Supplies are within easy reach and sterility is maintained.
12. Pour warmed sterile irrigating solution into sterile container. Amount may vary from 200 to 500 mL depending on size of wound.	This facilitates wound irrigation.

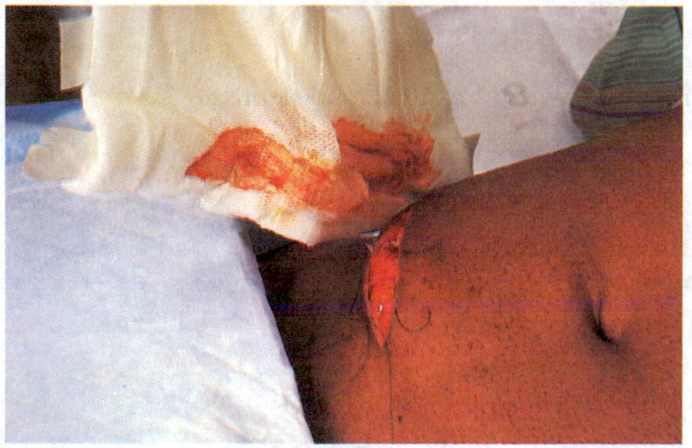

Action 9: Assessing wound drainage.

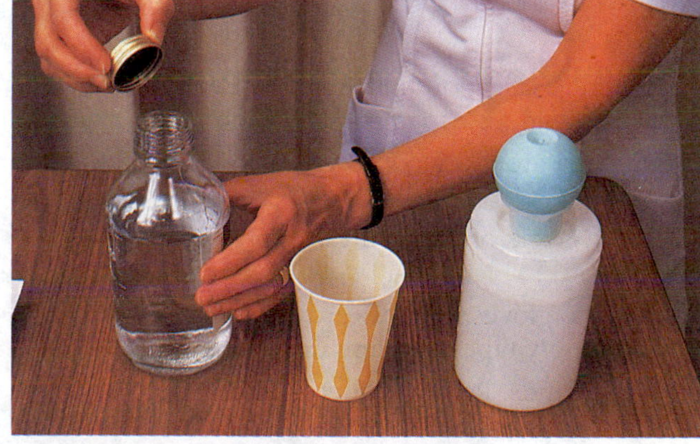

Action 12: Preparing sterile irrigating solution.

Action	Rationale
13. Put on sterile gloves (see Procedure 28-3).	This maintains surgical asepsis.
14. Position the sterile basin below the wound to collect irrigation fluid with nondominant hand.	Irrigation is facilitated and client and bed linens are protected from contaminated fluid.
15. Use dominant hand to fill syringe with irrigant. Gently direct a stream of solution into wound, keeping tip of syringe 1 inch (2.5 cm) above upper tip of wound. If using a catheter tip on syringe, insert it gently into wound to point of resistance.	Debris and contaminated solution flow from least contaminated to most contaminated area. Catheter allows introduction of irrigant into wound with small opening or one that is deep.

(continued)

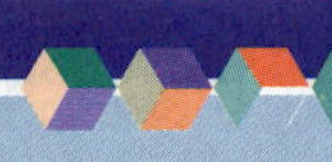

PROCEDURE 30-5 (continued)

Irrigating a Sterile Wound

Action	Rationale

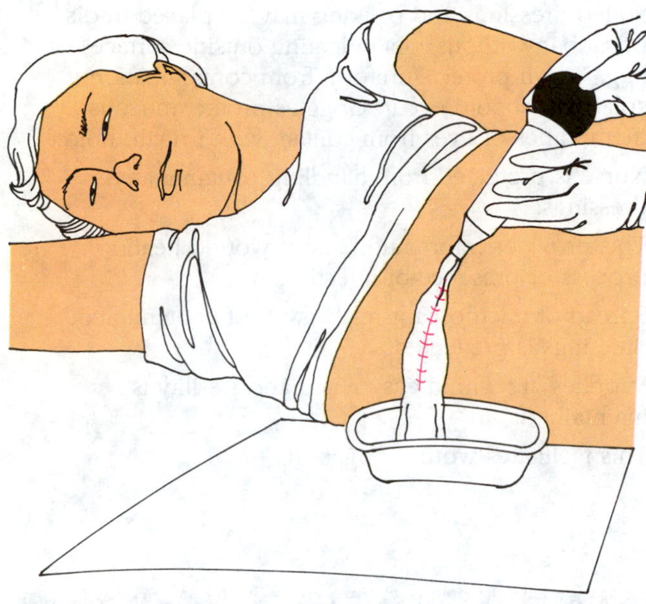

Action 15: Irrigating wound.

Action	Rationale
16. Continue irrigation until solution returns clear. Try to maintain a steady flow of solution.	Irrigation removes exudate and debris.
17. Dry area around wound with a sterile gauze sponge.	Moisture provides medium for growth of micro-organisms.
18. Apply layers of sterile dressing.	Drainage is absorbed and surrounding skin area is protected.
19. Remove gloves, and discard them in plastic waste bag. Apply tape to secure dressings.	Tape is easier to apply after gloves have been removed.
20. Wash hands. Remove all equipment, and make client comfortable.	This prevents spread of microorganisms.
21. Check dressing and wound site every shift. Record dressing change, appearance of wound, and describe any drainage in chart.	This provides for accurate documentation of procedure.

Special Considerations

If insertion of packing is ordered:

- Use sterile forceps to gently insert sterile packing into wound.
- Be careful not to pack wound excessively because this may impede blood flow and delay healing.
- Cut packing with sterile scissors if necessary.
- Allow a small strip of packing to protrude from small and deep wounds to facilitate removal.

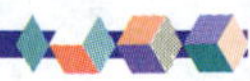

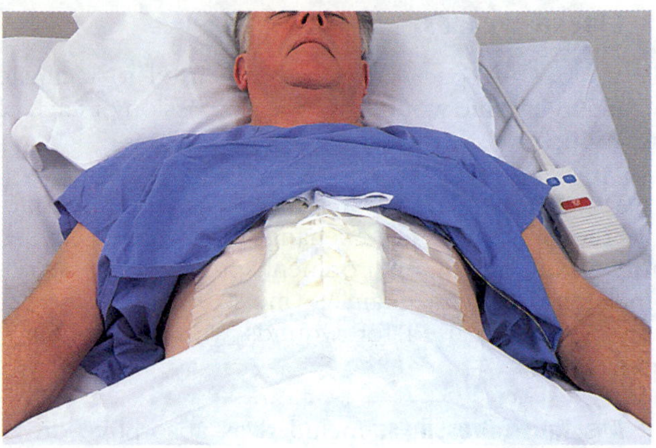

Figure 30-9
Montgomery straps make it possible to care for a wound without removing adhesive strips with each dressing change. (Photo © B. Proud.)

is recommended that Montgomery straps be used to secure the dressing (Fig. 30-9). These straps do not require changing with each dressing, as tape strips do. Montgomery straps can be made or are available commercially. The adhesive end of the strap is placed on the skin well away from the wound. The end of the strap near the wound remains free because the adhesive side is turned back on itself. Gauze or woven strips passed through eyelets are tied over the wound to secure the dressing. When the dressing is changed, the strips are untied and turned back to allow for wound care. After the fresh dressing is applied, the straps are retied to hold the dressing in place.

Preventing Infection and Promoting Healing. In caring for wounds, the nurse uses principles of both medical and surgical asepsis. Nurses should make certain that precautions are taken to prevent infection of the wound by following CDC guidelines.

Contamination occurs through a moist medium. Microorganisms can move from the external surface through the dressing to the wound if a dressing remains in place until it is saturated. In like manner, microorganisms can move from the wound to the outer surface of a saturated dressing. For this reason, dressings should not be allowed to become saturated. They should either be replaced with fresh dressings or be reinforced before drainage causes saturation.

A rubber tubular drain (Penrose), a sump tube, or a catheter may be placed in a wound to promote exudate drainage. Care must be used so that these devices are not dislodged when dressings are changed. A Penrose drain may be ordered to be shortened each day. This can be done by grasping the end of the drain with sterile forceps, pulling it out a short distance while using a twisting motion, and cutting off the end of the drain with sterile scissors. A sterile safety pin (or Klip) often is placed at the end of the drain so that it cannot slip down into the wound.

Closed drainage systems are used more often in place of incisional drains like the Penrose drain. Some studies show that the infection rate is cut nearly in half when drains are placed only when necessary and through a separate stab wound rather than in the incision itself. Closed drainage systems consist of a drain connected to an electric suction machine or a portable closed drainage suction system (Fig. 30-10).

Portable closed drainage systems have directions for their use printed on the container itself. The nurse should avoid touching the open port when emptying the drainage. Reflux of drainage from a contaminated port could contaminate the wound itself. The use of a closed drainage system eliminates a potential source of microorganisms. The frequent dressing changes needed with the open Penrose drain (which empties directly onto a dressing) are no longer necessary. Closed drainage systems also allow accurate measurement of drainage.

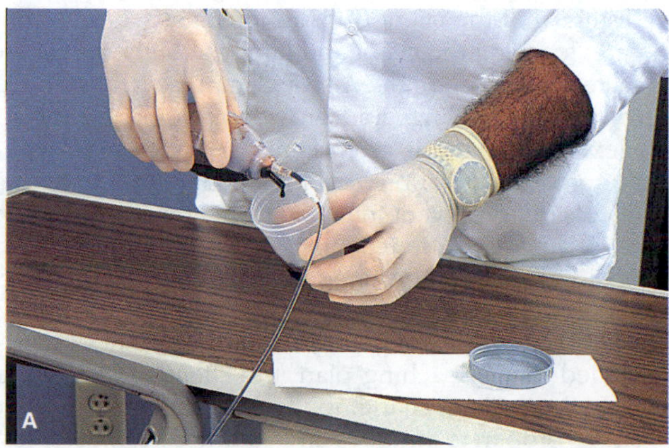

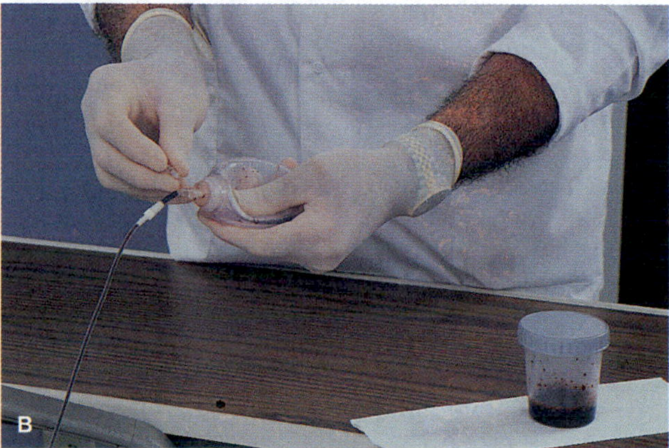

Figure 30-10
The Jackson-Pratt drain is a closed drainage system. The nurse empties the drain **(A)** and reapplies suction by compressing the drain **(B)**. (Photo © B. Proud.)

Changing Dressings in Special Situations

Infected Wounds

The CDC recommends special techniques for the care of extensive wounds with purulent drainage. In particular, wounds infected with *S. aureus*, beta-hemolytic streptococcus, and *C. perfringens* (gas gangrene) require the use of these special techniques. When information about the causative organism is unknown, the CDC advises the use of these techniques for all infected and extensive wounds with purulent drainage:

- Wash hands before wound care.
- Wear a gown while caring for the client's wound. This gown need not be sterile, unless there is danger of carrying organisms on a clean gown to an already debilitated client.
- Wear a mask while caring for the wound.
- Be prepared to use two pairs of sterile gloves, and change gloves between the removal of the old dressing and the application of the new dressing.
- Wash hands thoroughly between glove changes. An antimicrobial soap is recommended by many healthcare agencies.
- Use a no-touch technique when handling soiled dressings. Lift soiled dressings with a clamp or forceps. This prevents contamination of the hands.
- Place soiled dressings in a moisture-proof bag, which is then closed securely, double-bagged, and incinerated without being opened.
- Be sure to wash the hands again thoroughly after completing wound care. If organisms accumulate on the hands because proper technique was broken, the organisms not only are likely to be carried to others but eventually may also become resident flora on the nurse's hands.

Open Wounds

Recommendations for the treatment of open wounds focus on facilitating healing. Research supports the harmful effects of such treatments as the use of full-strength Betadine and of wet-to-dry dressings. In caring for wounds, each wound is individually evaluated, and one (or more) of a variety of choices for dressing might be made.

New trends are for a wet-to-damp packing for open wounds. Cellular migration needed for tissue repair and healing is enhanced by a moist surface. Packing material is soaked in a solution (with normal saline solution being the solution of choice) and then wrung out so it is only slightly moist. A wet packing slows wound closure, increases the risk of bacterial growth, and can macerate surrounding tissue. Packing is applied loosely and only to the edges of the wound; it is then covered with a secondary dressing to absorb drainage. If the packing dries, it should be soaked with saline solution before it is removed.

Chronic Wounds

Many types of special dressings are used to facilitate healing in chronic wounds. A brief discussion of each of these follows.

Transparent Adhesive Dressings. These semipermeable dressings allow an exchange of oxygen between the wound and the environment, protect against contamination, and maintain a moist wound environment. They are used for wounds with only minimal drainage.

Absorptive Dressings. Included as absorptive dressings are karaya powder, dextranomer beads, and copolymer starches. These dressings absorb drainage and maintain a moist surface by forming a gelatinous mass. Dextranomer and copolymer starch dressings are used for deep wounds with heavy drainage.

Hydrocolloid Dressings. Hydrocolloid dressings absorb drainage, maintain a moist wound surface, and decrease the risk of infection. They are used for shallow wounds that have minimal drainage. Polyurethane dressings are nonadhesive hydrocolloid dressings that must be taped down to prevent wound contamination because they do not adhere to the wound surface. They may be used in conjunction with packing for deep, open wounds.

Hydrogel Dressings. Hydrogel dressings are oxygen-permeable and nonadhesive and maintain moisture. They are used for wounds that are not deep.

Synthetic Barrier Dressings. These are pastes that dry to form transparent, semipermeable dressings. Pores in the dried paste allow drainage to move from the wound to an absorbent dressing.

Teaching for Home Care of a Wound

With the trend toward ambulatory surgery and earlier dismissal of the client from an inpatient setting to home care, teaching the client and family about wound care is increasingly important. Although a nurse may be needed to change dressings and provide wound care for complex situations, it is often family members who will do the procedure. To provide the continuity of care that is necessary to prevent infection and promote healing, the nurse must include teaching about wound care as part of discharge planning and in interactions with home care clients and families.

Each of the following components should be included in the teaching plan; the client or family member who will be changing the dressing should demonstrate proper techniques in wound care and dressing change.

- Dressing materials can be purchased from pharmacies, drug stores, discount stores, and medical

supply stores. Consideration of the cost and ease of use is important.
- Signs and symptoms of infection (increased body temperature; malaise; reddened wound edges; drainage that is thick, green, odorous, or increased in amount; increased pain) should be reported immediately to the healthcare provider.
- Eating well-balanced meals and drinking fluids are important to wound healing. The diet should be high in proteins, zinc, iron, and vitamins.
- Modifying activities of daily living and exercise patterns may be necessary until healing is completed.
- Disposable gloves should be worn when changing the dressing and hands should be washed before donning and after removing the gloves.
- The old dressing should be placed in a plastic bag or wrapped in several layers of newspaper before disposal in a trash container.

EVALUATING

As with any client, the plan of care for the surgical client is evaluated based on the expected outcomes. The plan has been effective if the client is discharged after surgery without complications, with a healing wound, and with knowledge of and ability for self-care.

Key Points

- Surgery is a stressful time for the client and family, imposing physical and psychosocial alterations and adaptations.
- The time before, during, and after surgery is called the perioperative period; it is divided into preoperative, intraoperative, and postoperative phases.
- Surgical procedures are categorized by urgency, risk, and purpose.
- Anesthesia may be general or regional. General anesthesia is given to induce narcosis, loss of reflexes, and relaxation of skeletal muscles; regional anesthesia produces sensory loss but the client remains awake.
- Clients agree to surgery by signing an informed consent form.
- Preoperative assessment identifies physical and psychosocial risk factors and strengths.
- Preoperative nursing interventions to prepare the client for the intraoperative and postoperative phases include therapeutic communications, preoperative teaching, and physical preparation.
- Intraoperative nursing roles are either as a scrub nurse or as a circulating nurse; each has specific client responsibilities.
- Immediate postoperative nursing care in the PAR area focuses on assessing and monitoring to prevent complications from anesthesia or surgery.
- Ongoing postoperative nursing care is planned to facilitate recovery from surgery and coping with alterations; both the client and the family are part of care.
- Ambulatory surgery is provided on an outpatient basis; preoperative assessment and teaching are critical elements in safe surgery and recovery.
- A wound is a disruption in the normal integrity of the skin.
- Wound healing is influenced by a variety of factors, including state of health; nature of the wound; age; and whether healing is by primary, secondary, or tertiary intention.
- Providing wound care requires knowledge and skill in assessing for complications, in using various supplies throughout the healing process, and in teaching clients or caregivers to provide self-care at home.
- The nursing process is used throughout the perioperative period to provide knowledgeable, holistic, individualized client care.

Study Questions

1. Mrs. Ogg requires surgery for treatment of a ruptured spleen as the result of an automobile accident. This type of surgery belongs in which of the following categories?
   a. minor, diagnostic
   b. minor, elective
   c. major, emergency
   d. major, palliative
2. A general anesthetic is given for specific purposes during a surgical procedure. Which one of the following purposes is *not* included?
   a. loss of consciousness
   b. relaxation of skeletal muscles
   c. reduction of reflex action
   d. localized loss of sensation
3. You have been asked to witness a client signature on an informed consent form for surgery. You would recognize that the document is valid for which one of these clients?
   a. a 92-year-old who is severely confused
   b. a 45-year-old who is oriented and alert
   c. a 10-year-old who is oriented and alert
   d. a 36-year-old who has had a narcotic
4. Although surgical clients may be taking any number of medications before surgery, which of the

following categories of drugs would be most likely to increase surgical risk?
   a. anticoagulants
   b. antacids
   c. laxatives
   d. sedatives
5. The obese client who has surgery is at risk for which of the following postoperative complications?
   a. hunger
   b. impaired wound healing
   c. hemorrhage
   d. gas pains
6. Which of these teaching methods would be most effective in preoperative teaching for ambulatory surgery?
   a. lecture
   b. discussion
   c. audiovisuals
   d. handouts
7. Mr. Ying is scheduled for surgery. He says to you, "I am so frightened—what if I don't wake up?" What would be your best response?
   a. "You have a wonderful doctor."
   b. "Let's talk about how you are feeling."
   c. "Everyone wakes up from surgery!"
   d. "Don't worry, you will be just fine."
8. A patient-controlled analgesia pump allows the postoperative client to
   a. be totally pain free
   b. take unlimited amounts of medication
   c. choose the type of pain medication
   d. administer his or her own analgesic
9. Mr. Moreno has had a surgical procedure that necessitated a thoracic incision. You anticipate that he will have a higher risk for postoperative complications involving which body system?
   a. respiratory system
   b. circulatory system
   c. digestive system
   d. nervous system
10. While assessing a client in the PAR, the nurse notes increased wound drainage, restlessness, a decreasing blood pressure, and an increase in the pulse rate. The most probable cause for these findings is
   a. thrombophlebitis
   b. atelectasis
   c. infection
   d. hemorrhage
11. Your client tells you she is having pain in her right lower leg. You assess the presence of thrombophlebitis by
   a. palpating the skin over the tibia and fibula
   b. measuring and documenting calf circumference daily
   c. taking and recording vital signs four times a day
   d. noting difficulty with ambulation
12. Gas pains are a common postoperative discomfort. Which of the following nursing actions implemented in the plan of care would be most likely to relieve gas pains?
   a. cough and deep breathe every 2 hours
   b. maintain NPO status for 48 hours
   c. encourage frequent ambulation
   d. take vital signs every 4 hours
13. Which of the following surgical clients would be at a greater risk for alterations in body image?
   a. female, aged 19, large facial laceration
   b. female, aged 42, gallbladder surgery
   c. male, aged 14, fractured clavicle
   d. male, aged 52, hernia repair
14. The older adult often has reduced vital capacity as a normal physiologic change. Which nursing action would be most important for the postoperative care of the older surgical client specific to this change?
   a. Take and record vital signs every shift.
   b. Turn, cough, and deep breathe every 4 hours.
   c. Encourage increased intake of PO fluids.
   d. Assess bowel sounds daily.
15. The rationale for the use of leg exercises after surgery is that leg exercises
   a. promote respiratory function
   b. maintain functional abilities
   c. provide diversional activities
   d. increase venous return

Answers With Rationale

1. The correct response is *c.* This surgery would involve a major body organ, has the potential of postoperative complications, requires hospitalization, and must be done immediately to preserve the client's life.
2. The correct response is *d.* Whereas *a, b,* and *c* are all purposes of a general anesthetic, a localized loss of sensation occurs with a regional anesthetic.
3. The correct response is *b.* A consent form is not legal if the client signing the form is confused, sedated, or a minor.
4. The correct response is *a.* Anticoagulant drug therapy would increase the risk of hemorrhage during surgery. The other categories of drugs normally would not increase surgical risk.
5. The correct response is *b.* Fatty tissue is more difficult to suture, less resistant to infection, and more prone to delayed wound healing.
6. The correct response is *d.* Although all of the responses might be useful in teaching clients and families before ambulatory surgery, written instructions are most effective in providing information.

7. The correct response is *b.* This response allows the client to talk about feelings and fears and is therapeutic. The other responses give false reassurance.
8. The correct response is *d.* A patient-controlled analgesia pump does allow the client to administer his or her own analgesic. Use of this device does not allow the client to take unlimited amounts of medication, choose the type of pain medication, or be totally pain free.
9. The correct response is *a.* A thoracic incision makes it more painful for the client to take deep breaths or cough. Shallow respirations and ineffective coughing increase the risk for respiratory complications.
10. The correct response is *d.* Increased wound drainage, restlessness, decreasing blood pressure, and increasing pulse rate are assessment findings that indicate hemorrhage.
11. The correct response is *b.* Inflammation from thrombophlebitis increases the size of the affected extremity and can be assessed by measuring circumference on a regular basis.
12. The correct response is *c.* Frequent ambulation stimulates peristalsis and relieves gas pains. The other responses are incorrect in this situation.
13. The correct response is *a.* The reaction of the client to an accidental or intentional incision is influenced by age, time to prepare for the change, and visibility of the trauma. Large facial wounds increase the risk of an alteration in body image.
14. The correct response is *b.* Reduced vital capacity in older adults increases the risk of respiratory complications, including pneumonia and atelectasis. Having the client turn, cough, and deep breathe every 4 hours maintains respiratory function and helps to prevent complications.
15. The correct response is *d.* Leg exercises in the postoperative period do increase venous return. As a result, the client has decreased risk of thrombophlebitis and emboli.

Bibliography

Agency for Health Care Policy and Research. (1992). *Acute pain management: Operative or medical procedures and trauma. Clinical practice guidelines.* DHHS Pub. No. (AHCPR) 92-0032. Silver Spring, MD: AHCPR.

Association of Operating Room Nurses. (1993). *AORN standards and recommended practices for perioperative practice.* Denver, CO: AORN.

Badger, J. (1994). Calming the anxious patient. *American Journal of Nursing, 94*(5), 46–50.

Bright, L., & Georgi, S. (1994). How to protect your patient from DVT. *American Journal of Nursing, 94*(12), 28–32.

Carpenito, L. J. (1995). *Nursing care plans and documentation: Nursing diagnoses and collaborative problems* (2nd ed.). Philadelphia: Lippincott.

Carpenito, L. J. (1995). *Nursing diagnosis: Application to clinical practice* (6th ed.). Philadelphia: Lippincott.

Cuzzell, J. (1993). The right way to culture a wound. *American Journal of Nursing, 93*(5), 48–50.

Erwin-Toth, P., & Hocevar, B. (1995). Wound care: Selecting the right dressing. *American Journal of Nursing, 95*(2), 46–51.

Fina, D. (1994). Ethical issues: A chance to say goodbye. *American Journal of Nursing, 94*(5), 42–45.

Fromm, C., & Metzler, D. (1993). Preparing your older patient for surgery. *RN, 56*(1), 38–43.

Good, M. (1995). A comparison of the effects of jaw relaxation and music on postoperative pain. *Nursing Research, 44*(1), 52–57.

Groath, L. (1990). *Operating room nursing: Perioperative practice* (2nd ed.). Norwalk, CT: Appleton & Lange.

Groath, L., & Howery, D. (1992). 25 predictions for perioperative nursing. *Nursing, 22*(1), 48–49.

Hawthorne, M. (1994). Gender differences in recovery after coronary artery surgery. *IMAGE: Journal of Nursing Scholarship, 26*(1), 75–80.

Hollinworth, H. (1995). Nurses' assessment and management of pain at wound dressing changes. *Journal of Wound Care, 4*(2), 77–83.

Jacobson, T. (1994). Obesity and the surgical patient: Nursing alert. *Ostomy Wound Management, 40*(2), 56–58.

Kane, A., & Kurlowicz, L. (1994). Improving the postoperative care of acutely-confused older adults. *MEDSURG Nursing, 3*(6), 453–458.

Krasner, D. (1995). Wound care: How to use the red-yellow-black system. *American Journal of Nursing, 95*(5), 44–47.

McConnell, E. (1994). Maintaining a closed wound-drainage unit. *Nursing 94, 24*(7), 26.

Meeker, M. H., & Rothrock, J. C. (1991). *Alexander's care of the patient in surgery* (9th ed.). St. Louis: Mosby.

Nash, C., & Jensen, P. (1994). When your surgical patient has hypertension. *American Journal of Nursing, 94*(12), 38–44.

Oberle, K., Allen, M., & Lynkowski, P. (1994). Follow-up of same day surgery patients. *AORN Journal, 59*(5), 1016–1025.

Porteous, A., & Tyndall, J. (1994). Yes, I want to walk to the OR. *Canadian Operating Room Nursing Journal, 12*(2), 15–16, 18–19.

Smeltzer, S. C., & Bare, B. G. (1996). *Brunner and Suddarth's textbook of medical–surgical nursing* (8th ed.). Philadelphia: Lippincott-Raven.

Spearing, C., & Cornell, D. J. (1988). Incentive spirometry: Inspiring your patients to breathe deeply. *Nursing, 17*(9), 50–51.

Walsh, J. (1993). Postop effects of OR positioning. *RN, 56*(2), 50–57.

Whittington, K. (1995). Debunking wound care myths. *RN, 58*(8), 32–33.

Willey, T. (1992). Use a decision tree to choose wound dressings. *American Journal of Nursing, 92*(2), 43–46.

Wooden, L. (1993). Cutting postop pain. *RN, 56*(8), 26–33.

Each individual is a composite of interrelated physiologic and psychosocial dimensions; alterations in one dimension affect all of the others. Unit VII discusses psychosocial considerations in holistic client care, focusing on self-concept; stress and adaptation; loss, grief, and dying; sensory stimulation; sexuality; and spirituality.

One's sense of self may contribute positively or negatively to health and self-care abilities. Similarly, stress can motivate or thwart growth and self-actualization. Nursing interventions to maintain, strengthen, or change self-concept and to promote healthy adaptation are basic to all aspects of client care.

Loss, grief, and dying are universal human experiences which most nurses encounter in some form on a daily basis. Effective nurses are competent and willing to assist people struggling with loss, grief, and dying.

Intact and functioning senses are necessary for life, normal growth and development, and pleasurable experiences. Alterations in any of the senses require caring, knowledgeable, and individualized nursing interventions to meet needs and prevent further overload or deprivation.

Sexuality and spirituality are important components of human functioning. These dimensions are an integral part of each person's identity and are critical elements in holistic client care. To facilitate sexual and spiritual wellness, nurses must develop self-awareness in these areas and become comfortable with values and practices different from their own. Nursing interventions and therapeutic interpersonal skills are used to elicit concerns, identify needs, implement teaching, make referrals, and demonstrate empathic acceptance and caring.

Unit VII provides the knowledge base for promoting healthy psychosocial responses in clients. Using the nursing process, interventions can be planned and implemented to meet needs and support strengths in both health and illness.

Promoting Healthy Psychosocial Responses

"The unique function of the nurse is to assist the individual . . . in the performance of those activities contributing to health or its recovery (or to peaceful death) that he would perform unaided if he had the necessary strength, will or knowledge . . . in such a way as to help him gain independence as rapidly as possible."

Virginia Henderson (1897–)
the "first lady of nursing," whose career spanned almost 70 years as both author and researcher; her works on nursing principles are research based and have been translated into 25 languages

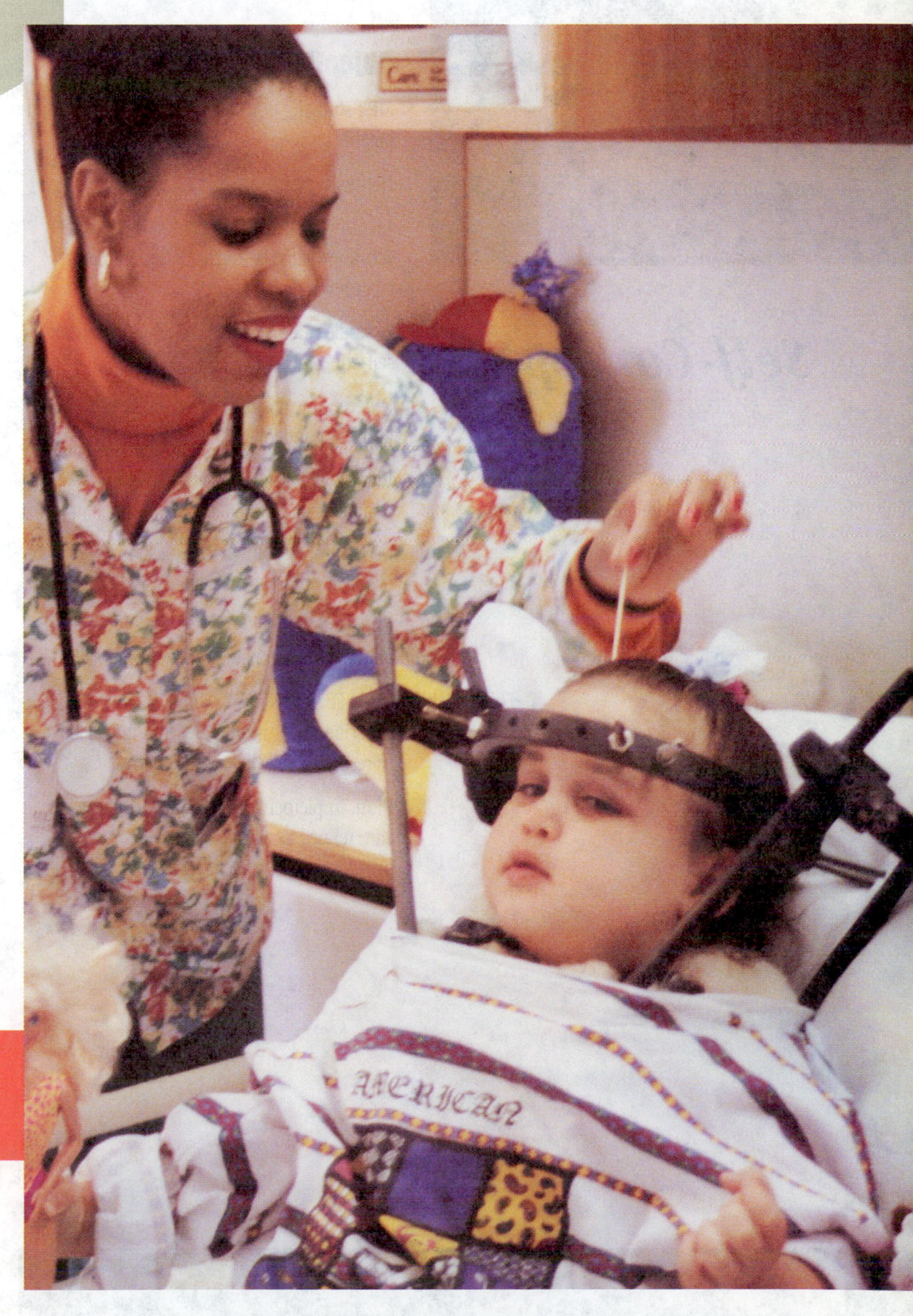

Unit VII

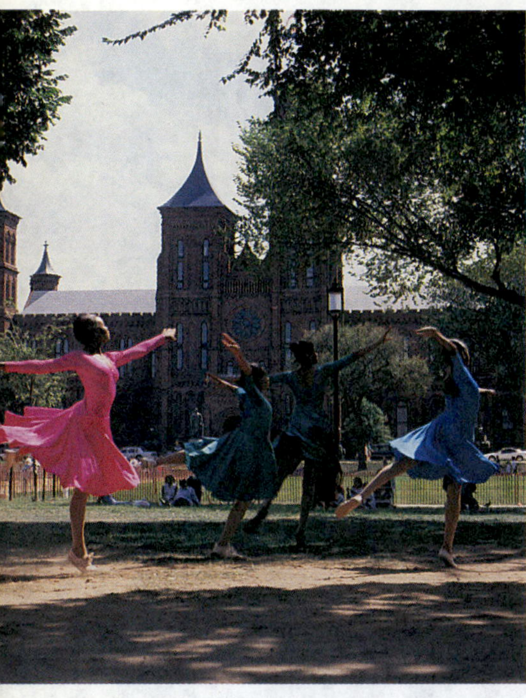

Chapter 31

Self-Concept

Objectives

After studying this chapter, the learner should be able to:

Define key terms used in the chapter.

Identify three dimensions of self-concept: self-knowledge, self-expectation, and self-evaluation (self-esteem).

Describe major steps in the development of self-concept.

Differentiate positive and negative self-concept and high and low self-esteem.

Identify six variables that influence self-concept.

Use appropriate interview questions and observations to assess a client's self-concept.

Develop nursing diagnoses to identify disturbances in self-concept (body image, self-esteem, role performance, personal identity).

Describe nursing strategies that are effective in resolving self-concept problems.

Plan, implement, and evaluate nursing care related to select nursing diagnoses for disturbances in self-concept.

Key Terms

body image
ideal self
personal identity
role performance
self-actualization
self-concept
self-esteem
social self
subjective self

As people move through the hierarchy of human needs to higher levels, needs for self-esteem and self-actualization arise as discussed in Chapter 2. The need for self-esteem is the need to feel good about oneself and to believe that others hold one in high regard. The need for **self-actualization** is the need to reach one's potential through full development of one's unique capability. A critical component of both of these needs is self-concept. One's self-image or self-concept has the power to either encourage or thwart personal growth.

People who think of themselves as born losers most likely will not be motivated to learn self-care behaviors in response to illness or trauma. Nursing efforts aimed at teaching such people are doomed to failure until the client values himself or herself enough to want to invest energy in self-care. On the other hand, clients may desperately want to modify their self-concept and self-care behaviors and have no idea how to do it. Nursing assistance can help them explore factors in self-esteem. The experience of illness, diagnostic testing, and treatment can severely threaten the self-concept of a client. Nurses sensitive to the self-concept needs of clients can use each nurse–client interaction to enhance the client's sense of self and to assist the client in resolving self-concept disturbances.

Study of this chapter provides knowledge of the dimensions of self-concept, formation of self-concept, and key factors affecting self-concept. Practical interview guides are offered for assessing self-concept (personal identity, body image, self-esteem, role performance). Strategies for enhancing the self-esteem of the nurse are provided. Numerous examples of nursing diagnoses are given, and specific nursing strategies for assisting clients to meet self-concept goals/outcomes are described. In the section Nursing Process in Clinical Practice, focused assessment, planning, implementation, and evaluation guides are offered for the nursing diagnosis Self-Concept Disturbance. Self-Concept Disturbance is not a North American Nursing Diagnosis Association diagnostic label but is often used initially as a broad diagnostic category until a client's problem can be further specified.

These guides and the concluding client care study illustrate how the nurse's knowledge of self-concept may be combined with skilled nursing interventions and caring to resolve successfully disturbances in self-concept.

Overview of Self-Concept

Dimensions of Self-Concept

Self-concept is the mental image or picture of self. All the feelings, beliefs, and values associated with "I" or "me" compose self-concept. Included in the notion of self-concept are the following:

Body image: How I experience my body
Subjective self: How I see myself, who I think I am
Ideal self: Self I would like to be or feel I should be
Social self: Way I feel others see me (Atwater, 1990)

The dimensions of self-knowledge, self-expectations, and self-evaluation describe self-concept. People with a positive self-concept have broad and diversified knowledge of the self, realistic expectations, and high self-esteem.

Self-Knowledge: "Who Am I?"

A person's self-knowledge includes basic facts (age, race, occupation), which place that person in social groups, and a listing of qualities or traits, which describe typical behaviors, feelings, moods, and other characteristics (generous, hot-headed, ambitious, intelligent, sexy). Although some labels cannot be changed (eg, sex, age, and race), most are unstable and subjective. *Global self* is the term used to describe the composite of all the basic facts, qualities, traits, and images one holds about oneself.

Self-Expectations: "Who or What Do I Want to Be?"

Expectations for the self flow from the ideal self, the self one wants to be or thinks one should be. These expectations often develop early in childhood and are based on the image of a role model. These expectations may be healthy or unhealthy. Many contemporary thinkers are expressing concern that many children currently identify as their heroes rock stars or pimps, prostitutes, and drug dealers rather than parents, government leaders, or other professional people.

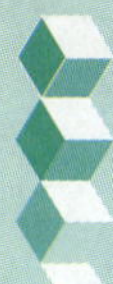

Research in Nursing: Making a Difference

Self-Concept and Nursing

The relationship between positive self-concept and health and well-being is often taken for granted. In the first study described below nurse researchers attempt to provide a theoretical understanding of self-concept. In the second study the authors compare the self-concepts of young adults with and without diagnoses of cancer.

Related Research

Stein, K. F. (1995). Schema model of the self-concept. *IMAGE; Journal of Nursing Scholarship, 27*(3), 187–193.
The centrality of the self-concept in maintaining physical and psychosocial well being is widely recognized in nursing. Despite its importance, progress in the development of an empirically supported and clinically relevant theoretical framework has been limited by difficulties in defining and measuring the construct. The schema model of the self-concept is presented as a theoretical framework that has the potential for explaining how the self-concept functions to influence emotional and behavioral responses to events relevant to health and well-being. In this model, the self-concept refers to a person's total collection of cognitions about the self including self-schemas, possible selves, and other less fully elaborated self-images.

Bello, L. K., & McIntire, S. N. (1995). Body image disturbances in young adults with cancer. *Cancer Nursing, 18*(2), 138–143.
The impact of the diagnosis of cancer and its treatment on the body image of young adults (18–29) diagnosed with cancer is relatively unknown. This descriptive, comparative study examined body image in scores of young adults diagnosed with cancer (n = 63) and young adults without cancer (n = 54). The conceptual framework for this study was taken from body image and developmental theory. A statistically significant difference was found between the mean scores reported by the young adults diagnosed with cancer for the body cathexis and self-cathexis scales. The *more* positive body image scores of the young adults with cancer may indicate that healthcare workers are making a difference.

Summary

More study of both the theoretical and practical dimensions of self-concept is needed so that nurses can better meet the self-concept and self-actualization needs of clients.

Self-Evaluation: "How Well Do I Like Myself?"

Self-esteem is the evaluative and affective component of the self-concept, sometimes termed self-respect, self-approval, or self-worth. According to Maslow (1954), all people "have a need or desire for a stable, firmly based, usually high evaluation of themselves, for self-respect or self-esteem, and for the esteem of others" (p. 90). Accordingly, he identified two subsets of esteem needs: (1) self-esteem needs (strength, achievement, mastery and competence, confidence in the face of the world, independence, and freedom) and (2) respect needs or the need for esteem from others (status, dominance, recognition, attention, importance, and appreciation). Research confirms that self-esteem comes from two major sources: how competent children think they are in various aspects of life and how much social support they receive from other people (Harter, 1990). There is growing recognition from authorities that one's self-esteem, like the various self-images that make up one's self-concept, varies considerably depending upon a specific relationship or situation (Atwater, 1996).

Coopersmith (1967) identified the four bases of self-esteem as (1) significance—the way a person feels he or she is loved and approved of by the people important to that person; (2) competence—the way tasks that are considered important are performed; (3) virtue—the attainment of moral–ethical standards; and (4) power—the extent to which a person influences his or her own and others' lives. According to Coopersmith, people with high, medium, and low self-esteem differ in their expectations of the future, in their affective reactions, and in their basic styles of adapting to environmental demands. People with high self-esteem are accustomed to being well received and successful. They are able to approach people, tasks, and new situations freely, with confidence in their ability to interact and to get along with people and to respond successfully to life's challenges.

Formation of Self-Concept

A person is not born with a self-concept. Rather, it is a social creation that develops as a result of interactions with others (Fig. 31-1). Steps in the formation of self-concept include the following:

1. An infant learns that the physical self is different from the environment. If basic needs are met and warmth and affection are experienced, the child begins life with positive feelings about self.
2. The child next internalizes (incorporates into self) other people's attitudes toward self. Parents play

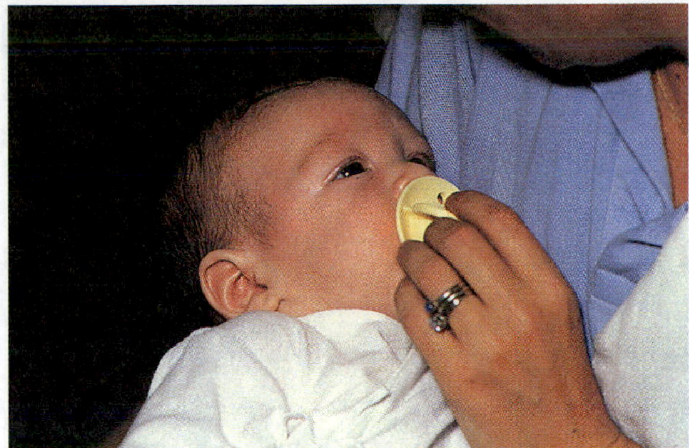

Figure 31-1
Interaction between parents and the infant are important to the child's development. Feeding, holding, cuddling, and cooing are forms of interaction.

the most influential role here; peers play the second most influential role.

3. The child or adult internalizes the standards of society.

Stages in the development of the self include self-awareness (infancy); self-recognition (18 months); self-definition (3 years); and self-concept (6–7 years).

Coleman, Morris, and Glaros (1990) identified the following psychologic conditions that foster healthy development of the self in children:

- Emotional warmth and acceptance
- Effective structure and discipline
    - Clearly defined standards and limits, so that children understand what goals, procedures, and conduct are approved
    - Adequately defined roles for both older and younger members of the family
    - Established methods of handling children that produce the desired behavior, discourage misbehavior, and deal with infractions when they occur
- Encouragement of competence and self-confidence
- Helping children meet challenges
- Appropriate role models
- A stimulating and responsive environment

Formation of self-concept is further described in developmental theories, especially in Erikson's stages of development, Piaget's cognitive developmental stages, and Havighurst's developmental tasks (see Chapters 8 and 9).

Threats to Self-Concept

Anxiety is a threat to self-concept. According to psychoanalysts, the ego uses many different methods to protect itself from anxiety. Among these methods are coping and defense mechanisms. Anxiety and coping and defense mechanisms are discussed in Chapter 32.

Factors Affecting Self-Concept

Almost any life experience can influence a person's self-concept. Key factors include developmental considerations, culture, internal and external resources, history of success and failure, stressors, and illness or trauma.

Developmental Considerations

As a person matures, the criteria that mark the experiences necessary for a positive self-concept change. (See the preceding discussion of formation of self-concept.) Although the infant needs a supportive environment in which all human needs are met, the growing child needs the freedom to explore and develop the ability to meet increasing personal needs. Table 31-1 highlights developmental changes affecting self-concept, related implications for nursing, and potential self-concept disturbances.

Culture

As a child internalizes the values of parents and peers, culture begins to influence a sense of self. If the culture is relatively stable, little tension may be experienced between what culture expects of the child and what the child expects of self. When parents, peers, and the adult world confront the child with different cultural expectations, the sense of self may be confused. For example, an adolescent may realize his or her parents live by the work ethic and believe it is necessary to rise early every day and put in a full day's work. The adolescent's peer group has few demands placed on it and encourages the adolescent to hang out with the group. The adolescent's vocational aptitudes, meanwhile, are leading him or her to consider a music career in a rock group, which will keep the adolescent out late many nights doing something the parents do not classify as work.

Internal and External Resources

The personal strengths an individual recognizes, develops, and uses are powerful but subjective determinants of self-concept. One person may use humor as both an effective coping mechanism and as a successful interpersonal tool. Another person may use humor to avoid facing conflict and may feel bad about being known as a joker or clown. External resources such as a network of support people, adequate finances, and organizational supports are also subjective determinants of self-concept. Generally, the more resources a person has and uses wisely, the better the feelings about self.

History of Success and Failure

People with a history of repeated failure (in school, friendships, work, or marriage) may perceive themselves as failures and actually perpetuate this image by unconsciously instructing others to treat them this way. They may come to fear success and actually find it easier to

Table 31-1
Developmental Changes Affecting Self-Concept

Developmental Period	Changes Affecting Self-Concept	Implications for Nursing	Potential Causes of Disturbances in Self-Concept
Infancy	• No self-concept at birth • Beginning differentiation of self and nonself	• Teach parents the critical importance of providing consistent and affectionate parenting • Assess if the parents have reasonable expectations of the infant: sleeping, eating, other awake behaviors	• Unmet basic human needs • Lack of adequate body and sensory stimulation • Parents' lack of acceptance of the infant's appearance or behavior
Childhood	• An intact body is important to the young child, who fears bodily mutilation • During middle childhood, a sense of being trusted and loved, of being competent and trustworthy develops • Differences between self and others are strong	• If invasive procedures are indicated, explain simply to the child what is being done and offer the child support • Assess the parents' ability to provide the type of developmental environment in which the child's self-concept can evolve positively	• Dysfunctional family • Too much or too little structure • Sensory perceptual impairments
Adolescence	• Development of secondary sex characteristics; rapid body changes • Emphasis on sexual identity • Parental influences on self-concept are often rejected; peers become more important; movement is toward development of own identity	• Assess adolescent's self-knowledge and understanding of body changes • Counsel adolescent regarding mature and healthy use of independence he or she craves • Provide anticipatory guidelines regarding hazards to life, health, human functioning	• Inability to accept body • Inability to resolve competing pulls to be both a child and an adult • Unhealthy peer pressure
Adulthood	• Society places emphasis on intactness of body, fitness, energy, sexuality, style, sophistication, beauty • Important to meet role expectations well	• Assess how realistic the adult's expectations are and the incentive they provide for growth and development • Assist client to deal constructively with negative influences in self-image • Preretirement counseling	• Inability to fulfill conflicting role expectations • Failure to accept role responsibility (eg, parenting responsibilities) • Unreasonable expectations • Irreversible body change related to trauma, illness • Unsatisfying job • Failure to develop new goals to give meaning and purpose to life
Later years	• Declining physical and possibly mental abilities	• Assess how the older person is adjusting to effects of aging • Counsel regarding meaningful use of time • Explore resources	• Loss of significant work (retirement); feelings of uselessness • Death of spouse, significant others • Diminished physical attractiveness, strength, overall health • Multiple stressors • Fear of dependency

fail even though they do not like themselves that way. Thus, failure influences an individual's self-concept negatively, and his or her self-concept instructs the person to continue to fail. On the other hand, one successful experience conditions a person to strive for the next success and a positive self-concept is forged that expects success and makes it happen.

Stressors

Life stressors (marriage, divorce, an exam, a new job, a gray hair, a fire) may call forth a personal response and mobilize an individual's talents, resulting in good feelings about oneself. Stressors may also evoke maladaptive responses that diminish the self-concept. Examples

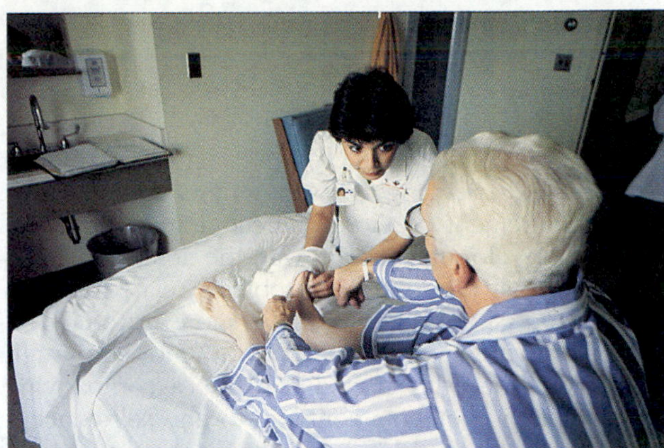

Figure 31-2
An illness or alteration in function may present a dilemma for the client and affect his or her self-concept.

of these include withdrawal, depression, extreme anxiety, and substance abuse. How the person perceives the stressor (threat, challenge, defeat) and his or her ability to mobilize personal strengths and other resources are determined largely by that person's self-concept, which in turn is influenced by the response the person chooses.

Aging, Illness, or Trauma

Because most people take a healthy body for granted, the diminishment of physical attractiveness or functioning, the suggestion of disease, or sudden impact of trauma may pose serious threats to the self (Fig. 31-2). People vary greatly in their response to aging, illness, and trauma.

The Nurse as Role Model

Before nurses can successfully identify and resolve self-esteem disturbances in clients, they must be comfortable with themselves and possess a certain measure of self-esteem. Important goals for the nurse's personal esteem are the following:

- Identify basic unmet human needs, exploring positive means to meet these needs.
- Schedule time every day to meet personal needs.
- Assess the effect of feedback from significant others on self-esteem.
- Describe personal strengths accurately.
- Develop a realistic plan to achieve goals for personal growth and development.

Specific strategies for developing self-esteem in relation to one's professional practice follow:

Dispel the myth that it is necessary to know all there is to know about nursing to be a good nurse. At no one point in time does any nurse ever have it all together. Acceptance of the need to learn new theories or new procedures frees you from having to practice defensively (ie, pretend to be on top of every new development) and is a great stimulus for professional growth and development.

Realistically evaluate strengths and weaknesses. Build a periodic review into your practice and be fair in your self-evaluation. "I think I'm giving better care than ever before and I know my clients are appreciative, but I'm sensing a lot of tension between myself and a couple of the other nurses. . . ."

Accentuate the positive. Many of us have a knack for forgetting the 99 things we did well and focusing

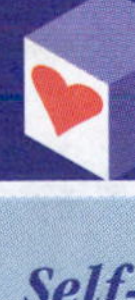

Promoting Wellness

Self-Concept

Use the assessment checklist to determine how well you are meeting your need for positive self-concept. Then develop a prescription for self-care by choosing appropriate behaviors from the list of suggestions.

Assessment Checklist

almost always	sometimes	almost never	
☐	☐	☐	1. I have established appropriate expectations and goals for myself.
☐	☐	☐	2. I have effective and satisfying relationships with others.
☐	☐	☐	3. I cope effectively with change and loss.
☐	☐	☐	4. I accept and feel good about myself.

Self-Care Behaviors

1. Accept normal variations in physical appearance and capabilities.
2. Use problem-solving and decision-making strategies to define expectations and set goals.
3. Set priorities and accept that no one person can be all things to all people.
4. Forget past mistakes; carrying around "excess baggage" is unhealthy.
5. Emphasize strengths and abilities in self.
6. Take an active part in group activities in school, work, church, or the community.
7. Volunteer time, talents, or services.
8. Avoid alcohol or drugs.
9. Live life one day at a time.

on our one error. Errors need to be taken seriously and evaluated but not to the exclusion of overlooking positive accomplishments.

Develop a conscious plan for changing weaknesses into strengths. Professional growth and development depend on strong motivation to become better at what you do. "Realizing that I never know what to say when a client receives bad news, I can try to avoid these clients or consciously plan to develop better interpersonal skills." Nurses are tremendous resources for each other. Tapping into each other's strengths is a great way to build self-esteem mutually. "You always seem to know the right thing to say or do with clients. Do you mind if I observe for a while and then 'try on' some of your behaviors?"

Work to develop team self-esteem. A basic interpersonal principle that seems to work well in practice is to offer to others what you want yourself. Because our sense of self is strongly influenced by the feedback we receive from others, positive reinforcement of our strengths and sincere offers to help correct deficiencies are needed by everyone.

Actively demonstrate your commitment to nursing and concern about nursing's public image. To feel good about yourself, you need to be able to experience pride in your profession. Active participation in professional organizations can offer many personal rewards—not the least of which is enthusiasm and pride in being a nurse. Monitoring the media's portrayal of nursing and providing appropriate feedback contributes to individual and corporate nursing self-esteem.

ASSESSING

The nurse assessing self-concept focuses on the client's personal identity, body image, self-esteem, and role performance. A general assessment of self-concept should be included in every comprehensive nursing assessment. It is as important to identify and label a client's positive self-concept as it is to note problems. Positive self-concept can be used as a key strength when working with clients to achieve other health goals. The following self-concept assessment was recorded on the nursing history of a 17-year-old single mother of a healthy newborn:

> Describes herself as a strong, healthy, fun-loving person who is "going to make it." Is unafraid of new parenting responsibilities. Identifies the following as strengths; experience with younger brothers and sisters; program for single parents in her high school; strong motivation to make something of herself (plans on getting an associate degree in x-ray technology); support of family and friends; and belief that "God will help me." Expresses concern about always being able to make the right decisions about going out with friends, dating, and so forth. Views motherhood as an achievement about which she is proud. Basically has positive self-concept with high self-esteem.
>
> M. LeBon, RN

Clients experiencing illness or trauma that results in body disfigurement or altered functioning or life crises that arrest development and thwart the achievement of life goals are at high risk for problems related to self-concept and should be assessed more carefully. If problems surface during the interview, a more thorough assessment should be carried out. The accompanying boxes highlight elements common to any self-concept assessment and high-risk factors. The discussion that follows offers specific interviewing guides for each element in the assessment.

It is important for the nurse conducting this assessment to realize the limitations of self-reporting. A client may give what he or she believes are the desired or socially acceptable responses to interview questions. "Why, of course I like myself. I'm a pretty good person. Yes, I have friends." For this reason the nurse must evaluate the client's responses in relation to observations made about the client and what is known about the client from other sources. The accompanying box outlines behaviors often associated with low self-concept. When the nursing assessment reveals a clustering of these behaviors, it is important to discuss this finding with the client. This is especially true when there is a discrepancy between the client's words and behavior.

High-Risk Factors for Self-Concept Disturbances

Personal Identity Disturbance

- Developmental changes
- Trauma
- Gender dissonance
- Cultural dissonance

Body Image Disturbance

- Loss of body part or function
- Disfigurement
- Developmental changes

Self-Esteem Disturbance

- Unhealthy interpersonal relationships
- Failure to achieve developmental milestones
- Failure to achieve life goals
- Failure to live up to personal moral code
- Sense of powerlessness

Altered Role Performance

- Loss of valued role
- Ambiguous role expectations
- Conflicting role expectations
- Inability to meet role expectations

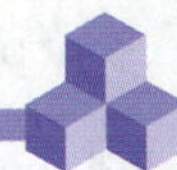

Focused Assessment Guide

Self-Concept

Factors to Assess	Questions and Approaches
Personal identity	How would you describe yourself to others? • Personal characteristics and traits • Strengths
Body image	Describe your body to me. What do you like most/least about your body? Is there anything about your body that you would like to change?
Self-esteem	Tell me something about your sense of satisfaction with yourself. Who would you like to be? Who or what has influenced your self-expectations? Are these expectations realistic? • Significance: What is your response when you feel unloved or unappreciated by those who are important to you? • Competence: How do you feel about your ability to do the things in life that are important to you? • Virtue: To what degree are you satisfied with the way you are able to live up to your moral standards? • Power: To what extent do you feel able to control what happens to you in life? How does this make you feel?
Role performance	How do you feel about your ability to do all the things your roles demand of you? Are these roles satisfying for you?

"You've told me that you feel in control of your situation right now and are committed to the treatment plan, but I notice you've broken three therapy appointments this month and you did mention that you are drinking more heavily. . . ."

Defining Characteristics of Low Self-Concept

Refusal to touch or look at a body part
Refusal to look into a mirror
Unwillingness to discuss a limitation, deformity, or disfigurement
Refusal to accept rehabilitation efforts
Inappropriate attempts to direct own treatment
Denial of the existence of a deformity or disfigurement
Increasing dependence on others
Signs of grieving—weeping, despair, anger
Refusal to participate in own care or take responsibility for self-care (self-neglect)
Self-destructive behavior (alcohol, drug abuse)
Displaying hostility toward healthy people
Withdrawal from social contacts
Changing usual patterns of responsibility
Showing change in ability to estimate relation of body to environment

(Carpenito, L. J. [1995]. *Nursing diagnosis: Application to clinical practice* [6th ed.]. Philadelphia: Lippincott, p. 794)

Personal Identity

When assessing self-concept, the information needed first is the client's description of self. **Personal identity** describes an individual's conscious sense of who he or she is. "How would you describe yourself to others?" The nurse pays special attention to the labels used by the client and the order in which they appear. Calhoun and Acocella (1989, p. 63) have recommended the following exercise:

> As an exercise in understanding how people organize knowledge about themselves, make a list of ten labels that you feel identify you (for example, "student," "Italian American," "opera fan," "premed major"). Put the most important label first and then list the others in order of decreasing importance. (What if the order were reversed?) To what extent do you think your way of organizing information about yourself affects your behavior?

It is important to discover if individuals are comfortable with their perceived identity. Developmental changes, trauma, and cultural and gender dissonance may all place a client at risk for personal identity disturbances.

Client Strengths. Many clients focus naturally on their deficiencies; asking pointed questions about personal strengths can help a client identify positive factors: "What are some of your personal strengths . . . qualities you are proud of . . . things you do well?"

"What special talents or abilities do you have?"
"What has helped you cope in the past when things were tough?"

Body Image

Once a body image disturbance is suspected, the nurse carefully interviews and observes the client to identify the nature of the threat to the person's body image (functional significance of the part involved, importance of physical appearance, and visibility of the part involved); the meaning the client attaches to the threat; the adequacy of the client's coping abilities; response of family members and significant others; and help available to the client and his or her family.

The client's response to the deformity or limitation is assessed, including changes in independence–dependence patterns and in socialization and communication.

Response to deformity or limitation

- *Adaptive responses:* Exhibits signs of grief and mourning (shock, disbelief, denial, anger, guilt, acceptance)
- *Maladaptive responses:* Continues to deny and to deal with the deformity or limitation, engages in self-destructive behavior, talks about feelings of worthlessness or insecurity, equates deformity or limitation with whole person, shows a change in ability to estimate relationship of body to environment

Independence–dependence patterns

- *Adaptive responses:* Assumes responsibility for care (makes decisions); develops new self-care behaviors; uses available resources; interacts in a mutually supportive way with family
- *Maladaptive responses:* Assigns responsibility for his or her care to others; becomes increasingly dependent or stubbornly refuses necessary help

Socialization and communication

- *Adaptive responses:* Maintains usual social patterns; communicates needs and accepts offers of help; serves as support for others
- *Maladaptive responses:* Isolates himself or herself; exhibits superficial self-confidence; unable to express needs (becomes hostile, ashamed, frustrated, depressed)

Self-Esteem

Once a client has shared perceptions of self, the nurse questions if the client likes himself or herself, if the client is pleased with his or her expectations, and the progress the client is making to realize these expectations.

"Tell me what you like about yourself."
"What would you change about yourself if you could?"

Using a graphic description of self-esteem as the discrepancy between the "real self" (what we think we really are) and the "ideal self" (what we think we would like to be or think we should be), the nurse can obtain a quick indication of a client's self-esteem by having the client plot two points on a line—real self and ideal self (Fig. 31-3). The greater the discrepancy, the lower the self-esteem; the smaller the discrepancy, the higher the self-esteem.

A person's ideal self may differ dramatically from the current sense of self and positively or negatively influence behavior and personal development. If indicated, the nurse questions the client about self-expectations:

"You've told me something about who you are, how you view yourself now. Tell me who you would like to be in the future."
"What life goals are important to you?"
"Where do you see yourself 5 years from now? In 10 years?"
"Are these expectations realistic?"
"Are your expectations stemming from who you would *like* to be or from who you think you *should* be?"
"Who or what has influenced your self-expectations?"

The nurse is assessing if the client possesses life goals that are positively motivating personal development. Unrealistic expectations need to be identified, and their source needs to be explored with the client. For example:

"You seem to feel that it is necessary to be all things to all people—no matter what this costs you. How might this belief have developed? Is it helpful to you?"
"What I'm hearing is that your performance must always be perfect, that although you allow others to make mistakes, you cannot allow yourself this luxury. . . . Tell me more about this."
"Then, unless you graduate at the top of your class you will not be satisfied? Why is this so important? Is this type of achievement realistic with your abilities? What will this success both benefit and cost you?"
"You state you have no goals for the future . . . when you wake up each morning what gets you out of bed? What keeps you moving?"

High self-esteem

Low self-esteem

Figure 31-3
The client who perceives his or her real self as relatively close to the ideal self has high self-esteem. The client who perceives his or her real self as far from the ideal self has low self-esteem.

If this exercise indicates the need for a more detailed assessment, the nurse next explores the concepts of significance, competence, virtue, and power.

Significance

"Are there people in your life with whom you share a close relationship?"

"Many people have 'people' problems. Are your relationships causing you any problems right now?"

"To what extent do you feel loved and approved of by the key people in your life?"

"Does it bother you when you feel unloved or when others fail to appreciate you?"

"In what ways do you let family members and friends know that you like them or are proud of their accomplishments?"

Competence

"What are the things you need to do to feel important?"

"Is anything interfering with your ability to execute these tasks?" ("How does this make you feel?")

"How important to you is it to feel that others value your work?"

Virtue

"Tell me something about the moral–ethical principles that govern your life."

"How must you live to describe yourself as a 'good' person?"

"How do you feel about your ability to live this way?"

"Describe any difficulties you experience in living up to your moral principles that you would like to discuss."

"In what ways can the nurses help you to better live according to your moral standards?"

Power

"How important is it to you to 'be in control' of your life (health)?"

"To what extent did you feel 'in control' of your life (health) before this illness (trauma, crisis, and so forth)?"

"To what extent do you feel 'in control' of your life (health) currently?"

"What is it that makes you feel not in control?"

"How might you change this? How can nurses help you to develop and gain more control?"

Role Performance

We all play many roles. Our ability to execute successfully societal expectations regarding role-specific behaviors, **role performance**, is easily compromised by illness and injury. If a nurse suspects this might be contributing to a self-concept disturbance, the following questions are indicated:

"What major roles describe you—son, daughter, spouse, parent, employer or employee, student, club member, and so on?"

"How important is it to you to be good in each of these roles?"

"Tell me how successful you think you are in each of these roles."

"What roles or expectations would you change if you could?"

"If you feel 'incompetent' or less than successful in some of these roles, why? What is preventing you from being more successful? What can you do about this? How might I help you?"

DIAGNOSING

Disturbances in Self-Concept as the Problem. Specific disturbances in self-concept that can be treated by independent nursing interventions receive one of four nursing diagnostic labels:

Body Image Disturbance: The state in which an individual experiences or is at risk to experience a disruption in the way one perceives one's body image

Self-Esteem Disturbance (Chronic Low Self-Esteem or Situational Low Self-Esteem): The state in which an individual experiences or is at risk of experiencing negative self-evaluation about self or capabilities

Altered Role Performance: The state in which an individual experiences or is at risk of experiencing a disruption in the way he or she perceives his or her role performance

Personal Identity Disturbance: The state in which an individual experiences or is at risk of experiencing an inability to distinguish between self and nonself (Carpenito, 1995)

Common etiologies and defining characteristics for these diagnoses are found in the accompanying box.

Disturbance in Self-Concept as the Etiology. Because disturbances in self-concept have the potential to affect so many other areas of human functioning, they may serve as etiologies for numerous problem statements. Examples of these follow:

Impaired Adjustment related to change in health status (increasing dependency, need for ongoing medical evaluation and treatment, and so forth)

Anxiety related to irreversible change in body image (eg, amputation, mastectomy, burn); delayed development of secondary sex characteristics (body image); discrepancy between real and ideal self (self-esteem); perceived incompetence in important roles; loss of key roles (child or spouse dies, separation, retirement, graduation)

Ineffective Individual Coping related to inability to identify personal strengths, low self-esteem, "I know I can't manage this"; role conflict

Anticipatory or Dysfunctional Grieving related to change in body image, loss of key roles

Altered Health Maintenance related to low self-esteem—"why bother?"

Hopelessness related to low self-esteem, overwhelming role demands, belief that nothing will change (destiny is controlled externally)

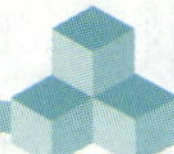

Nursing Diagnoses for Common Problems

Disturbances in Self-Concept

Problem	Related Factors	Sample Defining Characteristics
Body Image Disturbance	Irreversible changes in body image—amputation, mastectomy, hysterectomy, colostomy, scars, burns, disfiguring skin disorder	"Look at me. Nothing can ever be the same again. I feel less whole. When I look in the mirror all I see is my (stump, missing breast, scar). I know when others look at me they feel repulsed or at the very least pity me."
	Effects of treatment (eg, braces, casts)	Thirteen-year-old female adolescent with scoliosis wearing a Milwaukee brace (covers pelvic area and has rods in the front and back which extend up to the chin): "I feel dumb in this thing . . . it's bad enough that my back is crooked but this makes me look like a freak. Besides, it's hot. Must I wear it to school?"
	Difficulty accepting development of secondary sex characteristics or delayed development of same	Fifteen-year-old male adolescent, sophomore in high school, height 5′1″, weight 88 lb; "When am I going to grow up and start looking like the other guys in my class?" No pubic hair; penis, testes, and scrotum are the same size and proportion as in childhood.
	Extreme thinness or obesity	Twenty-year-old woman, height 5′7″; weight 98 lb; works out for 30 min three times a day in addition to 100 sit-ups a day: "When I look in the mirror I see fat!"
		Twenty-year-old woman, height 5′7″; weight 200 lb: "I hate my body . . . I've been fat all my life and I'm always on a diet. Why can't I be like everyone else?"
Self-Esteem Disturbance	Feeling unloved or unapproved of by significant others	Twelve-year-old son of parents in the process of getting a divorce: "No matter what I do to make my dad like me he acts like I don't exist. When he's home he fights with mom, but mostly he's away. I wouldn't even care if he yelled at me so long as he noticed me. I wonder why he doesn't like me?"
	Feelings of incompetence	Forty-two-year-old car salesperson, with company for 18 years: "What's wrong with me? I do my job, I'm also never absent, I have a good sales record, but I keep getting passed over for promotions. I think I'm too old to move to a different company, but I don't want to just sell cars for someone else for the rest of my life!"
	Failure to live according to personal moral ethical code	Thirty-three-year-old single female computer programmer: "I should have known I'd get pregnant—I deserve it. I knew I was wrong to go to bed with this guy. Basically I've tried to live the way I think I should all my life up until now. What if something's wrong with the baby because of my sin?"
	Powerlessness	Sixty-seven-year-old alert widow with degenerative joint disease: "It may be hard for me to move around now, but darn it—there's nothing wrong with my mind. The kids think they are helping me by making all my decisions but they aren't. I'm not a doddering old lady in a nursing home."
Altered Role Performance	Rejection of role	Twenty-two-year-old mother 2 days after birth of her second son (first son is 15 months old): "I don't know who my husband got to watch our son. I never wanted to be a mother anyway. My husband and I have never had any time for ourselves—and things aren't going to get any better."

(continued)

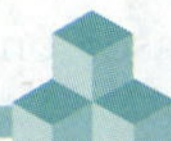

Nursing Diagnoses for Common Problems *(continued)*

Disturbances in Self-Concept

Problem	Related Factors	Sample Defining Characteristics
Altered Role Performance	Role conflict Role fatigue Multiple life stressors	Twenty-one-year-old, full-time junior nursing student who failed a major exam; is married and the mother of an 18-month-old daughter; works every other weekend in a hospital as an electrocardiogram technician: "I'm trying so hard to get my grades up, but I don't know what else I can do. My husband seems to be losing patience with me more and more and I sometimes feel awful about neglecting my daughter. I'd stop working but we need the money. I want nursing so bad but I'm getting awfully tired."
	Changing personal resources (physical health, mental abilities, motivation)	Fifty-year-old college chemistry teacher begins exhibiting signs of early Alzheimer's disease; forgets where she is and what she is doing; began rambling in class and saying things that made no sense—much to the class's amusement. Later cried and called herself "stupid."
Personal Identity Disturbance	Unresolved crisis	Eighty-eight-year-old man who lost his wife 6 months ago; wife took care of all his needs; sits alone in the house all day: "We always did everything together. I wish I had died first. What shall I do?"
	Declining physical, mental, or sensory abilities	Same 88-year-old man 3 months after admission to long-term care institution, medical diagnosis "rule out depression/dementia"; has become increasingly withdrawn, never initiates conversation; responses to questions are sometimes inappropriate: "What do you mean, what's my name? Who cares? I want to go home to my wife."
	Rejection of membership in minority group	Fifteen-year-old Cambodian girl recently emigrated to the United States with family; in constant conflict with parents as she rejects her family's culture in hopes of fitting in with peer group: "Sometimes I feel like I no longer know who I am or how I should act. I feel lonely inside and afraid."

Knowledge Deficit: How to help children develop high self-esteem, related to lack of experience with parenting

Noncompliance: (specify) related to low self-esteem

Altered Parenting related to disturbance in role performance (rejection of parent role)

Post-Trauma Response related to disturbance in personal identity

Self-Care Deficit related to learned helplessness, low self-esteem, "I can't"

Sensory/Perceptual Alterations related to disturbance in personal identity (ability to distinguish between self and nonself)

Altered Sexuality Patterns related to changed body image, disturbance in self-concept

Impaired Social Interaction or Social Isolation related to low self-esteem, disturbance in personal identity

Altered Thought Processes related to disturbance in personal identity

High Risk for Self-Directed Violence related to disturbance in self-concept, overwhelmed by failure to live according to moral–ethical standards

Important Distinctions

When assessment data point to an alteration in self-concept, the nurse's first task is to determine if the altered self-concept is the problem, the cause of the problem (etiology), or merely a sign that a problem exists (defining characteristics). Self-concept data seem to fit well in all three categories. It is important that an accurate determination be made because this directs the goals developed for the client and related nursing interventions. For example, the following three different diagnoses might be written for a 25-year-old woman who is recently divorced:

1. Self-Esteem Disturbance related to perceived failure in role of wife (recent divorce) as manifested by neglect of personal appearance and inability to accept positive reinforcement

   Assessment data point to a disturbance in self-esteem as the priority problem. Nursing energies will be directed to helping the client evaluate herself positively despite the stress of the divorce.

2. Altered Health Maintenance related to decreased self-esteem as manifested by failure to follow through on referrals (support group, stress-management class, and so forth); "Why bother? Nothing ever works for me anyway."

   Here, low self-esteem is contributing to the client's problem of failing to follow through with health-seeking behaviors. Nursing energies will be best directed to improving the client's use of health resources; one of the means used will be to help her to value herself enough to choose healthy behaviors.

3. Ineffective Individual Coping related to inability to accept recent divorce as manifested by low self-esteem statements: "I never should have gotten married—my mother said I'd be a rotten wife." "I know I can't make it on my own." "Why did he do this to me?"

   Here, low self-esteem statements are the cues that led to the identification of the problem statement. One of the criteria used to evaluate nursing intervention to increase the client's coping skills will be a reduction in or elimination of low self-esteem statements.

PLANNING: EXPECTED OUTCOMES

Whenever nurses care for clients, nursing interventions need to be supportive of the following client goals/outcomes. The client will:

- Describe self realistically, identifying both strengths and deficiencies
- Verbalize realistic expectations for self based on who he or she would like to be
- Verbalize that self is liked or at least okay
- Communicate his or her feelings and needs in a way that is comfortable and effective in meeting needs
- Nurture relationships in which needs for love and worth are mutually met (significance)
- Assume role-related responsibilities with confidence (competence)
- Express satisfaction with ability to live according to one's moral–ethical standards (virtue)
- Demonstrate confidence in ability to accomplish what is desired (power)

Home-bound clients are frequently at risk for alterations in self-concept because they are separated from many of the sources which affirmed their competence, worth, and lovableness. The accompanying box recommends strategies to address this potential problem.

Client goals for specific disturbances in self-concept and related nursing interventions are presented later in this chapter.

IMPLEMENTING

Nursing interventions to assist clients to develop and maintain a positive self-concept may vary tremendously from one client to another. Nurses must be comfortable with their own self-image before they can address image problems in clients. Specific nursing strategies addressed in this section include helping clients identify and use personal strengths, helping high-risk clients maintain a sense of self, changing the self-concept, de-

Home Care Considerations: Bridging the Gap

Newly homebound clients are at high risk for developing alterations in self-concept because they are often separated from the usual sources that affirm their worth, competence, and lovableness. Chronically homebound clients are uniquely vulnerable because their caregivers, who may be experiencing burn-out, are their major or sole source of determining personal worth. The clients' caregivers are also at high risk for developing alterations in self-concept because they may be overwhelmed by the clients' caregiving needs and feel chronically inadequate to meet these needs.

Assessment Priorities

Assess for alterations in self-concept whenever you detect the following:

- Client's inability to continue meaningful work
- Client's inability to continue usual patterns of social interaction: to visit with family, friends, and associates; to travel and recreate; to shop; to attend religious services; to participate in social gatherings, attend meetings
- Reduction of client's universe of meaning to one room and to one or several caregivers
- Client's dependence on uncaring caregivers who would prefer not to have to meet the client's needs
- Family caregivers who persistently feel overwhelmed and threatened by the needs of the client

Intervention Considerations

Pay attention to what you communicate merely by your person and manner of interacting. See the discussion of interpersonal competence in Chapter 15.

veloping a positive body image, and working with parents and educators to develop self-esteem in children and adolescents.

Helping Clients Identify and Use Personal Strengths

When confronted with a major stressor, many people forget that they have histories of successful coping and numerous personal strengths. Clients at high risk for giving up are those with low self-esteem or multiple stressors perceived as being overwhelming.

Although attributing strength to a client sounds like something nurses would do naturally, nurses frequently fall into the trap of doing for clients (ie, solving their problems, rather than helping them to identify and tap their personal power and strengths). Moreover, clients continually instruct nurses about how they should be perceived, and some clients successfully communicate a manipulative helplessness that encourages the nurse's taking charge. An appropriate nursing response in this case is, "I wonder why you want me to speak with your physician about treatment alternatives. I am sure you would feel much better hearing this information firsthand. If you'd like I will stay here while you talk with the physician."

Clients experiencing powerlessness may need help to recognize their strengths (Fig. 31-4). Examples of personal strengths include a healthy functioning body, cognitive abilities, emotional strengths, communication strengths, other interpersonal skills, a sense of meaning and purpose in life, a belief system, a social support network, meaningful work, hobbies, other interests, education, life experience, and a past history of effective coping. A good sense of humor, belief in a loving God, a healthy nutritional state, the ability to make decisions, and a sense of self-worth are all personal strengths that may better equip a person to respond to life's challenges.

Specific strategies nurses can use to help clients identify and use personal strengths include the following:

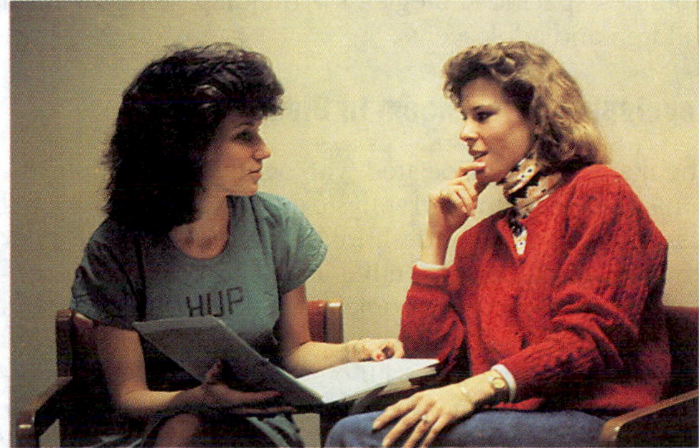

Figure 31-4
The nurse helps the client recognize his or her self-worth and strengths that he or she possesses. (Photo by Gates Rhodes, Courtesy of School of Nursing, University of Pennsylvania.)

- Encouraging clients to identify their strengths
- Replacing self-negation with positive thinking
- Noticing and reinforcing client strengths
- Encouraging clients to will for themselves the strengths they desire and to try them on

Helping High-Risk Clients Maintain a Sense of Self

People who are acutely ill are often separated not only from their strengths but also from any real sense of self. One client, a college president who was recovering from serious complications after surgery for ovarian cancer, shared the following:

> When I was very sick, I felt utterly weak and devoid of any personal strength. During this time, how I felt about myself was totally dependent on how the doctors and nurses approached me. My esteem was at their mercy. If they came into my room and did something to me without talking to me or talked as if I were not present, then I felt like a nonperson, unworthy of their care. But if they approached me gently and caringly and spoke with me, then I felt like a human again, worthy of human respect and care. Once I started feeling stronger, then I could fight feelings of depersonalization. But when I was really sick, my feelings of worth were totally determined by the behaviors of others.

Nurses can help clients maintain a sense of self and worth by doing the following:

- Using looks, touch, and speech to communicate worth
- Speaking respectfully to the client and addressing the client by preferred name whenever entering the client's room
- Offering the client a simple explanation before initiating any procedure
- Moving the client's body respectfully if the client is unable to do this
- Respecting the client's privacy and sensibilities

This type of caring does not require additional nursing time or energy. It does require from the nurse continual reaffirmation that nursing is a person-centered profession and that nothing is more important at any moment of a nurse's workday than the person being served.

Changing a Negative Self-Concept

The time is ripe for change when a client realizes that a negative self-concept is hindering personal development. A nurse working in a setting that allows long-term nurse–client relationships may intervene to assist the client in modifying self-concept. At the outset, it must be remembered that the self-concept is firmly entrenched and that by nature it resists change. See the interventions for the diagnosis of Self-Concept Disturbance at the end of this chapter.

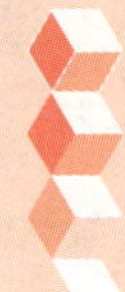

Helpscan

The following are resources for clients and health-care professionals. Many of these may be located by using the guide to human services in the phone book.

American Cancer Society and other medical societies

Community mental health centers/clinics

Self-help support groups (eg, Alcoholics Anonymous and AL-ANON, AIDS groups, Parents Without Partners and other Singles Groups)

Senior citizens' groups

University counseling centers

Developing a Positive Body Image

Interventions for body image disturbances vary according to the nature of the disturbance. Interventions may include any combination of the following:

- Establish a trusting relationship with the client. Allow the client to share his or her feelings openly. Sitting quietly by the client for a few minutes with a few words such as, "How are things?" or "Gee, it must be hard to lie there after all you've been through. . ." communicates to the client your willingness and readiness to share his or her experience.
- Support the client through the various stages of loss, grief, and mourning (shock, disbelief, denial, anger, guilt, acceptance), remembering that there is no one right way to proceed through these stages. Rather, clients may move fluidly in and out of various stages, sometimes returning to earlier stages. Some clients may need to learn that it is okay to cry, to be angry, to feel depressed.
- Use play therapy with children so they can describe their feelings and work through their grief using the nonthreatening medium of dolls or animals.
- Role-model for the client a healthy acceptance of the client's body. Be careful that facial expressions, words, or body positioning do not communicate to the client disgust, fear, or rejection.
- While communicating support to the client who is slow to develop and use appropriate self-care behaviors, firmly insist that the client participate in his or her care to the extent that the client is able. Whenever possible, provide the client with honest answers to his or her questions or put the client in touch with the appropriate person to give the answers.
- Strengthen the decision-making ability of the client by honestly exploring alternatives; help the client to imagine living with the consequences of different courses of action.
- Reinforce the client's personal strengths and help the client and family to identify all possible resources.
- Assess the response of the client's significant others and intervene if they negatively influence the client.

Teaching Adults How to Develop Self-Esteem in Children and Adolescents

Nurses who work in practice settings where they have access to groups of parents, adult caregivers, or teachers can offer specific guidelines for creating developmental environments that build high self-esteem. Children are most likely to develop high self-esteem when adults:

- Frequently communicate unconditional regard for the child (use body language and words to let the child know that he or she is *liked*)
- Communicate a range of acceptable behaviors
- Challenge the child to explore strengths and limitations
- Celebrate the child's competencies and accomplishments
- Assist the child to respond to mistakes responsibly and to learn from them

Because some parents and educators may not have experienced these helps to personal growth themselves, it is beneficial for the nurse to role-model these behaviors when interacting with children.

Important learning tasks for children include understanding and accepting oneself, feelings, and others; independence; goals and purposeful behavior; mastery, competence, and resourcefulness; emotional maturity; and choices and consequences. The accompanying box identifies specific strategies for building self-esteem in children and adolescents.

Developing Self-Esteem in Older Adults

The many losses associated with aging, for example, diminished strength and physical health, interpersonal losses, retirement, and shrinking income, make older adults especially vulnerable to disturbances in self-concept, particularly chronic low self-esteem. Society's generally negative view of aging compounds the problem. Nurses interacting with older adults need to understand that simple measures—such as addressing older clients respectfully, communicating that you take their concerns seriously, noticing and affirming their personal strengths, and interacting with them as individuals, as opposed to members of a homogeneous group—can greatly enhance the older person's self-esteem. The ac-

Building Self-Esteem in Children

Strategy One: Looking at the Positive and the Negative

Instruct parents to write an honest description of their child for a stranger. Next have the parents underline the child's positive and negative qualities.

To reinforce the positive qualities, (1) notice examples of ability in many different circumstances and point this out to the child; (2) find occasion to frequently and honestly praise the child; and (3) give the child an opportunity to show ability frequently.

To address the negative qualities constructively, ask: (1) What need is being expressed by this behavior? (2) Can I see a positive quality being expressed by this behavior? and (3) How can I help my child express this quality and meet her needs in a more positive way?

Reexamine the list of negative qualities and ignore those that are a matter of taste, preference, or personal style.

Strategy Two: Listening

The following guidelines can help parents to use listening to communicate to a child, "You are important. What you say matters to me. You matter to me."

1. Make sure that you are ready to listen.
2. Give your child your full attention.
3. Minimize distractions.
4. Be an active listener.
5. Invite your child to talk.

Listen for the point of a child's story ("What is she trying to tell me? Why is this important to him?"). Don't feel that you have to fix things. Listen for and respond to the feelings.

Strategy Three: Using the Language of Self-Esteem

Feedback that enhances self-esteem has three components: (1) a description of the behavior (describe the behavior without judging it); (2) your reaction to the behavior (language that shares something about yourself); and (3) acknowledgement of the child's feelings. For example, "Thanks for playing with your brother tonight [description]. I was wondering how I was going to pay attention to our guests if he got fussy and was really grateful when I noticed that you kept him occupied and happy [reaction]. I know that there were other things you might have enjoyed doing more [acknowledgement]."

To give correction using the language of self-esteem, (1) describe the problematic behavior, (2) state a reason for the behavior change, (3) acknowledge the child's feelings, and (4) offer a clear statement of what is expected.

Attacking communications: "Don't let me ever hear you talk that way to your mother again."

Language of self-esteem: "I overheard you telling your mom that she should 'Get a life and get off your case.' [description]. When you talk like that it just makes people angry or sad which isn't very helpful [reason for behavior change]. You probably feel like you are being picked on and we may have some expectations that are different from those of your friends' parents. I hope you know that this is because we love you and want the best for you [acknowledgement]. In the future try to talk to others with the same respect you'd like others to show you [statement of expectation]."

Avoid using the following destructive language styles, which tear down self-esteem: overgeneralizations ("You *never* come home on time!"), the silent treatment, and vague or violent threats.

Strategy Four: Helping Children Meet Expectations

To help children meet expectations, (1) be sure that your expectations are reasonable and appropriate for your child's age; (2) plan ahead; (3) be clear about your expectations; (4) focus on the positive; (5) provide choices when possible; and (6) provide rewards.

Strategy Five: Promoting a Feeling of Success

To help children have the courage to try new types of experiences, which results from successfully meeting challenges, (1) let a child know what to expect; (2) let your child practice the necessary skills; (3) be patient; and (4) make it safe to fail.

(Material adapted from M. McKay and P. Fanning (1992). *Self-esteem* [2nd ed.]. Oakland, CA: New Harbinger Publications.)

companying box describes nursing interventions to promote self-esteem in older adults.

EVALUATING

Nurses who are sensitive to the relation between self-concept and general well-being consistently evaluate the effect the nursing plan of care has on the client's self-concept. For example, while educating a client with hypertension for whom lifestyle counseling was recommended, the nurse may detect that the client is feeling extremely guilty about his or her smoking, dietary habits, and lack of exercise. "Why should I even try to change any of these things now. I made myself sick so I may as well live with the punishment." If the plan of care is to be effective, the nurse must first help this client value him or herself sufficiently to want to make the necessary changes.

When the plan of care includes specific interventions to assist clients with disturbances in body image, self-esteem, role performance, and personal identity, the

Focus on the Older Adult

Nursing Strategies to Promote Self-Esteem in Older Adults

Personal Identity

- When an older person's sense of self is threatened, assist him or her to find meaning in the experience, to regain mastery to the extent that this is possible, and to evaluate realistically the adequacy of his or her coping strategy.
- Teach older people to identify and develop a game plan for confronting anxiety-producing situations.
- Help to identify and secure intervention for treatable depressions.
- Remedy treatable causes of self-identity disturbances such as pain, abusive living arrangements, and substance abuse.

Body Image

- Notice and affirm positive physiologic characteristics of older adults.
- Teach preventive self-care measures that reduce discomforting signs of aging (eg, exercise, which maintains muscle mass and joint flexibility; proper nutrition; and basic hygiene and skin care measures).
- Explore new activities (including hobbies) that are within the changing physical capabilities of the older person.

Self-Esteem

- Assist older adults to identify and use personal strengths.
- Communicate that you value older people simply for who they are (unconditional affirmation)—know and use the name they prefer, ask them questions about their life, interests, or values.
- When appropriate, use the expertise of older people and ask their advice; let them know you value their life experience.
- Engage older people in activities in which they can be successful.
- Allow older people to make tough decisions and to confront challenging situations when appropriate; teach protective family members the value of older adults confronting situations that invite their continued growth.
- Empower older people to meet their own needs: provide necessary knowledge, teach new behaviors, instill the belief that they "can manage."

Role Performance

- Explore with older people the many roles they have fulfilled throughout their lifetime; invite reminiscences.
- Facilitate grieving over valued roles that are no longer able to be performed.
- Remedy, whenever possible, factors that prevent older people from engaging in valued roles.
- Explore new roles.

nurse listens carefully to the client's self-report and observes client behaviors to see if the disturbances are being resolved. Basically, the client should be able to meet the following outcomes:

- Comfortable with body image and able to use it effectively to meet human needs
- Able to describe self positively
- Able to meet realistic role expectations without undue anxiety and fatigue
- Capable of interacting appropriately with environment while recognizing self to be a separate and distinct entity

Nursing Process in Clinical Practice

When identifying and treating disturbances in self-concept categorized as nursing diagnoses, the nurse uses each phase of the nursing process. Quality care depends on the nurse's possession of the knowledge and skills described earlier in this chapter. What follows in outline format are the assessment priorities, expected outcomes, and nursing interventions for the diagnosis Self-Concept Disturbance. This diagnosis is not currently on the NANDA list but Carpenito (1995) recommends its use when the nurse does not have sufficient clinical data to validate a more specific diagnosis such as Chronic Low Self-Esteem or Body Image Disturbance.

> Self-Concept Disturbance: The state in which the individual experiences or is at risk of experiencing a negative state of change about the way he/she feels, thinks or views self. It may include a change in body image, self-ideal, self-esteem, role performance, or personal identity. (Carpenito, p. 794)

Many of the clients with whom nurses interact, especially on a long-term basis, may be interested in modifying some aspect of a negative self-concept that is related to faulty thinking. Common analogies of negative self-concepts include distortions and denials, faulty categorizing, and inappropriate standards—perfectionism, conventionality, "What the other guy thinks" (Calhoun & Acocella, 1989).

Distortions and Denials. A woman who was taught early in life that a woman's place is in the home may systematically have distorted or denied any talents or feelings that she thought were inconsistent with being a full-time wife and mother. For example, if she enjoyed math and did well in her math courses in high school, rather than feel good about this she might think it abnormal and consciously limit her study of math. If a guidance counselor recommended college to her, she might laugh off the suggestion.

Nursing diagnosis: Negative (Limited) Self-Concept related to a long history of distorting and denying her abilities and desires

Faulty Categorizing. A positive self-concept is characterized by a broad image of the self. The more labels we can attach to ourselves, the more self-information we are able to assimilate and make part of us. An adolescent who repeatedly hears from his or her father that he or she is no good and who consistently characterizes himself or herself this way may reject genuine affirmations of the adolescent's positive qualities and strengths from other family member, peers, teachers, and so forth. Moreover, the adolescent may choose to act in ways that reinforce his or her image of being no good.

Nursing diagnosis: Negative Self-Concept related to inability to recognize and "own" positive qualities, strengths ("I'm no good")

Inappropriate Standards. At the root of the negative self-concepts of some clients may be an unrealistic ideal self. With all the emphasis in society on being number one, many people hold *perfectionistic standards* that they will never be able to meet. In describing their self-expectations, these clients may reveal that they must always get an *A* to feel good about themselves, or always be the center of everyone's attention and love. Anything less is viewed as failure.

Conventionality offers another set of problems for the person who uncritically accepts all his or her culture dictates. When the person's feelings or preferred actions conflict with society's standards, then that person concludes that something must be wrong with him or her. Because sick-role behaviors are dictated by many cultures, the person who finds he or she cannot suffer in silence or, conversely, cannot express his or her pain or grief vocally, may feel alienated from his or her culture. An older person whose family is considering nursing home placement may find this more difficult to accept if the culture is one in which family members traditionally respect and care for aged members at home.

"What the other guy thinks" is the third faulty standard. Allowing others to define ideal behavior sets up a person for constant failure because it is impossible to please everyone. The young executive who tries to live up to the expectations of his or her boss, peer group at work, spouse and children, and college friends is bound to lose himself or herself in the process.

Nursing diagnosis: Negative Self-Concept related to unrealistic self-expectations (perfectionism, conventionality, "What the other guy thinks")

Assessment Priorities

- Assess how accurately the client is able to describe himself or herself; note in particular the use of negative labels and their significance for the client.
- Determine whether the client is motivated to modify the self-concept. Does the client see a relationship between a negative self-concept and self-defeating thoughts, feelings, and behaviors?
- Teach the client to choose a day on which he or she will write down every self-critical thought that enters his or her mind. At the end of the day, the client should review the list and ask three questions:
  - What is the standard (perfectionism, conventionality, other people's judgments) on which this self-criticism is based?
  - From whom do you think you picked up this standard?
  - Do you really subscribe to the standard wholeheartedly? (Calhoun & Acocella, 1989)

Expected Outcomes

By (specify date) the client will:

- Describe the relation between self-concept and behavior
- Identify faulty thinking that reinforces a negative self-concept (distortions and denials, faulty categorizing, inappropriate standards)
- Integrate positive self-knowledge into self-concept
- Report feeling better about himself or herself

Interventions

- See the box titled Changing the Self-Concept.
- Once the client has identified faulty thinking patterns (negative self-talk) that reinforce the negative self-concept, teach the client to "red flag" this behavior as soon as he or she is aware of it happening. The goal is to replace the negative self-talk with talk that will develop a more positive self-image.
- Help the client explore the positive dimensions of himself or herself that he or she wishes to develop, and incorporate this new knowledge into the self-concept. For an example, see the box titled Exploring and Developing the Positive.

Changing the Self-Concept

Analyzing the Problem

- Isolate the basic problem label.
- Describe your problem in situational terms.
- Search for correlations, watching out especially for negative self-talk.
- Review the background of your problem to check for causes:
  - Distortions and denials
  - Faulty categorizing
  - Perfectionism
  - Conventionality
  - Other people's judgments

Changing the Self-Concept

- Set a goal.
- Gather new information about this aspect of yourself.
- Engage in cognitive restructuring:
  - Listen to your old self-talk.
  - Talk back to this old self-talk, cross-examining it to get at the reality.
  - Act on your back-talk, substituting new behavior to accompany your new, more rational self-talk.

(Adapted from Calhoun, J. F., & Acocella, J. R. [1989]. *Psychology of adjustment and human relationships* [3rd ed.]. New York: Random House.)

Client Care Study

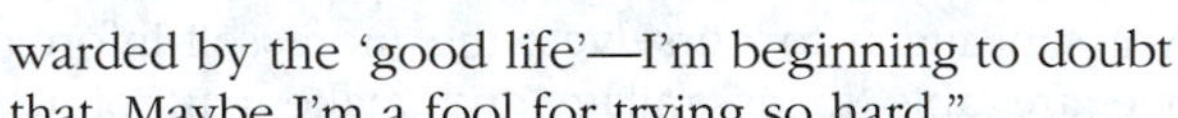

Melissa Motsky is a 31-year-old married woman, mother of three children (aged 12, 10, and 8), and junior-level nursing student. She works every other weekend as a nurse's aide. She has just received a letter from the nursing division head informing her that she is in academic jeopardy and will fail out of the program unless her grades improve. She presents this to her adviser.

After talking with Ms. Motsky, who calls herself a failure and who cries as she describes her situation at home, her faculty adviser suspects a serious self-esteem problem and helps her to list factors contributing to her current sense of failure and low self-esteem. The following list is generated:

Significance

– Receives little understanding, affection, approval from husband. "I stay with him because of the kids. I started back to school because I had to get out of the house and want to make something of myself. He doesn't understand this."

+ "Children are very supportive but get impatient when I have to study and can't spend time with them."

Competence

– Feels a failure in all the roles that are important to her—wife, mother, and, now, student. "I jeopardized everything to go back to school—if I fail, it's all over for me. There just isn't enough time or energy to do anything well."

+ "They do love me at work, though, which makes me feel like nursing is what I should be doing."

Virtue

– "I've always believed that hard work pays off and that if you were faithful to your duty you'd be rewarded by the 'good life'—I'm beginning to doubt that. Maybe I'm a fool for trying so hard."

+ "I do still try to live according to my beliefs and feel okay about this. I treat others as I'd like to be treated."

Power

– "I always believed I could do anything I put my heart and soul into. But I can't seem to change my marriage and if I fail out of school that will be the end of all my dreams."

Key indicators of low self-esteem that also surfaced in the interview included overeating (10-lb weight gain during the past year); difficulty sleeping; fatigue; new sensitivity to criticism; and expressions of feeling unloved, alone, and no longer able to manage. Personal strengths included history of "can do" mentality, high motivation to succeed, and past history of success as mother and nurse's aide.

See the Plan of Nursing Care developed to aid Ms. Motsky in accomplishing her goals.

Core Competencies

To assist Ms. Motsky in meeting her goals, the nurse needs the following specialized abilities:

Cognitive Competencies

- Knowledge of etiologies and defining characteristics for disturbances in self-esteem and specific nursing strategies to enhance self-esteem
- Belief that a person's self-esteem influences all aspects of his or her functioning and a commitment to addressing this human need (ie, holistic orientation)

- Ability to decide correctly that it is wise to encourage this student to continue in the nursing program, whereas another student of lesser ability would be assisted to reevaluate his or her career goals
- Teaching skills

Interpersonal Competencies

- Empathy for the multiple role expectations the client is experiencing and ability to identify and mobilize the client's inner strengths so that a *realistic* plan can be developed to assist the client to meet necessary role expectations *satisfactorily*
- Interpersonal skills to communicate to client that he or she is important, cared about, competent, and good, and that the client possesses within self the power and strength to turn the situation around
- Advocacy skills
- Counselling skills

Ethical/Legal Competencies

- Accountability (ability and willingness to encourage student and follow-up on the student's progress; celebrate goal achievement or make realistic plans if student should fail out of program)
- Advocacy skills
- Knowledge of students' moral and legal rights and of faculty adviser's professional responsibilities

Exploring and Developing the Positive

Example: Twenty-year-old mother who perceives herself as "a failure in everything I try"; states husband feels childrearing is the woman's responsibility and she is terrified.
Immediate goal: Develop confidence in parenting skills, see herself as a good mother

- Explore and reinforce the client's personal qualities and strengths that will help her to reach her goal.
  "You look like a natural mother when you hold your baby; some women are afraid at the beginning to even hold their infants."
  "That's good that you are talking with your baby. Babies quickly sense how a parent feels about them."
- Teach the client how to substitute positive self-talk for negative self-talk.
  Negative self-talk (mother during feeding): "She's awfully fussy tonight, I mustn't be doing this right. . . . It was probably dumb luck that she took to breast so well this morning. . . ."
  New positive self-talk: ". . . but she fed so well this morning and the nurse said her weight is good. I wonder what else might be making her fussy . . . maybe she's wet. . . ."

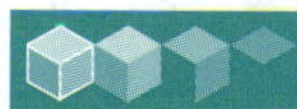

Nursing Plan of Care

for Mrs. Motsky

Nursing Diagnosis: Situational Low Self-Esteem related to decreased sense of significance, competence, virtue, and power as manifested by expressions of being a failure, powerlessness, fatigue, tears, weight gain, low academic performance (test grades 68, 74)

Expected Outcome: By this time next month, 11/2/98, the client will demonstrate increased self-esteem by:

- Expressing positive statements about herself

Nursing Interventions	Rationale	Evaluative Statement
Assist client to rediscover and "own" personal strengths: identify personal qualities and strengths that have pleased her in the past and explore why this has changed; recommend that she make at least one positive statement about herself each morning and evening.	Clients can lose touch with their strengths, especially when multiple stressors seem to create impossible demands.	11/3/98 Goal partially met. Client's statements are of the "This is good, *but* . . ." variety. "I think I'm doing better in school but I don't know if it will continue." *Recommendation:* Continue to identify and reinforce personal strengths. ***C. Taylor, RN***
Consistently interact with the client as if she had the power to weather the crisis successfully (ie, "will" strength to her). Role-model positive self-concept behaviors.	Once the client senses that an authority believes in her power and expects her to use it, she may internalize this knowledge and act on it.	

(continued)

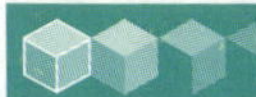

Nursing Plan of Care *(continued)*

for Mrs. Motsky

Expected Outcome: By this time next month, 11/2/98, the client will demonstrate increased self-esteem by:

- Reporting ability to receive negative feedback without falling apart

Nursing Interventions	Rationale	Evaluative Statement
Explore with client to what degree she allows the opinions of others to influence her self-concept.	Significance—sense of being loved and approved of by significant others—is a critical component of self-esteem.	11/3/98 Goal partially met. Client reports being able to handle everything except put-downs from her husband.
Teach how the self-concept filters life experiences; thus, if I feel that I am a failure, I may interpret the words and behaviors of others as confirming this, even though that was not their intention.	Principle of self-consistency: once I am down I may reinforce this by distorting what I feel, hear, and experience.	*Recommendation:* Explore origin of power she has given to her husband to influence her sense of self and what she wants to do about this. ***C. Taylor, RN***
Explore with the client ways she can enhance her self-concept independently of others (eg, take time each day for herself). Encourage client to draw on personal strengths.	This facilitates internal locus of control versus external. Spending time on self communicates that self is valuable.	
Teach the client how to analyze feedback constructively and respond appropriately; *cancel negative thinking.* For example, client receives care plan back with many corrections and the notation, "sloppy work." *Maladaptive response:* "She hates me. See, this proves I'll never be a good nurse. I wasted my time even doing this." *Adaptive response:* "I spent as much time as I had on this . . . now let me see what I did wrong. Maybe I should make an appointment with my instructor so she can show me how to improve."	It is important to break the cycle of negative thinking, which reinforces negative self-concept.	

Expected Outcome: By this time next month, 11/2/98, the client will demonstrate increased self-esteem by:

- Getting a passing grade on her next quarterly examination

Nursing Interventions	Rationale	Evaluative Statement
Explore study skills with client; recommend study group.	Poor study skills may also be contributing to her low academic performance. A study group will meet both her social and academic needs.	11/3/98 Goal met. Grade: 82 ***C. Taylor, RN***

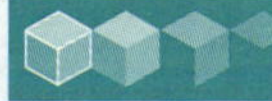

Nursing Plan of Care *(continued)*

for Mrs. Motsky

Nursing Interventions	Rationale	Evaluative Statement
Discuss importance of how she *perceives* present situation. If present failures are equated with *defeat,* she may be unable to mobilize her resources to succeed; if present failures represent *challenge,* it may call forth her best efforts and result in success.	The meaning given to present stressor can dramatically affect the client's response to it and condition her for success or failure.	
Discuss importance of breaking cycle of failure leading to another failure.	If this short-term goal is met, it will set the stage for future successes and contribute to the client's positive self-concept.	

Expected Outcome: By this time next month, 11/2/98, the client will demonstrate increased self-esteem by:

- Verbalizing that the way she is living her life is okay

Nursing Interventions	Rationale	Evaluative Statement
Assist client to examine her moral–ethical standards; explore sources of these standards and if the client feels comfortable with them.	Moral–ethical standards may be uncritically internalized and place the client in conflict.	11/3/98 Goal met. Client stated: "I guess I'm living the best way I know how right now. If things are meant to be different someone is going to have to show me how." *Recommendations:* Reinforce self-acceptance. ***C. Taylor, RN***
Identify unrealistic standards; client may need "permission" to be human.	Unrealistic standards (perfectionism, coventionality) may constantly undermine the client's self-esteem.	
Refer if appropriate for counseling.	Support groups on campus (counseling centers, ministries) may be able to meet client's needs.	

Expected Outcome: By this time next month, 11/2/98, the client will demonstrate increased self-esteem by:

- Reporting two recent instances when personal power was effective in accomplishing desired goals

Nursing Interventions	Rationale	Evaluative Statement
Identify and affirm client's use of personal power to accomplish goals.	A negative self-concept may deny or distort personal successes; outside intervention may be necessary to bring these to consciousness.	11/3/98 Goal met . . . with difficulty. Needed considerable prompting to identify successful use of her personal power. Was ready to attribute passing grade to luck rather than her own efforts. *Recommendation:* Have client make daily record of her use of personal power and results. ***C. Taylor, RN***

(continued)

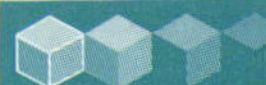

Nursing Plan of Care *(continued)*

for Mrs. Motsky

Sample Documentation

10/2/98

Melissa Motsky presented today after receiving academic jeopardy letter. She is strongly motivated to complete nursing program successfully and seems to have the ability to do this. Current multiple life stressors—lack of support from husband; need to mother three children (12, 10, 8); part-time nurse's aide job (necessary for financial reasons); and current academic jeopardy (test grades 68, 74) are all contributing to her low self-esteem and overwhelming sense of being a failure. We together developed a care plan that it is hoped will help her to do better academically as well as begin to feel better about herself. See attached. She will return 11/2/98 at 10 am for follow-up.

C. Taylor, RN

SOAP Format

10/2/98, 12:30 pm, nursing

Academic jeopardy—Melissa Motsky

S: "I jeopardized everything to go back to school—if I fail, it's all over for me." Reports lack of support from husband; grief that she does not have enough time for children; failure of personal work ethic ("hard work pays off"); and sense of powerlessness.

O: Nursing II quarterly exam grades: 68, 74; weight gain of 10 lb during past year; facial and body expressions of fatigue, profuse tears

A: Disturbance in Self-Esteem related to decreased sense of significance, competence, virtue, and power

P: See attached plan of care.

C. Taylor, RN

Key Points

- Self-concept is the mental image or picture of self. It has the power to encourage or thwart personal growth and development.
- Included in the notion of self-concept are body image ("how I experience my body"); subjective self ("how I see myself"); ideal self ("the self I want to be"); and social self ("the way I feel others see me").
- It is helpful to explore the self-concept by assessing self-knowledge, self-expectations, and self-evaluation or self-esteem. Self-esteem is a measure of a person's satisfaction with his or her significance, competence, virtue, and power.
- Self-concept is a social creation. An infant, born without a self-concept, develops positive feelings about self if basic needs are met and warmth and affection are experienced.
- A positive self-concept is characterized by stable and diversified self-knowledge, realistic self-expectations, and positive self-evaluation and acceptance of self.
- High self-esteem is characterized by positive expectations of the future, ability to approach others freely because of a history of being well received and successful, and ability to approach new tasks and situations freely—confident of own ability to get along.
- Life experiences both affect and are affected by a person's self-concept. Key factors influencing self-concept are developmental state, culture, internal and external resources, history of success and failure, stressors, and illness or trauma.
- Nurses who wish to meet the self-concept needs of clients effectively need to be comfortable with themselves and their own abilities and needs before they can interact therapeutically with clients. It is important for nurses to role-model positive self-concept behaviors.
- Because a client may offer the responses the interviewer wants rather than what is really felt, client responses should be evaluated in relation to observations the nurse makes of the client's behaviors.
- Nursing diagnoses may be written specifically addressing disturbances in self-concept (disturbances in self-concept, body image, self-esteem, role competence, and personal identity), or identifying the effect these disturbances have on other areas of human functioning (eg, coping, health maintenance, powerlessness).

Study Questions

1. Robert, aged 19, has Down's syndrome and is mildly mentally retarded with an intelligence quotient of 82. He told his nurse, "I'm a good helper. You see I can carry these trays because I am so strong. But I'm not very smart so I have just learned to help with the things I know how to do." Robert most likely has
   a. a negative self-concept and low self-esteem
   b. a negative self-concept and high self-esteem
   c. a positive self-concept and fairly high self-esteem
   d. a positive self-concept and low self-esteem
2. Jerry was having academic difficulty in all his college courses, and during a counseling session he was asked to make a list of 20 words that describe him. After 15 minutes, Jerry listed the following: 19 years old, male, named Jerry, and declared he couldn't think of anything else. Jerry has demonstrated
   a. lack of self-esteem
   b. deficient self-knowledge
   c. unrealistic self-expectation
   d. inability to evaluate himself
3. Jerry, who is in counseling because he is having academic difficulty, was able to list only three facts, traits, or qualities to describe himself. His counselor then asked him to list facts, traits, or qualities that he would like to be descriptive of himself or which he thinks he should have. Jerry quickly listed 25, all of which were characteristic of a successful man. When asked if he knew anyone like this, he replied, "My father." This discrepancy between Jerry's description of himself as he is and as he would like to be indicates
   a. positive self-concept
   b. Jerry's modesty (lack of conceit)
   c. body image disturbance
   d. low self-esteem
4. David and his wife have decided that she will get a job so that David can go to pharmacy school as he has wanted to do for some time. Their three teenagers, who were involved in the decision, are also getting jobs to buy their own clothes. David plans to work 12 to 16 hours weekly. He states, "I was always an *A* student, but I may have to settle for *B*s now because I don't want to neglect my family and I need to work a few hours so my wife won't have to work overtime." David's self-expectations are
   a. realistic and positively motivating his development
   b. unrealistic and negatively motivating his development
   c. unrealistic but positively motivating his development
   d. realistic but negatively motivating his development
5. Which of the following statements made by a parent of a child you are seeing in clinic needs to be followed up with teaching about how to foster healthy development of the self in children?
   a. "I love my child so much I 'hug him to death' every day."
   b. "I think children need challenges, don't you?"
   c. "My husband and I both grew up in very restrictive families. We want our children to be free to do whatever they want."
   d. "My husband and I have different ideas about discipline, but we're talking this out because we know it's important for Johnny that we be consistent."
6. Which intervention would you take first to assist a woman who states that she feels incompetent as a mother of a teenage daughter?
   a. recommend that she discipline her daughter more strictly and consistently
   b. make a list of things her husband can do to help her improve
   c. assist the mother to identify both what she believes is preventing her success and what she can do to improve
   d. explore with the mother what the daughter can do to improve her behavior
7. Which of the following clients is *least* likely to develop problems related to self-concept?
   a. 55-year-old female television news reporter undergoing a hysterectomy (removal of uterus)
   b. young clergyperson whose vocal cords are paralyzed following a motorbike accident
   c. 32-year-old accountant who survives a massive heart attack
   d. 23-year-old model who has just learned that she has breast cancer

For questions 8 to 11, read the client data below and use the following letters to indicate the diagnosis the data suggest (each response may be used only once):

a. Personal Identity Disturbance
b. Body Image Disturbance
c. Self-Esteem Disturbance
d. Altered Role Performance

8. Juanita Sanchez has only been in the United States 3 months and has recently suffered the loss of her husband and job. She states that nothing feels familiar, "I don't know who I am supposed to be here," and she misses home (Nicaragua) terribly.
9. Jim Boa, a sophomore in high school, has missed a great amount of school this year because of leukemia. He said he feels like he is falling behind in everything and misses "hanging out at the mall" with his friends most of all.
10. "Why did I have to be born into a family of big bottoms and short fat legs! No one will ever ask me out for a date . . . oh why can't I have long thin legs like everyone else in my class? What a frump I am."

11. Marissa Yule, a 33-year-old businessperson, is now in counseling attempting to deal with a long-repressed history of sexual abuse by her father. "I guess I should feel satisfied with what I've achieved in life but I'm never content and nothing I achieve makes me feel good about myself. . . . I hate my father for making me feel like I'm no good. This is an awful way to live."
12. Nancy, aged 36, who was divorced 5 years earlier, entered the emergency department with severe burns and cuts on her face after an auto accident in a car driven by her fiancé of 3 months. Three weeks later, her fiancé has not yet contacted her. Nancy states that he is so busy and she is too tired to visit anyway. Nancy frequently lies with her eyes closed and head turned away. These data suggest that
    a. there is no disturbance in self-concept
    b. this client has ego strength and high self-esteem but may have a disturbance of body image
    c. the area of self-esteem has very low priority at this time and should be ignored until much later
    d. it is probable that there are disturbances in self-esteem and body image
13. Which of the nursing interventions below is *least* likely to assist a severely ill client with cancer to maintain a positive sense of self?
    a. making it a point to address the client by name each time you enter the room
    b. fatiguing the client as little as possible by performing all procedures in silence
    c. continuing to respect the client's privacy and sensibilities
    d. offering the client a simple explanation before moving her in any way
14. Doris, aged 16, has a nursing diagnosis of Body Image Disturbance related to severe acne. In planning nursing care, an appropriate goal for this nursing diagnosis is, "The client will
    a. make above B grades in all tests at school"
    b. demonstrate by diet control and skin care increased interest in control of acne"
    c. report that she feels more self-confidence in her music and art, which she enjoys"
    d. express that she is very smart in school"
15. A 4½-year-old boy required stitches for a laceration on the eyebrow. After the doctor held him, visited with him, and explained what was going to be done and that his eye would get better and look just like it did before, the boy placed his hands under his hips as instructed and quietly permitted the procedure. He then expressed pride in himself. Evaluation of the effect of this healthcare experience is best expressed in which of the following?
    a. The doctor did an excellent job.
    b. The child's self-esteem was enhanced and fear of bodily mutilation decreased, and the parents were given an excellent role model.
    c. The child was made the center of attention and the situation exaggerated, thus encouraging the child to become self-centered.
    d. These interventions consumed too much physician time to be evaluated positively.

Answers With Rationale

1. The correct response is *c.* The data point to Robert's having a positive self-concept ("I'm a good helper") and fairly high self-esteem (realizes his strengths and limitations). The statement "But I'm not very smart" is accurate and is not an indication of a negative self-concept.
2. The correct response is *b.* Jerry's inability to list more than three items about himself indicates deficient self-knowledge. There are not enough data provided to determine if he lacks self-esteem, has unrealistic self-expectations, or is unable to evaluate himself.
3. The correct response is *d.* Low self-esteem is characterized by great discrepancy between the ideal and real selves. There are no data in this item to suggest that Jerry has either a positive self-concept or a body image disturbance. The data do indicate something more serious than modesty.
4. The correct response is *a.* David's self-expectations are realistic, given his multiple commitments, and seem to be positively motivating his development.
5. The correct response is *c.* Each option with the exception of *c* correctly addresses some aspect of fostering healthy development in children. Because children need effective structure and development, giving them total freedom to do as they please may actually hinder their development.
6. The correct response is *c.* The first intervention priority with a mother who feels incompetent to parent a teenage daughter is to assist the mother to identify what is preventing her from being an effective parent and then to explore solutions aimed at improving her parenting skills. The other interventions may prove helpful but they do not directly address the mother's problem with her feelings of incompetence.
7. The correct response is *a.* Based simply on the facts given, the 55-year-old news reporter would be least likely to experience a body image or role performance disturbance because she is beyond her childbearing years and the hysterectomy should not impair her ability to report the news. The young clergyperson's inability to preach, the 32-year-old's massive myocardial infarction, and the model's breast resection have much greater potential to result in self-concept problems.

8. The correct response is *a.* An unfamiliar culture coupled with traumatic life events and loss of husband and job has resulted in this client's total loss of her sense of self: "I don't know who I am supposed to be here." Her very sense of identity is at stake, not merely her body image, self-esteem, or role performance.
9. The correct response is *d.* Important roles for Jim are being a student and a friend. His illness is preventing him from doing either of these well. This self-concept disturbance is basically one that concerns role performance.
10. The correct response is *b.* Clearly, this client's concern is with his or her body image.
11. The correct response is *c.* Marissa's self-concept disturbance is mainly one of devaluing herself, and thinking that she is no good. This is a self-esteem disturbance.
12. The correct response is *d.* The traumatic nature of Nancy's injuries, her fiancé's failure to contact her, and Nancy's response, that is, her withdrawal, all point to potential problems with both body image and self-esteem. It is not true that self-esteem needs are of low priority.
13. The correct response is *b.* Each option with the exception of *b* should assist the client to maintain a positive sense of self. Working in silence with the client may be preferable to idle chatter but the ideal is to address the client by name, give simple explanations of procedures, and communicate that he or she is a person of worth by simple words of caring.
14. The correct response is *b.* All of these client goals may be appropriate for Doris, but the only goal that directly addresses her body image disturbance is *b.*
15. The correct response is *b.* The physician enhanced the child's self-esteem by teaching him how to participate effectively, decreased his fear of bodily mutilation by telling him that his eyebrow would heal and look normal, and gave the parents an excellent role model.

Bibliography

Atwater, W. E. (1990). *Psychology of adjustment* (4th ed.). Englewood Cliffs, NJ: Prentice-Hall.

Atwater, W. E. (1996). *Adolescence* (4th ed.). Upper Saddle River, NJ: Prentice-Hall.

Bello, L. K., & McIntire, S. N. (1995). Body image disturbances in young adults with cancer. *Cancer Nursing, 18*(2), 138–143.

Bensink, G. W., Godbey, K. L., Marshall, M. J., & Yarandi, H. N. (1992). Institutionalized elderly: Relaxation, locus of control, self-esteem. *Journal of Gerontological Nursing, 18*(4), 30–36.

Calhoun, J. F., & Acocella, J. R. (1989). *Psychology of adjustment and human relationships* (3rd ed.). New York: Random House.

Carpenito, L. J. (1995). *Nursing diagnosis: Application to clinical practice* (6th ed.). Philadelphia: Lippincott.

Coleman, J. C., Morris, C. G., & Glaros, A. G. (1990). *Contemporary psychology and effective behavior* (7th ed.). Glenview, IL: Scott, Foresman.

Coopersmith, S. (1967). *The antecedents of self-esteem.* San Francisco: Freeman.

Davidhizar, R. (1991). Ten strategies for increasing your self-confidence. *Imprint, 38*(3), 105–108.

Gilbert, R. (1983). The evaluation of self-esteem. *Family and Community Health, 6*(2), 29–49.

Harter, S. (1990). Processes underlying adolescent self-concept formation. In R. Montemayor, G. R. Adams, & T. P. Gulotta (Eds.). *From childhood to adolescence: A transitional period?* Newbury Park, CA: Sage.

Jenny, J. (1990). Self-esteem: A problem for nurses. *Canadian Nurse, 86*(11), 19–21.

LeMone, P. (1991). Analysis of a human phenomenon: Self-concept. *Nursing Diagnosis, 2*(3), 126–130.

Long, K. A., & Hamlin, C. M. (1988). Use of the Piers-Haris self-concept scale with Indian children: Cultural considerations. *Nursing Research, 37*(1), 42–46.

Maslow, A. (1954). *Motivation and personality.* New York: Harper & Row.

McKay, M., & Fanning, P. (1992). *Self-esteem* (2nd ed.). Oakland, CA: New Harbinger Publications.

Meisenhelder, J. B. (1986). Self-esteem in women: The influence of employment and perception of husband's appraisals. *IMAGE: Journal of Nursing Scholarship, 18*(1), 8–14.

Nystrom, A. E., & Segesten, K. M. (1994). On sources of powerlessness in nursing home life. *Journal of Advanced Nursing, 19*(1), 124–133.

Otto, H. (1965). The human potentialities of nurses and patients. *Nursing Outlook, 13*(8), 32–35.

Reasoner, R. W. (1983). Enhancement of self-esteem in children and adolescents. *Family and Community Health, 6*(2), 51–64.

Shell, J. A. (1995). Do you like the thing that life is showing you? The sensitive self-image of the person with cancer. *Oncology Nursing Forum, 22*(6), 907–911.

Stanwyck, D. J. (1983). Self-esteem through the life span. *Family and Community Health, 6*(8), 11–28.

Stein, K. F. (1995). Schema model of the self-concept. *IMAGE: Journal of Nursing Scholarship, 27*(3), 187–193.

Taylor, C. (1982). The need for self-esteem. In H. Yura & M. B. Walsh (Eds.). *Human needs 2 and the nursing process.* Norwalk, CT: Appleton-Century-Crofts.

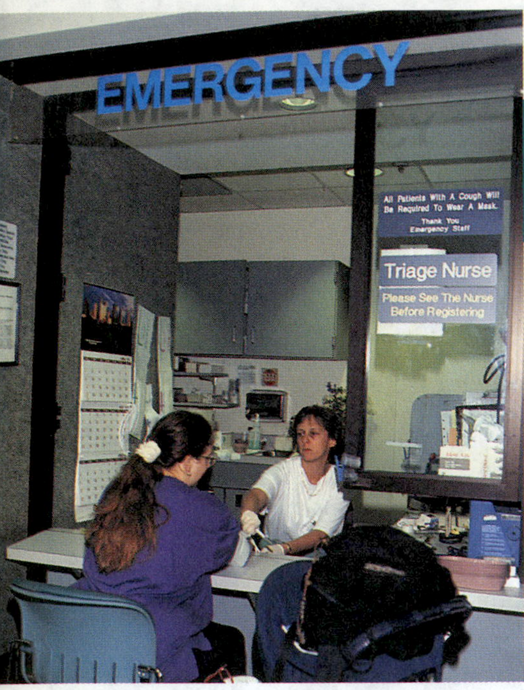
EMERGENCY
All Patients With A Cough Will Be Required To Wear A Mask.
Thank You
Emergency Staff
Triage Nurse
Please See The Nurse Before Registering

Chapter 32

Stress and Adaptation

Objectives

After studying this chapter, the learner should be able to:

Define key terms used in the chapter.

Describe the mechanisms involved in maintaining physiologic homeostasis.

Explain the interdependent nature of stressors, stress, and adaptation.

Compare and contrast developmental and situational stress, incorporating the concepts of physiologic and psychosocial stressors.

Describe the physical and emotional responses to stress, including mind–body interaction, local adaptation syndrome, general adaptation syndrome, and coping and defense mechanisms.

Discuss the effects of short- and long-term stress on basic human needs, health and illness, and the family.

Integrate knowledge of healthy lifestyle, support systems, stress management techniques, and crisis intervention into hospital-based and community-based care.

Recognize and effectively cope with stress unique to the nursing profession.

Key Terms

adaptation
anxiety
burnout
caregiver burden
coping mechanisms
crisis
crisis intervention
defense mechanisms
developmental crisis
fight-or-flight response
general adaptation syndrome
homeostasis
inflammatory response
local adaptation syndrome
psychosomatic disorders
reflex pain response
situational stress
stress
stressor

Stress is a part of life. Everyone uses the term at one time or another. Books and magazines are filled with articles about stress, discussing everything from the negative stressful effects that may be involved in performing one's job to the positive stressful effects of celebrating holidays. Television advertisements for over-the-counter remedies promise fast relief from stress headaches and upset stomachs. Stress is blamed for excessive weight gain, drinking, and smoking as well as for divorce and child abuse. Being "stressed out" is common, and taking "stress breaks" to do physical exercise is recommended in many work settings. With stress being so much a part of everyday life, it is easy to see that any additional problem—such as a health problem—increases the stress and its effects on the person experiencing the problem.

Stress is not only a part of everyday experiences, but a person's responses to stress are also necessary to life. Stress has both positive and negative effects and is produced by a change in the environment that is perceived as a challenge, a threat, or a danger (Smeltzer & Bare, 1996). Stress has a holistic effect—it affects the whole person in all the human dimensions (physical, emotional, intellectual, social, and spiritual). The perception of stress as well as the responses to it are highly individualized, not only from person to person but also from one time to another in the same person. Because stress is individualized and holistic, there is no commonly accepted definition or measurement. Most simply, **stress** is a condition in which the human system responds to changes in its normal balanced state.

A **stressor** is anything that causes a person to experience stress. It is a change in the person's balanced state. Stressors may be either internal (such as an illness, a hormonal change, or fear) or external (such as loud noise or cold temperature). As with stress, the perception and effects of the stressor are holistic and highly individualized. Stressors are neither positive nor negative, but rather have positive or negative effects as the person responds to change.

When a person is in a threatening situation, immediate responses are made. Those responses, which often are involuntary, are called *coping responses*. The change that takes place as a result of the response to a stressor is **adaptation**. Adaptation is, to some degree, an ongoing process as a person strives to maintain balance in both the internal and the external environment (Fig. 32-1). Although it is easier to explain coping and adaptation in terms of the individual, adaptation also occurs in families and groups. Adaptation results in the following:

- Optimal functioning in all dimensions
- Normal growth and development
- Normal reactions to physical and emotional stress
- Ability to tolerate changing situations

Stress, stressors, and adaptation are individualized and holistic. The process of adaptation to stress is constant and dynamic, and essential to physical, emotional, and social well-being. Stress and adaptation are major components in health and illness. It is important for nurses to understand the concepts and dimensions of stress as they provide nursing care to clients in all types of settings. Nurses themselves are subject to increased stress from the demands of their career, and they need to know healthy ways of responding. This chapter discusses stress from a holistic perspective, including both physical and psychologic stress. Major components to be discussed are homeostasis, stress and adaptation, and nursing actions to promote stress reduction. Examples of nursing diagnoses are included, and expected outcomes and nursing strategies to reduce the responses to stress are included. In the section entitled Nursing Process in Clinical Practice, focused assessment, planning, implementation, and evaluation guides are offered for Anxiety, the most common nursing diagnosis relevant to stress. These guides and the concluding case study illustrate how the nurse's knowledge of causes of and responses to stress is combined with specific nursing interventions to promote coping and adaptation.

Physiology of Stress and Adaptation

Our bodies are always interacting with a constantly changing environment. That environment can be divided into two parts: the external environment, which surrounds our bodies, and the internal environment, which includes the mechanisms that regulate body functions and the fluids that surround body cells. To maintain health, the body's internal environment must remain in balance within a fairly narrow range. Various physio-

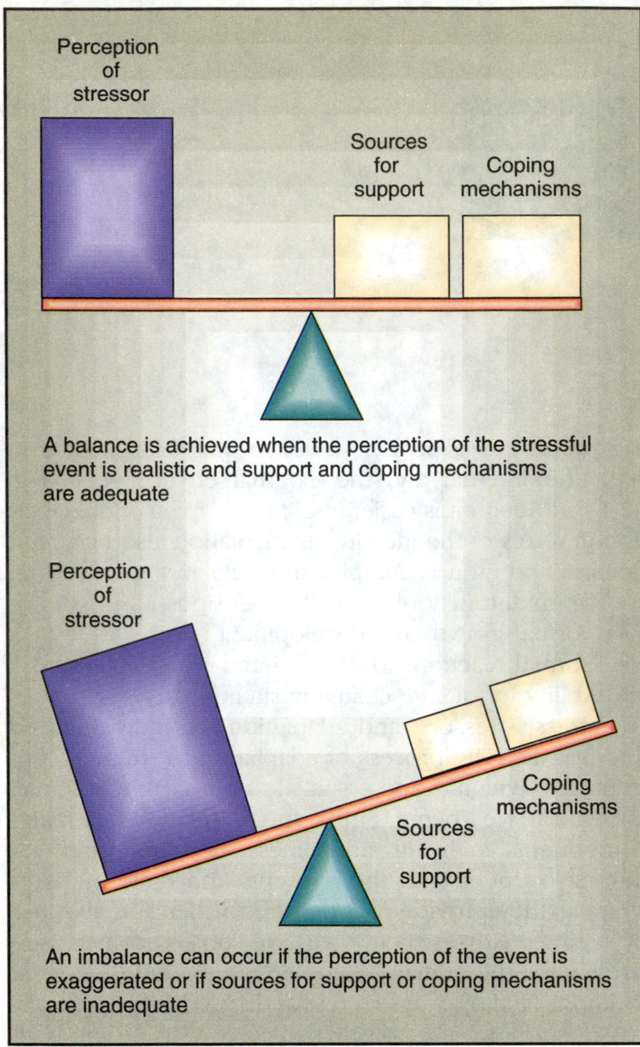

Figure 32-1
A realistic perception of a stressful event, sources for emotional support, and appropriate coping mechanisms are components of a system of balances during stress.

logic mechanisms within the body respond to internal changes to maintain relative constancy in the internal environment, called **homeostasis**.

Homeostasis

The concept of homeostasis was introduced by W. B. Cannon in 1939, but throughout history, the belief that health is the result of a balanced state has been present. This belief was written about and discussed by some of the most important people in medical history, including Hippocrates (the father of medicine) and Claude Bernard (the father of physiology). The knowledge that the human body responds to an ever-changing environment originally focused on the life processes that occur within the body, such as heart rate, blood pressure, and water balance. The definition of homeostasis has been expanded to include both the internal and the external environment, and physiologic *and* psychologic balance.

Physiologic Homeostasis

Long before you entered nursing you knew that sweating when you were hot and shivering when you were cold were ways to maintain a stable body temperature. This part of the chapter summarizes the homeostatic mechanisms that regulate the body's internal environment.

Regulation of the homeostatic mechanisms is primarily controlled by the autonomic nervous system and the endocrine system. Involved to a lesser degree are the respiratory, cardiovascular, gastrointestinal, and renal systems. These mechanisms are self-regulating, come into action without conscious thought, and usually function to correct abnormal conditions. They can be compared, on a simple level, to the relation of a thermostat to a furnace. When the temperature in a house falls below the preset temperature on the thermostat, the thermostat turns on the furnace, which heats the house to the desired temperature and then shuts off.

The regulatory mechanisms of the body are constantly reacting to change to maintain health. When a person is ill, injured, or subjected to long-term stress, the mechanisms continue to try to restore balance, but they may become ineffective. The result is increased illness or death. The body systems, with homeostatic mechanisms, are summarized in Table 32-1. They are important in understanding the consequences of both short- and long-term stress.

Psychologic Homeostasis

To remain healthy, humans also must maintain psychologic homeostasis, or a state of mental well-being. As discussed in Chapter 2, each person needs to feel loved and that he or she belongs, to feel safe and secure, and to have self-esteem. When these needs are not met or a threat to need fulfillment occurs, the person uses homeostatic measures in the form of coping or defense mechanisms to return to emotional balance. Additional information about psychologic homeostasis is included later in this chapter.

Adaptive Responses to Stress

Each person constantly encounters physical, psychologic, or social changes in the internal and external environment. The perception of these changes may be conscious or unconscious. If the person has the necessary resources, adaptation takes place, and balance is maintained. If the resources cannot reestablish balance, a state of stress will result. The responses that are made and the degree of stress that is produced depend on the nature, intensity, and duration of the stressor.

This section examines adaptive responses to stress, including the mind–body interaction, the local adaptation syndrome, the general adaptation syndrome, and coping/defense mechanisms.

Table 32-1
Homeostatic Regulators of the Body

System	Action	Effect
Autonomic Nervous		
Parasympathetic—Functions under normal conditions and at rest		
(Cranial and sacral nerves)	• Regulates heart rate • Stimulates secretion of digestive juices and digestive tract smooth muscle • Stimulates insulin secretion	• Slows rate • Improves digestion, increases peristalsis • Increases uptake of glucose by cells
Sympathetic—Functions under stress conditions to bring about the fight-or-flight response		
	• Stimulates heart rate and force • Dilates skeletal muscle blood vessels • Dilates blood vessels to the brain • Stimulates release of glycogen stores	• Increases rate, strengthens contractions, increases cardiac output • Increases muscle strength • Increases mental alertness • Increases blood glucose levels
Endocrine		
Pituitary	• Secretes hormones: Adrenocorticotropic hormone (ACTH) Thyroid-stimulating hormone (TSH)	• Stimulates the adrenal cortex • Stimulates the thyroid
Adrenals	• Medulla produces epinephrine and norepinephrine • Cortex secretes mineralocorticoids, glucocorticoids, and androgens	• Prepares the person for emergencies; supports the sympathetic system • Mineralocorticoid aldosterone regulates fluid and electrolytes • Glucocorticoids raise glucose levels (for energy) and increase resistance to physical stress
Thyroid	• Secretes thyroid hormone and calcitonin	• Regulates metabolic rate and growth
Other		
Cardiovascular	• Serves as transport system and pump	• Provides oxygen and nutrients and removes carbon dioxide and wastes from cells
Renal	• Filters, excretes, and reabsorbs metabolic products and water	• Maintains fluid, electrolyte, and acid–base balance
Respiratory	• Intake and output of oxygen and carbon dioxide	• Necessary for metabolism; helps maintain acid–base balance
Gastrointestinal	• Takes in food and fluids • Eliminates waste products	• Energy sources; maintains fluids and electrolytes

Mind–Body Interaction

Consider the following examples of mind–body interaction.

- Tomorrow you are scheduled to take a final examination, and you must make a passing score to pass the course and remain in the nursing program. After being awake most of the night, you are unable to swallow any food for breakfast, have a rapid heartbeat, are filled with feelings of apprehension, and have diarrhea.
- Since his wife was killed in a car accident, Tom Green has been the sole support of his 4-year-old son, who has developmental delay and is hyperactive. Tom has been coming to the neighborhood health clinic with increasing frequency the past 5 months, complaining of weight loss, headaches, and stomach pain.

These two examples illustrate the relation between psychologic stressors and the physiologic stress response and reinforce the holistic and individualized nature of stress. In the first example, as you begin the test and discover that you know most of the answers, your symptoms rapidly disappear. Tom's stress, however, is always present and long-term, causing increased risk for developing an illness.

Why does this happen? Although the exact cause is not well understood, it is thought that humans react to threats of danger as if they were real. A person perceives the threat on an emotional level, and the body prepares itself to either resist or run away and avoid the danger (the **fight-or-flight response**). Each person reacts in her or his own way. With prolonged stress, some may have chronic diarrhea, while others may develop headaches. The illnesses in these people are real but are called **psychosomatic disorders** because the physiologic alterations are thought to be at least partially caused by psychologic influences.

Another component of mind–body interaction is the impact of life change on a person. Researchers have

Helpscan

The following are resources for clients and healthcare professionals for information about mental health:

- American Mental Health Foundation, Inc.
  2 E. 86th St.
  New York, NY 10028
- National Clearinghouse for Mental Health Information
  National Institutes of Mental Health
  5600 Fishers Lane, Room 11A33
  Rockville, MD 20857
  (301) 443-4517
- Canadian Mental Health Association
  2160 Yonge St., Third Floor
  Toronto, ON M4S 2Z3
  (416) 484-7750

found that the number of changes a person has in his or her life (both positive and negative) has a positive correlation with the onset of illness. A life change can be defined as an event in a person's life that requires energy for adaptation. When energy is expended to adapt to the event, the person's resistance to illness is lowered.

Physiologic Responses to Stress

As we have seen, there are both physical and emotional components in the response—or adaptation—to stress. The physiologic responses are the local adaptation syndrome and the general adaptation syndrome.

Local Adaptation Syndrome. The **local adaptation syndrome** (LAS) is a localized response of the body to stress. It does not involve the entire body but rather involves a body part (tissue, organ) only. The stress precipitating the LAS may be traumatic or pathologic. LAS is an adaptive response, primarily homeostatic, and short-term. Although the body is capable of exhibiting many localized stress responses, two of the most common that influence nursing care are the reflex pain response and the inflammatory response.

The **reflex pain response** is a response of the central nervous system when pain is the stimulus. It is rapid and automatic, serving as a protective mechanism to prevent injury. The reflex depends on an intact, functioning neurologic reflex arc and involves both sensory and motor neurons. For example, if you step into a bathtub of hot water, your skin senses the heat and immediately sends a message to the spinal cord. In turn, the message is sent to a motor nerve, which activates the muscles in your leg, and you quickly withdraw your foot. All of this happens before you consciously realize that the water is too hot to be safe.

The **inflammatory response** is a localized response to injury or infection. It serves to localize and prevent the spread of infection and so promote wound healing. When you cut your finger, you often develop the symptoms of the inflammatory response: pain, swelling, heat, redness, and changes in function. There are three phases in the inflammatory response.

1. In the first phase, bleeding initially is controlled by vasoconstriction (or narrowing) of the blood vessels at the injury site. After the bleeding has been controlled, histamines are released and capillary permeability increases, allowing increased blood flow and white blood cells to the area. The blood flow then returns to normal, but the white blood cells remain to help resist infection.
2. During the second stage, exudate (made up of fluid, cells, and inflammatory by-products) is released from the wound. The amount of exudate depends on the size, location, and severity of the wound.
3. During the third and final stage, damaged cells are repaired by either regeneration (replacement with identical cells) or formation of scar tissue. Some body tissues (skin, bone) are easily reproduced, and regain their former function; others (nervous system, intestines) do not regenerate but rather form nonfunctional scar tissue.

General Adaptation Syndrome. The **general adaptation syndrome** (GAS) is a biochemical model of stress developed by Hans Selye (1976). The concept of stressors as factors that cause stress was also articulated by Selye. The GAS describes the body's general response to stress and serves as part of the knowledge base essential to all areas of nursing care.

There are three stages in the GAS (Fig. 32-2):

1. In the first stage, the *alarm reaction,* a person perceives a specific stressor, and various defense mechanisms are activated. The perception of threat may be conscious or unconscious. The autonomic nervous system initiates the fight-or-flight response, and hormone levels rise to prepare the body fully to react. This phase of the alarm reaction, called the *shock phase,* is characterized by an increase in energy levels, oxygen intake, cardiac output, blood pressure, and mental alertness.

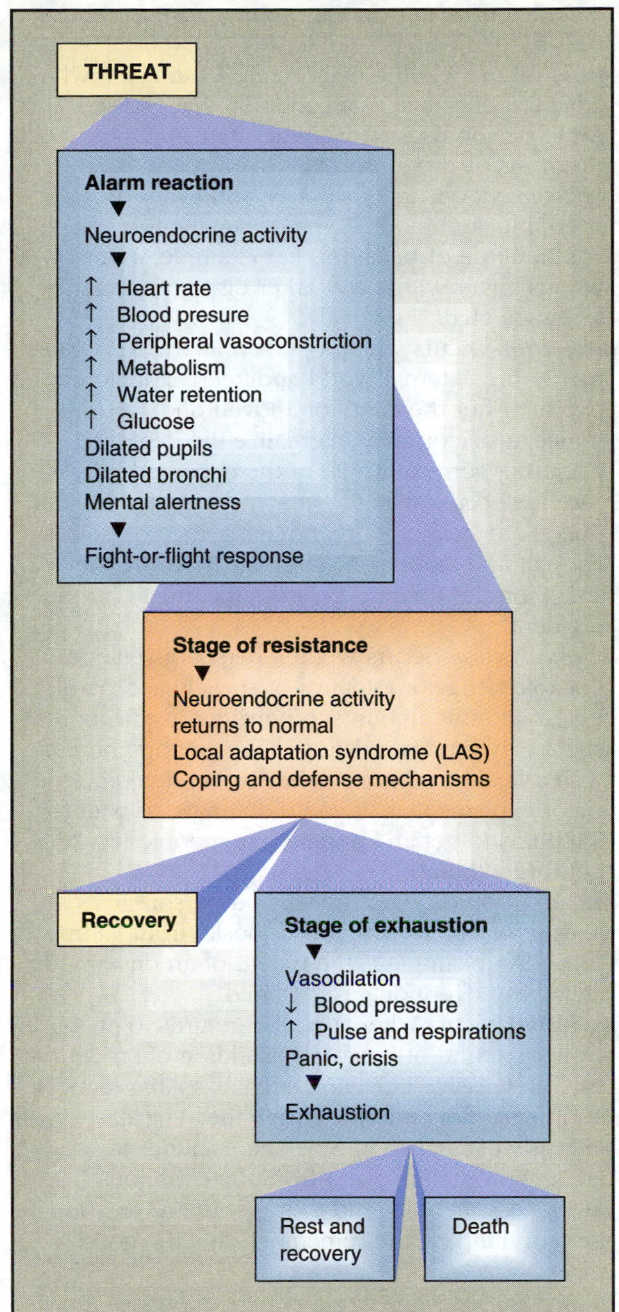

Figure 32-2
The general adaptation syndrome (general response to stress).

(If you think of the last time you narrowly missed wrecking your car, you will easily be able to identify these body reactions!) During the second phase of the alarm reaction, *countershock,* there is a reversal of body changes.

2. The second stage of the GAS is *resistance.* Having perceived the threat and mobilized its resources, the body now attempts to adapt to the stressor. Vital signs, hormone levels, and energy production return to normal. If the stress can be managed or confined to a small area (LAS), the body regains homeostasis. If the damage to the body is too great (for example, when there is severe injury and bleeding or a major illness such as cancer or a heart attack), the adaptive mechanisms fail, and the third phase of the GAS begins.
3. The third stage, *exhaustion,* is the result of exhaustion of the adaptive mechanisms. Without defense against the stressor, the body may either rest and mobilize its defenses to return to normal or reach total exhaustion and die.

Although the alarm stage is short-term (from minutes to hours), the length of the resistance and exhaustion stages varies greatly, depending on such variables as the severity and duration of the stressor, the previous health of the person, and the immediacy and effectiveness of healthcare interventions.

The GAS is a physiologic response to stress, but it is important to remember that the response is the result of both physical and emotional stressors. The stages occur in both physical and psychosocial damage to the body. Obvious examples are seen in clients after severe injury or in those who have an illness, but GAS also is a factor in mental illness, social isolation, and loss (or lack) of human relations.

Psychologic Responses to Stress

Humans respond to threat—and stress—psychologically as well as physically. Various emotional responses may occur, including depression and anger. The response most common in the human experience is anxiety. Anxiety is experienced from birth to death by all people, and involves one's body, self-perceptions, and social relationships (Stuart & Sundeen, 1995). **Anxiety** is a vague sense of impending doom or apprehension that appears to have no reason. In contrast, fear is a response to a real stressor. Anxiety is precipitated by the unknown and is present before all new experiences, serving as a threat to one's identity and self-esteem.

There are four levels of anxiety, each having different effects:

Mild anxiety: Present in day-to-day living; increases alertness and perceptual fields and motivates learning and growth. Although mild anxiety may interfere with sleep, it also facilitates problem solving.

Moderate anxiety: Narrows the person's perceptual fields so that the focus is on immediate concerns, with inattention to other communications and details.

Severe anxiety: Creates a very narrow focus on specific detail; causes all behavior to be geared toward getting relief. The person has impaired learning ability and is easily distractible.

Panic: Causes the person to lose control and experience dread and terror. The resulting disorganized state is characterized by increased physical activity, distorted perceptions and relations, and loss of rational thought. The person is unable to learn, concentrates only on the present situation, and often experiences feelings of impending doom. This level of anxiety can lead to exhaustion and death.

At a mild level, anxiety can have a positive effect. For example, mild anxiety about an upcoming examination can motivate you to do the required reading and review. Anxiety beyond that level is regarded as negative, with unpleasant effects. In an attempt to neutralize, deny, or counteract the anxiety, a person develops individualized patterns of coping (Stuart & Sundeen, 1995).

Coping Mechanisms. Mild anxiety often is handled without conscious thought through the use of **coping mechanisms** (behaviors used to decrease stress and anxiety). Typical behaviors include:

- Crying, laughing, sleeping, and cursing
- Physical activity and exercise
- Smoking and drinking
- Lack of eye contact and withdrawal
- Limiting relationships to those with similar values and interests

Moderate, severe, and panic levels of anxiety are greater threats and involve more complex coping mechanisms as the person strives to reduce the stress and anxiety. Coping mechanisms used at higher levels of anxiety are categorized as task-oriented reactions or defense mechanisms.

Task-oriented reactions involve consciously thinking about the stress situation and then taking action to solve problems, resolve conflicts, or satisfy needs. These reactions, as defined by Stuart and Sundeen (1995), are as follows:

Attack behavior: Occurs when a person attempts to overcome obstacles to attack a problem; may be constructive, with assertive problem solving, or destructive, with feelings and actions of aggressive anger and hostility

Withdrawal behavior: Involves physical withdrawal from the threat, or emotional reactions such as admitting defeat, becoming apathetic, or feeling guilty and isolated

Compromise behavior: Usually constructive; involves the substitution of goals or negotiation to fulfill one's needs partially

Many of these behaviors are learned and are based on past experiences and sociocultural influences and expectations.

Defense Mechanisms. Other unconscious reactions called **defense mechanisms** often are used to protect the self. These mechanisms protect one's self-esteem and are useful in mild to moderate anxiety. If used to an extreme degree, they distort reality and create problems with relationships. At that point, the mechanisms become maladaptive instead of adaptive.

Defense mechanisms are summarized here. You will learn more about them in the curriculum component that focuses on mental health and illness.

Compensation occurs when a person attempts to overcome a perceived weakness by strengthening other areas. A person may compensate for blindness by perfecting other senses.

Denial occurs when a person refuses to acknowledge the presence of a condition that is disturbing. An ill person uses denial when refusing to accept a diagnosis or prognosis.

Displacement occurs when a person can satisfy a need, blocked by one type of behavior, by using another type of behavior. For example, a person who is angry with a coworker displaces anger by kicking a chair.

Introjection occurs when a person internalizes some part of the external world and keeps it intact in the psyche. After the death of a loved one, for instance, a person may internalize the deceased person or some attribute of the deceased person.

Projection occurs when a person's undesirable impulses are attributed to another person or object. For example, a person carelessly trips over an article on the floor and blames the article for the accident.

Rationalization occurs when a person gives questionable behavior a logical or socially acceptable explanation. It amounts to behavior justification. A client may be rationalizing when an appointment with a healthcare practitioner is forgotten and the client explains that "if you didn't have to wait for 3 months to get an appointment, people would not forget them!"

Reaction formation occurs when a person gives a reason for behavior that is opposite from its true cause. An example is the parent of an unwanted child who overindulges the child.

Regression occurs when a person returns to an earlier method of behaving. Children often demonstrate regressive behavior, such as soiling diapers and demanding a bottle, when they are ill.

Repression occurs when a person excludes an anxiety-producing event from the conscious awareness. People tend to forget the unpleasantness of the past and remember only the good times.

Sublimation occurs when a person expresses an unacceptable or impossible impulse or feeling in a more acceptable way. A woman who has chosen to be celibate and forgo motherhood may sublimate her maternal drives by working with children, by breeding pets, or by nurturing plants.

Suppression occurs when a person consciously turns attention away from a perceived threat. "If I let myself give in to this headache, I'll never accomplish what I must do today."

Effects of Stress

Stress affects all of the human dimensions. It has a strong influence on the attainment of basic human needs; it is a factor in health and illness; and it becomes a component in family reactions to illness. Both long-term or prolonged stress and crisis situations may seriously affect a person's physical and emotional health. Each of these areas are discussed in this section.

Interactions With Basic Human Needs

Basic human needs, described in Chapter 2, are common to all people. Stress, too, is common to all people. Both need attainment and the adaptation to stress require energy, respond to internal and external environments, and motivate behaviors. As a person strives to meet basic human needs at each level, stress can serve as either a stimulus or a barrier.

Basic human needs and responses to stress are individualized; both are modified by sociocultural backgrounds, priorities, and past experiences. In all people, the failure to meet needs results in imbalance in homeostatic mechanisms and, eventually, illness. Stress affects a person and his or her attainment of basic human needs in different ways, as illustrated in the accompanying box.

Stress in Health and Illness

The health–illness continuum (described in Chapter 4) also integrates stress. Wellness and homeostatic balance are at one extreme of the continuum; exhaustion and death are at the other extreme.

Stress in a healthy person may promote health and prevent illness. For example, the fear of developing lung cancer may motivate a person to stop smoking, or anxiety about baby care may prompt prospective parents to attend prenatal classes and read child care books. Stressors in health also facilitate normal growth and development, provide the stimulus for learning constructive adaptive behaviors, stimulate problem-solving abilities, encourage social relationships, and help develop spiritual strength.

The effects of stress on a sick or injured person are, in contrast, usually negative. Stress can cause illness; illness causes stress. The presence of an illness or a disability demands new coping skills at a time when homeostasis is challenged. Additionally, people who enter the healthcare setting are subjected to stressors unique to the situation. Guidelines for nursing care of the client entering the healthcare setting are outlined in the accompanying box.

Adaptation to acute and chronic illness involves two sets of adaptive tasks: *general tasks* (as in the case of any situational stress) that involve maintaining self-esteem and personal relationships and preparing for an uncertain future, and *illness-related tasks,* which include the following (Moos, 1985):

- Losing independence and control
- Handling pain and incapacitation
- Facilitating body function recovery
- Dealing with the hospital environment
- Developing relationships with caregivers

Effects of Long-Term Stress on Basic Human Needs

Basic Human Need	*Effect of Stress*
Physiologic Needs	• Exhibits change in appetite • Demonstrates change in activity pattern • Experiences change in sleep pattern • Has altered elimination pattern • May have increased blood pressure, heart rate, and respiratory rate
Safety and Security Needs	• Feels threatened and nervous • Focuses on stressor, resulting in inattention, which may cause accidents • Uses ineffective coping mechanisms (smoking, drinking) that are harmful to physical and emotional health
Love and Belonging Needs	• Is withdrawn and isolated • Blames others for own faults • Becomes overly dependent on others • Demonstrates physical or verbal aggression toward others
Self-Esteem Needs	• Becomes a workaholic • Exhibits behaviors that draw attention to oneself • Has increasing complaints of physical illness
Self-Actualization Needs	• Refuses to accept reality • Centers on own problems • Demonstrates lack of control

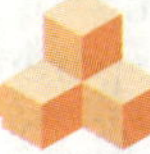

Guidelines for Nursing Care

Reducing Anxiety in the Client Entering the Healthcare Setting

Nursing Intervention	Rationale
• Assess physical status, sensory status, and cognitive status.	• Altered responses to illness or injury such as pain, nausea and vomiting, and dyspnea may increase anxiety and decrease the ability to be attentive and retain information. Impairments in function, such as vision, hearing, cognitive, or memory deficits, interfere with communications.
• Assess cultural/ethnic background, including beliefs about healthcare, dietary restrictions, and language spoken.	• Entering the healthcare system of a different culture is stressful; if a different language is used, communications and teaching are difficult.
• Assess past experiences with the healthcare system, including medical/surgical treatment for illness or injury.	• Expectations and perceptions of healthcare are influenced both positively and negatively by past experiences.
• Assess concerns and stressors.	• All people entering the healthcare system have an emotional response; additional stressors may increase anxiety.
• Assess amount and type of support systems available.	• Support from family, friends, and belief in a higher being can provide strength in handling new or unfamiliar stressors; a lack of support can increase stress and decrease coping.
• Provide information about the environment: a. All healthcare providers should introduce themselves by name and title. b. Explain policies and routines. c. If the hospital is the setting, provide verbal and written guidelines for use of equipment, telephone, television, meals, and visiting hours.	• Providing information decreases the unknown and thus lessens anxiety.
• Provide and discuss the patient's rights specific to care in the agency or institution.	• Knowing rights within an unfamiliar setting enhances a sense of control and helps decrease anxiety.
• Mutually determine expected outcomes of the plan of care.	• Coping is enhanced when the client participates in decision making; loss of control contributes to a feeling of powerlessness and increases anxiety.
• Provide information about all diagnostic procedures, surgical procedures, activity, and diet.	• Knowing the how, what, where, and why of what will be done allows a sense of control and decreases anxiety.
• Use verbal and nonverbal communication skills to convey genuine interest, concern for the client's well-being, and empathic understanding.	• Effective communications facilitate verbalization of concerns, allowing interventions to decrease anxiety and provide comfort.

(Adapted from Carpenito, L. (1995). *Nursing care plans and documentation: Nursing diagnoses and collaborative problems* (2nd ed.). Philadelphia: Lippincott, pp. 769–770.)

- Controlling symptoms
- Carrying out medical treatment
- Confronting economic and family problems

As a nurse, it is important to remember that each situation is different, that each person perceives and reacts to stressors in an individual manner, and that there is no one best way to cope with a given situation. Nursing considerations include the person's major concern, specific illness, sociocultural background, and available resources. For example, an older woman may be anxious about the cost involved in repairing her hip fracture, whereas her roommate, with the same injury, is seriously concerned about the care of her cats while she is in the hospital. As another example, two women (Mary and Jane) have entered the hospital with the medical diagnosis of breast cancer. Mary is worried about possible disfigurement and death, but she believes that with the help of surgery and chemotherapy, she can overcome the cancer. Jane, on the other hand, comes from a community that has strong fundamental religious beliefs. She believes that the cancer is a punishment from God and refuses treatment, even though she fears death.

Family Responses to the Stress of Illness

The stress that affects a person who is ill also affects the person's family members or significant others. Viewing the family as a system, the behavior of the individual is influenced by the family, and any alterations in the individual's behavior in turn affects the family. The family thus is an integral part in the assessment, planning, and nursing interventions for stress.

The family of a person with an acute or chronic illness is subjected to various stressors, including the following:

- Changes in family structure and roles
- Isolation from the loved person
- Loss of control over normal routines
- Anger and feelings of helplessness and guilt
- Lack of information about care
- Concern for future economic stability

The family, both as individuals and as a unit, uses many of the same coping and defense mechanisms previously described. Family members may be overly protective, deny the seriousness of the illness, or blame the hospital staff for the client's condition or behaviors. On the other hand, the family can provide the social support necessary to help the client manage and adapt to stress. Emotional support from family members allows open expression of feelings and meets love and belonging needs. The inclusion of family members in problem solving, teaching–learning activities, and physical care helps both the client and the family to maintain their self-esteem and feeling of worth.

Prolonged Stress

Prolonged or long-term stress is a serious threat to physical and emotional health. As the duration, intensity, or number of stressors increases, a person's ability to adapt is lessened. The failure of adaptive mechanisms also is influenced by a person's level of wellness and past experiences with stress.

Long-term stress affects physical status, increasing the risk of disease or injury; recovery and return to normal function also are compromised by prolonged stress. High levels of stress are associated with cardiovascular disease, gastrointestinal disorders, and cancer. It is believed that these diseases are the result of various factors, including the effects of the fight-or-flight response, eating patterns, lifestyle, and coping mechanisms. A person who reacts to stress by overeating, smoking, becoming chemically dependent, or becoming hyperactive puts additional strain on a body prepared to react to threat. Homeostasis cannot be maintained, and illness results.

Reactions to home care of family members for long periods also cause prolonged stress. Called **caregiver burden**, this stress response includes chronic fatigue, sleep problems, and increased incidence of stress-related illnesses, such as high blood pressure and heart disease.

Prolonged stress also can seriously threaten mental health. As coping or defense mechanisms become ineffective, a person may try less effective coping patterns or maladaptive defense mechanisms. As anxiety increases despite these measures, the person may experience difficulties on the job, with personal relationships, and with self-esteem. These problems in turn act as stressors, and mental illness may result.

Crisis

A **crisis** occurs when previous coping and defense mechanisms are no longer effective. This failure produces high levels of anxiety, disorganized behavior, and an inability to function adequately. A crisis situation is the result of a person's perception of and emotional response to a loss of self-esteem (or threat of a loss) from such events as illness, a change in status, a failure in school, or a verbal put-down.

The acute period of a crisis is self-limiting, lasting from 4 to 6 weeks. By that time, the threat is reduced, and the person has found some method of coping to reduce the emotional imbalance. A person in crisis needs immediate help. Crisis intervention is included below in the section on Implementing.

Factors Affecting Stress and Adaptation

Stress and adaptation are affected by both the sources of stress and the types of stressors experienced.

Sources of Stress

Although there are an infinite number of sources of stress, they can be categorized into two broad areas that create major demands for adaptive responses. The areas are developmental stress and situational stress.

Developmental stress or a **developmental crisis** occurs as a person progresses through the normal stages of growth and development from birth to old age. Within each stage, certain tasks must be achieved to resolve that crisis and reduce the stress. Examples of developmental stress include the following:

- The infant learns to trust others.
- The toddler learns to control elimination.
- The school-age child socializes with peers.
- The adolescent strives for independence.
- The middle adult accepts physical signs of aging.

Situational stress is different from developmental stress. It does not occur in predictable patterns as one progresses through life. Rather, situational stress can occur at any time, although the ability to adapt may be strongly influenced by a person's developmental level. Examples of situational stress (or crises), which may be either positive or negative, include the following:

- Illness or accidents
- Marriage or divorce
- Loss (belongings, relationships, family member)
- New job
- Role change

To further illustrate the positive or negative aspects of situational stress, consider pregnancy as an example. A young married couple may be overjoyed at the prospect of becoming parents, whereas an unmarried adolescent may be panic-stricken when she discovers she is pregnant. In this case, the situations and the developmental levels of the young couple and the adolescent will have a major impact on the adaptations made. The physical and psychosocial capacities to cope with the situation depend not only on the stage of maturation but also on the support systems available.

Types of Stressors

We are constantly bombarded with stressors, and we adapt to the changes to maintain a normal or healthy state. However, if the stressors increase in number or intensity, a person's physical or psychologic balance is impaired, and illness may result.

Physiologic stressors have both a specific effect and a general effect. The specific effect is seen in alteration of normal body structure and function. The general effect is the stress response. The accompanying box lists the agents considered to be primary physiologic stressors.

There is an almost infinite variety of *psychosocial stressors,* and they become so much a part of our daily lives that we often overlook them. To illustrate the many types of psychosocial stressors, consider the following categories, summarized from work by Antonovsky (1979):

- Accidents and their survivors, which cause stress for the victim, the person who caused the accident, and the families of both
- Experiences of family members and friends
- Horrors of history, such as Nazi concentration camps, famine in Africa, and the effects of the atomic bomb on Hiroshima
- Fear of aggression or mutilation from others, such as muggings, rape, murder, and terrorist attacks
- Events of history that are brought into our homes through television, such as wars, earthquakes, and violent threats to the lives of world figures
- Developmental and life crises
- Rapid changes in our world and the way we live, including changes in economic and political structures and technology

Psychosocial stressors may be either actual or the result of a person's perception of a threat. The person's responses are continuous and include the individualized coping mechanisms that are used to respond to anxiety, guilt, fear, frustration, and loss. The mechanisms serve to maintain psychologic homeostasis.

Primary Physiologic Stressors

Chemical agents
- Drugs
- Poisons
- Toxins

Physical agents
- Heat
- Cold
- Radiation
- Electric shock
- Trauma

Infectious agents
- Viruses
- Bacteria
- Fungi

Faulty immune system
Genetic disorders
Nutrition imbalances
Hypoxia

The Nurse as Role Model

Nurses who design care for clients to reduce stress must also examine themselves as a factor in the success of that plan of care. Clients use nurses as role models in achieving healthy lifestyles. Nurses dealing with stresses from professional and personal aspects of their lives sometimes make inappropriate responses. The nurse who wishes to encourage adaptation to stress must demonstrate behaviors that support a healthy lifestyle. With that goal in mind, the nurse will do the following:

- Follow the recommendations of the food pyramid for proper nutrition.
- Participate in regular exercise.
- Get adequate sleep and rest.
- Evaluate own use of drugs, nicotine, alcohol, and food as coping methods.
- Practice relaxation techniques regularly.
- Set aside time for activities that are fun.
- Emphasize his or her own strengths and abilities.
- Learn to say no without feeling guilty or offering an excuse.

The nurse can assess his or her own stress levels and adaptation with the checklist in the accompanying box.

ASSESSING STRESS

Stress and anxiety are client problems that nurses encounter no matter what the age of the client or the setting in which care is provided. Stress is assessed through a health assessment, with data from both the nursing history and the physical assessment. Risk factors for or indicators of stress may be identified by using standardized tests, or through the use of open-ended questions to elicit information. The client's willingness to share information is affected by the level of stress experienced as well as the coping or defense mechanisms in use. Examples of physiologic, psychologic, and social re-

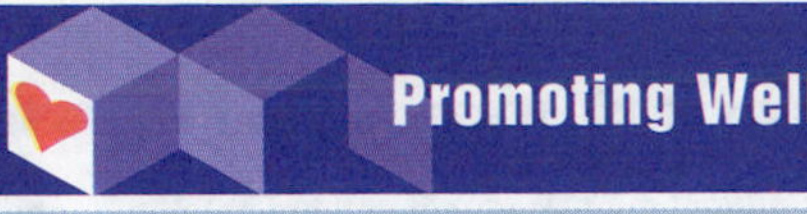

Promoting Wellness

Stress and Adaptation

Use the assessment checklist to determine how well you are adapting to stress. Then develop a prescription for self-care by choosing appropriate behaviors from the list of suggestions.

Assessment Checklist

almost always	sometimes	almost never	
☐	☐	☐	1. I have realistic perceptions of new situations, self, and others.
☐	☐	☐	2. I understand my own personal physical and emotional responses to stress.
☐	☐	☐	3. I anticipate and prepare for change.
☐	☐	☐	4. I have the ability to satisfactorily solve problems and make decisions.

Self-Care Behaviors

1. Accept as positive indicators of growth the changes that come with different parts and stages of life.
2. Maintain an open mind about change—change what you can, and accept what you cannot change.
3. Avoid self-defeating behaviors to cope with stress, such as smoking, alcohol, and drugs.
4. Practice methods of stress management that work best for you: relaxation techniques, exercise, hobbies.
5. Set realistic goals.
6. Develop problem-solving strategies for use in stressful situations.
7. Accept help from others.
8. Take life one day at a time.

sponses to anxiety are listed in the Focused Assessment Guide: Anxiety.

Nursing History

The questions asked in the nursing history assist the nurse in identifying stressors, perception of stressors, and how the person copes with stress. Questions and leading statements are listed in the Focused Assessment Guide: Stress. Indicators of stress may not be immediately apparent. If the nurse assesses manifestations of anxiety at any time, it is important to ask the client questions that identify problems. Questions or statements that may be used include:

You have been very quiet today . . . has anything happened since our last visit?

It must be very frightening to learn that you have cancer.

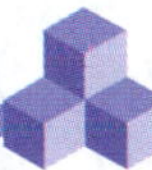

Focused Assessment Guide

Anxiety

Physiologic Responses

- Heart palpitations
- Dry mouth
- Difficulty breathing
- Nausea
- Increased perspiration
- Tremors
- Increased pulse rate
- Increased blood pressure
- Crying
- Sleep disturbances
- Eating disturbances

Psychologic Responses

- Expressions of sadness
- Expressions of apprehension
- Expressions of anger
- Mistrust of others
- Expressions of helplessness
- Expressions of hopelessness
- Inability to pay attention
- Alterations in sexuality

Social Responses

- Withdrawal from interaction with others
- Hostility toward others
- Inappropriate dress
- Alteration in communications

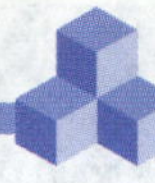

Focused Assessment Guide

Stress

Factors to Assess	Questions and Leading Statements
Present Problem	What is causing you a problem at this time? What emotions are you experiencing as a result of this problem? How does your body feel when you are nervous?
Past History	What has caused you to feel stressed in the past? What changes or losses have you experienced in the past? Do you use alcohol or drugs? If so, what do you use, how often, and when? Have you had treatment for arthritis, asthma, bowel problems, health problems, gland problems, headaches, skin disorders? If so, how did these health problems affect your life?
Self-Concept	If you had to describe yourself, what would you say? Do you have difficulty saying no to others? Whom do you share leisure time with?
Coping Mechanisms	What do you do for fun? Whom do you talk to if you feel stressed? What or who is your greatest source of comfort when you feel stressed? What did you do to feel better in the past when you had a similar problem?

I notice that you seem upset . . . would you like to talk about it?

Physical Assessment

There are no specific guidelines for physical assessment of stress. Rather, observations made during the assessment are indicators of stress and anxiety. Physical indicators of stress, in addition to those already described, may include cardiac dysrhythmias, chest pain, headache, hyperventilation, diarrhea, tense muscles, and skin lesions such as eczema (Fuller & Schaller-Ayers, 1994). These manifestations are the result of the mind–body interaction, described earlier in the chapter.

Other observations of stress might include one or more of the following:

- Disheveled appearance
- Slouched posture
- Poor eye contact
- Restlessness, pacing, wringing hands
- Expressionless vocal tone
- Rapid speech pattern
- Lack of facial expression

DIAGNOSING

When assessment data provides cues to a problem with stress that can be treated by nursing interventions, it receives the label *Anxiety.* Common etiologies for anxiety include conflicts about values and goals in life, threat to self-concept, threat of death, threat of or change in health status, threat to or change in environment or role, situational/maturational crisis, or unmet needs. Examples of other nursing diagnoses that are significant in clients or families having problems with stress are:

Ineffective Individual Coping related to inability to maintain marriage

Defensive Coping related to loss of job and economic security

Altered Thought Processes related to severe anxiety

Ineffective Denial related to continued smoking behavior

Decisional Conflict related to placement of parent in nursing home

Ineffective Family Coping: Disabling related to lack of knowledge about home care of child on ventilator

Stress may affect many other areas of human functioning. In the following nursing diagnoses, stress and anxiety are the etiologies of another problem.

Altered Nutrition: Less than body requirements related to inadequate caloric intake while striving to excel in gymnastics

Caregiver Role Strain related to long-term stress of care for parent with Alzheimer's disease

Social Isolation related to feelings of worthlessness and apprehension following failure in school

Spiritual Distress related to inability to accept diagnosis of terminal illness

Hopelessness related to presence of disabling physical injuries

Sleep Pattern Disturbance related to anxiety

Examples of nursing diagnoses for common problems are outlined in the accompanying box.

Nursing Diagnoses for Common Problems

Stress

Problem	Related Factors	Sample Defining Characteristics
Anxiety	Diagnosis of illness requiring surgery and fear of disfigurement	Newly diagnosed with breast cancer; pulse and respirations are increased above baseline; restless and unable to sleep; facial expression tense; states, "I can't get any rest because I'm so afraid of having surgery and losing my breast."
Impaired Adjustment	Myocardial infarction	Middle-aged man who had a serious myocardial infarction (heart attack) refuses to join a cardiac rehabilitation program and continues to smoke and eat high-fat foods.
Ineffective Individual Coping	Recent divorce and lack of support systems	"I just can't seem to handle things anymore. I know I smoke and drink too much, but I'm just so tired of being alone."
Ineffective Family Coping: Compromised	Spinal cord injury with loss of lower extremity function (paraplegia)	Mother of 19-year-old male who has paraplegia from a diving accident refuses to let him provide self-care. She states, "I know he will be able to walk soon and he needs me to take care of him now."
Ineffective Family Coping: Disabling	Developmental delay Childhood autism	10-month-old infant with severe mental retardation has obvious malnutrition and signs of neglect.
Family Coping: Potential for Growth	Joins a support group for lung cancer that includes a stop smoking program	Wife of husband with lung cancer attends support group and takes pride in her support of his success in stopping smoking.
Ineffective Denial	Changes in size, shape, and color of a mole	Older adult male has large black lesion on forehead, states "Oh, I've had that for a long time—it's just a pimple."
Defensive Coping	Obesity	"I don't care if I'm fat. It's not my fault that I can't lose weight. I just don't have time to exercise and I can't stand vegetables." Is 20% above standard weight for height.

PLANNING: EXPECTED OUTCOMES

The nurse plans and implements care to decrease anxiety and facilitate adaptation in the client with anxiety. The expected outcomes of the plan must be mutually determined with the client and/or family members. The expected outcomes of the plan of care are that the client will:

- Decrease the level of anxiety by verbalizing feelings and using support systems
- Develop effective coping skills through problem-solving skills and anxiety-reducing techniques
- Describe a reduction in anxiety and an increase in comfort

Expected outcomes for a client with anxiety are discussed further at the end of the chapter.

IMPLEMENTING

Nurses may use a variety of interventions to help clients decrease stress and to facilitate coping. If the client's anxiety seems too great or the nurse is uncomfortable with the interventions, referrals should be made to other sources. Referrals may be made, for example, to a professional counselor, to individuals who have experienced the same type of surgery or health problem, or to the client's rabbi, minister, or priest.

The following nursing interventions are discussed in this section: teaching healthy activities of daily living, encouraging use of support systems, and practicing stress management techniques. The methods used should be carefully selected, based on each person's physical and emotional characteristics, family and social structure, and previously used coping mechanisms.

Teaching Healthy Activities of Daily Living

A person's normal lifestyle greatly influences perceptions and reactions to stressors. The person who is overweight, sedentary, and chronically tired is at increased risk to develop an illness as a result of stress. These factors are stressors also, and further increase the risk. Exercise, rest, and good nutrition are important components in stress reduction.

Exercise. Regular exercise helps to maintain physical and emotional health. The benefits of exercise include an improved musculoskeletal system, more effective cardiovascular function, weight control, and relaxation. Exercise improves one's general sense of well-being, relieves tension, and enables one to better cope with day-to-day stressors. General health guidelines recommend that an exercise program consist of 30 to 45 minutes of activity three or four times a week. People

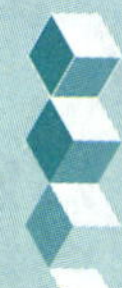

Research in Nursing: Making a Difference

Stress and Adaptation

The concepts of stress and adaptation are integrated into care as nurses provide interventions to promote wellness, maintain or regain health, and facilitate coping. A wide variety of studies have been conducted to determine how both clients and their caregivers respond to the stress of illness. Information from this research is used to improve the quality of care provided by nurses.

Related Research

Fink, S. (1995). The influence of family resources and family demands on the strains and well-being of caregiving families. *Nursing Research, 44*(3), 139–146.
This study was conducted to examine the strains and well-being of families providing care to older adult parents. Sixty-five families participated in the study. Family resources included social support and internal system resources. Demands examined were family life events, the amount of care provided, and the caregiver's appraisal of caregiving. Data from the study suggest that families are able to use resources to maintain overall family well-being despite the strain on the family system of older parent caregiving. These findings point out the importance of assessing the strengths and resources of families. They also suggest that interventions to either sustain or build resources for caregiving families may be the most important strategies in maintaining family well-being.

Narsavage, G., & Weaver, T. (1994). Physiologic status, coping, and hardiness as predictors of outcomes in chronic obstructive pulmonary disease. *Nursing Research, 43*(2), 90–94.
This study was conducted to examine the relationship of physiologic status, coping, and hardiness to exercise ability and functional status in 96 people with chronic obstructive pulmonary disease. The coping strategies of confrontation, seeking social support, and problem solving were significant. These problem-focused coping strategies were positively correlated with exercise ability as evidenced by distance walked. Challenge and commitment were significant components of hardiness (evidenced by a sense of control, involvement in what is happening, and belief that stress is a means for change) in people who used more problem-solving strategies. These findings provide additional information about how to help people cope with illness when planning nursing care.

Gulick, E. (1995). Coping among spouses or significant others of persons with multiple sclerosis. *Nursing Research, 44*(4), 220–225.
The purpose of this study was to identify coping strategies used by spouses/significant others of persons with multiple sclerosis (MS). Persons who used a systematic planning approach used systematic problem solving through activities such as obtaining accurate information about MS; obtaining support from family, friends, and clergy; and using assistive devices. Strategies within the confrontive coping dimension included aggressive efforts to alter the situation. The persons who used the ambivalence dimension of coping used a combination of worry, hope, and evasive behavior. The accepting dimension of coping was illustrated by people who proceeded with their lives as nearly normal as possible. The investigators suggest that nurses explore with persons with MS and their significant others the impact that meeting needs has on the family. The information gained can be used to provide essential information and counseling to help families cope more effectively with illness demands.

Summary

These studies are indicative of the trends in nursing care toward client self-care, family involvement in client care, aging, and chronic illnesses. They illustrate the stressors and coping methods used to provide care to older parents and to improve independence and meet needs in both clients and families of clients with chronic illness. All of the studies emphasize the importance of this knowledge to nursing care.

who are overweight, chronically ill, or over age 35 should have a thorough physical examination before beginning such a program. The type of exercise can be individualized to what one enjoys most—for example, walking, jogging, bicycling, swimming, or participating in sports such as golf or tennis.

Rest and Sleep. Rest and sleep allow the body to maintain homeostasis and restore energy levels. Adequate rest can provide "insulation" against stress, but stress may interfere with one's ability to sleep. Although each person has individualized needs, 7 to 8 hours sleep in each 24 hours is recommended. Relaxation techniques can be helpful in health and illness in facilitating rest and sleep. Hospitalized clients may require additional nursing interventions to relieve pain and promote comfort to get needed rest.

Nutrition. Nutrition plays an active role in maintaining the body's homeostatic mechanisms and in increasing resistance to stress. Obesity and malnutrition are major stressors, and greatly increase the risk of illness. People of all ages are encouraged to maintain a normal body weight and to follow guidelines established by the U.S. Senate Committee on Nutrition and Human Needs. These guidelines include the following recommendations:

- Reduce intake of salt, refined sugar, animal fat, and cholesterol.
- Eat more fruit, vegetables, and whole grains.
- Eat less red meat and more fish and poultry.

Nutrition is discussed further in Chapter 42.

Encouraging Use of Support Systems

Support systems provide emotional support that helps a person identify and verbalize feelings associated with stress. Other valuable contributions include providing information and services, maintaining positive self-concept, and establishing an avenue for new relationships and social roles. Additionally, families and support groups provide an accepting environment, allowing the person to explore problem-solving methods and try out new coping skills. There are support groups for almost every situation. Examples include:

Alcoholics Anonymous
Overeaters Anonymous

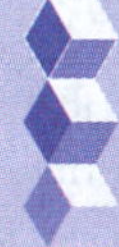

Through the Eyes of a Student

My First Non-English Speaking Patient

As an RN/BSN student with 5 years of clinical experience, I can emphatically say that I have had my share of frustrating moments. One in particular that comes to my mind happened not too long ago.

I was assigned to care for a 60-year-old gentleman who had had a coronary artery bypass graft operation a few days earlier. He was from Greece, spoke no English, and didn't have any family here in the United States. Communicating with this gentleman today was indeed going to be a challenge, I thought to myself as I got report from the night shift RN. I entered my patient's room to find him sitting on the side of his bed. Before I could even get a "hello" out of my mouth, he began speaking in his native language. It was obvious immediately that he was upset about something, so I quickly had to think of a creative way to calm him down.

In addition to drawing from my past clinical experiences, I remembered back to what I had learned about cardiac surgery patients in my AD program. I concluded that the stress level to which this patient was raising himself could possibly be very detrimental for him. Unfortunately, no amount of pantomime, body language, or theatrics was enough to calm him down. In fact, my efforts seemed only to frustrate him (and me) even more.

I can only imagine how scared this man was. He was away from his home, he had no family or friends nearby, he was in unfamiliar surroundings, and he was unable to communicate with anyone. No wonder he was so stressed!

Then I had an idea. I called the hospital's interpreting service hoping that there would be someone available who could speak his language. Unfortunately, no one did, so I was back to square one. Then, it hit me—*my sister-in-law is Greek!* I kept my fingers crossed as I dialed her home telephone number from my patient's room. Thankfully, she was home and agreed to talk to him. As he spoke with her, I could see his anxiety level decrease, and he even chuckled a few times during the course of their conversation.

As it turned out, he was *very* scared to be in the hospital. He didn't fully understand the implications of his coronary artery disease and what his postoperative course would be like. All he wanted was someone to talk to, and as hard as I tried to listen to him, very little was getting through.

My patient ended up going back to Greece after a clinically uncomplicated hospital stay. On the day he was to be discharged, we nurses thought it would be nice to surprise him with lunch from a local Greek restaurant. The owners of the restaurant felt very badly for him because of what he had been through, yet were so happy to know that he was going home, they gave him his lunch for free!

—Jeanne M. Tracby, RN
Georgetown University
Washington, DC

Weight Watchers
Parents Without Partners
Reach to Recovery (cancer)
Ostomy clubs
Child abuse support groups
Sudden infant death support groups
Stroke clubs
Assertiveness training groups

Encouraging Use of Stress Management Techniques

Stress creates emotional distress, often having outward symptoms. One person may have tension headaches; another becomes irritable; another clenches her fists. Many people take legal or illegal drugs, drink or smoke to excess, or eat compulsively. These behaviors can be modified and adaptive mechanisms strengthened through specific techniques aimed at managing stress. Only a few techniques are included here, but the literature is filled with stress reduction methods. Students are encouraged to learn different methods they can use for themselves and for varied clinical situations.

Relaxation. Relaxation techniques are useful in many situations—childbirth, pain, anxiety, sleeplessness, illness, anger—and other uses are being discovered. Relaxation promotes a body reaction opposite to that of the fight-or-flight response, decreasing respiratory, pulse, and metabolic rates; blood pressure; and energy use.

Relaxation can be taught to individuals or groups, and is especially helpful because it allows a person to control feelings and behaviors. Various techniques are used, but each involves rhythmic breathing, reduced muscle tension, and an altered state of consciousness (Stuart & Sundeen, 1995). Two relaxation activities are discussed in the accompanying box. Relaxation also is discussed as a pain relief measure in Chapter 41.

Meditation. Meditation has four components: quiet surroundings, a passive attitude, a comfortable position, and a word or mental image on which to focus. A person practicing meditation sits comfortably with closed eyes, relaxes each of the major muscle groups, and repeats the selected word silently with each exhalation. Alternatively, the person may focus on a pleasant scene and mentally place himself or herself in it while breathing slowly in and out. This exercise should be performed for 20 to 30 minutes twice a day.

Anticipatory Guidance. Anticipatory guidance focuses on psychologically preparing a person for an unfamiliar or painful event. Nurses use this technique to teach clients about procedures and the surgical experience. When clients know what to expect, their anxiety is reduced and their coping mechanisms are more effective. For example, before changing a dressing, teaching would include all the information about the pain involved—onset, severity, cause, and methods of relief. With this knowledge, the client feels less threat and tolerates the procedure more easily. A related process is anticipatory socialization, in which people prepare themselves for roles to which they aspire but do not yet occupy. This process may be used to prepare expectant parents for the role of parenting, thereby enhancing the potential of the child to experience normal growth and development.

Relaxation Activities

Deep Breathing

- Sit comfortably and place your hands on your stomach. Inhale slowly and deeply, letting your stomach expand as much as possible. Hold your breath for a few seconds.
- Exhale slowly through your mouth, blowing the air out through pursed lips. When your stomach feels empty, repeat the cycle.
- Repeat three or four times each session.

Progressive Muscle Relaxation

- Tighten your hand into a fist and notice how it feels; hold the tension for a few seconds.
- Loosen the grip on your muscles, relax your muscles, and let the tension slip away.
- Continue through each muscle group—hands, arms, shoulders, face, chest, back, stomach, legs, feet.

Guided Imagery. In guided imagery, a person creates a mental image, concentrates on the image, and becomes less responsive to stimuli (including pain). The nurse sits by the client and reads a description of a scene or an experience that the client has described as happy, pleasant, or peaceful. The client is then "guided" through the image. For example, using a soothing, soft voice, the nurse might start as follows: "You are floating in your swimming pool. The water is cool and comfortable. Birds are singing in the trees. The roses are perfuming the air." As the client becomes more and more focused on the scene, the nurse will need only to verbally "paint the picture" at intervals.

Biofeedback. Biofeedback is a method of gaining mental control of the autonomic nervous system and thus regulating body responses, such as blood pressure, heart rate, and headaches. A measurement device (eg, skin temperature sensors) is used, and the client tries to control the readings voluntarily through relaxation and conscious thought. The feedback from the change in readings teaches the person to control physiologic functions that normally are considered involuntary responses. The process is long-term and still being researched.

Providing Crisis Intervention

As defined earlier, a crisis is a situation that cannot be resolved by usual coping mechanisms. As a result, a person is unable to function normally and requires inter-

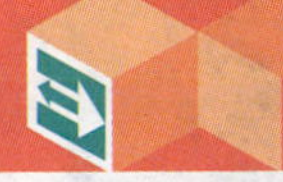

Developing Critical Thinking Skills

Situation

As part of your clinical course in medical–surgical nursing, you are assigned to visit, provide ongoing assessments, and teach self-care management to a 22-year-old man who was involved in a serious automobile accident last year and is paralyzed from the waist down. The client, Charles Obegide, is an African American. At first he willingly participated in rehabilitation and has managed independent living in his wheelchair. However, recently he has had problems with urinary tract infections and was unable to go to work; as a result he lost his job. When you made your last visit, Charles did little talking and seemed restless. When you knock on his door, Charles comes to the door. He is wearing dirty clothes and has a strong body odor. You also notice several empty beer cans in the room. Charles says, "I think I'm going to die. Please help me." What would you do?

1. ***Identify Goal of Thinking***
   Identify the level of anxiety experienced by Charles, and initiate interventions to help Charles decrease his level of anxiety.

2. ***Assess Adequacy of Knowledge***
   Pertinent Circumstances: Charles has had numerous losses in the past year, including loss of body function and body image. He has had physical illnesses (the urinary tract infections) and now has lost his job, a major source of economic support and self-concept. Under normal circumstances, Charles is always clean and well-groomed. There has been no previous evidence of drinking. His parents live nearby and are supportive and loving.

   Prerequisite Knowledge: Before you decide what to do in this situation, you need to assess the level of anxiety experienced by Charles. You will need to know the typical behaviors of each level and be able to recognize that Charles is in a crisis situation. You must recognize that a crisis is a situation that cannot be resolved by usual coping mechanisms and that the person requires interventions to regain equilibrium. You must also know that a person in crisis needs immediate help.

   Room for Error: Charles requires immediate help. You are unsure of your abilities to help him deal effectively with this crisis. You realize that his frustration with the situation could turn into anger against you simply because you are the one with him at the moment. You also know that depression and the potential for self-violence is a potential risk unless something is done to decrease his level of anxiety.

3. ***Address Potential Problems***
   There are several potential barriers to critical thinking in this situation. You feel responsible for Charles' physical and emotional safety, which causes you anxiety. You are also somewhat frightened by the client's appearance and behavior and by the fact that you are alone in the house with him until the home health aide arrives. Your own anxiety and fear make critical thinking more difficult. You do not believe your knowledge base in crisis intervention is strong enough to help Charles adequately, but at the same time you want to find someone to help him.

4. ***Consult Helpful Resources***
   Your best source of initial information is Charles himself. As he asked you for help and does not appear angry, you ask him to tell you how you can help. He replies, "Just get someone to help me." You ask his permission to call his parents, and tell him you need to talk to your instructor. With Charles' permission you call Mrs. Obegide, who tells you she will be there in 5 minutes. The home health aide arrives and sits quietly holding Charles' hand. You then call your instructor, and she tells you to call the home health agency for directions if Mrs. Obegide does not arrive quickly.

5. ***Critique Judgment/Decision***
   When Mrs. Obegide arrives, Charles starts to cry. His mother says she had no idea he was so distressed; she contacts his physician, who recommends medications to help calm Charles and makes a referral for professional counseling. You believe you made the right decisions: you identified that Charles needed immediate help, you contacted his mother (as a support person) to secure that help, and you remained calm throughout the situation despite your own anxiety.

ventions to regain equilibrium. **Crisis intervention** is a five-step, problem-solving technique designed to promote a more adaptive outcome, including improved abilities to cope with future crisis. The steps are as follows:

1. *Identify the problem.* This may be more difficult than it appears; the cause of the crisis often is difficult for the person to identify accurately. Until it is clear, a solution is impossible.
2. *List alternatives.* All possible solutions to the problem need to be listed. An appropriate solution to a problem is much more likely if a substantial number of options are considered.
3. *Choose from among alternatives.* Each option needs to be carefully considered, using a "what would happen if I . . ." approach. The alternative chosen will be highly individualized, based on priorities and values.
4. *Implement a plan.* The alternative chosen is put into action. It may be necessary to provide support and encouragement so that action is taken.
5. *Evaluate the outcome.* In this final step, the effectiveness of the plan needs to be carefully considered. If it did not work as well as expected, another alternative needs to be chosen. If it did work, it has the positive benefit of improving self-confidence and future problem solving.

The major factor in helping clients adapt to high levels of stress is to identify and plan for the individuality of each situation. The following suggestions are useful:

- Help the person recognize his or her own stress level and specific responses to stress.
- Encourage a philosophy of accepting what cannot be changed and changing what cannot be accepted.
- Encourage the person to accept help from others—and to give support to others when needed.
- Encourage active but deliberate involvement in problem solving and decision making.
- Be an active listener, increasing therapeutic relationships and communications.
- Provide health teaching about developmental crises and threatening events.

Addressing Stress in the Nursing Profession

Nursing involves activities and interpersonal relationships that often are stressful (Fig. 32-3). The activities identified as being most stressful include the following:

- Having to assume responsibilities for which one is not prepared
- Working with unqualified personnel
- Working in an environment in which supervisors and administrators are not supportive
- Caring for a client during a cardiac arrest or for a client who is dying
- Experiencing conflict with peers

The stress is even greater for two groups: new graduates, who must adjust to an environment different from what they experienced as students, and nurses who work in settings such as intensive care and emergency care. In the present healthcare reform climate, nurses are stressed by healthcare institutions downsizing and increased client care assignments. They worry not only about the future of their positions but also about the safety of their clients. The anxiety is further complicated by the expected behavior of nurses: Even though they may have strong negative feelings and reactions, their role does not include behaviors and verbal expressions that are less than positive and supportive.

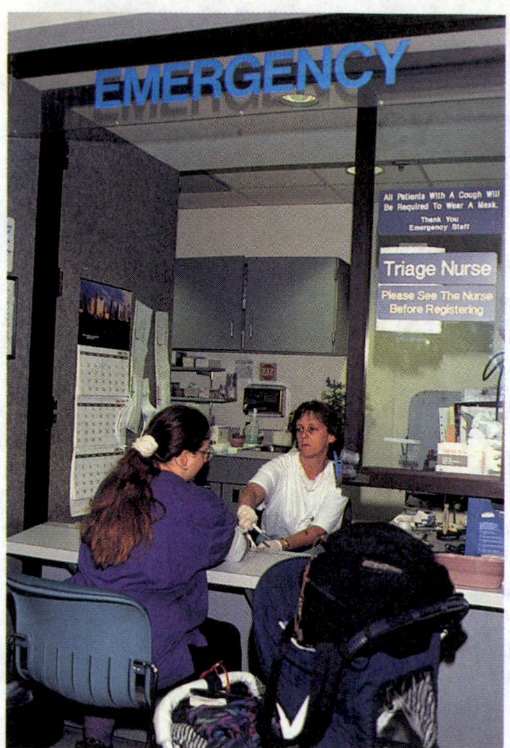

Figure 32-3
Some nursing specialties can be more stressful than others. To prevent burnout and alleviate personal stress, a nurse may need to work in another area of nursing temporarily or permanently. (Photo © Kathy Sloane.)

Most nurses thoroughly enjoy their work and cope with the physical and emotional demands effectively. Some, however, are overwhelmed and develop symptoms of anxiety and stress. The complex of behaviors is called professional burnout. **Burnout** can be compared with the exhaustion stage of anxiety and is characterized by a wide range of behaviors. Some nurses try to become "supernurses," expecting perfection in themselves and others. Some withdraw and do only minimal work; still others resort to drugs or alcohol. A large number of nurses who are unable to handle the stress leave the profession.

What can nurses do to help reduce stress and prevent burnout? The first step in preventing a stress level high enough to cause burnout is to identify and accept the stress. The same stress reduction techniques that are used for clients have positive benefits for nurses. Other suggested activities to reduce stress are as follows:

- Get involved in constructive change, particularly if organizational activities cause you stress.
- Be supportive of other nurses, other healthcare personnel, and student nurses; take time to give a compliment for something done well.
- Take time for relaxation—use break time to practice a relaxation technique that works, and go off the unit for lunch.
- Eat regularly, following recommended guidelines for nutrition.
- Carry out a regular exercise program—walk, jog, play tennis, play golf, play handball, join an aerobic dance class.
- Give yourself some time each day to unwind, relax, and do what you want—soak in a bubble bath, listen to music, read a novel.
- Learn something new—how to knit, cane chairs, speak a foreign language, cook gourmet food.
- Develop assertiveness skills—learn to say no to additional tasks (you don't have to have an excuse—just say, "no, I can't do that"). Accept the fact that no one person is perfect or indispensable.

Nurses must accept that they have the same needs and are as individual as their clients. By recognizing the early signs of stress and taking steps to reduce it, nurses will continue to be effective, productive, and self-satisfied in the profession.

EVALUATING

The evaluation of the plan of care is based on the mutually established expected outcomes. It is important to observe both verbal and nonverbal cues in evaluating the usefulness of the plan. In general, the plan is considered to be successful if the client (family):

- Verbalizes causes and effects of stress and anxiety
- Identifies and uses sources of support
- Uses problem-solving to find solutions to stressors
- Practices healthy lifestyle habits and anxiety-reducing techniques
- Verbalizes a decrease in anxiety and an increase in comfort

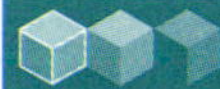

Nursing Process in Clinical Practice

Nursing Process in Clinical Practice

When identifying and treating responses to stress, the nurse uses each phase of the nursing process. Quality care depends on the nurse having the knowledge and skills described in this chapter. Following are the assessment priorities, expected outcomes, and nursing interventions for the most common response to stress—anxiety.

Anxiety

Anxiety is a vague, uneasy feeling whose source is often nonspecific or unknown to the individual (NANDA, 1994). Anxiety occurs in response to stress and has psychologic, physiologic, and social dimensions. A person experiencing anxiety uses interpersonal and interpsychic mechanisms to try to reduce or relieve the anxiety. The level of anxiety experienced depends on the severity of the perceived threat and how successful the individual is in coping and adaptation. Coping behaviors may be effective or ineffective. If the perceived threat is not resolved, anxiety levels may increase, causing more and more disruption in the individual's perceptions and responses. A further response to the frustration of an unresolved threat may be verbal or physical anger and aggression.

Assessment Priorities

- Identify the client's history of lifestyle, responses to stress, methods of coping, support systems, and medical care.
- Identify precipitating factors for, frequency of, duration of, and characteristics of physical sensations experienced from stress.
- Assess the client for manifestations of anxiety: verbalization of concerns, restlessness, tense muscles, tremors, diaphoresis, tachycardia, hypertension, difficulty breathing, inattention, withdrawal, anger.
- Ask the client to state in his or her own words feelings about self and others.
- Identify communication and interaction patterns with others, including the nurse and family members.
- Assess the client's usual lifestyle, including nutrition, exercise, and rest–sleep patterns. Instruct the client to complete a 24-hour recall or keep a diary for a specified time about foods eaten; prescribed and over-the-counter medications taken; times and amounts of alcohol, cigarette, and street drugs used; exercise completed; and hours slept each night. Use the client's information to relate factors that are effective and ineffective in handling stress.
- Assess the client's state of cleanliness and appropriate dress.

- Assess the client for manifestations of potentially aggressive behavior: restlessness, resentfulness, pacing, arguing, using a loud voice.

Expected Outcomes

The client will:

- Identify sources of stress and sources of support
- Use problem-solving to decrease the level of anxiety experienced as well as to decrease ineffective coping mechanisms
- Practice lifestyle changes to eliminate factors contributing to stress
- Practice techniques that decrease stress and anxiety
- Report that anxiety is decreased and manageable

Interventions

Interventions to reduce anxiety vary according to its cause and its level. In general, interventions include the following:

- Use therapeutic communications to encourage the client to verbalize feelings and concerns to help in identifying factors that cause or increase anxiety.
- Maintain a calm, supporting manner in interactions with the client to provide a sense of someone being in control of the situation and thus decreasing anxiety.
- Assist the client to reduce the level of anxiety by providing reassurance and comfort and decreasing sensory stimulation.
- Provide information about new experiences and situations to decrease anxiety from a lack of knowledge.
- Encourage the client to verbalize sources of support to facilitate stress management.
- Teach and have the client practice techniques to increase self-care in stress management.
- Teach and have the client practice problem solving to improve self-management of stress.
- Refer the client to appropriate support groups.

Client Care Study

Mei Fu is a 24-year-old graduate student. She is married and has two small children; her husband is also a graduate student. Although she lived in China until 3 years ago, she speaks English well. After several months of headaches and diarrhea, Mrs. Fu made an appointment at the student health clinic.

Assessment Findings

The nurse practitioner at the clinic conducted a health history and physical assessment of Mrs. Fu and noted the following data:

- Client is a thin woman who appears her stated age. She is currently in school and expects herself to make the highest grades. She also cares for her two children and her husband. Although her husband encourages her to go to school, he believes it is the wife's responsibility to provide all child and house care. She has had no previous serious illnesses or surgery.
- Client reports having frequent headache, rating the pain as a 3 on a scale of from 0 (no pain) to 10 (worst possible pain). She also reports having from 4 to 6 bowel movements each day, sometimes with abdominal cramping. The diarrhea does not seem to be related to any type of foods eaten. During the interview, the client appeared restless and talked rapidly. Questions often had to be repeated.
- Physical assessment reveals slight tachycardia, a fine hand tremor, and visible perspiration. Large muscle groups were tense and fists were clenched. No tenderness noted on abdominal palpation. Eye grounds normal. Nasal mucosa normal.

Core Competencies

In order to implement care, the nurse needs the following specialized abilities:

Cognitive Competencies: Critical Thinking

- Knowledge of how stress and anxiety affect one's physical, psychologic, and social dimensions
- The belief that people can learn to provide self-care in the management of stress
- Knowledge of which nursing interventions (such as relaxation techniques and the principles of anticipatory guidance) are most effective in reaching desired outcomes for Mrs. Fu
- Acceptance of each person's individualized responses to stress and coping
- Awareness of pertinent cultural considerations

Technical Competencies

- Strong assessment skills to identify normal and abnormal findings and differentiate between physical illness and the effects of stress

Interpersonal Competencies

- Effective interpersonal skills to establish rapport with Mrs. Fu and communicate the belief that she has the ability to manage her own life and stressors

- Counseling skills to facilitate Mrs. Fu's identification of concerns that are causing anxiety and the resulting physical responses, and identification of strengths and sources of support
- Teaching skills to enable Mrs. Fu to improve her lifestyle and to practice relaxation

Ethical/Legal Competencies

- Sensitivity to cultural factors in Mrs. Fu's situation that affect her ability to change her lifestyle
- Commitment to maintain competence to help Mrs. Fu reach the mutually established outcomes of the plan of care
- Competence in documenting nursing interventions and client responses

Documentation

10/06/98, 10 AM, nursing

Initial visit to student health center by Mrs. Fu to discuss physical problems of headache and diarrhea. History and physical assessment findings indicated large number of personal stressors, manifested by physical signs and symptoms. Assessment data supported nursing diagnosis: Anxiety related to stress of achievement in school and care of family. Discussion centered on identifying sources of stress, physical responses to stress, sources of support, and personal strength. Teaching strategies included diet, exercise, sleep, and progressive muscle relaxation. See care plan. Client's progress will be monitored at next visit on 10/20/98.

P. LeMone, RN

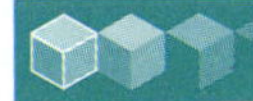

Nursing Plan of Care

for Mrs. Fu

Nursing Diagnosis: Anxiety related to stress of achievement in school and care of family as manifested by rapid speech, tachycardia, tremor, tense muscles, headache, and diarrhea.

Expected Outcome: By her return appointment in 2 weeks, 10/20/98, Mrs. Fu will:

- Identify sources of and responses to stress

Nursing Interventions	Rationale	Evaluative Statement
Ask Mrs. Fu to keep a diary of hours spent in school-related activities and family care, number and times of headaches, and circumstances that occurred before diarrhea.	Identifying sources of stress and the physical responses to stress is the first step in planning coping strategies to reduce stress.	10/20/98 Goal met. Mrs. Fu kept a diary as requested. She identified that she does not have any time for herself. Her headaches are worse during the week. She often has diarrhea when papers are due or when her husband and children are demanding of her time. *S. Aird, RN, FNP*

Expected Outcome: By her return appointment, 10/20/98, Mrs. Fu will:

- Identify sources of personal strength and support

Nursing Interventions	Rationale	Evaluative Statement
Ask Mrs. Fu to make a list of the persons who are important to her and provide her comfort. Ask her to discuss how these people can help her cope with her situation. Ask Mrs. Fu to describe her strengths as a woman, a mother, a wife, and a student.	Identifying support persons and areas of personal strength provides the client with the means to manage stress and enhances self-concept.	10/20/98 Goal met. Mrs. Fu stated that her family is her greatest source of support, but they are in China and she misses them very much. She does have a very good friend who is also a good listener. She identified her strengths as being a person who cares for others and a good student. She said she is also a good artist, but has not had time for art for months. *S. Aird, RN, FNP*

(continued)

Expected Outcome: By her return appointment, 10/20/98, Mrs. Fu will:
- Describe lifestyle changes that include eating a well-balanced diet with three meals a day, walking for 20 to 30 minutes four times a week, and sleeping restfully 7 hours a night

Nursing Interventions	Rationale	Evaluative Statement
Discuss with Mrs. Fu the food pyramid and the importance of eating foods from each group. Also discuss why she should eat three meals a day.	Adequate nutrition helps maintain the homeostatic mechanisms of the body and increases resistance to stress.	10/20/98 Goal met. Mrs. Fu was given a copy of the food pyramid, and food preparations were discussed. Although the Fu's have a healthy diet, Mrs. Fu often was too busy to eat more than a few bites. She said that she is making a big effort to eat three times a day.

Nursing Interventions	Rationale	Evaluative Statement
Discuss with Mrs. Fu the benefits of regular exercise in reducing stress.	Exercise improves well-being, relieves tension, and facilitates coping with daily stressors.	She is walking to school and enjoys the time by herself. She arranged this time by asking her husband to take the children to school.
Discuss with Mrs. Fu the importance of sleep in reducing stress.	Adequate rest and sleep restore energy and facilitate coping with stressors.	She is sleeping better, and averages 7 hours most nights. *S. Aird, RN, FNP*

Expected Outcome By her return appointment, 10/20/98, Mrs. Fu will:
- Practice relaxation for 20 minutes each day

Nursing Interventions	Rationale	Evaluative Statement
Teach and have Mrs. Fu practice progressive muscle relaxation. Suggest that she buy a tape to facilitate the technique (tapes for relaxation are widely available). Recommend that she plan a time when she can be alone and use 20 minutes to complete the technique.	Relaxation promotes a response opposite to the stress response; decreases heart rate, respiratory rate, blood pressure, and metabolic processes.	10/20/98 Goal met. Mrs. Fu said that at first she had difficulty in finding time to be alone, but she feels so much better after she relaxes that she insists on the time. She did buy a tape and says it helps her very much. *S. Aird, RN, FNP*

Expected Outcome: By her return appointment, 10/20/98, Mrs. Fu will:
- Report a decrease in headaches and diarrhea and an increase in her ability to provide self-care to manage stress

Nursing Interventions	Rationale	Evaluative Statement
Assess frequency and severity of headaches and bowel movements. Assess client's self-report of coping with stressors.	Decreasing stress in daily life often is effective in decreasing physical responses. Self-care of stress is critical in effective management.	10/20/98 Goal met. Mrs. Fu reports she has noticed fewer headaches in the past week, and the diarrhea is almost gone. Mrs. Fu verbalized the importance of continuing to practice a healthy lifestyle and relaxation. She said she has spent time with her friend and has gotten out her sketch pad. She stated that she believes she can manage her life much better now. *S. Aird, RN, FNP*

Key Points

- Homeostasis, or a healthy, balanced state, is maintained by various physiologic and psychologic mechanisms. Physiologic mechanisms are largely involuntary responses of the autonomic and endocrine systems, necessary to health maintenance. Psychologic balance is maintained through the use of coping or defense mechanisms.
- Stress, stressors, and adaptation are all interrelated parts of a process. *Stressors* (a challenge, a danger, or a threat) cause *stress* (a change in the balanced state). A person *adapts* through a series of responses. Each component is highly individualized and holistic in effect.
- Stress may be developmental or situational; stressors may be physiologic or psychosocial. Physiologic stressors have both a general and a specific effect. Psychosocial stressors affect us constantly in day-to-day living.
- The relation between physical and emotional stress is illustrated by the mind–body interaction, in which the perception of a threat on an emotional level results in the fight-or-flight response by the body. Resulting illnesses are called psychosomatic disorders.
- The LAS is a localized body response to traumatic or pathologic stress that helps to maintain homeostasis and adaptation. Two examples of the LAS are the reflex pain response and the inflammatory response.
- The inflammatory response occurs in response to injury or infection, serving to prevent the spread of infection and promote wound healing through regeneration of tissue or formation of scar.
- The GAS is a biochemical model that describes the body's general response to stress. There are three stages to the GAS: alarm reaction, stage of resistance, and stage of exhaustion. The stages occur in response to both physical and emotional stress.
- The most common psychologic response to stress is anxiety. Anxiety, precipitated by new experiences and the unknown, is a threat to self-esteem and identity. Anxiety has four levels: mild, moderate, severe, and panic.
- Coping mechanisms are largely unconscious methods of attempting to adapt to stress.
- Higher levels of stress may require psychologic adaptation by coping with task-oriented reactions (attack, withdrawal, or compromise behavior) or defense mechanisms. Many of these behaviors are learned, based on past experiences and sociocultural environment.
- Stress can interfere with basic need attainment, disrupting homeostasis and causing illness.
- Stress can promote health and learning, but the stress of illness imposes additional burdens on a person who is out of balance. Adaptation to illness involves general tasks and illness-related tasks. Nursing interventions to reduce the stress of illness must be individualized and holistic.
- Stress affects the family as well as the individual. Families use varied coping methods and provide an important support system for the ill person.
- Prolonged stress affects both physical and mental health.
- Crisis results from ineffective coping, leading to severe anxiety, disorganized behavior, and malfunction.
- Nurses can promote health by teaching stress reduction teaching methods, including healthy lifestyle, support groups, stress management techniques, and crisis intervention.
- Nursing is a stressful occupation. Nurses may become overwhelmed by the demands made on them and may develop symptoms of burnout. They can practice stress management techniques both on and off the job to help prevent stress and to improve career satisfaction.

Study Questions

1. Stress is a condition in which the human system
   a. becomes increasingly disorganized
   b. responds to changes in its normal balanced state
   c. responds to negative changes in its internal environment
   d. is less likely to respond appropriately to stimuli
2. Which of the following would be an external stressor?
   a. high environmental temperature
   b. changes in hormone levels
   c. fear of the dark
   d. having an infection of the intestine
3. The body maintains the internal environment at a constant state through
   a. internalization
   b. adaptation
   c. cellular integrity
   d. homeostasis
4. Which of the following would be classified as developmental stress?
   a. an infant learns to turn over
   b. a school-age child learns how to add and subtract
   c. an adolescent gets a job
   d. a young adult has a variety of friends

5. The reflex pain response and the inflammatory response are examples of
   a. localized responses of the body to stress
   b. negative responses of the body to stress
   c. generalized responses of the body to stress
   d. ways in which the body controls stress
6. What response would be expected during the shock phase of the general adaptation syndrome?
   a. decreasing pulse
   b. increasing sleepiness
   c. increasing energy levels
   d. slow respirations
7. A vague sense of impending doom or apprehension for no apparent reason is
   a. fear
   b. concern
   c. panic
   d. anxiety
8. Toward the end of the semester, as final examinations near, you find yourself sleeping more than usual. This behavior is probably your form of a
   a. coping mechanism
   b. defense mechanism
   c. offense mechanism
   d. adapting mechanism
9. Your client has just been diagnosed with cancer, but responds as though this is an impossibility. Which of the defense mechanisms is being demonstrated here?
   a. projection
   b. denial
   c. displacement
   d. repression
10. Home care of clients by family members for long periods of time can cause long-term stress and increased risk of illness. The name for this stress response is
    a. home care chronicity
    b. client burn-out
    c. residual stress
    d. caregiver burden
11. All but one of the following responses are typical of relaxation techniques. Which is *not* typical?
    a. rhythmic breathing
    b. an increased pulse rate
    c. reduced muscle tension
    d. an altered state of consciousness
12. Which type of stress reduction activity would probably be most useful for clients before an unfamiliar or painful event?
    a. progressive muscle relaxation
    b. meditation
    c. anticipatory guidance
    d. biofeedback
13. What is the first step in crisis intervention through problem-solving?
    a. identify the problem
    b. list alternatives
    c. implement a plan
    d. evaluate the outcome
14. Biofeedback is a method of gaining mental control of what part of the body?
    a. the skin
    b. the senses
    c. the autonomic nervous system
    d. the central nervous system
15. What type of setting is considered most stressful for nurses?
    a. cancer treatment centers
    b. nursing homes
    c. operating room
    d. intensive care units

Answers With Rationale

1. The correct answer is *b*. Individuals perceive and respond to stress in highly individualized ways. Stress evokes both positive and negative responses in response to changes in the internal and external environment.
2. The correct answer is *a*. Answers *b*, *c*, and *d* are all internal stressors.
3. The correct answer is *d*. To maintain health, the internal environment must remain in balance; this balance is maintained through various physiologic mechanisms as they respond to internal changes.
4. The correct answer is *c*. Although the other choices are milestones in a developmental age, the adolescent who gets a job is seeking independence, a major task for that level of growth and development.
5. The correct answer is *a*. The local adaptation syndrome is a localized response of the body to stress. These responses are homeostatic and short-term; the most common are the reflex pain response and the inflammatory response.
6. The correct answer is *c*. The body perceives a threat and prepares to respond by increasing the activity of the autonomic nervous and endocrine systems. The initial or shock phase is characterized by increased energy levels, oxygen intake, cardiac output, blood pressure, and mental alertness.
7. The correct answer is *d*. Panic is an experience of terror. A concern is a worry. Fear has a known cause. Only anxiety is a psychologic response to an unknown threat.
8. The correct answer is *a*. Mild anxiety is often handled without conscious thought through the use of coping mechanisms, which are behaviors used to decrease stress and anxiety. Sleeping is a coping mechanism.

9. The correct answer is *b*. Denial occurs when a person refuses to acknowledge the presence of a condition that is disturbing.
10. The correct answer is *d*. Reactions to home care of family members for long periods of time, called caregiver burden, include chronic fatigue, sleep disorders, and increased incidence of stress-related illnesses, such as hypertension and heart disease.
11. The correct answer is *b*. No matter what the technique, relaxation involves rhythmic breathing, reduced muscle tension, and an altered state of consciousness.
12. The correct answer is *c*. Anticipatory guidance focuses on psychologic preparation of the client for an unfamiliar or painful event. When clients know what to expect, their anxiety is reduced and their coping mechanisms are more effective.
13. The correct answer is *a*. Although identifying the problem may be difficult, a solution to a crisis situation is impossible until the problem is identified.
14. The correct answer is *c*. Biofeedback is a method of gaining control of the autonomic nervous system and regulating body responses to stress such as increased blood pressure, increased heart rate, and headaches.
15. The correct answer is *d*. Clients in intensive care units have complex needs and are at greater risk for death; their care often is stressful.

Bibliography

Antonovsky, A. (1979). *Health, stress and coping*. San Francisco: Jossey-Bass.

Badger, J. (1994). Calming the anxious patient. *American Journal of Nursing, 94*(5), 46–50.

Barsevick, A., Pasacreta, J., & Orsi, A. (1995). Psychological distress and functional dependency in colorectal cancer patients. *Cancer Practice, 3*(2), 105–110.

Bossert, E. (1994). Factors influencing the coping of hospitalized school-age children. *Journal of Pediatric Nursing: Nursing Care of Children and Families, 9*(5), 299–306.

Carpenito, L. (1995). *Nursing care plans and documentation: Nursing diagnoses and collaborative problems* (2nd ed.). Philadelphia: Lippincott.

D'Avanzo, C., Frye, B., & Froman, R. (1994). Stress in Cambodian refugee families. *IMAGE: The Journal of Nursing Scholarship, 26*(2), 101–105.

Fink, S. (1995). The influence of family resources and family demands on the strains and well-being of caregiving families. *Nursing Research, 44*(3), 139–146.

Fuller, J., & Schaller-Ayers, J. (1994). *Health assessment: A nursing approach* (2nd ed.). Philadelphia: Lippincott.

Grey, M., Cameron, M. E., & Thurber, F. W. (1991). Coping and adaptation in children with diabetes. *Nursing Research, 40*(3), 144–149.

Gulick, E. (1995). Coping among spouses or significant others of persons with multiple sclerosis. *Nursing Research, 44*(4), 220–225.

Johston, F. (1994). Stress can kill. *Today's OR Nurse, 16*(3), 5.

Kammer, C. (1994). Stress and coping of family members responsible for nursing home placement. *Research in Nursing and Health, 17*(2), 89–98.

Kelley, S. (1993). Caregiver stress in grandparents raising grandchildren. *IMAGE: The Journal of Nursing Scholarship, 25*(4), 331–337.

Moos, R. (1985). *Coping with physical illness* (2nd ed.). New York: Plenum.

Narsavage, G., & Weaver, T. (1994). Physiologic status, coping, and hardiness as predictors of outcomes in chronic obstructive pulmonary disease. *Nursing Research, 43*(2), 90–94.

North American Nursing Diagnosis Association. (1994). *Nursing diagnoses: Definitions & classification*. Philadelphia: NANDA.

Pollock, S. E., Christian, B. J., & Sands, D. (1990). Responses to chronic illness: Analysis of psychosocial and physiological adaptation. *Nursing Research, 39*(5), 300–304.

Roberts, C., Cox, C., Shannon, V., & Wells, N. (1994). A closer look at social support as a moderator of stress in breast cancer. *Health and Social Work, 19*(3), 157–164.

Rosella, J., & Albrecht, S. (1993). Toward an understanding of the health status of black adolescents: An application of the stress-coping framework. *Issues in Comprehensive Pediatric Nursing, 16*(4), 193–205.

Ryan-Wenger, N., & Copeland, S. (1994). Coping strategies used by black school-age children from low-income families. *Journal of Pediatric Nursing: Nursing Care of Children and Families, 9*(1), 33–40.

Selye, H. (1976). *The stress of life*. New York: McGraw-Hill.

Smeltzer, S., & Bare, B. (1996). *Brunner and Suddarth's Textbook of medical–surgical nursing* (8th ed.). Philadelphia: Lippincott-Raven.

Sorenson, E. (1994). Daily stressors and coping responses: A comparison of rural and suburban children. *Public Health Nursing, 11*(1), 24–31.

Stuart, G., & Sundeen, S. (1995). *Principles and practices of psychiatric nursing* (5th ed.). St. Louis: Mosby.

Topf, M. (1994). Theoretical considerations for research on environmental stress and health. *IMAGE: The Journal of Nursing Scholarship, 26*(4), 289–293.

Vines, S. (1994). Relaxation with guided imagery: Effects on employees' psychological distress and health seeking behaviors. *AAOHN Journal, 42*(5), 206–213.

Wakefield, M. (1992). Stress control for nurses. *Canadian Nurse, 88*(4), 24–25.

Walters, V. (1993). Stress, anxiety and depression: Women's accounts of their health problems. *Social Science and Medicine, 36*(4), 393–402.

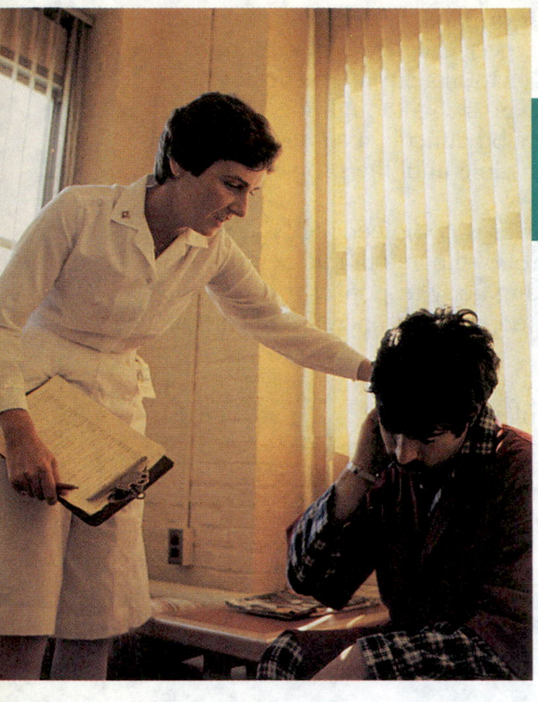

Chapter 33

Loss, Grief, and Death

Objectives

After studying this chapter, the learner should be able to:

Define key terms used in the chapter.

Differentiate the types of loss.

Describe the grief process and the stages of grief.

Describe Kübler-Ross's stages of dying.

Compare and contrast three definitions of death.

Identify ethical and legal issues concerning end-of-life care.

Identify six factors that affect loss, grief, and dying.

Describe physiologic, psychologic, and spiritual care of a dying client and family.

Use the nursing process to plan and implement care for dying clients and their families.

Articulate and defend a personal response to a client's plea, "Please help me die."

List the clinical signs of approaching death.

Outline nursing responsibilities after death.

Discuss the role of the nurse in caring for a client's family.

Key Terms

active euthanasia
actual loss
anticipatory loss
assisted suicide
bereavement
comfort measures only
death
do-not-hospitalize
do-not-resuscitate
dysfunctional grief
grief
hospice
loss
mourning
perceived loss
physical loss
psychologic loss
terminal illness
terminal wean

At any stage of one's life there is the potential for loss, grief, and death. This is especially true for the person experiencing altered health and for his or her family. A wide variety of losses may occur, including loss of a body part or function; loss of one's ability to care for oneself; loss of one's role as head of a family; and death, which may be the most difficult loss of all. Death may be as difficult for healthcare professionals as it is for surviving family members. The goals of nursing focus on health maintenance and health restoration, with an emphasis on facilitating maximum potential in wellness. One of the functions of the nurse is, however, to facilitate coping with disability and death. The nurse often is the key person in providing support and care when loss or death occurs. To provide effective care, the nurse must have accepted his or her own feelings about death and understand the stages of grieving and dying.

Loss and Grieving

Loss

Loss occurs when a valued person, object, or situation is changed or made inaccessible so that its value is diminished or removed. There are several types of loss, all of which everyone may experience at some time. **Actual loss** can be recognized by others as well as by the person sustaining the loss; loss of a limb, of a spouse, of a valued object such as money, and of a job are all examples of actual loss. **Perceived loss** is felt by the person but is intangible to others; loss of youth, of financial independence, and of a valued environment are examples of perceived loss. Directly related to actual and perceived loss are **physical loss** and **psychologic loss**. A person who loses an arm in an automobile accident suffers from both the physical loss of the arm and the psychologic loss that may be caused by an altered self-image and the inability to return to his or her occupation. These losses are simultaneously physical, psychologic, and actual. A person who is scarred but does not lose a limb may suffer a perceived and psychologic loss of self-image.

Another type of loss is **anticipatory loss**, in which a person displays loss and grief behaviors for a loss that has yet to take place. Anticipatory loss often is seen in families of terminally ill clients, and serves to lessen the impact of the actual loss of a family member.

Loss can have a tremendous impact on a person's development; conversely, age affects a person's reaction to loss (see Factors That Affect Grief and Death, later in this chapter). Although most adults can accept death on an intellectual level, they may have trouble dealing with it on an emotional level. The loss of a friend, a pet, or a job may help a person anticipate and cope with the loss of a spouse or other loved one.

Grieving

Grieving is the emotional reaction to loss. It occurs with loss caused by separation as well as with loss caused by death. Many people who divorce experience grief, and loss of a body part, a job, a house, or a pet may cause grief. **Bereavement** is the state of grieving during which a person goes through grief reaction. **Mourning** is the period of acceptance of loss and grief during which the person learns to deal with the loss.

Bereavement, which is experienced by both the client and the family, may have profound health consequences that require additional care. Bereaved people often neglect their health to an extreme, whereas mourning is characterized by a return to more normal living habits.

Grief Reactions. **Grief** is the emotional pain caused by a loss. Reactions to both grief and dying are similar. The stages of these reactions overlap and vary among individuals. One person may skip a reaction stage, whereas another may repeat an earlier stage. Each person is different, and clients and family members may be at different reaction stages.

Engel (1964) was among the first to define stages of grief. Engel's six stages are (1) shock and disbelief, (2) developing awareness, (3) restitution, (4) resolving the loss, (5) idealization, and (6) outcome. *Shock and disbelief* usually are defined as refusal to accept the fact of loss, followed by a stunned or numb response: "No, not me." *Developing awareness* is characterized by physical and emotional responses such as anger, feeling empty, and crying: "Why me?" *Restitution* involves the rituals

Grief and Death Reactions

Engel's Six Stages of Grief Reactions

1. Shock and disbelief
2. Developing awareness
3. Restitution
4. Resolving the loss
5. Idealization
6. Outcome

Five Stages of Kübler-Ross' Grief and Death Reactions

1. Denial and isolation
2. Anger
3. Bargaining
4. Depression
5. Acceptance

surrounding loss, and with death includes religious, cultural, or social expressions of mourning, such as funeral services. *Resolving the loss* is dealing with the void left by the loss, and *idealization* is the exaggeration of the good qualities of the person or object lost, followed by acceptance of the loss and a lessened need to focus on it. *Outcome* is the final resolution of the grief process, including dealing with loss as a common life occurrence.

Kübler-Ross (1969), considered a pioneer in the study of grief and death reactions, defined five stages of reaction similar to those of Engel: (1) denial and isolation, (2) anger, (3) bargaining, (4) depression, and (5) acceptance. Other works in the grief process literature include that of Clark (1984), who describes three stages of grief, and Martocchio (1985), who describes five grief groupings. More important than the actual stages of any given grief reaction is the idea that grief *is* a process and that it varies from person to person.

Normal Versus Dysfunctional Grief. Both normal and dysfunctional grief may be delayed, and normal grief may be either abbreviated or anticipatory. *Abbreviated grief* is of short duration but is genuine; *anticipatory grief* occurs before the actual loss, as in the extended terminal illness of a family member. **Dysfunctional grief** is abnormal or distorted; it may be either unresolved or inhibited. In *unresolved grief*, a person may have trouble expressing feelings of loss or may deny them; unresolved grief also describes a state of bereavement that extends over a lengthy period. In *inhibited grief*, a person suppresses feelings of grief and may instead manifest somatic symptoms.

Dying and Death

Dying may occur suddenly as a result of an accident, injury, or pathologic crisis such as a heart attack; or it may occur after a prolonged experience of debilitating disease such as cancer, AIDS, or multiple sclerosis. Whereas some welcome death and even hasten death, choosing the time and manner of their dying, others fear death and will try anything to delay it. Given the choice some die at home surrounded by loved ones, in what is called hospice care. Hallmarks of hospice care are:

Patients will be kept as free of pain as possible so that they may die comfortably and with dignity.

Patients will receive continuity of care and not be abandoned or lose personal identity.

Patients will retain as much control as possible over decisions regarding their care and be allowed to refuse further life-prolonging technological interventions.

Patients will be heard as individuals with personal fears, thoughts, feelings, values, and hopes (Catholic Health Association, 1993).

Others die alone or in intensive care units surrounded by healthcare professionals and technological equipment. A client's wishes should, if possible, be followed. Rights of dying persons are listed in the accompanying box.

Responses to Dying and Death

Although each person reacts to the knowledge of impending death or to loss in his or her own way, there are similarities in the psychosocial responses to the situation. Kübler-Ross has studied the emotional responses to death and dying in depth, and her findings have been used extensively by the nursing and other helping professions.

The stages of dying, much like the stages of grief, may overlap, and the duration of any stage may range from as little as a few hours to as long as a period of months. The process varies from person to person. Some people may be in one stage for such a short time that it seems as if they skipped that stage. Sometimes a person returns to a previous stage.

According to Kübler-Ross, the stages of dying are (1) denial and isolation, (2) anger, (3) bargaining, (4) depression, and (5) acceptance.

Denial and isolation: In the denial and isolation stage, the client denies that he or she will die, may repress what is discussed, and may isolate self from reality. The client may think, "They made a mistake in the diagnosis. Maybe they mixed my records with someone else's."

Anger: The client expresses rage and hostility in the anger stage and adopts a "why me?" attitude. "Why me? I quit smoking and I watched what I ate. Why did this happen to me?"

Bargaining: The client tries to barter for more time. "If I can just make it to my son's graduation I will be satisfied. Just let me live until then." Many clients put their personal affairs in order, make wills, and fulfill last wishes, such as trips, visiting relatives, and so forth. It is important to meet these wishes, if possible, because bargaining helps clients move into later stages of dying.

The Dying Person's Bill of Rights

I have the right to be treated as a living human being until I die.
I have the right to maintain a sense of hopefulness however changing its focus may be.
I have the right to be cared for by those who can maintain a sense of hopefulness, however changing this might be.
I have the right to express my feelings and emotions about my approaching death in my own way.
I have the right to participate in decisions concerning my care.
I have the right to expect continuing medical and nursing attention even though "cure" goals must be changed to "comfort" goals.
I have the right not to die alone.
I have the right to be free from pain.
I have the right to have my questions answered honestly.
I have the right not to be deceived.
I have the right to have help from and for my family in accepting my death.
I have the right to die in peace and dignity.
I have a right to retain my individuality and not be judged for my decisions which may be contrary to beliefs of others.
I have the right to discuss and enlarge my religious and/or spiritual experiences, whatever these may mean to others.
I have the right to expect that the sanctity of the human body will be respected after death.
I have the right to be cared for by caring, sensitive, knowledgeable people who will attempt to understand my needs and will be able to gain some satisfaction in helping me face my death.

(Created at the workshop *The Terminally Ill Patient and the Helping Person,* in Lansing, Michigan, sponsored by the Southwestern Michigan Inservice Education Council and conducted by Amelia J. Barbus, Associate Professor of Nursing, Wayne State University, Detroit.)

Depression: In the depression stage, the client goes through a period of grief before death. The grief is characterized by crying and not speaking much. "I waited all these years to see my daughter get married. And now I may not be here to see her walk down the aisle. I can't bear the thought of not being there for the wedding—and to see my grandchildren."

Acceptance: When the stage of acceptance is reached, the client feels tranquil. She or he has accepted death and is prepared to die. The client may think, "I've tied up all the loose ends—made the will, made arrangements for my daughter to live with her grandparents. Now I can go in peace knowing everyone will be fine."

Impact of Terminal Illness

In the case of a **terminal illness**, an illness in which death is expected within a limited space of time, the physician usually is responsible for deciding what and how much the client should be told. The nurse, clergyperson, and other healthcare professionals may be involved with this decision and in discussing the client's condition with him or her. Most clients want to know their diagnosis and prognosis as soon as possible, so that they can both come to grips with it and take care of business and personal affairs. Even more important is a description of how the disease is likely to play out and what this will mean for the client. All who are involved with the client's care should know exactly what the client and the family have been told; members of the client's healthcare team need to communicate among themselves. Cultural influences may dictate how much information is desired and which family members are to be informed.

Impact on Client. Many clients realize without being told that they are suffering from a terminal illness; this realization often is picked up from nonverbal communication by their families and by healthcare professionals. Clients must be allowed to go through the stages of the grieving process and to make decisions about their care, and must be supported in their decision making. Competent clients have the right to consent to and to refuse any and all indicated medical treatment—even that which is life-sustaining—and should be made aware of this right. In the past, clients and family members complained about receiving care they did not want and of not being allowed to die. In today's climate of cost-conscious decision making, some clients and family members are complaining that they are being denied costly life-sustaining treatment because of inadequate personal funds or insurance or because they are deemed a poor "investment" of scarce resources.

Impact on Family. The family and significant others of terminally ill clients should be encouraged to participate in planning the client's care. Healthcare personnel should be available to discuss the client's condition with family members and should offer support and care as the family begins the grieving process. The family may want to make arrangements with the client for funeral or memorial services; this is contingent on which stage of grief both client and family members have progressed to.

Signs of Impending Death

The clinical signs of *impending* or *approaching* death include inability to swallow; pitting edema; decreased gastrointestinal and urinary tract activity; bowel and bladder incontinence; loss of motion, sensation, and reflexes; elevated temperature but cold or clammy skin; cyanosis; lowered blood pressure; noisy or irregular respiration; and Cheyne-Stokes respirations. The client may or may not lose consciousness. It is often helpful to prepare family members and significant others for the transformations which signal impending death. Nuland's (1994) popular book entitled *How We Die* is a useful resource.

Definitions of Death

Death was defined in 1981 by the President's Commission for the Study of Ethical Problems in Medicine and Biomedical and Behavioral Research as follows:

> Death is present when an individual has sustained either (1) irreversible cessation of circulatory and respiratory functions, or (2) irreversible cessation of all functions of the entire brain, including the brain stem.

A Harvard University committee stated that the following characteristics must be present for at least 24 hours before death can be declared:

- Lack of receptivity and responsiveness
- Lack of movement or breathing
- Lack of reflexes
- Flat encephalogram

In the United States there are currently three definitions of death in the literature: the traditional heart–lung definition, the whole-brain definition, and the higher-brain definition. These are compared in Table 33-1.

Ethical and Legal Dimensions

Multiple treatment options and sophisticated life-support technologies may make it difficult to draw the line between promoting life and needlessly prolonging the dying process. In these cases healthcare decision making is complicated for clients and healthcare professionals alike. The increasing popularity of the "managed death" concept and calls to legalize physician-assisted suicide and physician-administered lethal injections ("aid in dying") pose new ethical challenges. As clients and families struggle with end-of-life treatment decisions, they are increasingly looking to nurses for information, advice, and support. Clients have a legally and morally protected right to consent to and to refuse any and all indicated medical therapies. Legal foundations for the client's freedom to choose include the common-law right of self-determination and the constitutionally

Table 33-1
Definitions of Death

Heart–Lung Death	Whole Brain Death	Higher Brain Death
The irreversible cessation of spontaneous respiration and circulation; the accepted criterion for death until the 1960s, this definition emerged from the historical idea that the flow of body fluids was essential for life.	The irreversible cessation of all functions of the entire brain, including the brain stem; this definition emerged in the 1960s from the belief that neocortical functioning is the key to the definition of a human being.[1] Most protocols require two separate clinical examinations including induction of painful stimuli, pupillary responses to light, oculo-vestibular testing, and apnea testing. To enhance accuracy standard practice is not to perform brain death testing while a patient is hypothermic, hypotensive, or under the influence of neuromuscular blocking agents or barbiturates.	The irreversible loss of all "higher" brain functions, of cognitive function;[2] this definition was suggested in the 1970s and emerged from the belief that the brain is more important than the spinal cord and that the critical functions are the individual's personality, conscious life, uniqueness, capacity for remembering, judging, reasoning, acting, enjoying, worrying.

[1] Report of the Ad Hoc Committee of the Harvard Medical School to examine the definition of brain death: A definition of irreversible coma. (1968). *JAMA, 205,* 337–340; President's Commission for the Study of Ethical Problems in Medicine and Biomedical and Behavioral Research. (1981). ***Defining death: medical, legal and ethical issues in the definition of death.*** Washington, DC: US Government Printing Office; Medical Consultants on the Diagnosis of Death to the President's Commission for the Study of Ethical Problems in Medicine and Biomedical and Behavioral Research. Guidelines for the determination of death. (1981). *JAMA, 246,* 2184–2186.

[2] Veatch, R. M. The whole-brain-oriented concept of death: an outmoded philosophical formulation. *Journal of Thanatology.* 1975;3(1):13–30; Truog, R. D., Fackler, J. C. Rethinking brain death. *Critical Care Medicine.* 1992;20(12):1705–1713.

(Material in this table adapted from Ott, B. B. [1995]. Defining and redefining death. *American Journal of Critical Care, 4*[6], 476–480.)

supported right of privacy. The ethical and legal implications of nursing are discussed in general in Chapters 6 and 7. Select counseling and advocacy responsibilities are described in Chapters 23 and 24. A discussion of nursing's ethical and legal responsibilities in end-of-life care follows.

Advance Directives

Decisions about healthcare are becoming increasingly complex. Clients, family members, and healthcare professionals alike are voicing frustration as they grapple with complex decisions about prolonging life. Some of the most difficult cases involve clients who are no longer able (competent) to indicate their treatment preferences. Two kinds of written **advance directives** can minimize difficulties by allowing individuals to state in advance what their choices would be for healthcare should certain circumstances develop. **Living wills** provide specific instructions about the kinds of healthcare that should be provided or foregone in particular situations. A **durable power of attorney for healthcare** appoints an agent the person trusts to make decisions in the event of the appointing person's subsequent incapacity. A combination directive is illustrated in Figure 33-1. In Canada, a public trustee is appointed on behalf of peo-

(text continues on page 789)

Computer Applications in Nursing

A Groundbreaking Web Site From Choice In Dying

Choice In Dying, a national, not-for-profit organization, has introduced a World Wide Web (WWW) site devoted to right-to-die issues and end-of-life decision making. The site features a wide range of educational materials as well as state-specific advance directives (living wills and medical powers of attorney) that can be downloaded from the site at no charge. These legal documents include a detailed instruction booklet that helps people execute the forms correctly.

The new web site includes sections dedicated to:

- *Advance Directives:* These documents (living wills and medical powers of attorney) allow individuals to record their wishes about end-of-life medical treatment. The site not only provides legal forms, it also provides important information to help people make informed decisions about the type of care they would like to receive. Choice In Dying staff are available through an e-mail link and by phone to help answer questions.
- *Honoring Final Wishes:* Information about getting healthcare providers to listen to and honor advance directives.
- *Legal Developments:* The legal landscape concerning the right to die continues to evolve rapidly. Summaries and analyses of major court cases and the most current information about right-to-die legislation are regularly updated.
- *Right-to-Die Issues:* What is the difference between active and passive euthanasia? Are there ethical or legal differences between withholding and withdrawing treatment? The CID-WWW site includes the answer to these and other questions about the right to die.
- *Choice In Dying Publications and Videos:* For those who need more information, the site includes a catalogue and order form for Choice In Dying's resources for professionals and the public, including the award-winning Question and Answer Series and the Right-to-Die Law Digest.

According to Karen Orloff Kaplan, ScD, Executive Director of Choice In Dying, "A study released just last month shows that physicians are ignoring patients' end-of-life wishes, and that many patients at the end of their lives continue to receive medical care they don't want but lack the adequate pain relief that they do want and deserve. The CID-WWW site helps to arm people with useful information. It focuses on all aspects of end-of-life decision making. The CID-WWW site gives professionals and consumers direct access to information and resources, based on their needs and specific areas of interest."

The CID-WWW can be accessed at: **http://www.choices.org.** Inquiries can be directed by e-mail to **choice\@choices.org.**

Choice In Dying (CID), a national, not-for-profit organization, is known as the creator of the first living will (1967) and it is now the only organization providing free counseling for families during end-of-life crises on its toll-free number, 1-800-989-WILL (9455). A the same 800 number, CID offers suggestions to ensure that healthcare providers honor end-of-life wishes as well as information about completing advance directives, selecting healthcare agents, and talking with physicians and family members about one's healthcare decisions. CID also provides award-winning educational booklets and videotapes, state-specific advance directives (living wills and medical power of attorney forms), public and physician education and ongoing monitoring of changes in state and federal right-to-die legislation.

For additional information, or if you do not have a computer and want to know more about advance directives and state law, call Choice In Dying toll-free at 1-800-989-WILL (9455) or 212-366-5540.

ADVANCE DIRECTIVE

Your Durable Power of Attorney for Health Care, Living Will and Other Wishes

This document has been prepared and distributed as an informational service of the District of Columbia Hospital Association.

INSTRUCTIONS AND DEFINITIONS

Introduction:

This form is a combined durable power of attorney for health care and living will for use in D.C., Maryland and Virginia. With this form, you can:

- Appoint someone to make medical decisions for you if you in the future are unable to make those decisions for yourself.

and/or

- Indicate what medical treatment you do or do not want if in the future you are unable to make your wishes known.

Directions:

- Read each section carefully.
- Talk to the person you plan to appoint to make sure that he/she understands your wishes, and is willing to take the responsibility.
- Place the initials of your name in the blank before those choices you want to make.
- Fill in only those choices that you want under Parts 1, 2, and 3. Your advance directive should be valid for whatever part(s) you fill in, as long as it is properly signed.
- Add any special instructions in the blank spaces provided. You can write additional comments on a separate piece of paper, but you should indicate on the form that there are additional pages to your advance directive.
- Sign the form and have it witnessed.
- Give to your family, and anyone else who might be involved in your care, a copy of your advance directive and discuss it with them.
- Understand that you may change or cancel this document at any time.

WORDS YOU NEED TO KNOW:

Advance Directive: A written document that tells what a person wants or does not want if he/she in the future can't make his/her wishes known about medical treatment.

Artificial Nutrition and Hydration: When food and water are fed to a person through a tube.

Autopsy: An examination done on a dead body to find the cause of death.

Comfort care: Care that helps to keep a person comfortable but does not make him/her better. Bathing, turning, keeping a person's lips moist are types of comfort care.

CPR (Cardiopulmonary Resuscitation): Treatment to try to restart a person's breathing or heartbeat. CPR may be done by pushing on the chest, by putting a tube down the throat, or by other treatment.

Durable Power of Attorney for Health Care: An advance directive that appoints someone to make medical decisions for a person if in the future he/she can't make his/her own medical decisions.

Life-Sustaining Treatment: Any medical treatment that is used to keep a person from dying. A breathing machine, CPR, and artifical nutrition and hydration are examples of life-sustaining treatments.

Living Will: An advance directive that tells what medical treatment a person does or does not want if he/she is not able to make his/her wishes known.

Organ and Tissue Donation: When a person permits his/her organs (such as eyes or kidneys) and other parts of the body (such as skin) to be removed after death to be transplanted for use by another person or to be used for experimental purposes.

Persistent Vegetative State: When a person is unconscious with no hope of regaining consciousness even with medical treatment. The body may move and eyes may be open but as far as anyone can tell, the person can't think or respond.

Terminal Condition: An on-going condition caused by injury or illness that has no cure and from which doctors expect the person to die even with medical treatment. Life-sustaining treatments will only prolong a person's dying if the person is suffering from a terminal condition.

Figure 33-1
Example of an advance directive. (Used with permission of District of Columbia Hospital Association, Washington, DC.)

D.C., Maryland and Virginia

ADVANCE DIRECTIVE

My Durable Power of Attorney for Health Care, Living Will and Other Wishes

I, ________________________________, write this document as a directive regarding my medical care.

Put the initials of your name by the choices you want.

PART 1. MY DURABLE POWER OF ATTORNEY FOR HEALTH CARE.

_______ I appoint this person to make decisions about my medical care if there ever comes a time when I cannot make those decisions myself:

NAME ________________________ PHONE HOME __________ WORK __________

ADDRESS ____

____

If the person above cannot or will not make decisions for me, I appoint this person:

NAME ________________________ PHONE HOME __________ WORK __________

ADDRESS ____

____

_______ I have not appointed anyone to make health care decisions for me in this or any other document.

I want the person I have appointed, my doctors, my family, and others to be guided by the decisions I have made below:

PART 2. MY LIVING WILL.

These are my wishes for my future medical care if there ever comes a time when I can't make these decisions for myself.

A. **These are my wishes if I have a *terminal condition:***
Life-Sustaining Treatments

_______ I do not want life-sustaining treatments (including CPR) started. If life-sustaining treatments are started, I want them stopped.

_______ I want life-sustaining treatments that my doctors think are best for me.

_______ Other wishes: ____

Artificial Nutrition and Hydration

_______ I do not want artificial nutrition and hydration started if it would be the main treatment keeping me alive. If artificial nutrition and hydration is started, I want it stopped.

_______ I want artificial nutrition and hydration even if it is the main treatment keeping me alive.

_______ Other wishes: ____

Comfort Care

_______ I want to be kept as comfortable and free of pain as possible, even if such care prolongs my dying or shortens my life.

_______ Other wishes: ____

B. **These are my wishes if I am ever in a *persistent vegetative state:***

Life-Sustaining Treatments

_______ I do not want life-sustaining treatments (including CPR) started. If life-sustaining treatments are started, I want them stopped.

_______ I want life-sustaining treatments that my doctors think are best for me.

_______ Other wishes: ____

Figure 33-1 *(continued)*

Artificial Nutrition and Hydration

_______ I do not want artificial nutrition and hydration started if it would be the main treatment keeping me alive.
If artificial nutrition and hydration is started, I want it stopped.

_______ I want artificial nutrition and hydration even if it is the main treatment keeping me alive.

_______ Other wishes: ______________________________

Comfort Care

_______ I want to be kept as comfortable as possible, even if such care prolongs my dying or shortens my life

_______ Other wishes: ______________________________

C. **Other Direction**

You have the right to be involved in all decisions about your medical care, even those parts not dealing with terminal conditions or persistent vegetative states. If you have wishes not covered in other parts of this document, please indicate them here.

____

____

PART 3. OTHER WISHES.

A. **Organ Donation**

_______ I do not wish to donate any of my organs or tissues.

_______ I want to donate all of my organs and tissues.

_______ I only want to donate these organs and tissues: ______________________________

_______ Other wishes: ______________________________

Autopsy

_______ I do not want an autopsy.

_______ I agree to an autopsy if my doctors wish it.

_______ Other wishes: ______________________________

If you wish to say more about any of the above choices, or if you have any other statements to make about your medical care, you may do so on a separate sheet of paper. If you do so, put here the number of pages you are adding: ______________________________

PART 4. SIGNATURES.

You and two witnesses must sign this document for it to be legal.

A. **Your Signature**

By my signature below I show that I understand the purpose and the effect of this document.

SIGNATURE ______________________________ DATE ______________

ADDRESS ______________________________

B. **Your Witnesses' Signatures**

I believe the person who has signed this advance directive to be of sound mind, that he/she signed or acknowledged this advance directive in my presence, and that he/she appears not to be acting under pressure, duress, fraud or undue influence. I am not related to the person making this advance directive by blood, marriage or adoption, nor, to the best of my knowledge, am I named in his/her will. I am not the person appointed in this advance directive. I am not a health care provider or an employee of health care provider who is now, or has been in the past, responsible for the care of the person making this advance directive.

Witness #1

SIGNATURE ______________________________ DATE ______________

ADDRESS ______________________________

Witness #2

SIGNATURE ______________________________ DATE ______________

ADDRESS ______________________________

Figure 33-1 *(continued)*

ple who do not have family support and who require financial and health decisions to be made.

Many means have been suggested to ensure that adult clients have an opportunity to learn about and use advance directives to indicate their wishes about life-prolonging treatment and to appoint surrogate decision makers should they lose decision-making capacity. Nurses have an important role to play in facilitating this dialogue. In the United States, the Patient Self-Determination Act of 1990 requires all hospitals to inform their clients about advance directives. Because the status of advance directives varies from state to state (or province to province) it is important for nurses to be familiar with federal and state (or province) law concerning these directives. Nurses can also be instrumental in developing institutional policies that ensure that clients on admission are encouraged to talk with family, significant others, and healthcare professionals about their treatment preferences.

Assisted Suicide and Direct Voluntary Euthanasia

Euthanasia may be simply defined as good dying. Until recently most societies maintained that the distinction between killing and allowing to die was morally relevant. This meant that withholding or withdrawing medically ineffective or disproportionately burdensome therapies was morally and legally justified even when this hastened or directly caused a client's death. On the other hand, killing a client by administering a lethal injection or carbon monoxide—even when performed with compassionate intent at the request of a client—was deemed both immoral and illegal. Some are questioning the validity of this distinction today and there are efforts to legalize assisted suicide and active euthanasia in numerous countries. In the United States many are expecting that the U. S. Supreme Court will soon decide whether legalization of assisted suicide is required, prohibited, or simply allowed by the Constitution.

It is important for nurses to understand the arguments for and against assisted suicide and direct voluntary euthanasia. These are briefly listed in the accompanying box.

The American Nurses' Association in 1994 issued position statements claiming that assisting in suicide and participating in active euthanasia are in violation of the *Code for Nurses* and the ethical traditions of the profession. See the accompanying box for a definition of these

Assisted Suicide and Direct Voluntary Euthanasia: Arguments For and Against

Arguments in Favor of Assisted Suicide and Direct Voluntary Euthanasia

1. It is a beneficent and compassionate act.
2. It respects autonomy by preserving the patient's control of the manner, method, and timing of death.
3. It takes the matter outside the reach of "medical power" and scrupulosity.
4. It prevents the injustice that allows some patients to choose death by refusal of life-support measures, while denying others the right to do so by active euthanasia.
5. In a pluralistic society, euthanasia must be accepted, whatever its intrinsic morality, since states have no moral justification for intruding into such private decisions.

Proponents of involuntary euthanasia argue, that in addition, it is irrational to afford rights of personhood to anencephalics or patients in a permanent vegetative state and unjust to deny them the right to die to which they are entitled. They argue that beneficence to patient, family, and healthcare professionals, as well as conservation of society's resources, make involuntary euthanasia a positive moral duty of physicians.

Arguments Against Assisted Suicide and Direct Voluntary Euthanasia

1. It undermines the value of, and respect for, all human life.
2. Guidelines cannot avoid sliding down the slippery slope to involuntary euthanasia and selective devaluation of the lives of the most vulnerable among us.
3. Euthanasia should be unnecessary since the major reasons for requesting it—intolerable pain and fear of overtreatment—can now be handled by better palliative care, analgesia, and advance directives.
4. A focus on euthanasia will deviate attention from other valuable palliative techniques.
5. If euthanasia is legal, it is predicted patients will feel a subtle pressure to conform so as to relieve the economic and emotional burdens they impose on family and friends.
6. Euthanasia is socially destructive: it undermines trust in physicians and healthcare professionals, desensitizes society to killing, and imperils the grounds already gained in legitimizing passive euthanasia.
7. Many Americans hold the religious belief that human life is the gift of the Creator and that humans are its stewards but not its absolute masters.

(Adapted from Pellegrino, E. D. [1991]. Ethics. *Journal of the American Medical Association, 265*[23], 3118-3119.)

American Nurses Association (ANA) Position Statements on Assisted Suicide and Active Euthanasia

Nurses, individually and collectively, have an obligation to provide comprehensive and compassionate end-of-life care which includes the promotion of comfort and relief of pain, and, at times, foregoing life-sustaining treatments. The ANA believes that the nurse should not participate in assisted suicide. Such an act is in violation of the *Code for Nurses* and the ethical traditions of the profession.

Terminology

Suicide is traditionally understood as the act of taking one's own life. **Assisting in suicide** entails making a means of suicide (eg, providing pills or a weapon) available to a patient with knowledge of the patient's intention. The patient who is physically capable of suicide subsequently acts to end his or her own life. Assisted suicide is distinguished from active euthanasia. In assisted suicide, someone makes the means of death available, but does not act as the direct agent of death.

Nurses have an obligation to provide timely, humane, comprehensive, and compassionate end-of-life care. The ANA believes that the nurse should not participate in active euthanasia because such an act is in direct violation of the *Code for Nurses,* the ethical traditions and goals of the profession, and its covenant with society.

Terminology

Active euthanasia means that someone other than the patient commits an action with the intent to end the patient's life, for example injecting a patient with a lethal dose. Sometimes euthanasia is subdivided into a situation in which a patient consents to euthanasia (voluntary), or a situation in which a patient refuses euthanasia (involuntary), or a situation when a patient is unable to consent to euthanasia (nonvoluntary). Active euthanasia is distinguished from assisted suicide. In active euthanasia someone not only makes the means of death available, but serves as the direct agent of death.

(American Nurses Association. [1994]. *Position statement on assisted suicide and on active euthanasia.* Washington, DC: ANA.)

terms and ANA recommendations. Nurses can expect to be confronted by clients who seek their assistance in ending their life. Unless nurses think through this issue carefully they will be unprepared to respond to the request, "Nurse, please help me die."

Do-Not-Resuscitate or No-Code Orders

To prevent the improper use of cardiopulmonary resuscitation, which is designed to prevent unexpected death, some physicians will write **do-not-resuscitate** (DNR), or no-code, on the chart of a terminally ill client if the client or surrogate has expressed a wish that there be no attempts to resuscitate the client in the event of cardiopulmonary resuscitation. Many physicians are reluctant to write these orders, especially when this issue is a source of conflict between the client and family or between individual family members. In these cases, a physician who believes the client will not benefit from resuscitative measures may verbally indicate to the nurse that only a slow-code should be called, that is, in the case of cardiopulmonary or respiratory arrest, calling a code and resuscitating the client are to be delayed until these measures will be ineffectual. Slow-codes are never good practice and many healthcare institutions now have policies forbidding their use. It is likely that a nurse could be charged negligent in the event of a slow-code and resultant client death.

The standard of care still obligates healthcare professionals to attempt resuscitation if a client stops breathing or his or her heart stops (cardiopulmonary arrest) and there is no order to the contrary. For this reason it is important for nurses to clarify a client's code status if the probable benefits of resuscitation are negligible or if the nurse has reason to believe a client would not want to be resuscitated. Many states now allow clients living at home to craft special orders that allow emergency technicians (EMTs) called to the home in the event of cardiopulmonary arrest to respect the client's wishes not to be resuscitated.

Comfort Measures Only and Other Special Orders

A do-not-resuscitate order means simply that—that no attempts are to be made to resuscitate a client who stops breathing or whose heart stops beating. When a discussion is taking place about resuscitation it is appropriate to question aggressive treatment in general, for example, the use of dialysis, ventilatory support, artificial nutrition and hydration, blood transfusions, antibiotics and other medications, and surgery. Whereas some clients may want aggressive treatment and such treatment is medically beneficial, other clients may be at a point in their illness where they choose to terminate all life-sustaining measures. There is no moral obligation to initiate or continue the use of life-sustaining treatment that is minimally effective or disproportionately burdensome. Law may place constraints upon who may decide to withhold or withdraw life-sustaining treatment for incompetent clients. Nurses should be familiar with pertinent federal and state (province) law and the policies in their institution or agency concerning the withholding or withdrawing of life-sustaining treatment. Nurses should also be familiar with the forms used to indicate client preferences about end-of-life care. A **comfort measures only** order is written to indicate that the goal of treatment is a comfortable, dignified death and that further life-sustaining measures are no longer indicated. A do-not-hospitalize order is being used by clients in nursing homes and other residential settings who have elected not to be hospitalized for further aggressive treatment.

Terminal Weaning

Terminal weaning is the gradual withdrawal of mechanical ventilation from a client with a terminal illness or an irreversible condition with poor prognosis. In some cases, competent clients decide that they wish their ventilatory support ended; more often, the surrogate decision makers for an incompetent client determine that continued ventilatory support is futile. Although it may be expected that a client will not be able to survive the weaning, death is never a certain outcome and it is not unusual for a client to initiate spontaneous respirations once ventilatory support is withdrawn and live for several hours to several days. Competent clients and family members should be prepared for all possibilities. Nursing's role in the event of a terminal weaning is to participate in the decision-making process by offering helpful information about the benefits and burdens of continued ventilation and a description of what to expect if terminal weaning is initiated. Supporting the client's family and managing sedation and analgesia are critical nursing responsibilities; unfortunately, many agencies and institutions do not have policies. If involved in terminal weaning, consult the literature (Campbell, 1994; Rushton & Terry, 1995).

Death Certificate

Both U.S. and Canadian laws require that a death certificate be prepared for each person who dies. The laws specify what information needs to be supplied. Death certificates are sent to local health departments, which compile many statistics from the information. The mortician assumes responsibility for handling and filing the death certificate with proper authorities. A physician's signature is required on the certificate, as well as that of the pathologist, the coroner, and others in special cases. The nurse's responsibility is to ensure that a death certificate has been signed by the physician.

Organ Donation

Clients who express a wish to donate functional organs, such as hearts, corneas, livers, lungs, and kidneys, can fill out an organ donor consent card (Fig. 33-2). The family of a deceased client also may decide to donate the client's functional organs. The nurse should be able to review options and provide consent forms to interested clients and their families. Until recently, most organs were retrieved from totally brain-dead clients. New protocols for retrieving organs from non–heart-beating cadavers are raising multiple practice concerns. Comprehensive attention to optimal client/family care at the time of withdrawal of life-sustaining therapy needs to remain nursing's priority.

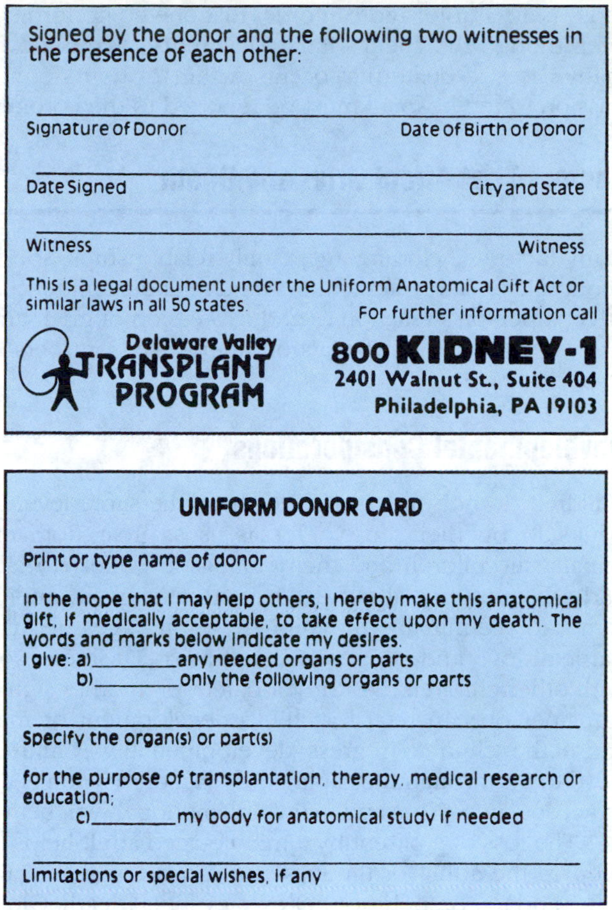

Signed by the donor and the following two witnesses in the presence of each other:

Signature of Donor | Date of Birth of Donor

Date Signed | City and State

Witness | Witness

This is a legal document under the Uniform Anatomical Gift Act or similar laws in all 50 states.

For further information call

Delaware Valley TRANSPLANT PROGRAM

800 KIDNEY-1
2401 Walnut St., Suite 404
Philadelphia, PA 19103

UNIFORM DONOR CARD

Print or type name of donor

In the hope that I may help others, I hereby make this anatomical gift, if medically acceptable, to take effect upon my death. The words and marks below indicate my desires.
I give: a)_______any needed organs or parts
b)_______only the following organs or parts

Specify the organ(s) or part(s)

for the purpose of transplantation, therapy, medical research or education;
c)_______my body for anatomical study if needed

Limitations or special wishes, if any

Figure 33-2
Example of an organ donor card.

Autopsy

An **autopsy** is an examination of the organs and tissues of a human body after death. Consent for autopsy is a legal requirement. The closest surviving family member or members usually have the authority to determine whether or not an autopsy is performed. Some religious groups prohibit autopsies except for legal purposes.

It commonly is the physician's responsibility to obtain permission for an autopsy. Sometimes the client may grant this permission before death. The nurse can assist by explaining the reasons for an autopsy. Many relatives find comfort when they are told that the knowledge gained from an autopsy may contribute to advancements in medical science as well as establish the exact cause of death.

If death is caused by accident, suicide, homicide, or illegal therapeutic practice, the coroner must be notified, according to law. The coroner may decide that an autopsy is advisable, and can order that one be performed, even though the client's family has refused consent. In many cases, a death that occurs within 24 hours of admission to the hospital must be reported to the coroner.

Factors That Affect Grief and Death

Many factors, including age, family relationships, socioeconomic position, and cultural and religious influences, affect a person's reaction to and expression of grief, and like the stages of grief reaction, they vary from person to person.

Developmental Considerations

Children do not understand death on the same level as adults do, but their sense of loss is just as great. Both terminally ill children and their siblings are likely to talk and ask questions about death in an attempt to understand it. Terminally ill children of all ages require parental love and support, as well as social interaction with other children. Death of a parent or another significant person can retard a child's development or may cause the child to regress developmentally. Children need to go through the same grief reactions as adults do to accept such a loss and maintain emotional well being.

The loss of a parent by a middle-aged adult helps to prepare the adult for the loss of a spouse or significant other and to accept his or her own eventual death. Older people may lose a spouse, or friends and relatives their own age. As this happens, they reminisce about life, put their lives and the purpose of living in perspective, and prepare themselves for their own inevitable death.

Family

Roles within families are important factors that affect reactions to and expressions of grief. For example, the eldest sibling may feel a need to "be strong," and therefore may not grieve openly; a person who loses a spouse may display the same type of behavior to "protect the children."

The death of a child usually is a devastating experience for her or his family. The family needs time to accept the reality of the situation, opportunities to talk and to be listened to, and the experience of expressing themselves behaviorally in a nonjudgmental environment. The family of a terminally ill child may express feelings of guilt by wondering if they were responsible for the impending death. A sibling may suppress a guilt feeling for having wished the ill child (or a parent) dead.

Socioeconomic Factors

A bereaved family may suffer more acutely if there is no health or life insurance or pension after the death of the family provider. Such families face not only the loss of a loved one, but also an economic loss that may further disrupt family life. Older people especially may be placed in a difficult position, since the death of a spouse may result in a source of retirement income for the surviving spouse being either diminished or cut off. This reduction in income may lead to loss of home, community, and support systems.

Cultural Influences

Both the physical and the emotional manifestations of grief may be culturally influenced. Schulz (1978) defined the clinical symptoms of grief as repeated somatic distress, tightness in the chest, choking or shortness of breath, sighing, empty feeling in the abdomen, loss of muscle power, and intense subjective distress. Other symptoms include vomiting, dizziness, fainting, fatigue, weight loss, headaches, and chest pains (Gonda & Ruark, 1984).

Culture also influences a person's expression of grief. In many families in the Western culture, grief is a private matter that is shared only with the family. As such, many people internalize their feelings of grief and may not express their grief or feelings of loss to others. On the other hand, cultural background may necessitate that the client's and family's public display be emotional and distressed, with loud weeping and moaning.

Although sex roles have become more unified in the past few decades, male and female reaction to death may differ. The widow who has a job may not be as emotionally distraught as the woman who has needed her husband for support. Likewise, the widower who has not taken care of the children or the house may view the future more bleakly than the man who has cooked meals and changed diapers. Some ethnic traditions may be ingrained in certain people, and the woman may be expected to be weak and need support, whereas the man may be expected to be emotionally supportive. This varies from culture to culture and from person to person.

Religious Influences

Faith and religious practices play an important role in the expression of grief, and provide comfort and solace to the person experiencing loss. Many people who have put spiritual matters in the background of their lives have found death to be an impetus for a return to earlier practices of religion. At the same time, others may blame God for the death of their loved one and turn away from God. (See Chapter 36.)

Cause of Death

Death may result from various causes, and the grief response often depends on the cause. Many deaths are sudden and involve shock as well as normal grieving in the survivors. *Death from disease* generates several types of response, including belief that the death is a punishment (for example, when acquired immunodeficiency syndrome was first diagnosed in homosexuals and drug users), terror and panic (when people are reminded of the devastation caused by plagues of earlier centuries), and guilt (when family and friends believe that they could have prevented the death). *Accidental death* often is associated with feelings of bad luck. The guilt response can be enormous, especially when children die as the result of an accident. *Death while defending a country* usually is viewed by most of society as honorable and necessary. *Violent deaths* occur daily, especially in the larger cities of North America. Suicide accounts for a great number of violent deaths; in fact, among teenagers, it has become a major concern. It also is believed that many accidental deaths are actually suicides.

The Nurse as Role Model

Holistic care of the terminally ill client and family almost always involves some personal emotional investment. It is unrealistic and unfair to expect nurses to handle circumstances surrounding death without feelings. The best policy seems to be taking the time to explore one's own feelings and express them. The nurse who neglects to deal with personal feelings about life, dying, and death is in a questionable position to analyze and consider the needs of clients facing death. Therefore, a nurse's own feelings play a major role in determining how he or she cares for a client with a terminal illness. The following are some personal questions the nurse should use to help clarify feelings about finiteness of self:

- If I could control the events that result in my own death, where would I want to be? What cause of death would I choose? Whom would I want to have present during my terminal illness?
- What fears do I have about death?
- How would I answer these same questions for a client for whom I have been caring?
- How could I improve the quality of care for a terminally ill client for whom I am caring?
- If I were a member of the client's family, what things would I want a nurse to do for me?

The nurse who cares for a client for an extended period will undergo a grief reaction when the client dies. Grief after the death of a client is natural, and the nurse should allow himself or herself to go through the grieving process rather than shut off the grief. The nurse also should address personal health needs.

Nurses caring for clients experiencing loss, grief, dying, and death will be effective role models if they can achieve the following goals:

- Identify personal losses that are influencing current state of well being and identify and utilize effective coping strategies
- Communicate openly with clients about their losses and invite a discussion of the adequacy of their coping mechanisms

Promoting Wellness

Use the assessment checklist to see how well you are responding to the losses in your life. Then develop a prescription for self-care by choosing appropriate behaviors from the list of suggestions.

Assessment Checklist

almost always	sometimes	almost never	
☐	☐	☐	1. I can name the personal losses which are presently influencing my state of well being.
☐	☐	☐	2. I have a plan for coping with these losses that is in place and helping me to cope.
☐	☐	☐	3. I understand the importance of grieving and I actually set time aside for this self-care measure.
☐	☐	☐	4. I am comfortable with my feelings and am able to give them expression.
☐	☐	☐	5. There is someone who knows and accepts me well enough to allow me to share openly and honestly.

Self-Care Behaviors

1. Make a list of the losses that are interfering with your present state of well being. These may include the loss of health; valued role, image/reputation, relationship; material object; job; person.
2. Determine whether or not you are addressing these losses in a conscious fashion, and identify coping strategies that may be of help.
3. Try implementing a "tried and true" or new coping strategy.
4. Talk about one of these losses with a friend, religious leader, or counselor/therapist. Assess your comfort level in sharing your feelings openly. Ask the person you are sharing with how they think you are responding.
5. Be honest about any maladaptive coping strategies you may be using to cope, eg, addictions, apathy ("Who cares?"), withdrawal and passivity, depression, acting out. Get any help you need to replace these maladaptive coping measures.

- Respond genuinely to the concerns and feelings of dying clients and their families; do not be afraid to cry with clients and to allow feelings to show
- Value time spent with clients and family members in which supportive presence is the primary intervention

ASSESSING

The nursing process is a helpful tool when caring for clients who are dying and their families and significant others. The needs of grieving family members are highlighted in the accompanying box. Focused assessment is directed to determining the adequacy of the client's and family's knowledge, perceptions, coping strategies (see Chapter 32), and resources. Pertinent interview questions are in the box on page 795. Physical assessment of both the dying client and of concerned family, friends, and family caregivers is essential to diagnosing some problems.

Needs of Grieving Families

Hope
- That the best care possible will be provided for their loved one
- That there is a place after death where suffering and pain cease

Participating
- In some way in what is happening
- By giving some form of care
- By feeling free to either stay at or leave the bedside
- By sharing in mutual decision making with the healthcare staff and the loved one

Being Informed
- By the medical and nursing staff on a regular basis
- So that choices and decisions can be made
- And having the right to ask questions

Support
- By having fears and concerns acknowledged, accepted, and understood
- So that anger, tears, denial, and decisions are accepted
- In coping with change
- To allow feelings of closeness and openness with the one who is dying

Spiritual Needs
- To be comforted by those who share a common faith
- To have prayer as a support
- To gain strength and comfort from God and from others

(Data from Carson, V. B. [1989]. *Spiritual dimensions of nursing practice.* Philadelphia: Saunders.)

DIAGNOSING

The data the nurse collects about how a client or the client's caregivers are responding to loss, actual or anticipated, or impending death, may lead to several different nursing diagnoses.

Response to Loss as the Problem

Nursing diagnoses that specifically address human responses to loss and impending death in the problem statement include the following: Impaired Adjustment, Caregiver Role Strain, Decisional Conflict, Ineffective Denial, Ineffective Coping, Anticipatory or Dysfunctional Grieving, Hopelessness, Ineffective Management of Therapeutic Regimen, and Powerlessness. Sample defining characteristics for these diagnoses appear in the box on page 796. The diagnoses Caregiver Role Strain, Decisional Conflict, and Grieving are worked up at the end of this chapter.

Response to Loss as the Etiology

Difficulty responding to loss or impending death may also affect other areas of human functioning and result in different diagnoses. Examples of nursing diagnoses for which the experience of loss is the etiology follow:

Anxiety related to inability to predict how the last stage of illness will play itself out
Altered Comfort related to complications of chemotherapy for end stage breast cancer
Altered Family Processes related to stress of caring for dying mother
Fatigue related to constant demands of caring for dying family member
Fear related to perceived loss of control and increasing need to be dependent in final stages of illness
Knowledge Deficit related to lack of experience of ever having to care for dying family member at home
Noncompliance related to denial of gravity of illness and impending death
Self-Esteem Disturbance related to inability to accept need for assistance as disease progresses
Spiritual Distress related to inability to reconcile diagnosis and pain with belief in a loving God
Self-Care Deficit related to waning strength as terminal illness progresses

PLANNING: EXPECTED OUTCOMES

Nursing care should be directed toward the achievement of the following goals or outcomes for dying clients and their families. The client will:

- Demonstrate freedom to express feelings, needs, fears, and concerns

Focused Assessment Guide

The Experience of Loss, Grief, Dying and Death

Assessment Priorities

Client and family's understanding of medical condition and prognosis

Client and family's attitude toward death and dying

Client's preferences concerning death: desire to be at home or in a hospital or hospice setting; decisions concerning aggressiveness of treatment, resuscitation, advanced life support, organ donation, etc.

For the incompetent client: existence of advance directive **[It is critical that the authorized decisionmaker be known to all members of the healthcare team]**

Religious beliefs

Cultural influences

Stage of grief and death reaction (denial and isolation, anger, bargaining, depression, acceptance)

Adequacy of coping behaviors

Adequacy of resources

Physiologic needs of the client: personal hygiene, pain control, nutritional and fluid needs, movement, elimination and respiratory care needs

Psychologic needs of the client and family: fear of the unknown, pain, separation, leaving loved ones, dependence; loss of dignity; unfinished business; powerlessness

Spiritual needs of the client and family: need for meaning and purpose, for love and relatedness, for forgiveness, for hope

Factors to Assess	Questions and Approaches
Adequacy of knowledge base	What have you been told about your condition? What do you know about this condition? Please describe what you have been told about your treatment options. Is there anything you don't understand about what your doctor is recommending? What else would you like to know about your present condition and treatment options? Do you know how to contact your doctor and to get the information you need/desire? *Objective is to identify whether or not the knowledge the client and family possess will allow them to make informed decisions that will serve their best interests.*
Realism of expectations/ perceptions	Have you had any previous experiences with this condition or with the death of someone you love? What are your expectations in this case? How do you see the next few weeks (days) playing out? What are your fears, hopes, concerns, worries? What good do you think might be happening in the midst of all this? *Objective is to discover if the client and family have unrealistic expectations or misperceptions about the diagnosis, prognosis, and care options that will interfere with their decision making and coping.*
Adequacy of coping strategies	Dealing with our own dying is a once-in-a-lifetime experience and sometimes we begin the process feeling totally unprepared. Tell me something about how you think you are coping with all this. How well do you think those around you are coping? How can I help you develop or tap the resources that will help you to cope better? *Objective is to identify whether the client and the client's family are using effective coping strategies. If you detect problems, try to identify coping strategies they have used effectively in the past. Also identify and address destructive habits that have not served them well in the past such as addictions, destructive relationships, passivity, acting out. Creatively problem-solve about new strategies they might try.*
Adequacy of resources	What is helping you to get through this? Do you think the resources available to you are adequate? If the sky was the limit, what help would you wish for? What is interfering with your getting the help you need? What are some of the community resources that might be of help to you? Are you using these? *Objective is to assess the adequacy of the human, financial, spiritual, and psychologic resources available to the client. Questions should be directed to determining what, if anything, is interfering with the client's using whatever resources are available to facilitate coping.*
Physical response	A physical assessment of the client and the client's family and caregivers should be performed to detect problems with coping that result in fatigue, decreased energy, decreased self-care (deficient grooming, unplanned weight loss), and other maladaptive responses.

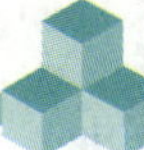

Nursing Diagnoses for Common Problems

Loss and Impending Death

Problem	Related Factors	Sample Defining Characteristics
Impaired Adjustment	Newly diagnosed terminal illness	"This can't be happening to me. . . . I know I'm going to die. . . . Why should I try and fight this? Mother fought this same diagnosis and died, why should I hope to be any different?"
Caregiver Role Strain	Hospital discharged dying client because of inadequate insurance	Spouse has dark circles under eyes, reports unable to sleep through night, decreased appetite, and general lack of energy. "I want to do everything I can for Tony, but I feel so overwhelmed. . . . I don't think anyone prepared me for everything I now find myself needing to do for him. . . . I'm always afraid that I'll hurt him or do something wrong." "I don't want to complain, but I miss being able to go out with my friends. Last week I didn't even get to church because Tony wasn't feeling well Sunday morning and asked me not to leave. . . . Sometimes I think I'll just go crazy."
Decisional Conflict	Repeat hospitalizations for aspiration pneumonia and new inability to swallow	Family has requested ethics consult because they are split about pending decisions for initiation of artificial nutrition and hydration and advisability of future hospitalizations and continued aggressive treatment; client has Alzheimer's disease and has been in a nursing home for last 5 years.
Ineffective Coping	Inability to accept death of 42-year-old son who died of a heart attack 2 years ago; failure of coping mechanisms that worked in the past	70-year-old widow who lived alone with son until his death 2 years ago has become a recluse and eats just enough to keep herself alive, seems to exist on gin, cigarettes, and chocolate. "Mothers aren't supposed to outlive their children . . . why didn't God take me first? I just want to die and be with Bernie. . . ."
Ineffective Denial	Inability to believe that she has AIDS and that husband was bisexual	Client who is just "getting her life back in order" (left abusive husband 1 year ago and is newly happily remarried) learns that she has AIDS. "This can't be happening to me . . . after all I've been through . . . I hear what you are saying but I don't believe you . . . there must be some mistake. . . ." Breaks next appointment and refuses to respond to repeated urgings to seek treatment.
Anticipatory Grieving	Knowledge that fetus is anencephalic	"I don't know how this can be happening to us. . . We've tried to do everything right. . . . We've waited for this baby for so long. . . . It's hard to believe that our baby won't be normal and that if what the doctors say is true she will only live for a few hours or days at most. . . ."
Dysfunctional Grieving	Inability to accept death of anencephalic infant; no grief resolution	Two years after birth of anencephalic infant who died 3 days after delivery, couple has failed to come to peace with child's death; divorce impending; wife has lost 15 pounds and her husband complains that she "really let herself go, she quit her job, mopes around the house all day, and isn't interested in anything anymore."

(continued)

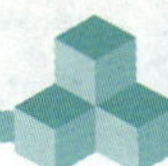

Nursing Diagnoses for Common Problems *(continued)*

Loss and Impending Death

Problem	Related Factors	Sample Defining Characteristics
Hopelessness	Inability to accept son's diagnosis of leukemia and favorable prognosis linked to knowledge of death of neighbor's son who had similar diagnosis	"Don't be leading us on. . . . We know what leukemia means, we have neighbors who lost a son to leukemia. . . . It's not true that you can treat this. . . ." Parents refuse to believe favorable prognosis; after hearing diagnosis they become apathetic and withdrawn. "Marge and Joe tried to do everything to save their son and failed, why should we even try? Nothing else in our lives has worked out."
Ineffective Management of Therapeutic Regimen (also, Powerlessness)	Suddenness of injury and inability to prepare sufficiently to provide needed in-home care	"One minute our life was perfect and then, WHAM, all of a sudden everything went wrong. If only my husband hadn't gone out that night and if only he could get his leg back. I should be doing more to help him but I just want to sit and cry. This isn't what I bargained for when we got married. I don't think I can spend the rest of my life with a cripple." Home health nurse notes that neither the client nor his wife is following through with recommended exercises, and he has broken several appointments at the rehabilitation center. Both the client and his wife seem to have given up and express no interest in therapeutic regimen.

- Identify and use effective coping strategies
- Accept need for help as appropriate and use available resources
- Make healthcare decisions reflecting personal values and goals
- Declare preferences regarding treatment options
- Report sufficient relief of pain to interact meaningfully with family and to attend to everyday concerns
- Experience a dignified and comfortable death
- (Family/significant others) resolve their grief after a suitable period of mourning and resume meaningful roles and daily activities

The client and the family should take an active role in planning for care. Such planning takes the client's preferences into consideration, facilitates the acceptance of death by the client and the family, and provides interventions to meet holistic needs. Client outcomes for specific problems related to loss, grieving, dying, and death follow later in this chapter.

IMPLEMENTING

The nurse's aims in caring for dying clients and their families include facilitating coping of the dying person and family and promoting wellness and preventing illness of the family. Specific intervention strategies follow.

Developing a Trusting Nurse–Client Relationship

Communication is a lifelong need up to the moment of death and should be maintained at all times with the client and family. To develop meaningful communications, the nurse must develop a trusting relationship with the client. This relationship is explored throughout this text. The nurse needs to develop listening skills and the ability to recognize both verbal and nonverbal cues given by the client and family. These skills are discussed in Chapter 22.

The nurse should be willing to discuss the client's fears and doubts openly and to serve as a nonjudgmental listener. A caring nurse feels at ease in crying with the grieving person and sharing experiences with fears, loneliness, and death. This allows the griever the freedom to express his or her deepest concerns. Nonverbal communication is equally important. A smile, a touching hand or stroke, and eye-to-eye contact are all meaningful. The warmth behind the gesture and the honest concern of the nurse are what count.

The sense of hearing is believed to be the last sense to leave the body; many clients retain a sense of hearing almost to the moment of death. It is kind and thoughtful of the nurse to speak to the comatose client and to encourage family members to do likewise. The nurse should explain to the client the nursing care being given and the noises in the unit.

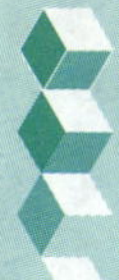

Research in Nursing: Making a Difference

Care for the Dying

Nurses committed to providing quality care for the dying and their family caregivers in both traditional and nontraditional healthcare settings face old and new challenges.

Related Research

Bramwell, L., MacKenzie, J., Laschinger, H., & Cameron, N. (1995). Need for overnight respite for primary caregivers of hospice clients. *Cancer Nursing, 18*(5), 337–343.
A major reason for admission of community hospice clients to the hospital is exhaustion of the primary caregiver. One way to prevent the problem of caregiver exhaustion may be the use of trained laypersons who remain overnight with the ill person, thereby providing respite that allows the caregiver to sleep. A survey was conducted to assess primary caregivers' appraisal of the need for overnight respite and their willingness to receive this support from trained laypersons. Thirty-seven primary caregivers who used the services of a community hospice were interviewed to determine primary caregivers' appraisals of problems, resources, and needs.

Dukes, C. S., Turpin, B. A., & Atwood, J. R. (1995). Hospice education about people with AIDS as terminally ill patients: Coping with a new epidemic of death. *American Journal of Hospice and Palliative Care, 12*(1), 25–31.
Hospice care for patients with AIDS differs from care for patients with other terminal illnesses, such as cancer. A seminar series was designed to educate regional hospice staff about these differences, and a study was designed to determine if the educational intervention was associated with improvement in AIDS-related knowledge, attitudes, or behaviors toward patients with AIDS. Quantitative and qualitative data were collected from seminar participants (n = 63) and a similar comparison group (n = 18). Findings suggest that cross-training in the cancer and AIDS hospice models of care benefits both providers and patients. Hospice staff who are trained in the AIDS care model will be equipped with the knowledge and skills needed to facilitate the care of patients with AIDS.

Henneman, E. A., Baird, B., Bellamy, P. E., Faber, L. L., & Oye, R. K. (1994). Effect of do-not-resuscitate orders on the nursing care of critically ill patients. *American Journal of Critical Care, 3*(6), 467–472.
The authors used a quasi-experimental design to compare nurses' attitudes about standards of care for critically ill patients with and without a do-not-resuscitate order. Nurses reported that they would be significantly less likely to perform a variety of physiologic monitoring modalities and interventions for patients with a do-not-resuscitate order than for patients without such an order. Patients with a do-not-resuscitate order were more likely to receive psychosocial interventions, including assessment of their spiritual needs and more flexible visiting practices. The findings suggest that "do not resuscitate" may be misinterpreted to include more than "no cardiopulmonary resuscitation" even if the patient is receiving aggressive medical management. Misinterpretation of orders not to resuscitate may be related to a variety of factors, including lack of understanding about hospital policy and ethical and moral values of the staff. The authors suggest replacing orders such as "do not resuscitate" with clearly defined resuscitation plans that are jointly determined by the multidisciplinary team, patient, and family.

Slone, M., & Stephany, T. (1995). Stressors of hospice home care nurses caring for AIDS patients: A pilot study. *American Journal of Hospice and Palliative Care, 12*(1), 32–36.
This exploratory study identified stressors of home care hospice nurses caring for hospice patients with AIDS. Five hospice home care nurses provided data obtained from demographic questionnaires and semistructured interviews. Results of this pilot study confirmed that experienced hospice nurses believe there is a difference between caring for AIDS hospice patients and non-AIDS hospice patients, and that nurses face increased stress when caring for AIDS hospice patients. Further research is needed to provide better care for the hospice patient with AIDS and to acknowledge and respond to the increased demand on the nurses who care for them.

Summary

The above studies demonstrate the difference research can make in identifying more effective ways to prepare and support caregivers of the dying. More research is needed on all fronts.

Explaining the Client's Condition and Treatment

All involved healthcare personnel should know exactly what the client and family have been told. Telling them different things puts the nurse and other team members at cross purposes and sets up distrust in the family. Because clients and families often direct questions about the client's prognosis to the nurse, it is up to the nurse to take the initiative in determining a means to be consistent in terminology, prognosis, and description of progress.

The client's condition and treatment should be explained to both the client and the family. Patience is required during explanations. They may be so grieved by the diagnosis that they do not hear all the information that is shared with them. The nurse can question them to learn how much they have retained. Then the information they missed can be repeated. Care options, as well as the expected outcomes of each option, should be fully explained.

Teaching Self-Care and Promoting Self-Esteem

The client should be encouraged to retain independence and decision making as long as possible. Personal hygiene practices and self-feeding also should be managed by the client as long as possible. Once the client is confined to bed, the creative nurse and family caregivers should attempt to find self-care activities the client can perform. When physical abilities fail, determining when to take medication (for example) may be all the control the client can retain.

Having familiar objects in view can help make the client feel more comfortable and secure. Whether the client is at home or in a healthcare agency, it is desirable to have the environment reflect personal preferences. This gives the client some degree of control when health and other activities of daily living have slipped out of the client's reach, and supports self-esteem.

In the transition from independence to interdependence and ultimately to dependence, the client may experience depression and express frustration and grief about "being a burden." It is critical for professional and nonprofessional caregivers to respond to the dying client as a person of worth whose life has meaning and value. Chapter 15 discusses practical ways nurses can use looks, touch, words, and actions to communicate respect and caring.

Teaching Family Members to Assist in Care

Preparing family members to assist in nursing care competently and confidently yields benefits to both the client and family members. The client is comforted by having loved ones near; family members are comforted by knowing that they helped comfort the client. Family members providing nursing care to the client must be supervised by the nurse.

Family members may not want to provide care themselves but want to know what to expect and how they can psychologically aid the client. The nurse can help by explaining the client's condition, what treatment the client is undergoing, and what result the family can expect from the treatment. Knowing the facts may help family members to better cope with impending loss. Bereavement resources for the survivors of a client are listed in the box on page 800.

Meeting the Needs of Dying Clients

Physiologic Needs

Physiologic care of the client involves meeting physical needs such as personal hygiene, pain control, nutritional and fluid needs, movement, elimination, and respiratory care. *Personal hygiene* includes cleanliness of the skin, hair, mouth, nose, and eyes. Frequent baths and linen changes may be necessary. The mouth and nose should be kept free of mucus, and secretions should be wiped from the eyes. The physician will determine the medication and dosage needed for *pain control*, but the client's wishes should be considered. (See Chapter 41 for a further discussion of pain control.) Some clients prefer and are able to control their own medication. Many dying clients suffer from malnutrition and dehydration, so *nutritional and fluid needs* must be addressed. The client may require nutritional support but should be encouraged to take sips of water if still able to swallow. The dying client may also elect to forego artificial nutrition and hydration since the burdens of feeding and hydrating artificially may outweigh the benefits. See the classic article by Zerwekh (1983) for a discussion of these benefits and burdens. Periodic *movement* also should be allowed; regular changes of position help prevent pressure ulcers. Problems with *elimination* include the development of incontinence, constipation, and urinary retention. Absorbent pads or a nearby bedpan may be used for incontinent clients; laxatives or enemas may be used for relieving constipation; and catheterization may be required for urinary retention. Bed linens should be changed often. *Respiratory care* can be provided by repositioning the conscious client in semi-Fowler's position; the unconscious client should be positioned in a semiprone position that allows drainage of saliva and mucus. Oxygen therapy may be necessary for some clients.

Psychologic Needs

When people speak of their fears of death, responses typically include fear of the unknown, pain, separation, leaving loved ones, loss of dignity, loss of control, and unfinished business. Kübler-Ross believes that there is still another, more overwhelming and more significant fear that often is repressed and unconscious: that of the catastrophic, destructive force that has befallen a person and that the person cannot change. Kübler-Ross points

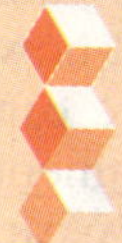

Helpscan

Bereavement Resources

The following may be of assistance to individuals who have lost loved family members or friends.

- Bereavement Publishing, Inc.
  8133 Telegraph Drive
  Colorado Springs, CO 80920
  (719) 282-1948

  Publishes *Bereavement Magazine,* which discusses grief situations through stories, articles, poems, and shared personal experiences.
- Centering Corporation
  1531 N. Saddle Creek Road
  Omaha, NE 68104-5064
  (402) 553-1200

  Offers a comprehensive list of books and pamphlets designed for those who care for the bereaved and are bereaved.
- Compassionate Friends
  P.O. Box 3696
  Oak Brook, IL 60522-3696
  (708) 990-0010

  A self-help organization offering friendship and understanding to bereaved parents and siblings.
- Pen Parents
  P.O. Box 8738
  Reno, NV 89507-8738
  (702) 826-7332
  (800) 484-1033

  A support network for those who have experienced pregnancy loss or the death of a child.
- Rivendell Resources
  P.O. Box 3272
  Ann Arbor, MI 48106-3272
  (313) 761-1960

  A quarterly bulletin of resources for the bereaved and caregivers.

out that terminally ill people communicate this fear of a destructive force but do so largely through symbolic language. A person may use nonverbal language, such as a facial expression, a particular kind of hand clasp, or, in the case of children, through drawings and manner of play with toys. Verbal communication also may be used symbolically. Two nurses, Maggie Callanan and Patricia Kelley, have provided an excellent study of the special awareness, needs, and communications of the dying (1992).

A fear of isolation, of having to face death alone, is a primary concern of the dying client. The nurse supports the client by indicating his or her presence, giving full attention, and showing that he or she cares. The presence of family members in the room should be encouraged. Reminiscences should be shared.

Spiritual Needs

Many terminally ill clients find great comfort in the support they receive from their religious faith. The nurse should aid in obtaining the services of clergy as each situation indicates.

Although not all clients follow specific spiritual or religious beliefs, most require some form of *spiritual care.* Most clients need to feel that their lives have meaning; many feel a need for hope in the face of death. The nurse should not impose his or her beliefs on the client, but should let the client know that the client's beliefs are important. The nurse should arrange for visits from a spiritual adviser if this is desired. Spiritual needs are discussed more fully in Chapter 36.

Meeting Family Needs

The nurse can provide care for the *family facing loss* by listening to the family's concerns. Family members need to verbalize their worries and fears, and nurses and other healthcare personnel can provide support by being nonjudgmental listeners. Likewise, nursing care of the *grieving family* involves communication and listening. Application of communication skills discussed in Chapter 22 and earlier in this section aids the nurse in being a nonjudgmental listener; feedback to the family can be provided by summarizing or paraphrasing, without questioning the validity of the family's emotions. All family members, including children, should be part of the grieving process.

In some instances, the nurse spends more time with the relatives than with the client, such as when the client becomes comatose. Family members may need to be reminded to get rest and to eat. Too many visitors may tire the client; when explanations are offered, most relatives readily understand this. When they want to remain at the hospital, they should be directed to a quiet place where they may relax.

The reality of death can be made less painful by preparing the family ahead of time. When the process has been explained to the family, they are better prepared to understand the needs of and to support the dying person.

The steps of the grieving process should be explained to all family members ahead of time, so that they will recognize the specific stages as they experience them and understand that the process is normal. They

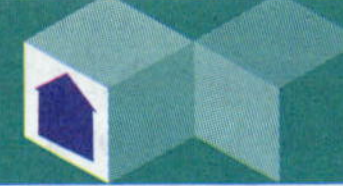

Home Care Considerations: Bridging the Gap

Assessment Priorities

When caring for clients in the end stage of a disease who are living at home, be alert for:

- Physiologic or behavioral changes in the client that signal the need for a change in the plan of palliative care
- Changes in the client's caregivers which indicate that they are becoming overwhelmed by their responsibilities in a way that places them or the client at risk
- Changes in the home environment which suggest the need for new safety considerations

When caring for clients in the end stage of a disease who are living at home and have not clarified their wishes for end-of-life care, initiate a discussion about advance directives and record their preferences regarding hospitalization, resuscitation, and life-sustaining treatment. Follow the agency's documentation guidelines. If indicated, assist in the preparation of a living will or durable power of attorney for healthcare.

Since needed changes in the plan of care may depend solely on your detection of new or developing problems, your assessment skills are critical. Always confer with an experienced colleague if you are uncertain about the significance of your findings.

Intervention Considerations

Assisted suicide may soon be a legal option in some states, and it is not unusual for nurses to receive requests to help a homebound client to die. The American Nurses Association has a position statement rejecting nurse-assisted suicide and nurse participation in direct voluntary euthanasia. It is critical for nurses caring for homebound clients to clarify their moral stance regarding suicide and direct voluntary euthanasia and to be familiar with pertinent legislation in their state/province. If this subject was not addressed in the orientation to your responsibilities, request an agency in-service or some other forum to explore how experienced nurses respond to these requests.

will be able to recognize that other members of the family are going through the same stages, perhaps at different times. This preparation allows for better understanding and communication within the family.

Death creates a change in family roles. As one person (the dying person) leaves a role, adjustments must be made within the family to compensate. Each member plays a part in that compensation. The nurse can help with these adjustments.

Responding to Requests for Suicide Assistance

Attempts to legalize assisted suicide and the media's portrayal of suicide as a defining heroic act are resulting in more and more nurses being confronted with requests for suicide assistance. Each nurse should carefully weigh the arguments for and against assisted suicide presented earlier in this chapter and know where he or she stands regarding the morality and legality of this intervention. What we believe influences what we do and do not say to clients and the way we say it. It also influences what we include in our range of therapeutic options.

Regardless of one's beliefs about the legality of assisted suicide, nurses must join other healthcare professionals in addressing the human responses that underlie requests for suicide assistance. Nursing is well positioned to offer leadership in meeting the following human needs:

Fear of losing control
Fear of not being "allowed" to die
Fear of intractable pain and overwhelming suffering
Fear of becoming increasingly dependent
Fear of loss of human dignity
Fear of an endless succession of meaningless days
Fear of dying alone
Economic fears

Providing Postmortem Care

When a client dies, the nurse's responsibilities include caring for the client's body, caring for the family, and discharging specific legal responsibilities. The latter involve ensuring that a death certificate is issued and signed, labeling the body, and reviewing organ donation arrangements, if any.

Care of the Body

After the client has been pronounced dead, the nurse is responsible for preparing the body for discharge. The body is placed in normal anatomic position to avoid pooling of blood, soiled dressings are replaced, and tubes are removed. In most cases, it is unnecessary to wash the body; the mortician normally attends to this. Some religions strictly forbid washing of the body, whereas in others, it must be performed by a special person. In cultures in which the family's washing of the deceased's body is considered the last service a family can give a loved one, the family should be given the necessary supplies and left alone in the room with the body. If an autopsy is to be performed, any tubes that were in place should not be removed. In such cases, the nurse should follow the hospital's policy.

The nurse is legally responsible for placing identification tags on both the shroud or garment the body is clothed in and the ankle to ensure that the body can be identified even if it is separated from its shroud. The nurse also should place an identification tag on the client's dentures or other prostheses to ensure that these are received by the mortician. The client's body may have to be placed in the hospital's morgue refrigerator if mortuary arrangements were not made before the client's death. *The importance of proper and complete identification cannot be overemphasized.*

If the client died of a communicable disease, the body may require special handling to prevent the spread of that disease. Requirements for such handling usually are specified by local law and are contingent on the disease-causing organism, mode of transmission, and other characteristics.

Care of the Family

After a client has died, the nurse provides support and care to the client's family. In most cases, this involves listening to the family's expressions of grief, loss, and helplessness. Because comforting words often are difficult to find, the nurse should offer solace and support by being an attentive listener. Family members may need to see the client's body to accept the death fully; in such cases, the nurse should arrange for family members to view the body before it is discharged to the mortician.

Sudden death creates unique problems for the family. In the case of sudden injury or illness, the physical needs of the client are paramount to the healthcare team. This means that family members are not provided as much emotional support or information as they would be if the client's illness were prolonged, nor are they permitted to exercise as many options regarding the client's care. The family that loses a member unexpectedly has not had an opportunity to begin the grieving process or to share in grieving with the deceased person. Family members should be allowed to express grief and given emotional support. Most often the family is in the emergency department waiting room when death is confirmed. They are stunned, bewildered, and numb. They should not be rushed from the waiting room, but rather provided a private place to begin their grieving. The nurse should acknowledge their shock and listen to their grief. The family needs guidance in making plans and help in making decisions.

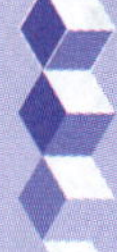

Through the Eyes of a Student

We had had several day-shift clinical rotations, but this was our first evening clinical experience. We were unsure as to what the evening would be like. We knew the evening would provide us with a new outlook on nursing, but we were not prepared for what unfolded.

I had been taking care of a client when another nursing student asked if I would check in on her client while she had her dinner break. This client was known to each of the students, because we all had the pleasure of caring for him. I was told he was lying in bed watching television and that his code status had been changed to "DNR" (do not resuscitate) just that day. When I went to check on him, I found him lying in bed but not watching television. His eyes were closed as if he were sleeping peacefully. I spoke his name several times without a response. At the same time, I was also checking for a radial pulse. When I couldn't find his pulse, I swiftly walked to find the instructor. Together we went back to him and assessed his condition. There were no radial or carotid pulses. His chest was not rising and the instructor listened to his heart with a stethoscope. There wasn't a heartbeat. I stood there feeling helpless and low-spirited. This was a man whom we had all grown close to. His family came to see him and to say a few final words. Tears were shed not only by his family but by those of us who had cared for him.

Our first evening clinical was an extremely emotional night. We were all quiet as we walked down the hallway to go home. The student who was caring for him that night was stopped by his daughter and two young granddaughters. One granddaughter was wearing his hat and the other was carrying his belt. This man's daughter was broken-hearted by his death, yet needed to know that he wasn't alone when he died. The student told her that I had been the one with him. The daughter seemed relieved to know that he was not by himself when he died.

As I look back on that evening, I'm sad that this man is no longer with us. I did not know him for very long, but he touched me in a way that helped me understand the true meaning of nursing: to care not only for the sick, disabled, or enfeebled, but also to be human and offer support for grieving families.

—Joyce A. Shearman, Delaware County Community College, Media, Pennsylvania

It is proper for the nurse who was caregiver or who took care of the client for a prolonged period to attend the funeral. It also is appropriate for the nurse to make a follow-up call to the client's family after the funeral or memorial service to offer both concern and care for the family's well being. Follow-up visits are important to give support to the family. If the nurse assesses that the family is not coping well (dysfunctional grief), appropriate referral should be made.

Care of Other Clients

Because it is not unusual for nurses in institutional settings to provide care to more than one client at a time, after the death of one client, the nurse must continue to provide care to the other clients. Other clients often are aware of a death and may need to be consoled; this is particularly true of a client who has shared a room with the deceased client. Other clients may have grief reactions and should be supported through the grief process by the nurse. Death of a client may cause depression in other clients and may make them more aware of their own future deaths.

EVALUATING

The plan of nursing care for dying clients is effective if clients meet the outcome of a comfortable, dignified death and family members resolve their grief after a suitable time of mourning and resume meaningful life roles and activities.

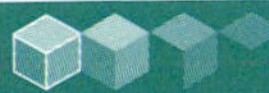

Nursing Process in Clinical Practice

The nurse uses the nursing process to address the grieving of dying clients and their families. The nursing care for two common diagnoses that address the needs of dying clients and their families follow.

Grieving

Grieving may be defined as the state in which an individual or family experiences a natural human response involving psychosocial and physiologic reactions to an actual or perceived loss (person, object, function, status, relationship). NANDA nursing diagnoses include:

Anticipatory Grieving: Intellectual and emotional responses and behaviors by which individuals work through the process of modifying self-concept based on the perception of potential loss (NANDA, 1994)

Dysfunctional Grieving: Extended, unsuccessful use of intellectual and emotional responses by which individuals attempt to work through the process of modifying self-concept based upon the perception of loss (NANDA, 1994)

Since nurses encounter clients dealing with anticipatory grieving more frequently than clients dysfunctionally grieving, assessment priorities, expected outcomes, and interventions will be given for anticipatory grieving.

Assessment Priorities

- Determine the exact nature of the anticipated or potential loss.
- Explore factors that are contributing to the importance or significance of the anticipated loss.
- Assess concerns, fears, feelings, and hopes related to the anticipated loss.
- Assess adequacy of knowledge and coping mechanisms.
- Recognize personal strengths and available resources, including present support system.

Expected Outcomes

The client(s) will:

- Express grief openly and progress through stages of grief with appropriate grief work
- Share concerns with significant others and seek needed help
- Make decisions about the future that advance best interests
- Demonstrate eventual resolution of grief by self-report, appearance, and resumption of usual activities of daily living

Interventions

Interventions for anticipatory grieving are determined by the type of loss (eg, body part; death of self, a significant other, or child), the extent of the loss to the individual and family, and what other support the individual or family has. Examples of interventions are the following:

- Use interpersonal skills to demonstrate empathy for client's situation and commitment to client's well being.
- Encourage the client to share concerns, feelings, fears, and hopes openly.
- Respond to inquiries honestly, compassionately, and in a manner that does not deprive the clients of realistic hope.
- Promote grief work through each stage of grieving (see accompanying box). Support the client and

Stages of Grief and Related Grief Work

Denial

- Initially support and then strive to increase the development of awareness (when individual indicates readiness for awareness)

Isolation

- Listen and spend designated time consistently with person and family
- Offer the person and family opportunity to explore their emotions
- Reflect on past losses and acknowledge loss behavior (past and present)

Depression

- Begin with simple problem solving and move toward acceptance
- Enhance self-worth through positive reinforcement
- Identify the level of depression and indications of suicidal behavior or ideas
- Be consistent and establish times daily to speak with the person and family

Anger

- Allow for crying to release this energy
- Listen to and communicate concern
- Encourage concerned support from significant others as well as professional support

Guilt

- Listen and communicate concern
- Allow for crying
- Promote more direct expression of feelings
- Explore methods to resolve grief

Fear

- Help the person and family recognize the feeling
- Explain that this will help cope with life
- Explore the person's and family's attitudes about loss, death, etc.

Rejection

- Allow for verbal expression of this feeling state to diminish the emotional strain
- Recognize that expression of anger may create a rejection of self to significant others

(Carpenito, L. J. [1995]. *Nursing diagnosis: Application to clinical practice* [6th ed.]. Philadelphia: Lippincott, pp. 421-422. Used with permission.)

"nudge" the client to begin the next stage of grieving as appropriate.

- Make appropriate referrals (see earlier listing of bereavement resources).
- Alert the client who is moving through the grief work slowly of the signs of dysfunctional grieving and instruct about how to obtain help should this happen; referral for counseling may be indicated.

Decisional Conflict

Clients and the surrogate decision makers for incompetent clients frequently feel overwhelmed when they need to make life-and-death decisions about end-of-life care. The NANDA diagnosis for this response follows:

Decisional Conflict: The state of uncertainty about course of action to be taken when choice among competing actions involves risk, loss, or challenge to personal life values (NANDA, 1994)

Assessment Priorities

The objective of assessment is to identify individuals and families who are at high risk for decisional conflict and to provide the support they need to make appropriate end-of-life care decisions that advance the client's interests before problems develop. Potential problems when this need is overlooked include postponement of decision making, which interferes with the client receiving optimal care; vacillation in decision making, which disturbs continuity of care for the client; and escalation of conflict concerning decision making, which may result in a stand-off between participating parties—the client, individual family members, and healthcare professionals.

- Detect difficulties with making decisions: fear; insufficient or erroneous information; inadequate support; conflict between religious convictions, personal moral beliefs, and choice one wants to make; reluctance to assume responsibility for making life-and-death decision.
- Identify what is causing the decision making to be hard for the client/family and what type of information or support could reverse this.
- Identify potential conflicts between what the client wants and what his or her family or caregivers believe should be done.
  - Observe the client or his/her surrogate decision makers for physical signs of distress which reflect feeling overwhelmed by the decision that needs to be made: signs of fatigue and general exhaustion; signs of agitation and distress; signs of growing anger and alienation.
  - Read the chart carefully to identify decisions that are pending and note the lack of movement toward a decision or toward resolution of existing conflict.

Expected Outcomes

The morally and legally valid decision-maker will:

- Describe care options (including the option of nontreatment), listing the advantages and disadvantages of each
- Seek clarification of options, if necessary, and whatever support is needed
- Express fears, concerns, and hopes
- Make an informed and voluntary choice
  - Make end-of-life decisions that reflect the client's values and goals, advancing his or her interests
  - Make end-of-life decisions that are consistent with the aims of medicine and nursing

Interventions

Nursing measures revolve around identifying and supporting the morally and legally valid decision-maker. The following should be considered:

- Competent clients—those who can (1) understand the information needed to make the decision, (2) reason in accord with a relatively consistent set of values, and (3) communicate a preference—have the right to consent to and to refuse any and all indicated medical treatment.
- Surrogates of previously competent clients are to be guided by what is known about the client's values and preferences. These surrogates may be designated in an advance directive or there may be state or province law designating a hierarchy of surrogates, eg, spouse, parent, adult child, sibling; the morally valid surrogate is the one who best knows the client and the client's preferences.
- Surrogates deciding for a never-competent client (child or profoundly retarded adult) must be guided by a determination of what is in the client's best interests by referring to more objective and socially shared values.

The nurse clarifies the goal of treatment (cure, stabilization of functioning, preparation for a comfortable and dignified death) and makes sure that treatment decisions are consistent with this goal. Nursing intervention may be helpful in making sure that everyone is clear about the goal of care and changes in the goal of care as the client's condition changes. Since some physicians are reluctant to accept preparation for a comfortable, dignified death as an appropriate goal of medicine, some clients have received unwanted care which needlessly prolonged their dying. Conversely, decisions are being made today for financial and other reasons which deprive clients of wanted end-of-life care.

The nurse serves as an advocate for the client and the family unless what the client/family wants violates the profession of nursing and nursing's code of ethics or one's own conscience. Interventions include:

- Providing whatever information and support the client/family needs to make an informed and voluntary decision
- Referring the client/family to sources that can clarify problematic aspects of the decision, eg, religious authority, ethicist, legal counsel
- Identifying and addressing coercive influences on decision making, being sensitive to cultural norms; for example, whereas a controlling husband may be violating his wife's freedom to make autonomous choices in one culture, in another it is customary for the husband (or male elder in the family) to make choices for a woman.

  Documentation of end-of-life care preferences of competent, or previously competent, clients is important. This includes a written record of communication, a living will, durable power of attorney for healthcare, and an advance medical directive. These preferences must be communicated to those who are ordering care.
- Mediating sources of conflict
- Refering client/family to ethics consult team or ethics committee if conflict cannot be resolved

Client Care Study

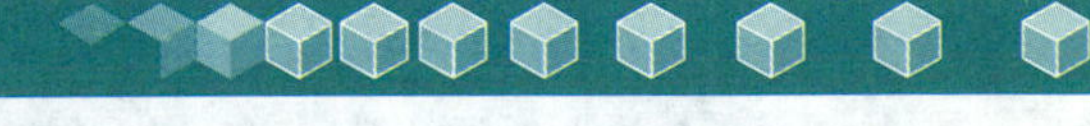

The Espositas have been married for 19 years and have two children, Jorge, who is 16, and Marita, who is 13. It has been 2 years since Mrs. Esposita was diagnosed with ovarian cancer, and this period has been difficult for the entire family. She has had several hospitalizations because of bowel obstructions and returned home more debilitated each time. At present she is extremely cachexic and in the end-stage of her illness. She initially tried aggressive treatment, and several chemotherapy regimens failed. During her last hospitalization 2 months ago, a decision was made not to continue aggressive therapy and Mrs. Esposita insisted on returning home to die.

The nurse who has been visiting Mrs. Esposita at home asked for assistance from her colleagues in devising a plan of care for Mr. Esposita. Until now, Mrs. Esposita wanted nothing to do with the local hospice because of a reported "bad experience" a neighbor had. Her insurance will not provide for all the home nursing care she needs, and her husband and children have been trying to meet her needs for nursing as well as run the house and meet their own needs. A demanding woman,

Mrs. Esposita never seems satisfied with anything anyone does, and the family is looking utterly frustrated, angry, and fatigued. Jorge is coping by "opting out"; he frequently spends the night with friends and doesn't even call home to report on his whereabouts. Marita's grades have fallen, and she has dropped out of cheerleading and other school activities so that she can take care of her mother. Mr. Esposita, who been silent until now, recently confided that he doesn't know how much longer he can go on this way, and seemed horrified to hear himself say, "I just wish she would die already and get this all over with!" He is very concerned about the changes in his children and feels powerless to change what is happening. For her part, Mrs. Esposita seems oblivious to her family's needs and, even in her weakened state, multiplies pleas for assistance. She seems to be afraid of dying and never wants to be left alone.

Core Competencies

To implement the plan of care for Mr. Esposita the nurse needs the following specialized abilities:

Cognitive Competencies

- Knowledge of the defining characteristics of caregiver role strain and the principles and rationale for nursing care of these caregivers

Interpersonal Competencies

- Ability to establish a trusting nurse–client relationship which communicates an understanding of the caregiver's burdens and respect for the positive choices the caregiver is making to meet his own needs and those of his family
- Ability to affirm the worth of the caregiver and to elicit and support new coping mechanisms
- Strong advocacy and counseling skills

Ethical/Legal Competencies

- Knowledge of professional responsibilities in this situation and execution of these responsibilities in a legally defensible manner
- Commitment to meet the needs of both Mrs. Esposita and her family, especially her husband
- Sense of personal accountability

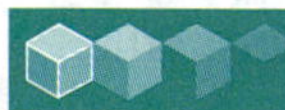

Nursing Plan of Care

for Mrs. Esposita and Her Family

Nursing Diagnosis: Caregiver Role Strain related to multiple losses and burdens associated with caregiving responsibilities as manifested by self-report, breakdown in family relationships, fatigue, and anger.

Expected Outcome:

- Mr. Esposita will talk openly about his feelings and share his frustrations about his present situation

Nursing Interventions	Rationale	Evaluative Statement
Plan visits for when there is time for private conversation with Mr. Esposita; initiate conversations by telling him that it is not unusual for family caregivers to feel fatigued, powerless, frustrated, angry, and emotionally distant. Encourage him to talk about what he is feeling: "You seemed surprised at yourself when you said that you wished your wife would 'just die.' This isn't an unusual wish for someone in your situation. . . . Tell me more about what you are feeling now. . . ."	This will normalize what Mr. Esposita is experiencing and communicate that someone cares about him and about what he is experiencing. Simply giving voice to what he is feeling and sharing this with a healthcare professional may help him to accept and address what he takes to be negative and possibly shameful feelings.	10/15/97 Goal partially met. Mr. Esposita states that he feels better now that he is sharing some of what he's been holding in for such a long time, but he still believes that if he was really a good husband he wouldn't feel this way. Also states that it is hard for him to find words to express everything that he is feeling. **Revision:** Continue to encourage Mr. Esposita to talk about what he is experiencing and provide a private opportunity for this to happen. *E. McLoughlin, RN*

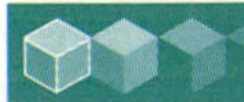

Nursing Plan of Care *(continued)*

for Mrs. Esposita and Her Family

Expected Outcome:

- By 10/17/97 Mr. Esposita will develop a realistic caregiving plan which matches his ability to care with his wife's need for care and which identifies other resources for his wife's unmet needs

Nursing Interventions	Rationale	Evaluative Statement
Assist Mr. Esposita to identify what his wife's actual needs for care are; how much of this care it is reasonable to expect the family to provide; and other potential caregiving sources.	Mr. Esposita may need "permission" to *not* meet his wife's unrealistic needs. The nurse's authority may be useful in helping him to believe that he can be a good and faithful husband and still fail to meet her expectations. Identifying other caregiving resources will ensure that Mrs. Esposita's needs will be met.	10/17/97 Goal not met. To date Mr. Esposita has been unable to identify any additional caregivers for Mrs. Esposita and continues to feel the need to assume all responsibility for her care when he is home. **Revision:** Bring list of community resources to Mr. Esposita including church group and plan with him to contact these sources. Reinforce that it is OK to ask for help. *E. McLoughlin, RN*
Explain to Mrs. Esposita that her family may not be able to meet all her needs for care but that every effort will be made to ensure these needs are met by other caregivers.	Even if the nurse's sympathies are with the family it is critical to communicate to the client that you are committed to her and intent on doing all in your power to ensure that her needs are met. If the client's needs are met it will improve her relationships with her family.	
Assist Mr. Esposita to identify and use new resources: identify at least one new support person who can sit with Mrs. Esposita and relieve the family of some of this burden; explore the family's reluctance to use hospice and evaluate other community resources. Use appropriate referrals.	The family may be feeling unnecessarily overwhelmed because they have failed to explore the availability of other resources. A gentle push may be needed to make this happen. If a "sitter" can be obtained for several hours in the evening, this would give Mr. Esposita time after work to do something with his children or for himself.	

Expected Outcome:

- By 10/20/97 Mr. Esposita will report feeling more in control and less depressed and angry

Nursing Interventions	Rationale	Evaluative Statement
Lead Mr. Esposita in a discussion that aims to identify everything that is making him feel powerless; then list those factors over which he has no control and those he can influence or change.	This will break the cycle of his thinking that there is nothing at present over which he can exert control. Simply making the list is a first step towards taking action.	10/20/97 Goal met. Mr. Esposita reports that even though most of his situation remains unchanged, he no longer feels powerless and is less depressed and angry. He expressed gratitude for this intervention and says it has given him new energy. *E. McLoughlin, RN*

(continued)

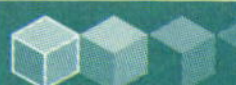

Nursing Plan of Care *(continued)*

for Mrs. Esposita and Her Family

Nursing Actions	Rationale	Evaluative Statement
Provide opportunities for Mr. Esposita to control decision making over those aspects of his life and his wife's care for which he can exert control. Affirm constructive decision making and ask him how it feels to be "back in control" of at least some aspects of his life. Discuss with Mr. Esposita those factors he can change and assist him in making decisions.	This is an example of "guided discovery"; you are allowing Mr. Esposita to experience himself as once again in charge and to allow this experience to define his self-image. Reinforcement of his success affirms his self-image of one who is in charge. Types of support that can be given to caregivers include emotional (concern, trust), appraisal (affirms self-worth), informational (useful advice), and instrumental assistance or tangible goods.	

Sample Documentation

10/17/97, 12 pm, Nursing

Met with Mr. Esposita this am and talked about the plan to identify other caregivers who might be able to "sit" with his wife on some evenings in order to give him time to do things for his children and himself. He reported no progress in identifying anyone but also stated that he hadn't really made any efforts to locate someone: "Who would want to help us? Besides, I wouldn't want to inflict my wife and her moods on anyone right now." I explained that there are many individuals and groups who provide exactly this type of assistance and that his wife's moods were not uncommon for someone in her situation. We then made a list of possible caregiver resources, including some family members who had earlier expressed an interest in helping out, the parish nurse service from his church, and finally the local hospice. If the first two sources do not work out, will explore family's reluctance to use hospice resources more carefully since this may be their best hope. Will evaluate progress made on 10-21-97.

E. McLoughlin, RN

Key Points

- Everyone experiences losses at various points in the life continuum. Such losses can be actual, perceived, physical, psychological, or anticipatory. Loss can have an effect on the developmental stages of the human life span, especially in children.
- Grief is the emotional response to loss, and grief reactions can be divided into identifiable stages. Grief can be manifested both emotionally and physically, and grief reactions are influenced by development, family and socioeconomic factors, and religious and cultural influences.
- Like grief, dying can be broken down into identifiable and overlapping stages.
- Nurses should be familiar with the clinical signs of approaching or impending death and three definitions of death.
- Clients and families increasingly look to nurses for information, advice, and support when making end-of-life treatment decisions. Nurses need to recognize the ethical, spiritual, and legal ramifications of these decisions.
- Stage of development, family, socioeconomic factors, culture, religion, and the cause of death can all influence an individual's experience of loss, grief, and dying.
- Dying clients have various needs, ranging from the need for open communication to physiologic, psychological, and spiritual needs. They should maintain self-care as long as possible.
- Families of dying clients also need open communication, and may want to assist the nurse in providing care. This is considered a healthy experience for both the client and family members.

- The nurse should provide emotional support for the grieving family by being an attentive, nonjudgmental listener and a good communicator.
- The nurse has specific responsibilities at the time of a client's death, including ensuring that a death certificate is issued, caring for the body, placing identification tags on the shroud and body, ensuring that the body is discharged to the proper party, and caring for the family.
- The nurse should provide care to other clients who are affected by the loss.

Study Questions

1. A woman who is firmly committed to natural childbirth and who has attended each natural childbirth class in preparation for her experience of labor and delivery undergoes a cesarean delivery when her fetus displays signs of distress. Inconsolable, she cries and calls herself a failure as a mother. Her loss may best be described as
   a. actual
   b. perceived
   c. psychological
   d. combination of above
2. The period of acceptance of loss and grief during which the person learns to deal with experienced loss is best termed
   a. anticipatory grieving
   b. bereavement
   c. mourning
   d. stages of death and dying
3. When you interview an 82-year-old resident in a nursing home, she tells you that she has never gotten over the death of her son who died 20 years ago. She reports that her life fell apart after that and she never again felt like herself or was able to enjoy life. This type of grief is best described as
   a. abbreviated
   b. anticipatory
   c. dysfunctional
   d. inhibited
4. A client with AIDS whom you have been visiting at home tells you "I'm no longer afraid of dying. I think I've made my peace with everyone and I'm actually ready to move on." This reflects his progress to which stage of death and dying?
   a. acceptance
   b. anger
   c. bargaining
   d. denial
5. When you next visit this dying client with AIDS he breaks down and cries and tells you that it is unfair that he should have to die now when he's finally made peace with his family and wants to live. You are shocked by this change in his mood. Your best reply would be
   a. "You can't be feeling this way. You have to proceed through the stages of dying in an orderly progression and you've just moved backwards."
   b. "It does seem unfair . . . tell me more about how you are feeling. . . ."
   c. "You'll be alright . . . who knows how much time any of us has to enjoy relationships with those we love. You are lucky to have had the opportunity to make your peace."
   d. "Tell me about your pain. Did it keep you awake last night?"
6. Which definition of death is gaining in popularity as more people believe that critical human functions are personality, conscious life, and the capacity for remembering, judging, reasoning, acting, enjoying, and worrying?
   a. heart–lung death
   b. higher-brain death
   c. personhood death
   d. whole-brain death
7. If your client tells you that he has no one he trusts to make healthcare decisions for him in the event that he becomes incapacitated, you should help him to prepare
   a. combination advance medical directive
   b. durable power of attorney for healthcare
   c. living will
8. Which of the following nurse responses would be endorsed by the American Nurses' Association?
   a. a nurse promises a dying client that he will do everything possible to keep her comfortable but that he cannot administer an injection or overdose to cause her death
   b. a nurse tells a dying client who is on a ventilator that under no condition can he be removed from the ventilator because this is active euthanasia and it is expressly forbidden by the Code for Nurses
   c. after exhausting every intervention in her bag of tricks to keep a dying client comfortable the nurse says, "I think you are now at a point where I'm prepared to do what you've been asking me. Let's talk about when and how you want to die."
   d. in response to a client who asks for assistance in committing suicide a nurse replies, "I'm personally opposed to assisted suicide but I'll find you a colleague who can help you."
9. You are caring for a comatose client whose primary diagnosis is breast cancer but who has suf-

fered multiple complications and who is now in the end stages of her illness. She has been in the medical intensive care unit for 3 weeks. Her husband tells you that he and his wife often talked about the end of her life and that she was very clear about not wanting aggressive treatment which would merely prolong her dying. You both agree that this seems to be all that therapy is now doing for her. Which of the following orders would you recommend the husband speak to her physician about
   a. comfort measures only
   b. do not hospitalize
   c. do not resuscitate
   d. slow code only
10. If you are involved in the terminal weaning of a client you will want to do all of the following *except*
   a. participate in the decision making process by offering the family information about the advantages and disadvantages of continued ventilatory support
   b. explain to the family what will happen at each phase of the weaning and offer support
   c. check the orders for sedation and analgesia and make sure that the anticipated death is comfortable and dignified
   d. tell the family that death will occur almost immediately after the client is removed from the ventilator
11. All of the following diagnoses may apply to a young couple who gave birth to a premature infant with serious respiratory problems who has been in the neonatal intensive care unit for the last 3 months. The couple has a 22-month-old son at home. Which diagnosis best fits the following set of assessment data: report of chronic fatigue and decreased energy, guilt about neglecting son at home, shortness of temper with one another, apprehension about continued ability to go on this way.
   a. anticipatory grieving
   b. ineffective coping
   c. caregiver role strain
   d. powerlessness
12. Which of the nursing actions described below would you correct if you saw a nursing assistant doing this?
   a. talking to a comatose client
   b. sitting on the bed of a dying client holding her hand and crying
   c. agreeing with the daughter of a dying resident with Alzheimer's disease that the burdens associated with artificially feeding her father may outweigh the benefits
   d. telling a dying client to sit back and relax and that she will wash him because it's easier that way
13. Which of the following nursing actions violates the standards of caring for the body after a client has been pronounced dead?
   a. keeping the client in a comfortable sitting position until the family has arrived and said their good-byes
   b. placing identification tags on both the shroud and the ankle
   c. removing soiled dressings and tubes
   d. preparing to transfer the body to the morgue
14. The family of a client who has just died requests to be alone with the body and asks for supplies to wash the body. You know that the mortician usually washes the body. Your best response is
   a. inform the family that there is no need for them to wash the body since the mortician does this
   b. explain that hospital policy forbids their being alone with the deceased client and that hospital supplies are only to be used by hospital personnel
   c. give the supplies but watch the family so that nothing unusual happens
   d. provide the requested supplies and ask if this request is linked to their religious or cultural customs and if there is anything else you can do to be of assistance
15. A 70-year-old woman who has had a number of strokes refuses further life-sustaining interventions including artificial nutrition and hydration. She is competent, understands the consequences of her actions, is not depressed, and persists in refusing treatment. Her doctor is adamant that she cannot be allowed to die this way and her daughter agrees. An ethics consult has been placed. Who is the appropriate decision maker?
   a. client
   b. daughter
   c. doctor
   d. ethics consult team

Answers With Rationale

1. The correct answer is *d.* Each of the above are only partially correct since there are elements of the loss of the type of delivery she values which are actual, perceived, *and* psychological.
2. The correct answer is *c.* Mourning is defined as the period of acceptance of loss and grief during which the person learns to deal with experienced loss. The text offers other definitions for anticipatory grieving, bereavement, and the stages of death and dying.
3. The correct answer is *c.* Abbreviated grief and anticipatory grief are both types of normal grief, and given the length of time this resident's grief has lasted and its effects on her life, it is not normal. Since she is able to give expression to her grief, inhibited grief is not the correct answer.

By a process of elimination the correct answer is dysfunctional grief.

4. The correct answer is *a*. The client's statement does *not* reflect anger, bargaining, or denial so by a process of elimination acceptance is the correct choice.
5. The correct answer is *b*; you want to validate that you have heard what the client is saying and invite him to share more of his feelings, concerns, and fears. You do *not* want offer false reassurance (*c*), nor use diversion (*d*): both of these strategies would communicate your lack of interest in what he is really feeling. It is simply not true that people have to move through these stages in an orderly fashion (*a*).
6. The correct answer is *b* because the functions described are controlled by the cortex, or higher brain. There is no such thing as personhood death.
7. The correct answer is *c*. The living will is a document whose precise purpose is to allow individuals to record specific instructions about the type of healthcare they would like to receive in particular end-of-life situations. Both the combination directive and the durable power of attorney involve appointing someone to make decisions—something this client is reluctant to do.
8. The correct answer is *a*. The ANA states that nurse-assisted suicide and participation in active euthanasia violates the Code for Nurses and the ethical traditions of the profession. This makes *c* and *d* incorrect, since it does not matter if a nurse's personal morality allows him or her to accept assisted suicide. Removing ventilatory support is not necessarily active euthanasia and is not expressly forbidden by the Code for Nurses.
9. The correct response is *a*, comfort measures only, since she would want all aggressive treatment to be stopped at this point and all care to be directed to a comfortable, dignified death. Since she is already in the hospital there is no need for *b* at this point, and a do-not-resuscitate order is not sufficiently comprehensive. One should never recommend performing a slow code since it violates good practice.
10. The correct answer is *d* since *a*, *b*, and *c* are all nursing interventions which should be carried out by the nurse involved in terminal weaning. Since there are no guarantees how any client will respond once removed from a ventilator and since it is very possible for the client to breathe on his or her own and live for hours, days, and, rarely, even weeks, the family should definitely *not* be told that death will occur immediately.
11. The correct answer is *c*; while it is true that each of the diagnoses listed might apply to the couple described, the defining characteristics for the NANDA diagnosis Caregiver Role Strain fit the set of assessment data provided.
12. The correct answer is *d*. *a* and *b* are acceptable and desirable nursing interventions and if the nursing assistant is experienced he/she may very well be in a position to do *c*. Since it is good to encourage dying clients to be as active as possible for as long as possible it is generally *not* good practice to perform basic self-care measures the client can perform simply because it is "easier" to do it this way.
13. The correct answer is *a*. *b*, *c*, and *d* are all indicated nursing interventions and consistent with standards of care. Since the body should be placed in normal anatomic position to avoid pooling of blood, leaving the body in a sitting position is contraindicated.
14. The correct answer is *d*. *a* ignores the needs of the family and reflects an ignorance of or insensitivity to cultural and religious practices. *b* is simply not true. *c* presumes that the family is up to no good purpose and, unless you have reason to suspect something out of the ordinary, is simply uncalled for.
15. The correct answer is *a*. Since this client is competent she has the right to refuse therapy which she finds to be disproportionately burdensome, even if this hastens her death. Neither her daughter nor her doctor have the authority to assume her decision-making responsibilities unless she asks them to do this. The ethics consult team is not a decision-making body; it can make recommendations but has no authority to order anything.

Bibliography

Amado, A. J., Grow, V., & Nofziger, J. (1995). An evaluation of hospice care with terminally ill cancer patients. *Caring, XIV*(11), 27–30.

Amenta, M. O., & Shubert, V. (1995). Hospice care can obviate the need for suicide. *Home Healthcare Nurse, 13*(4), 72–74.

American Geriatrics Society Ethics Committee. (1995). The care of dying patients: a position statement from the American Geriatrics Society. *Journal of the American Geriatrics Society, 43*, 577–578.

American Geriatrics Society Public Policy Committee. (1991). Voluntary active euthanasia. [Position statement]. *Journal of the American Geriatrics Society, 39*(8), 826.

American Nurses Association. (1991). Position statement on promotion of comfort and relief of pain in dying patients. Washington, DC: ANA.

American Nurses Association. (1995). *American Nurses Association position statement on assisted suicide.* Washington, DC: ANA.

Badger, J. M. (1994). Reaching out to the suicidal patient. *American Journal of Nursing, 94*(3), 24–31.

Baggs, J. G., & Schmitt, M. H. (1995). Intensive care decisions about level of aggressiveness of care. *Research in Nursing and Health, 18*(4), 345–355.

Beauchamp, T. L., & Veatch, R. M. (1996). *Ethical issues in death and dying* (2nd ed.). Upper Saddle River, NJ: Prentice Hall.

Bergevin, P. R. (1995). Hospice techniques: Creating the story of a life. *American Journal of Hospice and Palliative Care, 12*(6), 11, 27.

Bramwell, L., MacKenzie, J., Laschinger, H., & Cameron, N. (1995). Need for overnight respite for primary caregivers of hospice clients. *Cancer Nursing, 18*(5), 337–343.

Brown, P. S., & Sefansky, S. (1995). Enhancing bereavement care in the pediatric ICU. *Critical Care Nurse, 15*(5), 59–64.

Callanan, M., & Kelley, P. (1992). *Final gifts.* New York: Poseidon Press.

Campbell, C. S. (1992). Religious ethics and active euthanasia in a pluralistic society. *Kennedy Institute of Ethics Journal, 2*(3), 253–277.

Campbell, C. S., Hare, J., & Matthews, P. (1995). Conflicts of conscience: Hospice and assisted suicide. *Hastings Center Report, 25*(3), 36–43.

Campbell, M. L. (1994). Terminal weaning. *Nursing, 24*(9), 34–39.

Carpenito, L. J. (1995). *Nursing diagnosis: Application to clinical practice* (6th ed.). Philadelphia: Lippincott.

Carson, V. B. (1989). *Spiritual dimensions of nursing practice.* Philadelphia: Saunders.

Catholic Health Association. (1993 March). Care of the dying: A Catholic perspective. [Special Section]. *Health Progress,* 34–38.

Chabelewski, F., & Norris, M. K. G. (1994). The gift of life: Talking to families about tissue and organ donation. *American Journal of Nursing, 94*(6), 28–33.

Clark, M. D. (1984). Healthy and unhealthy grief behaviors. *Occupational Health Nursing, 32*(12), 633–635.

Curtin, L. (1994). DNR in the OR: Ethical concerns and hospital policies. *Nursing Management, 25*(2), 29–31.

Czerwiec, M. (1996). When a loved one is dying: Families talk about nursing care. *American Journal of Nursing, 96*(5), 32–36.

Dukes, C. S., Turpin, B. A., & Atwood, J. R. (1995). Hospice education about people with AIDS as terminally ill patients: Coping with a new epidemic of death. *American Journal of Hospice and Palliative Care, 12*(1), 25–31.

Dyer, I. D. (1993). Breaking the news: Informing visitors that a patient died. *Intensive Critical Care Nurse, 9*(1), 2–10.

Edwards, B. S. (1994). When the family can't let go. *American Journal of Nursing, 94*(1), 52–56.

Engel, G. L. (1964). Grief and grieving. *American Journal of Nursing, 64*(9), 93–98.

Eriksen, J., Rodney, P., & Starzomski, R. (1995). When is it right to die? *Canadian Nurse, 91*(8), 29–34.

Evans, J. (1993). Crisis, grief and loss. *Canadian Nurse, 89*(8), 40–43.

Ferdinand, R. (1995). "I'd rather die than live this way." *American Journal of Nursing, 95*(12), 42–48.

Finch, E., & Robins-Holm, E. (1994). Patients at risk of suicide. *Canadian Nurse, 90*(7), 31–34.

Furukawa, M.M. (1996). Meeting the needs of the dying patient's family. *Critical Care Nurse, 16*(1), 51–62.

Gonda, T. A., & Ruark, J. E. (1984). *Dying dignified: The health professional's guide to care.* Menlo Park, CA: Addison-Wesley.

Haight, B. K. (1995). Suicide risk in frail elderly people relocated to nursing homes. *Geriatric Nursing, 16*(3), 104–107.

The Hastings Center. (1987). *Guidelines on the termination of life-sustaining treatment and the care of the dying.* Bloomington, IN: Indiana University Press.

Hirsch, M. A. (1995). Uniquely hospice: Policies and procedures of terminal care at home. *Caring, XIV*(11), 20–26.

Irish, D. P., Lundquist, K. F., & Nelsen, V. J. (Eds.). (1993). *Ethnic variations in dying, death, and grief.* Washington, DC: Taylor & Francis.

Kass, L. R. (1993 January/February). Is there a right to die? *Hastings Center Report,* 34–43.

Kübler-Ross, E. (1969). *On death and dying.* New York: Macmillan.

Lauterbach, S. S. (Ed.). (1995). The experience of loss. *Holistic Nursing Practice, 9*(3).

Martocchio, B. C. (1985). Grief and bereavement: Healing through hurt. *Nursing Clinics of North America, 20*(2), 327–341.

McCue, J. D. (1995). The naturalness of dying. *Journal of the American Medical Association, 273*(13), 1039–1043.

Mulcahey, A. L., & Young, M. A. (1995). A bereavement support group for children: Fostering communication about grief and healing. *Cancer Practice, 3*(3), 150–156.

Murphy, P. A., & Price, D. M. (1995). "ACT": Taking a positive approach to end-of-life care. *American Journal of Nursing, 95*(3), 42–43.

Murry, M., & Neilson, L. (1994). Denial: Coping or cop-out. *Canadian Nurse, 90*(2), 33–35.

North American Nursing Diagnosis Association. (1994). *NANDA nursing diagnoses: Definitions and classifications 1995–1996.* Philadelphia: NANDA.

Nuland, S. B. (1994). How we die. NY: Alfred A. Knopf.

Orne, R. M. (1995). The meaning of survival: The early aftermath of a near-death experience. *Research in Nursing and Health, 18*(3), 239–247.

Ott, B. B. (1995). Defining and redefining death. *American Journal of Critical Care, 4*(6), 476–480.

Pellegrino, E. D. (1991). Ethics. *Journal of the American Medical Association, 265*(23), 3118–3119.

President's Commission for the Study of Ethical Problems in Medicine and Biomedical and Behavioral Research. (1981). *Defining death.* [Pub. No. 81-600150]. Washington, DC: U.S. Government Printing Office.

Quill, T. E. (1993). Doctor, I want to die. Will you help me? *Journal of the Americal Medical Association, 270*(7), 870–876.

Quill, T., Cassel, C. K., & Meier, D. E. (1992). Care of the hopelessly ill: Proposed clinical criteria for physician-assisted suicide. *New England Journal of Medicine, 327*(19), 1380–1383.

Rasmussen, B. H., Norberg, A., & Sandman, P. O. (1995). Stories about becoming a hospice nurse. *Cancer Nursing, 18*(5), 344–354.

Rushton, C., & Terry, P. B. (1995). Neuromuscular blockade and ventilator withdrawal: Ethical controversies. *American Journal of Critical Care, 4*(2), 112–115.

Saver, C. L. (1994). Decoding the ACLS algorithms. *American Journal of Nursing, 94*(1), 27–36.

Schulz, R. (1978). *The psychology of death, dying and bereavement.* Reading, MA: Addison-Wesley.

Shuster, E. (1995). My patient, my friend. *Home Healthcare Nurse, 13*(6), 70–71.

Slone, M., & Stephany, T. (1995). Stressors of hospice home care nurses caring for AIDS patients: A pilot study. *American Journal of Hospice and Palliative Care, 12*(1), 32–36.

Taylor, C. (1995). Medical futility and nursing. *IMAGE: Journal of Nursing Scholarship, 27*(4), 301–306.

Van Weel, H. (1995). Euthanasia: Mercy, morals and medicine. *Canadian Nurse, 91*(8), 35–40.

Vergara, M., & Lynn-McHale, D. J. (1995). Ethical issues: Withdrawing life support: Who decides? *American Journal of Nursing, 95*(11), 47–49.

Zerwekh, J. V. (1983). "The dehydration question?" *Nursing, 13*(1), 47–51.

Zerwekh, J. (1994). The truth-tellers. How hospice nurses help patients confront death. *American Journal of Nursing, 94*(2), 31–34.

Chapter 34

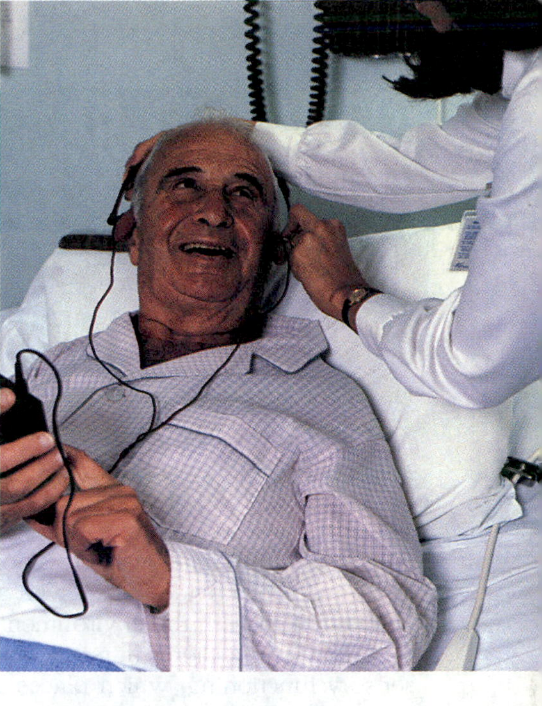

Sensory Stimulation

Objectives

After studying this chapter, the learner should be able to:

Define key terms used in the chapter.

Describe the four conditions that must be met in each sensory experience.

Explain the role of the reticular activating system in sensory experience.

Identify etiologies and perceptual, cognitive, and emotional responses to sensory deprivation and sensory overload.

Perform a comprehensive assessment of sensory functioning using appropriate interview questions and physical assessment skills.

Develop nursing diagnoses that correctly identify sensory/perceptual alterations that may be treated by independent nursing intervention.

Describe specific nursing interventions to prevent sensory alterations, to stimulate the senses, and to assist clients with sensory difficulties.

Develop, implement, and evaluate a plan of nursing care to help clients meet individualized sensory/perceptual outcomes.

Key Terms

arousal
auditory
cultural care deprivation
gustatory
kinesthesia
olfactory
perception
presbycusis
presbyopia
reception
reticular activating system
sensoristasis
sensory deprivation
sensory overload
sensory/perceptual alterations
stereognosis
stimulus
tactile
visceral
visual

A person's senses are vital to survival, growth and development, and the experience of bodily pleasure. For example, awareness of the intensities and sources of sound, ways to control noise, and the assessment of patients' perceptions of, and responses to sound, can provide nurses with a basis for therapeutic manipulation of the environment.

Many of the clients nurses encounter have impaired sensory functioning, which places them at high risk of injury and altered growth and development and decreases their well-being. Moreover, the stress of illness or trauma and the need for diagnosis and treatment may quickly result in sensory deprivation or overload with serious disturbances in visual, perceptual, cognitive, or emotional functioning.

Study of this chapter provides knowledge of the process of sensation, the role of the arousal mechanism, sensory alterations, and factors affecting sensory stimulation. Practical suggestions are given for performing an assessment of sensory functioning. Examples are given of nursing diagnoses identifying specific sensory/perceptual alterations, as are many diagnoses describing the effects of altered sensory functioning on other areas of human functioning. Client goals for preventing and managing sensory alterations are described. Specialized nursing interventions for vision- or hearing-impaired, confused, and unconscious clients are presented. In the section Nursing Process in Clinical Practice, focused assessment, planning, implementation, and evaluation guides are offered for selected nursing diagnoses of sensory deprivation related to inadequate parenting, to the effects of aging, and to unfamiliar culture.

The Sensory Experience

Components and Conditions

The two components of any sensory experience are reception and perception. **Sensory reception** is the process of receiving data about the internal or external environment through the senses. The senses by which individuals maintain contact with the external environment are vision (**visual**), hearing (**auditory**), smell (**olfactory**), taste (**gustatory**), and touch (**tactile**). The kinesthetic and visceral senses arise internally from muscles and hollow organs, respectively, and are the basic orienting systems. (**Kinesthesia** refers to awareness of positioning of body parts and body movement; **visceral** pertains to inner organs.) **Stereognosis** is the sense that perceives the solidity of objects, their size, shape and texture. **Sensory perception** is the conscious process of selecting, organizing, and interpreting data from the senses into meaningful information. Perception is influenced by the intensity, size, change, or representation of stimuli, as well as by past experiences, knowledge, and attitudes.

For a person to receive data necessary to experience the world, four conditions must be met:

- A stimulus—an agent, act, or other influence capable of initiating a response by the nervous system—must be present.
- A receptor or sense organ must receive the stimulus and convert it to a nerve impulse.
- The nerve impulse must be *conducted* along a nervous pathway from the receptor or sense organ to the brain.
- A particular area in the brain must receive and translate the impulse into a sensation.

Arousal Mechanism

To receive stimuli and respond appropriately, the brain must be alert or aroused. The **reticular activating system** (RAS), a poorly defined network that extends from the hypothalamus to the medulla, mediates arousal. The optimal arousal state of the RAS is a general drive state called **sensoristasis**. Nerve impulses from all the sensory tracts reach the RAS, which then selectively allows certain impulses to reach the cerebral cortex and be perceived. The mesencephalic portion of the RAS appears to be the center of the system, and stimulation of this area produces the most pronounced and long-lasting effects on the cerebral cortex (Fig. 34-1). With its many ascending and descending connections to other areas of the brain, the RAS serves to monitor and regulate incoming sensory stimuli and thereby maintain, enhance, or inhibit cortical arousal. States of awareness are described in the accompanying box.

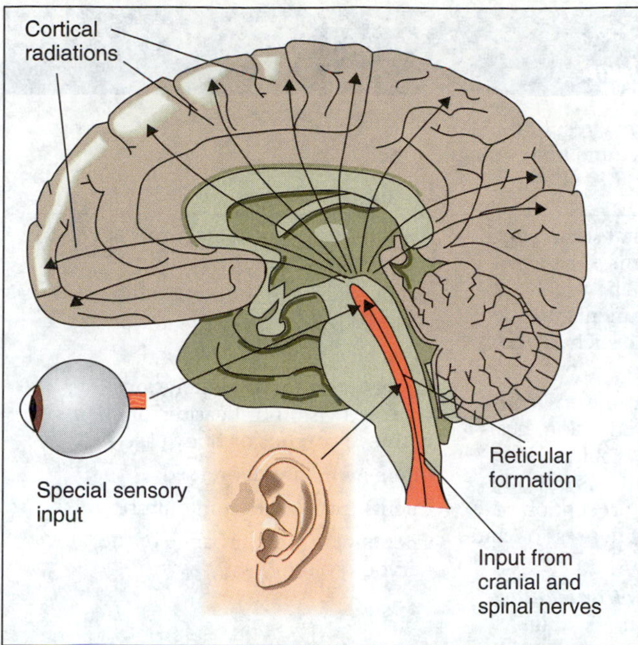

Figure 34-1
Nerve impulses from all the sensory tracts reach the reticular activating system (RAS), which then selectively allows certain impulses to reach the cerebral cortex and to be perceived.

A stimulus must be variable or irregular to evoke a response. The body quickly adapts to constant stimuli; thus the repeated stimulus of a continuing noise, such as city traffic, or a noxious odor eventually goes unnoticed. This phenomenon is termed *adaptation.* Impulses that are not acted on when received may be used at a later date. The memory process involves the storage of that material. For example, thought and memory are used when a new sensory experience occurs and the organism uses a response based on previous knowledge and experience.

Sensory Alterations

When a client is admitted to a health agency, he or she is confronted with stimuli that are different in quality and quantity to the accustomed stimuli. For example, a client confined to bed rest may receive many fewer stimuli, whereas one undergoing multiple diagnostic tests may receive a greater than normal level of sensory input. These and other typical experiences are likely to result in the client's having sensory alterations. Behavioral changes in hospitalized clients have been reduced because more attention is being paid to the use of color and sound and increased privacy and social interaction. Factors contributing to severe sensory alteration (intensive care unit psychosis) include sensory overload, sensory deprivation, sleep deprivation, and cultural care deprivation. Table 34-1 provides an overview of sensory deprivation and sensory overload with related nursing interventions.

Sensory Deprivation

Sensory deprivation results when a person experiences decreased sensory input or input that is monotonous, unpatterned, or meaningless. With decreased sensory input, the RAS is no longer able to project a normal level of activation to the brain and the individual may hallucinate simply to maintain an optimal level of arousal. Factors placing a client at high risk for sensory deprivation include the following:

(Text continues on p. 817)

States of Awareness

Conscious States	
Delirium	Disorientation, restlessness, confusion, hallucinations, agitation, alternating with other conscious states
Dementia	Difficulties with spatial orientation, memory, language, changes in personality
Confusion	Reduced awareness, easily distracted, easily startled by sensory stimuli, alternates between drowsiness and excitability; resembles minor form of delirium state
Normal consciousness	Aware of self and external environment, well-oriented, responsive
Somnolence	Extreme drowsiness, but will respond normally to stimuli
Chronic vegetative state	Conscious but unresponsive, no evidence of cortical function
Unconscious States	
Asleep	Can be aroused by normal stimuli (light touch, sound, etc.)
Stupor	Can be aroused by extreme and/or repeated stimuli
Coma	Cannot be aroused and does not respond to stimuli (coma states can be further subdivided according to the effect on reflex responses to stimuli)

Table 34-1
Overview of Sensory Deprivation and Sensory Overload

Sensory Deprivation Insufficient quantity or quality of stimuli; may result from decreased sensory input or monotonous, unpatterned, and unmeaningful input

Defining Characteristics	Contributing Factors	Clients at Risk
Physical behaviors: drowsiness, excessive yawning *Escape behaviors:* eating, exercising, sleeping, running away to escape the deprived environment *Changes in perception:* unusual body sensations; preoccupation with somatic complaints (dry mouth, palpitations, difficulty breathing, nausea); change in body image; illusions and hallucinations *Changes in cognitive behavior:* decreased attention span, inability to concentrate, decreased problem solving and task performance *Changes in affective behavior:* crying, increased irritability and annoyance over small matters, confusion, panic, depression	Decreased environmental stimuli: institutionalized environment; separation from significant others and usual sources of stimuli; treatments that decrease access to stimuli, such as bed rest or isolation *Impaired ability to receive environmental stimuli:* impaired vision, hearing, taste, smell, touch resulting from treatments such as bandages or body casts that interfere with reception of stimuli, or as a result of depression and other affective disorders *Inability to process environmental stimuli:* spinal cord injuries, brain damage, confusion, dementia, medications that depress the central nervous system	Institutionalized clients, especially those in long-term care settings Clients with communicable disease (eg, AIDS) Clients confined to bed Clients with sensory alterations (eg, impaired vision or hearing, or clients with eye patches or body casts) Clients who are depressed Clients from a different culture Clients with a disturbance of the nervous system

Nursing Interventions

Maintain sufficient level of arousal by increasing sensory stimuli from all sensory modalities:

- Instruct the client in self-stimulation methods: counting, singing, reading, reciting poetry.
- Structure meaningful tangible stimuli into client's external environment; include a variety of people, ideas, sensations; a pet may provide excellent stimulation.
  - *Visual stimulation*
    - Colorful sheets, pajamas, robes
    - Colorful uniform tops for the nurse
    - Face-to-face human contact
    - Clocks, calendars, wrist watches
    - Pictures, flowers, greeting card
  - *Auditory stimulation*
    - Call person by name
    - Conversation that communicates caring as well as orients client
    - Reading to the client
    - Television, radio
  - *Gustatory and olfactory stimulation*
    - Attention to oral hygiene and properly fitting dentures
    - Food of different textures, colors, temperatures served attractively
    - Smelling food before eating it and recalling pleasurable aromas from the past
    - Seasoning foods or having favorite foods brought from home
  - *Tactile stimulation*
    - Back rubs
    - Turning and repositioning
    - Passive range-of-motion exercises
    - Hair brushing, combing, washing
    - Foot soaks
    - Hugs
    - Touching of arms or shoulders
  - *Cognitive input*
    - Orient client to environment
    - Encourage client participation in self-care
    - Discuss current events or client's occupation, hobbies, or interests
    - Reinforce reality without arguing with a client who is hallucinating. "No, I don't see a man standing there but the linen hamper may be confusing you."
  - *Emotional input*
    - Encourage client to share fears, concerns, and perceptions; reassure client that illusions and misperceptions do occur with sensory deprivation

(continued)

Table 34-1 *(continued)*
Overview of Sensory Deprivation and Sensory Overload

- Incorporate culturally assistive, supportive, facilitative acts into nursing care.
- *Caution:* Because it can be difficult to distinguish the behavioral manifestations of sensory deprivation from sensory overload, introduce more stimulation cautiously. If the added stimulation only increases the client's maladaptive behaviors, consider reducing sensory input because the client may be experiencing sensory overload.

Sensory Overload Excessive stimuli over which an individual feels little control; brain is unable meaningfully to respond to or ignore stimuli

Defining Characteristics	Contributing Factors	Clients at Risk
Similar to those observed in sensory deprivation Elderly clients and clients who have suffered a stroke are more likely to experience confusion or agitation. Young clients are more likely to seek the comfort of their parents' embrace to block out sensory overload.	*Increased internal stimuli:* pain, pressure and discomfort of intrusive tubes (eg, intravenous lines [IVs], catheters; endotracheal tubes, nasogastric tubes), worry about state of health or need to make treatment decisions *Increased external stimuli:* unfamiliar healthcare environment, such as lights, noises, sounds, odors, movement, and constant presence of strangers, many of whom touch the body; intrusive procedures such as diagnostic tests and treatments; scratchy linens *Inability perceptually to disregard or selectively ignore some stimuli:* nervous system disturbances, medications such as caffeine that stimulate the central nervous system arousal mechanism	Any acutely or chronically ill client Clients in pain Client with intrusive monitoring or treatment equipment Hospitalized clients, especially those in critical care settings Clients with disturbances of the nervous system

Nursing Interventions

- Provide a consistent, predictable pattern of stimulation to help the client develop a sense of control over the environment.
- Offer simple explanations before procedures, tests, and examinations.
- Establish a schedule with the client for routine care such as eating, bathing, turning, positioning, coughing, and exercise.
- Speak calmly with the client and move slowly; communicate confidence.
- Explore with the client what stimuli are most distressing and develop a plan to reduce or eliminate these (eg, incoming phone calls, visitors); ear plugs or pain medication may be indicated.
- Be careful not to cause sensory deprivation.
- Identify and, wherever possible, eliminate culturally inappropriate stimuli.

(Adapted from Lee, K. A. [1991]. Sensory overload, sensory deprivation, and sleep deprivation. In M. L. Patrick, S. L. Woods, R. F. Craven, J. S. Rokosky, & P. M. Bruno [Eds.], *Medical-surgical nursing* [2nd ed.]. Philadelphia: Lippincott.)

- An environment with decreased or monotonous stimuli (institutionalized clients, clients confined to a small living area at home, clients on bed rest or in isolation, and so on)
- Impaired ability to receive environmental stimuli (clients with sensory alterations: impaired vision or hearing; clients with bandages or casts that interfere with vision, hearing, or tactile stimulation; clients with affective disorders who "close out" the environment, and so on)
- Inability to process environmental stimuli (clients with spinal cord injuries or brain damage, clients who are confused or disoriented, clients taking prescribed or recreational drugs that affect the central nervous system)

Effects of sensory deprivation include perceptual, cognitive, and emotional disturbances.

Perceptual responses—inaccurate perception of sights, sounds, tastes, smells, and body position, coordination, and equilibrium; mild to gross distortions ranging from daydreams to hallucinations

Cognitive responses—inability to control the direction of thought content; decreased attention span and ability to concentrate; difficulty with memory, problem solving, and task performance

Emotional responses—inappropriate emotional responses: apathy, anxiety, fear, anger, belligerence, panic, depression; rapid mood changes (see Table 34-1 for additional information)

Sensory Overload

Sensory overload is the condition that results when a person experiences so much sensory stimuli that the brain is unable meaningfully to respond to or ignore the stimuli. The person feels out of control and may exhibit all of the manifestations observed in sensory deprivation. The amount and quality of stimuli necessary to produce overload may differ greatly from one individual to another and are influenced by factors such as age, culture, personality, and lifestyle.

In some clients, especially those coming from a quiet environment with unvarying stimuli, the experience of being hospitalized quickly results in sensory overload. In such clients, the brain is assaulted by the constant presence of strangers who not only demand to be spoken to but who also touch and poke at the body; by the strange sights, odors, sounds, and feels of the unfamiliar environment; by the constant presence of pain or discomfort from dressings, IVs, drainage tubes, or endotracheal tubes; and by the ever-present worries about the meaning and course of the illness. Nursing assistance is directed to reducing distressing stimuli and helping the client to gain control over the environment (see Table 34-1).

Cultural Care Deprivation

Sensory deprivation, sensory overload, and sleep deprivation are all related to or affected by an individual's cultural practices, values, and beliefs. Kloosterman (1991) suggests that the concept missing in current practices concerning severe sensory alteration is "culturally congruent care." **Cultural care deprivation** is described as "a lack of culturally assistive, supportive, or facilitative acts" (p. 121). The nurse who is sensitive to the client's culture attempts to determine what constitutes acceptable levels of stimuli from the client's viewpoint. For example, in certain cultures touching is viewed as a natural and welcome custom whereas other cultures may view it as insulting or offensive. Kloosterman notes that different cultures have rules on how, where, and for what purpose the human body may be touched. Similarly, clients may find comfort in cultural and religious symbols of care and healing that are absent in a hospital environment.

Sensory Deficits

Impaired or absent functioning in one or more senses is termed **sensory deficit**. Examples of sensory deficits include impaired sight and hearing, altered taste, numbness and paralysis that results in altered tactile perception, and impaired kinesthetic sense. These deficits may be reversible or permanent, may occur gradually or all at once, and may be present at birth or evolve later. It is important for nurses to be aware of a client's sensory deficits and to determine if the client is able to compensate for the deficit. Illness and hospitalization may threaten a client's usual adapative patterns and require new self-care abilities. Clients with evolving deficits will require assistance in coping and in learning to skillfully compensate.

Factors Affecting Sensory Stimulation

There appears to be considerable variation in the amount of stimuli different individuals consider optimal. Factors influencing the amount and quality of stimuli needed to maintain cortical arousal include developmental considerations, culture, personality and lifestyle, stress, and illness and medication.

Developmental Considerations

Different types of sensory stimulation are needed for growth as sensory receptors and organs and the nervous system mature. Although the newborn is capable of rudimentary perceptual discriminations at birth, many neural pathways are immature and must be stimulated to develop, become refined, and function adequately. Appropriate stimulation includes soothing; holding; rocking and changes of position (tactile and kinesthetic sensations); singing and being talked to (auditory sensations); and changing patterns of light and shade, such as through the use of mobiles and bright objects (visual sensations). Developmentally appropriate play develops the child's muscles and coordination, provides an outlet for surplus physical energy, develops communication skills, furnishes sources of learning, acts as a stimulant to creativity, develops social skills, teaches sex roles, provides an outlet for the release of emotional energy, and develops self-insights.

Sensory functioning tends to progressively decline throughout adulthood as the result of aging or chronic illness. The adult may experience the need to compensate for the loss of one type of stimulation by increasing other sources of sensory stimuli.

Culture

An individual's culture may dictate the amount of sensory stimulation considered normal. For example, the amount of touching a child experiences in a Puerto Rican family may be different from that experienced by a child in a German family. Similarly, male and female roles may be culturally defined; for example, although the male is expected to respond to the challenge of out-of-the-home sensory stimuli, the female who attempts to do so may be scorned if her place is considered to be in the home. Ethnic norms, religious norms, income group norms, and the norms of subgroups within a culture all influence the amount of sensory stimulation sought by an individual and perceived as meaningful.

Personality and Lifestyle

Apart from a person's culture, different personality types demand different levels of stimulation. One person may thrive on a steady stream of fast-paced changes and excitement, whereas another may feel best when daily routines are rigidly structured and life sends no challenges necessitating changes. Lifestyle choices can dramatically influence the quantity and quality of stimuli received by an individual. The nurse who elects to work in the emergency room of a large city hospital is exposed to vastly different stimuli than the nurse making home visits in a rural setting.

Stress

Increased sensory stimulation may be sought during periods of low stress simply to maintain cortical arousal. During high-stress periods, multiple stressors may already be overloading the sensory system, and decreased sensory stimulation is desired. The stress of physical illness, pain, hospitalization, testing, surgery, and treatment may provide more stimulation than an individual can process and respond to without assistance.

Illness and Medication

Illness can affect the reception of sensory stimuli (eg, diminution of the sense of touch associated with diabetes and cerebrovascular disease) and their transmission and perception (eg, neurologic disorders, dementias). Medications that alert or depress the central nervous system may interfere with the perception of sensory stimuli. Certain medications also may contribute to impaired sensory functioning by decreasing reception (eg, captopril, an antihypertensive agent, can cause taste alteration; aspirin can cause tinnitus [ringing in the ears]).

The Nurse as Role Model

Sensitivity to the important role sensory functioning plays in a person's well-being guides the nurse to promote personal well-being. Awareness of one's own sensory functioning and the stimulation in one's own life is a stepping-stone to providing proper stimulation to clients. The nurse works to achieve the following goals. The nurse will:

- Evaluate the quantity and quality of sensory stimuli present in both the home and at work
- Identify stimuli important to self-development as a person (mental, physical, and spiritual health) and as a professional nurse
- Manipulate the environment to decrease distressing stimuli and increase positive stimuli
- When practicing nursing, be conscious of the need to promote optimal sensory functioning in clients

ASSESSING SENSORY FUNCTIONING

When assessing a client for sensory disturbances, the nurse interviews the client and examines him or her for sensory deficits and manifestations of sensory deprivation or overload. Examination of the client's environment is included in the assessment to determine whether it is providing adequate sensory stimulation for healthy development.

Assessing the Sensory Experience

The assessment may be structured using the components of the sensory experience—stimulation, reception, and transmission–perception–reaction. These components are outlined in the accompanying box (p. 821). Because clients may adapt to sensory impairments, it may be helpful to include someone the client knows well (eg, spouse or parent) in the assessment to see if that person has noticed behavioral characteristics in the client that suggest a sensory disturbance (eg, "I've noticed he turns the television volume much louder than ever before").

Stimulation

Assess if there have been any recent changes in sensory stimulation, for example, reduction of stimulation from one or more sensory modalities ("Since my husband died no one touches me anymore. It sounds crazy but I'm hungry to be touched!") or new or unusual stimulation ("Ever since my granddaughter moved in with me, my house is always noisy. I can't stand the constant noise and her smoking."). Assess if the type of stimulation present is developmentally appropriate. High-risk clients for problems related to stimulation include children in nonstimulating environments, older people, terminally ill clients, clients on bed rest, clients in isolation, and clients requiring intensive nursing in a critical care setting.

Reception

Assess for anything that may interfere with sensory reception and describe any corrective devices the client uses for sensory impairments (eyeglasses, contacts, hearing aids). The reception section of the Focused Assessment Guide highlights assessment strategies for each sense. High-risk clients for reception problems include people with visual, auditory, or other sensory impairments.

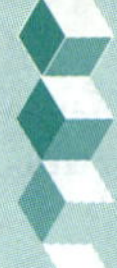

Research in Nursing: Making a Difference

Incorporating Sensory Experiences in Teaching

Knowledge of the sensory effects of new diagnostic and therapeutic modalities enables nurses to better prepare clients for these experiences.

McDaniel, R. W., Rhodes, V. A., Nelson, R. A. & Hanson, B. M. (1995). Sensory perceptions of women receiving tamoxifen for breast cancer. *Cancer Nursing, 18*(3), 215–221.
Tamoxifen has been used as adjuvant treatment in advanced and early-stage breast cancer for the past decade. Recently this synthetic antiestrogen drug assumed a new role of chemoprevention for women at risk of developing breast cancer. The commonly occurring side effects associated with tamoxifen administration contribute to the acceptance of this antineoplastic drug for palliation and cure. However, there are no data about its sensory effects. The purpose of this study was to elicit subjects' descriptions of sensory experiences while receiving tamoxifen. These descriptions are essential for developing nursing interventions to help patients use self-care behaviors and cope with the side effects of tamoxifen. Sensory data were collected from 20 women who had been receiving tamoxifen for at least 1 month and were not receiving other chemotherapy. The senses for which subjects most frequently provided descriptors were touch, taste and sight.

Poroch, D. (1995). The effect of preparatory patient education on the anxiety and satisfaction of cancer patients receiving radiation therapy. *Cancer Nursing, 18*(3), 206–214.
Facing treatment of cancer with radiation therapy causes anxiety for most prospective patients. The purpose of this study was to test the effectiveness of preparatory patient education in reducing anxiety and improving satisfaction during the course of treatment. A quasi-experimental time series design was used to compare two groups of 25 patients, matched according to treatment type and gender, who were commencing radiation therapy for the first time. The experimental group received two structured teaching interventions incorporating sensory and procedural information designed to familiarize the patient with the forthcoming experience. Sensory information is an important category of preparatory information. It attempts to create a realistic mental picture of the procedure, which assists patients in interpreting what is happening to them both before and during the procedure. The results indicated that the experimental group was significantly less anxious and significantly more satisfied during radiation therapy than their counterparts in the control group, and the effects were maintained throughout the treatment period of up to 7 weeks.

Summary

Nurses wanting to increase compliance with therapeutic regimens will be sensitive to the link between what clients experience with therapy, their ability to cope, and their continued compliance. Further research is needed to determine sensory effects and to identify which teaching and counseling interventions best prepare clients for these experiences.

Transmission–Perception–Reaction

High-risk clients for transmission–perception–reaction problems include confused clients and clients with nervous system impairments. Everyday interactions afford the nurse multiple opportunities to assess clients' abilities to transmit, perceive, and react to stimuli.

Defining Characteristics of Sensory Deprivation and Overload

Complete the assessment of the client's sensory functioning by assessing for specific indicators of sensory deprivation or overload (see Table 34-1), including boredom, inactivity, slowness of thought, daydreaming, increased sleeping, thought disorganization, anxiety, panic, illusions, and hallucinations. It is important to know the client's usual state to be able to identify changes stemming from sensory deprivation or overload.

Physical Assessment

Physical examination skills related to the senses are discussed in Chapter 26. Ear and eye tests, whether performed by a physician or nurse, should be considered when planning care. Problems with the neurologic system indicate the necessity of further assessment of the sensory experience.

DIAGNOSING

Sensory/Perceptual Alterations as the Problem. When assessment data point to sensory disturbances that can be treated independently by nursing interventions, nursing diagnoses are developed and labeled **sensory/perceptual alterations**. These alterations may be further specified as visual, auditory, gustatory, olfactory, tactile,

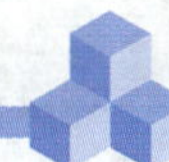

Focused Assessment Guide

Sensory Stimulation

Factors to Assess	Questions and Approaches
Stimulation	"Does your current environment overly, insufficiently, or appropriately stimulate you?" "Are you bored? Why?" "Are you able to read? Watch television? Knit? Why not?" "Are there other people in your home during the day? Do you spend much time together? How do you spend the time?" "Who visits you while you are in the hospital?" Note reduction in the patterns or meaningfulness of stimulation in each sensory modality; changes in stimulation other than decreases (eg, new or unusual stimulation); or developmental appropriateness of stimulation.
Reception	"Does anything interfere with the functioning of your senses?" "Describe any corrective devices you use for sensory impairments."
Assess for visual disturbances.	"Please read my name tag (or this page of print)." Note if the client can correctly identify objects directly in front of the eyes as well as those requiring peripheral vision. Note eye rubbing; squinting; movements indicating faulty vision (bumping into furniture, overreaching or underreaching for objects); changes in the appearance of the eye (cataracts, swelling); and complaints of eye pain, spots, halos, or other visual disturbances.
Assess for auditory disturbances.	"Repeat the words that I will speak softly close to each ear." Note if the client is able to hear equally well from both ears, distinguish voices, locate the direction of a sound, if the client needs to face the person speaking and relies on lip reading, if the client's responses to questions include blank looks, many nods, smiling, or inappropriate responses indicating faulty hearing. Note complaints of ringing or buzzing in ears.
Assess for gustatory (taste) disturbances.	"Close your eyes, stick out your tongue, and tell me if what I place on your tongue is sweet, sour, bitter, or salty." "Have you been experiencing any strange tastes (bitter, metallic) or aftertastes lately?" Note if the client is able to differentiate sweet, sour, bitter, or salty tastes or reports unusual, persistent taste sensations. Note deficient oral hygiene, ill-fitting dentures, braces, or anything else that might contribute to gustatory disturbances.
Assess for olfactory (smell) disturbances.	"Close your eyes and tell me what you smell." "Have you smelled odors lately that others cannot smell or have you been especially sensitive to odors?" Note if the client can correctly identify common odors (coffee, vanilla) or has noticed increased sensitivity to odors.
Assess for tactile (touch) disturbances.	"Close your eyes and tell me when you feel something (brush skin with cotton ball), if what you feel is dull or sharp (use both ends of safety pin), hot or cold (use items from food tray). Now, keep your eyes closed and tell me what I am placing in your hand (coin, cotton ball, paper clip)."

(continued)

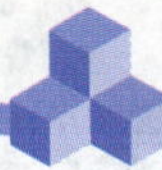

Focused Assessment Guide *(continued)*

Sensory Stimulation

Factors to Assess	Questions and Approaches
	Note if the client can correctly sense touch and distinguish sharp and dull, hot and cold, and different shapes.
	Note if the client reports decreased sensation in any part of the body; numbness, pins and needles, tingling; or abnormal sensitivity to pain or touch.
Assess for kinesthetic and visceral disturbances.	Note if the client withdraws from being touched.
	"Have you noticed any changes in the way you perceive your body?"
	"Do you feel any unusual pressure or pain inside your body?"
	Note if the client seems unsure of his or her body parts or body position and if he or she experiences new internal sensations (fullness, pressure, pain).
Transmission–perception–reaction	"Are you aware of any problems with your nervous system?"
	"Have you found it difficult to communicate verbally?"
	Note consciousness, orientation, appropriateness of responses, ability to perform usual self-care activities, ability to follow simple commands, decision-making abilities, pathology affecting central nervous system, or prescribed or recreational drug use that affects the central nervous system.
Behavioral manifestations of sensory deprivation or overload	
Perceptual responses	Mild to gross sensory distortions (illusions, hallucinations)
Cognitive responses	Thought disorganization, slowness of thought, decreased attention/concentration, difficulty with problem solving and task performance
Emotional responses	Rapid mood changes, anxiety, panic

or kinesthetic. *Sensory deprivation* and *sensory overload* may also be used to further specify the sensory/perceptual alteration and in some cases may be the etiology.

Common etiologies for sensory/perceptual alterations include the following:

- Altered environmental stimuli, excessive or insufficient
- Altered sensory reception, transmission, or integration
- Chemical alterations, endogenous (eg, electrolytes) or exogenous (eg, drugs)
- Psychologic stress

Sample nursing diagnoses in which the sensory/perceptual alteration is the problem are listed in the accompanying display.

Sensory/Perceptual Alterations as the Etiology. Because sensory/perceptual alterations affect many other areas of human functioning, they serve as etiologies for multiple problem statements. Examples of these follow:

- Activity Intolerance related to impaired balance and coordination (kinesthetic alteration)
- Anxiety related to paranoia stemming from hearing impairment, sensory deprivation (specify setting), sensory overload
- Impaired Verbal Communication related to difficulty receiving, transmitting, and perceiving sensory stimuli
- Ineffective Individual Coping related to sensory overload (multiple stressors)
- Diversional Activity Deficit related to impaired vision or hearing
- Altered Growth and Development related to nonstimulating home environment
- High Risk for Injury related to decreased or impaired sensation (specify visual, auditory, tactile, kinesthetic)
- Knowledge Deficit: Means to compensate for sensory impairment (blindness, deafness, and so forth), related to lack of previous experience with this problem, unavailability of resources
- Knowledge Deficit: Providing a developmentally stimulating environment, related to lack of experience with children's growth and development

Nursing Diagnoses for Common Problems

Sensory/Perceptual Alterations

Problem	Related Factors	Sample Defining Characteristics
Sensory/Perceptual Alteration: Sensory Deficit or Excess		
Visual	Eye patches following surgery	"I never realized before how sight-dependent I am. I don't know what time of day it is now unless I have the radio on or smell food coming in."
		"It's frightening not to know who is in my room and what they are doing."
		Client observed sitting in room with blank facial expression; frequently comments on how bored he or she is and how slowly time is passing; hesitant to move about room without assistance although he or she has been oriented repeatedly
Auditory	Effects of aging	"You're right. I don't always hear what people are saying anymore so I try not to get involved in conversations. If people insist on talking, I just nod and hope I'm giving the right response."
		Able to hear moderately spoken word close to right ear; cannot hear same from left ear; often startled when someone approaches from left side
		Sits close to television and radio; loud volume, no history of hearing testing
Gustatory or olfactory	Chemotherapy	"I always seem to have a bitter taste in my mouth now and can't stomach certain foods at all that I used to enjoy, like beef, tomatoes, coffee. . . . I also can't take sweets and I used to be a real sweets junkie."
		"Sometimes the very smell of certain foods or even the thought of eating nauseates me."
		Client has been receiving vincristine (cancer chemotherapeutic agent) for past 3 months; some nausea and vomiting; history of poor oral hygiene
Tactile	Psychologic stress	"I don't know why I feel this way, but I'm hypersensitive to any touch. If anyone even brushes against me I feel burning pain. Even the weight of my clothes against my skin bothers me. I'm trying to move my body as little as possible and keep it protected—but that's obviously impossible when even a breeze assaults me."
		Client observed holding the body stiffly looking like he or she does not know what to do with the arms and legs; dressed only in a loose-fitting outfit; reports that he or she sits at home all day afraid to go out
Kinesthetic	Clinitron bed therapy	"I've been in this bed for 2 weeks now and I've lost all sense of my body . . . it's a curious weightless feeling that I have . . . sort of like floating in Jell-O. I'm no longer sure where my body begins and ends, and when I try to lift an arm or leg I feel like I'm in slow motion. I hope I'll be able to walk when I get out of here."

(continued)

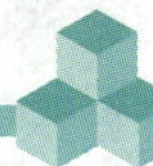

Nursing Diagnoses for Common Problems *(continued)*

Sensory/Perceptual Alterations

Problem	Related Factors	Sample Defining Characteristics
Sensory/Perceptual Alteration: Sensory Deprivation	Isolation	"One of the worst things that has happened to me since I found out I had AIDS is that everyone is afraid of me—and no one touches me. I'm so lonely. I've always needed a lot of people around." "Here in the hospital I think I'm going crazy. I can't leave this room. Everyone who comes in looks the same dressed in those yellow gowns. Lately I've seen some bizarre things that I know can't be real. I look at the clock and it turns into a swirling sun with a sad face that keeps coming closer and closer to me and I'm terrified I'll burn up if it gets too close. That's crazy, isn't it? I'm really losing it now." Disturbed sleep for past 2 weeks; during the day yawns excessively and catnaps; limited attention span; states he or she is unable to concentrate on anything.
Sensory/Perceptual Alteration: Sensory Overload	Trauma of rape and aftercare	"When is everyone going to stop touching me? First he wouldn't stop. Now everyone here is poking at me, looking at me, asking me hundreds of questions. . . . Why did I have to report this and come to the hospital? Oh please leave me alone. Get out of here everyone."

- Impaired Physical Mobility related to impaired balance and coordination (kinesthetic alteration)
- Altered Parenting: Failure to provide stimuli for growth related to lack of knowledge, decreased motivation to provide for child's growth and development
- Powerlessness related to inability to interact meaningfully with environment
- Self-Care Deficit: (specify) related to visual impairment, auditory impairment, tactile impairment
- Body Image Disturbance related to kinesthetic impairment (distorted sense of body parts), sensory deprivation
- Self-Esteem Disturbance related to sensory/perceptual alterations (specify visual, auditory, and so forth)
- Altered Role Performance related to sensory/perceptual alteration (blindness, deafness, and so forth)
- Personal Identity Disturbance related to sensory deprivation or overload
- Sexual Dysfunction related to decreased sensation
- Impaired Skin Integrity related to absent tactile sensation (injury)
- Sleep Pattern Disturbance related to sensory deprivation or overload
- Impaired Social Interaction related to inability to receive and process interactional stimuli
- Social Isolation related to visual or auditory impairment
- Altered Thought Processes (specify: illusions, hallucinations, decreased attention or concentration, and so forth) related to sensory deprivation or overload

PLANNING: EXPECTED OUTCOMES

In whatever setting nurses encounter and care for clients, optimal sensory stimulation is a priority and nursing care is supportive of the following client goals/outcomes. The client will:

- Live in a developmentally stimulating and safe environment
- Exhibit a level of arousal that enables the brain to receive and meaningfully organize patterns of stimulation
- Demonstrate intact functioning of the senses: vision, hearing, taste, smell, touch, kinesthetic and visceral awareness
- Maintain orientation to time, place, and person
- Respond appropriately (verbally and nonverbally) to sensory stimuli while executing self-care activities

Clients with impaired sensory functioning require individualized goals similar to the following. The client will:

- Report feeling safe and in control of the environment
- Describe different types of meaningful stimuli present in the environment

- Demonstrate (describe) appropriate self-care behaviors for visual impairment, hearing impairment, or other sensory impairment
- Verbalize acceptance of the sensory deficit

IMPLEMENTING

The nurse can assist clients to improve sensory functioning by teaching clients and significant others means to stimulate the senses, teaching clients with intact and impaired senses appropriate self-care behaviors, and interacting therapeutically with impaired clients. Safety is always a special concern for clients with sensory alterations. Nurses are responsible for ensuring that the client's environment is as free of danger as possible and for assisting the client to develop new self-care behaviors to compensate for sensory impairments. Safety considerations are discussed in Chapter 27. In this section, the nursing interventions described are preventing sensory alteration, stimulating the senses, meeting the needs of visually impaired and hearing impaired people, communicating with a confused person, and communicating with an unconscious person. Communication guidelines for clients with sensory deficits are also highlighted in Chapter 22.

Preventing Sensory Alteration and Stimulating the Senses

The most effective means by which sensory alteration can be managed is prevention. The key to prevention is, with the client's help, to create a functional and meaningful environment while keeping limitations in mind. The creation of such an environment requires careful observation, analysis, and creative planning.

Numerous nursing measures can be considered in planning care. Appropriate measures for implementing depend on the circumstances. Well-being is promoted by offering care that provides rest and comfort (see Chapters 40 and 41). Client discomfort should be controlled whenever possible. The nurse should be aware of the need for sensory aids and prostheses, such as eyeglasses, contact lenses, hearing aids, dentures, canes, and artificial limbs, and these should be made available as needed. Social activities, as shown in Figure 34-2, help to stimulate the senses and mind. Family members may participate in or encourage these activities. Physical activity and exercise, which help maintain normal sensory perceptions and decrease the likelihood of sensory alteration, should be encouraged (exercises are discussed in Chapter 39).

As many senses as possible should be stimulated. Varied sights, sounds, smells, body positions, and textures can be helpful in providing a variety of sensations. For example, music therapy was found to have beneficial effects for mechanically ventilated patients on selected psychophysiologic variables (heart rate, respiratory rate, and mood state). It was found that listening to music ameliorated the stress response and promoted nonpharmacologically induced relaxation for the study subjects. Critical care nurses can be confident in implementing this nonpharmacologic, independent intervention to promote relaxation without worry of untoward side effects, which are sometimes caused by pharmacologic sedation (Chlan, 1995). Cultural factors are taken

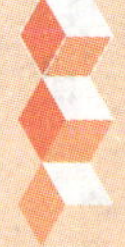

Helpscan

The following are resources for clients and health care professionals:

- Helpline for older adults without insurance or means to pay who need to see an ophthalmologist:
  National Eye Care Project
  PO Box 429098
  San Francisco, CA 94142-9098
  (800) 222-EYES
- For a free two-step screening test to encourage hearing-impaired people in the United States to get help:
  Dial-a-Hearing-Screening-Test (DAHST)
  (800) 222-EARS (between 9:00 AM and 5:00 PM EST)
- AT&T National Relay Center will relay messages between hearing-impaired and voice persons
  (800) 855-2880 (TTY—hearing impaired users)
  (800) 855-2881 (voice users)
- Resources for vision-impaired clients:
  National Eye Institute
  Box 2020
  Bethesda, MD 20892

  American Foundation for the Blind
  1615 M Street, NW, Suite 250
  Washington, DC 20036

  Guide Dog Foundation for the Blind
  (800) 548-4337

  Helen Keller National Center
  (301) 699-6256

  National Federation of the Blind
  (410) 659-9314

  (Deaf/Blind Division)
  (800) 859-4111

Consult the Guide to Human Services in your phone book to find a listing of local resources for hearing- and vision-impaired clients.

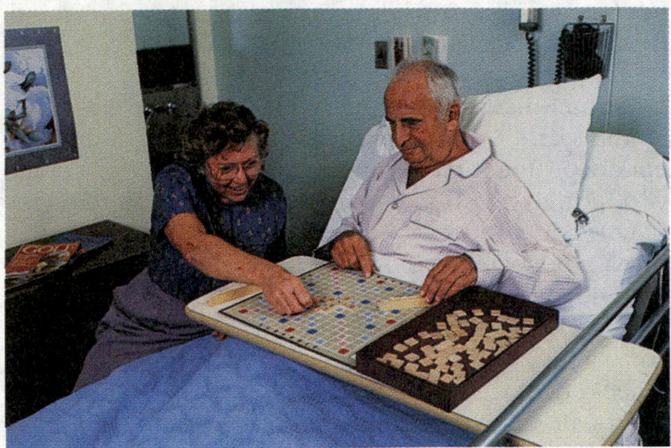

Figure 34-2
The nurse helps the client find methods for stimulating his or her senses. Family members may participate in sensory activities.

into consideration when stimulating senses and when offering nursing care. This is especially important when caring for clients from cultures different from the nurse's own culture.

Teaching About Sensory Experiences

Teaching is a significant nursing responsibility. The nurse can help prepare clients for sensory experiences. An informed client is better able to handle fears, frustration, and confusion; therefore procedures are explained before being instituted. Explanations also help prevent the client from feeling that his or her space and body are being invaded.

Individuals experiencing perceptual and thought distortions should have the opportunity to acknowledge that fact. To discuss such experiences and be reassured that they are normal and usually temporary generally eases anxiety.

Clients and family members can be guided in sensory self-stimulation, and parents can be aided in stimulation of newborns, infants, and children. The accompanying box gives helpful suggestions for teaching clients about sensory stimulation and includes suggestions that the nurse can use in a variety of situations.

Meeting the Needs of Visually Impaired Clients

It is necessary for the nurse to check with the physician to discover if a visual problem is temporary, permanent, partial, or complete and the degree to which the problem is likely to affect the client's everyday functioning. The nurse cannot develop a realistic teaching plan or plan of care without this information.

The nurse's first priority is to teach clients self-care behaviors to maintain vision and prevent blindness. Lindberg and Kruszewski (1983) offered the following suggestions:

- Avoid rubbing eyes.
- Avoid eyestrain.
- Avoid damage from ultraviolet rays.
- Protect eyes from foreign bodies.
- Keep eyeglasses clean, protected, adjusted.
- Avoid nonprescription eyedrops and seek attention for symptoms.
- Avoid cleaning eyes or contact lenses with soiled articles.
- Use caution with aerosol sprays.
- Use caution with ammonia, lye, and so on.
- Visit your physician frequently if you are prone to eye problems.
- Know the danger signals that indicate serious eye problems: persistent eye redness; pain or discomfort, especially after injury; visual disturbances; crossing eyes; growth on or near the eyes; discharge or increased tearing; and pupil irregularities.

The following guidelines are recommended for communicating with persons who are visually impaired:

- Acknowledge your presence in the client's room. Identify yourself by name.
- Speak in a normal tone of voice. Remember that the blind person is unable to pick up most nonverbal cues during communication.
- Explain the reason for touching the person before doing so.
- Keep the call light or bell within easy reach of the person and place the bed in the lowest position.
- Orient the person to sounds in the environment.
- Orient the person to the arrangement of the room and its furnishings. Clear pathways for the person and do not rearrange furnishings. Clarify this fact with housekeeping personnel also.
- Assist with ambulation by walking slightly ahead of the person, allowing the person to grasp your arm.
- Stay in the person's field of vision if he or she has partial or reduced peripheral vision.
- Provide diversions using other senses.
- Indicate to the person when the conversation has ended and when you are leaving the room.

Meeting the Needs of Hearing Impaired Clients

Temporary hearing losses are most often *conductive* in nature, that is, they are due to a problem with the external or middle ear (wax buildup, foreign body obstruction, infection). *Sensorineural hearing losses* are caused by inner ear or central nervous system problems and may not be totally correctable. Health teaching to prevent hearing problems includes the following recommendations from Lindberg and Kruszewski (1983):

- Avoid excessive noise.
- Avoid inserting sharp objects into ears.
- Avoid excessive cleaning of ears.
- Avoid practices that can cause infection; treat infection early.
- Know the symptoms of hearing loss: asking frequently that statements be repeated, inability to hear at a distance, need to see the person who is

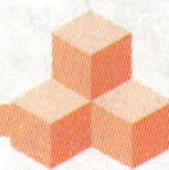

Guidelines for Nursing Care

Stimulating the Senses

	Teaching Clients	Nursing Interventions
Vision	Surround yourself with different colors and with an environment that changes (walk through a mall, sit by a window where you see people come and go). Develop a sensitivity to changes in nature (weather patterns, dawn to night cycle, changing seasons, changes in a plant or animal). Use visual devices to keep oriented (watches, calendars, newspaper, television). Use crossword puzzles and games to stimulate mental activities. Create favorite scenes in your mind, paying attention to tiny details.	Wear visually stimulating and comforting colors. Keep meaningful visual stimuli such as photos, greeting cards, toys, or flowers near client. Position clients with impaired mobility where they can see out a window or watch local traffic on the unit.
Hearing	Decrease or eliminate distressing auditory stimuli (change bedroom, talk with family members about noise of stereos and other such equipment, use earplugs, use headphones to listen to soft music). Develop sensitivity to different sounds (music, chirping birds, night sounds, different voices). Use the telephone to maintain contact with family and friends. Use television, radio, cassettes to keep current and to stimulate mental activities. Recall favorite sounds of the past with the situations in which they were heard.	Speak in a warm and pleasant tone and communicate caring to the client. Use your voice to orient client to environment and current situation (eg, procedure, treatment). Avoid speaking about the client to others within the client's hearing. Remember that clients overhearing snatches of conversation outside their room often presume it is about *them!* Decrease extraneous noise (intercom, movement of carts, loud conversations of staff); use carpets and sound-absorbing material whenever possible.
Taste	Experiment with foods of different tastes (seasonings), colors, temperature, and textures; realize that as taste buds age, things will no longer taste the same. Practice thorough oral hygiene and have regular dental examinations. Recall foods that tasted especially good in the past and the events surrounding these tastes (eg, grandparent baking cookies or homemade bread).	Consult with the dietitian about preparing meals with varied taste sensations; serve meals attractively. Perform routine oral hygiene for clients who are unable to do this for themselves.
Smell	Consciously savor smells that are pleasant; decrease or eliminate noxious odors. Recall pleasant aromas or smells from the past and the events surrounding them (eg, smell of the ocean as the vacation house was neared, smell of fresh pine in the house at Christmas, the body scent of a loved person or animal).	Keep the client's room well ventilated, using opportunities when the client is out of the room to air it out. Remove dressings, drainage, and any equipment with odors from the client's room as quickly as possible.

(continued)

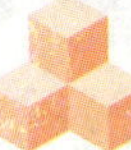

Guidelines for Nursing Care *(continued)*

Stimulating the Senses

	Teaching Clients	Nursing Interventions
		Encourage clients to focus on pleasant or familiar smells, such as coffee, newspaper, or flowers. Avoid wearing heavy perfumes.
Touch	Consciously surround yourself with different textures and let yourself feel and enjoy them (scratchy afghan; a puppy's moist, wet tongue; soft petal of a flower; smooth silk scarf; mug of hot chocolate). Allow these textures to evoke memories of past tactile experiences (grandchild's hug may bring back memories of hugs from own children, scrap of fabric may recall a prom dress or wedding gown or baby blanket). Recognize need to be touched and tell someone, "I need a hug today!" Receive tactile stimulation from a pet.	Include different textures in the client's environment (silky pillow sham from home, soft sheepskin, wooly blanket). Respect the client's need and desire to be touched or not touched (touch the client's forearm or shoulder, hug the client). Use physical care (bath time, foot soaks, hair care, back massages, turning and positioning, passive range of motion) to provide tactile stimulation. Limit intrusive procedures and times when the client needs to be uncomfortably manipulated.

General Nursing Strategies in the Hospital or Other Residential Care Setting

Encourage the client to participate in activities that require exploration of the environment (exercise, feeling, tasting, touching, moving, listening).

Use conversation to explore areas of interest to the client.

Encourage the client to share feelings.

Familiarize the environment by encouraging the client to wear own clothes and keep personal items nearby.

Suggest the use of self-stimulation techniques—humming, singing, whistling, reciting, memory review, and problem solving.

talking, leaning forward or turning an ear toward the speaker, answering inappropriately, talking too loudly, inability to carry on a phone conversation, strained facial expression (pp. 307, 312).

The following are recommended guidelines for communicating with people with hearing deficits:

- Orient the person to your presence before initiating conversation. This may be done by moving so you can be seen or by *gently* touching the person.
- Decrease background noises (television, radio) if possible before you speak.
- Position yourself so the light is on your face and the person can see your lips and expressions.
- Talk directly to the person while facing him or her or angle the chair so that your voice reaches the ear that hears best. If the person is able to lip-read, use simple sentences and speak in a quiet, natural manner and pace. Be aware of nonverbal communication.
- Do not chew gum, cover your mouth, or turn away when talking with the person.
- Demonstrate or pantomime ideas you wish to express, as appropriate.
- Use sign language or finger spelling, as appropriate.
- Write any ideas that you cannot convey to the person in another manner.

The accompanying box lists aids for hearing impaired clients.

Communicating With a Confused Client

The client who lacks the mental ability to process environmental stimuli may be aware of this inability and find it frustrating. This client needs the nurse's support to make adjustments to this limitation. Other clients may be oblivious of the deficiency. In both instances, the nurse must protect the safety of the client while providing optimal sensory stimulation. Nursing interventions include the following:

- Using frequent face-to-face contact to communicate the social process (use touch when appropriate, walk arm in arm, hug, give a back rub)
- Speaking calmly, simply, and directly to the client and allowing sufficient time for the client to think before responding

Communication Methods Available to Assist the Hearing Impaired

- Hearing aids
- Lip reading
- Signing
- TDD—telecommunication devices
- Infrared systems
- Computers
- Voice amplifiers
- Amplified telephones
- Low-frequency door bells and telephone ringers
- Closed-caption TV decoders
- Flashing alarm clocks
- Flashing smoke detectors

- Orienting and reorienting the client to the environment and filling the client's personal space with as many personal objects as possible
- Using conversation, watches, clocks, calendar, newspaper, television, radio, and other such devices to orient the client to time, place, and person
- Clearly communicating that the client is expected to perform all self-care activities of which the client is capable
- Keeping the emphasis on client strengths rather than on deficiencies and verbally reinforcing strengths
- Offering the client simple explanations for care, new activities, and so on
- Varying environmental stimuli gradually while keeping the environment structured enough that the client feels comfortable and at home
- Using objects from the client's past (baseball, picture of a train, photograph) to spark reminiscences and discussions
- Reinforcing reality if the client is delusional

Specific intervention suggestions for caring for confused older adults are given in the accompanying box.

Communicating With an Unconscious Client

The following are recommended guidelines for communicating with an unconscious client:

- Be careful of what is said in the person's presence. Hearing is believed to be the last sense lost in the unconscious person, and therefore the person is often likely to hear what is being said, even though there does not appear to be a response.
- Assume the person can hear you. Talk with the person in a normal tone of voice about things you would ordinarily discuss.
- Speak to the person before touching. Remember that touch can be an effective means of communicating with the unconscious person.
- Keep environmental noises at as low a level as possible. This helps the person focus on the communication.

EVALUATING

While implementing a plan of nursing care designed to decrease excessive sensory stimuli or increase meaningful stimuli, the nurse evaluates the effectiveness of the plan by observing for a decrease in the behavioral manifestations of sensory deprivation or overload. It may be concluded that the plan of care is working if a client who had begun to withdraw and spend most of the day lying in bed with a blank facial expression appears more alert and begins to initiate conversations and to take an interest in personal care. The nurse also evaluates the client's ability to interact appropriately with the environment while practicing necessary self-care behaviors. The client's achievement of desired outcomes is evaluated at established times.

The nurse also evaluates the client's need for nursing versus his or her ability to manage the plan of care independently. Ideally, the client and family learn to manipulate the environment to promote optimal sensory stimulation for growth and development. Clients with specific sensory impairments are evaluated for their knowledge of the impairment, acceptance and management of the treatment regimen, and ability to perform necessary self-care activities.

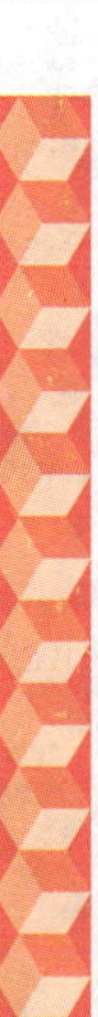

Focus on the Older Adult

A scientific basis is needed for nursing interventions that can be used in caring for persons with dementia who manifest agitation behavior. High stress is one of the possible causes of agitation behavior in persons with dementia; use of stress management interventions may be helpful in reducing the stress level.

Nurse researchers (Snyder, Egan & Burns, 1995) discovered that two nursing interventions—hand massage and therapeutic touch—were effective in producing a relaxation response in persons with dementia who had a history of agitation behaviors; they did not, however, decrease agitation behavior. Hand massage was more effective in producing relaxation than was therapeutic touch. In a study of 25 elderly nursing home residents, Moore and Gilbert (1995) found that residents who were subjected to comforting touch by their nurses perceived an increased feeling of affection and immediacy.

The conscious and intentional use of comforting touch by nurses and caregivers to elderly nursing home residents should be encouraged because of its beneficial effect of conveying love and belonging.

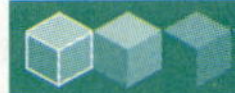

Nursing Process in Clinical Practice

The nurse uses each phase of the nursing process when identifying and treating sensory/perceptual alterations categorized as nursing diagnoses.

> Sensory Perceptual Alterations: A state in which an individual experiences a change in the amount or patterning of incoming stimuli accompanied by a diminished, exaggerated, distorted or impaired response to such stimuli. (NANDA, 1994)

Quality care depends on the nurse's knowledge and clinical skills as described earlier in this chapter. Following in outline format are the assessment priorities, client goals, nursing interventions, and evaluation criteria for two common types of age-related sensory deprivation problems:

Sensory/Perceptual Alterations: Sensory Deprivation related to parent's inability to provide a developmentally stimulating environment

Sensory/Perceptual Alterations: Chronic Sensory Deprivation related to effects of aging and institutionalization

In the client care study that follows the development of these diagnoses, nursing care is described for a non–English-speaking client who is experiencing mixed sensory deprivation and overload on admission to the maternity unit in a large teaching hospital.

Sensory Deprivation Related to Inadequate Parenting

Sensory organs and nerve fibers need early sensory stimulation to develop normally both structurally and functionally. Parents may fail to provide a developmentally stimulating environment for their child for many reasons:

- Lack of knowledge of the child's growth and development needs
- Lack of motivation to promote the child's development
- Inadequate resources—parenting skills, finances, and so on

Assessment Priorities

- Use well-baby/child visits to monitor the child's development (gross motor behavior, fine motor, adaptive, language, personal–social).
- Assess if the child is receiving the stimulation and interactional experiences with the environment necessary to develop optimally. For example, if an infant is slow to crawl, see if parents and caretakers are providing supervised time to explore the environment on the floor versus leaving the infant in a baby chair, swing, or some other device all day. Similarly, if a child's expressions are dull and the child's language development is slow, assess the quality of human interaction and communication the child is receiving.
- Assess if the child's sensory/perceptual abilities are intact; identify sensory impairments and make appropriate referrals.
- If a lack of environmental stimulation is suspected, assess for possible etiologies: parents' lack of knowledge, motivation, skill, or resources; inadequate child care outside the home; other such factors.

Expected Outcomes

The child will:

- Appear alert and interested in the environment
- Demonstrate improved sensory stimulation by achieving targeted developmental milestones (specify)

The parents will:

- Identify the relation between sensory stimulation and the child's development
- Suggest reasons for the child's limited sensory experiences to date
- Describe a realistic and developmentally appropriate plan to increase visual, auditory, olfactory, gustatory, and tactile stimulation for the child
- Verbalize commitment to the plan

Interventions

Interventions should be tailored to the etiology of the problem. If the parents are eager to participate in the care plan and simply lack knowledge:

- Offer suggestions for increasing environmental stimulation and role model appropriate interactional behaviors.
    - *Visual:* Vary colors in the child's environment, increase access to out-of-the-home stimulation (parks, stores, fire engines, and other such stimuli), offer the child books with interesting pictures, and limit television.
    - *Auditory:* Talk with and sing or hum to the child, read stories to the child, have the child join a storytelling group at the library, teach the child to become sensitive to nature's sounds or other sounds in the environment.
    - *Olfactory:* Allow the child to identify and distinguish different odors; role model for the child savoring special aromas (pizza coming out of the oven).
    - *Gustatory:* Encourage the child to experiment with foods of different tastes, shapes, colors,

textures, and temperatures; recognize that children enjoy finger foods and foods that are crispy, chewy, or bubbly.
- *Tactile:* Increase body contact with the child by means of games and sports as well as through demonstrative affection (hugs, holding child in lap, stroking face, and so on); if possible, allow the child to select a pet.

- Discuss with the parents developmentally appropriate play activities for children that will enable the child to learn social behavior, develop cognitive abilities, develop gross and fine motor skills, and work through emotional conflicts.
- Refer parents to parenting education group. If the parents lack the motivation to provide a developmentally stimulating environment for the child, intensive counseling is indicated with follow-up to ensure that the child is receiving adequate care. Counseling should explore the parents' experiences as children, the meaning the child holds for the parents, and the probability that the parents will learn and be motivated to use adequate parenting skills. If parents are resistant to counseling and child neglect is suspected, the nurse is legally responsible to report the family for evaluation.
- If lack of resources is contributing to the parents' difficulty in stimulating the child's development, available resources are explored. A referral to social services may be indicated.

Chronic Sensory Deprivation Related to Effects of Aging

Although the phenomenon of acute sensory deprivation has been carefully studied by nurses and other researchers, less attention has been paid to chronic sensory deprivation, a condition experienced by many elderly people. The elderly person who has multiple sensory deficits or who lives in a deprived environment is a prime candidate for chronic sensory deprivation. Symptoms of this disorder are most likely gradual in onset and all too often are mistaken for senility.

Assessment Priorities

To define the extent of the problem and its etiologies, Gioiella and Bevil (1985) recommend careful data collection in the following seven areas: (1) sensory status; (2) level of mobility; (3) preferred stimulation level; (4) sensory, perceptual, and social environment; (5) mental status; (6) behavioral changes; and (7) personal resources. Using assessment guidelines presented earlier in this chapter, the nurse assesses the elderly person's vision, hearing, taste, smell, touch, and kinesthetic and visceral awareness. It is critical to understand that some older people have a need to deny sensory impairment and may evolve remarkable compensatory abilities. Behavioral changes (eg, withdrawal or the paranoia that many hearing-impaired elderly clients demonstrate) may be the best indicator of an underlying sensory problem.

Sensory Status. The senses of vision, hearing, and touch (and to a lesser degree, taste and smell) all decline with age. Moreover, many of the chronic illnesses experienced by elderly people impair sensory functioning. Common sensory problems include vision problems such as cataracts; **presbyopia** (a condition of aging in which decreased elasticity of the lens hinders accommodation to close vision); glaucoma and macular degeneration; hearing problems such as **presbycusis** (age-related hearing loss in which there is decreased ability to distinguish higher frequencies); diminution of touch with diabetes and cerebrovascular disease; and altered body sense or awareness associated with restricted mobility and arthritis, cardiovascular and respiratory diseases, and neurologic disorders involving some degree of paralysis.

Level of Mobility. The less mobile an elderly client is, the more the client depends on the immediate environment and the more likely he or she is to experience sensory deprivation in an impoverished environment. The nurse needs to determine the client's physical ability to ambulate; the need for supportive devices (braces, canes, walkers, wheelchairs, railings, ramps); the client's motivation to be mobile; the presence of external factors hindering mobility ("I'm afraid if I go out of the house I'll be mugged"); and the need for support services (physical therapy, walking partner, transportation assistance, planned reinforcement).

Preferred Stimulation. Individuals vary greatly in the amount of stimulation they need. One older client sitting quietly may be enjoying reminiscences that effectively stimulate the brain whereas another client may be utterly bored and becoming disoriented.

Sensory, Perceptual, and Social Environment. The client's environment is assessed to determine if it presents a sufficient *variety* of meaningful sensory, cognitive, and emotional stimulation. Determine if each sense is being stimulated, if the client's mental abilities are being challenged, and if different emotions are being evoked. In caring families there often is a tendency to "do for" the older person, which may be counterproductive. The older person who has no need to meet everyday demands may feel useless and lose abilities not being used.

Mental Status. Changes in mental status or behavior may be the first indication of sensory deprivation. Assess for disorientation to time, place, or person; altered ability to concentrate or problem solve; and perceptual changes such as illusions or hallucinations.

Behavioral Changes. Significant behavioral changes include personality changes such as boredom and apathy, restlessness, withdrawal, and paranoia; alterations in sleep–wake patterns; decreased attention to personal hygiene and appearance; change in responses to others and communication patterns; and rapid mood swings.

Personal Resources. It is important to assess how well the client has coped with stresses in the past and the adequacy of supports currently available to him or her.

Expected Outcomes

The client will:

- Demonstrate orientation to time, place, and person
- Demonstrate interest in everyday self-care activities
- Demonstrate a decrease in the perceptual, cognitive, and emotional responses indicating sensory deprivation (specify)
- Actively participate in a plan to increase sensory stimulation

The client's caretakers (family, nursing staff) will:

- Identify factors contributing to sensory deprivation
- Develop a realistic plan to increase sensory, cognitive, and emotional stimulation

Interventions

- Make every effort to correct client's sensory impairments (eg, medical evaluation and treatment of sensory deficits; correct use and care of eyeglasses, contact lenses, hearing aids, ambulation aids).
- Ensure that the client has adequate periods of rest and that daytime activities prevent boredom and catnapping. Discourage the use of sedatives. Assess the effect on the central nervous system of any other medications the client is taking.
- Implement the plan to increase sensory stimulation (see Guidelines for Nursing Care earlier in the chapter). Homebound or institutionalized older people may benefit greatly from visits by children. Pet therapy is an excellent source of stimulation. Simple activities like rolling a colorful, large, soft ball among four people seated at a table can effectively stimulate multiple senses (vision, hearing, touch, kinesthetic) for confused clients. Exercise classes for elderly clients also provide excellent stimulation.
- Make a concerted effort to increase the client's mobility and encourage changes in the environment. Use family and community resources to get the homebound client out of the house. Implement a plan to assist institutionalized clients to visit other parts of the institution, to get outside, and to participate in scheduled social events. Volunteers may be extremely helpful once committed to a plan of action.
- When interacting with the older client, communicate that the client is important and valued and make your expectations known.
- Avoid endorsing confusion. Gently reorient the client to reality whenever delusional statements are made.
- Keep the environment safe for the client.

Client Care Study

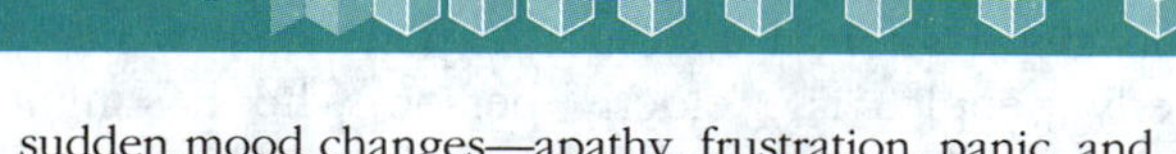

Two days ago, Mrs. Philomela Palikias delivered by cesarean birth a 32-week-old, small-for-gestational-age infant girl weighing 3 lb, 8 oz. Because of her size and respiratory distress, the infant was placed in the neonatal intensive care unit (NICU). Postpartal assessments indicate that Ms. Palikias's physical progress is satisfactory. However, the nurses are concerned about her mental status. Ms. Palikias arrived in the United States 3 months ago with her husband. Both speak only Greek and neither has family in the United States.

Recorded in the client's progress notes the evening of her second postpartal day is the following nursing assessment:

> 12/4/98, 9 pm, nursing
>
> Client refused to get out of bed again this evening—demonstrates no interest in seeing baby; to date has not ambulated to NICU. Refusing to learn and participate in self-care activities—expressing breast milk or performing perineal care. Nurses throughout the day reported sudden mood changes—apathy, frustration, panic, and hostility. Unable to find someone who speaks Greek to serve as translator. Husband does not speak English but appears concerned about his wife.
>
> N. Gable, RN

Core Competencies

The nurse needs the following specialized abilities in implementing the nursing plan of care.

Cognitive Competencies

- Knowledge of and respect for different cultures and their influence on health and human functioning
- Strong assessment skills and knowledge of factors contributing to sensory alterations and of nursing interventions to prevent and treat sensory alterations
- Knowledge and clinical skills of maternity nursing

- Teaching and counseling skills to prepare the client to assume new mothering role with confidence

Interpersonal Competencies
- Ability to empathize with a young woman experiencing multiple stressors (sensory overload) with few customary supports
- Strong interpersonal skills and creative ability to communicate well to non–English-speaking client using body language, services of interpreter, and so on
- Ability to communicate to client that what she is experiencing is understandable and that help is available
- Interpersonal and leadership skills to help the nursing staff view this client as a challenge and together to be committed to her care plan

Ethical/Legal Competencies
- Knowledge of professional responsibilities and ability and willingness to meet these responsibilities in a legally defensible manner
- Human caring, compassion, and strong sense of accountability for delivering quality care
- Ability and willingness to go the extra mile with this client to ensure that she is not lost in the system and discharged without receiving the assistance she needs

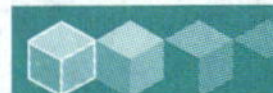

Nursing Plan of Care

for Mrs. Palikias

Nursing Diagnosis: Sensory/Perceptual Alteration: Mixed Sensory Deprivation and Overload related to unfamiliar hospital environment (different culture) and stress of cesarean birth and infant's prematurity as manifested by client not demonstrating interest in baby or self-care activities; limited ability to concentrate on new tasks (pericare, expressing breast milk); sudden mood changes—apathy, frustration, panic, hostility

Expected Outcome: Before discharge, the client will:
- Demonstrate increased comfort in the hospital environment (decreased or absent mood swings—apathy, frustration, panic, hostility)

Nursing Interventions	Rationale	Evaluative Statement
Secure assistance of an interpreter and work with the interpreter to do the following:		12/6/98 Goal met. Client is quiet but no longer apathetic, fearful, or hostile. Moving about in hospital with more confidence. ***N. Gable, RN***
• Orient the client to her surroundings (explaining reasons for equipment, procedures, treatment)	Sensory deprivation results from *meaningless,* unpatterned stimuli; once the client understands her environment she can respond to it appropriately.	
• Reassure the client that what she is experiencing is normal given her recent stresses (moving to new country, cesarean birth of first child, infant's prematurity)	Clients experiencing strange perceptual, cognitive, and affective responses to sensory deprivation and overload often fear they are going crazy and hesitate to share their feelings.	
• Determine the client's needs	The client herself is best able to voice her needs.	
Have the interpreter teach the nurse several Greek words and make recommendations about how the client can personalize her environment, such as having her husband provide her with usual food, music, and other familiar items.	Contributing to sensory deprivation is the absence of familiar sounds (native languages, sights, tastes, or scents). Having access to familiar food and the like may reduce sensory deprivation.	

(continued)

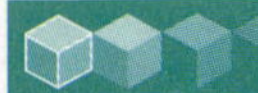

Nursing Plan of Care *(continued)*

for Mrs. Palikias

Nursing Interventions	Rationale	Evaluative Statement
See if the interpreter can explain usual customs regarding childbirth and aftercare in Greece.	Including culturally familiar childbirth and aftercare customs in the plan of care enhances client well-being and cooperation in the plan of care.	
Limit the number of nurses and other persons interacting with the client; attempt to have the same nurse caring for her each shift.	A trusting nurse–client relationship can develop.	
Schedule care to allow for uninterrupted periods of sleep and rest.	Sleep deprivation contributes to other sensory alterations.	

Expected Outcome Before discharge, the client will:

- Resume independent self-care activities

Nursing Interventions	Rationale	Evaluative Statement
Use services of interpreter to teach client importance of ambulating and becoming independent again in self-care measures.	Regaining independence enhances client's sense of well-being.	12/6/98 Goal partially met. Client is ambulating, but she resists pericare and is fearful when expressing breast milk. *Recommendation:* Continue teaching with assistance of interpreter. ***N. Gable, RN***
Have interpreter write simple directions for follow-up care, times when baby may be visited after client is discharged, and so on. Share these instructions with the client's husband.	Cognitive responses to sensory deprivation and overload include decreased attention span and concentration and problem-solving ability. Written instructions and husband's knowledge reinforce the client's learning.	
See if husband has bilingual friends or work acquaintances who might be willing to help the client when she gets home until she has established a comfortable routine of care for the baby and is knowledgeable about community resources.	Careful discharge planning is necessary to ensure that the client can manage new parenting responsibilities in an unfamiliar country.	

Expected Interventions Before discharge, the client will:

- Demonstrate interest in her baby by visiting the neonatal intensive care unit, holding the baby, expressing her milk, and other such activities.

Nursing Interventions	Rationale	Evaluative Statement
Learn and respect cultural norms for new mothering behaviors.	Nursing care that is not culturally sensitive is deficient.	12/6/98 Goal met. Client is now visiting baby in the unit on her own. ***N. Gable, RN***
Assist the client to ambulate to unit to see the baby; if interpreter is available, have the person explain equipment surrounding the baby and answer the client's questions about the baby.	The client may be refusing to visit the unit to protect herself from barrage of frightening stimuli (sensory overload); the goal is for her to become familiar with the unit so she is able to focus on bonding with her daughter.	

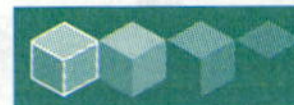

Nursing Plan of Care *(continued)*

for Mrs. Palikias

Sample Documentation

Traditional Note Format

12/5/98, 10 AM, nursing

First session with interpreter and client at 9 am. Client's face brightened as soon as she heard someone speak to her in Greek. Basically, client shared she did not care too much about what was happening to her but she was terrified about the baby and afraid of what everyone was doing to the baby. Directed interpreter to orient client to her environment, daily routine, and NICU. Client appeared anxious when she first saw baby but looked content when able to hold her. Scheduled teaching session for tomorrow am when interpreter will come for 1 hour. Client currently resting comfortably.

R. Traner, RN

SOAP Format

12/5/98, 9 PM, nursing

Sensory/Perceptual Alterations: Mixed Sensory Deprivation and Overload related to unfamiliar hospital environment stress of cesarean birth and infant's prematurity

S: —

O: Cried after husband left this evening; refused postpartal check; turned away from nurses

A: Still feels overwhelmed by newness of all that is happening to her and tries to shut out what she cannot handle

P: Continue to intervene with help of interpreter; focus on helping client develop more control over her situation; proceed at slow pace; referral to social services for follow-up care

N. Gable, RN

Key Points

- The senses of vision, hearing, smell, taste, and touch keep an individual in contact with the external environment. The kinesthetic and visceral senses arise from muscles and hollow organs, respectively, and orient the individual to the internal environment.
- The brain must be alert or aroused to receive stimuli and respond appropriately. The reticular activating system, with its many ascending and descending connections to other areas of the brain, monitors and regulates incoming sensory stimuli and thus maintains, enhances, or inhibits cortical arousal.
- Sensory alterations occur when a person experiences decreased sensory input or input that is monotonous, unpatterned, or meaningless (sensory deprivation), or excessive sensory input such that the brain is unable to respond meaningfully (sensory overload).
- Responses to both sensory deprivation and overload include perceptual changes (mild to gross distortions or hallucinations); cognitive changes (decreased attention and concentration, decreased problem-solving ability); and affective changes (apathy, anxiety, fear, panic, anger, depression, and rapid mood swings).
- Clients at high risk for sensory deprivation include those experiencing decreased environmental stimuli (homebound or institutionalized clients, clients on bed rest or in isolation) and those with impaired ability to receive or process environmental stimuli (clients with sensory deficits, clients from a different culture, clients with certain affective disorders and disturbances of the nervous system, clients with bandages or casts that interfere with sense reception, clients taking medications that affect the central nervous system).
- Clients at high risk for sensory overload include acutely ill clients, clients in critical care settings, clients in pain, clients with intrusive and discomforting monitoring or treatment equipment, and clients with disturbances of the nervous system.

- Factors affecting sensory stimulation include age, culture, personality and lifestyle, stress, illness, and medication.
- A comprehensive nursing assessment of sensory functioning includes an examination of the client for sensory deficits and manifestations of sensory deprivation or overload and an examination of the client's environment to see if it is providing adequate sensory stimulation for healthy development.
- Nursing diagnoses may be written specifically addressing sensory/perceptual alterations (visual, auditory, olfactory, gustatory, tactile, sensory deprivation, sensory overload) or identifying the effect sensory/perceptual alterations have in other areas of human functioning (eg, verbal communication, self-care, social interaction, thought processes).
- Small modifications in a client's environment and in the nurse's pattern of interacting may be all that is needed to prevent sensory alterations.
- Sensory deprivation during a child's formative years may yield permanent results because sensory organs and nerve fibers need early sensory stimulation to develop normally both structurally and functionally. Parents may fail to provide a developmentally stimulating environment for their child because of lack of knowledge, decreased motivation, or inadequate resources.
- The elderly person who has multiple sensory deficits or who lives in a nonstimulating environment is at high risk for chronic sensory deprivation. Symptoms of this disorder are frequently mistaken for senility.

Study Questions

1. The major components of any sensory experience are
   a. the kinesthetic and visceral senses
   b. reception and perception
   c. the intensity, size, change, or representation of stimuli
   d. vision, hearing, smell, taste, and touch
2. Four conditions necessary for a person to receive data and experience the world are
   a. a stimulus, a receptor, an intact nerve pathway, and a functioning brain
   b. the visual, auditory, olfactory–gustatory, and tactile senses
   c. the basic orienting systems arising from muscles, joints, hollow organs, and movement
   d. the reticular activating system, variable stimuli, memory, and motivation
3. By monitoring and regulating incoming sensory stimuli, this system maintains, enhances, or inhibits cortical arousal:
   a. general adaptation system
   b. kinesthetic/visceral system
   c. reticular activating system
   d. sensory/perceptual system
4. You notice that Mr. Wong, who has cataracts, is sitting closer to the television than usual. The etiology of his sensory problem is
   a. altered environmental stimuli
   b. altered sensory reception
   c. altered nerve impulse conduction
   d. altered impulse translation
5. Should you learn that Mr. Wong, who is 85 years old, also has presbycusis, you would want to
   a. obtain large print written material
   b. speak distinctly using lower frequencies
   c. decrease tactile stimulation
   d. initiate a safety program to prevent falls
6. Peter Almone is in the last stages of AIDS, which is now affecting his brain as well other major organ systems. He confides to you that he feels terribly alone because most of his friends are afraid to visit. The etiology of his sensory alterations is most likely related to
   a. stimulation
   b. reception
   c. transmission–perception–reaction
   d. all of the above
7. Which of the following factors is least likely to place a client at high risk for sensory deprivation?
   a. an environment with decreased or monotonous stimuli
   b. impaired ability to receive environmental stimuli
   c. impaired ability to process environmental stimuli
   d. impaired ability to respond to environmental stimuli
8. Which of the following clients is at greatest risk for sensory deprivation?
   a. an elderly man confined to bed at home after a stroke
   b. an adolescent in an oncology unit working on homework supplied by friends
   c. a woman in labor
   d. a toddler in a play room awaiting same-day surgery
9. A client in an intensive care burn unit for 1 week is in pain much of the time and has his face and both arms heavily bandaged. His wife visits every evening for 15 minutes at 6, 7, and 8 pm. A heart monitor beeps for a client on one side, and another client moans frequently. These data suggest that the client probably
   a. has sufficient sensory stimulation

b. has deficient sensory stimulation
c. has excessive sensory stimulation
d. has both sensory deprivation and overload

10. Richard's spinal cord was severed and he is paralyzed from the waist down. In making an assessment of this client, it is most important to assess which component of the sensory experience?
a. transmission of tactile stimuli
b. adequate stimulation in the environment
c. reception of visual and auditory stimuli
d. general orientation and ability to follow commands

11. An 11-year-old 6th grader whose grades have dropped has difficulty completing her work on time, frequently rubs her eyes, and squints. Her visual acuity on a Snellen's eye chart was 160/20. Based on these data, the most appropriate nursing diagnosis is
a. Knowledge Deficit related to visual impairment
b. Altered Role Performance (Student) related to visual impairment
c. Body Image Disturbance related to visual impairment
d. Altered Growth and Development related to visual impairment

12. Of the four items listed below, the best nursing intervention to prevent sensory alterations for a man with a severe hearing deficit who reads lips well is to
a. turn the radio or television volume up very loud and close the door to his room
b. prevent embarrassment and emotional discomfort as much as possible
c. provide daily opportunity for him to participate in a social hour with six or eight people
d. encourage daily participation in exercise and physical activity

13. In a boarding home where most clients have slight-to-moderate visual or hearing impairment and some are periodically confused, the nurse's first priority in caring for sensory concerns is to
a. maintain safety and prevent sensory deterioration
b. insist that every client participate in as many self-care activities as possible
c. emphasize and reinforce individual client strengths
d. encourage reminiscence and life review in groups

14. The nursing diagnosis for 8-month-old Sally was Sensory/Perceptual Alterations: Sensory Deprivation related to inadequate parenting. Since that time, both parents have attended parenting classes. However, both parents work while Sally stays with her 86-year-old grandmother who is visually impaired. The parents provide appropriate stimulation in the evening. At an evaluation conference at age 11 months, Sally lay on the floor sucking her thumb and rocking her body. Her facial expression was dull and she vocalized only in a low monotone ("uh-h-h"). Your best evaluation concerning Sally's sensory deprivation is that
a. her parents lack motivation to provide necessary stimulation
b. her grandmother is unable to improve Sally's care
c. Sally's sensory deprivation is still severe
d. this is normal behavior for a child of Sally's age

15. Which of the following nursing interventions should *not* have been implemented for an elderly woman in a nursing home who walked out the door unobserved and was hit by a car? The nursing diagnosis was Sensory/Perceptual Alterations: Chronic Sensory Deprivation related to the effects of aging.
a. Ignore when the client is confused or go along to prevent embarrassment.
b. Encourage self-care and independent decisions.
c. Take walks around the grounds and to the garden daily.
d. Provide daily contact with children, community people, and pets.

Answers With Rationale

1. The correct response is *b.* Reception and perception are the major components of any sensory experience. All other choices are merely part of the sensory experience.
2. The correct response is *a.* A stimulus, a receptor, an intact nerve pathway, and a functioning brain are the four conditions necessary for a person to receive data and experience the world.
3. The correct response is *c.* The reticular activating system maintains, enhances, or inhibits cortical arousal by monitoring and regulating incoming sensory stimuli.
4. The correct response is *b.* Cataracts are interfering with the client's ability to receive visual stimuli—altered sensory reception. The nature of incoming stimuli, the conduction of nerve impulses, and the translation of incoming impulses in the brain are not a problem here.
5. The correct response is *b.* Presbycusis is a normal loss of hearing as a result of the aging process. Speaking distinctly in lower frequencies is indicated. The other choices refer to interventions for other sensory problems.
6. The correct response is *d.* This client is receiving decreased environmental stimuli (eg, from his friends); is more than likely experiencing problems with reception because of major organ involvement; and his impaired brain function will impair impulse transmission–perception—reaction.

7. The correct response is *d.* The other options all pertain to components of the sensory experience that, if impaired, may place a client at high risk for sensory deprivation. An impaired ability to respond to environmental stimuli places a client at risk for problems other than sensory deprivation.
8. The correct response is *a.* The client confined to bed rest at home is at risk of having his environmental stimuli greatly reduced. The other clients are all in environments where environmental stimuli are at least adequate.
9. The correct response is *d.* This client's bandages may result in deficient sensory stimulation (sensory deprivation), and the monitors and other sounds in the intensive care burn unit may cause a sensory overload. All other options are incomplete responses.
10. The correct response is *a.* Below-the-waist paralysis makes the transmission of tactile stimuli a problem. Although the other options may be assessed, they are indirectly related to his paralysis.
11. The correct response is *b.* An important role for an 11-year-old is that of student. Her impaired vision is clearly disturbing her role performance as a student as evidenced by her lower grades. Although the other options may also represent accurate diagnoses for this client, they do not flow from the data that were presented.
12. The correct answer is *c.* Providing daily opportunities for this client to participate in a social hour builds on his strength of being able to lip-read and provides sufficient sensory stimulation to prevent sensory deprivation resulting from his hearing loss.
13. The correct answer is *a.* Safety is a basic physiologic need that must be met before higher-level needs such as love and belonging, self-esteem, and self-actualization can be met.
14. The correct response is *c.* Although the data show that the parents have been motivated to improve their parenting skills, it is clear from the data presented that Sally's sensory deprivation is still severe. The data suggest that the grandmother is not improving Sally's care, but there is nothing to suggest that she is *unable* to do so if shown how.
15. The correct response is *a.* Even if well motivated, ignoring a client's confusion to prevent embarrassment may be dangerous, as it was in this case in which the appropriate safety precautions were never implemented. The other options are all appropriate for this client.

Bibliography

Bolin, R. H. (1974). Sensory deprivation: An overview. *Nursing Forum, 13*(3), 240–258.

Broussard, A. B. (1990). Incorporating infant stimulation concepts into prenatal classes. *Journal of Obstetric, Gynecologic, and Neonatal Nursing, 19*(5), 381–387.

Brown, I. A. (1985). Sensory deprivation: An overview. *Journal of Neurosurgery Nursing, 17*(5), 273–279.

Chlan, L.L. (1995). Psychophysiologic responses of mechanically ventilated patients to music: A pilot study. *American Journal of Critical Care, 4*(3), 233–238.

Espezel, H. (1994). The visually impaired child. *Canadian Nurse, 90*(5), 23–25.

Fine, J.I. & Rouse-bane, S. (1995). Using validation techniques to improve communication with cognitively impaired older adults. *Journal of Gerontological Nursing, 21*(6), 39–45.

Gioiella, E., & Bevil, C. (1985). *Nursing care of the aging client.* Norwalk, CT: Appleton-Century-Crofts.

Glynn, N. J. (1992). The music therapy assessment tool in Alzheimer's patients. *Journal of Gerontological Nursing, 18*(1), 3–9.

Hancock, C.K., Munjas, B., Berty, K. & Jones, J. (1994). Altered thought processes and sensory perceptual alterations: A critique. *Nursing Diagnoses, 5*(1), 26–30.

Harrison, L. L., & Woods, S. (1991). Early parental touch and preterm infants. *Journal of Obstetric, Gynecologic, and Neonatal Nursing, 20*(4), 299–306.

Janken, J. K. (1990). Auditory sensory/perceptual alteration: Suggested revision of defining characteristics. *Nursing Diagnosis, 1*(4), 147–154.

Kloosterman, N. D. (1991). Cultural care: The missing link in severe sensory alteration. *Nursing Science Quarterly, 4*(3), 119–122.

Kolanowski, A. M. (1992). The clinical importance of environmental lighting to the elderly. *Journal of Gerontological Nursing, 18*(1), 10–14.

Koniak-Griffin D., & Ludington-Hol S. M. (1988). Developmental and temperament outcomes of sensory stimulation in healthy infants. *Nursing Research, 37*(2), 70–76.

Lindberg, J. B., & Kruszewski A. Z. (1983). Special senses and the environment. In J. Lindberg, M. Hunter, & A. Kruszewski (Eds.). *Introduction to person-centered nursing* (pp. 297–315). Philadelphia: Lippincott.

Lindblade, D.D. & McDonald, M. (1995). Removing communication barriers for the hearing-impaired elderly. *MEDSURG Nursing, 4*(5), 379–385.

McDaniel, R.W., Rhodes, V.A., Nelson, R.A. & Hanson, B.M. (1995). Sensory perceptions of women receiving tamoxifen for breast cancer. *Cancer Nursing, 18*(3), 215–221.

MacKinnon-Kesler, S. (1983). Maximizing your ICU patient's sensory and perceptual environment. *Canadian Nurse, 79*(5), 41–45.

Martini, F.H. & Timmons, M.J. (1995). *Human anatomy.* Englewood Cliffs, NJ: Prentice-Hall.

Moore, J.R. & Gilbert, D.A. (1995). Elderly residents: Perceptions of nurses' comforting touch. *Journal of Gerontological Nursing, 21*(1), 6–13.

Norris, C. M. (1985). Primitive pleasure as the basic human state. *Advances in Nursing Science, 8*(1), 25–43.

North American Nursing Diagnosis Association. (1994). *NANDA nursing diagnoses: Definitions and classifications 1995–1996*. Philadelphia: NANDA.

Oehler, J. M. (1991). Beyond technology: Meeting developmental needs of infants in NICUs. *Maternal–Child Nursing, 16*(3), 148–151.

Palumbo, M. V. (1990). Hearing access 2000: Increasing awareness of hearing impaired. *Journal of Gerontological Nursing, 16*(9), 26–31, 37–38.

Pope, D.S. (1995). Music, noise, and the human voice in the nurse–patient environment. *IMAGE: Journal of Nursing Scholarship, 27*(4), 291–296.

Poroch, D. (1995). The effect of preparatory patient education on the anxiety and satisfaction of cancer patients receiving radiation therapy. *Cancer Nursing, 18*(3), 206–214.

Seyfrit, M. (1995). Going blind. *American Journal of Hospice and Palliative Care, 12*(3), 31–40.

Snyder, M., Egan, E.C. & Burns, K.R. (1995). Interventions for decreasing agitation behaviors in persons with dementia. *Journal of Gerontological Nursinsg, 21*(7), 34–40.

Standley, J.M. & Moore, R.S. (1995). Therapeutic effects of music and mother's voice on premature infants. *Pediatric Nursing, 21*(6), 509–512.

Suedfeld, P. (1985). Stressful levels of environmental stimulation. *Issues in Mental Health Nursing, 7*(1/4), 83–104.

Wang, J.F. (1995). Caregiver–child interaction in Japan, Taiwan, and the United States. *JOGNN, 24*(4), 353–361.

Zahr, L.K. & Balian, S. (1995). Responses of premature infants to routine nursing interventions and noise in the NICU. *Nursing Researach, 44*(3), 179–185.

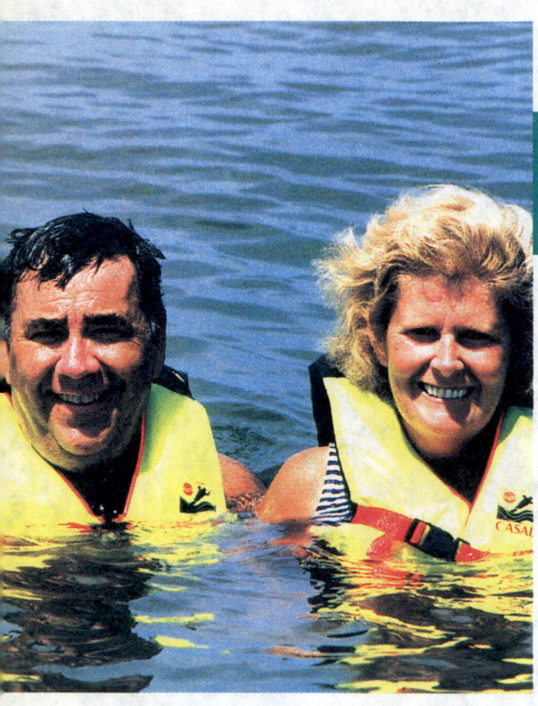

Chapter 35

Sexuality

Objectives

After studying this chapter, the learner should be able to:

Define key terms used in the chapter.

Describe male and female reproductive anatomy and physiology.

Describe the sexual response cycle, differentiating male and female responses.

Identify factors that affect an individual's sexuality.

Perform a sexual assessment using suggested interview questions and appropriate physical assessment skills.

Describe types of sexual dysfunctions and assessment priorities for each.

Develop nursing diagnoses identifying a problem with sexuality that may be remedied by independent nursing actions.

Describe five areas in which the nurse can provide the client with education to promote knowledge of sexuality.

Plan, implement, and evaluate nursing care related to selected nursing diagnoses involving problems of sexuality.

Key Terms

biologic gender
bisexuality
contraception
erogenous zones
gender identity
gender role behavior
heterosexuality
homosexuality
impotence
masturbation
menarche
menopause
menstruation
orgasm
premenstrual (tension) syndrome
rape
sexual dysfunction
sexual harassment
sexuality

Sexuality is a concern in professional nursing care because sexuality permeates an individual's life, both in illness and in wellness. **Sexuality** is the degree to which a person exhibits and experiences maleness or femaleness physically, emotionally, and mentally. Sexuality is defined not only by a person's genitalia but also by attitudes and feelings. It can also be defined as learned behaviors in how a person reacts to his or her own sexuality and by how one behaves in relationships with others. Culture profoundly influences learned behaviors about sexuality. Sexuality is an integral part of a person's identity and is present in one's demeanor through actions, communications, and physical appearances.

Biologic gender is the term used to denote chromosomal sexual development: male (XY) or female (XX). **Gender or sexual identity** is the inner sense a person has of being male or female, which may be the same as or different from biologic gender. **Gender role** is the behavior a person conveys about being male or female, which, again, may or may not be the same as biologic gender or gender identity (Pilliteri, 1995).

This chapter discusses reproductive anatomy and physiology, the sexual response cycle, and factors that affect sexuality. Obtaining a sexual history as part of a comprehensive client history is presented, as well as interview questions that specifically address a client with a sexual dysfunction. Nursing priorities with regard to assessment of the reproductive system are presented. Analysis of assessment data is discussed with examples of corresponding nursing diagnoses. The section Nursing Process in Clinical Practice provides the nurse with a format that uses assessment data, planning, interventions, and evaluations for nursing diagnoses that pertain to concerns with sexuality (Sexual Dysfunction: Inhibited Sexual Desire; Altered Sexuality Patterns: Change in Sexual Expression; Knowledge Deficit: Contraceptive Methods; and Body Image Disturbance: Surgical Removal of a Breast). The client care study and nursing plan of care provide the nurse with examples of how the information presented in the chapter can be used in a clinical setting to nurture and promote aspects of sexuality in clients.

Physiology

Female

The female genitalia are represented by both internal and external structures. The appearance of the external genitalia (illustrated in Fig. 26-47) varies slightly among individuals.

External Genitalia

The *mons pubis* is actually a pad of fatty tissue that lies over the part of the bony pelvis called the *symphysis pubis.* In the physically mature female, the mons pubis is covered with coarse *pubic hair.* It contains many nerve endings that make the mons pubis sensitive to touch and pressure. The *labia majora* consist of two rounded folds of fatty tissue. The outer lips separate downward from the mons pubis and meet again below the vaginal introitus. The labia majora contain a multitude of sebaceous and sweat glands. They respond to touch during sexual activity. The *labia minora* are the smaller lips located within the labia majora. They are thin and sensitive structures and are pale pink in color. When stimulated by touch, the labia minora may turn a darker pink or even red owing to the presence of many blood vessels. The labia minora have no hair and are smooth in texture.

The *clitoris* is found above the urinary meatus at the joining of the labia minora, called the *clitoral hood.* The clitoris is a small, button-like structure similar to the male penis in its reaction to stimuli. The clitoris contains erectile tissue, blood vessels, and nerves. It is extremely sensitive. The opening of the vagina lies between the urinary meatus and the anus. It may contain a structure called the *hymen,* which is a thick membrane with no apparent function. At one time, the hymen was thought to represent *virginity* (not having experienced sexual intercourse); however, this is erroneous. Remnants, or "tags," of the hymen may be noted at the vaginal introitus in both sexually active and inactive women.

Internal Genitalia

The internal genitalia—the ovaries, fallopian tubes, uterus, and vagina (Fig. 35-1)—are located deep within the pelvis of the female. The female body normally contains two ovaries, one on each side of the body. The ovaries closely resemble an almond in size and shape. At the time of a female child's birth, each ovary contains some 200,000 to 400,000 follicles. This number steadily decreases until puberty, when 100,000 to 200,000 follicles remain, and the number continues to decline over the reproductive years. The process of ovulation is discussed later in this chapter. The ovaries also secrete the hormones estrogen and progesterone.

The *fallopian tubes* are slender structures that extend from either side of the uterus and end in a fringed fashion near each ovary. Their function is to transport a mature *ovum* (female reproductive cell) from an ovary to the uterus. Fertilization of the ovum by a sperm usually occurs in the tube. The fertilized ovum then travels the rest of the way to the uterus, where it implants. An unfertilized ovum travels the same path but does not implant. It is eventually expelled from the body during the menses. Because the lumen of each tube is so narrow, it can easily be damaged by the effects of infection and surgery.

The *uterus* is a pear-shaped organ about 3 inches long located between the urinary bladder and the rectum. Its primary purpose is to house and nurture a *pregnancy* (the condition of carrying a developing embryo in the uterus). The uterus comprises three layers: the outermost layer, the *perimetrium*, consists of elastic tissue; the middle layer, the *myometrium*, is muscular; and the innermost layer, the *endometrium*, comprises tissue that thickens and sloughs off with the menses. The *cervix* is the structure at the lower portion of the uterus that connects the uterus and the vagina. The cervix is usually closed. However, during the birth process, it dilates and thins out extensively to permit the birth of a baby. The cervix is a smooth, pink-colored structure that possesses few nerve endings. When touched, the sensation resembles that of touching the end of one's nose.

The *vagina* is a tubular, hollow organ that lies between the urinary urethra and the rectum. Its size and shape are individual among women. The walls of the vagina are composed of rugae, or ribbed tissue. The vagina serves three purposes: it is (1) a receptacle for the penis during sexual intercourse, (2) a birth canal for the passage of a baby, and (3) an exit for menstrual flow from the uterus. During sexual activity the walls of the vagina secrete, or "sweat," a thin watery material, sometimes in copious amounts. This lubrication is necessary

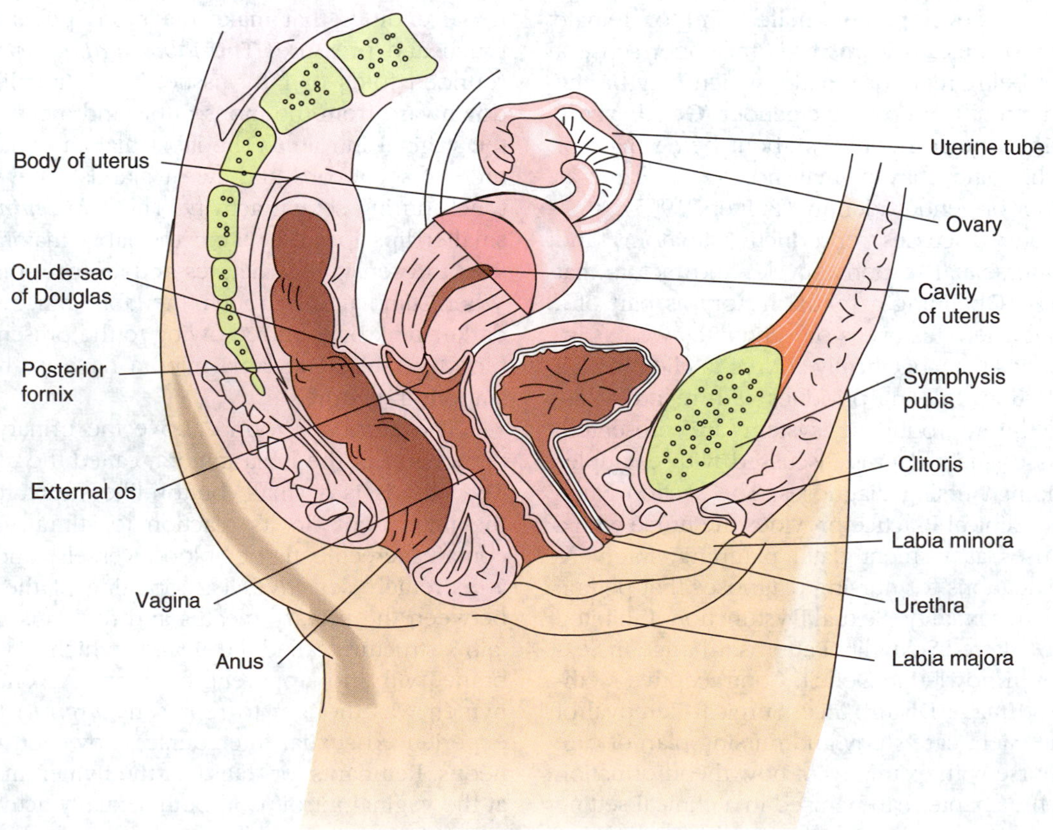

Figure 35-1
Sagittal section of the female reproductive organs.

for the comfortable placement and movement of the penis in the vagina.

Breasts

Although the breasts are not considered part of the internal or external genitalia, they are an important aspect of the female's physical sexuality. The breasts consist of fatty and glandular tissues and the nipples. Their size and shape vary widely among women. The nipples are pale to deep pink in color. Caressing of the breasts can be pleasurable during sexual activity, and many women can be brought to orgasm by this action alone.

Menstrual Cycle

Menstruation is a cycle during which the body prepares for the presence of a fertilized ovum. Each cycle is about 28 days long but may vary from as short as 21 days to as long as 40 days. The first menstrual period, called **menarche**, is experienced around age 12 years; again, the age of menarche is individual and may occur at age 8 years to age 17 years. **Menopause**, the cessation of a woman's menstrual activity, occurs between the ages of 45 and 55 years. The woman may experience irregular menses over time before menstruation ends.

The menstrual cycle is controlled by a series of reactions that rely on feedback from the ovaries to the pituitary gland. Actually two cycles occur simultaneously, one in the ovaries and one in the uterus (Fig. 35-2).

In the ovaries, in a typical 28-day cycle, the phase from day 4 to 14 is called the *follicular phase.* During this phase, a number of follicles mature but only one produces a mature ovum. At the same time, in the uterus, the endometrium is becoming thick and velvety in preparation for receiving a fertilized egg. This phase in the uterus is called the *proliferation phase.* Ovulation occurs on day 14. The mature ovum ruptures from the follicle and the surface of the ovary and is swept into the fallopian tube. If sperm are present, the ovum is fertilized at this time. Some women can detect ovulation by the presence of a sharp, cramping pain over the ovulating ovary; this pain is called *mittelschmerz,* or middle pain, because it occurs in the middle of the cycle. From day 15 to day 28, the phase in the ovaries is called the *luteal phase.* The leftover empty follicle fills up with a yellow pigment and is then called the *corpus luteum,* or yellow body. The purpose of the corpus luteum is to produce hormones that encourage a fertilized egg to grow. If fertilization does not occur, the corpus luteum begins to disintegrate. During the luteal phase in the ovaries, the uterus also undergoes changes. This phase is called the *secretory phase.* The endometrial lining becomes thick. However, in the absence of a fertilized egg, the corpus luteum dies and the endometrial lining disintegrates. At day 28, the *menses,* or the menstrual flow, begin as a result of the uterus shedding the useless portion of its endometrium.

The menses lasts for 3 to 7 days, the average length of flow being 5 days. The menstrual discharge is a

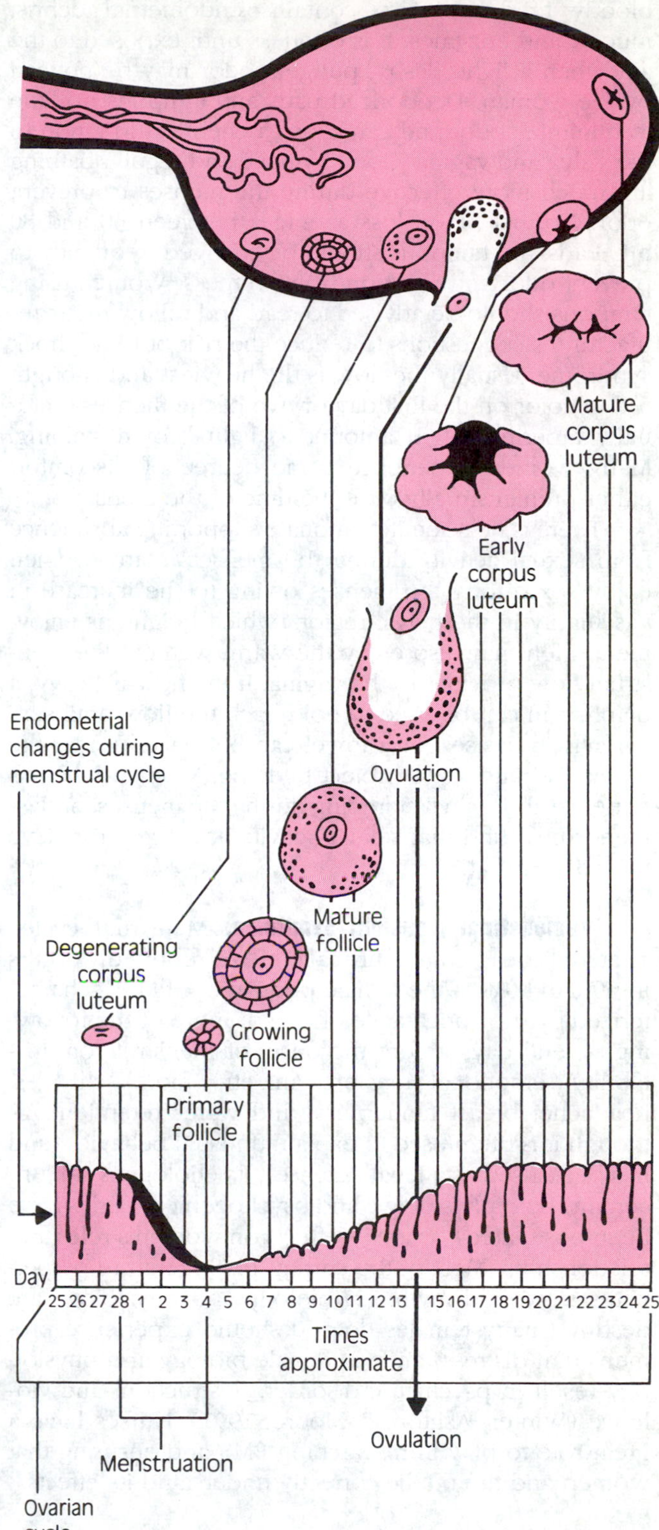

Figure 35-2
Schematic representation of one ovarian cycle and the corresponding changes in the endometrium.

bloody fluid that also contains endometrial debris, mucus, and enzymes. It is odorless until exposed to the air, when a light, fleshy, pungent odor may be noticed by the woman. Deodorized pads and tampons do little to minimize odor and can cause a chemical irritation to the vulva and vagina. Good hygiene and regular bathing are much more effective during the menses to prevent odor. Normal blood loss averages between 30 and 80 mL. Pads and tampons should be changed frequently to prevent odor and irritation from wetness. Women using tampons should be advised to read and follow the manufacturer's suggestions to reduce the risk of toxic shock syndrome. Usually the flow is the heaviest and is bright red in color on the first day or two of the menses, gradually tapering off in amount to light brown staining. Many women experience some degree of discomfort either premenstrually or at the time of the menses.

There is no scientific rationale supporting abstinence from sexual activity during the menses. Many women enjoy sex during the menses owing to the increase in vascularity in the pelvic region, which heightens enjoyment. Men may also enjoy the warm wetness the menstrual flow provides to the vagina. If the flow is heavy, a diaphragm can be used to hold back the flow until sexual activity ceases, or a towel can be placed under the woman's buttocks to protect bedding. Women who experience abdominal cramping during the menses, or dysmenorrhea, find that sexual activity and orgasm relieve their discomfort.

Premenstrual (Tension) Syndrome. Menstrual cycle–related distress, commonly called PMS, reportedly occurs in 50% to 90% of the female population. PMS is characterized by the appearance of one or more of the following several days before the onset of menstruation: irritability, emotional tension, anxiety, mood changes, headache, breast tenderness, and water retention. Although it is often used to explain unusual behavior (and has been used as a legal defense), its etiology is still uncertain (both physiologic and psychogenic theories have been postulated), as are its effects on women's roles and relationships. Most of the current PMS literature perpetuates a twofold myth: (1) biology and physiology are destiny (many females do and should experience premenstrual distress) and (2) female biology and physiology result in psychiatric disorder, destruction, and violence (Winter, Ashton, & Moore, 1991). Nurses have a great role to play in researching PMS and ensuring that women and the public correctly understand its effects.

Male

Unlike female genitalia, the male genitalia (illustrated in Fig. 26-48) are found primarily outside the body. The *testes*, which are about the size of walnuts, feel smooth and are freely movable within the scrotum. The *scrotum* is the loose, baglike structure that houses the testes. Normally two testes are present. The testes produce *sperm* and the hormones necessary for the maintenance of male sex characteristics. The primary hormone secreted by the testes is *testosterone*, which is responsible for a man's deep voice, beard growth, and body hair.

The scrotum hangs between a man's upper thighs. The area around the base of the penis and the scrotum is covered with pubic hair. The looseness of the scrotum is intentional to provide expansion and contraction. When exposed to cool temperatures, the scrotum contracts and draws the testes closer to the body for warmth. In warm temperatures, the scrotum become loose and allows the testes to hang farther away from the heat of the body. The testes are sensitive organs and can suffer discomfort, sometimes extreme, if handled roughly or jostled. It is important that a man wear a properly fitted athletic support, or jockstrap, when engaged in strenuous physical activity. However, the continuous use of a support can cause the temperature within the scrotum to rise and the delicate sperm to die because of constant exposure to high temperatures. Snug-fitting garments such as tight jeans can have the same effect on a man's fertility. The scrotum can be a source of sexual pleasure when lightly stroked, fondled, or caressed during sexual activity.

Tubules from the testes drain into the *epididymis*, which in turn drains into the *vas deferens* and *ejaculatory ducts*. These ducts then drain directly into the urethra. It is believed that the vas deferens acts as a reservoir for sperm between ejaculations.

The seminal vesicles, prostate gland, and Cowper's glands produce a liquid called *seminal plasma*. The seminal plasma and the sperm collectively make up the *semen*. The plasma aids in the transport of sperm and also provides energizing nutrients for the sperm. It contains a form of sugar (fructose), mucus, salts, water, base buffers, and coagulators to aid the sperm in their journey. Semen is a thick, creamy white fluid with the consistency of mucus or egg whites. The normal amount of semen per ejaculate is 2 to 6 mL. A fertile man dispels 120 to 160 million sperm per ejaculate. Cowper's glands produce small droplets of fluid during sexual activity that neutralize the acidity of the male urethra and aid in the transport of sperm. This fluid may contain sperm. Therefore, contraceptive measures, if used, must be taken before this fluid can be introduced into the woman's vagina.

The *penis* is a tubular structure located above the scrotum. It functions to eliminate urine from the bladder, to ejaculate semen and impregnate a woman, and as a sex organ for sexual pleasure. It consists of the shaft and the *glans* (head of the penis). In the uncircumcised male, the glans is covered by loose skin (*foreskin*) that can be retracted. In the circumcised male, the foreskin has been surgically removed and the glans is exposed. Penis size and shape vary among individuals. Normally the penis is soft and flaccid and 2½ to 4 inches long. The dimensions of the penis in no way dictate the man's ability to perform effectively during sexual activity. When an *erection* occurs, the blood vessels in the shaft of the penis become congested and the penis becomes hard and erect. The size of the penis during an erection may increase to 5½ to 7 inches in total length. The penis, particularly the glans, is extremely sensitive to stimulation.

Stroking and handling of the shaft of the penis are also pleasurable during sexual activity. Stimulation to prompt the penis to an erection is varied. A full bladder on awakening in the morning can cause an erection. Fantasy, memories of a past sexual encounter, and accidental brushing by an attractive stranger can all lead to an erection. An erection in the male does not always signify desire for sexual activity. Exposure of the male client by the nurse during a bed bath may cause an erection. An erection is a normal physiologic response and not something the man can voluntarily control. The erection ceases if no further stimulation is added.

Ejaculation is the expulsion of semen by the rhythmic contractions of the penis. The penis engages in short, jerky movements that produce a spurt of semen with each motion. The period of ejaculation is short, and the penis becomes flaccid after ejaculation. Many males, particularly adolescent boys, may experience a phenomenon known as *nocturnal emission*, or "wet dream." These ejaculatory episodes occur during sleep without physical stimulation. They are perfectly normal and do not represent any sort of deviation.

Male breasts contain little real breast tissue, but they still may be stimulated during sexual activity. Although the area of sensitivity is usually limited to the nipple and areola, its stimulation can be as pleasurable an experience for the male as it is for a female.

Sexual Response Cycle

The physiologic responses to sexual activity of female and male are more similar than different (Fig. 35-3). Also, body response is essentially the same regardless of the source of stimulation; that is, fantasy, masturbation, and sexual intercourse between two individuals can all bring about the same body reactions. The sexual response cycle is not limited to the genital organs but is a total body response that causes many physiologic changes throughout the body. The cycle has four

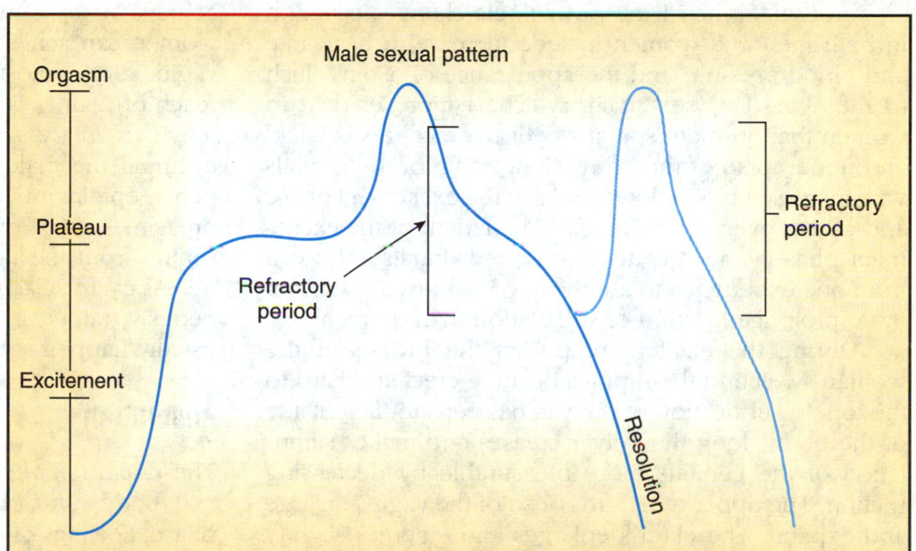

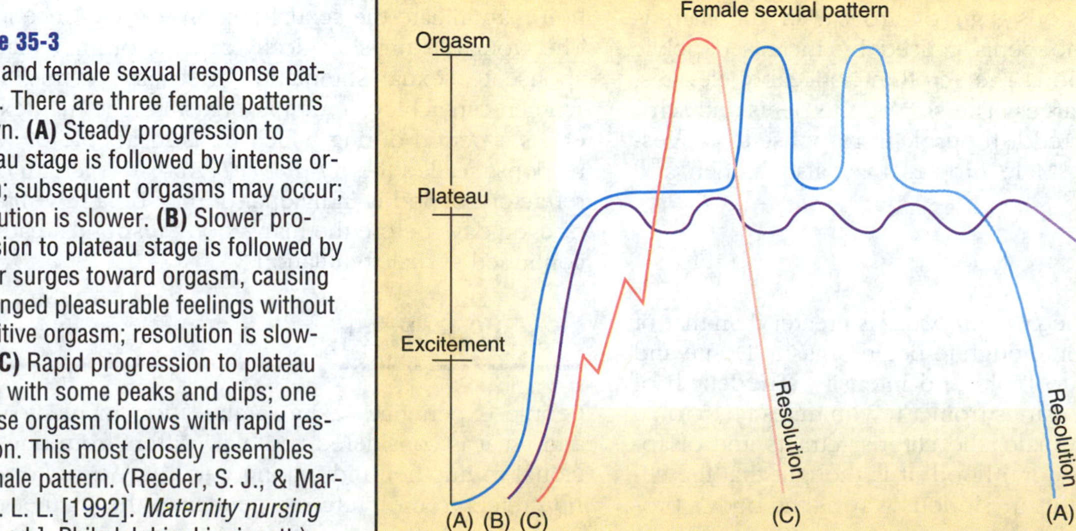

Figure 35-3
Male and female sexual response patterns. There are three female patterns shown. **(A)** Steady progression to plateau stage is followed by intense orgasm; subsequent orgasms may occur; resolution is slower. **(B)** Slower progression to plateau stage is followed by minor surges toward orgasm, causing prolonged pleasurable feelings without definitive orgasm; resolution is slowest. **(C)** Rapid progression to plateau stage with some peaks and dips; one intense orgasm follows with rapid resolution. This most closely resembles the male pattern. (Reeder, S. J., & Martin, L. L. [1992]. *Maternity nursing* [17th ed.]. Philadelphia: Lippincott.)

phases: (1) excitement, (2) plateau, (3) orgasm, and (4) resolution; there is a smooth progression from one phase to the next. Although only physiologic response is discussed here, the emotional and mental involvement of sexual response contributes a great deal to the pleasure and satisfaction of sexual activity.

The human body contains many **erogenous zones**, areas that, when stimulated, cause sexual arousal and desire. The genitals are an obvious source of sexual pleasure for both men and women, but other areas of the body are also considered erogenous zones. The skin of the body is the largest erogenous zone. Other areas include the ears, lips, thighs, and breasts. Some people can reach orgasm simply by stimulation of erogenous zones other than the genitals. The most important body organ for sexual arousal and stimulation is the brain. It allows individuals freedom to enjoy a sexual experience but also may prevent satisfaction by inhibitions, doubts, and guilt.

Excitement

The *excitement phase* is initiated by erotic stimulation and arousal. Some of the physiologic changes common in both men and women include increase in heart rate and blood pressure and the appearance of a pink flush to the skin. This sex flush, which is more evident in women than in men, spreads over the face, neck, back, and upper torso of the body. Congestion of the genitals with increased blood flow begins in the excitement phase and causes even more arousal. The length of the excitement phase varies greatly among individuals and even from one experience to another. Women usually enjoy a more prolonged period of stimulation than do men.

During the excitement phase, the breasts of the woman swell and the nipples become erect and hard to the touch. Lubrication of the vagina seeps to the outside of the body along the vulvar creases and makes stimulation of the genitals more pleasurable by decreasing friction. The upper two thirds or so of the vagina enlarge and expand. The clitoris enlarges and emerges slightly from the clitoral hood. The labia also enlarge and separate and turn a deep rosy red in color with arousal.

The first obvious sign of arousal in the man is an erection of the penis caused by increased pelvic congestion of blood. The scrotum noticeably elevates, thickens, and enlarges. The skin of the penis and scrotum turns a deep reddish-purple in response to congestion and arousal. Male nipples may also harden and become erect.

Plateau

The intensity of the *plateau phase* is greater than that of excitement but not enough to begin orgasm. Desire and arousal continue to build and intensify. The length of time of this phase varies from a few minutes to 15 to 20 minutes. In the female, the clitoris retracts and disappears under the clitoral hood. It is thought that the clitoris performs in this mysterious way as the body's protection against overstimulation. In the male, secretions from Cowper's glands may appear at the glans of the penis during the plateau phase.

Orgasm

The term **orgasm** defines the climax and sexual explosion of the tension built over the preceding phases. Orgasm lasts a matter of seconds, but it is an extremely intense reaction. Characteristic of the orgasm phase are the involuntary spasmodic contractions of the genital organs. The number of contractions felt by the individual depends on the intensity of the orgasm.

The orgasm phase in the female begins with a heightened feeling of physical pleasure followed by overwhelming release and involuntary contractions of the genitals. Loss of muscular control can also be seen in spastic contractions and twitching of the arms and legs. The number of contractions can be as few as 4 or as many as 20. Areas of the body that contract spasmodically are the uterus, anal sphincter, rectum, and urethral sphincter. It currently is believed that women achieve orgasm in a variety of ways. Although some women can achieve orgasm by penile thrusting in the vagina alone, most women need clitoral stimulation to reach orgasm.

Involuntary spasmodic contractions of the genitals occur in the male during orgasm. These occur in the penis, epididymis, vas deferens, and rectum. The male orgasm is most often accompanied by ejaculation of semen from the urinary meatus of the penis. It is not necessary for ejaculation and orgasm to occur simultaneously; rather, it is a coincidence that the two events usually happen at the same time.

Resolution

The *resolution phase* is characterized by a return to normal body functioning present before the excitement phase. Feelings of relaxation, fatigue, and fulfillment are common. Some people may also have a need to be held, fondled, and caressed. Physical demonstrations of affection may initiate the sexual response cycle once again. The woman is physiologically capable of immediate response to sexual stimulation. Because of this, many women can achieve multiple orgasms. The man experiences a period during which he is incapable of sexual response, called the *refractory period.* The length of the refractory period is individual; it may be a few minutes or even days before the man's body responds readily to continued sexual stimulation.

Sexual Orientation

People experience sexual gratification in many ways, and what is considered "normal" differs from one individual to another and among cultures. *Sexual orientation* refers to the preferred gender of the partner of an individual. The origins of sexual orientation are unknown, but there are studies claiming a genetic basis. Certainly some sexual preferences are culturally determined and may be dictated by opportunity.

A **heterosexual** is one who experiences sexual fulfillment with a person of the opposite gender. A **homosexual** is one who experiences sexual fulfillment with a person of the same gender. Homosexual males often use the term "gay"; homosexual females use the term "lesbian." Heterosexuality and homosexuality can be placed at opposite ends of a continuum with many variations in between. **Bisexuality** refers to a person who finds pleasure with both opposite-sex and same-sex partners. Homosexual or heterosexual people may have bisexual relationships at times.

A transsexual is a person of a certain biologic gender with the feelings of the opposite sex. The person feels trapped within the body of the wrong sex. The reason, or etiology, behind this is unknown, although many factors are believed to be involved. For many transsexuals, the solution is to change their bodies to match their inner feelings through surgery and hormone therapy. A transvestite is an individual who desires to take on the role or wear the clothes of the opposite sex. Most transvestites are heterosexual, and many keep their lifestyle hidden.

Sexual Expression

The methods by which people gain satisfaction through sexual stimulation are varied. Touch, smell, sight, sounds, feelings, thoughts, and fantasy can all contribute to sexual fulfillment in any form of expression chosen

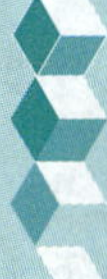

Research in Nursing: Making a Difference

The studies that follow demonstrate the commitment nurse researchers are making to discover better ways for nurses to meet the sexual needs of clients and themselves.

Steinke, E.E., & Patterson, P. (1995). Sexual counseling of MI patients by cardiovascular nurses. (1995). *Journal of Cardiovascular Nursing, 10*(1), 81–87.
Of 171 cardiac nurses from three midwestern hospitals surveyed by Wichita State University researchers, 75% said they offered to discuss sexual matters with fewer than 2% of post-MI patients. A similar percentage (78%) reported providing information or education on post-MI sex to fewer than 2% patients. Many respondents said that they never offered to talk about sexual concerns with their patients (42%) or that they never provided education or information (42%). Also, 71% reported that they had never referred patients to another professional for sex counseling. Of nurses who cited "barriers" to sex teaching, 14% mentioned lack of time; a similar number (11%) cited discomfort with the topic, a problem noted in other research. The study authors call for both formal education and informal efforts to increase nurses' knowledge of post-MI sexual concerns and their comfort in assessing for sexual problems and discussing them.

Cole, F. L. & Slocumb, E. M. (1995). Factors influencing safer sexual behaviors in heterosexual late adolescent and young adult collegiate males. *IMAGE: Journal of Nursing Scholarship, 27*(3), 217–223.
Heterosexual adolescents and young adults are at high risk for AIDS because many experiment with drugs and alcohol and are sexually active. Since behavioral changes are essential to preventing the spread of AIDS, this exploratory study examined variables characterized as predisposing to the practice of safe sexual behaviors. Findings identified three significant variables (attitude toward condoms, internal health locus of control, and self-esteem), each of which is amenable to intervention strategies to enhance the practice of safe sexual behaviors.

Kay, J., Donald, C. G., & Merker, S. (1994). Sexual harassment of critical care nurses: A costly workplace issue. *American Journal of Critical Care, 3*(6), 409–415.
In this descriptive study the federal government's definition of sexual harassment and a list of sexually harassing behaviors was mailed with a survey to 188 critical care nurses. Findings indicated that 46% of the respondents had been harassed. Offensive sexual remarks (56%), unwanted physical contact (53%), unwanted nonverbal attention (27%), requests for dates (16%), and sexual propositions (9%) were types of sexual harassment experienced. Harassers were physicians (82%), coworkers (20%), and immediate supervisors (7%). A majority of the incidents (69%) were not reported. Most nurses (80%) had not received training in reporting harassment, nor were there policies and procedures to follow in most cases. The authors conclude that sexual harassment training, policies, and procedures are needed to provide a safe, healthy work environment for critical care nurses.

Summary

In order to meet sexual needs, nurses must be comfortable about their own sexuality, develop competence in addressing and meeting client sexual needs, and be prepared to address workplace issues. Further research is needed in each of these areas.

by individuals. Feelings of love for another person are closely associated with desire.

Forms of sexual stimulation include kissing, hugging, stroking, squeezing, breast stimulation, manual stimulation of the genitals, oral–genital stimulation, and anal stimulation. Sexual stimulation may be physical or psychologic. Erotic stimulation through the use of films, magazines, and photographs is common. *Fetishism*, usually practiced by a male, is sexual arousal with the aid of an inanimate object not generally associated with sexual activity. Items such as shoes, leather, rubber, and women's undergarments may be used.

Masturbation

Masturbation is a technique of sexual expression in which an individual practices self-stimulation. Many myths and misinformation surround the issue of masturbation. Masturbation is a means of learning what is preferred by a person during stimulation and what feels good. Men masturbate by holding and stroking the shaft of the penis. Women find manual stimulation of the clitoris enjoyable, although variations of technique are numerous. People masturbate regardless of sex, age, or marital status. People may not masturbate because of a sense of guilt or wrongness associated with self-stimulation. Masturbation is not "dirty" and will not lead to blindness, nor will it cause insanity.

Sexual Intercourse

Heterosexual genital intercourse is the most common image that comes to mind when sexuality is mentioned. The act of intercourse (coitus or copulation) usually begins by stimulation of the senses in some way, followed by a period of activity known as foreplay. Petting is part of foreplay and can be simple stroking of the breasts, arms, back, and neck without genital involvement or may lead to mutual masturbation and orgasm.

The act of placing the penis in the vagina, penile–vaginal intercourse, can be accomplished by various positions. The most common position in Western cultures is the missionary position, which places the woman horizontally under the man. (This position was named *missionary* by the Polynesians because it was the preferred position used for intercourse by religious missionaries.) Other positions may be more stimulating and comfortable. Clitoral stimulation is difficult to achieve in the missionary position. Lying side by side, female on top, and rear entry are some examples of coital positions that make clitoral stimulation more successful. Some people are so inhibited they need permission to engage in alternative sexual positions.

When the penis is pushed into the vagina, the man begins rhythmic thrusting movements of his hips to stroke the penis back and forth along the vaginal walls. The woman may match her partner's hip movements with movements of her own body. These movements continue until orgasm is attained by one person or both. Simultaneous orgasms, or both people attaining orgasm at the same moment, are difficult to achieve. Preoccupation with attaining simultaneous orgasms may disrupt the ultimate intimacy and satisfaction possible during the coital experience. The period after coitus is just as significant as the events leading up to it. Caressing, hugging, and kissing actually deepen the intimacy shared by the couple and should be nurtured and not rushed.

Anal intercourse, the act of inserting the penis into the anus and rectum of a partner, is the other form of intercourse. Commonly practiced by gay men, it is also used by heterosexual couples. Once the penis (or any object) is placed in the rectum, it should not be introduced into the vagina without thorough cleansing, because many organisms present in the rectum can cause subsequent vaginal infections. Care should be exercised to avoid injury to the delicate rectal mucosa, and lubrication is essential for comfort. Condoms are now recommended for both types of intercourse to prevent sexually transmitted diseases.

Oral–Genital Stimulation

Stimulation by using the mouth and tongue on the genitals may be used during foreplay or as a method to reach orgasm. *Cunnilingus* is stimulation of the female genitals by licking and sucking the clitoris and surrounding structures. *Fellatio* is stimulation of the male genitals by licking and sucking the penis and surrounding structures. These techniques may be used singularly or simultaneously (*soixante-neuf*).

Celibacy

Celibacy is abstinence from genital sexual activity. Celibacy may be practiced for many reasons. Dissatisfaction with the harmful consequences of the "sexual revolution" of the 1960s is leading an increasing number of adolescents and adults to choose celibate lifestyles. Many members of religious orders and institutes live celibate lives in order to commit themselves to non-exclusive love relationships and to non-physical types of generativity.

Alternative Forms of Sexual Expression

Voyeurism is the achieval of sexual arousal by looking at the body of another. Some voyeurs develop complex means to spy on others that involve a violation of the observed's privacy rights.

Sadism refers to the practice of gaining sexual pleasure while inflicting abuse on another person. *Masochism* refers to gaining sexual pleasure from the humiliation of being abused. When practiced together, the act is called *sadomasochism*. It may involve being tied up, biting, hitting, spanking, whipping, pinching and other activities.

Pedophilia is a term used to describe the practice of adults gaining sexual fulfillment by sexual acts with children.

Factors Affecting Sexuality

Many factors influence and affect a person's sexuality and thus differentiate personal feelings regarding sexuality. That is, the brain, rather than the genitals, plays the most significant role in how people perceive themselves as sexual beings.

Developmental Considerations

The process of human development affects the psychosocial, emotional, and biologic aspects of life, and these in turn affect an individual's sexuality. Sexuality is the only distinguishing trait present at conception. From birth onward, gender, or sex, influences behavior throughout life. See Table 35-1 for a summary of sexuality throughout the life span and nursing implications for each stage.

Culture

The manner in which sexuality is perceived by a society in turn influences the individual. Every culture has its own norms regarding sexual identity and behavior. To some degree, culture dictates the duration of sexual intercourse, methods of sexual stimulation, and sexual positions. In some cultures, women may be expected merely to tolerate sex, whereas in others the woman's participation is encouraged.

Religion

Some view organized religion as having a generally negative effect on the expression of sexuality. Many forms of sexual expression other than male–female coitus are considered unnatural by some religions. Also, over time, the concept of virginity came to be synonymous with purity and sex became synonymous with sin. Double standards and rigid regulations have inflicted a considerable amount of guilt and anxiety on many individuals. A number of sexual dysfunctions can be related to the individual's anguish over the negative connotation of sex as dictated by some religious groups. Most major religions are currently reexamining their teachings on sexuality in response to challenges posed by their members. Many have recognized the importance of solid sex education within the realm of the church.

Ethics

Healthy sexuality depends on freedom from guilt and anxiety. What one person believes is wrong may be perfectly natural and correct to another. Some individuals, however, may feel that certain forms of sexual expression are bizarre and the people who participate in them are perverted. If the sexual expression is performed by consenting adults, is not harmful to them, and is practiced in privacy, it is not considered a deviant behavior. Individuals should personally decide with which aspects of sexual expression they are comfortable. Frequently, all an individual needs to alleviate guilt and consequently enhance sexual satisfaction is permission from a healthcare professional to engage in a different form of expression.

Lifestyle

Modern lifestyles greatly affect sexuality and its expression. Both men and women are exposed to stress, and many are under considerable strain to perform and function in the workplace as well as at home. Stressors may be external, such as job and financial demands, or internal, such as a competitive nature. These varied responsibilities place a time restraint on communication between a couple, as well as on the energy level and motivation for sexual satisfaction. Although some couples view sexual activity as a release from the stressors of everyday life, most place sex far from the top of the list of things to do. It is crucial to a relationship's survival that a couple set aside priority time—if not for lovemaking, then for intimate, quiet contact.

Health State

A healthy body, mind, and emotions are necessary for sexual wellness. Any trauma or stress that interferes with an individual's ability to perform daily functions certainly also affects the expression of sexuality. Illness is no exception.

Chronic Pain. Many chronic illnesses are accompanied by constant pain, and an individual with persistent pain may not desire any sexual contact. However, the desire for human warmth and contact does not cease because of pain. Altered or modified positions for coitus are sometimes necessary; these are discussed in more detail later in this section.

Diabetes Mellitus. Diabetes mellitus is a hormonal disease in which the body is deficient in the amount of insulin secreted by the pancreas. Although almost all hormonal disorders affect sexuality in some way, diabetes is the most prevalent and well known. *Erectile dysfunction*, or **impotence**, is a great concern among diabetic men. Treatment to date depends largely on the degree of erectile ability lost. Some men may be candidates for a penile prosthesis, which was developed in 1973. The prosthesis is surgically implanted below the base of the penis, and inflation of the device produces an erection when sexual activity is desired.

It is not uncommon for diabetic women to experience loss of capacity for orgasm (*orgasmic dysfunction*). Difficulty experiencing arousal and loss of vaginal lubrication have also been reported. Frequent *Monilia* infections of the vagina are also common and cause discomfort during coitus.

Table 35-1
Developmental Aspects of Sexuality Through the Life Span

Stage	Characteristics	Nursing Implications and Teaching Guidelines
Infancy: Birth to 18 mo	• Needs affection and tactile stimulation • Boys have penile erections and girls have orgasmic potential • Gradually can differentiate self from others • Obtain pleasure from touching genitals • Dressed according to gender • Toys are gender related	• Avoid early weaning to prevent oral deprivation. • Encourage parents to provide ample physical touch, deprivation of which may cause physical and mental underdevelopment. • Self-manipulation of genitals is normal behavior; avoid denoting this as "bad." • Avoid confusion of sex by consistent use of male or female role reinforcement.
Toddler: Age 1–3 yr	• Establishes control over bowels and bladder • Both sexes enjoy fondling genitals • Able to identify own gender • Develops vocabulary related to anatomy	• Allow toddler to designate his or her readiness to toilet-training. Strict measures may lead to compulsive behaviors later. • Punishment of genital fondling may lead to guilt and shame regarding sexual behavior later in life. • Use proper terms for body parts.
Preschool: Age 4–6 yr	• By age 6, sexuality has been internalized and preference for sexual partners determined • Methods of play and dress are in accordance with gender • Enjoys exploring body parts of self and playmates • Engages in masturbation	• Parents may cause anxiety in the child by intolerance of inconsistency of sex-role behavior. • Negative overreaction by parents of child's masturbating behavior can lead to a belief that the genitals and sex are bad and dirty.
School-age: Age 6–10 yr	• There is attachment to the parent of the opposite sex • Tendency toward having same-sex friends • Curiosity about sex and sharing of fears • Increasing self-awareness	• Same-sex preference for relationships is not related to heterosexual or homosexual tendencies. • Give child the information desired in a clear, factual form. May look to peers for information that may be incorrect.
Preadolescence: Age 10–13 yr	• Puberty begins for most boys and girls with development of secondary sex characteristics • Menarche takes place • May test behavioral limits	• Information is necessary regarding body changes to alleviate fears. This information should be given to the young person before pubertal changes begin. • Parents need to find a satisfactory middle ground for role setting. Rules that are either too rigid or too lenient can interfere with the development of self-confidence and internal value system. • Treat body image changes with a positive attitude to prevent poor self-image.
Adolescence: Age 13–19 yr	• Begins to develop opposite-sex relationships • Sexual fantasies are common • Masturbation is common • May begin to partake in sexual activity ranging from light to heavy petting to full genital intercourse • Girls concerned with reputations and self-image • Boys preoccupied with competitiveness of sexual activity • Incidence of adolescent pregnancies is increasing	• Parents share their beliefs and moral value systems with their children. • Teenagers may share their feelings with parents. If not taken seriously, may lead to lack of trust and communication gap. • Teens need information regarding contraceptive measures and the potential for contracting sexually transmitted diseases.

(continued)

Table 35-1 *(continued)*
Developmental Aspects of Sexuality Through the Life Span

Stage	Characteristics	Nursing Implications and Teaching Guidelines
Young adulthood: Age 20–35 yr	• Premarital sex is common • Although many young adults choose cohabitation instead of marriage, most marry and begin families before age 30 • Knowledge regarding sexual response and activity increases pleasure of relationship • May experiment with various sexual expressions • Develops own value system and respects values of other people • Many couples share financial responsibilities as well as household tasks	• Encourage communication between partners regarding sexual needs and differences. • Teach use of abstinence and contraceptive measures to prevent unwanted pregnancies. • Counsel against promiscuous behavior to guard against sexually transmitted diseases and loss of trust of partner • Daily communication is necessary to vent stresses and work out difficulties.
Adulthood: Age 35–55 yr	• Bodily changes as a result of menopause • Couples focus on quality rather than quantity of sexual experiences • Divorce is common • Grown children begin their own lives and sexual experiences • Sexual satisfaction may actually increase due to loss of fear of pregnancy	• Both men and women need positive reinforcement of what is good about themselves and their relationships. • Teach parents that *empty nest syndrome* (feelings of loss caused by children leaving) is common. Accentuate positive aspects of this situation. • Encourage couple to use this period as one of renewal for themselves.
Late adulthood and elderly: Age 55 yr and older	• Orgasms may become shorter and less intense in both men and women • Vaginal secretions decrease and period of resolution in men lengthens • May feel need to conform to stereotypes regarding the aging process and cease sexual activity • Fear of loss of sexual abilities	• Sexual activity need not be hindered by age. • Teach couples that adaptation to bodily changes is possible with use of comfortable positions for intercourse and increased time for stimulation. • Teach alternatives to coitus, such as caressing, hugging, and stroking, when coitus is impossible because of illness or disability. • Couples who have been consistently sexually active throughout their lives may continue their intimate relationship for as long as they desire.

Cardiovascular Disease. Cardiovascular disease is prevalent in North America. It is known that the sexual response cycle can greatly increase the demands of the heart and other structures. A person with a cardiovascular disease may experience much anxiety over the effect the illness will have on sexuality and sexual functioning.

Hypertension. The most significant difficulty a hypertensive person faces regarding sexuality is that the medication used to control the disease frequently causes a change in sexual functioning. These sexual dysfunctions may be relieved by modifying the dose of the medication or switching to a different medication.

Myocardial Infarction (Heart Attack). The primary goal after a myocardial infarction (MI) is to allow the heart ample time to heal. Activities of daily living, including sexual activity, should be resumed gradually, and stressors such as overexertion, alcohol consumption, and emotional upheavals should be avoided. In an uncomplicated MI, sexual activity may begin around week 3 of recovery, beginning with masturbation to partial erection in the male. Generally, this activity is gradually increased until 3 months after the MI when sexual intercourse may be resumed (Woods, 1984). A comfortable position that places the least stress on the affected partner should be assumed.

Diseases of the Joints and Mobility. Joint diseases and disorders affect young and old people. Pain, fatigue, stiffness, and loss of range of motion can accompany any of the dozens of known diseases of the joints. The disease itself does not affect sexual functioning, although the manifestation of it can cause discomfort and anxiety.

Surgery and Body Image. Surgery is performed to remove diseased tissue and repair body organs, usually requiring an incision with resulting scars. The most devastating kinds of surgery are those used to remove cancerous tissue and surrounding structures. The client is almost al-

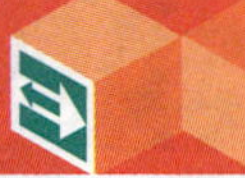

Developing Critical Thinking Skills

Situation

A 33-year-old Caucasian male with AIDS who is living alone at home asks you, the visiting nurse, about the nurse who was substituting for you during your vacation. "I don't like to complain, but he was overly friendly—if you get what I mean. . . . I wasn't comfortable with the way he was touching me and I'd rather not have help with my bath than have him back here." You have to decide how to respond.

1. ***Identify Goal of Thinking***
   Clarify what the client is saying and make a judgment about the behavior behind his concern so that you can respond appropriately.

2. ***Assess Adequacy of Knowledge***
   Pertinent circumstances: You have been visiting the client for the last 2 months following his discharge from a local hospital because of AIDS-related complications. Apart from his clinical picture you know very little about the client, who has always seemed private and reserved during your visits. You "feel sorry" that the client is as sick as he is at this point in his life, and your instinct is to trust him. You really don't know the colleague who was substituting for you because he is a "new hire."

   Prerequisite knowledge: Before you can make a judgment about the client's concern, you need to know more about what actually happened between him and your colleague. You do not know your colleague well since he is a "new hire" and has only been working in the agency for 3 months. You have heard reports that he is gay. You know that the client is single but do not know his sexual orientation. You will need to talk with your colleague to get his description of his encounter with the client. You will also need to know more about what touch means to both the client and your colleague, since culture and individual preference can profoundly influence the meaning different individuals give to touch.

   Room for error: Life and death do not hinge on how you respond to this client. However, the well-being of the client and your colleague's reputation are at stake, so the matter is grave.

   Time constraints: You must make some immediate response to the client. Since you do not have sufficient information to judge what happened, you should not feel pressured to make a definitive response. The client's well-being will not be jeopardized if you postpone a complete response until you have investigated the complaint.

3. ***Address Potential Problems***
   The most serious obstacles to critical thinking in this situation would be false assumptions you (and the client) might have about homosexuality in general and male homosexual nurses in particular, and the failure to reason carefully about the situation. Your tendency to "go to bat" for clients and to believe whatever a client tells you "no matter what" may result in your unfairly and prematurely judging a colleague.

4. ***Consult Helpful Resources***
   Your colleague is the first resource you should consult since you need to hear his side of the event before you can think critically about what happened. When you do meet with him, he thanks you for bringing up the subject because he was similarly disturbed by his encounter with this client. "I guess I'm a touchy-feely kind of guy and generally find that clients respond well to human touch. In the past, clients have told me how much it means to them to have someone massage their back, stroke a forearm, or greet them with a hug. Touch is certainly a big part of the 'therapeutic package' I give each of my clients. I did sense rather quickly, though, that Jim didn't like to be touched and modified my approach. My sense, from a few comments he made, is that he's probably homophobic [afraid of homosexuals]."

   After listening to your colleague you decide you need to learn more about touch, touch as a therapeutic intervention, and homophobia. You can consult the literature or local experts.

Critique Judgment/Decision

Wanting to explore the situation more fully, you responded to the client initially by saying, "I am sorry that you felt uncomfortable by my colleague's care. I want to talk with him about his sense of what happened and will then discuss this with you when I return on Wednesday." After talking with your colleague you are reasonably assured that he was not intending, inappropriately, to communicate anything of a sexual nature to the client. On your return visit to the client you inform him about your research and judgment and say, "Touch can mean different things to different people. My sense is

(continued)

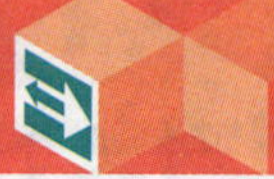

Developing Critical Thinking Skills *(continued)*

that Dave simply wanted to communicate that he cares. If he is going about this in the wrong way, he wants to know what he should be doing differently. We certainly don't want this to be a problem for you or any other client. Would you like to talk more about this or to file a report?"

You initially think you have three options: (1) to agree at the outset that your colleague has behaved in a sexually inappropriate and unprofessional manner, (2) to investigate the incident and conclude that your colleague was in the wrong, or (3) to investigate the incident and conclude that your colleague was in the right. You chose the third and are relieved when the client seems to accept your explanation. Two months later, when you receive a similar complaint from another male client, you are troubled. You realize now that there was a fourth option, and that this is the one you should have taken. Convinced by your colleague's sincerity and good intent, you might nonetheless have informed Dave that you need to communicate this client concern to your supervisor so that if future incidents are reported there will be a record of repeat complaints.

ways distressed over a diagnosis of cancer and possible death. After surgery, people need to cope and adjust to major alterations to their bodies. Changes in body image also affect a person's self-perception as a sexual being.

Mastectomy is a surgical procedure to remove a breast and its surrounding tissue. After such surgery, a woman's return to sexual functioning depends on many factors, such as support of her partner, the value placed on the breast by the man or woman, and fear of discomfort during sexual activity.

An *ostomy* is a surgical opening placed on the outside of the body to allow for the passage of secretions and elimination into a closed drainage bag. The grief over the loss of the natural means to eliminate waste, such as urine or feces, accompanies learning to live with an obvious artificial device. Many people are anxious as to how this apparatus will affect their sexual lives and how accepting sexual partners will be of it.

Spinal Cord Injuries. Thousands of people are victims of spinal cord injuries each year as a result of various types of accidents. This type of injury almost always results in some degree of permanent disability. Such people face multiple adaptations in normal living styles, including those related to mobility, bowel and bladder control, sexual functioning, and role expectations. The extent of remaining sexual response after a spinal cord injury depends primarily on the level and extent of the injury. Ejaculation and orgasm are most likely to remain with low spinal injuries. Women are more likely to experience orgasm than men but complain more about the lack of physical sensations during the excitement phase than do men. Many people find that other erogenous zones become more easily stimulated after the injury.

Mental Illness. Various psychologic and physical disorders can cause mental illness. The mind plays a powerful role in sexuality, and any disruption of its functioning will no doubt cause a disturbance in some way to sexual functioning. Even a disorder such as mild depression can affect desire and sexual functioning. Sometimes it is difficult for the partner of a client who has developed a mental illness to continue the sexual relationship. People afflicted with Alzheimer's disease can lose the memory of any contact with a partner or spouse. At times, clients with mental illness act out in a sexual manner, such as touching themselves or discarding their clothing at inappropriate times and places.

Sexually Transmitted Diseases. The term *sexually transmitted disease* (STD) is used to describe diseases that are almost always transmitted through direct sexual contact. Table 35-2 lists the more common types of STDs, their signs and symptoms, and corresponding treatment. The number of cases and varieties of STDs has increased over the years, and many currently are at epidemic proportions. STDs are hard to control because the partner or partners also need treatment; this is usually difficult if the partner is promiscuous or a one-time contact. It is believed that to have sexual contact with one person is also to have sexual contact with everyone else that person has had contact with in the past. The only clear way to avoid exposure to an STD is for a virginal person to have sexual contact with another virgin. Some STDs can be treated easily and effectively, whereas others have long-standing implications. For instance, women may suffer severe consequences from an STD by developing pelvic inflammatory disease (PID); the resulting adhesions cause much damage to delicate reproductive structures and may lead to infertility. Furthermore, other STDs, such as acquired immunodeficiency syndrome (AIDS), are deadly because there is no cure.

Medications

Medications are used to halt a disease, cure an illness, and promote and stabilize body functions. Some medications are necessary to prevent severe illness and even

Table 35-2
Sexually Transmitted Diseases

Disease	Characteristics	Treatment
Acquired immunodeficiency syndrome (AIDS)	• Human immunodeficiency virus (HIV) • Positive ELISA and Western Blot tests • Incidence high in IV drug users and homosexual and bisexual men; increased heterosexual transmission • Fatigue, diarrhea, weight loss, enlarged lymph nodes, fever, anorexia, and night sweats	• No cure, but treatment is directed toward delayed disease progression, opportunistic diseases, and relief of symptoms
Cervical intraepithelial neoplasia (CIN) Cervical cancer	• Abnormal Pap smears • Women with multiple sex partners, women who began sexual activity before age 18, and women whose partners have multiple female partners • Asymptomatic • Possible vaginal bleeding or spotting	• Depends on extent and stage of dysplasia • Surgical removal of cervix and other surrounding structures if severe; cryosurgery and laser treatment also used
Chlamydia trachomatis Nongonococcal urethritis (NGU) *Chlamydia*	• The most prevalent STD to date • Intracellular bacteria • Vaginal discharge, burning on urination, urinary frequency, dysuria, and urethral soreness • Many women are asymptomatic.	• Tetracycline, 500 mg PO qid for 7 days, or erythromycin, 500 mg PO qid for 7 days, for both partners; single dose azithromycin 1 g
Cytomegalovirus (CMV)	• A virus in the same family as herpes and Epstein-Barr • May be asymptomatic or may be confused with another disease such as pneumonia, mononucleosis, or hepatitis • Not exclusively sexually transmitted.	• No specific treatment; aimed at relief of symptoms; may be passed in utero and affect newborn
Nonspecific vaginitis *Gardnerella vaginalis*	• Mixed anaerobic bacteria • Foul-smelling, thin, grayish white vaginal discharge • Male partners are asymptomatic.	• Metronidazole (Flagyl), 500 mg PO bid for 7 days, for both partners; alcohol must not be consumed while taking medication.
Neisseria gonorrhoeae "The clap" or "the drip" Gonorrhea	• Gram-negative bacteria • Both men and woman may be asymptomatic. • Symptoms in men: purulent penile discharge, dysuria, frequency of urination • Symptoms in women: dysuria, abnormal menses, vaginal discharge, pelvic inflammatory disease • Symptoms of pharyngitis if oral sex practiced • May be accompanied by chlamydial infection • Detected by gonorrhea culture of cervix or penile discharge from men • Newborns exposed at birth are at risk for blindness and pneumonia. • Untreated gonorrhea can result in infertility, skin rash with lesions, and acute arthritis.	• Ceftriaxone, 250 mg IM (single dose) effective against PPNG, pharyngeal, and anorectal • Alternatively, tetracycline, 500 mg by mouth qid for 7 days, *plus* aqueous procaine penicillin G, 4.8 million units IM, *plus* probenecid, 1 g by mouth. • Cultures should be repeated 1 week after treatment.
Herpes simplex virus type 1 and 2 "Cold sores" *Herpes*	• A DNA virus • Lesions develop mostly in oral and genital areas. • Appear as single or multiple painful vesicles, which rupture and form ulcer-like lesions; these form scabs as they heal. • First infections last about 10 to 14 days, whereas subsequent infections are shorter in duration. • Recurrences are usually preceded by prodromal symptoms of tingling and fullness.	• No cure. • The antiviral drug acyclovir is used in treatment: acyclovir, 200 mg PO five times per day. • Areas of lesions should be kept clean and dry. • Use analgesics to reduce pain as well as topical anesthetics. • Avoid sexual contact while lesions are present. • May be transmitted to newborn at birth.

(continued)

Table 35-2 *(continued)*
Sexually Transmitted Diseases

Disease	Characteristics	Treatment
Human papilloma virus (HPV) Condylomata acuminata Genital warts Venereal warts	• A DNA virus • Pale, soft, papillary lesions found around the internal and external genitalia, and perianal and rectal areas of the body; vary in size • Profuse watery vaginal discharge, dyspareunia, intense pruritus, and vulvar irritation • Women with HPV are at risk for developing cervical cancer. • Male partner may or may not have lesions.	• Treat male partner if he has lesions. • Podophyllum 10% to 25% in tincture of benzoin may be applied to external lesions. Wash off in 1 to 4 hours. Repeat treatment until lesions are gone. • Cryosurgery and carbon dioxide laser surgery may also be used. • Use condoms or abstain from sex.
Treponema pallidum Syphilis	• A spirochete detected through serologic blood test (VDRL, RPR, STS) • Three stages to disease if left untreated *Primary:* Single painless genital lesion 10 days to 3 months after exposure *Secondary:* Generalized skin rash, enlarged lymph nodes, fever that may appear 2 to 4 weeks after appearance of primary lesion; may last for several years *Latent:* Usually no clinical symptoms present for as long as 20 years; may continue to involve and damage neurologic and cardiovascular organs; dementia, confusion, paralysis, and paresis may occur	• Treat both partners. • Benzathine penicillin G, 2.4 million units IM if of less than 1 year's duration; increase dosage and length of treatment if unknown duration of disease or longer than 1 year. • Repeat serology studies. • Avoid sexual contact or use condoms.
Trichomoniasis "Trich" *Trichomonas vaginalis*	• Protozoan with flagella • Identified on wet-mount microscopic examination of vaginal discharge • May be identified on Pap smear • Males usually asymptomatic • Foul-smelling vaginal discharge, thin, foamy, and green in color, causes itching of vulva and vagina, burning on urination and dyspareunia; "strawberry" cervix may be seen on speculum examination	• Treat both partners. • Metronidazole (Flagyl), 2 g PO at one time; avoid alcohol consumption. • Avoid sex or use condoms.

(Data from Baldwin, K., & Goodwin, K. [1985]. The Papanicolaou smear. *Journal of Nurse-Midwifery 30*[6]: 327–331; Bourcier, K., & Seidler, A. [1987]. *Chlamydia* and condylomata acuminata; An update for the nurse practitioner. *Journal of Obstetric, Gynecologic, and Neonatal Nursing 16*[1], 17–21; Fromer, M. [1983]. *Ethical issues in sexuality and reproduction.* St. Louis: Mosby; Hatcher, R. et al. [1986]. *Contraceptive technology.* New York: Irvington.)

death. Some medications have side effects that may affect sexual functioning. Illegal drugs are used by some people because of their reputed ability to heighten the sexual experience; these drugs can have serious and even deadly side effects of their own. Table 35-3 lists some of the categories of medications and their possible effects on sexual functioning.

The Nurse as Role Model

A nurse's attitudes, biases, and prejudice regarding sexuality are readily transmitted to clients through his or her actions, manner of speech, avoidance of certain circumstances, and types of discussion. The level of knowledge a nurse has about sexual issues can inhibit or promote discussion of sexual health. The nurse who does not have a sound knowledge base of reproductive anatomy and physiology, sexual response, sexual expression, and other issues surrounding sexuality will be unable effectively to assess, teach, or counsel the client with sexual concerns. The nurse must also feel comfortable with himself or herself as a sexual being.

Nursing goals to enhance interactions with clients and to promote individual sexual wellness are as follows. The nurse will be able to:

- Feel comfortable as a sexual being
- Develop self-awareness regarding sexual topics
- Develop communication skills that promote discussion of sexual concerns with clients

Table 35-3
Medications and Their Effects on Sexual Functioning

Drug	Effect on Sexual Functioning
Amyl nitrite	Peripheral vasodilator used in the past for treating angina; has become popular as sex enhancer among male homosexuals in particular; when inhaled at time of orgasm, the resulting vasodilation is felt to cause an intensified orgasmic release. Loss of erection, hypotension, and faintness may occur.
Anticonvulsants	Dilantin (phenytoin) has sedative effects, which may decrease desire and reduce sexual response.
Antidepressants	Similar to antihypertensive drugs. Male impotence is significant.
Tricyclic compounds	Male impotence and ejaculatory dysfunction in 25% to 30% of men.
Monoamine oxidase inhibitors	Decreases serum testosterone in men. Some antidepressants have been found to cause
Lithium carbonate	prolonged painful erections known as *priapism;* one such drug is trazodone.
Antihistamines	May have sedative effect that decreases desire; may also cause decreased vaginal lubrication.
Antihypertensives	
Methyldopa	May decrease desire in both male and female clients.
Clonidine	Erectile failure in 24% of men; no adverse effect on female clients.
Reserpine	Decreased desire in women; erectile and ejaculation dysfunctions in men.
Antipsychotics	Causes decreased desire in 10% to 20% of clients; may also cause erection and ejaculatory dysfunctions. Small amount of the antipsychotic drug may be found in the semen. The partner may experience resulting genital rash. Wear condoms while on therapy.
Antispasmodics	These drugs relax smooth muscle; male impotence may occur.
Barbiturates	In low initial doses, sexual pleasure may be increased due to loss of inhibitions. However, long-term use commonly causes decreased desire and orgasmic dysfunction. Male impotence is not uncommon.
Cocaine	Reported to increase quality of sexual experience. Chronic use, however, results in sexual dysfunction and loss of desire in both men and women.
Ethyl alcohol	In moderate amounts, decreases inhibitions and consequently improves sexual functioning. Continued consumption decreases sexual functioning. Chronic alcoholics are impotent and often sterile. Testicular damage and permanent dysfunction are common. Female alcoholics experience decreased desire and orgasmic dysfunction.
Marijuana	Release of inhibitions may cause feeling of increased sexual functioning. Marijuana users have increased incidence of decreased desire and male impotence.
Narcotics	Serious impairment of sexual functioning with increased dependence. Erectile and ejaculatory dysfunctions common in men. Testosterone levels and amount of semen decreased. High incidence of decreased desire occurs in both men and women.

(Data from Fuentes, R. [1983]. Sexual side effects. What to tell your patients, what not to say. *RN, 46*[2], 34–41; Woods, N. F. [1984]. *Human sexuality in health and illness.* St. Louis, MO: Mosby.)

- Identify clients with problems related to sexuality and competently and comfortably intervene to meet these needs
- Practice responsible sexual expression

Sexual Harassment

Nurses in different types of health care settings have experienced work-related sexual harassment. Sexual harassment may be defined as “any unwelcome verbal or physical advance or sexually explicit statement—such as leers, pats, grabs, jokes, requests for dates, and even rape—that interferes with your ability to do your job by making you feel humiliated, intimidated or uncomfortable” (Horsley, 1990, p. 69). It is important for nurses to recognize that harassment can often be effectively stopped when confronted early. Horsley gives the following specific measures to stop harassment:

Confrontation: Look the harasser in the eye and tell him or her you do not like this behavior and want it to stop.

Documentation: Document specific instances of harassment (words and acts, your response, date, time, place, and the names of any witnesses). Put the details of these incidents in a letter and send it to the harasser again, indicating that you do not like this behavior and want it to stop. Send the letter by way of registered mail.

Written complaint: If the behavior does not stop, submit a written complaint to administration (use appropriate channels).

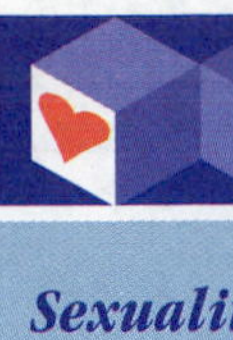

Promoting Wellness

Sexuality

Use the assessment checklist to determine how well you are meeting your sexuality needs. Then develop a prescription for self-care by choosing appropriate behaviors from the list of suggestions.

Assessment Checklist

almost always	sometimes	almost never	
☐	☐	☐	1. I feel good about my sexual identity.
☐	☐	☐	2. I have satisfying relationships with others.
☐	☐	☐	3. I accept sexual needs as a normal part of life.
☐	☐	☐	4. I am comfortable with physical actions that indicate love and belonging (such as touching and hugging).

Self-Care Behaviors

1. Avoid stereotyping typical gender roles.
2. Learn the biologic aspects of sexual functioning.
3. Ask questions about sexual needs and sexual activity when necessary.
4. Enjoy close relationships with others who love you.
5. Give a hug to someone you love.
6. Accept touch from others as a sign of caring and affection.
7. Practice safer sex (eg, use contraceptives or condoms, and choose partner carefully).
8. Recognize how age, illness, or disability influences sexual needs and expression.

Government complaint: If all else fails, file a complaint with the Equal Employment Opportunity Commission.

ASSESSING

Sexual History

The comprehensive health history should include information regarding a client's reproductive and sexual health, depending on the circumstances in which the client is receiving care. As a rule, three general categories of clients should have a sexual history recorded by the nurse:

- Any inpatient or outpatient client who is receiving care for pregnancy, STD, infertility, or contraception
- Any client who is currently experiencing a sexual dysfunction or problem
- Any client whose illness will affect sexual functioning and behavior in any way

Information is best obtained from the client by beginning with nonthreatening questions and progressing to more sensitive concerns (see the accompanying display). Clients usually have no difficulty answering questions regarding their bodies and general reproductive issues such as, "When did your menstrual periods first begin?"

Clients should understand why the nurse needs information about their intimate sexual functioning. Nurses should explain to clients that this information may be helpful in assisting them in the plan of care. The sexual history is a vital portion of the reproductive history. It also assists the nurse in identifying any sexual problems or concerns. It is an excellent opportunity for the nurse to teach by helping the client confront fears and allay myths. There are four general levels of sexual history suggested by Watts (1979):

Level 1: Sexual history as part of a comprehensive health history—obtained by a nurse

Level 2: Sexual history—obtained by a nurse with education and training in sexuality

Level 3: Sexual problem history—obtained by a sex therapist

Level 4: Psychiatric/psychosocial history—obtained by a psychiatric nurse clinician

Each level acquires more specific information from the client regarding sexual health and also requires the interviewer to have more sophisticated preparation and skills. The professional nurse usually performs a sexual history on level 1.

The nurse sets the tone or atmosphere for the interview. The nurse's attitudes will greatly affect the client's response to the sexual history, and clients will be more cooperative if they sense the nurse's security and ease during the interview. Privacy is essential for the sexual history; doors should be closed and no interruptions allowed. The nurse sits close to the client and speaks in a quiet, relaxed, objective tone of voice. Eye contact and open body posture are used. The client needs to know what will happen to this information and who will have access to it. The nurse needs to explain to the client that no one will have access to this information unless it is significant to the client's care. Reproductive health information should be obtained from the client first, followed by the client's sexual health history. The best approach is to begin with general open-ended questions and progress to more specific ones. The nurse should

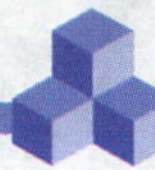

Focused Assessment Guide

Sexuality

Factors to Assess	Questions and Approaches
Reproductive history	Ask women their date of menarche, date of last menstrual period, duration and length of flow in days, number of pregnancies, living children, miscarriages, abortions, method of birth control. Ask men the number of children they have fathered and method of birth control used. Ask both men and women of childbearing age if they have any concerns about their fertility and determine if there is any interest in the new reproductive technologies and genetic testing options.
History of sexually transmitted diseases	"Do you or a sexual partner have a history of sexually transmitted diseases? Many people today have questions about sexually transmitted diseases that they are reluctant to express. Do you have any questions? Have you noticed any signs that might indicate a problem?"
History of sexual dysfunction	"Have you ever experienced a problem such as erectile dysfunction, failure to achieve orgasm, or pain during intercourse?"
Sexual self-care behaviors	"Do you perform the breast-self exam [testicular-self exam] on a monthly basis? When was your last gynecologic [urologic] examination (Pap smear, mammogram)? Is there a family history of breast disease, ovarian cancer, testicular cancer, colon cancer? With all the attention on safer sex today and responsible parenting, many people have questions about their sexual self-care behaviors. Do you have any such concerns?" [It is important for nurses to ascertain if clients possess the knowledge, attitudes, and skills necessary to promote their own sexual health and that of others.]
Sexual self-concept	
Sexual identity	"How do you feel about yourself as a man or woman? Is anything changing the way you feel about yourself?"
Sexual body image	"Many people have concerns about their sexual body image. Are you comfortable with your physical maleness or femaleness? Have you experienced any physical changes (eg, baldness, weight loss or gain, impotence, menopause, mastectomy, hysterectomy, sterilization) that are troubling to you?"
Sexual self-esteem	"We all have certain expectations of ourselves. Are you comfortable with the way you are currently expressing yourself sexually and meeting your sexual needs?"
Sexual role performance	"Has anything interfered with your ability to be a spouse, sexual partner, parent (any other valued sex-related roles)?"
Sexual functioning	"It's not unusual for people with health concerns [name specific medical problem, if appropriate] to have questions related to sexuality and sexual functioning. Do you have any questions or concerns that I can help you with? Has anything [if appropriate substitute the name of a specific disease, surgery, or medication] changed your ability to function sexually?" [Asking clients if they have questions about resuming their usual sexual activity is an appropriate part of discharge planning for many clients.]

use the language used by the client. If not, clients may be reluctant to tell the caregiver that they do not understand certain terms for fear of appearing ignorant or foolish. For example, the client may choose the term *come* to mean climax or orgasm.

It is useful to begin questions with "many people like" or "many people feel." This gives clients security in knowing they are not alone in how they feel and are encouraged to talk about their problems or concerns. An example of this type of questioning is the following: "Many people feel that it's helpful to discuss your concerns about sex with your partner. What do you think about this?"

One helpful means to obtain information about sexual problems follows:

- Description of the problem: "How would you describe the problem?"
- Onset and cause of the problem: "What do you think caused the problem or what was happening when you first noticed it?"

- Past attempts at resolution: "What have you tried in the past to correct the problem?"
- Goals of the client: "What do you wish to accomplish?"

A narrative form of recording a sexual history is generally used because it allows the interviewer to document the data in many of the client's own words. If a client is seeking help for a sexual problem, a more specific format will be used in recording information obtained by a skilled therapist.

Sexual Dysfunction

Sexual dysfunction is a problem that prevents an individual or couple from engaging in or enjoying satisfactory sexual intercourse and orgasm. Dysfunctions may occur as a result of physiologic malfunctions, conflicts with cultural norms, interpersonal problems, or any combination of these. Anxieties and fears concerning the sexual act are almost always present. Clients with severe sexual dysfunctions require intensive professional therapy from a qualified sex therapist. It is hypothesized that sexual dysfunctioning is a problem of considerable magnitude. A few of the major dysfunctions are briefly discussed here and in Table 35-4.

Male Sexual Dysfunctions. *Erectile failure*, also called **impotence**, is the inability of a man to attain or maintain an erection to such an extent that he cannot have satisfactory intercourse. Common causes of impotence include various illnesses, treatments for these illnesses, and personal anxieties.

Premature ejaculation is the condition when a man consistently reaches ejaculation or orgasm before or soon after entering the vagina. The result is that his partner usually does not have time to reach sexual satisfaction. Causes of the problem are rarely physical in nature.

Retarded ejaculation, also called *ejaculatory incompetence*, refers to a man's inability to ejaculate into the vagina or to suffer with delayed intravaginal ejaculation. The causes of this problem are similar to those of impotence. When it occurs after having experienced normal ejaculations, the cause is most probably due to interpersonal problems.

Female Sexual Dysfunctions. *Inhibited sexual desire* consists of an inhibition in sexual arousal so that congestion and vaginal lubrication are absent or minimal. Causative factors may be anxiety, negative emotions, fear, interpersonal problems, or physical factors.

Orgasmic dysfunction is defined as the inability of a woman to reach orgasm. The causes are similar to those of inhibited sexual desire.

Dyspareunia is painful intercourse. Although it is most often described by women, some men may also suffer from this disorder. The cause is usually physical in nature, although psychologic problems such as fear and anxiety can cause pain in some women.

Vaginismus is a rare condition in which the vaginal opening closes tightly and prevents penile penetration.

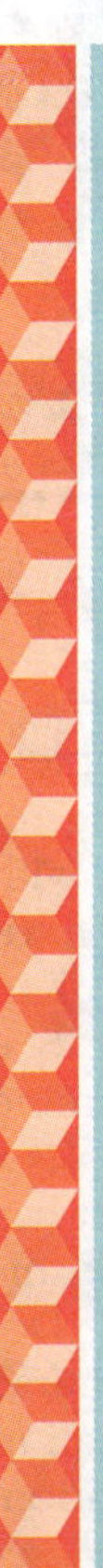

Focus on the Older Adult

Talking With Elderly People About Sexuality

The many losses associated with aging leave older people with special needs for love and affection. Unfortunately many healthcare professionals simply assume that older people have no health concerns related to sexuality. Factors that can inhibit sexual activity in older adults include the following:

- Societal expectations that sexual activity somehow belongs to the young and beautiful
- Rigid moral principles
- Decreased self-esteem
- Physical factors: age-related body changes, the effects of fatigue, illness, medications
- The attitudes of healthcare professionals who ignore or demean expressions of sexual needs by older people
- Institutional factors such as policies preventing sexual activity between competent, consenting older adults

Nurses who are sensitive to these factors can initiate a discussion about sexuality with older clients by asking the following questions. If questioning results in the older person's discomfort, do not press for information not needed for medical reasons.

"Many older people talk about feeling lonely. Are there people with whom you feel close who meet your needs for love and affection?"

"Are you sexually active currently?" [or] "Are you comfortable with your current level of sexual activity?"

"Is there anything interfering with your ability to be as sexually active as you would like? Physical limitations? Attitudes, beliefs, values? No partner?" [In a long-term care setting, institutional factors may inhibit sexual activity.]

"In what physical ways do you express and receive affection?" [kissing, hugging, hand-holding, coitus, oral or manual genital stimulation]

"Do you have concerns about sexually transmitted diseases?"

"Is there any information you would like from me that would help you to better meet your needs for love and affection?" "Are there any questions or concerns you have that we haven't addressed?"

Table 35-4
Sexual Dysfunction and Nursing Assessment

Sexual Dysfunction	Assessment Priorities
Male	
Erectile failure (impotence)	• History of diabetes, spinal cord trauma, cardiovascular disease, surgical procedure, alcoholism • Use of certain medications such as antihypertensives, antidepressants, or illicit drugs • Determine degree of mental depression that may be present • Obtain specific information regarding the degree of impotence, length of time of disorder, continuing life factors
Premature ejaculation	• Assess what client defines as his dysfunction and ability to control ejaculation • Assess any causative relationship factors, such as anxiety, guilt, lack of time, new partner, and so on
Retarded ejaculation	• History of neurologic disorders, Parkinson's disease, or use of certain medications • Same assessment priorities as for premature ejaculation
Female	
Inhibited sexual desire	• Use of oral contraceptives or other hormonal therapy, use of alcohol or certain medications • History of sexual abuse, rape or incest, depression, or other sexual dysfunctions • Assess any other contributing or relationship factors.
Orgasmic dysfunction	• Assess knowledge level regarding sexual response cycle and anatomy • Assess communication pattern between the client and her partner • Assess usual sexual pattern and behavior between client and her partner • Assess any other contributing factors
Dyspareunia	• History of diabetes, hormonal imbalance, vaginal infection, endometriosis, urethritis, cervicitis, or rectal lesions • Use of antihistamines, alcohol, tranquilizers, or illicit drugs • Assess client's ability for vaginal lubrication during sexual act • Assess client's use of coital positions • Assess use of cosmetic or chemical irritants to genitals such as deodorant tampons, contraceptive creams, or jellies or condoms • Physical assessment of internal and external genitalia • Assess any other contributing factors
Vaginismus	• Assess knowledge regarding anatomy and sexual response • Assess pattern of sexual activity: how often, level of arousal, orgasm • Assess presence of other sexual dysfunctions • History of sexual abuse, trauma, or rape • Assess client's feelings regarding her partner • Assess any other causative factors, such as fear of pregnancy, anxiety, guilt • Physical assessment of internal and external genitalia

Vaginismus is due to involuntary spastic contractions of muscles at and around the vaginal opening and the levator ani muscles. The cause of vaginismus may be physical, psychologic, or both.

Physical Assessment

Physical examination of the reproductive or genitourinary system for either male or female clients is necessary under the following circumstances:

- As part of a routine physical examination
- Annual women's health care, including Pap smear
- Suspicion of an STD
- Suspicion of pregnancy
- Work-up for infertility
- Unusual lump, discharge, or unusual appearance of the genital organs noticed by the client
- Request for birth control
- Change in urinary function

The examiner may routinely perform a complete physical examination along with assessment of the reproductive system if the client has not had contact with the healthcare system within 1 year or if assessment findings of a complete examination would be useful in diagnosing an ailment or complaint of the client. See Chapter 26 for a detailed description of how to examine the female and male genitalia.

The nurse should initially ask whether the client has experienced this type of examination in the past if this information is not evident by the client's records. Depending on the client's knowledge base, the nurse should explain the progressive steps of the examination and what the client may feel during the examination. This will give the client some feeling of control and security during the examination. The nurse's responsibilities during an examination of the reproductive system are as follows:

- To provide information to the client regarding the examination
- To teach the client
- To provide support for the client during the examination
- To assist the examiner, if appropriate, with any procedures or laboratory studies

Home Healthcare Alert

Sexual abuse of women, men to a lesser degree, and children is a common phenomenon in all socioeconomic groups. Nurses are responsible for knowing the signs of abuse and for reporting persons at risk of being in an abusive situation. Teaching self-help measures and empowering the victims of abuse to seek and utilize help are important nursing responsibilities. Nurses who work with children, adolescents, and young adults should be familiar with local resources to educate these vulnerable populations.

DIAGNOSING

Sexual Dysfunction as the Problem. Before a nursing diagnosis can be made regarding a sexual problem, the assessment data collected by the nurse must be carefully reviewed to determine if the situation can be corrected by independent nursing interventions. Although many problems of sexuality experienced by a client in a healthcare situation are amenable to nursing action, some require the expertise of other specialties. For example, an impotent diabetic client who would benefit from a penile implant needs medical consultation. A client with a serious sexual dysfunction or who practices a destructive sexual expression needs intensive therapy by a clinical psychologist, sex therapist, or counselor. Appropriate referrals by the nurse should follow the identification of such problems. Either of two diagnoses, *Sexual Dysfunction* or *Altered Sexuality Patterns*, is used to describe problems of sexuality amenable to nursing intervention. A related diagnosis is *Rape-Trauma Syndrome*.

Sexual dysfunction may be specified as erectile failure (impotence); premature ejaculation; retarded ejaculation; inhibited sexual desire; orgasmic dysfunction; vaginismus; or dyspareunia. Common etiologies for sexual dysfunction include effects of medication (specify); effects of alcohol consumption; effects of disease process (specify); history of abuse (specify rape, incest); feelings of depression; guilt; anxiety; fear of rejection; miscommunication with partner; fear of pain; effects of birth control method (specify); lack of knowledge; or effects of surgical procedure (specify). The nursing diagnosis Altered Sexuality Patterns can be further specified by loss of desire (to abstinence); increased desire (to promiscuity); or change in sexual expression. Common etiologies for Altered Sexuality Patterns include stress (lifestyle, job, family, finances, marital conflict); isolation from partner; effects of pregnancy (specify); feelings of depression; loss of privacy; loss of communication with partner; relationship change (new partner); effects of disease process (sexual position, frequency, mode of expression); change in body image; change in self-concept; or loss of partner. A representative sample of some nursing diagnoses concerning sexuality is given in the accompanying display.

Sexual Dysfunction as the Etiology. Changes in sexuality can affect other areas of human functioning. In the following nursing diagnoses, problems of sexuality are the etiology of another problem:

Impaired Adjustment related to loss of sexual partner, loss of sexual body part

Anxiety related to fear of pregnancy, loss of sexual functioning or desire, effects of disease process on sexual functioning

Pain related to sexual position, penile penetration, effects of genital surgery, lack of vaginal lubrication

Ineffective Individual Coping related to effects of body image on sexual expression, change in sexual partner

Fear related to pain during sexual intercourse, history of sexual abuse

Anticipatory Grieving related to loss of sexual functioning, effects of surgical excision of genital body part

Altered Growth and Development related to sexual exploitation or abuse, sexual guilt, effects of hormonal imbalance, lack of information about sexuality

Knowledge Deficit (specify: Contraceptive Methods, Spread of STDs, Sexual Response, Genital Anatomy, Modes of Sexual Expression, Self-Examination, Effects of Disease or Medications) related to misinformation, sexual myths, lack of interest in learning, cognitive limitation

Body Image Disturbance (specify: Surgical Excision of Genital Body Part, Loss of or Gain in Body Weight) related to fear of rejection

Impaired Social Interaction related to effects of marital separation or divorce

Social Isolation related to fear of contraction of STD, fear of sexual encounter

PLANNING: EXPECTED OUTCOMES

It is important for nurses to value sexuality as an important aspect of who the client is and how the client is identified as a unique human. Specific client goals/outcomes to promote sexual wellness will be determined. The client will:

- Define individual sexuality
- Establish open patterns of communication with significant others

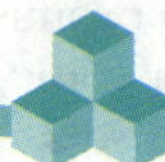

Nursing Diagnoses for Common Problems

Sexuality

Problem	Related Factors	Sample Defining Characteristics
Sexual Dysfunction: Erectile Failure	Use of antihypertensive medication	• 45-year-old man with 3-year history of hypertension • Maintained normotensive on reserpine, 0.25 mg daily • "I have had trouble keeping an erection. My wife and I haven't made love in months. We don't talk about it anymore. I guess that part of my life is over." • Client appears resigned and saddened.
Sexual Dysfunction: Dyspareunia	Effects of menopausal process	• 54-year-old female whose last menses was 1 year ago • "Whenever my husband and I make love, my vagina burns and stings." • States decrease in vaginal lubrication during past several months
Altered Sexuality Patterns: Change in Sexual Expression	Loss of privacy due to hospitalization	• 23-year-old man hospitalized for past 6 weeks with injuries resulting from car crash; has been in traction for fractured right femur • "I can't take this place anymore! Everyone barges in here whenever they want to—nobody cares about my feelings—a guy can't even act like a guy around here. I wish I could be alone with my wife for a while with no interruptions."
Altered Sexuality Patterns: Loss of Desire	Change in body image due to body-altering surgery	• Surgery for bowel cancer with construction of permanent colostomy 1 month ago • "I know the colostomy was necessary to save my life, but it is so disgusting. I'll never be able to have a relationship with my husband again. It's a real turn-off to me—just imagine what he'll think—how can I expect him to want to make love to a freak?"
Alteration in Comfort: Pain	Abduction of hips in sexual positioning	• 60-year-old woman with history of osteoarthritis for 6 years • "The act of intercourse hurts my hips so bad that I'm in pain the whole next day. I don't want to stop having intercourse with my husband, but I'm going to have to if this pain gets worse." • Client states that the missionary position is the only position used during sex with her husband throughout their 40-year marriage.

- Develop self-awareness and body awareness
- Describe responsible sexual health self-care practices, identifying appropriate resources
- Practice responsible sexual expression (eg, by 5/1/98, the client will use rubber condoms with all sexual encounters)

Specific client goals/outcomes will depend on the nature of the client's problem or concern. Expected outcomes should be client oriented, that is, something the client desires to do or has the ability to accomplish. For example, it is not enough to advise a method of birth control; rather, the nurse needs to know which method the client is motivated and able to use.

Implementing

Establishing a Trusting Nurse–Client Relationship

It is impossible to address or help a client's sexuality if trust has not developed between the nurse and the client. The nurse needs to project an objective, nonthreatening, and nonjudgmental attitude and an aura of confidentiality. Anticipating client concerns and needs through awareness of his or her behavior and verbal and nonverbal cues also helps the client trust the nurse later on with information of an intimate nature. It is important to establish respect for the individual and empathy before sexual topics are discussed. An empathic nurse considers all of an individual's circumstances and life experiences and views them from a therapeutic, not a pitying, approach. Only when the nurse is accepted as a trusted, caring person will the client relay details of private life, including concerns of a sexual nature.

Teaching About Sexuality and Wellness

Most nursing interventions pertaining to a client's sexuality encompass teaching to promote wellness. Major goals of client teaching are a change in knowledge, a change in client attitude, or a change in behaviors. In some situations, clients need assistance in defining or redefining their sexuality and its importance to their lives. Offering information, dispelling fears, and providing positive reinforcement are some ways nurses can assist clients to increase their knowledge about their bodies and sexual functioning. Clients may need assistance in modifying behaviors or learning new skills to increase the quality of sexual health and functioning. The accompanying box lists resources that may be accessed by clients and healthcare professionals.

Correcting Sexual Myths and Promoting Body Awareness

Many people believe things about sex that they have heard from family or friends or as part of their culture that are simply not true or not based on scientific data. The nurse may refute sexual myths (Table 34-5) and teach factual information during the assessment or while providing care.

Clients may need assistance in becoming familiar with what they believe and feel about their sexual selves. The nurse can be helpful in a situation in which a client has difficulty accepting or developing his or her sexuality by promoting self-confidence and a good self-concept in the client. When clients feel comfortable about themselves and their sensual feelings, they can begin to focus on how they feel about their sexual functioning and specific sexual expressions.

Getting to know one's physical body is important to healthy sexual development. Every man and woman, sexually active or not, needs to be aware of the appearance of his or her individual genitalia. Some people, because of their background, feel ashamed and repulsed by their bodies; others feel that touching the body is dirty and may feel guilt and anxiety in stimulating themselves. Clients need assistance in improving body awareness if any of these issues are present. Clients become accustomed to looking at their bodies by looking at nonthreatening anatomy first and then proceeding to the genitals. This can be done in the shower or with the use of a mirror. Knowing what looks normal can be of great importance in reporting the development of an unusual appearance later on. After clients have developed some degree of comfort in looking at their bodies, they can progress to experiencing touch. Again, clients should progress from nonthreatening parts of the body until the genitals can be touched without stress.

A good exercise for women in developing body awareness is the use of *Kegel exercises.* These exercises

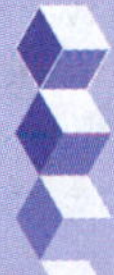

Through the Eyes of a Student

I knew it was going to happen sooner or later. Male nurses are not unheard of in this day and age, but some people just aren't yet ready for us. Especially Ethel, a 68-year-old black woman with a deep religious conviction. I concluded this because she called on Jesus for help when I told her that I was her student nurse for the day, and that I would be giving her a bath.

"You're my nurse?" she said. "Help me, Jesus . . . No, no, you just go on and help somebody else, honey. I've already had my bath," she insisted.

Accordingly, I told her she was mistaken and that I understood her anxiety. Then I proceeded to exaggerate the truth by saying that I had done this before, when really I had given baths before, but not to members of the opposite sex. She thought *she* was having anxiety!

Next I asked my instructor, Lynn, for help. She quickly assessed the situation and tried to comfort Ethel by vouching for my professional character and abilities, but still no go. Then I tried appealing to her logic.

"This is a hospital where male doctors examine you all the time. Why is this any different?" I asked. "Because you are *not* a doctor" was her logical reply.

I felt inadequate. I could not give this woman the care she needed because of my gender. Luckily, in the next bed, Michele was about to give her client a bath. She offered to give Ethel her bath if I would help her with her clients.

Consequently, Ethel got her bath, and I learned that a nurse has to be flexible as well as willing to ask for and accept help when the client's quality of care is at stake. This is something I hope to remember throughout my nursing career.

—Daniel E. Zirolli,
Delaware County Community College,
Media, Pennsylvania

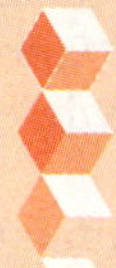

Helpscan

The following are resources for clients and healthcare professionals:

- American Association of Sex Educators, Counselors, and Therapists (AASECT)
  435 North Michigan Avenue, Suite 1717
  Chicago, IL 60611
  (312) 644-0828

  Can help you find resources for sex therapy in your area.
- Multi-Focus, Inc.
  1525 Franklin Street
  San Francisco, CA 94109
  (415) 673-5100

  Distributes films, videos, and slides on all aspects of sexuality. Send for free catalogue.
- SIECUS
  130 West 42nd Street, Suite 2500
  New York, NY 10036
  (212) 819-9770
  (617) 742-2100

  Publishes a bimonthly journal, annotated bibliographies, brochures, and other informational publications related to sexuality research, education, and legislation.
- *Women's Health Watch*, a newsletter offering information for enlightened choices from Harvard Medical School
  Harvard Women's Health Watch
  P.O. Box 420234
  Palm Coast, FL 32142
  (800) 829-5921

promote good vaginal tone by localizing and strengthening the *pubococcygeal* muscle. A woman can locate this muscle by stopping a stream of urine midway through urination. Contracting this muscle can be repeated at any time of the day in any circumstance because its performance is undetectable. Women who practice Kegel exercises have found that sexual satisfaction is greatly improved.

Teaching Self-Examination

It is important for both men and women to learn to examine themselves through inspection and palpation of sexual body parts. Many conditions, some life threatening, can be detected when self-examination is performed. Early detection of cancer is crucial to its control and cure. The presence of some STDs may also be detected by self-examination.

Breast Self-Examination. The importance of breast self-examination (BSE) lies in its routine monthly performance, which helps the person to become familiar with what is normal. BSE should be performed after each menses or once a month for a postmenopausal woman. Any contact with a female client in the healthcare delivery system should include assessment of her knowledge and practice of BSE.

The steps in performing BSE are shown in Figure 35-4 and are as follows:

1. Stand before a mirror with hands on hips to inspect the breasts. Look for the presence of indentations, dimpling, or odd position of a nipple. Any discharge from a nipple is abnormal unless the woman is nursing. Changes in size or shape of breasts should be reported.
2. Lie on the bed with a small pillow under the shoulder on the side of the breast to be examined and the arm over the head. Using the opposite hand, palpate the breast starting at the outer edge of the breast, using small circular motions of the flat portions of the fingers. Work inward in a clockwise manner toward the nipple. The nipple should be gently squeezed to detect the presence of any discharge. This procedure should be repeated for the opposite breast. Any unusual lump or tenderness should be reported to a healthcare professional.

Testicular Self-Examination. Male clients need to be taught to perform monthly assessment of the testicles. Although testicular cancer is not widespread, it can be easily detected and prognosis is good if found early. A good time to examine the testes is during a shower, when the scrotum becomes warm and loose. Men should also be taught the importance of examining their breasts.

The steps in TSE, shown in Figure 35-5, are as follows:

1. The thumb and the fingers of each hand are used to palpate each testicle simultaneously. The client should systematically palpate the testes for the presence of lumps or differences in texture. The testes should feel smooth.
2. The epididymis is palpated above each testicle. The epididymis feels soft and not as smooth as a testicle.
3. The spermatic cord, or vas deferens, extends upward from the scrotum toward the base of the penis and should be palpated for firmness and smoothness in texture.

Considering Contraception

Clients choose **contraception** for many reasons and may contact healthcare providers for information on birth control or contraceptive methods. Some people use

Table 35-5
Sexual Myths and Facts to Refute Them

Myths	Fact
Each person is born with a certain amount of sexual drive, which if overdrawn in youth leaves little reserve for later years.	Actually, the correlation between sexual activity and length of time it persists throughout life is just the opposite. The more consistently sexually active a person is, the longer the activity continues into the later years of life.
The need for expressing one's sexuality becomes less important in the latter half of one's life.	Physiologically, sexual desire and ability do not decrease markedly after middle age. The expression of one's sexuality, as an integral part of development, follows the overall pattern of health and physical performance.
Sexual abstinence is necessary in training for sports.	Physiologically, the achievement of orgasm is rarely more demanding than most activities encountered in daily life. The desire for sleep that often follows is most commonly due to factors other than physical exhaustion from sexual activities. There is no scientific evidence that sex "weakens" a person.
Excessive sexual activity can lead to mental illness.	The biologic significance of human sexuality has no greater effect on total development than any other necessary biologic function. There is no scientific basis for believing that one will develop a mental or physical illness with excessive or no sexual activity.
Wet dreams are indicators of sexual disorders.	Erotic dreams that culminate in orgasms are normal common physiologic phenomena in at least 85% of men. They can occur at any age after puberty. Some women also report in clinical studies that their sexual dreams culminate in orgasm. In women, this phenomenon is believed to increase with advancing age.
Because of the anatomic nature of the sex organs, women are passive and men are aggressive.	Physiologic studies disprove this myth by showing the woman to be far from passive. Maximum gratification requires each partner to be both passive and aggressive in participating mutually and cooperatively.
It is unnatural for a woman to have as strong a desire for sex as a man—women should not enjoy sex as much as men.	These myths have been reinforced by a society that has traditionally taught women that they are to suppress sexual desires to gain love, security, and society's respect, based on the assumption that it is the basic nature of women to be submissive, dependent, and subordinate. Physiologic studies indicate that, in some respects, the woman's sex drive is not only as strong but may be even stronger than that of the man.
Women who have multiple orgasms or who readily come to climax are nymphomaniacs or promiscuous.	Physiologic studies at this time suggest that we do not know women's sexual potential; these studies indicate that there is a wide range of intensity and duration of orgasmic experience, and the potential for multiple or frequent orgasms within a brief period is not at all uncommon. Therefore, women normally may have greater orgasmic capacity than men with regard to duration and frequency of orgasm.
There is a difference between vaginal orgasm and clitoral orgasm.	Physiologic misunderstanding has produced the myth of separate clitoral and vaginal orgasms rather than their interrelations. Female orgasm is normally initiated by clitoral stimulation, but because it is a total body response, there are marked variations in intensity and timing. There is no reason to believe that the female response to the sex act is due to a vaginal rather than a clitoral orgasm.
A mature sexual relationship requires the man and woman to achieve simultaneous orgasm.	Although simultaneous orgasm may be desirable, it is unrealistic. Often is is possible only under the most ideal circumstances, and is not a determinant of sexual achievement or of satisfaction (except to someone who accepts this as dogma).
It is dangerous to have intercourse during menstruation.	Because the source of the menstrual flow is from the uterus rather than the vagina, there is no basis for concern about tissue damage to the vagina. Actually, the desire for sex increases during the menses as a result of increased pelvic vasocongestion. There is no physiologic basis for abstinence during the menses.
The larger penis has greater possibilities for producing orgasm in the woman.	Physiologically, there is practically no relation between the size of a man's penis and his ability to satisfy a woman sexually. Furthermore, there is little correlation between penile size and body size and their relation to sexual potency.
The face-to-face coital position is the proper, moral, and healthy one.	Recent knowledge of human sexual practices dispels this myth with the recognition that there is no normal or single most acceptable sexual position. Whatever position offers the most pleasure and is acceptable to both partners is correct for them. Any variation is normal, healthy, and proper if it satisfies both partners.
The ability to achieve orgasm is an indicator of a person's sexual responsiveness.	Achievement of a satisfactory sexual response is the result of numerous physical, psychologic, and cultural influences. Too often the physical fact of orgasm (or lack of orgasm) is taken to be symbolic of sexual responsiveness and seen out of context of the entire relationship between man and woman.

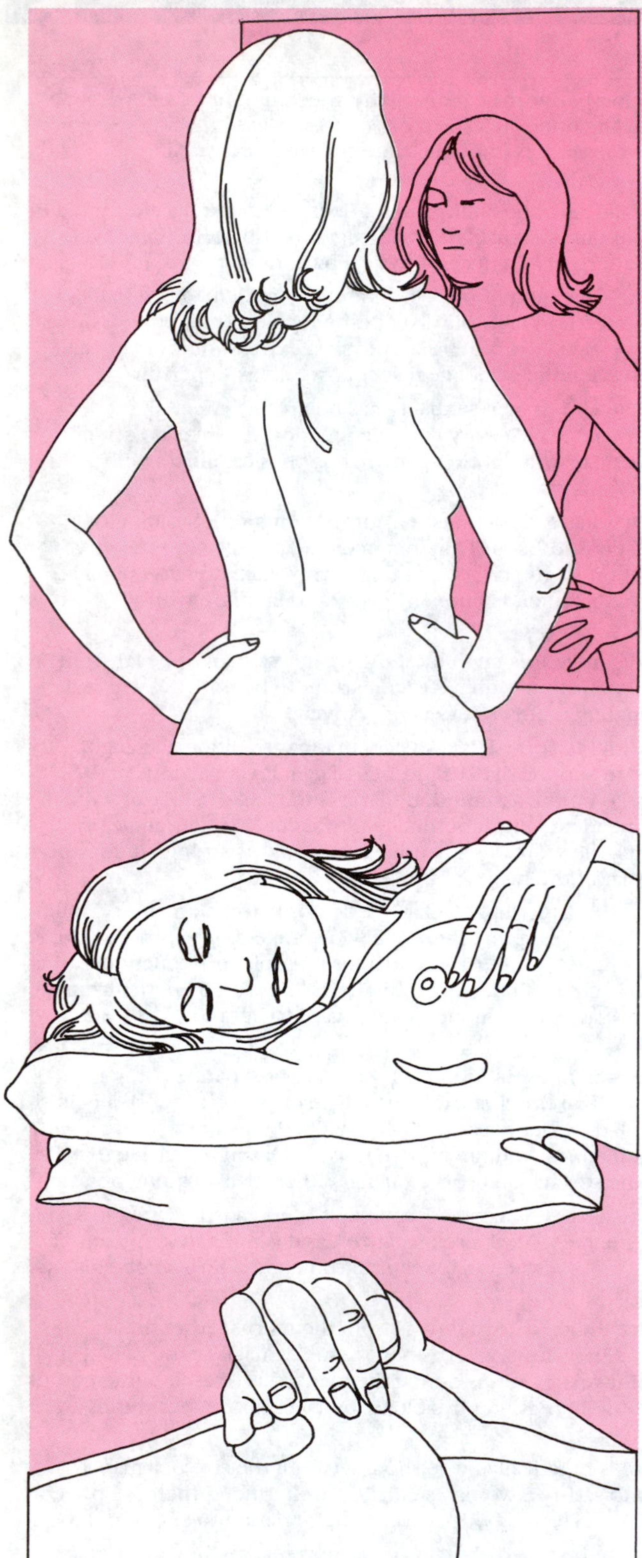

Figure 35-4
Breast self-examination is to be performed once a month. It is begun with inspection using a mirror. Attention is given to contours of the breast and to the skin. Pressing down on the hips serves to tense pectoralis major muscles to inspect for any retraction of the skin. Palpatory examination is performed in a supine position with the side to be examined elevated on a pillow or blanket. Self-examination is completed with a squeeze of the nipple to detect abnormal discharge.

contraception for the orderly spacing of pregnancies in a family. Others use a contraceptive method to prevent pregnancy from occurring until a family is desired. Some people choose a permanent method to prevent pregnancy from ever occurring. Factors that affect choice of a contraceptive method include age, marital status, desire for future pregnancy, religious beliefs, level of education, cost, and ease of use. Other considerations are the woman's knowledge about available methods, her perceptions of the various methods, and, in many cases, her previous experience with contraception.

The safest and most effective method available to prevent a pregnancy is sexual abstinence. For many people, however, this is not an acceptable method. All contraceptive methods have distinct advantages and disadvantages. It is the responsibility of the nurse to understand and explain thoroughly the available methods so the client can choose one that will best meet his or her unique situation and needs.

Natural Family Planning. Natural family planning methods are available to everyone, but using them effectively requires motivation and understanding of male and female reproductive anatomy and physiology. There are four basic natural family planning methods: calendar (rhythm method), basal body temperature (BBT), ovulation (Billing's method), and symptothermal.

The *rhythm* or *calendar* method is based on a woman's monthly menstrual cycle in determining safe and unsafe days. It is an inappropriate method for a woman with irregular cycles. The unsafe days are regarded as periods for sexual abstinence because they are optimal for conception. The *BBT* method is based on the body's response to hormones and ovulation. The woman takes and records her temperature on awakening every morning. A sudden drop in temperature indicates ovulation. This method restricts sexual activity to the second half of the menstrual cycle after ovulation has occurred. The *Billing's* method is based on the changes in the cervical mucus throughout the menstrual cycle. As ovulation occurs, the mucus changes considerably in consistency, becoming sticky, clear, and slippery like an egg white. This method requires the woman to be aware of and have the ability to assess her cervical mucus. The *symptothermal* method combines a number of signs of ovulation, including the rise in BBT, changes in cervical mucus, and variations of the cervix. Both the ovulation and symptothermal methods can be effective in avoiding pregnancy if mutual understanding, support, and motivation exist between the woman and her partner (Fehring, 1991).

Coitus interruptus, one of the oldest and most widely used contraceptive methods, is the withdrawal of the penis from the vagina before ejaculation. Its drawbacks include the possibility of the presence of sperm in Cowper's gland secretions before ejaculation and the stress it places on the man's sexual experience.

Barrier Methods. Barrier methods include the condom, diaphragm, cervical cap, and vaginal sponge used in

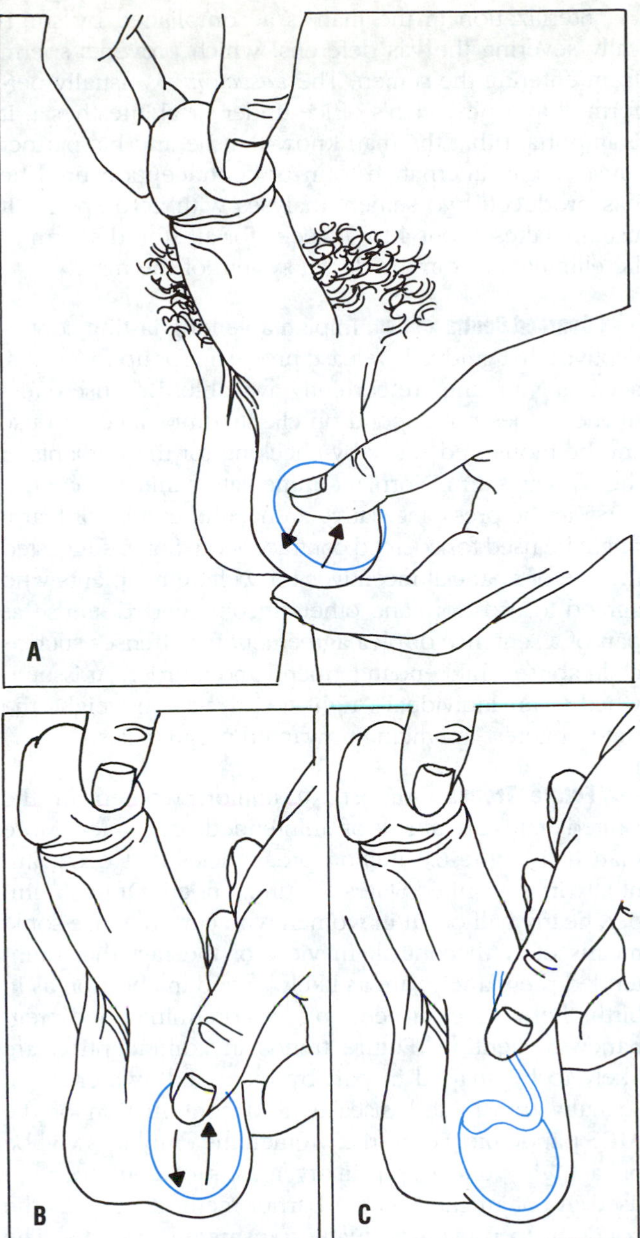

Figure 35-5
Testicular self-examination is to be performed once a month. A convenient time is after a warm bath or shower when the scrotum is relaxed. Both hands are used to palpate the testis; the normal testicle is smooth and uniform in consistency. **(A)** With the index and middle finger under the testis and the thumb on top, roll the testis gently in a horizontal plane between the thumb and fingers, feeling for any evidence of a small lump or abnormality. **(B)** Follow the same procedure for palpation in the vertical plane. **(C)** Locate the epididymis (cordlike structure on the top and back of the testicle that stores and transports sperm). Repeat the examination for the other testis; it is normal to find one testis larger than the other. Any evidence of a small, pea-size lump should be checked by a physician. It may be due to an infection or a tumor growth.

combination with a spermicidal agent. The *diaphragm* has been used in various forms since ancient times. It is currently marketed as a large, dome-shaped device made of latex rubber that mechanically prevents semen from coming into contact with the cervix. It is also used to hold a quantity of spermicidal jelly in place against the cervix. The diaphragm is placed in the vagina before sexual activity. It fits between the pelvic notch at the front of the vagina to behind the cervix at the back. It should not be detected by either the woman or her partner when correctly situated in the vagina. A diaphragm must be individually fitted at a pelvic examination. The woman needs to be familiar with her body and able to handle her genitals for diaphragm placement and removal. The diaphragm must be worn during each episode of sexual activity and consistently used with a spermicidal agent.

The traditional *condom*, or "rubber," is used by men, although it is appropriate for a woman to have them available for her partner's use. The condom is rolled over the erect penis and collects the semen after ejaculation occurs. If the condom does not have a nipple receptacle end, leave a small space at the end of the condom to collect sperm (this prevents breakage). Condoms are available over the counter and have had a surge of popularity with the recent increase in incidence of AIDS and other STDs among single people. A new female condom known as the *vaginal pouch* may offer women greater protection from STDs than male condoms and equal protection from unwanted pregnancy.

The *cervical cap* currently is not universally available. Its mechanism of action is similar to that of the diaphragm. The cervical cap is a thimble-shaped rubber device that is placed over the cervix and may be left there for up to 3 days at a time. Not all women can wear a cervical cap because of individual anatomic differences. There is some evidence to suggest that the cervical cap can cause cervical inflammation and increase risk of pelvic infection.

Spermicides are used with barrier methods but can also be used alone. Spermicides come in creams, jellies, foams, and suppositories. Although readily available, spermicides are not as effective alone as when combined with another method, such as a diaphragm or a condom.

The *vaginal sponge* is a barrier method that contains a spermicide. It has been available over the counter for several years. The sponge not only acts as a barrier between the semen and the cervix but also serves as a reservoir to hold semen. The vaginal sponge carries some risk of toxic shock syndrome (TSS) and is contraindicated for use in women who have a past history of TSS. It is important for women who use the vaginal sponge to follow package directions carefully and to remove the sponge within 24 hours. The vaginal sponge is about as effective as the diaphragm.

Intrauterine Device. The intrauterine device (IUD) is an object that is placed by a physician or nurse practitioner within the uterus to prevent implantation of fertilized ovum. The precise mechanism by which it works is unknown. Although it has a high effectiveness rate and requires little care or motivation on the part of the client, the IUD has many serious side effects and resulting complications. It is an excellent method for women who have completed their families but are not ready or willing to take the final step toward sterilization. Owing to the litigation resulting from complications caused by the IUD, it has been taken off the market by most IUD-producing pharmaceutical companies. Although the IUD may reappear in the future, all women who currently have an IUD in place should seek assistance from a healthcare provider to have it removed. Women wearing a Progestasert IUD should check for the presence of the string in the vagina after every menses and should have the IUD replaced every year.

Hormonal Methods. Hormonal methods are based on the feedback mechanism of hormones of the menstrual cycle. Synthetic estrogens and progestin chemical compounds are used in the form of a pill, shot, or implant to prevent ovulation.

The *oral contraceptive* ("the pill") is the most common contraceptive method and the most popular method for women in their twenties. Most of the harmful side effects and dangers associated with taking the pill are related to the estrogen component. However, most pills currently available contain a small dose of 35 µg of estrogen. The pill has many beneficial noncontraceptive effects. It has been shown to protect women against the development of breast, ovarian, and endometrial cancer (Dickerson, 1983). Taken consistently and as prescribed, the pill is almost 100% effective in guarding against pregnancy. However, the cost may be prohibitive to some women. The woman must also be motivated to take a pill every day at the same time. A health history and physical examination by a healthcare provider are necessary to obtain a prescription for oral contraceptives. Some women should not take the pill in the presence of certain physiologic disorders or diseases. Smoking increases the risks associated with oral contraceptives.

Vaccines. As this text goes to print there is news that a contraceptive vaccine is being developed that would make the woman's egg immune to sperm and confer immunity for about 3 years with an 85% effectiveness rate.

Sterilization. Although male and female sterilization methods can be surgically reversed, the results are not always satisfactory and these methods should therefore be regarded as permanent and irreversible. Sexual desire and ability are unaffected by sterilization.

Sterilization in the woman is accomplished by surgically severing the fallopian tubes. This procedure is known as a *tubal ligation* and prevents travel of the ovum down the tube. Tubal ligation is usually performed on an outpatient basis. Some physicians can also perform the tubal ligation under local anesthesia. Postoperative care and recovery time are required after a tubal ligation.

Sterilization in the man is accomplished by surgically severing the vas deferens, which prevents sperm from entering the semen. The *vasectomy* is usually performed in a physician's office under local anesthesia. It is important that the man know that he and his partner must use an alternative form of contraception until he has produced two semen analyses with zero sperm. It usually takes about 4 to 6 weeks for all stored sperm to be eliminated from the ductal system of the male.

Coerced Contraception. Implantable long-lasting contraceptives that gradually release progestin for up to 5 years, such as Norplant, are currently available. Because effectiveness does not depend on client compliance and use can be monitored easily by checking for the implants in the woman's arm, Norplant immediately initiated controversy in the press, legislative arena, and courts for fear it might be used for coerced contraception. Some suggested the use of financial incentives for welfare recipients who agreed to use Norplant; others recommended its use as part of a sentence or plea agreement for offenses such as child abuse, child endangerment, and murder. At issue is whether an individual's right to privacy outweighs the state's interest in limiting unwanted pregnancies.

Future Trends. Almost 40 million women in the United States are at risk of unintended pregnancy. More than half of the 6.3 million pregnancies that occur annually in the United States are unintended. Of this number, nearly half occur in women who currently use some means of birth control. In view of the fact that unintended pregnancies are as likely to end in abortion as in birth, there is a clear need to focus on unintended pregnancy prevention. Future trends in contraception are likely to be shaped in part by increased awareness of sexually transmitted diseases and continuation of the AIDS pandemic. For at-risk women the emphasis will be on a highly effective primary means of contraception used in conjunction with a barrier method, such as the condom, to prevent sexually transmitted diseases. The single factor having the most impact on future trends in contraceptive use may be the changing demographics of the U.S. population. From 1970 to 1987, the number of U.S. women aged 30 to 44 increased by 59%, from 17.7 million to 28.1 million, while the number of women who were childless at the age of 30 increased by 16% (Hillard, 1994, p. 142).

Facilitating Coping With Special Sexual Needs

The nurse can do much for clients to facilitate their coping with sexual concerns generated by diseases and their treatments. Anticipatory guidance and information should be offered to the client. The importance of open communication with the partner should be stressed. The nurse should include the partner in teaching. Discussion about possible sexual positions is useful and can aid in eliminating pain during coitus. The client can use drawings in selecting possible sexual positions. The client will also find that intercourse may be more comfortable if pain medication is taken before beginning any sexual activity.

When teaching clients about medications, it is important to include known possible sexual alterations to prevent future anxiety and also depression. Clients should alert their physicians if these side effects are experienced. Often a drug dosage can be modified or the drug changed if sexual functioning is affected; otherwise, clients may opt to discontinue the medication on their own rather than sacrifice optimal sexual functioning, if this is an important aspect of life.

Nurses also need to be aware of the special concerns and issues surrounding the care of a homosexual client. Homosexuals have the same right to health care, information, and confidentiality as do heterosexuals.

Teaching Responsible Sexual Expression

Clients need to know how best to gain satisfactory sexual experiences and yet behave responsibly in their activities. Responsible sexuality encompasses these major areas: the form of sexual expression, the prevention of unwanted pregnancy, the prevention of spread of STDs, and sex education.

The form of sexual expression used by clients should not inflict unwanted harm on themselves or others. When the sexual expression encroaches on the rights of others, it is neither healthy nor desirable. Sexual acts that violate another's rights are usually considered to be acts of aggression or hostility rather than stemming from sexual need or desire. Acts of rape in particular are motivated by the need to dominate and humiliate the victim.

The prevention of an unwanted pregnancy must be a conscious decision. Anyone considering the possibility of a sexual encounter who is unprepared for pregnancy should refrain from intercourse or seek out a contraceptive method either from a healthcare provider or from the pharmacy; it is too late to think about contraception during sexual intercourse. To practice responsible sexuality, the contraceptive method must be used consistently and according to instructions.

The incidence of the various STDs is widespread. The only absolute method to avoid an STD is to remain a virgin until marriage, to marry a person who is a virgin, and thereafter never to have sex with anyone else. When this is impractical, other practices that can decrease a person's exposure to STDs are the following:

- The client should limit the number of sexual partners. The risk of an STD rises with the addition of each new partner.
- If a partner has symptoms of an STD, the client should abstain from any sexual activity.
- If the client is in doubt about possible exposure, he or she should report to a healthcare facility for examination.
- If the client does contract an STD, all partners should be notified and advised to seek treatment.
- The use of condoms is advocated for protection against STDs as well as against pregnancy. The client should keep a box of condoms on hand if monogamy is not practiced within the relationship.

Sex education is critical to healthy sexual development and safe sexual behaviors. Information received from peers and friends is almost always inadequate and erroneous. Parents should be taught to answer children's questions immediately and accurately.

Advocating Sexuality Needs of Clients

A hospital experience or institutionalization puts a strain on a person's individuality and sexual self. Illness may diminish feelings of sexual desire. Therefore, it can be a sign of a client's improving health if sexual interaction is desired with the partner. This necessitates anticipatory guidance on the part of the nurse, because many clients may hesitate to make such a request for fear of being ridiculed. Often a client merely desires the privacy to hold and caress the partner. The intimacy of this act often fulfills feelings of longing to be needed and loved.

There are many ways nurses can advocate for a client's sexual needs. Some may seem obvious and commonplace, whereas others may necessitate nurses' coming to terms with their own sexuality (see the accompanying box).

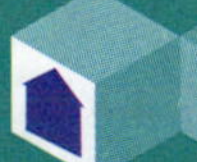

Home Care: Bridging the Gap

Those caring for a terminally ill sexual partner in a home setting may feel uncomfortable discussing care issues around sexual needs—their own or those of the client. Frequently they want to be physically intimate with their partner but are afraid of "hurting" him or her or are afraid that an open expression of sexuality is somehow "inappropriate" when someone is dying.

Sensitive nurses can help by encouraging discussion and by suggesting ways to be physically intimate that will meet the needs of both partners. A loving foot massage or tender, cradling body embrace may be exactly what a dying person needs in his or her last moments.

Advocating Clients' Sexual Needs

- All clients should be accepted as sexual beings with the right to be treated with dignity and with sensitivity to their feelings.
- All clients have the right to some degree of privacy.
  Anticipate the client's desire for privacy by the simple act of drawing a curtain or closing a door. Clients should be given the option of wearing their own sleepwear to promote sexual identity.
- Potentially shaming situations for the client should be anticipated.
  Give information regarding what the procedure is and why it needs to be done, and acknowledge that the client's embarrassment is normal and understandable.
- Health care providers should not simply take for granted that clients do not mind intrusive or embarrassing procedures performed on their bodies and private parts.
- Clients have a right to question the physician regarding sexual needs or future sexual functioning.
  Anticipate these questions for the client. Ask clients if they have any concerns regarding sexuality that can be answered by the nurse. Nurses can interface with the physician to obtain information required by the client.
- The atmosphere in healthcare settings needs to allow for sexual expression between clients and their partners.
- Confidentiality is a right of every client.
  Do not promise confidentiality if that promise cannot be kept.
  Allow no one access to the client's personal records who is not directly involved in the client's care.
  Allow no information regarding clients to escape into idle conversation.
- All clients should be referred to formally as Mr., Mrs., Miss, Ms., according to the client's preference.
- Visitors, including a visiting spouse, should be referred to as people with genders, rather than as "the visitor."
- Clients should be allowed to keep some personal possessions, if it is practical to do so.

Counseling the Client Regarding Sexuality

Not all clients with sexual concerns need intensive therapy. Some clients benefit greatly by the presence of another to listen to verbally expressed concerns. Voicing their concerns allows clients the opportunity to put information into perspective and gain a clearer focus on what the problem really is and how to solve it. Nurses counseling clients need to refrain from offering their own advice because what is right for one person may be wrong for another. Also, offering false reassurances, such as "It will be all right," is unproductive. Rather, the nurse needs to adopt an objective, empathic, and receptive attitude to facilitate an open communication between nurse and client.

Annon (cited in Hatcher et al., 1986) developed a model, termed PLISSIT, for counseling to be used by therapists and nontherapists for clients with sexual problems. The four stages to this model, each increasing in intensity with the seriousness of the client's problem, are listed in the accompanying box.

Model for Counseling Clients With Sexual Problems (PLISSIT)

P—*Permission giving:* The nurse may make a suggestion that the client can use. Permission giving is not the same as advice. Permission giving implies giving the client freedom to choose to do something that the authority figure (such as a nurse) deems to be a positive alternative. It may be something the client wanted to do all along. For example,

Client: "Aren't some sexual positions perverted?"

Nurse: "Many people enjoy using different positions for sex. Some positions are more pleasurable to some couples than others. You and your partner have the right to use any position for sex that you desire."

LI—*Limited information:* Specific factual information is required by the client. It often involves some aspect of anatomy and physiology or the specifics of certain sexual expressions.

SS—*Specific suggestions:* Clients need very specific instructions regarding a useful technique. Many clients have a sexual dysfunction for which they are seeking intervention and correction.

IT—*Intensive therapy:* Used primarily by therapists, it involves issues such as marriage, self-concept, and sexual desire, to name a few. If the first three levels of counseling presented were unsuccessful, intensive therapy is indicated.

EVALUATING

To evaluate the plan of care for the client's sexuality needs, the nurse needs to use information from the client for most client goals/outcomes. It is unrealistic and inappropriate for the nurse to evaluate the client by observing the client's expression of his or her sexuality. However, the nurse can evaluate how the client is progressing toward sexuality-oriented goals by appearance, level of self-confidence, and manner. For example, a client who has expressed feelings of anxiety in the past over a sexual concern should be observably more confident and free of anxiety if client goals are being met. The nurse also needs to question the client about progress toward goals. Some goals need to be steppingstones because not all problems are easily resolved with one-time intervention and direction.

One line of questioning when evaluating a client's progress is as follows: "In what ways have you been able to achieve [orgasm, increased desire, comfortable intercourse, erection]?" "What methods seemed most effective?" "Which were not?" "What do you think should be the next step?" The nurse should determine from this interaction with the client if something more needs to be accomplished. It is not enough to assume that because a set of goals has been met, the client is satisfied with the results.

Nursing Process in Clinical Practice

The nurse uses each phase of the nursing process when identifying and treating problems of sexuality categorized as nursing diagnoses. Quality care depends on the nurse's possession of the knowledge and clinical skills described earlier in this chapter. Nursing diagnoses written to address problems of sexuality belong to one of two categories:

Altered Sexuality Patterns: The state in which an individual experiences or is at risk of experiencing a change in sexual health. Sexual health is the integration of somatic, emotional, intellectual and social aspects of sexual being in ways that are enriching and that enhance personality, communication, and love.

Sexual Dysfunction: The state in which an individual experiences or is at risk of experiencing change in sexual function that is viewed as unrewarding or inadequate.

The four nursing diagnoses chosen for review here are examples of the types of diagnoses that can be developed.

Sexual Dysfunction: Inhibited Sexual Desire
Altered Sexuality Patterns: Change in Sexual Expression
Knowledge Deficit: Contraceptive Methods
Body Image Disturbance related to breast removal

The client care study in Chapter 37 addresses feminine hygiene concerns. In the client care study in this chapter, nursing care is described for an adolescent client with a knowledge deficit.

Sexual Dysfunction: Inhibited Sexual Desire

For information on inhibited sexual desire, the reader is referred to the section in this chapter on sexual dysfunctions. It is important to identify the causative factors of inhibited desire; this is difficult owing to the often complex nature of the problem. Therefore, an accurate and thorough assessment is crucial.

Assessment Priorities

- Assess the client's past ability for sexual arousal to determine if this is a new problem or a chronic one.
- Assess the client's interest in sexual activity.
- Assess for other contributing factors, such as change in relationship or stressors (lifestyle, finances, job, children).
- Assess medications the client is currently taking (prescription and nonprescription) and alcohol consumption.
- Assess the client's physical and mental status for presence of guilt, fear, anxiety, depression, fatigue.
- Assess the client's relationship with the current partner and the quality of communication patterns.
- Use Annon's set of questions during interviewing to determine specific data related to the problem.

Expected Outcomes

The client will:

- Report an increase in sexual desire
- Identify factors in lifestyle that may be affecting desire
- Promote changes in lifestyle to relieve factors contributing to decreased desire
- Initiate open communication pattern with partner

Nursing Interventions

The nursing interventions used for assisting the client to develop an increase in sexual desire actually stem from the causative factors involved in creating the problem initially. A thorough assessment is critical to identify these causative factors. The following interventions specifically address inhibited sexual desire caused by stressful lifestyle:

- Assist the client to identify the specific stressor.
- Assist the client to determine if the stressor can be modified or controlled.
- Plan sexual activity for the time of day when stressors are minimized. (It may be helpful to block out on a calendar a 1- or 2-hour period on specific days.)
- Advise the client to initiate honest dialogue with the partner regarding the plan.
- Use the blocked-out period for stroking and relaxing to focus in on partner.
- Stress that sexual intercourse need not always be the goal of this exercise and not to feel stressed if it does not occur, because this would defeat the purpose of the exercise.

Altered Sexuality Patterns: Change in Sexual Expression

Altered Sexuality Patterns is a broad diagnosis with many interpretations for use in nursing practice. Loss of desire, increased desire, and change in sexual expression are three dimensions of the problem that are defined more specifically as follows:

1. Loss of desire may also be interpreted as loss of opportunity or involuntary abstinence. The problem can be further specified by any number of causative factors.
2. Increased desire may also be interpreted as preoccupation with sexual activity. An example would be the beginning of a new sexual relationship. Although this in itself is rarely a problem for the individual, it could be if the desire leads to promiscuous or nondiscriminating behaviors.
3. A change in sexual expression may be a problem if it is involuntarily imposed on the client and the partner. Any disease process, the aging process, isolation from the partner, or life stressors can change the mode of sexual expression for the couple. Change in sexual expression is discussed in more detail in this section.

A disruption in a client's usual mode of sexual expression can cause stress and anxiety in his or her relationship. Although nursing actions cannot change medical conditions or reverse pathophysiology, nurses can assist clients to adapt to the changes in their lives.

Assessment Priorities

Assessment is important because it helps the nurse identify the specific etiologic factors that are amenable to nursing action. The reader is referred to the section "Diagnosing" for a list of possible etiologic factors. As an example of the nursing process in clinical practice, the effects of disease process on sexual expression are used.

- Use the three interview questions regarding relationships, feelings of sexuality, and sexual functioning to determine the significance of the problem (see the section "Sexual History" earlier in this chapter).
- Assess past sexual behaviors such as frequency, sexual positions, favored methods of foreplay, use of oral–genital sex, or sexual intercourse.
- Assess importance of each activity and what will remain the same or constant.
- Assess what has changed or will change for the client and partner as a result of the disease or surgery.
- Assess communication patterns between the client and partner.

Expected Outcomes

The client will:

- Identify positive aspects of the current sexual relationship
- Identify at least three viable alternatives to altered sexuality pattern
- Express satisfaction with change in sexual expression

Nursing Interventions

Nursing measures are needed to assist the client to discover possible alternatives to the change in sexual expression that will prove satisfying to the client and the partner.

If the preferred sexual position has been altered:

- Allow the client to voice any preferences regarding alternative sexual positions
- Give the client permission to use alternative sexual positions
- Teach the client regarding the use of alternative positions; use charts or diagrams and give specific instructions

If frequency of sexual activity has been altered:

- Review past frequency of sexual activity
- Identify options for increasing frequency (ie, increase desire, increase opportunity, increase privacy)
- Take pain medication, if indicated, before any sexual activity

If method of sexual activity has been altered:

- Review with the client and partner their feelings regarding the use of oral–genital stimulation and mutual masturbation
- Give the client permission to use alternative modes of sexual expression
- Give the client specific information about the use of alternative activities
- Encourage open communication between the client and partner to express their satisfaction or dissatisfaction with the activated care plan

Knowledge Deficit: Contraceptive Methods

Many areas of knowledge deficit can be identified and treated by nurses. Some examples as they pertain to sexuality are reproductive anatomy and physiology, sexual response cycle, modes of sexual expression, self-examination, spread of STDs, contraceptive methods, and the effect of disease and medications on sexual functioning.

To illustrate how the nursing process in clinical practice can be used for a knowledge deficit of a sexual concern, knowledge deficit about contraceptive methods is used as an example here. For a discussion of the various contraceptive methods currently available, the reader is referred to the pertinent section of this chapter.

Assessment Priorities

- Determine past use of contraceptive methods.
- Assess effectiveness and satisfaction with past methods.
- Assess the client's current knowledge of contraceptive methods.
- Assess frequency of the client's sexual activity.
- Identify any methods that are unacceptable to the client.
- Assess motivation of the client to use certain methods.
- Assess the client's level of comfort with manipulation of genital body parts.
- Obtain complete client history and perform a physical examination if indicated.

Expected Outcomes

The client will:

- Choose a contraceptive method that the client is motivated to use
- List the adverse effects or danger signs associated with the contraceptive method
- List the steps needed to use the contraceptive method effectively
- Use the contraceptive with every act of sexual intercourse
- Choose a back-up method
- Report back to the healthcare setting for follow-up as directed

Nursing Interventions

- Describe in terms at the client's level of understanding each contraceptive method for which the client needs information (give objective information in matter-of-fact manner to avoid bias by nurse).
- Describe the effectiveness of each method and side effects or possible complications.
- Instruct the client in the use of a chosen method, giving step-by-step instructions.
- Advise the client of the importance of having a back-up method on hand.
- Instruct the client in the use of the back-up method.
- Have the client obtain a physical examination if indicated by the chosen contraceptive method (eg, the pill).
- Instruct the client to report back in a specified period for follow-up of use of method if indicated (follow-up visits to a healthcare facility are important, particularly if a client elects to use the pill).

Body Image Disturbance Related to Breast Removal

Any change in one's physical body needs to be integrated into one's mental image of the body. Because the body plays such a large part in the expression of sexuality, any disturbance in body image will no doubt have some effect on the expression of sexuality.

In this section, a disturbance in body image as the result of the loss of a breast is illustrated. The effect of mastectomy on a woman's sexuality depends largely on how much significance she places on her breasts. Also, some women find stimulation of their breasts during foreplay a satisfying component of sexual activity. Some men place a great deal of sexual emphasis on women's breasts as well.

The fears experienced by some women after surgery include the fear of rejection by society and by the sexual partner. A woman may feel that she has been mutilated and is defective as a woman and sex partner. Some women may choose to hide the surgical site from their partners by undressing in the dark or by wearing a bra to bed. Although a stable marriage should not be threatened by illness and surgery, many marriages cannot bear the stress of the trauma of a mastectomy because of other contributing factors. The fear of causing revulsion in her partner and the possibility of the partner ending the relationship also cause much anxiety to the postoperative mastectomy client.

Assessment Priorities

Assessment should include review of preoperative relationship factors between the woman and her partner; these will be helpful in determining the causative factors of disturbed body image and provide clues for effective nursing intervention.

- Assess the client's feelings regarding herself as a woman, wife, and sexual partner (use the interview questions listed in the section "Sexual History" earlier in this chapter).
- Assess the client's fears regarding change in her femininity, sexual relationship, and images of herself as a person.
- Assess the client's concerns regarding the illness, treatment, and prognosis.
- Assess the value placed on the lost breast by the client (and by her sexual partner if appropriate).
- Assess the client's support system, including family and close friends.

Expected Outcomes

The client will:

- List positive aspects of her body
- List positive aspects of sexual relationship
- Maintain open communication patterns with her partner

- Enhance physical appearance and positive features with use of feminine clothing, make-up, and breast prosthesis if desired
- Report satisfactory sexual activity
- Verbalize integration of mastectomy into body image

Nursing Interventions

- Support the client as she examines her thoughts and feelings about her lost breast.
- Encourage the client to talk openly with her partner regarding her feelings and fears.
- Provide positive reinforcement by identifying the client's positive aspects.
- Instruct the client that as she recovers from surgery, desire for sexual closeness will return.
- Advise the client to strive to continue previous behaviors with partner.
- Inform the client that much attractive clothing is currently available to minimize the effects of mastectomy.
- Give the client information as desired regarding breast prosthesis and reconstructive surgery.
- Contact Reach for Recovery or other support people to assist client in adaptation to mastectomy.

Client Care Study

Pete is a 13-year-old adolescent boy attending the area health clinic. He is nervous as he explains to the nurse his need for health care. He has noticed "sticky white stuff" around his penis and bedclothes on arising some mornings and fears he may be ill. Pete has also expressed concern over his lack of knowledge regarding sexuality. He has heard a lot of stories from his friends but does not feel he can talk to his parents because the subject has never been broached at home. Also, although Pete is a virgin, he is beginning to feel pressured by his friends, who boast of many sexual experiences.

After spending time in conversation with Pete, the nurse gathered the following data:

- Pete is experiencing nocturnal emissions and has little scientific knowledge about their source.
- Pete is anxious over the stories regarding sex he has heard from his friends.
- There is no communication or dialogue at home with parents about issues of sexuality.
- Pete is having feelings of insecurity and anxiety over his present virginal status, which he feels he should change.
- Peer pressure from friends is also a concern.

Plan of Nursing Care

The nurse will work together with Pete to develop a plan of care to correct misinformation and relieve his anxiety. Planning will be directed toward correcting myths and supplying Pete with accurate information. Because Pete has a negligible knowledge base on sexuality, the plan of care will allow for ongoing sessions to augment the initial information. The nurse should outline this plan with Pete to be certain it is acceptable to him.

Core Competencies

In implementing the plan of care, the nurse needs the following specialized abilities:

Cognitive and Technical Competencies

- Strong knowledge base of human sexuality, including anatomy and physiology, growth and development, sexual myths, and current issues of sexuality
- Strong assessment skills of interviewing a client with concerns of sexuality
- Teaching skills to provide client with necessary information and skills

Interpersonal Competencies

- Interpersonal communication skills to build rapport with an adolescent client
- Nonjudgmental attitude to avoid bias, which would impede trusting nurse–client relationship
- Counseling skills to diffuse client anxiety over sexual growth and development
- Sense of own sexuality and comfort with sexual issues

Ethical/Legal Competencies

- Knowledge of professional responsibilities and ability and willingness to use these in a legally defensible manner to meet Pete's needs

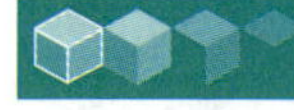

Nursing Plan of Care

for Pete

Nursing Diagnosis: Knowledge Deficit: Adolescent Sexuality Concerns related to misinformation and absent family-based sex education as manifested by self-report

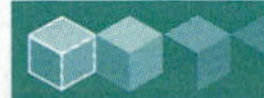

Nursing Plan of Care *(continued)*

for Pete

Expected Outcome: By the end of the teaching session, the client will:

- Describe the nature of nocturnal emissions

Nursing Interventions	Rationale	Evaluative Statement
Assess client's present knowledge base on nocturnal emission and the source of his information.	It is necessary to discover what the client does know and to build on that knowledge.	8/1/98 Goal met. Client able to describe the source of nocturnal emissions. *R. Gordon, RN*
Use terms that the client has used and language at the level of the client's understanding.	This facilitates comprehension.	
Teach the client about nocturnal emissions: • Nocturnal emissions, or "wet dreams," are normal in men of all ages, and they are particularly common in the teen years. They are not the result of disease. • They occur during sleep as the result of erotic dreams. The "white sticky stuff" is the result of ejaculation of semen from the penis. • This is an involuntary action over which the male has no control.	Knowledge decreases anxiety.	

Expected Outcome By the end of the teaching session, the client will:

- Differentiate sexual myths from sound knowledge

Nursing Interventions	Rationale	Evaluative Statement
Assess what client has heard from peers regarding sexual information:	The nurse can then specifically address the myths to which the client has been exposed.	8/1/98 Goal met. Client was able to differentiate between truth in sexual issues and what is myth. *R. Gordon, RN*
Myth 1: "A large penis is better for sex than a small one." *Truth:* No relation exists between the size of a penis and the man's ability to perform sexually. When a penis becomes erect, it reaches sufficient size to engage in sexual intercourse.	This enables the client to develop a positive sexual body image based on fact.	
Myth 2: "Jerking off causes blindness. It is a dirty habit." *Truth:* Masturbation or self-stimulation is a natural and healthy outlet for sexual urges. Men and women of all ages masturbate. Masturbation can also teach the person what feels good and what does not. Every person has the right to masturbate if he or she wishes to do so.	The client is given permission to engage in a sexual activity of a masturbatory nature.	

(continued)

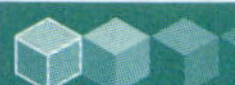

Nursing Plan of Care *(continued)*

for Pete

Nursing Interventions	Rationale	Evaluative Statement
Myth 3: "It looks bad for a guy to be a virgin—everybody's doing it." *Truth:* No one, whether male or female, should feel pressured into sexual activity at any age. Engaging in sexual activity carries with it a great deal of responsibility and concerns of pregnancy and spread of STDs. No one needs to know of another person's status if the person chooses not to discuss it.	The client is given permission to abstain from sexual activity and not to feel pressured by friends. Almost 39% of teens have had sex by age 16 years.	

Expected Outcome By the end of the teaching session, the client will:

- List the positive aspects of abstinence in a sexual relationship

Nursing Interventions	Rationale	Evaluative Statement
Assess the client including previous discussion of sexual myths and knowledge.	Giving the client all the information necessary allows him to make an informed decision.	8/1/98 Goal partially met. Client able to verbally list all positive aspects of abstinence but is still undecided. *Revision:* Reinforce to client that this is a personal decision that he can make for himself with a good knowledge base. Also, he does not have to make a firm decision for or against abstinence immediately. He should take time to think about this information. ***R. Gordon, RN***
Instruct the client on the positive aspects of abstinence, including the following: • Engagement in any sexual activity should be a personal decision and not the result of pressure from friends.		
• Abstinence will guarantee protection from pregnancy and from most sexually transmitted diseases.	Many young people think they are immune to the consequences of their actions. Therefore, it is important to stress that pregnancy and STDs are very probable results of sexual intercourse.	
• People can show affection for each other without sexual involvement.	It is difficult to understand and undertake all the implications of a sexual relationship during the teen years. The client learns that a successful sexual relationship requires intimacy, love, and sharing; it should not be merely an outlet for sexual feelings.	
• Every person has the right to say no.	The client has permission to refuse an activity in which he is not sure he wishes to engage.	

Expected Outcome By the end of the teaching session, the client will:

- Describe the correct use of rubber condoms

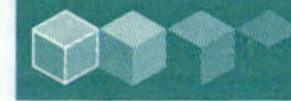

Nursing Plan of Care *(continued)*

for Pete

Nursing Interventions	Rationale	Evaluative Statement
Assess what the client knows about rubber condoms and their use.	Since client is undecided over whether to initiate a sexual relationship in the future, it is prudent to give him information to protect against pregnancy and STDs.	8/1/98 Goal met. Client successfully listed the steps in using a condom. ***R. Gordon, RN***
Inform the client that rubber condoms are available over the counter in drug stores. Prices will vary according to type and style.	Client should know where to purchase condoms and the variety available.	
Teach client the steps in using rubber condoms:	Client should know how to use condoms safely.	
• Roll condom onto the penis as soon as it becomes erect.	Protects against sperm from secretions from Cowper's glands	
• If condom does not have a nipple receptacle end, leave a small space at end of condom to collect semen.	Provides a pocket to collect semen and prevents breakage	
• Immediately after ejaculation, remove penis and condom from vagina by holding onto base of condom.	Prevents spillage of semen into the vagina	
• Discard condom.	Condoms are not meant to be used over. A new condom is used for each act of intercourse.	
Advise the client to use a condom with every act of intercourse. Spermicides used with condom increase effectiveness.	To be as effective as possible, the condom should be used with every act of intercourse. The rubber condom used with spermicide is effective against pregnancy and the spread of STDs. The woman's use of a spermicide foam in the vagina increases effectiveness.	

Expected Outcome By the end of the teaching session, the client will:

- Express a decrease in anxiety

Nursing Interventions	Rationale	Evaluative Statement
Assess client's anxiety level by verbal and nonverbal behavior.	Client was anxious when he came into clinic. It is important to evaluate level of anxiety before he leaves. If he is still anxious, reassessment should occur because plan of care may have been unsuccessful.	8/1/98 Goal met. Client expressed relief that he is normal. Would like to bring a friend to next session. Future teaching sessions to include these topics identified by client: • STDs, particularly AIDS • Pregnancy—occurrence and prevention • Sexual expression • Further discussion of sexual myths ***R. Gordon, RN***

(continued)

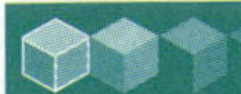

Nursing Plan of Care *(continued)*

for Pete

Sample Documentation

8/1/98, 11 AM, nursing

Nursing consultation with 13-year-old client regarding anxiety over cause and source of nocturnal emissions. Client also expressed concern about sexual myths he has heard from friends. Stated that much peer pressure exists to become sexually active. Client admits to possessing little knowledge regarding sexual issues. Feels he cannot discuss sexuality with parents, because it is not a topic that has been brought up in the past at home. Will conduct initial teaching session with client to provide information and decrease anxiety about priority concerns. Client is willing to return to clinic for at least three more teaching sessions to further expand knowledge base of sexuality.

R. Gordon, RN

Key Points

- Sexuality is a human component that is inadequately understood.
- Sexuality defines maleness and femaleness and is evident in behavior, physical appearance, and relationships with others.
- Nurses are concerned with clients' sexuality because individuals bring with them to a healthcare setting all aspects of what makes them human.
- A sound knowledge base of female and male reproductive anatomy and physiology, the sexual response cycle, and factors that affect sexuality is important for the nurse to be an effective teacher, counselor, and advocate in dealing with clients with sexual concerns.
- Factors that affect sexuality include developmental stage, culture, religion, ethics, lifestyle, sexual orientation, health state, and use of medications.
- Obtaining a comprehensive history and performing a physical assessment are paramount before nursing care can be planned for a client with a sexual concern. However, the collection of a sexual history is not appropriate in all healthcare situations. Clients who should have at least a brief sexual history recorded are those with concerns of a reproductive nature, those experiencing a sexual dysfunction, and those whose illness or treatment will affect their sexual functioning.
- The physical assessment of reproductive anatomy can be stressful and uncomfortable for both male and female clients. Because the major portion of female genitalia is internal, the examination is invasive and may be frightening. The nurse should provide support and information before and during a pelvic examination to create a positive experience for the woman.
- Problems associated with sexuality are rarely simple and clear-cut owing to the integral nature of sexuality. Clients may need assistance to talk through their concerns before definitive nursing diagnoses can be formulated.
- Nursing diagnoses can be written specifically to address Altered Sexuality Patterns and Sexual Dysfunction. The effect of sexual concerns on other areas of human functioning can also be identified (eg, Body Image Disturbance, Anxiety, Impaired Adjustment).
- Nurses who are good role models in promoting healthy sexuality have developed a definition of their own sexuality, have developed a self-awareness of their beliefs, and possess a knowledge base of sexual topics and issues.
- Nursing interventions that promote healthy sexuality include establishing a trusting nurse–client relationship, advocating for hospitalized clients' sexual needs, counseling clients regarding sexual concerns, and teaching clients about sexuality-related subjects.
- Client education, which includes topics of self-examination, contraceptive methods, and responsible sexual expression, can be implemented in many healthcare situations.

Study Questions

1. The female counterpart to a male penis is the
   a. clitoris
   b. vagina
   c. hymen
   d. labia majora
2. Fertilization of the ovum by the sperm usually occurs in the
   a. uterus
   b. fallopian tube
   c. ovary
   d. vagina

3. The primary hormone secreted by the testes is
   a. estrogen
   b. progesterone
   c. semen
   d. testosterone
4. The sexual response cycle is
   a. limited to the genitalia
   b. a total body response
   c. limited to the erogenous zone
   d. divided into two phases, excitement and resolution
5. Male orgasm always consists of
   a. ejaculation of semen
   b. 15 to 20 contractions
   c. involuntary spasmodic contractions of the genitals
   d. 4 to 10 contractions
6. A 16-year-old girl confides to the school nurse, "Something must be wrong with me. I'm the only one in my class who doesn't have her period yet." The nurse's best *initial* response is to
   a. recommend a thorough medical examination to rule out medical disease
   b. explain that menarche can be experienced as early as 8 years and as late as 17 years
   c. question her about life stresses that might be retarding the start of her period
   d. question her about the age at which her mother, maternal grandmother, and aunts experienced menarche
7. You are asked, "Is it okay to enjoy intercourse during menses?" Your answer is best based on the knowledge that
   a. there is no scientific rationale to support abstinence from sexual activity during menses
   b. intercourse during menses is more likely to damage sensitive tissues in the vagina
   c. women should not have intercourse during the time of the month when they are "unclean"
   d. women have been oppressed for too long and need to regain control of their bodies
8. When exposure of a male client during the bed bath results in an erection, the best nursing response is to
   a. explain that this is a natural physiologic response and offer to leave the room if the client wishes
   b. leave the room quickly to allow the client to regain control
   c. state firmly that this behavior makes you uncomfortable and that you expect it to stop
   d. ask that client if he is experiencing anxiety about his ability to be sexually active after his illness
9. When a young mother confides to you that she is concerned about her toddler who frequently fondles his genitals, you should
   a. explain that it is not too early to begin teaching the youngster what is "bad" or unacceptable behavior
   b. stress the importance of the parent's "setting limits" by using negative reinforcement
   c. explain that it is perfectly natural for toddlers to enjoy fondling their genitals
   d. stress that this may signal a medical/psychiatric problem that requires evaluation
10. A 77-year-old client asks you if you think it's wrong for her to masturbate. Your best response is
    a. "I thought you were too old for that!"
    b. "Do you really do that?"
    c. "How do you feel about it?"
    d. "Why don't you ask your physician?"
11. The statement below that reveals a correct knowledge of sexuality is
    a. "My small penis makes it hard for me to satisfy a woman sexually."
    b. "Because sex 'weakens a person,' the coach insists we abstain before big games."
    c. "Something must be wrong with me. I know women aren't supposed to enjoy sex as much as men."
    d. "I think all the attention being paid to achieving simultaneous orgasms is misplaced."
12. Which of the following statements indicates a need for contraceptive teaching?
    a. "Because breastfeeding isn't a foolproof contraceptive, we plan to use a condom as soon as we are sexually active again."
    b. "My partner always withdraws before ejaculation, so we are not worried about pregnancy."
    c. "My husband and I are highly motivated to make natural family planning work so that we can have our children when we are ready."
    d. "I understand that I should always use a spermicidal agent with my diaphragm."
13. When teaching young clients about sexually transmitted diseases, it is important to communicate
    a. abstinence is an unrealistic, old-fashioned idea
    b. having sexual contact with one person is to have contact with everyone else with whom that person has had sexual contact
    c. adolescents are less likely to contract a sexually transmitted disease because they are generally healthier than adults
    d. with prompt medical treatment, all sexually transmitted diseases can be cured without long-standing complications
14. In 1974, the American Psychiatric Association removed which of the following from the category of mental illness?
    a. transsexuality
    b. bisexuality
    c. homosexuality
    d. heterosexuality
15. During the admission history, Mrs. Victor tells you that she experiences extreme pain during intercourse. An appropriate nursing diagnosis would be
    a. Fear related to pain during sexual intercourse
    b. Body Image Disturbance related to painful intercourse
    c. Ineffective Individual Coping related to pain
    d. Pain related to dyspareunia

Answers With Rationale

1. The correct response is *a*. The clitoris is the female counterpart to the male penis because they are similar in their reaction to stimuli. The vagina, hymen, and labia majora are not similarly responsive to stimuli.
2. The correct response is *b*. Fertilization of the ovum by the sperm usually occurs in the fallopian tube, not in the uterus, ovary, or vagina.
3. The correct response is *d*. The primary hormone secreted by the testes is testosterone, not estrogen or progesterone (female sex hormones). Semen, seminal plasma, and sperm are not hormones.
4. The correct response is *b*. The sexual response cycle is clearly a total body response and is not limited to the genitalia nor to the erogenous zones. There are more than two phases in the sexual response cycle.
5. The correct response is *c*. By definition, the male orgasm always consists of involuntary spasmodic contractions of the genitals. The other options are all possible but unnecessary.
6. The correct response is *b*. The nurse's first priority is to inform the client that, at 16 years, she is still within the normal age span for experiencing menarche (8 to 17 years). Once this is done, a more detailed history may be taken.
7. The correct response is *a*. If a client asks about enjoying intercourse during the menses, it is important to base your response on fact (there is no scientific rationale to support abstinence from sexual activity during menses) rather than on a religious, cultural, or personal belief. Option *b* is simply false.
8. The correct response is *a*. Explaining to the client that this is a natural physiologic response and giving him time to regain control will decrease any embarrassment he is experiencing. Option *b* (leaving the room without comment) might be interpreted as signifying disapproval. Option *c* clearly communicates disapproval and option *d* is premature.
9. The correct response is *c*. The appropriate response to this mother's concern is the factual information that this is developmentally appropriate behavior. Options *a* and *b* communicate incorrectly that this is abnormal behavior that ought to be curbed. Option *d* is false.
10. The correct response is *c*. Option *a* is based on the myth that elderly people do not have any sexual needs. Option *b* implies disapproval. Option *d* refers to the physician a question the nurse should be able to answer. Asking the client how she feels (option *c*) opens the door for a frank discussion of the client's concerns and will surface any false information or negative beliefs the client holds.
11. The correct response is *d*. Placing too much attention on achieving simultaneous orgasm can detract from the overall sexual experience. The other options are all common sexual myths.
12. The correct response is *b*. Withdrawing before ejaculation is no guarantee that no sperm have been released because, during sexual activity, Cowper's glands produce small droplets of fluid that may contain sperm. The other options are all statements that reveal a correct understanding of contraceptive measures.
13. The correct response is *b*. Having sexual contact with one person is to have contact with everyone else that person has had contact with is the only factually correct response. Option *a* may be held by some nurses but is a personal belief that many would challenge. Options *c* and *d* are false.
14. The correct response is *c*. Homosexuality was removed from the category of mental illness in 1974 by the American Psychiatric Association.
15. The correct response is *d*. The data point to a nursing diagnosis of Pain related to dyspareunia (painful intercourse). The client has not mentioned fear, and no data point to a disturbance in body image or to ineffective coping.

Bibliography

Baldwin, K., & Goodwin K. (1985). The Papanicolaou smear. *Journal of Nurse–Midwifery, 30*(6), 327–331.

Bourcier K., & Seidler, A. (1987). *Chlamydia* and condylomata acuminata: An update for the nurse practitioner. *Journal of Obstetric, Gynecologic, and Neonatal Nursing, 16*(1), 17–21.

Buczny, B. (1992). Impotence in older men: A newly recognized problem. *Journal of Gerontological Nursing, 18*(5), 25–30.

Carter, J. & Verhoef, M.J. (1995). Efficacy of self-help and alternative treatments of premenstrual syndrome. *Women's Health Issues, 4*(3), 130–137.

Cholewinski, J. T., & Burge, J. M. (1990). Sexual harassment of nursing students. *IMAGE: Journal of Nursing Scholarship, 22*(2), 106–110.

Cole, F.L. & Slocumb, E.M. (1995). Factors influencing safer sexual behaviors in heterosexual late adolescent and young adult collegiate males. *IMAGE: Journal of Nursing Scholarship, 27*(3), 217–223.

Fehring, R. J. (1991). New technology in natural family planning. *Journal of Obstetric, Gynecologic, and Neonatal Nursing, 20*(3), 199–205.

Fromer, M. (1983). *Ethical issues in sexuality and reproduction* (2nd ed.). St. Louis: Mosby.

Fuentes, R. J., Rosenberg, J. M., & Marks, R. G. (1983). Sexual side effects. What to tell your patients, what not to say. *Registered Nurse, 46*(2), 34–41.

Gallup, R. (1993). Sexual contact between nurses and patients. *Canadian Nurse, 89*(2), 28–31.

Gruen, S. M., Hayes, E., & Fritsch-deBruyn, R. (1991). Setting up a school-based sexual education program to help prevent AIDS and other STDs. *Nurse Practitioner, 16*(8), 47–51.

Harbin, R.E. (1995). Female adolescent contraception. *Pediatric Nursing, 21*(3), 221–226.

Hatcher, R., Guest, S., Stewart, F., Stewart, G. K., Trussell, J., Cerel, S., & Kates, W. (1990). *Contraceptive technology* (15th ed.). New York: Irvington.

Hillard, P.A. (1994). Contraceptive use and attitudes among U.S. women. *Women's Health Issues, 4*(3), 138–143.

Horsley, J. E. (1990). Don't tolerate sexual harassment at work. *RN, 53*(1), 69, 72, 75.

Katzin, L. (1990). Chronic illness and sexuality. *American Journal of Nursing, 90*(1), 54–59.

Kaye, J., Donald, C.G., & Merker, S. (1994). Sexual harassment of critical care nurses: A costly workplace issue. *American Journal of Critical Care, 3*(6), 409–415.

King, J. (1992). Helping patients choose an appropriate method of birth control. *MCN, 17*(2), 91–95.

McGrory, A. (1995). Education for the menarche. *Pediatric Nursing, 21*(5), 439–443.

Pillitteri, A. (1995). *Maternal and child health nursing* (2nd ed.). Philadelphia: Lippincott.

Sarazin, S. K., & Seymour, S. F. (1991). Causes and treatment options for women with dyspareunia. *Nurse Practitioner, 16*(10), 30–41.

Staff. (1993). American Academy of Pediatrics Committee on Adolescence: Homosexuality and adolescence. *Pediatrics, 92*, 631–633.

Stockard, S. (1991). Caring for the sexually aggressive patient: You don't have to blush and bear it. *Nursing, 21*(11), 72–73.

Talashek, M. L., Tichy, A. M., & Eping, H. (1990). Sexually transmitted diseases in the elderly: Issues and recommendations. *Journal of Gerontological Nursing, 16*(4), 33–42.

Tillmann, J. (1992). Syphilis: An old disease, a contemporary perinatal problem. *Journal of Obstetric, Gynecologic, and Neonatal Nursing, 21*(3), 209–213.

Touchstone, D. M., & Davis, D. D. (1992). Consider chlamydia. *RN, 55*(2), 32–35.

Varnhagen, C. K. (1991). Sexually transmitted diseases and condoms: High school students' knowledge, attitudes, and behaviors. *Canadian Journal of Public Health, 82*(2), 129–132.

Watts, R. (1979). Dimensions of sexual health. *American Journal of Nursing, 79*(9), 1568–1572.

Weisberg, M. (1984). Physiology of female sexual function. *Clinical Obstetrics and Gynecology, 27*(3), 697–706.

Williams, A. B. (1992). The epidemiology, clinical manifestations and health maintenance needs of women infected with HIV. *Nurse Practitioner, 17*(5), 27–44.

Winter, E.J.S., Ashton, D. J. & Moore, D. L. (1991). Dispelling myths: A study of PMS and relationship satisfaction. *Nurse Practitioner, 16*(5), 34–45.

Woods, N. F. (1984). *Human sexuality in health and illness.* St. Louis: Mosby.

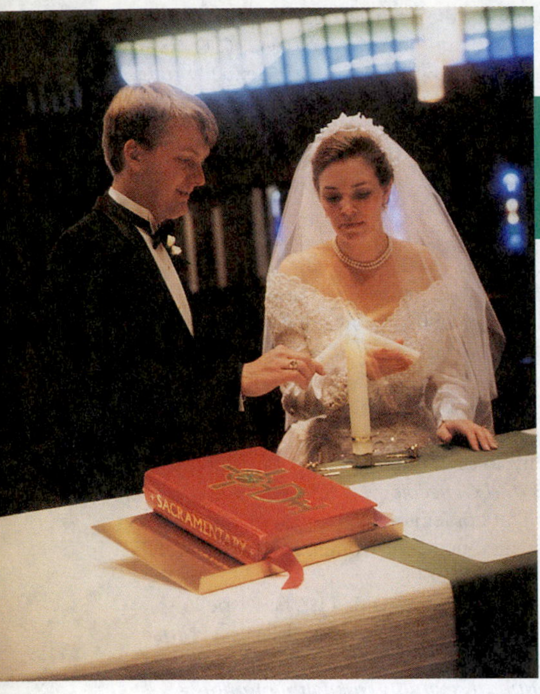

Chapter 36

Spirituality

Objectives

After studying this chapter, the learner should be able to:

Define key terms used in the chapter.

Identify three spiritual needs believed to be common to all people.

Describe the influences of spirituality on everyday living, health, and illness.

Differentiate life-affirming influences of religious beliefs from life-denying influences.

Distinguish the spiritual beliefs and practices of the major religions practiced in the United States and Canada.

Identify five factors that influence spirituality.

Perform a nursing assessment of spiritual health, using appropriate interview questions and observation skills.

Develop nursing diagnoses that correctly identify spiritual problems.

Describe nursing strategies to promote spiritual health and state their rationale.

Plan, implement, and evaluate nursing care related to select nursing diagnoses involving spiritual problems.

Key Terms

agnostic
atheist
faith
religion
spiritual beliefs
spiritual distress
spirituality
spiritual needs

The "spirit" dimension of the person was recognized in ancient cultures. "The dual roles of priest and physician were generally held by one individual, and thus the functions and dictates of religion (pertaining to the spirit) and medicine (pertaining to the body) were closely interwoven" (O'Brien, 1982, p. 85). Over the years, however, medicine and religion evolved separately. Not until the holistic health movement took root was the person once again viewed as an integrated whole of body, mind, and spirit. Healthcare practitioners began again to probe the relationships among physical, psychologic, and spiritual health.

Nursing has always had a strongly holistic tradition and nurses have practiced nursing sensitive to the physical, psychosocial, and spiritual needs of people. According to Fish and Shelly (1978), there are three **spiritual needs** underlying all religious traditions and common to all people: (1) need for meaning and purpose, (2) need for love and relatedness, and (3) need for forgiveness. Although nurses may differ in their beliefs about how involved they should become in meeting clients' spiritual needs, it is impossible to nurse individuals well while ignoring the spiritual dimensions of health. Nurses can assist clients to meet spiritual needs by offering a compassionate presence; assisting in the struggle to find meaning and purpose in the face of suffering, illness, and death; fostering relationships (with God/humans) that nurture the spirit; and facilitating the client's expression of religious or spiritual beliefs and practices.

Study of this chapter provides the student with a knowledge base of spirituality. Practical suggestions for performing a spiritual assessment are given, along with specific interview questions. Sample nursing diagnoses are developed for common problems of spiritual distress (spiritual pain, alienation, anxiety, guilt, anger, loss, and despair). Related client and nursing goals and specific nursing strategies for promoting spiritual health are described. In the section Nursing Process in Clinical Practice, focused assessment, planning, implementation, and evaluation guides are offered for clients experiencing spiritual distress related to challenged beliefs and value systems. These guides and the concluding client care study illustrate how the nurse's knowledge of spirituality may be combined with skilled nursing interventions and caring to resolve spiritual distress successfully.

Spirituality and Faith

Although the terms *spirituality, religion,* and *faith* are used interchangeably by some, there are distinctions. **Spirituality** is anything that pertains to a person's relationship with a nonmaterial life force or higher power. Whereas one person describes spirituality in terms of coming to know, love, and serve God, another speaks of transcending the limits of body and experiencing a universal energy. Spirituality may include **religion**, which refers to an organized system of beliefs about a higher power. Religions are often characterized by set forms of worship, spiritual practices, and codes of conduct. Thus a person may be deeply spiritual yet not profess a religion. The fact that people do not belong to an organized religion should not be interpreted by the nurse to mean that they have no spiritual needs. **Faith** generally refers to a confident belief in something for which there is no proof or material evidence. It can involve a person, idea, or thing, and it is usually followed by action related to the ideals or values of that belief.

An **atheist** is a person who denies the existence of a God; an **agnostic** is one who holds that nothing can be known about the existence of a God. The agnostic and the atheist are guided by philosophies of living that do not include a religious faith. They deserve respect for what they choose to believe, just as do those who accept a particular religious creed.

Spirituality and Everyday Living

Spiritual beliefs and practices are associated with all aspects of a person's life, including health and illness. Aspects of a person's life commonly influenced by spirituality and religion include relationships with others, daily living habits, required and prohibited behaviors, and the general frame of reference for thinking about oneself and the world.

Religious influences may be life affirming or life denying.

> Life-affirming influences enhance life, give meaning and purpose to existence, strengthen one's feelings of self-worth, encourage self-actualization, and are health-

Six Basic Spiritual Needs of Americans

George Gallup, who is chair of the George H. Gallup International Institute, recently identified six basic spiritual needs of contemporary Americans. His conclusions are based on a variety of religious research and were presented in a speech given at a meeting of the Theological Students Fellowship, Princeton Theological Seminary, on December 10, 1990.

The need to believe that life is meaningful and has a purpose. During a time when sociologists observe an obsession with self in America, 70% of Americans nevertheless believe it is important that life is meaningful and has a purpose. Yet as many as two thirds of people interviewed believe that "most churches and synagogues today are not effective in helping people find meaning in life." Here is a basic need apparently being only partially met. The fact is, significant numbers of people find churches irrelevant, unfulfilling, and boring.

The need for a sense of community and deeper relationships. "Radical individualism" continues to have a hold on the religious lives of Americans. Most Americans, for example, believe that one can be a good Christian or Jew if one does not attend church or synagogue. One of the poignant consequences of this separateness is loneliness. As we have discovered from surveys, as many as 3 people in 10 say they have been lonely "for a long period of time" in their lives, with half of these people saying this experience has affected their thoughts "a great deal."

The need to be appreciated and respected. This is certainly a basic and fundamental need, yet as many as one third of the American people have a low sense of self-worth or self-esteem, as a direct consequence of not being loved or appreciated. Low self-esteem brings with it a host of social problems, including alcohol and drug abuse, child and spouse abuse, lawlessness, and crime. Significantly, surveys suggest that the closer people feel to God, the better they feel about themselves. They are also more satisfied with their lives than are others, more altruistic, enjoy better health, and have a happier outlook. Furthermore, it has been found that experiencing the closeness of God is a key factor in the ability of people to forgive themselves and others.

The need to be listened to—to be heard. Americans overwhelmingly think the future of the church will be shaped to a greater extent by the laity than by the clergy. In specific terms, this means that the laity should play a greater role in the church, freeing up clergy to perform what the laity expects of them: to listen to people's religious needs and to provide spiritual counseling and inspiration. When the "unchurched" in one survey were asked what would most likely draw them back into the community of active worshippers, the lead reason given was "if I could find a pastor or rabbi with whom I could share my religious needs and doubts."

The need to feel that one is growing in faith. People like to feel that they are maturing spiritually; we go through passages in our faith lives, just as we do in our secular lives. It would appear that, basically, people aspire to lead good lives. Significant numbers of people have given thought to living a worthwhile life, to their relationship to God, to the basic meaning and value of their lives, and to developing their faith. People need help in understanding the significance of these experiences and in building on them.

The need for practical help in developing a mature faith. There is an urgent need to work toward closing the gap between belief and practice—to turn professed faith into lived-out faith.

(Used with permission.)

giving and life-sustaining. Life-denying influences restrict or enclose life patterns, limit experiences and associations, place burdens of guilt on individuals, encourage feelings of unworthiness, and are generally health-denying and life-inhibiting. (Larue, 1981)

Spirituality, Health, and Illness

Spiritual beliefs are of special importance to nurses because of the many ways they can influence a client's level of health and self-care behaviors.

Guide to Daily Living Habits. Certain practices generally associated with healthcare may have religious significance for a client. For example, many religions prescribe dietary requirements and restrictions. Acceptable birth-control practices are determined by some religious faiths, as are some types of medical treatments.

Source of Support. It is common for many people to seek support from their religious faith during times of stress. This support is often vital to the acceptance of an illness, especially if the illness brings with it a prolonged period of convalescence or indicates a questionable outcome. Prayer, devotional reading, and other religious practices often do for the person spiritually what protective exercises do for the body physically (Fig. 36-1).

Source of Strength and Healing. The values derived from religious faith cannot be enumerated or evaluated easily. However, the effects attributable to faith are constantly in evidence to healthcare workers. People have been known to endure extreme physical distress because of strong faith. Clients' families have taken on almost unbelievable rehabilitative tasks because they had faith in the eventual positive results of their effort.

Source of Conflict. There are times when religious beliefs conflict with prevalent healthcare practices. For example, the doctrine of the Jehovah's Witnesses prohibits blood transfusions. In the Islamic religion, humans are regarded as largely helpless in controlling their environment, and illness is accepted as their fate rather than something against which action might be taken. Some Navajo Indians use a lengthy religious ceremony to cure certain diseases, such as tuberculosis. For some people, illness is viewed as punishment for sin and therefore inevitable.

Such beliefs may require the healthcare worker to modify a treatment plan to accommodate the person's religion. In some instances, acknowledgment of the client's religious convictions and efforts by health practitioners to accommodate the client's beliefs can result in quality healthcare without violating the person's religious practices. In other situations, an objective explanation of alternative treatments and the predicted consequences of each may help the client determine acceptable therapy. Whatever the person's decision about healthcare, the nurse should remember that each person is unique and has a right to pursue his or her own convictions, even though they may differ from those of the healthcare provider.

Major Religions

Nurses care for people from many different religious traditions. Although it is impossible for nurses to be knowledgeable about all religions, nurses are better able to meet the spiritual needs of clients when they understand the client's religious beliefs and practices. These can directly influence the client's response to illness and suffering, self-care practices such as diet and hygiene, birth and death rituals, gender roles, spiritual practices, and moral codes. Nurses who are unfamiliar with a client's religion can gain valuable knowledge by reading (Carson's *Spiritual Dimensions of Nursing Practice* [1989] is an invaluable resource) and through discussion with the client and the client's family and spiritual adviser. A brief discussion of major religious traditions follows.

Religions With a Western Philosophy

The three major religions with a Western philosophy are Judaism, Christianity, and Islam. Each is monotheistic; central to their sacred scripture is one God who personally created the world and who reveals himself through events in human history. The moral codes of these religions stress the honor of parents, honesty, kindness, and generosity as important social concerns and reject lying, stealing, slander, covetousness, and adultery (Carson, 1989).

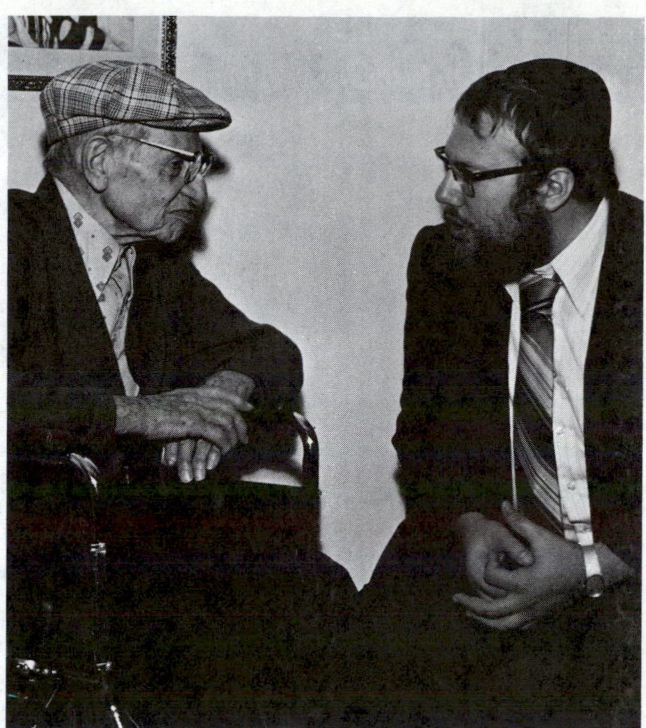

Figure 36-1
The rabbi's visit is important for this resident of a geriatric center.

Other Western faiths with which healthcare professionals should be familiar include Christian Science, Jehovah's Witnesses, Church of Jesus Christ of Latter-Day Saints (Mormons), Unification Church, and Unitarian Universalist Association of Churches and Fellowships (Table 36-1).

Judaism

Judaism, the oldest continuous religion still practiced in Western civilization, is the foundation on which both Christianity and Islam were built. The formation of the Jewish people is closely bound with a divine revelation and with the commitment of the people to obedience to God's will. The Jewish people have been called "the people of the Book," meaning that the Hebrew Bible has been the authority, guide, and inspiration of all the many forms that the religion of the Jews has taken in different periods and in different lands (Parrinder, 1983). There are currently three forms of Judaism: (1) Reform, (2) Conservative, and (3) Orthodox. Reform Judaism is more liberal than the other two in its beliefs, whereas Orthodox Judaism is the most traditional of the three.

Nurses caring for Orthodox Jews as well as some Conservative Jews need to be sensitive to their special needs in the areas of diet, birth rituals, male and female contact, and death. For observant Jewish clients, treatments and procedures should not be scheduled on the

Table 36-1
Beliefs and Healthcare Practices of Western Religions Other Than the Three Major Religions

Religion	Beliefs	Healthcare Practices
Adventist	Believe in the individual's choice and God's sovereignty. The body is believed to be the temple of the Holy Spirit.	• The taking of all narcotics and stimulants is prohibited because the body is the temple of the Holy Spirit and should be protected. Many groups prohibit meat. • Many regard Saturday as the Sabbath. • Approach to healthcare is holistic.
Christian Scientist	They deny the existence of health crises; sickness and sin are errors of the human mind and can be overcome by altering thoughts, not by using drugs or medicines.	• They will use orthopedic services to set a bone but decline drugs and, in general, other medical or surgical procedures. • They do not allow hypnotism or any form of psychotherapy, which alters the "Divine Mind." • A Christian Science Practitioner may be called to administer spiritual support. • Alcohol and tobacco are not used.
Church of Jesus Christ of Latter Day Saints (Mormons)	Devout adherents believe in divine healing through the "laying on of hands," though many do not prohibit medical therapy. The Church maintains an extensive and well-funded welfare system, including financial support for the sick.	• Disapprove of alcohol, tobacco, and caffeinated beverages. • A special undergarment worn by some members should be removed only in an emergency.
Jehovah's Witnesses	They oppose the "false teachings" of other sects; opposition often extends to modern science, including medicine.	• Blood transfusions violate God's laws and therefore are not allowed. Alternative treatments include use of nonblood plasma expanders, surgical techniques to decrease blood loss, and autotransfusions through use of a heart–lung machine. • The courts have not supported the right of Jehovah Witness parents to refuse life-saving treatment for their children. • Use of alcohol and tobacco are discouraged.
Unification Church	God is the living, eternal person who represents universal love and care. God created the world and humans to reflect his nature. The goal of the Unification Church is to unite Christians everywhere as one family under God.	• Most members are still healthy young adults. There is little information available on their interactions with the healthcare team.
Unitarian Universal Association of Churches and Fellowships	Encourage creativity, reason, and living an ethical life. No member is required to adhere to a given creed or set of religious beliefs. The inherent worth and dignity of every person is affirmed.	• Free to accept what they take to be best for their health.

Sabbath (sundown Friday to sundown Saturday) and important holy days, provided this will not harm the client.

Christianity

Christianity, the largest religion in the world, embraces adherents to Roman Catholic, Eastern Orthodox, and Protestant faiths. The Christian way of life is centered on worship of the one God revealed to the world through Jesus Christ of Nazareth (who lived in the 1st century AD), who is believed to be risen from the dead. Love of neighbor is a central tenet. Other beliefs include sin, redemption, salvation, and retribution or a final accounting with God at the end of life. The Christian tradition has always encouraged care for the sick. God, recognized as the author and giver and life, is also the healer. Most Christian clients accept medical science and many use prayer, faith healing, laying on of hands, and the sacraments in times of illness.

Roman Catholicism. Dating its beginning from the time when the apostles first began to preach about Jesus of Nazareth, the Roman Catholic Church governed the temporal world as well as the Church in the West until the 11th century. In AD 1054, theological differences resulted in the separation of Western and Eastern Orthodox traditions. However, in both the Roman Catholic and Eastern Orthodox Churches, there is a high regard and concern for human life as a gift of God. There is a prolife stance that honors and respects the life of each person as a divine gift that requires development and enhancement.

Nurses caring for Roman Catholic clients should be aware of the importance of the sacraments of baptism, Eucharist, penance, and the anointing of the sick; dietary habits; sexual ethical norms; and the potential importance of private devotions.

Eastern Orthodox. Factors contributing to the split between the Eastern and Western Churches include theological differences over the wording of the Nicene Creed regarding the Holy Spirit, the use of pictures and statues in the Churches, the sacraments, the marriage of priests, and the use of Greek or Latin in worship services. Patriarchs who rule the Eastern Orthodox Church are located in Istanbul, Alexandria, Antioch, and Jerusalem, as well as in Russia, Serbia, Romania, Bulgaria, and Georgia. Important concerns for the sick include the administration of sacraments, dietary practices, rituals regarding death, and calendar differences.

Protestant Faiths. Martin Luther, generally credited with starting the Protestant Reformation in 1517, concluded through his study of the Bible that a person's sins are forgiven by having a personal relationship with Jesus Christ and that God alone forgives through faith and not good works. The Protestant faith embraces a large number of denominations, most of which hold to Luther's beliefs in the final authority of the Bible, justification by faith, and the priesthood of all believers. Issues dividing diverse Protestant sects include ways of interpreting the message of the Bible, involvement of the Church with secular issues, and sacramental and worship differences. Nurses caring for Protestant clients need to assess how the client's beliefs and religious practices contribute to spiritual needs.

Islam

Islam, started by the prophet Muhammad in AD 580, is one of the largest and fastest-growing religions in the world. Nearly 500,000 Muslims are active in more than 1,000 Islamic centers in the United States and Canada. Major sects include the Sunni, the Shiites, and the Sufis. Followers of Islam believe in Allah, one God who is only one, all seeing, all hearing, all speaking, all knowing, all willing, and all powerful. Their religious duties include repetition of a creed; prayer five times each day facing Mecca preceded by washing, almsgiving, fasting during the sacred 9th month of Ramadan; and a pilgrimage to Mecca once during a lifetime. When caring for Muslim clients, it is helpful to understand the Koranic law and customs that influence birth, diet, care of women, death, and prayer rituals. Women are not allowed to make independent decisions, and husbands need to be present when informed consent is sought.

American Muslim Mission (Black Muslim)

Adherents of the American Muslim Mission trace their religious beginnings to Muslim slaves who came to the United States from Islamic West Africa but who were prevented from practicing Islam and consequently lost knowledge of the practices of their faith. Accepting the Koran as their sacred scripture, current members of "the Nation of Islam" stress the importance of cooperation among blacks in business and education to build self-esteem. Members are encouraged to obtain healthcare provided by the black community. Malcolm X was one of this sect's most charismatic leaders and with others preached an end to white domination and the establishment of an independent nation. Major tenets involve prayer rituals, dietary restrictions (prohibitions against pork and alcohol), hygiene (extreme cleanliness), lifestyle modifications, and marital faithfulness.

Religions With an Eastern Philosophy

Some areas of North America have citizens of Chinese, Korean, Japanese, and Indian descent, and people from Southeast Asia. It is thus helpful for nurses to have some understanding of religions with an eastern philosophy. Buddhism, Confucianism, Daoism (Taoism), and Hinduism are highlighted in Table 36-2.

There is a growing acceptance of therapies rooted in Eastern approaches to medicine such as acupuncture, biofeedback, yoga, and rolfing. In Eastern medicine, health is closely related to personal attitudes and actions.

> The healer's role is to impart deeper understanding of the ways of nature so that while promoting healing, he or she also educates clients in self-care. The client, in turn, needs to recognize that body and mind are intimately related to each other. To be in command of this crucial interaction requires a practiced sensitivity and response to the needs of body and mind. (Carson, 1989, p. 129)

The healthcare community continues to struggle to combine the ancient wisdom of Eastern health practices with the sophisticated scientific and technologic expertise of the West.

Native American Religions

The multitude of tribes in North America makes it difficult to generalize about Native American cultures and religions. There are, however, two basic and contrasting orientations—the old hunting religions (as seen among the Shoshoni) and the new horticultural religions (as among the Zuni). Although all Native Americans look to natural spirits, or the spirits of nature, for revelation and power, the Shoshoni look more to animals and the sky, whereas the Zuni look to plants and the underground.

Table 36-2
Healthcare Practices of Major Eastern Religions

Religion	Beliefs	Healthcare Practices
Buddhism	Buddha or "the Great Physician" taught the Four Noble Truths to indicate the range of "suffering," its "origin," its "cessation," and the "way" that leads to its cessation. The real cause of human suffering is ignorant craving. The Noble Eightfold Path, which consists of right views, aspirations, speech, conduct, mode of livelihood, effort, mindfulness, and concentration, leads to the cessation of suffering.	• Buddhist hospitals for sick humans and sick animals antedated anything similar found in the West. • Buddhists do not outwardly proclaim healing through faith. However, spiritual peace and liberation from anxiety attained through the awakening to Buddha's wisdom may be an important factor in expediting healing and the recovery process. • Accepts modern science. The doctrine of avoidance of extremes is applied to the use of drugs, blood, vaccines. • Buddhism does not condone taking lives of any form. • Check with the client about any special diet restrictions and the observance of holy days.
Confucianism	Inherent in Confucianism is the appreciation of life and the desire to keep the body from untimely or unnecessary death.	• Appreciate life and desire to keep the body from untimely or unnecessary death. • Historically emphasized public health solutions to impending health problems.
Daosim (Taoism)	Health is a manifestation of the harmony of the universe, obtained through the proper balancing of internal and external forces. Implicit throughout the Daoist tradition is the tendency to understand salvation in the biomedical sense of health and qualitative improvement and prolongation of human life. The universal principle of the Tao is the mysterious biologic and spiritual life rhythm or order of nature.	• There is a "medicinal" concern for maintaining and prolonging human health and life (*sheng*). Knowing and living a natural life—following the Tao—is the secret of both health and sagehood. • Long tradition of seeking pragmatic medical techniques, along with its religious techniques of meditation and ritual for establishing a harmony of body and spirit, humanity, and nature (holistic approach).
Hinduism	Doctrine of Transmigration. Moral factors, linked with the all-embracing doctrine of "karma" were believed to be significant in promoting health or causing disease.	• Hindu medicine shows a surprising openness to new ideas, at least in respect to practical treatment. • Many Hindu dietary restrictions conform to individual sect doctrine. • The nurse administering medications should avoid touching the client's lips. • Certain prescribed rites are followed after death; disposal of the body is by cremation.

(Data in part from Reich, W. T. [Ed.]. [1978]. *Encyclopedia of bioethics.* New York: Free Press.)

Features of the hunting religions include animal ceremonialism, quest for spiritual power, Male Supreme Being, annual ceremony of cosmic rejuvenation, few stationary cult places, shamanism, and life after death beyond the horizon or in the sky. Features of the horticultural religions include rain and fertility ceremonies, priestly ritual, goddesses and gods, yearly round of fertility rites, permanent shrines and temples, medicine society ritualism, and life after death in the underworld or among the clouds.

Unlike Western religions, Native American religions were handed down by tribes as oral traditions and have not been so dogmatically bound by what was inherited from the past. Most share a similar worldview, a notion of cosmic harmony, emphasis on directly experiencing powers and visions, and a common view of the cycle of life and death. Understanding time cyclically, Native North Americans view each individual's life as a cycle of time from birth to death, with rituals marking the important changes of life—birth ceremonies, puberty rituals, initiation rites, and death rituals. Death is not an end but the beginning of new life either on this earth (reincarnation as another human or transmigration into some animal) or in a transcendent hereafter. Medicine men and women have specialized spirits from whom they receive the mission to cure and who help to cure the diseases of clients. Instructions in the ways of doctoring are received in visions. Common therapeutic measures are sucking, blowing, and drawing out with a feather fan; all are designed to remove the agent of the disease. Medicine men and women who fall recurringly into deep trances to save a person's life are called *shamans* (Hultkrantz, 1987).

Religion and Law, Ethics, and Medicine

Christian Scientists, Jehovah's Witnesses, and members of faith-healing groups are among those challenging the intricate web of rights and responsibilities among individual, society, church, and state. These religious bodies are asking for protection, under the veil of religious freedom, of their right to exercise individual decisions in accordance with scriptural interpretations, even though those decisions may result in the individual's own death or that of a family member, including a child. The most troubling cases are those in which treatable problems such as bacterial meningitis, diabetes, and bowel obstruction resulted in the death of minors whose parents chose religious means of healing over traditional medicine. The American Pediatrics Academy is currently urging that all child abuse, neglect, and medical neglect statutes be applied without potential or actual exemption for religious beliefs.

Perhaps even more troubling for nurses are situations in which family members insist on care deemed medically futile (ie, the likelihood of medical benefit is virtually nonexistent) because they believe that God is going to work a miracle. In these cases, simple nursing measures such as turning or bathing clients become occasions of pain and torment to both the client and nurse. Nurses are forced to administer care that they take to be cruel and abusive to conscious clients whose agonized dying is being needlessly prolonged. Unfortunately, there are no clear guidelines for drawing the line between promoting life and prolonging the dying process. Although nurses always have the moral right to withdraw from administering care that violates their personal moral code, this does not resolve the problem for the client. More dialogue is needed on the interaction between religion and law, ethics, and medicine. Ideally, the religious freedom of clients and their families is respected as is the moral autonomy of caregivers and the integrity of the healing professions.

Cultural Care

After a year of legal struggles that took the case all the way to the U.S. Supreme Court, the parents of a Vietnamese refugee defeated an attempt by social workers to force their son to have corrective surgery on his two clubfeet. The surgery would have shattered the Hmong family's religious beliefs. They believe their son Kou was born with clubfeet so that a warrior ancestor whose own feet were wounded in battle could be released from a sort of spiritual entrapment. They do not regard Kou's clubfeet as a deformity but as a sign of good luck and they think their son is special because of it.

(Kurtzman, L. [1990, December 22]. Surgery for boy, 7, blocked. *Philadelphia Inquirer,* p. 3A.)

Factors Affecting Spirituality

Among the many factors that can influence a person's spirituality, the most important are developmental considerations, family, ethnic background, formal religion, and life events.

Developmental Considerations

Because spirituality has to do with the nonmaterial realm of being, a child must have some capacity for abstract thought before beginning to understand the spiritual self and to explore a relationship with a higher power. This is not to say that spirituality is meaningless for children.

David Heller (1985) interviewed 40 children, ages 4 to 12 years, affiliated with one of four major religions—Judaism, Roman Catholicism, Protestantism, or Hinduism—and discovered that the children had definite perceptions of God and preferred forms of prayer or spiritual exercises, which differed according to the age, sex, religion, and personality of the child. Central themes in all the children's descriptions of God included:

- Notion of a God who works through human intimacy and the interconnectedness of lives
- Belief that God is involved in self-change and growth and transformations that make the world fresh, alive, and meaningful
- Attributing to God tremendous and expansive power and then showing considerable anxiety in the face of this power
- Image of light

As the child matures, life experiences usually influence and mature spiritual beliefs. With advancing years, the tendency to think about life after death prompts some individuals to reexamine and reaffirm their spiritual beliefs. Chapter 8 describes the stages of faith development.

Family

A child's parents play a key role in the development of the child's spirituality. What is important is not so much what parents teach a child about God and religion, but rather what the child learns about God, life, and self from parents' behavior. Because the family is the first world the child experiences, his or her worldview is colored by experiences with parents and siblings.

Ethnic Background

Religious traditions differ among ethnic groups. There are clear distinctions between Eastern and Western spiritual traditions as well as among those of individual ethnic groups such as Native Americans. A person's culture and formal religion has much to do with whether the basic approach to religion is doing something, being someone, or continually striving for harmony.

Formal Religion

Each of the major religions discussed earlier in this chapter has several characteristics in common:

- Basis of authority or source of power
- A portion of scripture or sacred word
- An ethical code that defines right and wrong
- A psychology and identity so that its adherents fit into a group and the world is defined by the religion
- Aspirations or expectations
- Some ideas about what follows death (Murray & Zentner, 1989)

Life Events

Both positive and negative life experiences can influence spirituality and, in turn, are influenced by the meaning a person's spiritual beliefs attribute to them. For example, if two women who believe in a loving God both lose a child in a car accident, one may bitterly deny God's existence and stop going to church, whereas the other may spend more time in prayer asking God to help her understand and accept her loss. Similarly, a chain of successful life experiences (marriage, degree, promotion) may cause one person to assume success and experience no need for God, whereas for another it occasions deep gratitude and rejoicing.

The Nurse as Role Model

Three spiritual needs are common to all people—the need for meaning and purpose, the need for love and relatedness, and the need for forgiveness (Fish & Shelly, 1978). These needs are common to nurses, whether they observe an established religion, believe in a spiritual essence, or recognize a field of power. As the nurse develops plans to be a spiritual role model to clients, the nurse develops goals for self. The nurse will:

- Hold spiritual beliefs that meet his or her need for meaning and purpose, love and relatedness, and forgiveness
- Derive from these beliefs strength for everyday living, especially when confronting pain, suffering, and death in his or her professional practice
- Set aside regular periods to nurture his or her spiritual self
- Demonstrate in his or her interactions with others peace, inner strength, warmth, joy, caring, and creativity
- Respect the spiritual beliefs and practices of others even when they are different from the nurse's own
- Increase his or her knowledge of how the spiritual beliefs of clients influence their lifestyles, responses to illness, healthcare choices, and treatment options
- Demonstrate sensitivity to the spiritual needs of clients
- Develop successful nursing strategies to assist clients in spiritual distress

Use the assessment checklist in the accompanying box to see how well you are meeting your own spirituality needs.

ASSESSING SPIRITUALITY

Nursing History

Because a person's spirituality and religious beliefs have the potential to influence every aspect of being, an assessment of the client's spirituality should be included in each comprehensive nursing history. Helpful assessment guides are offered by Fish and Shelly (1978), Stoll (1979), and O'Brien (1982). Data are gathered about the client's spiritual beliefs and practices, the effect of these beliefs on everyday living, spiritual distress, and spiritual needs. Sample questions are listed in the accompanying box.

The following questions are from O'Brien's (1982) Spiritual Assessment Guide:

Spiritual pain: Do you ever feel hurt or pain associated with the spiritual or religious beliefs that you hold? Do you feel pain related to uncertainty or nonbelief?

Spiritual alienation: Do you frequently feel far away from God? Does it seem that he is remote and far removed from your everyday life?

Spiritual anxiety: Are you afraid that God might not take care of your needs? That he might not be there when you need him?

Spiritual guilt: Have you ever done things that God would be angry at you for? Are you feeling badly about things that you have done or failed to do in your life?

Spiritual anger: Are you angry at God for allowing you to be ill? Do you ever feel like blaming God for your illness? Do you think God is unfair to you?

Spiritual loss: Do you ever feel that you have lost God's love? That you have broken or weakened your relationship with God? Has God turned his back on you?

Spiritual despair: Do you ever feel that there is no hope of having God's love? Of pleasing him? That God does not love you anymore? (p. 102)

If the client shares a spiritual problem, remember to use interview questions to determine the specific nature of the problem, its probable causes, related signs and symptoms, when it first began and how often it occurs, how it affects everyday living, the severity of the problem and whether it can be treated independently by nursing or needs to be referred, and how well the client is coping with the problem.

Nursing Observation

Because many clients may find it difficult to talk about their spiritual beliefs and problems, the nurse also observes the client's behavior for signs of spiritual distress.

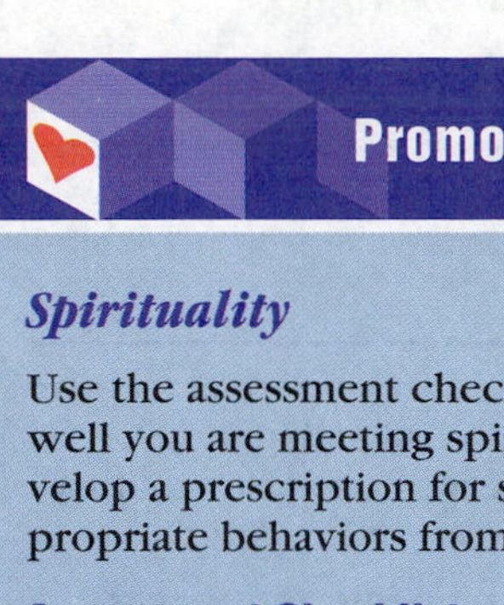

Promoting Wellness

Spirituality

Use the assessment checklist to determine how well you are meeting spirituality needs. Then develop a prescription for self-care by choosing appropriate behaviors from the list of suggestions.

Assessment Checklist

almost always	sometimes	almost never	
☐	☐	☐	1. I am comfortable with my spiritual beliefs and values.
☐	☐	☐	2. My beliefs meet my needs for love, belonging, forgiveness, meaning, and purpose.
☐	☐	☐	3. I respect the belief systems of others.
☐	☐	☐	4. I derive sufficient strength from my religious beliefs to meet each day's challenges.

Self-Care Behaviors

1. Explore personal values and beliefs of self and others.
2. Explore practices that are spiritually supportive.
3. Respect the belief systems of others.
4. Practice loving relationships with self and others.
5. Seek spiritual assistance to help cope with stress, crisis, or loss.

A family member or close friend may share significant observations.

"He's been awfully moody since his heart attack . . . I can't believe the change in him."

"I've never seen my father so depressed. He's never in his life been away from the synagogue at Passover. I don't know how to help him."

Significant behavioral observations include sudden changes in spiritual practices (rejection, neglect, fanatical devotion); mood changes (frequent crying, depression, apathy, anger); sudden interest in spiritual matters (reading religious books or watching religious programs on television, visits to clergy); and disturbed sleep. A nurse who observes these behaviors should follow up with appropriate interview questions. Often problems with spiritual distress do not surface until well after a client's admission history and examination. Effective questions include:

"You've been lying there so quietly . . . what are you thinking about?"

"After all you've been through you must have done a good bit of soul searching. . . . Experiences like these are enough to shake anyone's faith—how is yours holding up?"

DIAGNOSING

When assessment data point to a spiritual problem that can be treated by independent nursing intervention, it receives the label *Spiritual Distress.* This may be further specified as spiritual pain, alienation, anxiety, guilt, anger, loss, or despair (O'Brien, 1982). Common etiologies for spiritual distress include inability to reconcile current life situation (eg, illness, death of loved person, divorce) with spiritual beliefs ("God is all-powerful, all-loving, all-wise and he cares about me") or separation from the religious community or supports. Sample nursing diagnoses of spiritual distress are presented in the accompanying box.

Spiritual distress may affect other areas of human functioning. In the following nursing diagnoses, spiritual distress is the etiology of another problem.

- Impaired Adjustment to Illness related to inability to reconcile illness with spiritual beliefs
- Ineffective Individual Coping related to loss of religion as primary support (feels abandoned by God)
- Fear related to feeling unprepared for death and afterlife experience
- Dysfunctional Grieving: Despair related to belief that religion is meaningless
- Hopelessness related to belief that no one cares—including God
- Powerlessness related to feeling victimized by a tyrannical and arbitrary God
- Self-Esteem Disturbance related to failure to live according to dictates of religion
- Sexual Dysfunction related to values conflict
- Sleep Pattern Disturbance related to spiritual distress
- Risk for Self-Directed Violence related to feeling that life is meaningless

PLANNING: EXPECTED OUTCOMES

Nurses who are sensitive to the role spiritual beliefs play in influencing both a person's thoughts about self and the world and interactions with the world value spiritual

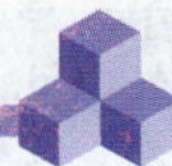

Focused Assessment Guide

Spirituality

Factors to Assess	Questions and Approaches
Spiritual beliefs	"Are there particular spiritual or religious beliefs that are important to you? Have these beliefs changed recently? Is your illness challenging these beliefs? Do your religious beliefs in any way dictate a course of action that puts you in conflict with what your physicians are recommending?"
Spiritual practices	"Describe your usual spiritual practices and anything interfering with your ability to perform them. Can I help in any way to secure the aids necessary for these practices (prayer shawl, Bible, crystals, beads, icon)?"
Relation between spiritual beliefs and everyday living	"Describe ways your spiritual beliefs affect everyday living (daily schedule, diet, hygiene, sense of self and the world, relationships). Do you find this influence to be healthy (life affirming) or destructive (life denying)?"
Spiritual deficit or distress	"Are your spiritual beliefs currently causing you any distress?"
Spiritual needs	"In what ways can I and the other nurses help you to meet your spiritual needs?" "Would you like me to contact your spiritual adviser or the hospital's pastoral care minister?"
Need for meaning and purpose	"In what ways do your religious beliefs help or hinder you to understand your current situation and face it with peace and courage?"
Need for love and relatedness	"In what ways do your religious beliefs help or hinder you to meet your need to love and be loved?"
Need for forgiveness	"In what ways do your religious beliefs help or hinder you to feel at peace?"
Significant behavioral observations	Be alert to sudden changes in spiritual practices, mood changes, sudden interest in spiritual matters, and sleep disturbances—all of which may point to unresolved spiritual needs.

health. Their interactions with any client who values spirituality are supportive of the following client goals/outcomes. The client will:

- Identify spiritual beliefs that meet needs for meaning and purpose, love and relatedness, and forgiveness
- Derive from these beliefs strength, hope, and comfort when facing the challenge of illness, injury, or other life crisis
- Develop spiritual practices that nurture communion with inner self, with God, and with the world
- Express satisfaction with the compatibility of spiritual beliefs and everyday living.

Goals/expected outcomes for clients in spiritual distress need to be individualized and may include some of the following. The client will:

- Explore the origin of spiritual beliefs and practices
- Identify factors in life that challenge spiritual beliefs
- Explore alternatives given these challenges: deny, modify, or reaffirm beliefs; develop new beliefs
- Identify spiritual supports (eg, spiritual reading, faith, community)
- Report or demonstrate a decrease in spiritual distress following successful intervention

IMPLEMENTING

There are a variety of interventions available to the nurse who wishes to help clients meet spiritual needs. Like other nursing skills, these interventions need to be practiced before the nurse is able to use them confidently, competently, and at the right moment. In this section, the following nursing interventions are presented: offering supportive presence, facilitating the client's practice of religion, nurturing spirituality, praying with a client, counseling the client spiritually, contacting a spiritual counselor, and resolving conflicts between treatment and spiritual beliefs.

Offering Supportive Presence

A nurse's gift of supportive presence must underlie all other types of intervention to meet spiritual needs. Supportive presence communicates value and respect

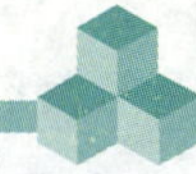

Nursing Diagnoses for Common Problems

*Spiritual Distress**

Problem	Related Factors	Sample Defining Characteristics
Spiritual pain	Inability to accept death of son	A 46-year-old woman, agnostic, only son died 6 months ago (lung cancer) "I've often wondered throughout my life if there is a God—thought maybe if I had tried harder I'd have recognized him. Now I don't care if God exists or not because if he allows this I don't want to know him." "My son was my whole life; there's nothing left for me to live for." Lost 10 lb in 6 months since son died; leaves home only when necessary to purchase food, go to bank, and engage in other routine activities.
Spiritual alienation	Separated from "faith community"	A 72-year-old Orthodox Jewish man, recently admitted to Protestant nursing home following 3-week hospitalization for stroke "I guess Yahweh has written me off; first the stroke that killed half my body and then I'm abandoned here where I can't even observe the Sabbath." "I want to go home."
Spiritual anxiety	Challenged belief and value system	A 37-year-old previously healthy male executive recovering from massive myocardial infarction "My parents were strict Methodists, but when I left home for college I stopped going to church . . . never gave it much thought . . . there was always something else to do. I started going again but it never meant much." "I haven't exactly done anything awful but I've also not been a saint and I find myself wondering if there is a God, what does he think of me." "Funny, I guess I thought I'd live forever. I sure never thought about dying and what happens after that." Often observed lying quietly in bed awake; asked to see minister.
Spiritual guilt	Failure to live according to religious rules	A 23-year-old, single, Baptist woman being treated for premenstrual syndrome "I was raised in a strict Baptist home but had to leave . . . I needed more room to be me. I like life here at the university but there's a restlessness in me I can't describe. I've dated several men, one or two I really liked, but I always do something to mess up the relationship. It would kill my mother if she knew I lived with Gary for 3 months." "What it really comes down to is my own sense of betraying myself, my family, and my religion. Who am I anyway?"
Spiritual anger	Inability to accept illness	A 38-year-old homosexual man recently diagnosed with AIDS "My parents are fundamentalists . . . all I ever heard at home was how much Jesus loves me . . . all the while my mom was beating the daylights out of me. . . . Does he love me? Does he love me so much that he had my parents throw me out when I finally told them I was gay? Does he love me so much that I got AIDS and now no one comes near me?" Facial features are tight; body held rigidly; speech is sharp, appears angry with God, the world, himself.

(continued)

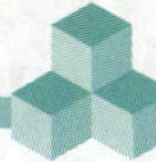

Nursing Diagnoses for Common Problems *(continued)*

*Spiritual Distress**

Problem	Related Factors	Sample Defining Characteristics
Spiritual loss	Terminal illness; anticipatory grieving; inability to find comfort in religion	A 40-year-old mother of three sons who was diagnosed with ovarian cancer 18 months ago; currently in advanced stage of disease I've tried hard to do it all right . . . I read my Bible, prayed every day, went to church each Sunday, loved my husband and kids . . . why is this all happening to me? Why must I lose it all? Where is God now that I need him? Some mornings I wish I could shoot myself and end it all—instead another day drags on. Who can help me?" Cries frequently, no longer interested in everyday activities of family, no interest in praying, told family not to have pastor call anymore. "No one can help now."
Spiritual despair	Feeling that no one (not even God) cares	A 92-year-old frail widow who lives alone in a two-room apartment; crippled with arthritis; has two married sons she has not seen for years. Says to community nurse who visits every week, "No one should have to live like this. If it weren't for the neighbor who comes on Saturday with a few groceries and you I'd be dead. I guess that would be for the best. It's been a long time since I felt like my living or dying would matter to anyone. Because I'm 92 now I guess even God doesn't want me. Couldn't you do something to put me out of my misery?"

*NANDA-approved nursing diagnosis label.

(Fig. 36-2). Chapter 22 presents basic communication skills helpful in establishing this type of presence.

The client who senses that the nurse is sincerely concerned and committed to helping meet human needs is better able to participate in the plan of care. Clients who experience respect and affirmation from other humans find it easier to hold spiritual beliefs that meet their needs for meaning and purpose, love and relatedness, and forgiveness.

Facilitating the Client's Practice of Religion

The following are means the nurse can use to help the client continue normal spiritual practices in the unfamiliar environment of the hospital or care center:

- Familiarize the client with religious services and materials available within the institution.
- Respect the client's need for privacy or quiet during periods of prayer.
- Assist the client to obtain devotional objects and protect them from loss or damage.
- Arrange for the client wishing to receive the sacraments to do so.
- Attempt to meet the client's religious dietary restrictions.
- Arrange for the client's minister, priest, or rabbi to visit if the client so wishes.

If the client has a conflict between spiritual beliefs and the proposed medical therapy, the nurse can assist the client in discussing this with the physician.

The ill client in the home may not be able to attend services or meetings to which the client is accustomed. The nurse can aid the client in finding ways to express his or her spiritual needs. Other sections in the remainder of this chapter can be used in the home, hospital, or care center in helping clients meet their spiritual needs.

Home Healthcare Alert

Recent research findings support the importance and value of caregivers' spirituality, yet as a resource it is often overlooked (Kaye & Robinson, 1994; Whitlatch, Meddaugh, & Langhout, 1994). Nurses should consider using interventions that enhance a caregiver's ability to take part in church activities to satisfy their spiritual needs and to work with church groups to secure helpful services. Using clergy, prayer, forgiveness, and spiritual reading materials as resources for caregivers may also be helpful.

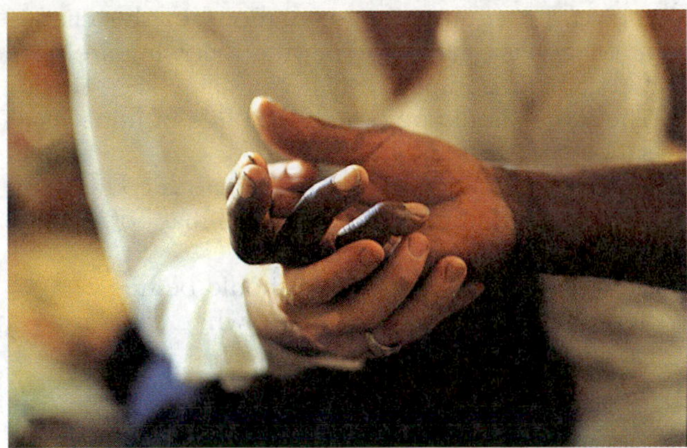

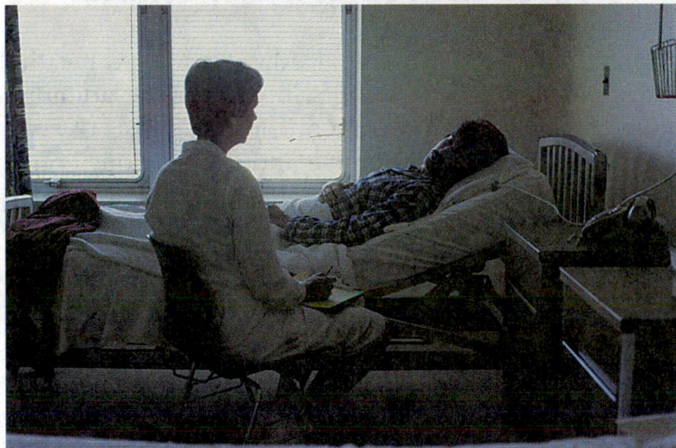

Figure 36-2
The nurse offers supportive presence by holding the client's hand to show that he or she is sincerely concerned or simply by being present to communicate value and respect.

Nurturing Spirituality

Some clients experiencing a need to get in touch with their spiritual self and to nurture their spiritual development may look to the nurse for direction. The person who lives life enmeshed in the action and noises of society may feel strangely uncomfortable when illness forces self-introspection. The nurse can be helpful in recommending means to develop a relationship with one's inner world and manifest spiritual energy in one's outer world (Hill & Smith, 1990). The accompanying box lists ways to develop one's inner world and to manifest this energy to the outside world.

Praying With a Client

Clients accustomed to regular periods of prayer but who feel too ill to pray as they would like or who enjoy praying with others may ask the nurse to pray with them or hope that the nurse will suggest this. Because there are many forms of prayer—quiet reflection, silent communion with God or higher power, reading or recitation of formal prayers, silent or loud calling on God or conversation with God, or reading the Bible—the nurse can take the lead from the client by asking, "How would you like us to pray?" The religious background of the client is considered along with the type of prayers that have been meaningful in the past. It is also helpful to ask the client if there is a particular prayer request.

The nurse unaccustomed to praying aloud or in public may find it helpful to have a Bible passage or formal prayer readily available. The prayer may also be a simple expression aloud of the client's needs and hopes. A sample follows:

> Lord God, our Creator and Healer, I entrust Mrs. Smith and her family to your loving care . . . bring peace to her mind and health and strength to her body. . . . Be with her [as her treatment begins today, as she goes for surgery, and so on]. . . . We remember all your blessings to us in the past and thank you. . . . We are confident of your help now as we claim your promises.

Prayer should not block communication with the client. Praying before a client feels ready to pray may communicate to the client a lack of interest in the client's feelings. Because prayer often evokes deep feelings, the nurse should be prepared to spend time with the client after sharing prayer to respond to these feelings (Fish & Shelly, 1978).

Counseling the Client Spiritually

The client who feels that the nurse is sensitive to spiritual needs and comfortable in his or her own spirituality may choose to share spiritual concerns with the nurse

Nurturing Spirituality

Ways to Develop a Relationship With One's Inner World

- Prayer
- Reflection or "quiet listening to one's essence"
- Communion with nature through walks in the park, woods, beach
- Enjoyment of music, drama, art, dance
- Inner dialogues with oneself or with a higher being
- Dream analysis

Ways to Manifest Spiritual Energy in One's Outer World

- Loving relationships with others
- Service to others in need
- Forgiveness of others
- Empathy, compassion, and hope
- Laughter, joyous expressions
- Participation in church services and activities and social gatherings

(Hill, L., & Smith, N. [1990]. *Self-care nursing* [2nd. ed.]. New York: Appleton & Lange.)

rather than with a religious counselor. The nurse who feels able to counsel the client may assist the client to:

- Articulate spiritual beliefs
- Explore the origin of the client's spiritual beliefs and practices
- Identify life factors that challenge the client's spiritual beliefs (cause spiritual distress)
- Explore alternatives given these challenges: modify lifestyle; deny, modify, or reaffirm beliefs; develop new beliefs
- Develop spiritual beliefs that meet needs for meaning and purpose, care and relatedness, forgiveness

To be an effective spiritual counselor, the nurse must be open to different spiritual beliefs and forms of spiritual expression and supportive of the client's efforts to nurture spiritual growth.

Contacting a Spiritual Counselor

Not every nurse feels comfortable in the role of spiritual counselor. The nurse may suggest the client talk to a spiritual counselor. When a client expresses a desire to speak to his or her spiritual counselor, the nurse helps make the appropriate referral. The nurse may offer to contact the client's own spiritual adviser. Other options are to contact the healthcare facility's pastoral ministry department or use a referral list of clergy in the local community. If a representative of the client's own religion is unable to visit within the hospital at a particular time, the nurse may suggest a visit from a clergyperson from another faith. Such a suggestion may be welcomed by the client, depending upon the situation and the immediacy of the need.

The nurse in a care center can assist the spiritual counselor by making the counselor feel welcome, answering questions about the client, directing the counselor to the client, and ensuring that the client is ready to receive the counselor. Preparations of the client's room for the visit may vary, but the following are generally recommended practices:

- The room should be orderly and free of unnecessary equipment and items.
- There should be a seat for the religious counselor at the bedside or near the client so that both can be comfortable during the visit.
- The top of the bedside table should be free of items and covered with a clean, white cover if a sacrament is to be administered.
- The bed curtains should be drawn to provide privacy if the client is in a unit with other clients and is unable to be moved to a more private setting.

Some clients and spiritual advisers may value the nurse's participation in prayers, rituals, or the administration of sacraments. When a nursing diagnosis of spiritual distress is made, the nurse and the religious counselor can often collaborate on the plan of care and reinforce each other's efforts to assist the client to meet goals/outcomes.

Resolving Conflicts Between Spiritual Beliefs and Treatments

Both the client and members of the client's family may experience conflict between a particular spiritual belief or religious law and a proposed medical treatment or health option. The client may want the nurse's assistance when conferring with the spiritual adviser about a particular procedure. The nurse's role is to assist the client in obtaining the information needed to make an informed decision and to support the *client's* decision making. Because what the nurse says and the way it is said may powerfully influence the client's decision, it is important for the nurse to maintain objectivity.

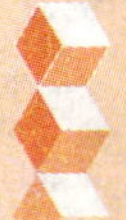

Helpscan

The following are resources for clients and healthcare professionals:

- *Healing Ministry*
  470 Boston Post Road
  Weston, MA 02193

  A new journal meant for those of all denominations who are actively providing care to the sick and terminally ill.
- Park Ridge Center
  211 E. Ontario, Suite 800
  Chicago, IL 60611
  (312) 266-2222
- The new Religious Traditions and Health Care Decisions series of booklets from the Park Ridge Center provides accessible and practical information on the values and beliefs of religious traditions. Each booklet has three sections: (1) a broad historical and theological context for the tradition, including its general views on health and illness, (2) the tradition's positions on a variety of clinical issues organized around the life cycle, and (3) information on special concerns relevant to the particular tradition.

EVALUATING

The nurse working with a client and family to achieve specified goals/outcomes to meet spiritual needs can use each client interaction to evaluate the plan of care. Necessary to the evaluation are sensitivity to what the client is saying and not saying and observation of the client when alone as well as when interacting with the family and nurses.

In general, the nurse evaluates the client's ability to:

- Find meaning and purpose in the client's current condition
- Interact honestly with family, friends, and others who meet the client's need for love and relatedness
- Derive strength and peace from the client's spiritual beliefs
- Reconcile any interpersonal differences causing the client anguish (religious belief or law in conflict with medical therapy)

The nurse helps the client to determine if spiritual beliefs are generally life affirming or life denying and if there is harmony between these beliefs and the client's everyday life experiences.

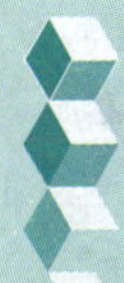

Research in Nursing: Making a Difference

The spiritual needs of clients and their caregivers are often overlooked by nurses and other members of the interdisciplinary team. In the first study described below, two nurse researchers examine the spiritual needs of clients in intensive care units and recommend specific nursing interventions. In the second study, a nurse expert on spirituality studies the relationship between prayer and healing and examines the question, "Does God answer prayer?" The last study examines religiosity as a coping strategy for caregivers of clients with Alzheimer's disease.

Related Research

Clark, C., & Heidenreich, T. (1995). Spiritual care for the critically ill. *American Journal of Critical Care, 4*(1), 77–81.
Spiritual well-being is the center of a healthy lifestyle and enables holistic integration of one's inner resources. However, the professional education process does not adequately provide socialization of nurses in the provision of spiritual care. The authors used a descriptive research design to identify factors that contribute to providing spiritual care for patients in intensive care units. Three themes were identified as integral to the spiritual well-being of critical care patients: care providers, family/friends, and religion/faith. Nursing interventions identified for the three themes include establishing trusting relationships, providing in-depth spiritual assessment, conveying technical competence, and acting as a facilitator among family, clergy, and other providers.

Fish, S. (1995). Can research prove that God answers prayer? *Journal of Christian Nursing, 12*(1), 24–27, 46.
This well-known nurse expert on spirituality examines the claim that if research on the role of religion and health is to receive respectability as a nonfringe area of study, it should have at least the following characteristics: methodological soundness, clinical relevance, and conceptual foundations—and that this is especially true when the study includes an exploration of prayer. She offers a list of resources on prayer research, which are highlighted in the accompanying box.

Whitlatch, A. M., Meddaugh, D. I., & Langhout, K. J. (1994). Religiosity among Alzheimer's disease caregivers. *Healing Ministry, 1*(1), 23–27, 32.
As a form of psychosocial support, religiosity has been related to the subjective well-being among middle-aged and older adults. In this study, the prominence of religious-related discussion in Alzheimer's Association family members during support group meetings indicates the need for further research regarding the extent and nature of religiosity as a coping mechanism among caregivers in general. The authors recommend collaboration between religious institutions, healthcare, and social service providers to preserve the religious practices and spiritual continuity of Alzheimer's disease caregivers and their families.

Summary

If nurses are to be both competent and comfortable in addressing the spiritual needs of clients and their caregivers, more research is required to define these needs and to identify a repertoire of effective nursing interventions. An investigation of how best to prepare nurses to meet spiritual needs is also indicated.

Resources on Prayer Research

- "The Effects of Prayer on Mental Well-Being" by Margaret M. Poloma. In *Second Opinion,* 1993, vol. 18, no. 3, pp. 37–51.
- "Empirical Studies of Christian Prayer: A Review of the Literature" by John R. Finney and H. Newton Malony Jr. In *Journal of Psychology and Theology,* 1985, vol. 13, no. 2, pp. 104–15.
- *The Human Side of Prayer* by L. B. Brown. Religious Education Press, 1994.
- "Patients' Spiritual Coping Strategies: A Study of Nurse and Patient Perspectives" by Kathy E. Sodestrom and Ida M. Martinson. In *Oncology Nursing Forum,* 1987, vol. 14, no. 2, pp. 41–46.
- "Preferences for Spiritually Related Nursing Interventions Among Terminally Ill and Nonterminally Ill Hospitalized Adults and Well Adults" by Pamela G. Reed. In *Applied Nursing Research,* 1991, vol. 4, no. 3, pp. 122–28.
- *Religion in Aging and Health: Theoretical Foundations and Methodological Frontiers* by Jeffrey S. Levin, ed. Sage, 1994.
- "Religious Cognitions and Use of Prayer in Health and Illness" by Lucille B. Bearon and Harold Koenig. In *The Gerontological Society of America,* 1990, vol. 30, no. 2, pp. 249–53.
- "Spiritual Needs and Interventions: Comparing the Views of Patients, Nurses and Chaplains" by Julia D. Emblen and Lois Halstead. In *Clinical Nurse Specialist,* 1993, vol. 7, no. 4, pp. 175–82.
- *What Americans Believe: An Annual Survey of Values and Religious Views in the U.S.,* by George Barna. Regal Books, 1991.

(Compiled by Sharon Fish [1995]. Can research prove that God answers prayer? *Journal of Christian Nursing, 12*[1], 24–27, 46.)

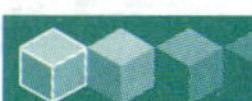

Nursing Process in Clinical Practice

The nurse uses each phase of the nursing process when identifying and treating spiritual problems categorized as nursing diagnoses. The NANDA diagnoses are:

Spiritual Distress: Disruption in the life principle which pervades a person's entire being and which integrates and transcends one's biological and psychosocial nature. (NANDA, 1994)

Potential for Enhanced Spiritual Well-Being: The process of an individual's developing/unfolding of mystery through harmonious interconnectedness that springs from inner strengths. (NANDA, 1994)

Quality care depends on the nurse's possession of the knowledge and skills described earlier in this chapter. Following in outline format are the assessment priorities, expected outcomes, and nursing interventions for spiritual distress. In the client care study, nursing care is described for a middle-aged male client who has not practiced any formal religion recently and who, following a heart attack, is concerned about his relationship with God.

Spiritual Distress

Spiritual distress may result when an individual is unable to meet one or more of the basic spiritual needs for meaning and purpose, for love and relatedness, or for forgiveness (Fish & Shelly, 1978). Possible etiologies for these spiritual deficits include the following:

Deficit: Meaning and purpose

Inability to reconcile spiritual beliefs with illness, pain, suffering, impending death

No prior need to explore life or its meaning and purpose

Deficit: Love and relatedness

Human relationships to date have been painful.

Belief that people are bad and best dealt with as little as possible

Belief that God is a distant and uncaring superpower

Deficit: Forgiveness

Inability to forgive oneself or others for human failings

Belief that God is a harsh taskmaster who desires nothing less than perfection

When identifying spiritual deficits, it is important to remember that individuals have different spiritual needs and meet them differently. The meaning one person attributes to life may be different from that of another. It must be sufficient that it enables the individual to face each day with renewed energy for living in pursuit of some good.

Assessment Priorities

- Use interview questions and observations of the client's behavior to identify defining characteristics of each spiritual deficit.
  - Meaning and purpose: Statements reflecting sense of despair, hopelessness, powerlessness ("What's the use?" "Nothing matters any more . . ." "Why should I bother?"); apathy,

indifference, listlessness, lethargy; decreased energy for daily living and for healing
- Love and relatedness: Statements indicating loneliness, desire for meaningful relationships with God and people; statements describing God and humans as overwhelmingly negative (evil, hurtful, distant, indifferent, uncaring); decreased ability to interact with others (withdrawal, behaviors that alienate others); absence of visitors for hospitalized client
- Forgiveness: Statements reflecting dissatisfaction with self, shame, guilt, desire for forgiveness, belief that one's failings are unforgivable; belief that God is punishing; anger, depression, cynicism; confessions of failings to others

- Identify attempts client has made or is making to resolve these deficits and their effectiveness.
- Assess the need for referral to a spiritual adviser.

Expected Outcomes

The client will:

- Identify some spiritual belief that gives meaning and purpose to everyday life
- Move toward a healthy acceptance of the current situation: illness, pain, suffering, impending death
- Develop mutually caring relationships
- Verbalize satisfaction with relationship with God (if this is important)
- Express peaceful acceptance of limitations and failings
- Express ability to forgive others and to live in the present
- Demonstrate an "interior state of peace and joy; freedom from abnormal anxiety, guilt, or a feeling of sinfulness; and a sense of security and direction in the pursuit of one's life goals and activities" (O'Brien, 1982, p. 98)

Interventions

Deficit: Meaning and Purpose

- Explore with the client what has given the client's life meaning and purpose up to the present, sources of meaning for other people, and possible meanings for the client's current experience of illness, pain, suffering, or impending death.
- Refer the client to a spiritual adviser if the client wishes this.
- Explore with the client spiritual practices from which strength and hope might be derived (eg, prayer or reading scripture or other spiritual books).
- Recommend that the client read spiritual biographies or Harold Kuschner's (1983) book *Why Bad Things Happen to Good People* (available in paperback in most bookstores).
- Refer the client to the appropriate support groups (eg, self-help groups for people with stroke, cancer, and so on).

Deficit: Love and Relatedness

- Treat the client at all times with respect, empathy, and genuine caring.
- Encourage the client to talk about relationships with others and to identify the origin of negative beliefs about people.
- Encourage conversation about God as the client knows and experiences God (if God is part of the client's spiritual beliefs). If appropriate, introduce or reinforce the belief that God is a loving and personal God who is concerned about the client.
- Whenever possible, encourage and facilitate visits from the client's family, friends, and spiritual adviser.

Deficit: Forgiveness

- Offer a supportive presence to the client that demonstrates your acceptance of the client.
- Explore with the client the importance of *learning* to accept oneself and others, including both strengths and limitations.
- Explore negative images of God and others that make it difficult for the client to seek forgiveness and to believe that the client is forgiven.
- Explore the client's self-expectations and assist the client to determine how realistic these are.
- Allow the client to verbalize shame, guilt, and anger and counsel about the importance of expressing negative emotions in healthy ways. Refer the client to a spiritual adviser, if appropriate.
- Offer the client examples of how feelings of unforgiving toward others can end up hurting only the one who cannot forgive.

Client Care Study

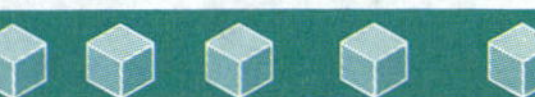

Mr. Gargan is a 38-year-old divorced man on a stepdown unit following treatment for a myocardial infarction. He owns a small car dealership. His religion is listed as Protestant. Frequently unable to sleep at night, Mr. Gargan often talks with the night nurse and once asked, "Did you ever give much thought to whether or not there is a God?" Sensing much concern behind this question, the nurse asks specific questions to determine if the client has spiritual needs that are not being met.

Assessment Findings

12/26/98, 2 AM

Client again unable to sleep and initiated discussion about God. States was raised in a Lutheran home where everyone went to church on Sunday and tried to live according to God's commandments. Upon leaving home, he stopped going to church (was never a value for his wife) and simply has not given much thought to religion—too busy running his business. Until now has not experienced any need for God. "But when I think how close I was to dying and that I've no idea what to expect after death—I'm actually scared. Do others feel this way?" Wants to explore religious beliefs—feels lack in his life. Said he would like to talk with hospital minister—will arrange for tomorrow.

E. Nolan, RN

Core Competencies

Successful implementation of the plan of care requires the following specialized nursing abilities:

Cognitive Competencies

- Holistic orientation to nursing, which values physical, psychologic, and spiritual health
- Respect for and knowledge of different spiritual beliefs (traditions) and the means people use to meet spiritual needs

Interpersonal Competencies

- Sensitivity to the spiritual needs of clients and the ability and willingness to address these needs
- Ability to offer the client a supportive nursing presence, including listening skills, empathy, vulnerability, humility, and commitment, as he struggles with his spiritual anxiety
- Willingness to refer the client to a spiritual adviser and to work collaboratively with this person
- Interpersonal and leadership skills to motivate the entire nursing staff to value spiritual health and to better understand its role in facilitating cardiac rehabilitation

Ethical/Legal Competencies

- Knowledge of professional responsibilities and competence and willingness to execute them in a legally defensible manner to meet the client's needs.

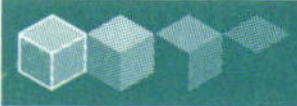

Nursing Plan of Care

for Mr. Gargan

Nursing Diagnosis: Spiritual Distress: Anxiety related to concerns about relationship with God as manifested by self report

Expected Outcome: Before discharge, the client will:

- Identify his religious beliefs

Nursing Interventions	Rationale	Evaluative Statement
Assist the client to (1) identify the spiritual beliefs he had as a child and the origin of these beliefs; (2) evaluate these beliefs in terms of his life experiences; and (3) reaffirm, modify, or reject these beliefs or develop new spiritual beliefs.	Life experiences may challenge religious beliefs that were uncritically held as a child.	12/30/98 Goal partially met. Client states he has a much clearer concept of God and no longer fears that God will reject him for ignoring him for so long . . . but believes he also has a lot to learn. *E. Nolan, RN*
Assist the client to assess whether his newly articulated spiritual beliefs are life-affirming or life-denying and the degree to which they meet his needs for meaning and purpose, love and relatedness, and forgiveness.	Because spiritual beliefs can exert positive (life-affirming) and negative (life-denying) influences on a person's life, individuals should have some criteria to use when evaluating their beliefs.	
Refer the client to the hospital minister for assistance with the above.	Client may value speaking with a minister.	

Expected Outcome Before discharge, the client will:

- Reconcile his life up until the present with God

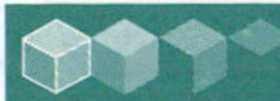

Nursing Plan of Care *(continued)*

for Mr. Gargan

Nursing Interventions	Rationale	Evaluative Statement
Reassure the client that many persons get involved in day-to-day living to the extent that they forget about God and that in some religions persons believe that God uses illness and other stressors to invite people to rethink their spiritual beliefs. In these traditions, God is often pictured with open arms waiting to welcome a child home.	Images of a stern and unyielding God ready to strike down transgressors may contribute to a client's spiritual distress.	12/30/98 Goal met. "This minister has really helped. I wish I had talked to him a long time ago. I've carried so much guilt about my divorce and some other things—thought God would never forgive me. I feel so much more at peace now." ***E. Nolan, RN***
Refer the client to a spiritual advisor for help in experiencing forgiveness if he mentions guilt feelings.	Guilt often inhibits persons from seeking and experiencing the forgiveness they desire.	
Communicate to the client the importance of people accepting themselves—with all their strengths and weaknesses.	Many persons have unrealistic self-expectations.	

Expected Outcome Before discharge, the client will:

- Verbalize that his spiritual beliefs have become a source of strength and peace rather than anxiety

Nursing Interventions	Rationale	Evaluative Statement
Encourage the client to compare the role of spiritual beliefs in his life before, during, and after hospitalization.	This highlights the positive and negative roles spiritual beliefs can play. It may motivate the client to continue searching if he values his present experience.	12/30/98 Goal met. "It's good to be able to feel more peaceful about whatever the future brings. I'm anxious to get out of here because there's a lot I want to do with God's help." ***E. Nolan, RN***

Expected Outcome: Before discharge, the client will:

- Increase night sleep to at least 6 undisturbed hours

Nursing Interventions	Rationale	Evaluative Statement
Nurse on the 11 to 7 shift checks on client at beginning of shift to make sure he is comfortable and ready for sleep.	Nursing supervision of the client at bedtime rules out other factors that may interfere with sleep.	12/30/98 Goal met. Client slept last night from midnight to 6 AM. Will continue to monitor. ***E. Nolan, RN***
Use power of suggestion to enhance sleep. "I'm sure when I check back you'll be sound asleep."	Suggestion has been shown to enhance the therapeutic effect of other interventions.	
If sleep remains disturbed, try relaxation exercises or guided imagery (see Chapter 32).	As spiritual anxiety decreases, sleep should improve. If sleep does not improve, other contributing factors and interventions will need to be explored.	

(continued)

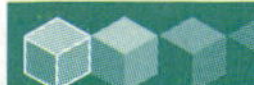

Nursing Plan of Care *(continued)*

for Mr. Gargan

Sample Documentation

12/27/98, 3 PM, Nursing

B. Hanks, Protestant minister, here to see client at 1 PM. Afterward, client said he felt "a whole lot better." Reported minister had assured him that many people in the hospital with a serious illness go through exactly what he is experiencing now—and this thought seemed to decrease much of his anxiety. Minister had reinforced nurse's suggestion that he explore his religious beliefs and he has already jotted down some thoughts. "I knew you fixed bodies in hospitals but didn't know you fix souls, too." Client looking forward to minister's visit tomorrow.

G. Paris, RN

Key Points

- The tradition of nursing has always been strongly holistic and nurses have practiced nursing sensitive to the physical, psychosocial, and spiritual needs of clients.
- Spiritual needs underlying all religious traditions and common to all people include need for meaning and purpose, need for love and relatedness, and need for forgiveness.
- Spiritual beliefs and practices are associated with all aspects of a person's life—health and illness, relationships with others, daily living habits, required and prohibited behaviors, the general frame of reference for thinking about oneself and the world.
- Spiritual beliefs during illness may be an important source of support, strength, and healing but may also be a source of anxiety when they conflict with proposed medical therapy.
- It is important for the nurse to be knowledgeable about and respect the spiritual beliefs of clients.
- The nurse who demonstrates peace, inner strength, warmth, joy, caring, and creativity in interactions with others will be most effective when assisting clients to meet spiritual needs.
- A comprehensive nursing assessment of spirituality addresses spiritual beliefs and practices, the relationship between spiritual beliefs and everyday living, indicators of spiritual distress, and unmet spiritual needs.
- Nursing diagnoses may be written that specifically address spiritual distress (spiritual pain, alienation, anxiety, guilt, anger, loss, or despair) or that identify the effect of spiritual distress on other areas of human functioning (Ineffective Individual Coping, Dysfunctional Grieving, Hopelessness, Powerlessness, Self-Esteem Disturbance).
- Nursing interventions that promote spiritual health include offering a supportive presence, facilitating the client's practice of religion, nurturing spirituality, praying with a client, spiritual counseling, referring a client to a religious counselor, and assisting clients to resolve conflicts between spiritual beliefs and treatment.

Study Questions

1. Which of the following statements most correctly differentiates between an agnostic and an atheist?
   a. The terms are used interchangeably, both believing there is no God.
   b. An agnostic denies that humans can know anything about God's existence, whereas an atheist denies God's existence.
   c. They both deny the need for a philosophy of living to guide their life.
   d. No aspect of an atheist's life is influenced by spirituality, whereas an agnostic has spiritual values.
2. A nurse who was raised a strict Roman Catholic stated she couldn't assist clients with their spiritual distress because she recognizes only a field power in each individual. She said, "My parents and I hardly talk because I've deserted my faith. Sometimes I feel real isolated from them and also God—if there is a God." Analysis of these data reveals which unmet spiritual need?
   a. need for meaning and purpose
   b. need for forgiveness
   c. need for love and relatedness
   d. need for strength for everyday living
3. Which statement is true concerning the influence of spirituality and religion on the various aspects of a person's life?
   a. All aspects of life may be influenced by spirituality.
   b. Activities of daily living (eating, bathing, sleeping, dressing) are rarely influenced by religion.

c. Work and recreation are not influenced by religion.
d. Whereas physical illness is seldom influenced by religion, mental illness frequently is.

4. A client whose last name was Goldstein was served on a paper plate a kosher meal ordered from a restaurant because the hospital made no provision for kosher food or dishes. Mr. Goldstein became angry and accused the nurse of insulting him. "I want to eat what everyone else does—and give me decent dishes." Analysis of these data reveals that
   a. the nurse should have ordered kosher dishes also
   b. the staff must have behaved condescendingly or critically
   c. Mr. Goldstein is a problem client and difficult to satisfy
   d. Mr. Goldstein was stereotyped and not consulted about his dietary preferences
5. You are *least* likely to encounter resistance to emergency life-saving surgery for a client from which of the following families?
   a. Christian Scientist family
   b. Faith Assembly Healer family
   c. Jehovah's Witness family
   d. Orthodox Jewish family
6. When the family desires baptism for an infant, it is imperative that the nurse provide for baptism to be done because
   a. baptism frequently postpones or prevents death or suffering
   b. it is legally required that nurses provide for this care when the family makes this request
   c. it is a nursing function to assure the salvation of the baby
   d. lack of baptism when desired may increase the family's sorrow and suffering
7. Because the capacity for abstract thought develops as a child grows older, spirituality is understood differently by children of different ages. Which of the following statements is *false?*
   a. Spirituality and perception of God is meaningless for the 4- to 5-year-old.
   b. Even young children, 4 to 5 years, have definite perceptions of God and forms of worship.
   c. Children's perceptions of their "spiritual self" mature as they mature.
   d. Children, 5 to 11 years, may show anxiety concerning the power they believe God has.
8. The most important source of learning about his or her own spirituality for a child is
   a. his or her church or religious organization
   b. what parents say about God and religion
   c. how parents behave in relationship to one another and their children, to others, and to God
   d. the spiritual adviser for the family
9. Even though a detailed nursing history in which spirituality is assessed is taken on admission, problems with spiritual distress may not surface until days after admission. The probable explanation is that
   a. clients usually want to conceal information about spiritual needs
   b. clients are not concerned about spiritual needs until after their spiritual adviser visits
   c. family members and close friends often initiate spiritual concerns
   d. illness increases spiritual concerns, which may be difficult for clients to express in words
10. When a client needs spiritual counseling, the nurse who is comfortable with his or her own spirituality should
    a. always call the client's own spiritual adviser
    b. consult with the client about the spiritual adviser with whom he or she wishes to counsel
    c. attempt to counsel the client and, if unsuccessful, make a referral
    d. advise the client and spiritual adviser concerning health options and the correct decision
11. When assessment data point to a spiritual problem that can be treated by independent nursing intervention, it receives the NANDA-approved diagnostic label
    a. Spiritual Alienation
    b. Spiritual Despair
    c. Spiritual Distress
    d. Spiritual Pain
12. A client states she feels so isolated from her family and church and even God "in this huge medical center so far from home." An appropriate goal for the client to relieve her spiritual distress is as follows. The client will
    a. express satisfaction with the compatibility of her spiritual beliefs and everyday living
    b. identify spiritual beliefs that meet her need for meaning and purpose
    c. express peaceful acceptance of limitations and failings
    d. identify spiritual supports available to her in this medical center
13. A man who is a declared agnostic is extremely depressed after losing his home, his wife, and his children in a fire. His nursing diagnosis is Spiritual Distress: Spiritual Pain related to inability to find meaning and purpose in his current condition. The most important nursing intervention to plan is to
    a. ask the client which spiritual adviser he would like you to call
    b. recommend that the client read spiritual biographies or religious books
    c. explore with the client what, in addition to his family, has given his life meaning and purpose in the past
    d. introduce the belief that God is a loving and personal God

14. After having an abortion, the client told the visiting nurse, "I shouldn't have had that abortion because I'm Catholic, but what else could I do? I'm afraid I'll never get close to my mother or back in the Church again." She then talked with her priest about this feeling of guilt. Which evaluation statement shows a solution to the problem?
    a. Client states, "I wish I had talked with the priest sooner. I now know God has forgiven me and even my mother understands."
    b. Client has slept from 10 PM to 6 AM for three consecutive nights without medication.
    c. Client has developed mutually caring relationships with two women and one man.
    d. Client has identified several spiritual beliefs that give purpose to her life.
15. Mr. Brown's teenage daughter had been involved in shoplifting. He expressed much anger toward her and stated he could not face her, let alone discuss this with her. "I just will not tolerate a thief." Which of the following nursing interventions would you take to assist Mr. Brown with his deficit in forgiveness?
    a. Assure him that many parents feel the same way.
    b. Reassure him that many teenagers go through this kind of rebellion and that it will pass.
    c. Assist the client to identify how unforgiving feelings toward others only hurt the one who cannot forgive.
    d. Ask him if he is sure he has spent sufficient time with his daughter.

Answers With Rationale

1. The correct response is *b*. It is factually correct that an agnostic denies that humans can know anything about God's existence, whereas an atheist denies God's existence. The other options are factually incorrect.
2. The correct response is *c*. The data point to an unmet spiritual need to experience love and belonging given her estrangement from her family and God following her leaving the church. The other options may represent other needs this client has, but the data provided do not support them.
3. The correct response is *a*. It is true that spirituality can influence all aspects of a person's life, including activities of daily living, work and recreation, and all types of illnesses. The other options are incomplete or false.
4. The correct response is *d*. The nurse jumped to the premature and false conclusion with this client on the basis of his name alone that he would want a kosher diet.
5. The correct response is *d*. There is no teaching in the Hebrew scriptures that prohibits emergency life-saving surgery. On the contrary, most Orthodox Jews would be highly motivated to have the surgery because of the high value attached to preserving life. All of the other groups mentioned might have religious grounds for refusing surgery.
6. The correct response is *d*. Failure to ensure that an infant baptism is performed when parents desire it may greatly increase the family's sorrow and suffering, and this is an appropriate nursing concern. Whether baptism postpones or prevents death and suffering (option *a*) is a religious belief that is insufficient to bind all nurses. There is no legal requirement regarding baptism; option *b* is false. Although some nurses may believe part of their role is to assure the salvation (option *c*) of the baby, this function would understandably be rejected by many.
7. The correct response is *a*. It is false that spirituality and perception of God is meaningless for the 4- to 5-year-old. All the other options are factually correct.
8. The correct response is *c*. Children learn most about their own spirituality from how their parents behave in relationship to one another, their children, others, and God. Less important sources of learning are each of the other options.
9. The correct response is *d*. It is factually correct that illness surfaces and may increase spiritual concerns, which many clients find difficult to express. The other options do not correspond to actual experience.
10. The correct response is *b*. Even when a nurse feels comfortable discussing spiritual concerns, he or she should always check first with clients to determine the spiritual adviser with whom they wish to counsel. Calling the client's own spiritual adviser (option *a*) may be premature if it is a matter the nurse can handle. Options *c* and *d* deny clients the right to speak privately with their spiritual adviser from the outset, if this is what they prefer.
11. The correct response is *c*. The only NANDA-approved nursing diagnosis among the options is *c*, Spiritual Distress. The other options may be further specifications of the broader diagnosis Spiritual Distress.
12. The correct response is *d*. Each of the four options represents appropriate spiritual goals. Identifying spiritual supports available to her in the medical center demonstrates a decreased sense of isolation.
13. The correct response is *c*. The nursing intervention of exploring with the client what, in addition to his family, has given his life meaning and purpose in

the past is more likely to correct the etiology of his problem, Spiritual Pain, than any of the other nursing interventions listed.

14. The correct response is *a*. Because this client's nursing diagnosis is Spiritual Distress: Guilt, an evaluative statement that demonstrates a diminishment of guilt is necessary. Only option *a* directly deals with guilt.
15. The correct response is *c*, as this is the only nursing intervention that directly addresses the client's unmet spiritual need concerning forgiveness. Options *a* and *b* may make him feel better initially, but neither option addresses his need to forgive. Option *d* is likely to make him feel guilty.

Bibliography

Andrews, M. M., & Hanson, P. A. (1995). Religion, culture, and nursing. In M. M. Andrews & J. S. Boyle, *Transcultural concepts in nursing care.* Philadelphia: Lippincott.

Berggren-Thomas, P., & Griggis, M. J. (1995). Spirituality in aging: Spiritual need or spiritual journey? *Journal of Gerontological Nursing, 21*(3), 5–10.

Burnhard, P. (1987). Spiritual distress and the nursing response: Theoretical considerations and counseling skills. *Journal of Advanced Nursing, 12*(3), 377–382.

Callahan, D., & Campbell, C. S. (Eds.). (1990). Theology, religious traditions, and bioethics: A special supplement. *Hastings Center Report, 20*(6), 18–19.

Carson, V. B. (1989). *Spiritual dimensions of nursing practice.* Philadelphia: Saunders.

Charnes, L. S. (1992). Meeting patients' spiritual needs: The Jewish perspective. *Holistic Nursing Practice, 6*(3), 64–72.

Clark, C., & Heidenreich, T. (1995). Spiritual care for the critically ill. *American Journal of Critical Care, 4*(1), 77–81.

Coles, R. (1990). *The spiritual life of children.* Boston: Houghton Mifflin.

Corinne, L., Baily, V., Valentin, M., Morantus, E., & Shirley, L. (1992). The unheard voices of women: Spiritual interventions in maternal–child health care. *MCN, 17*(3), 141–145.

Cutcliffe, J. R. (1995). How do nurses inspire and instill hope in terminally ill HIV patients? *Journal of Advanced Nursing, 22,* 888–895.

Dossey, B. (Ed.). (1989). Spirituality and healing. *Holistic Nursing Practice, 3*(3) [entire issue].

Dudley, J. R., Smith, C., & Millison, M. B. (1995). Unfinished business: Assessing the spiritual needs of hospice clients. *American Journal of Hospice & Palliative Care, 12*(2), 30–37.

Earhart, H. B. (Ed.). *Religious traditions of the world series.* San Francisco: HarperCollins.

Fish, S. (1995). Can research prove that God answers prayer? *Journal of Christian Nursing, 12*(1), 24–27, 46.

Fish, S., & Shelly, J. (1978). *Spiritual care: The nurse's role.* Downer's Grove, IL: InterVarsity Press.

Fitchett, G. (1993). *Assessing spiritual needs: A guide for caregivers.* Minneapolis: Augsburg.

Fitchett, G. (1995). Linda Krauss and the lap of God. A spiritual assessment case study. *Second Opinion, 20*(4), 41–49.

Fowler, J. W. (1981). *Stages of faith: The psychology of human development and the quest for meaning.* San Francisco: HarperCollins.

Gaskins, S., & Forte, L. (1995). The meaning of hope: Implications for nursing practice and research. *Journal of Gerontological Nursing, 21*(3), 17–24.

Goddard, N. C. (1995). "Spirituality as integrative energy": A philosophical analysis as requisite precursor to holistic nursing practice. *Journal of Advanced Nursing, 22*(4), 808–815.

Harrison, J. (1993). Spirituality and nursing practice. *Journal of Clinical Nursing, 2*(4), 211–217.

Hauerwas, S. (1990). *Naming the silences: God, medicine, and the problem of suffering.* Grand Rapids: Erdmans.

Heller, D. (1985). The children's God. *Psychology Today, 19*(12), 22–27.

Hill, L., & Smith, N. (1990). *Self-care nursing* (2nd ed.). New York: Appleton & Lange.

Hultkrantz, A. (1987). *Native religions of North America.* San Francisco: HarperCollins.

Hungelmann, J., et al. (1989). Development of the JAREL spiritual well-being scale. In NANDA (Eds.), *Classification of nursing diagnosis: Proceedings of the eighth conference* (pp. 393–398). Philadelphia: Lippincott.

Jamison, J. E. (1995). Spirituality and medical ethics. *American Journal of Hospice and Palliative Care, 12*(3), 41–45.

Kaye, J., & Robinson, K. M. (1994). Spirituality among caregivers. *IMAGE: Journal of Nursing Scholarship, 26*(3), 218–221.

Kuschner, H. S. (1983). *Why bad things happen to good people.* New York: Avon.

Larue, G. A. (1988). Religion and the aged. In I. M. Burnside (Ed.), *Nursing and the aged* (3rd ed.). St. Louis: Mosby.

Macrae, J. (1995). Nightingale's spiritual philosophy and its significance for modern nursing. *IMAGE: Journal of Nursing Scholarship, 27*(1), 8–10.

Mansen, J. J. (1993). The spiritual dimension of individuality: Conceptual development. *Nursing Diagnosis, 4*(4), 140–147.

Manson, C. H. (1995). Prayer as a nursing intervention. *Journal of Christian Nursing, 12*(1), 4–8.

Marty, M. E. (1990). The tradition of the Church in health and healing. *Second Opinion, 13,* 48–72.

Marty, M. E., & Vaux, K. L. (Eds.). *Health/medicine and the faith traditions.* New York: Crossroad.

Mayer, J. (1992). Wholly responsible for a part, or partly responsible for a whole? The concept of spiritual care in nursing. *Second Opinion, 17*(3), 26–55.

McHolm, F. A. (1992). A nursing diagnosis validation study: Defining characteristics of spiritual distress. In R. M. Carroll-Johnson (Ed.), *Classification of nursing diagnosis: Proceedings of the ninth conference* (pp. 112–119). Philadelphia: Lippincott.

Miller, M. A. (1995). Culture, spirituality and women's health. *JOGNN, 24*(3), 257–263.

Murray, R. B., & Zentner, J. P. (1989). *Nursing assessment and health promotion strategies throughout the lifespan* (4th ed.). New York: Appleton-Lange.

Narayanasamy, A. (1993). Nurses' awareness and educational responsibility in meeting their patients' spiritual needs. *Nurse Educator Today, 13*(3), 196–201.

North American Nursing Diagnosis Association. (1994). *NANDA nursing diagnoses: Definitions and classifications 1995–1996.* Philadelphia: NANDA.

O'Brien, M. E. (1982). The need for spiritual integrity. In H. Yura & M. Walsh (Eds.), *Human needs 2 and the nursing process* (pp. 81–115). Norwalk, CT: Appleton-Century-Crofts.

Parrinder, G. (Ed.). (1983). *World religions.* New York: Facts on File Publications.

Pumphrey, J. B. (1977). Recognizing your patients' spiritual needs. *Nursing, 8*(12), 64–69.

Ross, L. A. (1994). Spiritual aspects of nursing. *Journal of Advances in Nursing, 19*(3), 437–439.

Shaffer, J. L. (Ed.). (1989). Spirituality and healing. *Holistic Nursing Practice, 3*(3) [entire issue].

Smith, D. W. (1995). Power and spirituality in polio survivors: A study based on Rogeor's science. *Nursing Science Quarterly, 8*(3), 133–139.

Starck, P. L., & McGovern, J. P. (Eds.). (1992). *The hidden dimension of illness: Human suffering*. New York: National League for Nursing Press.

Stoll, R. I. (1979). Guidelines for spiritual assessment. *American Journal of Nursing, 79*(9), 1574–1577.

Widerquist, J. G. (1992). The spirituality of Florence Nightingale. *Nursing Research, 41*(1), 49–55.

Widerquist, J., & Davidhizar, R. (1994). The ministry of nursing. *Journal of Advanced Nursing, 19*(4), 647–652.

Whitlatch, A. M., Meddaugh, D. I., & Langhout, K. J. (1994). Religiosity among Alzheimer's disease caregivers. *Healing Ministry, 1*(1), 23–27, 32.

The art and science of caring are blended when nurses implement actions to meet basic human needs and to promote healthy physiologic responses. The chapters in Unit VIII focus on information and guidelines essential to nursing practice in a wide variety of clinical settings and involving both healthy and ill clients of all ages. Included are nursing interventions to promote safety and comfort and to meet basic physiologic needs—hygiene, activity and rest, nutrition, elimination, oxygenation, and fluid–electrolyte balance.

Each basic physiologic need is discussed first by reviewing concepts pertinent to the specific area of human function and response and then by presenting factors that affect need satisfaction. The steps of the nursing process are used to provide guidelines and information necessary for making accurate assessments; establishing goals; and planning, implementing, and evaluating specific nursing interventions to meet needs and promote wellness. A section entitled Nursing Process in Clinical Practice, at the end of each chapter, illustrates the application of knowledge by providing a client care study, selected nursing diagnoses, and a nursing plan of care, to show how skilled nursing interventions and caring are combined to resolve problems and meet ends.

The content of Unit VIII enables the beginning nurse caregiver to integrate the knowledge and skills necessary to promote healthy physiologic responses in clients in any practice setting. Nursing process skills are further refined to ensure that care is holistic, comprehensive, and individualized.

Promoting Healthy Physiologic Responses

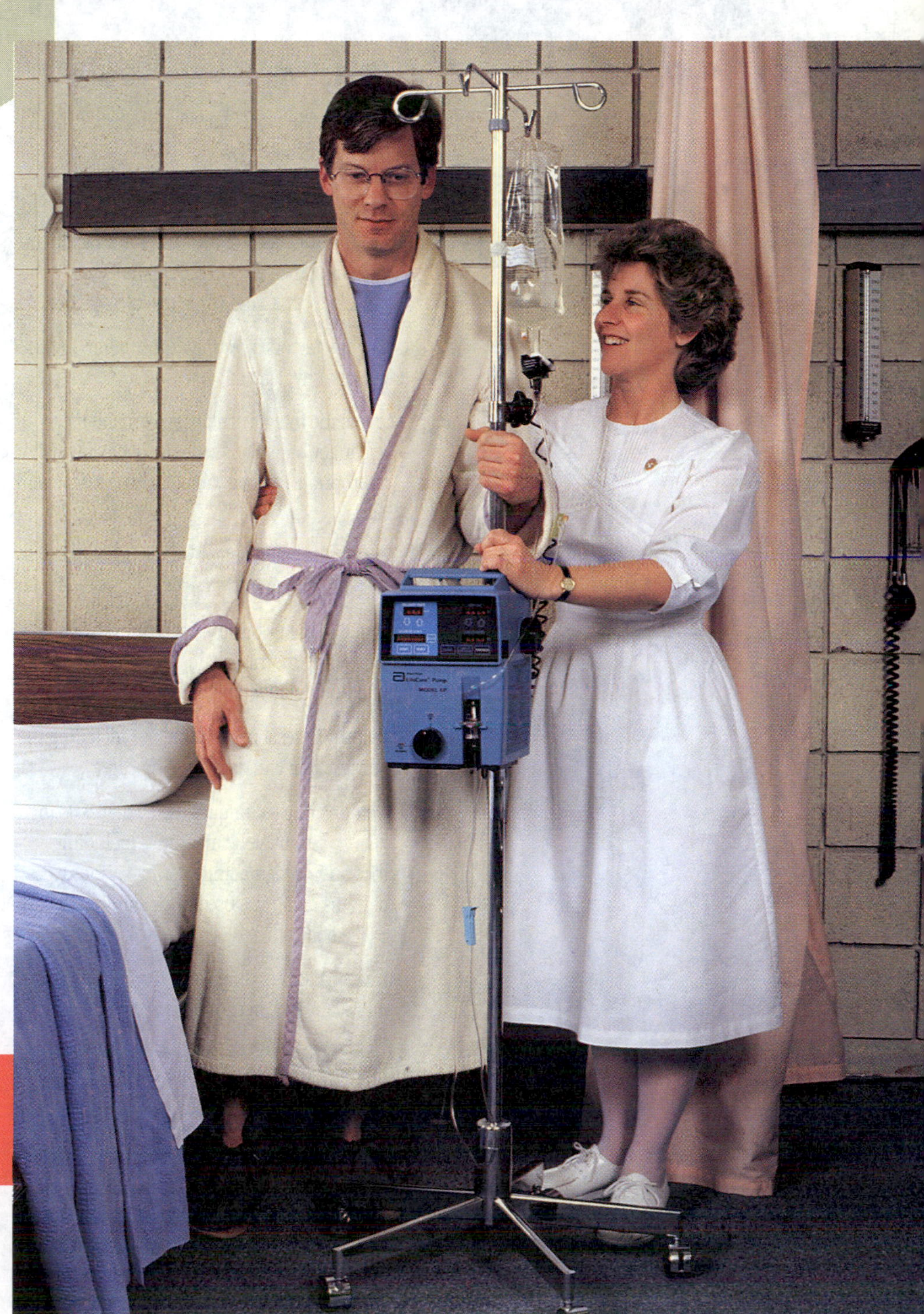

". . . what nursing has to do is to put the patient in the best condition for nature to act upon him."

Florence Nightingale (1820–1910)

a philosopher, theorist, statistician, humanitarian, and inspirational leader who founded modern nursing through a systematic method of training well-qualified nurses; also initiated important reforms in military sanitation and hospital construction that greatly improved patient survival

Unit VIII

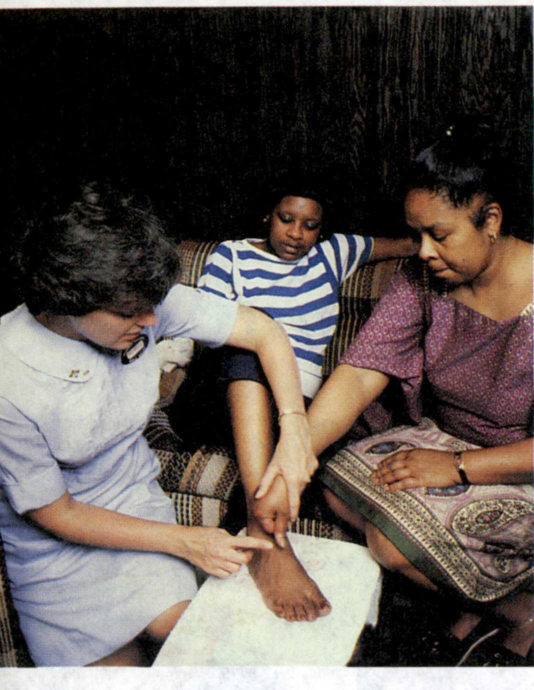

Chapter 37

Hygiene

Objectives

After studying this chapter, the learner should be able to:

Define key terms used in the chapter.

List five functions of the skin, three factors influencing the skin's condition, and four basic principles that guide practices of skin care.

Identify factors affecting skin condition and personal hygiene.

Assess the integumentary system and the adequacy of hygiene self-care behaviors using appropriate interview and physical assessment skills.

Develop nursing diagnoses related to deficient hygiene measures.

Describe the priorities of scheduled hygienic care, early morning care, morning care, afternoon care, and evening care.

Identify at least four reasons for including the back massage in daily nursing care.

Demonstrate techniques used when assisting clients with hygiene measures, including those used when administering various types of baths and those used in cleaning each part of the body.

Describe agents commonly used on the skin and scalp and precautions to observe in their use.

Plan, implement, and evaluate nursing care for common problems of the skin and mucous membranes.

Key Terms

alopecia
caries
cerumen
dermis
epidermis
erythema
gingivitis
halitosis
integument
ischemia
necrosis
pediculosis (lice)
plaque
podiatrist
pyorrhea
sebaceous glands
tartar

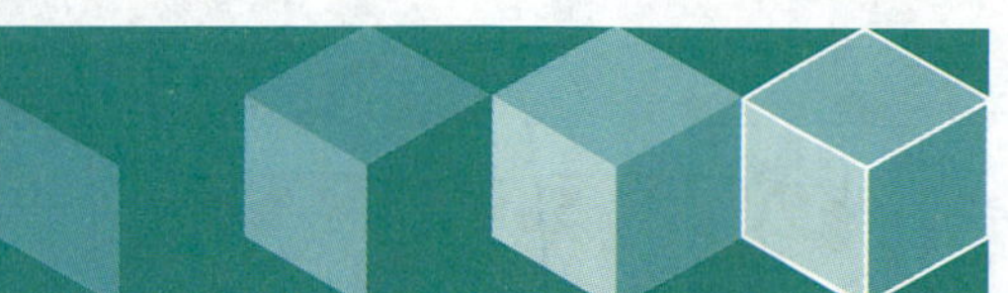

Measures for personal cleanliness and grooming that promote physical and psychologic well-being are called *personal hygiene*. Personal hygiene practices vary widely from one person to another. The time of day for bathing or the frequency of shampooing the hair and changing the bed linens and sleeping garments is relatively unimportant. What is important is that personal care be carried out conveniently and often enough to promote personal hygiene.

Ordinarily, the well person is responsible for self-hygiene. Through teaching, the nurse may assist the well person to develop personal hygiene habits the person may lack.

Illness, hospitalization, and institutionalization may demand modifications in hygiene practices. In these situations, the nurse helps the client to continue sound hygienic practices and has an opportunity to teach the client and family members regarding hygiene. The nurse who assists a client with basic hygiene respects individual client preferences and administers only that amount of care the client cannot or should not provide for himself or herself.

This chapter provides the nurse with knowledge of the multiple factors that affect personal hygiene and of nursing measures that promote personal hygiene. A practical guide for assessing the adequacy of personal hygiene behaviors is presented. Because the data the nurse collects when assisting with hygiene may lead to the identification of multiple nursing diagnoses and collaborative problems, samples of these are provided. Client goals are presented, as are descriptions of specific nursing strategies used when performing care of the skin; mouth; eyes, ears, and nose; feet; and perineal and vaginal areas.

In the section Nursing Process in Clinical Practice, assessment priorities, expected outcomes, and nursing interventions are presented for clients with a Self-Care Deficit associated with bathing and hygiene and Altered Oral Mucous Membranes. These guides and the concluding client care study on feminine hygiene illustrate how the nurse's knowledge of personal hygiene practices and the integumentary system is combined with specific nursing interventions to resolve nursing diagnoses successfully and promote the client's general sense of well-being.

Physiology of the Skin and Its Appendages

Integument refers to the skin. The *integumentary system* comprises the skin, the subcutaneous layer directly under the skin, and the appendages of the skin, that is, the hair, glands in the skin, and the nails. The skin is one of the body's vital organs and is essential for maintaining life.

The skin consists of two layers. The superficial portion, the **epidermis**, comprises layers of stratified epithelial cells. These cells are fused to form a protective, waterproof layer of keratin material. Epithelial cells have no blood vessels of their own and depend on underlying tissues for nourishment and waste removal. When well nourished, epithelium regenerates relatively easily and quickly.

The second layer of skin, the **dermis**, consists of smooth, muscular tissue; nerves; hair follicles; certain glands and their ducts; arteries; veins and capillaries; and fibrous, elastic tissue. Each hair consists of the shaft, which projects through the dermis beyond the surface of the skin, and the hair follicle, which lies in the dermis. The dermis rests on a subcutaneous fatty tissue layer that anchors the skin layers and serves as a heat insulator for the body. This fatty tissue layer contains blood and lymph vessels, nerves, and fat cells. The two main layers of skin and the subcutaneous layer comprise the integumentary system.

The skin covers the entire body and is continuous with the mucous membrane at normal body orifices. A cross-section of normal skin is illustrated in Figure 37-1. Glands in the skin include the sebaceous glands, the sweat glands, and the ceruminal glands. The **sebaceous glands** secrete an oily substance called *sebum*, which lubricates the skin and hair and keeps the skin and scalp pliant. The sweat glands secrete perspiration. The **cerumen** in the external ear canals, consisting of a heavy oil and brown pigment, is secreted by *ceruminal glands.*

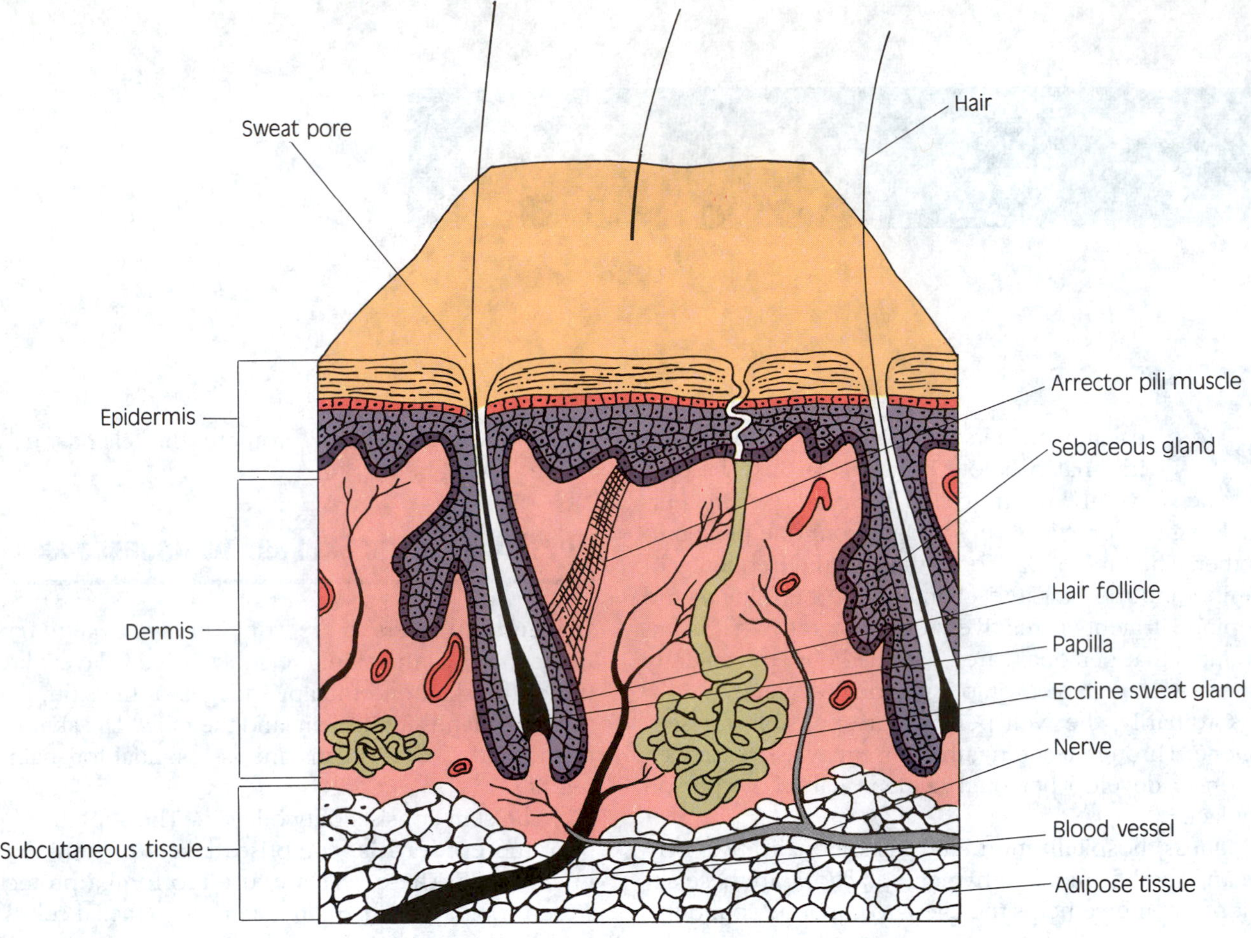

Figure 37-1
A cross-section of normal skin.

Functions of Skin and Mucous Membranes

The skin serves six major functions, described in Table 37-1:

- Protects the body
- Regulates body temperature
- Senses stimuli from the environment and transmits these sensations (ie, pain, temperature, pressure)
- Excretes waste products
- Helps maintain water and electrolyte balance
- Produces and absorbs vitamin D

Mucous membranes line body cavities that open to the outside of the body and can also be found in the digestive tract, the respiratory passages, and the urinary and reproductive tracts. Epithelium covers the mucous membrane surfaces and contains cells that secrete mucus. Connective tissue lies beneath the epithelium. Mucous membranes have receptors that offer the body protection; for example, an irritating substance in the upper respiratory tract causes a person to sneeze, and food caught in the larynx or trachea causes a person to cough. Sneezing and coughing are protective mechanisms that help rid the body of foreign materials. Mucous membranes are insensitive to temperature, except in the mouth and rectum, but are sensitive to pressure. Mucous membranes also function to absorb substances from their surface; for example, digested food is absorbed through the mucous membrane in the small intestine.

Principles of Skin Care

Knowledge of the functions of the skin and mucous membranes and of factors affecting them includes an understanding of certain basic principles that become important in the care of the skin and mucous membranes:

Unbroken and healthy skin and mucous membranes serve as the first lines of defense against harmful agents.

Resistance to injury of the skin and mucous membranes varies among people. Factors influencing resistance include a person's age, the amount of underlying tissues, and illness conditions.

Adequately nourished and hydrated body cells are resistant to injury. The better nourished the cell, the better its ability to resist injury and disease.

Adequate circulation is necessary to maintain cell life. The cells are inadequately nourished and wastes are poorly removed when circulation is impaired for any reason.

Table 37-1
Functions of the Skin

Function	Mechanisms
The skin protects the body	Invasion of the body by bacteria is prevented by intact skin. Injury to underlying tissues and organs is decreased by intact skin.
The skin helps regulate body temperature	The production of perspiration and its loss by evaporation help cool the body.
	Much heat is lost from the body by radiation and by conduction when the blood supply to the skin is increased by vasodilation.
	Lack of perspiration and vasoconstriction help the body retain heat.
	The phenomenon of producing gooseflesh, which is caused by contraction of pilomotor muscles in the skin, helps conserve body heat because the hair standing on end forms a layer of air on the body for insulation.
The skin is a sense organ	There are receptors for pain, touch, pressure, and temperature in the skin that help the body receive stimuli from the environment.
The skin is an excretory organ	Water, salts,and nitrogenous wastes are lost from the skin, although in much smaller quantities than are lost from the kidneys.
The skin helps maintain water and electrolyte balance	The escape of excess water and electrolytes from the body is prevented by the skin.
The skin produces and absorbs vitamin D	A precursor for vitamin D is present in the skin, which in conjunction with ultraviolet rays from the sun produces vitamin D.

Factors Affecting Skin Condition and Personal Hygiene

Skin Condition

A person's developmental stage and health condition influence the skin in various ways.

Developmental Considerations

- An infant's skin and mucous membranes are easily injured and subject to infection. Careful handling of infants is required to prevent injury and infection of the skin and mucous membranes.
- A child's skin becomes increasingly resistant to injury and infection. However, the skin requires special care because of the toilet and play habits of children.
- An adolescent's skin ordinarily has enlarged sebaceous glands and increased glandular secretions, caused by hormonal changes in the body. These characteristics predispose to acne, which is discussed later in this chapter.
- Secretions from the skin glands are at their maximum during adolescence and up to around age 50 years.
- Changes that occur in the skin with aging are discussed in the box, Focus on the Older Adult. These changes are irreversible. The skin becomes thinner, less elastic, and less supple with aging. Subcutaneous fat that normally helps absorb injury to the skin decreases. Wrinkles appear, most of which are deep in the dermis. The skin becomes dry, often scaly, and rough in appearance because less oil is secreted from sebaceous glands. Brown spots, called *liver spots,* often appear. They may begin appearing as early as age 35 years and tend to become more numerous and larger with aging. These spots result from exposure to the wind and sun and are not caused by liver disease.

Health State

- Very thin and very obese people tend to be more susceptible to skin irritation and injury.
- Fluid loss through fever, vomiting, or diarrhea reduces the fluid volume of the body and is called *dehydration.* Dehydration makes the skin appear loose and flabby.
- Excessive perspiration, often associated with being ill, predisposes to skin breakdown, especially in areas where the skin folds.
- *Jaundice,* a condition caused by excessive bile pigments in the skin, results in a yellowish skin color. The skin is often itchy and dry in the presence of jaundice.
- Diseases of the skin are usually characterized by various lesions that require special care to promote personal hygiene and to carry out therapeutic regimens.

Personal Hygiene

The nurse caring for clients from diverse backgrounds quickly learns that hygiene practices vary widely among individuals. The following factors may influence personal hygiene behaviors.

Culture. Many people in North America place a high value on personal cleanliness and feel unclean unless they shower or bathe at least once daily. They consider bathing incomplete without the use of multiple products to reduce or mask normal body odors. People from other cultures often find a weekly bath sufficient and feel no need to mask normal body odors. Culture may also dictate whether bathing is a private or communal activity.

Focus on the Older Adult

Older skin is different from younger skin. The visible changes may vary considerably based on intrinsic (natural aging) factors and extrinsic (environmental) factors.

Skin Alterations Due to Aging	Implications for the Older Adult
Subcutaneous and dermal tissue thins.	Skin is thinner, more easily injured, has less capacity to insulate, and wrinkles.
Activity of sebaceous and sweat glands decreases.	Perspiration is decreased, skin becomes dryer, and pruritus (itching) may occur.
Cell renewal is shorter.	Healing time is delayed.
Melanocytes (cells that make the pigment that colors hair and skin) decline in number.	Hair becomes gray-white and skin may be unevenly pigmented.
Vascularity decreases to the skin.	Skin temperature is cooler and pallor may be apparent.
Nail growth rate diminishes.	Nails become soft and tear easily.
Collagen fiber is less organized.	Skin loses elasticity.

Socioeconomic Class. Financial resources often define the hygiene options available to individuals. A single person renting one room in a boarding house may have limited or no access to tubs or showers and limited finances for the purchase of soap, shampoo, shaving cream, and deodorants. Homeless people, who often carry all their belongings in a car or shopping cart, may welcome the warm running water and soap available in a roadside or other public restroom. Other people may refrain from using public restrooms because they are perceived as being dirty.

Spiritual Practices. Religion may dictate ceremonial washings and purifications, which may be a prelude to prayer or eating. For example, in the orthodox Jewish tradition, ritual baths are required for women after childbirth and menstruation. In some religions, contact with a deceased person or a deceased animal may make a person "unclean."

Developmental Level and Knowledge Level. Children learn different hygiene practices while growing up. Family practices may dictate morning or evening baths, the frequency of shampooing, feelings about nudity, frequency of clothing changes, and so on. An adolescent may experience the need to change hygiene measures practiced throughout childhood and begin to take long, frequent, hot showers. Older people often experience the need to decrease bathing times and the use of deodorant soaps to avoid excessively drying the skin.

Health State. Disease or injury may adversely affect an individual's ability to perform hygiene measures or motivation to follow usual hygiene habits. Weakness, dizziness, and fear of falling may prevent an individual from entering a tub or shower or from bending to wash the lower extremities. Illness may also create a demand for new or modified hygiene measures.

Personal Preferences. Different people have different personal preferences with regard to hygiene practices. Showers versus tub baths, bar soap versus liquid soap, washing to wake oneself or to relax before sleep are personal preferences. One's self-concept and sexuality are also personal influences on hygiene.

The Nurse as Role Model

Nurses consistently serve as role models for clients in regard to personal hygiene. Before attempting to teach clients healthy hygiene practices, it is important that nurses evaluate their own practices. If unable to meet the following goals, you may wish to take the time now to examine your own hygiene practices.

- The nurse's physical appearance and body scents give evidence of adequate hygiene practices:
  - Hair is clean and neatly styled.
  - Skin is clean.
  - Mouth evidences satisfactory oral hygiene.
  - Nails are neatly manicured.
  - Body is free of unpleasant odors.
- The nurse's diet and exercise habits contribute to clean and intact skin.
- The nurse brushes teeth after each meal, flosses daily, and goes to the dentist for a checkup at least annually.
- The nurse's care of clients demonstrates an appreciation for the relationship between hygiene and overall well-being.
- The nurse consistently uses appropriate aseptic safeguards (ie, handwashing, use of gloves) to prevent the transmission of microorganisms.

A self-assessment checklist on feminine hygiene is included later in the chapter.

Basic Skin Care and Personal Hygiene

ASSESSING

A comprehensive assessment of the skin and appendages includes the following:

- Collection of data about usual hygiene practices:
  - Showering or bathing practices
  - Skin, hair, and scalp care
  - Eye, ear, nose, and mouth care
  - Nail and foot care
  - Perineal care
- Assessment of any sensory, cognitive, endurance, mobility, or motivation deficit that interferes with the individual's hygiene practices
- Identification of any existing problems of the skin or mucous membranes, as well as associated care and its effectiveness
- Nursing examination of the skin and mucous membranes

Skin and basic hygiene assessment guidelines follow. Focused assessment criteria for selected body parts appear later in the chapter.

Nursing History

While assessing hygiene practices, the nurse remembers that different individuals and families possess different ideas regarding personal cleanliness. Bathing practices and cleansing habits and rituals vary widely. A clear threat to health must exist before a nurse decides that an individual's hygiene practices are inadequate. The nurse assessing the adequacy of hygiene practices evaluates whether the individual possesses the knowledge, attitude, skills, and resources to care for the skin and mucous membranes (see the Focused Assessment Guide in the accompanying box).

The nursing history also includes data about problems of the integumentary system. The client should be questioned about any past or current problems such as rashes, lumps, itching, dryness, lesions, ecchymoses, masses, or specific changes in the hair or nails. When skin problems are present, the client should be asked the following:

How long have you had this problem?
Does it itch or bother you?
How does it bother you?
Have you found any care helpful in relieving these symptoms?

Sample entries in documentation of a nursing history follow:

Hygiene: "Showers twice daily, once in the AM and after working out in the evening. Skin tends to be

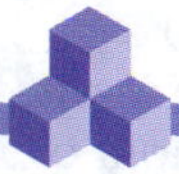

Focused Assessment Guide

Hygiene Practices

Factors to Assess	Questions and Approaches
Daily and weekly bathing habits	Tell me about your daily and weekly bathing habits. Are there special bathing or hygiene products you routinely use or cannot use? How can nurses best help you to meet your hygiene needs?
Factors interfering with hygiene practices (sensory, cognitive, endurance, mobility, or motivation)	What recently or in the past has interfered with your hygiene practices? Does anything interfere with your ability to be as clean as you would like?
History of skin or mucous membrane problems (nature, onset of problem and frequency, causes, severity, symptoms, interventions attempted, and results)	Describe any skin problems with rashes, lumps, itching, dryness, lesions, ecchymosis, or masses. Are you allergic to any cleansing or cosmetic products?
Special hygiene practices (eg, inflamed gums or menstruation)	I notice that your gums look inflamed. How do you clean your teeth and gums? Have you seen a dentist about this problem? Do you follow any special hygiene practices during menstruation? What type of feminine hygiene products (eg, pads, tampons, douches) do you use?

very dry, and moisturizing creams are used daily. Aveeno Oilated baths prn. Allergic to deodorant soaps."

Integument: "History of athlete's foot since high school days with outbreaks every 2 to 3 months. Knowledgeable about appropriate foot care. Uses Tinactin cream [topical fungicidal agent] and Mexsana medicated powder [topical protectant]."

Physical Assessment

The inspection and palpation skills used to assess the integumentary system are described in detail in Chapter 26. The nurse who assists a client with basic hygiene measures has an excellent opportunity to examine the client's skin carefully. Many individuals are unaware of skin lesions such as precancerous moles, which, if untreated, could prove fatal. Early detection and treatment of skin problems are important nursing functions.

In examining the skin, the nurse pays careful attention to cleanliness, color, texture, temperature, turgor, moisture, sensation, vascularity, and the presence of lesions. If a lesion is detected, the nurse documents the type, color, size, distribution and grouping, location, and consistency. Terminology helpful in describing these findings is presented in Chapter 26. General guidelines for assessing the skin are as follows:

- Proceed systematically in head-to-toe fashion.
- Use a good source of light, preferably daylight.
- Compare bilateral parts for symmetry.
- Use standard terminology to report and record findings.
- Allow data obtained in the nursing history to direct the skin assessment.
- Identify any variables known to cause skin problems, such as deficient self-care abilities; immobility; malnutrition; decreased hydration; decreased sensation; vascular problems (altered tissue perfusion or venous return); or presence of irritants (body secretions or excretions on the skin, other chemicals, mechanical devices).

Because lifestyle factors, changes in health state, illness, and certain diagnostic and therapeutic measures may adversely affect the skin, the nurse needs to identify high-risk populations and perform the appropriate skin assessment. Knowing *when* to perform the skin assessment and incorporating this into the client's plan of care is as important as knowing *how* to do this well. Table 37-2 identifies sample factors that place an individual at risk for skin alterations.

Sample entries under integumentary system in documentation of the nursing examination follow:

"Skin is pink, warm, dry, and elastic; no petechiae, lesions, or excoriation; multiple moles of small size and regular border and surface."

"Red, macular rash generalized over trunk and thighs; semiconfluent lesions measure 1 to 2 mm; abrupt onset."

DIAGNOSING

A careful assessment of the skin and mucous membranes may lead to the identification of numerous client problems that can be classified as nursing diagnoses. Problems concerning deficient hygiene are categorized as self-care deficits. Self-Care Deficit diagnoses address four specific activities necessary to meet daily needs—feeding, bathing and hygiene, dressing and grooming, and toileting. It is important to identify the cause of these problems correctly. If hygiene is deficient because of insufficient knowledge, health education can quickly remedy the problem. If, however, the individual attaches low priority to hygiene or lacks the physical ability to perform hygiene measures, these problems must be addressed before health education can be effective.

Sample nursing diagnoses related to hygiene and skin problems follow:

Bathing/Hygiene Self-Care Deficit related to sensory, cognitive, endurance, mobility, or motivation deficits

Pain related to skin or mucous membrane alterations

Ineffective Individual Coping related to chronic skin problems

Altered Health Maintenance (eg, dental caries, periodontal disease, halitosis) related to deficient oral hygiene practices

Knowledge Deficit related to new therapeutic regimen to manage skin or mucous membrane alteration

Impaired Physical Mobility related to painful foot condition (calluses, corns, plantar warts)

Altered Oral Mucous Membrane related to inadequate oral hygiene, stomatitis, malnutrition, or dehydration

Risk for Infection related to broken skin or traumatized tissue

Body Image Disturbance related to visible integumentary problems, body odors

Altered Sexuality Patterns related to fear of transmitting or acquiring sexually transmitted disease, painful genital lesions

Impaired Skin Integrity related to altered circulation, nutrition and fluid deficit or excess, impaired mobility, irritants (chemical, thermal, mechanical, radiation)

Risk for Impaired Skin Integrity related to immobility, use of physical restraints, use of aquathermia device, dehydration, bladder and/or bowel incontinence

Impaired Social Interaction related to negative body image (eg, acne, alopecia)

Impaired Swallowing related to reddened, irritated oropharyngeal cavity

Impaired Tissue Integrity (eg, cornea, mucous membrane, integumentary, or subcutaneous) related to altered circulation, nutrition or fluid deficit or excess, impaired mobility, irritants (chemical, thermal, mechanical, radiation)

Table 37-2
Factors Placing an Individual at Risk for Skin Alterations

Factor	Nursing Implications
Lifestyle Variables	
Homosexual male, with a history of multiple sexual partners; drug users; hemophiliacs; bisexual male; partners of the above	• High-risk profile for acquired immunodeficiency syndrome (AIDS). • Assessment needs to include careful examination of the skin for purple blotches that may be indicative of Kaposi's sarcoma.
Occupation that gives a fair, thin-skinned individual prolonged exposure to the sun	• Places individual at high risk for developing skin cancer, which has an excellent prognosis if detected and treated in its early stages but which may be fatal if treatment is delayed. • Assessment needs to include careful examination for a sore that does not heal or a change in size or color of a wart or mole.
Changes in Health State	
Dehydration or malnutrition	• If fluid, protein, and vitamin C intake is deficient, skin loses elasticity and becomes prone to breakdown. • Nursing care is directed toward preventing skin breakdown: frequent changes of client's position with skin assessment at each change, special mattresses and protection of bony prominences, use of lotions, attention to fluid and nutritional status.
Reduced sensation (paralysis, local nerve damage, circulatory insufficiency)	• Client's inability to sense temperature extremes, pressure, friction, and other such factors can easily result in injury. • Nursing care incorporates special attention to safety.
Illness	
Diabetes mellitus	• Numerous factors combine to cause skin problems in diabetics: cuts and sores that do not heal, lesions on the lower extremities that ulcerate and become necrotic, recurrent bacterial and fungal infections. • The diabetic must be taught special hygiene measures to prevent trauma to the skin and learn to assess the skin carefully to detect any alteration.
Diagnostic Measures	
Gastrointestinal (GI) series	• The GI cleansing preparations administered to clients having GI studies done may result in diarrhea, which irritates the sensitive skin in the perianal area—especially if the client had bouts of diarrhea before the studies; anticipating the problem, noting redness and inflammation, and beginning warm baths and ointments are welcome nursing measures that clients may be too embarrassed to seek.
Therapeutic Measures	
Bed rest	• Bed rest predisposes clients to skin breakdown; the harsh detergents used on hospital laundry compound this problem. • Pressure points need to be examined frequently and protected.
Casts	• Casts easily irritate the skin; careful assessment, covering the rough edges of the cast, and skin care indicated.
Aquathermia unit	• Wet heat has therapeutic benefit but if applied to the skin too long may macerate the skin; follow protocol in length of application, examine skin carefully between treatments, and allow to dry.
Medications	• Medications may cause allergic skin reactions, such as rashes. • When evaluating the client's response to a new drug, examine the skin for redness and itching.

In certain situations, a wellness nursing diagnosis may be appropriate as the client progresses toward an increased level of health awareness and wellness. An example of a wellness diagnosis is as follows:

Potential for Enhanced Oral Hygiene Practices

Additional diagnoses related to specific body parts are discussed later in this chapter.

Data collected during the nursing assessment may also lead to the identification of a collaborative problem. A nurse caring for a client receiving intravenous chemotherapy should carefully check the infusion site every shift, realizing that phlebitis commonly occurs with certain chemotherapeutic agents. Careful preparation and administration of the drug according to the manufacturer's instructions, adherence to nursing protocols for the maintenance of intravenous infusions, and ongoing nursing assessment may decrease the likelihood of phlebitis. If redness, warmth, tenderness, or swelling is noted with any intravenous infusion, immediate collaborative intervention is indicated.

Similarly, a nurse may notice a 1.5-cm mole with an irregular border on a client's back during a bath. Prompt reporting of this finding to the physician may lead to the detection and early, successful treatment of the medical diagnosis of malignant melanoma.

PLANNING: EXPECTED OUTCOMES

Each plan of nursing care identifies nursing measures to assist the client to develop or maintain hygiene practices that contribute to a sense of well-being. Appropriate expected outcomes include the following. The client will:

- Verbalize feeling comfortable and clean
- Participate fully in necessary hygiene measures according to cognitive, sensory, mobility, and endurance abilities
- Maintain intact skin and mucous membranes
- Demonstrate correct skin care measures (when indicated)
- Demonstrate signs of healing in existing lesions

Expected outcomes related to specific body parts are presented later in this chapter.

IMPLEMENTING

The nurse, in performing general personal hygiene skills, respects the client's personal preferences in hygiene measures, allows and encourages as much self-care as the client can perform, meets the client's needs for privacy, and promotes physiologic and psychologic wellness. In the following sections, general hygiene measures are discussed, including providing scheduled care, helping with bathing, massaging, bedmaking, and providing environmental care. Nursing care related to specific body parts is discussed later in this chapter.

Providing Scheduled Hygienic Care

When clients require nursing assistance with personal hygiene, it is important to schedule this care at regular intervals. In most hospitals and long-term care settings, the following types of hygienic care are provided. These are individualized according to the client's personal and cultural preferences.

Early Morning Care. Shortly after awakening, the client is assisted with toileting if necessary and then provided with comfort measures to refresh the client and prepare him or her for breakfast (or diagnostic tests). Nursing measures include washing the face and hands and providing mouth care. Agency policy dictates whether the nurses on night shift or day shift are responsible for early morning care. This is an excellent time to note if the supplies needed for morning care are available and to order any that are lacking.

Morning Care (AM Care). After breakfast, the nurse completes morning care. Depending on the client's self-care abilities, the nurse offers assistance with toileting; oral care; bathing; back massage; special skin care measures (eg, pressure ulcer); hair care (includes shaving if indicated); cosmetics (if desired); dressing; and positioning for comfort. Agency policies are followed in refreshing or changing bed linens, and the client's bedside area is tidied. When morning care is completed, the client should feel refreshed and be in a comfortable and safe environment. For some clients, this may mean positioning the call light within reach and using protective devices such as bed rails or restraints.

Morning care is often characterized as self-care, partial care, or complete care. *Self-care* clients are capable of managing their personal hygiene independently once oriented to the bathroom. These clients should still be offered a back massage and receive quality nursing time directed to assessing their day-to-day needs. *Partial care* clients most often receive morning hygiene care at the bedside or seated near the sink in the bathroom. Because of weakness, these clients may be able to wash only the parts of their bodies that are within easy reach. The nurse washes the back and legs and sometimes the axillae and perineum because these body parts have the most secretions and are difficult to reach. *Complete care* clients require nursing assistance with all aspects of personal hygiene. A complete bed bath is done or the client is taken to the shower or tub.

Afternoon Care (PM Care). Because hospitalized clients frequently receive visitors in the afternoon or evening or use this time to rest when not scheduled for tests, the nurse should ensure the client's comfort after lunch and offer assistance to nonambulatory clients with toileting, handwashing, and oral care. Straightening bed linens and helping clients with mobility problems to reposition themselves comfortably are other welcome nursing measures.

Hour of Sleep Care (hs Care). Shortly before the client retires the nurse again offers assistance with toileting, washing of face and hands, and oral care. Many clients find that a back massage helps them to relax and fall asleep and this should be offered routinely. Soiled bed linens or clothing should be changed and the client positioned comfortably. If protective devices are indicated for night hours (ie, side rails or restraints) these are applied at this time. The call light and any other objects the client desires (eg, urinal, radio, water glass) should be within easy reach.

As Needed Care (prn Care). In addition to scheduled care, the nurse offers individual hygiene measures as

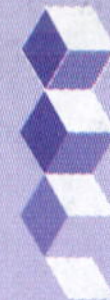

Through the Eyes of a Student

I entered the room with a feeling of dread. How could I possibly bathe the sick, elderly, helpless woman lying in this hospital bed? I had never bathed anyone older than age 2 years, other than myself, of course. How would I be able to move her limp, seemingly lifeless old body? What would an 85-year-old body look like? I could not imagine. I've read all the manuals that describe this procedure, I know what to do, so why am I so nervous? I must be worried that I will hurt her in some way. Maybe she has not been cared for properly before and her hygiene is poor. Well, I might as well get this over with because I'll be doing it the rest of my life. I've got to learn sometime.

I've mustered up enough courage to enter my client's room. Michelle, her primary nurse, offers to help me because the client is so difficult to move. Boy, am I relieved! Right before Michelle and I are about to begin, my client, Mrs. Ash, asks for her teeth. I assume this must mean her dentures and reassure her that I have not seen them but will be happy to look for them as soon as we have completed her bath. Michelle and I each take a side and begin to bathe her. It's truly amazing how those range-of-motion exercises come to mind so easily. I had thought they were long forgotten with the rest of the past semester. Wouldn't my instructors love to hear me now! Suddenly Mrs. Ash yells, "I need the bed pan!" "Oh no!" I thought, as I rushed to the bathroom with soapy gloved hands trying frantically to locate her bed pan before there could be an accident. Michelle, who remained calm during my frenzy, simply stated, "Don't worry, she has an indwelling catheter. She says that every time I bathe her." I knew she had a catheter, how did I forget? Somewhat humbled, I returned to the procedure. I really wanted to put some lotion on her skin because it was so dry. We are ready to do her back so we prepare to lift her. I pull her toward me and Michelle was to continue the bath. We were not prepared for what we saw underneath. Firmly cushioned in Mrs. Ash's lower left buttock were none other than her dentures! On removing them, Michelle and I had to smile at the periodontal grin implanted on Mrs. Ash's bottom. Michelle then asked her how her teeth had gotten to the location where we found them. All she seemed to know was that she needed those teeth back in her mouth STAT! She snatched the dentures from Michelle's hand and attempted to insert them. Michelle and I in unison blurted out, "*No,* Mrs. Ash, please wait until we clean your teeth before you put them back in your mouth!" Mrs. Ash, somewhat confused, begrudgingly handed over her teeth to be cleaned. Michelle had the honors while I finished the last touches of good hygiene for Mrs. Ash.

What a difference cleanliness can make, not only for the client but also for me, the student nurse. I felt better knowing that Mrs. Ash was clean and that this procedure was behind me. And to think that I was apprehensive! This was definitely an interesting learning experience.

—Marilyn Johnson,
Holy Family College, Philadelphia

needed. Some clients require oral care every 2 hours. Clients who are *diaphoretic* (sweating profusely) may need their clothing and bed linens changed several times a shift. At other times, a nurse may decide to forego hygienic measures because the client's need for undisturbed rest may take precedence.

Helping With Bathing

Bathing serves a variety of purposes, including the following:

- It cleanses the skin.
- It acts as a skin conditioner.
- It helps relax a restless person.
- It promotes circulation by stimulating the skin's peripheral nerve endings and underlying tissues.
- It serves as a musculoskeletal exercise through activity involved with bathing and thus improves joint mobility and muscle tonus.
- It stimulates the rate and depth of respirations.
- It promotes comfort through muscle relaxation and skin stimulation.
- It provides the person with sensory input.
- It helps improve self-image.
- It gives the nurse an excellent opportunity to strengthen the nurse–client relationship, to observe the client's physiologic and emotional status closely, to teach the client as indicated, and to demonstrate that the nurse cares for the client and is interested in the client's general welfare.

Shower and Tub Baths

Using a shower or a tub is the preferred method of bathing for hospitalized people who are ambulatory. Even though clients can, for the most part, do this on their own, the nurse still has responsibilities:

- Check to see that the bathroom is available, clean, and safe. Showers and tubs should have mats or nonskid strips to prevent the client from slipping and falling.
- Ensure that necessary articles, such as soap, a washcloth, a towel, and a gown, are available for the client.

- Provide for a place for a weak or physically disabled client to sit in a shower. Most health agencies have a stool or chair that can be used in a shower, and handheld shower heads may facilitate the process. Some nurses have reported that a commode chair with the pan removed serves effectively as a shower chair, and it offers the client more support than a stool or chair.
- Assist the client to the shower or bathroom, as indicated. Clients who are beginning ambulation need assistance to help prevent falling and fainting.
- Check to see that the water temperature is safe and comfortable, 43° to 46°C (110° to 115°F).
- Help the client get in and out of a bathtub, as indicated. Have the client grasp handrails at the side of the tub, or place a chair at the side of the tub. The client sits on the chair and eases to the edge of the tub. After putting both feet into the tub, it is then relatively easy for the client to reach the opposite side and ease down into the tub. The client may kneel first in the tub and then sit in it, and can leave the tub in the same manner. Use a hydraulic lift, when available, to lower and lift a helpless and heavy client in and out of a tub.
- Ensure privacy for the client who is safe to shower or bathe independently. See to it that a call device is handy so that the client can obtain help if necessary.
- Keep the bathroom door unlocked. Health personnel should be able to enter with ease if the client needs help. A sign hung on the door ensures privacy. Children should never be left alone in bathrooms.
- Help wash and dry areas of the body that the client cannot reach, such as the back.

Figure 37-2 illustrates several features that add to the safety of a client who takes a shower or tub bath.

Bed Baths

Some clients must remain in bed as a part of their therapeutic regimen, but they are able to bathe themselves. The nurse helps the client who takes a bath in bed in several ways:

- Provide the client with articles for bathing. Provide a basin of water that is of a comfortable and safe temperature. Place these items conveniently for the client on a bedside stand or overbed table.
- Provide privacy for the client. See to it that the call device is within reach.
- Remove top linens on the client's bed while replacing them with a bath blanket.
- Place cosmetics in a convenient place for the client's use. Provide a mirror, a good light, and hot water for the client who wishes to shave with a razor.
- Assist clients who cannot bathe themselves completely. For example, some clients are able to wash only the upper parts of the body. The remainder of the bath is then completed by nursing personnel.

Bathing procedures for the client who requires total nursing assistance vary among health agencies. The one described in Procedure 37-1 is offered as a guide. It assumes that the client is able to be raised or lowered in bed and that, although the client may have limited movement, it is possible for the nurse to manage the client alone.

Towel Baths

The in-bed towel bath, or lotion bath, uses a quick-drying solution containing a cleaning agent, a disinfectant, and a softening agent mixed with water that is 43.3° to 48.9°C (110° to 120°F). A commonly used solution developed cooperatively by a nurse and Vestal Laboratories is called Septi-Soft. A recommended procedure for giving the towel bath follows:

- Place a terry cloth towel, about 3 × 7 feet, in a plastic bag, and saturate it with the warmed cleaning solution.
- Wring out the towel well and unroll it over the client while simultaneously removing the upper bed linens.
- Fold an extra amount of the towel under the client's chin for later use.

(text continues on page 927)

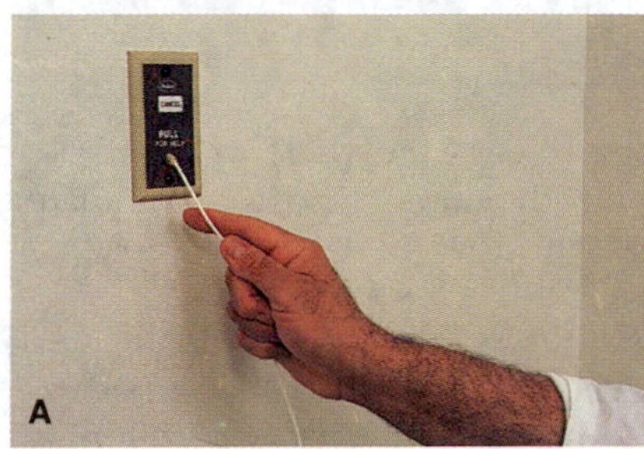

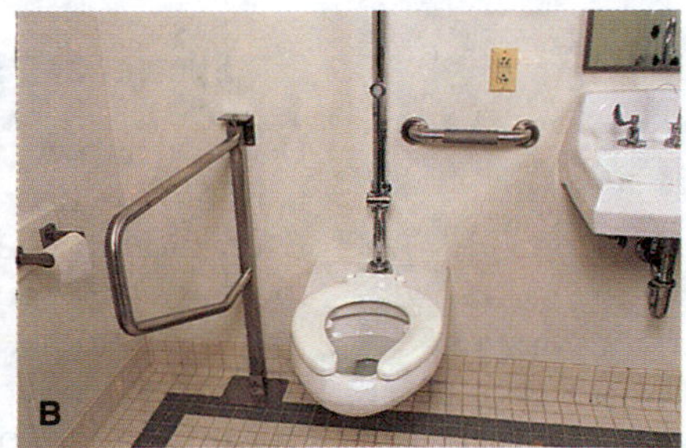

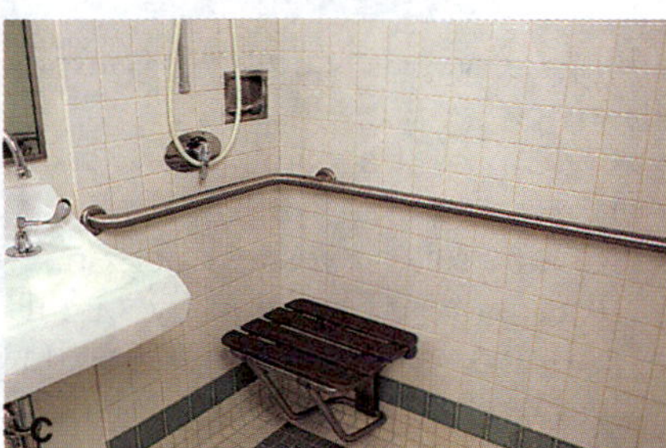

Figure 37-2
Examples of features that add to the safety of a client in bed: **(A)** a call bell equipped with a pull cord, **(B)** hand rails for use with the commode, and **(C)** a shower equipped with a safety seat. (Photos © B. Proud.)

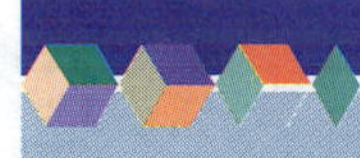

PROCEDURE 37-1

Giving a Bed Bath

Equipment

Wash basin
Soap and dish
Washcloths
Bath blanket
Gown or pajamas
Bed linen
Towels (2)
Disposable gloves—for anal and perineal care (optional for remainder of bath)
Personal hygiene supplies—deodorant, lotion, and others
Bedpan or urinal
Laundry bag or cart

Action	Rationale
1. Discuss procedure with the client and assess the client's ability to assist in the bathing process as well as personal hygiene preferences. Review the client's chart for any limitations in physical activity.	This discussion promotes reassurance and provides knowledge about the procedure. Dialogue also encourages client participation and allows for individualized nursing care.
2. Bring necessary equipment to the bedside stand or overbed table. Remove sequential compression devices and antiembolism stockings from lower extremities according to agency protocol.	Bringing everything to the bedside conserves time and energy. Arranging items nearby is convenient, saves time, and helps prevent unnecessary stretching and twisting of muscles on the part of the nurse. Most manufacturers and agencies recommend removal of these devices during the bath to allow for assessment.
3. Close the curtains around the bed and close the door to the room if possible.	This ensures the client's privacy and lessens the possibility of loss of body heat during the bath.
4. Offer the client the bedpan or urinal.	Voiding or defecating before the bath lessens the likelihood that the bath will be interrupted, because warm bath water may stimulate the urge to void.
5. Wash your hands.	Handwashing deters the spread of microorganisms.
6. Raise the client's bed to the high position.	Having the bed in a high position prevents strain on the nurse's back.
7. Lower the side rail nearer to you and assist the client to the side of the bed where you will work. Have the client lie on his or her back.	Having the client positioned near the nurse and lowering the side rail help prevent unnecessary stretching and twisting of muscles on the part of the nurse.
8. Loosen top covers and remove all except the top sheet. Place bath blanket over the client and then remove the top sheet while the client holds the bath blanket in place. If linen is to be reused, fold it over a chair. Place soiled linen in the laundry bag.	The client is not exposed unnecessarily and warmth is maintained. If a bath blanket is unavailable, the top sheet may be used in place of the bath blanket.
9. Assist the client with oral hygiene, as necessary, and as described in Procedure 37-5.	This helps maintain teeth and gums in good condition, alleviates unpleasant odor and taste, and may improve appetite. Some clients may prefer oral care after the bath is completed.
10. Remove the client's gown and keep the bath blanket in place. If client has an intravenous line, remove the gown from the other arm first. Lower the intravenous container and pass the gown over the tubing and the container. Rehang the container and check the drip rate.	This provides uncluttered access during the bath and maintains warmth of the client. Intravenous fluids must be maintained at the prescribed rate.

(continued)

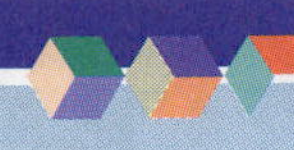

PROCEDURE 37-1 *(continued)*

Giving a Bed Bath

Action	Rationale
11. Raise the side rail. Fill the basin with a sufficient amount of comfortably warm water (between 43° and 46°C [110° to 115°F]). Change as necessary throughout the bath. Lower the side rail closer to you when you return to the bedside to begin the bath.	Warm water is comfortable and relaxing for the client. It also stimulates circulation and provides for more effective cleansing. Side rails maintain client safety.
12. Fold the washcloth like a mitt on your hand so there are no loose ends, as illustrated.	Having loose ends of cloth drag across the client's skin is uncomfortable. Loose ends cool quickly and will feel cold to the client.

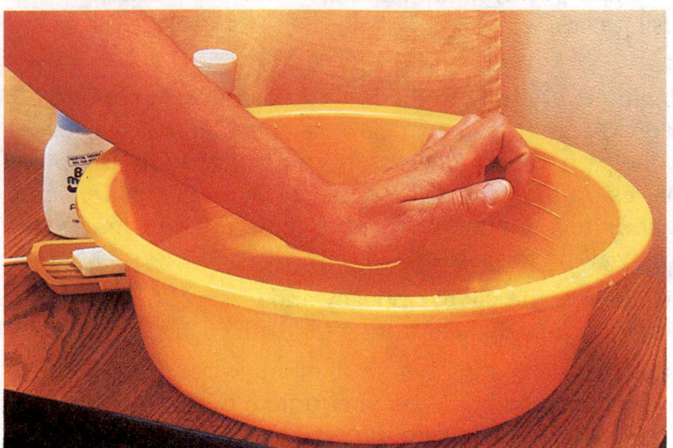

Action 11: Testing water temperature.

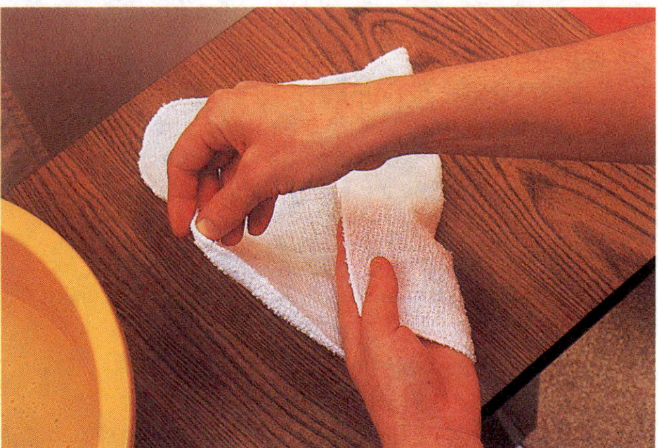

Action 12: Folding washcloth in thirds around hand to make a bath mitt.

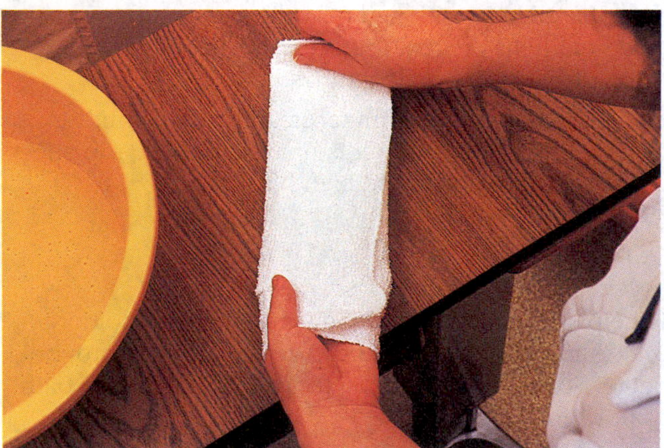

Action 12: Straightening washcloth before folding into mitt.

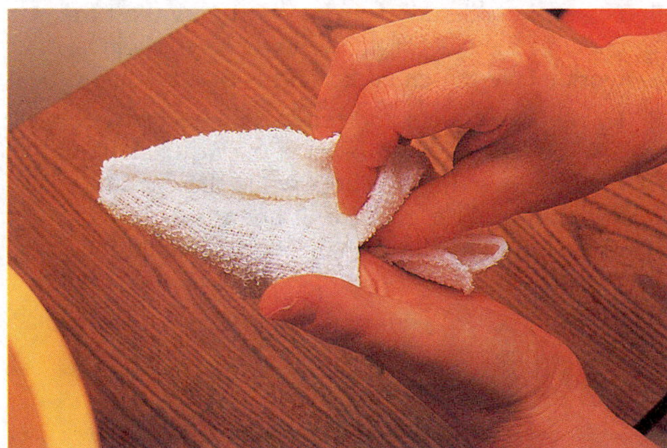

Action 12: Folding ends over and tucking ends under folded washcloth over palm.

Action	Rationale
13. Lay a towel across the client's chest and on top of the bath blanket.	This prevents chilling and keeps the bath blanket dry.

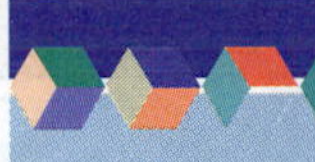

PROCEDURE 37-1 *(continued)*

Giving a Bed Bath

Action	Rationale
14. With no soap on the washcloth, wipe one eye from the inner part of the eye, near the nose, to the outer part. Rinse or turn the cloth before washing the other eye.	Rinsing or turning the washcloth prevents spreading organisms from one eye to the other. Soap is irritating to the eyes. Moving from the inner to the outer aspect of the eye prevents carrying debris toward the nasolacrimal duct.

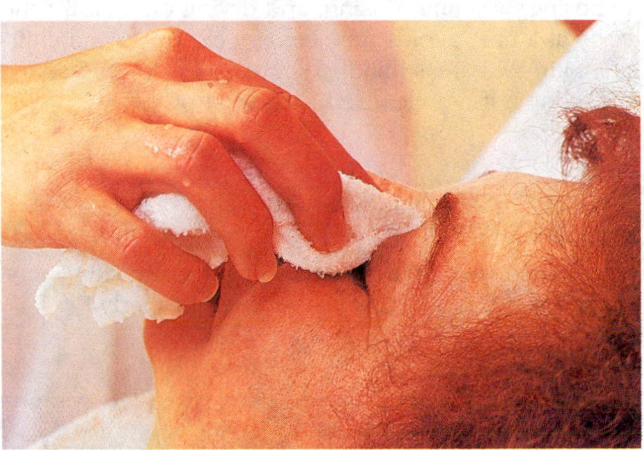

Action 14: Washing from the inner corner of the eye outward.

Action	Rationale
15. Bathe the client's face, neck, and ears, avoiding soap on the face if the client prefers.	Soap can be drying and may be avoided as a matter of personal preference.
16. Expose the far arm of the client and place the towel lengthwise under it. Using firm strokes, wash the arm and axilla, rinse, and dry.	The towel helps to keep the bed dry. Washing the far side first eliminates contaminating a clean area once it is washed. Gentle friction stimulates circulation and muscles and helps remove dirt, oil, and organisms. Long, firm strokes are relaxing and more comfortable than short, uneven strokes.
17. Place a folded towel on the bed next to the client's hand and put the basin on it. Soak the client's hand in the basin. Wash, rinse, and dry the hand.	Placing the hands in the basin of water is comfortable and relaxing for the client, allows for a thorough washing of the hands and between the fingers, and facilitates removal of debris from under the nails.

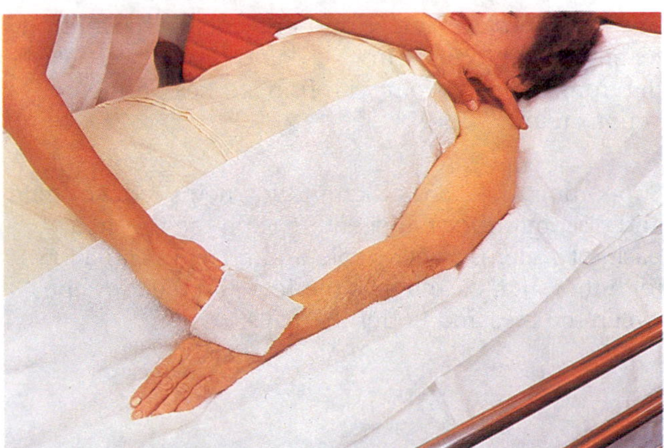

Action 16: Exposing the far arm and washing.

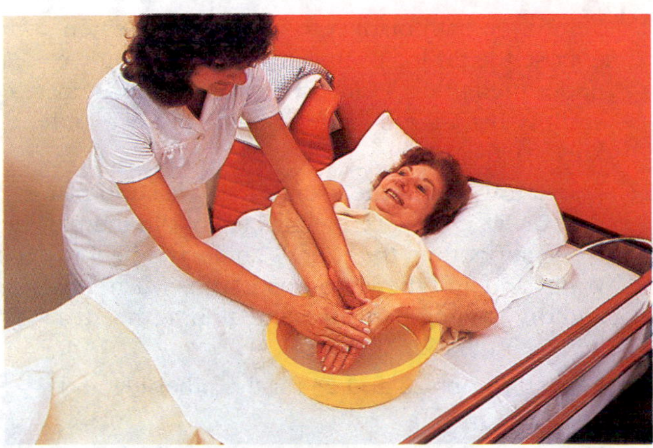

Action 17: Soaking hand in basin.

(continued)

PROCEDURE 37-1 *(continued)*

Giving a Bed Bath

Action	Rationale
18. Repeat actions 16 and 17 for the arm nearer to you. (An option for the shorter nurse or one prone to back strain might be to bathe one side of the client and move to the other side of the bed to complete the bath.)	
19. Spread a towel across the client's chest. Lower the bath blanket to the client's umbilical area. Wash, rinse, and dry the client's chest. Keep the client's chest covered with the towel between the wash and rinse. Pay special attention to skin folds under the breasts of clients.	Exposing, washing, rinsing, and drying one part of the body at a time avoids unnecessary exposure and chilling. Skin fold areas may be sources of odor and skin breakdown if not cleansed and dried properly.
20. Lower the bath blanket to the client's perineal area. Place a towel over the client's chest.	Keeping the bath blanket and towel in place avoids exposure and chilling.
21. Wash, rinse, and dry the client's abdomen. Carefully inspect and cleanse the umbilical area and any abdominal folds or creases.	Skin-fold areas may be sources of odor and skin breakdown if not cleansed and dried properly.

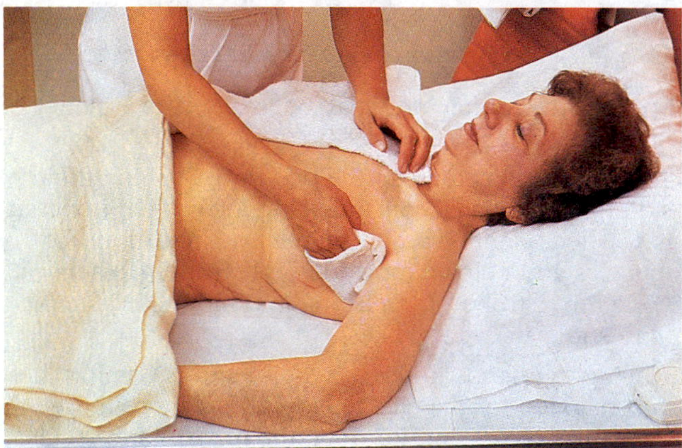

Action 19: Washing the chest area, including the axillae.

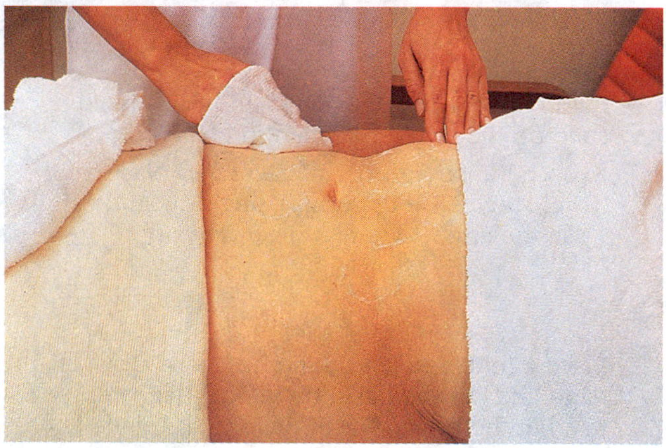

Action 21: Washing the abdomen, with perineal and chest areas covered.

Action	Rationale
22. Return the bath blanket to its original position and expose the far leg of the client. Place the towel under the far leg. Using firm strokes, wash, rinse, and dry the client's leg from ankle to knee and knee to groin.	The towel protects linens and prevents the client from feeling uncomfortable from a damp or wet bed. Washing from ankle to groin with firm strokes promotes venous return.
23. Fold a towel near the client's foot area and place the basin on it. Place the client's foot in the basin while supporting the client's ankle and heel in your hand and the leg on your arm. Wash, rinse, and dry, paying particular attention to the area between the toes.	Supporting the client's foot and leg helps reduce strain and discomfort for the client. Placing the feet in a basin of water is comfortable and relaxing and allows for a thorough cleaning of the feet and the areas between the toes and under the nails.
24. Repeat actions 22 and 23 for the other leg and foot.	
25. Make sure the client is covered with the bath blanket. Change water at this point or earlier if necessary. Assist the client onto his or her side.	The bath blanket maintains warmth and privacy. Clean, warm water prevents chilling and maintains the client's comfort.

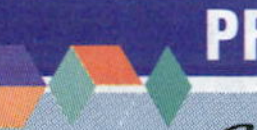

PROCEDURE 37-1 *(continued)*

Giving a Bed Bath

Action	**Rationale**

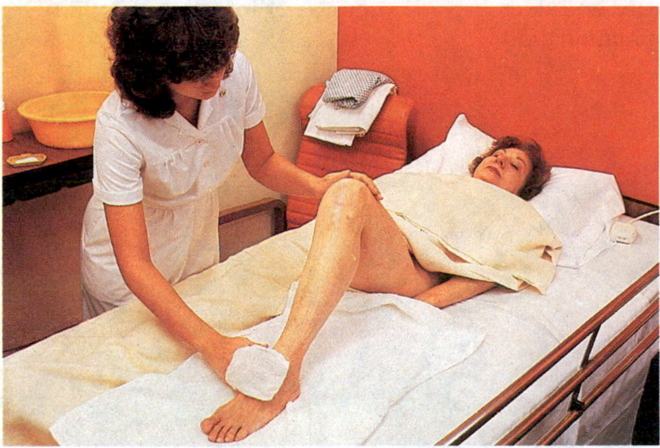

Action 22: Washing and drying far leg, keeping other leg covered.

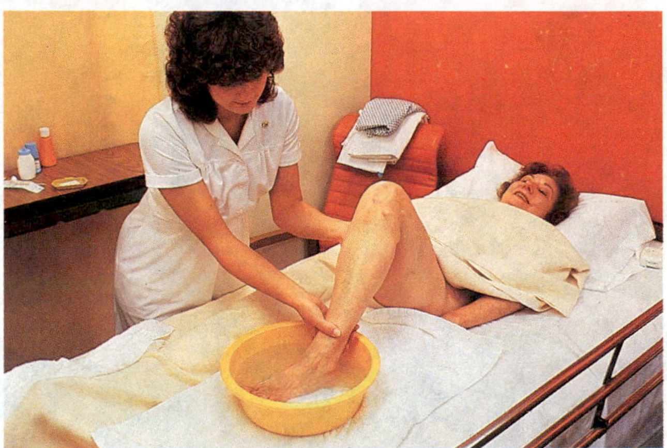

Action 23: Soaking the foot in basin.

Action	Rationale
26. Assist the client to a prone or side-lying position. Position the bath blanket and towel to expose only the back and buttocks.	Positioning of the towel and bath blanket protects the client's privacy and provides warmth.
27. Wash, rinse, and dry the client's back and buttocks area. Pay particular attention to cleansing between gluteal folds and observe for any indication of redness or skin breakdown in the sacral area.	Fecal material near the anus may be a source of microorganisms. Prolonged pressure on the sacral area or other bony prominences may compromise circulation and lead to development of decubitus ulcer.
28. If not contraindicated, give the client a back rub, as described in Procedure 41-1. Back massage may be given also after perineal care.	A back rub improves circulation to the tissues and is an aid to relaxation. A back rub may be contraindicated in clients with cardiovascular disease or musculoskeletal injuries.

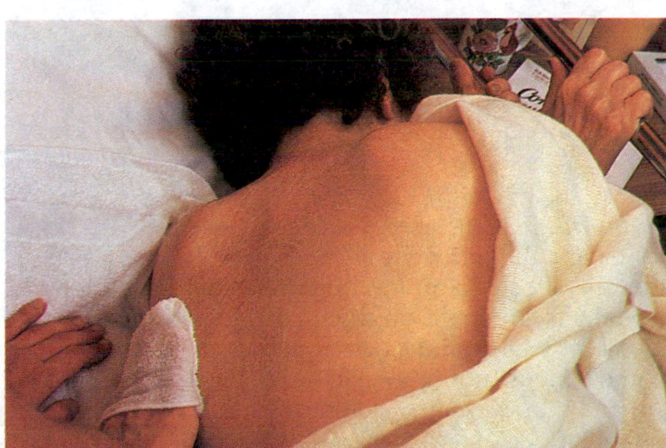

Action 27: Washing the upper back.

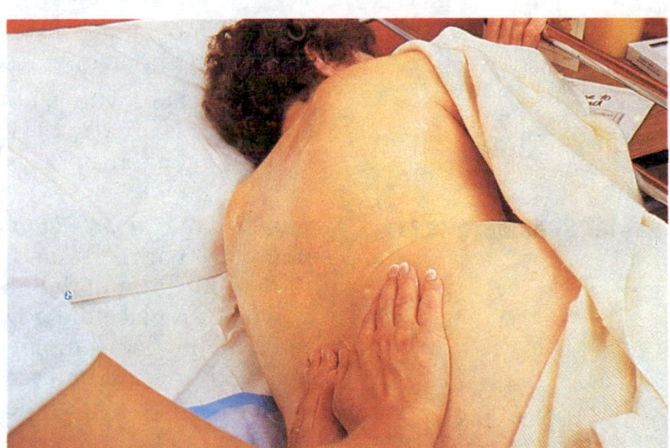

Action 28: Giving a backrub, after washing lower back.

Action	Rationale
29. Refill basin with clean water. Discard washcloth and towel.	The washcloth, towel, and water are contaminated after washing the client's gluteal area. Changing to clean supplies decreases the spread of organisms from the anal area to the genitals.

(continued)

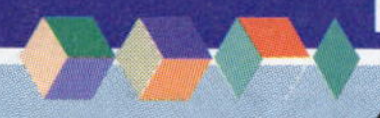

PROCEDURE 37-1 *(continued)*

Giving a Bed Bath

Action	Rationale
30. Clean the client's perineal area or set up the client so he or she can complete perineal self-care.	Providing perineal self-care may decrease embarrassment for the client. Effective perineal care reduces odor and decreases the chance of infection through contamination.

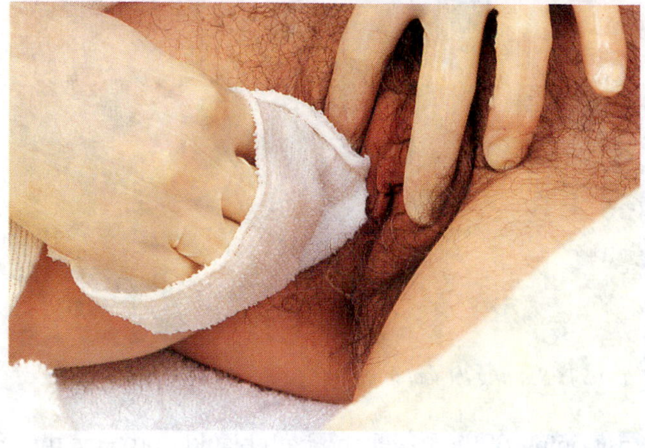

Action 30: Cleansing the perineal area.

Action	Rationale
31. Help the client put on a clean gown and attend to personal hygiene needs.	This provides for the client's warmth and comfort.
32. Protect the pillow with a towel, and groom the client's hair, as described in the text.	
33. Change bed linens, as described in Procedures 37-3 and 37-4.	
34. Record any significant observations and communication on the client's chart.	A careful record is important for planning and individualizing the client's care.

Age Considerations

When bathing an infant or young child, have supplies within easy reach and support or hold the child securely at all times to ensure safety. Never leave the child alone.

Check temperature of water, particularly before bathing an older client because sensitivity to temperature may be impaired.

An older client who is not incontinent may not require a full bed bath with soap and water every day. If dry skin is a problem, water and skin lotion or bath oil may be used on alternate days.

Special Considerations

Removal of gown if client has an intravenous line necessitates taking the gown off, uninvolved arm first, and then threading the intravenous tubing and bottle or bag through the arm of the gown after the affected arm has been removed from the gown. To replace the gown, place the clean gown on the unaffected arm first and thread intravenous tubing and bottle or bag from inside the arm of the gown on the involved side. *Never* disconnect intravenous tubing to change a gown because this causes a break in a sterile system and introduces the potential for infection.

Lying flat in bed during the bed bath may be contraindicated for certain clients. Position may have to be modified to accommodate their needs.

Perineal care for a client with an indwelling catheter may vary based on agency protocol. Refer to Chapter 43 for suggested techniques for care.

Change water as often as necessary to maintain at a comfortable temperature. Always change the water after performing perineal care or when the water is soiled.

Home Care Considerations

Evaluate the safety of the bathing area in the home. Tub mats, adhesive strips, grab bars, and shower stools are helpful accessories to prevent falls.

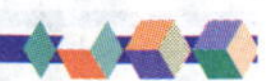

- Use a massaging motion to clean the body, beginning with the client's feet and working up the body.
- Fold the towel upward as the bath proceeds while a clean sheet is unfolded over the client.
- Cleanse the client's face, neck, and ears with the part of the towel that is folded under the chin.
- Fold the towel into quarters, soiled side turned in, and turn the client to the side. The folded towel is used to wash the back and buttocks.
- Remove the towel after finishing the bath. The back may then be rubbed.
- Place clean linen on the bed, and dress and position the client.
- The client need not be dried because the cleaning solution dries in a matter of seconds.

According to reports, the towel bath can be accomplished with little fatigue to the client; the towel remains warm during the short procedure; clients state that they feel clean and refreshed; and the oil in the bathing solution eliminates dry, itchy skin. Rader (1994) commented that cognitively impaired residents of a long-term care facility viewed the towel bath as a preferable alternative to the standard bathing experience. Miller (1994) also discovered that this population is more prone to display inappropriate behavior during the typical bath/shower routine because these residents may perceive it as a physical assault. The towel bath and linen change take about 10 minutes. The brevity of the bath may be its greatest disadvantage. The nurse has less time with his or her clients than when giving the traditional bath in bed, which is especially important for developing a helping relationship.

The "Bag Bath"

The "bag bath" developed by Skewes (1994) is a variation of the towel bath. Some healthcare agencies recommend this alternative as standard practice in their facility. Equipment for a bag bath consists of a plastic bag containing 10 wash cloths that have been moistened with a nonrinsable cleaner and water mixture and warmed for a short time (approximately a minute and a half) in the microwave. The nurse is advised to experiment to find the appropriate time that warms the contents of the plastic bag to a safe temperature. Each part of the client's body is cleansed with a fresh cloth. The skin is allowed to air dry (approximately 30 seconds), permitting the emollient ingredient of the cleaner to remain on the skin. Feedback about this procedure has been overwhelmingly positive. Staff value the time savings when compared with a traditional bed bath and find it effective and easy to perform. The majority of clients commented very favorably on the bag bath. Those clients with mild to moderate skin impairment demonstrated improvement in the condition of their skin when the bag bath was used consistently. Figure 37-3 demonstrates a nurse preparing to give a bag bath to a client.

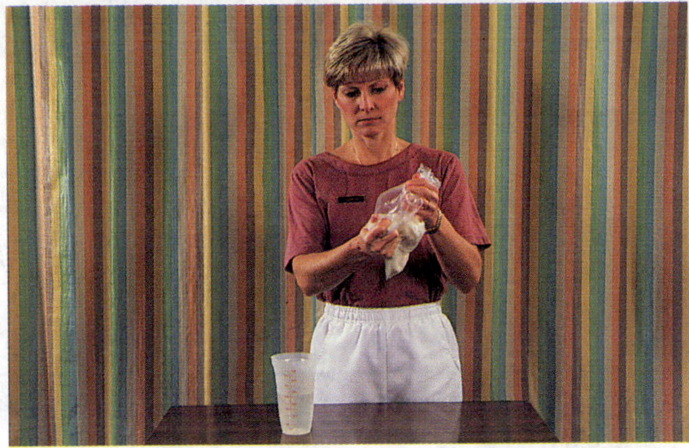

Figure 37-3
Bag bath. The nurse mixes the solution with the disposable cloths to distribute warmth evenly after bag bath has been warmed in the microwave. (Photo © B. Proud.)

Assisting With Antiembolism Stockings

Antiembolism stockings are often used for clients with limited activity to help prevent phlebitis and thrombi formation (these conditions are described in Chapter 39). They are made of elastic material, are manufactured by several companies, and are available in either knee-high or thigh-high length. Antiembolism stockings help force blood in superficial veins of the legs to deeper veins, prevent stagnation of blood in the veins of the legs, and promote venous return to the heart. A physician's order is required for their use.

Antiembolism stockings should always be removed during morning care, the legs inspected, and the stockings reapplied before the client is out of bed, as shown in Procedure 37-2. General nursing guidelines for assisting with antiembolism stockings follow:

- Measure the client's leg to ensure that a proper size stocking is used. The manufacturer whose stockings are being used gives directions for measuring. Some stockings fit either leg; others are designated right or left. An improperly fitting stocking is uncomfortable, ineffective, and may even harm the client.
- Be prepared to apply the stockings in the morning before the client is out of bed and while the client is supine. If the client is sitting or has been up and about, have the client lie down with legs and feet well elevated for at least 15 minutes before applying the stockings. After the leg vessels are congested with blood, the effectiveness of the stockings is defeated.
- Do not massage the legs. If a clot is present, it may break away from the vessel wall and circulate in the bloodstream.
- Be sure the client's heel is well positioned in the stocking. The purpose of the stocking is likely to be defeated if it is applied improperly.

(text continues on page 930)

PROCEDURE 37-2

Applying Antiembolism Stockings

Equipment

Elastic stockings (in correct size)

For knee-high stockings

- Measure from heel to popliteal space
- Measure circumference of calf at widest point

Measuring tape

Talcum powder (optional)

For thigh-high stockings

- Measure from heel to gluteal fold
- Measure circumference of calf and thigh at widest point

Action	Rationale
1. Explain the rationale for use of elastic stockings to the client	Explanation encourages the client's cooperation.
2. Wash your hands.	Handwashing deters the spread of microorganisms.
3. Assist the client to the supine position. If the client has been sitting or walking, it is necessary to have him or her lie down with the legs and feet well elevated for at least 15 minutes before applying the stockings.	Dependent position of legs encourages blood to pool in the veins.
4. Provide privacy. Expose legs one at a time, and powder lightly unless client has dry skin. If the skin is dry, a lotion may be used. Powders and lotions are not recommended by some manufacturers.	Powder and lotion reduce friction and make application of stockings easier.
5. Place hand inside stocking and grasp heel area securely. Turn stocking inside out to the heel area.	Inside-out technique provides for easier application and less compromising of circulation to the extremity from bunched elastic material.

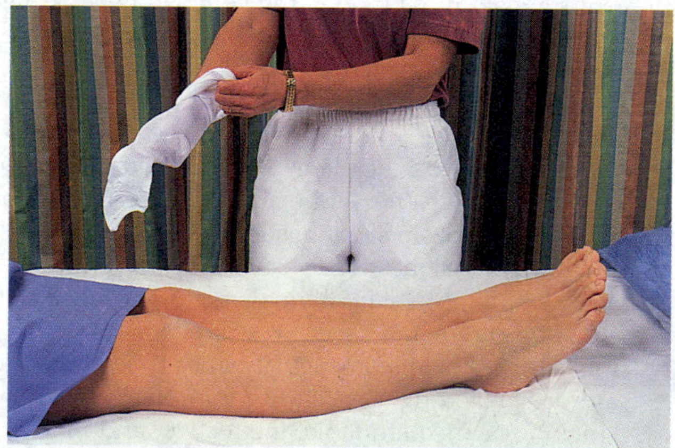

Action 5a: Inserting hand into stocking to grasp heel area.

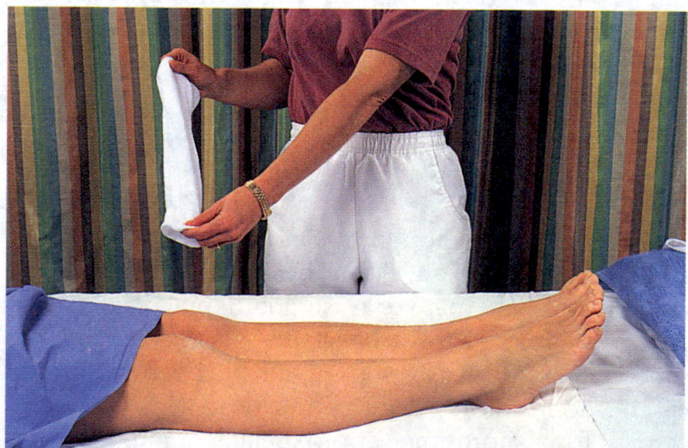

Action 5b: Turning stocking inside out to the heel pocket area.

Action	Rationale
6. Ease the foot of the stocking over the client's foot and heel. Check that client's heel is centered in heel pocket of stocking.	Wrinkles or improper fit interfere with circulation.
7. Using your fingers and thumbs carefully grasp the edge of the stocking and pull it up smoothly over the ankle and calf until entire stocking is turned right side out. Pull forward slightly on toe section. Repeat for the other leg. Caution the client not to roll stockings partially down.	Easing the stocking carefully into position ensures proper fit of the stocking to the contour of the leg. Rolling stockings may have a constricting effect on veins. Loosening the toe section provides for comfort in that area.

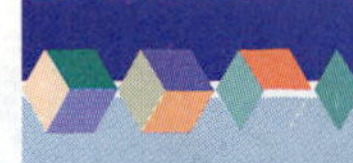

PROCEDURE 37-2 *(continued)*

Applying Antiembolism Stockings

Action	Rationale

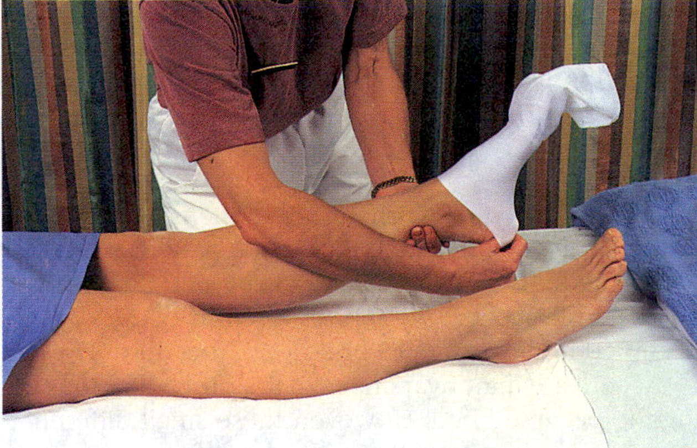

Action 6: Stretching stocking open and easing the foot of the stocking over the client's foot.

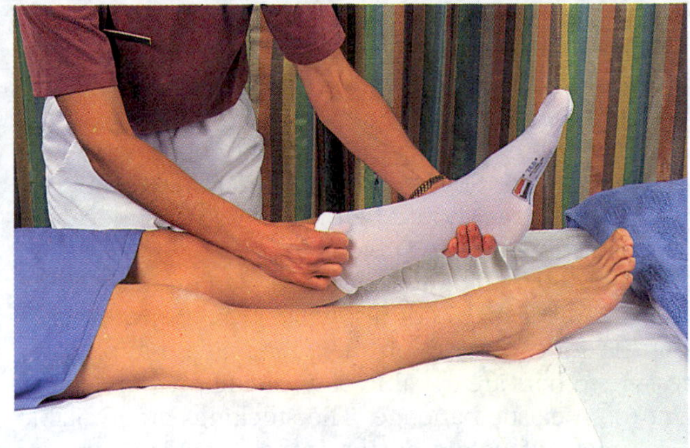

Action 7: Grasping top of stocking to pull up over calf.

Action	Rationale
8. Wash your hands.	Handwashing deters the spread of infection.
9. To remove stocking, grasp the top of the stocking with your thumb and fingers and smoothly pull the stocking off inside out to heel. Support the client's foot and ease stocking over it.	This preserves elasticity and contour of the stocking.
10. Remove stockings once every shift for 20 to 30 minutes. Wash and air dry as necessary (according to manufacturer's directions).	This allows observation of the client's circulatory status and condition of the skin on the lower extremity.
11. Record the application of elastic stockings as well as assessment of the client's circulatory status and skin condition.	This provides accurate documentation of the procedure.

Home Care Considerations

Make sure that the client has an extra pair of stockings ordered during the hospitalization before discharge (for payment and convenience purposes).

Stockings may be laundered with other "white" clothing. Avoid excessive bleach. Remove from dryer as soon as "low heat" cycle is complete to avoid shrinkage. May also be air dried.

Special Considerations

At times, despite the use of elastic stockings, a client may develop thrombophlebitis. A positive Homans' sign (pain on dorsiflexion of the foot) may be an indication of a deep thrombosis or development of a blood clot in the calf.

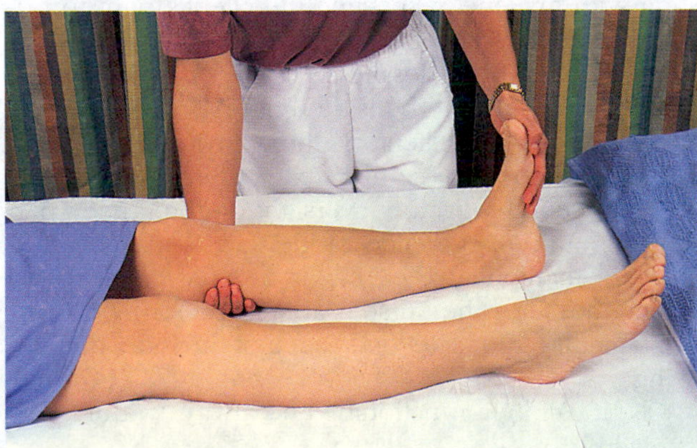

Special consideration: Checking of Homans' sign.

- Pull the toes of the stockings slightly to relieve pressure on the toes after the stockings are in place if they have no toe openings.
- Check the legs regularly for redness, blistering, swelling, and pain. Some people recommend checking the legs at least once every 8 hours; others recommend twice a day. The stockings should be removed completely once a day to bathe the legs and feet.
- Launder the stockings as necessary but at least every 3 days. Soiled stockings irritate the skin. The stockings should be dried on a flat surface to prevent them from stretching.

Several manufacturers produce men's and women's hose that are capable of applying pressure to the legs from the foot to midthigh or higher. Some apply mild pressure; others are capable of applying pressure equivalent to an elastic bandage. The stockings are available in a variety of colors so that other stockings are not needed to cover them for the ambulatory person. Many people who are on their feet or remain in one position a great deal, such as homemakers, nurses, salespeople, and business people, find them useful. The stockings should be fitted correctly to the person's measurements. Also, they should be applied immediately on awakening, before getting out of bed and before the legs are in a dependent position.

Applying Intermittent Pneumatic Compression Stockings

Intermittent pneumatic compression stockings may be used in conjunction with antiembolism stockings. They require a physician's order and are often prescribed for high-risk surgical clients, individuals with chronic venous disease, and clients at risk for deep venous disorders. They consist of a knee-length or thigh-high cuff that is connected to hoses and a pump apparatus. Sequential compression stockings promote venous return by simulating the normal muscle-pumping action in the legs. The stockings are described further in Chapter 30.

Massaging the Back

A back rub generally follows the client's bath. This acts as a general body conditioner. It can be used as a stimulant or a relaxant, or both. Meek (1993) commented on the importance of touch and back massage for the relaxation of terminally ill individuals. Giving a back rub provides an opportunity for the nurse to observe the skin for signs of breakdown. It improves circulation and provides a means of communication with the client through the use of touch.

Because some clients may consider the back rub a luxury and be reluctant to accept it, the nurse should simply say to the client, "Now it is time for your back massage." An effective back rub should take 4 to 6 minutes to complete. A lotion for massaging the back is usually used. For the comfort of the client, the lotion should be warmed before applying it to the back. The nurse should be aware of the client's diagnosis when a back rub is being considered. A back rub is contraindicated, for example, when the client has had back surgery or has fractured ribs. Position the client on the abdomen or, if this is contraindicated, on the side for a back rub. Recommended techniques for administering a back rub are outlined in Procedure 41-1.

Bedmaking

It is usual procedure to change bed linens after the bath but some agencies change linens only when soiled. The bed is made for the ambulatory client in the manner described in Procedure 37-3. If the client is bedridden, the occupied bed is made according to Procedure 37-4.

There are minor variations in the procedure for making the occupied bed. However, these small differences have no real effect on the client's comfort. In some instances it is necessary for nurses to devise unique ways to change the linens on a client's bed because of the nature of the client's condition, orthopedic appliances on the bed, or treatments that may be in progress.

Providing Environmental Care

Bedside Unit

Because the client's environment contributes positively or negatively to the sense of well-being, the nurse ensures that the *bedside unit*, the furnishings and equipment in the space surrounding the client's bed, is clean, safe, and pleasant. Basic furniture includes the bed, overbed table, bedside stand, and chairs. Standard equipment in the healthcare environment includes the call light, oxygen, suction, and electrical outlets; light fixtures; bath basin; emesis basin; bedpan or urinal; water pitcher and glass; and bed linens. A nursing responsibility is ensuring that necessary equipment and items are in their proper place and functioning properly.

Because the client's personal items are generally stored in the bedside stand, the nurse should request permission of the alert client before opening the stand to obtain the bath basin, lotion, or other items. When assisting with hygiene, respecting the client's right to privacy and ownership of personal goods decreases the client's sense of powerlessness.

Before leaving the bedside unit, it is good nursing practice to say to the client, "Is there anything else I can do to make you more comfortable?" Checking with the client compensates for any oversight on the nurse's part and communicates genuine caring. Limits may need to be set for manipulative clients as to what comfort and hygiene measures the nurse is able to perform.

Elements of a safe bedside unit include the following:

- Client call light functioning and always within reach

(text continues on page 939)

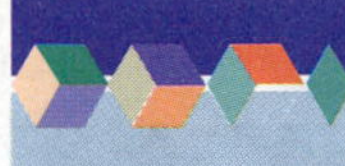

PROCEDURE 37-3

Making an Unoccupied Bed

Equipment

Two large sheets (or one large sheet and one fitted sheet)
Drawsheet
Blankets
Bedspread
Pillowcases
Linen hamper or bag
Bedside chair
Protective pad (optional)

Action	Rationale
1. Wash your hands.	Handwashing deters the spread of microorganisms.
2. Assemble equipment and arrange on a bedside chair in the order in which items will be used.	Organization facilitates performance of task.
3. Adjust the client's bed to the high position, and drop the bed side rails.	Having the bed in the high position and the side rails down reduces strain on the nurse while working.
4. Check bed linens for the client's personal items and disconnect call bell or any tubes from bed linens.	It is costly and inconvenient when personal belongings are lost.
5. Loosen all linen as you move around the bed from the head of the bed on the far side to the head of the bed on the near side.	Loosening linen helps prevent tugging and tearing on linen. Loosening the linen and moving around the bed systematically reduce strain caused by reaching across the bed.
6. Fold reusable linens, such as sheets, blankets, or spread, in place on the bed in fourths and hang them over a clean chair.	Folding saves time and energy when reusable linen is replaced on the bed. Folding linens while they are on the bed reduces strain on the nurse's arms. Some agencies change linens only when soiled.
7. Snugly roll all of the soiled linen inside of the bottom sheet and place directly into the laundry hamper. Do not place them on the floor or on furniture. Do not hold soiled linens against your uniform.	Rolling soiled linens snugly and placing them directly into the hamper helps prevent the spread of organisms. The floor is heavily contaminated; soiled linen will further contaminate furniture. Soiled linen contaminates the nurse's uniform, and this may spread organisms to another client.

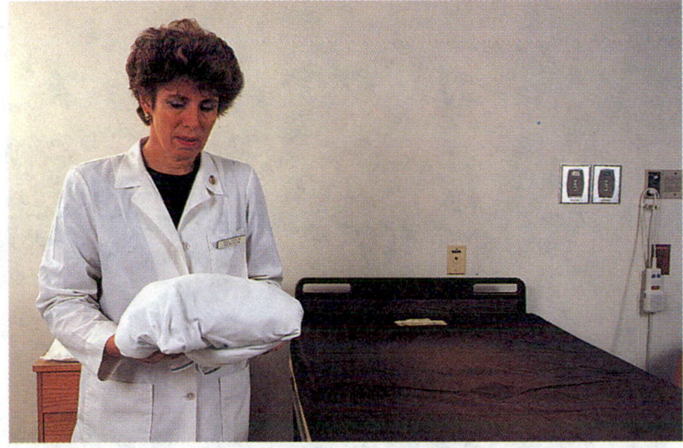

Action 7: Bundling soiled linens in bottom sheet and holding away from body.

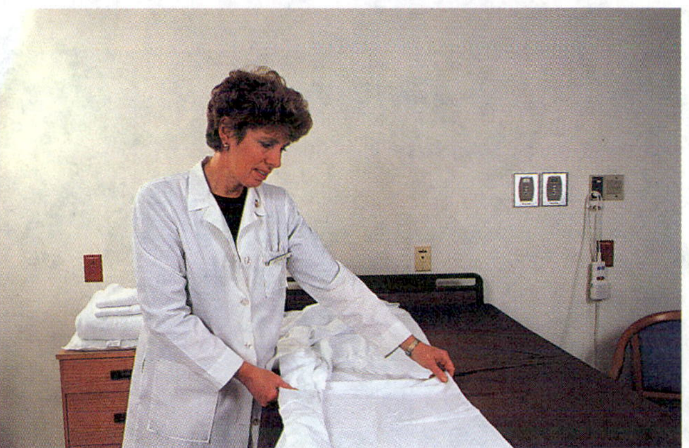

Action 9: Placing clean linens to begin bed making.

(continued)

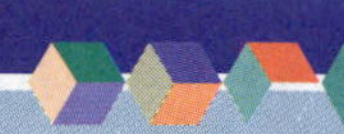

PROCEDURE 37-3 *(continued)*

Making an Unoccupied Bed

Action	Rationale
8. Grasp mattress securely and shift up to the head of the bed.	This allows more foot room for the client and moves the mattress against the head of the bed.
9. Place the bottom sheet with its center fold in the center of the bed and high enough to have a sufficient amount of the sheet to tuck under the head of the mattress.	Opening linens on the bed reduces strain on the nurse's arms and diminishes the spread of organisms.
10. Place the drawsheet with its center fold in the center of the bed and positioned so it will be located under the client's midsection. If a protective pad is used, place it over the drawsheet in the proper area. Not all agencies use drawsheets routinely. The nurse may decide to use one.	When a client soils the bed, drawsheets can be changed without the bottom and top linens on the bed. Having all bottom linens in place before tucking them under the mattress avoids unnecessary moving about the bed. A drawsheet also is an aid when moving the client in bed.
11. Tuck the bottom sheet securely under the head of the mattress on one side of the bed, making a corner according to agency policy. A mitered corner is shown in the illustrations. Using a fitted bottom sheet eliminates the need to miter corners. Tuck the remaining bottom sheet and drawsheet securely under the mattress. (At this point, before moving to the other side of the bed, top linens may be placed on the bed, unfolded, and secured, allowing the entire side of the bed to be completed at one time as shown in the illustrations.)	Making the bed on one side and then completing the bed on the other side saves time. Having bottom linens free of wrinkles reduces discomfort to the bedridden client.
12. Move to the other side of the bed to secure bottom linens. Secure top of sheet under the head of the mattress and miter the corner. Pull remainder of sheet tightly and tuck under mattress. Do the same for the drawsheet.	This rids bottom linens of any wrinkles that can cause discomfort for the client.

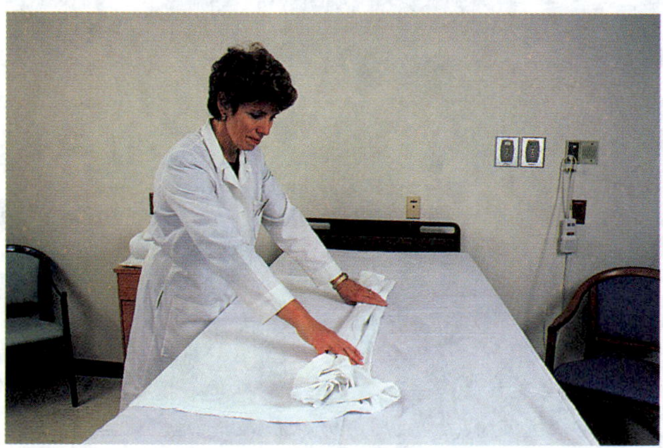

Action 10: Placing the drawsheet on the bed.

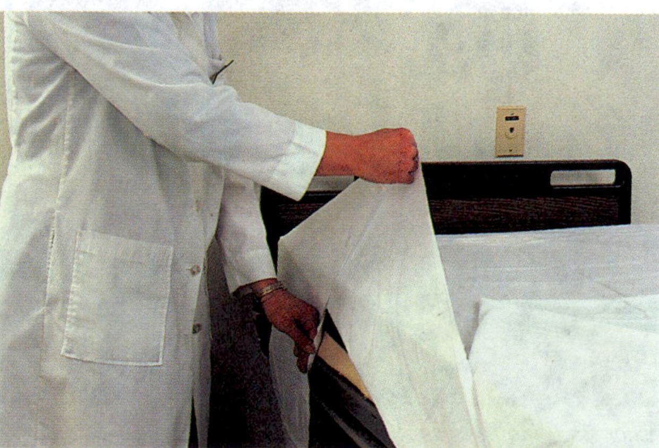

Action 11a: Beginning to make mitered corner by creating a triangular fold.

PROCEDURE 37-3 *(continued)*

Making an Unoccupied Bed

Action

Rationale

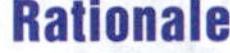

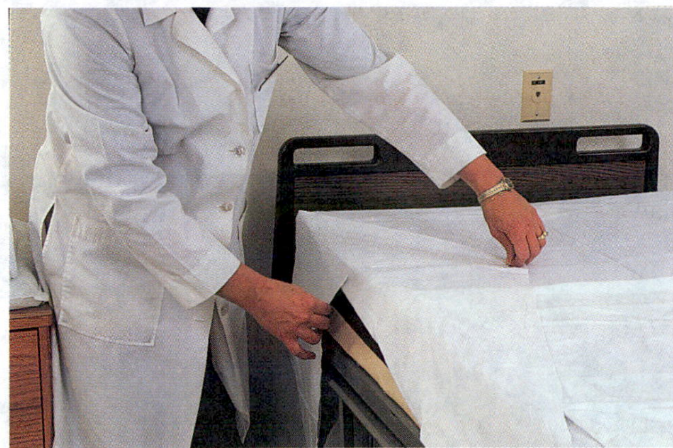

Action 11b: Laying triangular fold on top of bed.

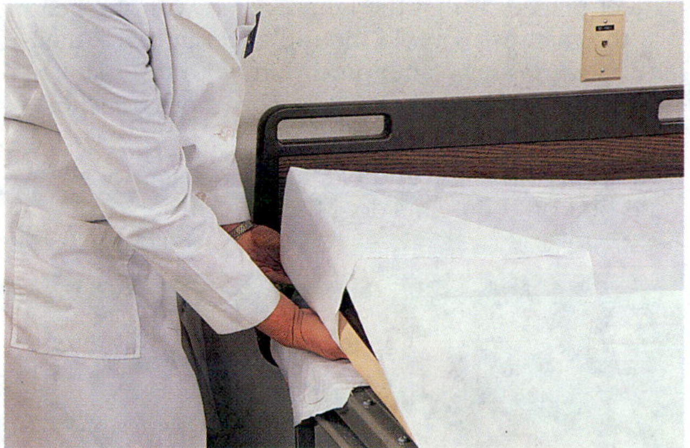

Action 11c: Tucking end of sheet under mattress.

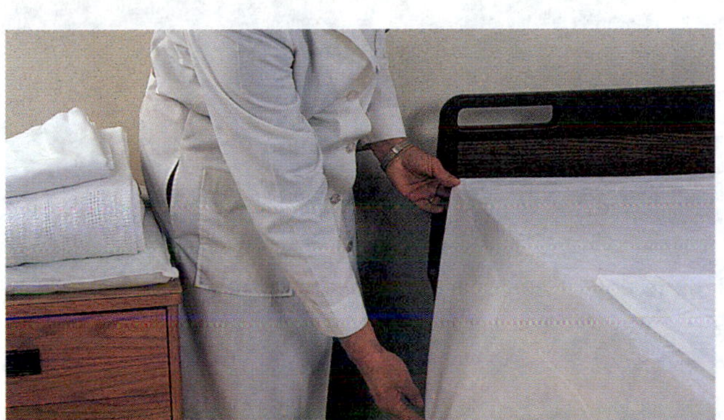

Action 11d: Folding triangular linen fold down over side of mattress.

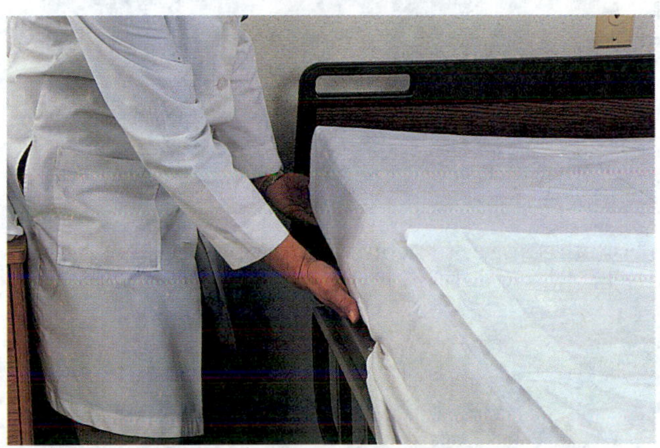

Action 11e: Tucking end of triangular linen fold under mattress to complete mitered corner.

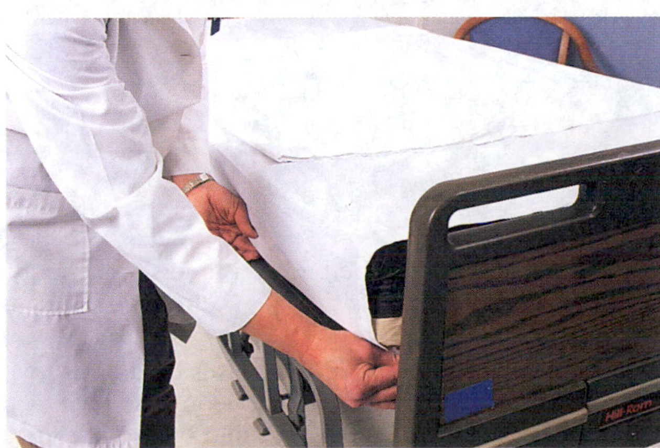

Action 11f: Tucking sheet snugly under foot of mattress.

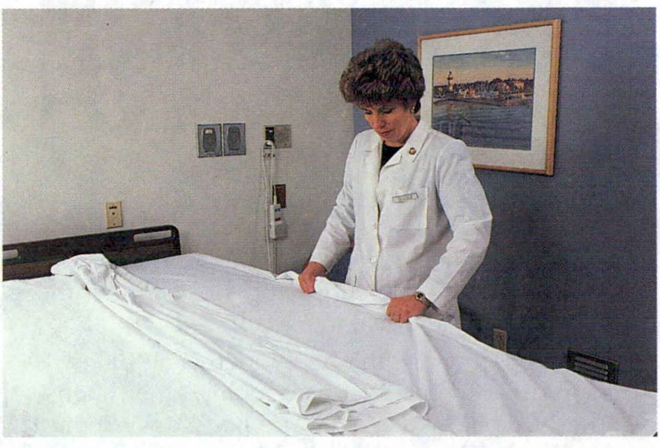

Action 12: Pulling bottom sheet tightly on opposite side of bed.

(continued)

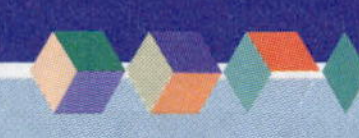

Making an Unoccupied Bed

Action	Rationale
13. Place the top sheet on the bed with its center fold in the center of the bed and with the top of the sheet placed so that the hem is even with the head of the mattress. Unfold the top sheet in place, as illustrated. Follow same procedure with top blanket or spread, placing the upper edge about 6 inches below the top of the sheet.	Opening linens by shaking them spreads organisms into the air. Holding linens overhead to open them causes strain on the nurse's arms.
14. Tuck the top sheet and blanket under the foot of the bed on the near side. Miter the corners.	This saves time and energy and keeps the top linen in place.

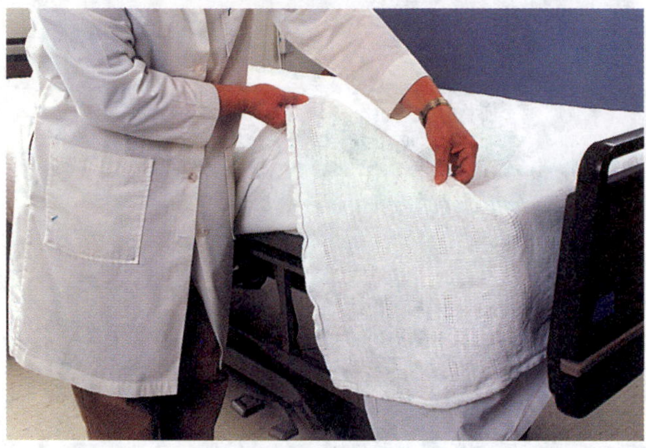

Action 14: Mitering the corner of the top sheet and spread.

Action	Rationale
15. Fold the upper 6 inches of the top sheet down over the spread and make a cuff.	This makes it easier for the client to get into bed and pull the covers up.

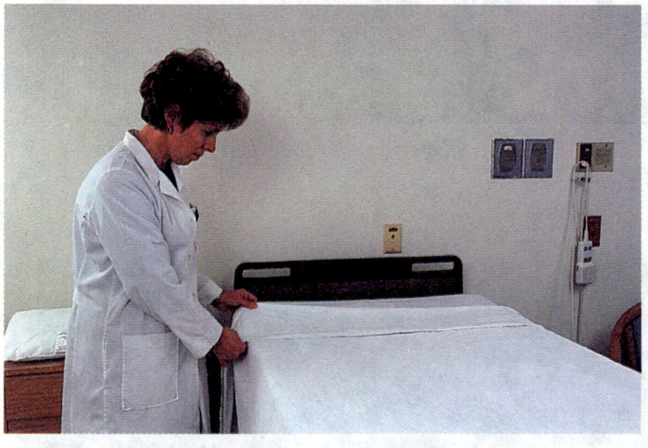

Action 15: Cuffing top linens.

Action	Rationale
16. Move to the other side of the bed and follow the same procedure for securing top sheets under the foot of the bed and making a cuff.	Working on one side of the bed at a time saves energy and is more efficient.
17. Place the pillows on the bed. Open each pillowcase in the same manner as opening other linens. Gather the pillowcase over one hand toward the closed end. Grasp the pillow with the hand inside the pillowcase. Keeping a firm hold on the top of the pillow, pull the cover onto the pillow.	Opening linens by shaking them causes organisms to be carried about on air currents. Covering the pillow while it rests on the bed reduces strain on the nurse's arms and back.

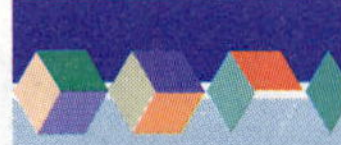

PROCEDURE 37-3 *(continued)*

Making an Unoccupied Bed

Action	Rationale
18. Place the pillow at the head of the bed with the open end facing toward the window.	This provides for a neater appearance.
19. Fan-fold or pie-fold the top linens.	Having linens opened makes it more convenient for the client to get into bed.
20. Secure the signal device on the bed according to agency policy.	Having the signal device handy for the client makes it possible for the client to call for assistance as necessary.

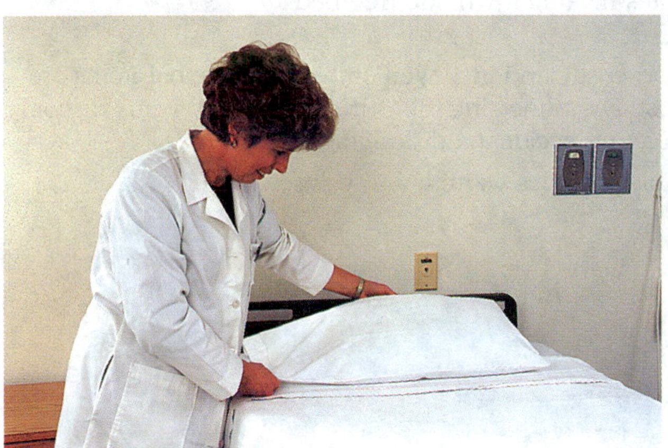

Action 18: Placing pillow on bed.

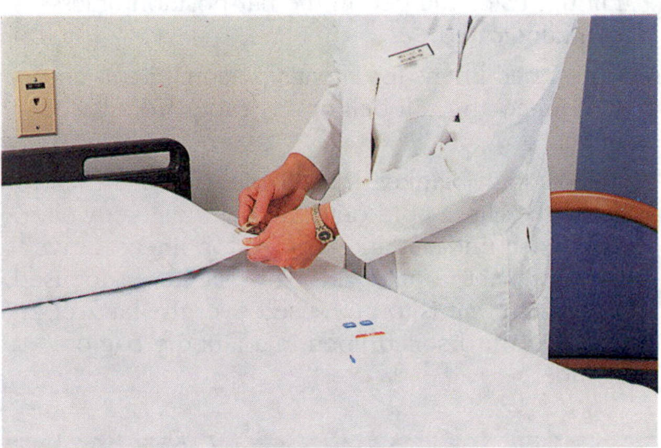

Action 20: Securing the signal device to the bed.

Action	Rationale
21. Adjust the bed to the low position.	Having the bed in the low position makes it easier and safer for the client to get into bed.
22. Dispose of soiled linen according to agency policy. Wash your hands.	This deters the spread of microorganisms.

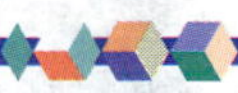

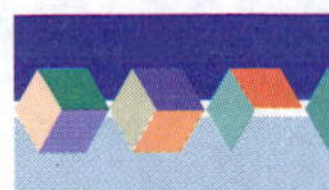

PROCEDURE 37-4

Making an Occupied Bed

Equipment

Two large sheets (or one large sheet and one fitted sheet)
Drawsheet
Blanket (optional)
Bedspread
Pillowcases
Linen hamper or bag (optional)
Bedside chair
Protective pad (optional)
Bath blanket (optional)

Action	Rationale
1. Explain the procedure to the client. Check the client's chart for limitations on the client's physical activity.	This facilitates client cooperation and determines level of activity.

(continued)

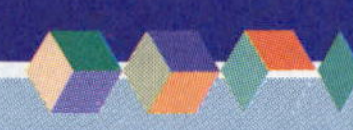

PROCEDURE 37-4 *(continued)*

Making an Occupied Bed

Action	Rationale
2. Wash your hands.	Handwashing deters the spread of microorganisms.
3. Assemble equipment and arrange on the bedside chair in the order the items will be used.	Organization facilitates performance of task.
4. Close door or curtain.	This provides for privacy.
5. Adjust the client's bed to the high position. Lower the side rail nearest you, leaving the opposite side rail up. Place the bed in the flat position unless contraindicated.	Having the bed in the high position reduces strain on the nurse while working. Having the mattress flat facilitates making a wrinkle-free bed.
6. Check bed linens for client's personal items and disconnect the call bell or any tubes from bed linens.	It is costly and inconvenient when personal items are lost. Disconnecting tubes from linens prevents discomfort and accidental dislodging of the tubes.
7. Place a bath blanket, if available, over the client. Have the client hold onto the bath blanket while you reach under it and remove top linens. Leave the top sheet in place if a bath blanket is not used. Fold linen that is to be reused over the back of a chair. Discard soiled linen in a laundry bag or hamper.	This provides warmth and privacy.

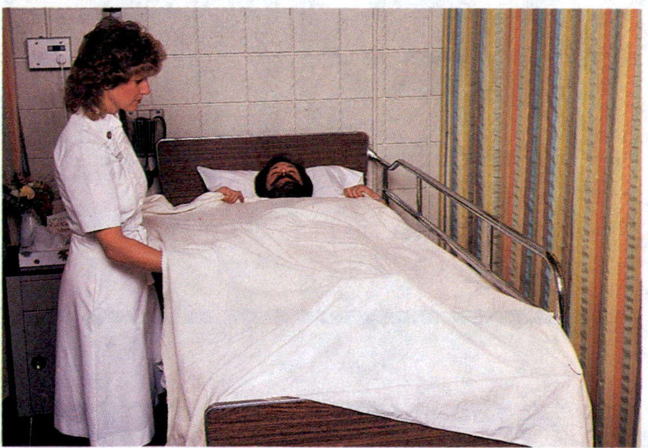

Action 7: Removing top linens from under bath blanket.

Action	Rationale
8. If possible and another person is available to assist, grasp mattress securely and shift it up to the head of the bed.	This allows more foot room for the client and positions the mattress against the head of the bed.
9. Assist the client to turn toward the opposite side of the bed and reposition the pillow under the client's head.	This allows the bed to be made on the vacant side.
10. Loosen all bottom linens from the head and sides of the bed.	This facilitates removal of linens.

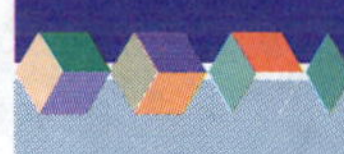

PROCEDURE 37-4 *(continued)*

Making an Occupied Bed

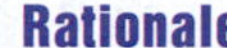

Action	Rationale
11. Fan-fold soiled linens as close to the client as possible.	This facilitates removal of linens when the client turns to the other side.
12. Use clean linen and make near side of bed following actions 9, 10, and 11 of Procedure 37-3. Fan-fold the clean linen as close to the client as possible.	This positions clean linen to make the side of the bed.

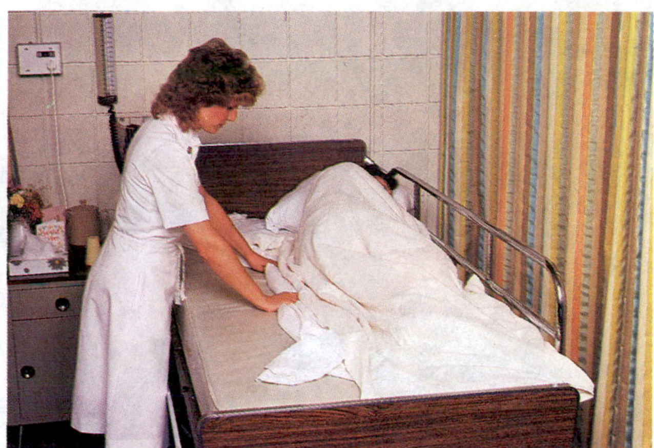

Action 11: Moving soiled linen as close to client as possible.

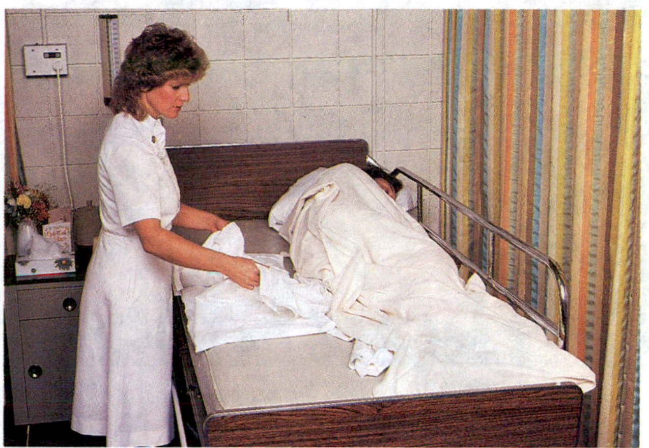

Action 12: Opening and folding clean linens.

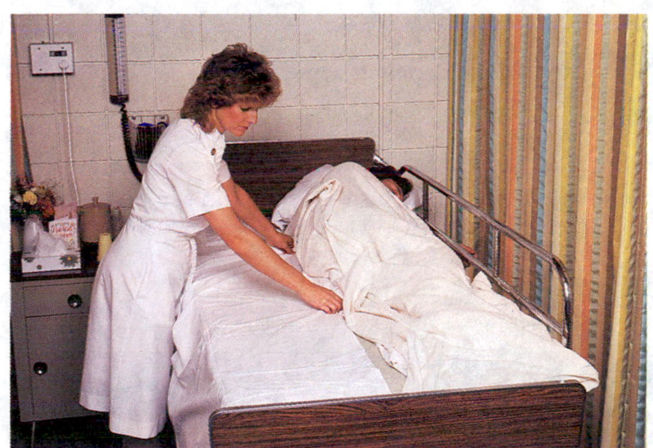

Action 12: Aligning clean bottom sheet on half of bed.

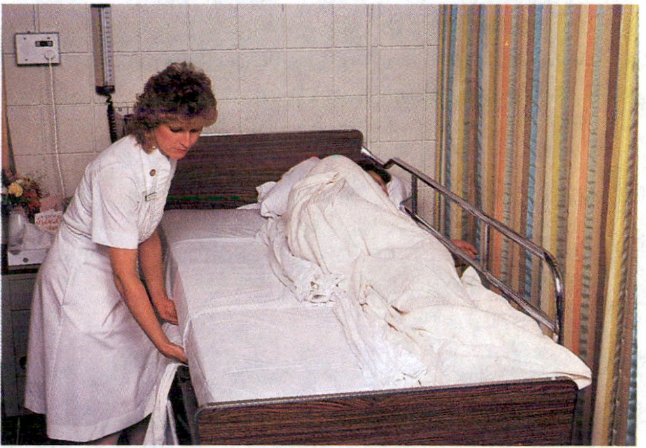

Action 12: Tucking bottom sheet and drawsheet tightly.

Action	Rationale
13. Raise the side rail. Assist the client to roll over the folded linen in the middle of the bed toward you. Reposition the pillow and bath blanket or top sheet. Move to the other side of the bed and lower the side rail.	This ensures client safety. The movement allows the bed to be made on the other side. The bath blanket provides warmth and privacy.

(continued)

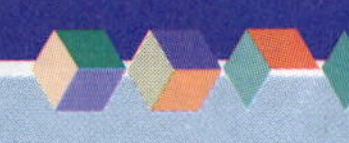

PROCEDURE 37-4 *(continued)*

Making an Occupied Bed

Action	Rationale
14. Loosen and remove all bottom linen. Place these in a linen bag or hamper. Hold soiled linen away from your uniform.	Proper disposal of soiled linen prevents spread of microorganisms.

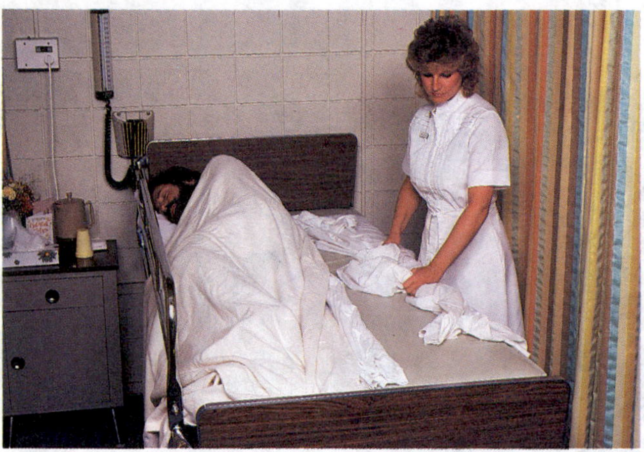

Action 14: Removing soiled bottom linens from other side of bed.

Action	Rationale
15. Ease the clean linen from under the client. Pull taut and secure the bottom sheet under the head of the mattress. Miter corners. Pull the side of the sheet taut and tuck under the side of the mattress. Repeat this with the drawsheet.	This removes wrinkles and creases in the linens, which are uncomfortable to lie on.
16. Assist the client to return to the center of the bed. Remove the pillow and change the pillowcase before replacing, with open end facing toward the window.	This provides for a neater appearance.
17. Apply top linen so that it is centered and top hems are even with the head of the mattress. Have the client hold onto the top linen so the bath blanket can be removed.	This allows bottom hems to be tucked securely under the mattress and provides for privacy.

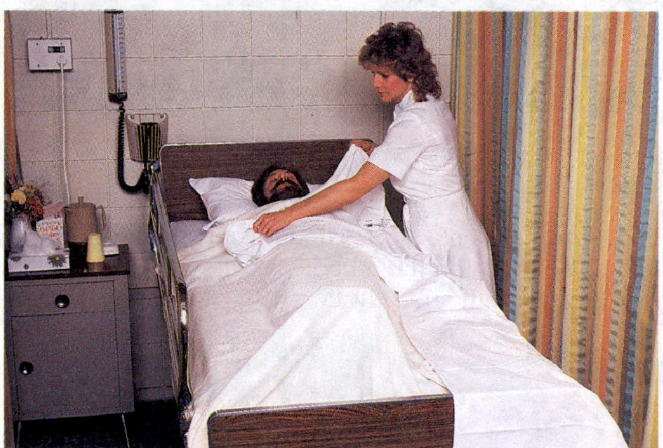

Action 17: Applying top linen over bath blanket.

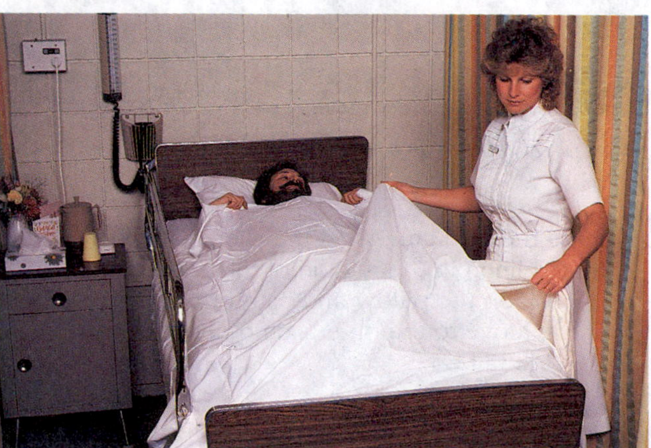

Action 17: Removing the bath blanket from under the top linens.

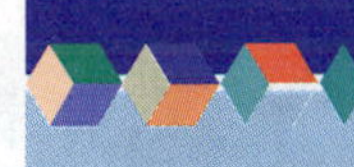

PROCEDURE 37-4 *(continued)*

Making an Occupied Bed

Action	Rationale
18. Secure top linens under the foot of the mattress and miter corners. Loosen top linens over the client's feet by grasping them in the area of the feet and pulling gently toward the foot of the bed.	This provides for a neat appearance. Loosening linens over the client's feet gives more room for movement.
19. Raise the side rail. Lower bed height and adjust the head of the bed to a comfortable position. Reattach call bell and drainage tubes.	This provides for the client's safety.
20. Dispose of soiled linens according to agency policy. Wash your hands.	This prevents spread of microorganisms.

Age Considerations Use of a synthetic sheepskin, a soft bath blanket, or flannelette blanket as a bottom sheet may solve the problem of "coldness" for elderly clients with vascular problems or arthritis.

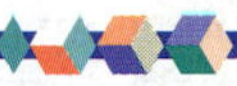

- Bed positioned properly and at the appropriate height
- Side rails and restraints safely used when indicated
- Principles of medical asepsis followed
- Electrical equipment safely grounded
- Uncluttered walk space

Elements of providing a comfortable bedside unit include attention to ventilation, odors, room temperature, lighting, and noise.

Ventilation and Odors. Because of pathogens and unpleasant odors associated with body secretions and excretions (ie, urine, stool, vomitus, draining wounds, or body odors), good ventilation in client rooms is imperative. Because many clients are sensitive to drafts, it is often wise to air the room during times when clients are absent for diagnostic or therapeutic procedures. Odors may be decreased by promptly emptying bedpans, urinals, and emesis basins and by being careful not to dispose of soiled dressings or anything with a strong odor in the waste receptacle in the client's room. Deodorizers may need to be used.

Room Temperature. Whenever possible, client preferences (which may vary widely) should be followed regarding room temperature. In general, the room temperature should fall between 20° and 23°C (68° and 74°F).

Lighting and Noise. Because many clients find it difficult to sleep in a healthcare facility and may need to be disturbed frequently for assessment or treatment purposes, the nurse should be careful to reduce harsh lighting and noises whenever possible. However, adequate lighting should be provided for all nursing procedures. Clients may enjoy sunlight or find it disturbing, and drapes may be arranged accordingly. Whenever possible, conversations should not be carried on immediately outside the client's room. Many clients find this stressful both because the noise disturbs them and because they believe whatever is being said involves them.

Beds

Because many people who are ill spend a large portion of the day—if not the entire day—in bed, the bed is an important part of the client's environment. Nursing responsibilities include ensuring a safe and comfortable bed.

Bed Safety. The typical hospital bed has a motorized metal frame in three sections, which allows the height of the bed to be raised or lowered as well as the head and foot of the bed to be adjusted. It is important that the nurse know how to operate the bed and explain this to the client. Bed positions are described in Chapter 39. Hospital beds can also be ordered for use in the home. Because certain positions may actually be harmful to some clients, the client and family should be instructed about advisable bed positions and use of the bed controls. Hospital beds are generally 66 cm (26 inches) from the floor. This is higher than most beds at home and enables the nurse or caregiver to reach the client without undue musculoskeletal strain.

Whenever the client's condition indicates the need for upper or lower side rails, these should be used to provide assistance with moving in bed and prevent dangerous falls in an unconscious client (refer to Chapter 27 for additional discussion about the use of side rails). The wheels (or casters) on the hospital bed should be locked whenever the bed is stationary to prevent the bed from slipping away from a client who is transferring from the bed to an upright position or to a stretcher. The headboard of most hospital beds is removable to allow close client contact in an emergency situation. Before leaving the client's bedside, ensure the following:

- The bed is in its lowest position.
- The bed position is safe for the client.
- The bed controls are functioning (bed is electrically safe).
- Side rails (upper and lower) are raised if indicated.
- The wheels or casters are locked.

Bed Comfort. The hospital mattress is firm and generally covered with a water-repellent material that can be easily wiped down with a bactericidal solution between clients. Many clients find it uncomfortable to rest with just a sheet between them and the rubberized mattress; thus, the nurse may need to find creative solutions—especially for clients at high risk for impaired skin integrity. Clients with arthritis and vascular problems often find the rubberized mattress cold; the use of sheepskin or a soft bath blanket or flannelette blanket used under or as a substitute for the bottom sheet may solve this problem. A variety of therapeutic beds and mattresses are available to reduce or relieve the effects of pressure on the skin (see Fig. 37-4 for an example) and are discussed in more detail in Chapter 39. Pillows covered with water-repellent material can be especially uncomfortable to clients. Clients spending many days in bed may find that having a pillow from home greatly aids their rest.

Agency policies usually dictate the availability and use of bed linens. Bed linens include mattress covers, sheets, drawsheets, incontinent pads, pillow cases, blankets, bedspreads, and bath blankets. Towels, washcloths, and client gowns are often included in linen packs. Devices to support and protect the client confined to bed are described in Chapter 39. In some settings, making the bed is not nursing's responsibility. However, ensuring client comfort is always a priority in nursing, and this often involves creating a comfortable bed environment. Before leaving a client, the nurse should ensure the following:

- Linens are clean and wrinkle free.
- The client feels comfortably warm.
- Pressure points on the client with a nursing diagnosis of Risk for Impaired Skin Integrity are protected from rough sheets, hem edges, and water-repellent materials.

Teaching Clients About Skin Care

Occasionally, clients ask for specific information; otherwise, the nurse can share information with the client during assessment and care procedures. The following section concerns skin care and skin problems.

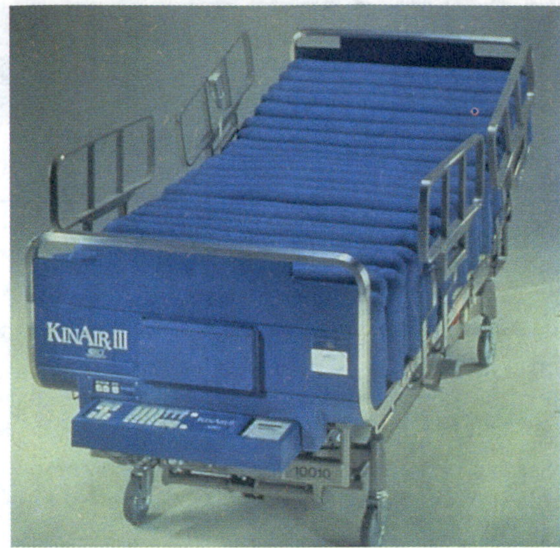

Figure 37-4
This special bed is an air-flotation, low-air-loss support surface that provides pressure relief. In this KinAir III there is a microprocessor computer control panel that controls air flow and temperature precisely. A built-in digital scale and heater are included. The bed also has a quick release level for CPR. (Photo courtesy of KCI Therapeutic Services, San Antonio, TX.)

Soaps, Detergents, and Creams

A great variety of soaps and detergents are available. Expensive cleansing agents have not been found to be superior to the less expensive ones. For most people, the best way to cleanse the skin is with soap or detergent and water. Soaps are often made from vegetable and animal fats. Most detergents are made from petroleum derivatives and are especially satisfactory when the water is hard, cold, or salty. People who are sensitive to soap often find they can use detergents without difficulty.

Cold creams usually consist of an oil or wax, water, and perfume. The cream feels cold because the water evaporates, producing a feeling of coolness. The oil and wax liquify on the skin and loosen and suspend dirt, oily secretions, perspiration, bacteria, cosmetics, dead cells, and other foreign material. They are then removed with a tissue or a soft cloth. Cleansing creams are similar to cold creams except they contain little or no water.

Deodorants and Antiperspirants

Perspiration is essentially odorless, although it contains some waste products, such as uric acid and ammonia. The odor of perspiration occurs when bacteria, normally present on everyone's skin, act on the skin's normal secretions.

Keeping the body and clothing clean is the prime requisite for preventing body odors. Deodorants and antiperspirants may be used *after* the skin is clean. Antiperspirants are intended to reduce the amount of perspiration. They act as astringents and tend to close the exits of the sweat glands. Antiperspirants and deodorants should be used with care and according to directions to prevent irritation of the skin.

Cosmetics

Cosmetics frequently enhance the appearance of clean and healthy skin, although certain cultural and religious groups may discourage their use. Cosmetics used judiciously help disguise blemishes, improve skin coloring, and make wrinkles appear less obvious. Creams and lotions made by reputable companies are safe to use.

Periodically, cosmetics containing harmful ingredients, such as various dyes, have appeared on the market. The nurse should be alert to such agents and help consumers avoid their use. The U.S. Department of Health and Human Services, Food and Drug Administration (FDA), enforces federal laws on the purity of foods, drugs, and cosmetics and on the advertising claims of their manufacturers. The FDA is a good source of information about these products. Similar agencies exist in Canada.

Cosmetics often become contaminated with bacteria and fungus. It is best to discard cosmetics after they are about 4 months old, especially those applied near the eyes. Make-up applicators and puffs should be kept immaculately clean. Cosmetics should not be shared.

Dry Skin

Dry skin is characteristically flaky and is easily susceptible to injury and irritation. Suggestions for people whose skin is dry and injured easily are the following:

- Bathe less frequently, especially when the outdoor temperature and humidity are low.
- Rinse off soaps or detergents well when they are used for cleansing the skin. Residue left on the skin predisposes to skin irritation and breakdown.
- Avoid defatting agents, such as alcohol, on dry and easily injured skin.
- Avoid wearing garments made of woolen fabrics because wool tends to irritate dry skin.
- Wash garments made of wrinkle-resistant fabrics once or twice before wearing them. The chemical impregnated in the fabric tends to irritate dry skin.
- Add moisture to the air through a humidifier when the skin is dry.
- Increase fluid intake when the skin is dry.
- Try using a bath oil when the skin is dry. These oils make bathtubs slippery, and care should be used to prevent falls. Bubble bath preparations, which often contain oil, should be mixed well in the bath water before the person sits in the tub.
- Use an *emollient*, an agent used to soften, soothe, and protect dry skin, after cleansing the skin. Emollient or moisturizing creams do not add moisture to the skin. Rather, the film they leave on the skin retards normal moisture evaporation and helps to hold down the scaly skin surfaces. Cocoa butter, petroleum jelly, and lanolin are examples of effective emollients that are used in many emollient creams.
- Use creams to clean skin that is dry or allergic to soaps and detergents.

Home Healthcare Alert

Remind clients that bubble bath preparations have been associated with the development of urinary tract infections.

Acne

Oily skin is especially bothersome during adolescence, when hormones cause enlargement of the sebaceous glands and increased glandular secretions. Blackheads and pustules appear when these secretions become dammed up in the sebaceous ducts, and inflammation with infection occurs. The condition is referred to as *acne* and most often appears on the face, neck, shoulders, and back. From a health standpoint, acne is not a serious condition, although it can lead to permanent scarring and psychologic problems for the person suffering from it. There are various recommended ways to help control acne and minimize scarring:

- The infected areas should not be squeezed or picked. This tends to cause a spread of the infection and scarring of the skin.
- The person with acne should wash the skin and shampoo hair with soap or detergent and hot water frequently to remove oil and debris.
- Oily cosmetics, cleansing creams, and emollients should be avoided. They tend to make the condition worse.
- Cosmetics should be used sparingly to avoid further blocking of sebaceous gland ducts.
- Exposure to an ultraviolet lamp may occasionally be prescribed to help keep acne under control. However, caution should be exercised to prevent burning the skin.
- Foods that are found to aggravate the condition should be eliminated from the diet. Chocolate, nuts, cola beverages, and foods containing iodine tend to make acne worse for some people.

In severe cases, the services of a physician are recommended. Treatment modalities vary.

Prescribed combination therapies that control the clinical manifestations of acne may result in **erythema** (redness) and skin peeling. Sun exposure during some of these treatments may be dangerous and cause an exaggerated sunburn.

Skin Rashes

Rashes are eruptions or inflammations of the skin that may be found anywhere on the body. Rashes may be precipitated by the skin's contact with an allergen (eg, chemicals in cleansers and soaps) or by overexposure to the sun or to moisture. They may also result from systemic causes such as the body's response to medications or to certain diseases. Rashes may be described as flat or raised, pruritic or nonpruritic, localized or systemic, dry or wet. Scratching a rash may result in inflammation and infection.

Interventions include the following:

- Wash the area thoroughly with a mild cleansing agent and rinse well.
- Use a moisturizing lotion on a dry rash to prevent itching and to promote healing.
- Use a drying agent on a wet rash.
- Tepid baths or soaks may relieve inflammation and itching.
- Antiseptic sprays or lotions may be useful in lessening itching, promoting healing, and preventing skin breakdown.
- A number of over-the-counter products such as Caladryl (benadryl hydrochloride) lotion and hydrocortisone creams may be useful, depending on the nature of the rash. Read the manufacturer's recommendations and cautions before testing a new product.
- If the causative agent is known, avoid exposure to it.
- Refer to a physician if symptoms do not respond to treatment.

Pressure Ulcers

Pressure ulcers are areas of cellular necrosis caused by the lack of blood circulation to the involved area. At best they are extremely painful and debilitating to clients; at worst they may be life-threatening. They offer a persistent challenge to even the most experienced nurse. Preventing pressure ulcers whenever possible and identifying and treating them at the earliest stage possible are critical nursing responsibilities. This topic is explored in detail in Chapter 38.

EVALUATING

Daily contacts with the client while hygiene measures are being performed enable the nurse to frequently evaluate whether the client is meeting hygiene goals. Evaluative criteria include the following:

- Level of client's participation in hygiene program
- Elimination, reduction in, or compensation for factors interfering with the client's independent execution of hygiene measures (eg, weakness, decreased motivation, lack of knowledge)
- Client's achievement of expected outcomes related to specific skin problems, by giving attention to the healing of skin lesions, the elimination or reduction of causative factors, and the client's ability to manage the prescribed treatment program independently

Oral Care

The mouth is the first part of the alimentary canal and is an adjunct of the respiratory system. The ducts of the salivary glands open into the vestibule of the mouth. The teeth and the tongue are accessory organs in the mouth and play an important role in beginning digestion by breaking up food particles and mixing them with saliva. Saliva is also important as a mechanical cleaner of the mouth.

General good health is as essential as cleanliness for maintaining a healthy mouth and teeth. The relationship, for example, between good teeth and a diet sufficient in calcium and phosphorus along with vitamin D, which is necessary for the body to use these minerals, is well established.

There are several benefits for maintaining good oral hygiene and dental care. There is aesthetic value in having a clean and healthy mouth. Having one's own teeth contributes to an intact body image. The beginning of the digestive process and gustatory pleasure are enhanced when the mouth and teeth are in good condition.

ASSESSING

Nursing History

Identify the client's normal oral hygiene practices—brushing, flossing, use of rinses, presence and care of dentures or other orthodontic devices, frequency of dental examinations, and variables influencing these practices. Note the history of any oral problems and related treatments.

Identify any variables known to cause oral problems, such as deficient self-care abilities, poor nutrition and excessive intake of refined sugars, family history of periodontal disease, or ingestion of chemotherapeutic agents that produce oral lesions. Clients at high risk for oral problems include those who are seriously ill, comatose, dehydrated, confused, depressed, or paralyzed. Clients who are mouth breathers, who can have no oral intake of nutrition or fluids, who have nasogastric tubes or oral airways in place, and who have had oral surgery are also at increased risk.

Physical Assessment

Examine the lips for color, moisture, lumps, ulcers, lesions, and edema. Examine the buccal mucosa for color, moisture, lesions, nodules, and bleeding. Examine the color of the gums and surface of the gums for lesions, bleeding, edema, and exudate. Examine for loose, missing, or carious (decayed) teeth. Note the presence of dentures or other orthodontic devices. Examine the tongue for color, symmetry, movement, texture, and lesions. Examine the hard and soft palates for intactness, color, patches, lesions, and petechiae. Examine the

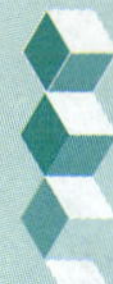

Research in Nursing: Making a Difference

Personal Hygiene

For clients who are unable to care for themselves or require assistance, personal hygiene measures provide personal cleanliness, promote comfort, and support feelings of well-being. A calm, professional approach by the caregiver, respect for client's individual preferences, and attention to privacy needs are integral to responsible nursing care. Nursing research has examined the many facets of hygiene both in health promotion and in disease prevention.

Related Research

Verderber, A., & Gallagher, K. (1994). Effects of bathing, passive range-of-motion exercises, and turning on oxygen consumption in healthy men and women. *American Journal of Critical Care, 3*(5), 374–381.
The morning care nursing routine of bathing, performing range-of-motion exercises, and turning the client from side to side to complete the bath may have an adverse effect on a client's oxygen consumption. Turning activities, regardless of when they occurred during the bathing routine, placed certain clients at risk for hypoxia because oxygen consumption was significantly increased. Nurses need to be aware of clients who have diseases that limit oxygen transport in order to determine how much activity the client can tolerate. Periods of rest during the morning routine may prove beneficial.

Corley, M., Ferriter, J., Zeh, J., & Gifford, C. (1995). Physiological and psychological effects of back rubs. *Applied Nursing Research, 8*(1), 39–43.
Few studies have substantiated nurses' belief that back rubs provide both physiologic and psychologic benefits. In this research study, back rubs improved the mood of the participants, although no significant physiologic changes occurred. Nurses, whether working in long-term care facilities or a hospital setting, need to assess the client's preferences regarding back rubs and observe individual responses to a back rub.

Miller, R. (1994). Managing disruptive responses to bathing by elderly residents: Strategies for the cognitively impaired. *Journal of Gerontological Nursing, 20*(11), 35–39.
The act of assisting a cognitively impaired client with a tub bath or shower can trigger disruptive and agitated behavior. The loss of privacy, inability to participate in care because of hurried approach by caregiver, and physical discomfort from being cold may cause frustration and confusion and impede communication with this client. Eliciting the resident's previous home routines and habits and combining these interventions with other effective preventive strategies outlined by the author reduced trauma and stress during these personal caregiving activities.

Summary

When assisting clients with hygiene needs, nurses need to incorporate the knowledge gained through nursing research into their daily practice to provide optimal client care. Careful assessment can determine client's personal hygiene routines and identify clients at risk for unexpected physiologic and psychologic responses. Nurses are in a unique position to foster a therapeutic environment where clients can have their individual hygiene needs met safely and respectfully.

oropharynx for movement of the uvula and condition of tonsils, if present. Note unusual mouth odors. Assess adequacy of mastication and swallowing. Chapter 26 has additional information concerning nursing assessment of the oral cavity.

When inspecting the oral cavity, the nurse frequently observes oral problems that at best are benign and only mildly annoying to clients but that may also be life threatening. It is imperative to identify the problem and its cause and to initiate the appropriate treatment. This may require consultation with a dentist or physician.

Dental Caries. The decay of teeth with the formation of cavities is called **caries**. Caries result from the failure to remove **plaque**, an invisible, destructive, bacterial film that builds up on everyone's teeth and eventually leads to the destruction of tooth enamel. A successful plaque-fighting program includes elimination of sweet snacks between meals, such as soft drinks, candy, gum, jams, and jellies; thorough cleansing; and regular dental checkups. The use of antiplaque, fluoride toothpastes and mouth rinses helps prevent dental caries.

Periodontal Disease. The major cause of tooth loss in adults older than age 35 years is gum disease. **Gingivitis** is an inflammation of the *gingiva*, the tissue that surrounds the teeth.

Pyorrhea, or *periodontal disease*, is a marked inflammation of the gums and also involves the alveolar tissues. Symptoms include bleeding gums; swollen, red, painful gum tissues; receding gum lines with the formation of pockets between the teeth and gums; pus that appears when gums are pressed; and loose teeth. If unchecked, plaque builds up and, along with dead bacteria, forms hard deposits called **tartar** at the gum lines. The tartar attacks the fibers that fasten teeth to the gums and eventually attacks bone tissue also. The teeth then loosen and fall out. A strong mouth odor (**halitosis**) or persistent bad taste in the mouth may be the first indication of periodontal disease. Regular dental treatment by a dentist is imperative.

Other Oral Problems. Other oral problems that the nurse may observe when inspecting the oral cavity include the following:

Stomatitis is an inflammation of the oral mucosa with numerous causes, such as bacteria, virus, mechanical trauma, irritants, nutritional deficiencies, and systemic infection. Symptoms may include heat, pain, increased flow of saliva, and halitosis. Manifestations include such diverse problems as aphthous ulcers; herpetic ulcers (fever blisters); fungal ulcers (*Candida albicans*–induced thrush); and chemotherapy-induced stomatitis.

Glossitis is an inflammation of the tongue.

Cheilosis is an ulceration of the lips (reddened fissures at the angles of the mouth) most often caused by vitamin B complex deficiencies (especially riboflavin).

Dry oral mucosa may simply be related to dehydration or may be caused by mouth breathing, an alteration in salivary functioning, or certain medications (eg, anticholinergic drugs).

Oral malignancies appear as lumps or ulcers; it is critical that these be distinguished from benign mouth problems because early detection may be the difference between cure and radical dissecting surgery or death. Teach clients if they notice white or red patches, persistent sores, swelling, bleeding, numbness, or pain in the mouth to see their dentist immediately.

DIAGNOSING

Make a judgment about the adequacy of the client's oral hygiene practices, identifying any factors contributing to deficiencies. An example is as follows:

Self-Care Deficit: Oral Hygiene, related to low value attached to regular brushing, flossing, and dental examinations

Identify actual or potential oral problems that nurses can treat, noting contributing factors. Identify unhealthy client responses to oral problems. Examples include:

Pain related to chemotherapy-induced oral ulceration

Risk for Infection related to breaks in oral mucosa and inadequate secondary defenses

Altered Nutrition: Less than body requirements, related to painful oral lesions (ill-fitting dentures, gingivitis)

Altered Oral Mucous Membrane related to dehydration (ineffective oral hygiene, medication)

Impaired Swallowing related to neuromuscular impairment

Body Image Disturbance related to loss of teeth, halitosis, or dental caries

PLANNING: EXPECTED OUTCOMES

Identify nursing measures that will assist the client to develop or maintain oral hygiene practices to promote oral health and general well-being and resolve identified nursing diagnoses. Plan to achieve the following client outcomes. The client will:

- Have lips, oral mucosa, gums, and tongue that are intact, moist, and free of inflammation and lesions
- Have clean teeth (or dentures)
- Demonstrate the ability to masticate and swallow food
- Demonstrate signs of healing of oral lesions
- Demonstrate correct oral hygiene measures—brushing and flossing
- Verbalize importance of fluoride use and regular dental examinations

Pertinent nursing measures to include in the plan of care are the following:

- Teach proper brushing and flossing techniques; instruct clients about fluoride use and the importance of regular dental examinations.
- Teach correct denture care or provide this when necessary.
- Perform mouth care for the unconscious client (clean the mouth with swabs dipped in dilute mouth rinse or in normal saline solution; suction as necessary to prevent aspiration; apply a petroleum jelly to the lips).
- Perform mouth care for clients with oral lesions (cleanse to prevent infection and numbing if indicated to encourage eating).

In the plan of care, identify any supplies needed to carry out the specified oral care and the timing and frequency of oral hygiene measures.

IMPLEMENTING

While carrying out the plan of care, the nurse uses each nurse–client interaction for ongoing assessment of the client's oral cavity and evaluation of the adequacy of the plan of care. Techniques for administering and teaching oral care are described in this section. Sample documentation of oral hygiene care follows:

> 10/20/98 Client generally breathes with mouth open. Sores present on palate, teeth, gums, and oral mucosa. Toothettes dipped in normal saline used for cleansing every 4 hours. Lubricating jelly to lips.
>
> D. Sadowski, RN

Administering Oral Hygiene

The mouth must be cared for even during illness. However, there are times when care must be modified to meet the specific needs of a client. If the client is able to assist with mouth care while bedridden, the nurse provides necessary materials (Procedure 37-5). If the client is helpless, the nurse needs to make certain that attention is given to the client's mouth as often as necessary to keep it clean and moist, as often as every hour or two, if necessary. This is especially true for clients who are unable or are not permitted fluids by mouth. Procedure 37-6 gives techniques for administering oral hygiene to the dependent client. Recent research by Tombes and Galluci (1993) confirmed findings from other studies indicating that hydrogen peroxide acts as an irritant and should not be used for mouth care. Use of this solution results in significant mucosal abnormalities and numerous complaints from clients about burning sensations, dryness, nausea, and "furry tongue." Normal saline solution is recommended when giving oral care to a dependent client. The nurse should wear disposable gloves to prevent exposure to blood and blood-borne infections such as AIDS and hepatitis B. Moisten the mouth with water, if allowed, and lubricate the lips sufficiently frequently to keep the membranes well moistened.

The procedure of cleaning the mouth thoroughly is more important than the agent used. This supports the personal experience of many people that no mouthwash, breath freshener, ointment, or paste replaces a thorough mechanical cleaning of the oral cavity.

Denture Care

Keeping dentures out of the mouth for long periods permits the gum line to change, thus affecting their fit. If the client has been instructed to remove dentures while sleeping, a disposable denture cup is convenient and easy to use. Dentures should not be wrapped in toilet tissue or disposable wipes because these are likely to be thrown away. It is recommended that dentures be stored in water to prevent drying and warping of plastic materials. A deodorant solution of water and a few drops of ammonia or white vinegar can be used. A few drops of essence of peppermint may be added also. Dentures made of vulcanite, which is a porous material, are especially prone to develop unpleasant odors.

The person with dentures is more likely to keep them in the mouth when dentures are kept clean. When the client is unable to care for them, the nurse is responsible for ensuring that dentures are clean. Care should be exercised when handling a client's dentures. They represent a considerable financial investment, and damage or loss becomes expensive. When cleaning dentures, the nurse should don gloves and hold them over a basin of water or a soft towel (Fig. 37-5) so that if they slip from the nurse's grasp, they will not fall onto a hard surface and break. Cool or lukewarm water should be used to cleanse them. Hot water may warp the plastic material from which most dentures are made. The use of a brush and a nonabrasive powder or paste is also recommended. There are also preparations in which to soak dentures to help remove stains and hardened particles. The dentures are rinsed well after cleaning. The client should be given the opportunity to rinse his or her mouth before the dentures are replaced.

Teaching Oral Hygiene

Toothbrushing and Flossing

A toothbrush should be small enough to reach all teeth. The bristles should be sufficiently firm to clean but not so firm that they are likely to injure tooth enamel and gum tissue. Brushes should be cleaned and dried between uses. There is a difference of opinion as to the best way to brush teeth. When assisting and teaching a client, the nurse should follow the preference of the client's dentist. One recommended brushing regimen is illustrated in Figure 37-6. Most damage is done by bacteria directly after eating. Therefore, it is ideal to brush the teeth immediately after eating or drinking. The tongue also should be cleaned with the brush.

Automatic toothbrushes, electric or battery operated, have been found to be simple to use and as good as hand brushes in removing debris and plaque. Water-spray units are available to assist with oral hygiene. However, if an undue amount of water pressure is used, particles of debris may be forced into tissue pockets and damage may occur to gum tissue. Therefore, it is recommended that their use be discussed with a dentist.

The toothbrush cannot effectively reach areas between the teeth where food lodges; hence, flossing once a day is recommended. The practice not only removes what the brush cannot but also helps to break up colonies of bacteria. Figure 37-7 illustrates a flossing technique. The following are additional recommended techniques for flossing the teeth.

- Wear gloves when flossing a client's teeth.
- Keep about 1 to 1½ inches of floss held taut between the fingers.
- Do not force the floss between the teeth, but insert it gently by moving it back and forth where teeth touch each other.
- Move the floss up and down while using both fingers, first on the side of one tooth and then on the side of the other tooth, until the surfaces are squeaky clean.
- Go to the gum tissue with the floss but not into the gum, because this may result in discomfort, soreness, or bleeding.
- Advance the floss from one hand to the other to bring up a fresh section of floss when it has become frayed or soiled.
- Rinse the mouth well with water after flossing to remove food particles and plaque that have been loosened. Also, rinse after eating when flossing or brushing is impossible.

(text continues on page 950)

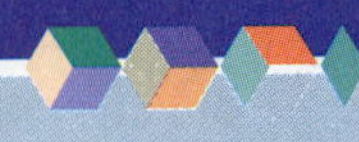

PROCEDURE 37-5

Assisting the Client With Oral Care

Equipment

Toothbrush
Toothpaste
Emesis basin
Glass with cool water
Disposable gloves
Towel
Mouthwash (optional)
Dental floss (optional)
Denture-cleansing equipment (if necessary)
Denture cup
Denture cleaner
4 × 4 gauze
Washcloth or paper towel
Petroleum jelly (optional)

Action	Rationale
1. Explain the procedure to the client.	Explanation facilitates cooperation.
2. Wash your hands. Don disposable gloves if assisting with oral care.	Handwashing deters the spread of microorganisms. Gloves protect the nurse from exposure to blood and blood-borne infections.
3. Assemble equipment on an overbed table within the client's reach.	Organization facilitates performance of task.
4. Provide privacy for the client.	Client may be embarrassed if cleansing involves removal of dentures.
5. Lower side rail and assist client to sitting position if permitted, or turn the client onto the side. Place the towel across the client's chest. Raise the bed to a comfortable working position.	The sitting or side-lying position prevents aspiration of fluids into the lungs. The towel protects the client from dampness.
6. Encourage the client to brush own teeth or assist if necessary:	
a. Moisten the toothbrush and apply toothpaste to bristles.	Water softens the bristles.
b. Place brush at a 45-degree angle to gum line and brush from gum line to crown of each tooth. Brush outer and inner surfaces. Brush back and forth across biting surface of each tooth.	This facilitates removal of plaque and tartar. The 45-degree angle of brushing permits cleansing of all surface areas of the tooth.

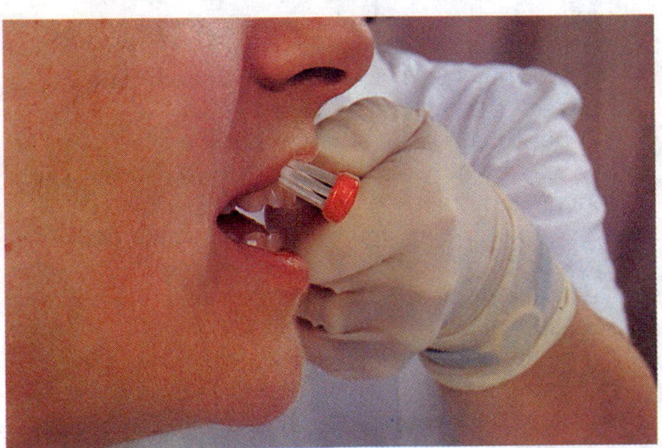

Action 6b: Placing brush at 45-degree angle to the gum line.

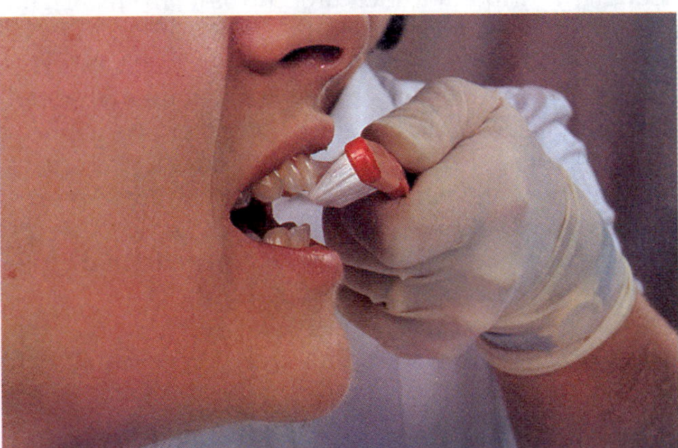

Action 6b: Brushing from the gum line to the crown of each tooth.

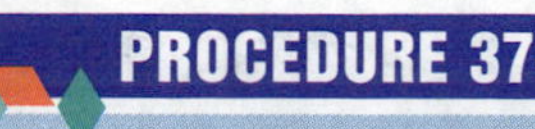

PROCEDURE 37-5 *(continued)*

Assisting the Client With Oral Care

Action	Rationale
c. Brush tongue gently with toothbrush.	This removes coating on the tongue. Gentle motion does not stimulate gag reflex.
d. Have the client rinse vigorously with water and spit into emesis basin. Repeat until clear. Suction may be used as an alternative for removal of fluid and secretions from mouth.	The vigorous swishing motion helps to remove debris. Suction is appropriate if swallowing reflex is impaired or absent.
e. Assist the client to floss teeth if necessary.	Flossing aids in removal of plaque and promotes healthy gum tissue.
f. Offer mouthwash if the client prefers.	Mouthwash leaves a pleasant taste in the mouth.
7. Assist the client with removal and cleansing of dentures if necessary:	
a. Apply gentle pressure with 4 × 4 gauze to grasp upper denture plate and remove. Place it immediately in the denture cup. Lift the lower denture using slight rocking motion, remove, and place in the denture cup.	Rocking motion breaks suction between the denture and gum. Using 4 × 4 gauze prevents slippage and discourages spread of microorganisms.
b. If the client prefers, add denture cleanser to the cup with water and follow directions on preparation or brush all areas thoroughly with toothbrush and paste. Place paper towels or washcloth in sink while brushing.	Dentures collect food and microorganisms and require daily cleansing. Paper towels or washcloth in the sink protects against breakage.
c. Rinse thoroughly with water and return dentures to the client.	Water aids in removal of debris and acts as a cleansing agent.
d. Offer mouthwash so client can rinse his or her mouth before replacing dentures.	Mouthwash leaves a pleasant taste in the mouth and removes food particles, thus permitting proper fit of dentures.
e. Apply petroleum jelly to lips if needed.	Petroleum jelly prevents cracking and drying of lips.
8. Remove equipment and assist the client to a position of comfort. Record any unusual bleeding or inflammation. Raise side rail and lower the bed.	This promotes oral hygiene and provides for oral assessment. Elevated side rails and lowered bed position maintain safety for bedridden clients.
9. Remove disposable gloves from inside out and discard appropriately. Wash your hands.	This protects the nurse from contact with any microorganism. Handwashing deters spread of microorganisms.

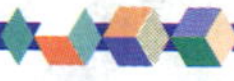

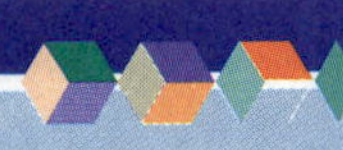

PROCEDURE 37-6

Providing Oral Care for the Dependent Client

Equipment

Toothbrush
Toothpaste
Emesis basin
Disposable gloves
Cup with cool water
Towel
Mouthwash
Normal saline solution
Denture-cleansing equipment (if necessary)
Denture cup
Washcloth or paper towel
Sponge toothette or tongue blades padded with 4 × 4 gauze sponges
Irrigating syringe with rubber tip (optional)
Petroleum jelly
Suction catheter with suction apparatus (optional)

Action	Rationale
1. Explain the procedure to the client.	Explanation facilitates cooperation.
2. Wash your hands and don disposable gloves.	Handwashing and disposable gloves deter the spread of microorganisms.
3. Assemble equipment on overbed table within reach.	Organization facilitates performance of task.
4. Provide privacy for the client. Adjust the height of the bed to a comfortable position. Lower one side rail and position the client on the side with head turned toward you and tilted toward the mattress. Place the towel across the client's chest and emesis basin in position under the chin.	The side-lying position with head turned down prevents aspiration of fluid into lungs. Towel and emesis basin protect client from dampness.
5. Open the client's mouth and gently insert a padded tongue blade between the back molars if necessary.	Padded tongue blade keeps mouth open for easier cleaning and prevents the client from biting the nurse's fingers.

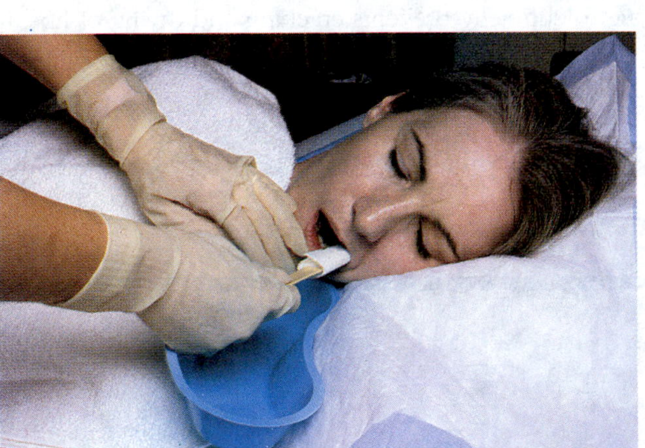

Action 5: Gently inserting padded tongue blade between back molars.

Action	Rationale
6. If teeth are present, brush carefully with toothbrush and paste. Remove dentures if present and clean before replacing (see action 7 of Procedure 37-5). Use toothette or gauze-padded tongue blade moistened with normal saline or dilute mouthwash solution to gently cleanse gums, mucous membranes, and tongue.	Toothbrush or padded tongue blade provides friction necessary to clean areas where plaque and tartar accumulate. Hydrogen peroxide is considered an irritant and no longer recommended. The mechanical action of cleansing is more important than the solution.

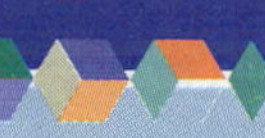

PROCEDURE 37-6 *(continued)*

Providing Oral Care for the Dependent Client

Action	**Rationale**

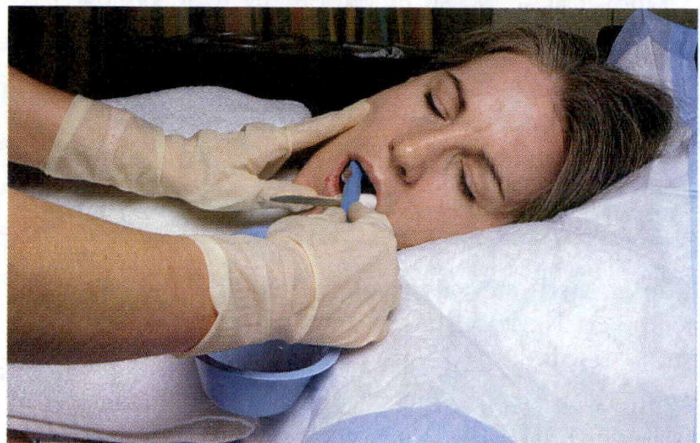

Action 6: Carefully brushing client's teeth.

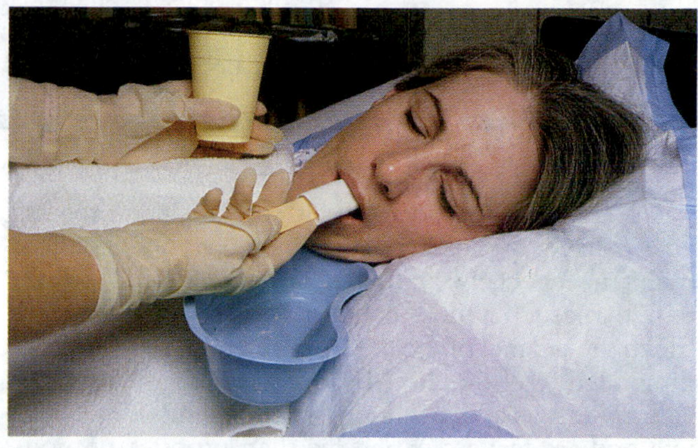

Action 6: Using moistened padded tongue blade to cleanse gums, mucous membranes, and tongue.

7. Use gauze-padded tongue blade dipped in mouthwash solution to rinse the oral cavity. If desired, insert the rubber tip of the irrigating syringe into the client's mouth and rinse gently with a small amount of water. Position the client's head to allow for return of water or use suction apparatus to remove the water from oral cavity.

   Rinsing helps to cleanse debris from the mouth. Solution that is forcefully irrigated may cause aspiration.

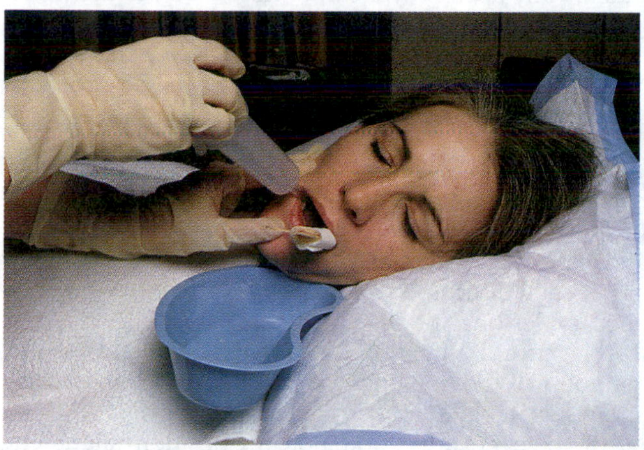

Action 7: Using irrigating syringe and a small amount of water to rinse mouth.

8. Apply petroleum jelly to the client's lips.

   This prevents drying and cracking of lips.

9. Remove equipment and return the client to a position of comfort. Raise the side rail and lower the bed. Record any unusual bleeding or inflammation.

   This promotes oral hygiene and provides for oral assessment. Raised side rail and lowered bed maintain client safety.

10. Wash your hands.

    Handwashing deters spread of microorganisms.

(continued)

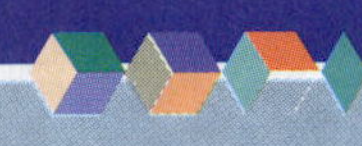

PROCEDURE 37-6 *(continued)*

Providing Oral Care for the Dependent Client

Special Considerations

A client receiving chemotherapy medication may have bleeding gums and extremely sensitive mucous membranes. Use a soft sponge toothette for cleaning or substitute a salt water rinse (1/2 teaspoon salt in 1 cup of warm water) for brushing of teeth.

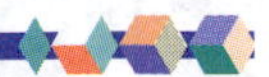

Toothpastes and powders aid the brushing process, usually have a pleasant taste, and often encourage brushing, especially among children. Most dentifrices are safe to use, but those containing harsh abrasives may scratch the enamel of the teeth and therefore are not recommended. Salt, sodium bicarbonate, or precipitated chalk are just as effective for cleaning the mouth and the teeth and are far less expensive than proprietary products on the market. Dentifrices containing stannous fluoride and antiplaque rinses have proven to be effective in helping to decrease dental caries and hence are recommended by many dentists.

Mouthwashes

An offensive breath odor or halitosis is often systemic in nature. For example, the odor of onions and garlic on the breath comes from the lungs, where the oils are being removed from the bloodstream and eliminated with respiration. A mouthwash cannot remove halitosis when odors are being eliminated by respiration.

If the cause of halitosis is poor oral hygiene, cleaning reduces the odor. Commercial mouthwashes may be helpful, and many people enjoy their fresh aftertaste. If concentrated mouthwashes are used frequently for debilitated clients, they may injure oral tissue, and infection and additional odor may result.

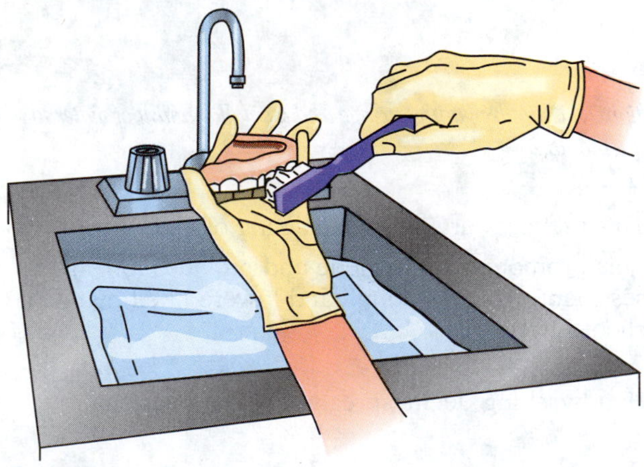

Figure 37-5
Proper method of cleaning dentures.

EVALUATING

At designated intervals, evaluate whether the client has met the goals established during planning and revise the care plan if indicated. An example follows:

> 10/26/98 Goal partially met. Client's oral mucosa is intact, but thick, dry secretions continue to build on oral mucosa and gums despite q [every] 4 hour care.
>
> *Revision*: Increase frequency of oral hygiene to q 2 hours. Instruct family.
>
> N. Glynn, RN

Care of the Eyes, Ears, and Nose

ASSESSING

Nursing History

Identify any special eye, ear, or nose care the client performs. Include the use and care of visual aids or prostheses (glasses, contact lenses, artificial eye) and hearing aids. Note any history of eye, ear, and nose problems and related treatments.

Physical Assessment

In the eye examination, note the position, alignment, and general appearance of the eye. Check that eyelashes are equally distributed and curl outward. Note the presence of lesions, nodules, redness, swelling, crusting, flaking, excessive tearing, or discharge of eyelids. Check the color of the conjunctivae, presence of blink reflex, and visual acuity (ability to read newsprint).

In the ear examination, note the position, alignment, and general appearance of the ear. Pay particular attention to a buildup of wax in the canal, dryness, crusting, or the presence of any discharge or foreign body. Check hearing acuity. Approximately one third of older adults have at least one ear obstructed by a wax build-up and this frequently causes hearing loss that can be reversed (Ney, 1993).

During examination of the nose, note its position and general appearance, patency of nostrils, and presence of tenderness, dryness, edema, bleeding, discharge, or secretions. Refer to Chapter 26 for additional information related to nursing assessment of the eyes, ears, and nose.

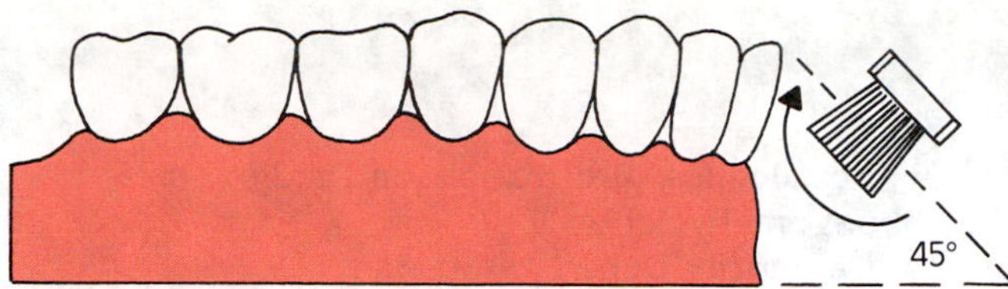

To clean gum line, surfaces, and between teeth, hold the toothbrush with the bristles at a 45° angle to the gum line and brush from the gum line to the crown of each tooth with a short, semicircular wrist action.

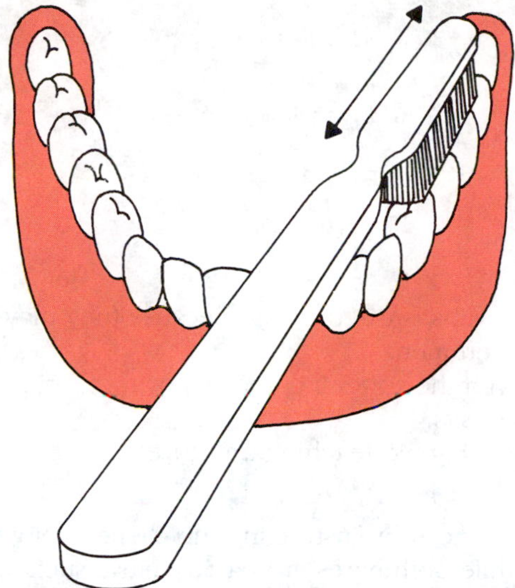

To clean biting and chewing surfaces of the teeth, hold the top of the bristles parallel to the tooth surface and brush back and forth.

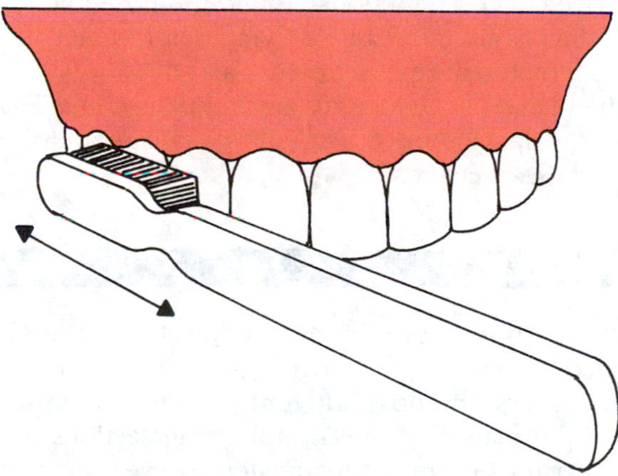

To polish the sides of the teeth, hold the brush bristles parallel to the surface of the teeth and gently brush back and forth.

Figure 37-6
Techniques for brushing teeth.

DIAGNOSING

Make a judgment about the adequacy of the client's self-care practices related to eye, ear, and nose care, identifying any factors that contribute to deficiencies. For example:

Self-Care Deficit: Artificial Eye Care, related to knowledge deficit

Identify actual or potential eye, ear, and nose problems that nurses can treat, noting contributing factors. Identify unhealthy client responses to eye, ear, and nose problems, for example:

Sensory/Perceptual Alterations (Visual, Auditory, or Olfactory) related to psychologic stress
Altered Health Maintenance related to perceptual impairment (visual or auditory)
Impaired Social Interaction related to visual or auditory impairment
Fear related to sudden loss of vision or hearing
Anticipatory Grieving related to increasing visual or auditory impairment
Risk for Injury related to visual impairment

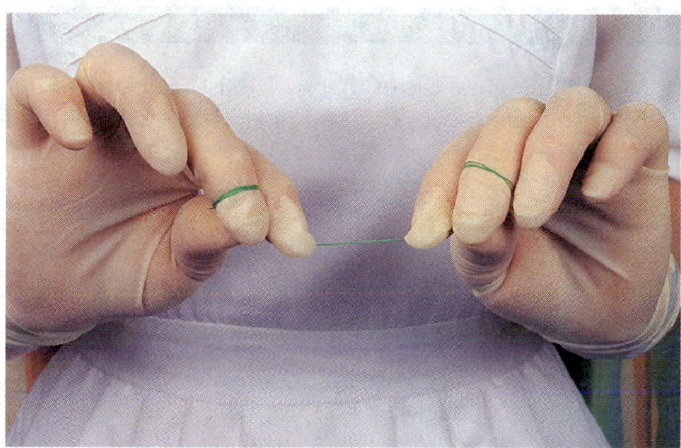

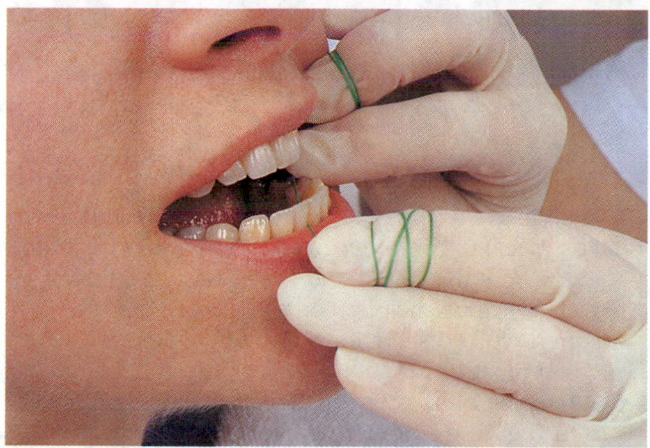

Figure 37-7
Dental flossing is necessary for removal of plaque and tartar between teeth. Flossing helps prevent gum disease as well as tooth decay by removing debris just below the gum line. Floss may be wrapped around the middle fingers of each hand or simply grasped in each hand in such a way that it can be stretched and held taut between the controlling fingers. Gently insert the floss between the teeth and move it with a sawing motion up from the gum line along the side of each tooth.

Helpscan

The following are resources for clients and health-care professionals:

- Helpline for older adults without insurance or means to pay who need to see an ophthalmologist
  National Eye Care Project
  PO Box 429098
  San Francisco, CA 94142-9098
  (800) 222-EYES
- For a free two-step screening test to encourage hearing-impaired people in the United States to get help
  Dial-a-Hearing-Screening-Test (DAHST)
  (800) 222-EARS between 9:00 AM and 5:00 PM EST
- For catalogues, information, and audiovisuals about oral hygiene
  American Dental Association
  211 East Chicago Avenue
  Chicago, IL 60611
  (312) 440-2500 (800) 947-4746

PLANNING: EXPECTED OUTCOMES

Identify nursing measures that will assist the client to develop or maintain eye, ear, and nose care measures that contribute to healthy eye, ear, and nose functioning and to the client's general sense of well-being. Plan to achieve the following client outcomes. The client will:

- Demonstrate healthy functioning of eyes, ears, and nose
- Have eyes, ears, and nose that appear clean
- Show signs of healing (if realistic, specify these signs) of sensory impairment (visual, auditory, olfactory), or seek aids appropriate to impairment
- Demonstrate correct eye, ear, and nose care measures, including the proper use and care of visual or auditory aids

Pertinent nursing measures to include in the plan of care are as follows:

Eye

- Clean the eye from the *inner canthus* (angle of the eye closest to the nose where the upper and lower lids meet) to the *outer canthus* (lateral angle of the eye where the upper and lower lids meet) using a wet, warm washcloth, cotton ball, or compress to soften crusted secretions. Carefully avoid cross contamination.
- When the blink (corneal) reflex is decreased or absent (eg, in the comatose client), use artificial tear solution or normal saline at least every 4 hours to keep the eyes moist and protected from drying; a protective shield may be necessary to keep the lids closed.
- Offer correct eyeglass, contact lens, or artificial eye teaching and care.

Ear

- Clean the external ear with a washcloth-covered finger, instructing the client never to insert objects into the ear for cleaning purposes. Use of cotton-tipped swabs is discouraged because they may impact cerumen.
- Assist with the softening and removal of excessive wax deposits.
- Offer hearing aid teaching and care.

Nose

- Clean the nose by instructing the client to blow the nose while both nares are patent (nasal suctioning with a bulb syringe may be indicated) unless contraindicated (eg, following brain surgery or head trauma).
- Remove crusted secretions around the nose and keep this tissue intact by applying a non–water-soluble ointment (eg, petroleum jelly).

In the plan of care, identify any supplies needed to carry out the specified eye, ear, and nose care and the timing of these measures.

IMPLEMENTING

Carry out plan of care, remembering to use each nurse–client interaction for ongoing assessment of the client's eyes, ears, and nose and for evaluation of the adequacy of the plan of care. The following sections describe select nursing measures related to eye, ear, and nose care. Sample documentation of eye care follows:

> 10/20/98 Client states, "I can't believe they expect me to take care of this eye. I don't want to touch it." Has not participated in artificial eye care to date. Client encouraged to verbalize concerns about artificial eye and assist with care.
>
> S. Cohen, RN

Cleaning the Eyes

Normally, the eyes are clear and kept clean with lacrimal secretions. During illness, the eyes may produce more secretions than they normally do and appear glasslike.

The following techniques are recommended when secretions adhere to the eyelashes and become dry and crusty or when discharge is present:

- Wear gloves during the cleaning procedure.
- Use water or normal saline and cotton balls or a clean washcloth or compress to clean the eyes. Boric acid solution, once popular for cleaning the eyes, is no longer recommended because of its toxicity when absorbed from mucous membranes. The eyes are never cleaned with soap because of its irritating effects on eye tissues.
- Position the client on the same side as the eye to be cleaned so that solution and debris do not run across the bridge of the nose and contaminate the other eye.
- Dampen a cotton ball with the solution of choice and wipe once while moving the cotton ball from the inner canthus to the outer canthus of the eye. This technique minimizes forcing debris into the area drained by the nasolacrimal duct. Discard the used cotton ball.
- Continue this technique, using one cotton ball for each stroke, until the eye is clean.
- Turn the client to the opposite side and clean the other eye in the same manner.
- Wipe the lashes dry with a paper tissue or a clean washcloth, exposing a clean area of the tissue or cloth with each stroke.

Caring for the Unconscious Client's Eyes

Clients with diminished or absent blink (corneal) reflexes and clients whose eyelids remain open require frequent eye care (at least every 4 hours). If the eye is not kept moist, corneal ulceration may result from excessive drying of the eye. Nursing measures include using saline or artificial tears to lubricate the eye and a protective eye shield to keep the eye closed.

Providing Care of Eyeglasses

Eyeglasses are essential for many people and represent a considerable financial investment. The nurse should take precautions to prevent their breakage or loss. Clients needing glasses should be encouraged to wear them to avoid eye strain.

Plastic lenses are popular because they are considerably lighter in weight than glass lenses and as accurate in correction as glass. One disadvantage of plastic is that the material scratches easily.

Eyeglasses should be cleaned over a terry towel so that if they slip they will not become scratched or broken. Glasses are cleaned with warm water and soap or using a special cleansing preparation. Hot water may warp plastic lenses and frames. The glasses should be rinsed well when cleansed with soap and water. They should be dried with a clean, soft cloth, such as a cotton handkerchief or cotton napkin. Paper products are made of wood pulp and are likely to scratch the lenses. Eyeglasses should not be cleaned with a dry paper tissue or cloth.

Providing Care of Contact Lenses

A contact lens is a small disc worn directly on the eyeball. It stays in place by surface tension of the eye's tears. Contact lenses are either hard or soft. The older hard lenses are not gas permeable, whereas newer ones are gas permeable and more comfortable because they allow oxygen to pass directly through the lens to the cornea. Soft lenses are of a plastic material that absorbs water to become soft and pliable. They are brittle when dehydrated and absorb water when placed in solution, usually normal saline, or when in contact with tears. Soft lenses may be used for daily wear or extended wear. Disposable soft lenses are also available.

People wearing contact lenses need to take special precautions to keep them free of microorganisms that may lead to eye infections and to use them in a manner that does not injure or scratch the surface of the eye. Hands must always be washed before touching eye surfaces and lenses. Lens wearers need to be cautious about eye irritation in the presence of noxious vapors or smoke. The lenses should not be in contact with cosmetics, soaps, or hair sprays because eye irritation may result. It is recommended that any adverse reaction to their use be reported to the prescribing physician immediately.

The cornea, which consists of dense connective tissue, does not have its own blood supply. It is nourished primarily by oxygen from the atmosphere and from tears. When wearing contact lenses, the cornea requires more than its normal supply of oxygen because its metabolic rate increases. To allow the cornea to receive a maximal supply of oxygen, hard lenses should be removed before sleeping and should not be worn more than 12 to 16 hours. Extended-wear soft lenses can be left in place for 1 to 30 days, depending on the manufacturer. It is recommended that extended-wear lenses be cleansed at least once weekly. The time that disposable soft lenses should be worn also varies according to the type and the manufacturer. A new disposable lens is replaced daily while other options include lenses that can be worn day and night for 7 days or those worn during waking hours only for 14 days. Excessive tearing, pain, and redness signal the need to remove lenses.

There may be times when the nurse may be required to remove lenses if a client cannot do so. To leave them in place for long periods could result in permanent eye damage. This may occur, for example, when the nurse is attending an unconscious client.

Before removing hard or gas-permeable lenses, the nurse should use gentle pressure to center the lens on the cornea. One method to remove this type of lens involves gently opening and spreading the eyelids past the upper and lower margins of the lens, causing it to shift slightly, and moving the eyelids toward each other, causing the lens to slide out between the eyelids. A small suction device can also be used in an emergency situation to remove gas-permeable or hard lenses.

Soft lenses are removed by gently grasping the lens near the lower edge, between the forefinger and thumb.

The lens folds up with this technique and is then lifted from the eye. Soft lenses are cleaned, rinsed, and placed in a container of solution for storage. The lenses should be identified as being for the right or left eye because the two lenses are not necessarily identical. The nurse should not try to remove lenses, however, if an eye injury is present, because of the danger of additional injury.

Providing Care of an Artificial Eye

Most clients who wear an artificial eye prefer to take care of it themselves, and they should be encouraged to do so when possible. The necessary equipment includes a small basin, soap and water for washing, and solution for rinsing the prosthesis. Normal saline or tap water can be used for rinsing. Most people have their own method for cleaning the eye socket and the area around it. The nurse should ask the client how he or she does this and make it possible for the client to continue with the usual practice. The client should be lying down so that the eye does not accidentally fall to the floor. The socket is ordinarily flushed with normal saline before the eye is replaced.

Providing Ear Care

Other than cleaning the outer ears, little is needed for routine hygiene of the ear. After the ears are washed, they should be dried carefully with a soft towel so that water and cerumen (wax) are removed by capillary action. Forcing the towel into the ear for drying or using a cotton-tipped applicator may aid in the formation of wax plugs.

If a wax plug is present in the auditory canal, it is easier to remove if a wax softening agent is used several days prior to irrigation. The stream of water should be directed toward the side of the canal to prevent injury to the drum (see Chapter 29 for the procedure for ear irrigations). A bulb syringe or an oral hygiene appliance (eg, a Water Pik) on a low setting may be used for this purpose. Using bobby pins, hairpins, paper clips, or fingernails to remove wax from the ear is extremely dangerous because these may injure or puncture the eardrum.

Hearing Aids. If the client uses a hearing aid, batteries should be checked routinely and the earpieces cleaned daily with mild soap and water. Refer to Chapter 22 for strategies nurses can use to facilitate communication with a hearing-impaired client. If hearing loss is mild and the client is not using a hearing aid, the following suggestions may help to improve hearing and should be included in any health teaching.

- Avoid noisy places for conversation.
- Choose well-lighted places where it is easier to look at the speaker's face, lips, and hands for cues to the conversation.
- Cup your hand behind your ear.
- Ask people to face you when they are speaking to you.
- Ask people to repeat what they said, if it was not clear to you, and to speak slowly.
- Consider buying amplitude devices so you can hear your television and radio without turning up the sound (Alberti et al., 1992).

Home Healthcare Alert

Remind clients and family members to ask the telephone company about special equipment that can help a hearing-impaired person hear the phone ringing and carry on a phone conversation more easily.

Figure 37-8 illustrates several types of hearing aids.

Providing Nose Care

The best way to clean the nose is to blow it gently. Both nostrils should be open while doing this. Closing one nostril adds to the danger of forcing debris into the eustachian tubes. Irrigations are usually contraindicated because of the possible danger of forcing material into the sinuses.

If the external nares are crusted, applying mineral or cottonseed oil helps to soften and remove the crusts. Disposable paper tissues are recommended for nasal secretions. A cotton applicator may be used to clean the nares, but with great care to avoid injury. The applicator should never be introduced into the nares.

EVALUATING

At designated intervals, evaluate whether the client has achieved the outcomes established during planning. Revise the plan of care if indicated. An example follows:

> 10/24/98 Goal met. Client demonstrated correct care (cleaning) of artificial eye for the past two mornings. States, "I guess I should be happy to be alive and still able to see."
>
> N. Glynn, RN

Hair Care

Hair is an accessory structure of the skin. Good general health is essential for attractive hair and skin, and cleanliness helps in keeping hair and skin attractive. Illness affects the hair, especially when endocrine abnormalities, increased body temperature, poor nutrition, or anxiety and worry are present. Changes in the color or condition of the hair shaft are related to changes in hormonal activity or to changes in the blood supply to hair follicles.

ASSESSING

Nursing History

Identify the client's usual hair and scalp care practices, including styling preferences. Note any history of hair or scalp problems; possible causes for changes in the distribution, texture, or amount of hair; and related treatments.

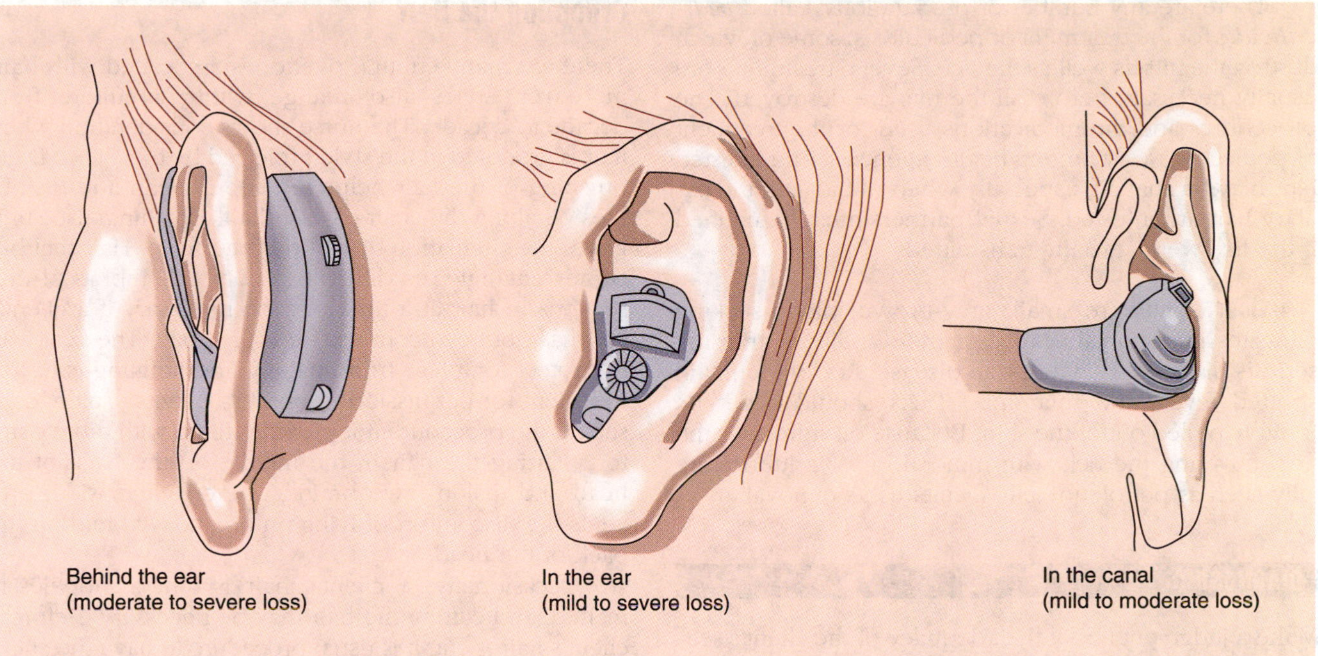

Figure 37-8
Several types of hearing aids.

Identify any factors known to cause hair or scalp problems or that require special care—deficient self-care abilities, immobility, malnutrition, treatments known to result in hair loss (eg, irradiation of the head, certain chemotherapeutic agents).

Physical Assessment

Assess the condition of the hair (texture, cleanliness, oiliness) and scalp (scaling, lesions, inflammation, infection). Common scalp and hair problems are discussed here.

Dandruff. *Dandruff* is a condition characterized by itching and flaking of the scalp that may be further complicated by the embarrassment it causes. Persistent, severe cases usually require medical attention. Daily brushing and shampooing with a medicated shampoo may be all that is needed to keep the scalp free of dandruff.

Hair Loss. Hair growth and hair loss are ongoing, daily processes. Hair loss from plaiting, excessive back combing and teasing, or the use of hair rollers is usually temporary, and hair returns when the tension on the hair shaft is halted. Some people experience hair loss owing to illness with high fever, certain medications, x-ray therapy of the head, childbirth, and general anesthesia. There appears to be no evidence that hair loss occurs as a result of wearing wigs or excessive shampooing. It is believed by some that an excessive intake of vitamin A may play a role in hair loss. Some permanent thinning of hair normally accompanies aging.

Baldness is called **alopecia**. It is common in men but rare in women, and it is believed to be hereditary. There is no known cure for baldness, although some external medications are currently in use and others are being developed. Their long-term efficacy is unknown. Hairpieces, frequently worn by people who are bald, require the same care as normal hair but less frequent washing.

A surgical procedure for baldness is the hair transplant. Hair is taken from donor sites, usually from the back or sides of the scalp, and transplanted to areas with no hair. The procedure is long and expensive but reportedly has decided benefits for people who find baldness psychologically unpleasant. Complications include serious scalp infections.

Pediculosis. Infestation with lice is called **pediculosis**. There are three common types of lice—*Pediculus humanus capitis*, which infests hair and scalp; *P. humanus corporis*, which infests the body; and *Phthirus pubis*, which infests the shorter hairs on the body, usually the pubic hair and the axillary hair. Lice lay eggs, called nits, on the hair shafts. *Nits* are white or light gray and look like dandruff, but they cannot be brushed or shaken off the hair. Frequent scratching and scratch marks on the body and the scalp suggest the presence of pediculosis. Although anyone may become infested with lice, the continued presence of pediculosis is usually a result of uncleanliness. Pediculosis can be spread directly by contact with infested areas or indirectly through clothing, bed linen, brushes, and combs. Teaching clients, especially children, not to share personal items is a good way to prevent transmission. The linens and personal-care items of a client with pediculosis require separate and careful handling to prevent spread from person to person.

There are any number of preparations, called *pediculicides* for the treatment of pediculosis, some of which destroy the nits as well as the lice. Several treatments are usually necessary before all the nits are destroyed. The procedures and the medications used for the treatment of pediculosis vary among health agencies. The infested hair may be shaved, especially when pubic hair and axillary hair are infested. Sexual partners must be notified if the lice were sexually transmitted.

Ticks. Ticks are small, gray-brown, blood-sucking parasites important because of their ability to transmit serious diseases such as Lyme disease, Rocky Mountain spotted fever, and tularemia. Ticks should never be forcibly pulled out of the skin. Because oil suffocates the tick, covering the tick with mineral oil or a lubricating jelly such as petroleum jelly facilitates its removal.

DIAGNOSING

Make a judgment about the adequacy of the client's self-care practices. Identify factors contributing to deficiencies, for example:

Self-Care Deficit: Hair Care, related to continuous bed rest

Identify actual or potential hair or scalp problems that nurses can treat, noting contributing factors. Identify unhealthy client responses to these problems, for example:

Risk for Infection related to hair transplant

Body Image Disturbance related to baldness

Impaired Skin Integrity related to scalp laceration (head bandages), pruritus

PLANNING: EXPECTED OUTCOMES

Identify nursing measures that will assist the client to develop or maintain needed hair and scalp care practices or that otherwise resolve nursing diagnoses. Specify any special products needed for hair care. Plan to achieve the following expected outcomes. The client will:

- Have clean and neatly styled hair
- Demonstrate decreased or absent scalp lesions (or infestation)
- Verbalize satisfaction with appearance
- Participate in hair and scalp care as able

IMPLEMENTING

Carry out the plan of care, remembering to use scheduled hygienic care interactions for ongoing assessment of the client's hair and scalp and for evaluating the adequacy of the plan of care. The following discussions give suggestions for grooming hair, shampooing hair, caring for beards and mustaches, and assisting with unwanted hair removal.

Grooming the Hair

There are many cultural overtones associated with hair; moreover, styles also change within a culture from decade to decade. The nurse shows consideration when hair is groomed in the style preferred by the client. Daily brushing of the hair helps to keep it clean and distributes oil along the shaft of each hair. Brushing also stimulates the circulation of blood in the scalp. Hair that becomes entangled is difficult to comb. Combing of tiny sections of hair at a time may be necessary if a client's hair has not been combed for even 1 day. The best way to protect long hair from matting and tangling is to ask the client for permission to braid it. Clients usually consent to the procedure if it provides them with more comfort. Parting the hair in the middle on the back of the head and making two braids, one on either side, prevents the discomfort of lying on one heavy braid on the back of the head.

Occasionally, a client's hair is almost hopelessly matted, and cutting the hair may be necessary. Before a client's hair is cut, it is usual procedure to have the client sign a written consent. It is also recommended that the nurse discuss the necessity for cutting the hair with an immediate member of the client's family.

The care of a person with kinky hair usually requires special attention. The hair is normally dry, curly, and becomes easily matted and tangled. The comb used for arranging the hair should have widely spaced teeth and is worked through the hair from the neckline upward toward the forehead.

Some individuals may choose to have their hair straightened. Even after this process, it may be difficult to untangle hair of a person who is confined to bed. African Americans may opt to style their hair in small braids. The braids are not undone for shampooing and may need to have a lubricant or oil applied daily to prevent hair strands from breaking.

Shampooing the Hair

The hair is exposed to the same dirt and oil as the skin. It should be washed as often as necessary to keep it clean. The comb and the brush should be washed each time the hair is washed and as frequently as necessary between shampoos. Many health agencies have beauticians and barbers to assist with the care of the client's hair, including shampooing it. However, this convenience does not relieve the nurse of responsibility.

Before shampooing the hair, it is recommended that the nurse, or the client, if able, brush and comb the hair well to stimulate the scalp and undo tangled hair. The client may then shampoo the hair while showering, if able. In some hospitals, a physician's order is required for shampooing a client's hair.

The following techniques are recommended for shampooing the hair of a client on bed rest (Fig. 37-9):

- Prepare several pitchers of water of a suitably warm temperature for a thorough washing and rinsing,

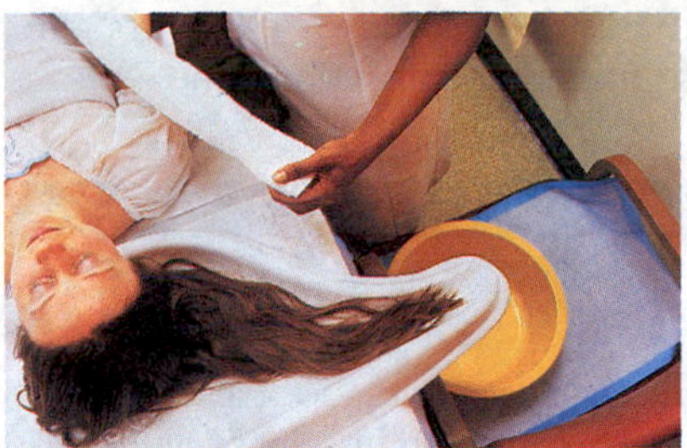

Place a waterproof pad under the client's shoulders, neck, and head. Position the shampooing trough under the client's head with the drainage spout extending over the edge of the bed. Place a recepticle below the spout to catch the water. Place a rolled towel under the client's neck at the edge of the trough.

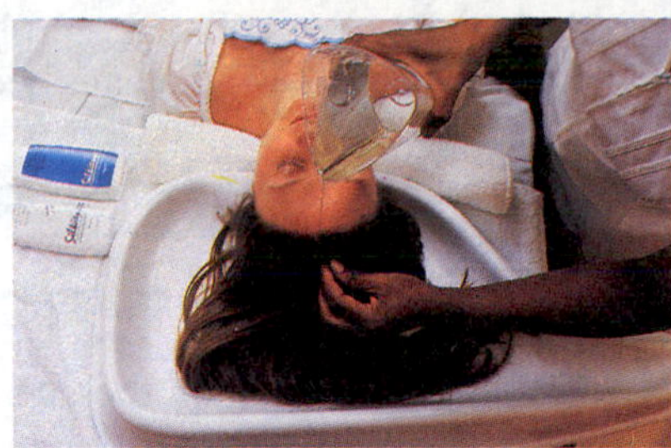

Using a pitcher of comfortably warm water, wet the client's hair completely.

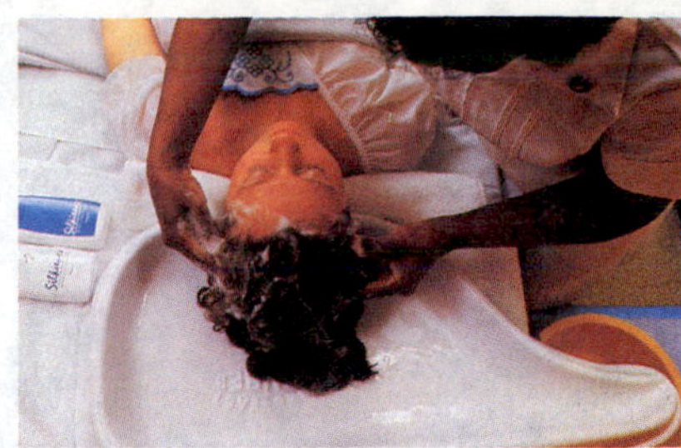

Apply shampoo and lather using both hands and working from the front to the back of the head.

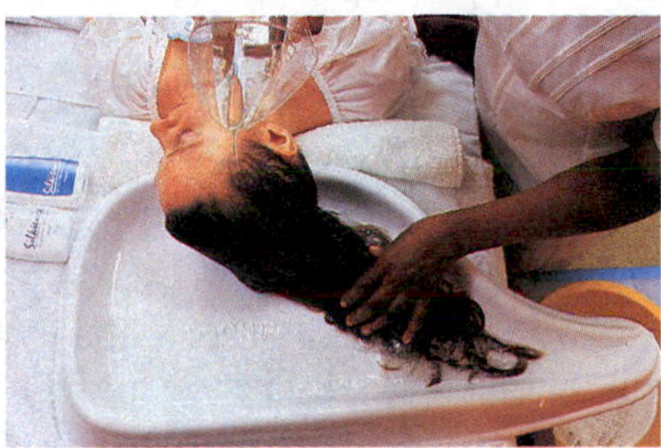

Rinse hair completely. Repeat shampooing and rinsing if necessary. Apply conditioner if requested and rinse again.

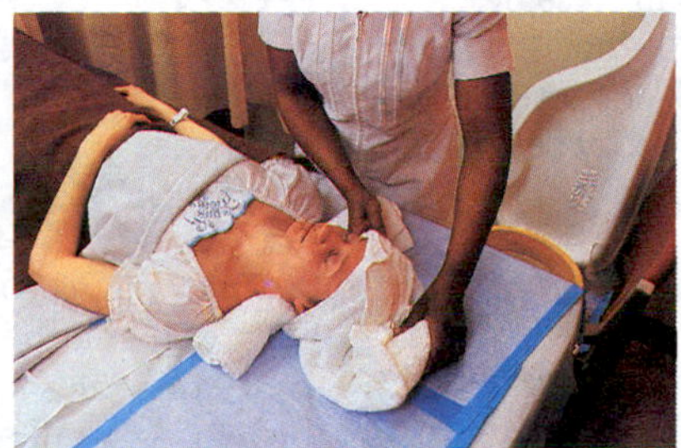

Wrap the client's head in towels to remove as much moisture as possible from the scalp and hair. Dry the client's face and neck.

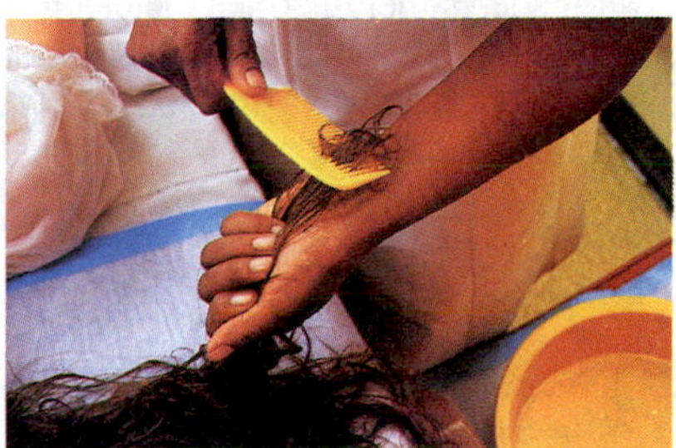

Comb gently to remove tangles. Complete drying of the hair using a dryer or towel according to agency policy.

Figure 37-9
Technique for shampooing a client's hair in bed.

shampoo soap, one or two towels for drying, and a receptacle to receive wash and rinse water.

- Place a protective pad under the head.
- Place the client in a position over the pad so that there is constant drainage of water directed into the receptacle.
- Wet the hair, apply soap, and massage the scalp well while washing the hair.
- Rinse the hair and apply soap for a second washing, if indicated.
- Rinse the hair thoroughly after washing it with soap and water.
- Apply conditioner if requested.
- Dry the hair as quickly as possible to prevent the client from becoming chilled, and arrange the hair according to the client's preference.

Dry Shampoo. Dry shampoos cannot replace the cleaning benefits of regular shampoos, but they are helpful in removing at least some of the dirt, oils, and odors from the hair of clients too ill or incapacitated to have a wet shampoo. Dry shampoos or powders are not recommended for people with kinky hair because of their normally dry hair and scalp. The dry shampoo or powder is applied and then combed or brushed from the hair. The teeth of a comb can be pulled through gauze, which helps remove and capture the powder.

Caring for Beards and Mustaches

Most clients with beards or mustaches are able to groom them independently. Dependent clients require nursing assistance to keep the beard and mustache clean, especially after eating. For no reason should a nurse trim or shave off a client's beard or mustache without the client's consent.

Shaving

Individual preferences for shaving methods are based on such factors as the type of skin, the quality of the beard, the frequency with which one shaves, the presence of skin problems, and convenience. An electric shaver is usually recommended when the client is on anticoagulant (blood thinning) therapy or has a bleeding disorder. Blade razors tend to give a closer shave than electric razors, but many clients find electric razors convenient and practical. They are especially convenient for the ill and bedridden client. The technique for shaving clients who are unable to shave themselves is described here and illustrated in Figure 37-10.

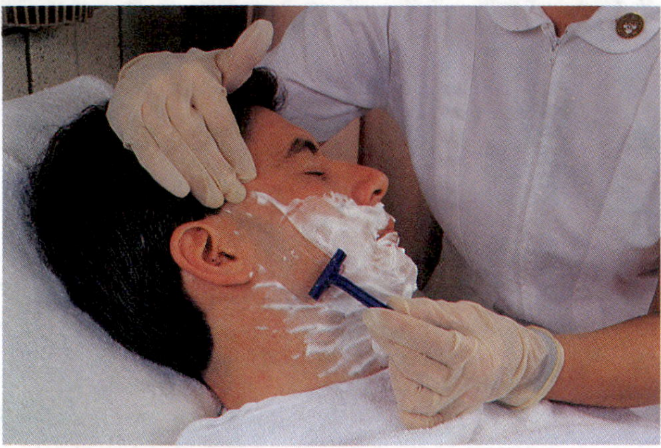

Figure 37-10
To shave a client's face with a razor, first apply shaving cream or warm soap lather to soften the beard. Shave the face by gently pulling the skin taut and using short, firm strokes in the direction of hair growth. After shaving, wash off any residual lather and dry the client's face. Aftershave lotion may be applied if requested.

- Glove use is optional but recommended because contact with blood is possible should any skin nicks occur.
- Shaving cream or a warm soap lather is first applied to the skin to soften the facial hair and prevent pulling.
- The skin of the face is pulled taut.
- Short, firm strokes in the direction of hair growth are used. Clients often can give suggestions on how they shave.
- Wash the client's face of residual lather and dry.
- Aftershave lotion may be applied. Aftershave preparations tend to make the face feel good and have a cosmetic rather than a therapeutic effect.

EVALUATING

At designated intervals, evaluate whether the client has achieved the outcomes established during planning and revise the plan of care if indicated. An example follows:

> 10/27/98 Goal partially met. Client reports that she is uncomfortable wearing a wig but feels better since its purchase.
>
> *Revision*: Because client still has many questions about effects of chemotherapy, continue teaching and use opportunities to build self-esteem.
>
> V. Henderson, RN

Nail and Foot Care

The nails are an accessory structure of the skin and comprise epithelial tissue. The body of the nail is the exposed portion; the root lies in the skin in the nail groove where the nail grows and is nourished. Healthy nails have a pink color and are convex and evenly curved. With certain pathologic conditions, and to some extent with aging also, the nails become ridged and areas become concave.

ASSESSING

Nursing History

Identify the client's normal nail and foot care practices, the type of footwear worn, and any history of nail or foot problems and their related treatments. The most important indication of a foot problem is a report from the client of a decreased ability to feel sensation in the feet (Brodbeck & Collier, 1994).

Identify any variables known to cause nail and foot problems, such as deficient self-care abilities, vascular disease, arthritis, diabetes mellitus, history of biting nails or trimming them improperly, frequent or prolonged exposure to chemicals or water, trauma, ill-fitting shoes, or obesity.

Physical Assessment

Examine nails for intactness and cleanliness; note capillary refill and the contour of the nailbed; observe the nail base for redness, swelling, bleeding, discharge, and tenderness. Examine the feet for cleanliness and intactness of skin, and note the presence of swelling, inflammation, lesions, tenderness, or orthopedic problems. Examine carefully the skin between the toes. Refer to Chapter 26 for additional information on techniques for assessing the nails and feet.

DIAGNOSING

Make a judgment about the adequacy of the client's self-care practices related to nail and foot care, identifying any factors that contribute to deficiencies. An example is as follows:

Self-Care Deficit: Diabetic Foot Care, related to knowledge deficit and weakened physical state

Identify actual or potential nail or foot problems that nurses can treat, noting contributing factors. Identify unhealthy client responses to these problems, for example:

Pain related to corns (calluses, plantar warts, ingrown nails) in foot

Impaired Physical Mobility related to painful foot condition (specify)

Risk for Infection related to traumatized nail base or deficient nail or foot care

Impaired Skin Integrity related to altered circulation to feet

PLANNING: EXPECTED OUTCOMES

Identify nursing measures that will assist the client to develop or maintain healthy nail and foot care practices. Plan to achieve the following expected outcomes. The client will:

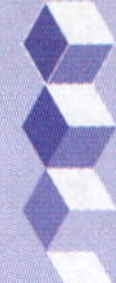

Through the Eyes of a Student

One of my first clients was a man in his late sixties who had suffered a stroke. I was assigned to care for him and his care included a bed bath and complete linen change—with him *in the bed.* I was determined to complete this task totally on my own, without asking anyone for help. This was my first mistake.

The client yelled obscenities at me and had very rough mannerisms. I kept thinking to myself, "I must treat him with gentle care and not show any fear." Inside I was shaking furiously.

I managed to complete his bath and then began to change the sheets. I helped the client to turn to one side, tucking the dirty linens close to him. I applied the fitted sheets to the upper portion of the bed . . . so far so good. Immediately going to the foot of the bed, I applied the bottom portion. The top portion popped off—I ran to the top of the bed, reapplied the top portion—the bottom portion popped off—I reapplied it. . . . I must have spent 15 minutes running back and forth trying to get both ends to stay on. By this time sweat was pouring off my face.

When I finally cried "Uncle," I discovered that certain fitted sheets just didn't fit all the mattresses. The usual routine in this case is to walk to the linen closet and get another fitted sheet. That probably takes about 15 seconds!

—Linda A. Keough, Delaware County Community College, Media, Pennsylvania

- Have intact, clean, and manicured nails
- Have intact, clean, and lesion-free foot skin
- Have reduced or absent nail and foot problems (specify: calluses, corns, plantar warts, ingrown nails, athlete's foot)
- Demonstrate correct nail and foot care measures
- Verbalize nails and feet contribute to general sense of comfort and well-being

Pertinent nursing measures to include in the plan of care are as follows:

- Soaking nails and feet and assisting with cleaning of nails and trimming nails (if not contraindicated)
- Massaging the feet to promote relaxation and comfort
- Teaching correct nail and foot care

In the plan of care, identify any supplies needed to carry out the specified nail and foot care and the timing of these measures.

IMPLEMENTING

Carry out the plan of care, remembering to use bath times to continually assess the status of the client's nails and feet and to evaluate the adequacy of the plan of care. Techniques for providing fingernail and foot care are described in this section. Sample documentation of foot care follows:

> 10/20/98 Client states "I guess I cut that nail too short—it's been hurting for 2 months now." Great toe on right foot is swollen, red, and painful. Skin at base of nail is white. Limps when walking. After bath, client soaked right foot and dried it carefully.
>
> A. Jones, RN

Providing Care of Fingernails

The following are recommended techniques for the care of fingernails:

- File the nails to form an oval at the ends. Do not trim so far down on the sides that injury to the skin and cuticle occurs.
- Remove hangnails, which are broken pieces of cuticle, by cutting them off. Take special care to avoid injury to tissue with the cuticle scissors.
- *Gently* push cuticles back off the nail after they are soft and pliable following a soaking in warm water.
- Push back cuticles with a blunt instrument or a terry cloth.
- Apply an emollient to the cuticle to help prevent hangnails.
- Clean under the nails with a blunt instrument or the large end of a toothpick, being careful to prevent injuring the area where the nail is attached to the underlying tissue.

Splitting and peeling of the nails are usually caused by dryness. It is helpful to avoid contact with soap and water as much as possible, use a good hand cream frequently, and avoid the use of nail polish and polish remover, both of which have a tendency to dry the nails.

Providing Foot Care

Proper foot care is important at any age. It becomes even more so with aging and when such conditions as circulatory disturbances or diabetes mellitus are present. Techniques for foot care follow:

- Bathe the feet thoroughly in a basin of soap or detergent and water solution. Be sure to clean the interdigital areas.
- Rinse the feet to remove soap or detergent residue, which irritates the skin if improperly removed.
- Continue to soak the feet in a basin of warm water if the toenails are brittle, thick, and striated before attempting to trim them. Or, wrap the feet in damp cloths and place them in plastic bags to soften the nails, if this is more convenient.

- Trim the nails straight across and not so short that tender areas of skin are exposed to the normal friction from shoes and stockings when the client is walking. In many institutions a physician's order is necessary for cutting nails.
- When trimming the nails, avoid digging into or cutting the toenails at the lateral corners. These practices predispose to ingrown nails. Clients with ingrown toenails, especially older people and clients with circulatory disorders or diabetes mellitus, may require the services of a physician or podiatrist.
- Clean under the nails with a blunt instrument or the large end of a toothpick, being careful to prevent injury to the area where the nail is attached to the underlying tissue.
- Apply powder to the feet and interdigital areas. If the skin is dry, use a lanolin cream instead.
- Bathe the feet at least daily but more often if they tend to perspire freely. Using a foot powder containing a nonirritating deodorant is helpful when foot odor is due to excessive perspiration. Foot powders are more absorbent than regular bath powders and often contain menthol, which makes the skin feel cool.

Improperly fitting and extremely worn or soiled hosiery contributes to foot problems. For some people with allergies or skin infections, nylon hosiery is contraindicated.

The nurse should be alert to any signs of foot problems, including infection, inflammation, ingrown nails, breaks in the skin in the interdigital areas, corns, calluses, bunions, and pressure areas, that may result in ulcerations. This is especially important for the client with diabetes.

Providing Foot Care for the Diabetic Client

A diabetic client is especially prone to foot problems owing to skin irritation, infection, and ulcers, which, without proper precautions, can result in gangrene. There are certain additional precautions that should be observed and taught to the client with diabetes:

- File the toenails. Scissors are too likely to slip and injure tissues.
- Do not cut off corns or calluses. Also, do not use commercial removers because they contain ingredients that often lead to irritation, infection, and ulcers. A physician who treats foot disorders, or **podiatrist**, should be consulted when corns and calluses are present.
- Do not use nonprescription preparations to treat athlete's foot and ingrown toenails because they may contain ingredients that lead to infection and ulcers. A physician or podiatrist should be consulted when athlete's foot or ingrown nails are present. The causative fungi of athlete's foot are species of *Trichophyton* or *Epidermophyton floccosum* and are capable of attacking the hair and nails as well as the skin.
- Avoid using heating pads and hot-water bottles applied to the feet because of the danger of blistering and burning the feet.
- Teach the client to avoid wearing round garters and stockings with elastic tops and not to sit with the knees crossed to prevent obstruction of circulation to the lower extremities and feet.
- Prop the feet up above the level of the hips a few minutes several times a day if the feet swell.
- Explain the dangers of going barefoot. The client may injure the skin of the feet or acquire athlete's foot in such places as public showers.
- Keep the feet dry and warm in shoes and stockings that provide plenty of room.
- Break in new shoes gradually; begin with a half hour of wear the first day and increase the time by about 1 hour a day. Improperly fitting shoes are a major cause of foot problems and can lead to corns, calluses, bunions, and blisters. The back of the shoe, or the counter, should fit snugly but not tightly. A heel offering safe support is recommended. When standing, there should be about 3/4 inch of space in the shoe beyond the great toe and also at the widest part of the shoe. In a shoe that fits well, the arch of the foot lies comfortably over the arch in the shoes. The soles should be flexible and nonslippery. Shoes with rough ridges, wrinkles, or tears in the linings should be discarded or repaired.

EVALUATING

At designated intervals, evaluate whether the client has achieved the expected outcomes established during planning and revise the plan of care if indicated. An example follows:

> 10/24/98 Expected outcome met. Client correctly verbalized rationale for diabetic foot care program and expressed interest in attending the diabetic classes.
>
> A. Diaz, RN

Perineal and Vaginal Care

The perineal area is dark, warm, and often moist, which favors bacterial growth. The client who is unable to clean the perineal area needs the nurse's assistance for this important part of personal hygiene. Neglecting cleaning the perineal area of the client who is unable to provide self-care often results in physical and psychologic discomfort for the client, a breakdown in the skin, and offensive odors.

ASSESSING

Nursing History

Identify any special perineal and vaginal hygiene practices the client performs, products used, and variables influencing these practices. Note any history of perineal or vaginal problems and related treatments.

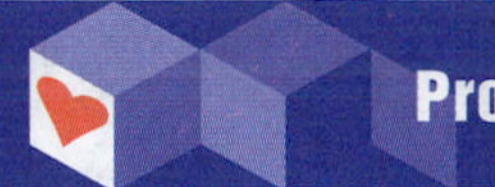

Promoting Wellness

Self-Care: Feminine Hygiene

Many women have concerns about feminine hygiene. Personal healthcare practices are influenced by past experiences, cultural knowledge, and societal expectations. It is important for women to feel comfortable with their bodies and to be knowledgeable about self-care practices that promote health and well-being and prevent infection and disease. If this is a concern for you, take a few minutes to respond to the questions below and read the accompanying information.

Assessment Guide (Check the phrase that best describes you)	Self-Care Knowledge, Attitude, Skills
☐ I feel comfortable with my body. I accept its uniqueness. ☐ My body often makes me feel uncomfortable (fearful, anxious, guilty).	A woman's health and sense of self can be uniquely influenced by her sexuality and its expression and by several changes in her physiology: the onset of menstruation, pregnancy, interruption of pregnancy, childbirth, postpartum, nursing, and menopause. By virtue of ownership, women have the right to control their own bodies. This includes *knowing* their bodies, accepting their uniqueness, and caring for their bodies appropriately. Distorted ideas that the genital area is somehow "dirty" and needs special deodorizing and scenting or that it is shameful to discuss problems in this area or to talk about related concerns need to be replaced by healthier attitudes.
☐ I am knowledgeable about feminine hygiene practices and products. I value preventive measures that promote health and reduce the likelihood of infections. ☐ I have never thought much about feminine hygiene nor discussed this with anyone.	Each woman can be an expert in the care of her own body. Feminine hygiene practices that promote health and prevent infection include the following: • Wash the perineal area at least once daily to remove perspiration and smegma accumulations; pat rather than rub the area dry; towels and washcloths should be clean and never shared. • Always wipe from front to back after voiding and defecation to avoid introducing bacteria into the vagina or urethra. • Sprays, soaps, powders, deodorants, and tampons and pads that are perfumed or irritating in any way should not be used; any chemicals that irritate the skin or vaginal mucosa or alter the vaginal environment should be avoided. • Avoid clothing that is too tight, does not allow free air flow to the perineum, or traps moisture; underpants and pantyhose should always a have a cotton crotch. • Douching should be avoided or kept to a minimum; douching can strip the vagina of its normal flora, introduce bacteria, and aggravate inflammation. • If tampons are used during menstruation, choose the smallest absorbency needed to absorb flow; change regularly (every 3 to 4 hours), and use good handwashing techniques before insertion; women who have had toxic shock syndrome should not use tampons until *Staphylococcus aureus* is no longer present in the vaginal flora. • Sexual partners should be clean; it is okay to discuss this with partners before intercourse; advise use of condoms; if any doubts exist about partner, refrain from contact; void before and after intercourse; if lubricant is needed during intercourse, a sterile, water-soluble type should be used.

(continued)

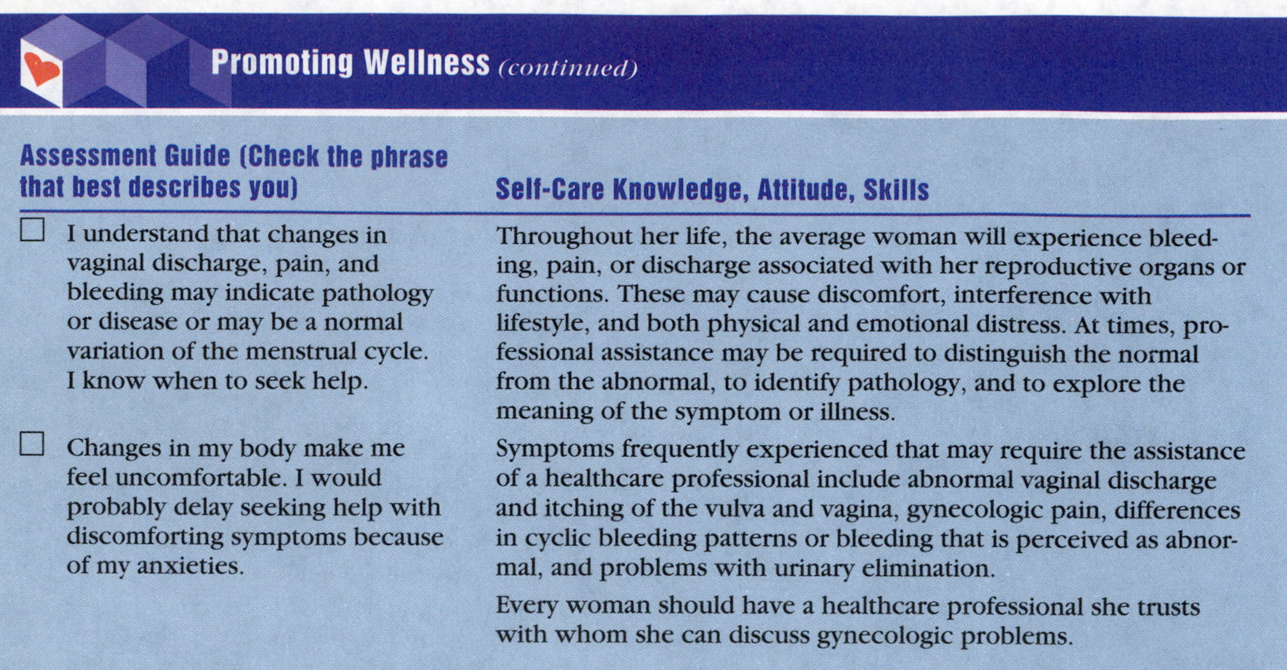

Promoting Wellness *(continued)*

Assessment Guide (Check the phrase that best describes you)	Self-Care Knowledge, Attitude, Skills
☐ I understand that changes in vaginal discharge, pain, and bleeding may indicate pathology or disease or may be a normal variation of the menstrual cycle. I know when to seek help.	Throughout her life, the average woman will experience bleeding, pain, or discharge associated with her reproductive organs or functions. These may cause discomfort, interference with lifestyle, and both physical and emotional distress. At times, professional assistance may be required to distinguish the normal from the abnormal, to identify pathology, and to explore the meaning of the symptom or illness.
☐ Changes in my body make me feel uncomfortable. I would probably delay seeking help with discomforting symptoms because of my anxieties.	Symptoms frequently experienced that may require the assistance of a healthcare professional include abnormal vaginal discharge and itching of the vulva and vagina, gynecologic pain, differences in cyclic bleeding patterns or bleeding that is perceived as abnormal, and problems with urinary elimination. Every woman should have a healthcare professional she trusts with whom she can discuss gynecologic problems.

(Adapted from Fogel, C. I., & Woods, N. F. [1981]. *Health care of women: A nursing perspective* [pp. 220–255]. St. Louis: Mosby).

Identify any variables known to cause perineal or vaginal problems or to create a need for special care: urinary or fecal incontinence; indwelling Foley catheters; childbirth; rectal or genital surgery; and diseases such as urinary tract infection, diabetes mellitus, and certain sexually transmitted diseases (STDs) such as herpes.

Physical Assessment

Examine the male genitalia (penis, scrotum, and perineum) for lesions, swelling, inflammation, excoriation, tenderness, and discharge (amount, color, odor, and source); examine the female genitalia (pubic area, labia, clitoris, urinary meatus, and perineum) for color, size, lesions, masses, swelling, inflammation, excoriation, tenderness, and discharge (amount, color, odor, and source). Examine the anal area for cracks, nodules, distended veins, masses, or polyps; note strong perineal odors. Refer to Chapter 26 for additional perineal assessment information.

DIAGNOSING

Make a judgment about the adequacy of the client's perineal (vaginal) self-care practices, identifying any factors that contribute to deficiencies. An example is:

Self-Care Deficit: Perineal Care, related to cognitive impairment

Next, identify actual or potential perineal and vaginal problems that nurses can treat, noting contributing factors, and identify unhealthy client responses to these problems. Examples of these are:

Pain related to excoriated perineal area
Risk for Infection related to client's deficient perineal hygiene
Knowledge Deficit: Advisability of using deodorized feminine hygiene products related to inexperience and a desire to "be clean"
Disturbance in Body Image related to genital lesions
Altered Sexuality Patterns related to painful genital lesions
Risk for Impaired Skin Integrity related to urinary and fecal incontinence

PLANNING: EXPECTED OUTCOMES

Identify nursing measures that will assist the client to develop or maintain healthy perineal (vaginal) care practices that will contribute to the client's general sense of well-being. Plan to achieve the following client outcomes. The client will:

- Demonstrate clean perineal area with skin intact
- Demonstrate signs of healing of perineal lesions or excoriations (discharge is decreased or absent)
- Demonstrate correct perineal and vaginal hygiene measures

The following are pertinent nursing measures to include in the plan of care:

- Cleaning the male genitalia (penis, scrotum, perineum, and rectal area) or the female genitalia

(pubic area, labia, clitoris, urinary meatus, perineum, and rectal area)

- Instructing the client on perineal hygiene practices

IMPLEMENTING

Carry out the plan of care, remembering to use bath time, when appropriate, for ongoing assessment of the client's perineum and for evaluation of the adequacy of the plan of care. Procedures for perineal and vaginal care are described in this section. Sample documentation of teaching care of genitalia follows:

> 10/20/98 Child presented with large amount of smegma under the foreskin and painful urination. Mother and child were instructed in the need and correct technique for cleansing the uncircumcised penis. Child correctly returned the demonstration.
>
> L. Woo, RN

Providing Perineal Care

It is not always possible for male nurses to attend to male clients and female nurses to attend to female clients. When the perineal cleaning is carried out in a matter-of-fact and dignified manner, clients generally do not find care by a person of the opposite gender to be offensive or embarrassing.

Some nurses use a sitz tub to clean the client's perineal and anal areas. The portable type is especially handy when it is cumbersome to move a client to a stationary sitz tub. The procedure may be carried out while the client remains in bed. The following techniques are recommended to administer perineal care to clients (Fig. 37-11):

- Assemble supplies and provide for privacy.
- Explain the procedure to the client and don disposable gloves.
- Wash and rinse the groin area for both the male and female client.
- Always proceed from the least contaminated area to the most contaminated area. For a female client, spread the labia and move the washcloth from the pubic area toward the anal area to prevent carrying organisms from the anal area back over the genital area. Use a clean portion of the washcloth for each stroke. For a male client, move the washcloth in a spiral motion from the tip of the penis down its length toward the pubic area.
- In an uncircumcised male client, retract the foreskin (prepuce) while washing the penis. Rinse well with plain water.
- Rinse the washed areas well with plain water.
- Pull the uncircumcised male client's foreskin back into place over the glans penis to prevent constriction of the penis, which may result in edema and tissue injury.
- Wash and rinse the male client's scrotum. Handle the scrotum, which houses the testicles, with care because the area is sensitive.
- Dry the cleaned areas and apply an emollient as indicated. Powder the area only if the client requests it. For the female client, powder may become a medium for the growth of bacteria, and studies currently are linking use of powder with increased risk of cervical cancer.
- Turn the client on his or her side and continue with cleansing the anal area. Continue in the direction of least contaminated to most contaminated

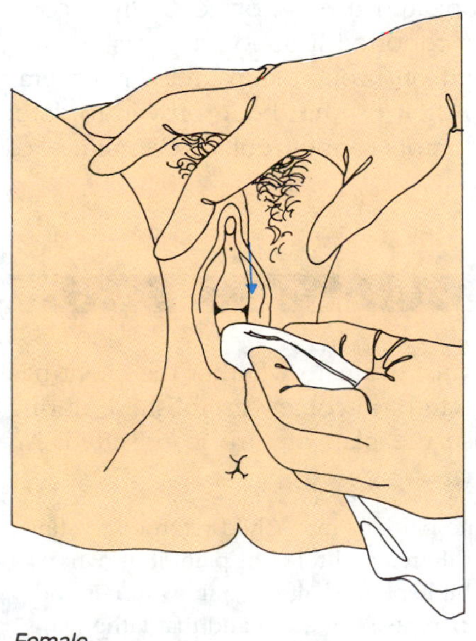

Female

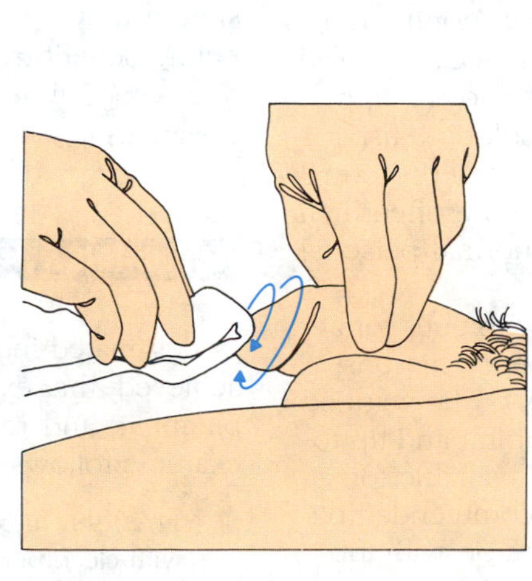

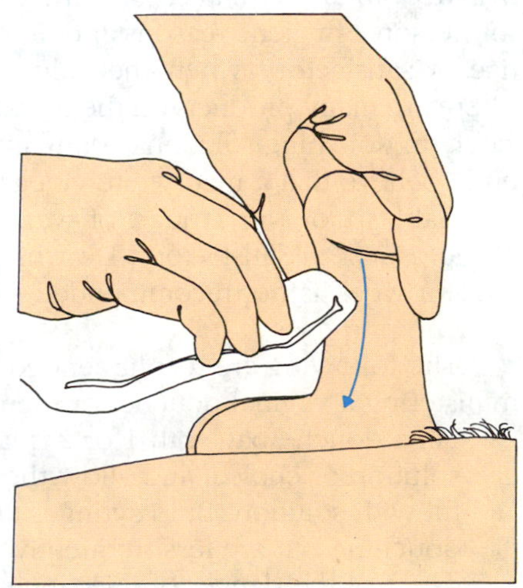

Male

Figure 37-11
Performing normal perineal care.

area. In the female, cleanse from the vagina toward the anus. In both female and male clients, change the washcloth with each stroke until the area is clean. Rinse and dry the area.

- If the client has an indwelling catheter and the agency recommends daily care for the catheter, it is usually done following perineal care. Agency policy may recommend use of an antiseptic cleaning agent (eg, povidone-iodine) or plain soap and water on a clean wash cloth. Put on clean gloves prior to cleaning the catheter. Cleanse 6 to 8 inches of the catheter, moving from the meatus downward. Be careful not to pull or tug on the catheter during the cleaning motion. Inspect the meatus for drainage and note the characteristics of the urine. A physician's order is required if antibiotic ointment is applied to the meatus after cleansing. Additional information involving care of an indwelling catheter is discussed in Chapter 43.

Home Healthcare Alert

Caregivers or clients at home with an indwelling catheter should be instructed to wash the urinary meatus and perineal area twice daily with soap and water. The anal area should also be cleansed after each bowel movement. Careful handwashing is imperative.

Providing Vaginal Care

In normal, healthy women, regular daily internal douching is believed to be both unnecessary and unwise. The practice tends to remove normal bacterial flora from the vagina, and if the solution is high in acid content, it may irritate or injure normal cells. Many women use douches for personal hygiene reasons after intercourse. The practice is satisfactory when the solution is nonirritating. There are many products on the market that can be used safely in douching solutions. Many gynecologists apparently believe that a mild white-vinegar solution, using 1 or 2 tablespoons in 1 quart of warm water, or normal saline, is just as satisfactory. Douching more often than twice a week is not recommended for normal personal hygiene purposes.

The following are recommended techniques for administering a vaginal douche for therapeutic reasons:

- Fill a douche bag with 1 or 2 quarts of the warmed solution of choice, and allow the tubing and tip to fill with solution. Bulb syringes are available for douching but are less frequently recommended because of the danger of injecting solution with too much force and forcing it into the cervix.
- Place the client on a bedpan. The client may lie in a bathtub if she is able to administer the douche herself. Standing up in the tub is not recommended because it requires too much force to carry solution to the vagina for thorough cleaning.
- Hold the bag or hang it on a standard so that it is about 24 to 36 inches (60 to 90 cm) above the level of the hips.
- Separate the labia with gloved fingers, and insert the douche tip by directing it downward and backward to follow the normal contour of the vagina. Allow the solution to begin flowing.
- Hold the vulva snugly to close the vaginal orifice or ask the client to contract her muscles around the orifice to allow solution to collect and distend the vagina; then allow the solution to escape. Repeat this procedure during the douche until all of the solution is used. This technique distends the vagina and permits better cleaning of its convoluted walls.
- Do not raise the level of the bag containing the solution during the douche because this may cause undue force that may result in the introduction of organisms into the cervix.

Medical attention is recommended when a discharge or irritation and itching about the vaginal orifice persist. Douching to relieve the symptoms may only tend to aggravate the cause of the problem. Before a vaginal examination, a douche is contraindicated because it removes secretions and discharge needed for specimens necessary for diagnostic procedures. Most authorities recommend not having a vaginal douche for 24 to 48 hours before a vaginal examination.

Deodorants to control odor around the vaginal orifice may be applied directly to the area or placed on sanitary napkins. Although these deodorants do not contain aluminum salts, which are irritating to the mucous membrane, they are intended for external use only. They should not be used on tampons. Some have been reported as possibly harmful when sprayed into the vagina. Repeated use is not generally recommended because of reported irritation and rashes, nor should they be used on broken skin areas. No therapeutic benefit from their use has been proven to date. These special deodorants cannot replace cleanliness of the area.

EVALUATING

At designated intervals, evaluate whether the client has achieved the expected outcomes established during planning, and revise the plan of care if indicated. An example follows:

> 11/20/98 Outcome partially met. Child returned to clinic with clean perineal area and relief of painful urination. Mother reports child spends half the time with her and half with father (parents separated) and that father is uncommitted to hygiene practices.
>
> *Revision:* Stress again to child importance of retracting foreskin during perineal care.
>
> C. Moser, RN

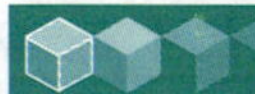

Nursing Process in Clinical Practice

Once a personal hygiene and oral care problem is identified, the nurse implements each phase of the nursing process to ensure its correct identification and treatment. The knowledge and clinical skills described in this chapter will enable the nurse to manage this situation correctly. The following section addresses specific assessment priorities, expected outcomes, and nursing interventions for two common nursing diagnoses for a client who requires assistance with personal care and oral hygiene measures:

Bathing/Hygiene Self Care Deficit
Altered Oral Mucous Membrane

Bathing/Hygiene Self Care Deficit

> A state in which the individual experiences an impaired ability to perform or complete bathing/hygiene activities for oneself. (NANDA, 1994)

Clients are unable to meet their own hygiene needs for a variety of reasons. Physical impairments (eg, a stroke or musculoskeletal problem) may interfere with their ability to move extremities in a coordinated manner. Clients may state that fatigue or pain limit their ability to complete such tasks. Decreased mental alertness may also be a contributing factor.

Assessment Priorities

- Use interview questions directed to the client and significant others to determine the nature and extent of the problem and its probable cause.
- Describe the client's self-care abilities including functional and mechanical skills.
- Assess the general condition of the skin.
- Determine the level of care required for this client.

Expected Outcomes

The client will:

- Complete personal hygiene measures according to ability on a daily basis
- Communicate feelings concerning limitations
- Express satisfaction with completion of personal hygiene measures
- Maintain skin integrity

Interventions

Nursing interventions include the following:

- Encourage maximum participation of client in personal hygiene activities.
- Assemble necessary equipment within easy reach of the client.
- Monitor client's ability to complete personal hygiene measures.
- Provide for privacy during bathing activities.
- Provide assistive devices based on client's need.
- Maintain safe environment during bath.
- Modify bathing routine according to client's ability.
- Instruct client or significant others in correct bathing procedure.
- Document client participation in bathing activities.
- Observe condition of skin while bathing or assisting with client's bath and document presence of any areas of skin breakdown.

Altered Oral Mucous Membrane

> The state in which an individual experiences disruptions in the tissue layers of the oral cavity. (NANDA, 1994)

Nurses play a key role in the assessment and prevention of oral health problems. According to Winkley et al. (1993), alterations in the oral mucous membrane of immobile clients may be related to a soft or liquid diet, effects of certain medications, circulatory deficit in the oral cavity, mouth breathing, or the presence of caries and periodontal disease. Frequent oral hygiene provides opportunity to assess for the development of any oral problems, reduces odors, and facilitates a healthy mouth. Whether the client performs his or her own care or requires assistance, has his or her own teeth or wears dentures, individualized nursing care can have a profound effect on the integrity of the oral cavity.

Assessment Priorities

- Use interview questions directed to client and significant others to determine history of oral surgery, dentures, braces, or other dental problems.
- Assess oral hygiene.
- Examine the oral cavity for signs of altered mucous membrane (eg, inflammation, dryness, lesions, ulcerations, white patches, bleeding).
- Assess presence of pain.
- Determine client's ability to perform oral care.
- Examine fluid, electrolyte, and nutritional status for additional information (eg, weight, intake and output, skin turgor, lab values, etc.)
- Explore the client's lifestyle and habits for contributing factors (eg, regular use of tobacco and/or alcohol, medication history).
- Assess client's ability to swallow.

Expected Outcomes

The client will:

- Demonstrate integrity of oral mucous membrane.
- Report improvement in comfort level.
- Relate need for improved oral hygiene.
- Perform or assist with oral hygiene activities according to ability.

Interventions

Nursing interventions include the following:

- Perform oral hygiene measures at frequent intervals for dependent client (eg, one who is unresponsive or who has altered level of consciousness).
- Teach preventive oral hygiene measures (eg, brushing, flossing techniques, regular dental examinations).
- Inspect oral cavity at regular intervals and document observations.
- Assist with oral hygiene before and after meals (eg, brush teeth, floss, provide mouthwash and lip lubricant).
- Discuss precipitating factors and planned alterations in habits.
- Encourage adherence to treatment regimen.

Client Care Study

Glenda Davis is a nurse practitioner who works in a campus health clinic at a state university. She is frequently approached by women who ask questions about feminine hygiene. Realizing that each woman who presents with a question probably represents many other women with similar unvoiced questions, she decides to develop an insert titled *Self Care: Feminine Hygiene* for the campus newspaper. The information she plans to include and the population she will address in her checklist are based on the following assessment data:

- Heterogeneous female population is of various ages, cultures, religions, sexual orientation, and family and lifestyle backgrounds.
- Knowledge about feminine hygiene varies widely from almost no knowledge to students who are well read or members of women's health professions.
- Students who present with questions are mostly concerned about dangers of certain products (eg, tampons and toxic shock syndrome) or have questions related to intercourse (eg, advisability of douching, how to avoid getting an STD, and so forth).
- Numerous students report to the clinic with vaginal infections and urinary tract infections.
- Interest is high; ability to comprehend written materials is high.

Core Competencies

In order to implement this plan of care, the nurse needs the following specialized abilities:

Cognitive Competencies

- Knowledge of feminine hygiene and advantages and disadvantages of various healthcare practices and products
- Teaching skills to work one-on-one with women who come to the campus health clinic
- Ability to develop nursing diagnoses that reflect the unique feminine hygiene needs of this student population
- Conviction that nursing can make a difference in the quality of life for these students

Technical Competencies

- Strong assessment skills (interviewing and physical assessment) to identify carefully gynecologic concerns and problems presented by these students
- Caregiver skills directed toward preventive hygiene measures that reduce the risk of acquiring a vaginal or urinary tract infection

Interpersonal Competencies

- Interpersonal skills to communicate concern for the health questions and fears of women of many different backgrounds
- Commitment to work with women to develop understanding of the female body and healthier self-care behaviors
- Attentive listening to assess correctly the healthcare needs of the population
- Ability to establish a trusting nurse–client relationship grounded in responsible caring
- Written communication skills to develop a self-care feature on feminine hygiene for campus publication

Ethical/Legal Competencies

- Accountability and willingness to act competently to help students recognize specific hygiene concerns and report problems and concerns promptly
- Competence in documenting nursing interventions
- Ability to serve as a trusted and effective client advocate

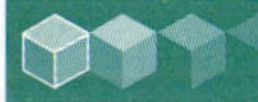

Nursing Plan of Care

for Female University Students

Nursing Diagnosis: Self-Care Deficit: Feminine Hygiene, related to knowledge deficit as manifested by: female students presenting to the campus clinic with questions about feminine hygiene; high incidence of vaginal and urinary tract infections; negative attitudes about feminine body frequently expressed.

Expected Outcome: Students will:

- Express positive body image, valuing their uniqueness

Nursing Interventions	Rationale	Evaluative Statement
With each student who presents at the clinic for help with a gynecologic concern or problem, take the time to assess her knowledge of the female body, and her acceptance of her body and comfort with it.	The women's health movement has encouraged women to feel ownership of their bodies, to appreciate their uniqueness as women, and to increase their awareness of their physical bodies and the feelings associated with them. Many women still feel that the genital area and cyclic phenomena such as the menstrual cycle and the female sexual response cycle are "dirty" and symptoms in this area may evoke fear, guilt, anxiety, and shame.	*Six-month evaluation:* 6/30/98 Goal partially met: students are beginning to discuss gynecologic concerns more freely yet great hesitancy persists. *Revision:* Continue to help women to know, understand, and accept their bodies and to talk about their bodies. Make this a priority of the nursing staff at the clinic. ***G. Davis, RN***
Counsel appropriately.	It is important for nurses to provide women with information about their bodies.	

Expected Outcome Students will:

- Correctly describe feminine hygiene self-care behaviors they are willing to incorporate into their daily lifestyles

Nursing Interventions	Rationale	Evaluative Statement
Assess with each client her knowledge of feminine hygiene practices (correct any misconceptions) and motivation to use them consistently.	Many women have never been instructed about feminine hygiene and harmful practices may be "picked up" from the media and other sources (eg, the use of frequent douching and deodorants to eliminate normal body odors).	6/30/98 Goal met. Following publication of the *Self-Care: Feminine Hygiene* feature and one-on-one counseling using this printed handout, clients are knowledgeable about preventive hygiene measures. ***G. Davis, RN***
Address specific concerns related to menstruation, intercourse, other maturational events.	Maturational events, such as menstruation, becoming sexually active, and pregnancy, may result in a need for new or modified hygiene practices.	
Teach the importance of using preventive hygiene measures to reduce the likelihood of acquiring a urinary tract or vaginal infection. Distribute the *Self-Care: Feminine Hygiene* handout and discuss this with the client.	It is better to prevent a genitourinary infection than to treat it.	

(continued)

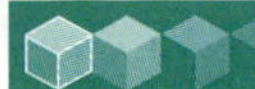

Nursing Plan of Care *(continued)*

for Female University Students

Expected Outcome

Campus health clinic records will:

- Demonstrate a reduction in both new and recurrent genitourinary infections

Nursing Interventions	Rationale	Evaluative Statement
Educate women regarding preventive hygiene measures (refer to the *Self-Care* handout).	It is better to prevent a genitourinary infection than to treat it.	6/30/98 Goal met. Six months after publication and use of the *Self-Care: Feminine Hygiene* handout, the incidence of genitourinary infections is reduced 10%. Will continue to keep education in this regard a priority. ***G. Davis, RN***
Educate women to distinguish normal from abnormal findings (vaginal discharge, pain, bleeding, problems with urination) and to seek help when appropriate. Nursing measures include teaching preventive measures, instructing in recognition of symptoms, and assisting with self-care activities to prevent and treat infections, including the securing of assistance when indicated.	Early treatment of genitourinary infections reduces the likelihood of residual problems.	
Document new and recurrent genitourinary infections; identify predisposing factors.	Documentation facilitates ongoing management of a recurring problem.	

Sample Documentation

6/15/98 Nursing

Student visited clinic and expressed need for information about feminine hygiene practices in general and, specifically, those specific hygiene measures for use after intercourse. Also related concern about contracting an STD from partners. Reported that she became sexually active this year and has sexual intercourse once or twice weekly. Stated that "many of my friends use douches" and questioned if any particular douche products are recommended. We discussed the *Self-Care: Feminine Hygiene* handout and reviewed various healthcare practices. Clarified for student her misconception regarding the advisability of douching. Also counseled her about her right to talk with a sexual partner about STDs and previous contacts with infected individuals. Advised that she refrain from contact or use a condom when she has intercourse. Student reported feeling more "in charge" of body and better able to care for it. Discussed all topics on plan of care and encouraged her to revisit clinic in 6 months for further clarification and evaluation.

G. Davis, RN

Key Points

- Personal hygiene refers to measures of personal cleanliness and grooming that promote physical and psychologic well-being.
- People differ in personal hygiene practices, which may be affected by culture, socioeconomic class, religion, developmental level, knowledge level, health state, and personal preferences.
- A comprehensive assessment of the skin and mucous membranes includes the collection of data about usual hygiene practices (showering or bathing practices; skin, hair, and scalp care; eye, ear, nose, and mouth care; nail and foot care; and perineal care); an assessment of any sensory, cognitive, endurance, mobility, or motivational deficit that interferes with the individual's hygiene practices; the identification of any existing problems of the skin or mucous membranes and associated care and its effectiveness;

and a physical examination of the skin and mucous membranes.

- Because lifestyle factors, changes in health state, illness, and certain diagnostic and therapeutic measures may adversely affect the skin, the nurse needs to identify high-risk populations and perform the appropriate skin assessment, teach the client how to examine and care for the skin, and institute preventive skin care measures.
- Nursing diagnoses may be written that specifically address problems of deficient hygiene (Self Care Deficit: Bathing/Hygiene) or that identify the effects problems of the skin, hair, scalp, eye, ear, nose, mouth, nails, feet, or perineum have on other areas of human functioning (comfort, mobility, nutrition).
- The individual with cognitive, sensory, endurance, mobility, or motivation deficits may require nursing assistance with any or all aspects of personal hygiene. The nurse promotes independence in these measures consistently. Whenever possible, the nurse offers assistance compatible with the individual's preferences and usual routines. When indicated, the client and family are taught necessary hygiene measures.
- Hospitalized clients receive scheduled hygienic care. This care includes careful attention to ensuring the safety and comfort of the client's bedside unit. Because of the long hours many ill clients spend in bed, the condition of bed linens is checked periodically throughout the day.

Study Questions

1. An older client's skin requires special care because
   a. subcutaneous fat increases
   b. sebaceous glands secrete more oil
   c. the skin becomes increasingly dry
   d. the skin thickens
2. An appropriate nursing intervention for a client wearing antiembolic stockings is to
   a. measure legs before applying stockings to assure proper fit
   b. apply stockings while the client is sitting in a chair
   c. massage the legs when the stockings are removed
   d. leave stockings in place for 1-week intervals
3. During a bath, the nurse observes that a client has dry skin. The nurse's best action is to
   a. bathe the client more frequently
   b. use an emollient on the dry skin
   c. massage the skin with alcohol
   d. discourage fluid intake
4. An adolescent client discusses her acne condition with the nurse. The nurse recommends that the client
   a. wash the skin frequently using soap
   b. use cosmetics liberally to cover blackheads
   c. use emollients on the area
   d. squeeze blackheads as they appear
5. A marked inflammation of the gums involving the alveolar tissue is referred to as
   a. glossitis
   b. caries
   c. cheilosis
   d. pyorrhea
6. A priority nursing action when administering oral care to a dependent client is
   a. assist the client to the dorsal recumbent position
   b. wear disposable gloves
   c. use a firm toothbrush to cleanse teeth and gums
   d. irrigate forcefully with hydrogen peroxide
7. Mr. James has an eye infection with a moderate amount of discharge. To clean his eyes, the nurse should
   a. use hydrogen peroxide
   b. wipe from the outer canthus to the inner canthus
   c. position him on the same side as the eye to be cleansed
   d. use only one cotton ball per eye
8. The nurse's responsibility when giving foot care to an older client includes
   a. using scissors to correct an ingrown toenail situation
   b. trimming toenails as short as possible
   c. using an alcohol rub if the feet are dry
   d. bathing the feet at least daily
9. Providing perineal care to a client requires that the nurse
   a. use a clean portion of the washcloth for each stroke
   b. proceed from most contaminated to least contaminated area
   c. use sterile gloves
   d. leave the foreskin undisturbed in an uncircumcised male
10. A nurse is caring for an 80-year-old client who requires total assistance with his personal and oral hygiene. He is thin, has few visitors, and prefers to remain in bed in a semi-sitting position. The priority nursing diagnosis is
    a. Risk for Impaired Skin Integrity related to immobility
    b. Bathing/Hygiene Self Care Deficit related to decreased strength and endurance
    c. Social Isolation related to lack of visitors

d. Activity Intolerance related to generalized weakness

11. An older client with an unsteady gait requests a tub bath. The nurse is aware that
    a. Alpha-keri oil should be added to the water to prevent dry skin
    b. the client should lock the door to guarantee privacy
    c. the client will require assistance in and out of the tub to prevent falling
    d. the water temperature should be very warm because the client chills easily
12. During morning care, the client asks the nurse to shave him with a disposable razor. Prior to shaving him, the nurse should
    a. have him sign a permission form
    b. check to see if the client is taking anticoagulants
    c. indicate that only a family member may shave a client
    d. position him flat in bed
13. To remove gas-permeable contact lenses from an unresponsive client, the nurse
    a. gently irrigates the eye with an irrigating solution from the inner canthus outward
    b. grasps the lens with a gentle pinching motion
    c. dons sterile gloves before attempting the procedure
    d. ensures that the lens is centered on the cornea before gently manipulating the lids to release the lens
14. To remove a client's gown when she has an intravenous line, the nurse
    a. temporarily disconnects the intravenous tubing at a point close to the client and threads it through the gown
    b. cuts the gown with scissors
    c. threads the bag and tubing through the gown sleeve keeping the line intact
    d. temporarily disconnects the tubing from the intravenous container and threads it through the gown
15. When making an occupied bed, it is important for the nurse to
    a. keep the bed in the low position
    b. use a bath blanket or top sheet for warmth and privacy
    c. constantly keep side rails raised on both sides
    d. move back and forth from one side to the other when adjusting the linens

Answers With Rationale

1. The correct response is *c.* With age the skin becomes increasingly dry, subcutaneous fat decreases, sebaceous glands secrete less oil, and the skin becomes thinner.
2. The correct response is *a.* The legs should always be measured according to manufacturer's directions before ordering antiembolism stockings. Stockings may be uncomfortable if applied while the client is sitting because leg veins are apt to be congested. Massage is dangerous because it may cause a clot to break away and circulate in the bloodstream. Stockings should always be removed once daily.
3. The correct response is *b.* An emollient soothes dry skin, whereas frequent bathing increases dryness, as does alcohol. Discouraging fluid intake leads to dehydration and, subsequently, dry skin.
4. The correct response is *a.* Washing the skin frequently with soap removes oil and debris, whereas liberal use of cosmetics and emollients can clog the pores. Squeezing blackheads is always discouraged because it may lead to infection.
5. The correct response is *d.* Pyorrhea is a marked inflammation of the gums, whereas caries refers to the presence of tooth decay. Cheilosis is ulceration of the lips and glossitis is an inflammation of the tongue.
6. The correct response is *b.* Disposable gloves provide a barrier to protect the nurse and client. The dorsal recumbent position is unsafe because the client may easily aspirate any secretions or fluids. A soft toothbrush is recommended to avoid causing irritation and bleeding, and forceful irrigation is never safe. Water would be the choice for any gentle irrigation.
7. The correct response is *c.* Positioning on the same side as the involved eye discourages any contamination of the other eye. Water or normal saline should be used for cleansing the eye of any discharge and one cotton ball should be used for each stroke. Always cleanse from the inner canthus to the outer canthus to avoid forcing debris into the nasolacrimal duct.
8. The correct response is *d.* An older client should have foot care once daily. Correcting an ingrown toenail situation should be done by a podiatrist and trimming the toenails may require a physician's order. Additionally, cutting the toenails as short as possible exposes tender areas to friction and may lead to the skin being cut during trimming. Alcohol is drying and should not be used when dry skin is usually already a problem.
9. The correct response is *a.* Using a clean portion of the washcloth for each stroke prevents contamination of other areas. Cleansing should always proceed from the least contaminated to the most contaminated area. Clean gloves, not sterile gloves, are used to provide perineal care, and the foreskin in

an uncircumcised male should be pulled back to allow cleansing underneath and then gently returned to its former position.

10. The correct response is *a.* While Bathing/Hygiene Self Care Deficit, Social Isolation, and Activity Intolerance may be appropriate nursing diagnoses for this client, the priority one at this time is Risk for Impaired Skin Integrity. A break in his skin, such as that from a pressure ulcer, may lead to infection. At his age, this could be life-threatening.
11. The correct response is *c.* Safe nursing practice requires that you assist a client with an unsteady gait in and out of the tub. Alpha-keri oil is dangerous for this client because it makes the tub slippery. Though privacy is important, if the client locks the door, the nurse cannot help if there is an emergency. The water temperature should be comfortably warm at 43 to 46°C. Older clients have an increased susceptibility to burns.
12. The correct response is *b.* A client who is taking anticoagulants should be shaved with an electric razor rather than a blade razor. Shaving a client does not require a permission and can be completed by either the caregiver or a family member. A shave is best completed with the client in a Fowler's or semi-Fowler's position to prevent soap and water from running behind the client's head.
13. The correct response is *d.* To remove hard contact lenses, the upper and lower eyelids are gently maneuvered to help loosen the lens and slide it out of the eye. The lens must be situated on the cornea, not the sclera, prior to removal. An attempt to grasp a hard lens might result in a scratch on the cornea. Clean gloves are optional if drainage is present.
14. The correct response is *c.* Threading the bag and tubing through the gown sleeve keeps the system intact. Opening an intravenous line causes a break in a sterile system and introduces the potential for infection. Cutting a gown off is not an alternative except in an emergency.
15. The correct response is *b.* Using the bath blanket or top sheet keeps the client warm and provides privacy. Keeping the bed in the low position and working over raised siderails may strain the nurse's back. Continually moving back and forth to tuck and arrange linen is time-consuming and disorganized.

Bibliography

Alberti, P., Ginsberg, I., Goode, R., & White, T. (1992). New reasons for hope in hearing loss. *Patient Care, 26*(6), 75–95.

Brodbeck, C., & Collier, J. (1994). Diabetic foot care: Focus on prevention. *Caring, 13*(11), 54–61.

Carpenito, L. (1995). *Nursing diagnoses: Application to clinical practice* (6th ed.). Philadelphia: Lippincott.

Eaglstein, W., McKay, M., & Pariser, D. (1994). The problems that plague aging skin. *Patient Care, 28*(7), 89–120.

Fenske, N., Grayson, L., & Newcomer, V. (1992). Tips for treating aging skin. *Patient Care, 26*(6), 61–72.

Mahoney, D. (1993). Cerumen impaction: Prevalence and detection in nursing homes. *Journal of Gerontological Nursing, 19*(4), 23–29.

Matteson, M. (1993). Vision and hearing screening in cognitively impaired older adults. *Geriatric Nursing, 14*(6), 294–297.

McGovern, M., & Kuhn, J. (1992). Skin assessment of the elderly client. *Journal of Gerontological Nursing, 18*(4), 39–43.

Meek, S. (1993). Effects of slow stroke back massage on relaxation in hospice clients. *IMAGE: Journal of Nursing Scholarship, 25*(1), 17–21.

Miller, C. (1995). *Nursing care of older adults* (2nd ed.). Philadelphia: Lippincott.

Miller, R. (1994). Managing disruptive responses to bathing by elderly residents: Strategies for the cognitively impaired. *Journal of Gerontological Nursing, 20*(11), 35–39.

North American Nursing Diagnosis Association. (1994). *NANDA nursing diagnoses: Definitions and classification 1995–1996.* Philadelphia: Author.

Ney, D. (1993). Cerumen impaction, ear hygiene practices, and hearing acuity. *Geriatric Nursing, 14*(2), 70–73.

Rader, J. (1994). To bathe or not to bathe: That is the question. *Journal of Gerontological Nursing, 20*(9), 53–54.

Skewes, S. (1994). No more bed baths! *RN, 56*(1), 34–35.

Taylor, K. (1993). Geriatric hearing loss: Management strategies for nurses. *Geriatric Nursing, 14*(2), 74–76.

Tombes, M., & Gallucci, B. (1993). The effects of hydrogen peroxide rinses on the normal oral mucosa. *Nursing Research, 42*(6), 332.

Walczak, M., Bernstein, A., Senzer, C., & Mohr, N. (1993). Elder hearing aids: Infrared listening device in a geriatric day center. *Journal of Gerontological Nursing, 19*(8), 5–8.

Webber-Jones, J. (1992). Doomed to deafness? *American Journal of Nursing, 92*(11), 37–39.

Winkley, G., Brown, J., & Stone, T. (1993). Interventions to improve oral care: The nursing assistant's role. *Journal of Gerontological Nursing, 19*(11), 47–48.

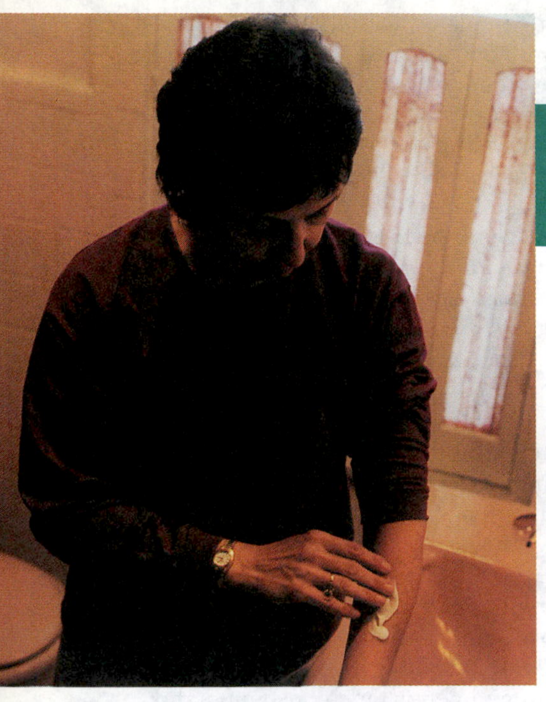

Chapter 38

Skin Integrity and Wound Healing

Objectives

After studying this chapter, the learner should be able to:

Define key terms used in this chapter.

Discuss the incidence and prevalence of pressure ulcers.

Identify clients at risk of developing a pressure ulcer.

Describe the four stages of pressure ulcers.

Discuss the assessment variables outlined in the Norton and Braden risk assessment tools.

Develop nursing diagnoses related to the development of a pressure ulcer.

Describe nursing interventions to prevent or minimize pressure ulcers in adults.

Discuss the guidelines for cleaning and dressing a pressure ulcer.

Develop a teaching program that addresses the needs of clients/family caregivers with altered skin integrity.

Key Terms

debridement
epithelialization
eschar
exudate
friction
granulation tissue
ischemia
necrosis
pressure ulcer
reactive hyperemia
shearing force

Because the skin is the body's first line of defense, an intact skin surface takes on added significance. Altered skin integrity is potentially dangerous and can be life threatening. It is especially serious among older adults, those who are immobile, those who have chronic health problems, and individuals in critical care settings.

Whereas the physiology of skin and skin care are discussed in Chapter 37 and wound healing is discussed in Chapter 30, this chapter deals with pressure ulcers, one of the most common skin disruptions. Care is taken by the nurse, the client, and the family in prevention of pressure ulcers. When pressure ulcers occur, aggressive intervention and treatment can spare the client unnecessary pain and discomfort, prevent further tissue deterioration, hasten wound healing, and save millions of healthcare dollars.

Development of Pressure Ulcers

A **pressure ulcer** is defined by the Agency for Health Care Policy and Research as any lesion caused by unrelieved pressure that results in damage to underlying tissue (USDHHS, 1994). The terms *pressure ulcer, decubitus ulcer,* and *bedsore* have been used synonymously. The term *decubitus* derives from a Latin word meaning lying down. However, lying down does not cause a decubitus ulcer, and a client need not be bedridden to develop one. Therefore, most people prefer the term *pressure ulcer* because pressure is the most prominent underlying cause.

Some 2.7% to 29.5% of hospitalized clients in the United States develop pressure ulcers, with older, quadriplegic, critical care, and older orthopedic clients with femoral fractures most at risk (Monaghan, 1993). Statistics for nursing homes indicate a prevalence rate of 23% for these residents (Burd et al., 1994). Canadian caregivers estimate that 25% of clients admitted to an acute care facility will develop a pressure ulcer (McNaughton & Brazil, 1995). Reliable figures are not yet available to indicate the scope of the problem in the home care setting.

As expected, the cost of treating clients with pressure ulcers is staggering. Carroll (1995) reports that healthcare facilities spend more than $6.5 billion a year, with estimates ranging from $14,000 to $75,000 per individual depending on the severity of the pressure ulcer. The threat these ulcers pose to the client's physical and mental well-being and the amount of nursing energy they consume make them one of nursing's persistent top-priority challenges.

Mechanisms of Development

Pathologic changes at a pressure ulcer site are the result of blood vessel collapse caused by pressure, usually from body weight. **Necrosis**, or death of cells, eventually occurs, leading to the characteristic ulcer.

Two mechanisms contribute to pressure ulcer development: external pressure that compresses blood vessels and friction and shearing forces that tear and injure blood vessels.

External Pressure

Pressure ulcers usually occur over bony prominences where body weight is distributed over a small area that does not have many subcutaneous tissues for cushioning damage to the skin. Common sites for pressure ulcers are illustrated in Figure 38-1. Of the susceptible areas, most pressure ulcers occur over the sacrum and coccyx, followed by the trochanter and the calcaneus (heel). One may form in as short a time as 1 to 2 hours if that individual is unable to move for an extended period of time.

The most formidable predisposing factor for a pressure ulcer is pressure over an area, which results in occluded blood capillaries and poor circulation to tissues. This lack of sufficient circulation causes necrosis and ulcer formation. The skin can tolerate considerable pressure without cell death, but for short periods only. Duration is more important than the amount of pressure in the formation of a pressure ulcer. Most pressure ulcers develop within 2 weeks of admission to a healthcare facility. By assessing a client's mobility and motivation to move, the nurse can estimate the length of time that a bony prominence is likely to be submitted to sustained pressure (Kemp & Krouskop, 1994).

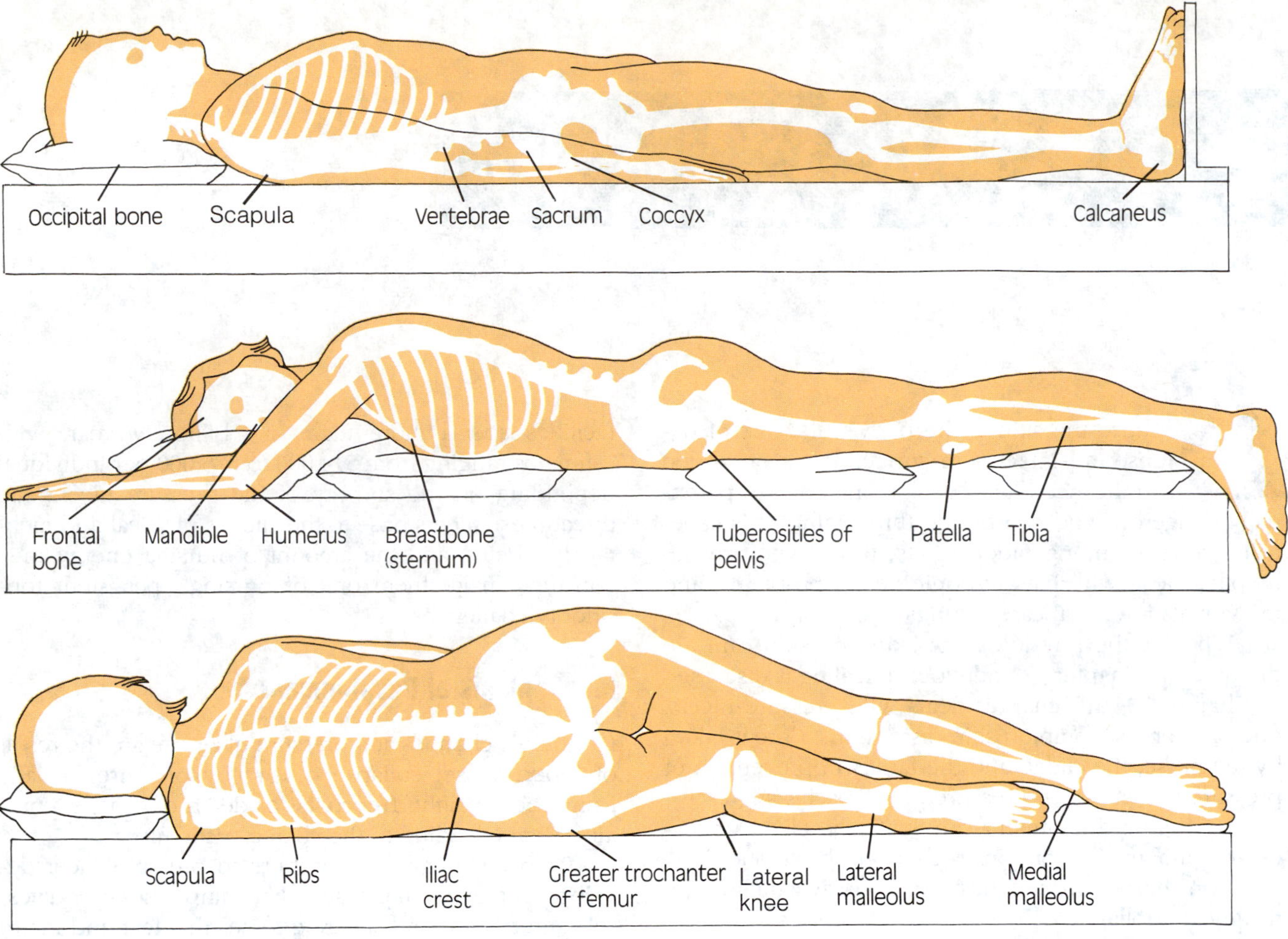

Figure 38-1
Common sites for development of pressure ulcers.

Friction and Shearing Forces

Friction occurs when two surfaces rub against each other. The injury resembles an abrasion and can also damage superficial blood vessels directly under the skin. The client who lies on wrinkled sheets is likely to sustain tissue damage due to friction. The skin over the elbows and heels often suffers injury when clients lift and help move themselves up in bed with the use of their arms and feet. Friction burns can also occur on the back when clients are pulled or slid over sheets when moved up in bed or transferred onto a stretcher.

Shearing forces are often responsible for deep pressure ulcers. A **shearing force** results when one layer of tissue slides over another layer. The small blood vessels and capillaries in the area are stretched and may even tear, thus resulting in poor circulation to the tissue cells under the skin. Figure 38-2 illustrates how shearing forces occur. Clients who are pulled rather than lifted when moved up in bed or from bed to chair or stretcher are at risk for injury from shearing forces. A client who is partially sitting up in bed is susceptible when skin sticks to the sheet and underlying tissues move downward with the body toward the foot of the bed. This may also occur in the client who sits in a chair but slides down.

Staging of Pressure Ulcers

Appropriate intervention is dependent upon early recognition of the stage of development of the pressure ulcer. The National Pressure Ulcer Advisory Panel (NPUAP) in 1989 adopted a four-stage classification system. Following this agreement, in 1992, the Agency for Health Care Policy and Research (AHCPR) published a clinical guideline for prediction and prevention of pressure ulcers (USDHHS, 1992). To improve the quality of healthcare and save healthcare dollars, AHCPR addressed the treatment of pressure ulcers in their most recent guideline (USDHHS, 1994). The staging of pressure ulcers used by AHCPR is consistent with the recommendations from NPUAP. Differentiation between the four stages and a visual representation of the difference between the stages are presented in Table 38-1.

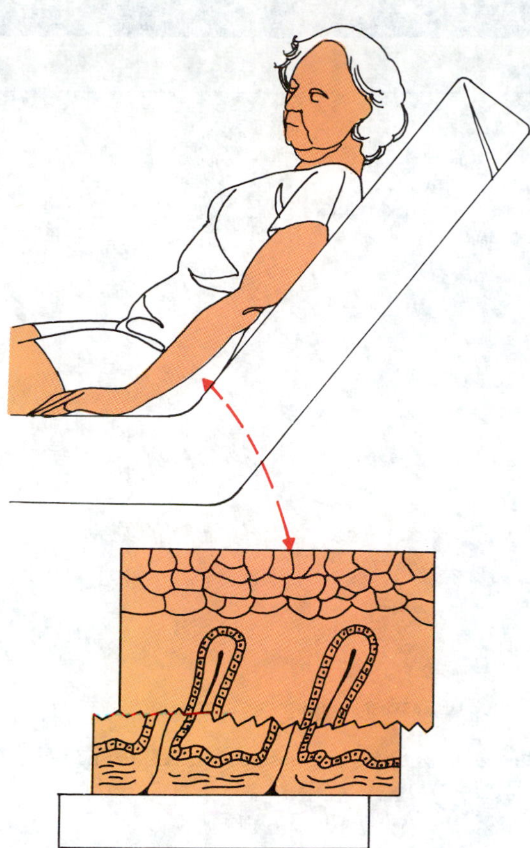

Figure 38-2
Shearing force can occur when a client is moved carelessly or slides down in bed. Friction causes resistance on the surface layers of the skin, while underlying tissue moves in the direction of the body movement. Capillaries in underlying tissue are stretched and torn in pressure areas by opposing forces of movements.

The first sign that a pressure ulcer may be developing is a blanching of the skin over the area under pressure. Instead of a healthy, pink color, the skin becomes pale and white. Insufficient blood circulation makes the skin appear pale when compared with areas where circulation is adequate. This local anemia resulting from poor circulation is called **ischemia.**

When pressure is relieved, ischemia is rapidly followed by *hyperemia*. The area appears red and feels warm. **Reactive hyperemia** is the occurrence of a blanchable reddening of the skin when pressure is removed. The body literally floods the area with blood to nourish and remove wastes from the cells. Reactive hyperemia is *not* a stage I pressure ulcer. With reactive hyperemia, once a client who has been lying on his or her back for 2 hours is repositioned onto the side, any reddened area should have faded within 1 to 1½ hours. In individuals with darkly pigmented skin, hyperemia may best be detected by touch. The skin feels warm or some change in color is detected. A stage II pressure ulcer is superficial and may present as a blister or abrasion. Damage to the subcutaneous tissue indicates a stage III lesion, and the extensive destruction associated with full-thickness skin loss is categorized as a stage IV pressure ulcer. This staging process has several limitations. If eschar is present, it may be difficult to stage a pressure ulcer. **Eschar** is a thick, leathery scab or dry crust that is necrotic and must be removed before staging can accurately be determined. As mentioned earlier, it is more difficult to identify a stage I pressure ulcer in an individual with darkly pigmented skin. Clients with casts, orthopedic devices, or support stockings require routine assessment of areas where inadequate circulation may be a contributing factor to development of a pressure ulcer.

Factors Affecting Skin Integrity

Factors affecting skin condition are discussed in Chapter 37. Several other factors predispose to pressure ulcers. Usually, a combination of causes, in addition to pressure, friction, and shearing, contribute to ulcer development.

Mobility and Immobility

The person who sits or lies most of the time is a candidate for a pressure ulcer because immobility predisposes to prolonged pressure on body areas. The ambulatory person does not develop this injury because no part of the body suffers from prolonged pressure. During sleep, the well person tends to move about in bed freely. Unconscious and paralyzed clients are subject to pressure ulcers if allowed to remain in any one position. So also are emotionally depressed people who do not ordinarily tend to move much. Additional factors that cause immobility and may result in this serious problem are lengthy surgery and the use of tranquilizers or sedatives.

Nutrition and Hydration

Malnutrition predisposes to pressure ulcer formation because poorly nourished cells are easily damaged. For example, vitamin C deficiency causes capillaries to become fragile, and poor circulation to the area results when they break. Protein deficiency leading to negative nitrogen balance, electrolyte imbalances, and insufficient caloric intake also predisposes the skin to injury. It is estimated that 25% of clients who develop pressure ulcers have a dietary deficiency (Eaglstein, McKay, & Pariser, 1994). The condition of the teeth or fit of dentures may also exacerbate the problem of inadequate dietary intake. Dehydration as well as the accumulation of excessive fluid in tissues can interfere with circulation and subsequent cell nourishment.

Moisture on the Skin

Prolonged moisture on the skin reduces the skin's resistance to trauma. Warmth increases the cells' demands for oxygen. Hence, moisture and warmth eventually lead to

Table 38-1
Comparison of Stages of Pressure Ulcers

Description of Stage	Treatment
Stage I	
Nonblanchable erythema of intact skin: the heralding lesion of skin ulceration. Note: Reactive hyperemia can normally be present for ½ to ¾ as long as the pressure occluded blood flow to the area. This should not be confused with a stage I pressure ulcer. 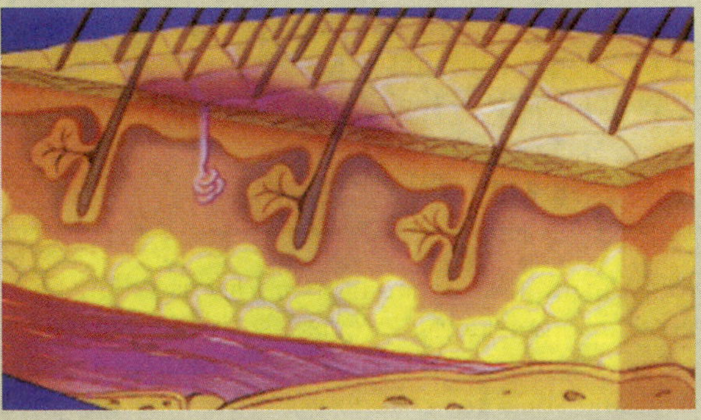	Pressure-relieving measures: • Frequent turning • Pressure-relieving devices • Positioning
Stage II	
Partial-thickness skin loss involving epidermis and/or dermis. The ulcer is superficial and presents clinically as an abrasion, blister, or shallow crater. 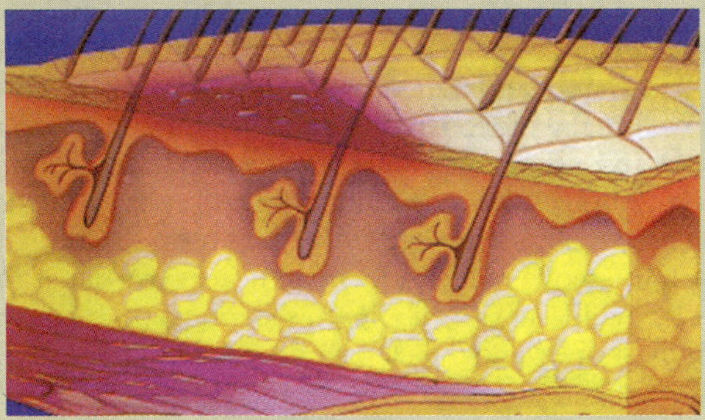	Maintenance of a moist healing environment: • Saline or • Occlusive dressing that promotes natural healing but prevents formation of a scar
Stage III	
Full-thickness skin loss involving damage or necrosis of subcutaneous tissue that may extend down to, but not through, underlying fascia. The ulcer presents clinically as a deep crater with or without undermining of adjacent tissue. 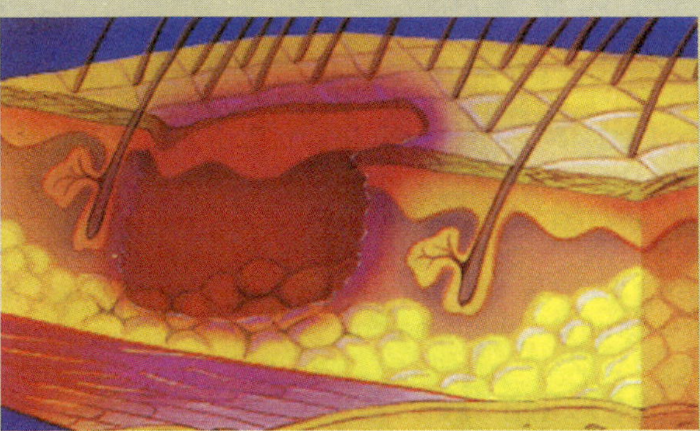	Requires debridement which can be accomplished by one of the following: • Wet-to-dry dressings • Surgical intervention • Proteolytic enzymes

(continued)

Table 38-1 *(continued)*
Comparison of Stages of Pressure Ulcers

Description of Stage	Treatment
Stage IV	
Full-thickness skin loss with extensive destruction, tissue necrosis, or damage to muscle, bone, or supporting structures (eg, tendon or joint capsule). Sinus tracts may also be associated with stage IV ulcers. 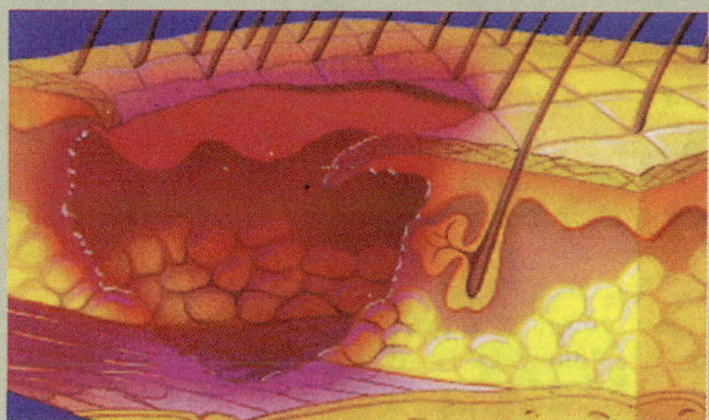	Wounds are treated in the following manner: • Covered with nonadherent dressing • Changed every 8–12 hours • May require skin grafts

(Source: U.S. Department of Health and Human Services, Agency for Health Care Policy and Research. [1992]. *Pressure ulcers in adults: Prediction and prevention.* Rockville, MD: DHHS. Porth, C. [1994]. *Pathophysiology: Concepts of altered health states.* Philadelphia: Lippincott.)

cell destruction, especially when pressure is present. When skin is damp, less friction is required to blister and abrade skin (Kemp, 1994). It is believed that the moisture associated with urinary incontinence increases the risk of skin damage more than is accounted for by the chemical irritation from the ammonia content of the urine. If personal hygiene is poor, the skin contains many organisms that thrive in the warm, moist environment. This adds to the danger of developing a pressure ulcer that will become infected.

Mental Status

The more alert an individual is, the more likely he or she is to protect skin integrity by relieving pressure periodically and managing adequate skin hygiene. Apathy, confusion, or a comatose state can diminish these self-care abilities and increase the likelihood of skin breakdown.

Age

Older people are good candidates for developing pressure ulcers because the skin is susceptible to injury. Refer to the box Focus on the Older Adult in Chapter 37, which outlines risk factors that predispose older individuals to pressure ulcers. Chronic and debilitating diseases, more common in this age group, may adversely affect skin nourishment. Destruction of tissues that leads to pressure ulcers becomes relatively easy when illness causes an elevated temperature and normal function of body cells is altered in any way. Figure 38-3 depicts changes that occur as the skin ages.

ASSESSING SKIN INTEGRITY

Most pressure ulcers in adults can be prevented. It is a nursing priority to perform a comprehensive assessment whatever the setting and identify the presence of a pressure ulcer or predisposing factors and clients at risk of developing one. A thorough nursing history and physical assessment provide the initial information for the data base.

All assessment data need to be reassessed regularly to ensure that clients receive healthcare interventions that prolong and enhance the quality of their life. The AHCPR, in the 1992 guideline, includes an algorithm (or visual display) summarizing their assessment strategy for predicting and preventing a pressure ulcer (Fig. 38-4). A wide variety of assessment tools are also available to assist the healthcare provider with pressure ulcer prevention.

Nursing History

Preventive strategy begins with a systematic assessment of the skin either in the home or upon admission to a healthcare facility. The nursing history includes questions that focus on the appearance of the skin and client activities that have the potential to contribute to altered skin integrity. It is often a combination of risk factors that

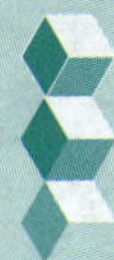

Research in Nursing: Making a Difference

Skin Integrity

Disruptions of the skin, especially over bony prominences, continue to plague the older client, the immobile client, and those with chronic health problems. In older adults, the incidence of alterations in skin integrity is staggering. Nursing research contributes significantly to an understanding of the causes of pressure ulcers and examines the prediction, prevention, and treatment of pressure ulcers from various perspectives.

Related Research

Bennis, S., & Davis, S. (1994). An effective approach to treating decubitus ulcers in home healthcare patients. *Home Healthcare Nurse, 12*(1), 47–52.
Pressure ulcers not only have an adverse effect on clients but can also have a negative impact on the family/caregivers and the professionals who are assigned to care for clients with these wounds. This study successfully used one skin care product and a simple monitoring system to improve wound healing significantly, reduce costs, and improve the client's self-image and quality of life. An additional secondary benefit was the feeling of self-satisfaction that caregivers experienced because of their positive contribution to the client's care.

Burd, C., Olson, B., Langemo, D., Hunter, S., Hanson, D., Osowski, K., & Sauvage, T. (1994). Skin care strategies: In a skilled nursing home. *Journal of Gerontological Nursing, 20*(11), 28–34.
Pressure ulcers are a major problem in nursing homes because they negatively impact on the physical condition and comfort of the client and pose a financial burden to the care facility. By identifying clients at risk, implementing a prevention plan, and employing ongoing assessment of skin integrity, nurses alleviated some of these problems. This study emphasized the effectiveness of these strategies in long-term care settings. In-service education for the staff also heightened awareness about pressure ulcers and facilitated transfer of this knowledge into effective treatment measures.

Gawron, C. (1994). Risk factors and prevalence of pressure ulcers among hospitalized patients. *Journal of Wound, Ostomy, and Continence Nursing, 21*(6), 232–240.
In the acute care setting, the incidence of pressure ulcers is higher because many of the clients are critically ill. The longevity of the current population of clients is also a factor. This author explored use of a risk assessment tool that identified moderate and high-risk clients and guided the initiation of an individualized plan of prevention. Additionally, results of this research indicated the need for further evaluation of the availability and use of pressure-relief devices.

Summary

Maintenance of skin integrity is one of the primary responsibilities of nurses. The results of these findings can help nurses determine the effectiveness of wound care strategies and risk assessment tools for a variety of client care settings. Participation in ongoing research promotes knowledge of healing strategies, prevents the recurrence of pressure ulcers, and is a pivotal role for nurses.

place the client at greatest risk for development of a pressure ulcer.

The nurse questions the client and caregiver about recent changes in the appearance or condition of the skin and any skin care regimens. It is important to assess activity status, nutritional state, changes in elimination patterns, and presence of pain associated with altered skin integrity. Nurses have long recognized that clients with a pressure ulcer experience pain. It is important to assess if dressing changes, position in bed or in a chair, or movement elicit any subjective or objective expressions of pain. Even if pain is never verbalized or expressed, the nurse should assume that pain is a definite possibility and focus on comfort needs when gathering information for the nursing history. Pain that is severe may actually slow the healing process by interfering with the immune system response (O'Hanlon-Nichols, 1995). Specific nursing assessments to validate the pain experience are included in Chapter 41.

Since stays in healthcare facilities are limited, the client is often cared for in the home environment. It is imperative that the nurse also assess the educational needs of the client and family and their ability to understand, participate in, and adhere to a treatment regimen. Assessment should include the following areas:

- Mental status, learning ability, and communication skills
- Social support systems
- Goals, values, and lifestyle
- Culture and ethnicity
- Stressors
- Personal strengths and resources

The accompanying box provides additional suggestions pertinent to gathering a nursing history.

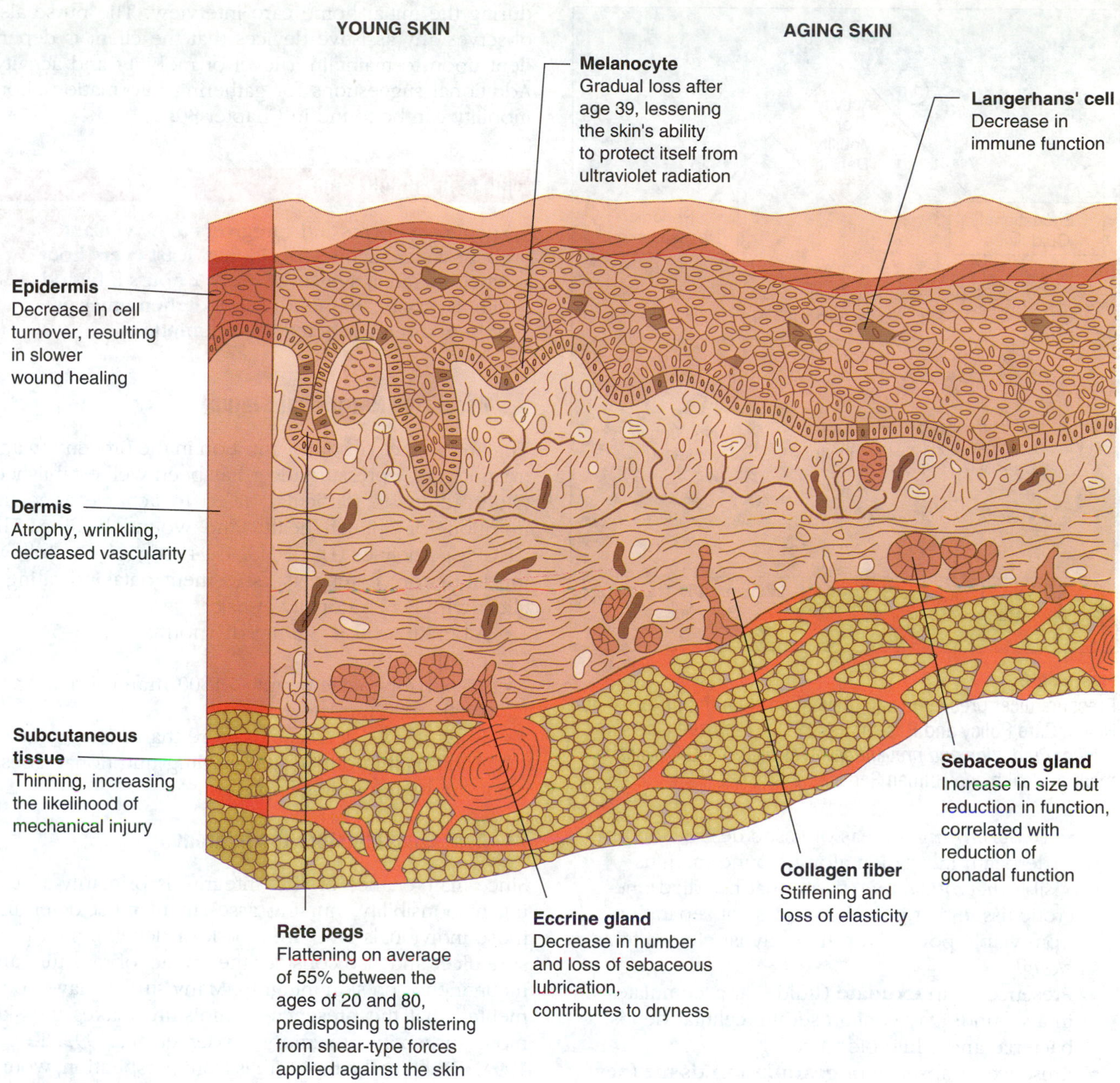

Figure 38-3
Changes that occur as the skin ages.

Physical Assessment

Physical assessment of the skin is included as part of the initial data base collection. In addition, all at-risk clients should have a systematic skin inspection, including bony prominences, at least once a day. Weekly inspections are recommended by AHCPR to monitor the progress and evaluate the effectiveness of treatment of a documented ulcer, whatever the setting. Documentation of these assessments ensures continuity of care and becomes the foundation for the skin care plan. All caregivers in the home or healthcare agency need to be aware of assessment criteria.

According to the AHCPR Clinical Practice Guideline (USDHHS, 1994) skin assessment for a pressure ulcer specifically includes inspection of the following:

- Location of any lesion or ulcer
- Estimation of the stage (based on the NPUAP and AHCPR classification)
- Dimensions of the ulcer (length, width, depth)
- Presence of any abnormal pathways in the wound:
  - *Sinus tract*—a cavity or channel underneath the wound that has the potential for infection
  - *Tunneling*—a passageway or opening that may be visible at skin level, but with most of the tunnel under the surface of the skin

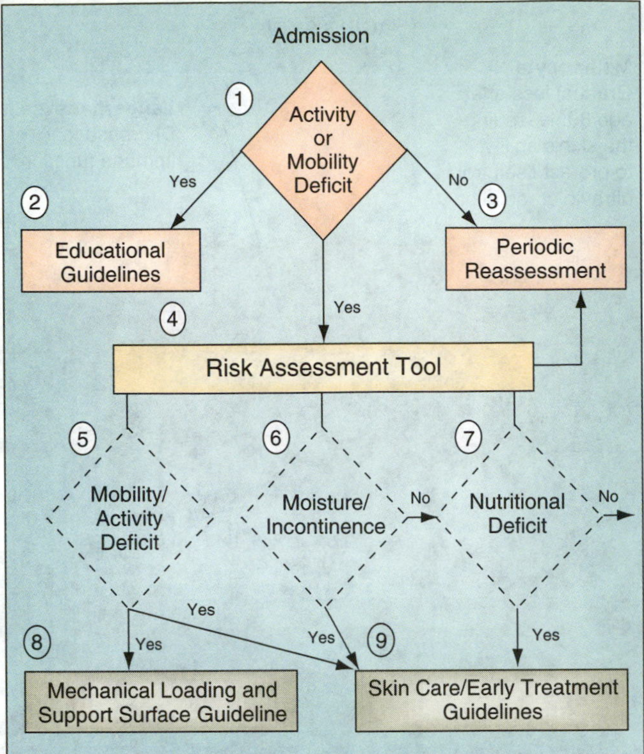

Figure 38-4
Pressure ulcer prediction and prevention algorithm. (Agency for Health Care Policy and Research,. [1992]. *Pressure ulcers in adults: Prediction and prevention.* Rockville MD: U.S. Department of Health and Human Services.)

- *Undermining*—areas of tissue destruction underneath intact skin along wound margins
- Visible *necrotic tissue* (tissue that has died); necrotic tissue that is in the process of separating from viable portions of the body is referred to as *slough*
- Presence of an **exudate** (fluid that accumulates in a wound; may contain serum, cellular debris, bacteria, and white blood cells)
- Presence or absence of **granulation tissue** (new tissue, pink/red in color, composed of fibroblasts and small blood vessels that fill an open wound when it starts to heal)
- Visible evidence of **epithelialization** (stage of wound healing in which epithelial cells move across the surface of a wound; tissue resembles the color of "ground glass" to pink)

Figure 38-5 demonstrates the various types of tissue the nurse may observe during assessment of a wound.

Assessing Mobility

Assessment of a client's mobility status includes checking his or her ability to move, turn, and reposition the body. A client who is confined to bed or a chair, or has limited range of motion, is at greater risk of developing a pressure ulcer. Nursing assessment of activity status is completed upon admission to the healthcare facility or during the initial home care interview. The nurse also observes any assistive devices that the client is dependent upon to maintain a level of mobility and activity. Additional suggestions for gathering information about mobility can be found in Chapter 39.

Home Healthcare Alert

Encourage clients and caregivers to be vigilant about changing body position at least every hour when seated in a chair or every 2 hours if bedridden. It may be helpful to use a kitchen timer or written turning schedule as a reminder.

Assessing Nutritional Status

The importance of sound nutrition in the prevention and treatment of a pressure ulcer has been well established. Older adults, in particular, need to achieve adequate nutrition for optimal health and wound healing. The AHCPR guidelines (USDHHS, 1994) suggest the following laboratory criteria as assessment data indicating a client who is nutritionally at risk:

- Albumin level < 3.5 mg/dL (normal = 3.5–5 mg/dL)
- Total lymphocyte count < 1800/mm^3 (normal = 1000–4000/mm^3)
- Body weight decrease of more than 15%

Additional information regarding nutritional assessment can be found in Chapter 42.

Assessing Moisture/Incontinence

Since maintenance of skin integrity is primarily a nursing responsibility, nursing assessment must determine those individuals who are at risk of developing a pressure ulcer and also consider the impact of moisture and incontinence on skin integrity. Many studies have documented that the presence of moisture makes the skin more susceptible to injury (Lyder et al., 1992; Kemp, 1994). Whether the moisture is from perspiration, wound drainage, urine, or stool, the skin is compromised. Moisture alone has the ability to create an environment where microorganisms can multiply and the skin is more likely to blister, suffer abrasions, and become *macerated* (softening or disintegration of the skin in response to moisture). Chapter 43 has additional assessment information related to incontinence.

Assessing Complications Associated With Pressure Ulcers

Numerous complications can accompany a pressure ulcer. Some are directly related to the impaired integrity of the body's first line of defense, while others may be associated with a particular treatment regimen. Many are related to the presence of an infection in the wound area. Chapter 30 includes information pertinent to assessment of wounds for signs of infection.

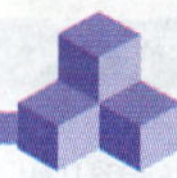

Focused Assessment Guide

Skin Integrity

Factors to Assess	Questions and Approaches
• Overall appearance of skin	Are there any areas of your skin that are discolored? Is there any difference in skin temperature anywhere on your body? How does your skin feel in relation to moisture? Dry? Clammy? Oily? Is this a change from normal? Are there any areas on your body where your skin seems paper-thin? Have you noticed any swelling in your feet? Around your ankles? In your fingers? Tell me about your bathing routine. Are there any skin products that you routinely use? Are there any that you are unable to tolerate? What happens?
• Recent changes in skin condition	Have you noticed any sores anywhere on your body? Do you ever notice redness over a bony area when you stay in one position for a while? Does the reddened area disappear after a short time? Is the skin broken? Do you have any drainage from this area? Has the sore changed in size?
• Contributing factors	
• Activity/Mobility	Do you need assistance to walk and move? Are you confined to a chair? Bed? Can you change your position whenever you want? Specifically, what kind of help do you need?
• Nutrition	Have you gained weight recently? Lost weight recently? Do you eat well-balanced meals? Do you drink adequate amounts of fluid every day? Do you take any vitamins? Food supplements? Has the doctor ever told you that you were anemic? Do you prepare your own meals? Do you need help to eat? Do you wear dentures? Do they fit? Do you have any difficulty swallowing?
• Pain	If you have a sore anywhere, is it painful? Does anything help relieve the pain? Are you currently taking any medication for pain?
• Elimination	Have you noticed any changes in your usual bowel and bladder patterns? Any problems with incontinence? Have you ever used any briefs or pads to help with an incontinence problem?

Assessment Measures

An aggressive approach to prevent a pressure ulcer or manage the care of a client who already has impaired skin integrity begins with the risk assessment tool, which must be simple to use, reliable, and cost-effective. The Norton scale (Fig. 38-6) was presented initially in 1962, (Norton, McLaren, & Exton-Smith, 1975). The Braden scale has been used and evaluated since 1987 (Bergstrom et al., 1987). Both scales rely on a numerical scoring system and have been tested extensively. In the Norton scale, a total score of 14 or less indicates risk of

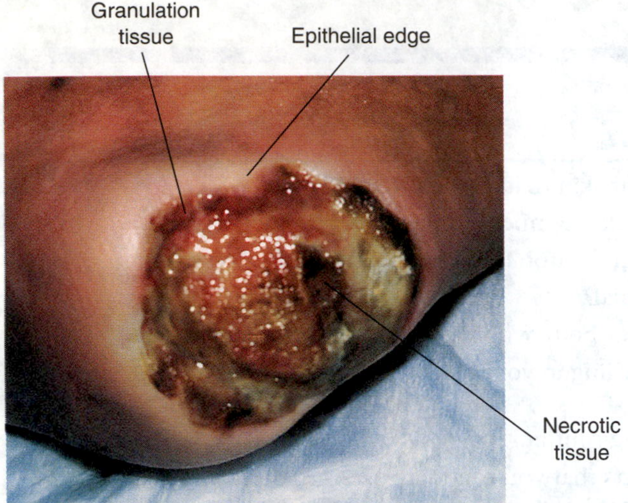

Figure 38-5
A chronic wound with various types of wound surface tissue.

pressure ulcer; a score under 12 indicates high risk. In the Braden scale, a total score of 16 or less indicates that the client is at high risk for pressure ulcer development. Initially, the Norton scale was criticized for its lack of attention to the role of nutrition in the development of a pressure ulcer. A modified version addresses this concern. The Braden scale (Fig. 38-7) incorporates priority risk factors and has been used in more diverse settings. Neither tool is considered ideal, but both efficiently and systematically identify those clients at high risk for developing a pressure ulcer.

Agencies use different approaches once a client "at risk" has been identified. Many healthcare facilities use a special pressure ulcer assessment form (Fig. 38-8 is a sample included in the AHCPR guideline). Signs placed outside the room or attached to medical records indicate the need for ongoing assessment and special attention to skin integrity.

DIAGNOSING

Impaired Skin Integrity is one of the more commonly used nursing diagnoses. The stage of the pressure ulcer, however, should be a factor in determining the nursing diagnosis. Stage I and II pressure ulcers have superficial skin damage, and Impaired Skin Integrity is the appropriate choice. Stage III and IV ulcers include full-thickness skin loss and damage to underlying tissue; therefore, the newer diagnosis Impaired Tissue Integrity is more appropriate. Impaired Skin Integrity is discussed later in the Nursing Process in Clinical Practice section.

Additional nursing diagnoses pertaining to the presence of pressure ulcers include:

Risk for Impaired Skin Integrity
Risk for Impaired Tissue Integrity
Risk for Infection
Impaired Physical Mobility
Altered Tissue Perfusion
Caregiver Role Strain
Pain
Altered Nutrition: Less than body requirements

PLANNING: EXPECTED OUTCOMES

Whenever nurses care for clients who have or are at risk for impaired skin integrity, nursing measures are supportive of the following client outcomes. The client will:

- Participate in the prescribed treatment regimen to promote wound healing
- Demonstrate progressive healing of the pressure ulcer
- Demonstrate increase in body weight and muscle size
- Remain free of infection at the site of the pressure ulcer
- Develop no new areas of skin breakdown

		Physical condition	Mental condition	Activity	Mobility	Continence	Total Score
		Good 4 Fair 3 Poor 2 Very poor 1	Alert 4 Apathetic 3 Confused 2 Stuporous 1	Ambulant 4 Walk/help 3 Sets in chair 2 Remains in bed 1	Full 4 Slightly limited 3 Very limited 2 Immobile 1	Good 4 Occasional incontinence 3 Frequent incontinence 2 Urine and fecal incontinence 1	
Name	Date						

Figure 38-6
The Norton scale for assessment and prevention of pressure ulcers in the older population.

Braden Scale for Predicting Pressure Sore Risk

Patient's Name ____________ Evaluator's Name ____________

					Date of Assessment			
Sensory perception Ability to respond meaningfully to pressure-related discomfort	**1. Completely limited:** Unresponsive (does not moan, flinch, or grasp) to painful stimuli, due to sensory diminished level of consciousness or sedation, OR limited ability to feel pain over most of the body surface.	**2. Very limited:** Responds only to painful stimuli. Cannot communicate discomfort except by moaning or restlessness, OR has a sensory impairment which limits ability to feel pain or discomfort over 1/2 of body.	**3. Slightly limited:** Responds to verbal commands but cannot always communicate discomfort or need to be turned, OR has some sensory impairment which limits ability to feel pain or discomfort in 1 or 2 extremities.	**4. No impairment:** Responds to verbal commands. Has no sensory deficit which would limit ability to feel or voice pain or discomfort.				
Moisture Degree to which skin is exposed to moisture	**1. Costantly moist:** Skin is kept moist almost constantly by perspiration, urine, etc. Dampness is detected every time the patient is moved or turned.	**2. Moist:** Skin is often but not always moist. Linen must be changed at least once a shift.	**3. Occasionally moist:** Skin is occasionally moist, requiring an extra linen change approximately once a day.	**4. Rarely moist:** Skin is usually dry; linen requires changing only at routine intervals.				
Activity Degree of physical activity	**1. Bedfast:** Confined to bed.	**2. Chairfast:** Ability to walk severely limited or non-existent. Cannot bear own weight and/or must be assisted into chair or wheel chair.	**3. Walks occasionally:** Walks occasionally during day but for very short distances, with or without assistance. Spends majority of each shift in bed or chair.	**4. Walks frequently:** Walks outside the room at least twice a day and inside room at least once every 2 hours during waking hours.				
Mobility Ability to change and control body position	**1. Completely immobile:** Does not make even slight changes in body or extremity position without assistance.	**2. Very limited:** Makes occasional slight changes in body or extremity position but unable to make frequent or significant changes independently.	**3. Slightly limited:** Makes frequent though slight changes in body or extremity position independently.	**4. No limitations:** Makes major and frequent changes in position without assistance.				
Nutrition Usual food intake pattern	**1. Very poor:** Never eats a complete meal. Rarely eats more than 1/3 of any food offered. Eats 2 servings or less of protein (meat or dairy products) per day. Takes fluids poorly. Does not take a liquid dietary supplement, OR is NPO[1] and/or maintained on clear liquids or IV[2] for more than 5 days.	**2. Probably inadequate:** Rarely eats a complete meal and generally eats only about 1/2 of any food offered. Protein intake includes only 3 servings of meat or dairy products per day. Occasionally will take a liquid dietary supplement, OR receives less than optimum amount of liquid diet or tube feeding.	**3. Adequate:** Eats over half of most meals. Eats a total of 4 servings of protein (meat, dairy products) each day. Occasionally will refuse a meal, but will usually take a supplement if offered, OR is on a tube feeding or TPN[3] regimen, which probably meets most of nutritional needs.	**4. Excellent:** Eats most of every meal. Never refuses a meal. Usually eats a total of 4 or more servings of meat and dairy products. Occasionally eats between meals. Does not require supplementation.				
Friction and shear	**1. Problem:** Requires moderate to maximum assistance in moving. Complete lifting without sliding against sheets is impossible. Frequently slides down in bed or chair, requiring frequent repositioning with maximum assistance. Spasticity, contractures, or agitation leads to almost constant friction.	**2. Potential problem:** Moves feebly or requires minimum assistance. During a move skin probably slides to some extent against sheets, chair, restraints, or other devices. Maintains relatively good position in chair or bed most of the time but occasionally slides down.	**3. No apparent problem:** Moves in bed and in chair independently and has sufficient muscle strength to lift up completely during move. Maintains good position in bed or chair at all times.					
					Total score			

[1]NPO: Nothing by mouth.
[2]IV: Intravenously.
[3]TPN: Total parenteral nutrition

Figure 38-7
Braden scale for predicting pressure sore risk. (Braden B., and Bergstrom, N. Copyright 1988. Reprinted with permission.)

Indicate Ulcer Sites:

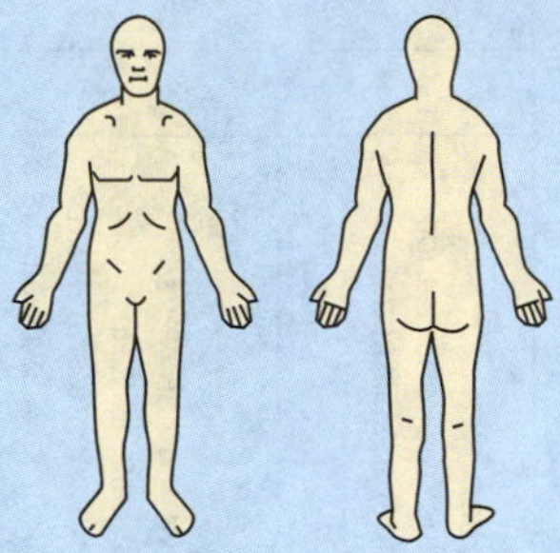

Anterior Posterior

(Attach a color photo of the pressure ulcer(s) [Optional])

Sample Pressure Ulcer Assessment Guide

Patient Name: ______________________ Date: ____________ Time: ___________

Ulcer 1:	No	Yes	Ulcer 2:	No	Yes
Site ________________			Site ________________		
Stage __________			Stage __________		
Size (cm)			Size (cm)		
Length _________			Length _________		
Width _________			Width _________		
Depth _________			Depth _________		
Sinus Tract	☐	☐	Sinus Tract	☐	☐
Tunneling	☐	☐	Tunneling	☐	☐
Undermining	☐	☐	Undermining	☐	☐
Necrotic Tissue	☐	☐	Necrotic Tissue	☐	☐
Slough	☐	☐	Slough	☐	☐
Eschar	☐	☐	Eschar	☐	☐
Exudate	☐	☐	Exudate	☐	☐
Serous	☐	☐	Serous	☐	☐
Serosanguineous	☐	☐	Serosanguineous	☐	☐
Purulent	☐	☐	Purulent	☐	☐
Granulation	☐	☐	Granulation	☐	☐
Epithelialization	☐	☐	Epithelialization	☐	☐
Pain	☐	☐	Pain	☐	☐
Surrounding Skin:					
Erythema	☐	☐	Erythema	☐	☐
Maceration	☐	☐	Maceration	☐	☐
Induration	☐	☐	Induration	☐	☐

Description of Ulcer(s):

Classification of pressure ulcers:

Stage I: Nonblanchable erythema of intact skin, the heralding lesion of skin ulceration. In individuals with darker skin, discoloration of the skin, warmth, edema, induration, or hardness may also be indicators.

Stage II: Partial thickness skin loss involving epidermis, dermis or both.

Stage III: Full thickness skin loss involving damage to or necrosis of subcutaneous tissue that may extend down to, but not through, underlying fascia. The ulcer presents clinically as a deep crater with or without undermining adjacent tissue.

Stage IV: Full thickness skin loss with extensive destruction, tissue necrosis, or damage to muscle, bone, or supporting structures (e.g., tendon or joint capsule).

Figure 38-8

Sample pressure ulcer assessment guide. (Agency for Health Care Policy and Research. [1994]. *Treatment of pressure ulcers.* Rockville, MD: U.S. Department of Health and Human Services.)

- Demonstrate self-care measures necessary to prevent development of a pressure ulcer (if able)

An additional expected outcome may be appropriate for family members who function as the primary caregivers for a person at risk for developing a pressure ulcer. The family members will:

- Demonstrate care measures necessary to prevent development of a pressure ulcer

IMPLEMENTING

Preventing Pressure Ulcers

Many pressure ulcers can be prevented, but some high-risk individuals may develop pressure ulcers that continue to worsen despite aggressive nursing intervention. The nurse, involved in preventing the human suffering and costly treatment associated with pressure ulcers, uses all phases of the nursing process to individualize care and achieve positive outcomes. The AHCPR (USDHHS, 1992) recommends a series of interventions to prevent injury to the skin and promote optimal health. These protocols, displayed in the accompanying box, also provide the basis for an educational program that promotes ongoing implementation of preventive measures by caregivers in the home setting.

Protecting the Skin From External Mechanical Forces

To protect clients at risk from the adverse effects of pressure, a turning schedule should be implemented every 2 hours (Jacobs, 1994). Some clinicians believe that older individuals have less tissue tolerance and should be repositioned more frequently if redness on bony prominences is noted (Maklebust, 1995). The oblique position is an alternative to the side-lying position and results in significantly less pressure on the trochanter area (refer to Chapter 39, Fig. 39-15). Positioning devices such as pillows or foam wedges can prove helpful to keep body weight off bony prominences. For example, a standard pillow placed under the calves effectively raises the heels off the bed and alleviates pressure. Ring cushions or donuts were previously thought to protect reddened areas from additional pressure; however, *donut-type devices cause increased venous pressure and should never be used.* The effects of shearing force can be minimized by limiting the amount of time the head of the bed is elevated (if this is possible). Positioning devices and techniques maintain posture and distribute weight evenly for clients in a chair. Using a trapeze or bed linen to assist transfer and position changes prevents friction on the skin. Pressure-relieving support surfaces are available but there is disagreement as to which device is most appropriate for a client at risk. Table 38-2 compares the various types.

Teaching Clients and Families About Prevention

Teaching clients and caregivers how to prevent pressure ulcers requires a comprehensive, organized educational effort. Initially the healthcare provider must present basic information that defines terms, identifies clients at risk, explains where pressure ulcers develop, and describes various prevention strategies and options. Written and illustrated instructions, presented at the level of the learner, are valuable resources. The AHCPR's booklet *Patient Guide for Preventing Pressure Ulcers* outlines specific care measures related to each risk factor; it emphasizes the importance of personal involvement in care and treatment decisions and is available for distribution to consumers. The previously mentioned protocols listed in the box Guidelines for Nursing Care can also serve as a model for development of a teaching plan that incorporates basic principles and targets individuals at risk. As new information becomes available, education for prevention of pressure ulcers should be updated.

Treating Pressure Ulcers

Despite prevention tactics, pressure ulcers may develop in certain high-risk individuals. Aggressive treatment measures by the nurse or caregiver are the key to effective management. Clients, family members and caregivers, and healthcare providers collaborate and communicate to decide on appropriate treatment goals. The 1994 AHCPR guideline on *Treatment of Pressure Ulcers* specifically outlines measures for treating a pressure ulcer that reflect current knowledge and research (USDHHS, 1994).

Home Healthcare Alert

If a dressing change or wound cleansing is painful, emphasize the value of taking pain medication (either prescription or OTC) 30 to 60 minutes before the procedure. Inform the physician or nurse if this is not effective.

Cleaning the Pressure Ulcer

For a wound to heal properly, it must be kept free of infection. Cleaning the wound facilitates removal of necrotic tissue, wound exudate, and metabolic wastes. A pressure ulcer that is clean and free of infection should demonstrate some degree of healing within 2 to 4 weeks (van Rijswijk, 1993). Experts agree on the following protocol for wound cleansing:

- Clean the wound with each dressing change.
- Use careful, gentle motion when using cleaning materials (eg, gauze) to minimize trauma.
- Avoid using harmful cleaners or antiseptic agents (eg, povidone-iodine, hydrogen peroxide) because they damage cells needed for healing.
- Use 0.9% sodium chloride to irrigate and clean most pressure ulcers.

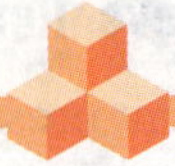

Guidelines for Nursing Care

Preventing Pressure Ulcers

Action	Rationale
Assess the skin of clients at risk on a daily basis. Pay particular attention to bony prominences.	Careful documentation of skin inspection is essential for formulating and evaluating an individualized plan of care.
Cleanse the skin routinely and whenever any soiling occurs. Use a mild cleansing agent, minimal friction, and avoid hot water.	Frequent cleansing limits exposure to environmental contaminants and the chemical irritants found in body waste products. Water that is just slightly warm causes less trauma to fragile skin and a mild cleansing product is less drying to the skin.
Maintain higher humidity in the environment and use skin moisturizers for dry skin.	Many older clients prefer overheated settings that promote dry skin. Humidification is effective in controlling dry skin. Moisturizers control the manifestations of dry skin and help to keep the skin intact (Frantz & Gardner, 1994a).
Avoid massage over bony prominences.	Massage, in general, promotes relaxation but massage over bony prominences may worsen soft tissue damage already present.
Protect the skin from moisture associated with episodes of incontinence or exposure to wound drainage.	Kemp (1994) has summarized research that indicates that the moisture associated with incontinence is responsible for skin breakdown. Underpads and briefs that absorb moisture and present a quick-drying surface to the skin can be used to keep the skin drier.
Minimize skin injury from friction and shearing forces by using proper positioning, turning, and transferring techniques. Use lubricants, protective films, dressings, and padding to diminish the effects of friction on the skin.	Proper positioning, turning techniques, lubricants, and protective dressings decrease friction between the skin and bed linens or contact surface, reducing the chance of injury.
Investigate reasons for inadequate dietary intake of protein and calories. Administer nutritional supplements or more aggressive nutritional intervention as needed.	Research has indicated that adequate dietary intake is a factor in preventing the development of a pressure ulcer and facilitating wound healing (Frantz & Gardner, 1994b).
Continue efforts to improve mobility and activity. If this is unrealistic, attempt to maintain current level of activity, mobility, and range of motion.	An individualized activity regimen is essential to promote intact skin and prevent the hazards of inactivity and immobility.
Document measures used to prevent pressure ulcers and the results of these interventions.	Documentation of interventions and outcomes ensures continuity of care and facilitates collaboration with other caregivers.

- Use an irrigating device that produces enough pressure to clean the wound adequately without damaging tissue (see accompanying box).
- Report when thick exudate or necrotic tissue is present in the wound. (Whirlpool treatments may be ordered until the ulcer is considered clean, or surgical excision of necrotic tissue may be necessary.)

Dressing the Pressure Ulcer

According to AHCPR (1994), the cardinal rule when dressing a pressure ulcer is to *keep the ulcer tissue moist and the surrounding skin dry*. Recommendations for wound dressing include:

- Use dressings that continuously keep the wound moist. Wet-to-dry dressings (see Chapter 30) should be used only for **debridement** (cleaning away of devitalized tissue and foreign matter from a wound; can be accomplished by various methods).
- Keep the intact, healthy skin surrounding the ulcer dry since it is susceptible to breakdown. Place the moist dressing only on the wound surface. Use a skin sealant or moisture-barrier ointment on the surrounding skin and the least amount of tape that is necessary.
- Select a dressing that absorbs exudate, if present, but still maintains a moist environment for healing.

Table 38-2

Description and Comparison of Support Surfaces

Type	Description	Increased Support Area	Low Moisture Retention	Reduced Heat Accumulation	Shear Reduction	Pressure Reduction	Dynamic	Cost Per Day
Foam overlay	Thick foam slab with textured surface designed to be placed on top of the standard mattress to reduce pressure by enveloping the body.	Yes	No	No	No	Yes	No	Low
Static flotation (air or water)	A vinyl mattress overlay composed of either interconnected air cells that are inflated with a blower before use or compartments that are filled with water. The shifting of air or water distributes pressure uniformly over the support area and creates a flotation effect.	Yes	No	No	Yes	Yes	No	Low
Alternating air mattress or overlay	Mattress or overlay with interconnecting air cells that cyclically inflate and deflate to produce alternating high and low pressure intervals.	Yes	No	No	Yes	Yes	Yes	Mod.
Low air loss bed	A series of interconnected woven fabric air pillows that allow some air to escape through the support surface. The pillows can be variably inflated to adjust the level of pressure relief.	Yes	Yes	Yes	?	Yes	Yes	High
Air-fluidized bed	Class of support surfaces that uses a high rate of air flow to fluidize fine particulate material (such as sand) to produce a support medium that has characteristics similar to a liquid.	Yes	Yes	Yes	Yes	Yes	Yes	High

(Source: U.S. Department of Health and Human Services, Agency for Health Care Policy and Research. [1994]. *Treatment of Pressure Ulcers.* Rockville, MD: DHHS.)

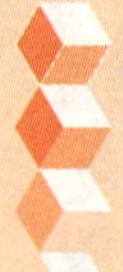

Helpscan

The following are resources for clients and health-care professionals:

- Clinical Practice Guidelines developed by the Agency for Health Care Policy and Research (AHCPR)

For Health Care Professionals

- Pressure Ulcers in Adults: Prediction and Prevention (May 1992)
- Treatment of Pressure Ulcers (December 1994)

For Consumers

- Preventing Pressure Ulcers: Patient Guide
- Treating Pressure Sores: Patient Guide
  AHCPR Clearinghouse
  (800) 358-9295
  or
  write to
  AHCPR Publications Clearinghouse
  PO Box 8547
  Silver Spring, MD 20907

- When choosing a dressing, consider the amount of nursing time that is involved for various types of dressings that maintain a moist wound environment.
- Pack wound cavities loosely with dressing material. Over-packing the wound may increase pressure and interfere with tissue healing.
- Tape the edges of a dressing that is near the anus (frame the dressing like a picture) to keep it intact and monitor it on a frequent basis.

Moisture-retentive dressings are recommended for pressure ulcers because they create a healing environment—one that allows epithelial cells to bridge the open surface of the wound more easily and close it. Previously, dressings that retained moisture were referred to as *occlusive,* but the more accurate term is *moisture-retentive* since some dressings keep the wound moist but still allow gas exchange to occur between the wound and the environment (Motta, 1995). These dressings also decrease the risk of infection and save healthcare dollars. Types of moisture-retentive dressings include transparent films, hydrocolloid dressings, and hydrogels. Table 38-3 outlines several types of wound dressings, and Figure 38-9 demonstrates a hydrocolloid dressing in place on a client. An abundance of dressing products exist and the nurse must rely on knowledge of the wound healing process to select that which is available for the client and will most effectively promote wound healing.

Effective Irrigation Pressure

- For irrigation to clean a wound effectively and safely, the pressure or force of the irrigation must measure between 4 and 15 pounds per square inch (psi).
- Irrigation pressure below 4 psi is ineffective (eg, using a bulb syringe).
- Irrigation pressure above 15 psi may cause trauma and force bacteria into the wound.
- The following types of equipment deliver from 4 to 15 psi, which is adequate to clean a wound:
  Piston irrigating syringe with catheter tip (60 mL)
  Syringe (35 mL) with a 19-gauge needle or angiocath
  Water Pic set at the lowest setting (#1)

(Source: U.S. Department of Health and Human Services, Agency for Health Care Policy and Research. [1994]. *Treatment of Pressure Ulcers.* Rockville, MD: DHHS.)

Controlling Infection

CDC guidelines or body substance isolation (BSI) precautions and good handwashing technique must be followed to prevent infection (refer to Chapter 28 for a review of barrier techniques and handwashing recommendations). AHCPR guidelines (USDHHS, 1994) state that clean gloves and clean dressings may be used to treat pressure ulcers as long as the agency infection control procedures are followed. Sterile instruments must be used for debridement purposes. Krasner and Kennedy (1994) reviewed an alternate method for dressing change that is a combination of sterile and nonsterile technique. Referred to as the "no-touch technique," it consists of the following steps:

- Use two pairs of nonsterile gloves, sterile 4×4s, and sterile saline.
- Discard first set of gloves after soiled dressing is removed. Wash hands.
- Open sterile supplies using sterile technique.
- Put on clean gloves and pour sterile saline directly on the wound using an emesis basin to collect drainage.
- Pick up sterile gauze and bunch ends backwards toward your hand, keeping the front center of the gauze untouched.
- Clean the wound moving from the center outward using a fresh gauze pad for each motion.
- Dry the surrounding skin also.
- Redress wound by picking up gauze sponges by the corner and placing the untouched side over the pressure ulcer.

Table 38-3
Wound Care Products: Dressings

Category	Sample Products	Description/Indications
Hydrocolloid	DuoDERM Tegasorb Restore Comfeel	Wafer-shaped dressings that come in many shapes and thicknesses Hydrophilic (water-loving) particles mix with exudate to form a gel that keeps the wound moist. Gel can have an offensive odor and be mistaken for infection. The wafer form is occlusive and not recommended for wounds with a large amount of exudate. May damage fragile surrounding skin. Can remain in place for 3–7 days
Transparent dressings	ACU-derm BIOCLUSIVE OpSite Tegaderm	Permit gas exchange between the wound and the environment, but prevent bacteria from invading the wound because of small pore size Nonabsorptive and fluid collection visible underneath is often mistaken for purulent exudate. Can damage skin surrounding wound and should not be used on infected wounds. Can remain in place 24–72 hours
Hydrogels	AQUASORB Biolex ClearSite Vigilon	Sheet or gel with a higher water content that enhances epithelialization Nonocclusive and can be used when infection is present Have limited ability to absorb exudate and should not be used if wound drainage is excessive Can remain in place for 8–48 hours
Absorption dressings	Bard Absorption Dressing DEBRISAN	May consist of beads, powders, or paste and absorb large amount of exudate Conform to the shape and size of the wound Must be irrigated from the wound bed when changed Can remain in place as long as 24 hours
Gauze dressings	"4×4s" Adaptic Vaseline gauze Xeroform	Woven or nonwoven dressing made of cotton or synthetic material. Can be impregnated with agents that promote healing. Limited ability to keep the wound bed moist Need a secondary dressing to keep them in place and protect from contamination Can remain in place for 8–24 hours, depending on if covered with a transparent dressing

(Data from Motta, G. [1993]. How moisture-retentive dressings promote healing. *Nursing, 23*[12], 26–33; and Hahn, J., & Olsen, C. [1994]. Wounds: Nursing care and product selection. *Nursing Spectrum,* October 31, 12–13.)

- Cover with a transparent dressing; secure edges with tape; and write date, time, and initials on the dressing.

This method allows sterile supplies to touch the wound but still saves nursing time and cuts costs without compromising client care. Refer to the accompanying box for comments pertinent to treating a pressure ulcer in the home environment.

Home Healthcare Alert

When removing a soiled dressing at home, the caregiver can use a small plastic sandwich bag instead of a glove to cover the hand. The dressing should be carefully lifted off the wound and the plastic bag turned inside out over the hand and the soiled dressing prior to careful disposal. It is always important to emphasize handwashing before and after any care measures.

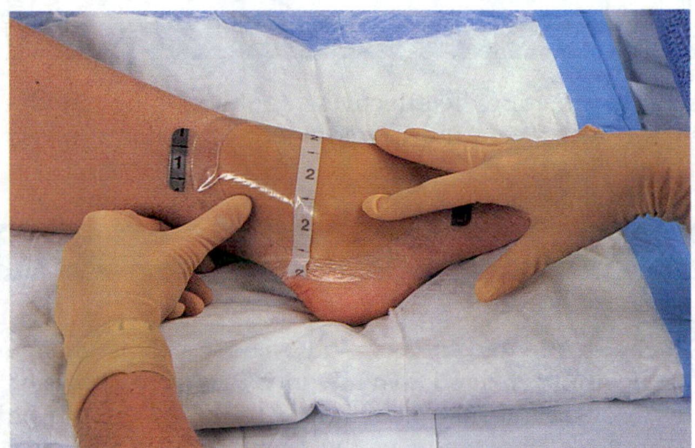

Figure 38-9
For proper wear, the hydrocolloid dressing must be sized generously, allowing at least a 1-inch margin of healthy skin around the wound. (Photo © B. Proud.)

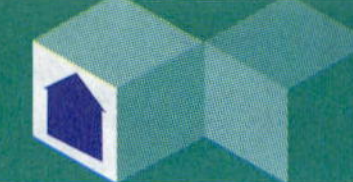

Home Care: Bridging the Gap

Treatment of a Pressure Ulcer

- Involve the home caregiver, as well as the client, in the plan of care.
- Provide the caregiver with a simple, easy-to-understand list of instructions about caring for the pressure ulcer. Include any special instruction for the particular product being used.
- Address the causative factor for the pressure ulcer before proceeding with the plan of care.
- Assess nutritional status of client and, if necessary, consult a dietician for nutritional recommendations.
- Consult frequently with the physician about the progress of wound healing and products being used.
- Use clean dressings in the home setting. Dispose of contaminated wound care materials according to Environmental Protection Agency guidelines and local regulations.
- Instruct the caregiver in good handwashing technique.
- Review signs of infection with the caregiver or signs of any other complications. Encourage caregiver to contact the physician or home health nurse about any problems with care.

Research has not supported the use of antiseptic agents to reduce bacteria in wounds. In fact, these antiseptics (eg, hydrogen peroxide, Dakin's solution) may prove harmful because they can be toxic to cells and thus delay healing.

Providing Care in Other Treatment Options

When other treatments have failed, surgery may be considered as an option. Direct closure of the wound, skin grafting, or various skin flap procedures are surgical procedures that can be selected based on the client's condition and the severity of the ulcer. Following surgery, the nurse must be vigilant about protecting the surgical site from pressure and contamination.

Several other treatment modalities are being considered and investigated at present. They include electrical stimulation, hyperbaric oxygen, laser irradiation, ultrasound, and miscellaneous topical agents and systemic drugs.

EVALUATING

When evaluating the effectiveness of a plan of care designed to prevent the development of pressure ulcers or treat those already present, the nurse uses each nurse–client interaction to check whether the client has met the individualized expected outcomes specified in the plan of care. Nursing care is considered effective if the client and/or family member or caregiver expresses satisfaction with prevention and treatment measures and is able to:

- Participate effectively in preventive and treatment regimens
- Prevent development of any additional areas of skin breakdown
- Demonstrate progressive healing of pressure ulcer
- Improve overall physical condition (including nutritional state and mobility status)
- Remain free of infection at any pressure ulcer site
- Communicate need for additional support (environmental, physical, psychosocial)
- Respond effectively to teaching strategies and plan

Color photographs can be an excellent method of evaluating progression of wound healing by comparing the pressure ulcer at the initial assessment with the recovery stages. Evaluation is a continuous process that leads to ongoing assessment and revised plans and implementations.

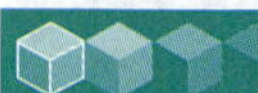

Nursing Process in Clinical Practice

When identifying and treating clients with a nursing diagnosis of Impaired Skin Integrity, the nurse uses each phase of the nursing process. Quality care depends on the nurse's possession of the knowledge and clinical skills described earlier in this chapter. What follows are the assessment priorities, expected outcomes, and nursing interventions for a client with a pressure ulcer.

Impaired Skin Integrity Related to Presence of Mechanical Factors

A state in which the individual's skin is adversely altered. (NANDA, 1994)

The nurse who is committed to decreasing the prevalence of pressure ulcers can have a serious impact on the quality of client care and healthcare costs. Older clients are particularly at risk for impaired skin integrity because their skin is much more prone to injury. The combination of age-related changes and some degree of immobility is devastating. Skin necrosis can develop quickly, and malnutrition further compounds the problem.

The sequence of events actually leading up to the development of a pressure ulcer and progression to a Stage IV ulcer is as follows: pressure → compression of small nutrient vessels of skin and underlying tissue → tissue anoxia and ischemia → necrosis of tissue cells → sloughing and ulceration → invasion by microorganisms → infection → sepsis → involvement of underlying fascia, muscle, and bone → rapidly irreversible condition (Smeltzer & Bare, 1996). Accurate, ongoing assessment of the pressure ulcer is essential. Most pressure ulcers can be prevented, and stage I ulcers can be treated effectively with a positive outcome. The nurse must be vigilant in the use of positioning, transfer, and support measures. Treatment is detailed earlier in this chapter. Documentation must be precise to facilitate continuity of care and collaboration with other caregivers.

Education is a vital component of the treatment strategy. The most effective educational approach stresses the involvement of the client and his or her family and caregivers. Information must be presented at an appropriate level and the client and caregiver, whenever possible, should participate in decisions regarding management and treatment strategies. Prevention or healing and recovery are optimal outcomes, but for a client in the latter stages of a terminal illness, promotion of comfort may be the primary goal. In this situation, pressure ulcer treatment goals such as frequent positioning or nutritional support may be secondary to the goal of keeping the client comfortable.

Assessment Priorities

A thorough assessment provides direction for interventions and also addresses the client's overall health and well-being. When a pressure ulcer is noted:

- Describe the pressure ulcer in terms of site, size, depth, undermining, edema, warmth, color, odor, eschar, slough, drainage, and surrounding skin. Description of the ulcer must be ongoing. Most agencies use a special pressure ulcer assessment form. See Figure 38-8 for a sample form, and refer to the box for specific techniques for measurement of a pressure ulcer.
- Describe the skin in general: turgor, dryness or moisture, sensation in pressure areas, and warmth.
- Describe contractures or any predisposing environmental factors (eg, casts, wrinkled linen).
- Describe the client's self-care abilities: hygiene, mobility, nutrition, continence, level of consciousness.
- Describe the current nursing care: special skin care, pressure-relief measures, nutritional support, and incontinence management or devices.

Measurement of a Pressure Ulcer

In addition to assessing location, stage, drainage, and types of tissue present in the wound, it is imperative that nurses accurately and consistently measure a pressure ulcer. Effective treatment is dependent on precise assessments. The nurse should document the following:

Size of the Wound

- **Draw the shape and describe it.**
- **Measure the length, width, and diameter (if circular).**

Depth of the Wound

- **Moisten a sterile swab with saline and insert it gently into the wound at a 90-degree angle with the tip down.**
- **Mark the point on the swab that is even with the surrounding skin surface.**
- **Remove the swab and measure the depth with a ruler.**

Presence of Undermining, Tunneling, or Sinus Tract

- **Insert a saline-moistened sterile swab under the wound edge.**
- **Apply gentle pressure and assess for any abnormal pathways.**
- ***Never use force when probing with the swab.***
- **Measure the location and depth of penetration.**

Expected Outcomes

The client will:

- Demonstrate signs of pressure ulcer healing
- Eliminate predisposing factors or reduce their effects
- Demonstrate appropriate self-care behaviors (if able):
  - Demonstrate satisfactory hygiene
  - Shift weight and change position every 1 to 2 hours
  - Eat nutritious diet (high in protein, iron, vitamin C; zinc supplements; sufficient fluids)
- State rationale for treatment measures
- Develop no new areas of skin breakdown

Interventions

Nurses and family members/caregivers may be the first line of defense to prevent the development of pressure ulcers. Nurses and educated caregivers also are responsible for measures to prevent further breakdown and skin care treatment interventions. These are addressed earlier in the chapter with rationales for each action. Interventions are as follows:

- Assess the stage of the pressure ulcer.
- Use measures to eliminate pressure on area of skin breakdown:
  - Communicate schedule for repositioning.

- Use positioning devices to protect area of skin breakdown.
- Keep head of bed in low position (if possible).
- Use an appropriate support surface (eg, *static support surface*, such as a foam overlay [pressure reduction remains constant], or *dynamic support surface*, such as an alternating air mattress [pressure reduction changes in a cyclical manner]).
- Change position at least every 2 hours, or more frequently based on skin assessments (redness on a bony prominence indicates the need for more frequent repositioning).
- Cleanse wound with each dressing change.
- Apply a moisture-retentive dressing to the wound.
- Monitor for possibility of infection.

Client Care Study

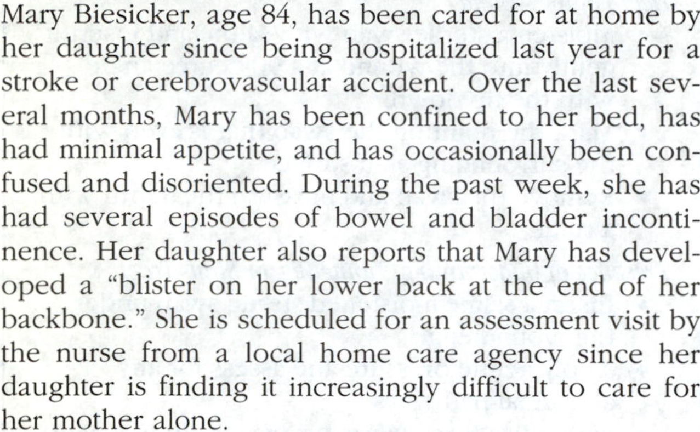

Mary Biesicker, age 84, has been cared for at home by her daughter since being hospitalized last year for a stroke or cerebrovascular accident. Over the last several months, Mary has been confined to her bed, has had minimal appetite, and has occasionally been confused and disoriented. During the past week, she has had several episodes of bowel and bladder incontinence. Her daughter also reports that Mary has developed a "blister on her lower back at the end of her backbone." She is scheduled for an assessment visit by the nurse from a local home care agency since her daughter is finding it increasingly difficult to care for her mother alone.

The nurse's initial assessment of Mary, relative to skin integrity, revealed the following:

Skin status: Presence of a nickel-sized open area on the sacrum (stage II pressure ulcer), 2 cm in diameter and 1 cm in depth. No abnormal pathways noted. Reddened area (0.5 cm) surrounding lesion. No drainage noted. Reddened area (2.5 cm) also noted on right elbow. Skin dry over all body surfaces.

Nutritional status: Daughter states "usual weight is 115–120 lbs and she has definitely lost some weight." Poor skin turgor.

Elimination status: Wearing "adult diaper," diaper damp with urine and small amount of light brown liquid stool.

Activity status: Lying quietly in bed, moans when area around lesion is palpated.

Core Competencies

In order to implement this plan of care, the nurse needs the following specialized abilities:

Cognitive Competencies

- Strong assessment skills and knowledge of wound healing concepts
- Knowledge of principles and practices related to infection control
- Knowledge of pertinent standards of care and agency/institutional policies
- Teaching skills to help Mary Biesicker and her daughter understand factors that place client at risk of developing pressure ulcers and develop ability to participate in care of the pressure ulcer

Technical Competencies

- Caregiver skills directed to preventing complications or deterioration of condition of wound as specified in Mrs. Biesicker's plan of care
- Ability to use a documentation system competently to communicate the client's plan of care

Interpersonal Competencies

- Ability to work collaboratively with the interdisciplinary caregiving team, client, and family to assess the client's need for healthcare
- Ability to establish a trusting nurse–client/family relationship grounded in responsible caring
- Interpersonal skills to communicate to Mrs. Biesicker and her daughter that pressure ulcers can be prevented and, in many cases, healed and that nursing is committed to helping

Ethical/Legal Competencies

- Commitment to do whatever is necessary and cost effective to successfully implement the plan of care by effective use of the nursing process
- Ability to serve as a trusted and effective client advocate
- Ability to practice nursing accountable to self, client, the profession, and society

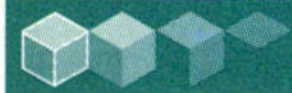

Nursing Plan of Care

for Mary Biesicker

Nursing Diagnosis:	Impaired Skin Integrity related to mechanical factors, inactivity, altered nutritional intake, and incontinence *as manifested by* Stage II pressure ulcer on sacral area and reddened area on right elbow

Nursing Plan of Care

for Mary Biesicker

Expected Outcome: 6/6/98—at daily observation (or weekly in the home setting), the client will:

- Experience reduction of pressure on bony prominences (absence of any additional reddened areas)

Nursing Interventions	Rationale	Evaluative Statement
Assess skin for development of any pressure areas (use agency tool).	Pressure results in poor circulation that causes skin breakdown.	6/13/98 Goal met. Client has been turned from side to side every 2 hours. Reddened area on right elbow measures 1.25 cm in diameter. No new reddened areas observed.
Avoid sitting or lying on a pressure ulcer.	This facilitates pressure relief in the area and allows blood to reenter capillaries and provide oxygen to the area.	
Reposition from side to side at least every 2 hours.	The duration of pressure is more devastating to skin than the amount of pressure.	
Use pillows to maintain side-lying or oblique position in bed and support right ankle off bed surface.	Pillows relieve pressure on lesion and areas at risk and promote improved circulation to those areas.	*Recommendation:* Arrange for delivery of hospital bed with overbed trapeze setup. Secure a home health aid for limited period of time to assist with repositioning during the night and allow daughter time to rest.
Place foam overlay mattress on bed.	Static device provides support and relieves pressure on skin surface.	***M. Lieb, RN***

Expected Outcome 6/6/98—at weekly observation the client will:

- Demonstrate a reduction in the size of the stage II pressure ulcer on sacrum

Nursing Interventions	Rationale	Evaluative Statement
Assess condition of pressure ulcer at time of dressing change (refer to previous assessments).	Signs of infection and deterioration can be recognized and treatment plan revised.	6/13/98 Goal met. Pressure ulcer has decreased slightly in size—1.7 cm in diameter, depth remains the same. No apparent infection noted. Will continue with present treatment regimen.
Irrigate wound with normal saline using a 60 mL piston syringe with a catheter tip.	Normal saline cleanses the wound without harming tissues.	***M. Lieb, RN***
Dry skin thoroughly surrounding the ulcer.	Moisture makes intact skin more susceptible to injury.	
Apply moisture-retentive dressing (Tegasorb).	Moisture-retentive dressings create a healing environment by allowing epithelial cells to bridge the wound gap and close it.	
Use clean technique for the dressing change.	In the home, the risk is minimal for cross-contamination of microorganisms.	

Expected Outcome 6/6/98—at weekly visit, the client/caregiver will:

- Demonstrate skills required to promote skin integrity and care for a pressure ulcer

(continued)

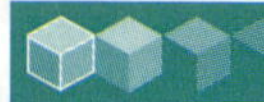

Nursing Plan of Care *(continued)*

for Mary Biesicker

Nursing Interventions	Rationale	Evaluative Statement
Assess caregiver's (daughter) motivation and ability to manage treatment regimen.	Motivation influences readiness to learn and contributes to positive learning outcomes.	6/13/98 Goal partially met. Daughter able to recognize appearance of pressure areas on skin. Stated she would like to review treatment routine again. Daughter performed assessment and dressing change satisfactorily with nurse in attendance. Clarified and reviewed written instructions again. Daughter states, "I feel much more confident now." ***M. Lieb, RN***
Instruct daughter about causes, skin assessment techniques, and individualized treatment regimen. Provide written instructions and illustrations where possible.	A clear, concise teaching guide provides consistent education and is available for reinforcement.	
Provide information about community resources available for assistance with care of mother.	Resources provide opportunity for support and problem solving.	

Sample Documentation

6/20/98 Home care visit (nursing)

Mrs. Biesicker was revisited in her home for continued assessment and treatment of pressure ulcer. Nursing diagnosis: Impaired Skin Integrity related to pressure, inactivity, inadequate nutritional intake, and incontinence. According to daughter, client was turned and repositioned every 2 hours. Foam mattress and pillow supports used for support and pressure reduction. Dressing on pressure ulcer changed. Wound cleansed with normal saline, intact skin dried surrounding wound, and Tegasorb dressing applied. Granulation tissue noted in wound bed, no evidence of drainage or reddened area around wound. Ulcer has decreased to 1½ cm in size. Reddened area not apparent on right elbow. Reviewed written instructions with daughter. Conference arranged with physician, dietician, client, and daughter for 6/23/98 to discuss health care options. Will continue current plan of care and visits every other day.

M. Lieb, RN

Key Points

- A pressure ulcer is caused by unrelieved pressure that results in damage to underlying tissue.
- Clients most at risk for developing a pressure ulcer include older adults, those who are immobile, and individuals living with chronic health problems.
- Family members who care for these individuals need information to effectively prevent pressure ulcers from developing.
- The most susceptible areas for development of a pressure ulcer are the sacrum, coccyx, trochanter, and heels.
- The Agency for Health Care Policy and Research (AHCPR) and the National Pressure Ulcer Advisory Panel (NPUAP) have adopted a four-stage classification system for pressure ulcers.
- The Norton scale and the Braden scale are risk assessment tools that have been used and tested extensively and are recommended for use in any healthcare setting.
- Skin assessment for a pressure ulcer includes a thorough nursing history and physical assessment describing the location, dimensions, and stage of the ulcer; presence of abnormal pathways, necrotic tissue, exudate, or granulation tissue; and occurrence of epithelialization.
- The nursing diagnoses that specifically address the presence of a pressure ulcer are Impaired Skin Integrity and Risk for Impaired Skin Integrity for stage I and II ulcers, and Impaired Tissue Integrity and Risk for Impaired Tissue Integrity for stage III and IV ulcers.
- Normal saline is the agent recommended for cleansing and irrigation of a pressure ulcer because it does not cause damage to tissue.
- A moisture-retentive dressing creates a healing environment that allows epithelial cells to bridge the open surface of a pressure ulcer more easily.

Study Questions

1. The most common site for a pressure ulcer to develop is the
   a. occipital area
   b. sacrum
   c. sternum
   d. humerus
2. The key factor contributing to the etiology of a pressure ulcer is
   a. moisture
   b. incontinence
   c. pressure
   d. malnutrition
3. Which hospitalized client is most at risk of developing a pressure ulcer?
   a. a 70-year-old client with a fractured hip
   b. a 45-year-old woman recovering from gallbladder surgery
   c. a 16-year-old male paraplegic who suffered a spinal cord injury
   d. a 50-year-old client who suffered a mild stroke
4. After an initial assessment, the nurse documents the presence of a reddened area that has blistered. According to recognized staging systems, this ulcer is classified as
   a. stage I
   b. stage II
   c. stage III
   d. stage IV
5. An older invalid client sits and slumps in her chair most of the day. She is most likely to develop a pressure ulcer because of
   a. malnutrition
   b. shearing forces
   c. edema
   d. a chronic disease
6. The nurse assesses a stage III pressure ulcer. The nurse has observed
   a. redness that persists when pressure is relieved
   b. an open lesion with subcutaneous tissue exposed
   c. a necrotic area extending through the fascia to bone
   d. a reddened area with an abrasion
7. A nurse assesses that a bedridden client is at risk for developing a pressure ulcer. As the nurse plans to change the client's position, the nurse is aware that
   a. a 30-degree turn to an oblique position is effective
   b. position should be changed once a shift
   c. the back-lying position should be used most frequently
   d. including position change in a care plan requires a physician's order
8. A priority nursing action to prevent a client from developing a pressure ulcer is
   a. use waterproof material on the bed
   b. massage any reddened area frequently
   c. use an air-inflated ring to relieve pressure on areas
   d. use a mild soap when cleansing the skin
9. During a dressing change, the nurse observes what appears to be reddish-pink tissue in the wound. This is most likely
   a. a sign of infection
   b. eschar
   c. exudate
   d. granulation tissue
10. Usual treatment for a stage II pressure ulcer is
    a. a moisture-retentive dressing
    b. surgical debridement
    c. exposure to a heat lamp four times daily
    d. whirlpool treatment twice daily
11. Ms. Sanchez is 80 years old, obese, has a stage III sacral pressure ulcer, and is being cared for at home by her family. The priority nursing diagnosis is
    a. Impaired Tissue Integrity
    b. Caregiver Role Strain
    c. Altered Nutrition: Less than body requirements
    d. Bathing/Hygiene Self Care Deficit
12. According to AHCPR, the cleansing agent that is least damaging to new tissue is
    a. hydrogen peroxide
    b. betadine
    c. Phisohex
    d. normal saline
13. A physician has ordered irrigation of a client's stage III pressure ulcer. To irrigate the wound effectively without damaging new tissue, the nurse selects
    a. a bulb syringe
    b. a 10 cc syringe without a needle
    c. a 35 mL syringe with a 19-gauge needle
    d. a spray bottle found at the bedside
14. Recent protocol from AHCPR recommends that when dressing a pressure ulcer, the caregiver should
    a. use sterile gloves
    b. keep healthy tissue dry that surrounds the ulcer
    c. pack wound cavities tightly with gauze
    d. apply wet-to-dry dressings
15. Which older, inactive client is nutritionally at risk and more likely to develop a pressure ulcer?
    a. Mr. Brown, whose albumin level is 4.5 mg/dL
    b. Ms. Green, who eats well but is a vegetarian
    c. Mr. Black, who has a lymphocyte count of $800/mm^3$
    d. Ms. White, who is 10 pounds overweight

Answers With Rationale

1. The correct response is *b.* All sites involve bony prominences but the sacrum is the most common area where pressure ulcers develop.
2. The correct response is *c.* Pressure interferes with circulation to the cell resulting in cell death. Moisture, incontinence, and malnutrition predispose a client to altered skin integrity, making the skin more susceptible to injury.
3. The correct response is *a.* An older client with a fractured hip already has age-related skin changes that, coupled with some degree of immobility, make that person a likely candidate. The two middle-aged clients should not suffer any extended period of inactivity. Even though a spinal cord injury may cause immobility, a 16-year-old is usually well-developed muscularly and in good health and is probably able to use his arms to aid in movement.
4. The correct answer is *b.* A stage II pressure ulcer is superficial and presents clinically as an abrasion, ulcer, or shallow crater.
5. The correct answer is *b.* Sitting slumped in a chair for an extended period can easily result in shearing force, causing a pressure ulcer. Malnutrition, edema, and the presence of chronic disease may certainly be risk factors for the development of a pressure ulcer, but the most likely cause in this situation is shearing force.
6. The correct answer is *b.* A stage III pressure ulcer is an open lesion that exposes subcutaneous tissue. Redness that persists is stage I, a reddened area that has an abrasion is stage II, and stage IV would involve a necrotic area extending through the fascia to the bone.
7. The correct answer is *a.* A 30-degree turn to the oblique position relieves pressure on vulnerable areas. Position needs to be changed at least every 2 hours and is an independent nursing action. The back-lying position should be avoided as much as possible because it places pressure on many vulnerable sites.
8. The correct answer is *d.* A mild soap is less irritating. The skin should be rinsed and dried thoroughly. Waterproof materials may cause the client to perspire; massage is not recommended for areas that are already traumatized; and air-inflated rings place additional pressure and compromise circulation to the area where they are used.
9. The correct answer is *d.* Granulation tissue is new tissue composed of many small blood vessels, is pinkish-red in color, and fills an open wound when it starts to heal. Eschar is thick, dry, necrotic tissue. An infection in a wound is usually accompanied by other signs of inflammation. A wound exudate is a fluid that accumulates in the wound.
10. The correct response is *a.* A moisture-retentive dressing provides a moist environment for wound healing. A heat lamp or irrigation with betadine is no longer recommended, and surgical debridement is used for stage III and IV pressure ulcers.
11. The correct response is *a.* Stage III pressure ulcers involve damage to underlying tissue and Impaired Tissue Integrity is the priority diagnosis. Her nutritional problem involves more than needed body requirements and the remaining two diagnoses may be appropriate but are not the priority diagnoses at this time.
12. The correct response is *d.* Normal saline is a physiologic solution that will not harm tissue and adequately cleanses most wounds. Betadine, hydrogen peroxide, and Phisohex may cause damage to tissue.
13. The correct response is *c.* This size syringe with a 19-gauge needle will effectively cleanse the wound without damaging tissue. The bulb syringe and the 10 cc syringe do not have enough pressure. The spray bottle found at the bedside may be contaminated and its irrigating pressure is not known.
14. The correct response is *b.* Moisture makes intact skin more susceptible to injury. Wet-to-dry dressings are no longer recommended because they do not maintain a moist environment and when removed can damage healthy tissue. According to AHCPR, there is no evidence to indicate that use of sterile dressings and gloves results in better outcomes.
15. The correct response is *c.* An albumin level of 4.5 mg/dL falls in the normal range, while a lymphocyte count of 800/mm^3 is below normal and places this client at risk. Both other clients appear to have adequate dietary intake and this is probably not a risk factor at this time.

Bibliography

Barnes, H. (1993). Wound care: Fact and fiction about hydrocolloid dressings. *Journal of Gerontological Nursing, 19*(6), 23–26.

Bennis, S., & Davis, S. (1994). An effective approach to treating decubitus ulcers in home healthcare patients. *Home Healthcare Nurse, 12*(1), 47–52.

Bergman-Evans, B., Cuddigan, J., & Bergstrom, N. (1994). Clinical practice guidelines: Prediction and prevention of pressure ulcers. *Journal of Gerontological Nursing, 20*(9), 19–26.

Bergstrom, N., Braden, B., Laguzza, A., & Holman, V. (1987). The Braden scale for predicting pressure sore risk. *Nursing Research, 36*(4), 205–210.

Burd, C., Langemo, D., Olson, B., Hanson, D., Hunter, S., & Sauvage, T. (1992). Skin problems: Epidemiology of pressure ulcers in a skilled care facility. *Journal of Gerontological Nursing, 18*(9), 29–38.

Burd, C., et al. (1994). Skin care strategies in a skilled nursing home. *Journal of Gerontological Nursing, 20*(11), 28–34.

Carpenito, L. (1995). *Nursing care plans and documentation* (2nd ed.). Philadelphia: Lippincott.

Carpenito, L. (1995). *Nursing diagnosis: Application to clinical practice* (6th ed.). Philadelphia: Lippincott.

Carroll, P. (1995). Bed selection: Help patients rest easy. *RN, 58*(5), 44–50.

Cleaned, dressed, and ready to heal. (1995). *Nursing, 25*(6), 32FF–32HH.

Eaglstein, W., McKay, M., & Pariser, D. (1994). The problems that plague aging skin. *Patient Care, 28*(7), 89–120.

Erwin-Toth, P., & Hocevar, B. (1995). Wound care: Selecting the right dressing. *American Journal of Nursing, 95*(2), 46–51.

Frantz, R., & Gardner, S. (1994a). Clinical concerns: Management of dry skin. *Journal of Gerontological Nursing, 20*(9), 15–18.

Frantz, R., & Gardner, S. (1994b). Elderly skin care: Principles of chronic wound care. *Journal of Gerontological Nursing, 20*(9), 35–44.

Goodridge, D. (1993). Pressure ulcer risk assessment tools: What's new for gerontological nurses. *Journal of Gerontological Nursing, 19*(1), 23–27.

Jacobs, B. (1994). Working on the right moves: Part 1. *Nursing, 24*(10), 58–62.

Jacobs, B. (1994). Working on the right moves: Part 2. *Nursing, 24*(11), 52–54.

Kemp, M. (1994). Protecting the skin from moisture and associated irritants. *Journal of Gerontological Nursing, 20*(9), 8–14.

Kemp, M., & Krouskop, P. (1994). Pressure ulcers: Reducing incidence and severity by managing pressure. *Journal of Gerontological Nursing, 20*(9), 27–34.

Krasner, D. (1995). Wound care: How to use the red-yellow-black system. *American Journal of Nursing, 95*(5), 44–47.

Krasner, D., & Kennedy, K. (1994). Using the no-touch technique to change a dressing. *Nursing, 24*(9), 50–52.

Lyder, C., Clemes-Lowrance, C., Davis, A., Sullivan, L., & Zucker, A. (1992). Structured skin care regimen to prevent perineal dermatitis in the elderly. *Journal of ET Nursing, 19*(2), 12–16.

Maklebust, J. (1995). Pressure ulcer: What works. *RN, 58*(9), 46–50.

McNaughton, V., & Brazil, K. (1995). Wound and skin team: Impact on pressure ulcer prevalence in chronic care. *Journal of Gerontological Nursing, 21*(2), 45–49.

Monaghan, J. (1993). Assessing risk and preventing pressure ulcers. *Patient Care, 27*(7), 36–66.

Motta, G. (1993). Dressed for success: How moisture-retentive dressings promote healing. *Nursing, 23*(12), 26–33.

Motta, G. (1995). Moistening up for good healing. *Nursing, 25*(4), 32H–32J.

North American Nursing Diagnosis Association. (1994). *NANDA nursing diagnoses: Definitions and classification 1995–1996.* Philadelphia: NANDA.

Norton, D., McLaren, R., & Exton-Smith, A. (1975). An investigation of geriatric nursing problems in hospital. London: Churchill Livingstone. Original work published 1962.

O'Hanlon-Nichols, T. (1995). Commonly asked questions about wound healing. *American Journal of Nursing, 95*(4), 22–24.

Singh, P. (1994). Wound healing in the home health arena. *Home Healthcare Nurse, 12*(1), 20–22.

Smeltzer, S., & Bare, B. (1996). *Brunner and Suddarth's textbook of medical-surgical nursing* (8th ed.). Philadelphia: Lippincott.

U.S. Department of Health and Human Services, Agency for Health Care Policy and Research. (1992 May). *Pressure ulcers in adults: Prediction and prevention.* Rockville, MD: DHHS.

U.S. Department of Health and Human Services, Agency for Health Care Policy and Research. (1994 December). *Treatment of pressure ulcers.* Rockville, MD: DHHS.

van Rijswijk, L. (1993). Full-thickness pressure ulcers: Patient and wound healing characteristics. *Decubitus, 6*(1), 16–21.

White, P. (1994). Skin rounds sharpen our focus. *RN, 55*(2), 19–20.

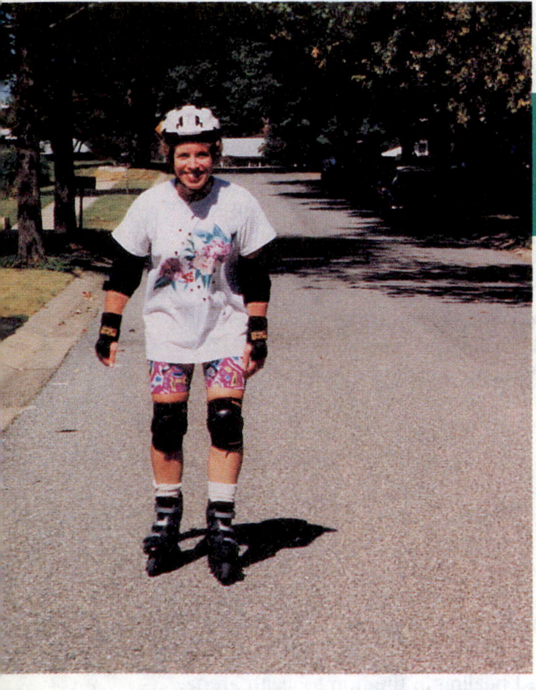

Chapter 39

Activity

Objectives

After studying this chapter, the learner should be able to:

Define key terms used in this chapter.

Describe the role of the skeletal, muscular, and nervous systems in the physiology of movement.

Identify seven variables that influence body alignment and mobility.

Differentiate isotonic, isometric, and isokinetic exercise.

Describe the effects of exercise and immobility on major body systems.

Assess body alignment, mobility, and activity tolerance, using appropriate interview questions and physical assessment skills.

Develop nursing diagnoses that correctly identify mobility problems amenable to nursing therapy.

Use proper body mechanics when positioning, moving, lifting, and ambulating clients.

Design exercise programs.

Plan, implement, and evaluate nursing care related to select nursing diagnoses involving mobility problems.

Key Terms

active exercise
ankylosis
atrophy
base of support
body mechanics
center of gravity
contractures
exercise
flaccidity
footdrop
isokinetic exercise
isometric exercise
isotonic exercise
line of gravity
osteoporosis
passive exercise
range of motion
spasticity
tonus

For most healthy individuals, the ability for movement is taken for granted. People simply expect our amazingly complex musculoskeletal and nervous systems to work together smoothly and on command to enable us to stand upright, to walk, and to reach for and grasp what we want. Often little thought is given to the need to care for the systems that promote and coordinate healthy movement until disuse, trauma, or illness cripples some aspect of movement. Although exercise and fitness are valued by some, many people live overwhelmingly inactive lifestyles that limit their ability to experience and enjoy life to its fullest and that openly invite degenerative and chronic diseases such as hypertension, ischemic heart disease, or diabetes.

The ability to move is closely related to the fulfillment of other basic human needs. Although breathing continues during rest, movement facilitates pulmonary functioning and increases peripheral blood flow. Because regular exercise contributes to the healthy functioning of each body system and, conversely, immobility negatively affects each body system, nurses actively promote exercise to promote wellness, prevent illness, and restore health. It currently is generally accepted that there are more serious health consequences related to a sedentary lifestyle than there are risks related to exercise.

Study of this chapter provides the student with knowledge of the physiology of movement, the principles of body mechanics, and factors affecting body alignment and mobility. A comprehensive section on exercise differentiates types of exercise, explores the role of exercise in disease prevention and health promotion, notes risks related to exercise, and allows the design of individualized exercise programs. The effects of immobility on body systems are presented with a full discussion of related nursing interventions. A practical guide to assessing body alignment and mobility states is offered with pertinent interview questions and physical assessment techniques. Analysis of mobility data may lead to the nursing diagnoses of Impaired Physical Mobility or Activity Intolerance or to diagnoses identifying the effect of mobility problems on other areas of human functioning. Examples of nursing diagnoses are included. Expected outcomes are identified and specific nursing strategies are presented. In the section entitled Nursing Process in Clinical Practice, focused assessment, expected client outcomes, and nursing interventions are offered for select nursing diagnoses of common mobility problems: Activity Intolerance; Impaired Physical Mobility; Risk for Injury: Complications of Immobility; and Altered Health Maintenance: Lack of Exercise Program. These guides and the concluding client care study illustrate how the nurse's knowledge of body mechanics and mobility is combined with specific nursing interventions and caring to promote fitness successfully and to resolve mobility problems.

Physiology of Movement

Purposeful, coordinated movement of the body requires the integrated functioning of the musculoskeletal and nervous systems. The following is a review of the physiology of movement.

Skeletal System

The framework of bones and cartilage that protects our organs and allows us to move is called the *skeletal system.* Functions of this system include the following:

- It supports the soft tissues of the body (maintains body form and posture).
- It protects the delicate structures of the body (brain, lung, heart, spinal cord).
- It furnishes surfaces for the attachments of muscles, tendons, and ligaments, which in turn pull on the individual bones and produce movement.
- It serves as storage areas for mineral salts and fat.
- It produces blood cells (hematopoiesis).

The 206 bones in the human body are classified on the basis of their shape. *Long bones,* which are found in the upper and lower extremities, contribute to height and length. *Short bones,* located in the wrist and ankle, contribute to movement. *Flat bones* are relatively thin (eg, ribs and several of the skull bones) and contribute to shape (structural contour). *Irregular bones* are all those bones not included in the preceding classifications (eg, bones of the spinal column and jaw).

Because bones are too rigid to bend without damage, all movements that change the positions of the bony parts of the body occur at joints. The terms *articulation* and *joint* refer to the area where bones come into close contact with one another. Joints are classified according to the amount of movement they permit. Of concern are the freely movable joints called *diarthroses* or *synovial joints*, in which there is a space between the articulating bones. Movements possible at diarthric joints include abduction, adduction, flexion, extension, and rotation. Special movements of the forearm, ankle, and clavicle include supination, pronation, inversion, and eversion. These movements are defined in Table 39-1 and illustrated in Figure 39-1. Types of freely movable joints include the following:

Ball-and-socket joint: Rounded head of one bone fits into a cuplike cavity in the other; flexion–extension, abduction–adduction, and rotation are permitted (eg, shoulder and hip joints).

Condyloid joint: Oval head of one bone fits into a shallow cavity of another bone; flexion–extension and abduction–adduction are permitted (eg, wrist joint).

Gliding joint: Articular surfaces are flat; flexion–extension and abduction–adduction are permitted (eg, carpal bones of wrist and tarsal bones of feet).

Hinge joint: Spool-like surface fits into a concave surface; only flexion–extension is permitted (eg, elbow, knee, and ankle joints).

Pivot joint: Ringlike structure that turns on a pivot; movement is limited to rotation, for example, turning a doorknob (eg, joints between the atlas and axis and between the proximal ends of the radius and the ulna).

Saddle joint: Bone surfaces are convex on one side and concave on the other; movements are side to side and back and forth (eg, joint between the trapezium and metacarpal of the thumb).

The strength and flexibility of the skeletal system also depend on ligaments, tendons, and cartilage. *Ligaments* are tough, fibrous bands that bind joints together and connect bones and cartilage. *Tendons* are strong, flexible, inelastic fibrous bands that attach muscle to bone. *Cartilage* is nonvascular connective tissue found in the joints as well as in the nose, ear, thorax, trachea, and larynx.

Table 39-1
Terms Commonly Used to Describe Body Positions and Movements

Term	Definition and Example
Abduction	Lateral movement of a body part away from the midline of the body. *Example:* A person's arm is abducted when it is moved away from the body.
Adduction	Lateral movement of a body part toward the midline of the body. *Example:* A person's arm is adducted when it is moved from an outstretched position to a position alongside the body.
Circumduction	Movement of the distal part of the limb to trace a complete circle while the proximal end of the bone remains fixed. *Example:* The leg is outstretched and moved in a circle.
Flexion	The state of being bent. *Example:* A person's cervical spine is flexed when the head is bent forward chin to chest.
Extension	The state of being in a straight line. *Example:* A person's cervical spine is extended when the head is held straight on the spinal column.
Hyperextension	The state of exaggerated extension. It often results in an angle greater than 180 degrees. *Example:* A person's cervical spine is hyperextended when looking overhead, toward the ceiling.
Dorsiflexion	Backward bending of the hand or foot. *Example:* A person's foot is in dorsiflexion when the toes are brought up as though to point them at the knee.
Plantar flexion	Flexion of the foot. *Example:* A person's foot is in plantar flexion in the footdrop position.
Rotation	Turning on an axis; the turning of a body part on the axis provided by its joint. *Example:* A thumb is rotated when it is moved to make a circle.
Internal rotation	A body part turning on its axis toward the midline of the body. *Example:* A leg is rotated internally when it turns inward at the hip and the toes point toward the midline of the body.
External rotation	A body part turning on its axis away from the midline of the body. *Example:* A leg is rotated externally when it turns outward at the hip and the toes point away from the midline of the body.
Special Movements	
Pronation	The assumption of the prone position. *Examples:* A person is in the prone position when lying on the abdomen; a person's palm is prone when the forearm is turned so that the palm faces downward.
Supination	The assumption of the supine position. *Examples:* A person is in the supine position when lying on the back; a person's palm is supine when the forearm is turned so that the palm faces upward.
Inversion	Movement of the sole of the foot inward (occurs at the ankle)
Eversion	Movement of the sole of the foot outward (occurs at the ankle)

Neck

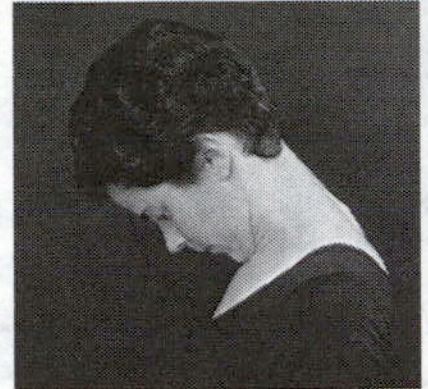
Flexion

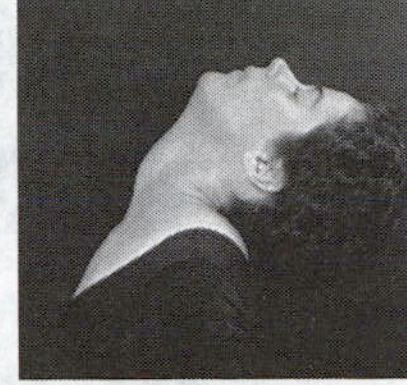
Hyperextension

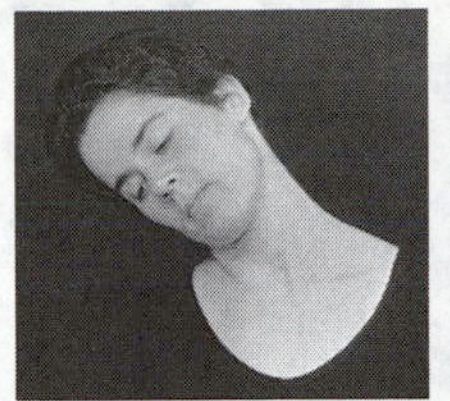
Lateral flexion

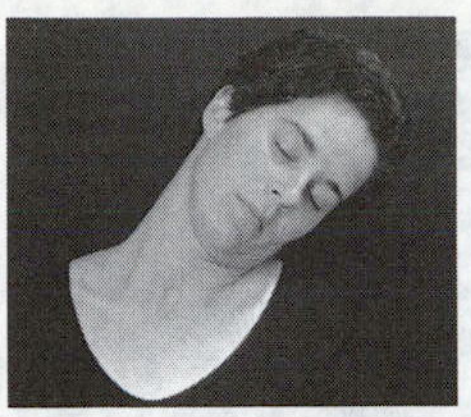

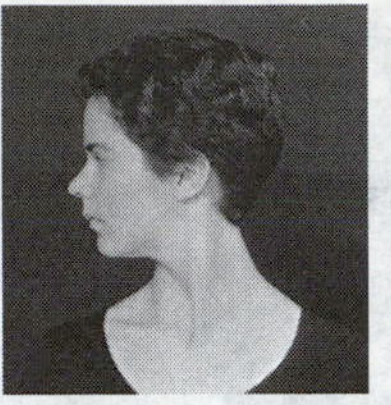
Rotation

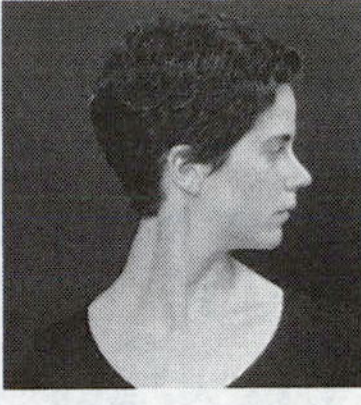

Shoulder

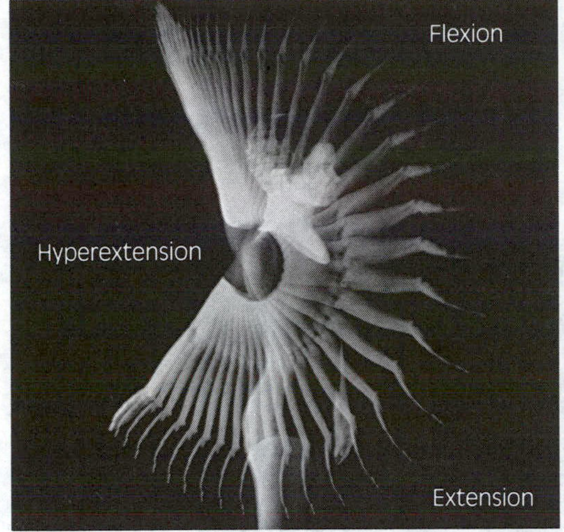

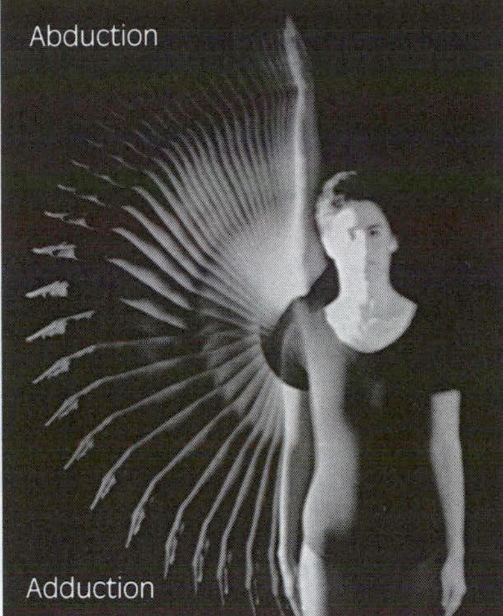

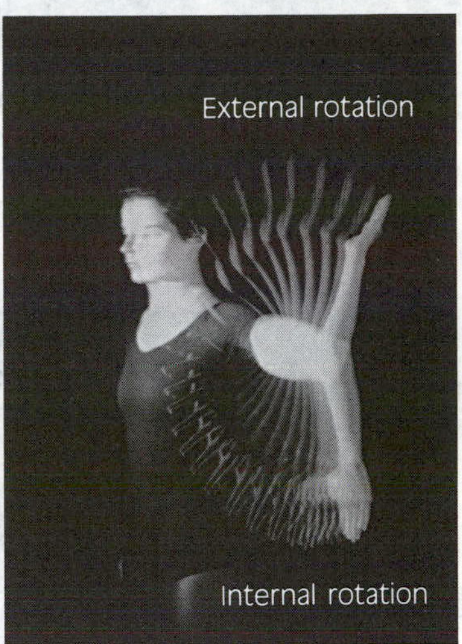

Elbow

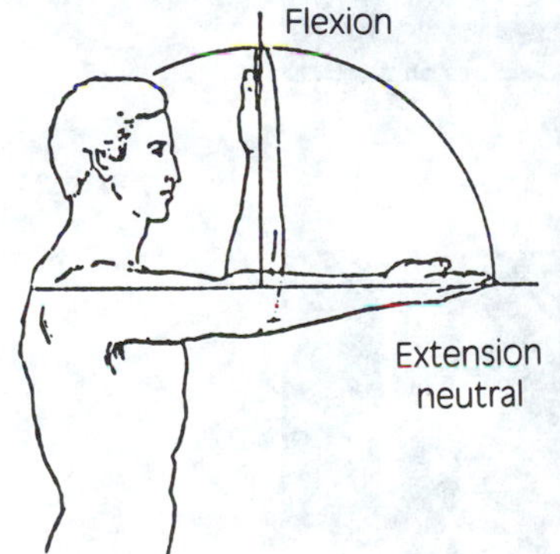

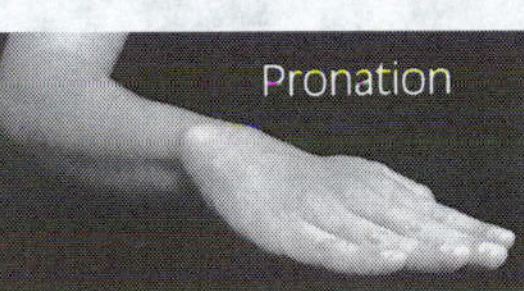

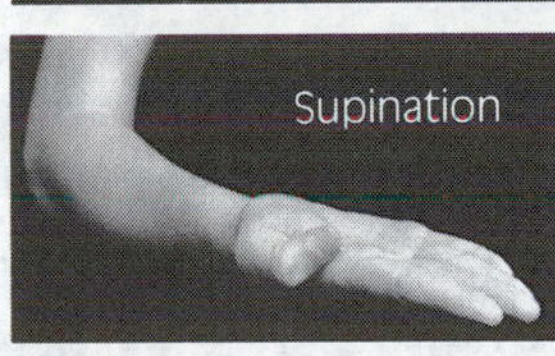

Wrist

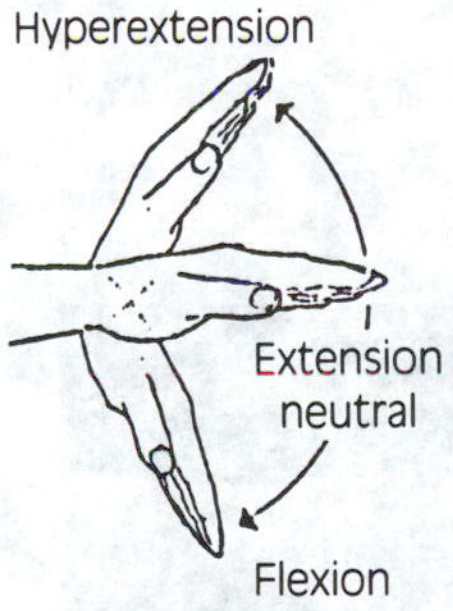

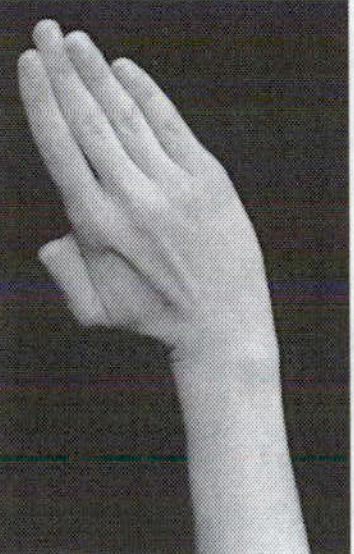
Radial deviation

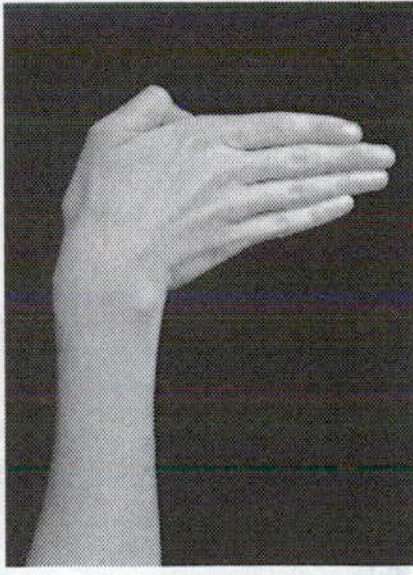
Ulnar deviation

Fingers

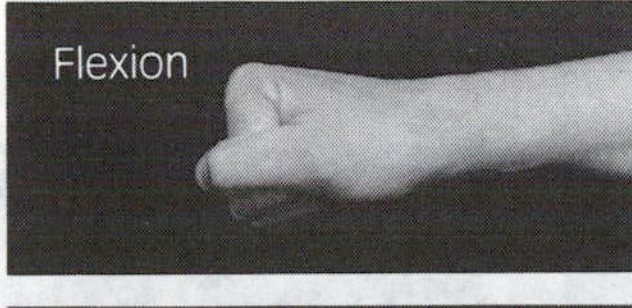

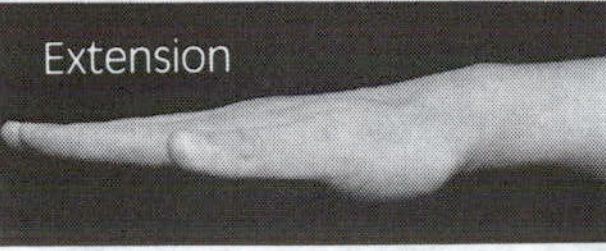

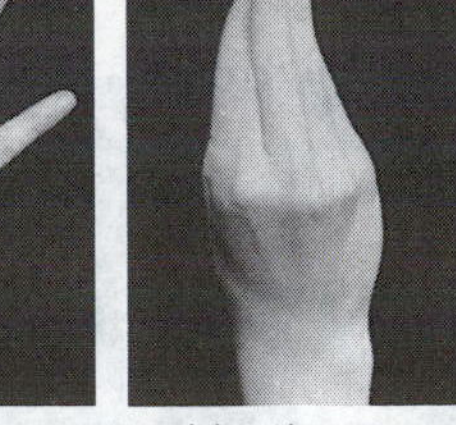
Abduction

Adduction

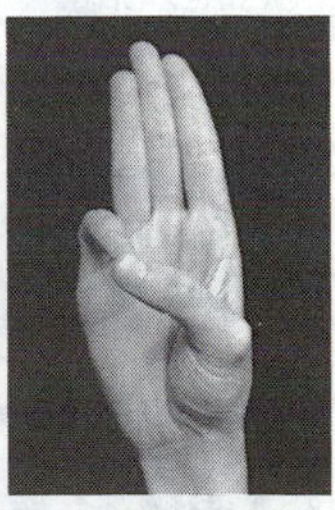
Apposition of thumb to finger

Figure 39-1
Normal range of motion of selected joints.

Hip

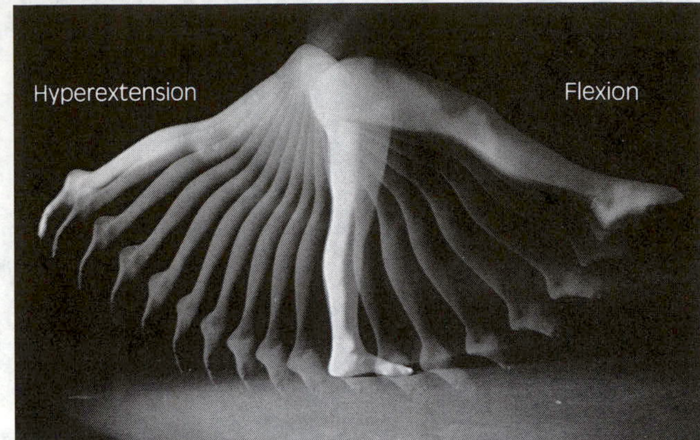

Extension

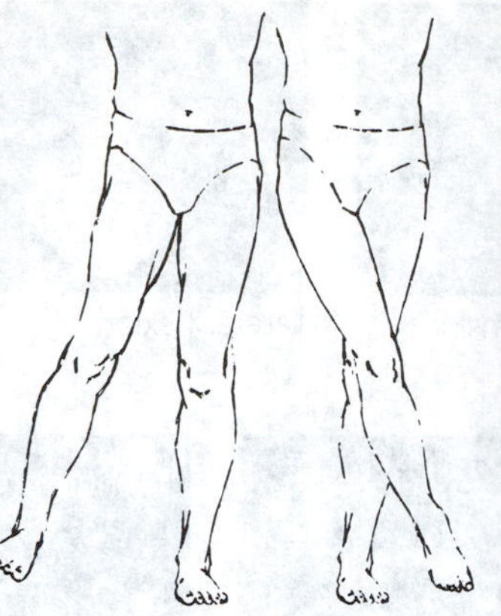

Abduction Adduction

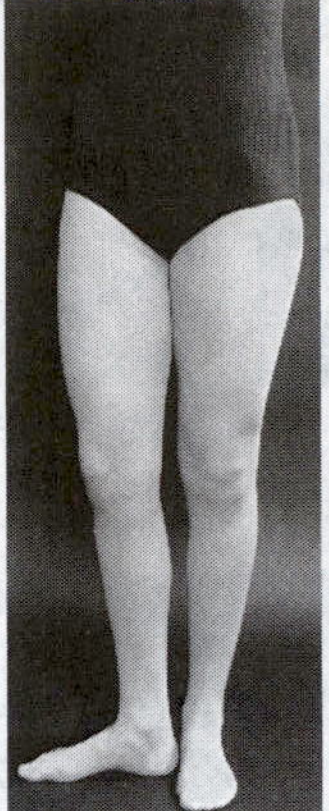

External rotation

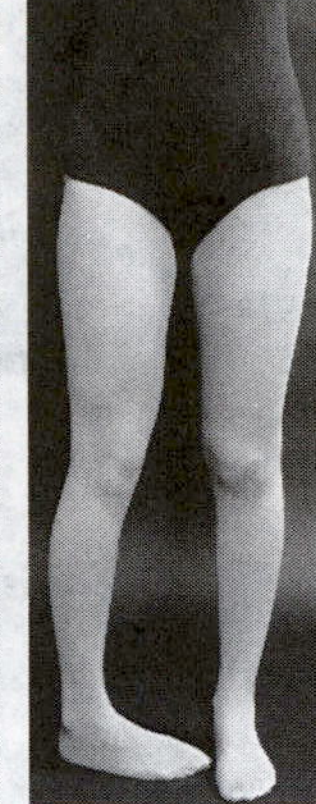

Internal rotation

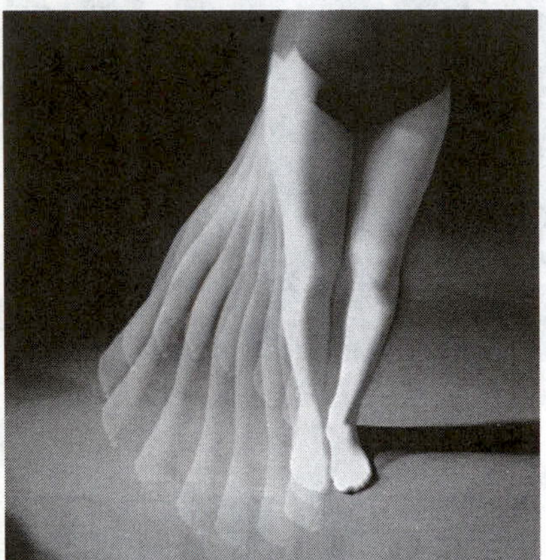

Rotation

Knee

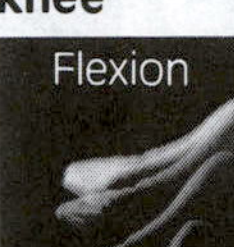

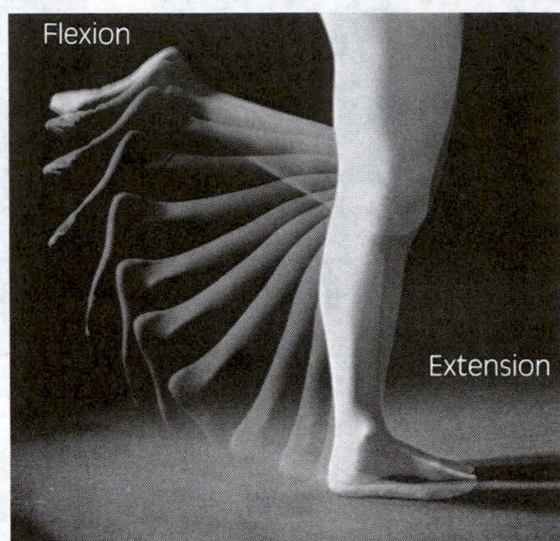

Ankle

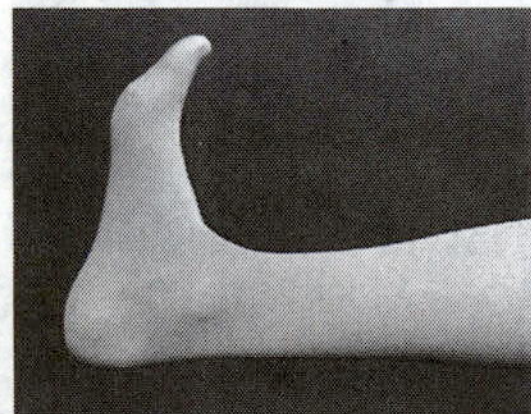

Dorsiflexion

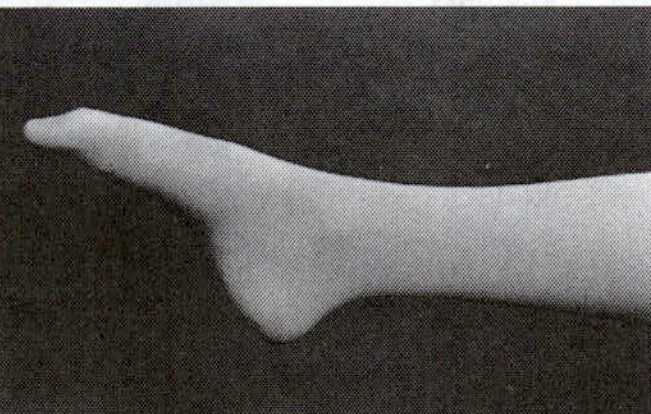

Plantar flexion

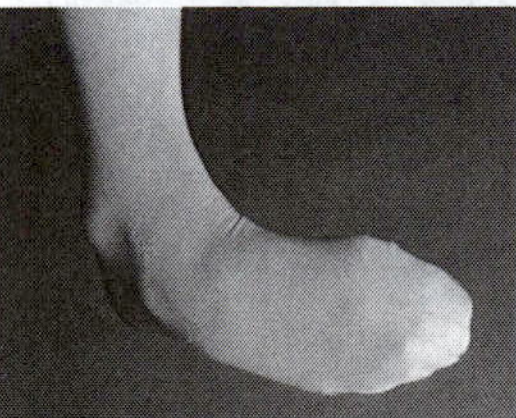

Inversion

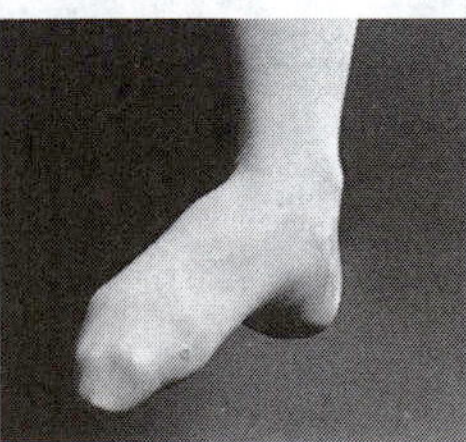

Eversion

Toes

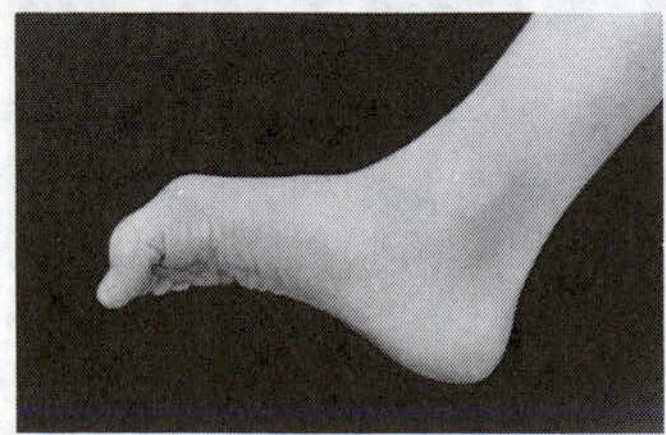

Flexion

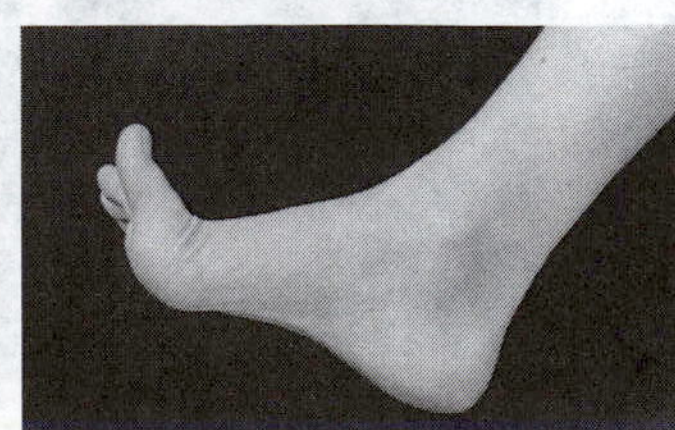

Extension

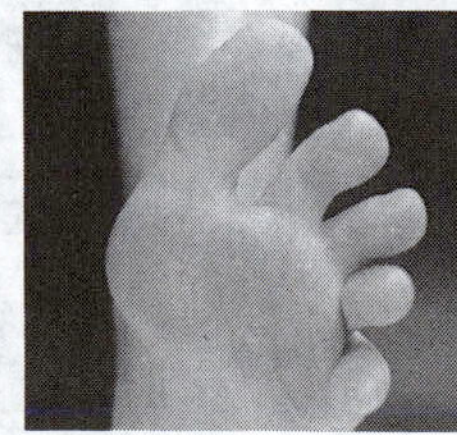

Abduction

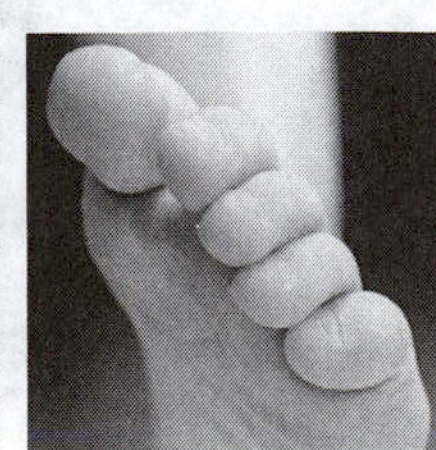

Adduction

Figure 39-1 ***(continued)***

Muscular System

Bones and joints provide form to the body and serve as the levers and fulcrums that make body movement possible. It is the contraction and relaxation of skeletal muscles, however, that actually produce movement by pulling on bones. The excitability, contractility, extensibility, and elasticity of muscles enable them to perform three important functions for the body through contraction:

- Motion
- Maintenance of posture (skeletal muscle contractions hold the body in stationary positions)
- Heat production (skeletal muscle contractions produce heat and help maintain body temperature)

There are actually three types of muscles: (1) skeletal, (2) cardiac, and (3) smooth or visceral. The skeletal muscle system includes the skeletal muscle tissue and connective tissue that compose individual muscle organs, such as the biceps. Movement is the result of a skeletal muscle contracting and exerting force on a tendon, which in turn pulls on a bone. Muscles have two differing points of attachment: (1) attachment of a muscle to the more stationary bone is called the *point of origin* and (2) attachment to the more movable bone is the *point of insertion*. Between these two points is the fleshy "belly" of the muscle. Figure 39-2 illustrates the relationship of skeletal muscles to bones and the use of bones as levers and joints as fulcrums to produce body movement.

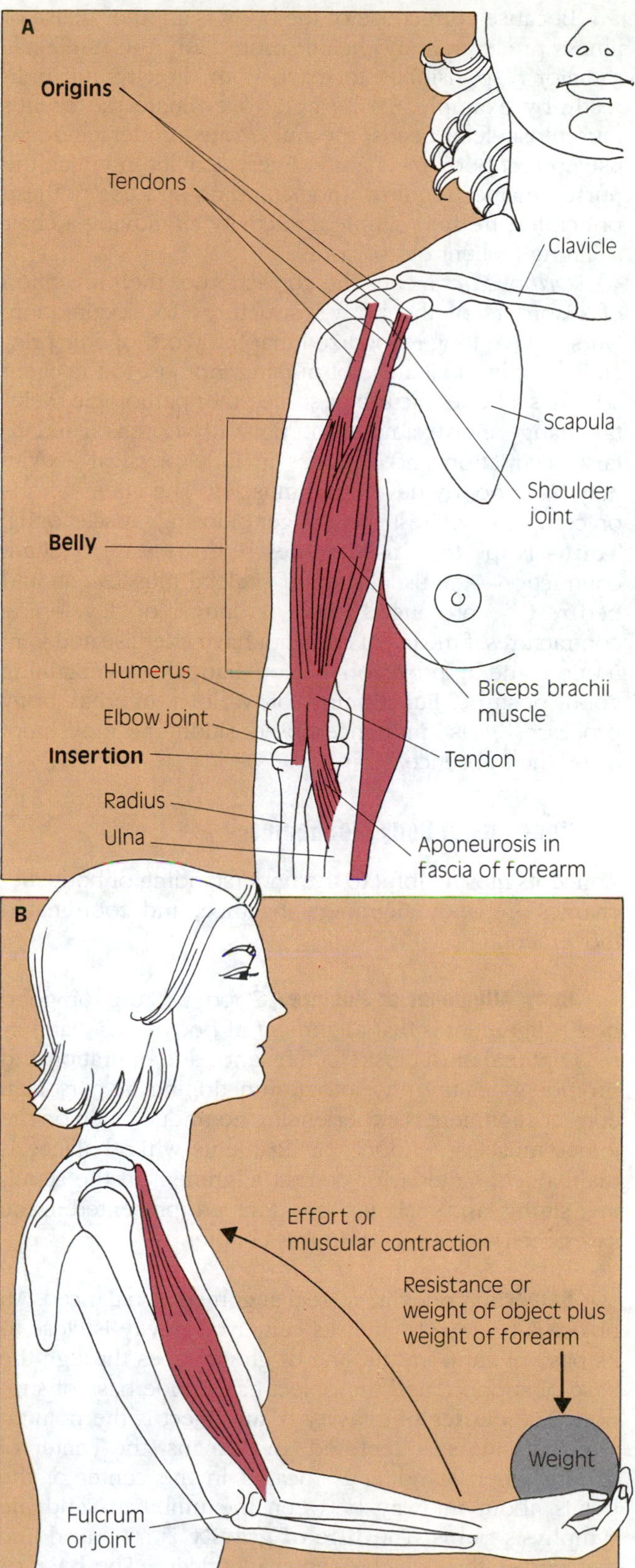

Figure 39-2
Relationship of skeletal muscles to bones. (*Top*) Skeletal muscles produce movements by pulling on bones. (*Bottom*) Bones serve as levers, and joints act as fulcrums for the levers. The lever and fulcrum principle is illustrated by the movement of the forearm lifting a weight.

Nervous System

The skeletal and muscular systems cannot produce purposeful movement without a functioning nervous system. It is a nerve impulse that stimulates muscles to contract. More specifically:

- The afferent nervous system conveys information from receptors in the periphery of the body to the central nervous system (eg, light pressure on nose).
- Nerve cells called *neurons* are responsible for conducting impulses from one part of the body to another.
- This information is processed by the central nervous system (CNS) and a response is decided on (eg, "There is a fly on my nose. I want to brush it off.").
- The efferent system conveys the desired response from the CNS to skeletal muscles by way of the somatic nervous system (eg, muscles in the arm, wrist, and hand contract and the fingers brush the fly from the face).

Body Mechanics

Body mechanics is the efficient use of the body as a machine and as a means of locomotion. Body mechanics is directly related to the effective functioning of the body. The correct use of body mechanics should be evident in every activity and even during rest periods.

Because correct use of the body is another phase of illness prevention and health promotion, the nurse has a major responsibility to teach both directly and indirectly by example. To be able to evaluate the client's musculoskeletal needs, the nurse must understand and use correct body mechanics. Every activity in which the nurse engages requires understanding and use of these principles, from as simple an activity as moving a chair to lifting a client out of bed.

Orthopedics means the correction or the prevention of disorders of the body's structures for locomotion. Nurses have long recognized that basic orthopedic principles apply to all areas of nursing, not just to the client who has a bone fracture or some other pathologic skeletal change. For example, the person who has a sedentary occupation and engages in little physical activity may have poorly developed muscles. The client who is on complete bed rest is in danger of losing muscle tonus. **Tonus** is the term used to describe the state of slight contraction—the usual state of skeletal muscles. Should bed rest be prolonged, there is danger of developing contractures if the client does not have exercise and joint motion and if provision is not made for maintaining good posture. Functioning of various internal body processes is also influenced by position and movement or by their absence.

Concepts of Body Mechanics

Concepts most helpful to the understanding of body mechanics are body alignment, balance, and coordinated movement.

Body Alignment or Posture. Good posture or good body alignment is that alignment of body parts that permits optimal musculoskeletal balance and operation and promotes healthy physiologic functioning. A person in correct alignment is experiencing no undue strain on the joints, muscles, tendons, or ligaments while balance is maintained. Criteria for correct alignment in the standing, sitting, and reclining positions are presented in the assessment section later in this chapter.

Balance. A body in correct alignment is balanced. An object is balanced when its center of gravity is close to its base of support, the line of gravity goes through the base of support, and the object has a wide base of support. The **center of gravity** of an object is the point at which its mass is centered. In humans, the center of gravity when standing is located in the center of the pelvis about midway between the umbilicus and the symphysis pubis. The **line of gravity** is a vertical line that passes through the center of gravity. The **base of support** is the foundation that provides for an object's stability. The wider the base of support and the lower the center of gravity, the greater the stability of the object. Figure 39-3 illustrates body balance.

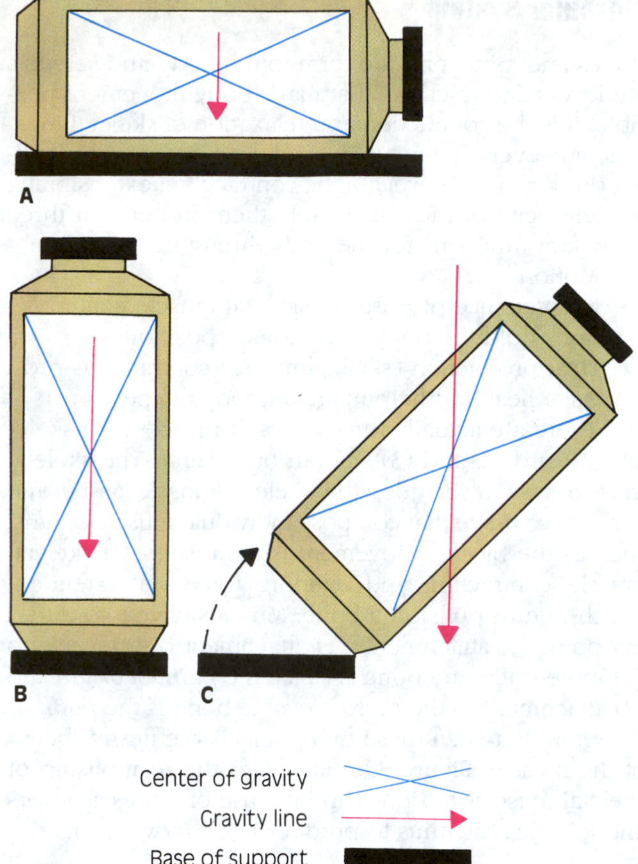

Figure 39-3
The effect of the base of support and gravity on balance is shown. (**A**) The line of gravity passes through the wide base of support. This object is the most stable of the three. (**B**) The line of gravity also passes through the base support, although the base is narrower. This object is less stable than the one above it. (**C**) The line of gravity does not pass through the base of support. This object is unstable.

Nurses can increase body balance when working by spreading their feet farther apart (broadening the base of support) and by flexing their hips and knees (lowering the center of gravity). These two simple maneuvers are important principles in body mechanics by which nurses can decrease musculoskeletal strain.

Coordinated Body Movement. Because the nurse providing direct client care must frequently use the body to assist in positioning, turning, and lifting both clients and equipment, it is important to do this knowledgeably to avoid musculoskeletal strain and injury. This work is facilitated when the nurse uses major muscle groups rather than weaker ones and takes advantage of the body's natural levers and fulcrums. For example, rather than attempt to push a client to the opposite side of the bed, the nurse flexes the knees, positions the forearms above and below the client's buttocks (preferably under a pull sheet), and rocks backward, sliding the client toward self. This one coordinated movement illustrates the following principles:

- The nurse is using major muscle groups—flexors, extensors, and abductors of the thighs; flexors and extensors of the knees; flexors and extensors of the upper and lower arms—rather than weaker ones.
- Use of the arm bones as levers and the elbows as fulcrums facilitates lifting a weight against resistance (force of gravity)—the lever and fulcrum principle.
- Using a pull sheet and smooth, dry, firm bed foundation decreases the effects of friction, which increases the amount of effort required to move an object. Rough, wet, or soiled surfaces contribute to friction's effect.
- By positioning the arms under the client's center of gravity (hips) and sliding the body back toward himself or herself, the nurse is working close to the object to be moved and decreasing the effort involved.

Postural Reflexes. Integrated functioning of the musculoskeletal and nervous systems is essential for body alignment and balance. Postural tonus, the sustained contraction of select skeletal muscles that keeps the human body in an upright position against the force of gravity, depends on the functioning of several postural reflexes:

Labyrinthine sense: This is provided by the sensory organs in the inner ear, which are stimulated by body movement (changes in head position) and transmit these impulses to the cerebellum.

Proprioceptor or kinesthetic sense: This informs the brain of the location of a limb or body part as a result of joint movements stimulating special nerve endings in muscles, tendons, and fascia.

Visual or optic reflexes: Visual impressions contribute to posture by alerting the person to spatial relationships with the environment (nearness of ceilings, walls, furniture, condition of floor, and so on).

Extensor or stretch reflexes: Conceivably, the force of gravity could exert enough force to flex the body at the hip and knees; when extensor muscles are stretched beyond a certain point (eg, when knees buckle under), their stimulation causes a reflex contraction that reestablishes erect posture.

Body Mechanics Used for Work

The following guidelines are offered for the use of body mechanics when the person is at work:

- Develop a habit of erect posture (correct alignment) and, whenever necessary, begin activities by broadening the base of support and lowering the center of gravity.
- Use the longest and the strongest muscles of the arms and the legs to help provide the power needed in strenuous activities. The muscles of the back are less strong and are easily injured when used improperly.
- Use the internal girdle and a long midriff to stabilize the pelvis and to protect the abdominal viscera when stooping, reaching, lifting, or pulling. The internal girdle is made by contracting the gluteal muscles in the buttocks downward and the abdominal muscles upward. It is helped further by making a long midriff. This is done by stretching the muscles in the waist. Figure 39-4 illustrates the internal girdle.
- Work as closely as possible to an object that is to be lifted or moved. This brings the body's center of gravity close to that of the object being moved, thereby permitting most of the burden to be borne by the leg and arm muscles. Figure 39-5 illustrates a proper and an improper way to pick up an object.
- Use the weight of the body as a force for pulling or pushing, by rocking on the feet or leaning forward or backward. This reduces the amount of strain placed on the arms and the back.
- Slide, roll, push, or pull an object rather than lift it to reduce the energy needed to lift the weight against the pull of gravity.
- Use the weight of the body to push an object by falling or rocking forward, and to pull an object by falling or rocking backward. Sliding a client in bed while rocking backward is illustrated in Figure 39-6.

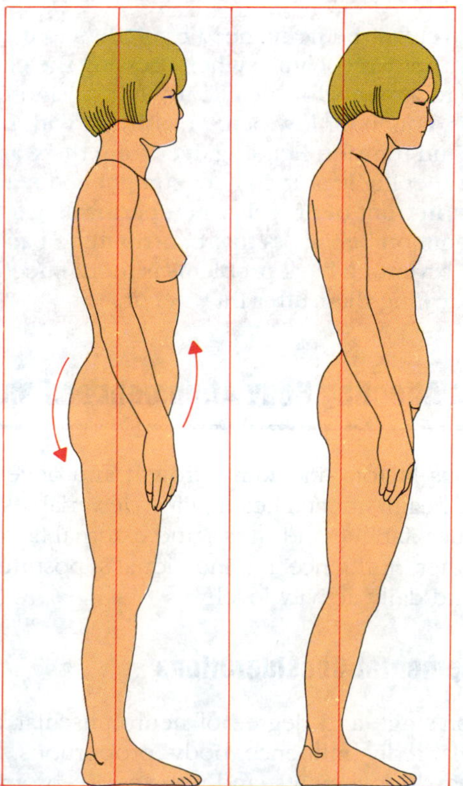

Figure 39-4
(*Left*) Internal girdle "on." Abdominal muscles contracted, giving a feeling of upward pull, and gluteal muscles contracted, giving a downward pull. (*Right*) Slouch position, showing abdominal muscles relaxed and body out of good alignment.

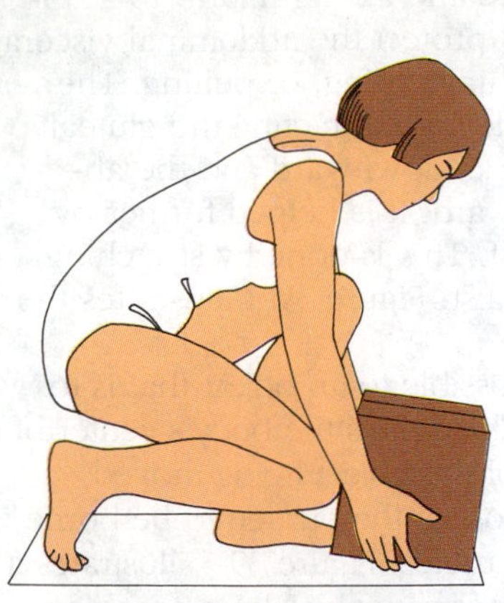

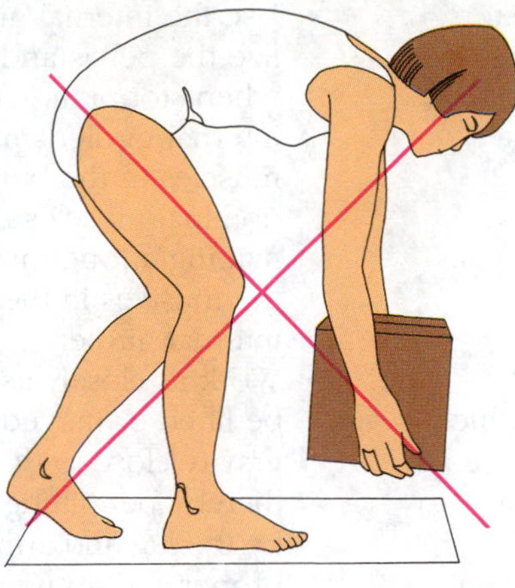

Figure 39-5
(*Left*) A good position for lifting is illustrated. This person is using the long and strong muscles of the arms and legs and holding the object so that the line of gravity falls within the base of support. (*Right*) This is an incorrect position for lifting because pull is exerted on the back muscles and leaning causes the line of gravity to fall outside the base.

- Place the feet apart to provide a wider base of support when increased stability of the body is necessary.
- Flex the knees, put on the internal girdle, and come down close to an object that is to be lifted.

The nurse can demonstrate to others the proper way of using the musculoskeletal system if good habits are consciously developed in the use of the musculoskeletal system.

Home Healthcare Alert

Caregivers in the home need reminders to use proper body mechanics when dressing the client; doing treatments for the client while positioned on a chair, couch, or low bed; or assisting with movement and transfer. Bending over from the waist while keeping legs and knees straight and reaching far out in front of oneself when performing a task are common behaviors that contribute to back injury. Preventing back problems is more effective than treating them after they occur.

Factors Affecting Body Alignment and Mobility

Numerous factors, including growth and development, physical health, mental health, lifestyle variables, attitude and values, fatigue and stress, and external factors, such as weather, influence an individual's posture, movement, and daily activity level.

Developmental Considerations

A person's age and degree of neuromuscular development markedly influence body proportions, posture, body mass, movements, and reflexes. To promote neuromuscular development in clients of all ages and to facilitate each client's use of the body to perform self-care actions, the nurse needs to be familiar with developmental variations in body proportions and neuromuscular development. These variations are presented in Table 39-2 with related nursing assessment priorities and nursing interventions.

Physical Health

Problems in the musculoskeletal or nervous systems can have a negative influence on body alignment and movement. Similarly, illness or trauma involving other body systems may also interfere with movement either because of the underlying pathology or the treatment regimen. Nurses need to develop sensitivity to how both acute and chronic health problems affect a client's general appearance (posture, body proportions, and movements) and to develop an ability to move purposefully to perform the activities of daily living. When assessing a client's response to a mobility deficit, the nurse:

- Reinforces behaviors that promote healthy functioning (eg, congratulates a client who manages transfers well despite left-sided weakness or paralysis)
- Corrects behaviors that compound the mobility deficit over time (eg, client with arthritis who severely restricts movement because of joint stiffness and tenderness learns successful adaptive strategies that can be shared with other clients and families; or energy conservation measures used by clients with emphysema who have greatly decreased activity tolerance)

Musculoskeletal Problems

Congenital or Acquired Postural Abnormalities. The newborn with congenital hip dysplasia or a clubfoot; the teenager with scoliosis (lateral curvature of the spine); and the older person with kyphosis (increased convexity in the curvature of the thoracic spine) are all experiencing postural abnormalities that affect appearance and mobility. Nursing responsibilities may include the following:

- Early detection and referral of these problems
- Exploration and selection of client education, counseling, and support as treatment options
- Careful attention to positioning, transfers, and exercise

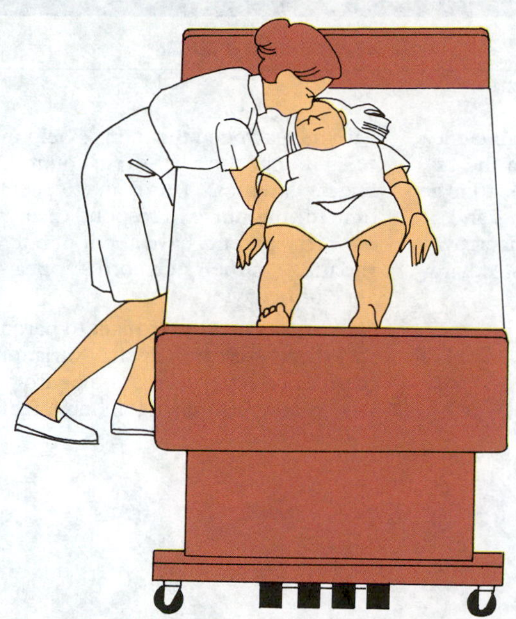

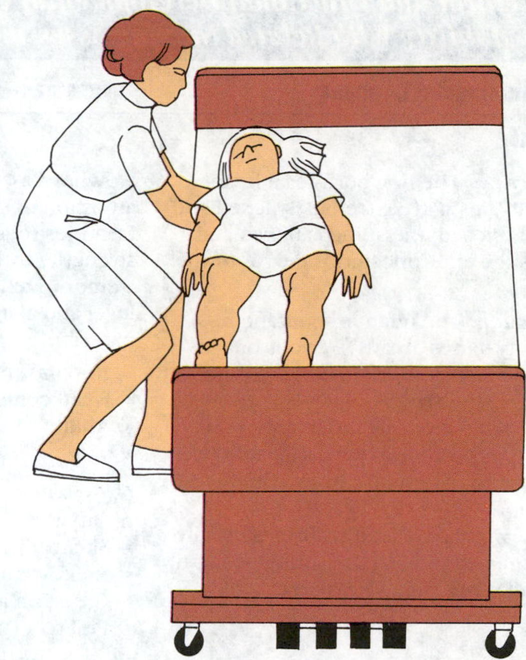

Figure 39-6
Before sliding a client to the edge of the bed, establish a wide base of support with one knee near the edge of the bed and both knees flexed. Place arms under the client as far as possible while close to and leaning over the client. Rock backward, using your own body weight to assist in moving the client toward you.

- Education of the client and family regarding safe self-care activities

Problems With Bone Formation or Muscle Development. Problems with bone formation may include any of the following:

- *Congenital*, such as achondroplasia, in which premature bone ossification leads to dwarfism, or osteogenesis imperfecta, which is characterized by excessively brittle bones and multiple fractures both at birth and later in life
- *Dietary related*, for example, vitamin D deficiency, which results in deformities of the growing skeleton (rickets)
- *Disease related*, such as in Paget disease, in which excessive bone destruction and abnormal regeneration result in skeletal pain, deformities, and pathologic fractures
- *Age related*, such as **osteoporosis**, in which bone destruction exceeds bone formation; the resultant thin, porous bones fracture easily

The muscular dystrophies are a group of genetically transmitted disorders that have in common progressive degeneration and weakness of skeletal muscles. They vary in terms of the muscle groups involved and their clinical course. Myasthenia gravis is a weakness of the skeletal muscles caused by an abnormality at the neuromuscular junction that prevents muscle fibers from contracting.

Nursing responsibilities with problems of bone formation and muscle development and functioning include the following:

- Careful collaboration with the physician and healthcare team to determine the motor capacities of the individual
- Client and family education aimed at developing optional mobility

The nurse must be knowledgeable about the underlying disease process and be able to position, lift, transfer, and exercise the client safely, with attention to client comfort.

Problems Affecting Joint Mobility. Inflammation, degeneration, and trauma can all interfere with joint mobility. The term *arthritis* describes more than 20 diseases, all characterized by inflammation in one or more joints and possibly pain and stiffness in adjacent body parts. *Degenerative joint disease*, also termed *osteoarthritis*, is a noninflammatory, progressive disorder of movable joints, particularly weight-bearing joints, characterized by the deterioration of articular cartilage and pain with motion. Spurs form, which restrict joint movement. Trauma to a joint may result in either a *sprain*, in which the wrenching or twisting of a joint results in a partial tear or rupture to its attachments, or a *dislocation*, that is, the displacement of a bone from a joint with tearing of ligaments, tendons, and capsules. Any condition restricting joint mobility has potentially crippling effects.

(text continues on page 1010)

Table 39-2
Structural and Functional Developmental Changes in Body Alignment and Mobility With Related Nursing Assessment and Intervention Priorities

Developmental Changes	Assessment Priorities	Nursing Interventions
Infant		
Structure: The newborn term infant usually lies with extremities flexed and hands closed; the spine is flexed and lacks the anteroposterior curves of the adult. *Function:* The infant's spontaneous activity varies greatly. Periods of activity and alertness alternate with quiet periods and sleep. • By age 3 months, the infant in the prone position is generally able to raise the chest and head from the floor. • By 5 months, head control is usually achieved in both the sitting position and when being held erect.	Newborn assessments should include attention to structure of spine and extremities (deformities); muscle tone and strength (abnormal movements and tremors); reflex responses; and activity level and alertness (jitteriness, lethargy, paresis). *3- to 6-month assessment* • Head control • Ability to sit *6- to 9-month assessment* *Gross motor* Ability to: • Sit steadily • Roll over adeptly • Creep on all fours • Pull to a standing position *Fine motor* • Improved hand–eye coordination *9- to 12-month assessment* *Gross motor* • Progress toward unassisted walking *Fine motor* • Skill in using hands—ability to pick up even tiny objects	Parents may need the nurse's help in "examining" their baby (eg, counting fingers and toes). This is an excellent time for the nurse to respond to any concerns parents have about minor variations in their newborn's appearance or behavior. Nurses may need to explain to parents that there is great individual variation in total activity patterns and neuromuscular development among infants and children.
Toddler		
Structure: The young toddler's long trunk, short legs, and undeveloped abdominal musculature (potbelly) give the toddler a top-heavy, sway-backed appearance. Growth during this period is rapid and faster in the legs than in the trunk. The young toddler walks on a broad base with flat feet that tend to toe in or out. Balance is achieved slowly. *Function:* Both gross and fine motor development continue rapidly. By 15 months, most toddlers can walk unassisted; they are running at age 18 months and jumping by 2 years. By age 3 years, most toddlers can stack blocks, string large beads, work simple puzzles, and dress themselves.	Assess progress in walking, running, and jumping. Assess small muscle coordination as evidenced in everyday skills: ability to dress themselves, wash hands, brush teeth. Distinguish slow developers who fall within normal ranges from those whose developmental lags may indicate deprivation of environmental stimulation or retardation.	Because individual differences in motor activity, balance, and grace become evident during this period, help parents to learn and accept their child's uniqueness. Teach parents the importance of providing a safe environment in which the toddler is free to explore, to satisfy curiosity, and to develop skill in motor control; that reinforcement, enthusiasm, and praise for progress stimulate the toddler's mastery of new skills; and that limits need to be set so the toddler does not overextend himself or herself in his or her newfound drive for mastery. The sense of mastery achieved through safe exploration and the practice of motor skills lays the foundation for all later physical, social, and intellectual pursuits.
Child		
Structure: Between ages 3 and 6 years, the child's arms and legs continue to grow rapidly relative to the trunk and the child develops better balance. By age 6 years, the child has replaced "baby fat" with muscle, developed increased tone in abdominal muscles (loss of potbelly), and developed a more prominent chest.	Use developmental charts to assess gross and fine motor development.	Because important attitudes about the body and exercise are developed during childhood, parents should be questioned about these during the nursing history. Teach or counsel as appropriate.

(continued)

Table 39-2 *(continued)*
Structural and Functional Developmental Changes in Body Alignment and Mobility With Related Nursing Assessment and Intervention Priorities

Developmental Changes	Assessment Priorities	Nursing Interventions
Child		
Function: Muscles, bones, and the nervous system are developing a harmony that allows greater gross and fine motor control. • By age 4 years, most children can negotiate stairs without using a hand rail, walk backward, and hop on one foot. • By age 5 years, most children have learned to skip, to play in running games, to jump rope, and to jump off heights of several steps. • Progress in fine motor development is reflected in the child's manipulation of writing materials. • By the time children enter school they have acquired all the basic mechanisms for physical locomotion they will use later in life.		
Adolescent		
Structure: There is considerable increase and change of the musculoskeletal system, resulting in increased size as well as the appearance of secondary sex characteristics. The adolescent growth spurt gives the adolescent an awkward, gangling appearance, and there is an increase in muscle mass and a decrease in fat, especially in boys. *Function:* For the physically fit adolescent this can be a time of boundless energy and great athletic performance. Lifestyle factors (inactivity, poor nutrition) may begin a lifelong unhealthy pattern of immobility and disuse.	Interview the client to determine current activity level and type of regular exercise. Evaluate safety of recreational choices. Note history of any musculoskeletal or neurologic problems. During the physical assessment, note posture and alignment. Screening for scoliosis (lateral curvature of the spine) should be made before the adolescent's peak growth velocity and a referral made when there is more than a 15-degree curvature of the spine. Examine muscle mass, tone, and strength and joint mobility.	Adolescents have many questions about their changing bodies and will often value nursing input, although they seldom seek professional advice. Lifestyle counseling regarding the importance of exercise and fitness is critical. Adolescents may need encouragement to exercise regularly or help in gauging their physical limits and a caution not to "push too hard."
Adult		
Structure: The healthy adult stands and sits erect and is capable of balanced and coordinated purposeful movement. During pregnancy, the developing fetus shifts the mother's center of gravity forward and she compensates by leaning backward and walking with a broader base of support. *Function:* Activity levels vary greatly among adults and are influenced by numerous factors explained in this chapter.	Assess the balance between activity and rest in the client's lifestyle and note any lifestyle factors or illnesses that interfere with the client's mobility or ability to carry out activities of daily living.	For most adults, the most important nursing intervention is fitness counseling, which includes clarifying misconceptions about exercise and designing and monitoring safe exercise programs. Clients with mobility alterations require special care.
Older Adult		
Structure: There is increased convexity in the thoracic spine (kyphosis) from disc shrinkage and decreased height, flexed posture, loss of muscle tone, and increased prominence of bony structure because of subcutaneous fat loss. Arthritic joint changes are often present. *Function:* General slowness of movement with progressive decrease in activity tolerance.	Assess general ease of movement and gait; alignment; joint structure and function; and muscle mass, tone, and strength.	Teach and counsel clients about: • Importance of regular exercise • Need to maintain appropriate weight to reduce stress on joints • Need for high protein, calcium, and vitamin D–enriched diet • To pace activities to compensate for decreased strength • To use assistive devices safely when needed • To safety-proof homes to reduce likelihood of falls

The nurse caring for clients with joint problems works collaboratively with the physician and physical therapist to maintain joint mobility. Client education is directed to the client's mastery of an exercise and care program, which fosters tissue repair and maximal independence in activities of daily living.

Problems Affecting the Central Nervous System

A problem in any of the principal parts of the brain or spinal cord concerned with skeletal muscle control can affect mobility:

Cerebral motor cortex: Assumes the major role of controlling precise, discrete movements. A cerebrovascular accident (stroke) or head trauma may damage the motor cortex and produce temporary or permanent voluntary motor impairment.

Basal ganglia: Integrate semivoluntary movements such as walking, swimming, and laughing. In Parkinson's disease, there is progressive degeneration of the basal ganglia of the cerebrum. Unnecessary skeletal movements result in tremors and muscle rigidity, which interfere with voluntary movement.

Cerebellum: Assists the motor cortex and basal ganglia by making body movements smooth and coordinated. In multiple sclerosis, the myelin sheaths of neurons in the CNS deteriorate to hardened scars or plaques. Plaque formation in the cerebellum may produce lack of coordination of one hand.

Pyramidal pathways: Voluntary motor impulses are conveyed from the brain through the spinal cord by way of two major pathways: (1) the pyramidal pathway and (2) the extrapyramidal pathway. With trauma to the spinal cord, transection of these motor pathways results in complete bilateral loss of voluntary movement below the level of the trauma.

The overwhelming complaint of clients with injury to the CNS is that no one talks with them (or with their families) about how the disease will progress and affect their functioning. Nurses caring for these clients need knowledge about the pathology and clinical course of these diseases so that appropriate client education and counseling can occur.

Trauma to the Musculoskeletal System

Injury to the musculoskeletal system can result in fractures and soft tissue injuries. A *fracture* is a break in the continuity of the structure of bone or cartilage. It may result from a traumatic injury or occur as a result of some underlying disease process. Healing requires realignment of the bone fragment, immobilization, and restoration of the bone's function. Soft tissue injuries include sprains, strains, and dislocations. (Dislocations and sprains are discussed above under Problems Affecting Joint Mobility.) A *strain*, the least serious of these injuries, is a stretching of a muscle. Nurses need to be knowledgeable in first-aid measures for musculoskeletal trauma as well as in acute and rehabilitative care.

Problems Involving Other Body Systems

The pathology of numerous other acute and chronic illnesses may also affect mobility. Chronic obstructive lung disease and conditions such as ascites may alter posture. Any illnesses that interfere with oxygenation at the cellular level decrease the amount of oxygen available to the muscles for work and thus decrease activity tolerance. These illnesses include anemia, angina, cardiac dysrhythmias, congestive heart failure, and chronic obstructive pulmonary disease. Diseases characterized by negative nitrogen balance (eg, anorexia nervosa and certain cancers) result in muscle wasting and decreased physical energy for movement and work. Symptoms accompanying many illnesses such as fatigue, muscle aches, and pain may also immobilize clients. Bed rest is an important component of the treatment regimen for many diseases or trauma states such as myocardial infarction, surgery, and fractures. Although rest is integral to the healing process, immobility may cause its own problems (Table 39-3). Nurses need to be vigilant in determining the effect any injury or illness will have on mobility and in providing care that facilitates optimal mobility.

Mental Health

Just as an individual's physical health influences body appearance and movement, so also does mental health. Bodily processes tend to slow down in depression and there is a lack of visible energy and enthusiasm. The depressed person often sits with the head bowed and shoulders slumped and may lack the energy to feed or even to toilet. Even facial movement may be decreased to the point where the individual's face registers no emotion (termed a *flat affect*). On the other hand, high-energy individuals have erect posture and animated facial features.

Lifestyle Variables

Whether an individual opts for an active or sedentary lifestyle is influenced by many factors. Among the most important are an individual's occupation, leisure activity preferences, and cultural influences. Because most professional occupations as well as many blue-collar jobs are sedentary in nature, individuals wishing to exercise regularly need to plan leisure activities that give the body a workout. Cultural influences may encourage or discourage exercise. For example, currently in North America it is popular for both male and female professionals to engage in some form of aerobic exercise. In the not-so-distant past, it was considered unladylike for women to be involved in most sports activities. The nurse, particularly one involved in community health activities, needs to consider appropriate forms of exercise and geographic location before making recommendations to clients from diverse cultures. Commonly pre-

(text continues on page 1015)

Table 39-3
Problems of Immobility With Related Etiologies, Assessment Priorities, Expected Outcomes, and Nursing Interventions

Problems Related to Immobility	Etiologies	Assessment Priorities	Expected Outcomes	Nursing Interventions
Cardiovascular				

Activity Intolerance: Increased Cardiac Workload	Supine position contributes to greater volume of circulating blood, which must be pumped by the heart; decreased vascular resistance	• Assess apical and peripheral pulses.
		• Note increased heart rate; presence of third heart sound; weakened peripheral pulses.
		• Note the presence of edema (check sacrum, legs, feet).
			Client will maintain baseline vital signs.	• When possible, encourage the client to sit in the Fowler position; avoid lying supine for prolonged intervals.
				• Avoid any activities that increase intrathoracic pressure:
				  • Discourage straining while moving or defecating (Valsalva maneuver).
				  • Exhale through mouth while exercising.

Altered Tissue Perfusion; Thrombus Formation	Venous stasis secondary to a lack of muscular contraction in the legs Calcium leaving bones and entering blood increases its coagulability External pressure on the veins (eg, that exerted by the knee gatch of the hospital bed) (Note: poor positioning can result in partial or total occlusion of the blood vessels.)	• Assess for complaints of pain, especially calf pain; signs of warmth, redness, swelling, tenderness—compare one extremity to the other. • Daily calf or thigh circumference measurements may be indicated (mark spot to be measured).	Client will show signs of adequate venous return (absence of dependent edema, thrombi, emboli).	• Encourage active exercise of legs (range of motion and quadriceps settings) three or four times daily. • Elevate legs periodically. • Position clients carefully, following agency guidelines; avoid prolonged knee and hip flexion. • Apply antiembolism stockings if ordered. • Assess for signs of thrombosis. *Never* rub or massage the legs—especially if the client complains of pain.
Risk for Injury: Orthostatic Hypotension	Skeletal muscle weakness and decreased vessel tone (failure of arteriole vasoconstriction on assuming an erect position) Hypovolemia	• Assess for complaints of light-headedness, dizziness, seeing spots or fainting. • Compare blood pressure before position change with that taken immediately afterward.	Client will change from a lying to a sitting or standing position safely, without injury.	• If not contraindicated, have client sleep sitting up or in an elevated position. • Encourage client to change position gradually and with support if needed: supine to Fowler's to sitting at edge of bed to standing (each change may require 15 to 20 minutes of stabilization time); instruct client never to jump to his or her feet and begin walking.

(continued)

Table 39-3 *(continued)*
Problems of Immobility With Related Etiologies, Assessment Priorities, Expected Outcomes, and Nursing Interventions

Problems Related to Immobility	Etiologies	Assessment Priorities	Expected Outcomes	Nursing Interventions
Cardiovascular				
				• Use waist-high antiembolism stockings. • Encourage leg exercises. • Encourage client to increase time out of bed as condition allows; gradually increase the frequency and duration of ambulation. • Remind client to get out of a hot bath slowly. • Teach the client to avoid the Valsalva maneuver or any activity involving holding the breath. • Encourage client to use a rocking chair to improve lower extremity circulation.
Respiratory				
Ineffective Breathing Pattern	Limited chest expansion: Prolonged sitting or lying position Muscle disuse—atrophy Loss of muscle coordination Depressant pharmacologic agents: analgesics, sedatives, anesthetics	• Assess rate, rhythm, and quality of respirations; note a decrease in the depth and rate of respirations. • Assess the symmetry of chest wall movements.	Client will maintain baseline respiratory rate and depth. Client coughs and deep breathes every 1 to 2 hours.	• Adhere to every-2-hour position change schedule. • If the client is allowed out of bed, encourage deep breathing when the client stands and ambulates. • Teach the client to cough and deep breathe every 1 to 2 hours. • If abdominal binders or rib supports are in place, remove them every 2 hours and encourage deep breathing.
Ineffective Airway Clearance	Altered function of mucous membranes and cilia Decreased position changes Ineffective coughing secondary to weakness, incisional pain, depressant pharmacologic action Dehydration Stasis of secretions	• Auscultate the entire lung region and note regions of diminished breath sounds, rales, rhonchi, or wheezes. • Percuss the chest and note any dull area. • Assess sputum (color, texture, odor); culture and sensitivity test may be ordered.	Client's lungs will be clear to auscultation. Client will remain free of signs of respiratory tract infection (fever, productive cough, chest pain)	• See nursing interventions for Ineffective Breathing Pattern. • Keep client well hydrated. • Initiate chest physiotherapy. • Suction as needed.

(continued)

Table 39-3 *(continued)*
Problems of Immobility With Related Etiologies, Assessment Priorities, Expected Outcomes, and Nursing Interventions

Problems Related to Immobility	Etiologies	Assessment Priorities	Expected Outcomes	Nursing Interventions
Respiratory				
Impaired Gas Exchange (O_2/CO_2 ratio)	Decreased respiratory movement Pooling of secretions	• Note any changes in the client's behavior, mental status. • Compare clinical picture with changes in arterial blood gas values, pulmonary function test values, or pulse oximetry.	Client will maintain an adequate O_2/CO_2 ratio.	• See nursing interventions for Ineffective Breathing Pattern and Ineffective Airway Clearance.
Musculoskeletal				
Risk for Activity Intolerance (self–care deficits) Impaired Physical Mobility	Decreased muscle mass, tone, and strength (atrophy) Contractures Stiffness and pain in the joints Limited range of motion Joint degeneration (ankylosis) Decreased stability Bone demineralization (disuse osteoporosis) Decreased endurance	• Assess for weakness, fatigue, complaints of muscle pain or joint pain or tenderness. • Assess for decreased muscle mass (anthropometric measurements, tape measurements), decreased muscle tone, and strength; test joint flexibility; note any contractures or ankyloses.	Client will maintain adequate muscle strength and joint mobility to perform basic self-care activities.	• Incorporate range-of-motion exercises (as client's condition permits) and isometric setting exercises into client's daily routine (at least three to four times daily).
Risk for Injury: Pathologic Fractures	Excessive bone demineralization (disuse osteoporosis)	• Bone demineralization is not detectable through physical assessment. • Relate clinical picture to blood chemistries (note elevated serum calcium and phosphorus levels).	Client will remain free of contractures, ankyloses, pathologic fractures.	• Increase client's activity tolerance gradually: • Participates in positioning in bed • Transfer from bed to chair • Ambulates • Gradually increases frequency and duration of sitting out of bed and frequency and distance of walks • Progresses to independence in all self-care activities
Metabolic				
Altered Nutrition: Less Than Body Requirements Altered Nutrition: More Than Body Requirements Fluid Volume Excess: Dependent Edema	Negative nitrogen balance Anorexia Imbalance between calories ingested and burned off Fluid shifts secondary to negative nitrogen balance	• Assess diet history and note problems with anorexia, digestion, or elimination. • Monitor intake and output and correlate client's clinical picture with laboratory studies that evaluate fluid and electrolyte status.	Client will maintain appropriate weight for height. Client's fluid output will approximately equal intake. Client's electrolyte values and serum protein will fall within normal range.	• Provide client with high-protein, high-calorie diet; explore parenteral and enteral (nasogastric, gastrostomy, or jejunostomy tubes) alternatives if the client is unable to eat. • Serve small, frequent feedings in a pleasant environment.

(continued)

Table 39-3 *(continued)*
Problems of Immobility With Related Etiologies, Assessment Priorities, Expected Outcomes, and Nursing Interventions

Problems Related to Immobility	Etiologies	Assessment Priorities	Expected Outcomes	Nursing Interventions
Metabolic				
		• Evaluate muscle atrophy by way of anthropometric measurements (height, weight, mid-upper arm circumference, and triceps skin-fold measurements). • Assess skin turgor and wound healing.	Client's skin will demonstrate adequate turgor.	• Monitor intake and output.
Gastrointestinal				
Constipation	Decreased gastric motility and muscle tone Decreased fluid intake	• Assess frequency and consistency of bowel movements (use of elimination aids). • Examine for bowel sounds, abdominal tone, and anal sphincter tone.	Client will have a formed, semisolid stool every 1 to 3 days. Client will be free of signs of fecal impaction (distended abdomen, no bowel movement for several days or liquid bowel movement, lethargy)	• Respect client's usual elimination schedule. • Offer assistance with the bedpan or commode if needed and provide privacy. • Increase fluid intake and roughage. • Caution about Valsalva's maneuver (straining with mouth closed).
Urinary				
Altered Urinary Elimination Urinary Retention Risk for Infection: Urinary Tract	Renal calculi Urinary stasis	• Assess voiding patterns—time and amount (note history of small, frequent voidings); question about urgency, dysuria, pain. • Monitor fluid output. • Examine for bladder distention. • Examine urine for cloudiness or odor (culture urine if indicated).	Client will maintain usual voiding pattern (frequency and amount). Client will be free of renal calculi. Client will be free of signs of urinary tract infection (urgency, burning, flank pain, fever).	• Keep the client well hydrated (aim is for client to void large amounts of dilute urine). • Maintain usual voiding pattern. • If needed, provide assistance with bedpan or urinal—respect client's privacy.
Skin				
Impaired Skin Integrity (pressure ulcer)	Decreased local blood circulation to the tissues Prolonged pressure on the skin	• Examine skin, especially pressure points, for beginning signs of breakdown with each position change (at least every 2 hours). • Assess for factors that place client at high risk for breakdown (malnutrition, incontinence, and so on).	Client's skin will show no sign of breakdown.	• Reposition client in correct alignment at least every 1 to 2 hours and ensure protection of pressure points where possible (eg, heel and elbow protectors). • Decrease effects of shearing forces. • Massage pressure points and keep skin clean and dry. • Keep bed linens dry and free of wrinkles.

(continued)

Table 39-3 *(continued)*
Problems of Immobility With Related Etiologies, Assessment Priorities, Expected Outcomes, and Nursing Interventions

Problems Related to Immobility	Etiologies	Assessment Priorities	Expected Outcomes	Nursing Interventions
Psychologic and Social				
Self-Esteem Disturbance Powerlessness Impaired Social Interaction Altered Thought Processes Knowledge Deficit Ineffective Individual Coping Ineffective Family Coping Sleep Pattern Disturbance	Inability to move body voluntarily Dependency on others Inability to fulfill role expectations Pain experience Skeletal deformities Exaggerated emotional and behavioral responses Loss of mobility to contact friends Decreased stimuli to maintain orientation Immobility-induced depression Decreased motivation to learn Decreased ability to learn and decreased retention Decreased motivation to solve problems Increased need for assistance with self-care abilities Exaggerated emotional responses Decreased physical exercise Increased bedtime and napping	• Assess client for changes in behavior, emotional status, and mental abilities. • Explore with the client and family possible reasons for these changes. • Assess the adequacy of the client's and family's coping strategies. • Assess sleep-wake patterns.	Client will identify personal strengths. Client will verbalize positive body image. Client will describe successful coping strategies. Client will demonstrate ability to problem solve.	• Use care contacts with client to explore immobility's effects on the client's mental status and behavior. • Explore means to meet client's needs for socialization. • Increase stimuli to maintain client's orientation. • Encourage client to be as independent as possible and to structure daily activities and schedule as closely as possible to preimmobilization; encourage wearing of personal clothes, use of cosmetics, and so on. • Challenge client intellectually. Communicate that you expect the client to reason, to problem solve. • Explore impact of client's illness on family and counsel appropriately.

scribed exercises such as jogging, tennis, or even walking may be viewed as white, middle-class choices and prove unsafe in a high-crime area. An exercise prescription for a Native American, for example, might suggest exploration of nearby mountain areas, hunting, or even participation in Native American dances as more acceptable methods to increase activity level. Other lifestyle variables that influence mobility include a person's diet and smoking history.

Attitude and Values

In some families, such as those that hike together, swim together, and play ball together, children learn early to value regular exercise. As these children mature, they often continue to value exercise and find new ways to incorporate regular exercise into their daily routine. Similarly, children may be raised in sedentary families where watching sports is the closest anyone comes to exercise. This attitude may also be internalized for a lifetime. Many individual values also explain the exercise options people make. Older people who integrate a planned exercise regimen into their daily routine benefit physiologically and report improved self-esteem.

Individuals who place a high value on physical attractiveness may be highly committed to regular exercise because it produces the body they want. Another individual may exercise because of the desire for physical strength, relating strength with power. Someone more disposed to intellectual pursuits may perceive body development as simply wasting time that could be better used to develop the mind.

Fatigue and Stress

Chronic stress may deplete body energy to the point that fatigue makes even the thought of exercise overwhelming. Ironically, regular exercise is energizing and can better equip a person to deal with daily stresses. At the same time, excessive exercise may stress the body and lead to injury as well as to fatigue.

External Factors

Many external factors can influence mobility. Among these, weather probably exerts the greatest influence. A brisk, clear day is invigorating and invites increased activity. High humidity and high temperatures, on the other hand, discourage any extra movement. Sufficient financial resources for exercise memberships and equipment, safe outdoor parks and sports areas, the availability of malls for early morning walkers, support people, and occupational or insurance rewards for exercise can all encourage regular exercise. Detractors include insufficient funds, air pollution, unsafe neighborhoods, and lack of support and reinforcement.

Exercise

Active exertion of muscles involving the contraction and relaxation of muscle groups is termed **exercise**. Each of the many different types of exercise has the potential to produce different physiologic and psychologic benefits.

Types of Exercise

Muscle Contraction. Exercise may be categorized according to the type of muscle contraction involved as being isotonic, isometric, or isokinetic (Fig. 39-7).

Isotonic exercise involves muscle shortening and active movement. Examples include carrying out activities of daily living, independently performing range-of-motion exercises, and swimming, walking, jogging, and bicycling. Potential benefits include increased muscle mass, tone, and strength; improved joint mobility; increased cardiac and respiratory function; increased circulation; and increased osteoblastic activity. When the nurse or family member performs passive range-of-motion exercises for a client, the client's muscles do not exert effort and potential benefits are reduced to improved joint mobility and increased circulation.

Isometric exercise involves muscle contraction without shortening (ie, there is no movement or a minimum shortening of muscle fibers). Examples include contractions of the quadriceps and gluteal muscles. Potential benefits are increased muscle mass, tone, and strength; increased circulation to the exercised body part; and increased osteoblastic activity. Nurses encourage both isotonic and isometric exercises for hospitalized clients with limited mobility.

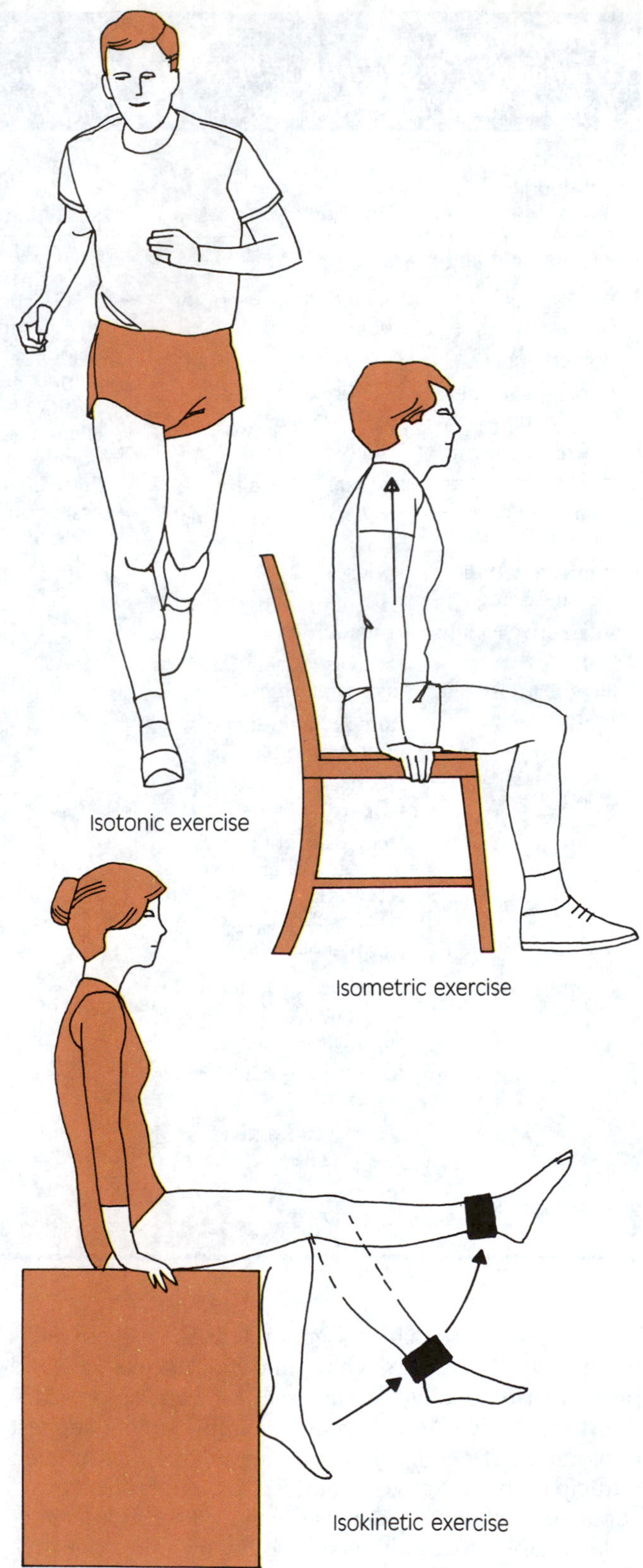

Figure 39-7
Three types of exercise: (1) isotonic, which involves muscle shortening and active movement; (2) isometric, which involves muscle contraction without shortening; and (3) isokinetic, which involves muscle contraction with resistance.

Isokinetic exercise involves muscle contractions with resistance, varying at a constant rate produced by a device with a capacity for variable resistance. Examples include rehabilitative exercises for knee and elbow injuries. Using the isokinetic device, the muscles and joint are taken through a complete range of motion without stopping, with resistance at every point.

Body Movement. Exercise activities may also be categorized according to the type of body movement involved and the health benefits they produce. Fuller and Schaller-Ayers (1994) discuss the following types:

Aerobic exercise. Sustained (often rhythmic) muscle movements that increase blood flow, heart rate, and metabolic demand for oxygen over time, promoting cardiovascular conditioning. Activities that may be aerobic are swimming, walking, jogging, cross-country skiing, aerobic dance, bicycling, jumping rope, and racquetball. (Aerobic exercise may be further distinguished as having high versus low impact. The number of injuries, such as shin splints, related to high-impact aerobic workouts led to the development of low-impact workouts that place less stress on the musculoskeletal system.)

Stretching exercises. Movements that allow muscles and joints to be stretched gently through their full range of motion increase flexibility. Specific warm-up and cool-down exercises, hatha yoga, and some forms of dance are examples. Benefits include increased range of joint movements, improved circulation and posture, and relaxation.

Strength and endurance exercises. A variety of muscle-building programs fall into this category. Weight training, calisthenics, and specific isometric exercises can build both strength and endurance, increasing the power of the musculoskeletal system and generally improving the whole body. They may or may not have aerobic benefit.

Movement and activities of daily living. Housecleaning, running after playful toddlers, climbing stairs instead of riding in elevators, all have an effect on health. Increased fitness does not require a gym.

Effects of Exercise and Immobility on Major Body Systems

The human body was designed for motion, and regular exercise is necessary for its healthy functioning. Individuals who choose inactive lifestyles or who are forced to inactivity by illness or injury place themselves at high risk for serious health problems. The effects of both regular exercise and immobility on major body systems are explored in this section and outlined in Figure 39-8. Just as individuals differ in the benefits they receive from exercise, complications resulting from immobility differ in their occurrence and severity according to the client's age and overall health state.

Cardiovascular System

Effects of Exercise. To meet the demand for oxygen created by the rhythmic contraction and relaxation of skeletal muscle groups, the supply of oxygenated blood to skeletal muscle needs to be increased. The cardiovascular system meets this challenge by increasing the heart rate, increasing the contractile strength of the myocardium, and increasing stroke volume (volume of blood ejected), thus increasing cardiac output. Arterial (systolic) blood pressure is increased and blood is shunted from the nonexercising tissues to the heart and muscles. Exercise also improves venous return because the contracting muscles compress superficial veins and push blood back to the heart against gravity. Over time, with cardiovascular conditioning, regular exercise produces the following benefits:

- Increased efficiency of the heart
- Decreased heart rate and blood pressure
- Increased blood flow to all body parts
- Increased circulating fibrinolysin (substance that breaks up small clots)

Effects of Immobility. The primary and serious effects of immobility on the cardiovascular system include increased cardiac workload, orthostatic hypotension, and venous thrombosis. Immobility results in an increased workload for the heart. It has been demonstrated that the heart works more when the person is resting, probably because there is less resistance offered by the blood vessels and because there is a change in the distribution of blood in the immobile person. As a result, the heart rate, cardiac output, and stroke volume increase.

Immobility predisposes to thrombi formation because of venous stasis, especially in the legs, where normal muscular activity helps move blood toward the central circulatory system. Thrombus formation is also caused by an increased rate in the coagulation of blood, one reason being that during periods of immobility, calcium leaves bones and enters the blood, where it has an influence on blood coagulation.

The immobile person is more susceptible to developing orthostatic hypotension. The person tends to feel weak and faint when the condition occurs. The phenomenon is probably due to a decrease in the neurovascular reflexes, which normally cause vasoconstriction, and to a loss of muscle tone. The result is that blood pools and does not squeeze from veins in the lower part of the body to the central circulatory system.

Pertinent nursing diagnoses and collaborative problems related to immobility include the following:

Altered Tissue Perfusion related to prolonged bed rest

Risk for Injury: Deep Vein Thrombosis related to venous stasis, hypercoagulability, and decreased muscle activity

Risk for Injury: Falls related to orthostatic hypotension

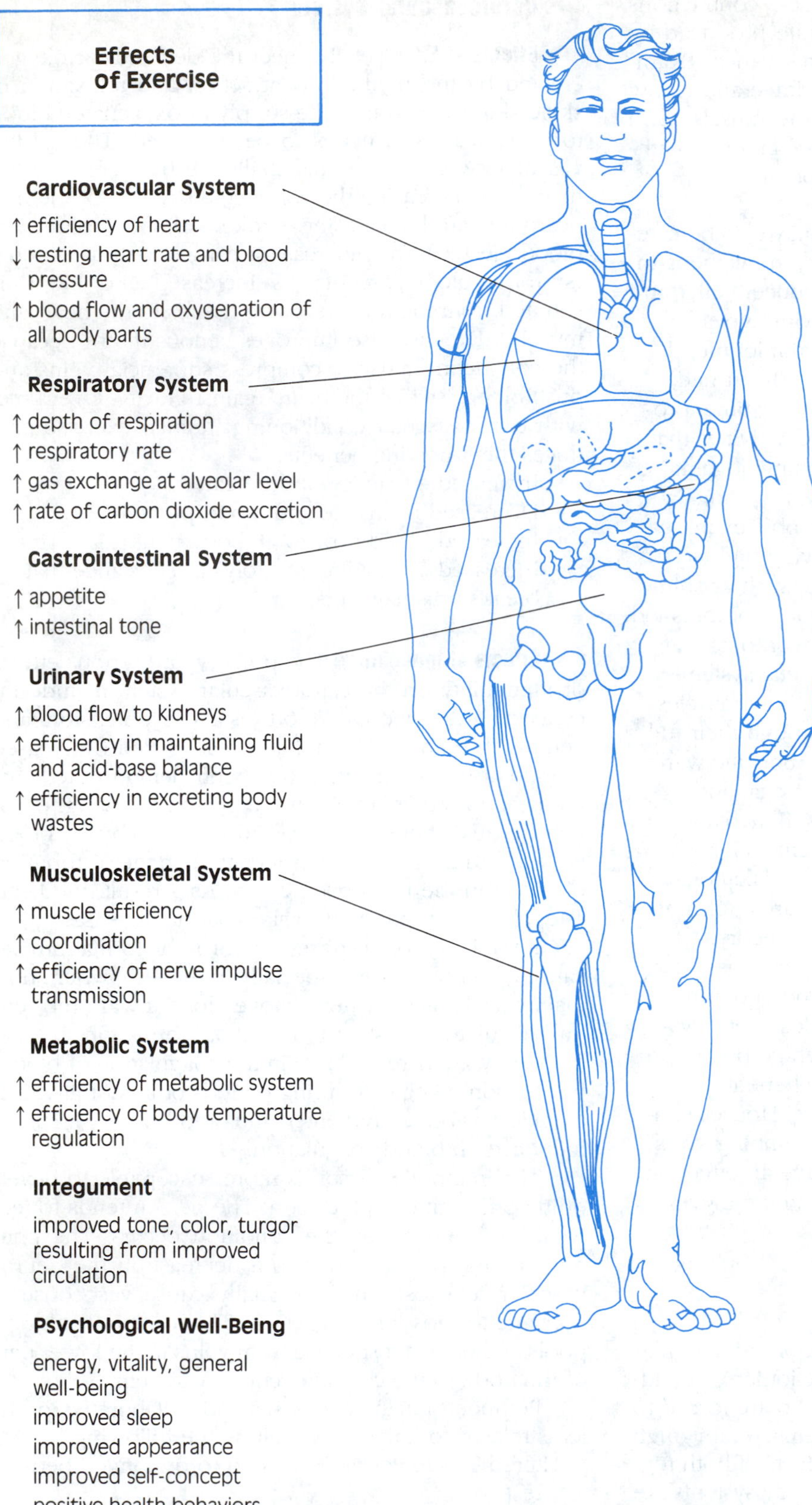

Figure 39-8
A summary and comparison of the effects of exercise and immobility by body system.

Activity Intolerance related to fatigue and inadequate tissue oxygenation

Impaired Tissue Integrity related to shearing force and prolonged bed rest

Several collaborative problems related to the effect of immobility on the cardiovascular system include the following:

Potential complication: thromboemboli/deep vein thrombosis

Potential complication: hypoxemia

Respiratory System

Effects of Exercise. The respiratory and cardiovascular systems work together to make increased oxygen available to the muscles. During exercise, the depth of respiration, respiratory rate, gas exchange at the alveolar level, and rate of carbon dioxide excretion are increased. Over time, regular exercise leads to improved pulmonary functioning.

Effects of Immobility. The effects of immobility on the respiratory system are related to decreased ventilatory effort and increased respiratory secretions. Immobility causes a decrease in the depth and rate of respirations owing at least partially to a reduced need for oxygen by body cells. When areas of lung tissues are not used over time, atelectasis may occur. *Atelectasis* is an incomplete expansion or collapse of lung tissue. Immobility results in a poor exchange of carbon dioxide and oxygen, upsets their balance in the body, and results eventually in an acid–base imbalance.

When a person is immobile, the movement of secretions in the respiratory tract is decreased, resulting in the pooling of secretions and in respiratory tract congestion. These conditions predispose to respiratory tract infections. *Hypostatic pneumonia* is a type of pneumonia that results from inactivity and immobility. The situation worsens when the person is dehydrated or using pharmaceutical agents that increase the tenacity of secretions, depress the coughing mechanism, and depress respirations.

Decreased movement in the thoracic cage during respirations also results from immobility. This decrease may be due to loss of tonus in muscles involved with respirations, to pressure on the chest wall owing to the client's position in bed, and to depression of the respiratory apparatus by various pharmaceutical agents.

Pertinent nursing diagnoses related to immobility include the following:

Ineffective Breathing Pattern related to limited chest expansion

Ineffective Airway Clearance related to decreased position changes, ineffective coughing, and stasis of secretions

Impaired Gas Exchange related to decreased respiratory movement (loss of muscle tonus)

Risk for Infection related to accumulation of secretions

A collaborative problem related to the effect of immobility on the respiratory system is the following:

Potential complication: hypoxemia secondary to pneumonia

Musculoskeletal System

Effects of Exercise. The rhythmic contraction and relaxation of muscle groups during exercise result in increased muscle mass, tone, and strength and increased joint mobility. The more a person exercises, the more strength he or she has to exercise or work in the future. Regular exercise produces the following benefits:

- Increased muscle efficiency (strength) and flexibility
- Increased coordination
- Increased efficiency of nerve impulse transmission

Regular exercise is also believed to slow the effects of aging (ie, it helps prevent osteoporosis associated with aging).

Effects of Immobility. Effects of immobility on the musculoskeletal system are rapidly seen in clients confined to bed. People attempting to walk after several days of bed rest are often surprised to find how weak their legs have become. Immobility (musculoskeletal disuse) leads to decreased muscle size (**atrophy**), tone, and strength; decreased joint mobility and flexibility; bone demineralization; and limited endurance, resulting in problems with activities of daily living.

Immobility is often the cause of **contractures**, which are permanent contraction states of muscle (muscle shortening), and **ankylosis**, which is a consolidation and immobilization of a joint. Contractures result from atrophy of muscles with resulting incompetence, and from a decrease in the muscle's strength, coordination, and endurance. A joint can be permanently fixed when ankylosed.

The process of bone demineralization (**osteoporosis**) is also increased in the immobile client. Normally the stress and strain of weight-bearing activity stimulate bone formation and balance destruction. With immobility, however, bone formation slows while breakdown increases, with a net loss of bone calcium, phosphorus, and matrix. This condition, *disuse osteoporosis*, is characterized by bones that may be either spongy or brittle. Bone demineralization may result in pathologic fractures related to the bone's brittleness; bone deformities related to the bone's sponginess; arthropathy (joint disease) related to calcium depletion in the joints; and renal calculi (stones) related to the excessive excretion of calcium through the kidneys and urinary tract.

Pertinent nursing diagnoses related to immobility include the following:

Activity Intolerance related to decreased muscle mass, tone, and strength

Impaired Physical Mobility related to muscle atrophy (contractures) and limited joint mobility (ankylosis)

Risk for Injury: Pathologic Fracture related to excessive bone demineralization (disuse osteoporosis)

Self-Care Deficit related to decreased muscle strength and decreased flexibility

Fatigue related to increased energy needed to perform activities of daily living

Metabolic System

Effects of Exercise. The metabolic rate increases during exercise so that sufficient glucose and fatty acids can be converted to provide the energy needed for increased muscle function. During strenuous exercise, the metabolic rate can increase to up to 20 times normal. Increased body heat and waste products are also produced. With regular exercise the body develops:

- Increased efficiency of metabolic system
- Increased efficiency of body temperature regulation

Effects of Immobility. Because the resting body requires less energy, the cellular demand for oxygen is decreased and this is reflected by a decreased metabolic rate. In many immobilized clients, however, factors such as fever, trauma, chronic illness, or poor nutrition can actually increase the body's metabolic demands and increase *catabolism* (the breakdown of the body's protein stores to provide energy to meet the body's energy requirements). If unchecked, this process results in muscle wasting. When more protein is being broken down than manufactured, the body excretes more nitrogen than it takes in and *negative nitrogen balance* occurs. Anorexia, or decreased appetite, often accompanies and compounds this problem. Negative nitrogen balance and poor nutrition thus worsen the muscle atrophy and weakness already resulting from immobility. Numerous fluid and electrolyte imbalances, alterations in the exchange of nutrients and gases at the cellular level, and gastrointestinal problems can all result from metabolic disturbances.

Pertinent nursing diagnoses related to immobility include the following:

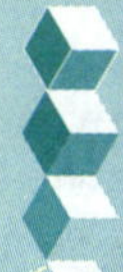

Research in Nursing: Making a Difference

Exercise

Exercise is an essential component in improving circulation and maintaining muscle strength and joint mobility. Nursing interventions traditionally have been carried out to prevent the complications associated with immobility. Recent nursing research has focused on analyzing the effects of participation in a regular exercise program for clients of various ages in home and healthcare settings.

Related Research

Ali, N., & Twibell, R. (1994). Barriers to osteoporosis prevention in perimenopausal and elderly women. *Geriatric Nursing, 15*(4), 201–205.
Women who participated in this study (n = 100) were asked to respond to questions about the use and importance of calcium, exercise, and hormone replacement therapy in relation to their activities of daily living. Researchers noted a chronically inadequate calcium intake coupled with a lack of recognition of the benefits of exercise and hormone replacement therapy for cardiovascular health. None of these women related regular exercise to the prevention of osteoporosis. Nurses need to design effective education strategies that emphasize adequate calcium intake and the importance of exercise in the delay or prevention of osteoporosis.

Spier, B., & Meis, M. (1994). Maintenance ambulation: Its significance and the role of nursing. *Geriatric Nursing, 15*(5), 277–281.
Nursing home residents who participated in a maintenance ambulation program were less likely to suffer the decreases in functioning and the problems of immobility common in more sedentary residents. Frail, older clients regained their mobility at varying rates when introduced to ambulation activities after periods of immobility. Continuing education programs for staff should emphasize the value of incorporating walking into clients' daily activities and discuss techniques for motivating residents to participate in these programs.

Felton, G., & Parsons, M. (1994). Factors influencing physical activity in average-weight and overweight young women. *Journal of Community Health Nursing, 11*(2), 109–119.
The sedentary lifestyle and poor nutritional practices of young women place them at risk for significant health problems. A group of variables were investigated as predictors of physical activity in a group of average-weight and overweight women. Three of the variables (race, personal control, and regular participation) were significant for both groups. In the overweight group, interpersonal support was also identified as positively influencing exercise participation. Nurses working in the community need to consider these variables when creating physical activity programs or working with existing ones.

Summary

Nursing research in the area of exercise, physical fitness, and daily activities has important implications for promoting wellness and preventing illness. Changing lifestyle behavior to include participation in regular physical exercise is also beneficial in improving clients' ability to function independently.

Altered Nutrition: Less Than Body Requirements, related to negative nitrogen balance and anorexia
Altered Nutrition: More Than Body Requirements, related to imbalance between calories ingested and burned off
Fluid Volume Excess: Dependent Edema related to fluid shifts (intravascular to interstitial compartments) secondary to negative nitrogen balance

Gastrointestinal System

Effects of Exercise. During exercise, blood is shunted away from the stomach and intestines to the exercising muscles—hence the advice never to exercise on a full stomach. With regular exercise:

- Appetite is increased.
- Intestinal tone is increased, which improves digestion and elimination.

Effects of Immobility. Immobility leads to disturbances in appetite, decreased food intake, altered protein metabolism, and poor digestion and utilization of food. If individuals increase food intake while decreasing energy expenditure, weight gain will result.

Normal muscular activity in the gastrointestinal tract also slows down in the immobile person, which often results in constipation, poor defecation reflexes, and an inability to expel feces and gas adequately.

Pertinent nursing diagnoses related to immobility include the following:

Constipation related to decreased gastric motility and muscle tone
Altered Nutrition: More Than Body Requirements, related to imbalance between food intake and activity (decreased energy expenditure)
Altered Nutrition: Less Than Body Requirements, related to anorexia and difficulty swallowing

Urinary System

Effects of Exercise. Regular exercise increases blood circulation, including improved blood flow to the kidneys. This allows the kidneys to more efficiently maintain the body's fluid balance and acid–base balance and excrete body wastes.

Effects of Immobility. In the nonerect client, the kidneys and ureters are level and urine stays longer in the renal pelvis before being expressed against gravity into the ureters and bladder. Urinary stasis favors the growth of bacteria that, when present in sufficient quantities, may cause urinary tract infections. Poor perineal hygiene, incontinence, decreased fluid intake, or an indwelling Foley catheter can increase the risk of urinary tract infection for an immobile client.

Immobility also predisposes to renal calculi, or kidney stones, which are a consequence of high levels of urinary calcium; urinary retention and incontinence resulting from decreased bladder muscle tone; the formation of alkaline urine, which facilitates growth of urinary bacteria; and decreased urinary volume.

Pertinent nursing diagnoses related to immobility include the following:

Pain related to inability to pass renal calculi
Urinary Retention related to prolonged immobility
Risk for Infection: Urinary Tract, related to urinary stasis and increased urine alkalinity

Skin

Effects of Exercise. Increased circulation resulting from regular exercise nourishes the skin and promotes its general health.

Effects of Immobility. In older or debilitated immobile clients, the impaired circulation that accompanies immobility may result in serious skin breakdown. Prolonged pressure over bony prominences produces areas of breakdown, or pressure ulcers, which can progress from stage 1, redness, to stage 4, destruction of subcutaneous tissue and muscle. Pressure ulcers are described in detail in Chapter 38.

Pertinent nursing diagnoses related to immobility include the following:

Impaired Skin Integrity (specify stage of pressure ulcer) related to decreased circulation and pressure on skin overlying bony prominences

Psychosocial Outlook

Effects of Exercise. Some of the most important benefits of regular exercise are psychologic:

- Increased energy, vitality, and general well-being
- Improved sleep
- Improved appearance (body image)
- Improved self-concept
- Increased positive health behaviors

Effects of Immobility. When a person can no longer move the body purposefully and needs to depend on someone else for assistance with simple self-care activities, the sense of self is often threatened. Skeletal deformities can influence body image; an inability to meet role expectations can decrease self-concept; and a prolonged period of lying dependent in bed can lead to feelings of worthlessness and diminished self-esteem.

Immobility can produce exaggerated emotional responses to the stresses of everyday living. People who become apathetic, possibly because of decreased sensory stimulation, often exhibit altered thought processes. Lack of mobility can also diminish an individual's opportunities to interact socially and deprive that person of normal support systems. Coping difficulties are common in both the immobilized client and the client's family. Furthermore, the amount of time the immobilized client spends resting often disrupts usual sleep–wakefulness patterns and may interfere with both the quantity and quality of sleep.

Pertinent nursing diagnoses related to immobility include the following:

Self-Esteem Disturbance related to immobility and need to depend on others (and other variables)

Powerlessness related to increasing dependency in basic self-care activities
Impaired Social Interaction related to immobility
Altered Thought Processes: Disorientation related to decreased stimulation to maintain orientation
Knowledge Deficit (specify) related to decreased motivation to learn
Ineffective Individual Coping related to prolonged bed rest and increasing activity intolerance
Sleep Pattern Disturbance related to increased bedtime or napping and decreased physical exercise

Role of Exercise in Preventing Illness and Promoting Wellness

Promoting exercise and emphasizing wellness behaviors are challenging opportunities for nurses. Nurses are committed to assisting and supporting clients to make lifestyle changes that improve the clients' health and well-being. As researchers focus on the potential of regular exercise activities to slow the aging process, nurses intervene to prevent the deleterious effects associated with decreased physical activity.

Positive physical benefits of exercise include the following:

- Improved cardiopulmonary function
- Decreased blood pressure
- Increased bone mineral content
- Increased muscle strength, coordination, and joint range of motion
- Improved fat and carbohydrate metabolism

Data also indicate that psychologic benefits of exercise can be identified:

- Improved sense of well-being
- A greater sense of control over life
- A decrease in fear, among older clients, of falling
- An improved body image

Although there is no evidence that exercise prevents the occurrence of chronic disease, clinical improvement has been noted when clients participate in regular exercise activities. See the accompanying box for a summary of the benefits of exercise and specific precautions related to exercise for this age group.

Risks Related to Exercise

Among the reasons many people offer for not exercising is fear of causing some personal harm. Nurses need to respond to these fears with realistic knowledge of the risks associated with exercise and specific prevention strategies.

Focus on the Older Adult

Exercise and Activity

Regular exercise is beneficial for all age groups. Older adults, particularly, demonstrate positive results from a program of regular physical activity that is appropriate for their age and health status.

Benefits that can result from regular physical activity include:

- Cardiovascular improvements
  - Decreased blood pressure
  - Decreased heart rate
  - Improved circulation
  - Decreased cholesterol level
  - Decreased body weight
- Respiratory improvements
  - Increased vital capacity
  - Increased endurance
- Musculoskeletal improvements
  - Increased muscle strength
  - Improved stability of gait
  - Improved range of motion
  - Increased flexibility
  - Decreased back and joint pain
  - Improved posture
- Psychosocial and cognitive improvements
  - Improved ability to manage stress
  - Improved memory
  - Increased self-esteem
  - Increased opportunities for socialization
- Other improvements
  - Improved sleep
  - Improved bowel function
  - Improved energy level

Special precautions for older adults prior to and during exercise include:

- Prior to exercise
  - Obtain physician's approval and directions for exercise program.
  - Wait until 2 hours after eating before exercising.
  - Perform warm-up exercises before beginning activity.
  - Wear proper footwear and appropriate clothing.
  - Provide for sufficient hydration.
  - Avoid extreme temperatures if exercising outdoors.
- During exercise
  - Avoid sudden position changes
  - Maintain heart rate at lower end of target zone specified by physician.
  - Check pulse at regular intervals while exercising.
  - Avoid exercise if weak or ill.
  - Stop exercising if chest pain or difficulty breathing occurs and consult with physician before resuming activity.

Avoiding Exercise. The greatest risk associated with exercise is viewing it as too much of a chore and avoiding it.

Precipitating a Cardiac Event. Although the risk of exercise precipitating a major cardiac event in a healthy individual is minimal, the risk is much higher for individuals with known or documentable cardiovascular disease. Thus, a preexercise medical examination, medical supervision during exercise, and an individually designed exercise plan are recommended for sedentary people older than age 35 years and for any person with a past or current cardiovascular condition.

Orthopedic Discomfort and Disability. The most common injuries associated with exercise are orthopedic in nature and are caused by irritation of bones, tendons, ligaments, and sometimes muscles. This irritation may result from added weight-bearing stress or from collision with the ground, an object, or another person. Teach clients when injured to rely on the acronym RICE—*r*est, *i*ce, *c*ompression, and *e*levation. A physician should be contacted immediately to diagnose the extent of the injury. Exercise should not be continued until the injury is healed; otherwise further damage may be done.

Other Health Problems. Many other types of health problems may be associated with different types of exercise, depending to a large extent on external factors (temperature on a given day, humidity, pollution index, safety of the neighborhood) as well as internal factors (age, history of previous injury, overuse, obesity, health history).

The Nurse as Role Model

Nurses who wish to role model healthy mobility behaviors to clients demonstrate a commitment to using the principles of body mechanics in both their leisure and work activities and to exercising regularly to promote fitness. Use the self-assessment checklist for exercise in the accompanying box to determine how well you are meeting your need for exercise. Because nurses who work closely with clients providing physical care are at high risk for developing musculoskeletal problems if they do not use their bodies properly, they also have a personal reason for being attentive to the use of good body mechanics. Similarly, the work of nursing places heavy demands on a nurse's psychic and physical energy; the nurse who is physically fit is better able to respond to these challenges. Nurses who are effective role models easily meet the following goals:

- Consistently use sound principles of body mechanics in both leisure and work activities
- Incorporate regular periods of physical exercise into lifestyle (minimum of three 30- to 45-minute exercise sessions weekly)
- Demonstrate a preference for an active versus a sedentary lifestyle (eg, use stairs in preference to elevators, walk rather than drive short distances, balance active leisure alternatives with sedentary options)
- Appear physically fit to clients and colleagues (appropriate weight for height; adequate muscle mass, tone, and strength; performs work activities without becoming short of breath or excessively fatigued)

It is not uncommon to hear nurses who are retiring or leaving the profession cite back injuries as an influencing factor. Nurses may incur back injuries as a result of poor body mechanics or become injured when a client falls. Back injuries are cited most frequently by nurses in workers' compensation claims and account for the greatest amount of lost work time in the hospital setting (NewsWatch, 1994). Many nurses report that although they had episodes of occupation-related back problems, they never filed an incident report and accept back pain as a routine consequence of the job. Transferring clients from a wheelchair to the bed, toilet, or scale-chair and any transfers related to bathing are listed as the most physically stressing tasks (Owen & Garg, 1993). Other variables that can lead to back injuries for healthcare workers include:

- Uncoordinated lifts
- Height–weight differential among the lifters
- Lifting when fatigued
- Lifting after recent recovery from a back injury
- Lack of training in proper body mechanics (NewsWatch, 1994)

Techniques to prevent back stress should be included routinely in injury prevention programs. Additional emphasis in the nursing curriculum on principles of body mechanics and client-lifting techniques may also be effective in improving the nursing environment.

ASSESSING

The nurse performing a comprehensive nursing assessment uses both interview and physical assessment skills to elicit data about the client's mobility status. When alterations in a client's physical or mental health state result in impaired mobility, more detailed assessment skills are needed.

Nursing History

During the nursing history the nurse interviews the client regarding daily activity level, endurance, exercise and fitness goals, mobility problems, physical or mental health alterations that affect mobility, and external factors affecting mobility. It is important to question clients about their fitness goals. This interviewing strategy communicates to clients that you expect them to be exercising and is itself a powerful teaching tool.

Promoting Wellness

Exercise

Use the following assessment checklist to determine how well you are meeting your need for exercise. Then develop a prescription for self-care by choosing appropriate behaviors from the list of suggestions.

Assessment Checklist

almost always	sometimes	almost never	
☐	☐	☐	1. My lifestyle demonstrates that I place a high value on exercise as a component of wellness (eg, I use stairs instead of elevators).
☐	☐	☐	2. I exercise for 30 to 45 minutes three or four times per week.
☐	☐	☐	3. I have sufficient energy for each day's tasks.
☐	☐	☐	4. I maintain my target weight.

Self-Care Behaviors

1. Decide to make the most of everyday opportunities for exercise: use stairs instead of elevators, walk instead of ride, park your car farther from your destination than usual and walk the distance briskly, and so forth.
2. Choose exercise activities you enjoy and plan three or four 30- to 45-minute exercise sessions weekly.
3. Obtain medical clearance for exercise if you fall in a high-risk group. Learn and observe the appropriate exercise safeguards (eg, wear running shoes with the proper support).
4. Alternate types of exercise to avoid boredom.
5. Use part of your lunchtime for brisk walking or other exercise.
6. Invite a friend to exercise with you so you have the added support of a buddy.
7. Join a spa, health club, or exercise group.
8. Build up exercise sessions gradually to avoid overexertion and injury to muscles.
9. Evaluate your lifestyle to see what prevents you from exercising regularly and address these factors (low value attached to health or exercise, low motivation, lack of time, lack of rest, or faulty nutrition).

The history of a client's mobility status is brief if initial questioning reveals no problems. The accompanying box illustrates elements common to a mobility status history. When a problem exists (eg, loss of joint mobility or decreased tolerance for physical activity), the nurse assesses the nature of the problem, onset and frequency, known causes, severity, symptoms, effect of problem on everyday functioning, and interventions attempted by the client and results obtained.

Physical Assessment

Physical assessment of mobility status includes an assessment of general ease of movement and gait; alignment, joint structure, and function; muscle mass, tone, and strength; and endurance. Table 39-4 provides normal findings and significant alterations. The nurse performing this assessment directs attention to both structure and function. The client's ability to stand, walk, sit up, and grasp are important because these enable the client to wash, dress, and feed himself or herself, and perform other basic activities of daily living.

General Ease of Movement and Gait

The nurse begins the examination of the ambulatory client the moment the client walks into the room. Voluntarily controlled, fluid, and coordinated body movements are keys to the integrated functioning of the skeletal, skeletal muscle, and nervous systems. Significant findings include the presence of any of the following involuntary movements (Bates, 1995, pp. 670–672):

Tremors—relatively rhythmic oscillatory movements
- *Resting tremors*—most prominent at rest and may decrease or disappear with voluntary movement
- *Intention tremors*—appear with activity and may increase in severity as the target is neared
- *Postural tremors*—appear when the affected part is maintaining a posture; may be aggravated by anxiety or fatigue

Tics—brief, repetitive, stereotyped, coordinated movements occurring at regular intervals (eg, repetitive winking, grimacing)

Chorea—brief, rapid, jerky, irregular, and unpredictable movements that occur at rest or interrupt

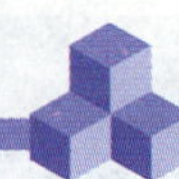

Focused Assessment Guide

Mobility and Exercise

Factors to Assess	Questions and Approaches
Daily activity level	Describe the activities you normally carry out during a routine day. What type of physical exercise is a part of your daily lifestyle? • Activities of daily living • Type, frequency, duration of physical exercise • Past history of activity and exercise; recent changes
Endurance	Describe how much and what type of activity makes you tired. • History of dizziness, dyspnea, frequent pauses in activity to rest, or marked increase in respiratory rate after moderate activity
Exercise/fitness goals	What exercise or fitness goals are you currently working on? • Attitudes about exercise and physical fitness • Knowledge of the benefits of exercise • Motivation to exercise • Current exercise and fitness goals
Mobility problems	Do you experience any problems with movement or with more vigorous activity or exercise? If yes, please describe these problems. • Nature of the problem • Onset of disturbance and frequency • Known causes • Severity • Symptoms • Effect of problem on everyday functioning • Interventions attempted and results
Physical or mental health alterations	Are there any physical or mental health problems that may be affecting your mobility? Tell me about them. • Decrease of strength or endurance (eg, myocardial infarction, congestive heart failure, cardiomyopathy, chronic obstructive pulmonary disease, cancer, gastrointestinal disorders) • Neuromuscular impairment (multiple sclerosis, Parkinson's disease, spinal injuries) • Musculoskeletal impairment (arthritis, fractures, muscular dystrophy) • Perceptual or cognitive impairment (cerebrovascular accident, brain tumor or trauma, vision disorders) • Pain or discomfort (burns, rheumatoid arthritis, chronic pain syndrome, postoperative pain) • Depression or severe anxiety (neurosis, schizophrenia)
External factors affecting mobility	Is there anything else you can think of that limits your ability to get around? • Environmental factors (stairs, lack of railings or other assistive devices, unsafe neighborhood) • Financial resources

normal, coordinated movements; seldom repeat themselves

Athetosis—movements that are slower, more twisting and writhing than chorea movements and have a larger amplitude; commonly involve the face and distal extremities

Dystonia—movements similar to athetosis but that involve larger portions of the body, including the trunk; may result in grotesque, twisted postures

Fasciculations—fine, rapid, flickering, or twitching movements originating in relatively small groups of muscle fibers; vary irregularly in frequency and extent, but rarely move a joint

Myoclonus—sudden, brief, rapid, unpredictable jerks, usually involving the limbs or trunk; may be single or repetitive

Orofacial dyskinesias—repetitive, bizarre movements that chiefly involve the face, mouth, jaw, and tongue

Table 39-4
Overview of the Physical Assessment of Mobility Status

Component	Normal Finding	Significant Alterations
General ease of movement	Body movements are: • Voluntarily controlled (purposeful) • Fluid • Coordinated	Involuntary movements: • Tremors • Tics • Chorea • Athetosis • Dystonia • Fasciculations • Myoclonus • Oral-facial dyskinesias
Gait and posture	• Head erect, vertebrae are straight • Knees and feet point forward • Arms at side with elbows flexed • Arms swing freely in alternation with leg swings • While one leg is in the stance phase the other is in the swing phase	Abnormalities of gait and posture: • Spastic hemiparesis • Scissors gait • Steppage gait • Sensory ataxia • Cerebellar ataxia • Parkinsonian gait • Gait of old age • Use of assistive devices for ambulation
Alignment	Independent maintenance of correct alignment: • In the standing and sitting position, a straight line can be drawn from the ear through the shoulder and hip • In bed, the head, shoulders, and hips are aligned	• Abnormal spinal curvatures • Inability to maintain correct alignment independently
Joint structure and function	Absence of joint deformities Full range of motion	• Limitation in the normal range of motion • Increased joint mobility • Swelling or tenderness in or around the joint • Heat or redness • Crepitation • Deformities • Muscle atrophy, nodules, skin changes • Asymmetry of involvement
Muscle mass, tone, and strength	Adequate muscle mass, tone, and strength to accomplish movement and work	• Atrophy, hypertrophy • Hypotonicity (flaccidity), spasticity • Paresis or paralysis
Endurance	Ability to turn in bed, maintain correct alignment when sitting and standing, ambulate, and perform self-care activities	Physiologic or psychologic inability to tolerate an increase in activity: • Significantly increased pulse, respiration, blood pressure after rest • Shortness of breath, dyspnea • Weakness • Pallor • Confusion • Vertigo

The nurse also notes if the body movements are quick and sure or slow and deliberate. These observations communicate both a sense of the person's emotional status and self-care abilities.

The gait of the ambulatory client is also noted. The client's movements while walking should be coordinated and the posture well balanced. The arms should swing freely in alternation with leg swings. Figure 39-9 illustrates stance and swing, the two phases of the normal gait. The heel of the right foot strikes the ground (stance) while the toe of the left foot pushes off and leaves the ground, moving the leg from behind to in front of the body (swing). While one leg is in the stance phase the other is in the swing phase.

Gait abnormalities should be noted because they may place the individual at risk for injury and also because they may be indicative of intoxication or a neuromuscular disorder. Common abnormalities of gait and posture are illustrated in Figure 39-10.

If a client uses a brace, cane, walker, or crutches to assist with ambulation, this should be noted. The nurse also determines if this aid is meeting the client's needs and is being used safely. The use of a wheelchair is also noted.

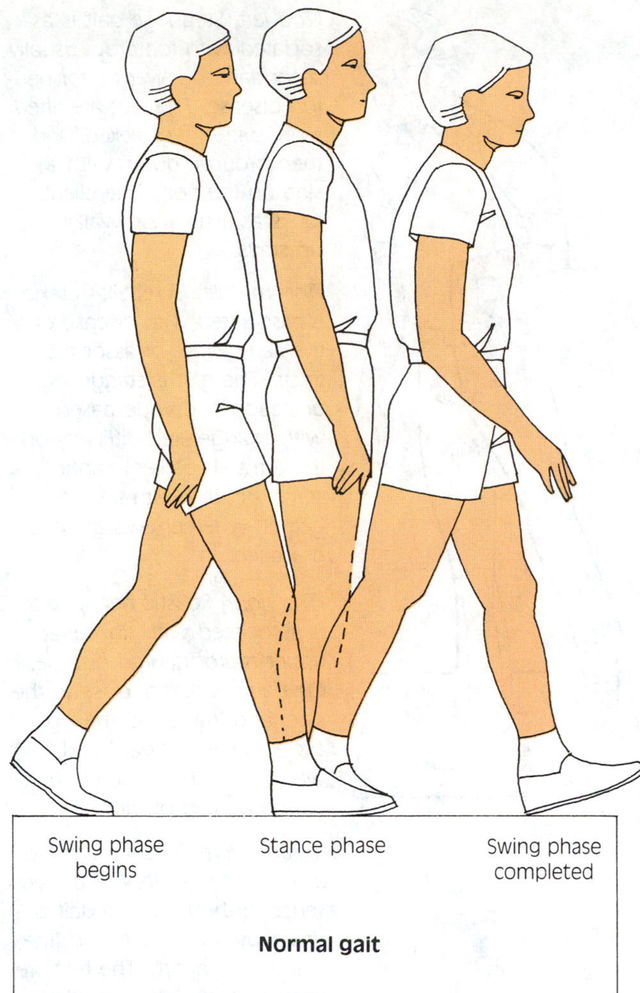

Figure 39-9
The stance and swing phases of normal gait.

Alignment

Correct body alignment permits optimal musculoskeletal balance and operation and promotes good physiologic functioning. Deviations in body alignment may result from chronic poor posture, trauma, muscle damage, or nerve dysfunction. Fatigue and a person's mental and emotional status may also influence alignment. Alignment may be observed when a client is standing, sitting, or lying (Fig. 39-11). The nurse notes whether the client is able to maintain correct alignment independently.

Correct body alignment when standing is as follows:

- The head is held erect.
- The face is in the forward position, in the same direction as the feet.
- The chest is held upward and forward.
- The spinal column is elongated, and the curves of the spine are within normal limits.
- The abdominal muscles are held upward and the buttocks downward.
- The knees are extended—not bent or hyperextended in the knee-locked position.
- The feet are at right angles to the lower legs.
- The line of gravity goes through the center of the knees and in front of the ankle joints.
- The base of support is on the soles of the feet and weight is distributed through the soles and heels.

Correct body alignment when sitting is similar to correct alignment when standing except the hips are flexed, the knees are flexed and not crossed, and the base of support is on the buttocks and upper thighs. The popliteal area should be free of the edge of the chair to prevent circulatory stasis and possible nerve injury.

Joint Structure and Function

The nurse uses inspection and palpation to examine joints, their range of motion, and the surrounding tissue. **Range of motion** is the complete extent of movement of which a joint is normally capable. See Figure 39-1, which illustrates the range of motion of selected joints. When assessing joint mobility, Bates (1995) has recommended nurses note the following:

- Any limitation in the normal range of motion or any unusual increase in the mobility of a joint (instability). Range of motion varies among individuals and decreases with aging.
- Any swelling in or around the joint. Swelling may involve the synovial membrane, which then feels boggy, or doughy, to your fingers, or may be produced by excessive synovial fluid within the joint space. Swelling sometimes originates not in the joint itself but in tissues around it, such as bones, tendons, tendon sheaths, bursae, and fat.
- Tenderness in or around the joint. Try to define the specific anatomic structure that is tender.
- Increased heat. Use the backs of your fingers to compare the joint with the symmetrical joint on the opposite side or, if both joints are involved, with the tissues near them.
- Redness of the overlying skin
- Crepitation, a palpable or even audible crunching or grating sensation produced by motion of the joint
- Deformities, such as bony enlargement, subluxation (partial dislocation), or contracture
- Condition of the surrounding tissues, including muscle atrophy, subcutaneous nodules, and skin changes
- Muscular strength
- Symmetry of involvement. Note whether arthritic changes involve several joints symmetrically on both sides of the body or affect only one or perhaps two joints (Bates, 1995, pp. 464–465).

Muscle Mass, Tone, and Strength

Adequate skeletal muscle mass, tone, and strength are prerequisites to body movement and work performance. Mass refers to muscle size. **Atrophy** describes muscle

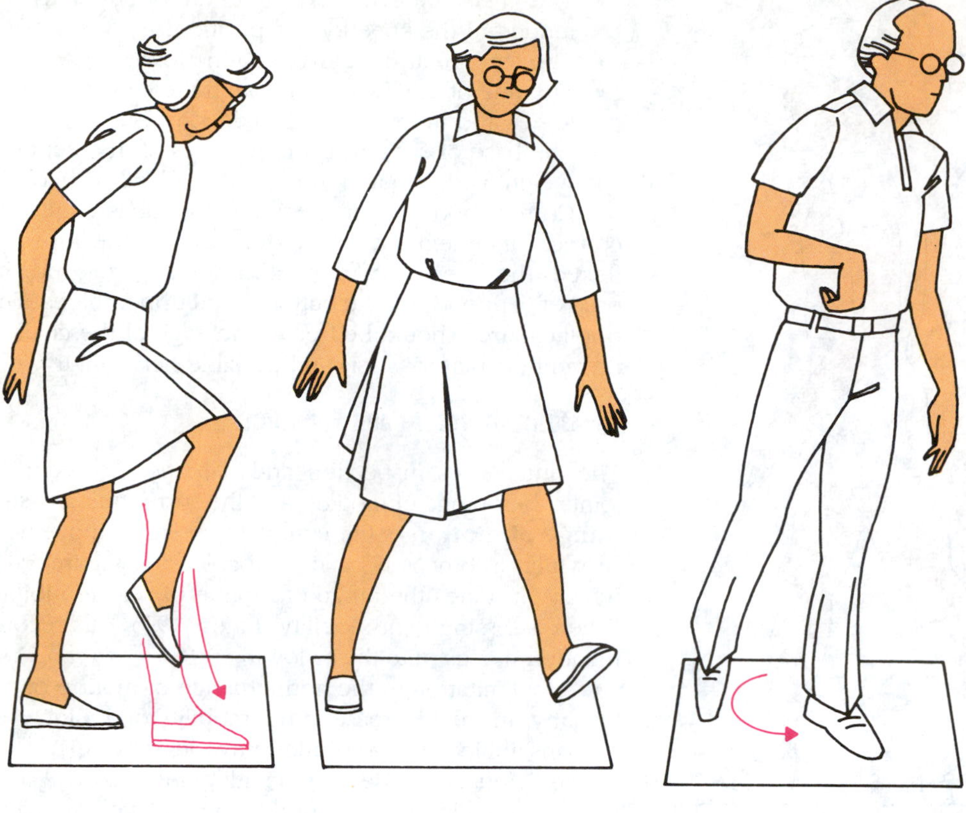

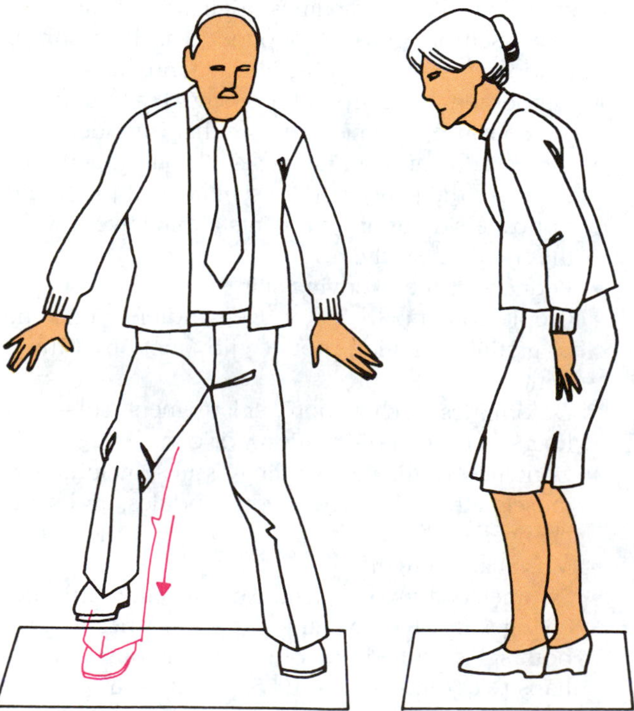

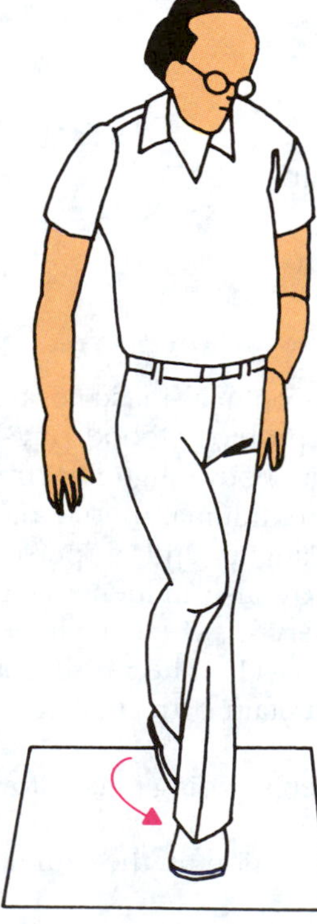

(*Top left*) Steppage gait is associated with footdrop, usually secondary to lower motor neuron disease. The feet are lifted high, with knees flexed, and then brought down with a slap on the floor. The client looks as if he were walking up stairs.

(*Top middle*) Cerebellar ataxia is associated with disease of the cerebellum or associated tracts. The gait is staggering, unsteady, and wide based, with exaggerated difficulty on the turns. The client cannot stand steadily with feet together, whether eyes are open or closed.

(*Top right*) Spastic hemiparesis is associated with unilateral upper motor neuron disease. One arm is flexed, close to the side, and immobile; the leg is circled stiffly outward and forward (circumducted), often with dragging of the toe.

(*Bottom left*) Sensory ataxia is associated with loss of position sense in the legs. The gait is unsteady and widebased (the feet are far apart). The feet are lifted high and brought down with a slap. The client watches the ground to guide his or her steps. He or she cannot stand steadily with feet together when the eyes are closed (positive Romberg's sign).

(*Bottom middle*) Parkinsonian gait is associated with the basal ganglia defects of Parkinson's disease. The posture is stooped, the hips and knees slightly flexed. Steps are short and often shuffling. Arm swings are decreased and the client turns around stiffly—"all in one piece."

(*Bottom right*) Scissors gait is associated with bilateral spastic paresis of the legs. Each leg is advanced slowly and the thighs tend to cross forward on each other at each step. The steps are short. The client looks as if he or she were walking through water.

Figure 39-10
Gait abnormalities.

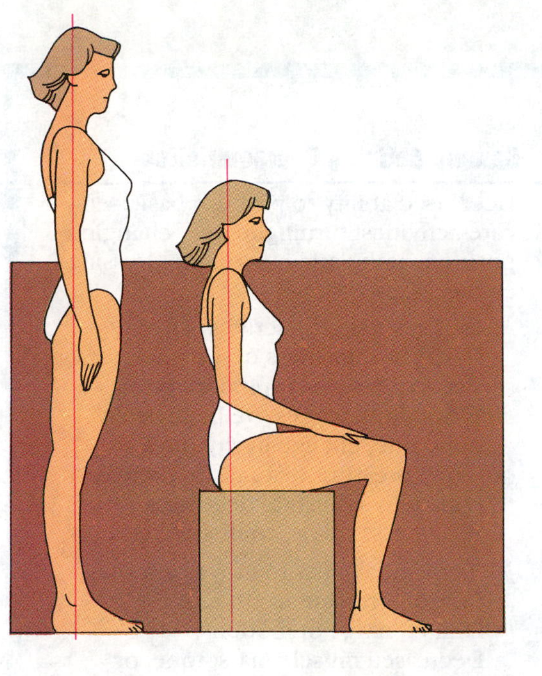

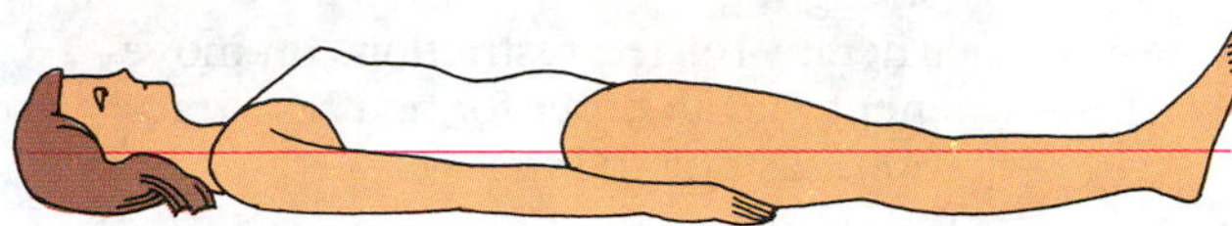

Figure 39-11
Adequate posture. In the sitting and standing positions, a straight line can be drawn from the ear through the shoulder and hip. In bed, the head, shoulders, and hips are aligned.

mass that is decreased through disuse or neurologic impairment. *Hypertrophy* refers to increased muscle mass resulting from exercise or training. The examiner assesses muscle mass throughout the body and may also compare one muscle group to another using tape measurements. Clients experiencing muscle wasting as a result of a chronic disease process such as cancer may report visible changes in muscle mass.

The slight residual tension that remains in a resting normal muscle with an intact nerve supply is termed *muscle tone*. Muscle tone may be assessed by flexing and extending the elbow or knee and noting the degree of resistance to these movements. Decreased tone, hypotonicity, or **flaccidity** results from disuse or neurologic impairments. **Spasticity**, increased tone that interferes with movement, is also caused by neurologic impairments.

Muscle *strength* varies greatly from one individual to another and within the same individual, and is affected by muscle use. Muscle strength is tested by asking the client to move actively against resistance. For example, the client may be instructed to push the examiner's palms apart or to push the foot against the examiner's palm. When comparing muscle groups it is important to remember that a person's dominant side tends to be stronger.

Impaired muscle strength or weakness is termed *paresis*. Absence of strength secondary to nervous impairment is *paralysis*. *Hemiparesis* refers to weakness of one half of the body, and *hemiplegia* to paralysis of one half of the body. *Paraplegia* is paralysis of the legs, and *quadriplegia* is paralysis of the arms and legs.

Nursing's concern is that the client's muscle strength is adequate for the performance of tasks the client deems necessary. For example, a client whose primary means of ambulation is a wheelchair requires upper body strength.

Endurance

When assessing *endurance*, the nurse evaluates the client's ability to turn in bed, maintain correct alignment when sitting or standing, ambulate, and perform self-care abilities. When a physical or psychologic factor is believed to be affecting endurance, the nurse:

- Takes the vital signs while the client is at rest
- Instructs the client to perform the activity (eg, ambulation)
- Observes the client's response during and after the activity
- Takes the vital signs immediately after the activity
- Reassesses the vital signs after the client has rested for 3 minutes

Significant findings include significantly increased pulse, respirations, and blood pressure; shortness of breath; dyspnea; weakness; pallor; confusion; and vertigo.

DIAGNOSING

The nurse must recognize cues that indicate both potential and actual problems when analyzing data about a client's mobility status. Because the problems accompanying immobility can seriously undermine well-being and often require complex and costly treatment, nursing energies are directed to preventing these problems whenever possible. The plan of care for the client with an alteration in mobility should contain nursing diagnoses that identify the complications of immobility for which the client is at greatest risk.

Nursing diagnoses specifically addressing problems of mobility include Activity Intolerance and Impaired Physical Mobility. Examples of pertinent etiologies and defining characteristics may be found in the accompanying box.

Examples of nursing diagnoses that describe the effect of mobility alterations on other areas of human functioning follow. This list is by no means exhaustive—multiple etiologies are possible for many of these problem statements.

Ineffective Airway Clearance related to prolonged bed rest, decreased position changes, ineffective coughing related to weakness

Constipation related to inactivity, decreased muscle tone

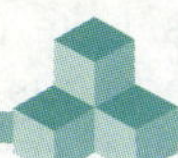

Nursing Diagnoses for Common Problems

Mobility

Problem	Related Factors	Sample Defining Characteristics
Activity Intolerance	Any condition that interferes with the transport of oxygenated blood to tissue (eg, cardiac problems such as congestive heart failure and arrhythmias; respiratory problems, especially chronic obstructive pulmonary disease; circulatory problems; diabetes mellitus) Any condition that causes fatigue (depression, pain, sleep disturbances, prolonged bed rest, sedentary lifestyle)	Decreased ability to perform basic self-care activities: turning in bed, changing position, ambulating, washing, dressing, eating, and so on Altered response to activity: • Dyspnea, shortness of breath, excessive increase in respiratory rate • Weak pulse, excessive increase in pulse rate, change in rhythm • Blood pressure that fails to increase with activity or that decreases • Weakness, pallor, confusion, vertigo
Impaired Physical Mobility	• Neuromuscular impairment (arthritis, stroke, Parkinson's disease) • Musculoskeletal impairment • Decreased strength and endurance • Pain or discomfort • Depression	• Physical inability to move purposefully or a reluctance to move • Limited range of motion • Decreased muscle mass, tone, or strength • Therapy-related restrictions on movement (eg, an order for bed rest, traction, cast, or splints)

Ineffective Breathing Pattern related to limited chest expansion (prolonged bed rest, muscle disuse, atrophy, loss of muscle coordination)

Pain related to inability to change body position independently

Pain: Joint, related to limited range of motion and muscle atrophy

Ineffective Individual Coping [or Ineffective Family Coping] related to loss of ability to move purposefully in environment, spouse's need for assistance with all self-care activities

Fluid Volume Excess related to prolonged bed rest

Impaired Gas Exchange related to decreased respiratory movement

Altered Health Maintenance related to lack of mobility to procure needed services—no support people

Impaired Home Maintenance Management related to immobility

Risk for Infection: Urinary Tract, related to urinary retention secondary to immobility

Risk for Injury: Falls related to orthostatic hypotension secondary to immobility

Risk for Injury: Venous Thrombosis related to immobility

Risk for Injury: Musculoskeletal Problems related to infrequent, excessive exercise

Knowledge Deficit: Exercise Program, related to having no previous experience with regular exercise

Noncompliance With Exercise Prescription related to decreased endurance, decreased motivation

Powerlessness related to inability to move self

Self-Care Deficit: Bathing/Hygiene, Feeding, Dressing/Grooming, Toileting, related to physical weakness (decreased muscle mass and strength), altered mobility (upper or lower extremities)

Self-Esteem Disturbance related to postural deviation, inability to perform self-care activities, inability to meet role expectations

Sexual Dysfunction related to neuromuscular impairment

Impaired Skin Integrity related to inability to change positions independently, prolonged bed rest

Sleep Pattern Disturbance related to lack of exercise (sedentary lifestyle)

Impaired Social Interaction related to decreased activity tolerance

Urinary Retention related to prolonged bed rest

Altered Tissue Perfusion (Cardiopulmonary) related to prolonged supine position and greater volume of circulating blood

For clients who are incorporating some form of exercise in their daily routine, the following wellness diagnoses may be appropriate:

Potential for Enhanced Activity Level

Potential for Enhanced Compliance With Exercise Regimen

PLANNING: EXPECTED OUTCOMES

If the client is not experiencing any mobility problems, expected client outcomes are directed toward the promotion of physical fitness. For example, the client will:

- Follow a program of regular physical exercise that improves cardiovascular function, endurance, flexibility, and strength

To achieve this long-term expected outcome, numerous short-term expected outcomes may be needed. An example follows.

By the next visit, 2/20/98, the client will:

- Identify four personal benefits of regular exercise
- Describe an exercise program (activities, frequency, duration) client is willing to follow
- Identify the target heart range
- Obtain medical clearance for the exercise program if at high risk for complications
- List support systems that will reinforce exercise efforts

Clients at high risk for developing specific mobility problems require different expected outcomes. The client will:

- Demonstrate correct body alignment whenever observed (alignment)
- Adhere to an every-2-hour positioning schedule (alignment)
- Demonstrate full range of joint motion (joint mobility)
- Demonstrate adequate muscle mass, tone, and strength to perform functional activities of daily living (muscle mass, tone, and strength)

Specific expected outcomes for the client at risk of developing complications related to immobility may be found in Table 39-3. Goals for more specific problems, for example, for the client learning to walk with crutches or needing to master transfer techniques with only upper body mobility, need to be individualized to the client.

IMPLEMENTING

Nursing strategies designed to promote correct body alignment, mobility, and fitness are described in this section. Techniques for positioning clients; performing range-of-motion exercises; moving, lifting, and ambulating clients; and designing exercise programs are highlighted.

Positioning Clients

Positioning that maintains correct body alignment and facilitates physiologic functioning contributes to the client's psychologic and physical well-being. The force of gravity pulls parts of the body out of alignment unless adequate support is provided. Various positions are therefore protective in nature only when the client is positioned properly.

Common Devices to Promote Correct Alignment

Many devices can help maintain good body alignment and muscle tonus while the client is in bed and alleviate discomfort or pressure on various parts of the body.

Pillows. Pillows are used primarily to provide support or to provide elevation of a part. Pillows of different sizes are useful for different body parts. Those intended for the head are usually full- or large-sized

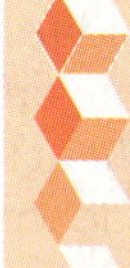

Helpscan

The following are resources for clients and health-care professionals:

- For a free "Lift It Safe" brochure call: (800) 824-BONES or (800) 824-2663 or, send a self-addressed, stamped business-size envelope to:
  LIFT IT SAFE
  American Academy of Orthopaedic Surgeons
  P.O. Box 1998
  Des Plaines, IL 60017
- For information on independent living for the older adult contact:
  National Voluntary Organization for Independent Living for the Aged
  c/o National Council on Aging
  West Wing, Suite 100
  600 Maryland Avenue SW
  Washington, DC 20024
- For "Age Pages" (short fact sheets developed by the National Institute on Aging to give older adults an overview of aging-related subjects, including tips and skills aimed at promoting health) contact:
  NIA Information Center
  Department AGS
  P.O. Box 8057
  Gaithersburg, MD 29898-8057
  (800) 222-2225

pillows. Small pillows are ideal for support or elevation of the extremities, shoulders, or incisional wounds. Specially designed heavy pillows are useful to elevate the upper part of the body when an adjustable bed is unavailable, such as in a home situation.

Mattresses. For a mattress to be comfortable and supportive, it must be firm but have sufficient "give" to permit good body alignment. A client who must remain in a bed with a nonsupportive mattress might well complain of backache and other discomforts.

A well-made and well-supported foam-rubber mattress retains a uniform firmness. This mattress is made of natural or synthetic rubber, or both in combination. A large volume of air is incorporated. The foam-rubber mattress conforms to the contours of the body and supplies support at all points. Its greatest advantage is that it does not form slopes and valleys as the innerspring mattresses are likely to do. Moreover, the foam-rubber mattress does not create as much pressure against bony prominences, such as the ankles, the elbows, the scapulae, and the coccyx. Special mattresses, pads, and types of beds used to help prevent pressure ulcers are discussed in Chapter 38.

Bed Board. If the mattress does not provide sufficient support, a bed board may help to keep the client in better alignment. Bed boards usually are made of plywood or some other firm composition. The size varies with the needs of the situation. For home use, full bed boards are available commercially or can easily be made at home from available materials.

Adjustable Bed. The head of an adjustable bed can be elevated to the desired degree. This positioning is discussed later in the chapter. The foot of an adjustable bed can also be elevated to the desired degree. Some adjustable beds allow the bed to be "broken," or gatched, so that the client can rest the knees over an elevated portion of the mattress. This position is rarely recommended or is used only for brief periods because it may cause nerve injury and decreased circulation.

The adjustable bed can also be changed so that the distance of the bed to the floor can be altered. The client can get in and out of bed easier when the bed is in the lowest position. The higher positions are used by healthcare workers so they do not strain their backs while giving bed care. General guidelines for safe use of beds are discussed in Chapter 37.

Circular Bed. The electric circular bed is a 6- or 7-foot metal frame with a diameter support for the client. The direction of the support can be changed so the client can be placed in a variety of positions. This bed is especially useful for the client who will be completely helpless for an extended period.

Stryker Frame. The Stryker frame is a narrow support that can be turned 360 degrees. The client can be alternated between the supine and prone positions without changing alignment. This bed is particularly useful for the totally immobilized client, such as one who is paralyzed.

Footboards. The greatest danger to the feet occurs when they are unsupported in the dorsal flexion position. The toes drop downward, and the feet are in plantar flexion. Because of the pull of gravity, this position of the feet occurs naturally when the body is at rest. If maintained for extended periods, plantar flexion can cause an alteration in the length of muscles, and the client may develop a complication called **footdrop**. In this position, the foot is unable to maintain itself in the perpendicular position, heel-toe gait is impossible, and the client will experience extreme difficulty in walking. The use of a foot support, such as the footboard, helps avoid this complication. Figure 39-12 demonstrates a foot in plantar flexion versus the dorsiflexion position maintained when a footboard is used. The footboard also provides a firm surface against which the feet of the bedfast client can be placed for proprioceptor stimulation.

Commercial footboards are generally adjustable for clients of different heights. The footboard must come far enough up from the foot of the bed so that the client's feet rest firmly against it without the client sliding down in bed. Also, the footboard should not be so far from the foot of the bed that the client's knees are flexed when the feet are against it.

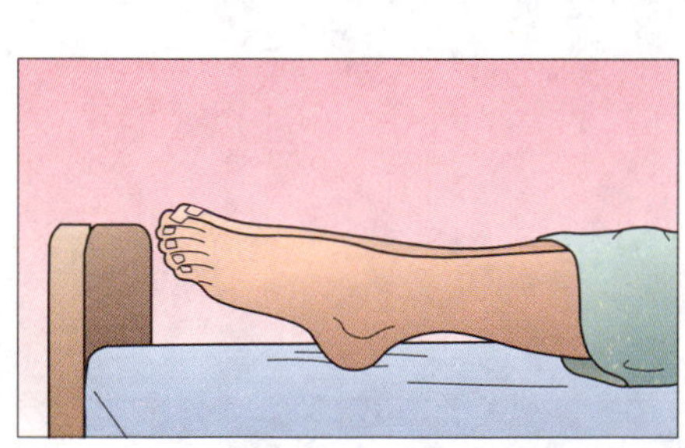

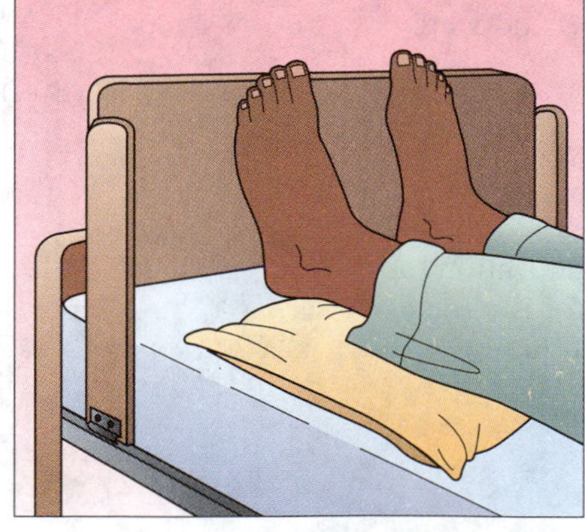

Figure 39-12
A footboard helps prevent footdrop in the unconscious client. (*Left*) Plantar flexion occurs when the foot is not supported. (*Right*) When a footboard is placed in support of the feet the dorsiflexion position is maintained.

If the client is in a sitting position while in bed, the footboard must be placed at an angle. This prevents hyperextension of the knees, which would result if the feet were kept in dorsiflexion while the trunk was flexed forward. Some clients at risk for developing footdrop are also being advised to wear high-top canvas sneakers while on bed rest, in conjunction with the footboard.

Cradle. If top bedding must be kept off the client's lower extremities, a device called a cradle is used. A *cradle* is usually a metal frame that supports the bed linens away from the client while providing privacy and warmth. There are any number of sizes and shapes of cradles. If used, the cradle should be fastened securely to the bed so that it does not slide or fall on the client.

Sandbags. Sandbags immobilize an extremity and support body alignment. Their value is enhanced if they are available in various sizes. When properly filled, they are not hard or firmly packed. They should be pliable enough to be shaped to body contours and to give support. They should be placed so they do not create pressure on a bony prominence.

Trochanter Rolls. Trochanter rolls are used to support the hips and legs so that the femurs do not rotate outward. Figure 39-13 illustrates and describes how to use trochanter rolls. Properly placed pillows can also be used to help prevent the thighs from turning outward, but they tend to slip out of place and require frequent adjusting to be effective.

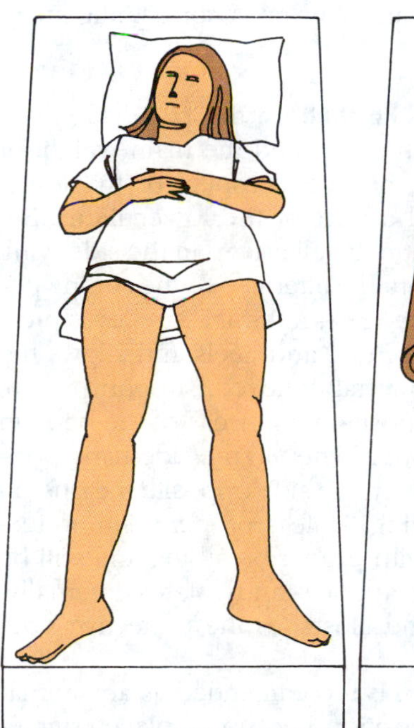

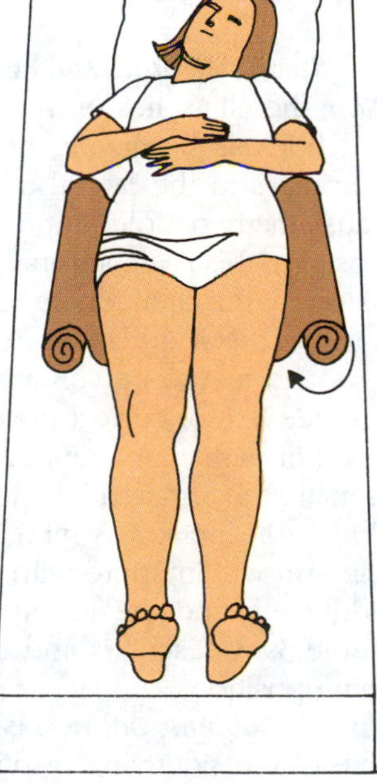

Figure 39-13
Trochanter rolls prevent the external rotation of the hips of a bedridden client. The client is placed on a folded sheet so that the top edge is at the hips and the lower edge is about one third of the way down the thighs. Towels or a bath blanket is rolled under each side until the roll is snugly against the client's hips and thighs. The support cannot unroll, and the weight of the client keeps it secure.

Hand–Wrist Splints. If a client is paralyzed or unconscious, it may be necessary to provide a means for keeping the thumb in the correct position, that is, slightly adducted and in apposition to the fingers. A commercial plastic or aluminum splint may be used to hold the thumb in place no matter what position the hand is in. Clients who are not moving their fingers should be encouraged to do finger exercises with special attention to having the thumb touch the tip of each finger.

Bed Side Rails. One of nursing personnel's greatest safety concerns is to prevent clients from falling out of bed. The use of side rails requires explanation to clients and their families and must follow the protocol of the healthcare agency. They help to remind clients that they are not in their usual environment, should they awaken during the night and wish to get out of bed. Side rails also make it possible for a client to roll from one side to the other or to sit up without calling for assistance. This in itself is a good activity: it helps the client retain or regain muscle efficiency.

Bed side rails may not deter some clients from getting out of bed. Many a client has crawled over the foot of the bed. It currently is recommended that side rails extend only for three fourths of the length of the mattress. Then, if side rails are in use and clients do attempt to get out of bed, they do not have to climb over the side rail or the foot of the bed and further increase the danger of falling. When a client sleeps restlessly or has frequent involuntary movements of the extremities and is in danger of harming himself or herself against the side rails, protective padding may be ordered. Safe use of side rails is discussed in Chapter 27.

Trapeze Bar. A *trapeze bar* (see Fig. 39-14) is a handgrip suspended from a frame near the head of the bed. The client can grasp the bar with one or both hands and then raise the trunk from the bed. The trapeze makes moving and turning considerably easier for many clients and facilitates transfers into and out of bed. It can also be used to perform exercises that strengthen some muscles of the upper extremities (eg, biceps).

Protective Positioning

Clients accustomed to an active lifestyle who generally only use a bed for sleep are often unaware of the importance of correct body alignment and regular position changes when on prescribed bed rest. Whenever possible, nurses should teach both the client and family the following:

- Correct positioning techniques
- The need to change positions frequently, at least every 2 hours

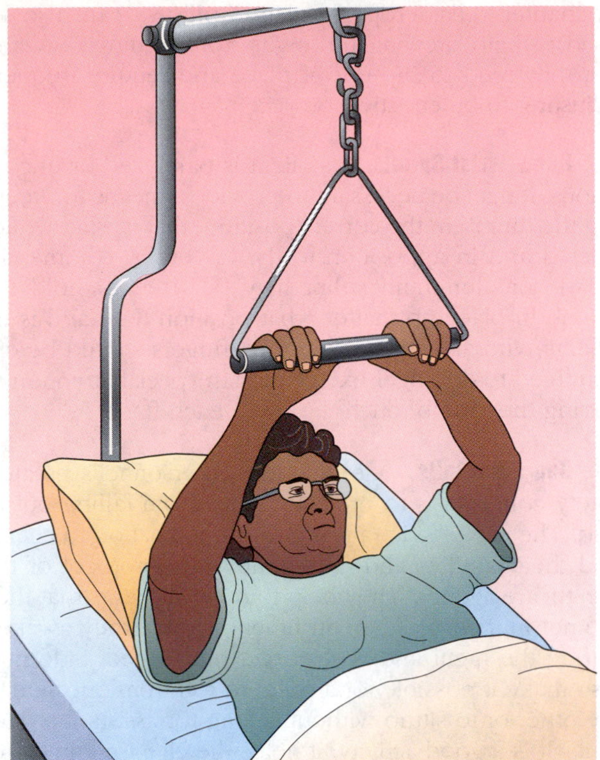

Figure 39-14
A trapeze device makes it possible for the client to lift part of the body from the bed, thus facilitating turning and moving up in bed.

- The importance of using the time allotted to position changes to exercise the extremities and to assess and massage pressure areas (Reddened areas should not be massaged.)

When the client is unable to change position independently, a turn schedule should be posted at the bedside so that nurses assist with and document the rotation of positions. Table 39-5 describes nursing measures to prevent complications associated with common bed positions.

Fowler's Position. The semisitting position is called *Fowler's position* and calls for the head of the bed to be elevated 45 to 60 degrees. This position is often used to promote cardiac and respiratory functioning because abdominal organs drop in this position and thereby provide maximal space in the thoracic cavity. This is also the position of choice for eating, conversation, vision, and urinary and intestinal elimination.

Variations of Fowler's position include high Fowler's and low Fowler's or semi-Fowler's position. In the high Fowler's position, the head of the bed is elevated 90 degrees. When a bedside table with a pillow on top of it is placed in front of the client in high Fowler's position, the client can lean forward and rest the arms on the pillow, assuming a posture that allows for maximal lung expansion. In the low or *semi-Fowler's position,* the head of the bed is elevated 30 degrees. In Fowler's position, the buttocks bear the main weight of the body. Other skin areas that require assessment and massage include the heels, the sacrum, and the scapulae.

The arms and feet need particular attention when the client is in a semisitting position. Unless properly supported, the arms fall to the bed and pull on the shoulders, and the feet fall into a footdrop position. Supportive devices may be necessary, including pillows supporting the upper back and head, the elbows and wrist joints, the lower back, the thighs, and the ankles; trochanter rolls; and a footboard. The correct positioning and nursing actions to prevent complications associated with the Fowler's position are presented in Table 39-5.

Supine or Dorsal Recumbent Position. In the *supine position,* the client lies flat on the back with the head and shoulders slightly elevated with a pillow unless contraindicated. The pillow under the head and upper shoulders may not be allowed following a spinal anesthetic or surgery on the spinal vertebrae.

The body areas in need of attention when in the supine position are the feet, elbows, and neck. Pillows are almost always used to support the head to tilt it forward so that the person's vision is improved. This causes flexion of the cervical spine. The feet will fall into a plantar flexion position unless support is provided. Elbow protectors may need to be applied on a restless client to relieve pressure on that area. Table 39-5 describes nursing actions to prevent complications associated with this position and illustrates correct alignment in the supine position.

Side-Lying or Lateral Position. In the *side-lying position,* the client lies on the side and the main weight of the body is borne by the lateral aspect of the lower scapula and the lateral aspect of the lower ilium. Because many people routinely fall asleep in the side-lying position, this is a comfortable alternate to the supine position for the client on bed rest. Although it relieves pressure on the scapulae, sacrum, and heels and allows the legs and feet to be comfortably flexed, support pillows are needed for correct positioning. Areas of the body in need of particular attention when in the side-lying position are the arm and leg on the side opposite the one on which the person is lying. Unless properly supported, the arm will interfere with proper breathing and will be adducted, and the leg adducts and rotates internally. Table 39-5 describes and illustrates the protective side-lying position.

The *oblique position* is recommended as an alternative to the side-lying position because it places significantly less pressure on the trochanter region. The client turns toward the side with the hip on the top leg flexed at a 30-degree angle and the knee flexed at 35 degrees. The calf of the upper leg is positioned slightly behind the body's midline. Pillows support the client's back and calf of the top leg (Fig. 39-15).

A variation of the lateral position is the *Sims' position.* In this position, the client again lies on the side but

Table 39-5
Common Bed Positions and Protective Nursing Actions

Position	Complication to Be Prevented	Suggested Preventive Actions
Fowler's Position		
	Flexion contracture of the neck	Allow the head to rest against the mattress or be supported by a small pillow only.
	Exaggerated curvature of the spine	Use a firm support for the back; position the client so the angle of elevation starts at the hips.
	Dislocation of the shoulder	Support the forearms on pillows to elevate them sufficiently so that no pull is exerted on the shoulders.
	Flexion contracture of the wrist	Support the hand on pillows so it is in natural alignment with the forearm.
	Edema of the hand	Support the hand so it is slightly elevated in relation to the elbow.
	Flexion contractures of the fingers and abduction of the thumbs	Provide hand–wrist splints if necessary.
	Impaired lower extremity circulation and knee contracture, pressure on heels	Elevate the knees for only brief periods; place one or two pillows under the lower legs from below the knees to the ankles; avoid pressure on the popliteal vessels; avoid using the knee gatch.
	External rotation of the hips	Use trochanter roll.
	Footdrop	Support the feet in dorsal flexion. Use footboard; high-top sneakers can also be used.
Protective Supine Position		
	Exaggerated curvature of the spine and flexion of the hips	Provide a firm supportive mattress; use a bed board if necessary.
	Flexion contracture of the neck	Place pillows under the upper shoulders, the neck, and the head so that the head and the neck are held in the correct position.
	Internal rotation of the shoulders and extension of the elbows (hunch shoulders)	Place pillows or arm supports under the forearms so that the upper arms are alongside the body and the forearms are pronated slightly.
	Flexion of the lumbar curvature	Place rolled towel or small pillow under lumbar curvature if needed.
	Extension of the fingers and abduction of the thumbs (clawhand deformities)	Use hand–wrist splints if appropriate.
	External rotation of the femurs	Place sandbags or a trochanter roll alongside the hips and the upper half of the thighs.
	Hyperextension of the knees	Place a pillow under the lower legs from below the knees to the ankles.
	Footdrop	Use a footboard or make an improvised firm foot support to hold the feet in dorsal flexion; high-top sneakers may also be recommended.

(continued)

Table 39-5 *(continued)*
Common Bed Positions and Protective Nursing Actions

Position	Complication to Be Prevented	Suggested Preventive Actions
Protective Side-Lying or Lateral Position		
	Lateral flexion of the neck	Place a pillow under the head and the neck.
	Inward rotation of the arm and interference with respiration	Place a pillow under the upper arm; lower arm should be flexed and positioned comfortably.
	Extension of the finger and abduction of the thumbs	Provide hand–wrist splint if necessary.
	Internal rotation and adduction of the femur	Use one or two pillows as needed to support the leg from the groin to the foot.
	Twisting of the spine	Ensure that the two shoulders are aligned with the two hips.
Protective Sims' Position		
	Lateral flexion of the neck	Place a small pillow under the head unless the drainage of oral secretions is desired.
	Damage to nerves and blood vessels in the axillae of the lower arm	Carefully position lower arm behind and away from the client's back.
	Internal shoulder rotation and adduction	Abduct the upper shoulder slightly so that shoulder and elbow are flexed; place a pillow between the chest and upper arm.
	Internal rotation and adduction of the hip; lumbar lordosis	Place a pillow under the upper flexed leg from the groin to the foot.
	Twisting of the spine	Ensure that the two shoulders are aligned with the two hips.
	Footdrop	Support the lower foot in dorsal flexion with a sandbag.
Protective Prone Position		
	Flexion on the cervical spine	Place a small pillow under the head.
	Hyperextension of the spine; impaired respirations	Place some suitable support under the client between the end of the rib cage and the upper abdomen if this facilitates breathing and if there is space there.
	Footdrop	Move the client down in bed so that the feet are over the mattress, or support the lower legs on a pillow just high enough to keep the toes from touching the bed.

the lower arm is behind the client and the upper arm is flexed at both the shoulder and the elbow. Because in this position the main body weight is borne by the anterior aspects of the humerus, clavicle, and ilium, the major pressure points differ from those in the lateral and other bed-lying positions (see Table 39-5).

Prone Position. In the *prone position*, the person lies on the abdomen with the head turned to the side. The body is straightened out in the prone position because the shoulders, head, and neck are in an erect position, the arms are easily placed in correct alignment with the shoulder girdle, the hips are extended, and the knees can be prevented from flexing or hyperextending. When clients on bed rest use this position periodically, it helps to prevent flexion contractures of the hips and knees. However, the pull of gravity on the trunk when the client lies prone produces a marked lordosis. The position is thus contraindicated for people with spinal problems. The pull of gravity on the feet may result in plantar flex-

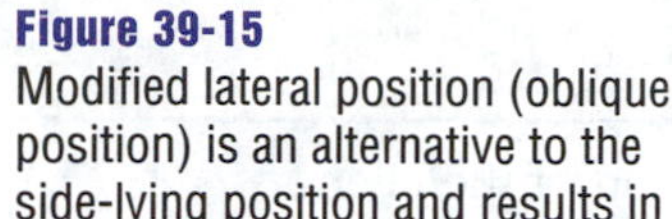

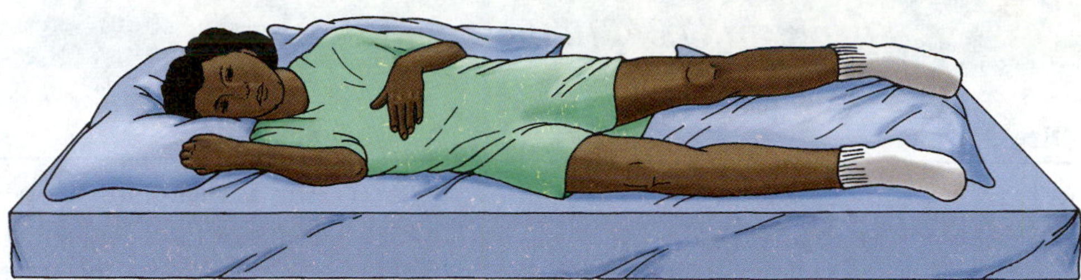

Figure 39-15
Modified lateral position (oblique position) is an alternative to the side-lying position and results in significantly less pressure on the trochanter area.

ion unless the legs and feet are positioned carefully. Table 39-5 illustrates correct alignment in the prone position and describes nursing activities to prevent complications. Placing a client in the prone position requires that the nurse and an assistant move the person as far as is safely possible onto his or her side, facing the direction that the person will be turned, and near the edge of the level bed. While maintaining the client securely in that position, pillows can be situated alongside the trunk and upper and lower extremities. Once the client is gently turned face down, the pillows can be readjusted for comfort and support.

Turning the Client in Bed

Frequently, the client is unable to turn in bed without assistance. Nurses need to use correct body mechanics and knowledge of correct alignment to turn the client from the back onto the side, from the back onto the abdomen, and from the abdomen onto the back. The technique for turning a client in bed is described and illustrated in Procedure 39-1. Mastering this turning technique will help the nurse to adhere to an every-2-hour turn schedule for an immobile client.

Assisting With Range-of-Motion Exercises

Range of motion is the complete extent of movement of which a joint is normally capable. Engaging in routine tasks, such as bathing, eating, dressing, and writing, helps use muscle groups that keep many joints in effective range of motion. When all or some of normal activities of daily living are impossible, attention should be given to the joints not being used at all or to those that are limited in their use.

Unless contraindicated, active, active-assistive, or passive range-of-motion exercises should be encouraged regularly and included in the client's plan of care. In **active exercise**, the client independently moves joints through their full range of motion (isotonic exercise). In *active–assistive exercise*, the nurse may provide minimal support, whereas in **passive exercise**, the client is unable to move independently and the nurse moves each joint through its range of motion. Both active and passive exercises improve joint mobility and increase circulation to the affected part, but only active exercise increases muscle mass, tone, and strength and improves cardiac and respiratory functioning. Thus, exercises should be as active as the client's physical condition permits. It is also helpful to teach isometric exercises to clients to increase muscle mass, tone, and strength.

Directives should be included in the nursing plan of care for range-of-motion exercises. The nursing orders should explain what, how, and when, so that all who care for the client observe the same routine. In some institutions, nurses work closely with physiotherapists in designing and implementing exercise programs. The following are basic guidelines for the nurse when helping to put the client's joints through range of motion:

- Teach the client what exercising is being undertaken, why, and how it will be done. Using a show-and-tell technique is often helpful.
- Avoid overexertion and using exercises to the point that the client develops fatigue. The exercises are not to exhaust or tax the client. Certain exercises may need to be delayed until the client's condition allows.
- Avoid neck hyperextension and attempts to achieve full range of motion in all joints with the older client. These movements may prove painful. Encourage adequate range of motion in those joints necessary to perform activities of daily living.
- Start gradually and work slowly. All movements should be smooth and rhythmic. Irregular and jerky movements are uncomfortable for the client.
- Move each joint until there is resistance but not pain. Uncomfortable reactions should be reported and exercises halted until further instructions are obtained.
- While exercising joints, use a variety of support measures to prevent muscle strain or injury to the client (Fig. 39-16):
  - *Cupping*—placing a cupped hand under the joint to support it (eg, under the elbow)
  - *Cradling*—supporting the joint with one hand while cradling the distal portion of the extremity with the remaining arm (eg, the calf or forearm might be cradled while the knee or elbow is supported)
  - *Supporting* the joint by holding the adjacent distal and proximal muscular areas (indicated when a joint is painful); grasping muscle groups or major tendons is likely to cause injury to the tissues.
- Return the joint to a neutral position, that is, its normal position of alignment, when finishing each exercise.

PROCEDURE 39-1

Turning a Client in Bed

Action	Rationale
1. Explain the procedure to the client.	This facilitates the cooperation of the client.
2. Wash your hands.	Handwashing deters the spread of microorganisms.
3. Raise the bed to your waist level. Adjust to flat position or as low as the client can tolerate. Lower side rail nearest you and raise the opposite side.	This position facilitates the turning maneuver and minimizes strain on the nurse yet keeps the client safe.
4. Position the client closer to the far side of the bed in the supine position.	The client will be in the center of the bed after turning is accomplished.
5. Place the client's arms across the chest and cross the client's far leg over the near one.	This facilitates the turning motion and protects the client's arms during the turn.
6. Stand opposite the client's center with your feet spread and one foot ahead of the other. Tighten your gluteal and abdominal muscles and flex your knees.	This positions the turner opposite the center of the body mass. It places the nurse in a stable position with good body alignment and prepared to use large muscle masses to turn the client.

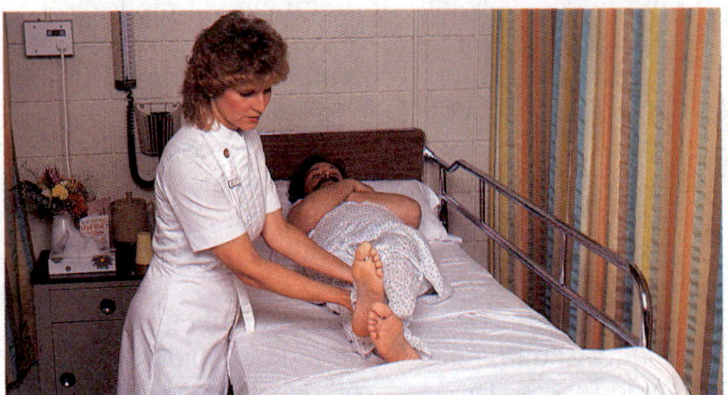

Action 5: Positioning client's arms and legs.

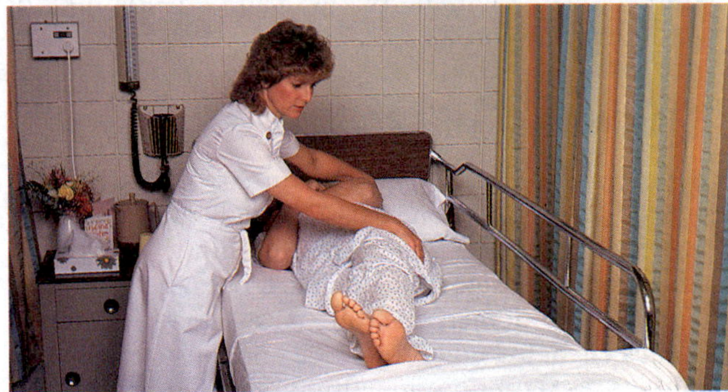

Action 6: Preparing to turn client.

Action	Rationale
7. Position your hands on the client's far shoulder and hip and roll the client toward you.	This maneuver supports the client's body and makes use of the nurse's weight to assist with turning.
8. Make the client comfortable and position in proper alignment.	This ensures that the client will be able to maintain desired position.

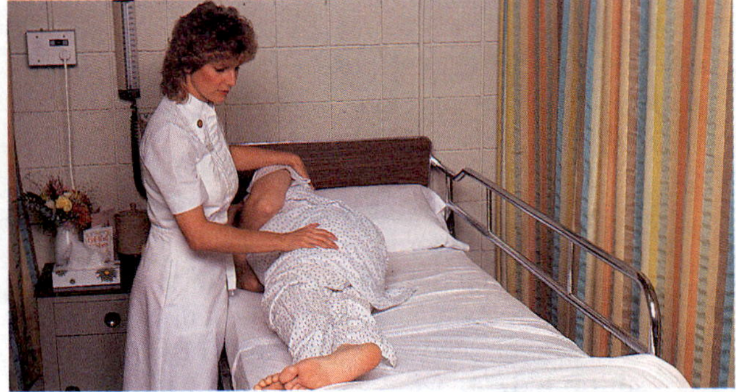

Action 7: Turning client.

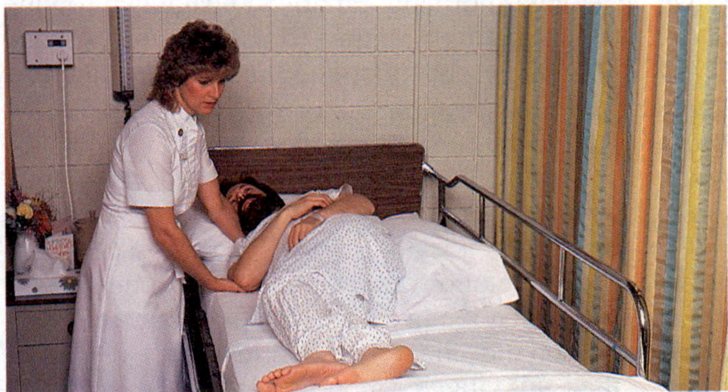

Action 8: Making client comfortable.

Action	Rationale
9. Readjust the bed height and position and raise side rail if appropriate.	This ensures the client's safety.
10. Wash your hands.	Handwashing deters the spread of microorganisms.

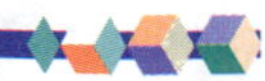

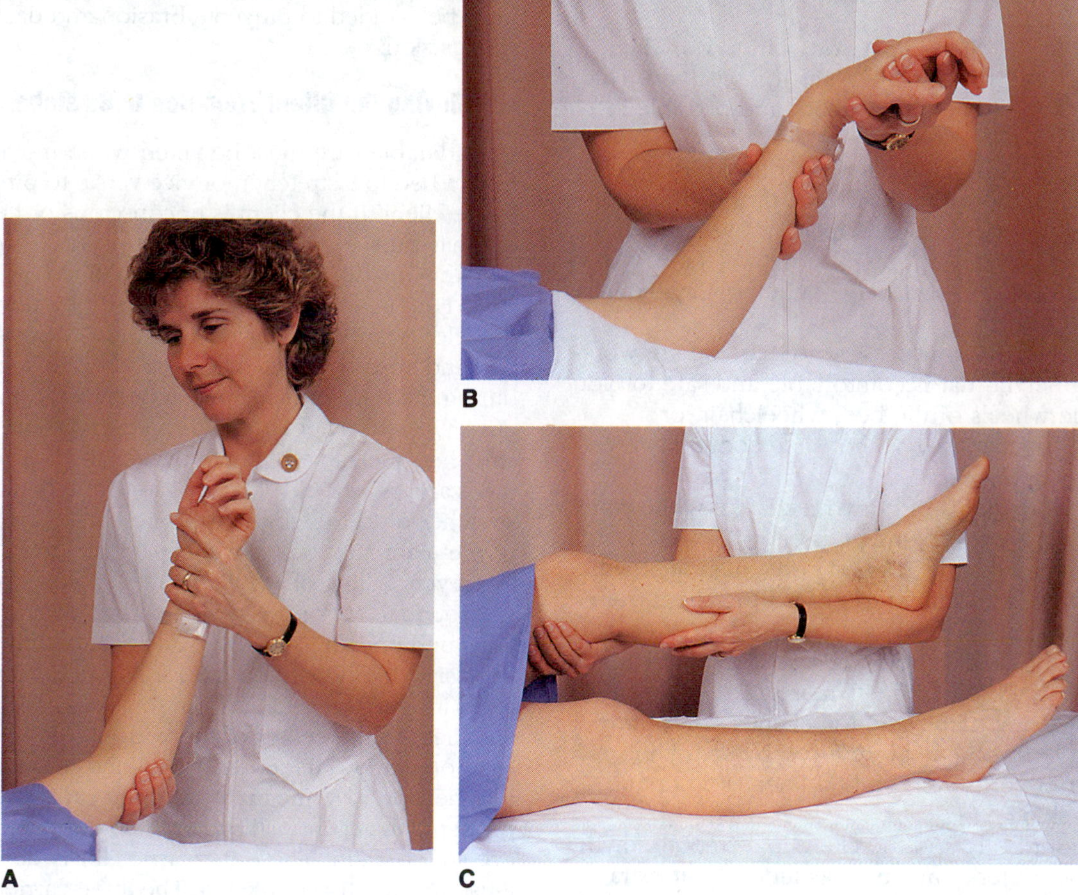

Figure 39-16
Support measures used to prevent muscle strain or injury to the client during range-of-motion exercises (**A**) using a cupped hand to support a joint; (**B**) cradling the distal portion of an extremity; and (**C**) supporting the joint by holding the distal and proximal areas adjacent to the joint.

- Keep friction at a minimum when moving extremities to avoid injuring the skin.
- Use range-of-motion exercises twice a day, and do the exercises regularly to build up muscle and joint capabilities. Each exercise is carried out two to five times. Many of the exercises can be carried out when the client is being bathed and become part of that procedure. Routine tasks, such as eating, dressing, self-bathing, and writing, also help to put certain joints through range of motion and should be encouraged.
- Expect the client's respiratory and heart rate to increase during exercising, which is good. These rates should return to normal within a few minutes. If they do not, the exercises are probably too strenuous for the client.
- Use passive exercises as necessary, but encourage active exercises of the same kind when the client is able to do so independently. Exercises should continue at home after a period of hospitalization, as necessary.

The goal of range-of-motion exercises is to keep the client in the best possible physical state while bed rest is necessary. When range-of-motion exercises are not considered as routine measures, the client's physician should be consulted. Figure 39-1 illustrates the normal movement incorporated in passive range-of-motion exercises.

Moving and Lifting the Client

Frequently it is necessary to move a helpless client. The client must be kept in good alignment and protected from injury while being moved. There are certain recommended guidelines the nurse should follow when moving and lifting clients:

- Know the client's diagnosis, capabilities, and any movement not allowed. Place braces or any device the client wears before helping from bed.
- Plan carefully what you will do before moving or lifting a client. Assess mobility of attached equipment. You may injure the client or yourself if you

have not planned well. If necessary, enlist the support of another nurse. This reduces the strain on all involved.

- Explain to the client what you plan to do. Then, use what abilities the client has to assist you. This technique often decreases work and possible injury to yourself.
- If the client is in pain, administer the prescribed analgesic sufficiently in advance of the transfer to allow the client to participate in the move comfortably.
- Remove obstacles that may make moving and lifting inconvenient.
- Elevate the bed as necessary so that you are working at a height that is comfortable and safe for you.
- Lock the wheels of the bed, wheelchair, or stretcher so that they do not slide about while you are moving the client.
- Observe principles of body mechanics while you work to prevent injuring yourself.
- Be sure the client is in good body alignment while being moved and lifted to protect the client from strain and muscle injury.
- Support the client's body well. Avoid grabbing and holding an extremity by its muscles.
- Avoid causing friction on the client's skin during moving. Friction can be reduced by sprinkling powder or cornstarch on bed linens and on the client's skin.
- Move your body and the client in a smooth, rhythmic motion. Jerky movements tend to put extra strain on muscles and joints and are uncomfortable for the client.
- Use mechanical devices such as a Hoyer lift or turning board when they are available for moving clients. Be sure that you understand how the device operates and that the client is properly secured and informed of what will occur. Clients who do not understand or are afraid may be unable to cooperate and may suffer injury as a result.
- Be realistic about how much you can safely do without injury. Two small people cannot lift or move an obese client without risking muscle strain and injury.

Moving the Client Up in Bed

Children and lightweight adults are relatively easy to slide toward the head of the bed without the assistance of a second person. A technique used to move a client up in bed when the client is able to assist is described and illustrated in Procedure 39-2. The procedure also describes and illustrates how two nurses can move the client up in bed.

Using a Sheet to Move the Client Up in Bed. Although the methods described may be convenient, the amount of effort expended by two nurses moving a client up in bed can be reduced. A drawsheet or a large sheet placed under the client's midsection can be used to lift the client safely. Friction between the lift sheet and the bed linen must be avoided to prevent abrasion and damage to the client's skin.

Moving the Client From Bed to Stretcher

Considerable care must be taken when moving a client from a bed to a stretcher, or vice versa, to prevent injury to the client. If the client is unconscious or helpless, additional nurses are needed to support the extremities and the head. The skills are explained in Procedure 39-3. For clients who are obese, use of a transfer board or roller board will facilitate the move from stretcher to bed and ensure that the client's body is properly aligned during the transfer (see Special Considerations in Procedure 39-3). When returning the client to the bed from the stretcher, the same techniques are observed. However, the carriers should first move the client from the stretcher onto the edge of the bed. Then, one member of the team supports the client on the edge of the bed to prevent falling off while the other two team members go around to the opposite side of the bed and place their arms underneath the client. After the two people on the opposite side of the bed have a good grip on the client, the third person is able to join them and assist in sliding the client to the center of the bed.

Sometimes clients must be lifted and carried. This can be done by means of a three-carrier lift. If done properly, the client will feel secure, and those lifting will not suffer strain. The three-carrier lift is described and illustrated in Procedure 39-4. The three-carrier lift is used in various other situations, such as lifting a client who has fallen to the floor and is unable to get up independently or lifting a client out of a chair into the bed.

For clients who present special problems because of their excessive weight or a cast, it may be necessary to have an additional person to support the heaviest or most cumbersome part of the client. The people distribute their arms while carrying so that the heaviest part is well supported.

Moving the Client From Bed to Chair

Safety and comfort are paramount concerns when the nurse assists the client out of bed. Preliminary assessment of vital signs provides baseline data and subsequent recordings can be used to determine the effect of this activity on the client. The position of the nurse as he or she prepares to move the client and placement of the chair are critical elements in the transfer. Client's apparel should be sufficient to prevent embarrassment and provide warmth yet not impede movement. The technique for assisting a client to transfer from bed to chair is described in Procedure 39-5.

It is possible for only one person to get a helpless client from a bed to a chair, although two people simplify matters. The one-person technique is valuable for nurses to know for the home care of invalids and for

(text continues on page 1048)

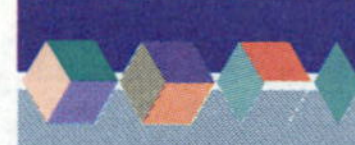

PROCEDURE 39-2

Moving a Client Up in Bed (One Nurse)

Action	Rationale
1. Explain the procedure to the client.	This facilitates cooperation of the client.
2. Wash your hands.	Handwashing deters spread of microorganisms.
3. Raise the bed to a comfortable position for you. Adjust the bed to flat position if the client can tolerate it. Lower the side rail nearest you.	This position facilitates moving the client upward and minimizes strain on the nurse.
4. Remove the pillow and place it at the head of the bed.	This reduces friction and protects the client's head from striking the top of the bed.
5. If able to assist, have the client flex the knees with the feet flat on the bed.	The client is prepared to push upward by using a major muscle group.
6. Assist the client to grasp the overhead trapeze bar or, if unable to assist, fold the client's arms across the chest.	This provides assistance and reduces friction.
7. Instruct the client to flex the neck with the chin on the chest.	This prevents hyperextension of the neck.
8. Stand opposite the client's center with your feet spread and turned toward the head of the bed. Position one foot slightly forward.	This positions the mover opposite the center of the body mass. It places the nurse in a stable position, with good alignment.

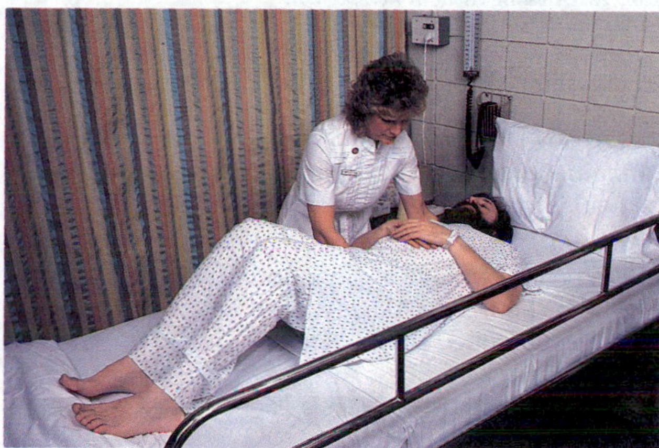

Action 5: Preparing client for move.

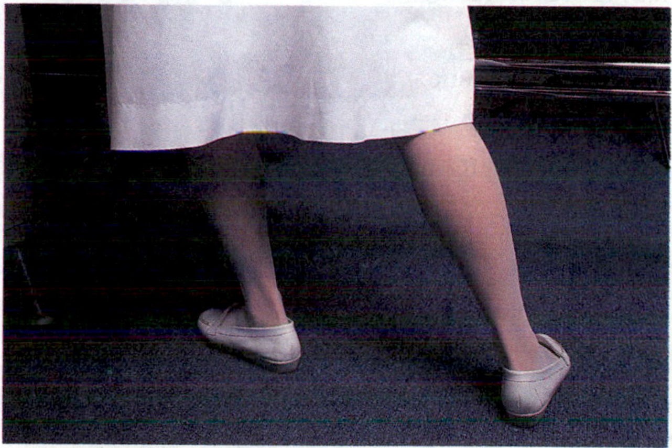

Action 8: Placing legs and feet for stable position.

Action	Rationale
9. Flex your knees and hips. Place one arm under the client's neck and shoulders, grasping the far shoulder with your hand. Place your other arm under the client's upper thighs. Pull the client closer to your side of the bed. Move the client's head and legs into alignment.	This prepares the nurse to use a large muscle mass to aid in lifting. The placement of the arms supports and evenly distributes the weight of the client.
10. Review the plan of movement with the client. Tighten your abdominal and gluteal muscles. Assume the position to move the client (see action 9).	These muscles stabilize the pelvis before the lifting maneuver.
11. Shift your weight back and forth from back leg to front leg, and on count of three, move the client upward in bed. If possible, the client should push with the legs and assist movement upward by grasping the trapeze. Repeat if necessary.	The rocking motion uses your weight to counteract the client's weight when moving the client up in bed. If the client assists, less effort is required by the nurse.

(continued)

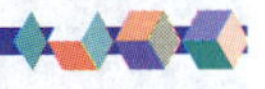

PROCEDURE 39-2 *(continued)*

Moving a Client Up in Bed (One Nurse)

Action	Rationale
12. Assist the client to a comfortable position in the center of the bed. Reposition the pillow. Raise the side rail and adjust the bed position, if necessary.	This ensures the client's safety.

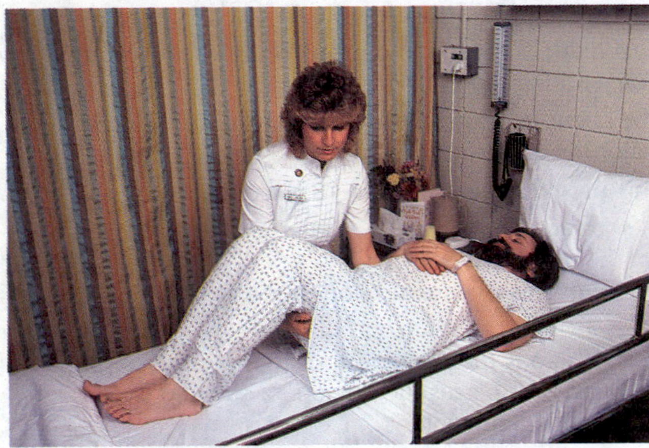

Action 11: Moving client.

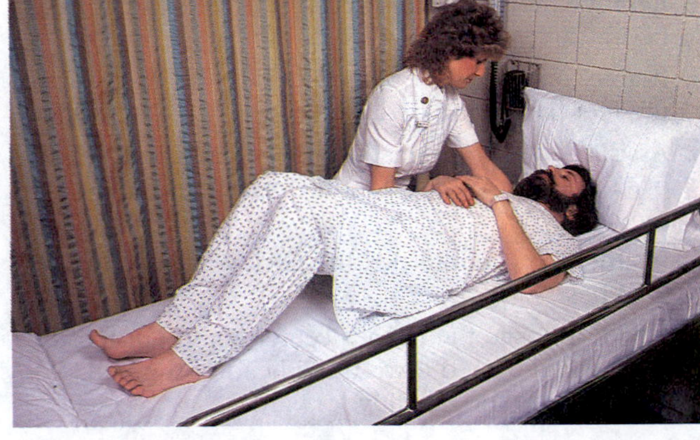

Action 12: Assisting client in new position.

Action	Rationale
13. Wash your hands.	Handwashing deters the spread of microorganisms.

Special Considerations

Two nurses on opposite sides of the bed may move a client up in bed by interlocking their arms under the client's shoulders and thighs and lifting as described previously.

Two nurses on opposite sides of the bed may move a client up in bed by using a drawsheet placed under the client from shoulder to thigh area. Fold or bunch the drawsheet close to the client and lift as described previously.

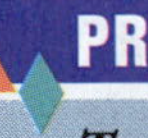

PROCEDURE 39-3

Transferring a Client From Bed to Stretcher

Action	Rationale
1. Explain the procedure to the client.	This facilitates the cooperation of the client.
2. Wash your hands.	Handwashing deters the spread of microorganisms.
3. Move the bed and equipment in the room to make room for the stretcher. Make sure that assistants are available. Close the door or curtain.	This facilitates transfer movement and provides for privacy.
4. Raise the bed to the same height as the stretcher and adjust the head of the bed to the flat position if the client can tolerate it. Lower side rails.	Pushing and pulling require less effort than lifting. This position facilitates moving the client.

Transferring a Client From Bed to Stretcher

Action	Rationale
5. Place a drawsheet under the client if one is not already there. Use the drawsheet to move the client to the side of the bed where the stretcher will be placed.	This facilitates movement of the client to the stretcher.
6. Position stretcher next to the bed and parallel to it. Lock wheels on the stretcher and bed. Remove the pillow from the bed and place it on the stretcher.	Positioning of the stretcher and locking the wheels facilitate safe transfer of client.
7. To move the client:	
a. The first nurse should kneel on far side of the bed away from the stretcher. Position the knee at the upper torso closer to the client than the other knee. Grasp the drawsheet securely.	The nurse uses a major muscle group to assist in movement. The nurse's flexed hips help avoid back injury.
b. The second nurse should reach across the stretcher and grasp the drawsheet at the head and chest areas of the client.	This promotes safe transfer by supporting the client's head and upper body.
c. The third nurse should reach across the stretcher and grasp the drawsheet at the client's waist and thigh area. Ask the client to fold arms across the chest.	This supports the lower part of the client's body for safe transfer.
d. At a signal given by the first nurse, the second and third nurses pull while the first nurse lifts the client from the bed to the stretcher.	Working in unison distributes the work of moving the client and facilitates the transfer.

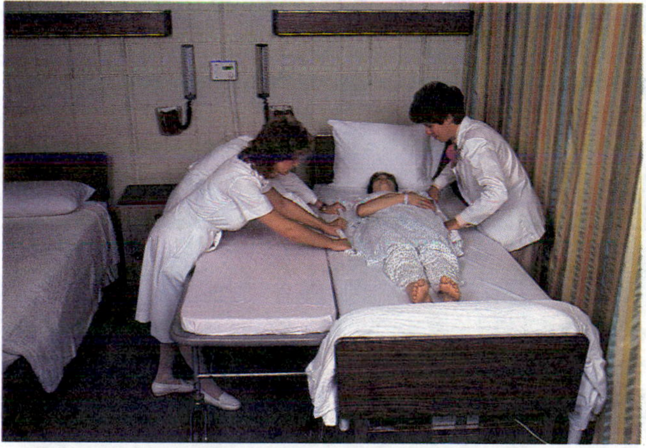

Action 5: Using drawsheet to move client to side of bed.

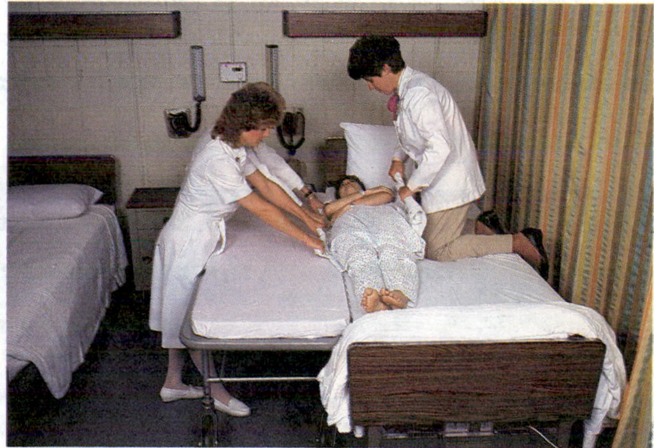

Action 7: Moving client to stretcher.

Action	Rationale
8. Secure the client on the stretcher until side rails are raised. Assist the client to a comfortable position with the covering in place. Leave the drawsheet in place for transfer back to bed.	This ensures client safety and comfort.
9. Wash your hands.	Handwashing deters the spread of microorganisms.

(continued)

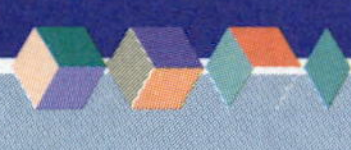

PROCEDURE 39-3 *(continued)*

Transferring a Client From Bed to Stretcher

Special Considerations

A long polyethylene board with handgrips on the edges may be used to assist with the transfer:

- Turn the client on his or her side with the back toward the stretcher.
- Position the transfer board lengthwise and midway between the bed and stretcher.
- Return the client to his or her back with a bottom sheet or drawsheet between the client and the board.
- Using the sheet, slide the client across the transfer board and onto the stretcher.
- Reposition the client on the stretcher, remove the board, and secure with safety belts and side rails.

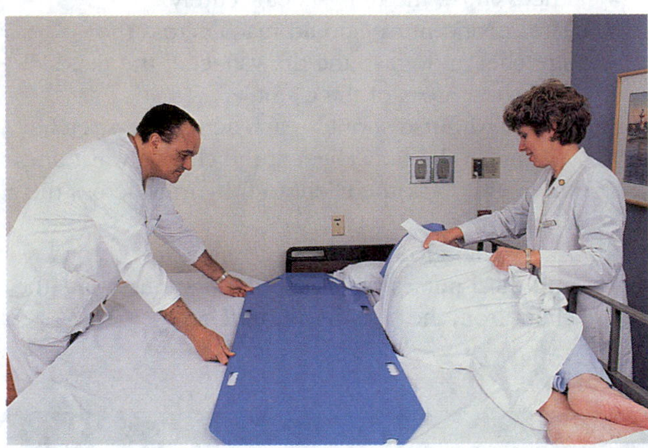

Special Considerations: Using a transfer board to facilitate moving the client from bed to stretcher.

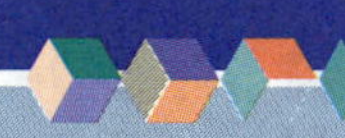

PROCEDURE 39-4

Transferring a Client From Bed to Stretcher (Three-Carrier Lift)

Action	Rationale
1. Explain the procedure to the client.	This facilitates the cooperation of the client.
2. Wash your hands.	Handwashing deters the spread of microorganisms.
3. Place the stretcher at a right angle to the foot of the bed. Lock the wheels of the stretcher. Raise the bed to the height of the stretcher.	The stretcher will be in position for the carriers after they pivot away from the bed.
4. Decide on responsibility for the lift. Each person must support one section of the body: a. Head, shoulders, and chest b. Hips c. Thighs and legs	Opinions differ about how to determine who lifts which area. The recommendations are that the strongest helper should support the heaviest body area or that the tallest person with the longest reach should support the client's head and shoulders.
5. In preparation for the lift, flex your knees and separate your feet, with the foot closest to the stretcher slightly forward.	Broad-based stance improves balance and lowers the lifter's center of gravity.

PROCEDURE 39-4 (continued)

Transferring a Client From Bed to Stretcher (Three-Carrier Lift)

Action	Rationale
6. Slide your arms under the client as far as possible and, on signal, all helpers should simultaneously roll the client toward their chests.	"Logrolling" the client onto the carriers brings the centers of gravity of all objects closer, thereby increasing the stability of the group and reducing strain on the carriers.
7. On signal, the helpers should stand up and steady the client securely against their chests.	Flexed knees and body position allow workers to lift with strong leg muscles.

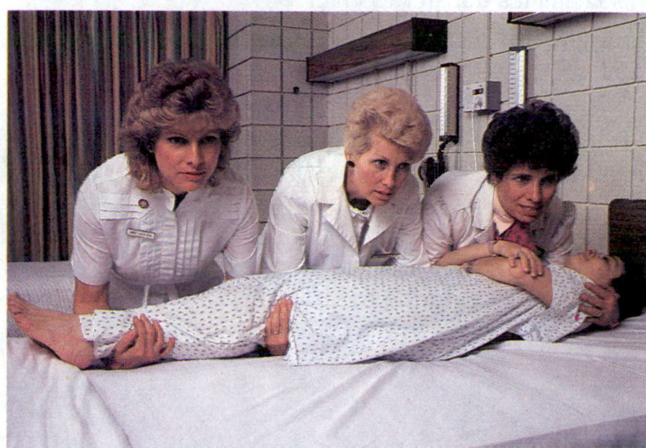

Action 6: Positioning client close to lifters.

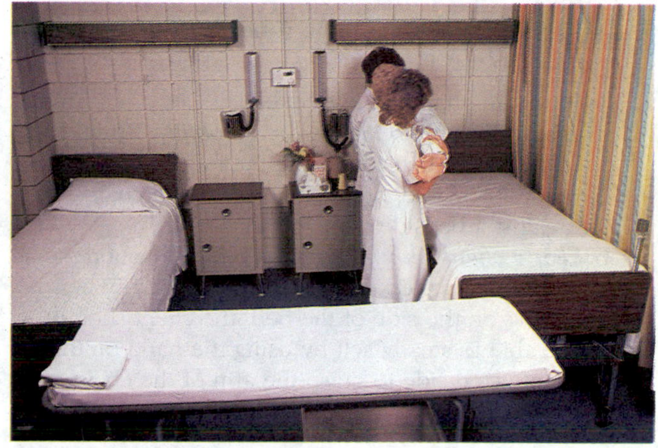

Action 7: Standing with client held to chest.

Action	Rationale
8. Helpers should step back together, pivot around to the stretcher, and, on signal, lower the client onto the stretcher.	This lets the large leg and arm muscles do the work of lowering the client.

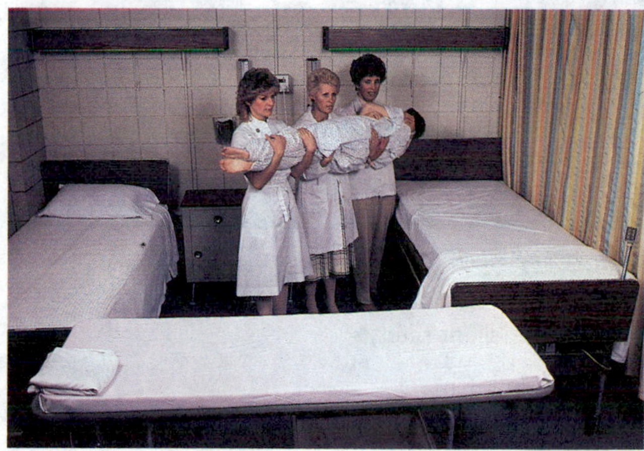

Action 8: Pivoting to stretcher.

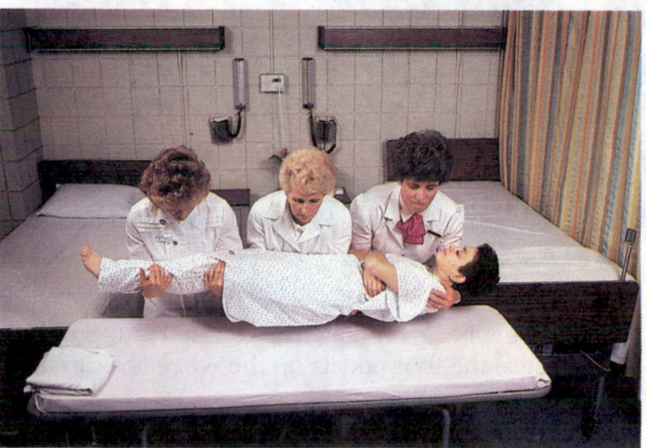

Action 8: Lowering client to stretcher.

Action	Rationale
9. The client should be covered with a sheet or blanket and positioned as necessary. Stretcher side rails should be raised.	This ensures comfort and safety of the client.
10. Wash your hands.	Handwashing deters the spread of microorganisms.

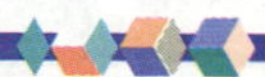

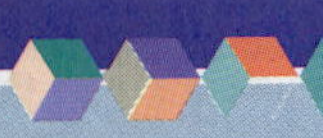

PROCEDURE 39-5

Assisting a Client to Transfer from Bed to Chair

Action	Rationale
1. Explain the procedure to the client. Offer bedpan.	This facilitates cooperation of the client. Empty bladder will increase client comfort.
2. Wash your hands.	Handwashing deters the spread of microorganisms.
3. Assess the client's ability to assist with transfer. Move equipment as necessary to make room for the chair. Close the door or curtain.	This ensures client safety and facilitates the transfer. Closing the door or curtain provides for privacy.
4. Place the bed in the low position.	This facilitates transfer to chair.
5. Assist the client to put on a robe and slippers with nonskid soles.	These provide warmth. Slippers provide protection and stability.
6. Position the chair at the bedside:	
a. *For a client with unimpaired mobility:* Bring chair close to the bedside facing the foot of the bed and, if possible, brace the back of the chair against a bedside table.	This increases stability and ensures client safety during the transfer.
b. *For a client with impaired mobility:* Position the chair facing the head or foot of the bed. When sitting on the side of the bed, the client should be able to steady self by using the hand on the unaffected side to grasp the arm of the chair.	This uses the strong side to provide balance and improve stability during the transfer.

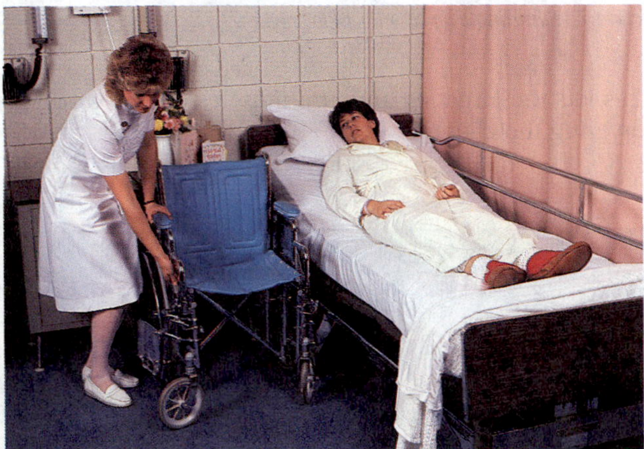

Action 6: Placing chair at bedside.

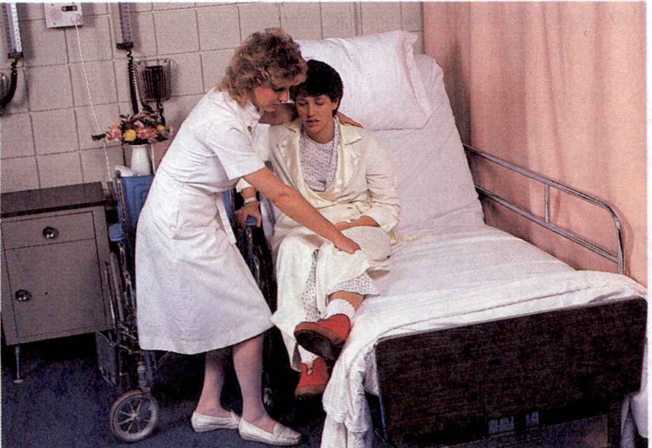

Action 9: Supporting client while moving legs off bed.

Action	Rationale
7. Lock the wheels on the chair and bed if appropriate. Raise the foot pedals on the wheelchair to the up position.	This ensures client safety.
8. Raise the head of the bed to the highest position.	Moving from the sitting to the standing position requires less energy.
9. Assist the client to sit on the side of the bed by supporting the client's head and neck while moving the client's legs off the bed to dangle. Steady the client in that position for a few minutes.	The sitting position facilitates transfer to the chair and allows the circulatory system to adjust to a change in position.

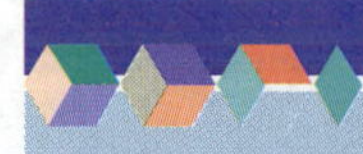

PROCEDURE 39-5 *(continued)*

Assisting a Client to Transfer from Bed to Chair

Action	Rationale
10. Assist the client to the standing position:	This provides for stability and for use of major muscle groups to facilitate movement. Allowing the client to grasp the nurse around the neck could injure the nurse if the client should fall.
a. *For a client with unimpaired mobility:* Face the client and brace your feet and knees against the client. Place your hands around the client's waist while the client holds onto you between the shoulders and the waist. Use your legs to help you raise the client to the standing position.	
b. *For a client with impaired mobility:* Face the client and brace your feet and knees against the client, especially against the affected extremity. Place your hands around the client's waist. The client may place the unaffected arm around your shoulder or use the unaffected arm to reach for the arm of the chair and to push up while raising to the standing position.	This provides for stability and makes use of the unaffected extremities to facilitate movement.
11. Pivot the client (on the unaffected limb if applicable) into position in front of the chair with legs positioned against the chair.	This provides security and proper position before sitting.

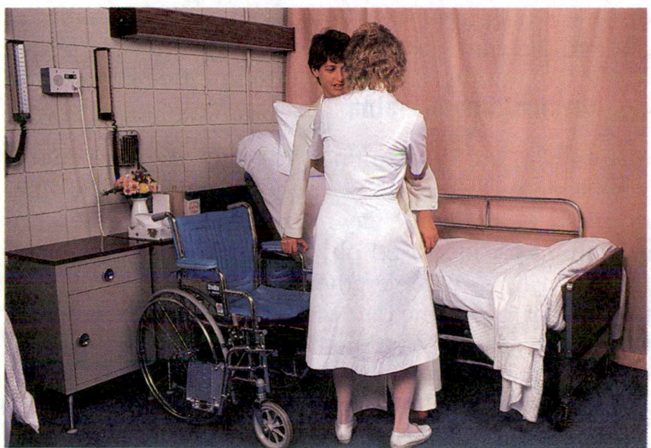

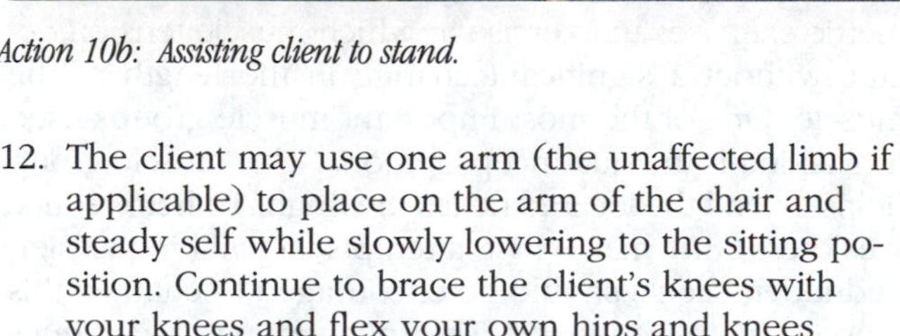

Action 10b: Assisting client to stand.

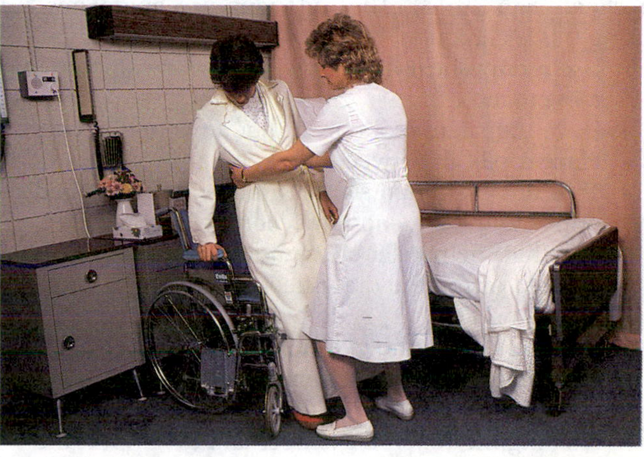

Action 12: Bracing client's knees while lowering client to chair.

Action	Rationale
12. The client may use one arm (the unaffected limb if applicable) to place on the arm of the chair and steady self while slowly lowering to the sitting position. Continue to brace the client's knees with your knees and flex your own hips and knees when seating the client.	The client uses own arm for support and stability. The nurse flexes the knees and hips to use a major muscle group to aid in movement and reduce strain on the back.
13. Adjust the client's position using pillows where necessary. Cover the client and use restraint if necessary. Position the call bell so it is available for use.	This maintains proper body alignment and provides for comfort and safety.
14. Wash your hands.	Handwashing deters the spread of microorganisms.
15. Document the client's tolerance of the procedure and length of time in the chair.	This provides accurate documentation and ensures continuity of care.

(continued)

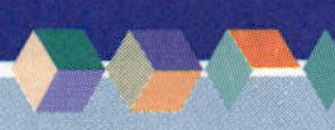

PROCEDURE 39-5 *(continued)*

Assisting a Client to Transfer from Bed to Chair

Special Considerations

- A walking or transfer belt may be used to assist the transfer. With the belt secure around the client's waist, the nurse can grasp the belt on both sides (or use handles if they are available) and assist the client to stand and move to the chair.
- A sliding board may also be used to ease the client who cannot stand into a chair.

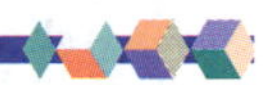

emergency use. More than one person should be available if the bed and chair seat are not the same height. The technique for transferring a client by two nurses is described in Procedure 39-6.

Logrolling a Client

When a client has a spinal injury or is recovering from neck, back, or spinal surgery, it is necessary to keep the body in straight alignment when turning him or her. Two or three nurses can accomplish this safely by logrolling a client (Fig. 39-17). The following are guidelines for using this technique:

- Use a drawsheet if possible to facilitate smooth movement.
- Have the client cross his or her arms on the chest.
- Place a pillow between the knees.
- Two nurses should stand on one side of the bed opposite the direction the client will be turned. The third helper should stand on the other side.
- Fanfold or roll the drawsheet tightly against the client and carefully slide him or her to the side of the bed toward the two nurses.
- One helper should then move to the other side of the bed.
- Holding the rolled drawsheet taut to support the body, turn the client as a unit toward the two nurses. Move on a predetermined signal.
- Use pillows to support the client on his or her side in straight alignment.
- Raise the side rails, lower the bed, and place the call signal within the client's reach.

Using a Hydraulic Lift

A hydraulic device, such as the Hoyer lift, can safely transfer an immobile or obese client from bed to chair. One person may operate the device but two are preferable. Manufacturer's instructions should be carefully reviewed before attempting the procedure. Generally, the client is positioned supine in the center of the sling. Chains or straps from the hydraulic mechanism are attached to the sling, the client is raised to a sitting position, lifted clear of the bed, and slowly lowered into the chair (Fig. 39-18). According to Owen and Garg (1993), the reasons caregivers cited for not using Hoyer lifts more frequently were: (1) the lift was not readily available, (2) the procedure is time-consuming, (3) the lift was viewed as unstable and unsafe, and (4) clients indicated they preferred not to use this device.

Helping Clients Ambulate

Fortunately for most clients, prolonged periods of bed rest are no longer considered necessary during most illnesses. Activity, even as mild as a stroll around the room, down the hall, from the bedroom to the living room, or out into the yard, is a protective measure for the body.

Physical Conditioning

Clients who are not confined to bed for long periods, who sleep well, and who experience possibly short periods of rest during the day may not require special considerations for increased physical activity in preparation for ambulation. However, there are others who will have to be prepared for the day when ambulation is resumed. Certain exercises that strengthen the overall efficiency of the musculoskeletal system can be done in bed.

Quadriceps Drills (Sets). *Quadriceps drills* are an isometric exercise, an exercise in which muscle tension occurs without a significant change in the length of the muscle. One of the most important muscle groups used in walking is the quadriceps femoris. This muscle group helps extend the leg and flexes the thigh. To help reduce weakness and make first attempts at walking easier, bedridden clients should be encouraged to contract this muscle group frequently. The following are techniques for quadriceps drills:

- Have the client contract the muscles on the front of the thighs by pulling the kneecaps toward the hips. The client has the feeling of pushing the knees downward into the mattress and pulling the feet upward.
- Have the client hold the position just described while counting slowly to four, and then relax the muscles for an equal amount of time. Emphasize that relaxation is important to prevent muscle fatigue.

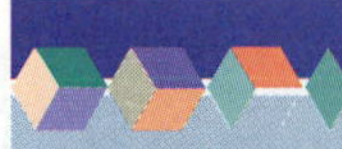

PROCEDURE 39-6

Transferring a Dependent Client From Bed to Chair (Two Nurses)

Action	Rationale
1. Explain the procedure to the client.	This facilitates cooperation of the client.
2. Wash your hands.	Handwashing deters the spread of microorganisms.
3. Move equipment as necessary to make room for the chair. Close the door or curtain. Assist the client to put on a robe and slippers.	This ensures client safety and facilitates transfer. It provides for privacy and warmth.
4. Move the client to the near side of the bed and cross the client's arms across the chest if possible. Lock the wheels of the bed.	This requires less effort to move the client. Locked wheels will prevent the bed from moving if the client leans against it.
5. Position the chair next to the bed near the upper end and with the back of the chair parallel to the head of the bed. (If wheelchair, remove the armrest closer to the bed if possible.) Lock the wheels if appropriate.	Positioning the chair next to the bed facilitates easier movement into the chair.
6. Adjust the bed to a comfortable level for nurses or at the level of the armrest if one is present on the chair.	This facilitates transfer with minimal muscle strain on the nurses.
7. Prepare to lift the client from the bed to the chair:	
a. The first nurse should stand behind the chair. Slip the arms under the client's axillae and grasp the client's wrists securely.	Two people lifting the client distributes weight and decreases the effort needed for transfer.
b. The second nurse should face the wheelchair and support the client's knees by placing the arms under them.	
c. On a predetermined signal, both nurses flex their hips and knees and simultaneously lift the client gently to the chair.	

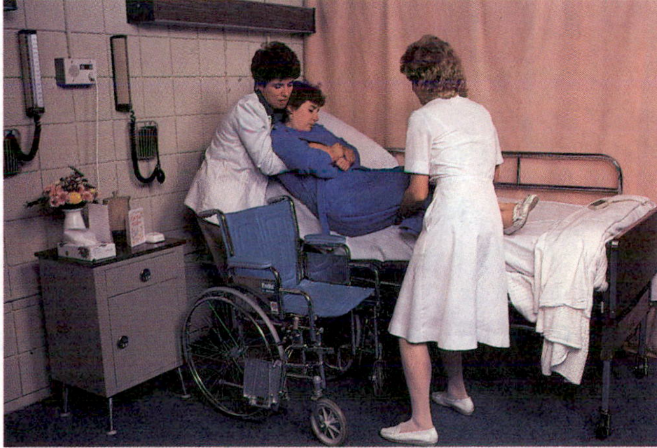

Action 7a & b: First nurse slips arms under client's axillae and grasps wrists; second nurse supports client's knees.

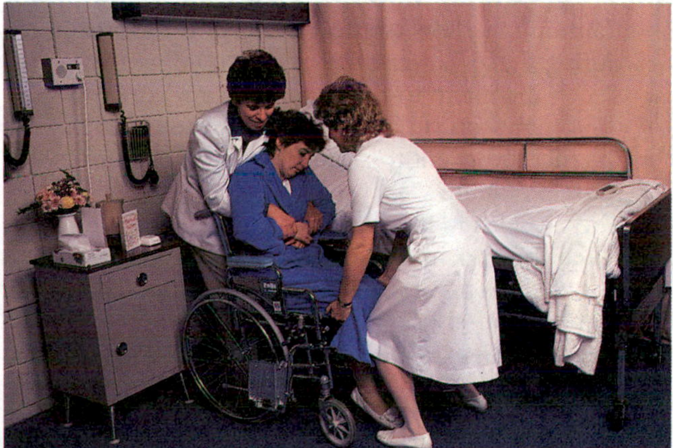

Action 7c: Lowering client into chair.

Action	Rationale
8. Adjust the client's position using pillows where necessary. Cover the client and use restraint if necessary. Position the call bell so it is available for use.	This maintains proper body alignment and provides for comfort and safety.
9. Wash your hands.	Handwashing deters the spread of microorganisms.
10. Document the client's tolerance of the procedure and length of time in the chair.	This provides accurate documentation and ensures continuity of care.

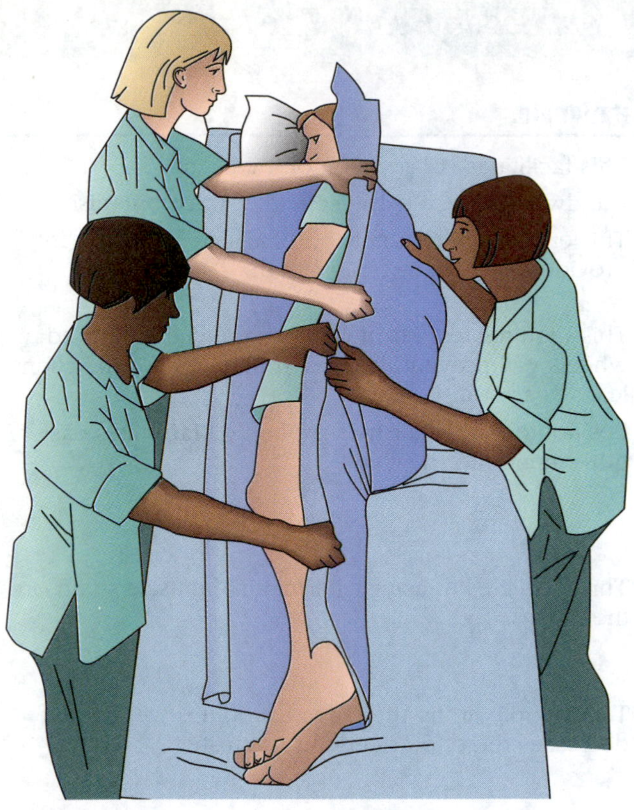

Figure 39-17
Logrolling by two or three nurses aids in turning a client with a spinal injury. One nurse stands on the side, holding the draw-sheet taut. The client is moved toward the other two nurses on a predetermined signal.

- Caution the client not to hold his or her breath during these exercises to avoid straining the heart.
- Teach the client to do quadriceps drills two or three times each hour, four to six times a day.
- Instruct the client to stop the exercise short of muscle fatigue.

The muscles in the buttocks can be exercised in the same way by pinching the buttocks together and then relaxing them. This is called gluteal settings. Tightening and holding the abdominal muscles for 6 seconds and then relaxing them also strengths this muscle group and facilitates walking.

Push-Ups. The muscle strength of the arms and shoulders also may need to be improved before the client is ready to be out of bed. Exercises should improve the strength needed to hold onto or get into a chair and to move about better. They are part of the preparation for clients who must learn to walk on crutches.

A trapeze attached to the bed of a client who has limited use of the lower part of the body helps the client to move about in bed and strengthens muscles in the upper part of the body. However, this does not strengthen the triceps, which is the muscle group necessary for crutch walking or for moving from a bed to a chair. More suitable exercises are push-ups, which are done as follows:

- Sitting up in bed without support is one type of push-up exercise. Instruct the client to lift the hips off the bed by pushing down with the hands on the mattress. If the mattress is too soft, a block of books can be placed on the bed under the client's hands.
- Push-ups may also be done with the client lying in bed on the abdomen. Instruct the client to place the hands near the outstretched body at about shoulder level, with palms down on the mattress and elbows bent sharply. Then have the client straighten the elbows while lifting the head and shoulders off the bed.
- Push-ups may also be done when the client sits in an armchair or wheelchair. The client places the hands on the arms of the chair and then raises the body out of the seat.

Push-ups are usually done three or four times a day, with the number increased as upper body strength is increased.

Dangling. *Dangling* refers to the position in which the person sits on the edge of the bed with legs and feet over the side of the bed. This exercise helps prepare the client for being out of bed also. It is carried out as follows:

- Place the client in the sitting position in bed for a few minutes. This will accustom the client to this position and help prevent feelings of faintness.

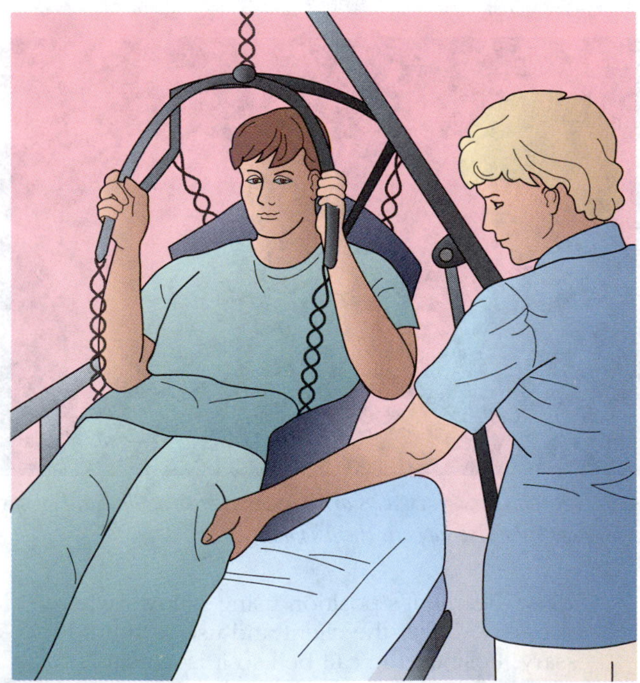

Figure 39-18
A hydraulic lift is used to transfer an immobile or obese client. The client is raised to a sitting position suspended just above the bed; then the client is transferred and the sling with the client is lowered onto the seat.

- Place the bed in the low position or have a footstool handy on which the client can rest the feet while dangling.
- Move the client toward the side of the bed near you so that you do not stretch and strain while turning the client.
- Pivot the client a quarter of a turn by supporting the shoulders and legs. Swing the client's legs over the side of the bed. The client may place his or her hands on your shoulders.
- Rest the client's feet on the floor or on a footstool. This gives a sense of security, and the client is less likely to slide from the bed.
- Have the client pick up and put down the feet alternately in a marching motion. This promotes circulation in the legs.
- Remain with the client, and be ready to put the client in a lying position if feeling faint so that the client does not fall out of bed.

Daily Activities for Purposeful Exercise. Many activities can be carried out with benefit to the client. These include placing the bedside stand so that the client must use shoulder and arm muscles to reach what is needed instead of placing it so that little effort is required to take things from it; placing the signal cord so that the client must engage in either arm or shoulder action to reach it; encouraging the client to sit up and reach for the overbed table, to pull it close, and then to push it back in place; encouraging a client to try to wash the back; and having the client put on socks while still in bed. There are innumerable ways in which clients can be helped to exercise, and when they understand the purpose, they often adopt other exercises for themselves.

Assisting the Client to Walk

Many clients who have been confined to bed for a long time find that they must almost learn to walk all over again. Often, it is the nurse who plays a major role in the client's recovery and mental outlook, hope, and faith, especially when the client must adhere to a rigid and often difficult schedule of reeducating muscle groups. A client able to raise the leg only 2.5 cm (1 inch) from the bed possesses sufficient power to permit walking.

When the major problem of muscle reeducation presents itself, the client will need the assistance of experts in physical medicine. However, nurses assist clients out of bed and help them to walk when a physical therapist is not present. The nurse should also plan to walk with a client who is using this activity for the first few times after a period of bed rest.

Before getting the client out of bed, the nurse does the following:

- Assesses the client's ability to walk and need for assistance (one nurse, two nurses, walker, cane, walking belt, or crutches)
- Explains to the client exactly what is to be done: transfer technique from bed to erect position, projected distance to be ambulated, assistance available and the correct manner of using it; the client is instructed to alert the nurse immediately if feeling dizzy or weak
- Ensures that the client has a clear path for ambulation

The nurse then slowly assists the client to an erect position and ambulation, pausing after the client is seated at the edge of the bed and again after the client first stands to ensure that the client feels steady. The nurse reminds the client to take deep breaths to promote good aeration of the lungs while walking. Clients who are fearful of walking often tend to look at their feet and may need to be reminded to stand erect and to hold the head high to achieve the full benefits of walking. Because it is not unusual for clients who are walking for the first time after prolonged bed rest to feel faint or weak, a short distance should be planned. As this distance is increased, it is helpful to have chairs readily available should the client need to rest. Should a client faint or begin to fall while walking, the nurse stands with feet apart to create a wide base of support and rocks the pelvis out on the side facing the client. With arms under the client's axillae and encircling the client, the nurse slides the client down the nurse's own body to the floor, carefully protecting the client's head. If the client is wearing a walking belt, the nurse can use the belt to ease the client backward against her own body and gently ease the client to the floor while protecting the client's head. This maneuver should be practiced before it is needed in an emergency situation.

Home Healthcare Alert

Clients and caregivers also need to be aware that lightheadedness and dizziness may occur when a client moves too quickly from a lying to a sitting or standing position. Encourage slow, gradual position changes to prevent falls.

One-Nurse Assist. The client who requires minimal nursing assistance may ambulate well with the nurse walking alongside. The nurse best supports the client by standing at the client's side and placing both hands at the client's waist. By supporting the client at the waist, the nurse helps the client maintain an erect posture and is prevented from pulling the client unintentionally to one side. Use of a walking belt snugly secured around the client's waist also facilitates this type of support. The nurse grasps the belt securely in the back and walks behind and slightly to the side of the client (Fig. 39-19).

Frequently it is necessary to assist the client to ambulate with intravenous (IV) therapy equipment. The nurse should secure a portable IV pole that moves easily. The client ambulates with the assistance of the nurse and the portable IV pole. The nurse needs to secure all the equipment before ambulating and be alert for any

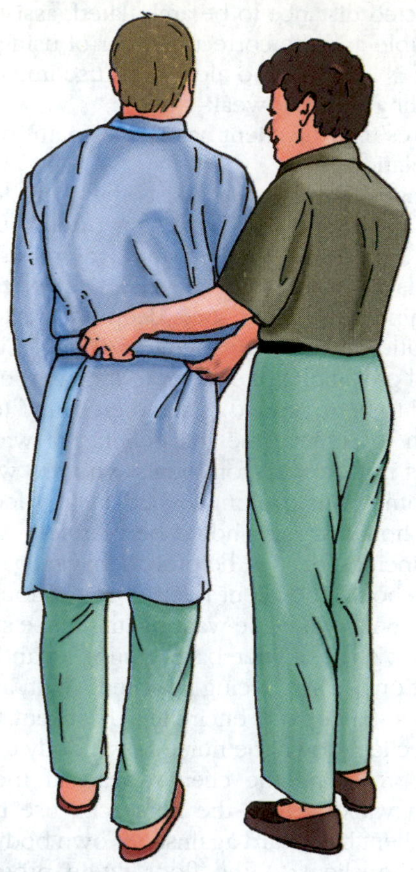

Figure 39-19
The nurse using a walking belt to support a client while walking.

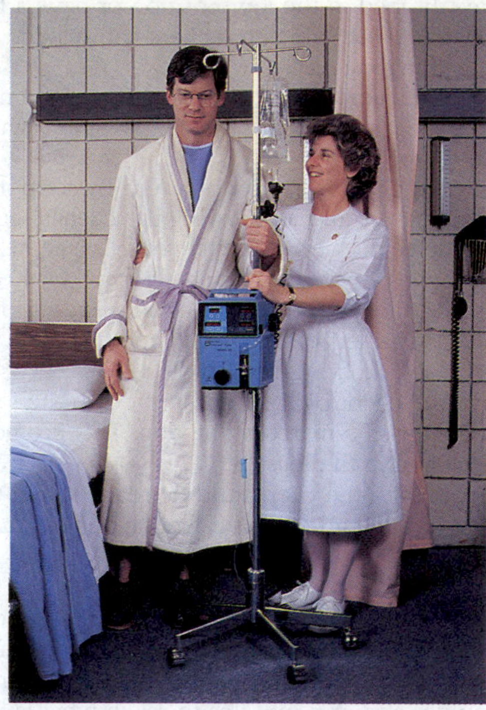

Figure 39-20
The nurse assists the client to ambulate with a portable IV pole. (Photo © B. Proud.)

tension or sudden action that might dislodge or interfere with the infusion (Fig. 39-20).

When a client has weakness or paralysis on one side, the nurse usually stands on the weaker or affected side and stabilizes the client by putting one arm around the client's waist. Support for the client's weak arm can be accomplished by placing the nurse's other arm around the inner aspect of the client's upper arm in the axilla area or using the nurse's hand to support the client's forearm and hand (Fig. 39-21). Supporting the client's weak arm in the axillary area allows the nurse to support the client's weight more easily and ease him or her to the floor should the client feel faint. A transfer belt should always be used with clients who are unstable. A two-nurse assist is the safer method when the nurse is uncertain of the client's ability to ambulate.

Two-Nurse Assist. There are two methods of ambulation that two nurses can safely use to support a client. In the first, the nurses stand at the client's sides with their near hands grasping the inferior aspect of the client's near upper arm and their far hands holding the client's lower arm or hand. The second position provides more support to the client but requires the three people involved to be of similar heights. The nurses again position themselves at the client's sides, slipping their near arms under the client's arms and around the client's back, grasping one another's wrists. The client stretches the arms around the nurses' shoulders and the nurses grasp the client's hands with their far hands. In both these positions, the nurses and the client step in unison (Fig. 39-22).

Using Mechanical Aids for Walking

Various devices can assist a client with walking. The most common are walkers, canes, braces, and crutches. Most often a client is fitted for these devices and instructed in their use in a department of physical medicine or physical therapy. In this instance, nursing's concern is chiefly to reinforce the teaching the client has received and to ensure the client continues to use the device properly to assist in safe ambulation. However, in some work settings, nurses may be responsible for fitting clients for these devices. Whenever a nurse assesses a client who has been using a walker, cane, brace, or crutches over time, it is important to determine if the device is still needed, if it continues to meet the client's needs, and if the client continues to use it properly.

General guidelines for helping clients who need the assistance of a walker, cane, brace, or crutches are the following:

- Whenever possible, instruct the client and family members in the correct use of the device before it is needed (eg, before surgery). If family members are knowledgeable, they can reinforce the teaching as needed.

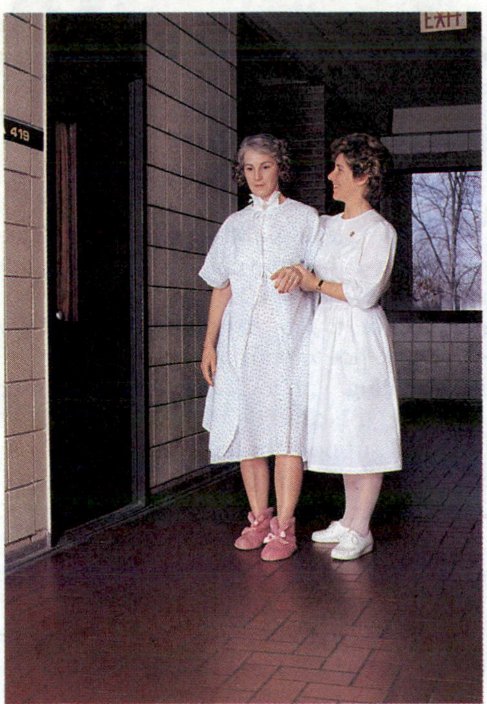

Figure 39-21
The nurse assists the client with weakness or paralysis on one side to ambulate by supporting the client on the affected side. (Photo © B. Proud.)

- When ready to begin ambulation with the new device, make sure the client is wearing rubber-soled, well-fitting shoes and that there is a clear path for ambulation (clean, flat, dry, and well lighted). If the client is at high risk for falls, use a walking belt for added support.
- Before moving, make sure the client is steady on the feet when standing; instruct the client to stand erect, looking straight ahead, and walk behind and slightly to one side of the client (in cases of hemiparesis or hemiparalysis, walk on the client's affected side). Should the client lose balance, be prepared to grasp the client's shoulder and the transfer belt to steady the client.

Walker. A *walker* is a lightweight metal frame (usually aluminum) with four legs (Fig. 39-23). The walker provides a sense of security and support. There are several variations of walkers, and they are specified according to the arm strength and balance of the client.

When the client stands between the back legs of the walker, the walker should extend from the floor to the client's hip joint; the client's elbows should be flexed about 30 degrees. Rubber tips should be intact to prevent slipping. Generally the client lifts the walker ahead of himself or herself and steps into it. Instructions for a client using a walker should include:

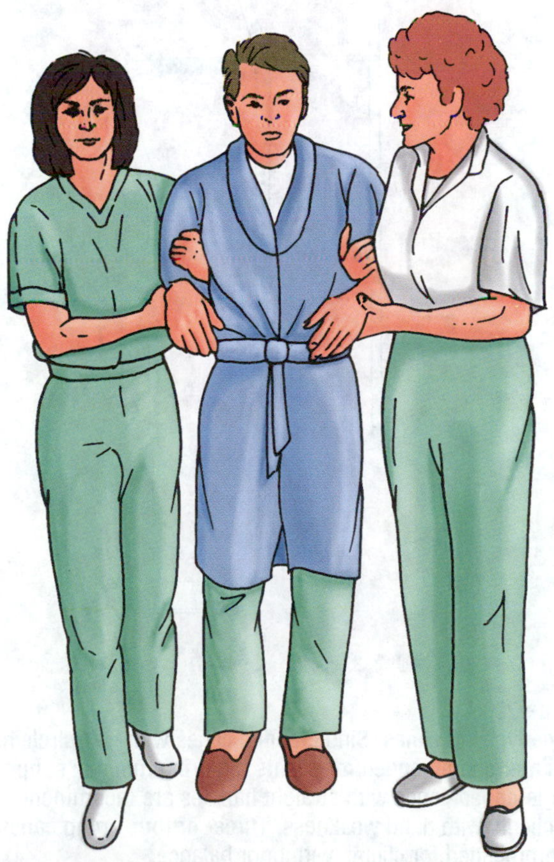

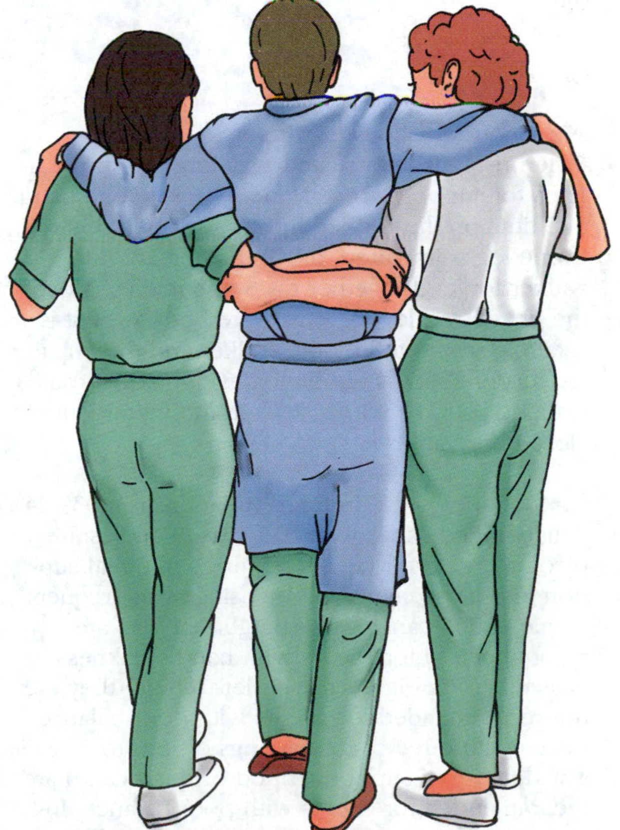

Figure 39-22
Two techniques for two nurses to safely assist a client to ambulate.

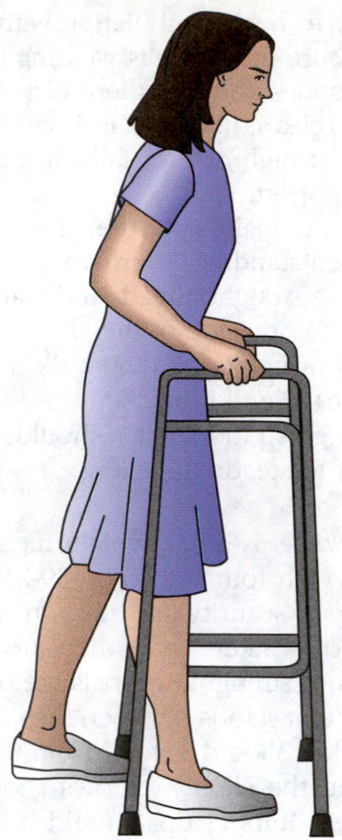

Figure 39-23
A walker is a lightweight metal frame with a broad, four-point base of support. The walker should be adjusted to the height of the client's hip joint so that the client's elbows are flexed about 30 degrees.

- Wear nonskid shoes or slippers.
- When rising from a seated position, use the chair arms for support. Once standing, place one hand at a time on the walker and move forward into it.
- If one leg is impaired, move that leg and the walker forward together for 6 to 8 inches. Move the unaffected leg forward once body weight is securely supported by the walker and the impaired leg. Older clients frequently develop dangerous walking patterns with a walker and may require close observation.

Canes. Canes come in three variations (Fig. 39-24):

- Single-ended canes with half-circle handles are recommended for clients requiring minimal support and if the client will be using stairs frequently.
- Single-ended canes with straight handles are recommended for clients with hand weakness because their handgrips are easier to hold; they are not recommended for clients with poor balance.
- Canes with three or four prongs or legs to provide a wide base of support (tripod or quad cane) are recommended for clients with poor balance. Instruct the client to use a cane with as small a base as possible, and eventually to progress to a single-ended cane if possible. The smaller the base, the less the client relies on the cane for support.

Many canes are adjustable and should be fitted so that when the client stands with the cane's tip 4 inches (10 cm) to the side of the foot, the cane extends from the floor to the client's hip joint. The elbow should be flexed at a 30-degree angle when holding the cane. Rubber tips on the cane prevent slipping and accidents. They should be inspected regularly for this reason. Clients should be taught to stand erect when walking with a cane and not to lean out over the cane.

When walking with a cane, clients are generally instructed to hold the cane on the unaffected side to provide additional support for the weaker leg. Ambulation proceeds in the following fashion:

- The client stands with weight evenly distributed between the feet and the cane.
- The cane is held on the client's stronger side and is advanced 4 to 12 inches (10 to 30 cm).
- Supporting weight on the stronger leg and the cane, the client advances the weaker foot forward, parallel with the cane.

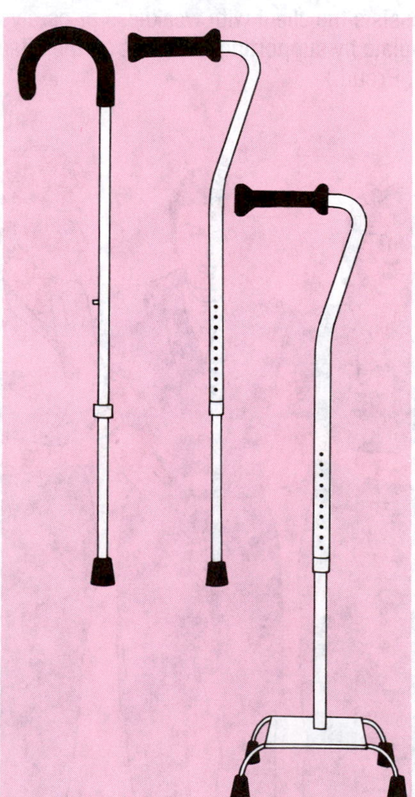

Figure 39-24
Three types of canes. Single-ended canes with half-circle handles are recommended for clients requiring minimal support. Single-ended canes with straight handles are recommended for clients with hand weakness. Three- or four-prong canes are recommended for clients with poor balance.

- Supporting weight on the weaker leg and the cane, the client next advances the stronger leg forward ahead of the cane (heel slightly beyond the tip of the cane).
- The weaker leg is moved forward until even with the stronger leg and the cane is once again advanced as in step 2.

When less support is required from the cane the client can advance the cane and weaker leg forward while the stronger leg supports the client's weight. Clients should be taught to position their canes within easy reach when they sit down so that they can rise easily.

Braces. Braces that support weakened leg muscles are available in many variations. Nursing responsibilities include learning with the client when the brace is to be worn and the correct technique for applying the brace; monitoring the client's correct use of the brace; and observing for any untoward problems the brace might be causing (eg, skin irritation). Muscle changes such as those occurring with growth and development or brought about by illness (atrophy) may result in the brace needing to be refitted to maintain its effectiveness.

Crutches. Sometimes, it is necessary for clients to use crutches for a time to avoid using one leg or to help strengthen one or both legs. This procedure is taught best by a physical therapist; however, there are numerous instances when the nurse is called on to measure clients for crutches and to teach them to use them. Even if a client is being taught to crutch walk by a physical therapist, it is necessary for the nurse to understand the client's progress and the gait being taught. The nurse must often guide the client at home or in the hospital after the initial teaching is completed. The two types of crutches most commonly used are the underarm or axillary crutches and the forearm support crutches (Fig. 39-25).

Measuring for Axillary Crutches. The following techniques are used to measure the client for axillary crutches:

- Have the client lie flat in bed on the back while wearing shoes to be used when walking.
- Measure the distance from the anterior fold of the axilla straight down to the heel, and then add 2 inches (5 cm). Or, measure the distance from the anterior fold of the axilla diagonally out to a point 6 inches (15 cm) away from the heel.
- Use the client's height and subtract 16 inches (40 cm) to obtain an approximate crutch length.
- After proper crutches are obtained, have the client stand to adjust the handgrips. Secure the handgrips while the client grasps them in the hands with elbows slightly bent and wrists bent backward.
- Teach the client that the support of body weight should come primarily on the hands and arms while using the crutches, not in the axillary areas, where pressure may damage nerves and cut off circulation. Also, the crutches should not be forced into the axillae each time the body moves forward.

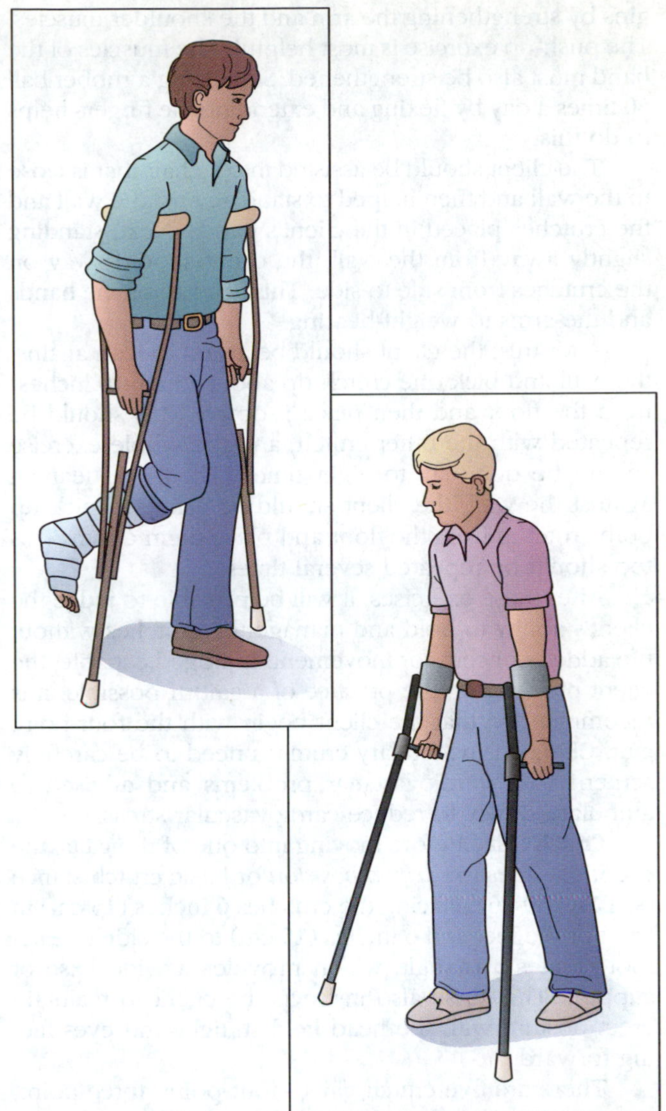

Figure 39-25
Axillary and forearm support crutches.

It is important that axillary crutches are properly fitted and used correctly to prevent damage to nerves and circulation in the axillae from being cut off, and to provide well-balanced support. There are crutches available that have no axillary support. A supportive frame extends beyond the handgrip for the lower arm to help guide the crutch. These crutches are more likely to be used by clients who have permanent limitations and will always need crutch assistance for ambulation.

Exercises to Prepare for Crutch Walking. Before being asked to use the crutches, several exercises will help the client to be more confident and skillful. The client begins by strengthening the arm and the shoulder muscles. The push-up exercise is most helpful. The muscles of the hand must also be strengthened. Squeezing a rubber ball 50 times a day by flexing and extending the fingers helps to do this.

The client should be assisted into a chair that is close to the wall and then helped to stand against the wall and the crutches placed in the client's hands. Next, standing slightly away from the wall, the client should sway on the crutches from side to side. This accustoms the hands and the arms to weight-bearing.

After this, the client should be asked to lean against the wall and pick one crutch up about 15 cm (6 inches) from the floor and then place it down. This should be repeated with the other crutch, and the whole exercise should be done six to eight times. Then, still leaning against the wall, the client should be asked to pick up both crutches from the floor and place them down. This too should be repeated several times.

After these exercises, it will be possible to judge the client's ability to hold and manage the crutches without the added concern for movement. If judged capable, the client proceeds to the practice of a gait. If possible, it is recommended that the client begin with the four-point gait. Clients using axillary crutches need to be carefully screened for cardiovascular problems and advised to ambulate slowly to reduce cardiovascular stress.

Crutch Gaits. Before moving into one of the gaits, the client assumes the *tripod position* or basic crutch stance (see Fig. 39-26). Placing the crutches 6 inches (15 cm) in front of the feet and 6 inches (15 cm) to the side of each foot creates a triangle which provides a wide base of support. The nurse also instructs the client to maintain erect posture with the head held straight and eyes facing forward.

There are five crutch gaits—four-point, three-point, two-point, swing-to, and swing-through. These gaits are described here with patterns outlined in Figure 39-27.

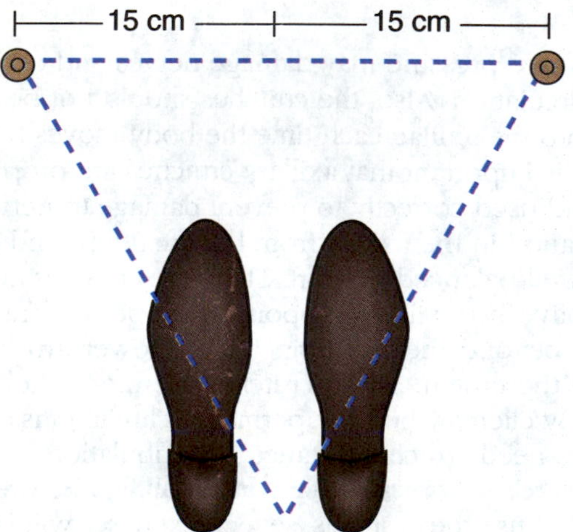

Figure 39-26
The tripod position is the initial crutch stance from which the person advances.

In *four-point gait*, weight-bearing is permitted on both legs. The pattern is shown in Figure 39-27, beginning at the bottom of the figure. In *two-point gait*, weight-bearing is permitted on both feet. The pattern is a speed-up of the four-point gait. In *three-point gait*, weight-bearing is permitted on only one foot; the other foot cannot support, but acts as a balance. The *swing-to gait* requires that both crutches move ahead together and the body weight is lifted by the arms and swung *to* the crutches. In *swing-through gait* the body weight is swung *through* and beyond the crutches. The swing gaits require strength and coordination and are frequently used by clients with hip and leg paralysis. A disadvantage of these two gaits is that they do not simulate normal walking. Extended use will lead to atrophy of the muscles in the lower extremity that are not being used.

Instructions for crutch walking should also include practice and demonstration of the safe technique for moving up and down stairs. One technique involves using a modified three-point gait. The unaffected leg is advanced first up the stairs and past the crutches. When coming down the stairs, move the affected leg and crutches first followed by the unaffected one (Fig. 39-28). An easy way to teach the client to remember this technique is the statement, "The good leg goes up, the bad leg goes down."

When a railing is available, the client can use another technique to climb and descend stairs. This technique involves using one hand to firmly grasp the railing while the other hand grasps both crutches together at the handgrips and uses them for support. While holding securely onto the rail, move the uninjured leg up one step, straighten it, and move the injured leg and the crutches onto the same step. When moving down the stairs, one hand should always be on the railing while the other hand again steadies both crutches under the arm using the handgrips. The crutches and the injured leg should move together down one step, followed by the uninjured leg.

Designing Exercise Programs

The benefits of exercise on each of the major body systems are so important that designing individualized exercise programs for clients is an important nursing responsibility. These programs incorporate activities of daily living and planned exercise sessions. Depending on the physical condition of the client, exercise is designed to promote optimal fitness.

An individual's commitment to a program of regular exercise rests on the following:

- Knowledge of the benefits of exercise and problems related to immobility
- Appreciation of the fact that in society, sedentary lifestyles are common and most people must consciously choose to exercise
- Belief that each person is responsible for self-health and that exercise is essential to well-being

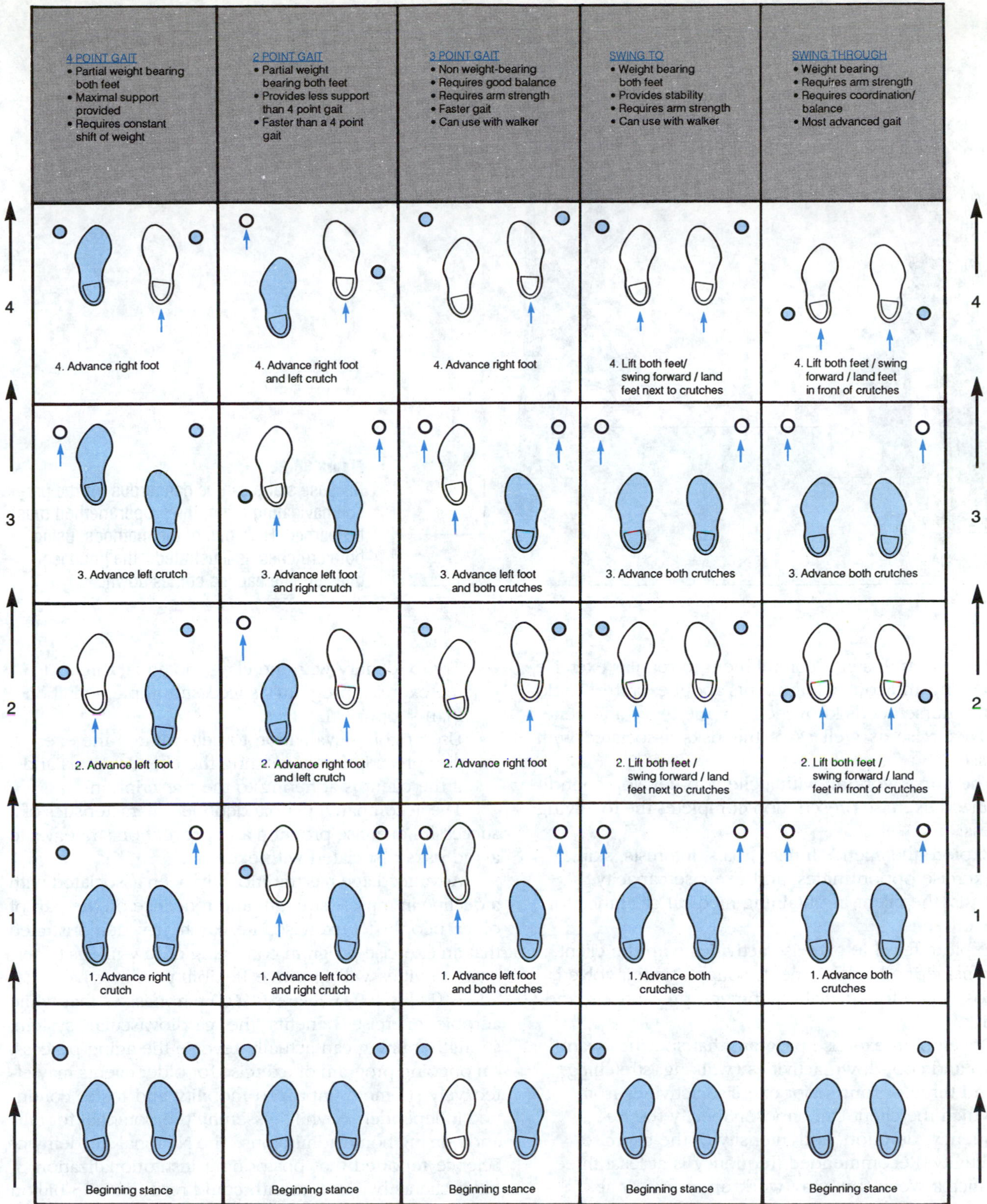

Figure 39-27

Crutch gaits. Shaded areas are weight-bearing ↑ indicates advance foot or crutch. (Smeltzer, S.C., & Bare, B.G. [1996]. *Brunner and Suddarth's textbook of medical–surgical nursing* [8th ed.]. Philadelphia: Lippincott.)

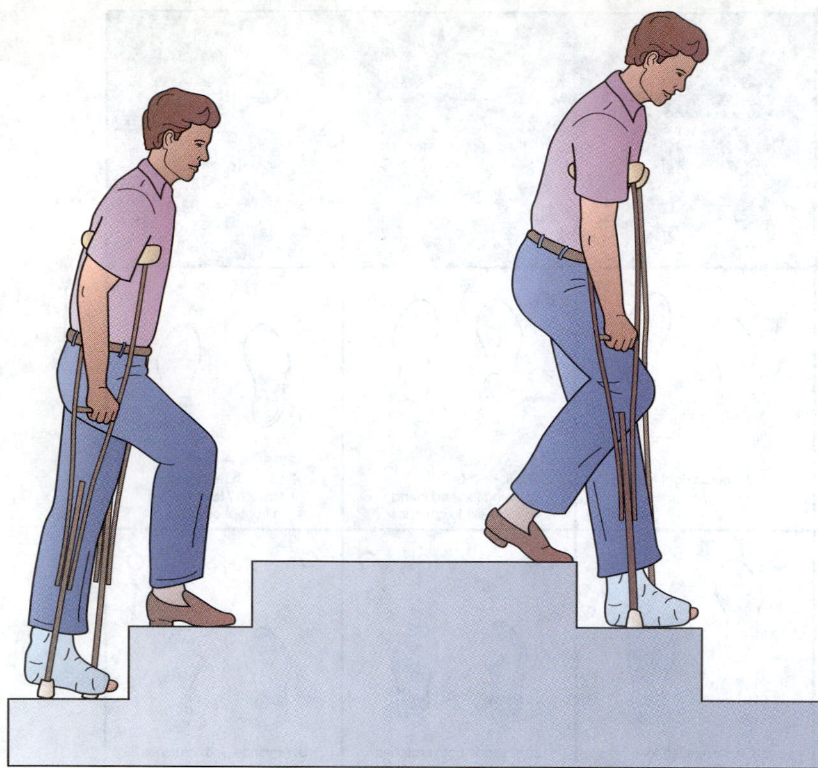

Figure 39-28
Because stairs can be dangerous for the person navigating them, the proper method must be learned. Here one of the methods, using both crutches, is illustrated: "the good leg goes up, the bad leg comes down."

Nurses can foster a commitment to regular exercise by teaching and counseling clients about exercise. To do this, the nurse needs knowledge of the types and benefits of exercise as well as of the risks associated with exercise.

The nurse working with a client to develop an individualized exercise prescription completes the following process:

- Explore the client's fitness goals, interests, skills, exercise opportunities, and exercise capacity.
- Assist the client in obtaining medical clearance for exercise.
- Explore feasible exercise activities with the client, considering health benefits sought, time involved, cost, need for special equipment, precautions, and risk.
- Develop an exercise program that specifies warm-up and cool-down activities (walking, stretching) and three or four major exercise activities from which the client can choose. Specify the frequency, duration, and intensity of the exercise activity. Recommended frequency is at least three times a week (but may work up to five or six times a week). For recommended duration and intensity, a person should be able to speak normally without getting out of breath or should maintain a *target heart rate* (60% to 90% of maximal heart rate [220 minus age]).
- Encourage the client to complement the exercise program with everyday activities that require exercise.
- Try to identify with the client potential threats to the exercise program's successful implementation. Plan support strategies.
- Use ongoing evaluation to determine if the exercise prescription is meeting the client's needs and if the client is adhering to the prescription.

The accompanying box identifies characteristics of a successful exercise program and prevention strategies to avoid risks associated with exercise.

Advanced age has traditionally been associated with a decline in muscle strength and reticence on the part of older people to exercise. Research has demonstrated that an exercise program consisting of low-intensity aerobic activities will improve flexibility in inactive older adults (Mills, 1994). Evans (1992) emphasizes that while aerobic exercise benefits the cardiovascular system, strength training can actually reverse the aging process. An ongoing program of exercise for older clients may effectively promote improved mobility and foster continued independence while lessening the potential for falls and nursing home admissions. The National Academy of Science reported that postponing institutionalization of older clients by just 1 month could result in a $3 billion savings in Medicare and Medicaid benefits (Evans, 1992).

Teaching Exercise Benefits to Populations at Risk

Health promotion and wellness are areas where the nurse can significantly contribute to the well-being of all populations. The emphasis remains on prevention. Assessment and intervention priorities that promote posi-

Characteristics of a Successful Exercise Program

- The program is individually designed (considers the individual's fitness goals, interests, skills, exercise opportunities, and exercise capacity.)
- The program specifies warm-up and cool-down activities and a variety of major exercise activities—variety is preferable to a single-exercise activity.
- The program specifies frequency, intensity, and duration of exercise.
- The program is convenient to perform, compatible with the individual's lifestyle, and fun!
- The individual in such a program should understand the program and feel confident that exercise will result in definite health benefits.

Prevention Strategies to Avoid Risks Associated With Exercise

People beginning exercise programs should be familiar with the following guidelines:

- Obtain a preexercise medical examination and medical supervision during exercise if older than age 35 years and sedentary or if there is any past or current cardiovascular condition.
- Begin a new exercise program slowly and allow your body's support structure time to accommodate to the new stress.
- Know your body and respect its limitations. Never force a joint beyond its natural range of motion.
- Respect fatigue. Whenever you feel tingling, pain, or burning in a muscle stop and rest the muscle for 15 minutes before continuing to exercise.
- Follow the safety guidelines for specific exercises; for example, joggers are advised to run on soft surfaces as opposed to cement or asphalt, to wear well-constructed shoes with thick soles and arch supports, and to run in a safe environment with a low pollution index.

tive health behaviors for each developmental stage are outlined in Table 39-2. As life expectancy increases, nursing activities will particularly focus on teaching that regular exercise is a positive factor contributing to longevity. In addition to improving the quality of life, exercise plays an important role in the prevention or slowing of osteoporosis. Nurses can help older clients use physical exercise to avert or alleviate the effects of this debilitating aging process.

EVALUATING

When evaluating the effectiveness of a plan of care designed to help clients enhance, maintain, or regain mobility and fitness goals, the nurse uses each nurse–client interaction to evaluate the client in the following respects:

- General ease of movement and gait
- Alignment
- Joint structure and function
- Muscle mass, tone, and strength
- Endurance

An excellent time to assess these essential ingredients of well-being is when the client is performing simple everyday tasks such as ambulating, undertaking hygiene measures, dressing, and eating. Because illness and enforced inactivity can affect these tasks negatively, ongoing evaluation is necessary if serious problems are to be avoided. Specific criteria for evaluating individualized plans of care follow.

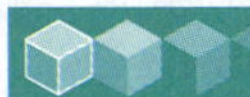

Nursing Process in Clinical Practice

Once a mobility problem is detected, the nurse implements each phase of the nursing process to ensure correct identification and treatment of the problem. The nurse who wishes to identify and manage the mobility problem correctly and to prevent complications related to immobility must possess the knowledge and clinical skills described earlier in this chapter. The following discussion outlines the assessment priorities, expected outcomes, and nursing interventions for the following nursing diagnoses:

Activity Intolerance
Impaired Physical Mobility
Risk for Injury: Complications of Immobility
Altered Health Maintenance: Lack of Exercise Program

In the client care study that follows, a nursing plan of care is developed to address the mobility needs of a client with left-sided hemiplegia following a cerebrovascular accident (stroke).

Activity Intolerance

A state in which an individual has insufficient physiological or psychological energy to endure or complete required or desired daily activities. (NANDA, 1994)

Nurses working with clients with chronic illnesses that affect oxygen transport or with immobilized clients will frequently observe in these clients a reduced ability to perform the activities of daily living. Activity intolerance is the diagnostic label describing the physical or psychologic inability to tolerate an increase in activity. For one client, this may translate into an inability to climb the four sets of stairs leading to an apartment, whereas for another client, it may mean the inability to walk the few steps from the bed to the bathroom without becoming winded.

Any factor causing fatigue or interfering with the amount of oxygen being delivered to the muscles for the work of contraction and relaxation can produce activity intolerance. Common etiologies include the following:

- Developmental factors (decreased strength in an older person)
- Pathophysiologic factors (illnesses altering oxygen transport: cardiac—congestive heart failure, arrhythmias, angina, myocardial infarction; respiratory—chronic obstructive pulmonary disease; circulatory—anemia, peripheral arterial disease; other chronic diseases; malnourishment)
- Situational (prolonged bed rest or inactivity, depression, decreased motivation, pain, anything causing fatigue)

Assessment Priorities

- Note complaints of fatigue, weakness, or an inability to perform usual tasks without dizziness, dyspnea, or frequent pauses to rest.
- Identify any contributing factors that increase fatigue or compromise oxygen transport.
- Assess the client's response to activity:
  - Take resting vital signs and note the client's mental status and skin characteristics.
  - Have the client perform an activity (eg, ambulation) and take the vital signs immediately after the activity and after the client rests for 3 to 5 minutes. Although it is customary for the pulse, blood pressure, and respiratory rate to rise with exercise, they should return to the baseline rate after rest. Weakness, pallor, diaphoresis, confusion, and vertigo may all signal activity intolerance.

Expected Outcomes

The client will:

- Identify factors contributing to activity intolerance
- Reduce or eliminate these factors to the extent possible
- Increase endurance to the point of being able to perform key activities of daily living (specify)
- Demonstrate energy conservation measures
- Demonstrate decreased signs of anoxia (sustained increases in pulse rate, blood pressure, respiratory rate, dyspnea, pallor)

Interventions

- Set daily realistic activity goals with the client and offer immediate reinforcement if the goal is met. Explore the client's motivation to increase the activity level.
- Assist the client to reduce or eliminate factors contributing to the decreased tolerance (eg, improve quantity and quality of sleep, offer pain medication before the client's activity, inspire client with a sincere "can do" mentality).
- Pace the activities according to the client's strength and intersperse activities with periods of rest.
- Teach the client and family how to progress activities gradually and how to conserve energy for priority activities.

Impaired Physical Mobility

> A state in which the individual experiences a limitation of ability for independent physical movement. (NANDA, 1994)

Because impaired physical mobility may interfere with an individual's ability to meet other human needs (eg, obtain, prepare, and eat food; bathe and dress self; toilet self) as well as with self-concept, it is important that problems affecting physical mobility be correctly identified and worked up in the plan of care. Mobility impairments may affect the upper or lower limbs, or both. Possible etiologies include the following:

- Developmental factors (muscle weakness or painful movement of joints in older clients)
- Pathophysiologic factors (neuromuscular or musculoskeletal impairment)
- Situational factors (need for bed rest; devices such as casts, splints, and braces; pain; nonfunctioning or missing limbs; effects of medications)

Assessment Priorities

- Observe the client to determine the precise nature of the mobility impairment:
  - Inability to maintain body alignment
  - Inability to execute coordinated, purposeful movements (includes bed mobility, transfers, ambulation—gait)
  - Decreased muscle strength or control (motor function in all four extremities—strong, weak, absent, spastic; weight-bearing potential)
  - Limited joint mobility
  - Impaired perception of position or presence of body parts
- Identify all etiologic factors. Carefully assess the client's motivation to be mobile and the effect of any secondary gains being derived from the immobility.
- When illness or trauma is causing the mobility problems, consult with the physician to determine both the immediate and future effects of the mobility deficit on human functioning so that realistic client counseling can be planned.

Expected Outcomes

Depending on the nature of the mobility impairment, the following goals need to be individualized. The client will:

- Maintain (or increase) muscle strength and control in the upper/lower/right/left extremities
- Demonstrate correct execution of isometric or isotonic exercise program
- Independently (or with the correct use of adaptive devices) demonstrate correct alignment, transfers, and ambulation
- Demonstrate correct use of safety measures to prevent injury
- Perform activities of daily living with greatest degree of independence possible

Interventions

- Whenever possible, reduce or eliminate factors contributing to immobility (fear of falling, apathy, effects of nonessential medications).
- If pain is contributing to immobility, administer the prescribed analgesic before the client's activity.
- Ensure that the client is positioned in correct alignment and changes position every 2 hours.
- Develop an exercise program that includes complete range-of-motion exercises, isometric setting exercises, and ambulation (as possible).
- Encourage maximal participation in activities of daily living.
- Provide the appropriate nursing care for casts, traction devices, slings, braces, and prosthetic devices.
- Teach the client how to transfer and ambulate safely using a cane, walker, crutches, or wheelchair.
- Be vigilant for the development of any of the complications of immobility. Identify high-risk clients and include preventive care in the plan of care (see Table 39-3).

Risk for Injury: Complications of Immobility

The state in which an individual is at risk of injury as a result of environmental conditions interacting with the individual's adaptive and defensive resources (NANDA, 1994).

The effects of immobility on major body systems as well as on an individual's psychosocial functioning are presented earlier in this chapter. Nursing's challenge is to identify clients at high risk for developing problems related to immobility and to institute nursing measures immediately to prevent these problems. Because the problems are multiple, they are presented in table format according to body system with specific etiologies, assessment priorities, client goals, and related nursing interventions (see Table 39-3). Nursing plans of care for immobilized clients should reflect nursing's concern to prevent immobility problems.

Altered Health Maintenance: Lack of Exercise Program

Inability to identify, manage, and/or seek out help to maintain health. (NANDA, 1994)

Although in recent years a fitness craze has prompted many individuals to develop more active lifestyles, many people still live overwhelmingly sedentary lives. Reasons for the lack of regular physical exercise are many:

- Science and technology have developed complex machines and services to aid in the performance of the activities of daily living, which formerly required an expenditure of physical energy. In the past, people who wished to survive had no choice but to be active. Currently, an individual must consciously choose to be active.
- Convenience (reduced energy expenditure) has come to be valued over activities requiring more effort.
- Children are quickly socialized into valuing sedentary activities such as watching television or listening to the radio.
- Society's fetish for cleanliness leads some people to abhor any activities that produce sweat.
- There is still lack of knowledge and much confusion about the benefits of regular exercise.
- Some individuals become discouraged from being more active following unsuccessful attempts.
- Physical injury or discomfort resulting from a poorly designed exercise program may cause a person to discontinue the activity.
- Some people believe that exercise is simply too much bother.
- Some people are unable to find the time for regular exercise.
- Embarrassment may be related to an individual's appearance, ability, or physical condition.
- Some people erroneously believe that the need for exercise decreases with age and eventually disappears.
- Some people overrate the benefits of light, sporadic exercise.
- Some people underrate their own abilities and exercise capacity.

Assessment Priorities

- Interview the client to determine past and present history of exercise; knowledge about the benefits of exercise; motivation to adhere to a regular program of exercise; exercise preferences; feasibility of these preferences (time involved, cost, need for special equipment, presence of support systems, safety concerns); any contraindications for beginning to exercise without medical supervision (eg, history of chest pain or pressure with activity, past or current cardiovascular or respiratory problems, degenerative joint diseases or other orthopedic problems); and ability to design and follow safe exercise program.

- Identify factors likely to sabotage the client's efforts to exercise (decreased motivation, multiple demands on time, lack of funds for child care, and so on).
- Perform a physical examination to rule out any physical contraindications (eg, obesity, high blood pressure, musculoskeletal problems) to exercising without medical clearance. (Stress testing is mandatory for sedentary people older than age 35 years and for anyone with a past or current cardiovascular condition.)

Expected Outcomes

The client will:

- Identify four personal benefits of exercise
- Identify personal factors that tend to prevent regular exercise
- Develop a feasible and safe exercise program, including specifics for the following:
  - Warm-up activities
  - A variety of exercise activities including aerobic and stretch exercises (type, frequency, duration)
  - Cool-down activities
- Identify the risks inherent in this program and the precautions that will be taken
- Obtain medical clearance for exercise program if needed
- Describe three means to reinforce exercise goals (reward system, exercise partner, use of other supports)

Interventions

- Teach the client:
  - Four components of fitness: (1) cardiovascular function; (2) endurance, (3) *flexibility* (ability to use a muscle through its entire range of motion); and (4) strength
  - Benefits of regular exercise
  - Types of exercise
- Assist the client to determine exercise preferences by comparing and contrasting different types of exercise: time required, place, equipment needed, cost, aerobic versus anaerobic value, advantages, disadvantages, and precautions and risks.
- Assist the client in developing an individualized exercise program:
  - Choose warm-up, major, and cool-down activities.
  - Set objectives for duration, intensity, and frequency.
  - Teach the client how to take a radial pulse and how to determine his or her target heart rate if necessary.
  - Consider the best setting for the activity and the equipment and money needed to perform the exercise safely.
  - Identify risks and safety factors.
  - Explore with the client potential threats to the exercise program and existing supports.
- Help the client to develop a strategy to evaluate the attainment of the exercise goals. A self-contract with or without additional nursing intervention may be sufficient.

Client Care Study

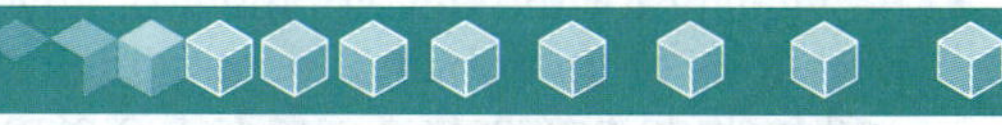

Quan Hong Nguyen is an alert, 57-year-old married man who was admitted to the hospital with a diagnosis of right cerebrovascular accident secondary to thrombosis. He has a history of hypertension. This is his second hospital day and the attending physicians have termed the stroke a *completed stroke*, that is, Mr. Nguyen's neurologic deficits have been unchanged for 2 days and he is believed to be ready for more aggressive rehabilitative treatment. On hospital day 2, an assessment of Mr. Nguyen's mobility status and ability to participate in activities of daily living revealed the following data:

- *Mental status*—basically alert and able to follow simple commands; expresses his needs verbally when encouraged but speech is slow; seems forgetful of usual routine for basic self-care activities
- *Neuromuscular status*—hemiplegia; severe motor and sensory deficits of the left side of the face and the left arm and leg
  - *Muscle mass, tone, and strength*—well-developed muscles in all extremities; history of a lifetime of sports, most recently played tennis two to four times weekly; decreased muscle tone (hypotonicity, flaccidity) in left arm and leg; motor function is absent in left arm and very weak in left leg; strong motor function on right extremities; incapable of weight-bearing on left side; incapable of independent turning, sitting, standing, transferring, or ambulation
  - *Joint mobility*—decreased on left side; otherwise full range of motion; no contractures
  - *Endurance*—fatigues quickly (eg, during complete bath)
  - Some deficit in spatial–perceptual orientation (eg, ignores objects on his left side) but difficult to assess this completely yet

Core Competencies

Cognitive Competencies

- Conviction that nursing can make a difference in the quality of this family's present and future life
- Knowledge of how the skeletal, muscular, and nervous systems function to produce purposeful and coordinated movement

- Knowledge of which nursing interventions are most likely to yield desired outcomes
- Awareness of pertinent cultural considerations

Technical Competencies

- Strong assessment skills to determine how the neurologic dysfunction is influencing Mr. Nguyen's mobility and coordination
- Caregiver skills directed to preventing complications and maintaining muscle strength and joint mobility to facilitate an optimal return to function
- Competent use of body mechanics when positioning Mr. Nguyen and assisting him with transfers (and when teaching these skills to the family)

Interpersonal Competencies

- Interpersonal skills to communicate to Mr. Nguyen and his family empathy for their situation and to mobilize their energies for the long process of rehabilitation
- Counseling skills to enable Mr. Nguyen to regain independence in self-care abilities
- Interpersonal and leadership skills to motivate the entire nursing staff to value Mr. Nguyen's rehabilitation
- Ability to work collaboratively with many other members of the healthcare team while coordinating all their efforts into a comprehensive plan of care
- Patience

Ethical/Legal Competencies

- Accountability: Commitment to maintain competence and willingness to use competence to help Mr. Nguyen reach his full rehabilitative potential
- Sensitivity to factors in Mr. Nguyen's situation which increase his risk for harm and concomitantly increase your risk of liability; ability to implement legal safeguards, eg, strong documentation skills

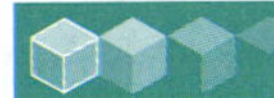

Nursing Plan of Care

for Quan Hong Nguyen

Nursing Diagnosis: Impaired Physical Mobility (turning in bed, sitting, standing, transferring, and ambulating) related to left hemiplegia and weakness as manifested by: motor function absent in left arm and weak in left leg, decreased joint mobility in left extremities, fatigue

Expected Outcome: 1/25/98 Whenever observed, the client will:

- Be in correct body alignment with (1) each joint on the left side higher than the joint proximal to it and (2) supportive devices in place (bed board, footboard, trochanter roll, hand–wrist splint, shoulder sling, pillows)

Nursing Interventions	Rationale	Evaluative Statement
At each position change (as dictated by every-2-hour turn schedule posted at the bedside), make sure that the client is in correct alignment. Follow agency positioning guidelines for the supine, side-lying (lies on unaffected side), and prone positions.	Correct positioning prevents contractures, relieves pressures, and maintains alignment. • Positioning each joint higher than the preceding one prevents edema and its resulting fibrosis. • Placing the client in the prone position for 30 minutes two or three times daily helps prevent knee and hip flexion contractures.	1/27/98 Goal being met. Every-2-hour positioning schedule being followed with client in correct body alignment to prevent contractures. *S. Beecher, RN*
Use the following supportive devices: firm mattress, footboard, trochanter roll, shoulder sling when client is in upright position, volar resting splint, and pillows.	Support devices aid in maintaining the client in correct positioning. • Firm mattress provides skeletal support.	

(continued)

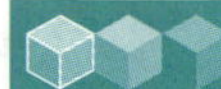

Nursing Plan of Care *(continued)*

for Quan Hong Nguyen

Nursing Interventions	Rationale	Evaluative Statement
	• Footboard during flaccid period prevents footdrop, heel cord shortening, and plantar flexion. • Trochanter roll prevents external rotation of hip when client is in dorsal position. • Shoulder sling during flaccid period prevents shoulder subluxation and shoulder–hand syndrome. • Volar resting splint supports the wrist and hand in a functional position. • A pillow in the axilla of the left side prevents adduction of the affected side.	
Teach both the client and family the importance of correct positioning.	Teaching promotes self-care and lays the foundation for successful rehabilitation.	
Allow the family to participate in helping the client to get comfortable in the different positions.	Involving the family in the client's care facilitates the coping process.	

Expected Outcome By hospital day 7, 1/30/98, the client will:

- Replace the passive range-of-motion exercises the nurse is now performing four times daily to all joints with (1) the client's active exercise of the left arm and left leg and (2) the client's active range-of-motion exercises for all other joints

Nursing Interventions	Rationale	Evaluative Statement
Assess the client's knowledge of the importance of exercise and ability and motivation to exercise.	Unless the client understands the reason for exercise and is physically, mentally, and attitudinally capable of exercise, he will not follow through.	1/30/98 Goal partially met. Client has successfully demonstrated complete set of range-of-motion exercises (to both left and right sides); however, he tires during the exercises and stops unless verbally encouraged. *Revision:* Monitor client's exercise four times daily; continue to enlist family's support. *S. Beecher, RN*
Teach the client how to exercise his left arm and leg by using his unaffected (right) extremities.	Active exercise maintains joint mobility, prevents contracture development in the paralyzed extremity, prevents further deterioration of the neuromuscular system, helps to regain motor control, and increases circulation.	
Demonstrate a complete set of range-of-motion exercises to the client and family and have the client return the demonstrations.	Involving the family helps ensure the success of the exercise program because it requires a big time and effort commitment.	

(continued)

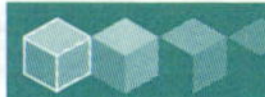

Nursing Plan of Care *(continued)*

for Quan Hong Nguyen

Expected Outcome

By hospital day 7, 1/30/98, the client will:
- Perform quadriceps, gluteal, and abdominal settings five times daily

Nursing Interventions	Rationale	Evaluative Statement
Teach the client and family how to tighten the quadriceps, gluteal, and abdominal muscles and hold them for 6 seconds (slow count to 4) before relaxing. A 2-minute rest should be allowed between contractions and the client cautioned not to hold his breath during these exercises because this places strain on the heart. The exercises should be stopped short of muscle fatigue.	These exercises will maintain muscle mass, tone, and strength (while the client is on bed rest); and prevent atrophy. They also increase circulation to the exercised body parts.	1/30/98 Goal partially met. Client has demonstrated exercises correctly; however, he needs to be reminded to perform them. Family is effective in this regard. *Revision:* Compliment family on excellent job they are doing and reinforce importance of exercise to maximize rehabilitative potential. *S. Beecher, RN*

Expected Outcome:

By hospital day 7, 1/30/98, the client will:
- Participate in the every-2-hour positioning schedule by assisting with turning to the degree he is able

Nursing Interventions	Rationale	Evaluative Statement
Teach the client how he can help to reposition himself by grabbing onto the side rail with his right hand and also by placing his unaffected leg under the left one to move himself.	The more the client can do independently, the more in control he will feel. These activities will pave the way to increasing independence in self-care activities.	1/27/98 Goal met. Client consistently assists in repositioning. Seems pleased to be able to help the nurses in this way. *S. Beecher, RN*

Expected Outcome

By hospital day 7, 1/30/98, the client will:
- Demonstrate a safe pivot transfer from bed to chair and chair to bed

Nursing Actions	Rationale	Evaluative Statement
Assess the stage of recovery of muscle function.	Most clients will begin to show signs of spasticity with exaggerated reflexes within 48 hours—this denotes progress. If muscles are still flaccid after several weeks, prognosis for regaining function is poor.	1/30/98 Goal met. Client can safely transfer from bed to chair and chair to bed but requires nursing assistance. *S. Beecher, RN*

Expected Outcome

By hospital day 7, 1/30/98, the client will:
- Demonstrate standing balance

Nursing Interventions	Rationale	Evaluative Statement
Assess activity tolerance by taking vital signs before attempting balance training and transfers.	Vital signs and the client's physical condition should be assessed before a new activity, during the activity, and shortly afterward to assess activity tolerance.	1/30/98 Goal not met. Client has not demonstrated standing balance; falls to left side without nursing support. *Revision:* Allow more time for goal achievement. *S. Beecher, RN*

(continued)

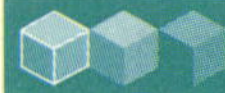

Nursing Plan of Care *(continued)*

for Quan Hong Nguyen

Nursing Interventions	Rationale	Evaluative Statement
Precede transfers with balance training. Assist the client to a sitting position at the edge of the bed and observe for steadiness and the ability to maintain an erect posture.	The client needs sitting and standing balance before progressing to harder tasks. Dizziness or syncope may signal vasomotor instability.	
Place the chair by the bed on the client's unaffected side and assist the client to dress. Initially the nurse helps the client to stand by placing his or her right knee against the client's strong knee, grasping the client around the waist with both arms, and pulling the client forward while rocking back on the left leg (nurse's knees are slightly flexed).	This prevents the client's knees from buckling and the pressure of the nurse's knee forces the client to straighten the strong knee and bear weight on it. In this position the client's feet cannot slip forward. In this position, the nurse is using good principles of body mechanics.	
Once the client is standing, assess standing balance and observe for signs of activity intolerance (pallor, shortness of breath, excessive increase in pulse rate, perspiration). Direct the client to (1) grab the far arm of the chair with his strong arm, (2) turn on his strong foot, and (3) sit down. The nurse's right leg and the client's strong leg are used as a pivot.	Using the unaffected extremity facilitates movement and provides stability.	
Pivot client out of bed to chair three times a day (may pivot out of bed to bedside commode). Gradually increase time in chair based on client's tolerance. Correctly align client in chair using supportive devices as necessary.	Increasing exercise to the client's tolerance level promotes improved muscle strength and maintenance of range of motion.	

Expected Outcome On discharge to rehabilitation center, the client will:

- Be free of contractures

Nursing Interventions	Rationale	Evaluative Statement
Implement previously stated nursing actions.	These actions promote independence and return to activities of daily living.	1/31/98 Goal met. Client has no contractures. *S. Beecher, RN*

Nursing Diagnosis: Self-Care Deficit (all basic self-care activities) related to decreased alertness and left-sided motor and sensory deficits as manifested by: inability to use left arm (is right-handed) inability to ambulate, forgetfulness, fatigue

(continued)

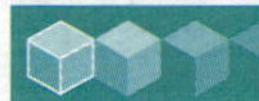

Nursing Plan of Care *(continued)*

for Quan Hong Nguyen

Expected Outcome: By hospital day 7, 1/30/98, the client will:

- Demonstrate beginning ability to resume self-care activities despite motor and sensory deficits of left side; use right arm to (1) assist in morning hygiene; (2) feed himself (finger foods, beverages); and (3) exercise

Nursing Actions	Rationale	Evaluative Statement
Continue to assess extent of client's motor and sensory deficits and ability to perform self-care activities.	This facilitates recognition of any recovery of function and allows setting of appropriate goals.	1/29/98 Goal met. For the past 2 days, client has washed his left arm, abdomen, and legs; combed his hair; fed himself; and performed range-of-motion exercises. *S. Beecher, RN*
Set realistic short-term goals for each session with client and reward progress: "This morning we'll see how much of your bath you are able to manage yourself!" "It must feel good to be able to do this for yourself again."	Adding *realistic* new tasks for each day gives the client a goal to work toward; a pattern of *noticed* success encourages continued efforts.	
Approach client from his unaffected side, and place call light, bedside table, phone, and so on, on this side.	This helps the client to compensate for alterations in sensory perception.	
Teach client how to transfer all self-care activities to the unaffected side and how to use one-handed techniques and adaptive equipment.	There is never only one way to do anything.	
Encourage client to brush his teeth, comb his hair, bathe and feed himself, and to assist in toileting. Explain to the family why it is critical to allow him to do these things himself, even if movements are tiring, clumsy, and initially frustrating.	This improves the client's sense of control of his own activities of daily living and improves morale.	
Continually reevaluate the client's need for gentle care versus firm, directive encouragement. Involve the family in this process.	Emotional lability is common after stroke. Clients fluctuate between heroic efforts toward independent self-care and whining demands to be totally cared for. The appropriate nursing response varies from moment to moment and runs the range of tender care to unrelenting firm direction. All nursing responses need to communicate the nurse's sincere care for the client and commitment to developing his best potential.	

Expected Outcome On discharge to rehabilitation center, the client will:

- Show signs of physical and mental readiness to acquire increasing independence in self care

(continued)

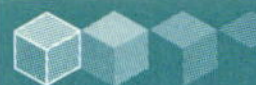

Nursing Plan of Care *(continued)*

for Quan Hong Nguyen

Nursing Interventions	Rationale	Evaluative Statement
Implement previously stated nursing actions.	These actions help the client toward regaining control of his daily living and improve morale.	1/31/98 Goal met. Client's muscle strength and joint mobility maintained during hospitalization. Client is now participating in self-care activities and is eager to learn skills to become more independent. *S. Beecher, RN*

Sample Documentation

1/25/98, 3 PM, Nursing

Dr. Steel examined the client at 1 PM and noted he is now in "completed stroke stage and ready for more aggressive rehabilitative treatment." This was explained to client, his wife, and son. The client smiled and seemed to understand that he is out of immediate danger. Initial instructions given to the client on how he can assist with position changes and actively exercise his left arm and leg. Correctly demonstrated these maneuvers with verbal cuing. Motor function still absent in left arm and weak in left leg. Plan of care revised to incorporate new exercise goals.

Susan Beecher, RN

Key Points

- The fulfillment of most human needs depends, at least partially, on the body's ability to move. Purposeful, coordinated movement of the body requires the integrated functioning of the skeletal, muscular, and nervous systems of the body.
- Bones and joints provide form for the body and serve as the levers and fulcrums that make body movement possible. It is the contraction and relaxation of skeletal muscles, however, that actually produce movement by pulling on bones, and it is nerve impulses that stimulate the muscles to contract.
- Good body mechanics is the efficient use of the body as a machine and as means of locomotion. To role model healthy body mechanics, the nurse pays special attention to body alignment, balance, and coordinated body movement during work and leisure activities.
- Factors that influence body alignment and mobility include developmental considerations, physical health, mental health, lifestyle variables, attitudes and values, fatigue and stress level, and external factors.
- The active exertion of muscles involving the contraction and relaxation of muscle groups is termed exercise. Isotonic exercise involves muscle shortening and active movement, and its potential benefits include increased muscle mass, tone, and strength; improved joint mobility; increased cardiac and respiratory function; increased circulation; and increased osteoblastic activity. Isometric exercise involves contraction without movement, and potential benefits are increased muscle mass, tone, and strength; increased circulation to the exercised body part; and increased osteoblastic activity.
- Individuals who choose to live inactive lifestyles place themselves at high risk for serious health problems. Problems of immobility include increased cardiac workload, thrombus formation, orthostatic hypotension, ineffective breathing patterns, ineffective airway clearance, impaired gas exchange, activity intolerance, pathologic fractures, nutritional alterations, fluid volume excesses, constipation, alteration in urinary elimination, potential for urinary tract infection, impairment of skin integrity, disturbances in self-esteem, powerlessness, impaired social interaction, altered thought processes, ineffective coping, and sleep pattern disturbances.
- People beginning exercise programs should be familiar with the following guidelines: Begin pro-

gram slowly and allow the body time to adjust to the new stress, know your body and respect its limitations, and follow the safety guidelines for specific exercises.

- When assessing mobility status, interview the client regarding daily activity level, endurance, exercise and fitness goals, mobility problems, physical or mental problems that affect mobility, and external factors that affect mobility. The physical assessment of mobility status includes an assessment of general ease of movement and gait; alignment; joint structure and function; muscle mass, tone, and strength; and endurance.
- Nursing diagnoses for mobility problems include Activity Intolerance and Impaired Physical Mobility. Both problem statements have multiple etiologies. Because mobility influences so many other areas of human functioning, many nursing diagnoses have as their etiology a problem with mobility.
- The aim of nursing care for both well and ill clients is that the client follow a program of regular physical exercise that improves cardiovascular function, endurance, flexibility, and strength.
- Nursing strategies that promote mobility for clients on bed rest include careful attention to positioning that maintains correct alignment and facilitates physiologic functioning, safe transfer of client from bed to chair or stretcher, and the early and safe ambulation of clients. The nurse may also play a key role in teaching clients to use mechanical aids for walking.
- Clients require specialized nursing care if they have the following mobility diagnoses: Activity Intolerance, Impaired Physical Mobility, Risk for Injury related to complications for immobility, and Altered Health Maintenance related to lack of exercise program.

Study Questions

1. The strong, flexible, inelastic fibrous bands that attach muscle to bone are
   a. tendons
   b. ligaments
   c. cartilage
   d. joints
2. The nurse spreads her feet apart as he or she prepares to help raise a client from a chair. The most important reason for doing this is to
   a. use the body's weight to assist movement
   b. make a long midriff
   c. provide a wide base of support
   d. facilitate use of the stronger back muscles
3. A client performs rehabilitative exercises with resistance after a knee injury. This type of exercise is referred to as
   a. isotonic
   b. isokinetic
   c. isometric
   d. aerobic
4. The expected result when more protein is broken down than is manufactured is
   a. fluid volume excess
   b. a contracture
   c. osteoporosis
   d. negative nitrogen balance
5. An immobile client experiences multiple urinary tract infections. Urinary bacteria are more likely to grow when urine is
   a. alkaline
   b. dilute
   c. aromatic
   d. acidic
6. Mr. Brown is experiencing some difficulty breathing. The nurse most appropriately assists him into the
   a. dorsal recumbent position
   b. lateral position
   c. Fowler's position
   d. Sims' position
7. While doing range-of-motion exercises with a bedridden client, the nurse is aware that
   a. neck hyperextension should be encouraged, particularly in older people
   b. exercises should be continued until the client is fatigued
   c. exercises should be done frequently so as to lessen pain for the client
   d. each joint is exercised to the point of resistance but not pain
8. The nurse is assisting a client with conditioning exercises to prepare for ambulation. The nurse correctly instructs the client to
   a. do full-body push-ups in bed six to eight times daily
   b. breathe in and out smoothly during quadriceps drills
   c. dangle on the side of the bed for 30 to 60 minutes
   d. allow the nurse to bathe the client completely to prevent fatigue
9. In many situations, a client has sufficient strength to walk if he or she can
   a. lie prone for 1 hour
   b. bathe himself or herself
   c. raise the foot off the bed 1 inch
   d. sit up in bed for 1 hour

10. Mrs. Eden tells the nurse she feels faint while walking in the corridor with the nurse. The nurse
    a. instructs the client to quicken her pace so they can return to her room
    b. leaves her momentarily to find another nurse to help
    c. advises her to look down at her feet to help maintain her balance
    d. guides her to a chair in the corridor and eases her onto it to rest
11. When using a cane for maximum support, the nurse is aware the client should
    a. hold the cane on the weaker side
    b. distribute weight evenly between the feet and the cane
    c. keep the elbow straight and stiff that is holding the cane
    d. advance the weaker foot ahead of the cane
12. When measuring a client for axillary crutches, the nurse should
    a. have the client lie flat on the back in bed while wearing walking shoes
    b. have the client stand with feet separated 12 inches and arms extended at shoulder height
    c. measure the distance from the shoulder to the heel and add 4 inches
    d. measure the distance from the anterior fold of axilla diagonally to a point 12 inches from the heel
13. When using the swing-through crutch gait, the client should
    a. bear weight on the unaffected foot
    b. bear weight on both feet
    c. simulate normal walking as closely as possible
    d. move the right crutch and left foot forward at the same time
14. When working with an older client to develop an exercise program, the nurse would recommend
    a. a frequency of six times a week
    b. exercising to the point of breathlessness when trying to speak
    c. maintaining a target heart rate of 220 plus age
    d. medical clearance before beginning the program
15. A bedridden client who is blind is admitted to a healthcare facility from his or her home with pressure ulcers on the sacral area. A priority nursing diagnosis is
    a. Risk for Altered Body Temperature related to stage 2 pressure ulcer
    b. Impaired Skin Integrity related to immobility
    c. Feeding Self-Care Deficit related to blindness
    d. Activity Intolerance related to prolonged bed rest

Answers With Rationale

1. The correct response is *a.* Tendons are the strong fibrous bands that attach muscle to bone. Ligaments bind joints together and connect bones and cartilage, whereas cartilage is nonvascular connective tissue found in the joints as well as in the nose, ear, thorax, trachea, and larynx.
2. The correct response is *c.* Spreading the feet apart broadens the base of support and lowers the center of gravity. The muscles of the back are not as strong as the long muscles of the arms and legs and making a long midriff is accomplished by stretching the muscles in the waist. Rocking on the feet or leaning forward or backward uses the weight of the body as a moving force.
3. The correct response is *b.* Isokinetic exercise involves muscle contraction with resistance, whereas isotonic exercise involves muscle shortening and active movement. Isometric exercise involves muscle contraction without shortening and aerobic exercise is sustained muscle movements that increase blood flow, heart rate, and metabolic demand for oxygen over time, promoting cardiovascular conditioning.
4. The correct response is *d.* Negative nitrogen balance results when the body excretes more nitrogen than it takes in. Contractures are permanent contraction states of muscles and osteoporosis involves bone demineralization. Fluid volume excess is indirectly related to protein manufacture or breakdown.
5. The correct response is *a.* Bacteria grow more easily in alkaline urine than acidic urine. Whether urine is dilute or aromatic is not a factor in bacteria growth.
6. The correct response is *c.* The Fowler's position promotes maximal breathing space in the thoracic cavity and is the position of choice when someone is having difficulty breathing. Lying flat on the back or side or Sims' position would not facilitate respiration and would be difficult for the client to maintain.
7. The correct response is *d.* Joints should never be exercised to the point of pain or fatigue. Joints should be exercised slowly, smoothly, and rhythmically. Neck hyperextension should be avoided in older clients and may prove painful.
8. The correct response is *b.* The client should never hold his or her breath during exercise drills because this places a strain on the heart. Push-ups are usually done three or four times a day and involve only the upper body. Dangling for 30 to 60 minutes is unsafe. The nurse encourages the client to be as independent as possible to prepare for return to normal ambulation and activities of daily living.

9. The correct response is *c.* Being able to raise the foot 1 inch off the bed frequently indicates sufficient strength for walking. Lying prone, bathing himself or herself, or sitting up in in bed do not necessarily indicate the muscle coordination and strength necessary in the lower limbs for walking.
10. The correct response is *d.* Guiding the client to a chair in the hall and easing her into it is the safest action. Asking her to walk faster or leaving her alone are definitely unsafe actions. If the client looks down at her feet, she may become dizzy and unbalanced.
11. The correct response is *b.* The client's weight should be evenly distributed between his or her feet and the cane. Holding the cane on the weaker side is difficult and unsafe. The elbow should be flexed at a 30-degree angle when holding the cane.
12. The correct response is *a.* Axillary crutches should be measured when the client is lying flat in bed with his or her walking shoes on. The distance is measured from the anterior fold of the axilla straight down to the heel, and then add 5 cm (2 inches). Or, measure the distance from the anterior fold of the axilla diagonally out to a point 15 cm (6 inches) away from the heel.
13. The correct response is *a.* With the swing-through gait, weight-bearing is permitted only on one foot. A disadvantage of this gait is that is does not simulate normal walking. Both crutches are brought forward at the same time and then both legs swing through and between the crutches with weight-bearing returning to the unaffected leg.
14. The correct response is *d.* Clients older than 35 years should always get medical clearance before initiating an exercise program. Frequency is initially three times a week and exercise should be maintained so that the client is able to talk without becoming breathless. The target heart rate is calculated as 60% to 90% of maximal heart rate (220 minus age).
15. The correct response is *b.* The priority nursing diagnosis for this client at this moment is Impaired Skin Integrity related to the pressure ulcer. The other nursing diagnoses may be appropriate but are not the priority on admission to the healthcare facility.

Bibliography

Ali, N., & Bennett, S. (1992). Postmenopausal women: Factors in osteoporosis preventive behaviors. *Journal of Gerontological Nursing, 18*(2), 23–32.

Ali, N., & Twibell, R. (1994). Barriers to osteoporosis prevention in perimenopausal and elderly women. *Geriatric Nursing, 15*(4), 201–205.

Bates, B. (1995). *A guide to physical examination and history taking* (6th ed.). Philadelphia: Lippincott.

Beck, C., Modlin, T., Heithoff, K., & Shue, V. (1992). Exercise as an intervention for behavior problems. *Geriatric Nursing, 13*(5), 273–275.

Carpenito, L. J. (1995). *Nursing diagnosis: Application to clinical practice* (6th ed.). Philadelphia: Lippincott.

Clinical News. (1992). Using muscle in the fight against falls. *American Journal of Nursing, 92*(9), 12.

Clinical News. (1994). Back belts don't enhance lifting power. *American Journal of Nursing, 94*(6), 10.

Evans, W. (1992). Give me strength: No rest for the aging. *Nutrition Action Health Letter, 19*(5), 1–7.

Fuller, J., & Schaller-Ayers, J. (1994). *Health assessment: A nursing approach* (2nd ed.). Philadelphia: Lippincott.

Gillett, P., Johnson, M., Juretich, M., Richardson, N., Slagle, L., & Farikoff, K. (1993). The nurse as exercise leader. *Geriatric Nursing, 14*(3), 133–137.

Hummer, A. (1993). Get your patient moving. *RN, 56*(6), 34–37.

Jacobs, B. (1994). Working on the right moves: Part 1. *Nursing, 20*(10), 58–62.

Jacobs, B. (1994). Working on the right moves: Part 2. *Nursing, 20*(11), 52–54.

McConnell, E. (1992). Using a stationary walker. *Nursing, 18*(10), 75.

McConnell, E. (1994). Logrolling a patient safely. *Nursing, 20*(9), 16.

McMahon, M., Peterson, C., & Schilke, J. (1992). Osteoporosis: Identifying high-risk persons. *Journal of Gerontological Nursing, 18*(10), 19–26.

Mills, E. (1994). The effect of low-intensity aerobic exercise on muscle strength, flexibility, and balance among sedentary elderly persons. *Nursing Research, 43*(4), 207–211.

NewsWatch. (1994). Back injuries reduced by lifting teams. *Geriatric Nursing, 15*(6), 293.

North American Nursing Diagnosis Association. (1994). *NANDA nursing diagnoses: Definitions and classification 1995–1996.* Philadelphia: NANDA.

Olsen, E., Johnson, B., & Thompson, L. (1967). The hazards of immobility. *American Journal of Nursing, 67*(4), 780–797.

Owen, B., & Garg, A. (1993). Back stress isn't part of the job. *American Journal of Nursing, 93*(2), 48–51.

Posner, J. (1992). Optimal aging: The role of exercise. *Patient Care, 26*(5), 35–63.

Spier, B., & Meis, M. (1994). Maintenance ambulation: Its significance and the role of the nurse. *Geriatric Nursing, 15*(5), 277–281.

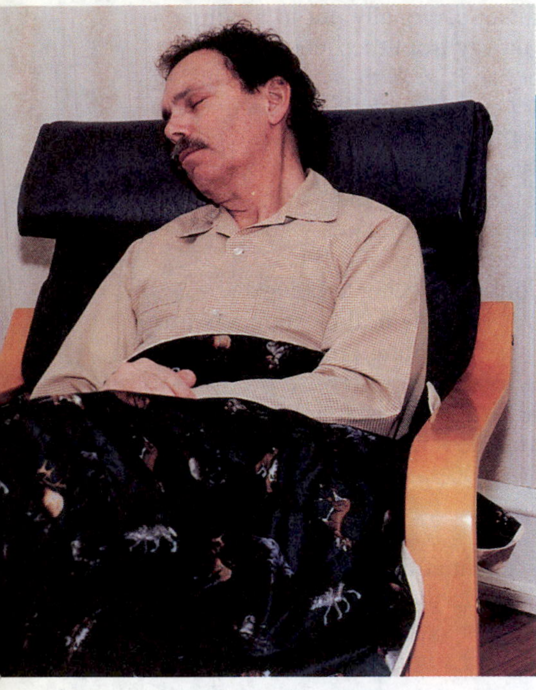

Chapter 40

Rest and Sleep

Objectives

After studying this chapter, the learner should be able to:

Define key terms used in this chapter.

Describe the functions and physiology of sleep.

Identify 12 variables that influence rest and sleep.

Describe implications for nursing for age-related differences in the sleep–wakefulness cycle.

Perform a comprehensive sleep assessment using appropriate interview questions, a sleep diary when indicated, and physical assessment skills.

Describe common sleep disorders, noting key assessment criteria.

Develop nursing diagnoses that correctly identify sleep problems that may be treated through independent nursing intervention.

Describe nine nursing strategies to promote rest and sleep, and identify their rationale.

Plan, implement, and evaluate nursing care related to select nursing diagnoses involving sleep problems.

Key Terms

circadian rhythm
delta sleep
electroencephalograph
electromyograph
electrooculogram
enuresis
hypersomnia
insomnia
narcolepsy
nocturnal myoclonus
non–rapid eye movement sleep
parasomnias
polysomnography
rapid eye movement sleep
rest
sleep
sleep apnea
sleep cycle
sleep deprivation
somnambulism

On the average, people spend one third of their lives asleep. Although the exact purpose of sleep is unclear, the functions of sleep are usually characterized as being protective and restorative. The advice that "everything will look better after a good night's sleep" is based on the belief that sleep:

- Restores physical well-being
- Relieves stress and anxiety
- Restores the ability to cope and to concentrate on activities of daily living

In this chapter, **rest** connotes a condition in which the body is in a decreased state of activity with the consequent feeling of being refreshed, and **sleep** means a state of altered consciousness, throughout which varying degrees of stimuli produce wakefulness. Sleep is an active and complex rhythmic state involving a progression of repeated cycles, each representing different phases of body and brain activity.

Most people can fall asleep easily and remain asleep until the desired waking time. On the other hand, some individuals rarely fall asleep without a struggle, and even then their sleep is fragmented. Many people have sleep disturbances that go undetected for years, progressively undermining energy and destroying their sense of self. Sleep loss that results in fatigue and decreased competence may be a contributing factor in accidents (Shaver & Landis, 1995). Most motor-vehicle accidents occurring from 2 to 7 AM are related to sleepiness (Leger, 1994). The discomfort produced by physical and mental illness and the need for hospitalization and treatment may interfere dramatically with a client's ability to sleep. Consequently, nurses need to be vigilant in detecting and treating sleep disturbances.

Study of this chapter provides the nurse with knowledge of the functions and physiology of sleep, dreams and dream theories, and factors affecting sleep. Practical suggestions for performing a comprehensive sleep assessment are given. Sample interview questions for both a general and focused sleep history are presented, along with information on sleep diaries and pertinent physical assessment data. The importance of analyzing these data is noted and numerous examples of nursing diagnoses are offered. Expected client outcomes and specific nursing strategies for promoting rest and sleep are described. In the section Nursing Process in Clinical Practice, guides to focused assessment, expected outcomes, and implementation are offered for select nursing diagnoses related to the sleep disturbances insomnia and sleep deprivation. These guides and the concluding client care study illustrate how the nurse's knowledge of rest and sleep, combined with skilled nursing interventions and caring, can successfully resolve sleep problems.

Physiology of Sleep

Two systems in the brain stem, the reticular activating system and the bulbar synchronizing region, are believed to work together to control the cyclic nature of sleep. The reticular formation (Fig. 40-1) is found in the brain stem. It extends upward through the medulla, the pons, the midbrain, and then into the hypothalamus. It comprises many nerve cells and fibers. The fibers have connections that relay impulses into the cerebral cortex and into the spinal cord. The reticular formation facilitates reflex and voluntary movements, as well as cortical activities related to a state of alertness. During sleep, the reticular system experiences few stimuli from the cerebral cortex and the periphery of the body. Wakefulness occurs when the reticular system is activated with stimuli from the cerebral cortex and from periphery sensory organs and cells. For example, an alarm clock awakens us from sleep to a state of consciousness when we realize that we must prepare ourselves for the day. Sensations such as pain, pressure, and noise produce wakefulness by means of periphery organs and cells. Wakefulness is activated by the cerebral cortex and body sensations. During sleep, stimuli from the cortex are minimal.

The hypothalamus has control centers for several involuntary activities of the body, one of which concerns sleeping and waking. Injury to the hypothalamus may cause a person to sleep for abnormally long periods.

It has been shown that some compounds play a role as neurotransmitters and are involved with the sleeping process. Norepinephrine and acetylcholine, followed by dopamine, serotonin, and histamine, are involved with excitation. Gamma-aminobutyric acid (GABA) appears to be necessary for inhibition. However, research has yet to prove exactly how biochemical changes and hormones function in sleep.

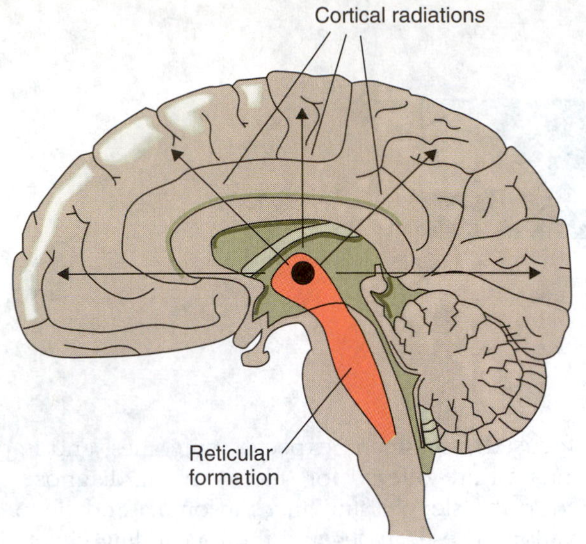

Figure 40-1
Reticular formation in brain stem and diencephalon with radiations to the cerebral cortex.

Circadian Rhythms

Rhythmic biologic clocks are currently known to exist in plants, animals, and humans. Influenced by both internal and external factors, they regulate select biologic and behavioral functions in humans. Some cycles are monthly, such as a woman's menstrual cycle. **Circadian rhythms** complete a full cycle every 24 hours. Fluctuations in heart rate, blood pressure, body temperature, hormone secretions, metabolism, and an individual's performance and mood depend in part on circadian rhythms.

Sleep is one of the body's most complex biologic rhythms. *Circadian synchronization* exists when an individual's sleep–wake patterns follow the inner biologic clock. That is, when physiologic and psychologic rhythms are high or most active, the person is awake, and when these rhythms are low, the person is asleep. Although light and dark appear to be powerful regulators of the sleep–wake circadian rhythm, they do not exert primary control. The regulating mechanism is an individualized biologic clock subject to occupational demands, social pressures, and so forth. The nurse who works the night shift may routinely sleep from 2 to 8 PM and peak physiologic activity may occur between 10 PM and 6 AM during work. Problems of desynchronization occur when sleep–wake patterns are frequently altered and an individual attempts to sleep during high activity rhythms and to work when the body is physiologically prepared to rest.

Stages of Sleep

Research illustrates that there are two major stages of sleep: **non–rapid eye movement** (NREM) and **rapid eye movement** (REM). These stages have been studied and analyzed with the help of the **electroencephalograph** (EEG), which receives and records electrical currents from the brain; the **electrooculogram** (EOG), which is a recording of eye movements; and the **electromyograph** (EMG), which records muscle tone (Fig. 40-2).

NREM Sleep. NREM sleep consists of four stages. Stages I and II, consuming about 5% to 50%, respectively, of a person's sleep, are light sleep, and the person can be aroused with relative ease. Stages III and IV, each composing about 10% of total sleep time, are deep-sleep states termed **delta sleep**, or slow-wave sleep (SWS). The arousal threshold (intensity of stimulus required to awaken) is usually greatest in stage IV NREM. Throughout the stages of NREM sleep, the parasympathetic branch of the autonomic nervous system dominates, and decreases in pulse, respiratory rate, blood pressure, metabolic rate, and body temperature are observed. Characteristics of the four stages of NREM sleep are summarized in Table 40-1.

REM Sleep. It is more difficult to arouse a person during REM sleep than during NREM sleep. In normal adults, the REM state consumes 20% to 25% of a person's nightly sleep. If people are awakened during the REM state, they almost always report that they have been

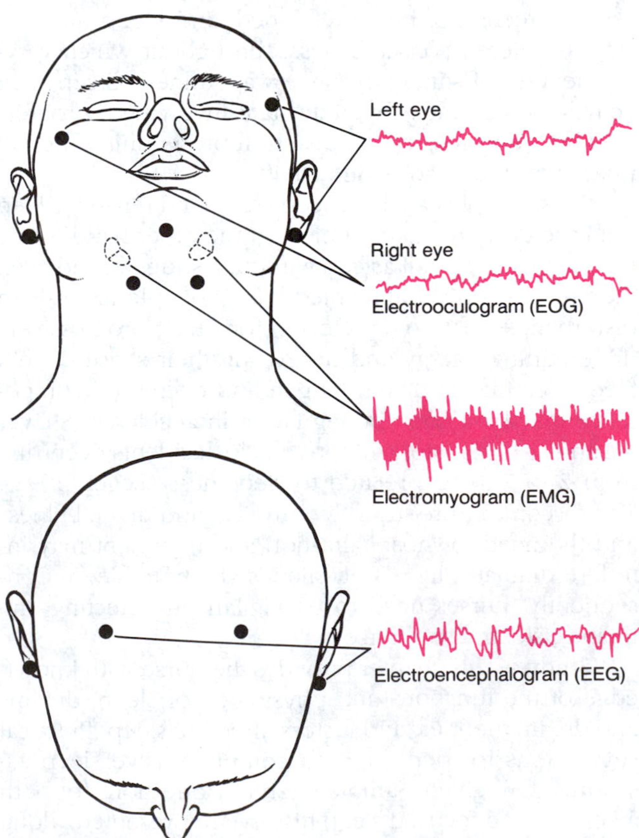

Figure 40-2
Sleep laboratory evaluation. Sleep is determined in the laboratory by measuring the electrical activity of the brain and muscles and the movement of the eyes, using techniques of electrooculography, electromyography, and electroencephalography.

Table 40-1
Characteristics of NREM Sleep

Stage	Characteristics
I	Is transitional stage between wakefulness and sleep
	The person is in a relaxed state but still somewhat aware of the surroundings.
	Involuntary muscle jerking may occur and waken the person.
	The stage normally lasts only for minutes.
	The person can be aroused easily.
	Constitutes only about 5% of total sleep.
II	The person falls into a stage of sleep.
	The person can be aroused with relative ease.
	Constitutes 50% to 55% of sleep.
III	The depth of sleep increases and arousal becomes increasingly difficult.
	Composes about 10% of sleep.
IV	The person reaches the greatest depth of sleep, which is called *delta sleep.*
	Arousal from sleep is difficult.
	Physiologic changes in the body include the following:
	Slow brain waves are recorded on an EEG.
	Pulse and respiratory rates decrease.
	Blood pressure decreases.
	Muscles are relaxed.
	Metabolism slows and the body temperature is low.
	Constitutes about 10% of sleep.

dreaming. Many researchers state that everyone dreams; those people who say they do not simply are unable to recall their dreams.

During REM sleep the pulse, respiratory rate, blood pressure, metabolic rate, and body temperature increase whereas general skeletal muscle tone and deep tendon reflexes are depressed. REM sleep is believed to be essential to mental and emotional equilibrium and to play a role in learning, memory, and adaptation.

When a person is deprived of REM sleep for several nights, he or she generally spends more time in REM sleep on successive nights. This phenomenon is termed REM rebound and allows the total amount of REM sleep to remain fairly constant over time. Characteristics of REM sleep are summarized in Table 40-2.

Sleep Cycle

Normally during a **sleep cycle**, a person passes consecutively through the four stages of NREM sleep. Then, the person reverses this pattern and returns from stage IV to stage III to stage II. Instead of reentering stage I and awakening, the person enters into the stage of REM

Table 40-2
Characteristics of REM Sleep

Item	Characteristics
Eyes	Dart back and forth quickly
Muscles	Small-muscle twitching, such as on the face
	Large-muscle immobility, resembling paralysis
Respirations	Irregular; sometimes interspersed with apnea
Pulse	Rapid or irregular
Blood pressure	Increases or fluctuates
Gastric secretions	Increase
Metabolism	Increases; body temperature increases
Brain waves	Encephalogram tracings active
Sleep cycle	REM sleep enters from stage II of NREM sleep and reenters NREM sleep at stage II: arousal from sleep difficult

sleep, after which he or she reenters NREM sleep at stage II and returns to stages III and IV. If a person is awakened from sleep at any time, he or she returns to sleep again by starting at stage I of NREM sleep.

It is typical to go through four or five cycles of sleep each night. On the average, each cycle lasts about 90 to 100 minutes. The cycles tend to become longer as morning approaches. Ordinarily, more sleep occurs in the delta stage in the first half of the night, especially if one is tired or has lost sleep.

Figure 40-3 illustrates the normal sleep pattern of young adults. Variations in the sleep cycle are observed according to age, as Figure 40-4 illustrates.

Sleep Requirements and Patterns

For no known reason, 8 hours of sleep every night has been the accepted standard, despite obvious variances shown in the general population. There is no rigid formula for normal periodicity and duration of sleep. It is important, however, that each person follow a pattern of rest that maintains well-being.

Despite variations, some generalities can be stated. On the average, infants sleep from 14 to 20 hours each day. Growing children require from 10 to 14 hours of sleep. Adults average 7 to 9 hours, although a 4-hour range has been observed in many normal adults. Those who are able to relax and rest easily, even while awake, often find that less sleep is needed, whereas others may find that more sleep is required to overcome fatigue. Fatigue can be considered a normal, protective body mechanism and nature's warning that sleep is necessary. Chronic fatigue is abnormal and is often a symptom of illness.

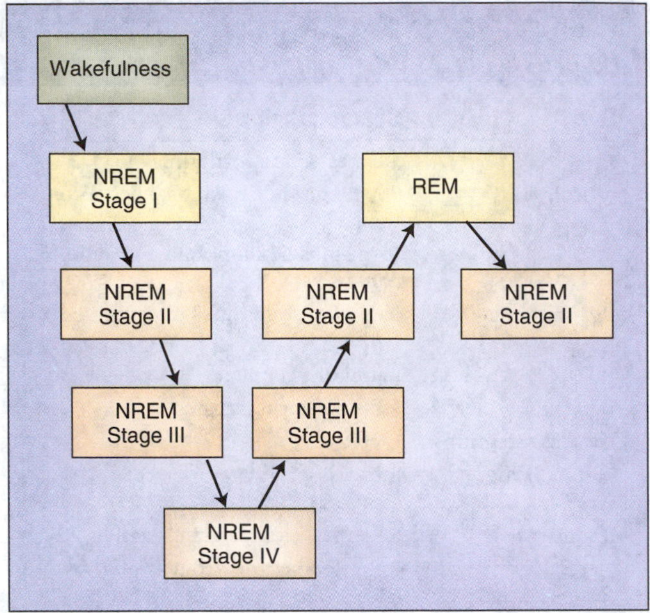

Figure 40-3
A single normal sleep cycle. In the normal nocturnal pattern, the shaded cycle is repeated four or five times. Periods of REM sleep generally increase in duration, and periods of deep sleep (stage IV) progressively decrease as morning approaches.

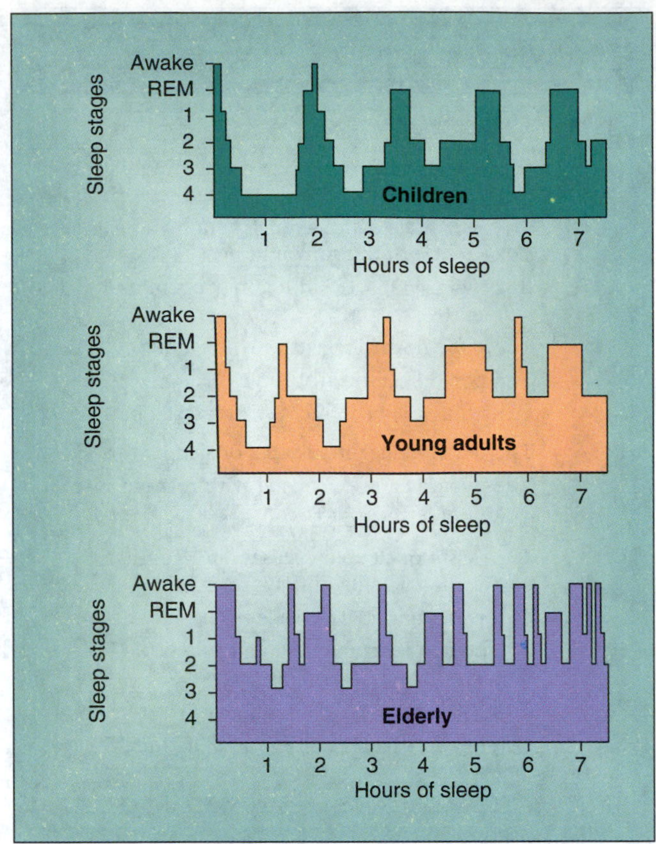

Figure 40-4
A comparison of developmental differences in NREM and REM cycles during nocturnal sleep for children, young adults, and older people.

Sleep patterns of older people vary. However, older people are characterized as requiring a longer time to go to sleep, waking earlier and more frequently during the night, and being less able to cope with changes in their usual sleep patterns than younger people. Older individuals tend to nap during the day, which often results in sleeping fewer hours at night.

Patterns of sleep periodicity appear to be learned. For example, most people learn to sleep at night and to be awake and work during the day. However, many night workers learn to sleep equally well during the day.

Factors Affecting Sleep

A variety of factors influence both the quality and quantity of sleep.

Developmental Considerations

Age variations exist in sleep–wakefulness cycles. These are presented with related nursing interventions in Table 40-3.

Physical Activity

Activity and exercise influence sleep by increasing fatigue and, in many instances, by promoting relaxation that is followed by sleep. It appears that physical activity increases both REM and NREM sleep.

Psychologic Stress

Illness and situations in daily living that cause psychologic stress tend to disturb sleep. Generally, psychologic stress affects sleep in two ways: (1) the person experiencing stress tends to find it difficult to obtain the amount of sleep he or she needs, and (2) REM sleep decreases in amount, which tends to add to anxiety and stress.

Motivation

A desire to be wakeful and alert helps overcome sleepiness and sleep. For example, a tired person may be wakeful and alert when at a party or when attending an interesting play or concert. The opposite is also true—when there is minimal motivation to be awake, sleep generally follows.

Cultural Implications

It is important for the nurse to recognize that cultural beliefs and practices can influence rest and sleep. Although developmental stages are similar, a child's bedtime rituals, sleeping place, and pattern of sleep may vary according to culture. An older Asian client may choose

(text continues on page 1080)

Table 40-3
Developmental Variation in the Sleep–Wakefulness Cycle

Sleep–Wakefulness Cycle	Nursing Implications
Infants	
The infant exhibits six states or levels of arousal 1. *Regular sleep*—Muscle tonus is low, eyelids are closed and still, respirations are about 36 breaths per minute, even, and of regular rhythm. 2. *Irregular sleep*—Muscle tonus is greater; movements follow no sequence, grimaces are frequent; there is intermittent gross mouthing (ie, chomping, chewing, and licking); respirations are irregular; and the mean rate is greater than during regular sleep. 3. *Periodic sleep* (intermediate between regular and irregular sleep)—respiratory rates are periodic (ie, bursts of rapid, shallow breathing alternate with bursts of deep, slow respirations similar to Cheyne-Stokes respiration). 4. *Drowsiness*—Less activity than in irregular or periodic but more activity than in regular sleep; the eyes have a dull, glazed appearance, open and close intermittently, and just before closing may roll upward; generally regular respirations may become tachypneic; there may be a high-pitched squeal. 5. *Alert inactivity*—The eyes are open and bright and make conjugate movements in the vertical and horizontal plane, the face is relaxed, respirations are more variable and faster than in regular sleep; not seen before 3½ weeks of age. 6. *Crying*—Vocalization accompanied by gross motor activity, open or closed eyes, tears can be seen as early as 24 hours after birth; characteristic patterns of crying identifiable as early as the first 5 days of life. In older infants, a state of active wakefulness is seen, during which they explore their world. This becomes increasingly evident as they mature. Each infant has a unique sleep pattern. Generally, by 8 to 16 weeks, the infant's biologic rhythms coincide with daytime and nighttime hours, and he or she will sleep through the night. The younger infant may sleep 17 to 20 hours a day. The 12- to 16-week-old infant will sleep 14 to 18 hours and by the end of the first year the infant may sleep from 12 to 16 hours a day. Young infants spend much time in irregular or REM sleep. This is believed to furnish great quantities of functional excitement to the higher brain centers.	Nurses may need to help parents understand the infant's sleep and wakefulness patterns. The eye movements, groaning, moving, grimacing, and irregular breathing and gasping are normal and require no attention. Research has indicated that sleeping in the prone position increases an infant's risk of SIDS (Sudden Infant Death Syndrome). Back or side sleeping positions are advocated. During waking hours, infants enjoy stimulation and play. The nurse should determine if the parents provide visual, auditory, and tactile stimulation for the infant when the child is awake. The parents' perception of the amount of sleep and activity the infant needs and the type of schedule provided should also be assessed. Guide and counsel as needed.
Toddlers	
The toddler averages from 10 to 15 hours of sleep in a 24-hour period. Two naps a day are more common in the early toddler period; the number and length of naps generally decline as the child approaches the preschool years. Awakening two or three times during the night occurs with most toddlers. This may be due to separation anxiety, loneliness, teething pains, illness, nightmares, or a stressful family situation. Often the toddler is able to fall back to sleep, but some toddlers may need attention and comfort from a parent. A circadian sleep–wakefulness rhythm can be identified by age 3 months, and a gradual maturation of this cycle occurs between the ages of 2 and 10 years in children. Thus, the toddler should manifest an individual pattern of night sleep, naps, and awake time in a 24-hour period.	Establishing a regular bedtime routine with the toddler will facilitate sleep. Routines can include a parent reciting or reading a story, singing a lullaby, rocking the child, or giving the child a bottle of water to suck on. Such activities provide the toddler with love and security and time to settle down after a busy day. To avoid behavioral or emotional disruptions caused by alterations in the toddler's cycle, it is important that parents learn to allow the child to follow a routine sleep pattern, with only occasional interruptions in the pattern.
Preschoolers	
Most authorities agree that by the age of 2 to 3 years, the child's sleep–wakefulness cycle, physiologic rhythms, and	When assessing the sleep–wakefulness cycle, it is essential that the nurse explore the parents' perception of the

(continued)

Table 40-3 *(continued)*
Developmental Variation in the Sleep–Wakefulness Cycle

hormonal cycles are established. The sleep–wakefulness cycle is fully developed by age 2 years; the REM sleep pattern is like an adult pattern by the preschool era. In children, naps represent about 12% of sleep for toddlers, 5% for 4-year-olds, and 0% for 5-year-olds. It is estimated that children from age 2 to 5 years need about 9 to 16 hours of sleep per day, which decreases as the child gets older.	amount of sleep the child needs and elicit information regarding the schedule the parents use for the child's sleep and rest times. Also, the sleeping patterns of the family should be determined so that congruency or conflict with the preschooler's pattern can be identified. If the child's primary caregiver is unable to obtain sufficient rest, the nurse needs to explore alternative ways to help her or him to get more rest so that health and caretaking responsibilities are not jeopardized. The nurse should determine if there are any external factors that might interfere with the child's sleep. Some significant factors include noise, heat, light, and disturbance from siblings. The nurse should offer the parents suggestions on how to change or eliminate any problem-causing environmental conditions.
School-Aged Children	
Normally children require an average of 8 to 10 hours of sleep, but this will vary with each individual. During periods of increased physical growth, the need for sleep may increase.	Parents may need reassurance that it is not uncommon for interruptions in sleep–rest patterns to occur at this age. Frequently, sleep disturbances are the result of increasing awareness of the concept of death. This knowledge, usually gained through television and books, can be frightening to the child, who views himself or herself as powerless in face of the perceived danger. Preparing the child for sleep in a relaxed manner (eg, through quiet talking or reading sessions) and establishing bedtime routines (eg, prayers) may help diminish anxiety. Adults, through their presence and support, can increase the child's own coping resources and help alleviate fears.
Adolescents	
Adolescent clients may have an unusual sleep–wakefulness cycle, especially if they live outside the family. Older adolescents tend to prefer sleeping late in the morning and going to bed late at night whenever possible. The sleep needs of different teenagers vary widely.	It is important to assess the amount of sleep the teenager needs and is able to obtain during each 24-hour period. Because adolescents may be sensitive about their personal habits, the nurse should always be careful to ask questions about these subjects in a nonjudgmental manner. Questions such as "Do you feel rested when you wake after sleeping?" or "Do you feel you get enough sleep?" or "How would you describe the way you sleep?" allow the client to describe personal perceptions (questions about dreams and waking during the sleep period should be included). A teenager may often have complaints about fatigue or inability to do well in school because of poor sleeping patterns.
Young Adults	
Of all the rhythmic patterns, the most important for the young adult is the sleep–wakefulness cycle. Many factors influence the need for rest and sleep, including physical health, type of occupation, and amount of daily exercise. The young adult is generally full of energy and participates in many activities—attending school, participating in family responsibilities, and working. All of these activities present new and exciting frontiers to explore as an adult, with minimal or no parental influence. The young adult often maintains an active lifestyle, interrupting sleep patterns along the way. Traditionally, it has been thought that the young adult requires 7 to 8 hours of sleep per night, but some members of this age group seem to do well with less. The percentage of time spent in each stage of sleep decreases with age; however, interestingly enough, the percentage of time spent in stage I REM sleep does not change	If there is a problem in sleep habits, the nurse needs to explore the client's current lifestyle to see if adequate time is being allocated for sleep. If stress is hindering sleep, means other than medication should be established for handling and decreasing the problem. The client might be encouraged to take a brief rest period during the day or to participate in stress-reduction exercises. Such activities may prevent sleepless nights. Brief periods of watching television, reading, or sewing may be just enough to bring easy rest at the end of the day. Whatever the prescription, the young adult needs to know the impact that a sustained, frantic, exhausting schedule will have over time. Good sleep habits established during the young adult years will not only have a significant impact on sustaining current health but on maintaining long-term wellness as the client ages.

(continued)

Table 40-3 *(continued)*
Developmental Variation in the Sleep–Wakefulness Cycle

throughout life, consistently composing 20% to 25% of total sleep time. This particular biologic rhythm is thought to be very important for maintaining a stable psychologic balance in each individual, no matter what age.

Frequently, the young adult will take medication to alter sleep patterns. Because of significant stress (eg, trying to achieve, to maintain a family, to establish meaningful relationships, to participate in extracurricular activities), the young adult may have difficulty falling asleep. He or she becomes overtired and increasingly worried about the inability to sleep. Medications may seem a logical way to get some rest quickly. All too often, the potential hazards of sleep medications are overlooked, and the young adult may become a prime target for some specific health problems.

Sleep medications significantly decrease REM sleep. If these medications are taken consistently, there is a gradual return to the normal amount of REM sleep. However, when the medication is stopped, the individual may undergo withdrawal symptoms, including insomnia, nightmares, fatigue, and increased sensitivity to pain. These symptoms may last up to 5 weeks.

Middle Adults

For the middle adult, gradual changes in the sleep patterns develop in earlier life and continue through middle adulthood. Specifically, total sleep time decreases, with a particular decrease in the amount of stage IV sleep. The number of sleep arousals increases, and the percentage of time in bed spent awake begins to increase. This will be exaggerated in people who follow previously established sleep patterns after their sleep requirements have decreased.

Because of the multiple changes and stresses in middle age, sleep disturbances are common. However, any sleep aberration should be investigated to exclude the possibility of underlying anxiety or depression that can be reflected by difficulty in falling asleep, early morning awakening, or alternatively, hypersomnia. Sleeping pills or other aids may be used by middle adults, and such use should be determined during the health history.

Older Adults

Sleep–wakefulness patterns are altered in the aged. Older people know they no longer sleep deeply. Many elders report that they have difficulty falling asleep and are more easily awakened once asleep. They are more likely to be disturbed by noise despite the fact that their sense of hearing is less acute. Even though older adults may spend more actual time in bed, they frequently comment that they feel less refreshed upon awakening in the morning. The proportion of REM and NREM sleep time changes with age. In elderly adults, stage I time increases, and less time is spent in stages III and IV. Some elder adults have no stage IV sleep—this decrease or loss of restorative sleep may result in signs and symptoms of sleep deprivation such as fatigue, daytime sleepiness, headaches, and poor concentration.

The amount of REM sleep decreases because the length of each episode shortens. Roberts (1990) summarized the possible reasons for abnormal sleep patterns in older adults:

- Decline in physical health that may result in pain or signs and symptoms of chronic disease
- Psychologic factors such as depressive disorders, mourning for a loved person or pet, or change in body image
- Undesirable effects of drug therapy such as nocturia
- Environmental factors (noise, temperature, familiarity of setting)

Sleep disturbances in older clients, although common, are not trivial. Age-related changes in sleep-wake patterns, concurrent medical or psychiatric disorders, and environmental changes may produce an array of sleep-related complaints. Comprehensive assessment and individualized intervention can be effective in the long-term care of these individuals.

(Data from Murray, R., & Zentner, J. [1993]. *Nursing assessment & health promotion strategies through the life span* [5th ed.]. Norwalk, CT: Appleton & Lange.)

herbal tea rather than a sleeping medication to promote relaxation and sleep. A cultural orientation toward privacy and quiet makes sleep difficult in a busy special care unit where male and female clients sleep in close proximity. Nursing interventions that are effective in preparing a culturally diverse client for an evening's sleep need to be included in the plan of care (Andrews & Boyle, 1995).

Diet

It has long been believed that the dietary amino acid L-tryptophan acts to promote sleep. A small protein snack before bedtime was frequently recommended for clients with insomnia. As nutritionists have studied the effects of various food substances on mood, new information has emerged. Protein may actually increase brain energy alertness and concentration, while carbohydrates appear to have an effect on brain serotonin levels and promote feelings of calmness and relaxation (Wardlaw & Insel, 1993).

Alcohol Intake

Alcoholic beverages, when used in moderation, seem to help induce sleep in some people. However, large quantities have been found to limit REM and delta sleep. This effect may partially explain the phenomenon of hangover after excessive alcohol consumption.

Caffeine-Containing Beverages

Caffeine is a central nervous system stimulant. For many people, beverages containing caffeine interfere with the ability to fall asleep. Examples of beverages containing caffeine include coffee, tea, and most cola drinks. Chocolate also contains caffeine.

Smoking

Nicotine has a stimulating effect, and smokers usually have a more difficult time falling asleep. They are more easily aroused once asleep and may describe themselves as light sleepers. Eliminating cigarette smoking after the evening meal seems to improve the smoker's ability to fall asleep, and people usually report improved sleep patterns once nicotine use is discontinued. It is also interesting to note that total withdrawal from smoking may be associated with sleep disturbances. Clients who stop smoking have an increase in periods of daytime sleepiness and report significantly more restlessness at night. Whether this is a short-term effect or possibly related to nicotine's effect on the central nervous system is uncertain.

Environmental Factors

Most people sleep best in their usual home environments. Sleeping in a strange or new environment tends to influence both REM and NREM sleep for most.

Lifestyle

Various lifestyles affect the ability to sleep well. People working a shift other than the day shift must reorganize their priorities. Alward and Monk (1995) describe the problems and outcomes experienced by the 33% of nurses who work rotating shifts. As expected, sleep difficulties are not uncommon. Sleep disorders are the major problem associated with shift work, but shift work can also result in anxiety, personal conflicts, loneliness, gastrointestinal symptoms, and substance abuse. Developing a sleep pattern is especially difficult if the shift changes periodically. The type of television watched in the evening, involvement in emotionally stirring outside activities, and the amount of activity or exercise in which one participates can all affect sleep. Moderate exercise is a healthy way to promote sleep, but excessive exercise can defeat sleep. One's ability to relax from work-related pressures and to disregard conflict in the home are important factors in the ability to fall asleep.

Illness

Illness acts as a physiologic and psychologic stressor and, as a result, influences sleep. Certain illnesses are more closely related to sleep disturbances than others. Several examples follow.

Gastric secretions increase during REM sleep. Many people with peptic ulcers awaken at night with pain. They find that eating a snack to help neutralize stomach acidity is often helpful to relieve discomfort and promote sleep.

The pain associated with diseases of the coronary arteries and the occurrence of myocardial infarctions is often associated with REM sleep. Seizure attacks owing to epilepsy are most likely to occur during NREM sleep and appear to be depressed by REM sleep. Liver failure and encephalitis tend to cause a reversal in day–night sleeping habits. Hypothyroidism tends to decrease the amount of NREM sleep, especially stages II and IV.

Chronotherapeutics is a growing field of study that involves investigation of the strategic use of time in medicine. Researchers have determined that certain treatments for disease are more effective when body rhythms are taken into account. The administration of a larger mid-afternoon dose of asthma medication may more effectively prevent attacks that commonly occur at night during sleep. Timing of antihypertensive medication may need adjustment to provide peak protection during early-morning hours, when heart attacks are more common. Cancer chemotherapy appears to be less toxic when administered at certain times of the day. Attention to biologic rhythms may influence drug tolerance and effectiveness of medication (Cowley, 1996).

Medications

Sleep quality is also influenced by certain drugs. Some examples of drugs that decrease REM sleep are barbiturates, amphetamines, and antidepressants. Bachman

(1992) implicated diuretics, anti-Parkinson drugs, some antidepressants and antihypertensives, steroids, decongestants, caffeine, and asthma medications as common causes of sleep interference. Chloral hydrate and zolpidem tartrate (Ambien) appear to influence the quality of sleep least and promote normal sleep.

Common Sleep Disorders

The nurse interviewing a client to obtain a sleep history needs to be knowledgeable about common sleep disturbances to recognize significant data. A brief description of these disturbances follows. Specific interview questions may be found in Table 40-4.

Primary Sleep Disorders

Primary sleep disorders are those in which the sleep disturbance is the main symptom or sign of the problem. Examples include insomnia, hypersomnia, narcolepsy, and sleep apnea.

Insomnia is characterized by difficulty in falling asleep, intermittent sleep, or early awakening from sleep. Usually, people complaining of insomnia have been observed to fall asleep more quickly and sleep more than they report they do. However, the condition can lead to such distress that further wakefulness results. It is the most common of all sleep disorders. Although it is difficult to determine the exact cause, research by Regestein and Dambrosia (1993) suggests that tense, anxious, and emotional individuals are more at risk for insomnia than those who remain calm and worry less during the day. **Hypersomnia** is a condition characterized by excessive sleep, particularly during the day. Although this may result from medical conditions, it is frequently used as a coping mechanism when someone has no desire or energy to face a new day.

Narcolepsy is a condition characterized by an uncontrollable desire to sleep. The person with narcolepsy can literally fall asleep standing up, while driving a car, in the middle of a conversation, or while swimming. It is considered to be a neurologic disorder. The condition usually begins in susceptible people during adolescence or early adulthood and continues through life. Sleepiness during the day is often the first symptom of narcolepsy and usually precedes by several years any difficulty with nighttime sleep (Shaver & Rodgers, 1994). Agrypnotic drugs that cause wakefulness are used to control narcolepsy. People using such drugs should take them faithfully because if they are discontinued, the uncontrollable desire to sleep returns.

Sleep apnea refers to periods of no breathing between snoring intervals. The person may not breathe for periods of 10 to 20 seconds to as long as 2 minutes. During long periods of apnea, there is a drop in the oxygen level of the blood, the pulse usually becomes irregular, and the blood pressure often increases. Although most commonly seen in middle-aged men, women and people of other ages may also experience it. Obstructive sleep apnea results when the airway is occluded due to collapse of the hypopharynx (Fig. 40-5). Fortunately, sleep apnea is not particularly common. Some investigators have theorized that sleep apnea may explain certain cases of death that occur during sleep. **Polysomnography** is the only certain method of diagnosing sleep apnea; this sleep study consists of an EEG recording of the stages of sleep and any episodes of apnea, continuous monitoring of arterial oxygen saturation, and an electrocardiogram (ECG) to detect any cardiac dysrhythmias.

Parasomnias

Parasomnias are patterns of waking behavior that appear during sleep. Common examples include **somnambulism** (sleepwalking); sleeptalking; nocturnal erections; bruxism (grinding of teeth during sleep); and **enuresis** (bedwetting during sleep).

Sleep Deprivation

Sleep deprivation refers to a decrease in the amount, consistency, and quality of sleep. It may result from decreased REM sleep or NREM sleep. Total sleep deprivation is rarely seen other than in an experimental setting. Causes are multiple, and manifestations progress from irritability and impaired mental abilities to a total disintegration of personality. In general, the effects of sleep deprivation become increasingly apparent after 30 hours of continual wakefulness (Shaver & Landis, 1994). Partial sleep deprivation may result in loss of concentration and pose serious safety risks. The strange environment of the hospital, physical discomfort and pain, the effects of medications, and the need for 24-hour nursing care may all contribute to sleep deprivation in the hospitalized client.

The Nurse as Role Model

It is difficult for clients to work collaboratively with a nurse to achieve sleep and rest goals when the nurse's appearance and behavior demonstrate inadequate rest and sleep. Because professional, personal, and family demands can all outrank sleep on a nurse's list of priorities, nurses often find themselves showing up for work with inadequate rest and energy. Nurses who value their own well-being and who wish to be role models of healthy sleep self-care behaviors must develop lifestyles supportive of the following goals. The nurse will do the following:

- Routinely obtain the amount of sleep necessary to provide energy for the next day's work (specify number of hours)
- Incorporate three to four periods of regular exercise into each week
- Perform some relaxing activity 1 hour before retiring
- Evaluate the use of nicotine, caffeine, alcohol, and any pharmacologic sleep aids
- When possible, limit shift rotations and working two shifts back-to-back to prevent disrupting usual circadian rhythm

Table 40-4
Common Sleep Problems: Description and Pertinent Interview Questions

Sleep Problem	Description	Sample Interview Techniques and Questions
Primary Sleep Disorders (sleep alteration is the only symptom or sign of a problem)		
Insomnia	Shortened sleep period; may be characterized by difficulty falling asleep (*initial insomnia*), frequent or prolonged awakening (*intermittent insomnia*), or early morning awakening with an inability to return to sleep (*terminal insomnia*).	*Initial insomnia* • Do you have difficulty falling asleep? • How long does it usually take to fall asleep? • What do you think prevents sleep? *Intermittent insomnia* • Do you find that you wake up after you have fallen asleep? • How often, on a usual night, does this happen? • What do you think causes you to awaken? *Terminal insomnia* • Do you awaken early and find that you can't go back to sleep? • Is this a regular occurrence? • Do you make up for the lost sleep by napping or retiring earlier?
Narcolepsy	A condition characterized by an uncontrolled and abrupt onset of "sleep attacks" during normally alert activities (eg, while eating, driving a car, talking). Undiagnosed, the narcoleptic is potentially dangerous to self or others. Clients with narcolepsy tend to fall asleep quickly, find it difficult to wake up, sleep fewer hours than others, and sleep restlessly. Common symptoms include sleep attacks, *cataplexy* (sudden loss of motor tone that may cause the person to fall asleep), *hypnagogic hallucinations* (nightmares or vivid hallucinations), and *sleep paralysis* (skeletal muscle paralysis that occurs during the transition from wakefulness to stage I).	• Do you ever fall asleep suddenly during the day? If yes, tell me more about that. • Has anyone ever teased you about falling asleep on them, right in the middle of a conversation, at work, or during a meal? • Have you ever had an attack of muscle weakness or paralysis? Wanted to move and couldn't? If yes, what were you doing when this occurred? How often does it happen? • Do you ever experience dreams right as you are falling asleep? What are they like? • Does sleep pose any particular problem for you?
Sleep apnea syndrome	Periods of no breathing during sleep—may last for 10–20 seconds or as long as 2 minutes; during periods of apnea, there is a drop in the oxygen level of the blood, the pulse may become irregular, and the blood pressure may increase. Many people experience sleep apnea without symptoms. Middle-aged men who are obese and have short, thick necks are most at risk. Repeated episodes may cause anginal attacks, cardiac arrhythmias, and pulmonary hypertension. It is currently thought that sleep apneas are related to mortality which occurs during sleep. Most types of sleep apnea are classified as *obstructive apnea,* which is caused by pharyngeal obstruction in the upper airway (see Fig. 40-5).	• Has anyone ever told you that there are times during sleep when you stop breathing for a while and then start up again? • If yes, tell me what this means to you. Do you have any concerns about this habit? • Do you snore? Is there someone who can describe your snoring? • Any recent problems with headache and nausea (related to low oxygen levels)? • Do you have a history of any heart or lung problems? Chest pain? • Are you aware of any changes in your mental abilities or any emotional changes? • Inspect body build. • Observe for airway deformities (short neck, thick tongue, deviated nasal septum). • In the hospitalized client, compare vital signs during apnea with baseline signs. • A report from a bed-partner or a tape recording of the client's sleep may be helpful in establishing a diagnosis.

(continued)

Table 40-4 *(continued)*
Common Sleep Problems: Description and Pertinent Interview Questions

Sleep Problem	Description	Sample Interview Techniques and Questions
Parasomnias (patterns of waking behavior that appear during sleep)		
Somnambulism (sleep walking)	Occurs during stages III and IV of NREM sleep; danger is that somnambulist may hurt self; protective environment is required	*These questions may be directed to the client:* • Has anyone ever told you that you walk in your sleep, talk in your sleep, and so forth? *Or the questions may be directed to a child's parent:* • Have you ever noticed your child walking in his or her sleep? Talking while asleep? • Does your child ever wake up screaming and terrified from a nightmare? *With yes to any of these questions:* • Are you aware of any stressful event or emotional conflict before these sleep events? • Describe a typical day and what you might have been feeling before one of these events. • Does this sleep activity pose any problems for you? Tell me how you are dealing with it.
Sleep talking	Occurs during NREM sleep; rarely presents a problem unless annoying to others	
Bruxism (grinding of teeth during sleep)	Usually occurs during stage II NREM sleep	
Nocturnal enuresis	Bedwetting during sleep (see Chapter 43)	
Pavor Nocturnis (night terrors)	Usually affects children under 6 years; child wakes up several hours after falling asleep and appears terrified from a nightmare; is difficult to awaken; usually occurs in stage IV sleep.	
Sleep deprivation	Sleep deprivation results in impaired cognitive function and leads to mental fatigue, impaired memory, inability to concentrate, perception changes, and poor judgment. It is also associated with lowered pain threshold and decreased production of hormones, which are essential to combat stress. Loss of REM sleep specifically has been associated with hyperactivity, mood swings, agitation, and decreased impulse control.	• In what way is your sleep shortened? • What might be causing this? • How do you feel when you get up? • In what ways do you think your lack of sleep is affecting you?

(Data from Fuller, J., & Schaller-Ayers, J. [1994]. *Health assessment: A nursing approach* [2nd ed.]. Philadelphia: Lippincott.)

Use the self-assessment checklist in the accompanying box to monitor how well you are achieving sleep and rest goals for yourself.

ASSESSING REST AND SLEEP

Sleep History

Because rest and sleep are important components of general health, a sleep history should be included in each comprehensive nursing history. Interview questions are used to identify the client's sleep–wakefulness patterns, the effect of these patterns on everyday functioning, sleep aids, and the presence of sleep disturbances and contributing factors. The sleep history may be brief (four questions) if the client's sleep is adequate and posing no problems, or it may be detailed. When the client's response to any of the interview questions indicates a potential problem, open-ended questions may be used to gather more data (see the accompanying box).

If the client is being admitted to a care facility, it is important to assess his or her usual times for retiring and waking, bedtime rituals, and preferences regarding sleep environment so that these can be incorporated into the plan of care, if possible. Sensitivity to small matters can make the difference between a good night's sleep and no sleep.

When a sleep disturbance is noted, the history should determine the following:

- The nature of the problem
- Its cause
- The related signs and symptoms
- When it first began and how often it occurs
- How it affects everyday living
- The severity of the problem and whether it can be treated independently by nursing or needs to be referred to another professional
- How the client is coping with the problem and the success of any treatments attempted

Interview questions may be directed to the client, to his or her bed partner, or to a caregiver. The client record may also contain pertinent information (eg, a history of illnesses that influence sleep or a history of drug dependency or withdrawal).

Sample recordings of a sleep history in a comprehensive nursing assessment are as follows:

Reports needs 8 to 9 hours of sleep to feel his best and usually gets this without problem. Generally retires at 11:30 PM and rises at 7:30 AM. No special sleep rituals.

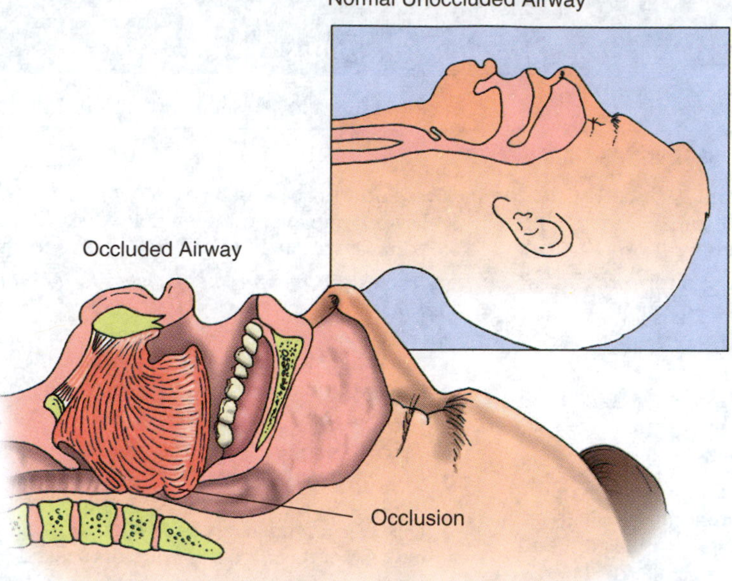

Figure 40-5
Obstructive sleep apnea occurs when the airway is occluded due to collapse of the hypopharynx. Normally the airway remains open during sleep *(see inset).*

Mother reports toddler has erratic sleep patterns. May nap at any time in the afternoon or evening and sleep from 1 to 3 hours. Depending on nap, goes to bed anywhere from 7 to 11 PM and sleeps about 11 to 13 hours. Resists falling asleep and wants "water, story, snack, kisses, etc." Parents' lifestyle is constantly changing—little consistency for the child regarding sleep expectations.

Sleep Diary

A sleep diary or log provides more specific data on the client's sleep–wakefulness patterns over a prolonged period. The diary generally is kept for 14 days and includes the following:

1. A graph of the total number of hours of sleep per day. Depending on the nature of the problem,

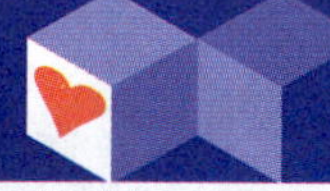

Promoting Wellness

Rest and Sleep

Use the assessment checklist to determine how well you are meeting needs for rest and sleep. Then develop a prescription for self-care by choosing appropriate behaviors from the list of suggestions.

Assessment Checklist

almost always	sometimes	almost never	
☐	☐	☐	1. I feel rested and refreshed when I get up in the morning.
☐	☐	☐	2. I have energy to carry out normal activities of daily living.
☐	☐	☐	3. I understand the normal changes in sleep and rest requirements and patterns that occur with aging.
☐	☐	☐	4. I set aside time for quiet recreation and restful activities each day.

Self-Care Behaviors

1. Follow a regular routine for bedtime and morning awakening.
2. Accept individual differences in need for sleep.
3. Use relaxation exercises to relax before bedtime, especially if feeling stressed.
4. Avoid caffeine, smoking, and alcohol before bedtime.
5. Adjust bedcoverings, room temperature, and lighting to your preferences.
6. Drink a glass of milk before going to bed.
7. Be aware of the potential dangers of sleeping pills.
8. Use some part of each day for quiet, enjoyable activities, such as crafts, hobbies, reading, watching television, listening to music, visiting with friends.

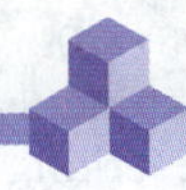

Focused Assessment Guide

Rest and Sleep

Factors to Assess	Questions and Approaches
Usual sleep-wakefulness pattern: Recent changes	
• Usual sleeping and waking times	How many hours of sleep do you usually get in a day? Do you wake up earlier in the morning than you would like and find it difficult to fall back asleep? Have there been any recent changes in your usual sleep-wake patterns? If yes, describe them and tell me if they are causing any problems for you. Do you usually go to bed and wake up about the same time each day?
• Number of hours of undisturbed sleep	How have you been sleeping? Do you have any difficulty falling asleep? Do you wake up frequently during the night? Do you dream at night? Are your dreams frightening?
• Quality of sleep	How much sleep do you think you need to feel rested?
• Number and duration of naps	Do you take naps throughout the day?
Effect of sleep pattern on everyday functioning	In what way does the sleep you get each day affect your everyday living? Has this sleep disturbance caused any change in your sex life?
• Energy level (ability to perform activities of daily living)	Do you feel rested and ready to start the day when you wake up? Are there times during the day or certain activities when you feel especially tired? What happens when you don't get enough sleep? Are you having difficulty concentrating?
Sleep aids	
• Means of relaxing before bedtime	What do you do to relax before you get ready for bed?
• Bedtime rituals	Describe what you usually do to help yourself fall asleep.
• Sleep environment	Tell me how you like your room (lights, noises, ventilation, position of door, temperature) and bed (mattress, pillows, blankets) when you are sleeping.
• Pharmacologic aids	Do you take any medications to help you sleep? Are you taking any medicine at all?
Sleep disturbances and contributing factors	
• Nature of the sleep disturbance	Tell me about your sleep problem.
• Onset of disturbance	How often does it occur?
• Causes (physical, psychosocial, medicine related)	Are you doing anything differently now that might be causing the problem?
• Severity	Do you wake up gasping for air?
• Symptoms	Do you snore? Do you recall changing your position frequently during the night?
• Interventions attempted and results	What have you been doing to deal with the problem?

graphs may be made of the number of undisturbed hours of sleep, number of awakenings, and so forth.

2. A daily record of the following:
    - Time client decided to retire
    - Time client actually tries to fall asleep
    - Approximate time client falls asleep
    - Time of any awakenings during the night and when sleep was resumed
    - Time of awakening in the morning
    - Presence of any stressors client believes are affecting his or her sleep
    - A record of any food, drink, or medication client believes has positively or negatively influenced his or her sleep (include time of ingestion)
    - Record of physical activities—type, duration, and time
    - Record of mental activities—type, duration, and time
    - Record of activities performed 2 to 3 hours before bedtime, bedtime rituals, changes in sleep environment
    - Presence of any worries or anxieties client believes are affecting his or her sleep

It is helpful if the client has a bed partner who can assist with the diary. It should be stressed to the client that the diary is simply a diagnostic tool. If keeping the diary causes too much stress for the client and further interferes with his or her ability to sleep restfully, it should be discontinued.

Physical Assessment

Physical findings during the nursing examination should either confirm that the client is getting sufficient rest to provide energy for the day's activities or validate the existence of a sleep disturbance that is decreasing the quantity or quality of sleep. Key findings include energy level (presence of physical weakness, fatigue, lethargy); facial characteristics (narrowing or glazing of eyes, swelling of eyelids, decreased animation); behavioral characteristics (yawning, rubbing eyes, slow speech, slumped posture). Data suggestive of potential sleep problems (eg, obesity, enlarged neck, deviated nasal septum) may also be noted.

If the nurse or a bed partner is able to observe the client sleeping, other sleep characteristics to assess include restlessness, sleep postures, and sleep activities such as snoring or leg jerking (nocturnal myoclonus).

Snoring. Snoring is caused by an obstruction to the air flow through the nose and mouth. Other than disturbing people sharing the same bedroom, snoring is ordinarily not considered to be a sleeping disorder. However, snoring accompanied by apnea can present a problem. When snoring changes from the characteristic "sawing wood" sound to a more irregular silence followed by a snorting, this is indicative of obstructive apnea.

Nocturnal Myoclonus. Observed in 10% to 20% of chronic insomniacs, **nocturnal myoclonus** involves marked muscle contraction that results in the jerking of one or both legs during sleep. The jerking lasts about 28 seconds and may arouse the sleeper. *Restless leg syndrome* is a different condition in which the awake individual is unable to lie with his or her body, and especially the legs, still long enough to fall asleep. Both conditions may contribute to insomnia.

DIAGNOSING

Sleep Pattern Disturbance as the Problem. When assessment data point to a sleep problem that is amenable to nursing therapy, it receives the label Sleep Pattern Disturbance and may then be further specified:

Insomnia: Difficulty falling asleep
Insomnia: Difficulty remaining asleep
Insomnia: Premature awakening
Hypersomnia: Excessive daytime sleeping
Sleep deprivation
Altered sleep–wake patterns

Common etiologies for sleep pattern disturbances include the following:

Physical discomfort or pain
Emotional discomfort or pain caused by anxiety and stress
Changes in bedtime rituals or sleep environments
Disruption of circadian rhythm
Exercise just before sleep
Caffeine, nicotine, or alcohol after dinner
Drug dependency and withdrawal
Symptoms of physical illness

Sample nursing diagnoses in which the sleep disturbance is the primary problem are presented in the accompanying box.

Sleep Pattern Disturbance as the Etiology. Sleep pattern disturbances may affect many other areas of human functioning. In the nursing diagnoses that follow, the sleep pattern disturbance is the etiology of another problem:

Anxiety related to inability to fall asleep, inability to control behavior while asleep, sleep apnea—threat of death
Activity Intolerance related to sleep deprivation
Fatigue related to prolonged excessive role demands
Ineffective Individual Coping related to insomnia: Insufficient quantity and quality of sleep
Fear related to narcoleptic's potential to harm self or others
Impaired Gas Exchange related to sleep apnea (oxygen saturation of the blood)
Risk for Injury related to somnambulism, narcolepsy, sleep apnea
Knowledge Deficit (specify: eg, nonpharmacologic remedies for insomnia) related to misinformation, lack of interest in learning, cognitive limitation

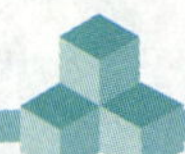

Sleep

Problem	Related Factors	Sample Defining Characteristics
Sleep Pattern Disturbance: Difficulty Falling Asleep	Worries about family and lack of destressing rituals	• "At least four or five nights a week I lay in bed awake for 3 or 4 hours before I finally fall asleep. Sometimes it is 2 or 3 in the morning and I'm still awake worrying about the kids. I've tried getting up and reading or paying my bills, but even that doesn't make me sleepy." • Reports problem falling asleep for past 6 months; is widowed and very concerned about two teenage sons. Never sleeps until both sons are home. States she does nothing special to relax. Feels her worries are "her business"—no support person with whom she shares these.
Sleep Pattern Disturbance: Difficulty Remaining Asleep	Noise of hospital environment and need for periodic treatments	• Admitted to hospital 3/6/98; cholecystectomy 3/7/98 • "I don't think I've had one decent night's sleep since my surgery. I've been falling asleep about 9 PM and then someone wakes me up for my medicine. I just about get back to sleep and someone's putting the light on to poke at my dressing or to check this tube. I know I'm getting grouchy." • Orders include every-4-hour vital signs; nursing assessment of the incision, nasogastric tube, intravenous therapy; and medication for pain and for sleep.
Sleep Pattern Disturbance: Premature Awakening	Barbiturate dependency and lack of knowledge of nonpharmacologic aids for insomnia	• Client has history of mild to moderate depression, related to loss of job and perceived role inadequacy, for the past 3 years; has been taking secobarbital (Seconal), a barbiturate hypnotic, 100 mg by mouth nightly for the past year and a half. • "I seem to be waking up earlier and earlier, can't fall back asleep, and I start each day feeling like I have a hangover." • "I'd like to get off these drugs, but I'm terrified that without them I won't sleep at all."
Sleep Pattern Disturbance: Excessive Daytime Sleeping	Altered sleep cycle and inability to cope with multiple stresses	• Only child, first-year college student who is living away from home for the first time. Shares a dormitory room with a roommate. Sleep patterns are erratic and depend on school and social demands. Has recently broken up with high school boyfriend. Fears she is failing three courses. Has no desire to do anything but sleep. "When I get up my only thought is: When can I go back to bed? I often sleep through class."
Sleep Pattern Disturbance: Excessive Daytime Sleeping	Effects of biologic aging (moderate increase in stage I and II sleep; slow-wave sleep, stages III and IV, decreases by 50% or more)	• Male client, aged 74, complains during his annual physical that he seems to be napping more during the day, yet when he tries to fall asleep at night he often cannot. • "I'm spending more time in bed, but I'm less rested. Worst of all is not knowing whether or not I'll be awake enough to drive my car or enjoy a good card game."

(continued)

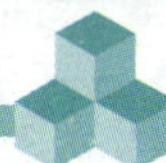

Nursing Diagnoses for Common Problems *(continued)*

Sleep

Problem	Related Factors	Sample Defining Characteristics
Sleep Pattern Disturbance: Altered Sleep–Wake Patterns	Frequent rotations of shift and overtime	• Graduate nurse, 24 years old, who has been working on a busy medical floor for 6 months; rotates 11-7 and 7-3 shifts; recently a problem with staffing has necessitated frequent rotations. Client often volunteers (two or three times a week) for overtime. • "I don't know what is wrong with me. I'm so tired anymore and don't feel at all like myself. All I want to do when I'm off is to sleep—but often I can't fall asleep when I lay down. Please help!"

Self-Esteem Disturbance related to effects of sleep deprivation (hypersomnia or sleep apnea syndrome)

Anxiety related to nocturnal enuresis

Impaired Social Interaction related to excessive daytime sleeping, sleep deprivation

Altered Thought Processes related to chronic insomnia, sleep deprivation

Important Distinctions. Because the *problem statement* of the nursing diagnosis identifies what is wrong with the client and suggests the expected outcomes and the *etiology* of the problem directs nursing interventions, it is important for the nurse analyzing the assessment data to decide if the sleep data are indicative of the problem, are contributing to a different problem, or are signs or symptoms of the problem. Sleep data potentially fit well in all three categories. For example, when altered sleep–wake patterns are noted in the graduate nurse who is getting adjusted to a new full-time job, shift work, and increased independence, three different diagnoses might be written:

Sleep Pattern Disturbance: Altered sleep–wake pattern (insomnia) related to shift work and stress of new job as manifested by complaints of always feeling tired and never getting enough sleep anymore

Altered sleep–wake patterns are the problem statement; priority nursing energies are directed to changing these patterns and to helping the client achieve both the necessary quantity and quality of sleep.

Ineffective Individual Coping related to multiple stresses of new job and altered sleep–wake patterns (→ sleep deprivation) as manifested by statements such as, "I don't know how much longer I can do this," "I'm always tired anymore and all I want to do is sleep," "I'm so grouchy—people must hate me!"

Here, the altered sleep–wake pattern is just one of the factors contributing to the client's problem of ineffective coping; priority nursing energies are directed toward improving the client's coping skills by teaching the client how to increase the quantity and quality of sleep.

Ineffective Individual Coping related to multiple stressors and lack of destressing rituals as manifested by inability to fall asleep (altered sleep–wake patterns); excessive fatigue; and feelings that personality is changing

In this instance, altered sleep–wake patterns are merely a symptom of the client's actual problem—ineffective coping; it is expected that when the coping problem is resolved, the symptom will disappear.

None of the preceding diagnoses is more correct than the others. With each client, the nurse must make a decision with each cluster of significant data and pull out the key problem, contributing factors, and related signs and symptoms. How the diagnosis is developed directs the nursing interventions.

PLANNING: EXPECTED OUTCOMES

Rest and sleep are essential components of well-being. Planning for client care, especially in a healthcare facility, involves planning with the client suitable measures to promote rest and sleep. Whenever nurses care for a client, nursing measures support the following expected client outcomes. The client will:

- Maintain a sleep–wake pattern that provides sufficient energy for the day's tasks
- Demonstrate self-care behaviors that provide a healthy balance between rest and activity
- Identify stress-relieving rituals that will enable him or her to fall asleep more easily
- Demonstrate decreased signs of sleep deprivation

- Verbalize feeling less fatigued and more in control of life activities

IMPLEMENTING

Usually sleep problems are not the primary reason for a client's interaction with the healthcare system. The key to detection of a sleep problem is often the attitude the nurse communicates to the client. Clients who believe the nurse is generally concerned about their well-being are not reluctant to discuss insomnia or voice concern about a child who is a bedwetter. Fundamental to the success of any nursing measure to correct a sleep problem is the client's belief that the nurse cares and is readily available for extra help to promote rest and sleep.

Home Healthcare Alert

Nurses need to emphasize to older clients that it is normal for sleep pattern changes to occur, and thc quality of sleep is different at every stage of life.

Preparing a Restful Environment

Having a comfortable bed helps promote rest and sleep. The bottom linen should be tight and clean. The upper linen, while secure, should allow freedom of movement and should not exert pressure, especially over the legs and feet. Having the body in good alignment is conducive to relaxation. For clients who must assume unusual positions because of their illness, ingenuity and skill are necessary to keep muscle strain and discomfort at a minimum. For example, the client who must remain in the orthopneic position to aid breathing should be well supported in a manner that relieves muscle strain.

A quiet and darkened room, with privacy, is relaxing for nearly everyone. In a strange environment, unfamiliar noises, such as people walking or entering and leaving the room and the closing of elevator doors, bring complaints from most hospitalized clients. Although some of these sources are difficult for the nurse to control, every effort should be made toward reducing disturbances to promote relaxation and sleep.

The temperature of the room, the amount of ventilation, and the quantity of bed covering are matters of individual choice. The client's wishes should be met when at all possible. Refer to the accompanying box for additional suggestions pertinent to this age group.

Home Healthcare Alert

Many older clients are unable to sleep if they feel cold. Warming the bed using thermal blankets or comforters, insulated bed socks, cotton flannel sheets, leg warmers, long underwear, and a stockinette cap create the sensation of warmth and help to promote comfort and sleep.

Promoting Bedtime Rituals

Most people have bedtime rituals to help relaxation and promote sleep. Reading, listening to the radio, watching television, talking to a family member, and praying are common before-sleep activities. Children may search out a favorite doll, stuffed toy, or blanket before going to bed; insist on a bedtime story; kiss everyone goodnight; and say prayers before bed. Readiness for sleep is preceded by a personal hygiene routine for many people, such as brushing teeth, washing hands and face, voiding, or taking a bath or shower. Snacks are important elements in the bedtime rituals of many children and

Focus on the Older Adult

Promoting Sleep

Nonpharmacologic measures to promote improved sleep in older clients include:

- Establish a daily schedule for waking and sleeping.
- Exercise daily, preferably not near bedtime.
- Avoid napping during the day.
- Avoid food, beverages, or OTC medications that contain caffeine in the evening.
- Consume alcohol only in small amounts and not before bedtime.
- Refrain from cigarette smoking in the evening.
- Eat a light meal for dinner.
- Eat a light carbohydrate snack at bedtime if hungry.
- Use relaxation methods at bedtime (eg, deep breathing, relaxation exercises, soothing music, massage, reading).
- Maintain comfortable temperature and reduced noise level in sleeping area.
- Keep to usual waking time every day even if previous night's bedtime was later than usual or sleep was restless.
- Get out of bed if unable to fall asleep within 30 minutes and go into another room. Engage in a nonstimulating activity such as reading and return to bed when drowsy.
- Use bed only for sleeping or sexual activity.

adults. Although it is true that eating the wrong foods may produce a bad night's sleep, going to bed hungry may also interfere with sleep.

The nurse should be alert to the client's bedtime rituals and make every effort to observe them as far as possible to aid in promoting relaxation and sleep. These rituals should appear in the client's plan of care so that all health personnel can observe them.

Offering Appropriate Bedtime Snacks and Beverages

Because carbohydrates seem to help promote sleep, there currently appears to be justification for offering a snack or beverage high in carbohydrates before bedtime, such as toast, a small bagel, crackers, or a glass of fruit juice, when this is allowed in the client's regimen. An alcoholic beverage helps to promote sleep for some people, but generally alcohol after dinner should be avoided. For most, beverages containing caffeine should be avoided for at least 4 to 5 hours before bedtime. It is best that the client take fluids during the day and avoid excessive fluid intake before bedtime to help prevent the necessity of using the bathroom during sleeping hours.

Promoting Relaxation

One can relax without sleeping, but sleep rarely occurs until one is relaxed. Stress and anxiety-producing situations tend to interfere with a person's ability to relax, rest, and sleep. Effective means for dealing with worries include dealing with problems as they arise; conditioning oneself to worry only during preset times; teaching oneself that worrying never solves problems and is counterproductive; and giving the worries over to another (eg, a trusted family member, friend, caregiver, or God). The distraction and relaxation techniques described in Chapters 32 and 41 may be beneficial when counseling a client whose worries are contributing to a sleep disturbance. Back rubs, warm baths, and face washing if the client is bedridden are typical nursing measures to help the client relax. The technique for back massage is given in Procedure 41-1.

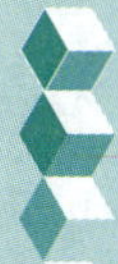

Research in Nursing: Making a Difference

Rest and Sleep

The human body uses sleep for rest, recuperation, and adaptation to physical and emotional stress. Although sleep disturbances may occur at any age, it has been documented that the older adult often experiences difficulty in achieving restful sleep. Nursing research has explored the topic of sleep, identified factors that interfere with sleep, and developed strategies that may effectively promote rest and sleep.

Related Research

Johnson, J. (1994). Sleep and alcohol use in rural old-old women. *Journal of Community Health Nursing, 11*(4), 211–218.
In this study, rural older women over the age of 85 routinely used over-the-counter medications and alcohol to promote a restful sleep. Although 95% of these women also took prescription drugs, most were unaware of the possible adverse effects when combined with OTC medications and alcohol. The most frequently cited reason for seeking healthcare was the need for a stronger medication. This suggests that effective nursing interventions to promote sleep in this population should include careful assessment of sleep patterns and encouragement to seek healthcare earlier and explore nonpharmacologic measures to enhance sleep.

Floyd, J. (1995). Another look at napping in older adults. *Geriatric Nursing, 16*(3), 136–138.
This investigation examined the many myths about the adverse effects of naps on nighttime sleep behavior and daytime well-being in older adults. Even though nappers do complain about the quality of their sleep and the number of nighttime awakenings, no relationship appears to exist between napping and being awake all night. Until more knowledge is available, nurses working with older clients need to encourage them to explore the effect of napping on the quality of their life.

Southwell, M., & Wistow, G. (1995). Sleep in hospitals at night: Are patients' needs being met? *Journal of Advanced Nursing, 21*(2), 1102–1108.
These authors interviewed clients and nurses and both groups agreed that clients who are hospitalized do not get enough sleep. Noise level on the nursing unit and interruption of sleep for treatments were viewed as interfering with normal sleep patterns. It was suggested that nurses need to question clients about their perception of factors that disturb sleep, initiate appropriate nursing measures to enhance sleep, and be more aware of the noise they make while performing nursing tasks. Client-focused care requires that nurses weigh the benefits of intervention versus undisturbed sleep.

Summary

Implications from nursing research about sleep in older clients include creating a physical environment that is conducive to a restful night, assessing for symptoms of sleep deprivation, and incorporating measures for a healthy sleep cycle into the nursing plan of care.

Promoting Comfort

One of the greatest deterrents to rest and sleep is pain; it is not an uncommon experience when illness is present. Depending on the cause and severity of the discomfort or pain, appropriate nursing measures include remaining with a lonely and frightened child or adult, using the simple strategy of caring presence and touch, offering a back massage, obtaining an extra blanket, or administering an analgesic. These and other nursing techniques to promote comfort are described in Chapter 41. However, the nurse must be sensitive to the client's discomfort before he or she can relieve it.

Respecting Normal Sleep–Wake Patterns

Every effort should be made to observe the client's normal periods of sleep. In many instances, it is hardly necessary to insist that all clients retire and awaken at specific times. For example, is there a good reason to wake a client at 7 AM when the client ordinarily sleeps until 9 AM? It is also recommended that a client's normal napping habits be followed when possible. It has been observed that REM sleep is common during morning naps whereas NREM sleep is common during naps later in the day. With this knowledge, the nurse can help the client plan napping periods that best fit individual needs and that interfere least with nighttime sleeping.

Scheduling Nursing Care to Avoid Unnecessary Disturbance

Common client complaints are that they are awakened to take sleeping pills and are aroused at early morning hours to prepare for breakfast long before it is served. These common observations should be considered when planning care that will help most to promote rest and sleep.

Every effort should be made to time care during periods when the client is normally awake. When this cannot be done, it is preferable to avoid awakening the client during REM sleep, when the rapid eye movements can be observed. Because a client's need for sleep is important, priorities should be examined. For example, the nurse should ask if checking a vital sign or carrying out a particular nursing measure is more important than the client's sleep.

Using Medications to Produce Sleep

Medications for sleep are often ordered for clients. Sedative-hypnotics induce sleep; antianxiety drugs reduce anxiety and tension. The sleep produced by sedative-hypnotics is an unnatural sleep. All these drugs disturb either REM or NREM sleep to some degree. Although most sedative-hypnotics provide several nights of excellent sleep, the medication often loses its effect after a week or two. At this point, many people increase the dosage of the medication or complement the drug with alcohol. The combination of a sedative-hypnotic and an over-the-counter antihistamine (eg, Benadryl) may intensify depression of the central nervous system leading to additional safety concerns (Gorbien, 1993). Vigorous nursing intervention is needed to prevent a client from developing a pattern of drug dependency and alcohol abuse.

Nurses also need to be alert to the dangers of withdrawal symptoms that can accompany the abrupt cessation of barbiturate sedative-hypnotics. Progressive withdrawal symptoms include weakness, tremulousness, restlessness, insomnia, increased pulse and heart rates, anxiety, convulsions, psychosis, continued seizures, and death.

Medications used to induce sleep may produce daytime drowsiness and the morning hangover effect. Some people counteract this side effect by taking amphetamines, or uppers. The antianxiety medications, once hoped to be the answer to the sleeping pill dilemma, are increasingly implicated in physical and psychologic dependence.

Many times these medications are ordered on a prn (as needed) basis. The nurse should administer these medications only when indicated and always with full knowledge of their limitations. Thorough client teaching should accompany their use. Nurses should aid clients in developing other self-care strategies, including developing healthy sleep and lifestyle behaviors.

Teaching About Rest and Sleep

A well-informed person is better able to cope with distressing situations. Helping clients and their families understand the nature of rest and sleep and their importance to well-being through teaching is an important nursing function. Teaching should include aspects of normal variations in sleep patterns and common measures to promote relaxation and sleep. Also, the plan of care should be discussed with the client for acceptability. When sleep disorders become a problem and common nursing measures are inadequate, the nurse can assist and teach by recommending the services of health practitioners especially prepared to deal with them.

EVALUATING

The nurse evaluates the effectiveness of a plan of care to promote rest and sleep by checking whether the client has met the individualized expected outcomes specified in the plan. Nursing care is considered effective if the client is able to:

- Verbalize feeling rested or having had a restful night's sleep
- Identify factors that interfere with or disrupt the normal sleep pattern
- Use techniques that effectively promote sleep and provide a restful environment
- Concentrate and function effectively during waking hours
- Eliminate behaviors related to sleep deprivation

Developing Critical Thinking Skills

Situation

You have just arrived on the unit and checked your clinical assignment. You have two clients today and approximately 30 minutes before preconference. Your routine is to review their charts for pertinent information, go and introduce yourself to them, and take their morning vital signs before preconference. With 10 minutes to spare, you visit your second client and find that he is sound asleep. Remembering that he had a fractured hip repaired 2 days ago and that the night nurse had stated in his note that the client was restless and awake until 4:00 AM, you are reluctant to awaken him. On the other hand, at your midterm conference your instructor commented that you need to improve your organizational skills. If you don't have your vital signs recorded until after preconference, then breakfast arrives, doctors make rounds, and you're that much further behind in your morning care and documentation. When you look at the flow sheet at the foot of the bed, you note that the last set of vitals were taken at 12 midnight and were within normal limits. You're attempting to reconcile several things—the importance of these morning vital signs, the client's need for sleep, and your need to accomplish your tasks on time and receive a good evaluation. What should you do?

1. ***Identify Goal of Thinking***
   Determine whether it is more important to awaken your client for morning vital signs or let him sleep at least until after your preconference.

2. ***Assess Adequacy of Knowledge***
   Pertinent circumstances: Your client had major surgery 2 days ago, did not have a restful night, but is sleeping peacefully now. You realize that his vital signs can be an important indicator of a complication. You also need to accomplish your tasks in a timely and organized manner.

   Prerequisite knowledge: In order to make your decision, you need knowledge about his postoperative condition, and assessment data that indicate he is recovering or developing a complication. You are aware that sleep is vital to promote tissue repair, physical recovery, and mental well-being. You also need to review the tasks that you need to accomplish this morning and decide how and if priorities could be shifted.

   Room for error/Time constraints: Will a delay in taking vital signs cause injury to this client? You are not planning to omit this task but just questioning whether to postpone it and allow the client to have some additional sleep.

3. ***Address Potential Problems***
   Waking your client for vital signs may be disturbing for him and interfere with his need for rest. A decision to postpone morning vital signs might also cause several problems. If the client has developed a complication such as an infection, his elevated temperature may go undetected for at least another hour. By the time you come out of preconference, the client may be eating his breakfast, which further delays recording of vital signs. You perceive that you are already falling behind on your schedule and are really intent on completing your responsibilities on time today.

4. ***Consult Helpful Resources***
   Before you make your decision you should check the client's flow sheet and note if the previous set of vital signs were within normal limits. The primary nurse and your instructor may also help you sort through your priorities in this situation.

5. ***Critique Judgment/Decision***
   You have two choices here. If you wake your client up and take his vital signs, you are disturbing him when he is sleeping soundly, risking the fact that he may be angry with you, but are on schedule for the day's activities. By postponing his vital signs at least until after postconference, you provide additional rest for the client but know that you are already behind schedule and worry that your instructor will view you as disorganized. After reviewing your options and checking his chart again, you decide to allow him to sleep and plan to take them as soon as possible after your preconference. During preconference, when your instructor reviews your priorities for the day, she comments positively that you have individualized care based on your particular client's needs at the moment. In your mind, you determine that the vital signs are your next priority and will take minimal time, and you should still be able to complete care and documentation in a competent manner and on time.

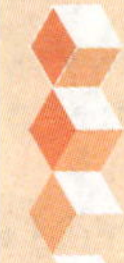

Helpscan

The following are resources for clients and health-care professionals:

- The American Sleep Disorders Association
  604 2nd St., SW
  Rochester, MN 55902
  (507) 287-6006
- The National Sleep Foundation
  122 S. Robertson Blvd., 3rd Floor
  Los Angeles, CA 90048
  (Please contact by letter only)
- The Canadian Association for Narcolepsy
  PO Box 223, Station "S"
  Toronto, ON M5M 4L7
  (416) 398-1627

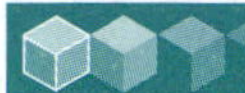

Nursing Process in Clinical Practice

When identifying and treating sleep disturbances categorized as nursing diagnoses, the nurse uses each phase of the nursing process. Quality care depends on the nurse's possession of the knowledge and clinical skills described earlier in this chapter. What follows are the assessment priorities, expected outcomes, and nursing interventions for two common types of sleep problems treated by nurses: (1) insomnia and (2) sleep deprivation.

Sleep Pattern Disturbance: Insomnia (difficulty falling asleep, difficulty remaining asleep, or premature awakening)

Sleep Pattern Disturbance: Sleep deprivation

Sleep Pattern Disturbance: Insomnia

Disruption of sleep time causes discomfort or interferes with desired life style. (NANDA, 1994)

An inability to obtain the quantity or quality of sleep that is essential for an individual's healthy functioning is insomnia. The knowledge base for insomnia was discussed in Table 40-4. Insomnias may also be classified as transient, short-term, or chronic (Shaver & Landis, 1995). Transient insomnia is a difficulty in falling asleep or staying asleep, which lasts for only a few days and is associated with significant life change. Insomnia is referred to as short-term when it is related to the death of a loved one or a major emotional upheaval and lasts for no more than 3 to 4 weeks. Nursing intervention is directed to helping the client understand the relationship between the sleep problem and the stressor. Chronic insomnias last for longer than 3 to 4 weeks and may continue throughout life. They are the most common complaint reported by clients seen in sleep disorder centers.

Assessment

- Use interview questions directed to the client and his or her bed partner and direct observation when possible to determine if the insomnia is caused by difficulty falling asleep, periodic awakenings, or early morning awakenings. Determine if the client's perception of his or her sleep–wakefulness pattern corresponds to reality.
- Explore the client's lifestyle and physical and mental health for contributing factors. Because problems in sexual adjustment or functioning may contribute to insomnia, a sexual history may be indicated.
- Instruct the client to keep a sleep diary that may include a graph of undisturbed hours of sleep per night. Use the diary to relate factors causing or correcting the insomnia to sleep–wakefulness patterns.
- Assess for signs of sleep deprivation.
- Assess the actual and perceived degree of control the client has over his or her insomnia.
- Assess the safety and effectiveness of aids client has used to deal with insomnia.

Expected Outcomes

The client will:

- Report that his or her regular pattern is reestablished or that a new pattern characterized by ease in falling asleep and diminished or absent nighttime and early morning awakenings is established
- Identify the reversible causes of the insomnia
- Institute lifestyle changes to eliminate factors contributing to insomnia (eg, decrease caffeine intake)
- Incorporate appropriate destressing rituals into pre-bedtime activities (eg, listening to soothing music, progressive relaxation, prayer)

Interventions

Interventions for insomnia vary according to its cause and severity. Lifestyle counseling includes the following recommendations, when appropriate:

- Eating a light carbohydrate snack before bedtime, such as crackers, toast, or fruit juice, which is thought to induce sleep
- Eliminating caffeine and alcohol in the evening because both are known to disrupt the normal sleep cycle

- Decreasing or stopping smoking because nicotine withdrawal can occur 3 hours after the last cigarette and cause sleep restlessness, altered sleep cycle, and early awakening to obtain a cigarette
- Incorporating a period of regular exercise into each day—but not before bedtime; avoiding any stimulating activity before attempting to fall asleep
- Setting aside time for destressing rituals (relaxation exercises, music, conversation, prayer) immediately before retiring; having someone with whom one can share fears, worries, and anxieties is often helpful
- Trying to sleep only when sleepy and not when wakeful
- Observing a regular bedtime hour and awakening hour because biologic clocks are affected by staying up later or rising later in the day
- Avoiding naps during the day and evening because, for some people, the ability to fall asleep is related to the time interval since the last sleep period
- Leaving the bed and bedroom when awake; even if this occurs during the night, the client should take up a quiet, nonstimulating activity (reading, television, music) in another room, so that the bed remains firmly associated with sleep

Independent nursing measures for insomnia may include all those described earlier in the chapter. The nurse may also need to collaborate with the physician in determining the best course of action if the client's insomnia is drug related. Clients who have used hypnotic medications for a long time will probably benefit most from a gradual program of withdrawal and will value nursing support throughout this process. On the other hand, a short course of treatment with a sedative-hypnotic or antianxiety agent may be indicated, in which case the nurse works collaboratively with the prescribing physician and teaches the client the action of the drug, the reason it is being used, safe administration particulars, side effects to watch for and to report, and potential dangers of overreliance on medication.

For severe problems of insomnia, referral for psychiatric evaluation and treatment may be necessary. Clients may also be referred to a sleep disorder clinic.

Sleep Pattern Disturbance: Sleep Deprivation

Shortchanging one's sleep rarely results in any serious problems, but a prolonged pattern of sleep deprivation produces symptoms progressing from irritability and fatigue to generalized personality disintegration. There are basically three types of sleep deprivation:

REM deprivation (absence of dreaming): Caused by certain drugs (especially alcohol and barbiturates), general sleep disturbances (eg, shift work, travel, or hospitalization—especially in intensive care setting). When people are denied dreaming during normal REM sleep, they become irritable, insecure, and anxious. Also, their sensitivity to pain increases, they are unable to concentrate, and they exercise poor judgment. Relationships with other people suffer. Depression is a common mental symptom, and in extreme cases, a person's ethical standards have been known to deteriorate. Symptoms of psychoses have appeared in rational people after prolonged REM sleep deprivation. These same subjects, when allowed to sleep uninterrupted, experience more frequent REM periods, as if the body were trying to make up for losses. It has been observed that when people are denied REM sleep for whatever reason, REM sleep with dreaming, often including nightmares, increases. Similarly, when stage IV NREM sleep is denied, the person tries to catch up on lost NREM sleep. If both REM and NREM sleep are insufficient, stage IV NREM sleep increases.

NREM deprivation (delta sleep or SWS deprivation): Causes may be the same as for REM deprivation, and also may include continual interruption of the sleep cycle (eg, with frequent treatments); certain medications (eg, diazepam [Valium], flurazepam [Dalmane], and morphine); and conditions such as sleep apnea, hypothyroidism, and diseases causing respiratory distress. Older people frequently experience lack of NREM sleep. Symptoms include fatigue, lethargy, depression, and difficulty in executing the repetitive tasks of everyday living.

Total sleep deprivation: Rarely occurs except in controlled laboratory situations. Symptoms of total sleep loss occur in a relatively slow but predictable pattern, mounting as time goes on. As weariness begins, normal performance fades off with lapses in attention and concentration. Unpleasant sensations, such as blurred vision, glazed and itching eyes, nausea, and headache are common symptoms of fatigue. Hallucinations and illusions eventually become vivid, and mental confusion and inability to determine reality occur. There may be a lack of memory, a decrease in intellectual effort, and an attitude of not caring what happens.

Exactly why sleeplessness leads to ill effects is unknown. It is unknown whether irreversible damage to body tissue results from prolonged or chronic sleep deprivation. However, that sleep deprivation produces changes in physical and mental functioning supports observations that sleep is essential for well-being.

Assessment Priorities

- Use interview questions directed to the client and family and observation skills to determine the type of sleep deprivation, its probable causes, its effect on everyday functioning, and the severity of the problem.
- Instruct the client to keep a sleep diary and note increases or decreases in quality sleep and the factors that contribute to or detract from quality sleep.

- Assess the actual and perceived amount of control the client has over his or her sleep–wakefulness patterns.

Expected Outcomes

The client will:
- Keep a sleep diary (if feasible) until factors causing sleep deprivation and factors that facilitate sleep are identified
- If indicated, change or eliminate lifestyle behavior contributing to sleep deprivation
- Increase REM and NREM sleep until usual sleep cycle is reestablished (specify)
- Increase REM and NREM sleep until behaviors indicating sleep deprivation (specify) are no longer present

Interventions

As soon as the cause of the sleep deprivation has been identified, nursing measures are instituted to eliminate the cause or to modify either it or the client's response:
- If insomnia is the cause, the nurse institutes the interventions for insomnia described earlier.
- If hospitalization is the cause, appropriate nursing measures include the following:
  - Familiarizing the client with the hospital environment
  - Recreating the client's usual sleep environment as much as possible: favorite pillow, dim light or darkness, ventilation, door open or closed, child's favorite toy
  - Respecting the client's pre-sleep habits and rituals when these are sleep producing—eating a carbohydrate, watching the 11 PM news, listening to music, taking a warm shower or bath, using relaxation exercises, praying
  - Using good nursing care measures to ensure the client's comfort before he or she falls asleep: body is repositioned and in good alignment, supported if necessary; bed linens are clean and straightened; client is free of pain; tubes are patent and draining; equipment is functioning optimally (if frequent checks are needed throughout the night [eg, with an intravenous line], keeping a soft night light on continuously may be less distressing than having each nurse fumble for a light); finally, if pharmacologic aids are to be used to promote sleep, a determination should first be made that they are not negatively interfering with REM or NREM sleep
  - Carefully evaluating the need for nursing interventions throughout the night that are likely to awaken the client and to schedule nursing care to allow the client the longest periods of undisturbed rest; careful assessment of the sleeping client also allows the nurse to determine when a sleep cycle is completed and when it might be best to awaken the client
- If medications are contributing to sleep deprivation, the nurse needs to consult with the physician regarding the advisability of their use and possible substitutes.
- When alcohol is contributing to sleep deprivation, the nurse needs to teach the client about alcohol's effects in the body and counsel the client about decreasing or eliminating alcohol intake.
- When sleep deprivation results from shift work, travel, and so forth, the nurse must explore with the client the need for this activity and suggest means to compensate if the activity is necessary.

Client Care Study

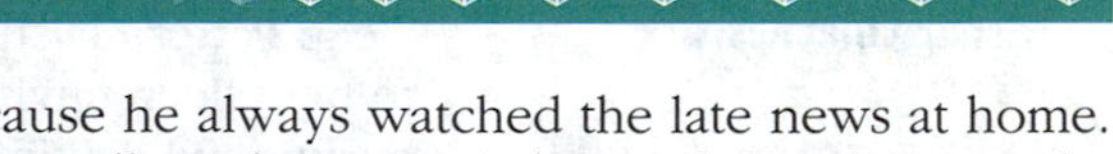

Mr. Bitner is an alert, widowed, 86-year-old African-American man who was admitted to a nursing home 2 months ago. He is ambulatory and performs most of his self-care. Admitting medical diagnoses included diabetes mellitus and hypertension. He adds to this list "a touch of arthritis." His daughter complains to the charge nurse that her dad seems to be spending more and more time during the day napping and that he says he does not sleep well at night. A comprehensive sleep assessment of Mr. Bitner following his daughter's expression of concern revealed the following data.

Sleep–Wakefulness Pattern
- Client goes to bed between 8 and 9 PM and gets out of bed between 7 and 8 AM because the staff are getting his roommate out of bed at this time. He states he never falls asleep before midnight because he always watched the late news at home. He usually wakens twice during the night to void and often cannot go back to sleep.
- During the day, client is frequently observed dozing in his chair. If not discouraged, he returns to his room midmorning and afternoon for a 1-hour nap.

Effect of Sleep Pattern on Everyday Living
- Client states: "I'm always tired. I don't seem to have much energy anymore."
- Client has not socialized yet with other residents, and without strong encouragement does not participate in group activities.
- From his point of view, life holds little reason for him to be awake. "I worked for the railroad for almost 50 years and I never overslept once."

Sleep Aids

- Client denies ever using medication to fall asleep. States he often relaxed at home in the evening with a couple of beers.
- Client likes a dim light on during the night so he can find the bathroom easily and likes his bedroom door ajar.
- Client sleeps with two blankets and is often still cold.

Sleep Disturbances and Contributing Factors

- Client states: "Ever since my wife died, I'm just not getting enough sleep and since I came here it's worse. I don't know why I don't fall asleep when I go to bed or why I wake up so much. It sure makes the nights long."
- Client has no regular periods of exercise and drinks black coffee with every meal and one or two diet colas in the evening.

Core Competencies

Cognitive Competencies

- Knowledge of how aging affects sleep–wakefulness pattern
- Knowledge of the multiple factors that contribute to insomnia and successful treatment strategies
- Teaching skills to meet the needs of Mr. Bitner and his family
- Ability to develop nursing diagnoses that reflect the unique factors interfering with Mr. Bitner's sleep
- Knowledge of which nursing interventions are most likely to yield desired outcomes

Technical Competencies

- Strong assessment skills to identify carefully the factors causing Mr. Bitner's sleep disturbance
- Caregiver skills directed to strengthening Mr. Bitner's sleep–wake cycle rhythm

Interpersonal Competencies

- Strong interpersonal skills to communicate to both Mr. Bitner and his daughter that something can be done to improve the duration and quality of his sleep and that the nursing staff is committed to helping
- Interpersonal and leadership skills to motivate the nursing staff to value Mr. Bitner's expected outcomes and to work collaboratively with the social worker and activities director
- Ability to establish a trusting nurse–client relationship grounded in responsible caring

Ethical/Legal Competencies

- Willingness to assume responsibility for ensuring that the plan of care successfully assists Mr. Bitner in achieving his sleep/rest goals
- Competence in documenting nursing interventions
- Ability to serve as a trusted and effective client advocate

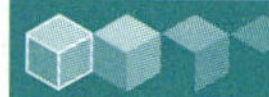

Nursing Plan of Care

for Mr. Bitner

Nursing Diagnosis: Sleep Pattern Disturbance: Difficulty Falling Asleep and Remaining Asleep related to new sleep environment and schedule, evening caffeine intake, and insufficient meaningful daytime activity

Expected Outcome: By the next monthly assessment, 1/20/98, the client will:

- Retire after viewing the 11 PM news in the TV room with Mr. Sparter

Nursing Interventions	Rationale	Evaluative Statement
Assess advisability of reestablishing Mr. Bitner's usual retiring pattern of going to bed after the 11 PM news. Assess how client spends the time from the evening meal to 11 PM—explore relaxing alternatives with him. Investigate possibility that he and Mr. Sparter might become social partners.	Strengthens the natural rhythm of his sleep-wake cycle. Elimination of evening naps will facilitate his falling asleep more easily.	1/18/98 Goal met. Client does not go to bed until after the news and has been observed talking with Mr. Sparter. *Recommendation:* Continue to develop evening activities with him—he finds that the time after supper "drags." *M. LeBon, RN*

(continued)

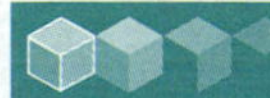

Nursing Plan of Care *(continued)*

for Mr. Bitner

Expected Outcome: By the next monthly assessment, 1/20/98, the client will:

- Report that he falls asleep within 1 hour of getting into bed

Nursing Interventions	Rationale	Evaluative Statement
Continue to assess how long it takes client to fall asleep after getting into bed.	In elderly clients, stage I time is increased.	1/18/98 Goal partially met. Three or four nights a week he falls asleep within 30 minutes of going to bed. States he really misses comfort of his wife. *Revision:* Investigate client's sense of loss and need for touch. May be a good candidate for pet therapy program. *M. LeBon, RN*
Explore with client means to relax before falling asleep—deep breathing, imagery, prayer.	Activities that calm and relax the person prepare the body for sleep.	
Teach the importance of using the bed only as a place to sleep. Advise client when he cannot sleep to get out of bed and to go to another room where he can perform some monotonous activity (watching television, listening to radio).	This maintains the bed as a powerful stimulus for sleep and helps to prevent "conditioned" insomnia ("Well, here I am in bed now and I know sleep won't come").	

Expected Outcome: By the next monthly assessment, 1/20/98, the client will:

- Decrease nighttime awakenings to one after which he returns to a sound sleep

Nursing Interventions	Rationale	Evaluative Statement
Assess and manipulate factors that contribute to nighttime awakenings: • Need to void (time of day diuretic is taken, amounts of fluid intake in the evening) • Roommate's wakefulness, snoring, or need for care • Uncomfortableness in strange environment • Comfort (eg, temperature)	Individualizing the client's bedtime environment and meeting comfort needs (warmth, soft light, and so forth) promote sleep onset and maintenance.	1/18/98 Goal partially met. Nighttime awakenings vary from none to three nightly. See previous revision. *M. LeBon, RN*
Teach client how, on awakening, to concentrate on breathing until he falls back to sleep.	This uses the power of positive thinking to facilitate return to sleep.	

Expected Outcome: By the next monthly assessment, 1/20/98, the client will:

- Attend the center's exercise sessions Monday through Friday at 10 AM

Nursing Interventions	Rationale	Evaluative Statement
Assess whether client understands the relation between daily exercise and his ability to sleep.	Regular exercise throughout the day is known to increase physical fatigue and to promote sleep. Exercise or stimulating activities immediately before retiring interfere with sleep's onset.	1/20/98 Goal met. Client has become an enthusiastic participant in exercise sessions—attends daily. *L. Fox, RN*
Determine how his exercise needs can best be met (ie, through a group program or an individualized program of walking, or other program)	Exercise program must be individualized based on physical state and interests of client.	
Use positive verbal reinforcement to communicate to client that someone cares that he is using positive means to remedy his sleep disturbance and increase his well-being.	Activity provides the opportunity for socialization and improvement of a self-image.	

(continued)

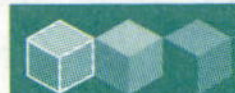

Nursing Plan of Care *(continued)*

for Mr. Bitner

Nursing Interventions	Rationale	Evaluative Statement
Encourage client's daughter to go for walks with him when she visits and to question him about his exercise program.	Communication and interaction with family members helps the elderly client to maintain self-esteem and to feel valuable and loved.	

Expected Outcome

By the next monthly assessment, 1/20/98, the client will:

- Substitute caffeine-free beverages for coffee and cola at supper and evening snack

Nursing Actions	Rationale	Evaluative Statement
Assess client's willingness to substitute caffeine-free beverages for coffee and cola.	Caffeine is a stimulant that can cause difficulty sleeping.	1/20/98 Goal met. Client now drinks decaffeinated coffee with meals and milk in the evening. Dislikes caffeine-free sodas. *M. LeBon, RN*
Consult with dietary department and his daughter about options. Experiment with options until his preferences are determined.	Caffeine-free versions of beverages are often available and can be used based on client acceptance.	
Gradually reduce his caffeine intake, especially from evening meal onward. Offer a carbohydrate evening snack.	Carbohydrate snack appears to promote sleep	

Sample Documentation

12/20/97 Nursing

Family conference to discuss Mr. Bitner's sleep disturbance—initiated by daughter's concern. Present were Mr. Bitner and his daughter (A. Jelner), K. Behner (social worker), W. Quing (activity director), and M. LeBon (primary nurse). Primary nurse presented findings from comprehensive sleep assessment: Nursing diagnosis: Sleep Pattern Disturbance: Difficulty falling asleep and remaining asleep related to new sleep environment and schedule, evening caffeine intake, and insufficient meaningful daytime activity. Discussion centered on strategies to help Mr. Bitner develop interests in the center, including possibilities for increased physical exercise; decrease his evening caffeine intake (daughter to bring noncaffeine colas); and reestablish usual retiring and waking times. See plan of care. Client's progress will be evaluated at next monthly assessment, 1/20/98.

M. LeBon, RN

Key Points

- Most people spend about one third of their lives asleep; sleep of some quality and duration is an essential component of well-being.
- Sleep is a state of altered consciousness throughout which varying degrees of stimuli produce wakefulness. It is an active and complex rhythmic state, a progression of repeated cycles.
- The cyclic nature of sleep is controlled by the reticular activating system and bulbar synchronizing region in the brain stem. Biochemical changes and hormones also influence the sleep process.
- Circadian synchronization occurs when an individual's sleep–wake patterns follow the inner biologic clock. Shift work, traveling across time zones, and irregular sleep–wake patterns can easily lead to desynchronization, poor quality sleep, and decreased work performance.
- There is both NREM sleep and REM sleep. During a sleep cycle, a person passes through the four stages of NREM sleep and through REM sleep. The average person has four or five complete sleep cycles each night.

- Factors affecting sleep include age, physical activity, psychologic stress, motivation, diet, alcohol intake, caffeine intake, nicotine use, environment, lifestyle, illness, and medications. Most people with sleep disturbances can initiate lifestyle changes that will improve sleep.
- Nurses should explore parents' perceptions about the amount of sleep their infant or child needs and the schedule the parent uses for sleep and rest times. Development variations and the need for consistent sleep-wake patterns and bedtime rituals may need to be taught.
- For the young adult, the sleep-wakefulness cycle is the most important of all the rhythmic patterns and the one most likely to be abused. Multiple stressors can interfere with the young adult obtaining sufficient rest and sleep and can encourage the use of alcohol or sleep medications. Teaching needs to include the importance of developing good sleep habits to promote long-term wellness.
- The nurse who wishes to be an effective role model in promoting rest and sleep uses appearance and energy level to communicate to clients the value of proper rest and sleep self-care behaviors.
- A comprehensive sleep history includes data on sleep-wakefulness pattern, the effect of the sleep pattern on everyday functioning, sleep aids, sleep disturbance, and contributing factors.
- When a sleep disturbance exists, the assessment attempts to identify the nature of the problem, its cause, related signs and symptoms, onset and frequency, effect on everyday living, severity, whether the problem can be treated independently by nursing, and the coping means the client has used and their success. A sleep diary and information from a bed partner may be needed to establish a diagnosis.
- Common sleep problems include insomnia, narcolepsy, sleep apnea, parasomnias (sleep walking, sleep talking, enuresis), and sleep deprivation.
- Nursing diagnoses may be written to address sleep pattern disturbances specifically (insomnia: difficulty falling asleep, difficulty remaining asleep, or premature awakening); or to identify the effect sleep pattern disturbances have on other areas of human functioning (eg, anxiety, comfort, coping, alteration in thought process).
- Nursing interventions to promote rest and sleep include establishing a trusting relationship, preparing a restful sleep environment, attending to bedtime rituals, offering appropriate bedtime snacks, promoting relaxation and comfort, respecting normal sleep-wake patterns, scheduling nursing care to avoid disturbances, using medications to promote sleep, and teaching the client about rest and sleep.

Study Questions

1. A client's body temperature is 99°F (37.2°C) in the late afternoon. This is most likely
   a. a sign of an infection
   b. normal circadian rhythm
   c. hyperpyrexia
   d. due to a warm environment
2. Muscle tone is recorded by the
   a. electroencephalograph (EEG)
   b. electrocardiogram (ECG)
   c. electrooculogram (EOG)
   d. electromyograph (EMG)
3. The nurse observes some involuntary muscle jerking in her sleeping client. The client is most likely in
   a. stage I NREM sleep
   b. stage II NREM sleep
   c. stage IV NREM sleep
   d. REM sleep
4. The nurse observes a slight increase in her client's vital signs when she assesses them while the client is sleeping during the night. According to his stage of sleep, the nurse expects that
   a. he is aware of his surroundings at this point
   b. he is in delta sleep at this time
   c. it would be most difficult to awaken him at this time
   d. this is most likely an NREM stage
5. How many cycles of sleep does a person typically go through each night?
   a. 2
   b. 4 or 5
   c. 10
   d. 20 to 25
6. While discussing factors that induce sleep with an older client, the nurse teaches her that
   a. a cup of regular tea may induce sleep
   b. large quantities of alcohol promote a deep sleep
   c. the amount of REM sleep decreases with age
   d. physical activity decreases REM and NREM sleep
7. A client falls asleep in the middle of a conversation. This disorder is called
   a. hypersomnia
   b. narcolepsy
   c. somnambulism
   d. sleep apnea
8. A sleep diary is a diagnostic tool that
   a. is generally kept for one week

b. includes a record of daily physical activity
c. includes a record of body temperature taken each evening
d. reports only subjective information about sleep activities

9. To help Mr. Yang get to sleep, the nurse suggests that he
a. follow his usual bedtime routine if possible
b. drink two or three glasses of water at bedtime
c. have a large snack at bedtime
d. take a sedative-hypnotic every night at bedtime

10. The most common complaint of clients visiting sleep disorder clinics is
a. hypersomnia
b. narcolepsy
c. chronic insomnia
d. enuresis

11. A prolonged pattern of REM deprivation may result in
a. symptoms of psychosis
b. increased episodes of dreaming
c. decreased sensitivity to pain
d. increased mental alertness

12. Active dreaming occurs during
a. stage II NREM
b. stage III NREM
c. stage IV NREM
d. REM sleep

13. Illness is a stressor and can influence sleep during various stages. An example is
a. asthma attacks appear to occur less frequently during stage IV NREM sleep
b. a person with heart disease is more likely to have chest pain during NREM sleep
c. an epileptic is more likely to have seizures during REM sleep
d. an increase in gastric secretion in a person with an ulcer will most likely occur in NREM sleep

14. Caffeine is a known stimulant and intake should be
a. avoided at least 30 minutes before bedtime
b. combined with milk to counteract its effect
c. avoided at least 4 to 5 hours before bedtime
d. encouraged during waking hours to counteract effects of sleeplessness

15. Medications that induce sleep (sedative-hypnotics) may disturb REM or NREM sleep. The nurse should be aware that
a. they should be taken with alcohol for increased effect
b. these medications usually become ineffective after several weeks
c. they can usually be given at intervals during the night
d. they should be combined with daytime use of amphetamines to counteract any hangover effect

Answers With Rationale

1. The correct response is *b*. A slight increase in body temperature in the late afternoon is a normal circadian rhythm. This slight variation from normal does not necessarily mean an infection is present nor is it hyperpyrexia (high fever). A warm environment might possibly cause an elevation in body temperature, but the most likely cause is normal circadian rhythm.
2. The correct response is *d*. An EMG measures muscle tone whereas an EEG records electrical currents from the brain. An EOG is a recording of eye movements and an ECG records cardiac activity.
3. The correct response is *a*. Involuntary muscle jerking occurs in stage I NREM sleep. In the other stages, the muscles proceed from a relaxed state to large muscle immobility.
4. The correct response is *c*. During REM sleep, it is difficult to arouse a person and the vital signs increase. Delta sleep is NREM stage III and IV.
5. The correct response is *b*. A person goes through probably four or five cycles of sleep each night with each cycle lasting 90 to 100 minutes.
6. The correct response is *c*. Regular tea has caffeine and increases alertness, and large quantities of alcohol limit REM and delta sleep. Physical activity increases both REM and NREM sleep.
7. The correct response is *b*. Narcolepsy is an uncontrollable desire to sleep. Hypersomnia refers to excessive sleep, somnambulism is sleepwalking, and sleep apnea is a period where breathing ceases between snoring.
8. The correct response is *b*. A sleep diary includes activities during the day since they have an effect on sleep, usually is kept for at least 14 days, and is more helpful if objective comments from a bed partner are included. A record of body temperature is insignificant.
9. The correct response is *a*. Drinking two or three glasses of water at bedtime will probably awaken the client during the night to void. A large snack may be uncomfortable right before bedtime and taking a sedative-hypnotic every night disturbs REM and NREM sleep. The sedative also loses its effectiveness shortly.
10. The correct response is *c*. Chronic insomnia is the most common reason why people visit a sleep disorder clinic.
11. The correct response is *a*. Prolonged episodes of REM deprivation may cause symptoms of psychosis. REM deprivation results in an absence of episodes of dreaming, sensitivity to pain increases, and the person is less mentally alert.

12. The correct response is *d*. Active dreaming occurs during REM sleep.
13. The correct response is *a*. Chest pain occurs more frequently during REM sleep. Epileptic seizures occur more frequently during NREM sleep and gastric secretions increase during REM sleep.
14. The correct response is *c*. Caffeine should be avoided at least 4 to 5 hours before bedtime. Milk does not counteract its effect, and caffeine use is never recommended, even during waking hours.
15. The correct response is *b*. Sedative-hypnotics should never be taken with alcohol because it potentiates their effect. They are usually ordered only at bedtime and may have one repeat order if the client cannot fall asleep. However, they are not given at intervals during the night. Amphetamine use is never recommended.

Bibliography

Alward, R., & Monk, T. (1995). Sleep as a circadian rhythm: The impact of shiftwork. *American Nurse, 27*(2), 20–21.

Andrews, M., & Boyle, J. (1995). *Transcultural concepts in nursing care* (2nd ed.). Philadelphia: Lippincott.

Bachman, D. (1992). Sleep disorder with aging: Evaluation and treatment. *Geriatrics, 47*(9), 53–61.

Carpenito, L. (1995). *Nursing diagnosis: Application to clinical practice* (6th ed.). Philadelphia: Lippincott.

Cowley, G. (1996). Timing is everything. Newsweek (March 11), 68.

Feinsilver, J. (1993). Sleep in the elderly patient. *Clinics in Chest Medicine, 14*(3), 405–411.

Fuller, J., & Schaller-Ayers, J. (1994). *Health assessment: A nursing approach* (2nd ed.). Philadelphia: Lippincott.

Gorbien, M. (1993). When your older patient can't sleep: How to put insomnia to rest. *Geriatrics, 48*(9), 65–75.

Knapp, M. (1993). Night shift: The restorative sleep specialists. *Journal of Gerontological Nursing, 19*(5), 38–42.

Lankford, S. (1994). Sleep loss in the elderly: Understanding the reasons. *Journal of Gerontological Nursing, 20*(8), 49–52.

Leger, D. (1994). The cost of sleep related accidents: A report for the National Commission on Sleep Disorders Research. *Sleep, 17*(1), 84–93.

Miller, C. (1995). *Nursing care of older adults: Theory and practice* (2nd ed.). Philadelphia: Lippincott.

North American Nursing Diagnosis Association. (1994). *NANDA nursing diagnoses: Definitions and classification 1995–1996.* Philadelphia: NANDA.

Regestein, Q., & Dambrosia, J. (1993). Daytime alertness in patients with primary insomnia. *American Journal of Psychiatry, 150*(10), 1529.

Roberts, A. (1990). Senior systems: Older patients and their medications. *Nursing Times, 86*(11), 14–20.

Rosa, R. (1993). Napping at home and alertness on the job in rotating shift workers. *Sleep, 16*(8), 727–735.

Shaver, J., & Landis, C. (1994). Understanding the behavior of sleep. *American Nurse, 26*(7), 16–17.

Shaver, J., & Landis, C. (1995). Helping people manage primary insomnia. *American Nurse, 27*(1), 22–23.

Shaver, J., & Rodgers, A. (1994). Screening for sleep-related disorders: Sleep apnea and narcolepsy. *American Nurse, 26*(8), 24–25.

Spenceley, S. (1993). Sleep inquiry: A look with fresh eyes. *IMAGE: Journal of Nursing Scholarship, 25*(3), 249–256.

Stanley, M., & Beare, P. (1995). *Gerontological nursing.* Philadelphia: Davis.

Topf, M. (1992). Effects of personal control over hospital noise on sleep. *Research in Nursing and Health, 15*(1), 19–28.

Wardlaw, G., & Insel, P. (1993). *Perspectives in nutrition* (2nd ed.). St. Louis: Mosby.

Webb, W. (1994). Sleep as a biological rhythm: A historical review. *Sleep, 17*(2), 188–194.

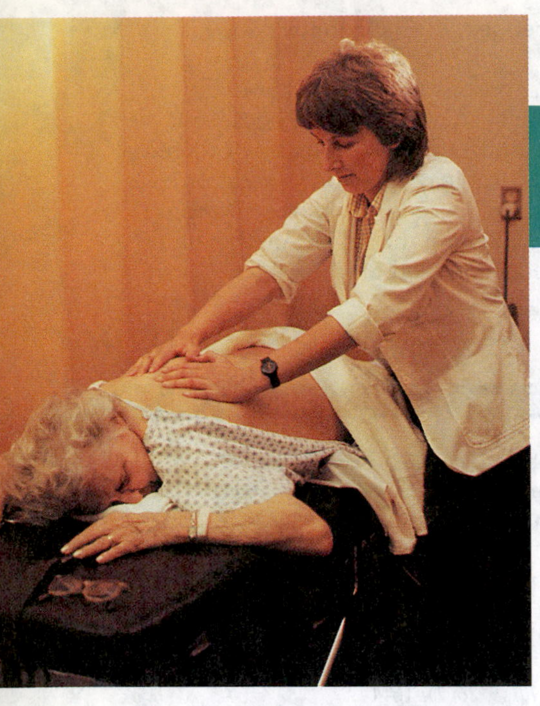

Chapter 41

Comfort

Objectives

After studying this chapter, the learner should be able to:

Define key terms used in the chapter.

Describe specific elements in the pain experience.

Compare and contrast acute and chronic pain.

Identify factors that may affect an individual's pain experience.

Obtain a complete pain assessment using appropriate interviewing and physical assessment skills.

Develop nursing diagnoses that correctly identify pain problems and demonstrate the relation between pain and other areas of human functioning.

Demonstrate the correct use of nonpharmacologic pain-relief measures.

Administer analgesic agents safely to produce the desired level of analgesia without causing undesirable side effects.

Collaborate with the members of other health disciplines using different treatment modalities to promote pain relief.

Use teaching and counseling skills to empower clients to direct their own pain management programs.

Key Terms

acute pain
analgesic
chronic pain
cutaneous pain
endorphins
enkephalins
gate control theory
intractable
neuromodulators
neurotransmitters
nociceptors
opioid
pain threshold
pain tolerance
phantom pain
placebo
psychogenic pain
referred pain
somatic pain
visceral pain

A person in pain often experiences pain as an all-consuming reality and wants only one nursing intervention—pain relief. If pain relief were as simple as rubbing a back or administering a prescribed analgesic, nursing's task would be easy. However, no two people experience pain exactly the same way. Differences in individual pain perception and response to pain as well as the multiple and diverse etiologies of pain require highly specialized abilities of the nurse seeking to promote comfort and relieve pain. The most essential of these are the nurse's belief that the client's pain is real, willingness to become involved in the client's pain experience, and competence in developing effective pain management regimens. Although pain is often an all-consuming priority for clients, it is frequently a low priority for nurses because it is an intangible commodity. Unfortunately, it is easier to ignore a client's poorly communicated pain than it is to ignore a dressing that needs to be changed, a client who requires assistance with ambulation, or a prescribed medication. Nurses who somehow manage to practice nursing while remaining insensitive to the comfort needs of their clients do a grave disservice to these clients and to the nursing profession itself.

Nurses are not alone in undervaluing the need for pain management. Although pain is the second most common reason for seeing a physician following colds and upper respiratory infections and the number one reason why people take medication, medical science is still ill equipped to deal with this widespread occurrence (Batten, 1995). Despite its prevalence, limited information on pain and its management is included in educational programs for physicians and nurses. However, new advances in understanding and treating pain have focused on the real possibility of controlling most human pain and made pain management a priority for healthcare workers.

Study of this chapter will provide the student with knowledge of the pain experience and factors that influence it. A detailed guide to assessing alterations in comfort is presented. Numerous examples of nursing diagnoses are accompanied by specific nursing strategies for promoting comfort and assisting clients to achieve pain management goals. The recently published guidelines for acute pain management and management of cancer pain developed by the Agency for Health Care Policy and Research are presented as standards for effective pain management by nurses (AHCPR, 1992; AHCPR, 1994).

In the section Nursing Process in Clinical Practice, focused assessment, expected outcomes, implementation, and evaluation guides are offered for nursing diagnoses of acute and chronic pain problems. These guides and the concluding client care study illustrate how the nurse's knowledge of and sensitivity to the client's pain experience may be combined with specific nursing interventions to resolve pain problems successfully.

The Pain Experience

Definition

Pain is an elusive and complex phenomenon, and despite its universality, its exact nature remains a mystery. It is one of the human body's defense mechanisms that indicates the person is experiencing a problem. The definition of pain that is probably of greatest benefit to nurses and their clients is that offered by Margo McCaffery (1979): "Pain is whatever the experiencing person says it is, existing whenever he (or she) says it does" (p. 11). This definition rests on the belief that the only one who can be a real authority on whether an individual is experiencing pain is that individual.

Pain is present whenever a person says it is, even when no specific cause of the pain can be found. Health practitioners must rely on the client's description of the pain because it is a subjective symptom that only the client can identify and describe.

Origins of Pain

Pain is categorized as cutaneous, deep somatic, or visceral in origin. **Cutaneous** (or superficial) **pain** usually involves the skin or subcutaneous tissue. A paper cut that produces sharp pain with a burning sensation is an example of cutaneous pain. Deep **somatic pain** is diffuse or scattered and originates in tendons, ligaments, bones, blood vessels, and nerves. Strong pressure on a bone or damage to tissue that occurs with a sprain causes deep somatic pain. **Visceral pain** is poorly localized and originates in body organs in the thorax, cranium, and abdomen. This pain may be **referred** or perceived in an area that is distant from its point of origin. Pain associated with a myocardial infarction, or heart attack, is frequently referred to the neck, shoulder, or arms (often the left arm).

Pain may originate from physical causes, that is, a physical cause for the pain can be identified. Pain may also have a psychogenic origin (**psychogenic pain**), that is, a physical cause for the pain cannot be identified. However, it has been observed that a pure origin is probably rare, and pain usually has both physical and psychogenic components. Furthermore, pain that results from a mental event can be just as intense as pain that results from a physical event.

When the threshold of perception for pain has been reached and when there is injured tissue, it is believed that the injured tissue releases chemicals that excite nerve endings. A damaged cell releases histamine, which excites nerve endings. Lactic acid accumulates in tissues injured by lack of blood supply and is believed to excite nerve endings and cause pain or to lower the threshold of nerve endings to other stimuli (eg, heat or pressure). Other substances are also released that stimulate **nociceptors** or pain receptors. These include bradykinin, prostaglandins, and substance P.

- *Bradykinin*, a powerful vasodilator that increases capillary permeability and constricts smooth muscle, plays an important role in the chemistry of pain at the site of an injury even before the pain message gets to the brain. It also triggers the release of histamine, and in combination with histamine produces the redness, swelling, and pain typically observed when an inflammation is present.
- *Prostaglandins* are hormonelike substances that send additional pain stimuli to the central nervous system.
- *Substance P* is believed to act as a stimulant at pain receptor sites and may also be involved in the inflammatory response in local tissues (Fuller & Schaller-Ayers, 1994).

Prostaglandins, substance P, and serotonin (a hormone that can act to stimulate smooth muscles, inhibit gastric secretion, and produce vasoconstriction) are **neurotransmitters**, or substances that either excite or inhibit target nerve cells.

Receptors in the skin and superficial organs, although incapable of responding selectively, are stimulated by mechanical, thermal, chemical, and electrical agents. Friction from bed linens and pressure from a cast are mechanical stimulants. Sunburn and cold water on a tooth with caries are thermal stimulants. An acid burn is the result of a chemical stimulant. The jolt of a static charge is an electrical stimulant.

Stretching of the hollow viscera, pulling on the omentum, and muscle spasms result in pain. Some investigators believe that at least some of the deep-lying organs have their own individual pain receptors, the uterus being an example. Some organs, such as the lungs, are insensitive to pain because of the absence of nociceptors or pain receptors.

It has been observed that pain may be present without injury and may not be present with injury. Therefore, tissue injury does not necessarily accompany pain in all instances. For example, tissue injury is present when the client experiences pain because of a first- or second-degree burn. On the other hand, although physiologic changes do occur, tissue injury or destruction is not necessarily present when the client has a headache owing to psychologic tension. In addition, intensity of pain may not accurately relate to the seriousness of a particular condition giving rise to the pain. Thus, the client may not experience pain until the ravages of a malignancy are beyond control, whereas the severe pain that usually accompanies a bunion is not in keeping with the degree of pathology involved.

Pain Syndromes. Although the causes of pain are many, certain major pathologic pain syndromes have been identified to describe the conditions most frequently associated with producing severe or prolonged pain. Common pain syndromes highlighted in Table 41-1 include peripheral pain syndromes (causalgia, postherpetic neuralgia, and phantom limb pain); central pain syndromes (thalamic syndrome, trigeminal neuralgia); and pain with underlying pathology syndromes (musculoskeletal pain syndromes, headache, cancer pain syndrome). Because appropriate treatment of these syndromes is often delayed because of misdiagnosis, nursing can play an important role in their early detection.

Transmission of Pain Stimuli

Pain sensations are conducted along pathways that have been rather clearly defined in certain areas but are still somewhat questionable in other areas. There are no specific pain organs or cells in the body. Rather, an interlacing network of undifferentiated free nerve endings receives painful stimuli. Free nerve ending pain receptors include *A delta-fibers*, for fast-conducting, acute, well-localized pain, and *C fibers*, for slow-conducting, diffuse, chronic pain. It is estimated that there are several million of these nerve endings in the body. They are numerous in the layers of the skin and in some internal tissues, such as the joint surfaces. In the deeper tissues of the body, the pain receptors are diffusely but unevenly spread.

Somatic sensation is carried to the dorsal gray horn cells of the spinal cord, then to the spinothalamic tract, and eventually to the cerebral cortex. Although the autonomic nervous system is an *efferent* system—that is, it carries impulses from the central nervous system—pain sensations from the viscera apparently course along the autonomic system. Through that system, these sensations from deep-lying structures reach the spinal cord by way of the dorsal roots and then continue along the same pathways as sensations from the skin and superfi-

Table 41-1
Common Pain Syndromes

Pain Syndrome	Description
Peripheral Pain Syndromes	
Causalgia	Pain occurs in the area of a partially injured peripheral nerve (the most common lesions are of the brachial plexus or median or sciatic nerve). The pain is described as burning, severe, diffuse, and persistent, and occurs most commonly on the palms of the hands, soles of the feet, and in the digits. Hyperalgesia (excessive sensitivity to pain) and hyperesthesia (excessive sensitivity to stimuli) are often so severe that any stimuli (eg, contact with clothing) can trigger the dreaded pain.
Postherpetic neuralgia	Pain syndrome that follows an acute central nervous system infection primarily of the dorsal root ganglia by the varicella zoster (herpes) virus. The herpes syndrome is characterized by a vesicular eruption and neuralgic pain, which is usually unilateral and encircles the body in bandlike clusters. The severity of the pain may be mild to severe and the quality may be burning, sharp, or dull. In the postherpetic syndrome, severe, intractable pain persists for months and years, with episodes of lightning-like pain in the area of the original eruption.
Phantom limb pain	May occur in any person who has had a body part amputated either surgically or traumatically. Pain varies and may be a severe, burning, fiery sensation; crushing; cramping; a sense that the limb is edematous; or a sensation that the limb is being twisted and distorted. It may be triggered by the sensation of touching the stump, the occurrence of another illness, fatigue, atmospheric changes, and emotional stress.
Central Pain Syndromes	
Thalamic syndrome	Syndrome characterized by severe, spontaneous, and often continuous pain and hyperesthesia on the contralateral side of the lesion in the thalamus. This pain syndrome is often accompanied by a myriad of symptoms resulting from a disturbance in the major relay function of the thalamus.
Trigeminal neuralgia	Paroxysms of lightning-like stabs of intense pain in the distribution of one or more divisions of the trigeminal nerve, the fifth cranial nerve. Pain is usually experienced in the mouth, gums, lips, nose, cheek, chin, and surface of the head, and may be triggered by everyday activities like talking, eating, shaving, or brushing one's teeth. Serious consequences of this syndrome are dehydration, wasting, and exhaustion because clients will refrain from anything that triggers the pain.
Pain With Underlying Pathology Syndromes	
Musculoskeletal pain syndromes	Many conditions are capable of causing severe pain in the musculoskeletal structures—the bones, joints, cartilage, synovial membranes, fibrous sheath, muscles, and tendons. Clients may present with pain that is acute or chronic and local or referred, and that varies in intensity.
Myofascial pain syndrome	Pain in the muscles and fascia; these syndromes are among the most frequent causes of severe, disabling pain; characterized by the presence of trigger points in muscles or connective tissue together with a specific syndrome of pain: muscle spasm, tenderness, stiffness, limitation of motion, weakness, and occasionally autonomic dysfunction. Pain is described as dull and aching and its intensity varies from mild to severe and disabling.
Intervertebral disc syndrome	Pain syndrome caused by ruptured, herniated, or prolapsed intervertebral discs; most often occurs in the lower back or cervical area. Pain and limitation are the most frequent symptoms.
Arthritis	Chronic, systemic, often painful disease of connective tissue; one of the major disabling chronic diseases in North America. Rheumatoid arthritis (joint and muscle involvement) is characterized by pain, inflammation, swelling, tenderness, and stiffness in the involved joints. In contrast, osteoarthritis occurs primarily in weight-bearing joints and is benign and slowly progressive.
Headache	The most common type of deep, somatic pain; experienced by about 90% of the population in some form or another. Headaches have multiple intracranial and extracranial causes. A careful analysis of the quality of the pain (dull, deep aching; sharp, throbbing; pressure, tightness); its location; its onset, duration, frequency, and time course; and prodromal signs and symptoms is important in accurately diagnosing the headache.
Cancer pain syndrome	Pain syndromes in cancer patients may develop due to the progression of the disease, as a result of the therapy directed at the control or cure of the disease, or unrelated to the disease.

All of these pain syndromes are capable of causing severe pain.

(Adapted from Meinhart, N.T., & McCaffery, M. [1983]. *Pain: A nursing approach to assessment and analysis.* Norwalk, CT: Appleton-Century-Crofts.)

cial body structures. Pain impulses are also carried by the cranial nerve to the central nervous system. There is integration of the sensory impulses of pain along its entire central nervous system route, but the highest level of integration occurs in the cortex. Figure 41-1 illustrates the transmission of the pain sensation and the initiation of response.

Referred pain is transmitted to a cutaneous (skin) site different from where it originated. This is possible because *afferent neurons,* or those carrying impulses from the pain receptors toward the brain, enter the spinal cord at the same level as the cutaneous site to which the pain has been referred. Figure 41-2 illustrates cutaneous areas to which pain from various organs is usually referred.

Stimulation of sensory receptors and intactness of their nerve supply are neither necessary nor sufficient conditions for pain. It would seem that a receptor for pain and a nerve route that eventually carries the impulse to the brain are necessary when pain is present, yet it is well-known that this is not always necessary. The pain that is often referred to an amputated leg where receptors and nerves are clearly absent is a real experience for the client. This type of pain is called **phantom pain** or phantom limb pain and is without demonstrated physiologic or pathologic substance.

Gate Control Theory of Pain. The **gate control theory** of pain is related to the transmission of painful stimuli and recognizes a relation between pain and emotions.

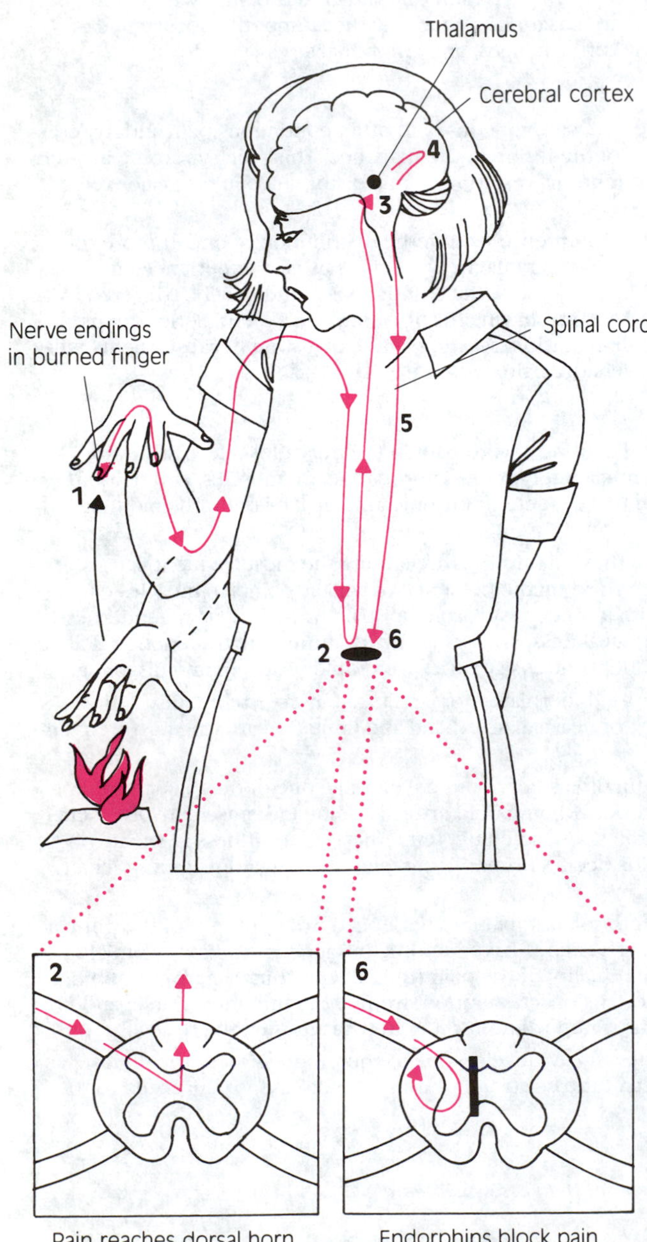

Figure 41-1
Pain sensation and relief. (1) Pain's path begins as a message is received by nerve endings in a burned finger. Potent chemicals (substance P, bradykinin, prostaglandins) are released, sensitizing the nerve endings, helping to transmit the pain message from the injured finger toward the brain, and setting the stage for healing (inflammatory response). (2) The pain signal from the burned finger travels as an electrochemical impulse along the length of the nerve to the dorsal horn on the spinal cord (a region that runs the length of the spine and receives signals from all over the body). (3) The message is relayed to the thalamus, a sensory center in the brain where sensations like heat, cold, pain, and touch first become conscious. (4) It then travels on to the cortex, where the intensity and location of pain are perceived. Little is known about factors that influence the individual's perception of pain at this point, the meaning attributed to the pain, and the voluntary responses elicited. (5) Pain relief begins as a signal from the brain descends by way of the spinal cord. (6) In the dorsal horn, chemicals like endorphin S are released to diminish the pain message from the injured finger. (Adapted from Unlocking pain's secrets. [1984, June 11]. *Time,* pp. 58–66.)

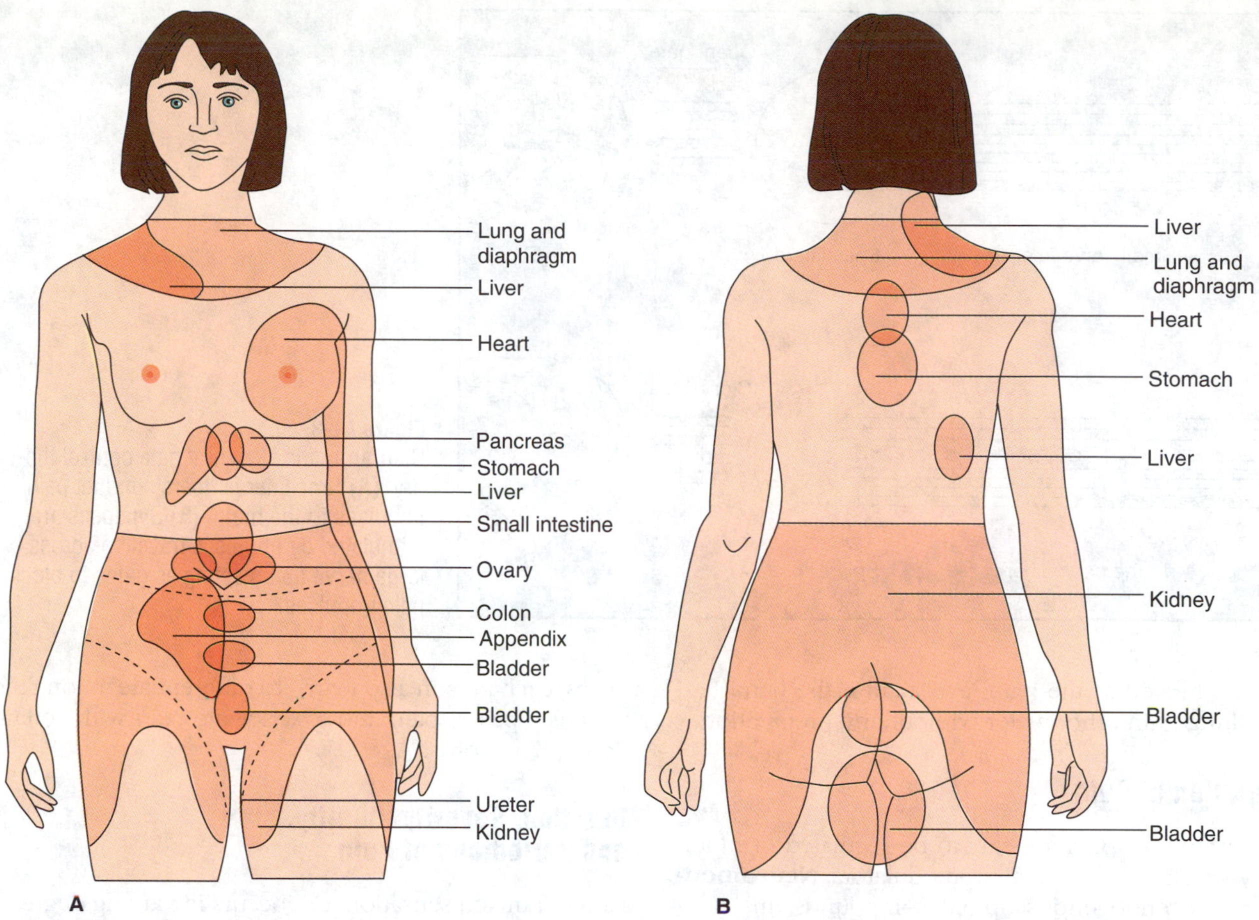

Figure 41-2
These drawings representing the anterior **(A)** and posterior **(B)** views of the body illustrate areas to which various organs refer pain.

The theory states that certain nerve fibers, those of small diameter, conduct excitatory pain stimuli toward the brain, but nerve fibers of a large diameter appear to inhibit the transmission of pain impulses from the spinal cord to the brain. There is a gating mechanism that is believed by some to be located in substantia gelatinosa cells in the dorsal horn of the spinal cord. The exciting and inhibiting signals at the gate in the spinal cord determine the impulses that eventually reach the brain. Thus, only a limited amount of sensory information can be processed by the nervous system at any given moment. When too much information is sent through, certain cells in the spinal column interrupt the signal as if closing a gate. The brain also appears to influence the gating mechanism. Past experiences and learned behaviors, which are interpreted by the brain, have the effect of regulating or adjusting the eventual behavioral responses to pain. This helps explain why similar painful stimuli are interpreted differently by different people. Although not everyone accepts the gate control theory, it appears to explain why mechanical and electrical interventions or heat and pressure may effectively relieve pain. Nursing measures such as a massage or a warm compress to a painful lower back area stimulate large nerve fibers to close the gate, thus blocking pain impulses from that area. Figure 41-3 outlines the gate control theory of pain.

Perception of Pain

The perception of pain involves the sensory process when a stimulus for pain is present. It includes the person's interpretation of the pain. The threshold of perception is the lowest intensity of a stimulus that causes the subject to recognize pain. This threshold is remarkably similar for everyone. Still, it is theorized by at least some authorities that the phenomenon of adaptation does occur; that is, the **pain threshold** can be changed within certain ranges. This phenomenon has been studied, for example, when prisoners of war reported that the pain of repeated torture was not as acute as it would have been under different circumstances. Many factors might well have played a role, but at least some adaptation appears likely.

Adaptation may also be present when a person's hand is immersed in warm water. A sensation of pain eventually occurs as the water is heated. However, the person can tolerate a higher temperature as water is

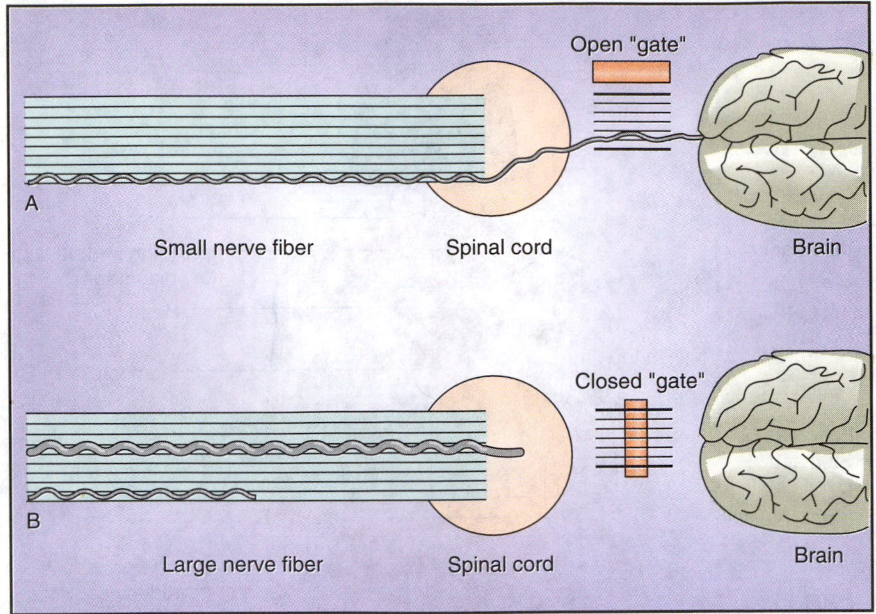

Figure 41-3
Diagrammatic sketch of gate control theory. **(A)** Small nerve fibers conduct pain impulses to the brain. **(B)** Synapses are stimulated by impulses traveling across large nerve fibers acting as gates to block pain impulses.

gradually heated to the pain level than if the hand had been plunged into hot water without any preparation.

Modulation of Pain

The sensation of pain appears to be regulated or modified by substances called neuromodulators. **Neuromodulators** are endogenous opioid compounds, meaning they are naturally present, morphinelike chemical regulators that are found in the spinal cord and brain. They appear to have analgesic activity and alter the perception of pain. It is believed that these endogenous opioid compounds produce their analgesic effects by binding to specific opioid receptor sites throughout the central nervous system and blocking release or production of pain transmitting substances. Both pain and stress seem capable of activating the endogenous opiate system.

Endorphins and enkephalins are opioid neuromodulators. **Endorphins** are produced at neural synapses at various points in the central nervous system pathway. They are powerful pain-blocking chemicals that have prolonged analgesic effects and produce euphoria. It is suggested that endorphins may be released when certain measures are used to relieve pain, such as skin stimulation and relaxation techniques, and when certain pain-relieving drugs are used. Many questions remain about endorphins. **Enkephalins,** which are widespread throughout the brain and dorsal horn of the spinal cord, are considered less potent than endorphins. It is believed that enkephalins reduce pain sensation by inhibiting the release of substance P from the terminals of afferent neurons.

Pain is a highly personal experience. A person learns to know what causes unpleasantness and what to interpret as pain. Each person's interpretation is influenced by background, such as how he or she has experienced and dealt with pain in the past and what cultural factors have taught about pain. Through past experiences, each person also learns to differentiate among the various types of pain and to associate pain with certain descriptive words.

Duration, Severity, Quality, and Periodicity of Pain

Pain is a mixed sensation and occurs in varying degrees. It is also associated with other sensations, such as the sensations of stretching, pulling, pressure, squeezing, heat, or cold. Terms commonly used to describe the duration, severity, quality, and periodicity of pain are listed in Table 41-2. Usually, the more intense the stimulation, the more likely it will produce pain and the more likely the pain will be severe. For example, there normally is pressure from a cast on the body part to which it has been applied but the sensation of the pressure is not painful. However, if there is abnormal swelling of the body part within the cast, the pressure may exceed the pain threshold and be perceived as pain. Pain perception is sharply increased if tissue injury results from unrelieved cast pressure.

Responses to Pain

The three types of responses to pain are physiologic, behavioral, and affective. These responses are summarized in Table 41-3.

The severity of pain and its duration affect responses to pain. Mild pain experienced briefly may produce little or no behavioral responses, whereas intense pain experienced briefly usually results in reflex action to escape the cause. Pain that continues for a relatively short time, such as for a few days or a week, is often accepted by the client without its being all-consuming. The client expects relief and believes the cause is self-limiting. However, anxiety is ordinarily present. On the other hand, chronic pain tends to consume the entire person.

Table 41-2
Terms Used to Describe the Duration, Severity, Quality, and Periodicity of Pain

Duration	
Acute	An episode that lasts for seconds to fewer than about 6 months
Chronic	An episode of pain that lasts for 6 months or longer. The pain may be intermittent or continuous.
Quality	
Sharp	Pain that is sticking in nature and that is intense
Dull	Pain that is not as intense or acute as sharp pain, possibly more annoying than painful. It is usually more diffuse than sharp pain.
Diffuse	Pain that covers a large area. Usually the client is unable to point to a specific area without moving the hand over a large surface, such as the entire abdomen.
Shifting	Pain that moves from one area to another, such as from the lower abdomen to the area over the stomach.
Other terms used to describe the quality of pain include sore, stinging, pinching, cramping, gnawing, cutting, throbbing, shooting, viselike pressure.	
Severity	
Severe or excruciating Moderate Slight or mild	These terms depend on the client's interpretation of pain. Behavioral and physiologic signs help assess the severity of pain. On a scale of 1 to 10, slight pain could be described as being between about 1 and 3; moderate pain, between about 4 and 7; and severe pain, between about 8 and 10.
Periodicity	
Continuous	Pain that does not stop
Intermittent	Pain that stops and starts again
Brief or transient	Pain that passes quickly

It demands total attention so that the client has limited resources to take care of other matters of daily living. It is physically and emotionally exhausting and tends to result in depression and irritability. Chronic fatigue usually accompanies chronic pain.

Lack of an obvious response to pain does not mean the client is without pain. Careful assessment is especially important to understand what the client is experiencing.

Acute Versus Chronic Pain

Pain is classified in many ways. Perhaps the most common distinction is between acute and chronic pain. **Acute pain** is generally rapid in onset, varies in intensity from mild to severe, and may last from a brief period up to any period less than 6 months. Acute pain is protective in nature, that is, it warns the individual of tissue damage or organic disease. Once its underlying cause is resolved, acute pain disappears. Causes of acute pain include a pricked finger, sore throat, or surgery.

Chronic pain is pain that may be limited, intermittent, or persistent, but that lasts for 6 months or longer and interferes with normal functioning. Pain associated with cancer or other progressive disorders is termed *chronic malignant pain* and pain in people whose tissue injury is nonprogressive or healed is termed *chronic nonmalignant pain.* When pain is resistant to therapy and persists despite a variety of interventions, it is referred to as **intractable.** Clients have difficulty describing chronic pain because it may be poorly localized and healthcare personnel have difficulty assessing it accurately due to the unique responses of individual clients to persistent pain. Most pain researchers agree that one fourth of the population may have persistent or recurrent chronic pain and many of these individuals are over 65 years of age (Ignatavicius, Workman, & Mishler, 1995). According to Ferrell, Ferrell, and Osterweil (1990), about 70% of elder clients residing in nursing homes have significant pain and one third of these are in constant pain. Unlike acute pain, chronic pain is often perceived as meaningless and may lead its host to withdrawal, depression, anger, frustration, and dependency.

Management of clients with chronic pain can be adversely affected by the misconceptions and personal biases of caregivers. Individuals with chronic pain may be viewed in general by healthcare personnel as hysterical personalities, malingerers, or hypochondriacs. On the other hand, nurses who have experienced chronic pain or struggled through the experience with a loved one have a special awareness of its debilitating, destructive nature. McCaffery and Ferrell (1992) summarized how gender affects pain control and reported that nurses may be more sensitive to reports of pain from clients of the same gender. Nurses need an awareness of their own personal feelings toward pain and the factors that affect pain if they are to assess and manage their client's pain creatively and effectively.

Factors Affecting the Pain Experience

Many factors influence the comfort status of a person at any given moment. When an individual experiences pain, almost anything can influence how the painful stimulus is transmitted to the brain, how it is perceived, and the response that is made to it.

Culture

Because cultural norms dictate much of our daily behavior, attitudes, and values, it is natural to assume that culture influences the individual's response to pain. It is important for nurses to understand that there are ways other than their own of responding to pain. Nurses, as a subculture, value self-control and the ability to function under stress and may expect clients in pain to display a

Table 41-3
Common Responses to Pain

Response	Comments
Behavioral (Voluntary) Responses	
Moving away from painful stimuli	The person moves self or a part of the body away from the source of pain. It is one of the body's protective mechanisms.
Grimacing, moaning, and crying	These responses are normal in many cultures when they are in keeping with the amount of pain the client experiences.
Restlessness	Restlessness keeps the person alert and probably also serves as a distraction from pain (eg, pacing the floor).
Protecting the painful area and refusing to move	The person assumes a posture to protect the painful area, such as holding a painful hand or drawing the knees up when abdominal pain is present. The client may assume a posture and then refuse to move.
Physiologic (Involuntary) Responses	
Typical Sympathetic Responses When Pain Is Moderate and Superficial Increased blood pressure Increased pulse and respiratory rates Pupil dilation Muscle tension and rigidity Pallor (peripheral vasoconstriction) Increased adrenalin output Increased blood glucose	These signs are the body's responses to promote homeostasis; the body is preparing for emergency action, or the fight-or-flight phenomenon, as described in Chapter 32.
Typical Parasympathetic Responses When Pain Is Severe and Deep Nausea and vomiting Fainting or unconsciousness Decreased blood pressure Decreased pulse rate Prostration Rapid and irregular breathing	The body shows signs of being unable to cope with the stressor of pain.
Affective (Psychologic) Responses	
Exaggerated weeping and restlessness Withdrawal Stoicism Anxiety Depression Fear Anger Anorexia Fatigue Hopelessness Powerlessness	A person's previous experience with pain and sociocultural background play an important role in the emotional responses to pain. Emotional responses differ according to whether pain is acute or chronic. Anxiety is most often associated with acute pain and is frequently present when pain is anticipated. Depression is most often associated with chronic pain. Emotional responses tend to intensify the reactions to pain, causing a vicious cycle that may be difficult to break. Emotional responses help explain why some people experience pain that seems to be without physiologic cause or why some tend to complain of pain more than others when circumstances are similar. Pain is real as reported by the person, but for some, pain may help relieve feelings of guilt or serve as a way to gain attention and relieve loneliness.

similarly calm, objective, uncomplaining approach to pain (Andrews & Boyle, 1995). It is particularly important to avoid stereotyping responses to pain since the nurse frequently encounters clients who are in pain or anticipating that it will develop. A form of pain expression that is frowned on in one culture may be desirable in another cultural group. The nurse studies cultural variations to develop an understanding of cultural influences on pain tolerance, expressions of pain, and alternative practices used to manage pain.

Ethnic Variables. Much research has been done on cultural influences on pain. The classic study on behavioral responses to pain present in groups of people of similar ethnic origin was done by Zborowski (1969). He studied males in four cultural groups—Old American (American-born, white, Protestant, and without identification with any foreign group), Jewish, Italian, and Irish. A summary of his findings follows.

Old American. A man of this background describes his pain efficiently to healthcare practitioners, minimizes his pain when with family and friends, carefully controls his expression of pain, and tends to withdraw when his pain is severe—he wants to be alone. The Old American finds little value in pain and expects to have it relieved.

Jewish. A man of Jewish background tends to be more vocal about his pain and uses pain to elicit sympathy and support from others. Like the Old American, he is future oriented and concerned with the significance of his pain but he is less confident that modern medicine can cure the cause of the pain. He often seeks the advice of several physicians, including specialists.

Italian. The Italian man finds it natural to respond to pain with cries, moans, complaints, gestures, and body movements. Unlike the Old American and Jewish men, the Italian man is oriented to the present and is concerned with the sensation of pain itself rather than with its significance. The Italian wants quick pain relief and willingly accepts pain-relief measures.

Irish. Like the Old American, the Irish man is calm and unemotional about pain, believing that complaining serves no purpose; he wants to be alone with his pain. He takes pride in his ability to handle pain, generally using two strategies—relaxing and fighting. The Irish male may struggle with his pain for a long time before consulting a physician.

Other. The nurse working with other ethnic groups can find pertinent studies in the literature. Additional information on cultural influences on pain can be found in Chapter 3.

Family, Gender, and Age Variables. Variables related to culture are family, gender, and age. Snelling (1990) studied the role of the family in relation to chronic pain and reported the following:

- There is a tendency for individuals with chronic pain to come from families that include a member suffering from pain.
- Spouses may reinforce pain behavior in their partners.
- Family size and birth order are not significant in distinguishing chronic pain sufferers.

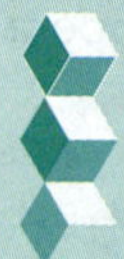

Research in Nursing: Making a Difference

Comfort

The relief of pain has long been a subject of study. Pain is a physical response to malfunction of an organism but can also occur in the absence of an organic cause. Individual responses to pain, whether acute or chronic, are unique, and effective nursing measures to relieve pain are varied. Nursing research continues to explore interventions that promote comfort, communicate empathy, and reduce the helplessness that clients in pain frequently experience.

Related Research

Ryan, P., Vortherns, R., & Ward, S. (1994). Cancer pain: Knowledge, attitudes of pharmacologic management. *Journal of Gerontological Nursing, 20*(1), 7–13.
This study compared responses from oncology nurses and long-term care facility (LTCF) nurses to determine impediments to effective pain management. Both groups agreed that clients with cancer pain are frequently undermedicated but LTCF nurses were more likely to believe that clients overexaggerate their pain. Although oncology nurses indicated more knowledge about pharmacologic measures, LTCF nurses expressed willingness to expand their knowledge base and improve their pain assessment skills as preparation for assuming a leadership role in pain management in their institutions.

Vallerand, A. (1995). Gender differences in pain. *Image: Journal of Nursing Scholarship, 27*(3), 235–237.
This author reviewed research about pain in women and suggested implications for clinical practice. Even though research findings indicate there is no difference in how men and women experience pain, it is treated less aggressively when present in women. Women may be more likely to communicate the presence of pain but men receive opioid analgesics more frequently as treatment for pain. Nurses need to be aware that pain in women may be inadequately managed and rely on individualized assessments to develop a plan of care for pain relief.

Sloman, R. (1995). Relaxation and the relief of cancer pain. *Nursing Clinics of North America, 30*(4), 669–709.
This study suggests that guided imagery combined with progressive muscle relaxation has the potential to aid in relief of cancer pain. These techniques are easy to learn and can be taught by nurses in all settings. Teaching these strategies provides the client with the ability to take partial control over his or her pain by promoting a relaxation response.

Summary

These studies demonstrate several implications for clinical nursing practice. Pain relief is more effective when nurses expand their pain assessment skills, address the impact of gender on pain control, and use additional noninvasive techniques to relieve the anxiety associated with unrelieved pain. It is the responsibility of the nurse to promote maximum well-being for all clients and to accept that pain is a unique and individual response deserving appropriate therapeutic interventions.

Children growing up in different families may quickly learn to ignore pain, to exploit pain as a means to secure the attention and services of family members, or to value pain as a means the body uses to teach important truths. Similarly, children may learn that there are gender differences in pain expression; whereas it may be acceptable for a little girl to run home crying with a scraped knee, a little boy may be told that he should be brave and not cry. Adult men and women may hold onto gender expectations regarding pain communication and incorrectly interpret the presence or absence of pain expressions in others. In addition, different age groups have different beliefs and norms regarding pain sensation and response. At one time, the infant's inability to communicate pain led healthcare practitioners to the erroneous assumption that pain sensation was diminished or absent. It is now generally believed that infants and small children are sensitive to and experience pain.

Among older people, pain has often been viewed as a natural component of the aging process and may be ignored or undertreated by healthcare providers. On the other hand, conditions normally painful in young adults (eg, myocardial infarction) may present minimal pain complaints in older people. That an older person does not complain of pain may indicate that he or she fears the treatment for the pain or just refuses to give in to the pain (AHCPR, 1992). These variables, which influence pain sensation, perception, and response, make pain assessment a complex task for the nurse.

Religious Beliefs

Religious beliefs may powerfully influence the individual's experience of pain. In some religions, individuals view pain and suffering not as good in themselves but as a means of purification or of making up for individual and community sin. This meaning helps the individual to cope with pain and becomes a source of strength. Clients with this belief may refuse analgesics and other pain-relief measures, feeling that this lessens their offering. On the other hand, illness and pain may also be viewed as punishment from a vengeful God. Individuals may find their faith shaken and question the existence of a loving God. How can belief in a loving God be compatible with their present experience of pain? Anger, resentment, and depression may then compound the pain experience. Clients may find it helpful to confer with a spiritual adviser about their pain experience.

Environment and Support People

An individual's environment and the presence or absence of caring support people may also influence the experience of pain. Many people find that the strangeness of the healthcare environment, and especially the lights, noise, and constant activity of a critical care unit, compound the experience of pain. The sense of powerlessness that accompanies admission to an institution may decrease the individual's ability to cope with pain. Depersonalization or separation from a favorite pillow, pet, or source of music may further decrease the person's sense of comfort. For some, the presence of a loved family member or friend is essential to their sense of well-being. Others prefer to be alone when in pain and may become agitated in the presence of a family member.

Some clients may use their pain to acquire secondary gains, such as special attention and services from their families. Because this tendency, if unchecked, usually leads to resentment and anger in family members and their eventual avoidance of the client, the nurse should intervene and attempt an honest discussion of this problem when noting its occurrence.

Anxiety and Other Stressors

Anxiety, which is almost always present when pain is anticipated or being experienced, tends to increase the perceived intensity of pain. The threat of the unknown is ordinarily more devastating and anxiety producing than a threat for which one has been prepared. Studies have indicated that clients who were taught preoperatively about what to expect postoperatively did not require as much medication for pain as those who had similar operative procedures but were not taught preoperatively.

Pain is ordinarily aggravated when anxiety, muscular tension, and fatigue are present. A vicious circle can easily develop when pain interferes with rest and relaxation, and tension and fatigue almost always aggravate the discomfort. The rested and relaxed person can often cope with great discomfort.

The individual who is greatly fatigued and who has no competing demands requiring attention may experience pain acutely. For example, many people have discovered that the pain of a footache or ingrown toenail that was only mildly annoying during the day's work became unbearable at night when there was nothing else to distract the mind from the pain. Similarly, athletes can be so determined to win a game that they are oblivious to the pain of a serious sports injury. After the game, and particularly if the game was lost and the effort seemingly useless, the pain becomes overpowering.

Past Pain Experience

Whether an individual has experienced pain in the past and the qualities of that experience profoundly affect new pain experiences.

- Some clients have never known severe pain and have no fear of pain, not realizing how intense the sensation can be.
- Some clients have experienced severe acute or chronic pain in the past but received immediate and adequate pain relief. These clients are generally unafraid of pain and initiate appropriate requests for assistance.
- Some clients have known severe pain in the past and were unable to secure relief. Even the sug-

gestion of new pain can throw these clients into a frenzy of fear and feelings of despair and hopelessness.

- The individual whose past pain experience led to correction of unhealthy behavior and produced a greater sense of health and well-being may respect and value pain and study the meaning and significance of a new pain carefully.
- In general, people who have experienced more pain than usual in their lifetimes tend to anticipate more pain and to exhibit increased sensitivity to pain.
- Some pain memories are virtually unerasable and new contact with conditions similar to those that caused the earlier pain can provoke a violent response.

The Nurse as Role Model

The nurse who wishes to role model healthy pain management behaviors to clients does the following:

- Balances work and leisure activities to promote optimal personal well-being (consistently communicates to self "I care about you!")
- Respects pain as the body's means of signaling that all is not well
- Treats what is producing pain as opposed to simply trying to eradicate pain
- Uses an effective coping model (pain view and view of self) when responding to personal pain
- Routinely incorporates comfort measures into nursing care
- Practices nursing sensitive to the pain needs of clients and is committed to pain relief:
  - Communicates to clients the belief that their pain experience is real and that help is available
  - Assigns high nursing priority to assisting clients (and family members) to develop effective pain management strategies compatible with their belief systems
  - Designs varied pain management programs that incorporate noninvasive and invasive interventions; works collaboratively with other health professionals
  - Supports pain management programs with attention to the client's overall nutrition, hydration, elimination, rest, activity, and stimulation
- Continuously updates knowledge of pain theories, assessment strategies, and treatment modalities

Use the self-assessment checklist in the accompanying box to monitor your progress in learning to meet comfort needs.

ASSESSING THE PAIN EXPERIENCE

Because the pain experience is unique to each individual, the nurse who wants to understand a client's pain to help the client achieve pain control needs sophisticated pain assessment skills. It is necessary to assess all factors that affect the pain experience—psychologic,

Promoting Wellness

Comfort

Use the assessment checklist to determine how well you are meeting comfort needs. Then develop a prescription for self-care by choosing appropriate behaviors from the list of suggestions.

Assessment Checklist

almost always	sometimes	almost never	
☐	☐	☐	1. I seek medical attention when pain persists.
☐	☐	☐	2. I am aware of my usual behavioral responses to pain.
☐	☐	☐	3. I use stress reduction techniques regularly.
☐	☐	☐	4. I am able to have a restful sleep at night
☐	☐	☐	5. I have a positive outlook about my present situation.
☐	☐	☐	6. I am aware of how to use distraction strategies to deal with pain

Self-Care Behaviors

1. Obtain a medical evaluation when acute or chronic pain is present.
2. Control stress in the environment.
3. Avoid excessive fatigue.
4. Practice stress reduction or diversionary behaviors when pain is present.
5. Become aware of personal preconceived notions that affect your perception of pain in others.

emotional, and sociocultural as well as physiologic. Pain is complex and difficult to interpret and requires a reliable assessment tool.

Misconceptions

Many client misconceptions interfere with the client's ability to communicate pain:

- The nurse will know when I am in pain and will do something to relieve it if possible.
- The doctor has ordered pain-relieving medication for me, which I will be given routinely.
- If I ask for something for my pain, I may become addicted to the medication.
- Sometimes it's better to put up with the pain than to deal with the side-effects of the pain medication.
- I should somehow be able to control my pain. It is immature to talk about pain.
- It is better to wait until the pain gets really bad before asking for help. If I take the medication now for moderate pain, it won't relieve severe pain later on.
- I don't want to bother anyone—I know how busy they are.
- It's natural to have pain as you get older. It's just something I've learned to live with.
- It's natural for me to have pain after surgery. After a few days, I should notice it lessening.

Misconceptions and prejudices about pain and pain relief that hamper the nurse's assessment of the client with pain have been summarized by McCaffery and Beebe (1989) and are presented in Table 41-4.

Table 41-4
Misconceptions About Assessment of Patients Who Indicate They Have Pain

Misconception	Correction
The health team is the authority about the existence and nature of client's pain sensation.	The person with pain is the only authority about the existence and nature of that pain, because the sensation of pain can be felt only by the person who has it.
Our personal values and intuition about the trustworthiness of others is a valuable tool in identifying whether a person is lying about pain.	Personal values and intuition do not constitute a professional approach to the patient with pain. The client's credibility is not on trial.
Pain is largely an emotional or psychologic problem, especially in the patient who is highly anxious or depressed.	Having an emotional reaction to pain does not mean that pain is caused by an emotional problem. If anxiety or depression is alleviated, the intensity of pain will not necessarily be any less.
Lying about the existence of pain, malingering, is common.	Few people who say they have pain are lying about it. Outright fabrication of pain is considered rare.
The client who obtains benefits or preferential treatment because of pain is receiving secondary gain and does not hurt as much as he or she says or may not hurt at all.	The client who uses pain to his or her advantage is not the same as a malingerer and may still hurt as much as the client says he or she does. Also, secondary gain may be an inaccurate diagnosis.
All real pain has an identifiable physical cause.	All pain is real, regardless of its cause. Almost all pain has both physical and mental components. Pure psychogenic pain is rare.
Visible signs, either physiologic or behavioral, accompany pain and can be used to verify its existence and severity.	Even with severe pain, periods of physiologic and behavioral adaptation occur, leading to periods of minimal or no signs of pain. Lack of pain expression does not necessarily mean lack of pain. How must the client act for us to believe he or she has pain?
Comparable physical stimuli produce comparable pain in different people. The severity and duration of pain can be predicted accurately for everyone on the basis of the stimuli for pain.	Comparable stimuli in different people do not produce the same intensities of pain. Comparable stimuli in different people will produce different intensities of pain that last different periods. There is no direct and invariant relation between any stimulus and the perception of pain.
People with pain should be taught to have a high tolerance for pain. The more prolonged the pain or the more experience a person has with pain, the better is his or her tolerance for pain.	Pain tolerance is the individual's unique response, varying among clients and varying in the same client from one situation to another. People with prolonged pain tend to have an increasingly low pain tolerance. Respect for the client's pain tolerance is crucial for adequate pain control.
When the client reports pain relief following a placebo, this means that the patient is a malingerer or that the pain is psychogenic.	There is not a shred of evidence anywhere in the literature to justify using a placebo to diagnose malingering or psychogenic pain.

(McCaffery, M., & Beebe, A. [1989]. *Pain: Clinical manual for nursing practice.* St. Louis: Mosby.)

Components of Pain Assessment

Various forms used to help guide the assessment of pain have been described in the nursing literature. The primary purposes of using a guide to assess pain are to eliminate guesswork and biases when dealing with the client's pain, to understand what the person is experiencing, and to analyze findings that will help prepare an appropriate nursing response to the client's pain.

Characteristics of pain generally assessed include the following:

- The client's verbalization and description of the pain
- Duration of the pain
- The location of the pain
- The quantity and intensity of the pain
- The quality of the pain
- Chronology of the pain
- Aggravating factors
- Physiologic indicators of pain
- Behavioral responses
- The effect of the pain experience on activities and life-style.

Gordon and Ward (1995) suggest that a comprehensive pain assessment must also include discussion of the client's expectations for pain relief. The client and healthcare team need to select a realistic goal or numerical number on the pain scale that is acceptable and facilitates recovery. This helps the client recognize and report pain that is unacceptable and also allows caregivers to evaluate more readily the effectiveness of their pain management techniques. See the accompanying box that suggests questions or approaches helpful in assessing the various pain factors.

Pain centers commonly ask clients to complete a self-questionnaire. The McGill-Melzack Pain Questionnaire is an example of such a questionnaire and requires that an individual check words that fit the description of the pain experience. Marks on a body figure also designate the location of the pain. Comparison of changes on subsequent questionnaires aid in determining an individual's improvement or regression. This comprehensive pain assessment is time-consuming and should be performed when the client is more comfortable and better able to respond to questions. The AHCPR (1994) in their clinical practice guideline suggests use of an initial pain assessment tool (see Fig. 41-4) which is brief and easily administered. For continual assessment of pain and evaluation of pain control measures, a pain scale allows the client to rate effectively the pain he or she is experiencing on a continual basis. Figure 41-5 displays an example of several pain intensity rating scales.

Nurses working in a hospice setting created a Pain Intensity Flow Sheet (PIFS) for a more objective evaluation of their clients' pain. They developed a pain rating scale of 0 to 5 that also includes the client's report of the nature and location of the pain, medication that relieves the pain, time of day when the pain usually worsens, and the level of pain they are willing to accept. Staff on each shift document the client's pain rating on a flow sheet in addition to their observations of the client's mental status and level of awareness. This ongoing graphic recording of pain intensity facilitates communication between staff and is also used by the agency's quality improvement committee as documented proof of effective pain management (Kohr, 1995). Figure 41-6 is a sample of a portion of the PIFS.

Assessment in the Cognitively Impaired Client. Assessment of pain in people who are cognitively impaired presents special challenges to nurses. It currently is generally recognized that cognitively impaired individuals are frequently undertreated because they may be unable to report pain verbally or express concepts such as pain magnitude. Special efforts are needed to identify accurate means of assessing their pain. Marzinski (1991) conducted pain assessments on an Alzheimer's unit in a nursing home and expressed concern about the lack of an operational definition of pain and reliable assessment tools for use with this population. Although these tools are being developed, to manage pain effectively, nurses must rely on their own careful assessments, their empathetic qualities, and the expectation that a client will experience pain if a verbal client usually reports this event as painful.

Assessment in a Child. In recent years, healthcare personnel have become more concerned about children and their response to pain. It was formerly believed that young children lacked the neurologic development to sense pain the way adults do and pain relief was not a priority when children were hospitalized. Young children frequently received no treatment for pain during entire hospital stays. New methods of assessing and measuring children's pain frequently involve use of more than one technique for assessment. A pain history provides information about the language the child uses to indicate pain, how and to whom this pain is usually reported, and indications of previous pain experiences and coping strategies. Self-report is usually the most reliable account of pain but observation of facial expressions, body positions, and whether children cry as well as physiologic responses also provide additional information. Communication with parents, guardians, or other important family members is vital for accurate pediatric pain assessment and management. One commonly used pain assessment scale asks children to compare their pain to a series of faces ranging from a broad smile to a tearful grimace. (Fig. 41-7 is an example of a pediatric pain assessment scale.) Children may also be asked to record their pain experiences in a daily diary. Detecting and accurately assessing pediatric pain has resulted in new and innovative approaches toward pain control in children.

Assessment in the Older Client. Because many older people have chronic disease, pain is a prevalent occurrence. Visual or hearing impairments may influence the assessment format. Multiple drug regimens that are common in older people can also affect reliable reporting of

(text continues on page 1119)

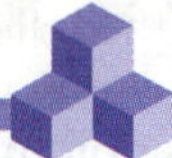

Focused Assessment Guide

The Pain Experience

Factors to Assess	Questions and Approaches
Characteristics of the pain	
Location	"Where is your pain? Is it external or internal?" (Asking the client with acute pain to point to the painful area with one finger may help to localize the pain. Clients with chronic pain may have difficulty trying to localize their pain, however.)
Duration	"How long have you been experiencing pain? How long does a pain episode last? How often does a pain episode occur?"
Quantity	Ask the client to indicate the degree (amount) of pain currently experienced on the scale below: 0 No pain — 1 — 2 Mild — 3 — 4 Moderate — 5 — 6 — 7 Severe — 8 — 9 — 10 Pain as bad as it can be It is also helpful to ask how much pain the client has (on the same scale) when the pain is at its least and at its worst: Least ________ Worst ________
Quality	"What words would you use to describe your pain?" (Useful in research, this characteristic is least useful in day-to-day clinical practice.)
Chronology	"How does the pain develop and progress?" (If pattern can be identified, interventions early in a pain sequence will often be far more effective than those used after the pain is well established.) "Has the pain changed since it first began? If so, how?"
Aggravating factors	"What makes the pain occur or increase in intensity?"
Alleviating factors	"What makes the pain go away or lessen? What methods of relief have you tried in the past? How long were they used? How effective were they?" (Methods of relief currently in effect for hospitalized clients should be apparent from the chart. It is important to verify the use of current orders and their effectiveness with the client. Outpatients may need to be asked to record a medication profile, a thorough and accurate account of all medications they are taking.)
Associated phenomena	"Are there any other factors that seem to relate consistently to your pain? Any other symptoms that occur just before, during, or after your pain?"
Physiologic responses Vital signs (blood pressure, pulse, respirations) Skin color Perspiration Pupil size Nausea	Signs of sympathetic stimulation commonly occur with acute pain. Signs of parasympathetic stimulation (decreased blood pressure and pulse, rapid and irregular respirations, pupil constriction, nausea and vomiting, and warm, dry skin) may be present, especially in prolonged, severe pain, visceral, or deep pain.
Muscle tension	Observe. Ask the client if he or she is aware of any tight, tense muscles.
Anxiety	Are signs of anxiety evident? (May include decreased attention span or ability to follow directions, frequent asking of questions, shifting of topics of conversation, avoidance of discussion of feelings, acting out, somatizing.)

(continued)

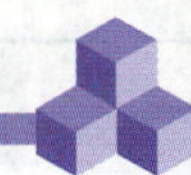

Focused Assessment Guide *(continued)*

The Pain Experience

Factors to Assess	Questions and Approaches
Behavioral responses	
Posture, gross motor activities	Does client rub or support a particular area? Make frequent position changes? Walk, pace, kneel, or assume a rolled-up position? Does client rest a particular body part? Protect an area from stimulation? Lie quietly? (In acute pain, postural and gross motor activities are often altered; in chronic pain, the only signs of change may be postures characteristic of withdrawal.)
Facial features	Does the client have a pinched look? Are there facial grimaces? Knotted brow? Overall taut, anxious appearance? (A look of fatigue is more characteristic of chronic pain.)
Verbal expressions	Does the client sigh, moan, scream, cry, repetitively use the same words?
Affective responses	
Anxiety	"Do you feel anxious? Are you afraid? If so, how bad are these feelings?"
Depression	"Do you feel depressed, down, or low? If so, how bad are these feelings? Are your feelings about yourself mostly good or bad? Do you have feelings of failure? Do you see yourself or your illness as a burden to those you care about?"
Interactions with others	How does the client act when he or she is in pain in the presence of others? How does the client respond to others when he or she is not in pain? How do significant others and caregivers respond to the client when the client is in pain? When the client is not in pain?
Degree to which pain interferes with client's life (use past performance as baseline)	"Does the pain interfere with sleep? If so, to what extent? Is fatigue a major factor in the pain experience? Is the conduct of intimate or peer relationships affected by the pain? Is work function affected? Participation in recreational-diversional activities?" (An activity diary is often helpful—sometimes crucial. One to several weeks of hourly activity recorded by the client may be necessary. Levels of pain, intake of food, and sleep-rest periods are noted along with activities performed. Separate diaries for inpatient and outpatient episodes may be necessary, because hospitalization markedly affects the nature and type of activities performed.)
Perception of pain and meaning to client	"Are you worried about your illness? Do you see any connection between your pain and the nature or course of illness? If so, how do you see them as related? Do you find any meaning in your pain? If so, is this beneficial or detrimental to you? Are you struggling to find some meaning for your pain?"
Adaptive mechanisms used to cope with pain	"What do you usually do to relieve stress? How well do these things work? What techniques do you use at home to help cope with the pain? How well have they worked? Do you use these in the hospital? If not, why not?"
Goals	"What would you like to be doing right now, this week, this month, if the pain were better controlled? How much would the pain have to decrease (on the 0 to 10 scale) for you to begin to accomplish these goals?"

(Adapted from Donovan, M.I., & Girton, S.E. [1984]. *Cancer care nursing* [2nd ed.]. Norwalk, CT: Appleton-Century-Crofts.)

Initial Pain Assessment Tool

Date ______

Patient's name ______ Age ______ Room ______

Diagnosis ______ Physician ______

Nurse ______

I. Location: Patient or nurse marks drawing.

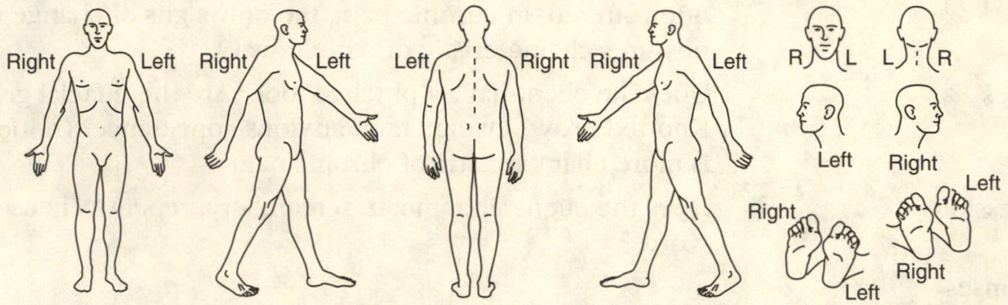

Right Left Right Left Left Right Right Left R L L R Left Right Left Right Right Left

Intensity: Patient rates the pain. Scale used ______

Present: ______

Worst pain gets: ______

Best pain gets: ______

Acceptable level of pain: ______

III.Quality: (Use patients's own words, e.g., prick, ache, burn, throb, pull, sharp)

IV. Onset, duration, variation, rhythms:

V. Manner of expressing pain: ______

VI. What relieves the pain? ______

VII. What causes or increases the pain? ______

VIII. Effects of pain: (Note decreased function, decreased quality of life.)

Accompanying symptoms (e.g., nausea) ______

Sleep ______

Appetite ______

Physical activity ______

Relationship with others (e.g., irritability) ______

Emotions (e.g., anger, suicidal, crying) ______

Concentration ______

Other ______

IX. Other comments ______

X. Plan: ______

Figure 41-4
Sample of an initial pain assessment tool. (McCaffery, M., Beebe, A., [1989]. *Pain: Clinical manual for nursing practice,* St. Louis: Mosby.)

Pain Distress Scales

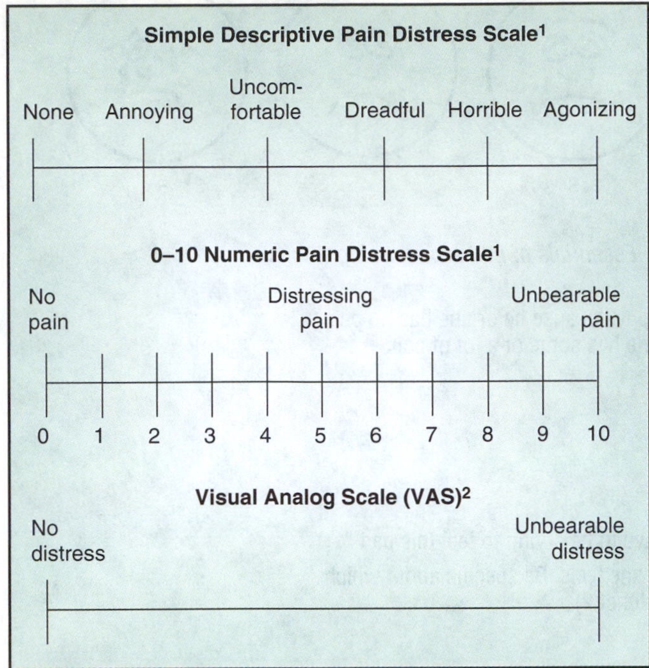

[1] If used as a graphic rating scale, a 10 cm baseline is recommended.
[2] A 10-cm baseline is recommended for VAS scales.

Figure 41-5
Pain distress scales. (AHCPR, Acute Pain Management Guide Panel, 1992.)

pain. The AHCPR guidelines for management of acute and chronic pain (1992, 1994) summarize reasons why pain assessment is more complex in older people:

- There is a common belief that pain is an expected outcome of aging.
- Some caregivers mistakenly believe that older clients have a decreased sensitivity to pain and heightened pain tolerance.
- There is a fear among older clients that the admission of pain may limit independence.
- Pain is frequently considered an ominous sign—a forecast of serious illness or death.
- Terminology describing pain may vary significantly.
- The expression and interpretation of pain varies according to culture or ethnic group.
- Changing patterns or presentations of pain have been observed in older people.
- Boredom, loneliness, and depression may affect an older person's perception and report of pain.

Home Healthcare Alert

Caregivers/family members need to be reminded that older adults with chronic pain may be less active, sleep more, or appear confused when pain is unrelieved.

Research by Brockopp et al. (1993), based on responses by practicing nurses and student nurses to a pain questionnaire, supports the need for ongoing education about pain assessment and management for this population. Special attention and consideration of an older client's pain can positively affect the nurse's ability to assess pain accurately.

DIAGNOSING

Pain is such a complex phenomenon that its analysis often requires the collaboration of different members of the health team. Although nursing has much to offer individuals experiencing both acute and chronic pain, the data collected by the nurse during the comprehensive pain assessment will most benefit the client when shared with physicians and other members of the healthcare team.

Attempting to intervene before an accurate assessment has been completed may mask the real cause of the client's pain and lead to false assumptions and even further progression of symptoms and the disease process. The nurse who notes a pattern of headaches in a client and relates this to the client's description of recent stress (divorce, relocation, new job) may erroneously assume that the headaches are merely stress re-

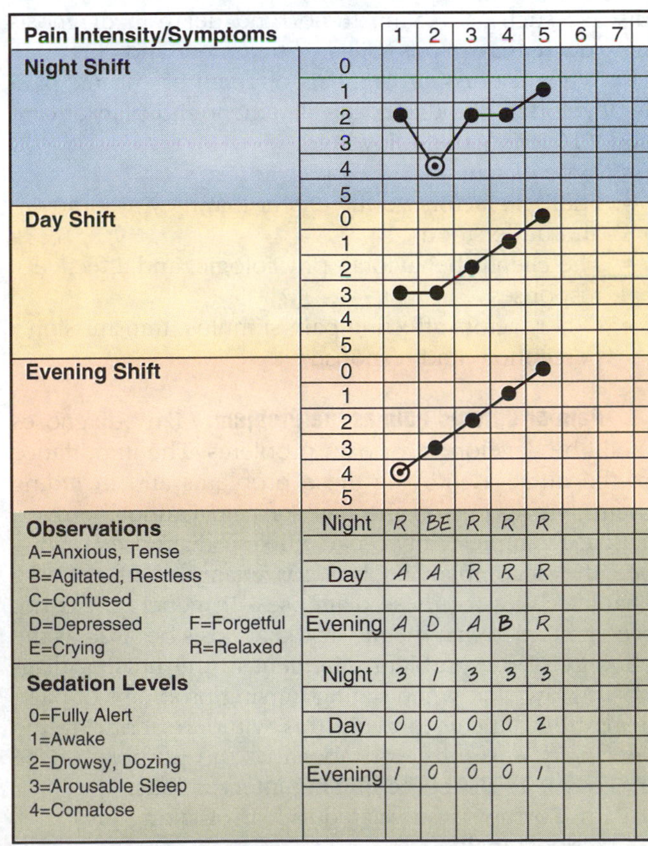

Figure 41-6
Sample of a portion of the pain intensity flow sheet. (Kohr, J. [1995]. Measuring your patient's pain. *RN, 58*(4), 40.)

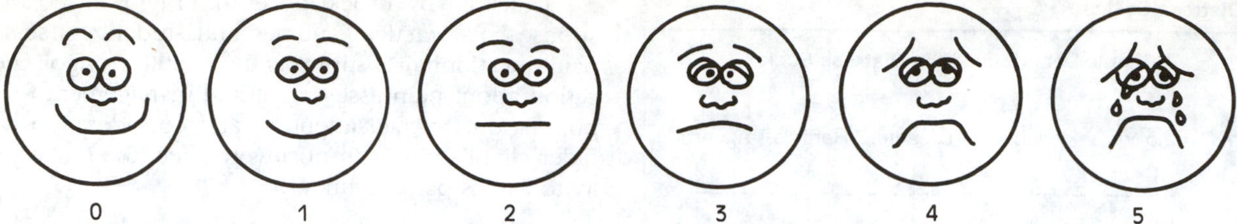

Figure 41-7
Wong/Baker Faces Rating Scale for use with children. (Wong, D. *Essentials of pediatric nursing* [4th ed.]. St. Louis: Mosby.)

1. Explain to the child that each face is for a person who feels happy because he or she has no pain (hurt, or whatever word the child uses) or feels sad because he or she has some or a lot of pain.
2. Point to the appropriate face and state, "This face . . .":
   0—"is very happy because he [or she] doesn't hurt at all."
   1—"hurts just a little bit."
   2—"hurts a little more."
   3—"hurts even more."
   4—"hurts a whole lot."
   5—"hurts as much as you can imagine, although you don't have to be crying to feel this bad."
3. Ask the child to choose the face that best describes how he or she feels. Be specific about which pain (eg, "shot" or incision) and what time (eg, Now? Earlier before lunch?)

lated and devise and implement a plan of relaxation exercises. A more careful analysis of client data, however, may reveal that the headaches are of vascular origin, migraine in nature, and medical intervention is indicated. The headaches may also be symptomatic of intracranial disease such as a brain tumor and delay in diagnosis may decrease the possibility of treatment and cure.

When a nursing diagnosis of acute or chronic pain is developed, the diagnostic statement and plan of care should identify the following:

- Type of pain
- Etiologic factors, to the extent that they are known and understood
- The client's behavioral, physiologic, and affective responses
- Other factors affecting pain stimulus, transmission, perception, and response

Pain or Chronic Pain as the Problem. Many diagnoses could be developed for pain problems. The importance of the nurse identifying these problems and including them as priorities in the plan of care cannot be overstated. Examples of two-part nursing diagnoses follow. See the accompanying box for examples of defining characteristics for these diagnoses. In general, it is not recommended that the medical diagnosis be used as the etiology of the problem statement in the nursing diagnosis. However, when stating nursing problems of pain, it may be difficult to avoid this without sacrificing the specificity desired. Remember that the purpose of the etiology is to direct the nursing interventions.

Pain: Postoperative related to fear of taking prescribed analgesics

Pain related to fractured femur and multiple lacerations and unsuccessful attempts to determine effective analgesic

Pain related to prolonged labor (dystocia) and commitment to natural childbirth

Anxiety related to heightened pain anticipation from child's history of undergoing frequent painful procedures

Pain related to decreased blood supply to myocardium (angina)

Chronic Pain: Headache related to inadequate pain management secondary to belief that client somehow "deserves" this pain

Chronic Pain related to inadequate pain management of metastatic cancer involving bone

Chronic Pain related to rheumatoid arthritis

Pain or Chronic Pain as the Etiology. Because the experience of pain affects so many other aspects of human functioning, pain may be the etiology of numerous other nursing diagnosis statements:

Ineffective Airway Clearance related to postoperative incisional pain

Anxiety related to pain anticipation and inadequate pain management in the past

Constipation related to chronic use of narcotic analgesics

Ineffective Family Coping: Disabling, related to father's inability to allow family to share his pain experience

Ineffective Individual Coping related to failure of chronic pain management strategies to date

Altered Health Maintenance related to loss of will to live secondary to prolonged chronic pain

Hopelessness related to belief that present pain means imminent death

Risk for Injury related to decreased pain sensation

Knowledge Deficit: Angina Pain Management, related to belief that nothing will help the pain

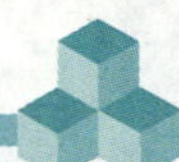

Nursing Diagnoses for Common Problems

Pain

Problem	Related Factors	Sample Defining Characteristics
Pain: Acute Postoperative	Fear of taking prescribed analgesics	• Recent cholecystectomy • Face is pale and drawn; vital signs elevated from baseline. • States, "I don't like to ask for anything for pain because I know people often get addicted."
Pain: Left Leg	Fractured femur and multiple lacerations; unsuccessful attempts to determine effective analgesic	• Recent motor vehicle accident • Grimaces whenever left leg is moved • Directs abusive language to anyone who touches left leg • Refused to have dressing changed on left leg • Reports analgesic "only takes the edge off" the pain
Pain	Prolonged labor (dystocia) and commitment to natural childbirth	• Admitted to labor unit 18 hours ago with moderate contractions 2 minutes apart • Strength of contractions weakening; progress of dilatation and effacement slow; failure to progress • "I'll feel like a failure if I take anything for pain. I want to 'go natural.' I know I can do it. Besides, the drugs would only hurt my baby."
Pain: Heightened Anticipation	Child's history of undergoing frequent painful procedures	• Child diagnosed at age 3 years with acute non-lymphoid leukemia • History of bone marrow aspirations, spinal taps, platelet transfusions, chemotherapy, and other such procedures • Child "freezes" when unfamiliar healthcare worker enters room
Pain: Chest	Decreased blood supply to myocardium (angina) and fear	• "I never know when it will grab me next. I get this crushing pain in my chest and can't do anything. Usually one or two of those nitro tablets bring me relief. I'm always scared, though, that the pain won't go away."
Chronic Pain: Headaches	Inadequate pain management secondary to belief that somehow client "deserves this pain"	• Reports history of migraine headaches for past 5 years • Never sought treatment • "My mother told me that we all get the pain in life that we deserve—and goodness, I've been no saint."
Chronic Pain	Inadequate pain management of metastatic cancer involving bone	• "I can't help feeling, though, that no one is meant to live like this." • Diagnosed with cancer of bladder 2 years ago; presently metastatic spread to spine • Rates pain 10 on a scale of 1 (minimal) to 10 (greatest) • "I haven't been taking as much of this pain medicine as the doctor said I could because if I get used to it now nothing will work when the pain gets even worse later." • "When I told the nurse in the hospital about my pain she said I'd have to get used to it." • "I don't want to burden my wife and kids with my pain."
Chronic Pain	Rheumatoid arthritis and inappropriate activity during exacerbations	• Stiffness of joints, limitation of motion, heat, swelling, and tenderness • States pain is often intense after activity • "I can't accept not being able to do all I want to do for my husband and children."

Fatigue related to lack of relief from chronic pain
Fear related to possible significance of pain
Impaired Physical Mobility related to arthritic pain
Altered Nutrition: Less Than Body Requirements, related to gastrointestinal distress
Self-Care Deficit: Dressing/Grooming, related to painful movement of joints
Altered Sexuality Patterns related to painful intercourse
Sleep Pattern Disturbance: Inability to Fall Asleep related to pain's worsening at night
Spiritual Distress related to belief that God is unfairly causing this pain as some sort of undeserved punishment
Altered Thought Processes related to effects of chronic pain and overmedication
Risk for Self-Directed Violence related to loss of will to live with unrelieved chronic pain

PLANNING: EXPECTED OUTCOMES

Once the diagnosis of a pain problem is made, it is critical for nurses to develop a plan of care that, when implemented, demonstrates nursing's commitment to assist the client to develop effective pain management strategies. Table 41-5 illustrates possible outcomes of two different nursing responses to a client with a diagnosis of low back pain most likely due to a herniated lumbar disc.

Nursing measures are directed toward the achievement of the following client goals for the client whose pain is acute in nature (ie, it is expected that with healing the pain will subside and eventually disappear). The client will:

- Describe a gradual reduction of pain using a scale ranging from 0 (no pain) to 10 (pain as bad as it can be)
- Demonstrate competent execution of successful pain management program (specify)

Chronic Pain

For the client whose pain is chronic in nature, an expected outcome may be contacting a hospice or a pain clinic.

IMPLEMENTING

Once the plan of care is developed, the nurse implements the nursing strategies that are most likely to assist the client to achieve pain-relief goals. Nursing interventions described in this chapter include establishing a trusting nurse–client relationship; manipulating factors that affect the pain experience; initiating nonpharmacologic pain relief measures; managing pharmacologic interventions; reviewing additional pain control measures; considering ethical/legal responsibility to relieve pain; and teaching the client about pain.

Establishing a Trusting Nurse–Client Relationship

Most clients with pain feel better, suffer less, and experience less anxiety when they believe that a competent nurse cares about their experience of pain and is available for help and support. Without the confidence developed in a good nurse–client relationship, nothing seems to work. With it, often amazing results have been obtained by using measures that ordinarily are only modestly effective. Measures that help strengthen the nurse–client relationship and promote pain relief include discussing pain with the client, allowing the client to help decide on a method of pain relief, and visiting and remaining with the client in pain. These measures promote a collaborative relationship in which the client's pain is treated with respect.

Manipulating Factors Affecting the Pain Experience

Removing or Altering the Cause of Pain. Removing or altering the cause of the pain is ideal and sometimes possible. Ways of doing this include removing or loosening a tight binder, if permissible; seeing to it that a distended bladder is emptied; taking steps to relieve constipation and flatus; changing body positions and ensuring correct body alignment; and changing soiled linens and dressings that may be irritating the skin. The hungry or thirsty client may need a snack or a drink to feel more comfortable.

Certain drugs are useful for removing or altering the intensity of painful stimuli. For example, drugs that decrease smooth muscle spasms in the gastrointestinal tract and those that decrease contractions of skeletal muscles reduce discomfort.

Altering Factors Affecting Pain Tolerance. As a result of the pain assessment and the trusting relationship he or she has established, the nurse is better able to identify those factors that are increasing the client's pain experience and decreasing his or her pain tolerance. **Pain tolerance** is the point beyond which a person is no longer willing to endure pain. These factors should be alleviated whenever possible. For example, clients whose families have never acknowledged their pain and who have repeatedly been told that their pain is all in their head may experience a greater ability to deal with their pain when someone finally takes the pain seriously. Nursing measures include communication to the client that responses to pain are acceptable as well as education of the client's family.

Fatigue tends to increase pain, and promoting rest is then helpful. The client in pain usually feels more comfortable when the environment is quiet and restful. Although sensory restrictions such as eliminating unnecessary noise, bright lights, and so on are usually indicated, it is rarely helpful to leave the client alone in an environment with little sensory input. The client then is more likely to focus on self and the discomfort.

Table 41-5
Different Outcomes for a Client With Low Back Pain

Client

A 32-year-old married man, father of two, presents to the hospital with complaints of knife-like, continuous low back pain, weakness, and stiffness. Bed rest, heat treatments, antiinflammatory medication, and analgesics are ordered.

Situation A	Situation B
Nursing Priorities During Client's Hospitalizations	
• Administer medications. • Assist with assuming comfortable position in bed. • Inquire how heat treatments are going. • No detailed pain assessment is performed.	• Nursing and medicine collaborate in detailed pain assessment. • Once a diagnosis of degenerative disc disease is made the nurses teach the client about the disease and related self-care measures (eg, alternate methods of pain control, including use of heat, activity, massage, and progressive relaxation). • Intensive inhospital care includes use of bed rest, measurement for a brace, administration of medications, and heat treatments.
Typical Nursing Comments	
• "Did you injure your back to get a couple of days off? I've often thought of doing that myself." (Some nurses are upset about understaffing and angry with two nurses claiming work-related back injuries.)	• "Gee, it must be awfully hard for someone as healthy as you've been to suddenly find yourself in bed with all this pain. How's it going?" • "How do you think your back problem will affect you once you get home?"
Client's Discharge and Evaluation of Care	
• Client withdrawn during hospitalization; discharged after 2 days of treatment reporting relief of symptoms. • Tells family: "No one in there believed I had pain—or if they did, they sure didn't care. I wish someone would have wanted to help me. I won't go that route again!"	• While hospitalized, client experiences an increased sense of self-respect and worth as well as hope that relief from pain will be found. • Many years later when the disc herniates, the client returns to the hospital confident in the healthcare team's ability and willingness to help him.
Aftermath of Hospitalization	
• Client tries to ignore pain when it recurs. • Irreversible musculoskeletal damage occurs from prolonged muscle spasm. • Weakness, endocrine imbalance (loss of weight), and sleep disturbance are frequent. • Client experiences irritability, depression, feelings of worthlessness, powerlessness, personality changes, decreased motivation, suicidal ideation. • Client is unable to meet role expectations as spouse, father, friend, and employee—results in divorce, unemployment, and destruction of the quality of his life and that of his family.	• Early treatment and lifelong care of back complemented by general health behaviors (eg, good nutrition, regular exercise, stress management), prevent the development of symptoms related to the gradual buildup of paravertebral spasms. • Health status and quality of life are actually improved following client's hospitalization.

Lack of knowledge, finding no meaning in the pain, being pessimistic about its relief, and fear may also interfere with the client's ability to deal with pain. Common fears include a fear of losing control and embarrassing oneself by being unable to deal with the pain maturely, and the fear of taking pain-relief medication because this may be viewed as a sign of weakness, may become addictive, or will lose its effectiveness later. Older clients, in particular, are frequently frustrated by similar concerns about pain management.

Initiating Nonpharmacologic Relief Measures

Distraction

Conscious attention often appears to be necessary to experience pain, whereas preoccupation with other things has been observed to distract the client from pain. Distraction requires the client to focus attention on something other than the pain. It is not entirely clear whether distraction raises the threshold of pain or increases pain tolerance. Many clients whose pain is relieved by distraction report being able to place pain in the periphery

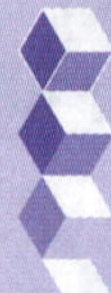

Through the Eyes of the Client

I've always thought of myself as a "take charge" kind of person. It's important for me in my business to be calm and always in control of my emotions. The "big C" changed everything for me. A recent hospitalization made me take time to think about what's happening to me.

Even in the hospital, I had a steady stream of visitors—some friends and some business associates. Even the mayor stopped by to see me! For all of them, I was my usual self—smiling, joking, and acting as if everything was normal. I made sure I took my pain medicine before they came. I kept all my fears about cancer and dying hidden behind my smiling face. I never broke down—not even in front of my wife! Men aren't supposed to cry, you know!

One nurse's simple gesture changed all that. One evening after all my visitors, my wife, my son had left, she must have sensed something. She came over, stood next to me, put her arm around my shoulders and quietly said, "You know, Bob, it's alright to cry." It was like the dam opened up. I looked at her, my face cracked, and all of a sudden I couldn't stop sobbing. She must have known that I needed to talk about what was happening to me. I needed to say those words out loud to someone—"I'm afraid the pain will get too bad! I'm afraid of dying. I can't let my family see me this way!" She just let me cry, kept holding my hands, and just by being there and listening, helped me at that particular moment in ways that you will never know.

of awareness. This is compatible with the theory that if the reticular formation in the brain stem receives sufficient sensory input it can ignore or block out select sensations such as pain. The Lamaze method of childbirth illustrates one common use of distraction.

Distraction alone may relieve mild pain but is best used before pain begins or soon thereafter. It has also proven effective when used with analgesics for treatment of a brief episode of severe pain (eg, pain that accompanies a diagnostic procedure). When distraction is attempted for longer periods of time, the end result may be an increased sense of pain and fatigue at its completion.

Distraction may be used successfully with children. For distraction to be effective, the individual must be aware of activities or situations that are the most exciting, interesting, or absorbing. Distractions may be visual, auditory, tactile, kinesthetic, or "project" (see the accompanying box).

Imagery

The client who uses *imagery*, an example of mind–body interaction, to decrease pain sensation imagines something that involves one or all of the senses, concentrates on that image, and gradually becomes less aware of the pain. Imagery may be as simple as a child thinking of "happy things" (a beloved pet, lollipops, Christmas morning, grandmom's lap) or as involved as an adult recreating a favorite place and then experiencing the healing presence or touch of a loved person or the healing energies of nature in that setting. Imagery has also been used to create an image in which the cause of the pain is visualized and then overcome, or counteracted, by some more powerful image.

Imagery has been found to be more effective for the client with chronic pain than for the client with acute, severe pain. The nurse can teach a client to use imagery by performing guided imagery. Dossey (1995) suggests four guidelines for successfully guiding the client to use imagery:

- Help the client to identify the problem or goal.
- Suggest beginning the imagery with several minutes of focused breathing, relaxation, or meditation.
- Help the client to develop images of the problem as well as personal internal resources (eg, coping strategies) and external healing therapies (eg, medications, treatments).
- Encourage images of the desired state of well-being at the end of the session.

If the client becomes restless or upset, the imagery experience is terminated and attempted later when the client seems better disposed. Guided imagery is also discussed in Chapter 32.

Techniques That Distract Attention

Visual Distractions
- Staring at an object or spot and describing it in detail
- Counting objects
- Reading or watching television

Auditory Distractions
- Listening to music

Tactile Kinesthetic Distractions
- Holding or stroking a loved person, pet, or toy
- Rocking
- Slow, rhythmic breathing

Project Distractions
- Playing a challenging game (puzzles, card game, computer game)
- Performing meaningful play or work (hobby, vocational work, creative work, such as writing a journal, taping memoirs, and other such projects)

Relaxation

Relaxation techniques reduce skeletal muscle tension and lessen anxiety. By assisting the client with relaxation techniques, the nurse acknowledges the client's pain and expresses a willingness to help the client relieve the distress caused by his or her pain. The positive effects of relaxation for the person with pain include the following:

- Improved quality of sleep
- Improved problem-solving ability
- Decreased fatigue
- Increased confidence and sense of self-control in coping with pain
- Lessening of the detrimental physiologic effects of continued or repeated stress from pain
- Distraction from pain
- Increased effectiveness of other pain relief measures
- Improved ability to tolerate pain
- Decreased distress or fear during anticipation of pain
- Reassurance that the nurse is aware of his or her problem and wants to help (McCaffery & Beebe, 1989)

Most relaxation techniques can be learned with little practice and with relative ease. Some require the help and guidance of a person experienced in the technique, such as Zen or yoga. Practices producing relaxation generally have four elements in common:

- Assuming a comfortable position with the body in good alignment
- Being in quiet surroundings
- Repeating a certain word, sound, phrase, or prayer
- Adopting a passive attitude when distracting thoughts enter the individual's consciousness

Relaxation is most effective as a pain alleviator when combined with slow, deep, easy breathing from the abdomen or diaphragm while the eyelids are closed or with the individual focusing on a real or imagined fixed spot. Relaxation techniques are also discussed in Chapter 32.

Other methods to promote relaxation include listening to restful music or nature sounds while concentrating or relaxing; thinking about something that is relaxing, such as lying on a beach while listening to the roar of the waves; or techniques such as meditation, yoga, Zen, biofeedback, systematic desensitization, and operant conditioning. Good (1995) reported that tape-recorded music selected by clients before surgery effectively reduced painful sensations when ambulating postoperatively for 88% of the clients in a study group. Relaxation strategies appear to be more effective in chronic pain situations.

Cutaneous Stimulation

The success of *cutaneous stimulation*—techniques that stimulate the skin's surface—in relieving pain is often explained on the basis of the gate control theory. The gate control theory of pain postulates that cutaneous nerve fibers are large-diameter fibers carrying impulses to the central nervous system. When the skin is stimulated, pain is believed to be controlled by closing the gating mechanism in the spinal cord. This decreases the number of pain impulses that reach the brain for perception. According to Meintz (1995), massage, one form of cutaneous stimulation, successfully reduced anxiety and the perception of pain in clients with cancer.

Cutaneous stimulation techniques include the following:

- Massage (with or without analgesic ointments or liniments containing menthol); see Procedure 41-1
- Application of heat or cold, or both intermittently (explained in detail in Chapter 30)
- Acupressure
- Contralateral stimulation

Acupressure is a modern-day Western descendant of acupuncture. It involves the application of pressure or massage, or both, to usual acupuncture sites. The effectiveness of acupressure may be explained on the basis of the gate control theory.

Contralateral stimulation is a technique that involves stimulating an area opposite the painful area. For example, if the left arm is painful, skin stimulation is used on the right arm. The reason contralateral stimulation works is not understood.

Cutaneous stimulation is limited in that unless the pain can be localized, it is most likely too diffuse to benefit from these techniques. In addition, most individuals cannot tolerate stimulation of the painful area; they may, however, be helped by stimulation of the surrounding or contralateral area.

Transcutaneous Electrical Nerve Stimulation

Transcutaneous electrical nerve stimulation (*TENS*) is a noninvasive alternative technique that involves electrical stimulation of large-diameter fibers to inhibit transmission of painful impulses carried over small-diameter fibers. The TENS unit consists of a battery-powered portable unit, lead wires, and electrodes that are applied to the painful area (Fig. 41-8). It requires a physician's order. TENS therapy has reportedly been effective in reducing postoperative pain and improving mobility following surgery (AHCPR, 1992). Positive results have also been noted when it is used as an adjunct with physical therapy and for clients with low back pain. The TENS unit may be applied intermittently throughout the day or worn for extended periods of time based on the physician's order.

Acupuncture

Acupuncture is a technique that uses needles of various lengths to prick specific parts of the body to produce insensitivity to pain. After the needles are inserted into the body, they are twirled or used to conduct a mild electrical current. The technique was developed in China and has been used for centuries in many Asian countries. It is beginning to gain acceptance in the Western world and is being investigated as a possible tool to help control discomfort. The relief of pain by acupuncture is gen-

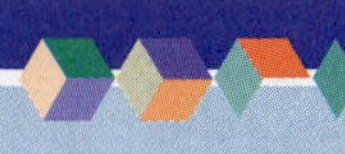

PROCEDURE 41-1
Giving a Back Massage

Equipment

Massage lubricant or lotion	Bath blanket
Powder	Towel

Action	Rationale
1. Explain the procedure and offer back massage to the client.	Back massage can facilitate circulation and promote relaxation.
2. Wash your hands.	Handwashing deters the spread of microorganisms.
3. Close the curtain or door.	Privacy increases relaxation.
4. Assist the client to the prone position or side-lying position with the back exposed from the shoulders to the sacral area. Use the bath blanket to drape the client. Raise the bed to the high position and lower the side rail closest to you.	This position exposes an adequate area for massage with privacy and warmth maintained. Having the bed in the high position reduces back strain for the nurse.
5. Warm the lubricant or lotion in the palm of your hand or place the container in warm water.	Cold lotion causes chilling and uncomfortable sensation.
6. Using light gliding strokes (*effleurage*), apply lotion to client's shoulders, back, and sacral area.	Effleurage relaxes the client and lessens tension.
7. Place your hands beside each other at the base of the client's spine and stroke upward to the shoulders and back downward to the buttocks in slow, continuous strokes. Continue for several minutes.	Continuous contact is soothing and stimulates circulation and muscle relaxation.
8. Massage the client's shoulders, entire back, areas over iliac crests, and sacrum with circular stroking motion. Keep your hands in contact with the client's skin. Continue for several minutes, applying additional lotion as necessary.	A firmer stroke with continuous contact promotes relaxation.
9. Knead the client's skin by gently alternating grasping and compression motions (*pétrissage*).	Kneading increases blood circulation to areas.
10. Complete the massage with additional long stroking movements.	Long stroking motion is soothing and promotes relaxation.
11. During massage, observe the client's skin for reddened or open areas. Pay particular attention to the skin over bony prominences.	Pressure may interfere with circulation and lead to development of decubitus ulcers. Back rub stimulates circulation to these areas.
12. Use the towel to pat the client dry and to remove excess lotion. Apply powder if the client requests it.	This provides additional comfort for the client.
13. Wash your hands.	Handwashing deters the spread of microorganisms.
14. Assess the client's response and record your observations on the client's chart.	This provides accurate documentation of the procedure and condition of the client's skin.

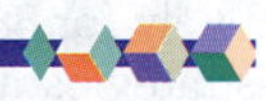

erally explained on the basis of the gate control theory. The needles are believed to stimulate large-diameter nerve fibers and thereby the gating mechanism is closed and pain impulses do not reach the brain for perception. Self-hypnosis may also account for some of acupuncture's success. Repeated treatments are often needed.

Hypnosis

Hypnosis, a technique that produces a subconscious condition accomplished by suggestions made by a hypnotist, has been used successfully in many instances to control pain. The person's state of consciousness is al-

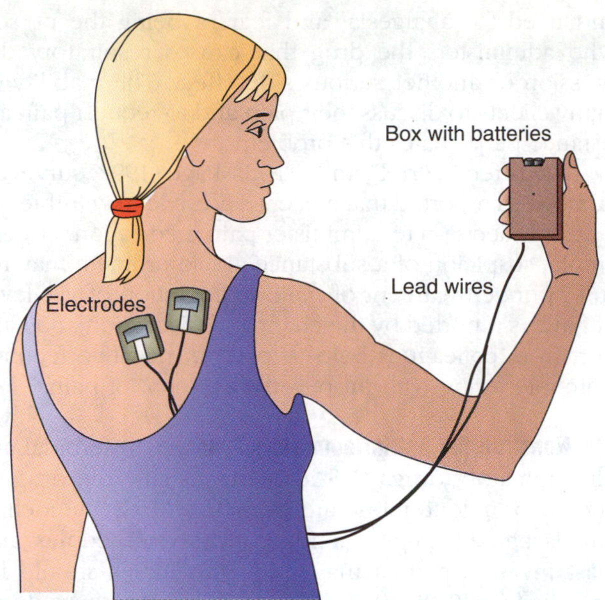

Figure 41-8
Three major components of a TENS unit with two electrodes placed on the upper back of the patient to relieve shoulder pain. This shows the size of the TENS unit in relation to an adult body, illustrating that it is small and portable. (McCaffery, M., & Beebe, A. [1989]. *Pain: Clinical manual for nursing practice.* St. Louis: Mosby, p. 158)

tered by suggestions so that pain is not perceived as it normally would be. According to many hypnotists, it also alters the physical signs of pain. Many people can be taught autohypnosis, that is, self-induced hypnosis, for the control of pain. It is generally believed that a successful response to hypnosis is related to the individual's openness to suggestion, belief that hypnosis will work, and emotional readiness.

Biofeedback

Biofeedback is a technique that uses a teaching machine with a feedback signal to help a client learn by trial and error to control the supposedly involuntary body mechanisms (eg, poor circulation, muscle spasms) that may cause pain. The technique decreases the individual's pain by reducing the anxiety associated with lack of control over bodily functions, by distracting the person's attention from the pain to concentration on the person's inner state and the feedback signal, and by reducing the cause of the pain. Limitations for this method include the high degree of motivation needed and difficulty of maintaining control at the end of the training program.

Therapeutic Touch

Therapeutic touch is viewed by many as a powerful adjunct to pain relief therapy. Clients who have received therapeutic touch report feeling relaxed and require less pain medication with longer periods of pain relief (Mackey, 1995; Schmidt, 1995). It is derived from the ancient practice of laying on of hands, but nurses skilled in therapeutic touch never actually touch their clients when administering this modality. *Therapeutic touch* was developed by nurses, does not require a physician's order, and can be used in any setting. This alternative therapy involves using one's hands to consciously direct an energy exchange from the practitioner to the client to facilitate healing or pain relief. The accompanying box summarizes the four basic steps involved in therapeutic touch. In addition to being used for pain relief and to facilitate the healing process, nurses caring for clients with terminal diseases relate that therapeutic touch complements their efforts to alleviate suffering and promote comfort during the final stages of life.

Managing Pharmacologic Relief Measures

Whether pain is acute or chronic, measures exist to control most pain experiences. However, many misconceptions still exist about pain relief and, because of this, many people still receive inadequate pain treatment and suffer needlessly. The recent AHCPR guidelines focus on

> ### Therapeutic Touch
>
> The four basic steps necessary to perform therapeutic touch include:
>
> 1. Centering yourself
>   - Caregiver reaches a meditative state where inner peace is obtained and the practitioner is very sensitive to the client's needs
>   - May be the most difficult step to master
> 2. Assessing differences in the client's energy flow
>   - Involves scanning the client's energy field for subtle bilateral differences
>   - Hands are placed on each side of the client, 2 to 6 inches above the face, and moved slowly down toward the feet
>   - Signs of congestion or deficiency are evident in bilateral differences in temperature, texture, rhythm, or energy flow
> 3. Restoring balance to the client's energy field (also known as treatment, rebalancing or intervention)
>   - Facilitates recovery of client's own healing powers
>   - Vivid visualization is vital for reestablishing energy flow within the field
> 4. Evaluating when the treatment is completed
>   - Caregiver senses that initial cues indicating an imbalance are no longer present or that client desires end of treatment
>
> (Adapted from: Mackey, R. [1995]. Discover the healing power of therapeutic touch. *American Journal of Nursing, 95*(4), 27–33); and Schmidt, C. [1995]. The basics of therapeutic touch. *RN, 58*(6), 50–54.)

individualizing pain relief strategies and aggressively using pharmacologic measures. In order to make informed decisions and individualize care, nurses need updated information and ongoing education about drug therapy, the cornerstone of many pain treatment regimens. The AHCPR guidelines are a valuable resource for current knowledge and research on using drugs to control pain.

Analgesic Administration

An **analgesic** is a pharmaceutical agent that relieves pain. Analgesics function to reduce the person's perception of pain and to alter the person's responses to discomfort. There are three general classes of drugs used for pain relief:

- NSAIDs or nonsteroidal antiinflammatory drugs (eg, aspirin, acetaminophen, ibuprofen)
- Opioids or narcotic analgesics (all controlled substances; eg, morphine, codeine, meperidine, methadone); **opioid** is the more correct term for narcotic analgesics because these drugs act by binding to opiate receptor sites in the central nervous system (McCaffery & Beebe, 1989)
- Adjuvant drugs (anticonvulsants, antidepressants, and others)

The nurse administering analgesics needs to combine a healthy respect for the drug being administered with thorough knowledge of its mechanism of action, side effects, and administration guidelines. This respect for the drug should result in analgesics being used wisely to produce their desired effect. Knowledge of common analgesics enables the nurse to tailor the client's regimen and communicate professionally with physicians about a client who is being undermedicated or who needs a different drug or route of administration.

At no time should analgesics be used as a substitute for good nursing care that includes other measures to relieve discomfort. If the administration of painkillers is the only treatment strategy a nurse consistently uses to deal with pain, then care is grossly deficient. On the other hand, nurses should not refrain from using analgesics or reduce their doses because of an unrealistic fear of their potency and side effects.

Repeated studies have demonstrated that pain is frequently undertreated. Physician, nurse, and client variables all contribute to this outcome. Physicians often prescribe insufficient analgesic doses because of a tendency to overestimate the efficacy and duration of analgesics, underestimate the pain experience, and worry excessively about the possibility of respiratory problems and addiction. Nurses who ideally spend the most time with the client and who are supposed experts in human responses, for example, such as the response to pain, often compound this problem by further reducing the insufficient analgesic dose or by not administering the medication at all. Nurse variables include the low priority nurses give to pain management; arbitrary pain assessments and erroneous judgments about a client's pain and need for analgesia; and fear of being the person who administers the drug that causes respiratory depression or another serious side effect. The inability of many clients to discuss their pain and to request pain assistance perpetuates this problem.

McCaffery, Ferrell, and O'Neill-Page (1992) surveyed nurses and reported that a client's lifestyle may influence a nurse's decision to administer pain medication. For example, suspicion of a substance abuse problem may result in undertreatment of pain. Recognition of the level of pain as reported by the client and discussion and support from colleagues help to prevent negative feelings from interfering with proper management of pain.

Nonsteroidal Antiinflammatory Drugs. Nonsteroidal antiinflammatory drugs (NSAIDs) are usually the drug of choice for mild to moderate pain. The AHCPR guideline panels agree that the simplest dosage schedules and least invasive pain management modalities should be used first (AHCPR, 1992; 1994). Many times, these drugs alone can provide adequate pain relief. NSAIDs produce analgesia via peripheral mechanisms outside of the nervous system (eg, by way of interfering with the biosynthesis of prostaglandins). Many of these medications are over-the-counter products; some are available by prescription only; and others are prepared in an injectable form. Some can cause gastric side-effects, but these symptoms may be preventable if the drug is taken with food or antacids. Individual responses to NSAIDs vary but they are contraindicated in clients with bleeding disorders (their action may interfere with platelet function) or probable infections (NSAIDs can mask the signs of an infection). The combination of NSAIDs and opioids provides more analgesia than either drug taken alone.

Opioid Analgesics. According to the AHCPR panel, "opioids are the major class of analgesics used in the management of moderate to severe pain because of their effectiveness" (AHCPR, 1994, p. 49). In sufficient dosage, opioids are considered capable of relieving pain of virtually every nature. They produce analgesia by central nervous system (eg, brain and spinal cord) mechanisms that are not fully understood. The "multiple opioid receptor theory" suggests that these drugs provide analgesia by binding to, turning on, or occupying certain opioid receptor sites at the ends of nerves (Blake, 1995; McCaffery & Beebe, 1989). Morphine is a commonly used opioid because it is available in multiple dosage forms, its action is fairly predictable, and it is relatively inexpensive. The most common side effects associated with morphine use are sedation and constipation, but nausea, vomiting, confusion, and respiratory depression have also been reported.

Many myths and irrational fears persist concerning the use of opioid analgesics. Clients and caregivers cite fear of addiction as a reason for ineffective treatment of pain. Because of this, nurses are concerned about administering prescribed doses of opioids, physicians underprescribe pain medication, and clients refuse or take less than prescribed of the drugs. Physical dependence and tolerance are frequently confused with addiction. The accompanying box defines these terms. Batten (1995) reports that 0.5% of all individuals with cancer pain and other severe types of pain will become addicted to opioids, yet half of the nurses in one survey seriously overestimated the likelihood of addiction when opioids are used for pain relief (McCaffery & Ferrell, 1994). Opioid tolerance and physical addiction are common with chronic opioid use, but this is not the same as the psychologic dependence of addiction. It is also a fact that doses of morphine and morphine-like drugs can be increased in increments of 25% to 50% to control pain that is unrelieved (McCaffery, 1994a).

Respiratory depression is a commonly feared side effect with opioid use. In reality, it is an uncommon occurrence in long-term therapy because clients have usually developed a tolerance to the drug and its respiratory depressant effects. Those most at risk are clients receiving their initial dose of an opioid. In the past, a respiratory rate of less than 10 was cause for alarm, but respiratory depression with opioid use is now recognized as a decrease in rate or depth of respirations and not necessarily a specific number of respirations per minute (Pasero & McCaffery, 1994). If respiratory depression is suspected, it is usually preceded be sedation. The analgesic can be withheld or the client may be physically stimulated by shaking or using a loud sound, along with reminders every few minutes to breathe deeply.

Home Healthcare Alert

A client who is taking around-the-clock opioid medication but can easily be aroused from sleep has an acceptable level of sedation.

Addiction, Physical Dependence, and Tolerance

Addiction or psychologic dependence: pattern of compulsive drug use characterized by continued craving for an opioid and the need to use the opioid for effects other than pain relief

Physical dependence: physical phenomenon in which the body physiologically adapts to the presence of an opioid and suffers withdrawal symptoms if the opioid is suddenly withdrawn

Tolerance: a common physiologic result of chronic opioid use; it means that a larger dose of opioid is required to maintain the same level of analgesia

(From AHCPR, Management of Cancer Pain Guideline Panel: Management of Cancer Pain. (1994 March). *Clinical practice guideline.* AHCPR Pub No 94-0592. Rockville, MD. Author.)

Sedation Scale

S Sleep, easily aroused
1 Awake and alert
2 Occasionally drowsy, easy to arouse
3 Frequently drowsy, arousable, drifts off to sleep during conversation
4 Somnolent, minimal or no response to stimuli

(Pasero, C., & McCaffery, M. [1994]. Avoiding opioid-induced respiratory depression. *American Journal of Nursing, 94*(4), p. 29.)

Nursing assessment using a numeric sedation scale (see accompanying box) can determine those clients at risk for respiratory depression. A sedation level of 3 indicates the need for a decrease in dose or discontinuance of the opioid. NSAIDs can be used to manage the pain during this interval. A sedation level of 4 requires immediate intervention and may involve use of naloxone (Narcan), which is an antagonist that reverses the respiratory-depressant effect of an opioid.

Constipation is a common occurrence when opioid therapy is long-term. It may occur slowly and respond to treatment with increased fluids and fiber and use of a mild laxative.

Adjuvant Drugs. Adjuvant drugs or analgesics are used to enhance the effect of opioids by providing additional pain relief. In addition, they may also reduce side effects from prescribed opioids or lessen anxiety about the pain experience. Commonly used adjuvant drugs include corticosteroids, anticonvulsants, antidepressants, and antihistamines.

General Principles for Administering Analgesics

Goals for Pain Relief. When using medications for pain relief, the nurse must first assess the client's pain and understand the client's goals for pain relief. McCaffery and Beebe (1989) recommend the following guidelines for effective, individualized pain management:

- Try various pain control measures.
- Use pain control measures before pain increases in severity.
- Ask the client what has proved effective for pain relief in the past.
- Select and modify pain control measures based on the client's response.
- Encourage the client to try the pain treatment several times before labeling it ineffective.
- Be open-minded about pain relief strategies.
- Be persistent.
- Be a safe practitioner.

Various organizations and groups have made recommendations for pain control in a variety of settings. These include the American Pain Society, the NIH

National Center for Nursing Research, and the ANA. The Agency for Health Care Policy and Research is the major federal agency responsible for health services research and has issued guidelines for management of acute pain and cancer pain (see Figs. 41-10 and 41-12 later in this chapter) accompanied by pain control plans that facilitate participation of clients and their families as members of the healthcare team. These guidelines will be updated regularly to reflect the most current information on pain control. Quality assurance techniques have also been recommended to monitor the effectiveness of pain management by healthcare agencies (Jacox et al., 1992).

Ongoing Assessment. Just as the pain experience of each client is unique, so is the response of each client to a prescribed analgesic. The nurse continually needs to evaluate whether the medication is producing the desired analgesic effect; identify changes in the client's condition (correction or worsening of pathology, increased drug tolerance) that necessitate changes in the analgesic agent, dose, or route of administration; and identify the development of side effects of the analgesic that may warrant its discontinuance. As long as the client's pain exists, the need for ongoing assessment is imperative. The flow sheet in Figure 41-9 facilitates this assessment. Fundamental to this assessment is the knowledge of the basic action, doses, routes of administration, side effects, and administration guidelines of the analgesic being administered.

Timing. Timing is an important consideration when administering analgesics. Their effect is usually greatest when administered before pain occurs or becomes severe. To time analgesics appropriately, the nurse needs to know the average duration of action for the drug and time administration so that the peak analgesic effect occurs when the pain is expected to be most intense. For example, an analgesic would be offered before ambulating a client postoperatively.

A prn (as-needed) drug regimen has not proved effective for people experiencing acute pain. In the early postoperative period, when pain is expected, this protocol may result in an intense pain experience for the client. The duration between the request for pain medication and the administration of the analgesic may result in unnecessary pain and frustration for both parties. Later, though, in the postoperative course, a prn schedule may be acceptable to relieve occasional pain episodes. Continuous intravenous infusion of opioids has also proved effective for the relief of acute postoperative pain. Patient-controlled analgesia (PCA) and epidural analgesia are discussed later in the chapter.

The prn protocol is totally inadequate for clients experiencing chronic pain. Regular administration of analgesics or ATC administration (around the clock at regularly scheduled intervals) has been shown to offer superior pain management for chronic pain.

Pain Treatment Regimens

Acute Pain Management. The AHCPR guideline (1992) on acute pain management places strong emphasis on the need for aggressive, individualized postoperative pain control. It addresses strategies that can minimize or eliminate acute pain and promote positive client outcomes. Preventing pain is easier than treating it once it has occurred. Treating acute pain requires a collaborative effort between clients who must accurately report pain and indicate personal goals for pain relief, and healthcare providers who must adjust pain relief strategies to fit individual needs of clients. The pain treatment flow chart outlined in the AHCPR guideline (1992), as shown in Figure 41-10, represents a comprehensive interdisciplinary approach to relieve postoperative pain and provide comfort and support.

Cancer or Chronic Pain Management. Individuals with cancer suffer needlessly from pain. This pain, surprisingly, remains undertreated in both children and adults while the disease becomes increasingly more prevalent. The American Cancer Society (1994) reported that in 1994, one in five deaths in the United States were caused by cancer. The AHCPR guideline on management of cancer pain (1994) aggressively supports treatment of the chronic pain associated with this disease using pharmacologic and nonpharmacologic approaches. Some of the reasons why relief of cancer pain continues to be inadequate are:

- Clients, families, and caregivers have unfounded fears of addiction to opioid drugs.
- Caregivers have inadequate knowledge of current pain treatment modalities.
- Clients are reluctant to report pain and caregiver's pain assessments are often incomplete and infrequent.
- Clients express concerns about side effects of prescribed medication and worry about becoming tolerant to these drugs.
- Pain control has not been a priority in healthcare institutions. (AHCPR, 1994)

In an effort to alleviate this unnecessary pain and suffering, the World Health Organization (WHO) has devised a three-step analgesic ladder (Fig. 41-11) that recommends the appropriate progression of drugs and dosages that should be used to manage chronic pain effectively. Emphasis is on individualizing treatment, using noninvasive measures for initial treatment (NSAIDs), providing medication around-the-clock with additional prn coverage when necessary, and using the analgesic ladder to provide attentive, aggressive pain relief. The AHCPR flowchart (1994) for treatment of cancer pain (Fig. 41-12) incorporates these recommendations from WHO.

Pain Treatment in Special Populations

Children. Effective pain management in children requires careful assessment; good communication be-

Pain Flow Sheet

Patient ______________________________ Date ____________

Pain rating scale used* ______________________________

Purpose: To evaluate the safety and effectiveness of the analgesic(s).

Analgesic(s) prescribed: ______________________________

Time	Pain Rating	Analgesic	R	P	BP	Level of Arousal	Other[†]	Plan & Comments

** Pain rating: A number of different scales may be used. Indicate which scale is used and use the same one each time. For example, 0 to 10 (0 = no pain, 10 = worst pain).*

† Possibilities for column: bowel function, activities, nausea and vomiting, other pain relief measures. Identify the side effects of greatest concern to the patient, family, physician, and nurses.

Figure 41-9

Flow sheet for pain. (McCaffery, M., & Beebe, A. [1989]. *Pain: Clinical manual for nursing practice.* St. Louis: Mosby.)

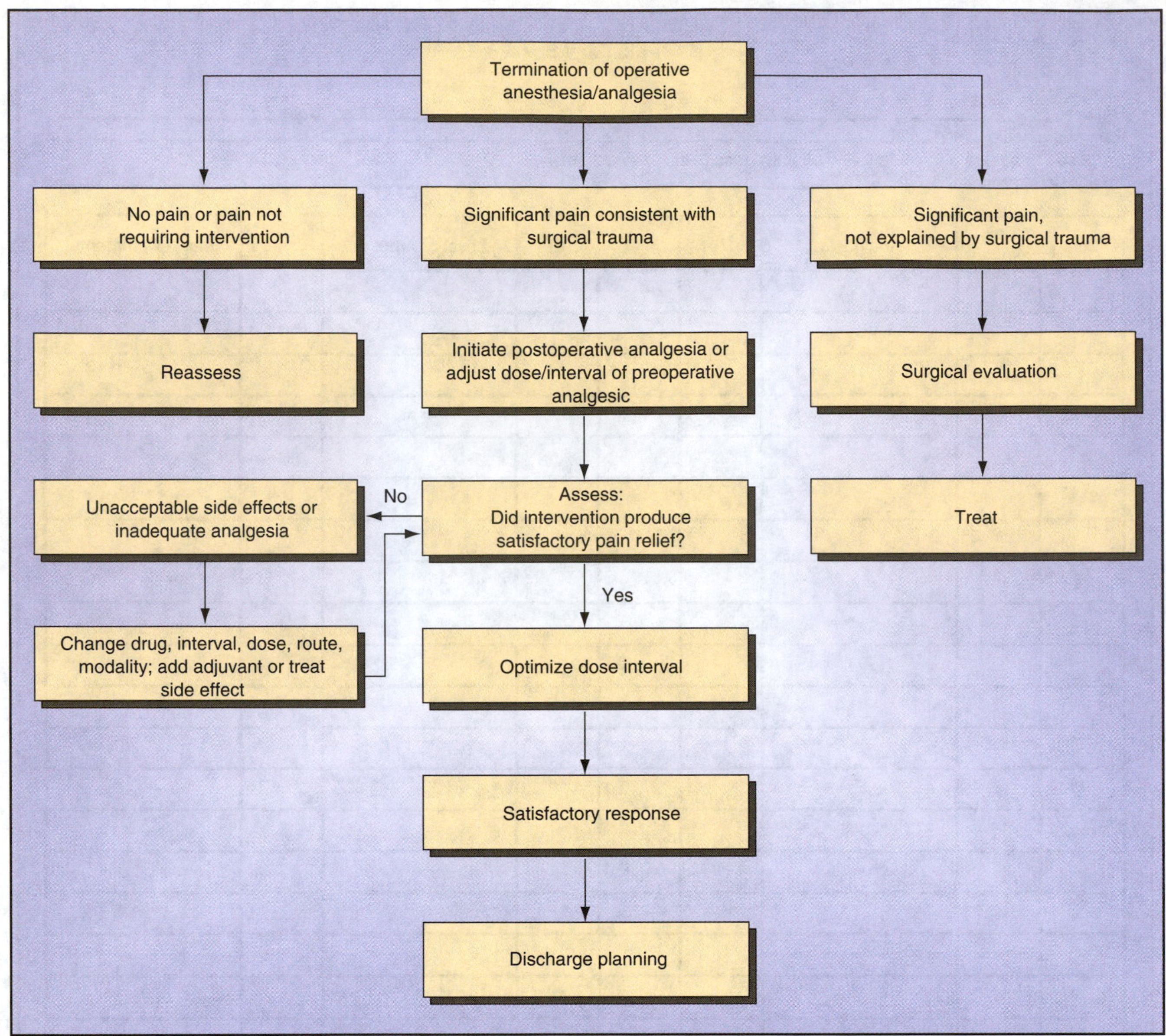

Figure 41-10
Pain treatment flow chart: postoperative phase. (AHCPR, Acute Pain Management Guideline Panel, 1992.)

tween client, family, and caregivers; and understanding of the actions and side effects of drugs used to relieve pain. The child is still the best source of information about the pain and various assessment tools help to measure the intensity of the pain. In postoperative situations, children need analgesics around the clock or by continuous infusion and opioids are the drug of choice for moderate to severe pain. Pain management for cancer pain or chronic pain in children follows the prescription outlined in the WHO analgesic ladder. Withholding opioid drugs from children with cancer because of fear of addiction is unjustified since current knowledge does not indicate they are vulnerable to chemical dependence. Children also require pain management to minimize or alleviate the pain and distress associated with some procedures. Adequate education prior to the procedure and using drug and nondrug therapies to complement each other can take the pain and fear out of the experience. This is especially important for children with a chronic disease who must undergo multiple procedures as part of the treatment regimen (Schmidt et al., 1994).

Older Clients. Little research exists about pain management in older adults. According to Melding (1991), less than 1% of published research articles on treatment of pain focus on older clients. Many healthcare givers, and older individuals as well, expect that pain is a natural outcome of the aging process. The AHCPR guidelines on acute and chronic pain emphasize a vigilant, attentive approach to pain management in this age group. Opioid drugs can be used safely for these clients as long

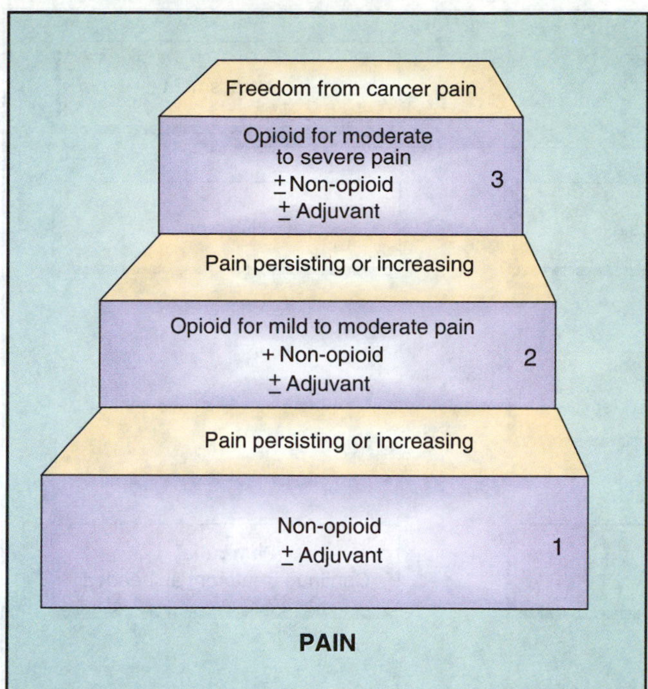

Figure 41-11
The WHO three-step analgesic ladder. (World Health Organization. [1990]. Cancer pain relief and palliative care: Report of a WHO expert committee. WHO Tech Rep Series, No. 804. Geneva: *WHO.*)

as appropriate precautions are taken and pain is conscientiously assessed and potential side effects are monitored. Refer to the accompanying box for additional strategies pertinent to this age group.

Alternative Methods for Administering Analgesics

Patient-Controlled Analgesia. *Patient-controlled analgesia* (PCA) provides effective individualized, client-controlled analgesia and comfort. This drug delivery system may be used to manage acute and chronic pain in a healthcare facility or in the home setting. Patient-controlled analgesia effectively relieves pain associated with operative procedures, labor and delivery, trauma situations, and cancer. This device is most commonly used to deliver analgesics intravenously, but the subcutaneous route is also an option. The most frequently prescribed drug for PCA administration is morphine. The PCA system consists of a portable infusion pump containing a reservoir or chamber for a syringe that is prefilled with the prescribed opioid. When the sensation of pain occurs, the client pushes a button that activates the PCA device to deliver a small preset bolus dose of the analgesic. A lockout interval that is programmed into the PCA unit (usually 5–15 minutes) prevents reactivation of the pump and administration of another dose during that period of time. The pump mechanism can also be programmed to deliver only a specified amount of analgesic within a given time interval (either every hour or every 4 hours). These safeguards limit the possibility that a client may overmedicate and provide time for the client to evaluate the effect of the previous dose. Most pumps also have a locked safety system that prohibits any tampering with the device.

Patient-controlled analgesia has many advantages:

- Consistent analgesic blood level is maintained rather than the inconsistent analgesia obtained with periodic intramuscular injections, which results in sharp rises and falls of serum opioid levels.
- The analgesic is delivered intravenously so that absorption is faster and more predictable than with the intramuscular route.
- The client is in charge of the pain management program.
- The client tends to use less medication because it is self-administered before the pain becomes too severe.
- The client is more satisfied and has improved pain relief.

Nursing responsibilities include educating the client about the purpose and operation of the PCA. Clients need instruction preoperatively if they are expected to utilize the PCA device postoperatively. Suitable candidates for this type of delivery system include individuals who are alert and capable of controlling the unit. Setting up the PCA system and ensuring that it is functioning properly are additional nursing activities. It is also vital that the nurse assess and document effectiveness of pain relief, monitor the client's response to the medication, and observe carefully for any side effects of the therapy. Figure 41-13 demonstrates a PCA device.

A broader definition of PCA is advocated by McCaffery and Beebe (1989), for whom PCA encompasses any drug administration method (oral, PCA pump, intravenous, subcutaneous, or spinal route) that allows the client to exercise control. They recommend that all analgesics be given on the basis of this concept, provided the client is able and willing to participate and safe limits are set. Pasero and McCaffery (1993) also suggest several unconventional situations where patient-controlled analgesia may be considered a valid option. An individual or child who is cognitively or physically unable to operate the PCA device may rely on a family member to act as pain manager. The nurse may also function in this role if a client is incapable of managing PCA yet requires the consistent pain relief that this delivery system offers. A chemically dependent client may qualify as a candidate for this pain relief strategy provided that expectations for its use are clearly stated. All these adaptations of traditional PCA require the approval of the healthcare provider and careful documentation indicating specifically who is responsible and how the individual's pain is being managed.

Epidural Analgesia. *Epidural analgesia* is being used with increasing frequency to provide pain relief during the immediate postoperative phase (particularly after thoracic, abdominal, orthopedic, and vascular surgery) and for chronic pain situations. The anesthesiologist usually inserts the catheter in the midlumbar region into the epidural space. For temporary therapy, the catheter exits

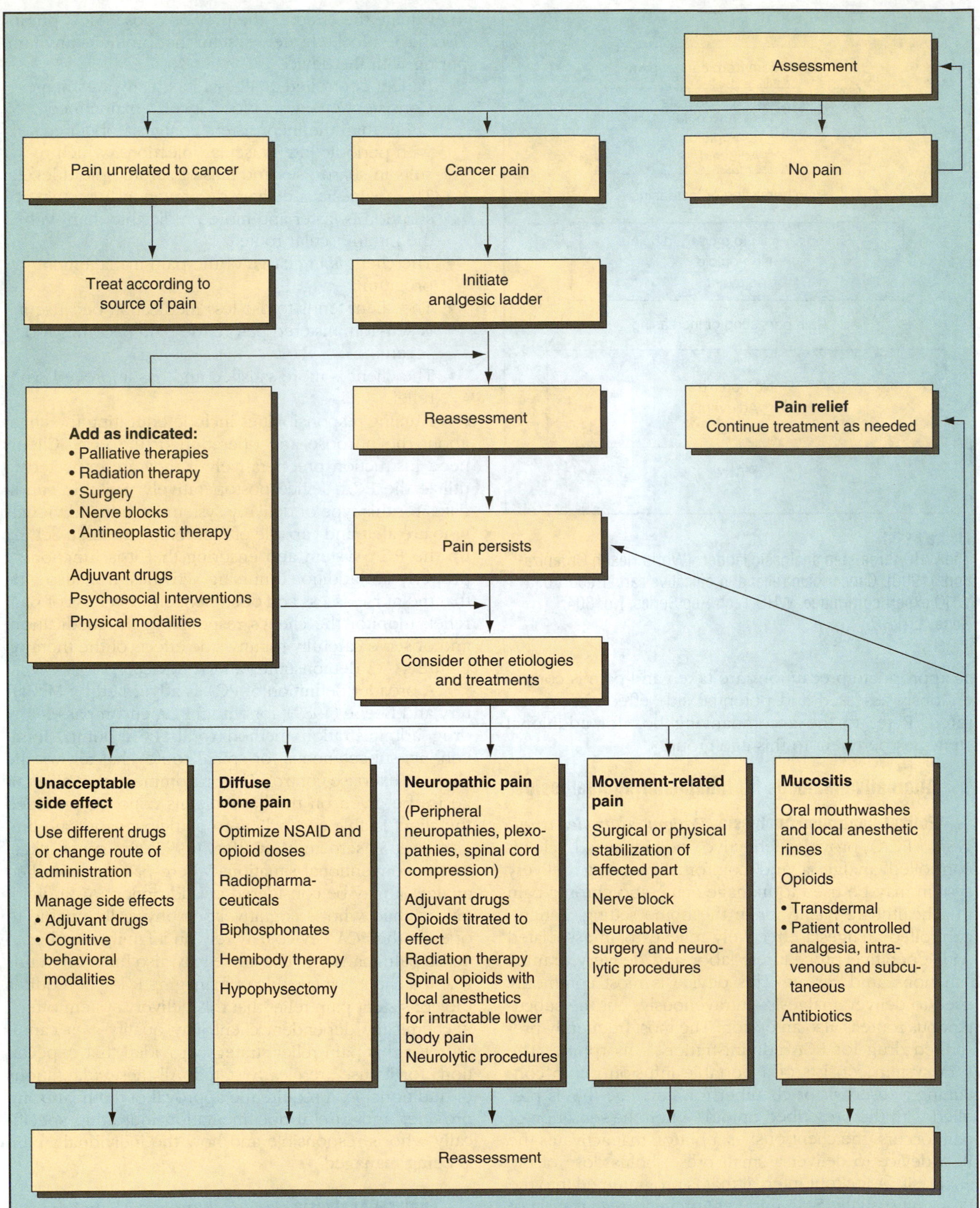

Figure 41-12
Flowchart: Continuing pain management in patients with cancer. (AHCPR: Management of Cancer Pain Guideline Panel, 1994.)

Focus on the Older Adult

Nursing Strategies for Pain Affecting Older Adults

Communication Difficulties

- Observe carefully for any behavioral manifestations or indications of pain (eg, change in activity level or grimacing with movement).
- Use open-ended questions to solicit information about pain.
- Rely on family or caregiver to assist with information gathering process.
- Monitor for any behavior changes or confusion after medication has been taken.

Denial of Pain

- Clarify terms used to describe pain or discomfort.
- Emphasize importance of reporting pain to caregivers.
- Express concern about pain and willingness to help. Explain that pain is not a normal consequence of aging.

Altered Physiologic Response to Analgesics

- Be aware of dosage and frequency to avoid oversedation and toxicity.
- Monitor carefully for oversedation and respiratory depression.
- Explain side effects of analgesics to client.
- Use memory aid if necessary to avoid overdosing.
- Discourage self-medication.
- Caution about use of alcohol with analgesics.
- Caution about driving when taking analgesics.

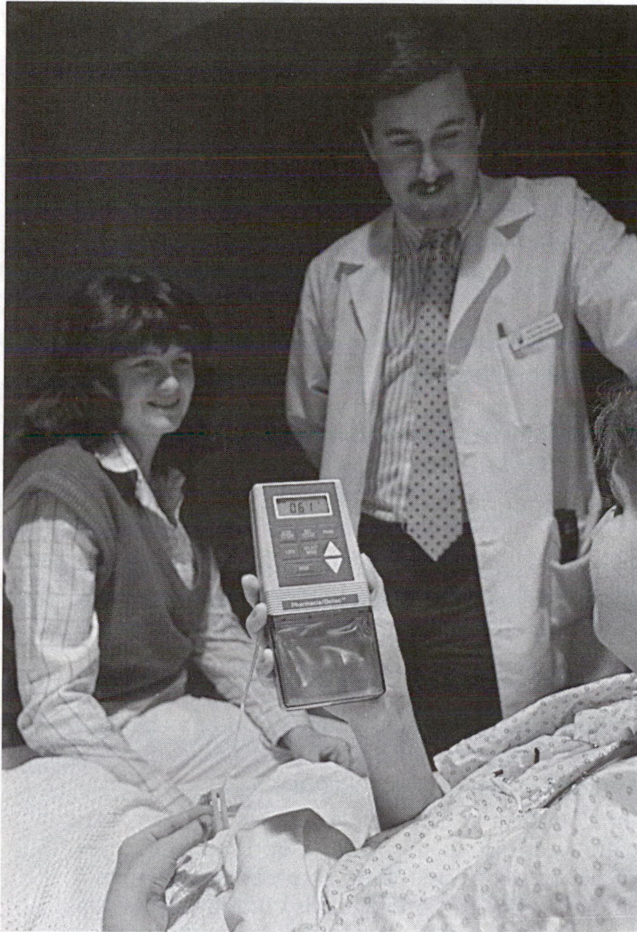

Figure 41-13
A patient-controlled analgesia unit allows the client to regulate the intravenous infusion of small amounts of analgesic as needed. (Photo by Don Walker, courtesy of Thomas Jefferson University, Philadelphia.)

directly over the spine, whereas for long-term therapy, the catheter usually is tunneled subcutaneously and exits on the side of the body or on the abdomen (Fig. 41-14). Epidural catheters used for the management of acute pain are typically removed between 36 to 72 hours after surgery when oral medication can be substituted for relief of pain. The narcotic or opioid acts directly on the opiate receptors in the spinal cord and pain relief is achieved with smaller doses and less severe side effects. The drug of choice is usually preservative-free morphine

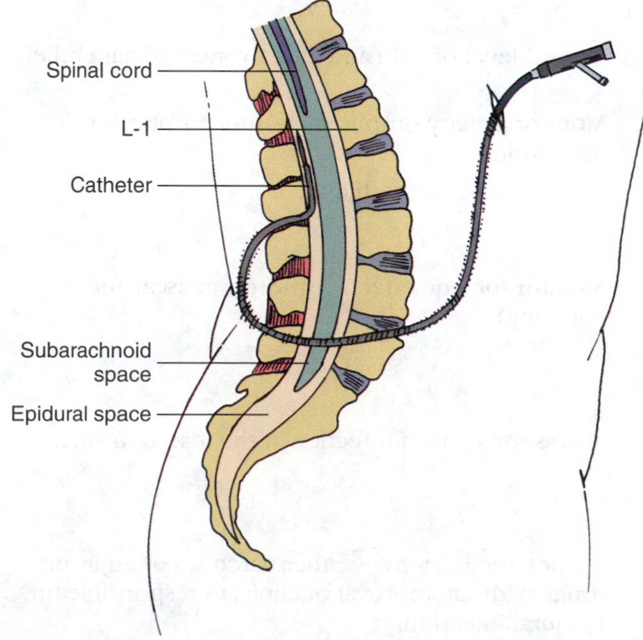

Figure 41-14
Placement of an epidural catheter for long-term use.

or fentanyl and the medication can be administered via a single dose, intermittent bolus injections, or continuous infusion. Pasero and Vanderveer (1994) noted that some institutions are allowing clients to self-administer pain medication using patient-controlled epidural analgesia (PCEA).

Nursing responsibilities vary at each institution but must include careful monitoring of the client's response to therapy, with particular attention to the respiratory rate and pattern (refer to the accompanying box for specific nursing interventions). Too much narcotic or a displaced catheter may allow the medication to exert its depressant effect on the brainstem center, causing life-threatening respiratory depression. Other potential side effects include infection or contamination, pruritus, urinary retention, and nausea and vomiting (Hambleton, 1994). Research has yet to determine the ideal client and specialized situations that are most appropriate for this type of analgesia.

Local Anesthesia. Anesthetic agents may be applied topically to the skin or mucous membranes or injected into the body to produce a temporary loss of sensation and motor and autonomic function in a localized area. The agents work by chemically blocking the nerve pathways involved in pain sensation and response and are sometimes called *nerve blocks.* Many people have experienced nerve blocks during dental work, when having a wound sutured, during delivery of a newborn, and for some minor surgical procedures. Nursing measures in-

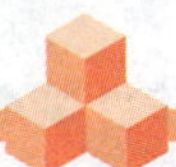

Guidelines for Nursing Care

Caring for Clients Receiving Epidural Opioids

Nursing Action	Rationale
Verify the physician's order for analgesia, drug preparation, and rate of infusion with another RN.	Verification provides for safe administration of the correct dose at the correct rate.
Keep an ampule of 0.4 mg of naloxone (Narcan) and a syringe at the bedside.	Naloxone reverses the respiratory depressant effect of opioids.
Label tubing and pump apparatus "For Epidural Infusion Only."	Labeling prevents inadvertent administration of other IV medications through this set-up.
Assess and record sedation level (using a sedation scale) and respiratory status q1h for the first 24 hours followed by q4h intervals (or according to agency policy). Notify MD for the following: sedation rating of 3, ↓ in depth and respiratory rate below 8/min.	Opioids can depress respiratory center in the medulla. Change in level of consciousness is usually the first sign of altered respiratory function.
Keep head of bed elevated 30 degrees unless this is contraindicated.	Elevation of the client's head minimizes upward migration of opioid in the spinal cord, thus decreasing risk of respiratory depression.
Record level of pain and effectiveness of pain relief.	Referencing helps in determining need for subsequent "breakthrough" pain medication.
Monitor urinary output and assess for bladder distention.	Opioids can cause urinary retention.
Assess motor strength q4h.	Catheter may migrate into the intrathecal space and allow opioids to completely block transmission of nerve impulses through the spinal cord to the brain.
Monitor for side effects (pruritus, nausea, and vomiting).	Opioids may spread into the trigeminal nerve causing itching or result in nausea and vomiting due to slowed GI function or stimulation of a chemoreceptor trigger zone in the brain. Medications are available to treat these side effects.
Assess for signs of infection at the insertion site.	Inflammation or local infection may develop at the catheter insertion site. Strict aseptic technique and sterile dressing and tubing changes according to agency policy can prevent this complication.
Do not administer any other narcotics or adjuvant drugs without approval of clinician responsible for epidural injection.	Additional medication may potentiate the action of the opioid, thus increasing the risk for respiratory depression.

clude noting any allergic responses the client has had in the past to anesthetic agents, alerting the client to the pain the initial injection of the anesthetic may cause if the physician does not numb the area first, offering emotional support to the client during the procedure and observing for any untoward effects, and protecting the client from injury until sensory and motor functions return.

Home Care Considerations. In the home setting, oral morphine is still the drug of choice to control chronic pain and moderate to severe acute pain. This method is less expensive and easy to administer but requires that the client can swallow and retain food and fluids. Accurate documentation is imperative to determine effectiveness of the current regimen or the need to change pain control measures if relief is not obtained. Effective client and family teaching is the cornerstone of pain relief therapy in the home setting. Important points to be covered include:

- Review the pain scale of choice thoroughly. All caregivers coming into the home should use the same tool.
- Discuss the benefits of using a pain scale. The client can more accurately define the pain level and indicate satisfaction with pain relief measures.
- Review the meaning of the word "pain." The client's definition may not include the entire scope of sensations that can be used to indicate and qualify pain.
- Encourage the client to practice using the pain scale. Rate previous painful experiences on the pain scale.
- Establish the client's personal goal for pain relief. Home health nurses provide quality nursing care when they empower clients to take charge of their pain relief measures (McCaffery, 1994b).

Reviewing Additional Pain Control Measures

Pain conduction pathways can be interrupted permanently by surgical measures. Because the destruction is permanent, it is usually used only as a last resort for intractable pain. In people for whom psychologic elements contribute heavily to the pain experience, the pain may persist after nerve transection. These procedures require highly skilled neurosurgeons and anesthesiologists and their execution varies from one healthcare facility to another.

Neurectomy

Neurectomy is a partial or total excision of a peripheral or cranial nerve to relieve localized pain. It may result in total loss of sensation and some paralysis of the affected area.

Rhizotomy

Rhizotomy is an interruption (by surgical resection) of the posterior root just outside the posterior horn cells of the spinal cord. This procedure offers the benefit of relief of both localized acute pain and deep visceral pain (interrupts sensory function) while preserving motor function. A surgical rhizotomy is indicated for localized pain in the neck, chest, back, and perineum if the client is in good physical condition.

Cordotomy

Cordotomy is a surgical resection of the spinal and cerebral tracts carrying painful impulses and is used for advanced disease and intractable pain. Ideally, pain and temperature sensation below the level severed are obliterated whereas the sense of touch and awareness of position are retained. This procedure carries a heavy risk of complications, and permanent paralysis may result from accidental resection of the motor nerves. This open surgical procedure has been largely replaced by percutaneous thermoregulation.

Sympathectomy

Sympathectomy is a severing of the sympathetic afferent nerve pathways that is used primarily for causalgias, phantom pain, and pain due to vascular disorders.

Considering the Ethical/Legal Responsibility to Relieve Pain

Quality pain management results when clients have access to safe, effective pain relief measures. Healthcare givers, in addition to monitoring, delivering, and documenting administration of analgesics, also have responsibility to inform clients that effective pain relief is vital to their treatment. Clients also have the right to expect that their statements of pain will be heeded quickly. Institutions must assign and educate clinicians to address these issues in a timely, knowledgeable manner. The Joint Commission on Accreditation of Healthcare Organizations, as part of their review process, checks medical records to affirm that pain is being adequately managed in each institution. The first legal case involving nursing management of an individual's pain resulted in a multimillion-dollar award to a client's family for failing to relieve the increased pain that the client suffered prior to his death in a healthcare facility (Cushing, 1992; Weiler, 1992). The "Pain Patient's Bill of Rights" (displayed in the accompanying box) recognizes the multidimensional aspects of the pain experience and an individual's right to have pain controlled as soon as possible.

The Placebo Controversy

The term **placebo** is a Latin word meaning "I shall please." It consists of an inactive substance often given to satisfy a person's demand for a drug. The person, unaware of the placebo's properties, may find it to be effective for the relief of pain because of the perception that it will provide comfort and because of belief in the person administering it. It is an injustice to judge a per-

Pain Patient's Bill of Rights

You have the right to:

- Have your pain prevented or controlled adequately.
- Have your pain and pain-medication history taken.
- Have your pain questions answered freely.
- Develop a pain plan with your doctor.
- Know what medication, treatment or anesthesia will be given.
- Know the risks, benefits and side effects of treatment.
- Know what alternative pain treatments may be available.
- Sign a statement of informed consent before any treatment.
- Be believed when you say you have pain.
- Have your pain assessed on an individual basis.
- Have your pain assessed using the 0 = no pain, 10 = worst pain scale.
- Ask for changes in treatments if your pain persists.
- Receive compassionate and sympathetic care.
- Receive pain medication on a timely basis.
- Refuse treatment without prejudice from your doctor.
- Seek a second opinion or request a pain-care specialist.
- Be given your records on request.
- Include your family in decisionmaking.
- Remind those who care for you that your pain management is part of your diagnostic, medical or surgical care.

(Balton, M. [1995]. Take charge of your pain. *Modern Maturity, 38*(1), p. 80. Adapted from Cowles, J. [1994]. *Pain relief!* MasterMedia.)

son experiencing relief from pain after the use of a placebo as a malingerer or as mentally ill. Various researchers have reported that a positive placebo effect may be related to a physiologic response (release of endorphins) or the client's cultural expectations, attitudes, health beliefs, or anticipation of a positive response.

The use of placebos, however, raises serious ethical questions. Is lying to a client justifiable? The nurse who administers a placebo must be willing to risk the possible consequence of the client becoming aware of the duplicity and then refusing to trust the nurse or any other healthcare professional again. Clients who feel themselves to be in pain are vulnerable. If such a client discovers a seeming plot to trick him or her into feeling better, it is unlikely that the client will respect or appreciate the good intentions of the physicians and nurses involved. The long-term effects of this practice far outweigh any of its benefits. Fox (1994) conducted a computer search of the literature and was unable to find a single article recommending the use of placebos to control pain. The consensus of the AHCPR Management of Cancer Pain Guideline Panel (1994) also clearly states that placebos should *not* be used in the management of cancer pain. The nurse has firm legal and ethical grounds for refusing to administer a placebo.

Teaching the Client About Pain

The well-informed person can often cope better with the distress of pain and tends to experience less anxiety about pain. Teaching about pain should include family members so that they understand and may help the person in pain.

The following are examples of information to share with the client and family when pain is present:

- Function of pain
- Cause of pain
- When pain can be anticipated and when it need not be anticipated
- Quality and duration of pain to expect
- Assurance that it is acceptable to express feelings about pain
- What pain-control measures can and will be used
- Teaching about fears related to addiction, tolerance, and side effects of various medications
- Knowledge about nondrug methods that can also provide effective relief
- Assurance that the client's complaints about pain are believed
- Knowledge that it is easier to control pain before it is allowed to become severe (Ferrell & Rhiner, 1994)

Play may often be used effectively to discover a child's experience of pain and to teach the child how to cope with pain. Children are usually receptive to using dolls to act out pain experiences.

EVALUATING

As soon as a pain problem is identified and a treatment plan developed and implemented, evaluation becomes ongoing. Evaluation is directed toward the changing nature of the pain experience; the treatment modalities (pain management program); and the client and family's response to the plan of care, all of which overlap.

The Pain Experience

The pain the client is experiencing may change in many ways and the nurse must be careful not to make a judgment about this too quickly. For example, if the pain lessens in intensity or disappears, it may mean that the underlying cause of the pain is diminished or absent and that treatment should be stopped, or it may mean that the pain management program is effective and should be continued. When pain intensity is increased, it may

Helpscan

The following are resources for clients and healthcare professionals:

- To order AHCPR guidelines or obtain further information on their availability:
  Center for Research Dissemination and Liaison
  AHCPR Clearinghouse
  P.O. Box 8547
  Silver Spring, MD 20907
  (800) 358-9295
- To attend support group meetings and receive the quarterly newsletter, free of charge, write to:
  American Chronic Pain Association (ACPA)
  P.O. Box 850
  Rocklin, CA 95677
- The National Chronic Pain Outreach Association (NCPOA) can refer pain sufferers to healthcare professionals or support groups that concentrate on specific pain conditions. NCPOA also provides publications and audiotapes for pain sufferers and healthcare professionals (membership fee required). Write to:
  NCPOA
  7979 Old Georgetown Road, Suite 100
  Bethesda, MD 20814
- Other organizations in the United States and Canada that supply information about pain and pain-relief centers include:
  The American Pain Society
  5700 Old Orchard Road, 1st Floor
  Skokie, IL 60077-1057
  (708) 966-5595

  North American Chronic Pain Association of Canada (NAC-PAC)
  6 Handel Court
  Brampton, Ontario, Canada L6S 14
  (416) 793-5230

  National Committee on Treatment of Intractable Pain
  P.O. Box 9553
  Friendship Station
  Washington, D.C. 20016-1553
  (202) 944-8140

simply indicate the need for more aggressive therapy, or it may be a warning that the underlying pathology has changed or worsened and that new medical intervention is required. Often a new problem amenable to treatment is masked by "old pain" and its detection may be delayed to the point that treatment is useless.

Treatment Modalities

The use of both noninvasive and invasive therapies must be continually evaluated to determine if they are the best possible means the client could use to obtain pain relief and if they are effective with only minimal risk to the client. Too often a client stays with the first analgesic prescribed without questioning if it is the most effective drug for the particular pain, if the dosage and timing guidelines are correct for the client, and if the analgesic is perhaps producing annoying or even harmful side effects that another drug would not produce. Similarly, one client may take to progressive relaxation exercises and find them helpful, whereas another client may obtain similar benefits from a daily walking program. Nursing time spent evaluating the effectiveness of each pain-relief therapy is well spent and results in a pain management program that is truly individualized to the client.

Client and Family Response

Ultimately, the plan of care is unsuccessful unless the client and family are satisfied with the results. A successful plan of care results in the achievement of specified client goals that the client values. Whenever possible, nursing care should terminate when the client and family can independently direct the pain management program with the assistance of appropriate resources.

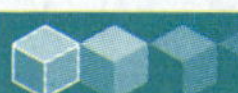

Nursing Process in Clinical Practice

Once a pain problem is suspected, the nurse implements each phase of the nursing process to ensure its correct identification and treatment. The knowledge and clinical skills described in this chapter will enable the nurse to manage these problems successfully. The following section outlines specific assessment priorities, expected outcomes, and nursing interventions for nursing diagnoses representative of the two major classifications of pain—acute and chronic:

Pain: Acute Postoperative
Chronic Pain: Malignant

The client care study that follows the discussion of these diagnoses presents a woman suffering from the discomforts of premenstrual syndrome (PMS). Although her symptoms considered individually hardly constitute a pain problem, together they afford the client sufficient discomfort to interfere with her everyday functioning. This case illustrates the close relation between an individual's comfort level and functional abilities.

Pain: Acute Postoperative

A state in which an individual experiences and reports the presence of severe discomfort or an uncomfortable sensation (NANDA, 1994)

Once the anesthesia administered during surgery begins to wear off, the surgical client generally experiences pain. Etiologies for the preceding diagnosis vary. The nature and degree of surgical trauma, the physical and mental health of the client, and the presence of other discomforting conditions (eg, nausea and vomiting, flatulence, drains and dressings, multiple tubes and equipment) contribute to the client's pain experience. The client's lack of knowledge of pain-relief measures and self-imposed restrictions on pain expression or use of relief measures, as well as deficient pain management skills of healthcare professionals, may compound the client's pain.

Assessment Priorities

Initiate this assessment preoperatively and continue postoperatively.

- Conduct a thorough assessment of the client's pain experience (see the Focused Assessment Guide for the pain experience). Note in particular the accuracy of the client's knowledge about pain (ie, its protective function) and assess the client's ability to manage pain appropriately by using both invasive (drug) and noninvasive treatment modalities.
- Never rely on the client to communicate the need for pain medication or assistance with pain relief. Anticipate the client's need for help and initiate a pain assessment during times when pain is probable. Communicate that the client's pain responses are "okay."

Expected Outcomes

The client will:

- Identify pain as the body's means to protect itself
- Request prescribed analgesic or initiate appropriate noninvasive relief modalities before pain becomes severe and before beginning a painful activity
- Report a gradual reduction in pain and its eventual elimination

Interventions

- Teach the client preoperatively about the purpose of pain and its value in alerting us to certain body conditions. Inform the client that pain-relieving medications will be available and that they are most effective when taken before the pain becomes severe. Review the management of patient-controlled analgesia (PCA) if that will be used or discuss expectations and assessments necessary when epidural analgesia is ordered by the physician for control of postoperative pain. Correct any misconceptions the client has and counsel regarding fears.
- During the immediate postoperative period, carefully assess the lessening of anesthetic effect and the need for pharmacologic analgesia. Initial doses of opioids may need to be reduced if the client is hypotensive; however, the pain may also be causing the hypotension.
- Use good nursing care to keep the client as comfortable as possible. This includes assistance with turning, positioning, and ambulation (as ordered); assistance with coughing and deep breathing; assistance with hydration and nutrition (mouth care for the client who is allowed no oral intake of nutrition or fluids); wound care; massage; help with bathing; and attention to bed linens and elimination needs. Family members may be shown how to comfort clients through massage, repositioning, feeding, and other comfort measures.
- Administer analgesic medications as needed, carefully assessing whether they are producing the desired analgesia without producing undesired side effects. Collaborate with physicians, noting when doses need to be increased or decreased or when a different medication is needed.
- Assist the client to develop a repertoire of noninvasive pain-relief modalities (distraction, relaxation, cutaneous stimulation) that he or she can use both during hospitalization and at home.

Chronic Pain: Malignant

A state in which the individual experiences pain that continues for more than six months in duration (NANDA, 1994)

Clients frequently describe chronic malignant pain as hopeless, cyclical, all consuming, and meaningless, and as leading to fear, anxiety, depression, and helplessness. Common causes include cancers involving infiltration of nerves, blood vessels, or lymphatic channels; pathologic fractures; and obstruction of hollow organs. The untoward side effects of the treatment for cancer may contribute to the severity of this chronic pain. The client's inability to communicate effectively the severity of the pain or the need for analgesia, coupled with possible insensitivity to the pain by healthcare personnel, may compound the problem. Managing this type of pain most often involves the energies of a multidisciplinary healthcare team and the active involvement of the client and family. Many nursing interventions are collaborative in nature.

Assessment Priorities

- Conduct a thorough assessment of the client's pain experience and update this as necessary. Note any difficulty the client has in communicating or expressing pain or the need for pain relief.
- Assess:
  - Characteristics of the pain (location, duration, quantity, quality, chronology, aggravating and alleviating factors, associated phenomena)
  - Physiologic responses
  - Behavioral responses
  - Affective responses
  - Interactions with others
  - Degree to which pain interferes with the client's life
  - Perception of pain and its meaning to the client
  - Adequacy of adaptive mechanisms used to cope with pain
- Collaborate with the medical team to identify the physiologic reasons for the client's pain.
- Continually assess the client's response to treatment modalities and note any changes in the client that would necessitate a change in the plan of care; be especially sensitive to the development of discomforting or harmful side effects.
- Assess the effect of the client's pain on the family and note the family's coping strategies.

Expected Outcomes

The client will:

- Relate ability to draw strength (sense of control) from the conviction that the pain will be treated
- Identify people and resources that can be used to secure assistance with pain relief
- Describe a gradual reduction of the pain using a scale ranging from 0 (no pain) to 10 (pain as bad as it can be)
- Demonstrate competent execution of pain management program
  - Analgesics (produce desired pain relief with minimal side effects—sedation, respiratory depression, gastrointestinal problems)
  - Noninvasive pain-relief measures
- Demonstrate the ability to control pain by managing and enjoying key elements of everyday living

The family will report feeling better able to deal with the client's pain.

Interventions

- Establish a trusting nurse–client/family relationship within which the client can freely express pain, fears, and concerns. Be alert to misconceptions about pain and specific fears (fear of losing control, of being abandoned, of addiction; the family's fear that the client will use pain for secondary gains). Whenever possible, assure the client that he or she need never (or never again) feel overwhelmed by pain, and then work to make this promise real.
- Work closely with the physician to develop effective pain control with narcotic analgesics or opioids. Realize that addiction is usually not a problem. Continual experimentation with drug dosage is frequently necessary to keep the dose in the zone between oversedation and recurrence of pain. Use of the pain flow sheet (see Fig. 41-9) is helpful. The client in severe pain needs relief with opioids before noninvasive treatment modalities can be helpful. When in severe pain, the client does not have sufficient psychic energy for hypnosis, imagery, or progressive relaxation.

Analgesic options are varied. For rapid and flexible control initially, morphine has been unsurpassed and around-the-clock (ATC) administration has proved most effective. Because the goal for maintenance management is an oral drug, opiate cocktail mixtures were used for years but are no longer considered effective. More recently, a sustained-release oral morphine and analgesia administration via percutaneous absorption (patch) have been used quite successfully.

Home Healthcare Alert

Instruct family caregivers about safe techniques when applying an opioid analgesic patch. Apply patch according to directions, fold patch in half with adhesive area on the inside for disposal, and keep all patches out of the reach of children and pets.

Severe, intractable cancer pain has also been treated with morphine administered by continuous intravenous drip, and epidural analgesia is used with increasing frequency for long-term therapy. With the continuous drip route, more uniform pain control is achieved with lower doses of the drug. Safe administration is facilitated with use of an infusion pump and requires close monitoring of vital signs. A narcotic antagonist, for example, naloxone (Narcan), should be readily available to reverse respiratory depression if needed. Depending on the client, other narcotic and nonnarcotic analgesics may become the drug of choice. Nursing responsibilities with all drug therapy include client education, safe administration, and the reduction or elimination of drug side effects.

- Identify other factors that compound the client's pain experience and work with the healthcare team to resolve these problems. Common disturbances include the following:
  - *Anxiety and depression*: Interventions include simple psychologic support; attention to social, financial, and legal problems; and administration of low doses of tricyclic antidepressants or anxiolytic agents.
  - *Gastrointestinal symptoms*: Common problems include anorexia and dysphagia, mouth problems, nausea and vomiting, intestinal obstruction, constipation and diarrhea, and ascites; because each of these problems can cause discomfort to the client, nursing needs to identify them quickly and initiate measures for their management and control.
  - *Skin problems*: pressure ulcers, other open lesions, pruritus
  - *Fever*
  - *Weakness*
  - *Respiratory symptoms*
- Collaborate with the client and family in initiating appropriate noninvasive pain-relief measures—distraction, relaxation, cutaneous stimulation; remember that these may have little effect on severe, intractable pain.
- Work with the client and family to improve the self-care abilities that promote the lifestyle they desire.
- Assist the family to respond optimally to the client's pain experience.
- If necessary, refer the client and family to a hospice or a pain clinic for assistance.

Client Care Study*

Patti Potter is a 26-year-old white woman. She is unmarried and has no children. She is employed at a large company as a computer programmer. During the past 7 months, Patti has been experiencing periodic fatigue, anxiety, irritability, depression, and mood swings. Her general health is excellent. The nurse practitioner at the gynecologist's office believes Ms. Potter may be suffering from PMS. The nurse practitioner who interviewed Ms. Potter noted the following data:

- Client has generalized discomfort—fatigue, anxiety, irritability, depression, and mood swings—about 1 week before her menses; discomfort subsides after onset of menses.
- Discomforts are believed to be heightened by stress at work but do not depend on this. Client denies any new or unusual stress in life currently but believes symptoms are affecting her job performance and relationships.
- Client relates history of "bad cramps" ever since periods started. Client lacks knowledge of appropriate dietary and stress management techniques.
- Client relates she has occasionally taken some of her friend's "tranquilizers" to ease her through a bad day—but she prefers not to take medication.

*Client care study and accompanying nursing plan of care contributed by Ruth E. Gordon, RNC, CRNP, DEd, Assistant Professor, Department of Nursing, Millersville University, Millersville, PA.

Core Competencies

Cognitive Competencies

- Knowledge of women's health and of current modes of treatment of PMS
- Teaching skills to provide Ms. Potter with the knowledge she needs to control discomforts of PMS
- Ability to develop nursing diagnoses that reflect Ms. Potter's unique health problems
- Knowledge of which nursing interventions are most likely to yield desired outcomes

Technical Competencies

- Strong assessment skills to determine how the discomfort associated with PMS is affecting Ms. Potter's lifestyle
- Caregiver skills directed toward relieving the discomfort that Ms. Potter is experiencing

Interpersonal Competencies

- Interpersonal skills to collaborate with Ms. Potter on a plan of care that will work for her
- Counseling skills to listen and empathize with Ms. Potter regarding her symptoms and how they are affecting her job performance and relationships
- Ability to establish a trusting nurse–client relationship grounded in responsible caring

Ethical/Legal Competencies

- Ability to serve as a trusted and effective client advocate
- Commitment to maintain competence to help Ms. Potter reach her full wellness potential
- Competence in documenting nursing interventions

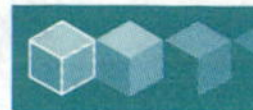

Nursing Plan of Care

for Ms. Potter

Nursing Diagnosis: Ineffective Individual Coping related to discomforts of premenstrual symptoms as manifested by reports of fatigue, anxiety, irritability, depression, and mood swings

Expected Outcome: By the next monthly assessment, 10/30/98, client will:

- Use relaxation techniques during periods of anxiety

Nursing Interventions	Rationale	Evaluative Statement
Assess client's knowledge of relaxation techniques and motivation to use them.	Effective use of relaxation techniques requires a motivated client.	10/30/98 Goal partially met, client used relaxation techniques during two periods of anxiety. Was driving on expressway during another period of anxiety, which made relaxation difficult. *R. Gordon, RNC*
Instruct client regarding the use of progressive relaxation exercises and controlled breathing during periods of anxiety. For example, "Find a quiet, comfortable place and sit down. Consciously contract and relax the muscles of the whole body starting at the head and neck and working down to the feet until completely relaxed. At the same time, take slow, rhythmic breaths. Continue until anxiety passes."	Relaxation and controlled breathing are used to decrease anxiety and increase coping mechanisms.	

Expected Outcome By the next monthly assessment, 10/30/98, the client will:

- Use a meal plan that includes three balanced meals per day and excludes caffeine, sugar, and sodium

Nursing Interventions	Rationale	Evaluative Statement
Assess client's nutritional intake. Have client identify current food preferences high in caffeine, sugar, and sodium and discuss substitutes. Teach client rationale for decreasing intake of caffeine, sugar, and sodium.	Refined sugar and caffeine contribute to feelings of tension and irritability. Sodium contributes to water retention in the body.	10/30/98 Goal met. Client used meal plan for three balanced meals per day and eliminated all sugar, caffeine, and sodium from diet. *R. Gordon, RNC*
Instruct client in developing a meal plan that includes three balanced meals per day.	Balanced meals provide optimal nutrition.	

Expected Outcome By the next monthly assessment, 10/30/98, the client will:

- Incorporate exercise into routine

Nursing Interventions	Rationale	Evaluative Statement
Assess value client attaches to physical fitness and regular periods of aerobic exercise; explore preferences.	Exercise can alleviate symptoms of depression, tension, anxiety, fatigue, and irritability. Exercise also serves as a distraction from discomforts.	10/30/98 Goal met. Client includes daily brisk walk around her neighborhood in her routine. *R. Gordon, RNC*
Instruct client in use of regular daily exercise; design exercise prescription.	The fitness produced by regular exercise contributes to self-esteem.	

(continued)

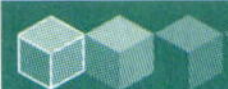

Nursing Plan of Care *(continued)*

for Ms. Potter

Expected Outcome

By the next monthly assessment, 10/30/98, the client will:

- Supplement her diet with 50 mg of vitamin B_6 daily

Nursing Interventions	Rationale	Evaluative Statement
Instruct client on daily use of vitamin B_6.	Vitamin B_6 may be effective in relieving symptoms of irritability, fatigue, and depression.	10/30/98 Goal met. Client supplements her diet daily with 50 mg of vitamin B_6. *R. Gordon, RNC*

Expected Outcome

By the next monthly assessment, 10/30/98, the client will:

- Continue use of daily record of PMS symptoms

Nursing Interventions	Rationale	Evaluative Statement
Instruct client to continue use of daily record of PMS symptoms throughout the menstrual cycle.	Record keeping allows evaluation of the effectiveness of care plan.	10/30/98 Goal met. Client continued daily record, which illustrated drastic reduction in occurrence of PMS symptoms. Client expressed delight in greater feeling of control she now has over how she feels. "I never realized that so many things affect my comfort level and health." *R. Gordon, RNC*

Sample Documentation

8/13/98 Nursing

Consultation with client regarding apparent symptoms of PMS. She stated she experiences fatigue, anxiety, irritability, depression, and mood swings about 1 week before her menses. She states these symptoms interfere with her job performance and relationships. She also states that these symptoms seem to subside after onset of her menses. Client admits to use of tranquilizers but prefers not to use medication. Advised client to keep daily record of symptoms for one complete menstrual cycle. Client indicated understanding of all instructions. She will return to office after completion of daily record for its analysis and to begin treatment, if indicated.

R. Gordon, RNC

Key Points

- Pain is a universal human experience, yet no two individuals experience and respond to pain exactly the same way. The most important services nurses offer a client experiencing pain are belief that the client's pain is real, willingness to become involved in the client's pain experience, and competence in developing effective pain management regimens.
- Pain may originate from physical (cutaneous, somatic, or visceral) causes or mental or emotional (psychogenic) causes. Most often pain is a blend of both. There is no direct and constant relation between a stimulus for pain and its perception. Little is understood about what causes individuals to perceive pain differently.
- The transmission of pain stimuli is a complex process involving the release of potent chemicals that sensitize the nerve endings, help transmit the pain message, and set the stage for healing; transmission of the pain signal as an electrochemical impulse along the length of the nerve to the dorsal horn of the spinal cord; and relay of the pain signal to the thalamus and eventually to the cortex.

- The gate control theory of pain transmission postulates that only a limited amount of sensory information can be processed by the nervous system at any given moment. The effectiveness of many nursing measures to relieve pain (cutaneous stimulation, imagery) may result from their overstimulation of nerve fibers and the "closing of the gate" to pain stimuli.
- Pain is a mixed sensation and occurs in varying degrees. Pain characteristics include duration, severity, quality, and periodicity. Pain responses may be physiologic, behavioral, or affective.
- Many factors influence the pain experience. Among these are culture, religion, environment, support people, anxiety and other stressors, and past experience with pain.
- Numerous misconceptions about pain by both clients and healthcare professionals interfere with the client's communication of pain and relief needs and with pain assessment and management.
- It is helpful for nurses to assume that all clients are experiencing some degree of discomfort or pain and to initiate a pain assessment rather than waiting for the client to indicate experiencing pain.
- Pain flow sheets clearly demonstrate the effectiveness of treatment modalities and the development of undesirable side effects.
- Multiple nursing diagnoses may be written that specifically address pain problems or identify the effect of pain problems on other areas of human functioning. Nursing diagnoses developed for pain problems should identify type of pain; etiologic factors; client responses; and other factors affecting pain stimulus and transmission, perception, and response.
- Expected client outcomes regarding pain are directed toward the reduction and elimination of discomfort and pain and, whenever possible, to the client's management of a pain-relief program that allows the client to resume his or her normal lifestyle pattern.
- Nurses are often reluctant to become involved in pain management because of a natural tendency to avoid pain and because pain in the past has evoked in them feelings of fear, frustration, inadequacy, uselessness, and incompetence.
- The unique relationship that can be developed between a client, the family, and the nurse makes the nurse a critical member of the pain management team. Nursing skills are ideal for developing in the client and family the needed self-care behavior to direct an effective pain management program.
- Nursing interventions for pain relief include education, empowerment, manipulating factors that affect the pain experience, initiation of nonpharmacologic treatment modalities (distraction, relaxation, cutaneous stimulation), safe and effective administration of analgesics, and participation in alternate methods of administering analgesics.
- Cancer pain requires specialized nursing skills. The chief objective with severe cancer pain is to prevent rather than treat the pain and this most often involves regular doses of opioid analgesics. Until the client with cancer pain trusts that the pain can be effectively managed, he or she has little psychic energy for other life activities. The nurse's vigilant control of newly developing symptoms can contribute greatly to the client's comfort.
- Evaluation of the plan of care necessitates the nurse's ongoing attention to the client's pain experience and the continual modification of pain therapies as needed. Integral to evaluation is feedback from the client and family regarding their feelings about themselves and their current ability to deal with pain.

Study Questions

1. Abdominal pain that is difficult to localize is most likely categorized as
   a. causalgia
   b. visceral
   c. superficial
   d. psychogenic
2. Pain that is transmitted to a cutaneous site different from where it originates is termed
   a. transient pain
   b. superficial pain
   c. phantom pain
   d. referred pain
3. A client who has fallen and injured his or her wrist carefully cradles it with the other hand. This response to pain is referred to as
   a. behavioral
   b. affective
   c. physiologic
   d. involuntary
4. To help relieve her pain, Ann concentrates on a favorite vacation setting. This is known as
   a. distraction
   b. relaxation
   c. recall
   d. imagery
5. Intractable pain is best described as being
   a. intermittent in nature
   b. resistant to treatment
   c. excruciating
   d. widespread

6. According to the gate control theory of pain, an effective nursing intervention for a client with lower back pain is
   a. encouraging regular use of analgesics
   b. applying a K-pad to the area at prescribed intervals
   c. reviewing the pain experience with the client
   d. ambulating the client after medicating him or her
7. A physiologic response to moderate pain is
   a. increased blood pressure
   b. restlessness
   c. decreased pulse rate
   d. protection of the painful area
8. The nurse medicates Mr. Kim, an Asian client, for pain. Her assessment that he required an analgesic was most likely based on
   a. nonverbal manifestations of pain
   b. verbal expressions of pain
   c. his previous history of pain
   d. exaggerated weeping
9. When assessing pain in a child, the nurse needs to be aware that
   a. immature neurologic development results in reduced sensation of pain
   b. inadequate or inconsistent relief of pain is widespread
   c. reliable assessment tools are currently unavailable
   d. narcotic analgesic use should be avoided
10. Mr. Wright is recovering from abdominal surgery. When the nurse assists him to ambulate, she observes that he grimaces, moves stiffly, and becomes pale. She is aware that he has consistently refused his pain medication. A priority nursing diagnosis would be
    a. Acute Postoperative Pain related to fear of taking prescribed medications
    b. Impaired Physical Mobility related to surgical procedure
    c. Anxiety related to outcome of surgery
    d. Risk for Infection related to surgical incision
11. When planning strategies for pain control in older clients, the nurse should be aware that
    a. pain is a natural outcome of the aging process
    b. sensitivity to pain increases with age
    c. narcotic use should be avoided
    d. denial of pain may occur
12. Chronic pain is most effectively relieved when analgesics are administered
    a. on a prn (as-needed) basis
    b. conservatively
    c. at regularly scheduled intervals
    d. intramuscularly
13. Using a placebo for pain control is
    a. a widespread practice
    b. consistently effective
    c. deceptive and unethical
    d. justified to determine if the pain is real
14. The client receiving epidural analgesia requires careful monitoring to prevent the occurrence of
    a. pruritus
    b. urinary retention
    c. nausea and vomiting
    d. respiratory depression
15. When assessing a client receiving a continuous opioid infusion, the nurse immediately notifies the physician when the client has
    a. a respiratory rate of 10 with respirations of normal depth
    b. a sedation level of 4
    c. mild confusion
    d. reported constipation

Answers With Rationale

1. The correct response is *b.* Visceral pain is poorly localized and can originate in body organs in the abdomen. Causalgia is pain that occurs in the area of injured peripheral nerves whereas cutaneous pain is superficial and usually involves the skin or subcutaneous tissue. When a physical cause for the pain cannot be identified, it is known as psychogenic pain.
2. The correct response is *d.* Referred pain is perceived in an area distant from its point of origin, whereas transient pain is brief and passes quickly. Superficial pain originates in the skin or subcutaneous tissue. Phantom pain may occur in a person who has had a body part amputated, either surgically or traumatically.
3. The correct response is *a.* Protecting or guarding a painful area is a behavioral response. Affective responses are psychologic ones and examples of a physiologic or involuntary response would be increased blood pressure and dilation of the pupils.
4. The correct response is *d.* Imagery is a mind–body interaction that decreases pain sensation by focusing on pleasurable images. Distraction involves preoccupation with other things to relieve pain and relaxation is a technique that reduces skeletal muscle tension and lessens anxiety. Recall is not a noninvasive relief measure.
5. The correct response is *b.* Intractable pain is severe pain that is resistant to relief measures. The other terms do not describe this resistance to treatment.
6. The correct response is *b.* Nursing measures such as applying warmth to the lower back stimulate the large nerve fibers to close the gate and block

the pain. The other choices do not involve attempts to stimulate large nerve fibers that interfere with pain transmission as explained by the gate control theory.

7. The correct response is *a.* Increased blood pressure is a physiologic or involuntary response to moderate pain, whereas decreased pulse rate occurs when pain is severe and deep. Restlessness and protection of the painful area are behavioral responses.
8. The correct response is *a.* Members of the Asian culture rarely complain about what is bothering them. The nurse must rely on nonverbal cues that indicate pain is present. Exaggerated weeping is also atypical of this culture and a previous history of pain does not necessarily affect this current experience.
9. The correct response is *b.* Healthcare personnel are only now becoming aware of pain relief as a priority for children in pain. The evidence supports the fact that children do indeed feel pain and reliable assessment tools are available specifically for use with children. Opioid analgesics may be safely used with children as long as they are carefully observed.
10. The correct response is *a.* Mr. Wright's immediate problem is his pain that is unrelieved because he refuses to take his pain medication for an unknown reason. The other nursing diagnoses are plausible but not a priority in this situation.
11. The correct response is *d.* Older people frequently deny pain because they view it as an ominous sign that may interfere with their independence. Pain sensitivity may decrease with age but even this assumption is unsafe and it is not a natural outcome of the aging process. Opioid medications can be used if the older client's response is carefully monitored and evaluated.
12. The correct response is *c.* The prn protocol is totally inadequate for clients experiencing chronic pain. Regularly scheduled doses of analgesic are more effective, whereas conservative pain management for whatever reason may also prove ineffective. Intramuscular administration is not practical on a long-range basis for a client with chronic pain.
13. The correct response is *c.* Using a placebo to control pain creates distrust in the nurse–client relationship and is considered unethical behavior. It is not a widespread practice, is ineffective, and is never used to determine if pain is real. Pain exists when the client says it does.
14. The correct response is *d.* Too much of an opioid drug given by way of an epidural catheter or a displaced catheter may result in the occurrence of respiratory depression. Pruritus, urinary retention, and nausea and vomiting may occur but are not life-threatening.
15. The correct response is *b.* Sedation level is more indicative of respiratory depression because it usually precedes it. A sedation level of 4 calls for immediate action because the client has minimal or no response to stimuli. A respiratory level of 10 with normal depth of breathing is usually not a cause for alarm. Mild confusion may be evident with the initial dose and then disappear; additional observation is necessary. Constipation should be reported to the physician but is not the priority in this situation.

Bibliography

AHCPR, Acute Pain Management Guideline Panel. (1992 February). *Clinical practice guideline, acute pain management: Operative or medical procedures and trauma.* AHCPR Pub. No. 92-0032. Rockville, MD: USDHHS.

AHCPR, Management of Cancer Pain Guideline Panel. (1994 March). *Clinical practice guideline, management of cancer pain.* AHCPR Pub. No. 94-0592. Rockville, MD: USDHHS.

American Cancer Society. (1994). *Cancer facts and figures—1994.* Atlanta: ACS.

American Nurses Association. (1991). *Position statement on promotion of comfort and relief of pain in dying patients.* Kansas City, MO: ANA.

American Pain Society. (1990). *Principles of analgesic use in the treatment of acute pain or chronic cancer pain* (3rd ed.). Skokie, IL: APS.

Andrews, M., & Boyle, J. (1995). *Transcultural concepts in nursing care* (2nd ed.). Philadelphia: Lippincott.

Batten, M. (1995). Take charge of your pain. *Modern Maturity, 38*(1), 35–37.

Blake, G. (1995). Close-up on opioid receptor subtypes. *Nursing, 25*(2), 55.

Brockopp, D., Warden, S., Colclough, G., & Brockopp, G. (1993). Nursing knowledge: Acute postoperative pain management in the elderly. *Journal of Gerontological Nursing, 19*(11), 31–36.

Brockopp, D., Warden, S., Colclough, G., & Brockopp, G. (1994). Postoperative pain: Getting a grip on the facts. *Nursing, 24*(6), 49–50.

Carpenito, L. (1995). *Nursing diagnosis: Application to clinical practice* (6th ed.). Philadelphia: Lippincott.

Cushing, M. (1992). Pain management on trial. *American Journal of Nursing, 92*(2), 21–23.

Dossey, B. (1995). Using imagery to help your patient heal. *American Journal of Nursing, 95*(6), 41–46.

Ferrell, B. A., Ferrell, B. R., & Osterweil, D. (1990). Pain in the nursing home. *Journal of the American Geriatric Society, 38*(4), 1–5.

Ferrell, B., & Rhiner, M. (1994). Managing cancer pain: A three-step program. *Nursing, 24*(7), 57–59.

Fox, A. (1994). Confronting the use of placebos for pain. *American Journal of Nursing, 95*(9), 42–45.

Fuller, J., & Schaller-Ayers, J. (1994). *Health assessment: A nursing approach* (2nd ed.). Philadelphia: Lippincott.

Fulton, J., & Johnson, G. (1993). Using high-dose morphine to relieve cancer pain. *Nursing, 23*(2), 32–40.

Good, M. (1995). Relaxation techniques for surgical patients. *American Journal of Nursing, 95*(5), 39–42.

Gordon, D., & Ward, S. (1995). Correcting patient misconceptions about pain. *American Journal of Nursing, 95*(7), 42–45.

Hambleton, N. (1994). Dealing with complications of epidural analgesia. *Nursing, 24*(10), 55–57.

Herr, K., & Mobily, P. (1991). Complexities of pain assessment in the elderly. *Journal of Gerontological Nursing, 17*(4), 12–19.

Ignatavicius, D., Workman, M., & Mishler, M. (1995). *Medical-surgical nursing* (2nd ed.). Philadelphia: Saunders.

Jacox, A., Heidrich, G., Hester, N., & Miaskowski, C. (1992). Managing acute pain: A guideline for the nation. *American Journal of Nursing, 92*(5), 49–55.

Kohr, J. (1995). Measuring your patient's pain. *RN, 58*(4), 39–40.

Mackey, R. (1995). Discover the healing power of therapeutic touch. *American Journal of Nursing, 95*(4), 27–33.

Marzinski, L. (1991). The tragedy of dementia: Clinically assessing pain in the confused, nonverbal elderly. *Journal of Gerontological Nursing, 17*(6), 25–28.

McCaffery, M. (1979). *Nursing management of the patient with pain* (2nd ed.). Philadelphia: Lippincott.

McCaffery, M. (1994a). Ensuring pain relief. *Nursing, 24*(9), 81–82.

McCaffery, M. (1994b). Home health care update 94: Pain control—keeping current. *Nursing, 24*(6), 51–52.

McCaffery M. (1996). Analgesics: Mapping out pain relief. *Nursing, 26*(1), 41–46.

McCaffery, M., & Beebe, A. (1989). *Pain: Clinical manual for nursing practice*. St. Louis: Mosby.

McCaffery, M., & Ferrell, B. (1992). Does the gender gap affect your pain control decisions? *Nursing, 22*(8), 48–51.

McCaffery, M., & Ferrell, B. (1994). Understanding opioids and addiction. *Nursing, 24*(8), 56–59.

McCaffery, M., Ferrell, B., & O'Neill-Page, E. (1992). Does lifestyle affect your pain-control decisions? *Nursing, 22*(4), 58–61.

Meinhart, N., & McCaffery, M. (1983). *Pain: A nursing approach to assessment and analysis*. Norwalk, CT: Appleton-Century-Crofts.

Meintz, S. (1995). Whatever became of the back rub? *RN, 58*(4), 49–56.

Melding, P. (1991). Is there such a thing as geriatric pain? *Pain, 46*(2), 119–121.

North American Nursing Diagnosis Association. (1994). *NANDA nursing diagnoses: Definitions and classification 1995–1996*. Philadelphia: NANDA.

Pasero, C. (1995). Pain control: Managing pain from pressure ulcers. *American Journal of Nursing, 95*(6), 22–24.

Pasero, C., & McCaffery, M. (1993). Unconventional PCA: Making it work for your patient. *American Journal of Nursing, 93*(9), 38–41.

Pasero, C., & McCaffery, M. (1994). Avoiding opioid-induced respiratory depression. *American Journal of Nursing, 94*(4), 25–30.

Pasero, C., & Vanderveer, B. (1994). Pain control: Epidural infusions—not just for labor anymore. *American Journal of Nursing, 94*(12), 51–52.

Schmidt, C. (1995). The basics of therapeutic touch. *RN, 58*(6), 50–54.

Schmidt, K., Holida, D., Kleiber, C., Petersen, M., & Phearman, L. (1994). How to apply the AHCPR's pediatric pain guideline. *American Journal of Nursing, 94*(3), 69–74.

Snelling, J. (1990). The role of the family in relation to chronic pain: Review of the literature. *Journal of Advanced Nursing, 15*(7), 771–776.

Sternback, R. (1968). *Pain: A psychophysiological analysis*. New York: Academic Press.

Strangio, L., & Brudner, C. (1995). When pain cuts to the bone. *RN, 58*(6), 28–29.

Weiler, K. (1992). Pain management as a legal responsibility. *Journal of Gerontological Nursing, 18*(10), 46.

Woodin, L. (1993). Cutting postop pain. *RN, 56*(8), 26–33.

Zborowski, M. (1969). *People in pain*. San Francisco: Jossey-Bass.

Chapter 42

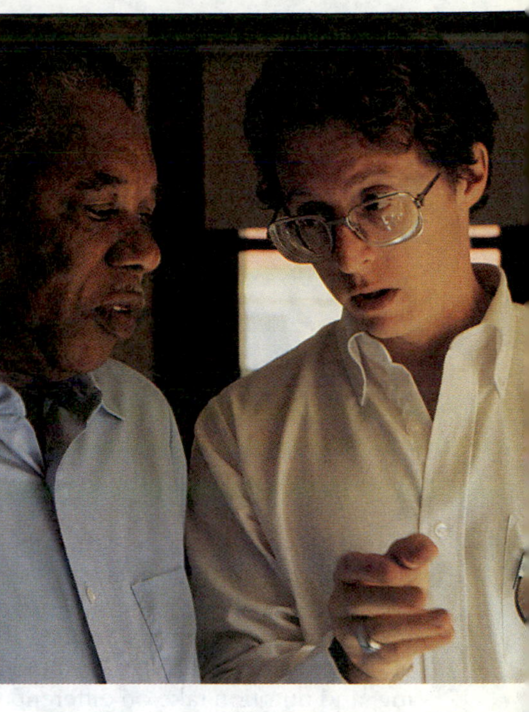

Nutrition

Objectives

After studying this chapter, the learner should be able to:

Define key terms used in the chapter.

List the six classes of nutrients and explain the significance of each.

Evaluate a diet using the food guide pyramid.

Identify risk factors for poor nutritional status.

Describe nutritional implications of growth and development throughout the life cycle.

Discuss the components of a nutritional assessment.

Develop nursing diagnoses that correctly identify nutritional problems that may be treated by independent nursing intervention.

Describe nursing interventions to help clients achieve their nutritional goals.

Plan, implement, and evaluate nursing care related to selected nursing diagnoses that involve nutritional problems.

Differentiate between enteral and parenteral nutrition.

Key Terms

anorexia
anthropometric
basal metabolism
calorie
carbohydrate
cholesterol
enteral nutrition
lipid
minerals
nasogastric tube
nasointestinal tube
nutrient
nutrition
obesity
percutaneous endoscopic gastrostomy tube (PEG)
protein
recommended dietary allowance (RDA)
total parenteral nutrition (TPN)
triglycerides
vitamins

Nutrition is a basic human need that changes throughout the life cycle and along the wellness–illness continuum. Food provides nutrition for both the body and the mind. Eating has evolved from being simply a necessity; it may be a source of pleasure, a pastime, a social happening, a political statement, a religious symbol, a cultural emblem, or an integral component of medical treatment. As such, food, eating, and nutrition take on different meanings to different people, and changing a person's eating behaviors may be a difficult and slow process. Because nutrition is vital for life and health, and because poor nutrition can seriously decrease one's level of wellness, it is a vital component of nursing.

This chapter provides a knowledge base of basic nutrition theory, focusing on the six classes of nutrients, energy balance, choosing an adequate diet, food patterns and habits, and factors that affect nutrition. Components of simple screening and in-depth nutritional assessments are outlined. Two sets of nursing diagnoses are provided, and client goals for healthy nutrition are discussed. In the section titled Nursing Process in Clinical Practice, assessment priorities, expected outcomes, and interventions are offered for select nursing diagnoses related to Altered Nutrition: More Than Body Requirements or Less Than Body Requirements, and Knowledge Deficit related to a new therapeutic diet. These guides and the concluding client care study illustrate the significance of nutrition in nursing care.

Principles of Nutrition

The science of **nutrition** encompasses the study of nutrients and how they are handled by the body, as well as the impact of human behavior and environment on the process of nourishment. As such, this discipline includes physiology, psychology, and socioeconomics.

Nutrients are specific biochemical substances used by the body for growth, development, activity, reproduction, lactation, health maintenance, and recovery from illness or injury. Because the metabolic processes involved in these functions are complex, most nutrients work better together than they do alone. Also, nutrient needs change throughout the life cycle in response to changes in body size, activity, growth, development, and state of health.

Some nutrients are considered essential because they are either not synthesized in the body or made in insufficient amounts; essential nutrients must be provided in the diet or through supplements. Essential nutrients that supply energy and build tissue (such as carbohydrates, fats, and protein) are referred to as *macronutrients. Micronutrients*, such as vitamins and minerals, are required in much smaller amounts to regulate and control body processes.

Nonessential nutrients do not have to be supplied through exogenous sources because they either are not required for body functioning or are synthesized in the body in adequate amounts. Some nutrients can be converted to others in the body. For instance, the body converts excess carbohydrates and protein into fat, and stores them as triglycerides.

Of the six classes of nutrients, three supply energy (carbohydrates, protein, and lipids) and three regulate body processes (vitamins, minerals, and water).

Energy Balance

Energy in the diet is measured in the form of kilocalories, commonly abbreviated as **calories** or cal (kilojoule [KJ] in Canada). Only carbohydrates, protein, and fat provide energy; vitamins and minerals are needed for the metabolism of energy but do not provide calories. Total energy intake for a meal, a day, or longer can be calculated by using food composition tables: the values given for total calories for each food eaten can simply be added, or the grams of carbohydrate, protein, and fat for each food eaten can be added and multiplied by the appropriate calorie level (4, 4, and 9 cal, respectively).

Energy in the body is used to carry on any kind of activity, whether voluntary or involuntary. A person's total daily energy expenditure is the sum of all the calories used to perform physical activity, maintain basal metabolism, and digest, absorb, and metabolize food.

Basic Metabolic Requirements. Basal metabolism is the amount of energy required to carry on the involuntary activities of the body at rest, such as maintaining body temperature and muscle tone, producing and releasing secretions, propelling food through the gastrointestinal tract, inflating the lungs, and beating the heart. As the amount of energy used on physical activity declines, the proportion of calories used for basal metabolism increases; it accounts for more than half of most people's total energy requirements. Because of their larger muscle mass, males have a higher basal metabolic rate (BMR) than females. Other factors that increase BMR include growth, infections, fever, emotional tension, extreme environmental temperatures, and elevated levels of certain hormones, especially epinephrine and thyroid hormones. Aging, prolonged fasting, and sleep all decrease BMR. Most nutritionists agree that fasting or following a very low-calorie diet (VLCD) defeats a weight loss plan because the body interprets this eating pattern as starvation and compensates by slowing down the resting metabolic rate, making it even more difficult to lose weight. BMR is about 1 cal/kg of body weight per hour for men and 0.9 cal/kg/hr for women.

Body Weight Standards. Ideal body weight (IBW) or healthy body weight is an estimate of optimal weight for optimal health. A general guideline, often called the rule of thumb (ROT) method, is to allow 100 lb (45.4 kg) for the first 5 ft (152.4 cm) of height and add 5 lb (2.3 kg) for each additional inch (2.54 cm) for adult women. A range spanning 10% below and above is considered normal, depending on body frame size. For men, the guidelines suggest 106 lb (48.1 kg) for the first 5 ft (152.4 cm) of height, with an additional 6 lb (2.7 kg) for each additional inch (2.54 cm). Again, this weight can be adjusted up or down by 10%, depending on body frame. Using this method can result in unrealistically low figures for adults who are very short or very tall. (Height and weight tables commonly are used for infants and children.)

The 1983 Metropolitan Life Insurance Company height and weight table has consistently been the standard reference that nurses use for healthy body weight (Table 42-1). The weight standards on the chart represent survey results of Americans who purchased life insurance, and are adjusted according to height and frame size for the 25- to 59-year age bracket. The height range may be limiting for some, and the calculated weights do not reflect body fat stores. A person usually is considered overweight if he or she weighs 10% to 20% more than ideal, and obese if he or she weighs more than 20% above ideal weight for his or her height. Ongoing research, however, seems to indicate that health risks are equally as great in each age group for those who are extremely thin as for those considered obese.

Although numerous tables and approaches have been devised for determining healthy body weight, many health experts now consider the body mass index (BMI) to be the most precise parameter. The BMI is a ratio of height to weight, and more accurately reflects total body fat stores in the general population. The BMI does not differentiate according to sex, and is calculated in the following manner:

Table 42-1
1983 Metropolitan Life Insurance Company Height and Weight Table

	Weight (lb)		
Height	*Small Frame*	*Medium Frame*	*Large Frame*
Men*			
5′ 2″	128–134	131–141	138–150
5′ 3″	130–136	133–143	140–153
5′ 4″	132–138	135–145	142–156
5′ 5″	134–140	137–148	144–160
5′ 6″	136–142	139–151	146–164
5′ 7″	138–145	142–154	149–168
5′ 8″	140–148	145–157	152–172
5′ 9″	142–151	148–160	155–176
5′ 10″	144–154	151–163	158–180
5′ 11″	146–157	154–166	161–184
6′ 0″	149–160	157–170	164–188
6′ 1″	152–164	160–174	168–192
6′ 2″	155–168	164–178	172–197
6′ 3″	158–172	167–182	176–202
6′ 4″	162–176	171–187	181–207
Women†			
4′ 10″	102–111	109–121	118–131
4′ 11″	103–113	111–123	120–134
5′ 0″	104–115	113–126	122–137
5′ 1″	106–118	115–129	125–140
5′ 2″	108–121	118–132	128–143
5′ 3″	111–124	121–135	131–147
5′ 4″	114–127	124–138	134–151
5′ 5″	117–130	127–141	137–155
5′ 6″	120–133	130–144	140–159
5′ 7″	123–136	133–147	143–163
5′ 8″	126–139	136–150	146–167
5′ 9″	129–142	139–153	149–170
5′ 10″	132–145	142–156	152–173
5′ 11″	135–148	145–159	155–176
6′ 0″	138–151	148–162	158–179

* Weights at ages 25 to 59 are based on lowest mortality. Weight in pounds is according to frame (in indoor clothing weighing 5 lb, shoes with 1-inch heels).

† Weights at ages 25 to 59 are based on lowest mortality. Weight in pounds is according to frame (in indoor clothing weighing 3 lb, shoes with 1-inch heels).

(Courtesy of Statistical Bulletin, Metropolitan Life Insurance Company.)

$$\text{BMI} = \frac{\text{weight in kilograms}}{\text{height}^2 \text{ in meters}} \quad \begin{matrix}(2.2 \text{ lb} = 1 \text{ kg}) \\ (39.37 \text{ inches} = 1 \text{ m})\end{matrix}$$

A quick method of determining BMI is displayed in Figure 42-1. Many health practitioners use this more accurate weight calculation as an initial assessment of nutritional status.

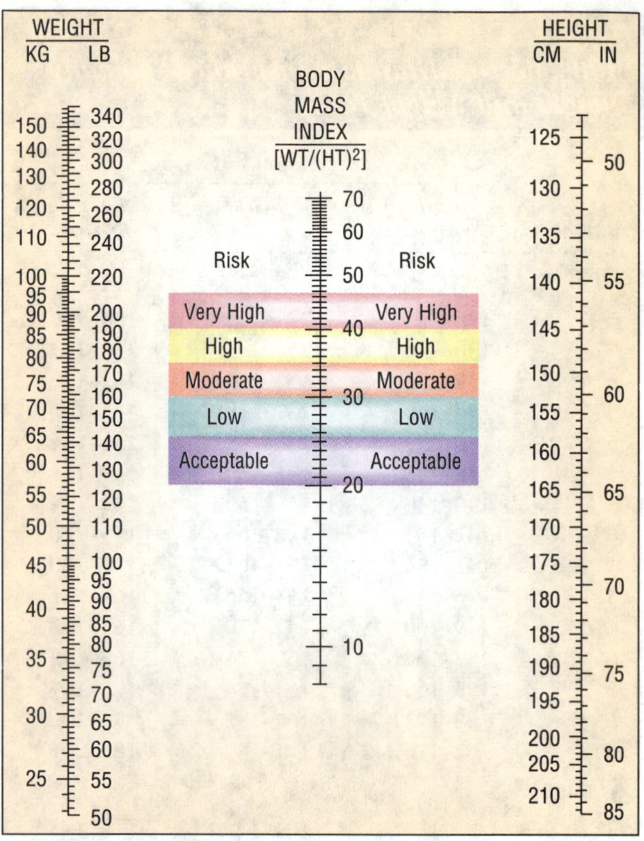

Figure 42-1
A quick way for determining BMI. Lay a straightedge across the figure, connecting your weight and height values. The point where the straightedge crosses the BMI line is the BMI in metric units (kg/m^2). (Wardlaw, G. & Insel, P. [1993]. *Perspectives in Nutrition* [2nd ed.] St. Louis: Mosby, p. 250.)

Caloric Requirements. Just as healthy body weight or IBW can be determined in a variety of ways, so can a person's calorie requirements. Three methods appear in the accompanying box. The Food and Nutrition Board, National Research Council, has published recommended energy intake ranges based on age and sex. The Bureau of Nutritional Sciences of the Department of National Health and Welfare (Canada) has developed a similar energy requirement table (see Appendix D). After calorie requirements have been determined, adjustments can be made for weight gain or loss as needed. For instance, 1 lb (0.45 kg) of body fat equals about 3500 cal. Therefore, to gain or lose 1 lb (0.45 kg) in a week, daily calorie intake should be increased or decreased, respectively, by 500 cal (3500 cal divided by 7 days = 500 cal/d). Similarly, a weight gain or loss of 2 lb (0.9 kg) per week would require an adjustment of 1000 cal/d. Because it becomes increasingly difficult to plan an adequate diet as the calorie level drops, diets that result in more than a 2-lb (0.9-kg) weight loss per week are not recommended.

Energy Nutrients

Carbohydrates

Significance. Carbohydrates, commonly known as sugars and starches, are organic compounds composed of carbon, hydrogen, and oxygen. They serve as the structural framework of plants; the only animal source of carbohydrate in the diet is lactose, or "milk sugar."

The significance of carbohydrates cannot be overstated. Because they are relatively easy to produce and store, carbohydrates are the most abundant and least expensive source of calories in the diet worldwide. In fact, carbohydrate intake is correlated to income: as income

Three Methods of Calculating Caloric Requirements

Method I

Adults

Multiply ideal body weight (IBW) by 10 to determine basal body requirements. Depending on activity level, multiply IBW by the appropriate number indicated below and add to the basal body requirement.

Activity	Calories
Sedentary	Basal calorie needs × 3
Moderate	Basal calorie needs × 5
Heavy	Basal calorie needs × 10

Children (under 12 years old)

Generally allow 1000 calories plus 100 calories per year of age. For example, a 4-year-old child needs about 1000 + (100 calories × 4) = 1400 calories.

Method II

Depending on activity level, multiply IBW in pounds by the appropriate number of calories.

Activity	Cal/lb of IBW
Sedentary	11-12
Light	13-14
Moderate	15-16
Heavy	18-19

Method III: USDA Guidelines for Calculating Caloric Requirements

Based on activity level, multiply IBW in pounds by the appropriate number of calories per pound according to sex.

	Cal/lb of IBW	
Activity	Males	Females
Sedentary	16	14
Moderate	21	18
Heavy	28	22

(Adapted from Dudek, S. G. [1993]. *Nutrition handbook for nursing practice* [2nd ed.]. Philadelphia: Lippincott.)

increases, carbohydrate intake decreases and protein intake, a more expensive form of energy, increases. In countries where grains are the dietary staple, carbohydrates may contribute as much as 90% of total calories. In the United States, the average person consumes about half of his or her total calories from carbohydrates, an amount many healthcare professionals think should be higher. In Canada, the recommended amount is 55% (Murray & Beare-Rogers, 1990).

Classification. Depending on the number of molecules within the structure, carbohydrates are classified as either simple sugars (monosaccharides and disaccharides) or complex (polysaccharides). *Monosaccharides* are composed of only one sugar molecule; as the simplest sugar, they are absorbed without undergoing digestion. Monosaccharides with nutritional significance include glucose (dextrose), fructose, and galactose.

Disaccharides are double sugars composed of glucose and one other monosaccharide. Disaccharides (ie, sucrose, lactose, and maltose) must be broken down by enzymes within the intestinal tract before they can be absorbed.

Polysaccharides, such as starch, glycogen, cellulose, and other types of fiber, are complex molecules composed of hundreds to thousands of glucose units. They are not sweet, and vary in their degree of digestibility. Table 42-2 summarizes the sources, functions, and significance of dietary carbohydrates.

Metabolism. Carbohydrates are more easily and quickly digested than protein and fat. Ninety percent of carbohydrate intake is digested; the percentage decreases as fiber intake increases.

Although a small amount of cooked starch may begin to be digested in the mouth, the primary site of chemical digestion is the small intestine. Polysaccharides and disaccharides are broken down into monosaccharides through the action of pancreatic and intestinal enzymes, which are complex protein molecules that facilitate chemical reactions without undergoing change themselves. Monosaccharides are absorbed through the intestinal mucosa and transported to the liver through the portal blood circulation. Cellulose and other undigestible fibers cannot be broken down by human enzymes and are, therefore, excreted in the feces unchanged.

In the liver, monosaccharides are converted to glucose, which may then be released into the bloodstream to keep serum glucose levels within a normal range (Fig. 42-2). Under normal conditions, certain tissues, particularly the central nervous system, rely on glucose as their sole source of fuel; therefore, a constant supply of glucose is necessary. Hormones, especially insulin and glucagon, are responsible for keeping serum glucose levels fairly constant during both feasting and fasting.

Through a series of steps, cells oxidize (burn) glucose to provide energy, carbon dioxide, and water. Depending on a person's state of energy balance, the period between carbohydrate consumption and when it is used for energy may vary from minutes to months or longer. Unlike protein and fat, glucose is burned efficiently and completely, and does not leave a toxic product for the kidneys to excrete.

When the supply of glucose exceeds what is needed for energy and to maintain serum levels, it is stored. If muscle or liver glycogen stores are deficient, glucose is converted to glycogen and stored (glycogenesis). Conversely, glycogen is broken down in time of need to supply a ready source of glucose (glycogenolysis). When glycogen stores are adequate, the body converts excess glucose to fat and stores it as triglycerides in adipose tissue.

Functions and Recommended Dietary Allowance. The primary function of carbohydrates is to supply energy. Except for undigestible fiber, all carbohydrates provide 4 cal/g, regardless of the source. Carbohydrates also function to spare protein (ie, using carbohydrates for energy spares protein so it can be used to carry on functions specific for protein, such as building and repairing tissue). Carbohydrates also are needed to burn fat efficiently for energy and thereby prevent ketosis. Research has indicated that carbohydrate intake may also affect a person's mood, resulting in increased fatigue and relaxation or mood elevation and lessening of depression depending on individual sensitivities to this nutrient (Cerrato, 1992).

The **recommended dietary allowance (RDA)** of essential nutrients refers to recommendations for average daily amounts that healthy population groups should consume over time. Although an exact requirement for carbohydrates has not been established, at least 50 to 100 g is needed daily to prevent ketosis. In terms of an optimal diet, most health experts recommend that carbohydrates provide 50% to 60% of the diet's total calories, mostly in the form of complex carbohydrates.

Protein

Significance. Protein is a vital component of every living cell. Within the human body, more than a thousand different proteins are made by combining various amounts and proportions of the 22 basic building blocks known as *amino acids*. Although amino acids, like carbohydrates, contain carbon, hydrogen, and oxygen, they differ in that amino acids also contain nitrogen. Nine amino acids are classified as essential because they cannot be synthesized in the body; the remaining amino acids are no less important, but because the body can make them if a supply of nitrogen is available, they are termed nonessential.

Classification. Dietary proteins may be labeled complete (high quality) or incomplete (low quality), based on their amino acid composition. *Complete proteins* con-

Table 42-2
Sources, Functions, and Significance of Carbohydrates, Protein, and Fat

Nutrient	Sources	Functions	Significance
Carbohydrates			
Simple sugars and starch	Fruits Vegetables Grains: rice, pasta, breads, cereals Dried peas and beans Milk (lactose) Sugars: white and brown sugar, honey, molasses, syrup	Provide energy Spare protein so it can be used for other functions Prevent ketosis from inefficient fat metabolism	Provide about 46% of the calories in the typical American diet (40% in Canadian); many believe carbohydrate intake should be increased to 50%–60% of total calories Low carbohydrate intake can cause ketosis; high simple sugar intake increases the risk of dental caries
Cellulose and other water insoluble fibers	Whole wheat flour and wheat bran Vegetables: cabbage, peas, green beans, wax beans, broccoli, brussels sprouts, cucumber skins, peppers, carrots Apples	Absorb water to increase fecal bulk Decrease intestinal transit time	Is nondigestible; therefore, it is excreted Helps relieve constipation North Americans are urged to eat more of all types of fiber Excess intake can cause gas, distention, and diarrhea
Water-soluble fibers	Oat bran and oatmeal Dried peas and beans Vegetables Prunes, pears, apples, bananas, oranges	Slow gastric emptying Lower serum cholesterol level Delay glucose absorption	Help improve glucose tolerance in diabetics
Protein	Milk and milk products Meat, poultry, fish Eggs Dried peas and beans Nuts	Tissue growth and repair Component of body framework: bones, muscles, tendons, blood vessels, skin, hair, nails Component of body fluids: hormones, enzymes, plasma proteins, neurotransmitters, mucus Helps regulate fluid balance through oncotic pressure Helps regulate acid–base balance Detoxifies harmful substances Forms antibodies Transports fat and other substances through the blood Provides energy when carbohydrate intake is inadequate	Most North Americans consume twice the RDA (RNI) for protein Experts recommend that we eat less animal protein and more vegetable protein. Protein deficiency is characterized by edema, retarded growth and maturation, muscle wasting, changes in the hair and skin, permanent damage to physical and mental development (in children), diarrhea, malabsorption, numerous secondary nutrient deficiencies, fatty infiltration of the liver, increased risk of infections, and high mortality Except for elderly people, fad dieters, hospitalized clients, and people of low income, protein deficiency is rare in the United States and Canada
Fat	Butter, oils, margarine, lard, salt pork, salad dressings, mayonnaise, bacon Whole milk and whole milk products High-fat meats Nuts	Provides energy Provides structure Insulates the body Cushions internal organs Necessary for the absorption of fat-soluble vitamins	Fat supplies about 37% of total calories in the typical North American diet; experts suggest a reduction to 30% or less of total calories High-fat diets increase the risk of heart disease and obesity, and are correlated with an increased risk of colon and breast cancers

(Dudek, S. G. [1993]. *Nutrition handbook for nursing practice* [2nd ed.]. Philadelphia: Lippincott.)

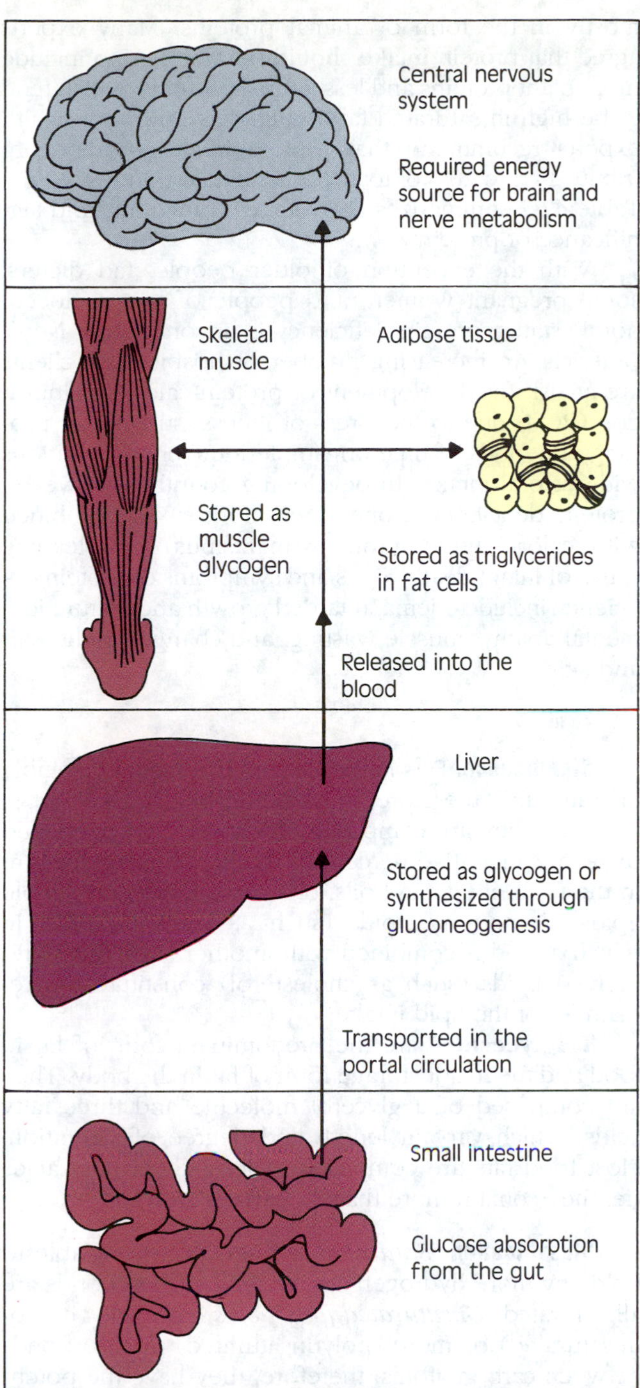

Figure 42-2
Glucose is an efficient fuel on which certain tissues, particularly the central nervous system, rely almost exclusively as an energy source. Glucose ingested in the diet is transported from the gastrointestinal tract, through the portal vein, to the liver. The liver stores glucose and regulates its entry into the blood. (Adapted from Porth, C. M. [1994]. *Pathophysiology: Concepts of altered health states* [4th ed.] Philadelphia: Lippincott.)

tain sufficient amounts and proportions of all the essential amino acids to support growth, whereas *incomplete proteins* are deficient in one or more essential amino acids. Generally, animal proteins (eggs, dairy products, and meats) are complete, and plant proteins (grains, legumes, and vegetables) are incomplete. Because different sources of plant proteins lack different amino acids, a plant protein can be complemented and its quality made high by combining it with a different plant protein or by adding a small amount of an animal protein. Examples of complementary vegetable proteins include corn tortilla and refried beans and lentil rice soup. Complementary proteins that use a small amount of animal protein are cereal with milk, rice pudding, and a cheese sandwich.

Metabolism. Chemical digestion of protein begins in the acid medium of the stomach; however, most protein digestion occurs in the small intestine through the action of pancreatic and intestinal proteases. Amino acids are absorbed through the intestinal mucosa into the portal blood circulation for transport to the liver. Neonates are uniquely able to absorb whole proteins—antibodies from breast milk—which affords them a certain degree of immunity from infections. Only a small amount of ingested protein normally remains undigested and is excreted in the feces.

Once in the liver, amino acids can then be recombined to form new proteins, or may be released into the bloodstream and carried to tissues and cells for protein synthesis (Fig. 42-3). The body's protein tissues are in a constant state of flux: tissues are continuously being broken down (catabolism) and replaced (anabolism). *Nitrogen balance*, a comparison between catabolism and anabolism, can be measured by comparing nitrogen intake (protein intake) and nitrogen excretion (nitrogen lost in urine, urea, feces, hair, nails, and skin). When catabolism and anabolism are occurring at the same rate, as in healthy adults, the body is in a state of neutral nitrogen balance (ie, nitrogen intake equals nitrogen excretion). A positive nitrogen balance occurs when nitrogen intake is greater than excretion—for example, during periods of growth, pregnancy, lactation, and recovery from illness. A negative nitrogen balance, an undesirable state such as starvation and the catabolism that immediately follows surgery, illness, trauma, and stress, indicates that more nitrogen is being excreted than consumed.

Functions. The major function of protein is to maintain body tissues that break down from normal wear and tear and to support the growth of new tissue. Protein also is a component of the body's framework (bones, muscles, tendons, blood vessels, skin, nails, and hair), many essential secretions and fluids (hormones, enzymes, neurotransmitters, breast milk, mucus, sperm, and bile acids), and body compounds, such as the blood-clotting factor thrombin. Protein plays a role in fluid and acid–base balance, helps to detoxify harmful foreign substances, and forms antibodies to help the

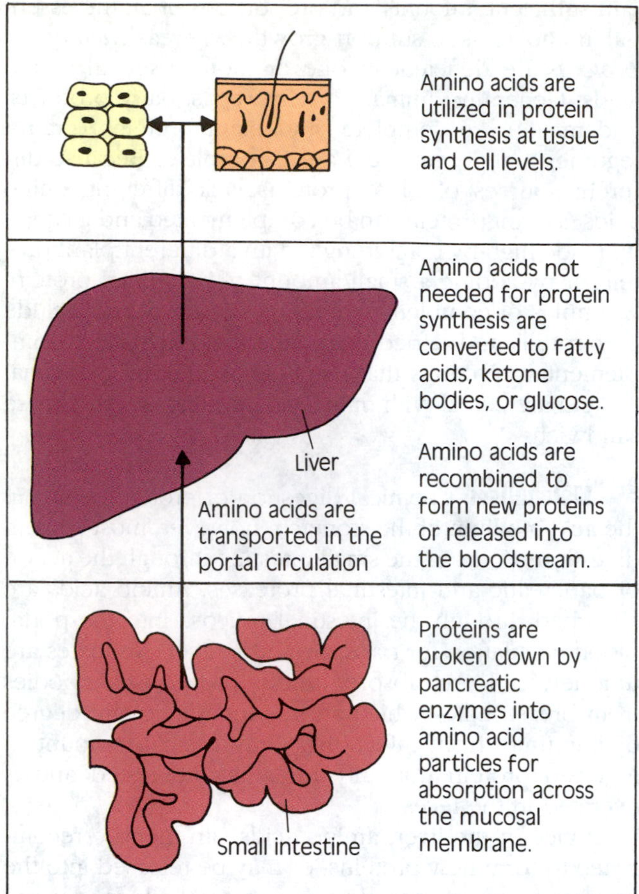

Figure 42-3
Dietary protein is broken down into amino acid particles by pancreatic enzymes in the small intestine and absorbed through the intestinal mucosa for transportation to the liver. In the liver, amino acids are recombined into new proteins or are released into the bloodstream for use in protein synthesis by tissues and cells. Excess amino acids are converted to fatty acids, ketone bodies, or glucose, and stored or used as metabolic fuel. Proteins are essential for the formation of all body structures, including genes, enzymes, muscle, bone matrix, and hemoglobin. Amino acids are the building blocks of protein.

body resist infection and certain diseases. It helps move fat, fat-soluble vitamins, minerals, and other substances through the blood. Lastly, protein can be oxidized to provide 4 cal/g. Using protein for energy is more expensive both financially and physiologically than using carbohydrates; the nitrogen remaining after protein is metabolized burdens the kidneys and requires energy to be excreted. Like carbohydrates, protein consumed in excess of need can be converted to and stored as fat.

Recommended Dietary Allowance. The recommended daily dietary allowance (RDA) for protein for adults is 0.8 g/kg of desirable body weight, or about 44 g for the average woman and 56 g for the average man. (Canadian protein requirements are listed in Appendix D.) Most Americans consume twice as much protein as this, mostly in the form of animal proteins. Many experts agree that protein intake should be modified to include more plant proteins and less animal proteins, which tend to be high in saturated fat and cholesterol. Most health experts recommend that protein intake should contribute 10% to 20% of total caloric intake (Dudek, 1993). Table 42-2 summarizes the sources, functions, and significance of protein.

With the exception of older people, fad dieters, some pregnant women, and people of low socioeconomic status, protein deficiency is uncommon in North America. An increasing number of hospitalized clients are at risk for development of protein-calorie malnutrition (PCM) due to the stress of illness, surgery, or prolonged periods of time on simple intravenous solutions without oral intake. In developing countries, however, protein deficiency alone (kwashiorkor) or combined with calorie undernutrition (marasmus) is a leading cause of infant death. Signs and symptoms of protein deficiency include edema, retarded growth and maturation, mental apathy, muscle wasting, and changes in the hair and skin.

Fats

Significance. Fats in the diet, or **lipids**, are insoluble in water and, therefore, insoluble in blood. Like carbohydrates, they are composed of carbon, hydrogen, and oxygen. Ninety-five percent of the lipids in the diet are in the form of fats and oils, otherwise known as simple lipids. Compound lipids (such as phospholipids, in which a lipid is combined with another substance) and derived lipids (such as cholesterol) constitute the remainder of the lipid intake.

Triglycerides are the predominant form of fat in food and the major storage form of fat in the body. They are composed of a glycerol molecule and three fatty acids, which vary in length and degree of saturation. Most food fats are composed of long-chain fatty acids (ie, they contain more than 12 carbon atoms).

Classification. *Saturated fatty acids* are not able to hold any more hydrogen atoms; their carbon bonds are all saturated. *Unsaturated fatty acids* have one (monounsaturated) or more (polyunsaturated) double bonds between carbon atoms; therefore, they have the potential to hold more hydrogen atoms if the double bonds are broken. Food fats contain mixtures of saturated and unsaturated fatty acids. Most animal fats are considered saturated because they contain proportionately more saturated fatty acids and have a solid consistency at room temperature. Conversely, most vegetable fats are considered unsaturated because they contain more unsaturated than saturated fatty acids. Unsaturated fats are liquid at room temperature and referred to as oils. Commercially, the addition of hydrogen atoms to unsaturated fats (hydrogenation) makes a fat more saturated and thereby increases its shelf life and stability. Saturated fats tend to raise serum cholesterol levels, whereas unsaturated fats lower serum cholesterol levels.

Cholesterol is a fatlike substance found only in animal products. It is not essential that cholesterol be provided in the diet because the body synthesizes about twice as much cholesterol as most people in North America eat. Cholesterol is an important component of cell membranes and is especially abundant in brain and nerve cells. It also is used to synthesize bile acids and is a precursor of the steroid hormones and vitamin D. Although cholesterol serves many important functions in the body, high serum levels are clearly associated with an increased risk of atherosclerosis. To help lower serum cholesterol levels, researchers recommend limiting cholesterol intake, eating less total fat—especially saturated fat—eating more unsaturated fat, and increasing fiber intake, which increases fecal excretion of cholesterol.

Linoleic acid is the only fatty acid the body cannot synthesize; therefore, it is labeled essential. Linoleic acid is important for capillary strength and cell membrane structure, is a precursor of prostaglandins, and helps decrease serum cholesterol levels. Because the requirement for linoleic acid is so small (about 2% to 3% of total calories), a deficiency is rare. The best sources of linoleic acid are polyunsaturated vegetable oils, such as sunflower, soybean, and corn.

Metabolism. Fat digestion occurs largely in the small intestine. Bile, secreted by the gallbladder, emulsifies fat to increase the surface area so that pancreatic lipase can break down fat more effectively. Through a complex series of events, most fats are absorbed into the lymphatic circulation with the help of a protein carrier and are transported to the liver (Fig. 42-4). Of 100 g eaten, only about 3 g are excreted in the feces.

Functions. Fats are the most concentrated source of energy in the diet, providing 9 cal for every gram. Fat increases the palatability of the diet (eg, to most people, filet mignon tastes better than flank steak) and has a high satiety value because it delays gastric emptying time. In the body, fat aids in the absorption of the fat-soluble vitamins and provides insulation, structure, and temperature control. Table 42-2 summarizes the source, functions, and significance of fat.

Recommended Dietary Allowance. Because fat can be synthesized in the body from carbohydrates and protein, an RDA for fat has not been established. Americans consume about 37% of their total caloric intake in the form of fat. Most experts agree that fat should not contribute more than 30% of the day's caloric intake, and saturated fat intake should be limited to 10% or less of total fat calories (Dudek, 1993).

Regulatory Nutrients

Vitamins, minerals, and water are regulatory nutrients because they are needed by the body for the metabolism of energy nutrients.

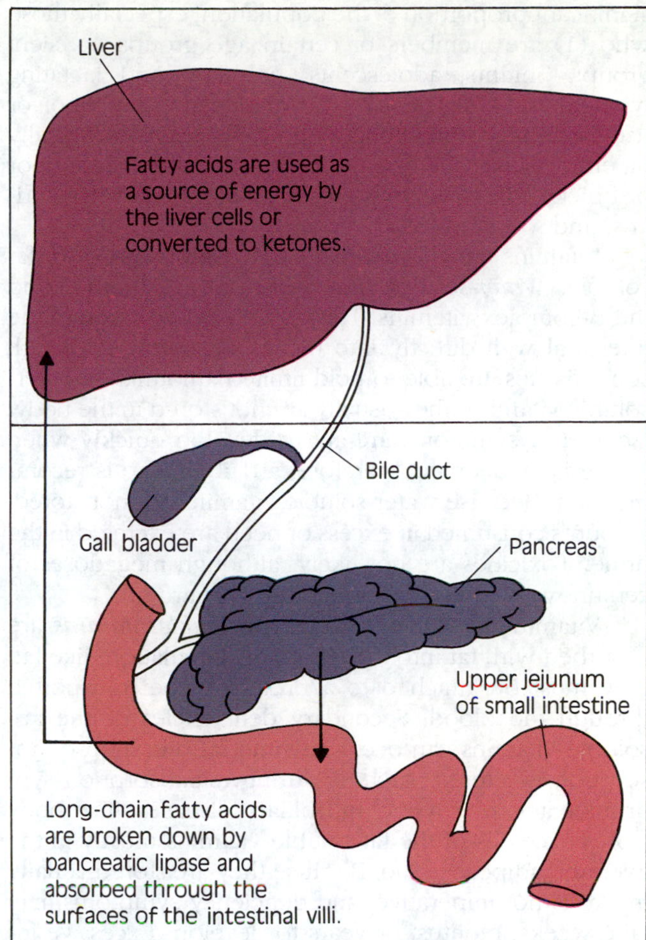

Figure 42-4
The average adult consumes 60 to 100 g of fat daily, mostly as triglycerides. These triglycerides are broken down by pancreatic lipase and are absorbed primarily in the upper jejunum. Fatty acids transported to the liver are used by the liver cells as a source of energy or are converted to ketones.

Vitamins

Vitamins are organic compounds needed by the body in small amounts. Most vitamins are active in the form of coenzymes, which together with enzymes facilitate thousands of chemical reactions in the body. Although vitamins do not provide energy (calories), they are needed for the metabolism of carbohydrates, protein, and fat. Because most vitamins are either not synthesized in the body or made in insufficient quantities, they are essential in the diet.

Vitamins are present in foods in only small amounts. Because vitamins may be destroyed by light, heat, and air and during preparation, fresh foods are higher in vitamins than processed foods. The exception is in the case of fortification, when vitamins that do not naturally occur in a food are added (eg, vitamin D–fortified milk).

In North America, severe vitamin deficiencies are uncommon. Mild or subclinical deficiencies of vitamin A, vitamin C, folate, and vitamin B_6, however, may affect a significant proportion of the population, especially those who (1) are members of certain age groups or client groups (infants, adolescents, pregnant and lactating women, and older people); (2) smoke, abuse alcohol, or use medications on a long-term basis; (3) are chronically ill, either physically or psychologically; and (4) are poor or finicky eaters, such as chronic dieters, strict vegetarians, and food faddists.

Vitamins are classified as either water soluble or fat soluble. *Water-soluble vitamins* include vitamin C and the B-complex vitamins. They are absorbed through the intestinal wall directly into the bloodstream. Although some tissues are able to hold limited amounts of water-soluble vitamins, they usually are not stored in the body. Deficiency symptoms are apt to develop quickly when intake is inadequate; therefore, a daily intake is recommended. Because water-soluble vitamins are not stored, amounts consumed in excess of need are excreted in the urine. Toxicities are not likely, although megadoses of certain water-soluble vitamins can be harmful.

Vitamins A, D, E, and K, the *fat-soluble vitamins*, are absorbed with fat into the lymphatic circulation; like fat, they must be attached to a protein to be transported through the blood. Secondary deficiencies of the fat-soluble vitamins can occur anytime fat digestion or absorption is altered, such as during malabsorption syndromes and pancreatic and biliary diseases. The body stores excesses of the fat-soluble vitamins mostly in the liver and adipose tissue. Because they are stored, a daily intake is not imperative, and deficiency symptoms may take weeks, months, or years to develop. Excessive intakes, particularly of vitamins A and D, are toxic.

Vitamins have been promoted as a cure-all by many enthusiasts. In addition to promoting improved health and vitality, vitamins have been touted as protection against birth defects, heart disease, and cancer. Many researchers fall short of endorsing these claims but agree that vitamin supplements may be valuable in certain situations. Many nutrition experts still believe that adequate amounts of most vitamins can be obtained from a healthy diet. While scrutiny and research continue about vitamin supplements and their long-term effects, most nutritionists agree that vitamins will never be a substitute for good nutrition and healthy lifestyle practices.

Table 42-3 summarizes water- and fat-soluble vitamins. (Canadian Recommended Nutrient Intakes [RNI] are listed in Appendix D.)

Minerals

Minerals are inorganic elements found in all body fluids and tissues in the form of salts (eg, sodium chloride) or combined with organic compounds (eg, iron in hemoglobin). Some minerals function to provide structure within the body, whereas others help to regulate body processes. Because they are elements, minerals are not broken down or rearranged in the body but are contained in the ash that remains after digestion. Although excessive soaking and cooking in water can cause loss of minerals from food, minerals commonly are not destroyed by food processing. Calcium, phosphorus, and magnesium are considered *macrominerals* because they are needed by the body in amounts greater than 100 mg/day. Required intake of *microminerals* or trace elements is less than 100 mg/day. Iron, zinc, manganese, and iodine are examples of microminerals. Trace elements with an established RDA or RNI (Canada) include iron, iodine, and zinc. Ranges of estimated safe and adequate daily intakes have been suggested for copper, manganese, fluorine, chromium, selenium, and molybdenum; no recommendations have been made for cobalt, nickel, vanadium, arsenic, and silicon. Macrominerals and microminerals are summarized in Table 42-4. (Canadian RNIs are listed in Appendix D.)

Water

As the major body constituent present in every body cell, water accounts for between 50% and 60% of the adult's total weight; infants have proportionately more water. About two-thirds of the body's water is contained within the cells (intracellular fluid [ICF]); the remainder is called extracellular fluid (ECF), and includes all other body fluids, such as plasma and interstitial fluid. Total body water and ECF decrease with age; ICF increases with an increase in body mass.

Water is more vital to life than food because it provides the fluid medium necessary for all chemical reactions, it participates in many reactions, and it is not stored in the body. Water acts as a solvent that dissolves many solutes, thereby aiding digestion, absorption, circulation, and excretion. Through evaporation from the skin, water helps to regulate body temperature. As a lubricant, water is needed for mucous secretions and between moving joints.

Sources of water in the diet include not only beverages but also solid foods, which contain from 10% to 98% water. Water also is produced through the metabolism of carbohydrates, protein, and fat. It leaves the body through urine, feces, expired air, and perspiration. Water intake (an average of 1500 to 3000 mL/day) usually equals water output. Water balance may be seriously affected when either intake (eg, in comatose states) or output (eg, in altered renal function, profuse perspiration, diarrhea, vomiting, fistulas, drainage tubes, hemorrhage, and severe burns) is altered.

How to Choose an Adequate Diet

An adequate diet provides a balanced intake of all essential nutrients in appropriate amounts; what constitutes an adequate diet is less obvious. Although a major problem in developing countries, malnutrition related to poor dietary intake is uncommon in North America. Rather, nutritional concerns focus more on problems of overnutrition. Tools for planning or evaluating a diet for adequacy include the Food Guide Pyramid, the RDA or

Table 42-3
Summary of Vitamins

Nutrient and Adult RDA*	Sources	Functions	Signs and Symptoms of Deficiency	Signs and Symptoms of Excess
Water-Soluble Vitamins				
Vitamin C (ascorbic acid) 60 mg (60–100 mg for smokers)	Citrus fruits, broccoli, green pepper, strawberries, greens	Collagen formation, antioxidant, enhances iron absorption	Scurvy, hemorrhaging, delayed wound healing	Kidney stones, scurvy on withdrawal, nausea, diarrhea
Vitamin B Complex				
Thiamin 1–1.4 mg	Pork, liver, whole and enriched grains, legumes	Co-enzyme in key reactions that produce energy from glucose	Beriberi, mental confusion, fatigue	None known
Riboflavin 1.2–1.7 mg	Milk, organ meats, enriched grains, greens	Carbohydrate, protein, and fat metabolism	Ariboflavinosis—symptoms related to inflammation and poor wound healing	None known
Niacin 13–19 mg	Kidney, grains, lean meat, nuts	Carbohydrate, protein, and fat metabolism	Pellagra, dermatitis	Flushing and itching, nausea, vomiting
B_6 (pyridoxine) 1.6–2 mg	Yeast, banana, cantaloupe, broccoli, spinach	Co-enzyme in protein, fat, carbohydrate metabolism	Anemia, CNS problems	Difficulty walking, numbness of feet and hands
Folate 180–200 μg	Green leafy vegetables, liver	RNA and DNA synthesis, formation and maturation of RBC	Macrocytic anemia: fatigue, weakness, pallor	None known
B_{12} (cobalamin) 2 μg	Only animal foods: organ meats, seafood	Co-enzyme in protein metabolism and formation of heme portion of hemoglobin	Pernicious anemia (B_{12} deficiency related to impaired absorption due to lack of intrinsic factor)	None known
Pantothenic acid 4–7 mg	Liver, egg yolk, yeast	Carbohydrate, protein, and fat metabolism	None known	None known
Biotin 30–100 μg	Liver, egg yolk	Carbohydrate, protein, and fat metabolism	Deficiency produced by adding large amounts of raw egg white to a biotin-deficient diet	None known
Fat-Soluble Vitamins				
Vitamin A (retinol, retinal, retinoic acid) 800–1000 RE	Liver, carrots, egg yolk, fortified milk	Visual acuity in dim light, formation and maintenance of skin and mucous membranes	Night blindness, rough skin	Anorexia, loss of hair, dry skin, bone pain
Vitamin D (cholecalciferol, ergosterol) 5–10 μg	Sunlight, fortified milk, fish liver oils	Calcium and phosphorus metabolism, stimulates calcium absorption	Retarded bone growth, bone malformation	Excessive calcification of bones, renal calculi, nausea, headache
Vitamin E (tocopherol) 8–10 mg	Vegetable oils, wheat germ, whole-grain products	Antioxidant, protects vitamin A, heme synthesis	Increased RBC hemolysis and macrocytic anemia in premature infants	Relatively nontoxic, although large doses can cause fatigue, diarrhea
Vitamin K 65–80 μg	Dark, green leafy vegetables; synthesized in intestines from gut bacteria	Synthesis of certain proteins necessary for blood clotting	Hemorrhagic disease of newborn, delayed blood clotting	Hemolytic anemia and liver damage with synthetic vitamin K

* See Appendix D for Canadian RNIs.

(Dudek, S.G. [1993]. *Nutrition handbook for nursing practice* [2nd ed.]. Philadelphia: Lippincott; and Williams, S. [1994]. *Essentials of nutrition and diet therapy* [6th ed.]. St. Louis: Mosby.)

Table 42-4
Summary of Macrominerals and Microminerals

Nutrient and Adult RDA*	Sources	Functions	Signs and Symptoms of Deficiency	Signs and Symptoms of Excess
Macrominerals				
Calcium 800 mg (18–24 yr: 1200 mg)	Milk and dairy products, canned fish with bones, greens	Bone and tooth formation, blood clotting, nerve transmission, muscle contraction	Tetany, osteoporosis	Renal calculi in susceptible people
Phosphorus 800 mg (11–24 yr: 1200 mg)	Milk and milk products, soft drinks, processed foods	Bone and tooth formation, acid–base balance, energy metabolism	Hypophosphatemia: anorexia, muscle weakness	Hyperphosphatemia: symptoms of hypocalcemic tetany
Magnesium 280–350 mg	Green leafy vegetables, nuts, beans, grains	Bone and tooth formation, protein synthesis, carbohydrate metabolism	Hypomagnesemia: weakness, muscle pain, poor heart function	Hypermagnesemia: CNS depression, coma, hypotension
Sulfur (provided by adequate amounts of protein)	Meat, eggs, milk, dried peas and beans, nuts	Promotes certain enzyme reactions and detoxification reactions	None known	None known
Sodium 500 mg	Salt, processed foods	Major ion of extracellular fluid, fluid balance, acid–base balance	Hyponatremia: muscle cramps, cold and clammy skin	Edema, weight gain, high blood pressure if susceptible
Potassium 1600–2000 mg	Whole grains, fruits, leafy vegetables	Major ion of intracellular fluid, fluid balance, acid–base balance	Hypokalemia: muscle cramps and weakness, irregular heart beat	Hyperkalemia: irritability, anxiety, cardiac arrhythmia, heart block
Chlorine 750 mg (minimum requirement)	Salt	Component of HCI in stomach, fluid balance, acid–base balance	Hypochloremia: muscle spasms, alkalosis, depressed respirations	Hyperchloremia: acidosis
Microminerals				
Iron 10–15 mg	Liver, lean meats, enriched and whole-grain breads and cereals	Oxygen transport by way of hemoglobin, constituent of enzyme systems	Microcytic anemia, pallor, decreased work capacity, fatigue, weakness	Hemosiderosis; acute iron poisoning from accidental overdose leads to GI symptoms and possible shock
Iodine 150 mg	Iodized salt, seafood, food additives	Component of thyroid hormones	Goiter	Acne-like skin lesions
Zinc 12–15 mg	Oysters, liver, meats, dried peas and beans, nuts	Tissue growth, sexual maturation, immune response	Impaired growth, sexual maturation, immune system functioning	Anorexia, nausea, vomiting, diarrhea, muscle pain, lethargy
Copper 1.5–3 mg	Liver, shellfish, grains, dried peas and beans	Aids in iron metabolism and activity of some enzymes	Anemia, altered bone formation, hypercholesterolemia	Nervous system disturbances, vomiting
Manganese 2–5 mg	Whole grains, nuts, dried peas and beans, fruit	Part of enzymes needed for protein and energy metabolism	Poor reproductive performance, growth retardation	None known
Fluoride 1.5–4 mg (estimated safe, adequate intake)	Fluoridated water, fish, tea	Tooth formation and integrity, bone formation and integrity	Tooth decay; may increase risk of osteoporosis	Mottling and discoloration of tooth enamel

(continued)

Table 42-4 *(continued)*
Summary of Macrominerals and Microminerals

Nutrient and Adult RDA*	Sources	Functions	Signs and Symptoms of Deficiency	Signs and Symptoms of Excess
Chromium 50–200 μg	Whole grains, meats	Cofactor for insulin, proper glucose metabolism	Impaired glucose tolerance, insulin resistance	None known
Selenium 55–70 μg	Wheat (if grown in high selenium soil), organ meats	Antioxidant	None known	Loss of hair, brittle fingernails, fatigue
Molybdenum 75–250 μg (estimated safe, adequate intake)	Liver, whole grains, dried peas and beans, organ meats	Oxidizes sulfur and products of sulfur metabolism	None known	Interferes with copper metabolism
Cobalt Unknown—apparently minute	Organ meats	Essential component of vitamin B_{12}	None known	None known

* See Appendix D for Canadian RNIs.

(Dudek, S.G. [1993]. *Nutrition handbook for nursing practice* [2nd ed.]. Philadelphia: Lippincott; and Williams, S. [1994]. *Essentials of nutrition and diet therapy* [6th ed.]. St. Louis: Mosby.)

RNI, dietary recommendations and guidelines issued from health and U.S. governmental agencies, Nutrition Recommendations for Canadians, and Canada's Food Guide. The task of promoting health through proper nutrition has been made easier by new labeling regulations that provide specific information about food contents and their comparison to recommended daily intakes.

Food Guide Pyramid

In response to the concerns of nutritionists and health officials coupled with public interest in fitness and health, the U.S. Department of Agriculture developed the Food Guide Pyramid (Fig. 42-5). This graphic device places the grain and cereal group at the base of the pyramid followed by the fruit and vegetable group, the meat and dairy groups, and a fat, oil, and sweets group at the peak. The intent of the pyramid is to emphasize the grain and cereal group as the basic food in the diet with the less desirable groups playing a much smaller nutritional role. Each of these groups provides some nutrients, but all are required, in proper proportions, for a healthy diet. Initially, representatives of the meat and dairy industries were critical of the food pyramid and temporarily stalled its adoption. After minor design changes, however, the final version of the Food Guide Pyramid was adopted in April 1992.

The Food Guide Pyramid was designed to represent a total diet and to provide a firm foundation for health. It represents a focus on wellness and recognition of the role that food plays in prevention of such chronic disease threats as heart disease, high blood pressure, some types of cancer, diabetes, and obesity. To use the Food Guide Pyramid effectively, consumers should do the following:

- Make an effort to eat at least the minimum number of recommended servings from each of the lower five groups.
- Learn what constitutes a serving size in each group (typical serving sizes are displayed in the box accompanying Fig. 42-5).
- Understand that children over 6 years should use adult serving sizes, whereas children between 2 and 5 years of age should consume two-thirds of adult serving recommendations. Diet for younger children should follow physician's recommendations (Nurses' Guide to Good Nutrition and Sensible Weight Loss, 1993).

Recommended Dietary Allowance and Recommended Nutrient Intakes

The RDA, prepared by the Committee on Dietary Allowances of the Food and Nutrition Board (see Appendix C), and the RNI, prepared by the Health Promotion Directorate, National Health and Welfare in Canada (see Appendix D), are recommendations for average daily amounts of nutrients considered to be adequate to meet the known nutritional needs of practically all healthy people. Unlike a requirement, which is the amount of a nutrient needed to prevent a deficiency, an allowance has a safety factor built in to account for individual variations. Because the RDA and the RNI are intended for populations and not individuals, some people may not be able to meet their individual requirements, despite consuming the RDA or RNI. Likewise, it is possible for some people to eat less than the RDA or RNI and still avoid deficiencies. Although RDAs and RNIs are defined for age and sex and are revised about every 5 years as new information becomes available, they have not been

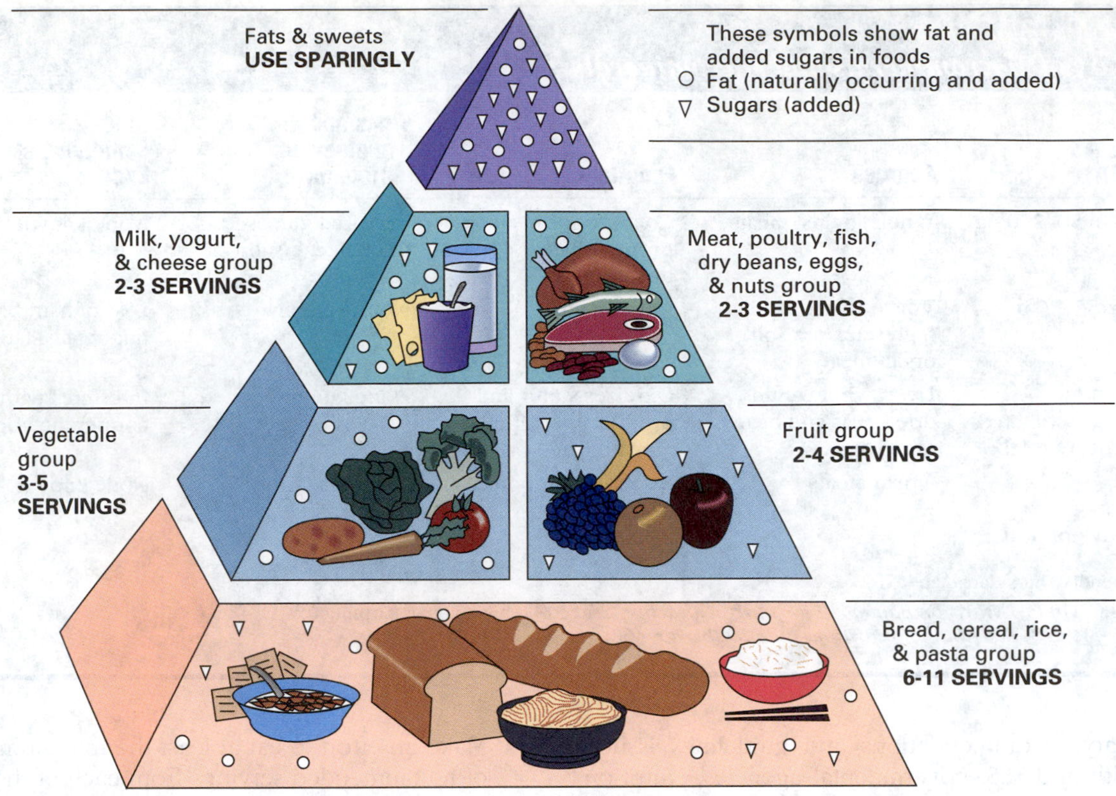

Figure 42-5
The Food Guide Pyramid. (Source: U.S. Department of Agriculture, April 1992.)

established for all nutrients. Like the food pyramid approach, variety is recommended.

Dietary Recommendations

The diet recommendations and guidelines proposed by numerous governmental and health agencies complement the food pyramid approach to diet planning and the RDAs and RNIs through their focus on avoiding nutritional excesses. Although these diet recommendations are not guaranteed to prevent diseases, many experts believe that most Americans and Canadians can reduce their risk of chronic diet-related diseases, such as diabetes, certain types of cancer, and heart disease, by modifying the typical diet. The U.S. Department of Health and Human Services Public Health Service re-

Food Guide Pyramid: Typical Serving Size

Bread, Cereal, Rice, & Pasta Group

1 slice of bread
½ cup of cooked rice, pasta, or cereal
1 ounce of ready-to-eat cereal
½ English muffin

Vegetable Group

½ cup of chopped raw or cooked vegetables
1 cup of leafy raw vegetables

Fruit Group

1 medium piece of fruit or melon wedge
¾ cup of juice
½ cup of canned fruit
¼ cup of dried fruit

Milk, Yogurt, & Cheese Group

1 cup of milk or yogurt
1½ ounces of natural cheese
2 ounces of processed cheese

Meat, Poultry, Fish, Dry Beans, Eggs, & Nut Group

2½ to 3 ounces of cooked lean meat, poultry, or fish
Count ½ cup of cooked beans, or 1 egg, or 2 tablespoons of peanut butter as 1 ounce of lean meat.

Fats & Sweets

Limit calories from these, especially if you need to lose weight.

(U.S. Department of Agriculture and the U.S. Department of Health and Human Services)

leased a report in 1990 with expanded goals for promoting healthy lifestyle habits into the next decade. This document, titled *Healthy People 2000*, included seven broad nutritional challenges as part of overall strategies for health promotion. These guidelines were updated in 1995 (see accompanying box). Canadian standards are similar to U.S. standards.

Food Labeling

Regulations that control food labels have always been controversial. In 1975, the *Food and Drug Administration* (FDA), a federal agency charged with protecting the U.S. food and drug supply, enacted legislation for a standardized label format that was considered a positive step toward educating the consumer about nutrition. Confusion and misinformation resulted as food manufacturers oversimplified or exaggerated health claims for their products. In the fall of 1990, Congress passed the Nutritional Labeling and Education Act, which requires all foods, including fruits and vegetables, to be clearly labeled. Four broad categories are addressed in this legislation. They include nutrition labeling, serving sizes, descriptors, and health claims (Couig, 1993). Consumers will easily be able to identify the amount of saturated fat and dietary fiber included in a product, in addition to viewing a listing of other nutritional information. Figure 42-6 illustrates a sample label with explanation of terms. Canadian food products are labeled by content (not necessarily the amounts), and the breakdown lists the amount of protein, carbohydrate, fat, sugar, starch, dietary fiber, sodium, and potassium (given in milligrams or grams and percentage of recommended daily allowances). All professional organizations agree that the food label is primarily a tool to educate the public about nutrition, and they expect the new law to go a long way toward ensuring that nutritional labeling is responsible and accurate.

Dietary Guidelines for Americans

- Eat a variety of foods.
- Balance the food you eat with physical activity; maintain or improve your weight.
- Choose a diet with plenty of grain products, vegetables, and fruits.
- Choose a diet low in fat, saturated fat, and cholesterol.
- Choose a diet moderate in sugars.
- Choose a diet moderate in salt and sodium.
- If you drink alcoholic beverages, do so in moderation.

(Report of the Dietary Guidelines Advisory Committee on the Dietary Guidelines for Americans. [1995]. U.S. Department of Agriculture and the U.S. Department of Health and Human Services.)

Factors Affecting Nutrition

Although nutritional adequacy is an important consideration in planning a diet, a person's food patterns and habits may have a greater impact on overall food intake. Food habits are a product of many evolving variables, such as physical factors (eg, geographic location, food technology, and income), physiologic factors (eg, health, hunger, and stage of development), and psychosocial factors (eg, culture, religion, tradition, education, politics, social status, food ideology, and learned aversions). Although not static, conservative traditional influences, like culture, geographic region, and religion, have a stabilizing effect on food habits.

Physiologic Factors That Influence Nutrient Requirements

Developmental Considerations. Throughout the life cycle, nutrient needs change in relation to growth, development, activity, and age-related changes in metabolism and body composition. Periods of intense growth and development, such as during infancy, adolescence, pregnancy, and lactation, cause an increase in nutrient needs. Nutrient needs stabilize during adulthood, although older people may need more or less of some nutrients. Older women, for example, are candidates for specific dietary interventions related to an increased risk for coronary heart disease, breast cancer, and osteoporosis. Yen (1994b) suggests the following dietary recommendations to protect this population from chronic disease:

- Reduce dietary fat intake to 30% or less.
- Eat 25 g of fiber daily.
- Include 5 to 9 servings of fruits and vegetables daily (emphasize vitamins A & C).
- Ensure an intake of 1000 to 1500 mg of calcium daily.
- Use alcohol and caffeine sparingly.

Refer to the box for general nutritional problems that affect older adults.

Age influences not only nutrient requirements but also food intake. The consistency of food, eating patterns, and the significance of food change with physical and psychosocial development. Nutrient needs and developmental landmarks are summarized in Table 42-5.

Sex. Men have somewhat different nutrient requirements than women related to differences in body composition and reproductive function. Their larger muscle mass translates into higher caloric and protein requirements (and therefore slightly higher needs for B vitamins that metabolize calories and protein) because it is more metabolically active than adipose tissue, of which women proportionately have more. Women of childbearing age have higher iron requirements related to menstruation.

(text continues on page 1168)

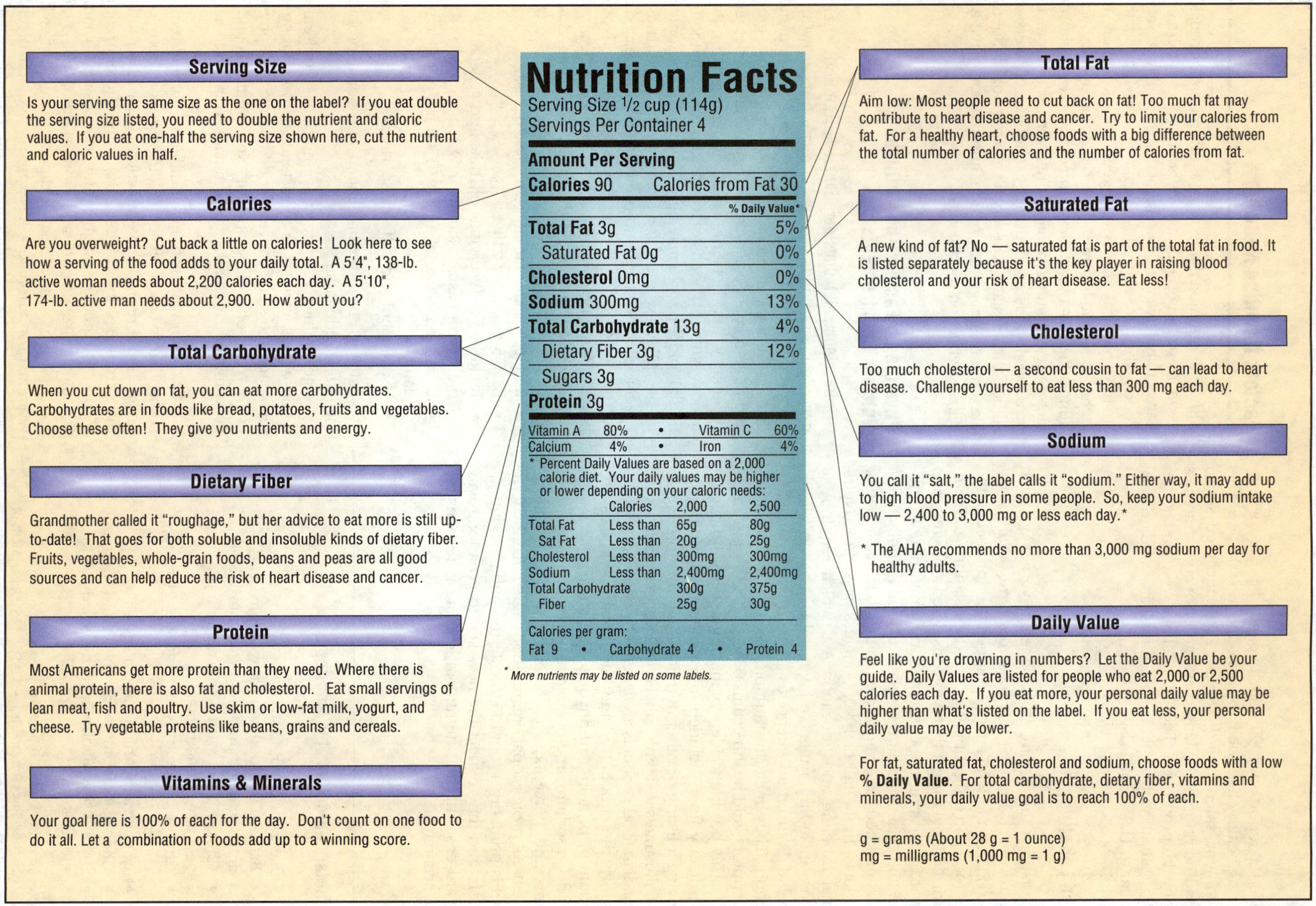

Serving Size

Is your serving the same size as the one on the label? If you eat double the serving size listed, you need to double the nutrient and caloric values. If you eat one-half the serving size shown here, cut the nutrient and caloric values in half.

Calories

Are you overweight? Cut back a little on calories! Look here to see how a serving of the food adds to your daily total. A 5'4", 138-lb. active woman needs about 2,200 calories each day. A 5'10", 174-lb. active man needs about 2,900. How about you?

Total Carbohydrate

When you cut down on fat, you can eat more carbohydrates. Carbohydrates are in foods like bread, potatoes, fruits and vegetables. Choose these often! They give you nutrients and energy.

Dietary Fiber

Grandmother called it "roughage," but her advice to eat more is still up-to-date! That goes for both soluble and insoluble kinds of dietary fiber. Fruits, vegetables, whole-grain foods, beans and peas are all good sources and can help reduce the risk of heart disease and cancer.

Protein

Most Americans get more protein than they need. Where there is animal protein, there is also fat and cholesterol. Eat small servings of lean meat, fish and poultry. Use skim or low-fat milk, yogurt, and cheese. Try vegetable proteins like beans, grains and cereals.

Vitamins & Minerals

Your goal here is 100% of each for the day. Don't count on one food to do it all. Let a combination of foods add up to a winning score.

Nutrition Facts

Serving Size 1/2 cup (114g)
Servings Per Container 4

Amount Per Serving	
Calories 90	Calories from Fat 30
	% Daily Value*
Total Fat 3g	5%
Saturated Fat 0g	0%
Cholesterol 0mg	0%
Sodium 300mg	13%
Total Carbohydrate 13g	4%
Dietary Fiber 3g	12%
Sugars 3g	
Protein 3g	

Vitamin A	80%	•	Vitamin C	60%
Calcium	4%	•	Iron	4%

* Percent Daily Values are based on a 2,000 calorie diet. Your daily values may be higher or lower depending on your caloric needs:

	Calories	2,000	2,500
Total Fat	Less than	65g	80g
Sat Fat	Less than	20g	25g
Cholesterol	Less than	300mg	300mg
Sodium	Less than	2,400mg	2,400mg
Total Carbohydrate		300g	375g
Fiber		25g	30g

Calories per gram:
Fat 9 • Carbohydrate 4 • Protein 4

* *More nutrients may be listed on some labels.*

Total Fat

Aim low: Most people need to cut back on fat! Too much fat may contribute to heart disease and cancer. Try to limit your calories from fat. For a healthy heart, choose foods with a big difference between the total number of calories and the number of calories from fat.

Saturated Fat

A new kind of fat? No — saturated fat is part of the total fat in food. It is listed separately because it's the key player in raising blood cholesterol and your risk of heart disease. Eat less!

Cholesterol

Too much cholesterol — a second cousin to fat — can lead to heart disease. Challenge yourself to eat less than 300 mg each day.

Sodium

You call it "salt," the label calls it "sodium." Either way, it may add up to high blood pressure in some people. So, keep your sodium intake low — 2,400 to 3,000 mg or less each day.*

* The AHA recommends no more than 3,000 mg sodium per day for healthy adults.

Daily Value

Feel like you're drowning in numbers? Let the Daily Value be your guide. Daily Values are listed for people who eat 2,000 or 2,500 calories each day. If you eat more, your personal daily value may be higher than what's listed on the label. If you eat less, your personal daily value may be lower.

For fat, saturated fat, cholesterol and sodium, choose foods with a low **% Daily Value**. For total carbohydrate, dietary fiber, vitamins and minerals, your daily value goal is to reach 100% of each.

g = grams (About 28 g = 1 ounce)
mg = milligrams (1,000 mg = 1 g)

Figure 42-6
Sample nutritional label with explanation of terms. (Source: American Heart Association.)

Focus on the Older Adult

Nursing Strategies for Nutritional Problems Affecting Older Adults

Altered Ability to Chew Related to Loss of Teeth, Ill-Fitting Dentures, and Gingivitis

- Encourage and instruct client to care for and retain own teeth and dentures.
- Encourage proper tooth-brushing and use of special toothpaste if gums and teeth are sensitive.
- Chop, shred, or puree foods that are difficult to chew.
- Select ground meat, fish, or poultry as protein sources more easily chewed.

Loss of Senses of Smell and Taste

- Serve food that is attractive and at proper temperature.
- Eat one food at a time rather than mixing foods.
- Serve foods with different textures and aromas.

Decreased Peristalsis in the Esophagus

- Avoid cold liquids.
- Avoid emotional upsets and stress-producing situations.
- Take anticholinergic drugs as ordered by physician.

Gastroesophageal Reflux

- Avoid overeating.
- Avoid juices, chocolate, and fat.
- Avoid alcohol and smoking.
- Elevate the head of the bed 30 to 40 degrees when sleeping.
- Lose weight if necessary.
- Avoid bending over.
- Take antacids or other medications as ordered by physician.

Decreased Gastric Secretions

- Chew food thoroughly.
- Eat meals on a regular schedule.
- Use antacids or other medications as prescribed by physician.
- Be alert for symptoms of deficiency of nutrients, particularly iron, calcium, fat, protein, and vitamin B_{12}.
- Ensure adequate intake of vitamin D for calcium absorption.

Slowed Intestinal Peristalsis

- Eat a high-fiber diet.
- Remain as active as possible.
- Increase fluid intake.
- Avoid laxative use.
- Eat meals at a regular time.
- Drink prune juice or eat prunes every morning.

Lowered Glucose Tolerance

- Eat more complex carbohydrates.
- Avoid sugar-rich foods.

Reduction in Appetite and Thirst Sensation

- Offer fluids at regular intervals and at preferred temperature.
- Be alert for symptoms of dehydration and electrolyte imbalance.
- Offer small meals at frequent intervals.

Nutritional Deficiencies Related to Alcohol Intake

- Encourage diet high in protein and carbohydrates.
- Offer small, frequent meals to maintain caloric intake.
- Restrict sodium and fluids if edema is present.
- Take multivitamin supplements as ordered by physician.

Loss of Appetite Associated with Depression and Loneliness

- Promote mealtime as a social event.
- Set an attractive table in a pleasant setting.
- Eat outdoors whenever possible.
- Invite guests as often as possible.
- Participate in special programs for senior citizens.

Physical Handicaps

- Open cartons and assist with setup of meal.
- Arrange for home-delivered meals.
- Conserve energy when preparing meals (sit on a stool, and so forth).
- Provide transportation and assistance to obtain food.

Low Income

- Buy specials when available at food store.
- Use generic brands.
- Use coupons.
- Cook larger quantities than necessary and freeze the leftovers for future use.
- Substitute eggs, skim milk powder, and beans for meat.

Malnutrition

- Eat essential foods first.
- Select nutrient-dense foods.
- Monitor for signs of nutritional deficiencies.
- Encourage eating by planning special events.

Drug–Nutrient Interactions

- Avoid unnecessary drugs.
- Be aware of drug actions and interactions.
- Check with pharmacist to determine if medication may or may not be taken with food.
- Assess for confusion and inability to manage medication regimen.

Table 42-5
Nutritional Implications of Characteristic Developmental Landmarks Throughout the Life Cycle

Age and Characteristic Development	Nutritional Implications
Infants (birth to 1 year)	
• Most rapid period of growth after birth; birth weight doubles in 4 to 6 months and triples by age 1 year; length increases 50% in first year.	• Nutritional needs per unit of body weight are greater than at any other time in life cycle.
• Inborn reflexes, such as rooting, sucking, swallowing, and gagging, disappear between 4 and 6 months.	• Milk feedings are most appropriate for the first 4 to 6 months. • Breastfeeding is recommended as the major source of nutrition for the first 6 months; supplements of vitamins C and D, fluoride, and iron may be prescribed.* • A variety of routine and special infant formulas are available if mothers choose not to breastfeed or if breastfeeding is contraindicated because of medical problems in the infant or mother.
• Muscle control of the head, neck, jaw, and tongue develops, as does hand–eye coordination and the ability to sit and self-feed.	• Spoon-feeding becomes possible. Solids may be introduced between ages 4 and 6 months. • Common progression is iron-fortified infant cereals followed by strained vegetables, noncitrus fruits, noncitrus fruit juices. • Texture increases gradually to table food at 1 year. • Finger foods and drinking from a cup may begin around 6 months.
• Stomach capacity is limited at birth, peristalsis is rapid.	• Initially, small frequent feedings are necessary.
• Pancreatic amylase (starch-digesting enzyme) is limited at birth until age 3 months.	• Starch digestion (ie, cooked cereal) does not develop until age 3 months.
• Iron stores present at birth start to become depleted between 3 and 4 months.	• Exogenous iron is necessary. Cow's milk given too early (ie, before the infant is eating the equivalent of 1½ jars of baby food a day) contributes to iron deficiency anemia.
• Immune system matures between 4 and 6 months.	• Solid foods given too early may trigger allergic reactions. • New foods should be introduced one at a time for 5 to 7 days so that allergic reactions can be noted. • Egg whites should not be given until age 1.
Toddlers and Preschoolers	
• Decrease in growth rate is dramatic.	• Appetite dramatically decreases and becomes erratic; caloric needs per unit of body weight decline.
• Maturation of biting, chewing, and swallowing continues.	• A variety of textures are eaten.
• Mobility, autonomy, and coordination increase.	• Self-feeding is complete by age 2 years. Food is sought independently. Food may be used to manipulate parents; food jags begin around 15 months.
• Muscle mass and bone density increase.	• Adequate amounts of protein, calcium, and phosphorus are needed.
• Language skills increase.	• Food is associated with name; food likes and dislikes are verbalized.
• Food attitudes develop between ages 3 and 5.	• Inappropriate use of food (ie, to punish, reward, bribe, or convey love) may lead to inappropriate food attitudes.
School-Aged Children (6- to 12-year-olds)	
• Erratic, uneven growth pattern; wide variations in growth rate among individuals.	• Appetite improves but may still be irregular; caloric needs per unit of body weight gradually decline.
• Digestive system matures.	• Can eat larger meals and eat less frequently.
• Permanent teeth erupt.	• Fluoride, vitamins A and D, calcium, and phosphorus are important for dental health.
• Socialization and independence increase.	• Parents' role as primary gate keepers of what their children eat diminishes; advertising impacts on food choices; variety of food eaten increases.
• Reserves are laid down for upcoming adolescent growth spurt.	• Nutrient needs increase toward the end of school-aged period in preparation for growth spurt.

Table 42-5 *(continued)*
Nutritional Implications of Characteristic Developmental Landmarks Throughout the Life Cycle

Age and Characteristic Development	Nutritional Implications
Adolescents	
• Period of rapid physical, emotional, social, and sexual maturation.	• Nutrient needs, especially for calories, protein, calcium, and iron, increase to support growth.
• Growth spurt begins at different ages among individuals, begins earlier for girls than boys.	• Physiologic age is a more valid indicator of need than chronologic age.
• Boys experience an increase in muscle mass, lean body tissue, and bones.	• Iron needs increase; boys have higher caloric needs than girls to maintain larger muscle mass.
• Girls begin menstruation and experience fat deposition.	• Iron needs increase; body fat requires fewer calories to be maintained, so girls need fewer calories than boys. • Weight consciousness becomes compulsive in 1 of 100 teenaged girls and results in *anorexia nervosa,* an eating disorder characterized by extreme weight loss, muscle wasting, arrested sexual development, refusal to eat, and bizarre eating habits. • An estimated one in five teenage girls suffers from *bulimia,* an eating disorder characterized by gorging followed by purging with self-induced vomiting, diuretics, or laxatives. • Teenage pregnancy occurring within 3 to 4 years after menstruation begins places mother and fetus at increased nutritional risk.
• Period of intense psychosocial growth, family conflict, social and peer pressure.	• Nutritional needs may be hard to meet because fewer meals are eaten at home, because of peer influence and busy schedules, and because independence may be expressed through diet.
Adults	
• Growth ceases.	• Nutrient needs level off.
• Basal metabolic rate (BMR) declines each decade.	• Fewer calories are required for BMR; weight gain occurs if adjustments in intake are not made.
• Physical activity may decline.	• Also contributes to weight gain if caloric intake does not decrease.
Pregnant Women	
• Fetus, maternal tissues, and placenta grow dramatically.	• Nutrient needs increase to support growth and maintain maternal homeostasis. • Key nutrients include protein, calories, iron, folic acid, calcium, and iodine. Iron and folic acid supplements are necessary to meet needs. • Actual nutrient needs increase little during the first trimester in a well-nourished mother but increase steadily throughout the remainder of pregnancy.
• Weight gain occurs.	• Recommended pattern: 2 to 4 lb (1 to 3 kg) during the first trimester; 0.8 to 0.9 lb (0.45 kg) per week during second and third trimesters; underweight women may need more, overweight women less. • Pattern of weight gain is more significant than total amount.
• GI changes occur that may cause nausea, vomiting, heartburn, or constipation.	• Dietary changes may help relieve unpleasant symptoms.
• The quantity of milk produced is dependent on an adequate supply of nutrients.	• Caloric needs are higher for lactation than pregnancy, as are the requirements for vitamin A, niacin, riboflavin, iodine, zinc, and fluid. Calcium and protein also are important. • Calories may come from diet or fat mobilized from adipose tissue.
• The quality of milk is not affected by maternal diet, with the exception of vitamin C, riboflavin, thiamine, and fat.	• The nutritional quality of breast milk is maintained at the expense of maternal nutrition if the diet is inadequate.

(continued)

Table 42-5 *(continued)*
Nutritional Implications of Characteristic Developmental Landmarks Throughout the Life Cycle

Age and Characteristic Development	Nutritional Implications
Older Adults	
• Energy expenditure decreases related to a decrease in BMR, decrease in physical activity, and loss of lean body mass.	• Caloric needs decrease.
• Loss of teeth, periodontal disease, and jaw bone disease may result in difficulty chewing.	• Food intake may be limited to soft, easy-to-chew foods; meat is the food most commonly eliminated.
• Constipation is a common problem related to decreased activity, decreased peristalsis due to a loss of abdominal muscle tone, inadequate fluid and fiber intake, or secondary to drug therapy.	• Increasing fiber and fluid may help relieve constipation.
• Digestive disorders may occur related to normal changes in GI function.	• Diet modifications may be necessary to relieve discomfort.
• Loss of taste begins between ages 55 and 59; people lose tastes of sweet and salt; bitter and sour remain.	• Taste threshold increases, which may lead to an increase in sugar and salt intake or anorexia.
• Sensation of thirst decreases.	• Elderly people are prone to dehydration.
• Physical disabilities related to arthritis or strokes may develop.	• Food preparation may be difficult or impossible.
• Income becomes fixed.	• Most-sacrificed items on a limited food budget are milk and meats.
• Degenerative diseases and the use of medications are more common with aging.	• Nutrient intake, digestion, absorption, metabolism, or excretion may be altered.
• Social isolation, poor self-esteem, or being institutionalized may affect intake.	• Lack of interest in eating is common.

*In Canada, vitamin B_{12} may be prescribed if mothers are strict vegetarians.

(Dudek, S. G. [1993]. *Nutrition handbook for nursing practice* [2nd ed.]. Philadelphia: Lippincott.)

State of Health. The alteration in nutrient requirements that results from illness and trauma varies with the intensity and duration of the stress. For instance, fevers increase the need for calories and water. However, unlike fevers related to septicemia, fevers caused by a mild case of the flu require few dietary adjustments.

Trauma, like major surgery, burns, and crush injuries, is followed by hormonal changes that profoundly affect the body's use of nutrients. To preserve or replenish body nutrient stores and to promote healing and recovery, nutrient requirements increase dramatically in the adaptive phase after stress. In some cases of severe trauma, such as major burns, the rehabilitative phase of recovery, characterized by the gradual normalization of nutrient needs, may last for years.

Chronic disorders, like diabetes mellitus, renal disease, hypertension, heart disease, gastrointestinal disorders, and cancer, can alter nutrient requirements by influencing nutrient intake, digestion, absorption, metabolism, utilization, or excretion.

Alcohol Abuse. Alcohol can alter the body's use of nutrients, and thereby its nutrient requirements, by numerous mechanisms. The toxic effect of alcohol on the intestinal mucosa interferes with normal nutrient absorption: thus, requirements increase as the efficiency of absorption decreases. Need for B vitamins increases because they are used to metabolize alcohol. Alcohol also can influence nutrient metabolism by impairing nutrient storage, increasing nutrient catabolism, and increasing nutrient excretion. Alcohol abuse that results in liver damage has profound effects on the body's nutrient metabolism and requirements.

Medication. Many drugs have the potential to influence nutrient requirements. *Nutrient absorption* may be altered by drugs that (1) change the pH of the gastrointestinal tract, (2) increase gastrointestinal motility, (3) damage the intestinal mucosa, or (4) bind with nutrients, rendering them unavailable to the body. *Nutrient metabolism* can be altered by drugs that (1) act as nutrient antagonists, (2) alter the enzyme systems that metabolize nutrients, or (3) alter nutrient degradation. Some drugs alter the renal reabsorption of nutrients, and therefore may increase or decrease *nutrient excretion.*

Megadoses of Nutrient Supplements. Because some nutrients compete against each other for absorption, an excess of one nutrient can lead to a deficiency (or increase the requirement) of another, especially if one is absorbed preferentially. For instance, a delicate balance exists between zinc and copper. People who take therapeutic levels of zinc run the risk of developing a copper deficiency—which is otherwise rare—unless they also increase their intake of copper.

Sociocultural and Psychologic Factors

Religion. Nurses need to be aware of dietary restrictions associated with the various religions that might affect a client's nutritional requirements. During the lenten season, Roman Catholics, for example, fast on Ash Wednesday and Good Friday in addition to abstaining from meat on every Friday, and the nurse may recommend alternative food choices or meal patterns. Kosher dietary laws require special food preparation techniques and prohibit intake of pork and shellfish. The nurse must be conscious of the client's religious affiliation and its impact on his or her nutritional regimen. Kosher diets and other special diets are available in hospitals, nursing homes, retirement homes, and programs such as Meals on Wheels.

Economics. The adequacy of the food budget affects dietary choices and patterns. The increasing cost of food coupled with limited purchasing power may result in a decrease in the nutritional quality of the diet. Many variables influence the types of foods that are purchased. Creative use of the food dollar means using unit pricing to determine cost per serving (eg, comparing the unit price of $.39 per serving with a similar product's $.42 per serving), selecting foods that contain adequate nutrients, and buying seasonal foods that are more economical and can be prepared easily at home. Avoiding convenience foods and meals purchased away from home saves food dollars.

Psychosocial Factors. Food plays multiple roles in the lives of most people. In addition to satisfying hunger and providing nutrition, food may signify a celebration, a social gathering, or a reward. Some people use various foods to indicate caring or to give comfort and reassurance during times of stress or unhappiness. Mealtime may evoke memories of family discussions, laughter, and enjoyable times. Some may remember conflicts associated with eating or avoid eating because it reminds them of their loneliness and isolation. Others, because of society's emphasis on being thin, may resort to fad or crash-reducing diets to resolve eating conflicts and lose weight rapidly. This initial weight reduction seldom is sustained for an extended period, and a cycle of yo-yo dieting frequently results. Drastic weight loss is followed by an eating binge that causes the dieter to regain all the lost weight and, possibly, some additional weight each time the sequence occurs. Nutritional deficiencies may occur and place them at risk for other diseases. Losing weight and keeping it off require a change in eating habits as part of the overall commitment to health. Nurses can help by being aware of the multitudes of meanings that food has for people.

Two common eating disorders with psychologic components are anorexia nervosa and bulimia. Although contrasts exist, there is also some overlap between these diseases. *Anorexia nervosa* is an eating disorder characterized by the denial of appetite and bizarre eating patterns. It may result in an extremely dangerous physical condition leading to an early death. The typical individual with this disease is an adolescent girl from the middle or upper socioeconomic class who tends to be competitive and obsessive and has a distorted image of her body. It is not uncommon for an individual with anorexia nervosa to also develop bulimic symptoms. *Bulimia* is abnormal eating behavior that is characterized by episodes of gorging followed by purging. It is frequently observed in college students who fear gaining weight but are overwhelmed by periods of intense hunger. A bulimic fixates on food in times of stress while an anorectic turns away from food during a crisis. Most likely, they are both depressed and feel like their behavior is out of control. Both conditions are serious health and nutritional problems and individuals with these disorders require professional help.

Cultural Factors. Nutritional diversity is common among cultural or ethnic groups. The variety and selections are unique to each group and represent their personal beliefs and customs. Culture determines what is eaten, how it is prepared, and what combinations of food are permitted. The variations in food choices within a culture also are dependent on income levels and availability of foods. Cerrato (1993) mentions the necessity of including "culture-specific" food choices in any therapeutic diet to improve compliance with the prescribed dietary modifications. Table 42-6 summarizes the food preferences for common ethnic groups.

Home Healthcare Alert

Investigate a client's 24-hour food intake to identify culturally specific choices that may be included on a prescribed therapeutic diet.

Decreased Food Intake

Food intake may decrease for various reasons. **Anorexia**, or the lack of appetite, may be related to systemic and local diseases; numerous psychosocial causes, such as fear, anxiety, and depression; pain; and impaired ability to smell and taste, or it may occur secondary to drug therapy or medical treatments. Others who may have limited food intake include those who have difficulty chewing and swallowing, those who experience chronic gastrointestinal problems or undergo certain surgeries, and those on inadequate food budgets.

The Nurse as Role Model

A nurse's credibility as a health practitioner may be severely questioned if he or she appears badly nourished, or displays poor eating habits, weight problems, or other clinical signs of nutritional deficiencies. As a role model

Table 42-6
Cultural Variations on Nutrition

Culture	Milk	Meat	Bread and Cereals	Fruits and Vegetables	Additional Variations
Italian	Seldom use milk; cheese is calcium source	Chicken, beef, veal, fish—baked, simmered, or browned in olive oil	Bread and pasta basic foods	Squash, tomatoes, salad; fruit used as dessert	Drink red or white wine with dinner; use garlic for seasoning
Chinese	Use little milk or cheese	Pork, lamb, chicken, fish—cooked in combination with vegetables	Rice with most meals	Cabbage, snow peas, squashes, mushrooms; fruit usually eaten fresh	Fresh foods prepared by stir-frying; unsweetened green tea
Japanese	Little milk or cheese	Seafood main protein source, especially raw fish	Rice is basic grain; white and wheat bread being increasingly used	Steamed and served with soy sauce; tray of fruit served at main meal	Soy sauce main seasoning; soybean oil main cooking fat; traditionally, dinners follow specific sequence of courses; tea is main beverage
Greek	Little milk; yogurt popular; cheese a favorite food	Lamb favorite meat; little beef eaten	Bread center of every meal; rice commonly served	Large amounts of vegetables, cooked and seasoned, preferably fresh; large quantities of fresh fruit	Meal is family ritual; holidays are special occasions with great variety of foods
Puerto Rican	Little milk	Most cannot afford meat; may use dried codfish; legumes good protein source	Rice	Almost all eat viandas, which are starchy vegetables and fruits, such as plantain and green bananas; other fruits and vegetables used in limited quantity	Simple daily diet that contrasts with holiday meal; economy major factor in food selection
Mexican	Little milk	Little meat used	Corn basic grain used in bread and cereal; oatmeal popular cereal	Corn, fresh or canned, and chili peppers; fruit use depends on availability	Drink large amounts of coffee; common seasonings chili pepper, onions, and garlic; lard basic cooking fat
African American	Low intake of milk and dairy foods	Diet usually high in protein; favorite meats pork and chicken; most meats fried or barbecued	Sweet potatoes and hominy grits	High intake of dark, leafy green vegetables; fruits used in limited quantity	Diet high in fat and sodium because of methods of preparation

for health behaviors, the nurse should adopt the following goals:

- Attain and maintain ideal body weight.
- Use RDA guidelines for adequate nutrient intake.
- Maintain appropriate balance between food intake and exercise.
- Limit intake of alcohol, fats, sugar, salt, caffeine, and red meats.
- Eat foods high in fiber (refer to the accompanying box).

ASSESSING NUTRITIONAL STATUS

Nutritional status has a significant impact on both health and disease. For well clients, good nutritional status can help to maintain health, promote normal growth and de-

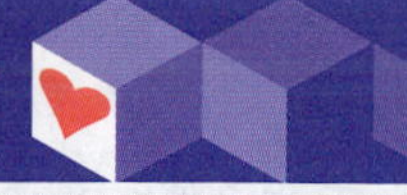

Promoting Wellness

Nutrition

Use the assessment checklist to determine how well you are meeting your nutritional needs. Then develop a prescription for self-care by choosing appropriate behaviors from the list of suggestions.

Assessment Checklist

almost always	sometimes	almost never	
☐	☐	☐	1. I know and use the recommended dietary guidelines and servings.
☐	☐	☐	2. My weight is within 10% of the ideal for my height and body frame.
☐	☐	☐	3. I maintain an appropriate balance between exercise and food intake.
☐	☐	☐	4. I limit my fat, sugar, salt, and red meat intake.
☐	☐	☐	5. I limit my caffeine intake.
☐	☐	☐	6. I use alcoholic beverages in moderation.

Self-Care Behaviors

1. Maintain desirable weight, eating a variety of foods in adequate amounts from each of the four food groups.
2. Eat slowly, take smaller portions, and avoid second helpings if trying to control overeating.
3. Eat a variety of foods low in calories and high in nutrients to lose weight.
4. Obtain medical clearance before starting a weight-loss program.
5. Avoid too many foods high in cholesterol (milk, egg yolk, organ meats, fats, oils); instead choose lean meat, fish, poultry, and beans.
6. Eat foods high in fiber: whole-grain breads and cereals, fruits, vegetables, dry beans.
7. Avoid excess use of salt and sugar.
8. Begin an exercise program, and maintain it.
9. Learn healthy eating habits; read labels, become familiar with healthy fast-food and restaurant menus, drink alcohol moderately (if at all).
10. Substitute healthy rewards for yourself that do not include high-calorie, low-nutrition snacks and beverages.

velopment, and protect against disease. During illness, good nutritional status can reduce the risk of complications and speed recovery time. Conversely, poor nutritional status can increase the risk of illness or death.

The nature of the nurse–client relationship affords nurses the opportunity to incorporate nutritional assessment in the nursing process. Like other aspects of nursing care, nutritional assessment is a systematic approach used to identify the client's actual or potential needs, formulate a plan to meet those needs, initiate the plan or assign others to implement it, and evaluate the effectiveness of the plan. As such, nutritional assessment is appropriate for all clients, although the level of assessment may range from simple screening to a comprehensive, in-depth assessment, depending on individual circumstances (see accompanying box). Nurses can collect assessment data through history taking (dietary and medical–socioeconomic data), physical assessments (anthropometric and clinical data), and laboratory data. An awareness of specific changes in older people that may reflect on the accuracy of the assessment process is necessary (see accompanying box).

Discussion continues among health experts about determining what is the most effective method to assess for risk of developing nutritionally related complications. Some nutritionists state that a thorough physical assessment and nutritional history can more accurately determine the presence of malnutrition than a series of laboratory test results (Lutz & Przytulski, 1994). Williams (1994) supports a basic nutritional assessment known as the *ABCD approach*. This strategy includes: *A*nthropometrics, *B*iochemical tests, *C*linical observations, and *D*iet evaluation and personal histories. Nurses, by nature of their caring role and personal encounters, are ideally situated to identify nutritional needs and assess and monitor for nutritional risks.

Dietary Data

Dietary data may be collected from the client or family and can be evaluated according to the food group approach, dietary guidelines, or the RDA (RNI in Canada), depending on the purpose of the assessment. Statistics indicate that only 26% of older individuals discuss diet or nutrition with their physician, yet a large majority (85%) of illnesses common to this population are nutrition-related and preventable (Cope, 1994). The Nutrition Screening Initiative is a national project with a nutritional home healthcare focus. It was designed to incorporate routine screening and intervention to improve nutrition care available to older adults (Nutrition Screening Manual for Professionals Caring for Older Americans, 1992). The Nutritional Health Checklist (Fig. 42-7), included in this manual, is a simple, self-administered assessment

Elements of a Nutritional Assessment

Dietary Data

Screen
- 24-hour food recall
- Food frequency record

In-depth
- Food diary
- Diet history

Medical–Socioeconomic Data

Screen
- Brief personal and family history

In-depth
- Sequential history, including current and past health status, social history, and family history

Anthropometric Data

Screen
- Height
- Weight
- Ideal body weight (IBW)
- Usual body weight (UBW)

In-depth
- Triceps skinfold (TSF)
- Midarm circumference (MAC)
- Midarm muscle circumference (MAMC)
- Body mass index (BMI)

Clinical Data

Screen and in-depth
- Observe for signs and symptoms of malnutrition

Biochemical Data

Screen
- Serum hemoglobin and albumin levels and hematocrit
- Total lymphocyte count (TLC)

In-depth
- Serum transferrin level
- Antigen skin testing
- 24-hour urinary creatinine excretion
- Urinary urea nitrogen (UUN)

tool that can be used to easily identify clients at risk. Specific interventions are suggested depending on the client's individual score. When combined with other methods of assessing nutritional status, the nurse is better prepared to coordinate a focused strategy to combat malnutrition.

24-Hour Recall Method. The easiest way to collect dietary data is to obtain a 24-hour recall of all food and beverages the client normally consumes during an average day. It includes the client's usual portion sizes, meal and snack patterns, meal timing, and the place where food is eaten. Because this method relies on memory and accurate interpretation of portion sizes, the information may not be reliable.

Food Diaries. Food frequency questionnaires or food diaries may provide a better overall picture of nutrient intake because the client records all food and beverages consumed in a specified period, usually 3 to 7 days.

Diet History. A more comprehensive approach to diet assessment is taking a full diet history. In addition to a 24-hour food recall and food frequency record, interview questions are geared to provide information on past and present food intake and habits. Sample questions are included in the accompanying box.

The following findings are considered dietary risk factors for poor nutritional status:

- Inadequate food intake, fad dieting, numerous food intolerances or allergies
- Use of inadequate modified diet (ie, clear liquid) for more than 3 days without adequate supplementation
- NPO with simple IV therapy (eg, 5% dextrose and water) for longer than 3 days
- Inadequate tube feedings
- Difficulty chewing or swallowing
- Changes in taste, smell, or appetite

Nutritional Assessment Considerations for Older Adults*

Biochemical Data

- Low serum albumin level (below 3.5 mg/dL) may be a reflection of the aging process rather than a nutritional risk factor. Albumin synthesis declines with age.
- Hemoglobin levels that are lower than normal may only reflect anemia observed in elderly people as part of the aging process.

Anthropometric Data

- Because of age-related changes in body composition, skin fold measurements should be taken from several body sites.

Dietary Data

- Dietary recall may be inaccurate because of vision and memory problems.
- Question use of vitamin and mineral supplements.
- Gather information concerning medication regimen (prescribed and over-the-counter) to assess for food–drug interactions and adverse effects of medications.

* Specific clinical data for older people may be found in the Focus on the Older Adult display.

The Warning Signs of poor nutritional health are often overlooked. Use this checklist to find out if you or someone you know is at nutritional risk.

DETERMINE YOUR NUTRITIONAL HEALTH

Read the statements below. Circle number in the yes column for those that apply to you or someone you know. For each yes answer, score the number in the box. Total your nutritional score.

	YES
I have an illness or condition that made me change the kind and/or amount of food I eat.	2
I eat fewer than 2 meals per day.	3
I eat few fruits or vegetables, or milk products.	2
I have 3 or more drinks of beer, liquor or wine almost every day.	2
I have tooth or mouth problems that make it hard for me to eat.	2
I don't always have enough money to buy the food I need.	4
I eat alone most of the time.	1
I take 3 or more different prescribed or over-the-counter drugs a day.	1
Without wanting to, I have lost or gained10 pounds in the last 6 months.	2
I am not always physically able to shop, cook and/or feed myself.	2
TOTAL	

Total Your Nutritional Score. If it's —

0-2 **Good!** Recheck your nutritional score in 6 months.

3-5 **You are at moderate nutrional risk.** See what can be done to improve your eating habits and lifestyle. Your office on aging, senior nutrition program, senior citizens center or health department can help. Recheck your nutritional score in 3 months.

6 or more **You are at high nutritional risk.** Bring this checklist the next time you see your doctor, dietitian or other qualified health or social service professional. Talk with them about any problems you may have. Ask for help to improve your nutritional health.

These materials developed and distributed by the Nutrition Screening Initiative, a project of:

AMERICAN ACADEMY OF FAMILY PHYSICIANS

THE AMERICAN DIETETIC ASSOCIATION

NATIONAL COUNCIL ON THE AGING, INC.

Remember that warning signs suggest risk, but do not represent diagnosis of any condition. Turn the page to learn more about the Warning Signs of poor nutritional health.

DETERMINE

The nutrition checklist is based on the following warning signs. Use the word DETERMINE to help you remember them.

D-Disease
E-Eating Poorly
T-Tooth Loss/Mouth Pain
E-Economic Hardship
R-Reduced Social Contact
M-Multiple Medicines
I-Involuntary Weight Loss/Gain
N-Needs Assistance in Self Care
E-Elder Years Above Age 80

Figure 42-7
Nutritional health checklist. (Cope, K. [1994]. Nutritional status: a basic vital sign. *Home Healthcare Nurse, 12*[*2*], 31.)

Medical–Socioeconomic Data

Medical, social, and economic factors, as well as cultural and psychologic influences, should be evaluated for their impact on nutritional requirements and food choices. Table 42-7 outlines medical–socioeconomic data for assessment.

The following findings are considered medical–socioeconomic risk factors for poor nutritional status:

- Medical conditions that alter intake or nutrient requirements—cancer, malabsorption, diarrhea, hyperthyroidism, severe infection, recent surgery, hemorrhage, physical or mental disabilities, multiple wounds or fractures, extensive burns
- Persistent fever above 37°C (98.6°F) for more than 2 days
- Chronic use of drugs that affect nutritional status
- Alcohol abuse
- Inadequate food budget

Anthropometric Data

Anthropometric measurements are used to determine body dimensions. In children, anthropometric measure-

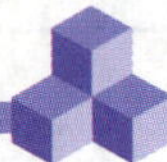

Focused Assessment Guide

Nutrition

Factors to Assess	Questions and Approaches
Usual dietary intake	Does your current intake differ from your usual intake? If so, is the reason a loss of appetite, changes in smell or taste, difficulty chewing and swallowing, hospitalization, a modified diet?
Food allergies or intolerances	Do you have any food allergies or intolerances?
Food preparation and storage	Who does the food shopping? Who prepares the meals? How is the food normally prepared? For instance, is food usually fried, baked, or broiled? Do you have adequate food storage space and preparation equipment?
Type of diet	Do you now or have you in the past followed a modified diet prescribed by a physician?
Dietary practices	Do you now or have you in the past used a fad diet, health foods, or self-prescribed supplements?
Eating disorder patterns	Do you view yourself as overweight? Do you weigh yourself frequently during one day? How is your appetite? Do you binge on large amounts of food in a short period? Have you ever caused yourself to vomit after eating a meal? Have you used laxatives, diuretics, or over-the-counter weight loss pills to lose weight?

ments are used to assess growth rate; in adults, they can give indirect measurements of body protein and fat stores. For the data to be accurate and reliable, standardized equipment and procedures must be used and the data must be compared with the appropriate reference standards for the client's age and sex.

Height and weight, the most common anthropometric measurements, should be determined when the client is admitted to the healthcare facility and periodically thereafter. A client should be weighed on the same scale each time and at the same time of day, preferably before breakfast. Weight should be compared with IBW and usual body weight. Because actual weight may be inflated if the client has edema, hydration status should be considered. Although self-reported weight may be recorded when actual weight is unobtainable, it is highly inaccurate and should be duly noted.

In-depth anthropometric measurements include triceps skin fold measurements, a measure of subcutaneous fat stores (Fig. 42-8); midarm circumference, a measure of skeletal muscle mass; and midarm muscle circumference, a measure of both skeletal muscle mass and fat stores.* Reference standards have been determined for men and women for all three measures, as have figures representing 90%, 80%, 70%, and 60% of standard.

The following findings are considered anthropometric risk factors for poor nutritional status:

- Weight 20% greater or 10% less than ideal
- Recent unintentional weight loss greater than 10% of weight
- Arm muscle circumference or triceps skin fold less than 85% of standard
- Inconsistent growth rates in children or abnormal weight for height

Clinical Data

Although signs and symptoms of malnutrition may be observed during a physical assessment (Table 42-8), they usually do not appear until malnutrition is advanced. In addition, further investigation is necessary to determine whether abnormal findings are actually caused by a nutritional deficiency, possibly related to a nutritional deficiency, or unrelated to nutritional status.

Biochemical Data

Laboratory tests, which measure blood and urine levels of nutrients or biochemical functions that are dependent

*In Canada the Quetelet, or body mass, index is calculated as:

$$\text{BMI} = \frac{\text{weight (kg)}}{\text{height m}^2}$$

Table 42-7
Medical–Socioeconomic Data for Nutritional Assessment

Collect	Evaluate
Medical Data	
Medical history: type of disorder, treatment (including diet and drug)	Effect on intake, digestion, absorption, metabolism, and excretion of nutrients
Current illness or chief complaint	Need for diet modifications
Family medical history	
Surgical history: type, date, length of hospitalization, development of complications	
Past and current drug history: name of prescription and non-prescription drugs used on a regular basis, purpose, dosage, duration of use	Potential or actual effects on nutritional status; need for diet modification
History of drug dependence; drug abuse	
Ability to chew and swallow (Does the client have missing teeth? Full or partial dentures? Do the dentures fit?)	Impact on food intake
Appetite, food intolerances and allergies, bowel habits	Normal pattern, recent changes, impact on intake and nutritional status, need for diet modification
Social Data	
Age, gender	Effect on nutritional requirements
Position in family; number in family; lifestyle	Outside support systems; social aspects of eating
Occupation; frequency and intensity of physical exercise; usual number of hours of sleep per day	Effect on caloric requirements and meal timing
Religious affiliation, cultural and ethnic background	Effect on food choices and aversions
Educational background	Ability to comprehend diet instruction; appropriate teaching materials and methods
Use of alcohol and tobacco	Effect on food intake, food budget, and nutrient requirements
Economic Data	
Source of income	Reliability and adequacy; eligibility for social assistance
Food budget	Adequacy

(Dudek, S. G. [1993]. *Nutrition handbook for nursing practice.* [2nd ed.]. Philadelphia: Lippincott.)

on an adequate supply of nutrients, can objectively detect nutritional problems in their early stages. Most routine biochemical tests measure protein status; measures of body vitamin, mineral, and trace element status also are available.

Hemoglobin, the oxygen-carrying protein of the red blood cells, and hematocrit, the volume of red blood cells packed by centrifugation in a given volume of blood, are measures of plasma protein also used to assess iron status. Protein status also can be determined by measuring serum albumin and transferrin levels and by a total lymphocyte count. The total lymphocyte count reflects immune status and is directly impacted by impaired nutritional states. Albumin is the single most important laboratory value to assess over a period of time (Cope, 1994). The albumin level does not change with increasing age but malnutrion and various disease states will cause its level to decrease.

Twenty-four-hour urine tests used to measure protein metabolism are urine creatinine excretion and urine urea nitrogen. Urea, a breakdown product of amino acids, can be measured in the urine and blood. It reflects protein intake and the body's ability to detoxify and excrete this metabolic by-product. Creatinine levels are directly proportional to the body's muscle mass and a reduction in this value reflects severe malnutrition. These biochemical indicators with nutritional implications are summarized in the accompanying box.

DIAGNOSING

Assessment data may reveal actual or potential nutritional problems.

Altered Nutrition as the Problem

Altered Nutrition: Less Than Body Requirements, related to NPO, inadequate tube feeding, prolonged use of a clear liquid diet, numerous food intolerances or allergies, excessive dieting, anorexia,

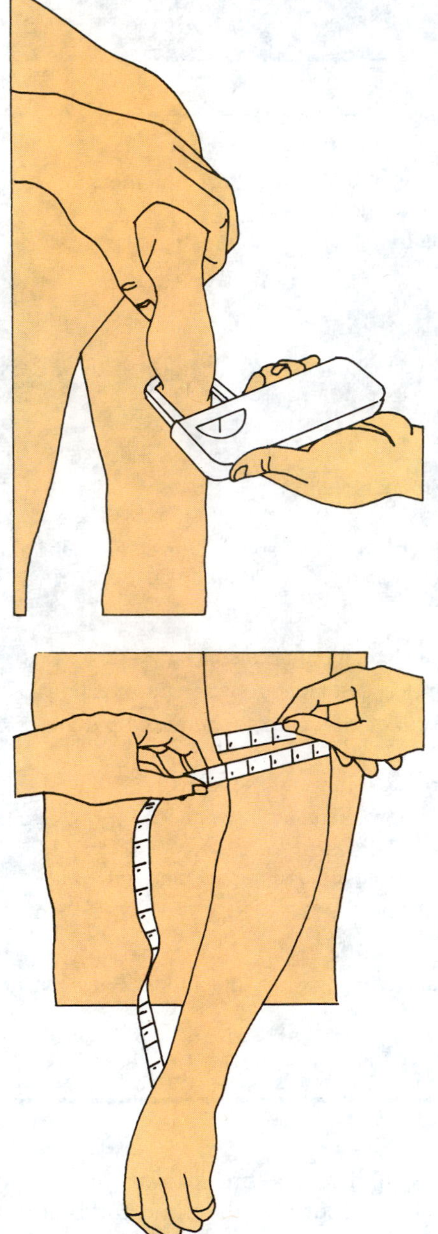

Figure 42-8
Two anthropometric measurements to assess nutritional status—tricips skin fold measurement (*top*) and midarm muscle circumference (*bottom*).

chewing or swallowing difficulties, nausea, vomiting, chronic diarrhea, malabsorption, psychologic eating disorders (anorexia nervosa, bulimia), alcoholism, metabolic and endocrine disorders, inappropriate use of supplements

Altered Nutrition: More Than Body Requirements, related to overeating, inactivity, metabolic and endocrine disorders, inappropriate use of supplements

Altered Nutrition: Risk for More Than Body Requirements, related to inappropriate eating, closely spaced pregnancies, metabolic and endocrine disorders, inappropriate use of supplements

Samples of three of these diagnoses are given in the accompanying box.

Altered Nutrition as the Etiology. Nutritional problems may affect other areas of human functioning. In the following nursing diagnoses, the nutritional problem is the cause of another problem.

Activity Intolerance related to inadequate caloric intake, obesity, iron deficiency anemia

Altered Health Maintenance related to lack of knowledge about adequate nutrition

Anxiety related to obesity

Constipation related to inadequate fluid or fiber intake

Diarrhea related to overeating, excessive fiber intake, excessive sorbitol intake (sugar alcohol)

Fluid Volume Deficit related to inadequate fluid intake

Risk for Infection related to inadequate calorie intake, inadequate protein intake

Impaired Home Maintenance Management related to inability to purchase, store, or prepare food for family

Impaired Skin Integrity related to protein malnutrition, vitamin A deficiency

Knowledge Deficit related to new medical diet, nutrition misinformation, lack of interest in nutrition, intellectual deficit

Noncompliance to a particular diet order related to lack of motivation, misinformation

Self-Esteem Disturbance related to obesity

Sleep Pattern Disturbance related to excessive caffeine intake

Social Isolation related to obesity

Wellness Diagnosis

For clients who are incorporating sound nutritional practices in their daily routine, the following wellness diagnosis may be appropriate:

Potential for enhanced compliance with low-fat diet regimen

PLANNING: EXPECTED OUTCOMES

Expected outcomes evolve from the actual or potential nutritional problems diagnosed. General client goals follow. The client will:

- Attain and maintain ideal body weight
- Eat a diet adequate but not excessive in all nutrients
- Eat a variety of food in each of three or more meals
- Follow the appropriate modified diet, when necessary, to restore health, avoid disease recurrences, and prevent or delay potential complications

Table 42-8
Clinical Observations for Nutritional Assessment

Body Area	Signs of Good Nutritional Status	Signs of Poor Nutritional Status
General appearance	Alert, responsive	Listless, apathetic, and cachexic
General vitality	Endurance, energetic, sleeps well, vigorous	Easily fatigued, no energy, falls asleep easily, looks tired, apathetic
Weight	Normal for height, age, body build	Overweight or underweight
Hair	Shiny, lustrous, firm, not easily plucked, healthy scalp	Dull and dry, brittle, loss of color, easily plucked, thin and sparse
Face	Uniform skin color; healthy appearance, not swollen	Dark skin over cheeks and under eyes, flaky skin, facial edema (moon face), pale skin color
Eyes	Bright, clear, moist, no sores at corners of eyelids, membranes moist and healthy pink color, no prominent blood vessels	Pale eye membranes, dry eyes (xerophthalmia); Bitot's spots, increased vascularity, cornea soft (keratomalacia), small yellowish lumps around eyes (xanthelasma), dull or scarred cornea
Lips	Good pink color, smooth, moist, not chapped or swollen	Swollen and puffy (cheilosis), angular lesion at corners of mouth or fissures or scars (stomatitis)
Tongue	Deep red, surface papillae present	Smooth appearance, beefy red or magenta colored, swollen, hypertrophy or atrophy
Teeth	Straight, no crowding, no cavities, no pain, bright, no discoloration, well-shaped jaw	Cavities, mottled appearance (fluorosis), malpositioned, missing teeth
Gums	Firm, good pink color, no swelling or bleeding	Spongy, bleed easily, marginal redness, recessed, swollen and inflamed
Glands	No enlargement of the thyroid, face not swollen	Enlargement of the thyroid (goiter), enlargement of the parotid (swollen cheeks)
Skin	Smooth, good color, slightly moist, no signs of rashes, swelling, or color irregularities	Rough, dry, flaky, swollen, pale, pigmented, lack of fat under the skin, fat deposits around the joints (xanthomas), bruises, petechiae
Nails	Firm, pink	Spoon shaped (koilonychia), brittle, pale, ridged
Skeleton	Good posture, no malformations	Poor posture, beading of the ribs, bowed legs or knock-knees, prominent scapulas, chest deformity at diaphragm
Muscles	Well developed, firm, good tone, some fat under the skin	Flaccid, poor tone, wasted, underdeveloped, difficulty walking
Extremities	No tenderness	Weak and tender, presence of edema
Abdomen	Flat	Swollen
Nervous system	Normal reflexes, psychologic stability	Decrease in or loss of ankle and knee reflexes, psychomotor changes, mental confusion, depression, sensory loss, motor weakness, loss of sense of position, loss of vibration, burning and tingling of the hands and feet (paresthesia)
Cardiovascular system	Normal heart rate and rhythm, no murmurs, normal blood pressure for age	Cardiac enlargement, tachycardia, elevated blood pressure
GI system	No palpable organs or masses (liver edge may be palpable in children)	Hepatosplenomegaly

(Worthington-Roberts, B.S., & Williams, S.R. [1993]. *Nutrition in pregnancy and lactation* [5th ed.]. St. Louis: Mosby-Year Book.)

IMPLEMENTING

Providing proper and adequate nourishment to the client is a team effort implemented in a variety of settings: Diet orders are written by the physician, confirmed by the dietitian, and frequently explained to the client by the nurse. The nurse also may be responsible for screening clients at home who are at nutritional risk, observing intake and appetite, evaluating the client's tolerance, assisting the client with eating, administering enteral and

Biochemical Data With Nutritional Implications

- Hemoglobin (Normal = 12–18 g/dL)
  decreased → anemia
- Hematocrit (Normal = 40–50%)
  decreased → anemia
  increased → dehydration
- Serum albumin (Normal = 3.3–5 g/dL)
  decreased → malnutrition (prolonged protein depletion), malabsorption
- Transferrin (Normal = 240–480 mg/dL)
  decreased → anemia, protein deficiency
- Total lymphocyte count (Normal = greater than 1800)
  decreased → impaired nutritional intake, severe debilitating disease
- Blood urea nitrogen (Normal = 17–18 mg/dL)
  increased → starvation, high protein intake, severe dehydration
  decreased → malnutrition, overhydration
- Creatinine (Normal = 0.4–1.5 mg/dL)
  increased → dehydration
  decreased → reduction in total muscle mass, severe malnutrition

(Fischbach, F. [1992]. *A manual of laboratory and diagnostic tests* [4th ed.]. Philadelphia: Lippincott.)

parenteral feedings, consulting with the dietitian and physician when dietary problems arise, addressing the potential for drug–nutrient reactions, obtaining more food or snacks for the client when appropriate, monitoring food brought by visitors, and participating in nutrition education efforts.

Teaching Nutritional Information

For the greatest chance of success, diet instructions should be individually tailored to the client's lifestyle, intellectual ability, and level of motivation. Although strict guidelines and printed handouts may be viewed as the

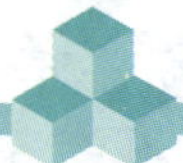

Nursing Diagnoses for Common Problems

Nutrition

Problem	Related Factors	Sample Defining Characteristics
Altered Nutrition: Less Than Body Requirements	Malabsorption	• "I seem to eat all day long and yet I keep losing weight." • Reports losing 15 lb within the past 3 weeks. Has 8 to 10 bowel movements daily of frothy, odorous stools that float. Fecal fat excretion test indicates steatorrhea. Client appears fatigued and undernourished; muscle wasting is evident. Laboratory data reveal low serum albumin level (protein deficiency) and iron deficiency anemia.
Altered Nutrition: More Than Body Requirements	Decreased thyroid function leading to a decrease in metabolism	• "I don't eat enough to keep a bird alive, but I just keep getting fatter and fatter. I don't know what else to do unless I stop eating altogether." • Client reports a 10-lb weight gain within the past month despite following a 1200-calorie diet. Other symptoms noted include fatigue, amenorrhea, and dry skin. Laboratory data indicate low serum thyroxine (T_4) level, protein-bound iodine, and elevated serum thyroid-stimulating hormone and cholesterol levels. Radioactive iodine uptake was low.
Altered Nutrition: High Risk for More Than Body Requirements	Inappropriate use of supplements	• "I sent a sample of my hair away for a nutritional analysis, and the report came back saying that I should take supplements of zinc, iron, potassium, and magnesium." • For the past week, client has been taking supplements of 500% of the RDA for zinc and magnesium. She takes twice as much iron as recommended, and large doses of potassium ad lib.

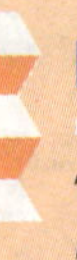

Helpscan

The following are resources for clients and healthcare professionals:

- For information on all nutrition topics:
  Call the National Center for Nutrition & Dietetics
  (800) 366-1655
- For information on diet, nutrition, and cancer:
  Call the American Institute for Cancer Research Nutrition Hotline
  (800) 843-8114
- For information on eating disorders:
  National Eating Disorder Information Centre
  Toronto General Hospital
  200 Elizabeth St.
  College Wing 1-318
  Toronto, ON M5G 2C4
  (416) 340-4156
- For a free newsletter subscription (10 issues/year) write to:
  Contemporary Nutrition, General Mills
  P.O. Box 5588
  Dept. N93
  Stacy, MN 55079

ideal, in practice, simplicity and compromise often are the keys to client compliance. Specific instructions vary according to the diet order; however, the following guidelines are applicable for all types of diets:

- Provide simple verbal instructions. When appropriate, include family members and provide written teaching aids.
- Advise the client to eliminate any foods not tolerated.
- Advise the client to alert the physician if the diet conflicts with religious beliefs, if adverse effects develop, or if special foods required are too costly or difficult to locate.
- Offer support and encouragement.
- If possible, spread diet instructions out over a period of days or weeks, so as not to overwhelm the client with too much information at one time and to allow the client time to internalize the information and form questions.
- Evaluate the client's level of understanding; assess the need for reinforcement or elaboration.

Monitoring Nutritional Status

Nurses are aware that malnourished clients are more likely to have slower wound healing and develop complications. Prevention of malnutrition can have a positive effect on client outcomes. In the hospital, shortened stays limit the time available for nutritional screening and intervention. Clients are often acutely ill and uninterested or unable to absorb and retain any nutritional instruction. It may also be difficult to include a family member or caregiver responsible for food preparation in scheduled teaching sessions. In many situations, the home healthcare nurse has the opportunity to have significant impact on nutritional health. Instruction can be provided in a relaxed setting that allows insight into a client's cultural orientation and family patterns and traditions. This environment also encourages modification and adjustments in the nurse's approach to nutritional instruction.

Home Healthcare Alert

Investigate the variety of community services and programs available to provide nutritional support to clients at home.

Stimulating Appetite

Pain, illness, anxiety, and medications can contribute to anorexia and poor intake when in a healthcare facility or in the home. To the hospitalized client, food and eating may take on much greater meaning. Loss of control over food choices, the way food is prepared, when and how food is served, and eating alone may do little to encourage normal eating. Every effort must be made to ensure that the proper food is not only served but also eaten. The additional time and attention nurses and caregivers spend when encouraging a person to eat may have a positive impact on dietary intake (Yen, 1994a). The following measures may help to stimulate appetite in any setting:

- Serve small, frequent meals to avoid overwhelming the client with large amounts of food.
- Solicit food preferences and encourage favorite foods from home or prepared when at home, if possible.
- Provide encouragement and a pleasant eating environment.
- Be sure the client's tray looks attractive.
- Schedule procedures and medications at times when they are least likely to interfere with appetite.
- Control pain, nausea, or depression with medications.
- Offer alternatives for items the client cannot or will not eat.
- Encourage or provide good oral hygiene.
- Remove clutter from area in which client is eating.
- Keep eating area free from irritating odors.

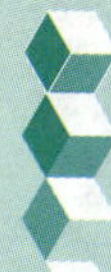

Research in Nursing: Making a Difference

Nutrition

Current research in nutrition and fitness has created a focus on the dietary behavior of our society. Despite emphasis on developing healthy eating habits, nutrition for older persons continues to be a widespread problem. Nurses need an awareness of relevant health concerns, familiarity with successful nursing interventions, and a willingness to explore relevant nutritional issues.

Related Research

Dellasega, C., Brown, R., & White, A. (1995). Cholesterol-related health behavior in rural elderly persons. *Journal of Gerontological Nursing, 21*(5), 6–12.
Findings from a survey conducted by the investigators indicated that the rural older population in this study were concerned about their cholesterol levels but generally unaware of cholesterol-reduction strategies. Since traditional resources for healthcare may not be available for this population, the community health nurse is in an ideal position to explain and reinforce nutritional interventions. Written materials that can easily be understood, newspaper articles, and telephone contact were viewed as effective methods of promoting nutritional health in older people living in a rural setting.

Gilmore, S., Robinson, G., Posthauer, M., & Raymond, J. (1995). Clinical indicators associated with unintentional weight loss and pressure ulcers in elderly residents of nursing facilities. *Journal of the American Dietetic Association, 95*(9), 954–992.
Older clients residing in extended care facilities are likely candidates for unintentional weight loss and development of pressure ulcers. The most common reasons for unintentional weight loss in this group were reduced functional ability, a 50% decrease in food intake for three consecutive days, and chewing problems. The most frequently identified indicator for pressure ulcer development was a serum albumin level of less than 35 g/L with normal hydration status. Nurses working with older clients need to be aware of risk factors and initiate nutritional health teaching and interventions appropriate for this population and these health concerns.

Van Ort, S., & Phillips, L. (1995). Nursing interventions to promote functional feeding. *Journal of Gerontological Nursing, 21*(10), 6–14.
Results of this study indicated that by modifying the environment, nurses were able to promote self-feeding for residents in a long-term care facility as well as increase the amount of food they consumed without extending meal time. Effective nursing actions included reducing meal-time distractions, seating residents at a dining table, using placemats, and placing finger foods directly in front of the residents. This increase in independence provided autonomy for the residents and enhanced meal-time environment for the client and caregiver.

Summary

Nursing research about nutritional concerns is valuable as nurses intervene to improve the health prospects of older clients in a variety of settings. Linking theory to the practice setting may positively affect the ability to influence the behavior of clients and improve the quality of their lives.

- Arrange food tray so that client can easily reach food.
- Provide a comfortable position.
- Involve the person as much as possible. Solicit his or her preferences with regard to the order of items eaten and the eating pace.
- Engage the individual in pleasant conversation to ease tension.
- Place a napkin, not a bib, over the person's clothes for protection.
- Use straws or special eating utensils whenever possible.

Home Healthcare Alert

To increase caloric intake, instruct the client or caregiver to add nonfat dry milk powder to any food containing liquid.

Assisting With Eating

The loss of independence that comes with the inability to self-feed can be a severe blow to a person's self-esteem. The following measures may help a person maintain dignity while being fed:

Providing Nutrition in Special Situations

A variety of normal and modified diets are available in the healthcare setting and may be prescribed for use at home. Normal or house diets are designed to maintain optimal nutritional status by providing adequate amounts of all nutrients. The diet's actual composition varies with the quantity and types of food selected; the average calorie content ranges from 1400 to 2500 cal.

Liquid diets are used most often as transitional diets when eating resumes after acute illness, surgery, or parenteral nutrition. *Clear liquid diets* contain only foods that are clear liquids at room or body temperature—gelatin, fat-free broth, bouillon, ice pops, clear juices, carbonated beverages, regular and decaffeinated coffee, and tea. Because clear liquid diets are inadequate in calories, protein, and most nutrients, they should be progressed as soon as possible. *Full liquid diets* contain milk, plain frozen desserts, pasteurized eggs, cereal gruels, and milk and egg substitutes in addition to clear liquids. A full liquid diet contains liquids that can be poured at room temperature. High-calorie, high-protein supplements are recommended if the diet is used for more than 3 days.

Soft diets usually are regular diets that have been modified to eliminate foods that are hard to digest and to chew, including those that are high in fiber, high in fat, and highly seasoned. Soft diets are adequate in calories and nutrients and may be used on a long-term basis.

Some clients may prefer a *vegetarian diet.* Over 7 million Americans follow some type of vegetarian food pattern (Williams, 1994). Meats are usually replaced with legumes, grains, and vegetables and, if well planned, this type of diet can satisfy all nutritional requirements. People may choose to be vegetarians for a variety of reasons: religious preference, ethical belief that killing animals for food is unjust, fear of contamination with pesticides, or health concerns about the cholesterol and saturated fats found in meats. Vegetarian diets have a variety of formats and are more commonly followed by younger people. An individual who will eat any animal product except red meat and a Zen macrobiotic who consumes only brown rice and herb tea represent both ends of the spectrum. Vitamin B_{12}, vitamin A, and iron are nutrients that may require supplementation in a vegetarian diet. The nurse can support clients who follow a vegetarian diet by assisting them or their caregiver to select nutritious food items from the large variety of foods available within their dietary framework.

Clients may be ordered NPO (nothing by mouth) for several reasons. Food is prohibited before surgery to prevent aspiration related to anesthesia, and after surgery until bowel sounds return. NPO also may be necessary for clients undergoing certain medical tests and for clients experiencing severe nausea and vomiting, an inability to chew or swallow, coma, various acute or chronic gastrointestinal abnormalities, and labor and delivery.

Well-nourished clients can easily withstand the stress of NPO for a short period but, in reality, over 50% of clients admitted to a healthcare facility are malnourished (Messner & Stephens, 1994). Clients with increased nutritional requirements or those who will be NPO for more than 2 days may require nutritional support from enteral or parenteral nutrition.

The following measures may provide comfort to clients who are NPO:

- Encourage or provide good oral hygiene.
- Provide the client with ice chips, sips of water, hard candies, or gum, as allowed.
- Let the client chew favorite foods without swallowing.
- Urge the client to avoid watching others eat. Suggest alternate activities at mealtimes.

Providing Enteral Nutrition

Oral feeding is the preferred and most effective method of feeding clients. The next best method is the enteral route. **Enteral nutrition** involves passing a tube into the gastrointestinal tract to administer a formula containing adequate nutrients. This alternate feeding method may deliver total or supplemental nutrition over a short-term period or for longer intervals.

Providing Short-Term Nutritional Support

For short-term use (less than 6 weeks), a nasogastric or nasointestinal route is usually selected. A **nasogastric (NG) feeding tube** is inserted through the nose and into the stomach while a **nasointestinal (NI) tube** is passed through the nose and into the upper portion of the small intestine. Nasogastric feedings have the advantage of allowing the stomach to be used as a natural reservoir, regulating the amount of foods and liquids released into the small intestine. It is also thought that the presence of gastric acid in the stomach may decrease the risk of infection. The possibility of aspiration of tube feeding solution into the lungs is a disadvantage of this route. Clients with a dysfunctional gag reflex or those who are unable to have the head of the bed elevated during feedings are not candidates for nasogastric feeding. Occasionally, a smaller, softer, more pliable tube (eg, Dobbhoff tube) may be placed in the stomach or small intestine. The advantage of increased client comfort with this tube is offset by difficulty checking tube placement. The nasal method of inserting a feeding tube, discussed in Procedure 42-1, requires skill and accuracy, and is frequently done by the nurse.

A client with a nasointestinal tube has minimal risk for aspiration. When formula is delivered directly into the intestine, a type of *dumping syndrome* may develop because the pyloric valve in the stomach, which normally slows transit of food into the intestine, is bypassed. The volume of feeding distends the intestine, and combined with a hypoglycemic reaction, may result in symptoms of gas, bloating, crampy pain, weakness, and dizziness. Some medical conditions (delayed gastric emptying, gastric tumor) also necessitate the use of a nasointestinal tube.

Providing Long-Term Nutritional Support

When enteral feeding is required for a long-term period, an opening may be created into the stomach (gastrostomy) or into the jejunum (jejunostomy). The methods of accomplishing long-term feeding into the stomach in-

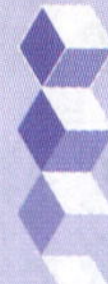

Through the Eyes of a Student

She looked lost in that big hospital bed, so thin and frail. Her hair was as white as her pillowcase and blankets, and her skin looked almost transparent. And then I saw it. Snaking under her blankets into her belly was the feeding tube surrounded by thick, green, smelly discharge.

During preconference my instructor had told me that I needed to check residual every 2 hours to monitor her absorption rate. The first time, with my instructor standing beside me like my guardian angel (or my patient's guardian angel, I'm not sure which), the procedure naturally went off without a hitch. I could do this, I thought, feeling more confident.

Because my patient had chronic diarrhea as well as skin breakdown at her sacrum, the next 2 hours flew by in a whirlwind of bathing. But now the time had come. This is it, I thought. I'm on my own for the second residual check. And, again, I breathed a sigh of relief when the procedure was completed with no problems.

As the day progressed, I got myself a little behind schedule because I was determined to remove the hardened crusts from underneath her nails. Before I knew it, I got the message from another student that it was postconference time. Oh no! I didn't do my last residual check yet. Quickly, I emptied the basin I was using on her fingernails and grabbed the plunger. I reached into my pocket for my hemostat to clamp off the line and the next thing I saw was Jevity squirting all over the bed, my patient, the clean Chux and me! I had cut the line instead of clamping it!

I quickly pinched both ends to stop the Jevity from squirting and frantically called for help. While waiting for rescue, I checked on my patient response, not knowing how she was going to react. Thankfully, she was sound asleep, soothed by her recent nail massage. It seemed like forever before my instructor rushed in. With my eyes filling up, I attempted to explain that I had grabbed the scissors from my pocket instead of the hemostat. Guardian angel that she was (I think she was both of ours), my instructor calmly and efficiently proceeded to attach both ends of the tube together with the use of an adapter.

Many lessons were learned that day, such as don't attempt a procedure in haste and have all your supplies readily at hand. But the one thing I'll never, ever forget is that the scissors are the crooked ones!

—Eileen Cooper
Delaware County Community College, Media, PA

clude **percutaneous endoscopic gastrostomy (PEG)** or a surgically or laparoscopically placed gastrostomy tube. PEG tube insertion is popular because, unlike a gastrostomy tube, it usually does not require general anesthesia, can be safely inserted and removed at the bedside or in an outpatient setting, and is, therefore, more economical (Thompson, 1995). Simply stated, positioning a PEG tube involves local anesthesia, passage of an endoscope into the stomach, a small incision or stab wound through the skin of the abdomen, pushing a cannula through the small incision, insertion of a guide wire or suture material through the cannula, and introduction and placement of the PEG tube via one of several methods (Fig. 42-9 indicates a PEG tube in place in the stomach). Use of a PEG tube or other type of gastrostomy tube requires an intact, functional GI tract. In long-term feeding situations when gastric problems exist, the jejunostomy is an alternate method through which nutrition can be delivered. These tubes may be inserted surgically or through a laparoscopy. Gastrostomy or jejunostomy tubes are not easily dislodged.

Confirming Placement of Tubes

After the initial insertion of a feeding tube, before beginning a feeding or instilling liquids, and at regular intervals during continuous feedings, the placement of a nasogastric or nasointestinal tube must be verified. A misplaced feeding tube in the lungs or pulmonary tissue places the client at risk for aspiration. X-ray examination is usually the standard procedure to verify initial placement of a feeding tube (Eisenberg, 1994c). This is especially a priority when a small-bore tube has been used or when clients are at high risk for aspiration. Once placement has been confirmed, the tube should be marked with indelible ink at the exit point from the nose and the length of the tube measured and documented for future reference (Bockus, 1993). Since X-ray exposes the client to radiation, must be interpreted by a physician, and may be inaccessible, other methods are utilized to check tube placement. These include aspirating gastric contents, measuring the pH of the aspirate, and insufflation (or injection) of air into the tube coupled with auscultation (refer to the box for a summary of these methods).

Following x-ray examination, measurement of pH is the recommended method for determining correct placement of a feeding tube. A pH of 4 or less is acidic and indicative of gastric acid. Certain medications (eg, antacids) and certain diseases (eg, pernicious anemia) reduce gastric acidity and may be responsible for a higher pH value. To obtain accurate results, check the pH before each feeding. Checking pH following a feed-

(text continues on page 1186)

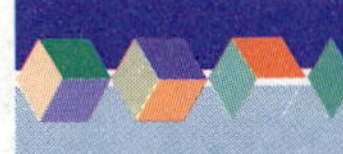

PROCEDURE 42-1

Inserting a Nasogastric Tube

Equipment

- Nasogastric tube of appropriate size (8 to 18 French)
- Small basin filled with ice or warm water (optional)
- Water-soluble lubricant
- Tongue blade
- Flashlight
- Topical analgesic (optional)
- Stethoscope
- Normal saline solution (for irrigation only)
- Asepto bulb syringe or Toomey syringe (20 to 50 mL)
- Nonallergenic tape (1 inch wide)
- Tissues
- Glass of water with straw
- Suction apparatus (if ordered)
- Bath towel or disposable pad
- Safety pin and rubber band
- Clamp
- Emesis basin
- Disposable gloves
- Tincture of benzoin

Action	Rationale
1. Check physician's order for insertion of nasogastric tube.	This clarifies procedure and type of equipment required.
2. Explain procedure to client.	Explanation facilitates client cooperation.
3. Gather equipment.	This provides for organized approach to task.
4. If nasogastric tube is rubber, place it in a basin with ice for 5 to 10 minutes or place a plastic tube in a basin of warm water.	Cold stiffens the rubber tube, making it easier to insert. Plastic tube may be placed in warm water to make it more flexible.
5. Assess client's abdomen.	Assessment determines presence of bowel sounds and amount of abdominal distention.
6. Wash your hands. Don disposable gloves.	Handwashing deters the spread of microorganisms. Gloves protect from exposure to blood or body fluids.
7. Assist the client to high Fowler's position, or 45°, if unable to maintain upright position, and drape chest with bath towel or disposable pad. Have emesis basin and tissues handy.	Upright position is more natural for swallowing and protects against aspiration, if the client should vomit. Passage of tube may stimulate gagging and tearing of eyes.
8. Check the nares for patency by asking the client to occlude one nostril and breathe normally through the other. Select the nostril through which air passes more easily.	Tube passes more easily through the nostril with the largest opening.
9. Measure the distance to insert the tube by placing tip of tube at client's nostril and extending to tip of earlobe and then to tip of xiphoid process. Mark tube with a piece of tape.	Measurement ensures that the tube will be long enough to enter the client's stomach.

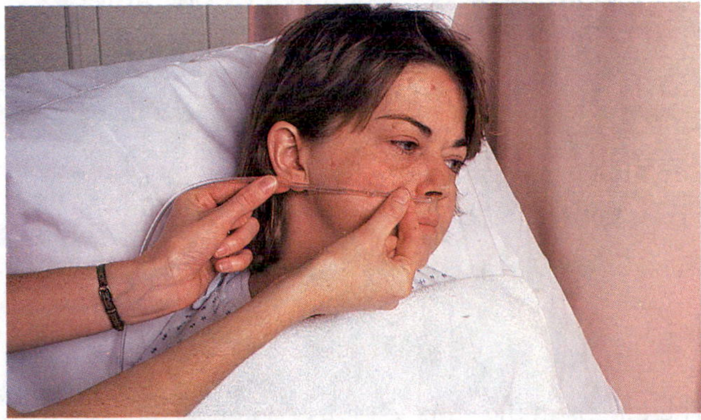

Action 9a: Measuring distance from nostril to tip of earlobe.

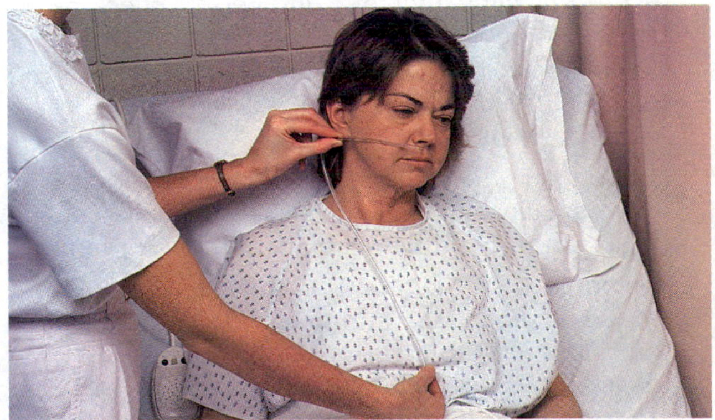

Action 9b: Measuring distance from earlobe to tip of xiphoid process.

(continued)

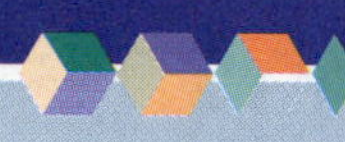

PROCEDURE 42-1 *(continued)*

Inserting a Nasogastric Tube

Action	Rationale
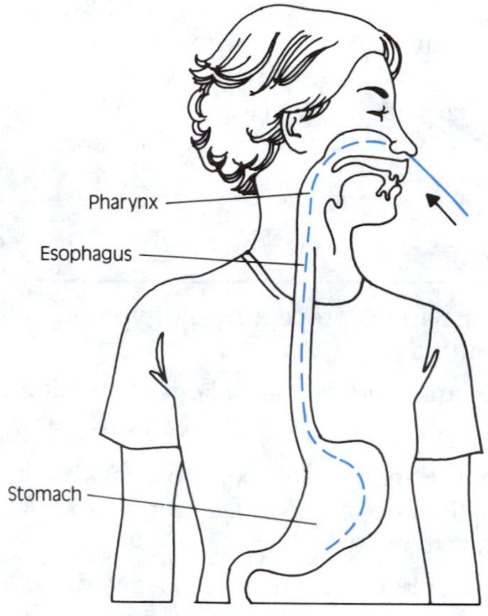	*Path of the tube.*
10. Lubricate the tip of the tube (at least 1–2 in) with a water-soluble lubricant. Apply topical analgesic to nostril and oropharynx or ask client to hold ice chips in mouth for several minutes (according to physician's preference).	Lubrication reduces friction and facilitates passage of the tube into the stomach. Water-soluble lubricant will not cause pneumonia if tube accidentally enters the lungs. Topical analgesic or ice acts as a local anesthetic, reducing discomfort.
11. Ask the client to lift the head, and insert the tube into the nostril while directing the tube downward and backward. The client may gag when the tube reaches the pharynx.	Following the normal contour of the nasal passage while inserting the tube reduces irritation and the likelihood of mucosal injury. The gag reflex is readily stimulated by the tube.
12. Instruct the client to keep head in upright or normal eating position. Encourage him or her to swallow even if no fluids are permitted. Advance the tube in a downward and backward direction when the client swallows. Stop when the client breathes. Provide tissues for tearing or watering of eyes. If gagging and coughing persist, check placement of tube with a tongue blade and flashlight. Keep advancing the tube until the tape marking is reached. Do not use force. Rotate the tube if it meets resistance.	Bringing the head forward helps close the trachea and open the esophagus. Swallowing helps advance the tube, causes the epiglottis to cover the opening of the trachea, and helps to eliminate gagging and coughing. Tears are a natural response as the tube passes into the nasopharynx. Excessive coughing and gagging may occur if the tube has curled in the back of throat. Forcing the tube may injure mucous membranes.
13. Discontinue the procedure and remove the tube if there are signs of distress, such as gasping, coughing, cyanosis, and the inability to speak or hum.	The tube is not in the esophagus if the client shows signs of distress and is unable to speak or hum.
14. Determine that the tube is in the client's stomach (these methods are appropriate for large-bore tubes but may be ineffective to check placement of small-bore, pliable tubes):	
a. Attach the syringe to the end of the tube and aspirate 10 to 20 mL of stomach contents.	The tube is in the stomach if its contents can be aspirated; pH of aspirate can then be tested to determine gastric placement.

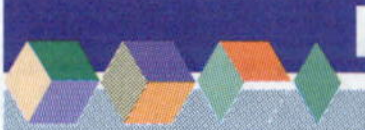

PROCEDURE 42-1 *(continued)*

Inserting a Nasogastric Tube

Action	**Rationale**
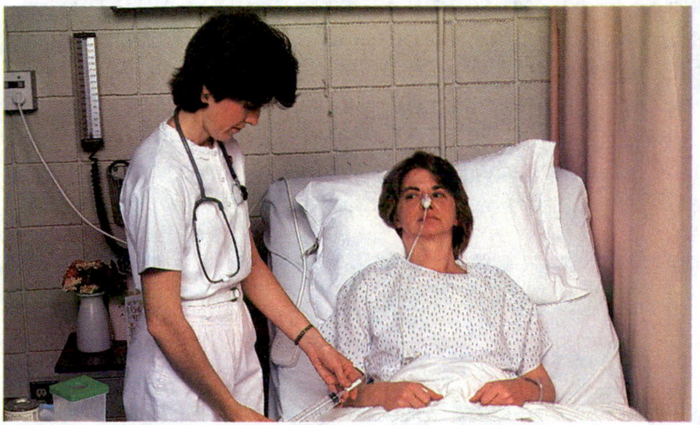	*Action 14a: Aspirating gastric contents.*
b. Measure the pH of aspirated fluid using pH paper or a meter.	The pH of gastric contents is acidic (4 or less), compared with an average pH of 7.0 or greater for respiratory fluid. Because pH of intestinal fluid also is slightly basic, this method will not effectively differentiate between intestinal fluid and pleural fluid.
c. Obtain x-ray of placement of tube (as ordered by physician).	X-ray visualization is the most definitive measure to determine tube placement.
15. Apply tincture of benzoin to tip of nose. Secure the tube with tape to the client's nose. Be careful not to pull the tube too tightly against the nose: a. Cut a 4-inch piece of tape and split bottom 2 inches or use packaged nose tape for NG tubes. b. Place unsplit end over bridge of client's nose. c. Wrap split ends under the tubing and up and over onto the nose.	Tincture of benzoin facilitates attachment of tape. Constant pressure of the tube against the skin and mucous membranes causes tissue injury.
16. Attach tube to suction or clamp the tube and cap it according to the physician's orders.	Suction provides for decompression of stomach and drainage of gastric contents.
17. Secure tube to the client's gown by using a rubber band or tape and a safety pin. If double-lumen tube is used, secure vent above stomach level. Attach at shoulder level.	This prevents tension and tugging on the tube. Securing the double-lumen tube above stomach level prevents seepage of gastric contents and keeps the lumen clear for venting air.
18. Assist with or provide client with oral hygiene at regular intervals.	Oral hygiene keeps mouth clean and moist and promotes comfort.
19. Wash hands. Remove all equipment and make client comfortable.	Handwashing deters the spread of microorganisms.
20. Record the insertion procedure, type and size of tube, description of gastric contents, and client's response.	This facilitates documentation and provides for comprehensive care.

(continued)

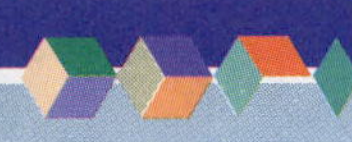

PROCEDURE 42-1 *(continued)*

Inserting a Nasogastric Tube

Special Considerations

For insertion of a nasointestinal tube:

- Measure tube from tip of nose to ear lobe and from ear lobe to xiphoid process. Add 8 to 10 inches for intestinal placement. Mark tubing at desired point.
- Place client on his or her right side. NI tube is usually placed in the stomach and allowed to advance via peristalsis through the pyloric sphincter (may take up to 24 hours).
- Test pH of aspirate when tube has advanced to marked point to confirm placement in the intestine. Check position via x-ray. Tape in place when confirmed.

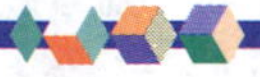

ing or administration of medications requires the following: flush the tube with water, wait at least one hour, instill 30 mL of air, and aspirate for gastrointestinal contents. A pH meter or pH paper may be used to test the aspirate. Some feeding tubes now have pH sensors on the tip to aid in assessment of proper location, but this should not be the sole method of determining placement (Viall, 1994).

Small-bore tubes offer greater resistance during aspiration than larger feeding tubes. Since they are less rigid, they may be more likely to collapse when *negative* pressure is applied during aspiration. More than likely, the difficulty is due to a blocked tube or the fact that the ports on the tip of the tube are not positioned in fluid. Research by clinicians has demonstrated a successful method for aspirating fluid from small-bore tubes. The steps are:

- Use a large syringe (30-mL or greater or according to manufacturer's directions) and insert 20 mL of air. *This moves the tube away from the GI mucosal wall and clears the tube of any fluid or feeding residual.*
- Pull back on the syringe and aspirate the air or GI fluid. If fluid is obtained, measure its volume and pH and flush the tube with water. *Removing the air prevents gastric distention and clearing the tube with water after obtaining aspirate keeps it patent.*
- If fluid was not obtained, instill 20 more mL of air, remove the large syringe, attach a smaller syringe (10 or 12 mL) and attempt to aspirate. *The smaller syringe may result in less negative pressure and make the tube less likely to collapse.*
- If still unsuccessful, instill air again with the larger syringe, remove it, attach the smaller syringe, and leave in place and attached to the tube for a 15-minute interval before attempting to aspirate gastric fluid. *This allows time for fluid to accumulate.*
- A final helpful maneuver might be to change the client's position. *Turning from side to side or raising the head of the bed up or down may facilitate movement of the tube to an area where fluid has accumulated* (Metheny et al., 1996).

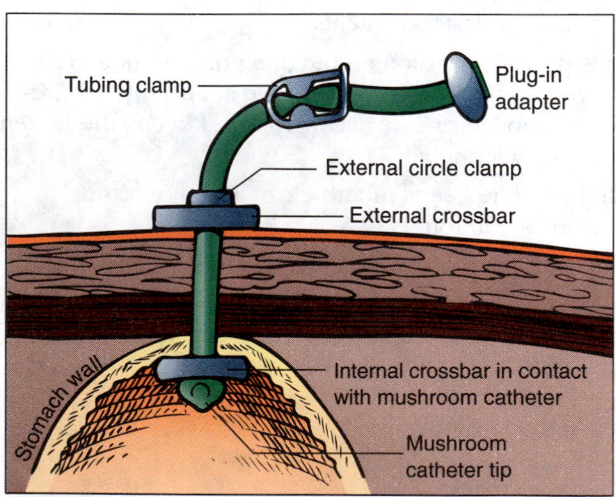

Figure 42-9
PEG tube in place in the stomach. (Smeltzer, S.C., & Bare, B. G. [1996]. *Brunner and Suddarth's textbook of medical–surgical nursing* [8th ed.]. Philadelphia: Lippincott.)

Checking placement of a gastrostomy or jejunostomy tube requires regular comparisons (according to agency policy) of the tube length to the measurement that was documented after insertion. An indelible marker can be used to identify the exit point of the tube from the abdomen (Bockus, 1993).

Administering the Feeding to the Client

Feeding Schedule. Based on the client's physical, medical, and nutritional condition, the nutritionist usually makes recommendations concerning the feeding pattern or schedule. *Continuous feedings* allow gradual introduction of the formula into the gastrointestinal tract, promoting maximum absorption. They require use of an enteral feeding pump which limits the client's mobility and increases cost. Feedings into the intestine are always

Guidelines for Nursing Care

Checking Placement of a Feeding Tube

Methods of checking placement of feeding tubes, once there has been initial verification of placement by x-ray, are controversial. Placement may have to be checked several times, and if any coughing or choking is observed or the caregiver has any doubt that the tube is properly placed, the feeding should be discontinued and the tube position checked via x-ray visualization. Other common methods to check placement include the following:

- Aspirate 10 to 20 mL of gastrointestinal fluid. Small-bore tubes offer the greatest resistance. Specific techniques are reviewed in the accompanying text.
- Measure the pH of aspirated gastrointestinal fluid. Gastric fluid is acidic (0–4), whereas intestinal and pleural fluid usually are slightly basic (>6). According to research by Metheny et al. (1993a), measuring the pH of aspirate correctly identified position of NG tubes 8 times out of 10 and of NI tubes 9 times out of 10. Their studies also indicate that it is probably safe for nurses to assume that a feeding tube is not in respiratory tissue if the pH of aspirated fluid is definitely acidic (≤4). This is the recommended method for subsequent monitoring of tube placement following x-ray verification.
- Inject 10 to 20 cc of air into the tube (insufflation) while simultaneously auscultating over the epigastric area with a stethoscope. A whooshing sound may indicate that the tube is in the gastric area. This method is considered less reliable because research has demonstrated that it is difficult for nurses to differentiate accurately between sounds in the lungs and sounds in the GI tract (Eady, 1993). Insufflation of air in the feeding tube should not be relied upon as the primary method to determine accurate placement of a feeding tube.

continuous to avoid triggering the dumping syndrome. Continuous feeding into the stomach is controversial because of the risk of reflux and aspiration.

Intermittent feedings are delivered at regular intervals using a gravity drip or a feeding pump to introduce the formula gradually over a set period of time. Bolus intermittent feedings, where a syringe is used to deliver the formula quickly into the stomach, may place the client at risk for aspiration or cause distention. They are usually not recommended but may be used in long-term situations if tolerated by the client. Another option is *cyclic feeding*. This involves administering continuous feeding for a portion of the 24-hour period. The usual routine is to feed the client for 12 to 16 hours, most often overnight. Cyclic feeding allows the client to attempt eating regular meals during the day, if this is possible, and makes ambulation and activity easier (Forloines-Lynn, 1996). The basic method for administering a tube feeding is outlined in Procedure 42-2.

Feeding Formulas. The nutritional composition of tube feedings depends on the feeding route, the client's ability to digest and absorb nutrients, and his or her nutrient and fluid requirements. Other considerations include the availability and cost of the formula, medical conditions that require diet modifications, food intolerances, and allergies. The typical feeding formula has the following caloric breakdown: 16% protein, 54% carbohydrate, and 30% fat (Eisenberg, 1994a). Protein is the most critical component; the client's needs will determine the complexity of the protein that is required. Many enteral feeding formulas are available. In addition to being nutritionally balanced, formulas may be high caloric, contain fiber, contain additional protein, or be especially formulated for clients with respiratory, renal, or other health problems. Detailed information on their composition and caloric value (most formulas contain 1 cal/mL) can be obtained from the product label.

Enteral Feeding Pumps. An enteral feeding pump regulates the amount of feeding solution that is delivered to the client. The newer pumps are user-friendly, have built-in safeguards that protect the client from risk of complications, and can be used in institutional and homecare settings. Safety features include automatic tube flush, cassettes that prevent free-flow of formula, safety tips that prevent accidental attachment to an IV set-up, and various audible and visible alarms (Viall, 1994; Gruver, 1993). Most pumps can operate for up to eight hours on battery, but manufacturers recommend that whenever the client is seated or resting for a period of time, the pump should be plugged into an electrical outlet for recharging.

Nursing Considerations

Agency protocols may differ and should be followed, but nursing actions that contribute to successful tube feedings include the following.

Promote Client Safety

- Check tube placement (for techniques refer to box given earlier in this section on enteral nutrition). The practice of adding food dye or coloring to the tube feeding as a means of detecting aspirated

(text continues on page 1191)

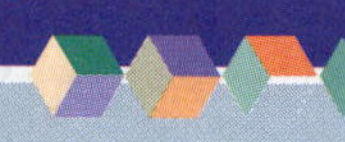

PROCEDURE 42-2

Administering a Tube Feeding

Equipment

Tube feeding at room temperature
Stethoscope
Feeding bag or prefilled tube feeding set
Alcohol preps
Clamp (Hoffman or butterfly)
Disposable pad or towel
Sterile water for irrigation
Asepto or Toomey syringe
Rubber band
Enteral feeding pump (if ordered)
IV pole
Disposable gloves

Action	Rationale
1. Explain procedure to client. Use stethoscope to assess bowel sounds.	This facilitates cooperation and provides reassurance for client. Presence of bowel sounds indicates functional GI tract.
2. Assemble equipment. Check amount, concentration, type, and frequency of tube feeding on client's chart. Check expiration date of formula.	This provides for organized approach to task. Ensures that correct feeding will be administered. Outdated formula may be contaminated.
3. Wash your hands. Don disposable gloves.	Handwashing deters the spread of microorganisms. Gloves protect from exposure to blood or body fluids.
4. Position client with head of bed elevated at least 30 degrees or as near normal position for eating as possible.	This position minimizes possibility of aspiration into trachea.
5. Unpin tube from client's gown and check to see that the nasogastric tube is properly located in the stomach, as described in Procedure 42-1, Action 14.	Even when initially positioned correctly, a nasogastric tube left in place can become dislodged between feedings. The instillation of water or nourishment could lead to serious respiratory problems if a gastric tube is in the trachea or a bronchus, rather than in the stomach.
6. Aspirate all gastric contents with a syringe and measure. Return immediately through tube. Flush tube with 30 mL of sterile water for irrigation. Proceed with feeding if amount of residual does not exceed policy of agency or physician's guideline. Disconnect syringe from tubing.	This indicates gastric emptying time. A residual more than 100 mL or more than 10% to 20% above the hourly feeding rate must be reported to physician. Fluid should be returned to stomach so as not to cause any fluid or electrolyte losses.
For Intermittent Feedings	
7. When using a feeding bag (open system):	
a. Hang bag on IV pole and adjust to about 12 inches above the stomach. Clamp tubing.	Formula displaces air in the tubing.
b. Cleanse top of feeding container with alcohol before opening it. Pour formula into feeding bag and allow solution to run through tubing. Close clamp.	Cleansing container top with alcohol minimizes risk of contaminants entering feeding bag. Formula displaces air in tubing.
c. Attach feeding set-up to feeding tube, open clamp, and regulate drip according to physician's order or allow feeding to run in over 30 minutes.	Introducing the formula at a slow, regular rate allows the stomach to accommodate to the feeding and decreases gastrointestinal distress.

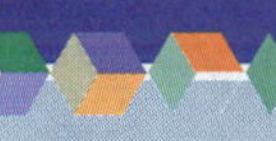

PROCEDURE 42-2 *(continued)*

Administering a Tube Feeding

Action | **Rationale**

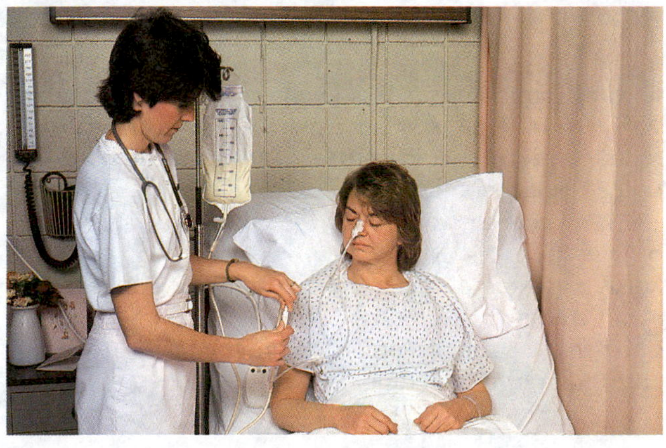

Action 7c: Attaching feeding-bag tubing to tube.

d. Add 30 to 60 mL (1–2 oz) of sterile water for irrigation to feeding bag when feeding is almost completed and allow it to run through tube.

Water rinses the feeding from the tube and helps to keep it patent.

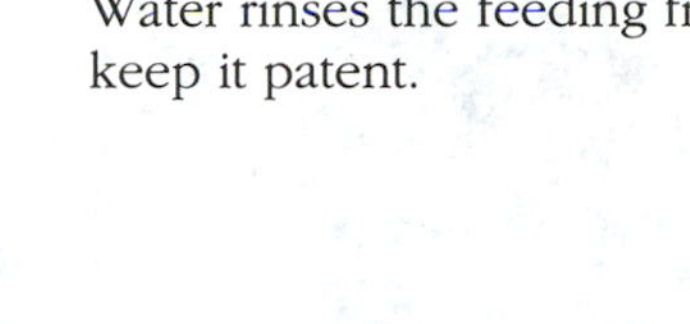

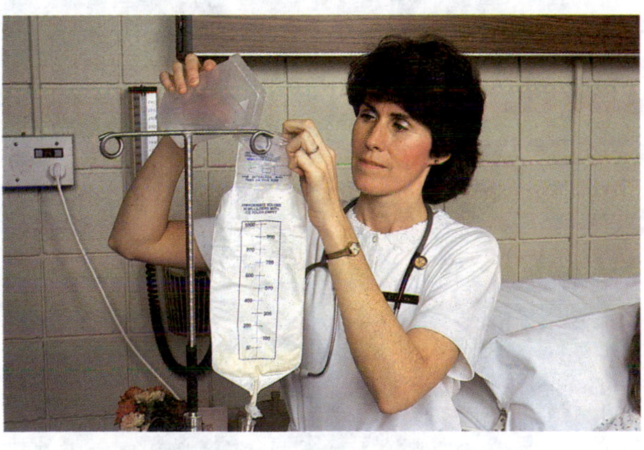

Action 7d: Adding water to rinse feeding tube.

e. Clamp the tubing immediately after water has been instilled. Disconnect from tube. Clamp tube and cover end with sterile gauze secured with a rubber band or apply cap.

Clamping the tube prevents air from entering the stomach. Cover on end of tube deters entry of microorganisms and protects client and linens from fluid leakage from tube.

8. When using prefilled tube feeding set-up (closed system):
   a. Remove screw-on cap and attach administration setup with drip chamber and tubing. Hang set on IV pole and adjust to about 12 inches above the stomach. Clamp tubing and squeeze drip chamber to fill one-third to one-half of capacity. Release clamp and run formula through tubing. Close clamp.

   Formula displaces air in tubing.

   b. Follow Actions 7c, 7d, and 7e. Feeding pump may be used with tube feeding set-up to regulate drip.

(continued)

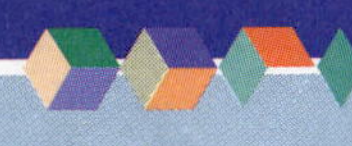

PROCEDURE 42-2 *(continued)*

Administering a Tube Feeding

Action	Rationale
For Continuous Feedings	
9. When using a feeding pump:	
a. Close flow regulator clamp on tubing and fill feeding bag with prescribed formula. The amount used depends on agency policy. Place label on container.	Feeding intolerance is less likely to occur with smaller volumes. Hanging smaller amounts of feeding also reduces risk of bacteria growth and contamination of feeding at room temperature.
b. Hang feeding container on IV pole and allow solution to flow through tubing.	This prevents air from being forced into the stomach or intestines.
c. Connect to feeding pump following manufacturer's directions. Set rate.	Smaller volume of feeding is infused continuously and is more easily tolerated by client.
d. Check residual every 4 to 8 hours.	Checking verifies placement of the tube and proper absorption of the feeding.

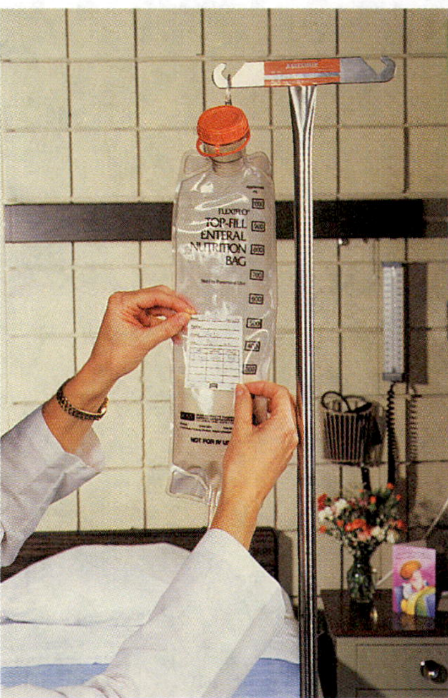

Action 9a: Placing label on container. (Photo © B. Proud.)

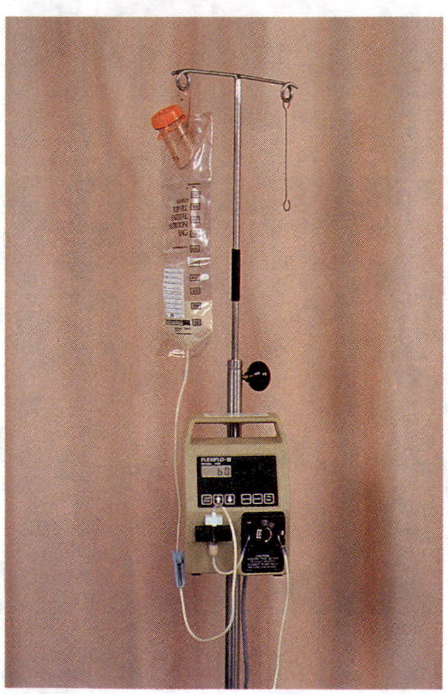

Action 9c: Feeding pump with feeding.

Action	Rationale
10. Observe client's response during and after tube feeding.	Pain may indicate stomach distention, which may lead to vomiting.
11. Have client remain in upright position for at least 30 minutes to 1 hour after feeding.	This position minimizes risk of backflow and discourages aspiration, if any vomiting should occur.
12. Wash and clean equipment or replace according to agency policy. Remove gloves and wash your hands.	This prevents contamination and deters spread of microorganisms.
13. Record type and amount of feeding and client's response. Monitor blood glucose, if ordered by physician.	This provides accurate documentation of procedure. Many feedings contain high amounts of carbohydrates.

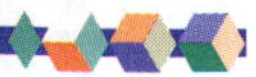

fluid is not recommended (Eisenberg, 1994a). The coloring may be contaminated with bacteria since it usually sits by the bedside, cause diarrhea because it contains sorbitol, and interfere with guaiac testing of stool.

- Check *residual* (feeding remaining in the stomach) before each feeding or every 4 to 8 hours during a continuous feeding. Record residuals on flow sheet or progress notes. Check agency procedure, but a residual of more than 100 mL or more than 10% to 20% above the hourly rate for the feeding usually indicates that the feeding should be interrupted or delayed for ½ to 1 hour (Bockus, 1993).
- Assess for bowel sounds at least once per shift to ensure presence of peristalsis and a functional intestinal tract.
- Prevent contamination during enteral feedings by maintaining the integrity of the feeding system and using proper technique. Kinsey (1995) states that a *closed system* reduces the opportunity for bacterial contamination. A closed system consists of a sterile, prefilled, ready-to-hang container, while an *open system* exists when formula from a can or bottle is added to a feeding set-up. The expiration date of formula should always be checked, hands should be washed before touching the equipment, sterile water should be used for flushing the tube, and disconnected tubing should be capped or covered.

Monitor Client for Presence of Complications. A summary of common complications and preventive nursing measures is given in the accompanying box.

- Prevent tube from becoming clogged or obstructed. Common causes of clogged enteral tubes include aspirated stomach contents, residue from medications, feeding flow rate of less than

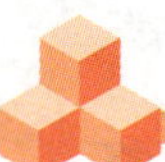

Guidelines for Nursing Care

Preventing Complications in Enteral Feeding

Potential Complication for Aspiration

- Use appropriate measures to check tube placement.
- Elevate head of bed at least 30 degrees during feeding and for 1 hour afterward.
- Give small, frequent feedings.
- Avoid oversedation of client.

Potential Complications for Clogged Tube

- Flush tube before and after feeding, every 4 hours during continuous feeding, and after withdrawing aspirate.
- Instill 30 mL of water with 50 mL syringe.

Potential Complication for Nasal Erosion with NG or NI Tubes

- Check nostrils every shift for signs of pressure.
- Clean and moisten nares every 4 to 8 hours.

Potential Complication for Diarrhea

- Start feeding at slow rate.
- Prevent contamination in both open and closed systems:
  - Change delivery set every 12 to 24 hours according to agency policy.
  - Refrigerate opened cans of formula and discard after 24 hours.
  - Limit hang time to 8 hours when using open system.
- Use aseptic technique for clients who are immunosuppressed or acutely ill (Znerneman, 1995).
- Assess for fecal impaction.

Potential for Other GI Symptoms (Nausea, Vomiting, Distention)

- Check residual prior to intermittent feedings and every 4 hours during continuous feedings.
- Avoid oversedating client (delays gastric emptying).

Potential Complication for Unplanned Extubation

- Anchor tube adequately with tape.
- Check on client frequently.
- Measure external length of tubing at regular intervals.

Potential Complication for Gastrostomy or Jejunostomy

"Buried Bumper" Syndrome (bumper or retaining disc presses too tightly against abdominal wall)

- Notify physician for complaints of bloating, abdominal discomfort, or signs of tube malfunction or bleeding.

Potential Complication for Stoma Infection

- Clean skin every shift with soap and warm water. Dry thoroughly.
- Use topical antibiotics as ordered.
- Assess for signs of infection.
- Request consult with wound care specialist.

50 mL/h, infrequent or inadequate addition of water to the system, and using a tube with a small lumen (Webber-Jones et al., 1992). Flush tube using at least a 30 mL syringe with 30 to 60 mL of water or irrigant recommended by facility. The use of carbonated cola or cranberry juice is controversial but many nurses feel these effectively clear feeding tubes of obstructions.

- Irrigate tube before and after feeding or administration of medications, at least every 4 hours during a continuous feeding, and after aspirating a tube for gastric contents.

Provide Comfort Measures

- Administer oral hygiene frequently to prevent drying of tissues and to relieve thirst. Offer the client the opportunity to rinse the mouth with warm water and mouthwash solution frequently. Lubricate the lips generously.
- Keep the nares clean, especially around the tube where secretions tend to accumulate. Using a lubricant after cleaning the nares is recommended.
- Help control local irritation from the tube in the throat. Analgesic throat lozenges or anesthetic sprays may be effective.
- Encourage client, if able, to verbalize concerns about tube feeding and presence of tube. A visit from another person who has learned to cope with this alternate feeding method may prove helpful.

Provide Instruction

- Provide health teaching to client and caregivers if enteral feedings will continue in the home setting. The accompanying discharge planning box re-

Discharge Planning for the Tube-Fed Patient

Here are actions you need to take and patient-specific information you should relay to the new caregivers when tube feeding will continue beyond discharge—at home or at an extended care facility.

When the patient is going home, caregivers need to know what supplies will have to be on hand when he arrives. That includes formula, administration set, tape, dressings, and syringes for irrigation. If they need help arranging for delivery, contact the social worker.

In addition, document the following information in writing:

- ☐ The name of the formula, and how much and how often it's given
- ☐ How the formula is stored, and for how long
- ☐ Proper handwashing technique
- ☐ How to mix or prepare the formula, if needed
- ☐ How to fill and hang the administration bag
- ☐ How to use an enteral pump, if indicated
- ☐ Proper patient positioning during and after feedings
- ☐ The type of irrigant and flushing fluid, as well as a schedule
- ☐ Which medications to administer through the tube
- ☐ The type and location of the tube and when it was inserted
- ☐ The measurement of the length of feeding tube outside the body
- ☐ How the skin at the insertion site should normally look, and how to care for it
- ☐ How to monitor temperature and pulse
- ☐ How to keep records such as I&O and weight
- ☐ When to see the physician for a follow-up visit
- ☐ Signs and symptoms to report, such as increased breathing rate, fever, decrease in urine output, altered level of consciousness, and increased stool frequency
- ☐ Emergency telephone numbers for the home-care agency, nursing agency, and physician
- ☐ How to dispose of equipment
- ☐ Whether and what the patient can eat by mouth

Although such detailed—and in some cases, basic—information isn't usually necessary if the patient is going to an extended care facility, you should at least send:

- ☐ A prescription for the formula as well as the feeding rate
- ☐ The type and location of tube, and the date of insertion
- ☐ Irrigation fluid and schedule

If you have most of the home care information on a prepared sheet, however, it won't hurt to just send it along to the extended care facility.

Before discharge, request the following consults:

- ☐ Social work
- ☐ Pharmacy
- ☐ Psychologic counselor
- ☐ Support groups
- ☐ Other, as applicable

(Eisenberg, P. [1994]. Feeding formulas. *RN, 57*(12), 51.)

views the nurse's planning for discharge of a client who needs a tube feeding and is returning home or to an extended care facility.

Removing the Tube

The tube must be removed as carefully as it is inserted to provide as much comfort as possible to the client. Oral hygiene follows removal of the tube. This is especially important to remove disagreeable tastes and odors, and should be done thoroughly when the tube has been in the intestinal tract and in contact with intestinal contents. Directions for removing the nasogastric tube are given in Procedure 42-3.

Using Nasoenteric Tubes for Decompression

In addition to providing enteral feedings, nasogastric tubes can be used for other purposes. They may be inserted to decompress or drain the stomach of fluid and air, allowing it to rest, or pre- or postoperatively, to promote healing after surgery. Nasogastric tubes also may be used to monitor gastrointestinal bleeding and prevent intestinal obstruction. Single- and double-lumen tubes (the lumen is the inner open space) are available. A single-lumen Levin tube lacks a venting system and mucosal damage can occur when suction is applied continuously. Double-lumen sump tubes are a tube within a tube (eg, the Salem sump tube). One lumen empties the stomach while the second lumen provides for a continuous flow of air. The airflow lumen controls suction by preventing the drainage lumen from pulling stomach mucosa into the tube's eyes and irritating the stomach lining. Suction can be continuous rather than intermittent, as is required when a single-lumen tube is used. Nasogastric tubes used for decompression require irrigation with 30 to 60 mL of normal saline solution (0.9% sodium chloride) to compensate for electrolytes that are lost in the gastric fluids removed by suction (McConnell, 1994). This is different from tubes used for feeding purposes, which are cleared before and after use with sterile water or tap water according to the physician's order. Procedure 42-4 outlines techniques for irrigating a nasogastric tube that is being used for decompression.

Providing Parenteral Nutrition

Clients who have nonfunctional gastrointestinal tracts, who are comatose, or who cannot consume a nutritionally adequate diet enterally (eg, clients undergoing aggressive cancer therapy, or those recovering from extensive burns, surgery, sepsis, or multiple fractures) may require parenteral nutrition. **Total parenteral nutrition (TPN)** bypasses the gastrointestinal tract for clients who are unable to take fluid orally, and meets the client's nutritional needs by way of nutrient-filled solutions administered intravenously through a central line, usually the subclavian or internal jugular veins. *Hyperalimentation* is another term used synonymously with parenteral nutrition.

TPN therapy is costly, requires constant monitoring, and has the potential for causing infectious, metabolic, and mechanical complications (see the accompanying box for complications). It should be used only when enteral intake is inadequate or contraindicated, and should be gradually discontinued as soon as possible. *Partial parenteral nutrition or peripheral parenteral nutrition* (PPN) is prescribed for clients who have an inadequate intake of oral feedings and require supplementation of nutrients through a peripheral vein. Isotonic solutions may be delivered peripherally (PPN) while hypertonic solutions must be administered through a central vein (TPN).

Identifying the Client Who Needs Parenteral Nutrition

Assessment of serum albumin level is the best indicator of a client in need of TPN. Clients whose levels are 2.5 g/dL or less are at severe risk of malnutrition. Total parenteral nutrition contains the three primary components necessary to maintain nutrition: proteins, carbohydrates, and fats. Additional components of parenteral nutrition include electrolytes, vitamins, and trace elements. Medications such as insulin (since TPN contains large concentrations of glucose) and heparin (to prevent formation of a blood clot on the tip of the catheter) may also added to the solution. The concentration of glucose in TPN is usually about 25%, yielding a hypertonic solution that, because of its concentration, must be delivered via a central vein. Fat or lipid emulsions may be administered separately or can also be added to a compatible glucose/amino acid solution to create a total nutrient admixture (TNA) which simplifies the administration of parenteral nutrition (Viall, 1995). TPN can be given for extended periods of time (up to 3 months) via a PICC or peripherally inserted central catheter (refer to Chapter 46 for additional discussion of PICCs). PPN solutions provide fewer calories and supplement a client's inadequate oral intake. This solution usually contains 10% glucose, which is suitable for administration into a peripheral vessel.

Nursing Considerations

Guidelines for the nurse to follow with parenteral nutrition therapy include the following:

- Use a pump to control accurate infusion of TPN or PPN.
- Compare the client's daily weight to fluid intake and output. Total weight gain should not be greater than 3 pounds per week.
- Assess serum protein and electrolyte levels for signs of imbalance. Check these values daily initially.
- Monitor blood glucose levels every 6 hours initially. Many clients on TPN therapy will continue to have their blood glucose level monitored at least every 8 hours throughout the duration of this treatment. Check agency policy. Because of the added glucose, be on the alert for hyperglycemia. Procedure 42-5 explains the technique for monitoring serum blood glucose.

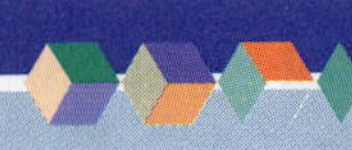

PROCEDURE 42-3

Removing a Nasogastric Tube

Equipment

Tissues
Bath towel or disposable pad
Disposable plastic bag
50-mL syringe (optional)
Normal saline solution for irrigation (optional)
Disposable gloves

Action	Rationale
1. Check physician's order for removal of nasogastric tube.	This ensures correct implementation of physician's order.
2. Explain procedure to client and assist to semi-Fowler's position.	Explanation facilitates client cooperation. Sitting position decreases risk of aspiration, if vomiting should occur.
3. Gather equipment.	This provides for organized approach to task.
4. Wash your hands. Don clean disposable gloves.	Handwashing deters the spread of microorganisms. Gloves protect hands from contact with abdominal secretions.
5. Place towel or disposable pad across client's chest. Give tissues to client.	Precautions protect client from contact with gastric secretions. Tissues are necessary if client wants to blow his or her nose when tube is removed.
6. Discontinue suction and separate tube from suction. Unpin tube from client's gown and carefully remove adhesive tape from client's nose.	Disconnecting tube allows for its unrestricted removal.
7. Attach syringe and flush with 10 mL normal saline solution or clear with 30 to 50 cc of air (optional).	Air or saline solution clears the tube of feeding or debris.
8. Instruct client to take a deep breath and hold it.	This prevents accidental aspiration of gastric secretions in tube.
9. Clamp tube with fingers by doubling tube on itself. Quickly and carefully remove tube while client holds breath.	Careful removal minimizes trauma and discomfort for client. Clamping prevents drainage of gastric contents in tube.
10. Place tube in disposable plastic bag. Remove gloves and place in bag.	This prevents contamination with microorganisms.
11. Offer mouth care to client and make client comfortable.	Provides for comfort.
12. Measure nasogastric drainage. Remove all equipment and dispose according to agency policy. Wash your hands.	Measuring nasogastric drainage provides for accurate recording of output. Proper disposal deters spread of microorganisms.
13. Record removal of tube, client's response, and measurement of drainage.	Facilitates documentation and provides for comprehensive care.

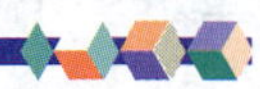

- Monitor liver and kidney function for signs of intolerance by assessing appropriate laboratory values. Common blood tests include the ALT and AST, which indicate the status of liver enzymes, and the BUN, which measures renal function.
- Use aseptic technique when changing solution, tubing, or dressings according to agency policy. Most infection control practitioners recommend changing infusion administration sets every 24 hours although some healthcare facilities recommend 48 to 72 hours (Viall, 1995).
- Be alert for signs of inflammation, infection, or sepsis, which are common complications of parenteral nutrition therapy.

Although the benefits of parenteral nutrition are extensive, return to oral or enteral nutrition is recommended as soon as possible. This lessens the risk of sepsis and prevents wasting and deterioration of the gas-

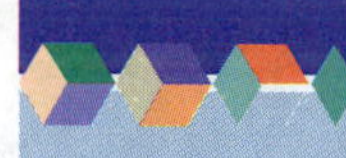

PROCEDURE 42-4

Irrigating a Nasogastric Tube Connected to Suction

Equipment

Nasogastric tube connected to continuous or intermittent suction
Irrigation set (Asepto or Toomey syringe and container for irrigating solution)
Normal saline solution (0.9% sodium chloride solution) for irrigation
Stethoscope
Disposable pad or bath towel
Clamp
Disposable gloves

Action	Rationale
1. Check physician's order for irrigation. Explain procedure to client.	This clarifies schedule and irrigating solution. An explanation encourages client cooperation and reduces apprehension.
2. Gather necessary equipment. Check expiration dates on irrigating saline solution and irrigation set.	This provides for organized approach to task. Agency policy dictates safe interval for reuse of equipment.
3. Wash your hands.	Handwashing deters the spread of microorganisms.
4. Assist client to semi-Fowler's position, unless this is contraindicated.	This position minimizes risk of aspiration.
5. Check placement of nasogastric tube (refer to Procedure 42-1, Action 14).	
6. Clamp suction tubing near connection site. Disconnect tube from suction apparatus and lay on disposable pad or towel.	This protects client from leakage of nasogastric drainage.
7. Pour irrigating solution into container. Draw up 30 mL of saline solution (or amount ordered by physician) into syringe.	This delivers measured amount of irrigant through tube. Saline solution compensates for electrolytes lost through nasogastric drainage.
8. Place tip of syringe in tube. If Salem sump or double-lumen tube is used, make sure that syringe tip is placed in drainage port and not in air vent. Hold syringe upright and gently insert the irrigant (or allow solution to flow in by gravity if agency or physician indicates). Do not force solution into tube.	Position of syringe prevents entry of air into stomach. Gentle insertion of saline solution (or gravity insertion) is less traumatic to gastric mucosa.

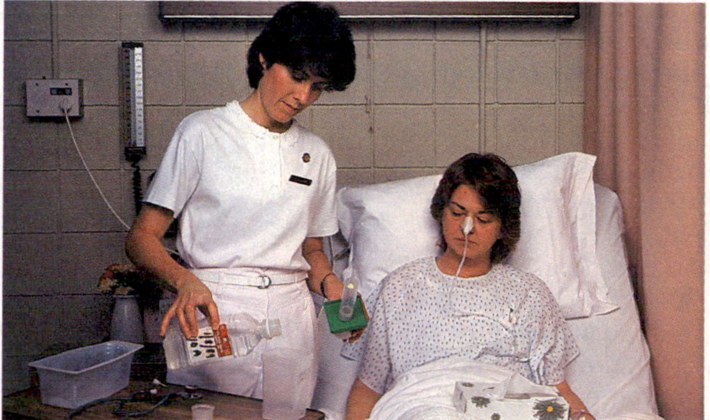

Action 7: Preparing irrigant.

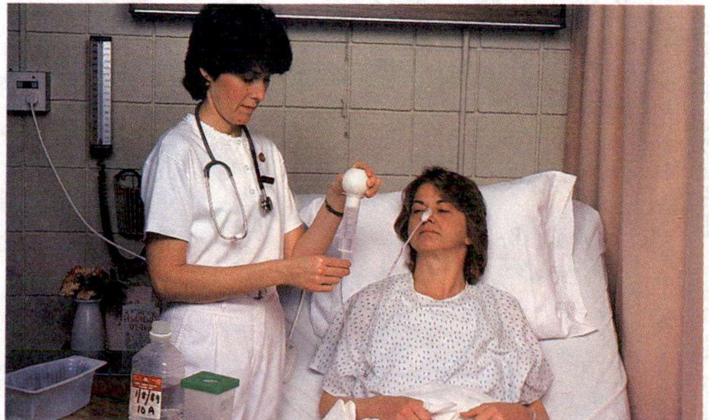

Action 8: Introducing irrigant into tube.

(continued)

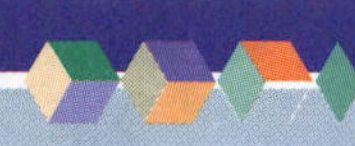

PROCEDURE 42-4 *(continued)*

Irrigating a Nasogastric Tube Connected to Suction

Action	Rationale
9. If unable to irrigate tube, reposition client and attempt irrigation again. Check with physician if repeated attempts to irrigate tube fail.	Tube may be positioned against gastric mucosa, making it difficult to irrigate.
10. Withdraw or aspirate fluid into syringe. If no return, inject 20 cc of air and aspirate again.	Injection of air may reposition the end of tube.
11. Reconnect tube to suction. Observe movement of solution or drainage.	Observation determines patency of tube and correct operation of suction apparatus.
12. Measure and record amount and description of irrigant and returned solution.	Irrigant placed in tube is considered intake; solution returned is recorded as output.
13. Rinse equipment if it will be reused.	This promotes cleanliness and prepares equipment for next irrigation.
14. Wash your hands.	Handwashing deters the spread of microorganisms.
15. Record irrigation procedure, description of drainage, and client's response.	This facilitates documentation of procedure and provides for comprehensive care.

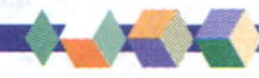

trointestinal tract. Many clients, however, require long-term parenteral nutrition and continue this therapy in the home setting. Individuals with AIDS, advanced cancer, difficulty swallowing, or chronic bowel problems are candidates for this type of nutritional support. Nurses are involved in educating the client and caregiver about the techniques and responsibilities associated with parenteral nutrition, providing technical and psychologic support, and documenting the assessments that allow parenteral nutrition to be continued in the home setting.

Potential Complications of Total Parenteral Nutrition

Infection and Sepsis Related to:
- Catheter contamination during insertion
- Long-term indwelling catheter
- Catheter seeding from blood-borne or distant infection
- Contaminated solution

Metabolic Complications
- Dehydration
- Hyperglycemia
- Rebound hypoglycemia
- Hyperosmolar, hyperglycemic nonketotic coma
- Azotemia
- Electrolyte disturbances
  - Hypocalcemia
  - Hypophosphatemia, hyperphosphatemia
  - Hypokalemia
  - Hypomagnesemia
- High serum ammonia levels
- Deficiencies of
  - Essential fatty acid
  - Trace elements
- Altered acid–base balance
- Elevated liver enzymes

Mechanical Complications Related to Catheterization
- Catheter misplacement
- Hemothorax (blood in the chest)
- Pneumothorax (air or gas in the chest)
- Hydrothorax (fluid in the chest)
- Hemomediastinum (blood in the mediastinal spaces)
- Subcutaneous emphysema
- Hematoma
- Arterial puncture
- Myocardial perforation
- Catheter embolism
- Air embolism
- Endocarditis
- Nerve damage at the insertion site
- Laceration of lymphatic duct
- Chylothorax
- Lymphatic fistula
- Thrombosis

(Dudek, S. G. [1993]. *Nutrition handbook for nursing practice* [2nd ed.]. Philadelphia: Lippincott.)

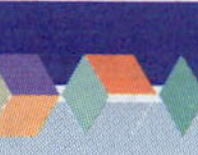

PROCEDURE 42-5

Monitoring the Blood Glucose Level

Equipment

Blood glucose meter
Testing strips
Sterile lancet
Cotton balls
Alcohol swab or soap and water
Disposable gloves

Action	Rationale
1. Check physician's order for monitoring schedule.	This confirms times for checking blood glucose.
2. Gather equipment.	This provides an organized approach to the task.
3. Explain procedure to client.	Explanation encourages client cooperation.
4. Wash hands. Don disposable gloves.	Handwashing deters the spread of microorganisms. Gloves protect from exposure to blood or body fluids.
5. Prepare lancet.	Aseptic technique maintains sterility.
6. Remove test strip from the vial and recap container immediately. Turn monitor on and check that code number on strip matches the code number on the monitor screen.	Immediate recapping protects strips from exposure to light and discoloration. Matching code numbers on the strip and glucose monitor ensure that machine is calibrated correctly.
7. Massage side of finger for adult (or heel for child) toward puncture site.	Massage encourages blood flow to the area.

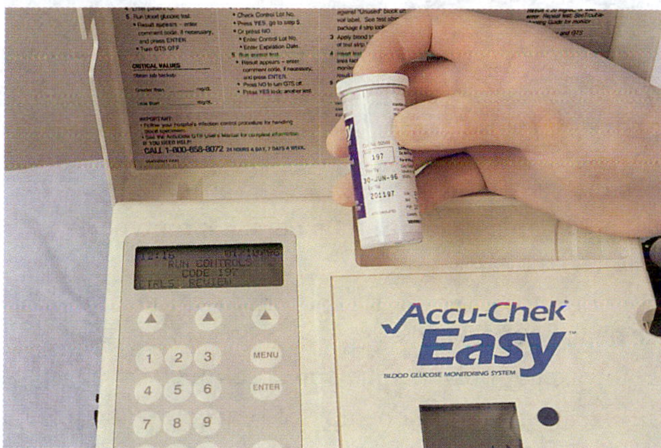

Action 6: Comparing the code number on the strip to the code number on the monitor screen.

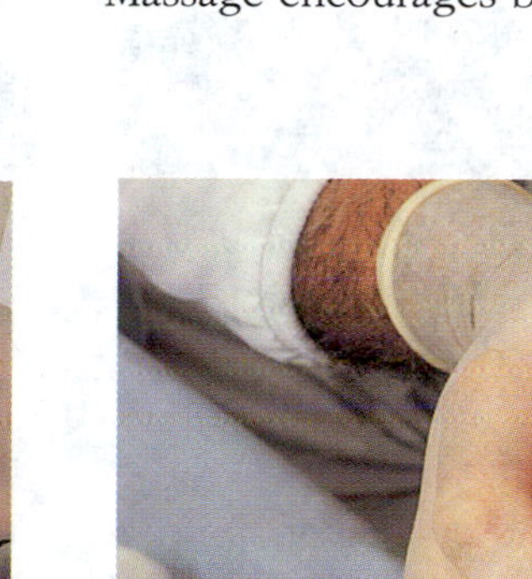

Action 7: Massaging side of finger toward puncture site.

Action	Rationale
8. Have client wash hands with soap and warm water or cleanse area with alcohol. Dry thoroughly.	Washing with soap and water or alcohol cleanses the puncture site. Warm water also helps to cause vasodilation.
9. With finger in dependent position, hold lancet perpendicular to skin and prick site with the lancet.	Dependent position increases blood flow to the site. Holding lancet in proper position facilitates proper skin penetration.
10. Wipe away first drop of blood with cotton ball if recommended by manufacturer of monitor.	Some feel first drop of blood may be contaminated by serum or cleansing product and produce an inaccurate reading.

(continued)

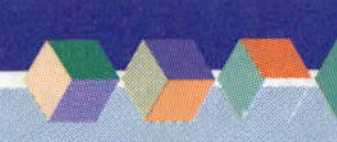

PROCEDURE 42-5 *(continued)*

Monitoring the Blood Glucose Level

Action	Rationale
11. Lightly squeeze or milk the puncture site until a hanging drop of blood has formed (check instructions for monitor).	Large droplet facilitates accurate test results.
12. Gently touch drop of blood to pad on test strip without smearing it.	Smearing blood on strip may result in inaccurate test results.
13. Insert strip into the meter according to directions for that specific device.	Correctly inserted strip allows meter to read blood glucose level accurately.

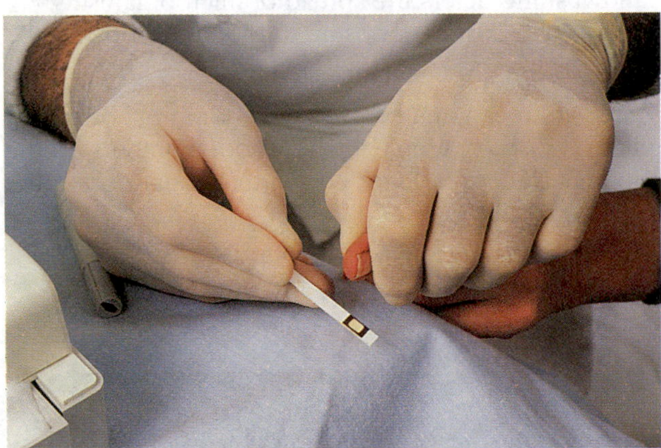

Action 12: Placing drop of blood on strip pad.

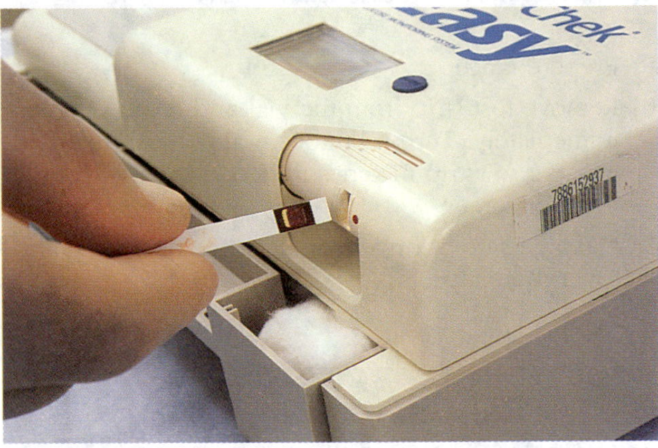

Action 13: Preparing to insert strip into monitor. (Photos © B. Proud.)

Action	Rationale
14. Apply pressure to puncture site.	Pressure causes hemostasis.
15. Read blood glucose results and document appropriately at bedside. Inform client of test result.	Timing when awaiting results depends on type of meter.
16. Turn meter off, dispose of supplies appropriately, and place lancet in sharps container.	Proper disposal prevents exposure to blood and accidental needle sticks.
17. Remove gloves and wash hands.	Handwashing prevents the spread of microorganisms.
18. Record blood glucose on chart or medication record.	This facilitates documentation of procedure and provides for comprehensive care.

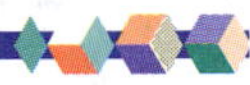

Home Healthcare Alert

A client on home TPN needs to be instructed to check weight and temperature regularly. Recordings should be documented on a form provided for this purpose.

EVALUATING

The effectiveness of the plan of care is evaluated as the last step in the nursing care process. On an ongoing basis, the nurse should:

- Evaluate the client's progress toward meeting nutritional goals
- Evaluate the client's tolerance and adherence to the diet, when appropriate
- Assess the client's level of understanding of the diet and the need for further diet instruction or reinforcement
- Communicate findings to other members of the healthcare team
- Revise the plan of care, as needed, or terminate nursing care

Nursing Process in Clinical Practice

Nursing diagnoses related to the client's nutritional status can be made after assessment data have been collected and analyzed. Nursing diagnoses may cite actual or potential nutritional problems, deal with how nutritional problems affect other areas of human functioning, or be related to nutritional knowledge deficits. The following three examples of nutritional diagnoses include assessment priorities, expected outcomes, and nursing interventions.

Altered Nutrition: More Than Body Requirements—Obesity

> The state in which an individual is experiencing an intake of nutrients which exceeds metabolic needs
> (NANDA, 1994)

Obesity is defined as body weight 20% or more above ideal weight (Fuller & Schaller-Ayers, 1994). A positive caloric balance, resulting from an excess caloric intake or a decrease in energy expenditure, leads to the gradual accumulation of weight. Although society assumes that obese people gorge themselves with food, studies have shown that obese people actually eat less than their thin counterparts. The cascading effect of increased weight gain leading to a decrease in activity and social isolation perpetuates the problem of obesity.

About 30% to 40% of adult Americans are obese (Burrel, 1992). One Canadian fitness study indicated that almost 24% of the participants had BMIs above 27 (obesity) and 16% fell into the overweight BMI range of 25 to 27 (Nutrition Recommendations, 1990). Obesity strikes all segments of society, although an increase in socioeconomic status is related to an increased risk of obesity in men and a decreased risk of obesity in women.

Obesity is probably multifactorial in origin, with different factors contributing to its development in different people. Numerous theories have been proposed. According to *genetic theories*, a low resting metabolic rate and an inherited family tendency contribute to obesity. *Physiologic factors* that have been implicated include an increased number of fat cells; the set-point theory, whereby the hypothalamus lowers the metabolic rate to maintain body weight; presence of decreased amounts of brown fat which burns kilocalories; ineffective insulin or "insulin resistance"; and hormonal imbalances. A food and family environment that encourages overeating or a work environment where exercise is minimal are *environmental theories* that have been introduced. Additionally, many identify *psychologic reasons* for obesity including compulsiveness, using food to satisfy emotional needs, relying on food for compensation for lack of affection and companionship, and overeating as a release mechanism for boredom, anxiety, and feelings of inadequacy.

Obesity presents a serious health problem physically, socially, and emotionally. It increases the risk of numerous medical problems, such as hypertension, hyperlipidemia, cardiovascular and respiratory disorders, diabetes mellitus, and osteoarthritis; increases the risks associated with surgery; increases the risk of complications during pregnancy, labor, and delivery; and increases morbidity and mortality. Obese people often are discriminated against in social, educational, and employment settings. And in a society that values thinness, obesity can cause one to feel desperate, frustrated, and rejected and to perceive oneself as being a failure.

Obesity is resistant to treatment, and weight loss usually is temporary at best. Current statistics indicate that approximately 90% of dieters who lose more than 25 pounds regain the lost weight within 2 years and only 1 in 50 are able to maintain the weight loss for 7 years (Shuman, 1993).

The following assessment criteria, expected outcomes, and nursing interventions are for a client diagnosed with obesity related to overeating.

Assessment Priorities

A thorough assessment to determine not only the degree of obesity but also whether the client is likely to succeed in a weight loss program must be performed before a plan of care can be devised. Although all obese clients have the potential to benefit from weight loss, not all clients are motivated enough to lose weight and to keep it off. Only the individual can determine if he or she is willing to permanently change behavior and food selections and exercise consistently to maintain the weight loss.

To determine the severity of the obesity and the client's level of motivation:

- Use interview questions to assess pertinent dietary factors, such as the pattern and frequency of eating; the social environment surrounding eating; the client's actual and perceived reasons for eating; the client's previous use of weight loss diets; cultural, familial, religious, and ethnic influences on eating habits and their relative importance to the client; and nutritional knowledge.
- Explore the client's lifestyle and physical and mental health for factors that contribute to obesity.
- Instruct the client to keep a food diary for 3 to 7 days to determine level of motivation as well as to gain knowledge about his or her eating habits.
- Compare the client's current weight and IBW and determine the percentage of excess body weight.
- Obtain body measurements, such as bust or chest, waist, hips, and thighs, for use in ongoing evaluation. Skin fold measurements also may be helpful in determining body fat and measuring weight loss progress.
- Assess for complications—hypertension, diabetes, heart disease, osteoarthritis.

- Assess the duration of obesity—age of onset, family history.
- Assess activity patterns and how activity is affected by obesity.
- Assess the actual and perceived degree of control the client has over food.
- Assess the client's feelings about obesity and weight loss diets and his or her sense of body image and self-esteem.
- Determine if outside support systems are present.
- Assess the safety and effectiveness of weight loss aids the client has used in the past.

Expected Outcomes

The client who undertakes a weight control program will:

- Identify eating attitudes and behaviors that contribute to obesity
- Practice behavior modification techniques to control factors that contribute to overeating
- Incorporate some type of physical activity into his or her daily routine, gradually increasing the intensity and duration of activity
- Enlist the support of family and friends, and attend group weight loss sessions, if possible

Interventions

Interventions for obesity vary according to its cause and severity. Weight loss programs should combine dietary changes, social support, exercise, and behavior modification.

Dietary Interventions

- Decrease calories for a gradual, weekly weight loss of about 1 to 2 lb (about 0.5 to 1 kg/wk).

Low caloric intake can be achieved by several methods, depending on the amount of weight the client has to lose and his or her level of motivation. For clients who do not have a lot of weight to lose, simply eliminating second helpings and snacks may be adequate. Counting total calories consumed throughout the day may work, but it does not ensure nutritional adequacy. A more effective and realistic approach uses exchange lists that state the size and number of servings allowed daily from each of six or more food group lists.

Traditional low-calorie diets may produce too gradual a weight loss for clients who are moderately to morbidly obese (ie, greater than 40% and 100% above ideal weight, respectively). In such cases, a medically supervised VLCD (very low-calorie diet) may be indicated. They generally provide between 400 to 800 calories per day and are designed to promote weight loss while preserving lean body mass. Supplemental vitamins and minerals are given, based on the client's laboratory data, and the client is closely monitored for tolerance, weight loss, and complications. Although the average weight loss in a 12-week period is about 45 lb (20.4 kg), the loss tends to be poorly maintained after the diet is discontinued.

Social Support

- Enlist the support of family and friends.
- Encourage the client to enroll in a group weight loss program. Such programs usually are more successful than individual programs.

Exercise

- Incorporate an exercise period into each day, gradually increasing its intensity and duration. Eating less and exercising more is absolutely essential for losing weight and maintaining the weight loss.

Behavior Modification Techniques. Behavior modification techniques encourage adopting desirable behaviors and eliminating undesirable ones, rather than stipulating rules.

- *Think thin.* List reasons why the client wants to lose weight, set long-term weight loss goals, reward successes periodically with nonfood items, and avoid talk about food.
- *Plan strategies.* Keep food only in the kitchen and avoid the kitchen except for mealtime. Cook only as much food as is needed for each meal, and avoid tasting food while cooking. Position low-calorie food in the front of the refrigerator and higher-calorie items in the back. Keep tempting items out of sight, preferably out of the house. Limit the list of forbidden foods.
- *Change eating habits.* Wait 10 minutes after feeling the urge to eat. Eat slowly. Never skip meals. Eat only in one designated place, and do not do anything else while eating. Eat low-calorie foods first. Use a small plate, and leave some food on your plate. Chew food thoroughly and eat slowly.
- *Modify shopping habits.* Never shop while hungry. Always shop from a list. Buy only as much food as needed. Do not buy items that you know are your weakness.
- *Incorporate lifestyle changes.* Keep busy with projects and hobbies. Accept changes in eating as a way of life, not a short-term hurdle to overcome. Trim recipes of extra fat and sugar. Do not weigh yourself too frequently. Accept setbacks or infrequent cheating without giving up on the plan—they are inevitable.

Although numerous prescription and over-the-counter drugs are promoted as diet aids, they are inappropriate and ineffective when used alone. At best, some drugs may be useful on a short-term basis when combined with other weight loss measures. If drugs are prescribed, the nurse instructs the client about the action of the drug, the reason for its use, adverse effects to be aware of and to report, and the potential dangers of the drug.

Surgical intervention, such as gastroplasty or gastric stapling, may be used as a last resort in clients who cannot lose weight by nonsurgical methods or are at increased risk of illness because of obesity. In certain clients, obesity poses a greater risk than the risk of surgery. Intestinal bypass procedures which use staples to reduce the size of the stomach and connect it to the jejunum via a small intestinal loop produce a dumping syndrome accompanied by weight loss.

Clients who suffer from compulsive overeating may benefit from Overeaters Anonymous, a self-help program designed to identify and cope with feelings that lead to overeating. Other options include referral for psychiatric evaluation.

Altered Nutrition: Less Than Body Requirements—Iron Deficiency Anemia

> The state in which an individual experiences an intake of nutrients that is insufficient to meet metabolic needs (NANDA, 1994)

One of iron's major functions in the body is to form heme, the pigment that combines with the protein globin in the blood to form hemoglobin. Hemoglobin is responsible for carrying oxygen from the lungs to the tissues, and therefore it is needed by all body cells for the release of energy.

Iron deficiency anemia, characterized by small (microcytic), pale (hypochromic) red blood cells, is a nutritional deficiency disorder that is found worldwide. Without sufficient iron, the body cannot produce enough hemoglobin, which hinders oxygen transport and leads to fatigue, weakness, and pallor.

The incidence rate in the United States for iron deficiency anemia is 10% to 50% (10% to 60% in Canada) among those in high-risk groups who simply do not consume enough dietary iron to meet their requirements—infants and children under age 2, menstruating women, older people, people in low-income groups, and vegetarians. Iron deficiency anemia commonly is related to an inadequate intake for two reasons. First, iron is not plentiful in the diet, and there are few excellent sources—liver and other organ meats, muscle meats, clams, liver sausage, oysters, pork loin, sardines, shrimp, and dark poultry meat. These animal sources are known as heme iron. Nonheme sources of iron include enriched and fortified grains and cereals, dried fruit, dried peas and beans, nuts, and leafy green vegetables. Second, only about 10% of dietary iron is absorbed, with a 15% to 35% absorption rate for heme iron and a 3% to 8% absorption rate for nonheme iron. Unlike heme iron, nonheme iron absorption is greatly influenced by other dietary factors. For instance, vitamin C, heme iron, and certain animal proteins enhance nonheme iron absorption, whereas tea, coffee, bran, phosphates, oxalates, phytates, and antacids inhibit its absorption.

Iron deficiency anemia also may occur secondary to an increase in iron requirement related to the following:

- Chronic blood loss—bleeding ulcers, gastritis, cancer, parasites, closely spaced pregnancies
- Inadequate absorption—chronic diarrhea, malabsorption syndrome, partial or total gastrectomy, pica, poor iron bioavailability of foods consumed
- Accelerated growth—pregnancy, infancy, and puberty

The following assessment priorities, expected outcomes, and nursing interventions are for a toddler diagnosed with iron deficiency anemia related to inadequate intake.

Assessment Priorities

To determine the severity of the iron deficiency anemia and contributing factors:

- Observe for signs and symptoms of iron deficiency anemia, which vary with severity and chronicity—fatigue, weakness, pallor, sensitivity to cold, anorexia, dizziness, headaches, thin and spoon-shaped fingernails, sore tongue and mouth, and pica (ingestion of nonfood substances, such as dirt, clay, or laundry starch).
- Interview the primary caregiver to determine the amount and sources of iron normally consumed. Be aware that toddlers who consume more than a quart of milk daily are at risk of iron deficiency anemia because milk displaces the intake of foods rich in iron.
- Assess intake for the influence of nonheme iron inhibitors and enhancers.
- Assess medical–socioeconomic data to determine whether the child's inadequate intake is related to low socioeconomic status or compounded by another medical problem.
- Interview the primary caregiver to determine whether the client has ever or is currently taking iron supplements; symptoms of iron overload may mimic iron deficiency anemia.

Expected Outcomes

The client will:

- Increase iron intake, especially heme iron
- Eat a source of heme iron at every meal
- Include a rich source of vitamin C at each meal (ie, citrus fruits and juices, broccoli, tomatoes, strawberries, cantaloupe, green pepper, brussels sprouts)
- Avoid tea and coffee immediately before and after eating because of their inhibitory effect on nonheme iron absorption

Interventions

- Instruct the family on ways to increase the iron content of the diet:
  - Use iron-fortified infant cereals until the child is 18 months old, if possible, because the iron in these cereals is absorbed more readily than the iron in other cereals.
  - Eat more organ meats, muscle meats, and poultry dark meat.
  - Eat meat at every meal, if possible.
  - Limit milk intake to less than 1 qt (0.95 L) a day to avoid displacing other iron-rich foods.
  - Add dried fruits to cereals and cookies; use as a snack or dessert.

- Use crushed iron-fortified cereals as a breading for meat, fish, poultry, and vegetables; mixed with butter for a casserole topping; as a meat extender in meatloaf, meatballs, and burgers; sprinkled on ice cream, fruit salad, yogurt, pudding.
- Substitute whole grains for refined products.
- Cook in iron pots whenever possible, especially acidic foods (tomatoes, foods with vinegar or lemon).

- Instruct the family on ways to increase iron absorption:
  - Eat meat at every meal, if possible.
  - Include a rich source of vitamin C at every meal.
  - Do not give a child tea or coffee.
- Instruct the family that if the client is anorexic or a finicky eater, small, frequent meals may be better tolerated.
- Advise the family to avoid giving the client acidic and salty foods, strong spices, coarse breads, raw vegetables, and hot foods and beverages if the oral mucosa is inflamed.
- If an inadequate food budget is contributing to poor iron intake, refer the family to the appropriate social service.
- If iron supplements are prescribed, teach the family when they should be taken, possible adverse effects to watch for, and the dangers of overuse.

Knowledge Deficit—New Therapeutic Diet

Absence or deficiency of cognitive information related to specific topic (NANDA, 1994)

The following assessment priorities, expected outcomes, and nursing interventions may be used for a client who is being discharged from a healthcare facility on a high-fiber diet (for diverticulum) that he has been receiving for 3 days.

Assessment Priorities

Through interview questions, obtain a diet history to determine the following:

- Quantity and sources of fiber in the client's usual diet
- Client's tolerance of a high-fiber diet while in the hospital: potential adverse effects of initiating a high-fiber diet too quickly include flatus, distention, cramping, and diarrhea
- Client's willingness to make the appropriate dietary changes
- Who shops and prepares the client's meals

Expected Outcomes

The client will:

- Eat a variety of high-fiber foods daily
- Substitute high-fiber foods for foods of lower fiber content
- Add bran to the diet slowly to decrease the likelihood of developing flatus and distention
- Drink six to eight glasses of water daily
- Recognize the signs and symptoms of eating too much fiber

Interventions

- Instruct the client that a high-fiber diet will increase stool bulk, stimulate peristalsis, and reduce pressure within the bowel to avoid aggravating the diverticulum.
- Instruct the client that many types of fiber exist in the diet; some are effective as laxatives, and others tend to lower serum cholesterol levels and may lower glucose levels in diabetics.
- Advise the client and family that the following dietary changes should be incorporated gradually:
  - Eat more raw vegetables and fresh fruit, preferably with the skin on.
  - Substitute whole-grain breads and cereals for those that contain refined grains.
  - Add up to 3 tbsp of coarse bran to the diet. The fiber in bran is the type most effective as a laxative. Bran can be sprinkled over cereal, applesauce, or eggs; added to muffins, quick breads, casseroles, and meatloaves before baking; and mixed with fruit juice or milk.
  - Drink eight to ten glasses of water daily; fiber absorbs water in the gut to increase fecal bulk.
- Inform the client about the potential adverse effects of eating too much fiber too quickly—flatus, distention, cramping, and diarrhea. Advise the client to reduce fiber intake if symptoms appear.

Client Care Study

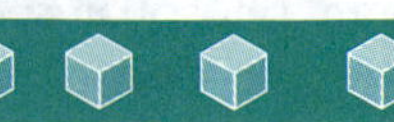

Susan Oakland, a 21-year-old student, was seen at the prenatal clinic for her first pregnancy at 5 weeks' gestation. On her next visit, 4 weeks later, she complained of nausea and vomiting and had lost 3 lb (1.4 kg).

Assessment Findings

A comprehensive nutritional assessment revealed the following data:

Anthropometric Data

Usual body weight: 112 lb (50.8 kg)
Weight at 9 weeks' gestation: 109 lb (49.4 kg)
Height: 5 feet 5 inches (165.1 cm)
Ideal body weight: 125 lb (56.7 kg; range is 113 to 137 lb [51.3 to 62.1 kg])
Expected weight gain for 9 weeks' gestation: 1 to 2 lb (0.45 to 0.9 kg)

Biochemical Data

- Laboratory data revealed low hemoglobin level and hematocrit.

Medical–Socioeconomic Data

- Client complains of nausea and vomiting, which begin in the morning and continue until midafternoon. Her appetite is poor. She also states, "I'm always tired."
- Client and her husband are first-semester graduate students; their source of income is graduate assistantships, so their food budget is limited.
- Client states that she did not intend to become pregnant, but both she and her husband are excited about becoming parents. She plans to take a leave of absence from school for one semester when the baby is born; she wants to breastfeed.

Clinical Data

Client appears pale. No other abnormal physical findings were noted.

Dietary Data

- Client's 24-hour recall revealed an inadequate intake from the milk group and a marginal intake from the grain and meat groups. She skips breakfast because of a hurried schedule, which is now complicated by nausea; lunch comprises soup, salad, and fruit; dinner usually comprises chicken; cooked vegetables; pasta, rice, or potatoes; and fruit. Client dislikes red meat and eats it only once or twice a month. She also dislikes milk and substitutes sugar-free soft drinks and water. Before becoming pregnant, she drank five or six cups of black coffee a day, but now she avoids it. Her snacks usually consist of fresh fruit and vegetables.
- Client is very weight conscious; she periodically crash diets to maintain her weight at 112 lb (50.8 kg).
- Client does not take vitamins, medications, or drugs; she drinks socially.
- Nutritional problems and contributing factors include the following:
    - Inadequate intake of milk and calories contributed to by nausea and vomiting, dislike for milk, limited food budget, weight consciousness
    - Poor iron intake contributed to by lack of good sources of iron in her diet, no supplemental iron intake
    - Meal-skipping contributed to by nausea and vomiting, hurried schedule
    - Underweight or weight loss contributed to by weight consciousness, nausea and vomiting

Core Competencies

In order to implement this plan of care the nurse needs the following specialized abilities.

Cognitive Competencies

- Knowledge of basic nutritional theory and the factors and variables that affect nutrition
- Awareness of pertinent economic considerations related to Ms. Oakland's nutritional needs
- Ability to develop nursing diagnoses that reflect Ms. Oakland's unique nutritional health problems
- Knowledge of which nursing interventions are most likely to yield desired outcomes
- Teaching skills to help Ms. Oakland and her husband understand need for nutritional modifications

Technical Competencies

- Strong assessment skills to determine Ms. Oakland's risk factors for nutritional alterations
- Caregiver skills directed toward maintaining adequate nutritional intake for Ms. Oakland and the developing fetus
- Ability to use a documentation system competently to communicate the prioritized list of nutrition-related nursing diagnoses

Interpersonal Competencies

- Interpersonal skills to communicate to Ms. Oakland that you are concerned about her priorities and committed to her well-being
- Ability to establish a trusting nurse–client relationship grounded in responsible caring
- Ability to work collaboratively with members of the caregiver team to meet common nutritional goals for Ms. Oakland

Ethical/Legal Competencies

- Willingness to assume responsibility for ensuring that the plan of care successfully assists Ms. Oakland in achieving her nutritional goals
- Competence in documenting nursing interventions
- Ability to serve as a trusted and effective client advocate

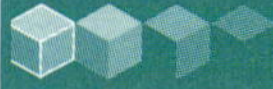

Nursing Plan of Care

for Susan Oakland

Nursing Diagnosis:	Altered Nutrition: Less Than Body Requirements, related to increased requirements imposed by pregnancy, nausea and vomiting, weight consciousness, hurried schedule, food dislikes as manifested by: reports of anorexia, fatigue, 3-pound weight loss in 4 weeks' time, pale color, and low hemoglobin and hematocrit values.

(continued)

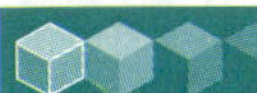

Nursing Plan of Care *(continued)*

for Susan Oakland

Expected Outcome: By the next monthly assessment, 6/26/98, the client will:
- Eat three or more small meals a day

Nursing Interventions	Rationale	Evaluative Statement
Determine how the client's schedule may be altered to allow time for meals. Encourage the client to have easy-to-eat foods available for quick snacks, like cartons of yogurt, cheese and crackers, muffins, and fresh fruit.	Client complained that her current schedule prevents regular meals. Easy-to-eat foods may be more acceptable and can be nutritionally comparable to traditional meals.	6/26/98 Goal met. Client eats three meals daily. Tries snacking on easy-to-eat foods when possible. *Recommendation:* Encourage more snacking to increase overall food intake. *L. Swift, RN*
Advise the client that nausea may be lessened by avoiding periods of hunger, and that later in the pregnancy, avoiding hunger will help ensure a steady supply of nutrients to the fetus.	Low blood glucose may contribute to nausea early in pregnancy; later in pregnancy, low blood glucose and resultant ketosis may be harmful to the fetus.	

Expected Outcome: By the next monthly assessment, 6/26/98, the client will:
- Eat dry crackers, bread sticks, or dry cereal 30 minutes before rising

Nursing Interventions	Rationale	Evaluative Statement
Advise the client to eat a source of dry carbohydrates before getting up in the morning.	Eating dry carbohydrates 30 minutes before rising helps avoid nausea.	6/26/98 Goal met. Client eats dry crackers every morning 30 minutes before getting out of bed. Reports that it prevents morning nausea. *L. Swift, RN*

Expected Outcome: By the next monthly assessment, 6/26/98, the client will:
- Drink water between meals

Nursing Interventions	Rationale	Evaluative Statement
Advise the client to avoid fluid with meals. Recommend fluids be consumed 1 hour before or 2 hours after eating.	Fluid with meals may contribute to nausea.	6/26/98 Goal met. Client avoids liquids with meals. Nausea is occurring less frequently throughout the day. *L. Swift, RN*

Expected Outcome: By the next monthly assessment, 6/26/98, the client will:
- Avoid diet soft drinks

Nursing Interventions	Rationale	Evaluative Statement
Advise the client to avoid diet soft drinks. Recommend acceptable nutritional alternatives to the client.	Saccharin and aspartame have not been proven safe for the fetus.	6/26/98 Goal partially met. Client reports that she drinks two or three cans of diet soft drinks a week at school to relieve thirst because nothing else is available.

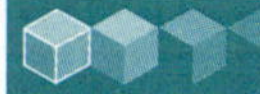

Nursing Plan of Care *(continued)*

for Susan Oakland

Nursing Interventions	Rationale	Evaluative Statement
		Recommendation: Encourage the client to bring something to drink during the day from home, such as frozen drink boxes of 100% fruit juice, which will thaw at room temperature, or an insulated container of ice water or milk flavored with vanilla (dislikes plain milk). *L. Swift, RN*

Expected Outcome: By the next monthly assessment, 6/26/98, the client will:

- Eat the recommended number of servings from each food group as suggested by the daily food guide for pregnancy

Nursing Interventions	Rationale	Evaluative Statement
Provide the client with a daily food guide for pregnancy, and explain the rationale for the increased recommendations. Investigate acceptable alternatives for red meat and milk, which the client normally does not consume.	Because this is the client's first pregnancy, she is not aware of the recommendations for eating during pregnancy. Although no one particular food is essential during pregnancy, red meat is essential during pregnancy and an excellent source of iron, and milk is an excellent source of calcium, two minerals important for the developing fetus. If the client is not provided with nutritionally equivalent alternatives, her diet may not be optimal, even if she consumes the recommended number of servings from the meat and milk groups (ie, client may not be getting as much iron as she can from her diet if she relies on fish, cheese, and white-meat poultry to satisfy the meat group recommendations).	6/26/98 Goal partially met. Client's intake is improved: intake from the grain and meat groups is adequate instead of marginal. However, the client still has difficulty consuming enough items from the milk group. *Recommendation:* Continue encouraging the client to consume more items from the milk group, such as cheese, yogurt, and pudding. Will advise the client to add skim milk powder whenever possible to fortify home-cooked and home-baked products. Will recommend that the client increase her intake of nondairy sources of calcium, such as broccoli, spinach, and greens. *L. Swift, RN*

Expected Outcome: By the next monthly assessment, 6/26/98, the client will:

- Gain 1 to 2 lb

(continued)

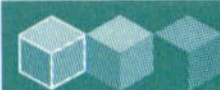

Nursing Plan of Care *(continued)*

for Susan Oakland

Nursing Interventions	Rationale	Evaluative Statement
Advise the client on the recommended rate and amount of weight gain. Stress the importance of quality weight gain.	Client needs to understand that a 25- to 35-lb gradual weight gain is considered optimal for fetal development, and results in little gain in maternal fat tissue. However, because the fetus and maternal tissues require nutrients along with calories, it is essential that the weight gain comes from eating nutrient-dense calories instead of empty calories.	6/26/98 Goal met. Noting a relief from nausea and an increase in the number of daily meals, the client gained 2 lb. *L. Swift, RN*

Expected Outcome: By the next monthly assessment, the client will:

- Take prenatal vitamins as prescribed by the physician

Nursing Interventions	Rationale	Evaluative Statement
Advise the client to take the supplement as prescribed and that the supplements are not a substitute for an adequate diet.	Supplements are intended to be used in conjunction with an optimal diet, not in place of one, because they do not provide optimal amounts of all required nutrients. Because the requirements for folic acid and iron during pregnancy are usually not met through diet alone, supplements of these two nutrients in particular are necessary.	6/26/98 Goal met. Client reports taking supplement as prescribed. No adverse effects noted. *Recommendation:* Will continue to monitor client's tolerance of supplement. Will continue to implement plan and reassess at next monthly appointment, 7/28/98. *L. Swift, RN*
Advise the client that the iron content in the supplements may cause constipation and the stools to become black.	Common adverse effects of large iron doses are constipation and black stools.	

Sample Documentation 5/22/98 Nursing

Mrs. Oakland was seen for routine prenatal checkup at 9 weeks' gestation. Assessment findings reveal that the client is underweight, has lost 3 lb (1.4 kg) in the past 4 weeks, is experiencing nausea and vomiting, has a deficient hemoglobin and hematocrit, and is fatigued. Other contributing factors include weight consciousness, hurried schedule, and food dislikes. Discussion centered on maintaining good dietary habits, improving overall intake and meal patterns to meet the demands of pregnancy and subsequent lactation, initiating dietary changes aimed at avoiding nausea and vomiting, and increasing iron intake. See plan of care. Client's progress will be evaluated at the next monthly visit, 6/26/98.

L. Swift, RN

Key Points

- A person's state of energy balance can be determined by comparing caloric intake with caloric expenditure, which is the sum of calories used during physical activity, for basal metabolism, and for specific dynamic action.
- The six classes of nutrients needed by the body are carbohydrates, protein, fats, vitamins, minerals, and water.
- Carbohydrates provide most of the calories in the diet. Glucose, the only carbohydrate present in

systemic circulation, may be burned for energy, stored as glycogen, or converted to fat and stored as adipose.

- Protein is broken down by the body into amino acids, which are then recombined to form proteins. Eight or nine amino acids are considered essential because they cannot be made in the body and must be supplied in the diet. Protein is used in the body for tissue growth and repair, as well as for the production of enzymes, hormones, antibodies, blood and other substances, and secretions; it also may be oxidized for energy. Excess protein is converted to fat and stored as adipose.
- Lipids provide more than twice the calories per unit of either carbohydrates or protein. Essential fatty acids cannot be made by the body, and therefore must be supplied through the diet. Dietary fat not used for immediate energy is stored as adipose.
- Vitamins and minerals do not provide calories but are needed for the metabolism of energy.
- Water provides the medium for all chemical reactions within the body; it is more vital to life than food.
- Tools used to evaluate a diet for adequacy include food groups and RDAs or RNIs. Dietary guidelines issued by health and governmental agencies focus on avoiding excesses rather than on obtaining sufficient quantities of nutrients. Most experts recommend that Americans and Canadians eat a variety of food; maintain their ideal weight; reduce their intake of fat, saturated fat, cholesterol, salt, and alcohol; and eat more complex carbohydrates and fiber.
- A person's food habits are a product of many variables, such as physical factors (eg, geographic location, food technology, income), physiologic factors (state of health, hunger, stage of development), and psychosocial factors (culture, religion, tradition, education, politics, social status, food ideology).
- Factors that influence nutrient requirements include age, sex, state of health, alcohol abuse, the use of medications, and megadoses of nutrient supplements. Nutrient intake can be affected by numerous physiologic and psychologic factors.
- A systematic approach is used to identify the client's actual or potential needs, formulate a plan to meet those needs, initiate the plan or assign others to implement it, and evaluate the effectiveness of the plan.
- Nutritional assessment data can be collected through history taking (dietary data and medical–socioeconomic data), physical examination (anthropometric data and clinical data), and laboratory data.
- Nursing diagnoses may be written to address nutritional problems specifically (Altered Nutrition: Less Than Body Requirements, More Than Body Requirements, Risk for More Than Body Requirements) or to identify the effect nutritional problems have on other areas of human functioning (eg, Activity Intolerance, Anxiety, Constipation, Diarrhea).
- Implementing a plan of care may involve nursing actions that are concerned with stimulating appetite, providing special diets, assisting with eating, withholding food, feeding by tube, feeding by vein, and conducting diet instructions.
- A nasogastric or nasointestinal tube is used to provide enteral nutrition for short-term use (less than 6 weeks) while a gastrostomy or jejunostomy tube can be used to supply nutrients via the enteral route for long-term use.
- Total parenteral nutrition (TPN) is a hypertonic, nutrient-rich solution that is administered intravenously through a central vein. Partial or peripheral parenteral nutrition (PPN) is an intravenous supplement for clients who have inadequate intake of oral nutrition and is delivered through a peripheral vein.

Study Questions

1. The most concentrated source of energy in the body is
   a. protein
   b. carbohydrates
   c. fat
   d. macrominerals
2. The Food Guide Pyramid that is a replacement for the food group wheel
   a. puts meat and dairy products at the peak
   b. gives equal emphasis to all food groups
   c. initially met with resistance from the meat and dairy industries
   d. focuses on deficiencies in our diet
3. Which laboratory test result indicates that a client is at risk for poor nutritional status?
   a. decreased serum albumin level
   b. increased lymphocyte count
   c. decreased blood urea nitrogen level
   d. increased platelet count
4. Mr. Yow is refusing to eat. What nursing action may stimulate his appetite?
   a. administer pain medication after meals
   b. encourage food from home when possible
   c. schedule his respiratory therapy before each meal
   d. reinforce the importance of his eating exactly what is delivered to him

5. Mrs. James has progressed to a full liquid diet. The nurse expects to see what items on her tray?
   a. apple juice and bouillon
   b. water ice and ginger ale
   c. pureed beef and cream of broccoli soup
   d. custard and a glass of milk
6. Parenteral nutrition provides nutrients to the client by way of the
   a. gastrostomy tube
   b. intravenous route
   c. nasointestinal route
   d. jejunostomy tube
7. The nurse completing anthropometric measurements for a client collects the following information
   a. height and weight
   b. serum hemoglobin/hematocrit levels
   c. diet history
   d. intake and output
8. The nurse and Mrs. Young discuss a weight reduction plan. The nurse teaches Mrs. Young that 1 lb of body fat is equal to about
   a. 1500 cal
   b. 2400 cal
   c. 3500 cal
   d. 5000 cal
9. Mr. White has been admitted to the alcoholic referral unit in the local hospital. Nutritionally, he will most commonly be prone to
   a. vitamin B malnutrition
   b. obesity
   c. dehydration
   d. vitamin C deficiency
10. A client has a nasogastric tube inserted for feeding purposes. Using the stomach as a reservoir for food is advantageous in preventing what complication?
    a. dumping syndrome
    b. duodenal ulcers
    c. hyperglycemia
    d. gastric ulcers
11. Intermittent suction is used in the client with a single-lumen nasogastric tube for the purpose of
    a. draining the stomach more effectively
    b. preventing electrolyte losses
    c. helping to prevent dumping syndrome
    d. helping to prevent the tube from suctioning the mucosa
12. Mr. Lang is receiving continuous tube feedings by way of a nasogastric tube. The nurse checks the tube's placement once a shift because
    a. the physician ordered it to be done
    b. the tube could be misplaced in the ileum
    c. the tube should be in the esophagus for feeding
    d. the tube can become dislodged and enter the trachea
13. Saline solution is used to irrigate a nasogastric tube used for decompression. The rationale for this is
    a. irrigating with water is a contaminated procedure
    b. saline solution is a hypertonic solution
    c. saline solution replaces electrolytes lost through nasogastric suction
    d. saline solution is less irritating to the gastric mucosa
14. Gorging followed by purging with self-induced vomiting describes the disorder of
    a. anorexia
    b. morbid obesity
    c. bulimia
    d. cachexia
15. Protein helps to regulate fluid balance by
    a. oncotic pressure
    b. hydrostatic pressure
    c. secretion of antidiuretic hormone
    d. retention of sodium

Answers With Rationale

1. The correct response is *c.* Fat provides 9 cal for every gram compared with 4 cal/g of protein and carbohydrates. Macrominerals are regulatory nutrients, not energy nutrients.
2. The correct response is *c.* The meat and dairy industries believed that their products were deemphasized in the Food Guide Pyramid and exerted pressure that blocked initial acceptance of it in April 1991. Fats are at the peak of the pyramid, while the greatest focus is on grains and cereals as the basic food group.
3. The correct response is *a.* A decreased serum protein level places a client at nutritional risk. The other test results do not represent a nutritional risk.
4. The correct response is *b.* Food from home that the client enjoys may stimulate him to eat. Pain medication should be given before meals, respiratory therapy should be scheduled after meals, and telling the client what he must eat is no guarantee that he will comply.

5. The correct response is *d.* Custard and milk are items found in a full liquid diet. Apple juice, bouillon, water ice, and ginger ale are clear liquids, and pureed beef and cream of broccoli soup are more likely to be found in a soft diet.
6. The correct response is *b.* Parenteral nutrition is given intravenously. Gastrostomy tube, nasointestinal route, and jejunostomy tube are routes for enteral feedings.
7. The correct response is *a.* Intake and output measurements indicate fluid balance, hemoglobin and hematocrit are biochemical data, and a diet history is used to complete dietary data.
8. The correct response is *c.* One pound of body fat is equal to about 3500 cal.
9. The correct response is *a.* The need for B vitamins is increased in alcoholics because they are used to metabolize alcohol.
10. The correct response is *a.* When the stomach is used as a reservoir, the formula is released at a controlled rate, preventing the occurrence of the dumping syndrome.
11. The correct response is *d.* Intermittent suction prevents damage to the mucosa of the stomach, and that is the primary purpose for using it with a single-lumen tube.
12. The correct response is *d.* Checking tube placement verifies that the tube is in the stomach and has not slipped into the trachea. The nurse's concern is to prevent aspiration of the feeding, leading to severe respiratory problems.
13. The correct response is *c.* Saline solution compensates for electrolytes lost during nasogastric drainage and is, therefore, the irrigant of choice.
14. The correct response is *c.* Bulimia is the only eating disorder mentioned that involves the cycle of gorging and purging.
15. The correct response is *a.* Serum proteins are responsible for maintaining oncotic pressure, which exerts a "pull" pressure.

Bibliography

Bockus, S. (1993). When your patient needs tube feedings: Making the right decisions. *Nursing, 23*(7), 34–42.

Burrell, L. (1992). *Adult nursing in hospital and community settings.* East Norwalk, CT: Appleton & Lange.

Capozza, C., & Sousa, A. (1994). Preventing malnutrition in the home care patient. *Caring, 13*(11), 68–71.

Carpenito, L. (1995). *Nursing diagnosis: Application to clinical practice* (6th ed.). Philadelphia: Lippincott.

Cerrato, P. (1992). Pasta: The perfect pick-me-up? *RN, 55*(5), 79–92.

Cerrato, P. (1993). Suggest diets with a difference. *RN, 56*(2), 67–72.

Cope, K. (1994). Nutritional status: A basic "vital sign." *Home Healthcare Nurse, 12*(2), 29–34.

Couig, M. P. (1993). The new food label. *American Journal of Nursing, 93*(2), 68–72.

Dudek, S. (1993). *Nutrition handbook for nursing practice* (2nd ed.). Philadelphia: Lippincott.

Eady, B. (1993). Dispelling the swoosh myth. *American Journal of Nursing, 93*(6), 16.

Eisenberg, P. (1994a). Feeding formulas. *RN, 57*(12), 46–53.

Eisenberg, P. (1994b). Gastrostomy and jejunostomy tubes. *RN, 57*(11), 54–60.

Eisenberg, P. (1994c). Nasoenteral tubes. *RN, 57*(10), 62–69.

Forloines-Lynn, S. (1996). How to smooth the way for cyclic tube feedings. *Nursing, 26*(3), 57–60.

Fuller, J., & Schaller-Ayers, J. (1994). *Health assessment: A nursing approach* (2nd ed.). Philadelphia: Lippincott.

Gruver, J. (1993). Selecting an enteral feeding pump. *American Journal of Nursing, 93*(6), 66–68.

Kestel, F. (1994). Blood glucose meters. *Nursing, 24*(8), 32P–32R.

Kinsey, G. (1995). Preventing contamination during enteral feedings. *Nursing, 25*(3), 20.

Lutz, C., & Przytulski, K. (1994). *Nutrition and diet therapy.* Philadelphia: Davis.

McConnell, M. (1994). Managing a nasoenteric decompression tube. *Nursing, 24*(3), 18.

Messner, R., & Stephens, N. (1994). Myths & facts about malnutrition. *Nursing, 24*(2), 25.

Metheny, N., Rud, L., Wiersema, L., McSweeney, M., Wehrle, M., & Clark, J. (1993a). Effectiveness of pH measurements in predicting feeding tube placement: An update. *Nursing Research, 42*(6), 324.

Metheny, N., Reed, L., Worseck, M., & Clark, J. (1993b). How to aspirate fluid from small-bore feeding tubes. *American Journal of Nursing, 93*(5), 86–88.

Miller, D., & Miller, H. (1995). Giving meds through the tube. *RN, 58*(1), 44–48.

Murray, T., & Beare-Rogers, J. (1990). Nutrition recommendations, 1990. *Journal of the Canadian Dietetic Association, 51*(3), 391–395.

North American Nursing Diagnosis Association. (1994). *NANDA nursing diagnoses: Definitions and classification 1995–1996.* Philadelphia: NANDA.

Nurses' guide to good nutrition and sensible weight loss. (1993). *Nursing, 23*(5), 67–74.

Nutrition recommendations: Report of the Scientific Review Committee. (1990). Minister of Supply and Services Canada, Cat. No. H49-42/1990E.

Nutrition screening manual for professionals caring for older Americans. (1992). (Project of the American Academy of Family Physicians, The American Dietetic Association, National Council on Aging.) Washington, DC: Nutrition Screening Initiative.

Ricciardi, E., & Brown, D. (1994). Managing PEG tubes. *American Journal of Nursing, 94*(10), 29–31.

Shuman, J. (1993). Weight-loss programs. *Nursing, 23*(5), 70–73.

Shuster, M., & Mancino, J. (1994). Ensuring successful home tube feeding in the geriatric population. *Geriatric Nursing, 15*(2), 67–81.

Steel, L. (1994). Identifying technique errors: Self-monitoring of blood glucose in the home setting. *Journal of Gerontological Nursing, 20*(2), 9–12.

Thompson, L. (1995). Taking a closer look at percutaneous endoscopic gastrostomy. *Nursing, 25*(4), 62–63.

Tomky, D. (1995). Advances in monitoring. *RN, 58*(3), 38–44.

U.S. Department of Health and Human Services. (1990). *Healthy people 2000: National health promotion and disease prevention objectives.* Washington, DC: DHHS.

Viall, C. (1994). Enteral feeding technology. *Nursing, 24*(8), 32J–32K.

Viall, C. (1995). Taking the mystery out of TPN: Part 1. *Nursing, 25*(4), 34–41.

Wardlaw, G., & Insel, P. (1993). *Perspectives in nutrition* (2nd ed.). St. Louis: Mosby.

Webber-Jones, J., Sweeney, K., Winterbottom, A., Fontneau, L., Johnson, K., & Fradette, M. (1992). How to declog a feeding tube. *Nursing, 22*(4), 63–64.

Williams, S. (1994). *Essentials of nutrition and diet therapy* (6th ed.). St. Louis: Mosby.

Yen, P. (1994a). Boosting intake when appetite is poor. *Geriatric Nursing, 15*(5), 284.

Yen, P. (1994b). Focus on women's nutrition. *Geriatric Nursing, 15*(4), 225–226.

Zwerneman, K. (1995). Use aseptic technique for tube feedings. *American Journal of Nursing, 95*(2), 58.

Chapter 43

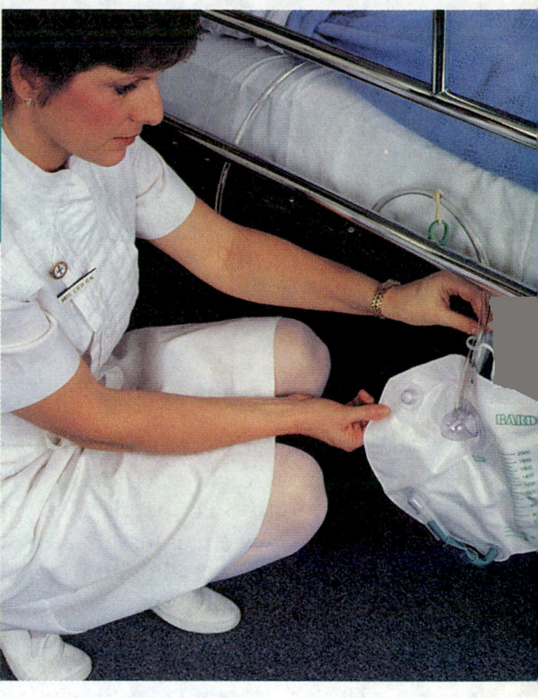

Urinary Elimination

Objectives

After studying this chapter, the learner should be able to:

Define key terms used in the chapter.

Describe the physiology of the urinary system.

Identify seven variables that influence urination.

Assess urinary elimination, using appropriate interview questions and physical assessment skills.

Execute the following assessment measures: measure urine output, collect urine specimens, determine the presence of select abnormal urine constituents, determine urine specific gravity, and assist with diagnostic tests and procedures.

Develop nursing diagnoses that correctly identify urinary problems amenable to nursing therapy.

Demonstrate how to promote normal urination; facilitate use of the toilet, bedpan, urinal, and commode; perform catheterizations; and assist with urinary diversions.

Describe nursing interventions that can be used to manage urinary incontinence effectively.

Plan, implement, and evaluate nursing care related to select nursing diagnoses associated with urinary problems.

Key Terms

condom catheter
enuresis
frequency
functional incontinence
hematuria
hesitancy
ileal conduit
indwelling urethral catheter
Kegel exercises
micturition
nocturia
oliguria
overflow incontinence
post-void residual (PVR)
stress incontinence
suprapubic catheter
urge incontinence
urgency
urinary incontinence
urinary retention

Elimination from the urinary tract helps to rid the body of waste products and materials that exceed bodily needs. The proper functioning of the urinary system is essential to the body's physical well-being, to life itself, and to a person's general sense of well-being. The nurse assisting a client with urination or intervening to resolve health problems related to urination needs many specialized abilities.

This chapter provides the student with knowledge of the physiology of the urinary system and the multiple factors that affect urination. A practical guide to assessing urinary elimination is presented, including detailed information on specific assessment measures, such as monitoring fluid intake, collecting urine specimens, testing urine, and assisting with other diagnostic procedures. Analysis of urinary data may lead to the identification of multiple nursing diagnoses or, when reported to the physician, to the early detection of a medical problem. Numerous examples of nursing diagnoses are offered. Expected client outcomes are established in planning care, and specific nursing strategies are presented. The section Nursing Process in Clinical Practice offers assessment priorities, expected outcomes, and nursing interventions for select nursing diagnoses of common urinary problems (Altered Urinary Elimination related to dysuria and maturational enuresis; Urinary Retention; Risk for Infection related to indwelling urinary catheter). These guides and the concluding client care study illustrate how the nurse's knowledge of the urinary system and urinary pathology is combined with specific nursing interventions to resolve urinary problems successfully.

Physiology

Kidneys and Ureters

The kidneys are located on either side of the vertebral column behind the peritoneum and in the posterior portion of the abdominal cavity. One of the more significant functions of the kidneys is to maintain the composition and volume of body fluids. They perform this function in a selective manner by filtering and excreting blood constituents that are not needed and retaining those that are. It is estimated that the total blood volume passes through the kidneys for waste removal about every half hour. Despite varying kinds and amounts of food and fluids ingested, body fluids remain relatively stable if there is proper kidney functioning. The waste product that the kidneys excrete, called *urine,* contains organic, inorganic, and liquid wastes.

The nephron is the basic unit of kidney structure. There are about 1 million nephrons in each kidney. Urine from the nephrons empties into the pelvis of each kidney. From each kidney, urine is transported by rhythmic peristalsis through the ureters to the urinary bladder. The ureters enter the bladder obliquely, and a fold of membrane in the bladder closes the entrance to the ureters so that urine is not forced up the ureters to the kidneys when pressure exists in the bladder. Figure 43-1 shows views of the male and female urinary systems and shows the position of the kidneys and ureters in the abdominal cavity.

Bladder

The urinary bladder is a smooth muscle sac that serves as a reservoir for urine. There are three layers of muscle tissue in the bladder—the inner longitudinal layer, the middle circular layer, and the outer longitudinal layer. These three layers are called the *detrusor muscle.* At the base of the bladder, the middle circular layer of muscle tissue forms the internal, or involuntary, sphincter, which guards the opening between the urinary bladder and the urethra. The urethra conveys urine from the bladder to the exterior of the body.

The urinary bladder muscle is innervated by the autonomic nervous system. The sympathetic system carries inhibitory impulses to the bladder and motor impulses to the internal sphincter. These impulses cause the detrusor muscle to relax and the internal sphincter to constrict. This, in turn, causes urine to be retained in the bladder. The parasympathetic system carries motor impulses to the bladder and inhibitory impulses to the internal sphincter. These impulses cause the detrusor muscle to contract and the sphincter to relax. The male and female urinary bladders are shown in Figure 43-1.

The bladder normally contains urine under very little pressure, and as the volume of urine increases, the

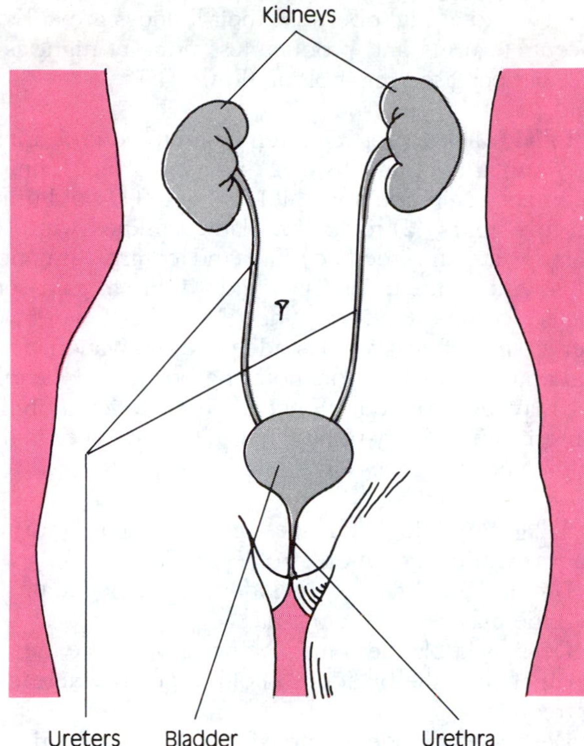

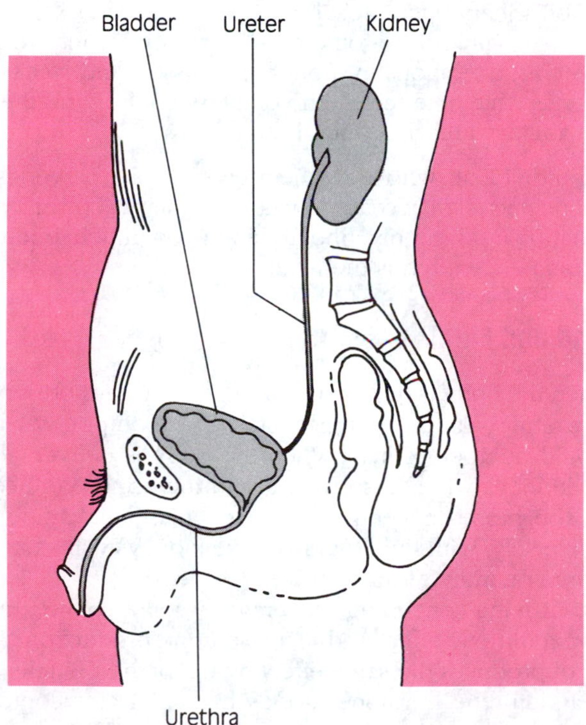

Figure 43-1
Frontal view of the female urinary tract (*top*) and lateral view of the male urinary tract (*bottom*).

pressure increases only slightly. This adaptability of the bladder wall to pressure is believed to be due to the characteristics of muscle tissue in the bladder, and makes it possible for urine to continue to enter the bladder from the ureters against low pressure. When the pressure becomes sufficient to stimulate stretch receptors located in the bladder wall, the desire to empty the bladder becomes apparent.

Urethra

The urethra differs in males and females. The male urethra is common to both the excretory system and the reproductive system. It is about 13.7 to 16.2 cm (5½–6¼ in) long and consists of three parts—the prostatic, the membranous, and the cavernous portions. The external urethral sphincter consists of striated muscle, and is located just beyond the prostatic portion of the urethra. The external sphincter is under voluntary control.

The female urethra is about 3.7 to 6.2 cm (1½–2½ in) long. Its function is to convey urine from the bladder to the exterior. The external, or voluntary, sphincter is located about midurethra. No portion of the female urethra is external to the body, as is true in the male. Most literature refers to muscle at the meatus in the female as the external sphincter.

Act of Micturition

The process of emptying the bladder is known as **micturition**; it also is called *voiding* or *urination.* Nerve centers for micturition are situated in the brain and the spinal cord. Voiding is largely an involuntary reflex act, but its control can be learned.

After stimulation of the stretch receptors in the bladder as the urine collects, the desire to void is experienced. Usually this occurs when about 100 to 200 mL for the child and 200 to 300 mL for the adult has collected. If micturition is initiated, the detrusor muscle contracts, the internal sphincter relaxes, and urine enters the posterior urethra. The muscles of the perineum and the external sphincter relax, and micturition occurs. The act consists of relaxation of the internal sphincter, contraction of the detrusor muscle, slight contraction of the muscle of the abdominal wall, and lowering of the diaphragm. The act of micturition normally is painless. During micturition, the pressure within the bladder is many times greater than it is during the time the bladder is filling. The voluntary control of voiding is limited to initiating, restraining, and interrupting the act.

Restraint of voiding is believed to be subconscious when the volume of urine in the bladder is small. But when voiding is delayed, the bladder continues to fill. Discomfort may then be felt when undue distention occurs, and the urgency to void becomes paramount.

Sometimes increased abdominal pressure, as occurs with coughing and sneezing, forces the escape of urine involuntarily, especially in the female, since the urethra is shorter. Any involuntary loss of urine that is sufficient to cause a problem is referred to as **urinary incontinence**. Strong psychic factors, such as marked fear, also may result in involuntary urination. Under certain conditions, it may be difficult to relax the restraining muscles sufficiently to void, such as when a urine specimen is requested from a shy or an embarrassed person.

When the higher nerve centers develop after infancy, the voluntary control of micturition develops also. Until that time, voiding is purely reflex. People whose bladders are isolated from control of the brain because of injury or disease also void by reflex only. This is called *autonomic bladder.*

Frequency of Micturition

The frequency of micturition depends on the amount of urine being produced. The more urine produced, the more often voiding is necessary, and vice versa. Unless the fluid intake is very large, most healthy people do not void during normal sleeping hours. The first voided urine of the day usually is more concentrated than urine excreted during the remainder of the day. The nurse should remember that because the first voiding of the day is not fresh, but rather an accumulation of a number of hours of kidney output, this urine may or may not be used as a specimen for certain tests.

Some people normally void small amounts at frequent intervals because they habitually respond to the first early urge to void. This habit is insignificant and not necessarily an indication of disease. Conversely, if this pattern is not a habit but a change in urination routine, it can be an indication of illness.

Other people have habits that result in infrequent voiding. For example, some people go 8 to 12 waking hours or longer without urinating. Factors such as a habitual low fluid intake owing to environmental conditions or age may be the reason. The inaccessibility of toilet facilities owing to travel, work circumstances, or illness, and limitations of mobility also can be the cause of infrequent urination. People who habitually urinate infrequently develop more urinary tract infections and kidney disorders than those who urinate at least every 3 to 4 hours. The reason is believed to be stagnation of urine in the bladder, which serves as a good medium for bacterial growth. Infrequent voiding that is a change in one's urination pattern also can be indicative of a decreased production of urine owing to kidney or circulatory disorders. **Urinary retention** occurs when urine is produced normally but not appropriately excreted from the bladder.

Factors Affecting Micturition

Numerous factors affect the amount and quality of urine produced by the body and the manner in which it is excreted.

Developmental Considerations

Infants are born without voluntary control of micturition and with little ability to concentrate urine. Most children develop urinary control between ages 2 and 5 years. Daytime control precedes nighttime control, and most girls develop control earlier than boys. Older children and adults control urination voluntarily and seldom wake to void at night because their kidneys are able to concentrate urine and produce less urine at night as a result of decreased renal blood flow.

Toilet Training. Most children begin to control urination voluntarily at age 18 to 24 months. Toilet training should not begin until the child is able to (1) hold urine for 1 to 2 hours, (2) recognize bladder fullness, and (3) communicate the need to void and control urination until seated on the toilet. The child's desire to gain control also is important. Wanting to be like a parent or older sibling often provides adequate motivation. Lifelong attitudes toward urination, the body, and cleanliness may develop during the time of toilet training. (Enuresis, involuntary urination, is discussed later in the section Nursing Process in Clinical Practice.)

Aging. Physiologic changes that accompany normal aging may affect urination in older adults:

- Diminished ability of the kidneys to concentrate urine may result in nocturia.
- Decreased bladder muscle tone may reduce the capacity of the bladder to hold urine and increase frequency.
- Decreased bladder contractility may lead to urine retention and stasis, which increase the likelihood of urinary tract infection.
- Neuromuscular problems, degenerative joint problems, alterations in thought processes, and weakness may interfere with voluntary control and the ability to reach a toilet in time.

Individuals who view themselves as old, powerless, and neglected may cease to value voluntary control over urination and simply find toileting too much bother. Incontinence often is the result.

Food and Fluid

When the body is functioning well, the kidneys preserve a careful balance of fluid intake and output, which should be about equal. When the body is dehydrated, the kidneys will reabsorb fluid and the urine produced will be more concentrated and decreased in amount. Conversely, with fluid overload, the kidneys will excrete a large quantity of dilute urine.

Caffeine-containing beverages (cola, coffee, tea) have a diuretic effect and increase urine production. Alcohol produces the same effect by inhibiting the release of antidiuretic hormone. Foods high in water content may increase urine production. Foods and beverages with high sodium content cause sodium and water reabsorption and retention, thereby decreasing urine formation. Also, certain foods may affect the odor of the urine (asparagus, onions) or its color (beets).

Lifestyle

Many individual, family, and sociocultural variables influence a person's normal voiding habits. For some people, voiding is a personal and private act, something one

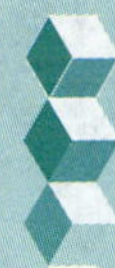

Research in Nursing: Making a Difference

Urinary Elimination

Urinary incontinence is an embarrassing, potentially disabling, and costly health problem that affects clients of all ages, but it is particularly devastating for older adults. Rather than being viewed as an inevitable outcome of aging, it is now recognized as a symptom of an underlying medical, psychologic, or environmental problem. In recent research, nurses have examined urinary incontinence in various settings and from various perspectives. Implications from this research can be incorporated into nursing practice.

Related Research

Gray, M., Rayome, R., & Anson, C. (1995). Incontinence and clean intermittent catheterization following spinal cord injury. *Clinical Nursing Research, 4*(1), 6–18.
A large majority of clients with spinal cord injury use clean, intermittent catheterization for management of bladder functions. Some experience leakage between catheterizations but none of the clients in this study related this leakage to the possible presence of a urinary tract infection. They were also unaware of the diuretic effect of some liquids and the possible relationship between fluid intake and the occurrence of incontinent episodes. Ongoing education is of paramount importance in assisting these clients to manage any persistent leakage and attain their optimal quality of life.

Flynn, L., Cell, P., & Luisi, E. (1994). Effectiveness of pelvic muscle exercises in reducing urge incontinence among community residing elders. *Journal of Gerontological Nursing, 20*(5), 23–27.
A group of incontinent older adults living in the community were visited weekly by continence nurses and taught how to perform pelvic strengthening exercises. This educational effort resulted in a significant reduction of incontinent episodes in clients with urge as well as stress incontinence. The assimilation of these restorative interventions into nursing practice had a beneficial impact on the lives of this particular population.

Colling, J., Owen, T., & McCreedy, M. (1994). Urine volumes and voiding patterns among nursing home residents. *Geriatric Nursing, 15*(4), 188–192.
Although older adults are prone to fluid imbalance, it is sometimes difficult to keep an accurate output record due to their urinary incontinence. When voiding patterns for a group of incontinent nursing home residents were carefully examined, two major findings were reported. One third of these residents were underhydrated and the largest amount of urine output occurred between midnight and 8:00 AM despite the fact that the majority of their fluid intake occurred earlier in the day. Additional hydration and a toileting program that continues through the night were recommended to resolve dehydration and lessen incontinence.

Summary

Incontinence research presents implications for changing current methods of nursing practice. The diverse causes of urinary incontinence and the various environmental settings must be considered as nurses strive to identify the most successful and clinically realistic methods of significantly improving urinary incontinence.

does not talk about. Needing assistance with a bedpan or urinal thus provokes great embarrassment and anxiety, which can be compounded when the bedpan is offered by a nurse of the opposite sex. For others, voiding is a natural act, and these people readily excuse themselves to void whenever the urge presents.

Toilet training is a developmental milestone that is taught a variety of ways according to cultural patterns. Initiation of toilet training may begin in some cultures before the child is 1 year old and in others may not be considered until the child is near 5 years of age. The nurse must recognize cultural influences on this parenting responsibility while promoting the concept of flexibility. It is always reassuring for parents to hear that any regression of toileting skills that may occur during a hospitalization is not unexpected and is usually short-lived (Andrews & Boyle, 1995).

Psychologic Variables

Many people who experience stress will void smaller amounts of urine at more frequent intervals. Stress also can interfere with the ability to relax perineal muscles and the external urethral sphincter. When this happens, the urge to void is present but emptying the bladder completely becomes difficult or impossible.

Activity and Muscle Tone

Among the many benefits of regular exercise are increased metabolism and optimal urine production and elimination. With prolonged periods of immobility, decreased bladder and sphincter tone can result in poor urinary control and urinary stasis. People with indwelling urinary catheters lose bladder tone because the bladder muscle is not being stretched as the bladder fills with urine. Other causes of decreased muscle tone include childbearing, menopausal muscle atrophy, and damage to muscles from trauma.

Pathologic Conditions

Certain renal or urologic problems can affect both the quantity and the quality of urine produced. Diseases known to be associated with renal problems include congenital urinary tract abnormalities, polycystic kidney disease, urinary tract infection, urinary calculi (kidney stones), hypertension, diabetes mellitus, gout, and certain connective tissue disorders.

Diseases that reduce physical activity or lead to generalized weakness, such as arthritis, Parkinson's disease, and degenerative joint disease, may interfere with toileting. Cognitive deficits and certain psychiatric problems can interfere with a person's ability or desire to control urination voluntarily. Fever and diaphoresis (profuse perspiration) result in the kidney's conservation of body fluids. Urine production is decreased, and the urine is highly concentrated. Other pathologic conditions, such as those present in congestive heart failure, may lead to fluid retention and decreased urine output.

Medications

Medications have numerous effects on urine production and elimination. Of gravest concern are the many prescription and nonprescription drugs known to be nephrotoxic (capable of causing kidney damage). Abuse of analgesics, such as aspirin, has resulted in nephrotoxicity; some antibiotics, such as kanamycin, can be nephrotoxic.

Diuretics (water pills), which commonly are used in the treatment of hypertension and other disorders, prevent the reabsorption of water and certain electrolytes in the tubules. Depending on their strength, they cause moderate to severe increases in production and excretion of dilute urine. *Cholinergic* medications stimulate contraction of the detrusor muscle and produce urination. Some *analgesics* and *tranquilizers* that suppress the central nervous system interfere with urination by diminishing the effectiveness of the neural reflex.

Certain drugs cause urine to change color (Table 43-1). Anticoagulants may cause **hematuria** (blood in the urine).

The Nurse as Role Model

Before intervening to help clients develop healthy urinary elimination patterns, it is important for nurses to assess the adequacy of their own urinary elimination habits and patterns. If you are unable to meet the following goals, you may want to take the time now to revise your own health practices, so that you will be an effective role model for clients. The nurse:

Table 43-1
Urine Color Changes Commonly Seen With Medications

Urine Color	Medication
Pale yellow	Diuretics
Orange, orange-red, or pink	Pyridium (urinary tract analgesic)
	Sulfonamides (antiinfectives)
	Dilantin (anticonvulsant)
	Rifampin (antitubercular)
Green or blue-green	Elavil (antidepressant)
	B-complex vitamins
Brown or black	Levodopa (antiparkinsonian)
	Injectable iron compounds

- Empties the bladder completely at regular intervals
- Responds to the urge to void (ie, does not routinely postpone voiding because of being too busy)
- Drinks 8 to 10 glasses of water daily
- Responds to changes in urinary characteristics (or frequency) by seeking their cause and getting medical assistance when necessary

ASSESSING

A comprehensive nursing assessment of the functioning of the urinary system includes the following:

- Collection of data about voiding patterns, habits, and difficulties and a history of current or past urinary problems
- Physical examination of the kidneys, bladder, and urethral meatus; assessment of skin integrity and hydration; and examination of the urine
- Correlation of these findings with the results of diagnostic tests and procedures for examining urine and the urinary tract

Nursing History

In the initial nursing history, the nurse questions the client (or the caregiver) about usual voiding habits and the current or past occurrence of voiding difficulties. Terminology should be used that the client understands. Elements of a urinary elimination history that should be incorporated into the initial nursing assessment are suggested in the accompanying box.

With infants and young children, it is important to assess whether the child has achieved bladder control and if a toileting schedule has been established. The nursing history and plan also should note the words the child uses to indicate the need to void.

With older adults, decreased bladder tone may be a problem, and the nursing history should note any

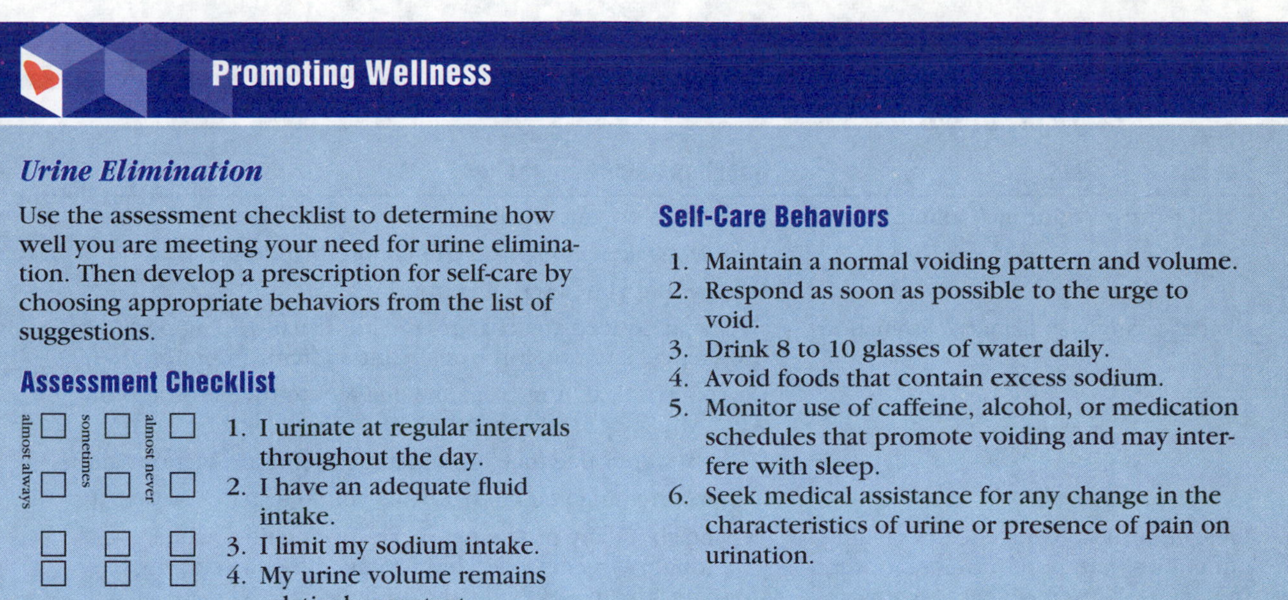

Promoting Wellness

Urine Elimination

Use the assessment checklist to determine how well you are meeting your need for urine elimination. Then develop a prescription for self-care by choosing appropriate behaviors from the list of suggestions.

Assessment Checklist

almost always	sometimes	almost never	
☐	☐	☐	1. I urinate at regular intervals throughout the day.
☐	☐	☐	2. I have an adequate fluid intake.
☐	☐	☐	3. I limit my sodium intake.
☐	☐	☐	4. My urine volume remains relatively constant.

Self-Care Behaviors

1. Maintain a normal voiding pattern and volume.
2. Respond as soon as possible to the urge to void.
3. Drink 8 to 10 glasses of water daily.
4. Avoid foods that contain excess sodium.
5. Monitor use of caffeine, alcohol, or medication schedules that promote voiding and may interfere with sleep.
6. Seek medical assistance for any change in the characteristics of urine or presence of pain on urination.

problems, how the person normally handles these problems, and nursing judgments about the adequacy of the solution.

People with limited or no bladder control as well as those with urinary diversions usually have well-established routines for emptying the bladder. The procedures and equipment used should be assessed to make sure they follow accepted guidelines and are not predisposing the person to infection or other risk. Any special routine, equipment, or supplies used for urinary elimination should be noted in both the history and the nursing plan of care.

When a problem with voiding is reported, its duration, severity, and precipitating factors should be explored (see the accompanying box for definitions of terms used to describe such problems). It also is important to note the client's perception of the problem and the adequacy of the client's self-care behaviors.

Physical Assessment

Physical assessment of urinary functioning includes an examination of the kidneys, urinary bladder, urethral meatus, skin, and urine.

Kidneys

In the normal adult, the kidneys are well protected by a considerable amount of fat and connective tissue and are difficult to palpate. The right kidney is at the level of the 12th rib and is lower than the left kidney. The right kidney may at times be palpated by the nurse if pushed down by the diaphragm when the client inhales. The nurse stands to the right of the supine client and places the left hand under the client's flank while the right hand palpates the abdominal wall. This technique requires deep palpation and should be practiced under supervision. The left kidney is palpated similarly. The contour and size of the kidneys are noted, as is any tenderness or lumps.

An examination of the kidneys includes checking for *costovertebral tenderness.* The costovertebral angle is formed by the 12th rib and the spine. When the kidneys are inflamed, the client experiences pain when this angle is percussed or struck. The nurse places one palm flat over the costovertebral angle and strikes the back of this hand with the other fist.

Bladder

The bladder normally is positioned below the symphysis pubis and cannot be assessed by the nurse when it is empty. Once the bladder becomes distended, it rises above the symphysis pubis and may reach to just below the umbilicus. At this point the nurse observes the lower abdominal wall, noting any swelling, and palpates this area for tenderness, also noting the smoothness and roundness of the bladder. The height of the edge of the bladder above the symphysis pubis may be measured, and the bladder also may be percussed. A full bladder produces a dull sound.

Urethral Orifice

The urethral orifice is inspected for any signs of inflammation or discharge. In the female, the urethral meatus is a pink, slitlike opening below the clitoris and above the vaginal orifice. The female needs to be in the dorsal recumbent position with the inner labia retracted for good visualization of the meatus. In the male, the meatus is at the tip of the penis. If the male is uncircumcised, the foreskin may need to be retracted for visualization of the meatus. Foul odors should be noted.

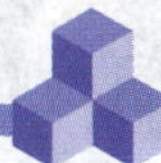

Focused Assessment Guide

Urinary Elimination

Factors to Assess	Questions and Approaches
Usual patterns of urinary elimination	How often do you urinate (pass your water) during the day?
	Do you awaken at night to empty your bladder?
	How would you describe your urine?
Recent changes in urinary elimination	Have you noticed any changes in your usual voiding patterns (frequency, amount, force of stream, difficulty, comfort)?
	Do you ever leak urine (eg, on your way to the bathroom or when you sneeze or cough)?
	Do you ever notice that your undergarments are wet or damp?
Aids to elimination	Is there anything you do that helps you to urinate?
Present or past occurrence of voiding difficulties (nature of problem, onset, frequency, causes, severity, symptoms, intervention attempted, and results)	Tell me about any problems you are having now when you urinate (urgency, pain or burning, difficulty starting or stopping stream, dribbling, incontinence).
	If there is a problem, describe what you feel like before you urinate and while you are urinating.
	Have you had any urinary problems in the past (any history or urinary tract infections, kidney or bladder disease or problems)?
	Do you use any type of absorbent pad or product to protect your clothes?
Presence of artificial orifices (normal routine, history of problems)	Tell me about your usual routine with your ureterostomy.

Skin Integrity and Hydration

Because problems with urinary functioning may result in disturbances in hydration and excretion of body wastes, the skin should be carefully assessed for color, texture, turgor, and the excretion of any wastes. The integrity of the skin in the perineal area also should be assessed. Problems with continence may result in severe excoriation.

Urine

Each time a client's urine is handled it should be assessed for color, odor, clarity, and the presence of any sediment. Abnormalities should be noted. In select clients, the pH and specific gravity of the urine will be monitored as well as the presence of abnormal constituents, such as protein, blood, glucose, ketone bodies, and bacteria. Normal characteristics of urine and special considerations for observation are detailed in Table 43-2.

Assessment Measures

In addition to interviewing the client and performing the physical examination, the nurse gathers data about urinary elimination by carrying out the following assessment measures: measuring urine output, collecting urine specimens, determining the presence of abnormal constituents in the urine, and assisting with diagnostic procedures. Discussions of the nursing responsibilities related to each of these measures follow.

Measuring Urine Output

Measuring the client's intake and output is an important nursing responsibility. Accuracy of the total fluid intake and output from all sources is essential for the planning of the client's nursing and medical care. The measurement of intake and output is described further in Chapter 46. Wearing gloves when handling urine is required because they protect the nurse from possible exposure to pathogenic microorganisms or blood that may be present in the urine.

The Voiding Client. The procedure for measuring the urine output of the client who is voiding is as follows:

- Have the client void into a bedpan or urinal, either in bed or in the bathroom. Urinary devices used to collect or measure urine are shown in Figure 43-2.
- Pour urine voided into a bedpan or urinal into the appropriate measuring device provided by the agency. The devices are calibrated in milliliters.
- Place the calibrated container on a flat surface, such as a shelf, for an accurate reading. Note the

Common Urinary Problems

Anuria: Technically, no urine voided; 24-hour urine output is less than 100 mL; synonyms are complete *kidney shutdown* or *renal failure*
Dysuria: Difficulty in voiding; may or may not be associated with pain; a feeling of warm local irritation occurring during voiding is called *burning*
Enuresis: Most often used to refer to the child who involuntarily urinates during the night
Frequency: Increased incidence of voiding
Glycosuria: Presence of sugar in the urine; if due to an unusually large intake of sugar or to marked emotional disturbances and is temporary, there is little cause for alarm
Hematuria: Blood in the urine; if present in large enough quantities, urine may be bright red or reddish brown
Hesitancy: Delay or difficulty in initiating voiding
Incontinence: Inability voluntarily to control the discharge of urine
Nocturia: Frequency of urination during the night
Oliguria: Scanty or greatly diminished amount of urine voided in a given time; 24-hour urine output is 100 to 400 mL
Orthostatic albuminuria: Presence of albumin in urine that is voided after periods of standing, walking, or running; phenomenon of the circulatory system and not necessarily a symptom of kidney disorders
Pneumaturia: Passage of urine containing gas
Polyuria: Excessive output of urine (diuresis)
Proteinuria: Albumin in the urine; indication of kidney disease
Pyuria: Pus in the urine; urine appears cloudy
Retention: Inability to void although urine is produced by the kidneys and enters the bladder; excessive storage of urine in the bladder
Suppression: Stoppage of urine production; normally the adult kidneys produce urine continuously at the rate of 60 to 120 mL/h
Urgency: Strong desire to void

amount of urine voided, read at eye level, and record it on the appropriate form. Figure 43-3 shows a form commonly used for recording urine output. The form is usually kept at the client's bedside. The total amount voided during each shift and 24-hour period is recorded on the client's permanent record.

- Do *not* discard the urine if a specimen is required. Otherwise, the urine is discarded in the toilet.
- Tell clients who are ambulatory when their urine output is to be measured and recorded, so that they do not use the bathroom without measuring output. A specimen hat can be placed under the toilet seat to collect and measure voided urine. Clients who are willing and able can be taught to measure and record their own output.

The Client With an Indwelling Catheter. When a client has an indwelling urinary catheter, the procedure for measuring urine output is as follows:

- Wear clean gloves.
- Bring a calibrated measuring device to the bedside and place it beneath the collection bag.
- Place the drainage spout from the collection bag above, but not touching, the calibrated measuring device and open the clamp.
- Allow urine to flow from the collection bag into the measuring device.
- Reclamp the drainage tube, wipe the spout of the tube with an alcohol pad, and replace the tube into the slot on the drainage bag. Then proceed as described above.

For catheterized clients who are acutely ill, urine may need to be measured hourly. This is facilitated by using a special collection bag with a built-in calibrated measuring chamber. After the nurse assesses and records the amount of urine produced hourly, the measuring chamber is tilted, and this urine empties into the general collection bag. The measuring chamber is now ready to collect the next hour's urine.

Collecting Urine Specimens

Nurses have specific responsibilities for diagnostic tests pertinent to urinary elimination. They routinely collect clean and sterile urine specimens, measure specific gravity of urine, and assess urine for abnormal constituents.

Routine Urinalysis. The collection of urine specimens for urinalysis is a nursing responsibility. A sterile urine specimen is not required for a routine urinalysis. Urine is collected by having the client void into a clean bedpan, urinal, or receptacle in the toilet bowl. Care must be taken to avoid contamination with feces. If a woman is menstruating when a urine sample is obtained, this must be noted on the laboratory slip because red blood cells may appear in the urine. If voiding into a bedpan or collection device on the toilet, female clients need instruction not to place toilet tissue into the urine since this makes analysis more difficult. Strict aseptic technique, according to OSHA and institution guidelines, must be used when collecting and handling urine specimens. The urine is poured into an appropriate container; labeled with the client's name, date, and time of collection; packaged appropriately; and sent to the laboratory for examination. Urine should not be left standing at room temperature for a long period before being sent to the laboratory because this may alter both the appearance and chemistry of the urine.

Specimens From Infants and Children. Plastic disposable collection bags are available for infants and young children who have not yet achieved voluntary bladder

Table 43-2
Characteristics of Urine

Characteristic	Normal Findings	Special Considerations
Color	A freshly voided specimen is pale yellow, straw-colored, or amber, depending on its concentration.	Urine is darker than normal when it is scanty and concentrated. Urine is lighter than normal when it is excessive and diluted. Certain drugs, such as cascara, L-dopa, and sulfonamides, alter the color of urine.
Odor	Normal urine smell is aromatic. As urine stands, it oftens develops an ammonia odor because of bacterial action.	Some foods cause urine to have a characteristic odor; for example, asparagus causes urine to have a strong, musty odor. Urine high in glucose content has a sweet odor. Urine that is heavily infected has a fetid odor.
Turbidity	Fresh urine should be clear or translucent; as urine stands and cools, it becomes cloudy.	Cloudiness observed in freshly voided urine is abnormal and may be due to the presence of red blood cells, white blood cells, bacteria, vaginal discharge, sperm, or prostatic fluid.
pH	The normal pH is about 6.0, with a range of 4.6 to 8. (Urine alkalinity or acidity may be promoted through diet to inhibit bacterial growth or urinary stone development or to facilitate the therapeutic activity of certain medications.) Urine becomes alkaline on standing when carbon dioxide diffuses into the air.	A high-protein diet causes urine to become excessively acid. Certain foods tend to produce alkaline urine, such as citrus fruits, dairy products, and vegetables, especially legumes. Certain foods tend to produce acidic urine, for example, meat and cranberry juice. Certain drugs influence the acidity or alkalinity of urine; for example, ammonium chloride produces acidic urine, and potassium citrate and sodium bicarbonate produce alkaline urine.
Specific gravity	This is a measure of the concentration of dissolved solids in the urine. The normal range is 1.010 to 1.025.	Concentrated urine will have a higher than normal specific gravity and diluted urine will have a lower than normal specific gravity. In the absence of kidney disease, a high specific gravity usually indicates dehydration and a low specific gravity indicates overhydration.
Constituents	*Organic* constituents of urine include urea, uric acid, creatinine, hippuric acid, indican, urene pigments, and undetermined nitrogen. *Inorganic* constituents are ammonia, sodium, chloride, traces of iron, phosphorus, sulfur, potassium, and calcium.	*Abnormal constituents* of urine include blood, pus, albumin, glucose, ketone bodies, casts, gross bacteria, and bile.

control (Fig. 43-4). The manufacturer's instructions should be followed and care taken in application and removal so as not to irritate the sensitive perineal skin.

Clean-Catch or Midstream Specimen. A clean-catch specimen of urine is required in some situations. Most health agencies specify that a clean-catch specimen be collected during midstream. This means that the client voids a little urine, which is discarded; the specimen is then collected during midstream in a sterile specimen container; and the last urine in the bladder also is discarded. The first voided urine helps to flush away organisms that may be near the meatus. The urinalysis findings may be inaccurate if these organisms enter the specimen. Also, it is generally thought that urine voided at midstream is most characteristic of the urine the body is producing. A clean-catch midstream specimen from a male is sterile. The female may be catheterized if a sterile specimen is required. Catheterization is discussed later in this chapter.

The client who can carry out proper techniques may collect his or her own clean-catch midstream urine specimen and often prefers to do so. The nurse should provide the appropriate equipment and instructions to carry out the procedure.

Guidelines for obtaining a clean-catch midstream urine specimen from a female client and from a male client are as follows:

Female Client

- Wear clean gloves.
- Clean the area at the external meatus with soap and water. Studies since the mid-1980s have indicated that special meatal cleansing and separating the labia in the female are no longer necessary

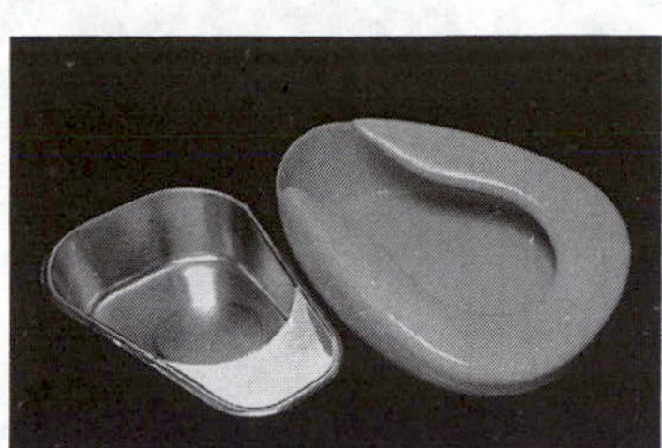

Bedpan and fracture pan
Containers used to collect urine from nonambulatory clients

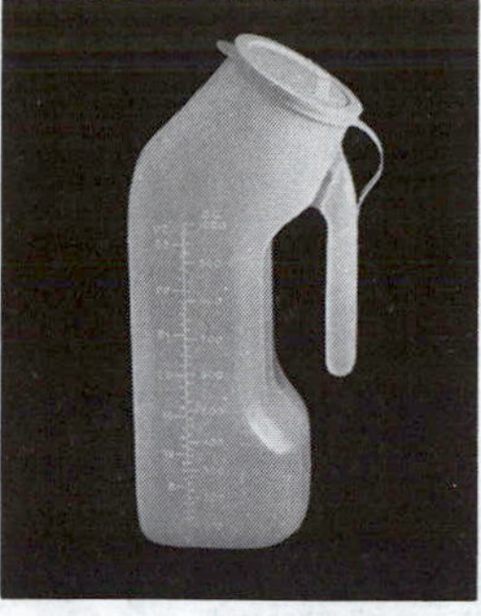

Urinal
Container used to collect urine from nonambulatory male clients

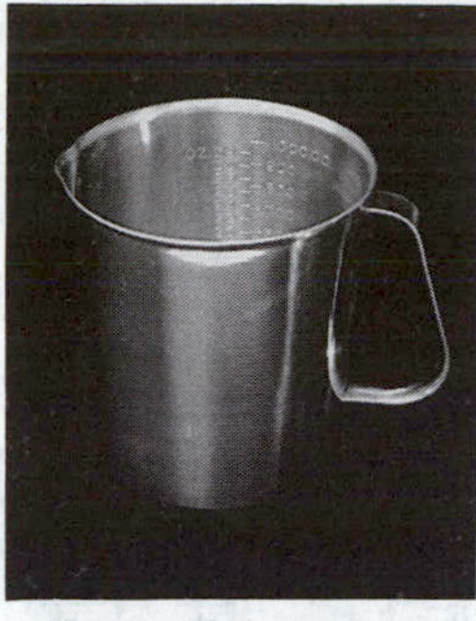

Calibrated measuring device
Device which makes possible the recording of an accurate urine output

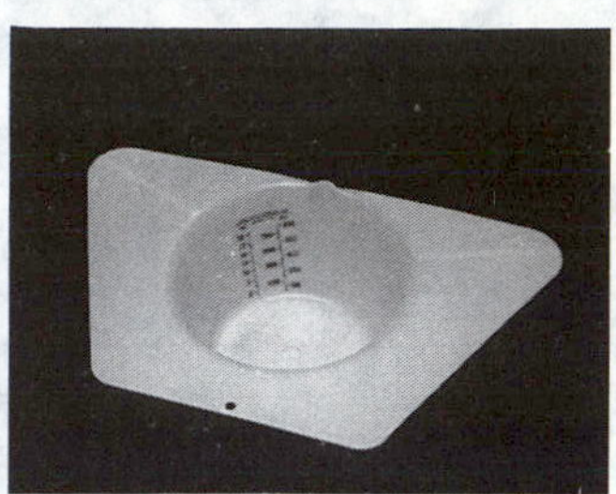

Specimen hat
Container which when placed anteriorly in the toilet, underneath the seat, collects urine for measurement or study

Straight catheter and specimen container
Single lumen catheter which drains urine from the bladder—here into a sterile urine specimen container

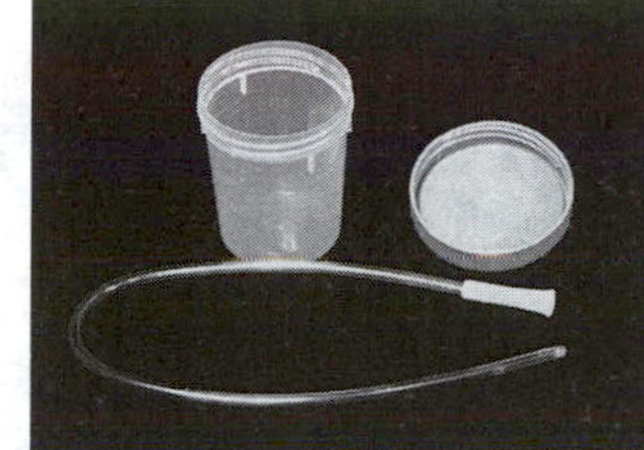

Small urine collection bag well-suited to ambulatory clients; may be easily emptied in the toilet; easily concealed in pants or a skirt

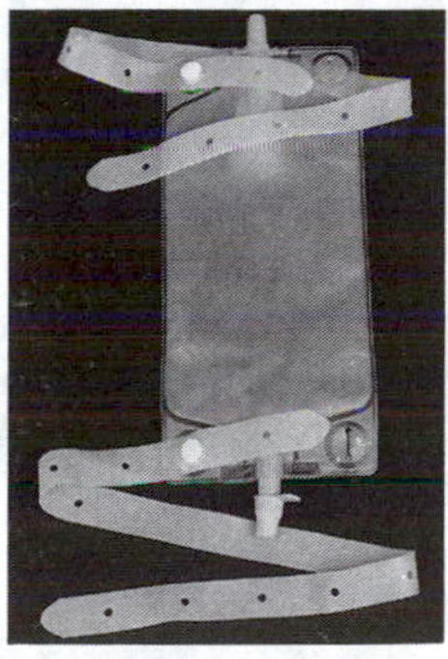

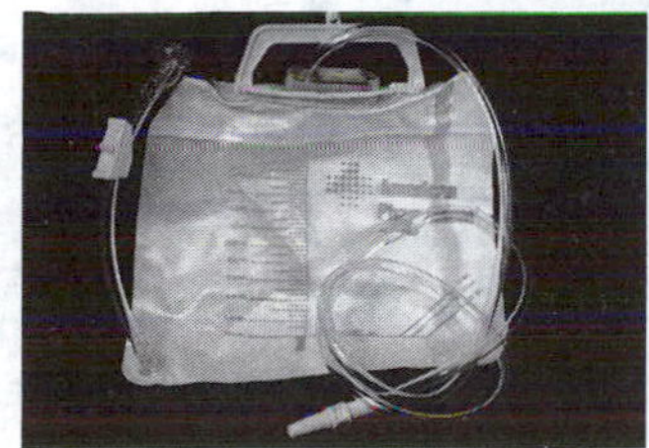

Large urine collection bag—generally emptied once each eight-hour shift; provides an approximate measure of urine

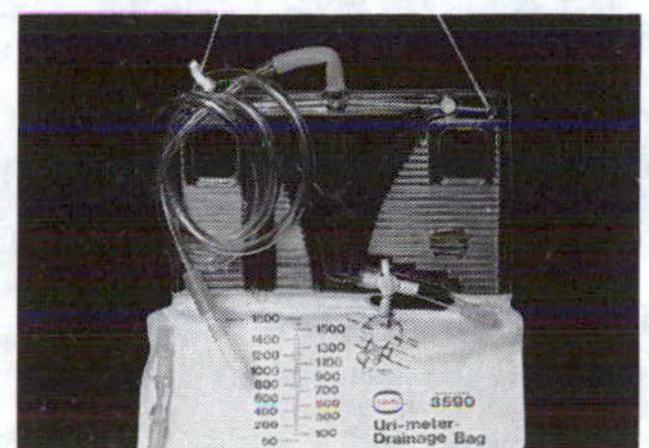

Large urine collection bag with accurately calibrated small chamber for determining precise hourly urine outputs

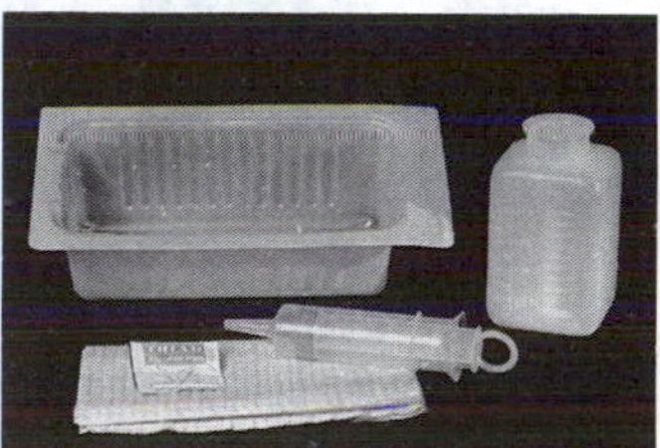

Irrigation tray containing a sterile piston syringe, a sterile container for holding the irrigation fluid, and a sterile tray for collecting the solution which returns from the catheter

3000 cc bag of irrigation fluid for continuous bladder irrigation

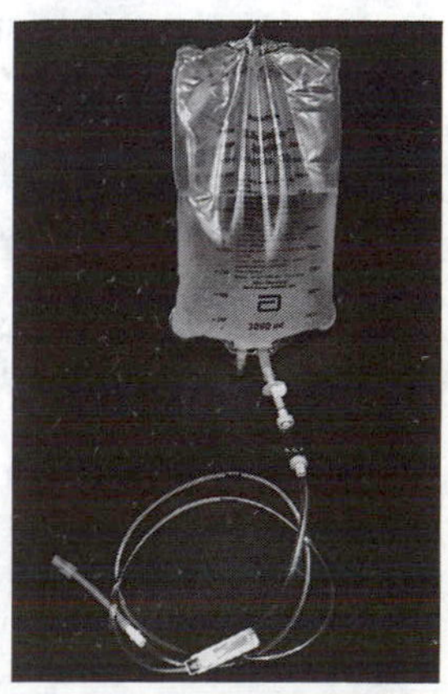

Figure 43-2
Devices for collecting and measuring urine.

Intake and Output Chart

7:00 AM 11-18 to 7:00 AM 11-19

	Intake						Output							
	Oral	I.V.		Blood	Other	Comments	Urine	Stool	Gastric tube	Drainage tubes		Vomitus	Other	Comments
7-8	250					Force fluids to 1100cc/shift	300							
8-9														
9-10	120													
10-11	60													
11-12	100						250							
12-1	300													
1-2	240													
2-3	100						200							
8 hr Tot	1170						750							voiding s̄ discomfort
3-4														
4-5														
5-6														
6-7														
7-8														
8-9														
9-10														
10-11														
8 hr Tot														
11-12														
12-1														
1-2														
2-3														
3-4														
4-5														
5-6														
6-7														
8 hr Tot														
24 hr Tot														
	Total intake						**Total output**							

Figure 43-3
An example of a form commonly used for recording intake and output.

when collecting a midstream urine specimen (Winslow, 1993a).

- Have the client void about 30 mL and discard this urine.
- Position the sterile specimen container near, but not touching, the meatus, and ask the client to void forcibly if she is lying down. This prevents collecting a specimen that has dribbled down and across the perineal area.
- Stop collecting urine before the client empties her bladder. Allow the client to continue emptying her bladder, and discard the urine not needed for the specimen.
- Use a sterilized bedpan to collect the midstream specimen if the client has difficulty voiding into the container, and then transfer the urine into the sterile specimen container.
- Label the specimen container, package it appropriately, and send the specimen to the laboratory.

Male Client

- Wear clean gloves.
- Retract the foreskin to expose the glans penis in the uncircumcised male client.
- Clean the area of the external meatus with soap and water.
- Have the client void about 30 mL and discard this urine.
- Have the client void directly into the sterile container.
- Stop collecting urine before the client empties his bladder. Allow the client to empty his bladder, and discard this urine. Return the foreskin to its normal position to prevent swelling and irritation of the glans penis.
- Use a sterilized urinal to collect the midstream specimen if the client has difficulty voiding into the container, and then transfer the urine into the sterile specimen container.

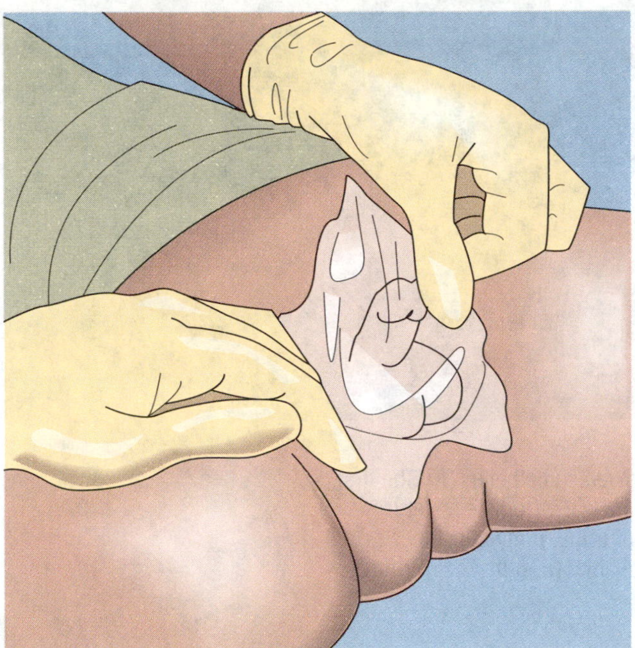

Figure 43-4
Urine collection device for infants.

- Label the specimen container appropriately and send the specimen to the laboratory.

Sterile Specimen From an Indwelling Catheter. Sterile urine specimens may be obtained by catheterizing the client's bladder (see Procedures 43-2 and 43-3 later in this chapter) or by withdrawing the specimen from an indwelling catheter already in place.

When it is necessary to collect a urine specimen from a client with an indwelling catheter, it should be done from the catheter itself using the special port for withdrawing specimens. A specimen from the collecting receptacle (drainage bag) may not be fresh urine, and its use could result in an inaccurate analysis. Sterile technique must be observed.

The size of the syringe is determined by the specific laboratory test. A urine culture requires about 3 mL, whereas routine urinalysis necessitates the collection of at least 10 mL of urine. A sterile 21- to 25-gauge needle, an antiseptic swab, a specimen container, and, possibly, a clamp complete the list of necessary equipment. Wearing gloves protects the nurse from any accidental contact with the specimen.

If urine is not present in the tube, it may be necessary to clamp the tube below the collection port briefly (not to exceed 30 minutes) to allow urine to accumulate. Most catheters have a self-sealing area that tolerates a needle puncture. It is unsafe to puncture a Silastic or plastic catheter, as leakage will probably occur. Clean the entry port with an antiseptic swab, and carefully insert the sterile needle into the catheter. Aspirate urine into the syringe, remove the syringe, release the clamp if one was used, and transfer the specimen into the appropriate container. The uncapped needle and syringe should be placed in the "sharps" container and the specimen is then packaged and transported according to agency policy.

Figure 43-5 shows how urine is removed from an indwelling catheter.

Collecting 24-Hour Urine Specimens. For some types of laboratory studies, 24-hour specimens are required. It is critical that the client and the entire nursing team understand the importance of collecting *all* the urine voided in a 24-hour period. A sign posted on the client's bathroom door is a helpful reminder not to discard urine. The collection is initiated at a specific time (which is recorded) by having the client empty his or her bladder. This urine is discarded. All urine excreted for the next 24 hours is collected.

Depending on the type of examination used, the urine from each voiding may be kept in a separately marked container and the time of each voiding recorded,

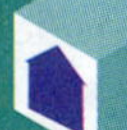

Home Care Considerations

Assessment Priorities

When caring for clients with altered urinary elimination who are living at home, be alert for:

- Any change in the appearance of voided urine or urine that is collected in a drainage bag (eg, cloudy, red-tinged, concentrated appearance)
- Any previously unobserved evidence of incontinence
- Physical disabilities or mechanical barriers that limit access to toileting facilities
- Presence of a distended bladder when the abdomen is palpated
- Any indication that voiding is painful
- Responses of caregivers/family members as they attend to elimination needs of the client

Since needed changes in the plan of care may depend solely on your detection of new or developing problems, your assessment skills are critical. Always confer with an experienced colleague if you are uncertain about the significance of your findings.

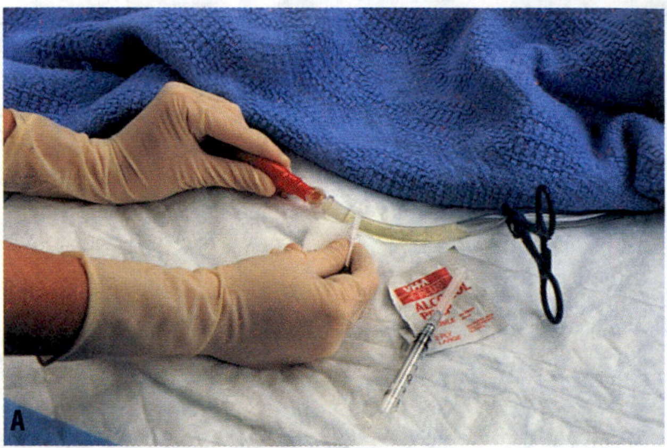

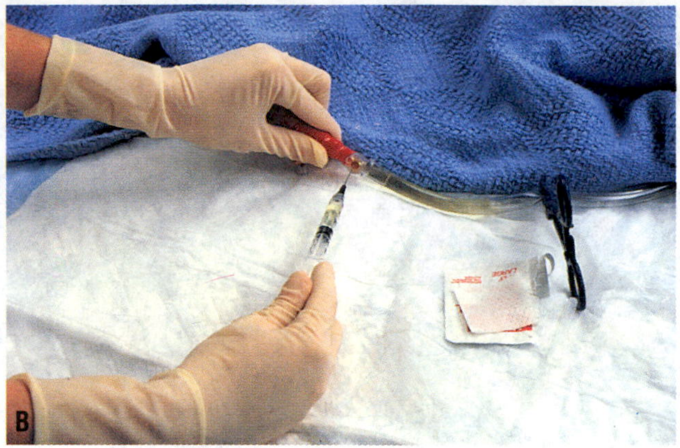

Figure 43-5
The nurse is obtaining a urine specimen from a patient using an indwelling catheter. (**A**) She first uses a swab moistened with an antiseptic to clean the area where she will introduce a sterile needle. (**B**) She then inserts the needle and withdraws a specimen of urine. Body substance precautions require that gloves be used when contact with urine is probable. (Photos © B. Proud.)

or all voidings may be collected in a common receptacle. The laboratory should be contacted to determine whether a preservative is needed to retard decomposition and if the specimens are to be refrigerated or kept on ice. Many laboratories have a transport service to pick up specimens from a client's home and return them to the laboratory within the appropriate time frame.

Determining Abnormal Constituents in the Urine. In some situations the nurse may perform tests on urine specimens, especially when specimens are being tested repeatedly for known abnormalities, when screening tests are being used, or when laboratory facilities are not readily available. For example, a nurse may test urine for the presence of glucose, protein, bilirubin, and blood. The results of the test are recorded on the client's record. Many types of commercially prepared diagnostic kits are available for determining the presence of abnormal substances in the urine and can be used in the home setting or a healthcare facility. Although the performance of these tests is economical and fast, laboratory analysis is recommended when more precise results are needed.

Most diagnostic kits contain needed equipment and the appropriate reagent, a substance used in a chemical reaction to detect another substance. Reagents are prepared in the form of tablets, fluids, impregnated paper, and plastic strips with a special coating. When the reagent is brought in contact with urine, a chemical reaction occurs, which causes a color change. The reaction is then compared with an accompanying chart that describes the significance of the color.

The precise directions for the amount of the specimen, the time allowance for the chemical reaction, and the significance of the colors vary with the manufacturer. Therefore, it is important to read the directions accompanying the diagnostic kit carefully and to follow them exactly.

Determining Specific Gravity. Determining the specific gravity of urine requires an instrument called a *urinometer* or *hydrometer.* The urinometer has a calibrated scale for the measurement of specific gravity. Urine is placed in a cylindrical container, and the urinometer is inserted in a circular motion without touching the bottom or side of the container. The reading on a urinometer should be made at eye level at the bottom of the meniscus formed by the urine (Fig. 43-6). The density of the urine supports the urinometer. If the urine is concentrated, the urinometer will be buoyed up high in the urine container and will register high on the measurement scale. If the urine is diluted, the urinometer will be supported low in the urine, and a low specific gravity reading will result.

Assisting With Diagnostic Procedures

Various diagnostic procedures, ordinarily performed in a hospital operating room or outpatient facility, are used to study the urinary system. The nurse is responsible for preparing the client and giving appropriate aftercare. Anxieties the client may have tend to be reduced when the nurse explains the procedure. Some common diagnostic procedures used to study the urinary system include cystoscopy, intravenous pyelogram, retrograde pyelogram, computed tomography (CT or CAT scans), and ultrasound examination. A *cystoscopy* provides a direct visualization of the bladder, the ureteral orifices, and the urethra. The instrument used is a cystoscope. *Intravenous pyelography,* or *excretory urography,* involves the injection of a contrast material intravenously, followed by x-ray examination of the kidney and urethra. In a *retrograde pyelogram,* x-ray films are taken of the kidney and ureters after a contrast material is injected into the renal pelvis through the ureter. *Computed tomography* provides a clear, computerized, cross-

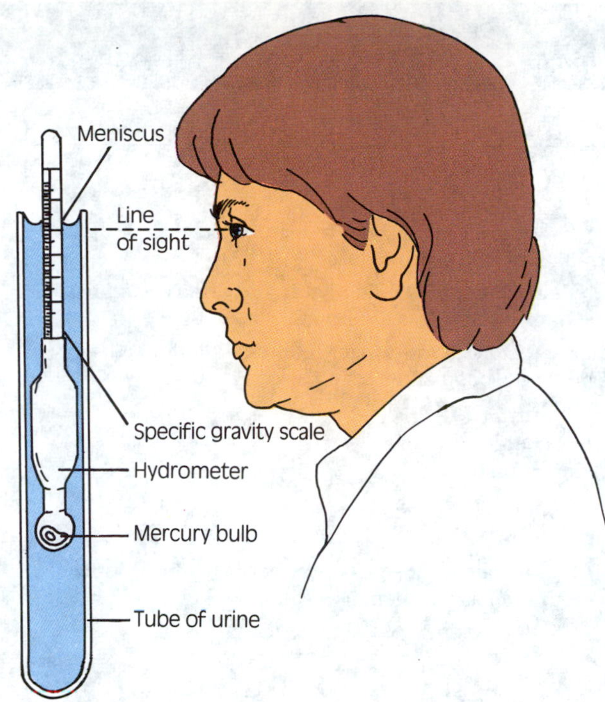

Figure 43-6
To determine specific gravity, the urinometer should be read at eye level at the base of the meniscus formed by the urine.

sectional image of the body organ or area by scanning it from different angles with an x-ray beam. It is particularly effective in diagnosing an early stage of a disease. *Ultrasonography* or *ultrasound* is a noninvasive procedure that involves the use of high-frequency sound waves to produce an image or photograph of an organ or tissue. Ultrasound waves penetrate and bounce back, or echo, according to the density of the tissue. This test is commonly used to examine the kidneys. Descriptions of the preparation and aftercare of the client for each of these procedures are presented in Table 43-3.

DIAGNOSING

The data the nurse collects about the client's urinary functioning may lead to the development of one or several nursing diagnoses. Some data are appropriately reported to the physician and may contribute to the physician's identification of a medical diagnosis. It is important that nurses detect significant urinary findings, record these appropriately, and report them to the proper people.

Urinary Functioning as the Problem. Nursing diagnoses that specifically address problems in urinary functioning include problems of incontinence, pattern alteration, and urinary retention. Sample defining characteristics for these diagnoses appear in the accompanying box.

Urinary Functioning as the Etiology. Difficulty with urination or changes in normal voiding patterns may affect other areas of human functioning. Examples of nursing diagnoses that may be related to urinary problems include the following:

- Anxiety related to incontinence, diagnostic procedures
- Caregiver Role Strain related to incontinence of family member
- Risk for Infection related to indwelling urinary catheter
- Impaired Skin Integrity (Actual, Risk for) related to incontinence
- Knowledge Deficit related to any existing or new urinary disease or disorder, lack of information about personal hygiene
- Noncompliance with Medication Regimen related to misunderstanding of the need to finish all doses of medication for urinary tract infection
- Pain related to bladder spasms, dysuria, urinary retention, cancer of the bladder, diagnostic procedures
- Self-Esteem Disturbance related to urinary incontinence, urinary diversion
- Sexual Dysfunction related to urinary incontinence, urinary diversion
- Sleep Pattern Disturbance related to nocturia
- Toileting Self-Care Deficit related to parent's lack of knowledge or motivation to toilet-train child, neuromuscular impairment or musculoskeletal disorders, immobility, trauma or surgical procedures, confusion, disorientation

The nurse's challenge is to correctly identify human responses to alterations in urinary elimination that pose specific health problems for the client and his or her family.

PLANNING: EXPECTED OUTCOMES

When the client is ambulatory and not experiencing difficulties with the urinary system, the promotion of normal voiding is not a problem. Trauma or illness may result in the client's need for nursing assistance with voiding. Nursing interventions (which follow) should be supportive of planned client goals.

The client will:

- Produce urine output about equal to fluid intake
- Maintain fluid and electrolyte balance
- Empty the bladder completely at regular intervals
- Report ease of voiding
- Maintain skin integrity

Client goals for specific urinary problems follow later in this chapter.

IMPLEMENTING

Any alteration in urinary elimination invariably invokes anxiety and fear in individuals. Nursing interventions

(text continues on page 1228)

Table 43-3
Common Diagnostic Procedures Used to Study the Urinary Tract

Preparation	Aftercare
Cystoscopy: The direct visual examination of the bladder, ureteral orifices, and urethra with a cystoscope	
The client is allowed liquids on the morning of the examination. Sedation and analgesics are usually prescribed before the procedure. A signed consent form is required for the procedure. The procedure is ordinarily painless.	Tissue swelling, dysuria, and hematuria may occur owing to trauma from the procedure. Encourage a generous fluid intake, and observe and measure urine output for at least 24 hours. Observe the client for urinary retention and for signs of infection; nosocomial infection after a cystoscopy is common.
Intravenous Pyelography (excretory urography): The x-ray examination of the kidney and ureter after a contrast material is injected intravenously	
No fluids or food are given for at least 12 hours before the examination so that contrast material will concentrate in the urinary system. Elderly, debilitated, or young clients may not tolerate this dehydration, and compromises may need to be made. A laxative the evening before the examination and an enema the morning of the examination are given so that stool and gas do not interfere with visualization. The client should void before the examination.	Fluids and food may be given immediately after the examination. Observe the client for signs of a reaction to the contrast material, such as a rash, nausea, and hives.
Retrograde Pyelography: The x-ray examination of the kidney and ureters after a contrast material is injected into the renal pelvis through the ureter	
No fluids and food are given after midnight before the examination. A laxative the evening before the examination and an enema the morning of the examination are given so that stool and gas do not interfere with visualization. The client should void before the examination. A signed consent form is recommended for the procedure.	Foods and fluids may be given, but if anesthesia has been used, this is delayed for several hours. Check the vital signs regularly if anesthesia has been used. Observe the client for signs of a reaction to the contrast material, such as a rash, nausea, and hives. Ureteral catheters may be in place and should be connected to drainage receptacles so that the amount and character of drainage from each catheter can be noted.
Ultrasonography: A noninvasive procedure that involves the use of ultrasound to produce an image or photograph of an organ or tissue	
A signed consent form is required. Food and fluids are restricted for 8–12 hours before an abdominal ultrasound. The client should not smoke or chew gum prior to the procedure to prevent swallowing air. The procedure is painless.	No special care is required after the test. Inform client that results are usually available 1–2 days after the study.
Computed tomography (CT scanning): A noninvasive x-ray procedure whereby a body part can be scanned from different angles with an x-ray beam and a computer that calculates varying tissue densities and records a cross-sectional image on paper	
A consent form should be signed. The client is usually NPO for 8 hours prior to the test if a contrast dye is used. Check for any history of allergic reaction or hypersensitivity to shellfish, iodine, or any contrast dyes. All metal objects need to be removed before the test. Medications may usually be taken until 2 hours before the test.	Observe for a delayed reaction to the contrast dye (skin rash, urticaria, headache, vomiting). An oral antihistamine may be given for mild reactions. Be supportive to client and family. Test can be frightening. Instruct client to resume usual diet and activity unless otherwise indicated.

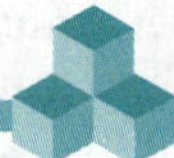

Nursing Diagnoses for Common Problems

Urinary Elimination

Problem	Related Factors	Sample Defining Characteristics
Altered Urinary Elimination	Enuresis (maturational) Dysuria	Parents report 6-year-old son wets bed three or four times a week. Small bladder capacity, less than 300 mL. "It hurts when I pass my water." Urinalysis reveals hematuria and proteinuria.
Functional Incontinence	Altered environment Sensory, cognitive, or mobility deficits	"I don't know why Johnny started wetting since he's been hospitalized. He has been toilet trained for 6 months now." "When I remember to take mother to the toilet she urinates fine. But if I don't remember, I find her wet."
Reflex Incontinence	Neurologic impairment	Client with spinal cord lesion reports no awareness of bladder filling, no urge to void or feelings of bladder fullness, involuntary loss of urine at somewhat regular intervals.
Stress Incontinence	Age-related degenerative changes High intraabdominal pressure Incompetent bladder outlet Overdistention between voidings Weak pelvic muscles and structural supports	Obese mother of four reports involuntary dribbling of urine with coughs, sneezes, hearty laughter. Client "too busy to void" during day reports involuntary leakage of urine with sudden movement, cough, and so on.
Total Incontinence	Neurologic impairment Trauma or disease affecting spinal cord nerves	Constant flow of urine at unpredictable times without distention or uninhibited bladder contractions. Nocturia
Urge Incontinence	Decreased bladder capacity Bladder spasms Increased intake of caffeine or alcohol Increased urine concentration Overdistention of bladder	"I can never make it to the bathroom in time." Urgency, frequency, nocturia, bladder contracture or spasm
Urinary Retention	High urethral pressure caused by weak detrusor Inhibition of reflex arc Strong sphincter Blockage	Elderly male diagnosed with benign prostatic hypertrophy complains of inability to urinate despite feeling bladder is full. Woman 6 hours after delivery has had no urine output since labor; 800 mL IV fluids infused; fundus of uterus is displaced to the right by a full bladder.

focus on maintenance and promotion of normal urinary patterns regardless of the healthcare setting, vigorous efforts to improve or cure urinary incontinence, prevention of potential problems associated with bladder catheterization, and assistance with care of urinary diversions. Nurses who are actively involved in designing and implementing effective nursing interventions can assist the client and family to achieve mutually desirable outcomes related to urination needs.

Promoting Normal Urination

Maintaining Normal Voiding Habits

If the client's voiding habits are adequate, the nurse provides care or teaches the client to maintain these habits to ensure comfort and satisfactory urine output. Attention to the following variables is helpful:

Schedule: Some clients will report voiding on demand in no apparent pattern. Others have inflexible patterns that have developed over the years, and become anxious if these are interrupted. Some clients need assistance voiding and may experience urgency. Nursing actions should support the client's normal voiding pattern as much as possible.

Privacy: Many adults and children cannot void in the presence of another person. Unless the client is extremely weak and requires assistance, privacy should be offered in the healthcare facility and in the home setting.

Position: Helping clients assume *normal* voiding positions may be all that is necessary to resolve an inability to void. Some males cannot use a urinal while lying down or sitting; the nurse should encourage them to void while standing at the bedside unless this is contraindicated. Similarly, some females cannot void easily on a bedpan and respond favorably to the use of a bedside commode.

Hygiene: Clients who are confined to bed will find it difficult to perform their usual genital hygiene. Careful cleansing of the perineal and genital areas is needed to promote client comfort and prevent infection. This is easily accomplished for clients on bed rest by placing them on a bedpan and then pouring warm soapy water over the perineal area followed by clear water. Families providing care for ill members at home may be taught this technique.

Because many people customarily wash their hands after toileting, clients confined to bed should be offered a moistened towelette or soap and water to wipe their hands after the nurse removes the bedpan. Specific recommendations for urinary elimination problems that affect the older adult are listed in the accompanying box.

Promoting Fluid Intake

Many people routinely drink less fluid than is optimal to promote healthy urinary functioning. The adult who has no disease-related fluid restrictions should drink 2000 to 2400 mL (8 to 10 8-oz glasses) of fluid daily. A common misperception is that drinking this much fluid causes water retention and contributes to weight gain. If a good proportion of the daily fluid intake is water, the kidneys and urinary structures will be well flushed and waste products will be removed, including potentially harmful bacteria. Fluid intake should be monitored for potentially harmful excesses of caffeine-containing beverages, high-sodium beverages such as diet sodas, and high-sugar beverages.

Fresh water and juices and fluids of preference should be made available to clients confined to bed. Confused clients and children may need to be reminded to drink. Fluid restrictions may be ordered by the physician in certain diseases. In others, forced fluids (above-average intake of fluids) are prescribed. This needs to be incorporated in the plan of care and explained to the client.

Strengthening Muscle Tone

Strengthening perineal and abdominal muscle tone can facilitate voluntary control of urination and significantly reduce or eliminate problems with stress incontinence. Weakening of the pelvic-floor muscles is a common cause of urinary incontinence. **Kegel exercises**, or pelvic muscle exercises, target the inner muscles that lie under and support the bladder. These muscles can be toned, strengthened, and actually made larger by a regular routine of tightening and relaxing them. Often, clients have difficulty determining the muscles to exercise. These are the same muscles that you contract to stop urinating midstream or control defecation. Clients are instructed to contract the pelvic floor muscles for 10 seconds and to relax them for 10 seconds. Kegel exercises should be performed without involving the muscles in the abdomen, inner thigh, and buttocks. Once the client is familiar with these sensations, these exercises should be performed 30 to 80 times a day for at least 6 weeks and possibly longer, depending on the response (Agency for Health Care Policy and Research [AHCPR], 1992). The exercises can be done anywhere, and clients should be assisted to incorporate them into their daily activities.

Stimulating Urination

Urinary retention, the inability to void even though the bladder is full, is discussed later in this chapter. Many people experience **hesitancy**, a delay, or difficulty in initiating voiding. This problem may be resolved by resorting to simple measures that are appropriate for the nurse to use in a healthcare facility or caregivers to use at home:

- Assist the client to void when the urge to void is first experienced. Routine delaying of urination may result in difficulty initiating a stream.
- Make use of the factors noted earlier to provide a natural environment for voiding—relaxed and pri-

Focus on the Older Adult

Nursing Strategies for Urinary Elimination Problems Affecting Older Adults

Nocturia, Frequency, and Urgency

- Ensure easy access to the bathroom or commode.
- Discourage fluid intake at bedtime.
- Discourage alcohol use before bedtime.
- Evaluate medication regimen and schedule, particularly diuretics and drugs that produce sedation or confusion.
- Use a night light.
- Use clothing that is easily removed for voiding.
- Keep assistive ambulatory devices (walkers, canes, etc.) readily available.
- Provide call bell if assistance is necessary.
- Evaluate gait and ability to ambulate safely.
- Assess for urinary tract infection.

Incontinence

- Maintain a fluid intake of 1500 to 2000 mL/day.
- Discourage use of alcohol, NutraSweet, and caffeine.
- Provide easy access to the bathroom.
- Assess factors that influence voiding.
- Use assistive devices when necessary (raised toilet seat, grab bars, walker).
- Use collection devices when necessary (urinal or bed pan).
- Ensure safety when ambulating (eg, skid-proof slippers).
- Encourage use of whole, unprocessed, coarse wheat bran to prevent constipation and fecal impaction.
- Perform Kegel exercises several times daily.
- Encourage participation in a bladder retraining program.
- Consider insertion of an indwelling catheter as the *last resort*.

Urinary Tract Infections

- Maintain a liberal fluid intake.
- Encourage shower instead of tub bath to decrease opportunity for bacteria in bath water to enter urethra.
- Void at frequent intervals.
- Void immediately after sexual intercourse.
- Assess for signs of urinary tract infection (may be nonspecific in elderly client).
- Use dipstick (Microstix) if recommended to monitor bacteria count in urine.
- Continue antimicrobial therapy as ordered.

vate setting and normal position. Squatting or leaning forward may assist by putting pressure on the suprapubic area.

- Run tap water within the client's hearing.
- Use a warm bedpan.
- Pour warm water over the perineal area. Measure the amount of water if the voided specimen needs to be measured.
- Pour warm water over the client's fingers.
- Stroke the client's leg or thigh.
- Exert gentle downward pressure over the bladder to facilitate bladder emptying. This technique differs from Credé's maneuver, in which manual bladder compression is used to stimulate urination by creating a sensation of bladder fullness and relaxing the urethral sphincter. The nurse places one hand on top of the other over the client's bladder (between the umbilicus and the symphysis pubis, fingers pointing downward) and exerts downward pressure to compress the bladder walls and forcefully expel urine. This maneuver should be performed only when bladder flaccidity exists and the client is not expected to regain voluntary control. It usually requires a physician's order.
- If urination is being stimulated for the purposes of obtaining a urine specimen and the client is cooperative, sometimes having the client forcefully cough will create sufficient intra-abdominal pressure to stimulate the micturition reflex.
- Ask the client to blow bubbles through a straw in a glass of water.

Assisting With Toileting

Toilet. Despite the client's ability to use the bathroom toilet, the nurse may be responsible for noting any abnormalities of elimination. In some instances, clients may need to be taught to report abnormalities to the nurse and instructed not to flush the toilet until the nurse checks the urine. In other instances, when the urine volume is to be calculated, the client may need to urinate in a bedpan or some other receptacle placed on the toilet so the urine can be measured before it is discarded. Although many clients can easily be taught to measure their urine output, the nurse should observe the urine at least once during a work shift and more frequently if warranted.

A weak client should be assisted to the bathroom. Someone should remain in attendance if there is any danger of the client's falling. Bathrooms should not be locked, and, especially in healthcare facilities, a signal bell should be within easy reach of the client so that help can be summoned easily if the client feels weak and needs assistance. A hand rail near the toilet is helpful.

Commode. Commodes can be used for clients who are able to be out of bed but unable to use the bathroom toilet. Commodes are chairs, straight-back chairs, or wheelchairs with open seats under which there is a shelf or a holder on which a bedpan is placed. The commode can be placed adjacent to the bed, and the client can be assisted to it with minimal exertion.

Bedpan and Urinal. Male clients confined to bed usually use the urinal for voiding and the bedpan for defecation; female clients use the bedpan for both. When a female client is unable to sit up in bed—for example, when she is in a body cast—a female urinal may be used. The bedpan and the urinal are difficult to use and embarrassing to many clients. Privacy is important to almost all clients when they use a bedpan or urinal.

A special bedpan called a fracture bedpan is frequently used by people with fractures of the femur or lower spine. Smaller and flatter than the ordinary bedpan, it is helpful for clients who cannot easily raise themselves to use the regular bedpan.

Figure 43-2 displays the types of bedpans and urinals, and Procedure 43-1 shows how to help a client use a bedpan or urinal.

Safety Considerations. Many dangerous situations have been created in the absence of a signal bell or bedpan. Clients confined to bed have gotten up to go to the bathroom to void, sometimes climbing over or around bed side rails or removing oxygen masks or infusion tubings. Offering a bedpan or urinal frequently can save clients from fracturing their hips, dislodging an intravenous infusion, or being embarrassed by soiled linen. A recent study involving a prompted voiding program in nursing homes resulted in a 26% decrease in wet episodes for older incontinent women who were encouraged to void and helped to the bathroom at regular intervals. The additional attention from a caregiver and praise when the client voided or remained continent was a significant factor in minimizing incontinence (Winslow, 1993b). A very ill or sedated client may not think to ask in time. As a precaution, family members of clients at home may need to be made aware of this. The nurse is responsible for the client's safety.

Teaching Feminine Hygiene. Female clients often need to be taught the proper technique for perineal care after urination. Drying or washing of the perineal area should be from the front to the back, or from the urethra toward the rectum. A reverse cleaning motion can result in fecal organisms being introduced into the urethra or vagina. This type of contamination is a common cause of urinary tract and vaginal infections.

Caring for an Incontinent Client

Urinary incontinence is widely underreported and underdiagnosed. This inability to retain urine in the bladder is a common but treatable health problem that is not, as widely believed, an inevitable result of growing old or bearing children. Many people self-manage this life-altering condition for at least 5 years before seeking assistance from a healthcare provider (Gerhard, Nichols, & Smith, 1995). Conservatively, at least 15% to 30% of the American population over age 60 and 50% of those individuals who live in extended-care facilities or receive home care are incontinent (AHCPR, 1992; Newman et al, 1995). Canadian statistics indicate that 5% to 40% of individuals living at home and 50% of clients in healthcare facilities are believed to be incontinent (Lukaz, 1995). Twice as many women as men are incontinent, and healthcare costs related to managing incontinent episodes are staggering.

According to 1993 figures, the annual cost of incontinence care in the United States was estimated at $11.2 billion for persons living in the community and $5.2 billion for nursing home residents (Newman et al, 1995). Sales of absorbent products continue to increase 25% per year with approximately a $1.5 billion expenditure for these items in 1994. As the number of older persons increases, the cost of managing urinary incontinence will continue to escalate. The Agency for Health Care Policy and Research (AHCPR), in its 1992 guideline on urinary incontinence in adults, recognized the role of nurses, as healthcare professionals, in delivering quality care and ensuring long-term improvement, thus reducing the cost and personal suffering caused by urinary incontinence.

As statistics indicate, urinary incontinence is a special problem for older adults who may experience decreasing control over micturition and who may find it more difficult to reach a toilet in time to void because of mobility problems or dexterity problems in undressing. The discomfort, odor, and embarrassment of urine-soaked clothing can greatly diminish a person's self-concept and cause the individual to feel like a social outcast. Certainly there are age-related changes that affect urinary function, but urinary incontinence can be treated, and individualized interventions can help the client to lead a normal life. Advertisements for adult disposable undergarments have increased public awareness about urinary incontinence, but they fail to mention possible treatment strategies.

Types of Urinary Incontinence. The AHCPR guidelines (1992) recognized four types of urinary incontinence: stress, urge, overflow, and functional incontinence. **Stress incontinence** occurs when there is an involuntary loss of urine related to an increase in intra-abdominal pressure following coughing, sneezing, laughing, or other physical activities. Childbirth, menopause, obesity, or straining from chronic constipation can result in urine loss (Thayer, 1994). The leakage usually does not occur when the person is supine. **Urge incontinence** is the involuntary loss of urine associated with an abrupt and strong desire to void (urgency). It is usually associated with instability or involuntary contractions of the detrusor muscle that may or may not be associated with a neurologic disorder. With **overflow incontinence**, the

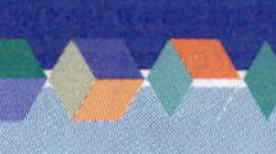

PROCEDURE 43-1

Offering and Removing a Bedpan or Urinal

Equipment

Bedpan or urinal
Toilet tissue
Handwashing supplies
Disposable gloves
Cover for bedpan or urinal (use Chux or disposable cover if others not available)

Action	Rationale
1. Bring the bedpan or urinal and equipment to bedside. Don disposable gloves.	Having equipment on hand saves time by avoiding unnecessary trips to the storage area. Gloves protect against exposure to blood and body substances.
2. Warm the bedpan, if it is made of metal, by rinsing it with warm water.	A cold bedpan feels uncomfortable and may make it difficult for the client to void. Plastic bedpans do not require warming.
3. Place an adjustable bed in the high position.	Having the bed in the high position reduces strain on the nurse's back while assisting the client onto the bedpan.
4. Place the bedpan or urinal on the chair next to the bed or on the foot of the bed. Fold the top linen back just enough to allow for placement of bedpan or urinal.	Folding back the linen in this manner prevents unnecessary exposure while still allowing the nurse to place the bedpan or urinal.
5. If the client needs assistance to move onto the bedpan, have him or her bend the knees and rest some of his or her weight on the heels. Lift the client by placing one hand under the lower back, and slip the bedpan into place with the other hand.	The client uses less energy as the nurse assists by lifting him or her onto the bedpan. The nurse uses less energy when the client can assist by placing some of his or her weight on the heels.

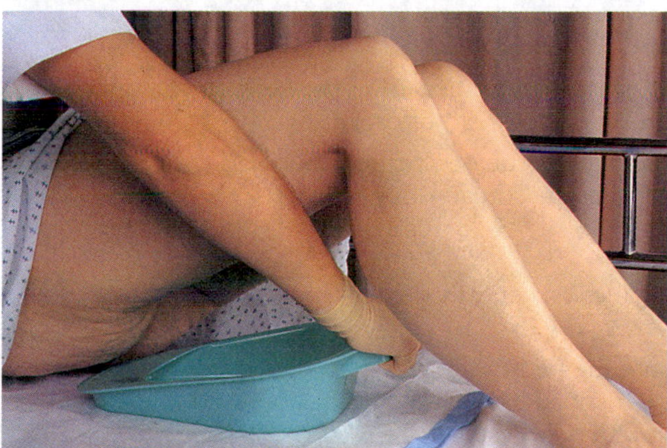

Action 5: Placing a fracture pan under buttocks.

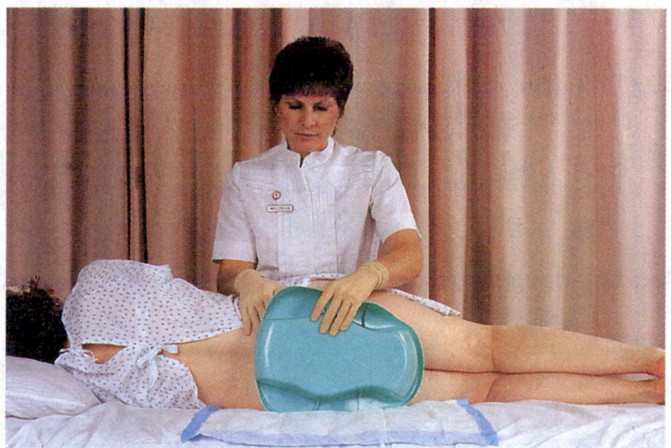

Action 6: Placing bedpan against buttocks while client is on his side. (Photos © B. Proud.)

Action	Rationale
6. If the client is helpless, two people may be required to lift him or her onto the bedpan. Or, the client may be placed on his or her side, the bedpan is placed against the buttocks, and the client is rolled back onto the bedpan, as shown.	Having two people lift a helpless client causes less strain on the nurse's back. Rolling the client takes less energy than lifting the client onto a bedpan.

(continued)

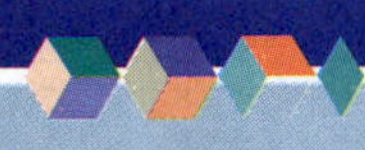

PROCEDURE 43-1 *(continued)*

Offering and Removing a Bedpan or Urinal

Action	Rationale
7. When the bedpan is in the proper place, the client's buttocks rest on the rounded shelf of the bedpan, as shown. For male clients, the urinal is properly placed between slightly spread legs with the penis positioned in it and with the urinal resting on the bed.	Having the bedpan or urinal in the proper place prevents spilling contents onto the bed and prevents injury to the skin from a misplaced bedpan.
8. If permitted, raise the head of the bed as near to the sitting position as tolerated.	This position makes it easier for the client to void or defecate, avoids strain on the client's back, and allows gravity to aid in elimination.
9. Place call device and toilet tissue within easy reach. Leave the client if it is safe to do so. Use side rails appropriately.	Falls can be prevented when the client does not have to reach for items he or she needs. Side rails are an additional safety precaution. Leaving client alone, if possible, promotes self-esteem and respects privacy.
10. Remove the bedpan in the same manner in which it was offered, being careful to hold it steady. If necessary to assist the client, don disposable gloves, wrap tissue around the hand several times, and wipe the client clean, using one stroke from the pubic area toward the anal area. Discard tissue, and use more until the client is clean. Place the client on his or her side, and spread the buttocks to clean the anal area. Cover bedpan.	Holding the pan steady prevents spilling its contents. Cleaning an area from front to back minimizes fecal contamination of the vagina and urinary meatus. Cleaning the client after he or she has used the bedpan prevents offensive odors and irritation to the skin.
11. Do not place toilet tissue in the bedpan if a specimen is required or if measurement of elimination is required. Have a receptacle handy for discarding the tissue.	Toilet tissue mixed with a specimen makes laboratory examination more difficult and interferes with accurate output measurement.
12. Offer the client supplies to wash and dry his or her hands, assisting as necessary.	Washing hands after using the bedpan or urinal helps prevent the spread of organisms.
13. Empty and clean the bedpan and urinal. Wash your hands. Record according to agency procedure.	Provides adequate documentation. Handwashing helps prevent the spread of organisms.

Nursing Considerations

A fracture bedpan may be substituted when it is difficult or uncomfortable to use a regular bedpan.

If it is difficult to slide client onto the bedpan, powder may be used on the resting surfaces of the pan to eliminate friction. Powder should not be used if a specimen is required because contamination could result.

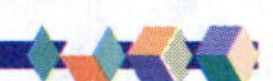

involuntary loss of urine is associated with overdistention and overflow of the bladder. The signal to empty the bladder may be underactive or absent, the bladder fills, and dribbling occurs. It may be due to a secondary effect of some drugs, fecal impaction, or neurologic conditions. **Functional incontinence** is urine loss caused by factors outside the lower urinary tract such as chronic impairments of physical and/or cognitive functioning (AHCPR, 1992). It can usually be treated effectively by identifying medical conditions, medications, or other physical or environmental barriers that interfere with normal voiding.

Diagnostic Evaluation. In addition to assessment strategies mentioned earlier in the chapter, physical examination and specific diagnostic tests aid in identification of urinary incontinence. The nurse examines the client's abdomen for a distended bladder, any masses, or

Developing Critical Thinking Skills

Situation

You have been assigned to care for an 80-year-old client who was admitted with a recurrent leg ulcer and is due to be discharged the following day. Her nursing notes indicate that she has had two or three episodes of urinary incontinence every day while in the hospital and her plan of care states "use adult diapers." You go into the room to answer Mrs. Bartowski's call bell and help her into the bathroom. She is wearing an adult diaper and a half-used package of diapers is on the chair. After voiding 150 cc of urine, she tearfully begs, "Please don't put that diaper back on me; I'm not a child." According to her chart, Mrs. Bartowski is mentally alert, lives at home with her daughter who visits frequently, and appears able to identify her need to urinate. You're aware that there are effective alternative therapies to resolve or minimize urinary incontinence rather than relying on absorbent products. However, the nurses have obviously made a decision to use diapers in this situation. You prefer to leave the diaper off, try some other measures, and, possibly, discuss this with her daughter; but you're only a student who is here for 2 days. You want to be a client advocate and do the right thing. What should you do?

1. ***Identify Goal of Thinking***
   Determine whether it is more important to replace the diaper against the client's wishes or leave it off and discuss the possibility of using behavioral strategies with the staff.
2. ***Assess Adequacy of Knowledge***
   Pertinent circumstances: Mrs. Bartowski is alert and oriented and obviously upset that diapers are being used. She has used her call light when she feels the urge to urinate but incontinent episodes have also been documented. The nursing staff have decided that diapers are appropriate for this client. Her daughter, with whom she lives, appears supportive and attentive. Discharge is scheduled for tomorrow.

   Prerequisite knowledge: Before you decide what to do in this situation, you need to discuss your options with your instructor. Of primary importance is whether the client and her daughter are interested in pursuing alternatives. They can also provide invaluable information about her elimination pattern at home. The physician must be consulted to determine the etiology of the incontinence and validate that her urinary tract is intact and functioning adequately. You will also need to review the various treatment options for incontinence since these will have to be communicated to the client and her daughter prior to discharge.

   Room for error/time constraints: Absorbent products can provide a sense of security and are widely used for incontinence. There is, however, an 80% chance that continence can be restored once incontinence is assessed, recognized, and addressed. Early dependence on absorbent products can remove motivation to seek treatment and promote acceptance of the condition. The treatment options should be discussed with Mrs. Bartowski and her daughter prior to discharge tomorrow.
3. ***Address Potential Problems***
   Continuing to use absorbent products offers a temporary solution to the problem. They protect the client from embarrassment and provide a sense of security, although they do nothing to prevent incontinent episodes. Using behavioral techniques to control incontinence will require health teaching before discharge and a long-term commitment to follow-up in the home.
4. ***Consult Helpful Resources***
   The client's motivation to restore continence is your most valuable resource. The primary nurse or case manager, the physician, and your instructor can also help you sort through your priorities in this situation. The AHCPR Guideline on Urinary Incontinence in Adults reflects the latest research and recommends use of behavioral techniques first to treat incontinence.
5. ***Critique Judgment/Decision***
   If you decide to reapply a diaper against the client's wishes, you may, in fact, be supporting the myth that incontinence is inevitable and untreatable. Long-term use of absorbent products can place the client at risk for skin breakdown and a urinary tract infection if used improperly. You decide to leave the diaper off and establish regular intervals for voiding for the 2 days you will be caring for Mrs. Bartowski. In this short time, you hope to demonstrate to the client, her daughter, and the staff that it is possible for Mrs. Bartowski to maintain a pattern of continence. Since she will most likely be discharged tomorrow, you also discuss the possibility of referral to home care or a continence expert who will instruct, support, and follow through with the necessary components of care. When you discuss your situation at postconference, your clinical group supports your decision.

tenderness. Pelvic and rectal examinations can determine muscle and sphincter tone and detect any irregularities. Measurement of the **post-void residual (PVR)** urine can be accomplished by catheterization and indicates the amount of urine remaining in the bladder immediately following the completion of urination. A PVR less than 50 mL is adequate, a volume greater than 200 mL is considered inadequate bladder emptying, and results between these two numbers indicate the need for further evaluation. A *provocative stress test* can also verify urinary incontinence. The client is instructed to cough before voiding in the toilet while holding a paper towel or folded toilet tissue over the urinary meatus. Any leakage of urine indicates stress incontinence (Mondoux, 1994). A voiding record or diary provides information about frequency, timing, and amount of voiding. Urodynamic tests that evaluate the anatomy and functional status of the urinary bladder and urethra also provide valuable information.

Treatment. Many clients believe that surgery is the only treatment option for urinary incontinence. Surgical intervention is considered only after behavioral and pharmacologic measures have proved ineffective. According to the urinary incontinence guideline (AHCPR, 1992), treatment can significantly improve or cure 80% of the clients with this condition. Nursing skills and creativity can help clients become continent again. The accompanying box summarizes the recommended treatment regimen for urinary incontinence.

Clients frequently turn to absorbent products for protection when they are incontinent of urine and have not had this condition properly diagnosed and treated. Protective products help the client feel more secure but may lead to acceptance of their condition and lack of motivation to seek further treatment (McCormick et al., 1992). When used improperly they may cause skin breakdown and place the client at risk of developing a urinary tract infection (UTI). Many types of products are available including adult diapers, liners, pads, pant systems, and drip collectors. Long-term use of these products is not recommended in the AHCPR guideline until the following factors are considered and discussed with a healthcare provider:

- Functional disability of the client
- Type and severity of incontinence
- Gender
- Availability of caregivers
- Failure with previous treatment programs
- Client preference

Home Care Considerations. Urinary incontinence is among the ten principal diagnoses of clients requiring home care services (Flynn, Cell, & Luisi, 1994). It is also the second most commonly cited reason for placing a client in a nursing home (McDowell et al., 1994). Through careful assessment and planned interventions, the nurse can restore a client's continence and help to postpone a caregiver's decision to place a family member in a costly healthcare facility. Environmental factors

Summary of Treatment Options for Urinary Incontinence

Behavioral Techniques

Bladder training—a substantial retraining effort consisting of education, scheduled voiding, and positive reinforcement that requires resisting the sensation of urgency, postponing voiding, and urinating according to a timetable.

Habit training—a program that focuses on voiding at regular intervals with an attempt to match the scheduled toileting to the person's natural elimination pattern.

Prompted voiding—a strategy that includes monitoring of continence status, prompting to try to void, and praise for remaining dry and for attempting to void.

Pelvic muscle exercises—Kegel exercises that strengthen the voluntary periurethral and pelvic muscles.

Vaginal cones—a structured exercise program involving insertion of cones that are identical in shape and volume but of increasing weight, and retention of the cone for up to 15 minutes twice daily.

Biofeedback—use of electronic or mechanical instruments to relay information to clients about physiologic activity.

Electrical stimulation—involves stimulating the pelvic viscera, the pelvic muscles, or the nerve supply to these structures.

Pharmacologic Treatment

This depends on the type of incontinence and involves a medication regimen for detrusor overactivity (urge incontinence) or drugs to improve urethral sphincter insufficiency (stress incontinence).

Surgical Intervention

Proper client selection is necessary prior to surgical intervention. The type of surgery depends on the specific etiology related to the incontinence.

Source: Urinary Incontinence Guideline Panel. *Urinary Incontinence in Adults: Clinical Practice Guideline.* AHCPR Pub. No. 92-0038. Rockville, MD: Agency for Health Care Policy and Research, Public Health Service, U.S. Department of Health and Human Services.

are of paramount importance and require careful assessment. It may be necessary to provide equipment that ensures improved access to toileting facilities (eg, walker, cane, wheelchair, Velcro closings on clothing). Dietary habits such as excess caffeine intake and insufficient fluid intake indicate the need for nutritional health teaching. Caffeine and concentrated urine irritate the bladder and may contribute to incontinence. The home setting is ideally suited to the use of noninvasive, low-risk behavioral interventions that are the first line of therapy. Nurses can identify clients who are incontinent and use these techniques or refer them to nurse or physician continence experts in the community. All nurses caring for older adults need to be familiar with education about urinary incontinence.

Catheterizing the Client's Bladder

Urinary catheterization is the introduction of a catheter through the urethra into the bladder for the purpose of withdrawing urine. A *catheter* is a tube for injecting or removing fluids. Catheterization is considered the most prominent cause of nosocomial infections, that is, an infection acquired in a hospital. Whenever possible, it is recommended that catheterization be avoided. When deemed necessary, it should be performed with careful technique. (See Nursing Process in Clinical Practice, later in this chapter.)

Types of Catheters. If a catheter is to remain in place for continuous drainage, an **indwelling urethral catheter** is used. Indwelling catheters also are called *retention* and *Foley catheters*. The indwelling urethral catheter is designed so that it does not slip out of the bladder. These catheters are used for the gradual decompression of an overdistended bladder, for intermittent bladder drainage and irrigation, and for continuous bladder drainage.

An indwelling catheter has a balloon, which is inflated after the catheter is inserted into the bladder. Several types of indwelling catheters are available, but the principles on which they operate are similar.

The indwelling catheter has more than one lumen. In a double-lumen catheter, one lumen is connected directly with the balloon, which is distended with solution, and the other is the lumen through which the urine drains. The triple-lumen catheter provides an additional lumen for the instillation of irrigating solution. Figure 43-7 shows a triple-lumen, a double-lumen, and a straight catheter. Wear gloves to protect against possible exposure to blood and body substances.

Intermittent or *straight catheters* are used to drain the bladder for shorter periods (5–10 min). Clients can be taught to insert and remove intermittent catheters themselves. Intermittent catheters are discussed later in this section.

A **suprapubic catheter** occasionally is used for continuous drainage. This type of catheter is inserted through a small incision above the pubic area. Care of the client with a suprapubic catheter is more appropriately discussed in clinical texts.

When a client has a urinary tract obstruction and is not a candidate for surgery, a *urologic stent* may be inserted. These devices may be temporary (when placed in the ureters) or permanent (when positioned in the

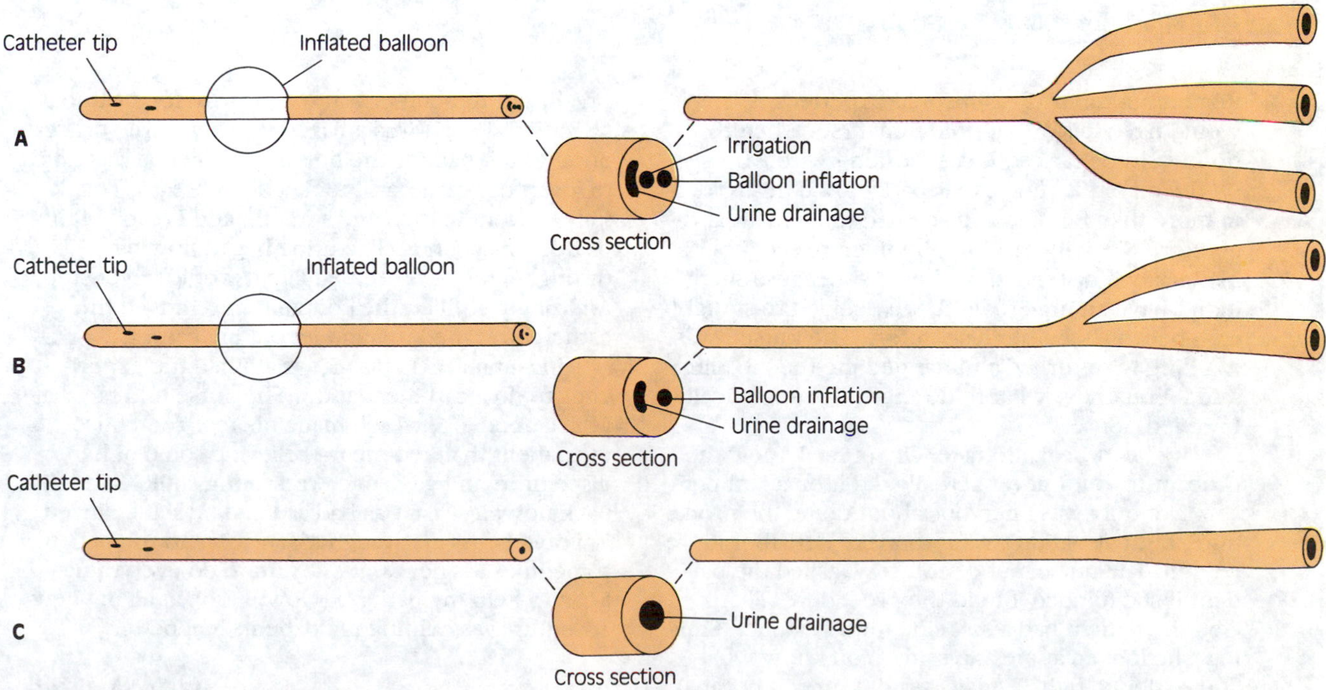

Figure 43-7
(A) Triple-lumen indwelling catheter. **(B)** Double-lumen indwelling catheter. **(C)** Straight catheter.

urethra). Temporary stents are usually made of a pliable material such as radiopaque silicone while permanent stents require a stronger material and typically are made of a flexible metal mesh. They are inserted during a cystoscopic procedure and, in most cases, the client receives only a local anesthetic and sedation. Urologic stents relieve urinary obstructions and provide a path for the flow of urine. Major nursing responsibilities include assessment, measurement, and documentation of urinary output. The nurse should never irrigate a blocked stent (Dunne, 1994).

Home Healthcare Alert

The client with a urologic stent must be instructed to notify the physician *immediately* if urine becomes bright red in color, severe pain occurs, the drainage pattern changes, or there is any sign of infection. The client should also be encouraged to wear a medical alert bracelet at all times.

Facts About the Lower Urinary Tract System. The following basic facts about the lower urinary tract system should be borne in mind when considering catheterization:

- The bladder normally is a sterile cavity.
- The external opening to the urethra can never be sterilized.
- The bladder has defense mechanisms. It empties itself of urine regularly and maintains an acidic environment, which has antibacterial advantages. These help to maintain a sterile bladder under normal circumstances and also help in clearing an infection if it occurs.
- Pathogens introduced into the bladder can ascend the ureters and lead to bladder and kidney infection.
- A normal bladder is not as susceptible to infection as an injured one. A client's lowered resistance, present in many diseases and stressful situations, predisposes to urinary infection.

Reasons for Catheterization. The following are common reasons for performing a urinary catheterization:

- To relieve urinary retention
- To obtain a sterile urine specimen from a woman
- To measure the amount of post-void residual (PVR) urine in the bladder. The client is first asked to void and is then catheterized to determine how much urine stays in the bladder after normal voiding.
- To obtain a urine specimen when a specimen cannot be secured satisfactorily by other means. Examples include collecting an uncontaminated specimen from a woman who is menstruating and from an incontinent client.
- To empty the bladder before, during, and after surgery and before certain diagnostic examinations.

Hazards of Catheterization. The hazards of introducing an instrument or a catheter into the bladder are sepsis and

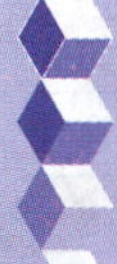

Through the Eyes of a Student

Remembering my first hospital experiences, I would have to say that doing my first catheterization was the scariest. I was working with a nurse on the maternity floor. Our patient had not voided in more than 8 hours and seemed to be in great discomfort. We palpated her abdomen to see if her bladder was distended, and it was. Because she didn't have an urge to void, we decided to straight cath her to lessen her discomfort. The nurse I was working with turned and handed me the kit. She said, "You know what to do, right?" Automatically I replied, "Sure."

My heart began to race. Of course I knew the procedure, but I never actually did it on a real person. Not only was I nervous about doing the procedure, but I also didn't want to make her labor more painful. The nurse, out of courtesy, asked the patient if she minded if I did the procedure. Thank God the patient had a soft side for a beginner. Smiling, she looked at me and said, "You know what you're doing, right?" Again I said, "Sure." I began setting up to begin my mission. To my amazement, I really did remember how to prepare for a catheterization. I even was amazed that my sterile procedure wasn't bad for the first time. When it was time to insert the catheter, I took a deep breath. Thankfully, it went in nice and smooth, and I reached the bladder in seconds. The urine began flowing through rapidly. It seemed like it would never stop. Amazingly, it filled the container. I removed the catheter, cleaned up, and let out my breath.

In summary, I was glad that I had the experience to do a catheterization. The nurse told me that I did a good job, which made me feel good. Also, my patient thanked me for relieving some of her discomfort and gave me a reassuring smile. As I look back now, it wasn't as bad as I had myself believed it would be. Even though it's invasive to the patient, sometimes it's necessary. I want to do everything I can to help my patients. Now, I look at all my new adventures as helping my patients feel better.

—Alysia Paxson,
Holy Family College, Philadelphia

trauma. The male urethra is especially vulnerable to injury because of its length. An object forced through a stricture or an irregular opening from the wrong angle can seriously damage the urethra. Although the urethra in the female is shorter than that in the male, it also is susceptible to damage if a catheter is forced through it. The mucous membrane lining the urethra is delicate and easily damaged by the friction resulting from the insertion of a catheter. Bacteria can enter the bladder when the catheter is inserted. When the catheter is left in place, the organisms may move up the catheter lumen or the space between the catheter and the urethral wall. This asymptomatic condition is known as *bacteriuria*. Most clients with an indwelling catheter in place for more than 2 weeks will develop bacteriuria (DeGroot-Kosolcharoen, 1994).

Intermittent catheterization may be necessary for clients with spinal cord injuries or other neurologic conditions. It may be done by the client or a caregiver in the home setting. Although the risk of developing a urinary tract infection is always present, most research supports the use of clean rather than sterile technique in this environment.

Equipment. The equipment used during a catheterization usually is prepackaged in a sterile, disposable tray. Most kits already contain a standard-size catheter. The trays used for catheterizing male and female clients are the same. Catheters are graded on the French scale according to lumen size. For the female adult, 14 and 16 French catheters commonly are used. Smaller catheters usually are not necessary, and the size of the lumen is so small that it increases the length of time necessary for emptying the bladder. Larger catheters distend the urethra and increase the discomfort of the procedure. For the male adult, 18 and 20 French catheters commonly are used, but if these are too large, a smaller catheter should be used. Size 8 and 10 French catheters commonly are used for children.

Client Preparation. Before the catheterization, the client should be given an adequate explanation of the procedure and the reason for it. A catheter being inserted produces a sensation of pressure and some discomfort, and this should be explained to the client. In addition, the client should be assured that every measure to avoid exposure and embarrassment will be taken. The more relaxed the client can be, the easier it will be to insert the catheter.

The most common position for the client is the dorsal recumbent, preferably on a solid surface, such as a firm mattress or a treatment table. Catheterizing a client in a bed with a soft mattress, especially for the female client, is not as satisfactory because the client's pelvic surfaces are not firmly supported, and visualization of the meatus is difficult. Also, the client may sink into the bed, causing the bladder to be lower than the outlet of the catheter. If the client is in bed, supporting the buttocks on a firm cushion is helpful.

The Sims', or lateral, position can be an alternate position for the female client. This position may allow for better visualization and be more comfortable for the client, especially if hip and knee movements are difficult. A reduced area of exposure also can result in less psychic discomfort for the client. The client may lie on either side, depending on which position is easiest for the nurse and best in terms of the client's comfort. The client's buttocks are placed near the edge of the bed with her shoulders at the opposite edge and her knees drawn toward her chest. The nurse lifts the upper buttock and labia to expose the urinary meatus. This positioning is shown in Figure 43-8.

Procedure. Catheterization of the urinary bladder for female and male clients is described in Procedures 43-2 and 43-3. Techniques of surgical asepsis are of extraordinary importance when catheterizing a client to help prevent urinary tract infection.

Indwelling Catheters

Inserting and Connecting to the Drainage System. The procedure for inserting an indwelling catheter is the same as for inserting a straight, single-lumen catheter with the following differences:

- Inflate the balloon with the prefilled syringe before inserting the catheter, to check for balloon patency. Aspirate the fluid back into the syringe when it is determined that the balloon is patent.
- Insert the catheter 1 to 2 inches beyond the point where urine flow occurred. Trout et al. (1993) recommend inserting the catheter in a male client to the bifurcation of the catheter tubing. Then the balloon can be safely inflated and the catheter can be gently pulled back into place.
- When the balloon is inflated, usually 4 to 5 mL *more* sterile water than the size of the balloon is used. This additional water remains in the tube leading to the balloon.
- If the client complains of pain after the balloon is inflated, allow it to empty and replace the catheter with another one. The balloon is probably located in the urethra and is causing discomfort owing to distention of the urethra.

Technique to Complete a Closed Urinary Drainage System. The following technique is used to complete the closed urinary drainage system:

- Check to see that the drainage tubing is not kinked. Do not place it under the leg, where it may be compressed. Also, do not place it in a manner so that it moves above the level of the bladder. This may cause the client's bladder to drain by suction rather than by gravity, risking injury to the bladder mucosa.
- Clip the drainage tubing to the bottom bed linen to help hold the drainage tube in the proper place while the client is in bed. This helps prevent pooling of urine in the drainage tubing.

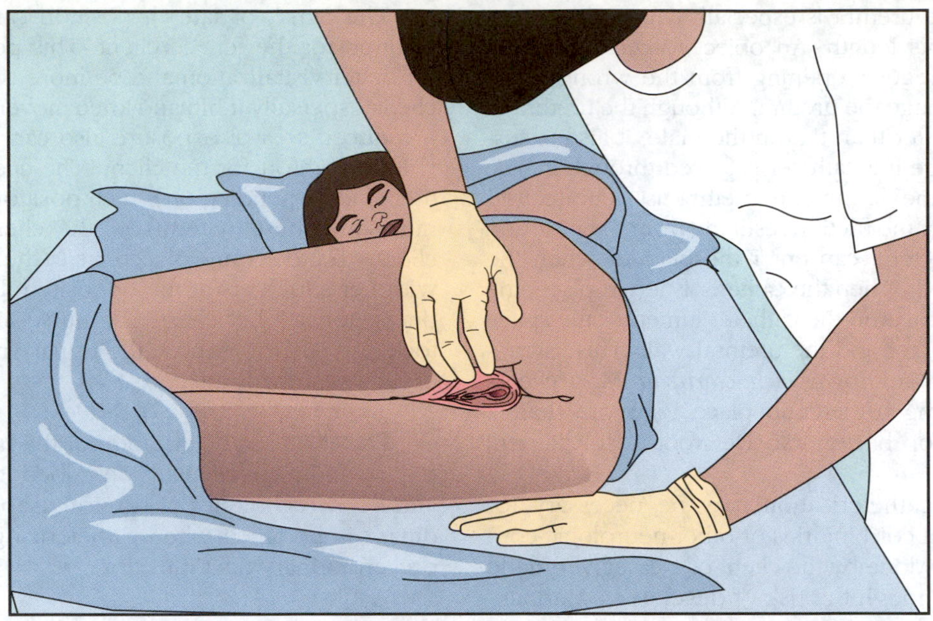

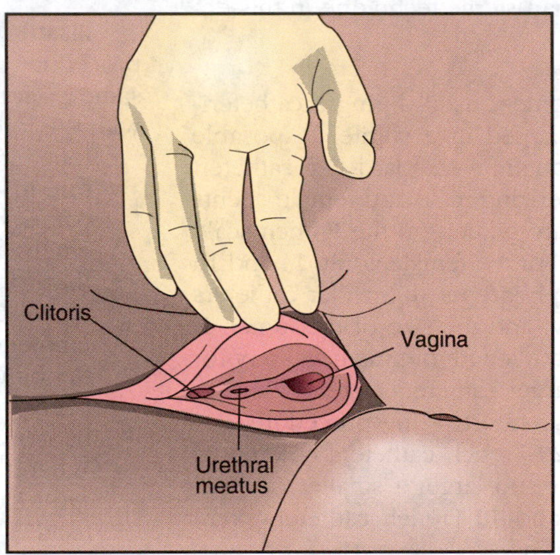

Figure 43-8
Demonstration of the side-lying position (*top*) and of how to expose the urinary meatus when catheterizing a female patient (*bottom*).

- Keep the drainage bag off the floor at all times to reduce the risk of infection. The floor is grossly contaminated!

Irrigating the Indwelling Catheter. The flushing of a tube, canal, or area with solution is called *irrigation*. The purpose of a catheter irrigation is to restore or maintain its patency. Procedure 43-4 describes how to irrigate an indwelling catheter using the closed system.

Continuous or frequent irrigations may be ordered when blood clots or other debris threaten to block the catheter. In the past, the open procedure was done routinely for almost all indwelling catheters, but because

(text continues on page 1246)

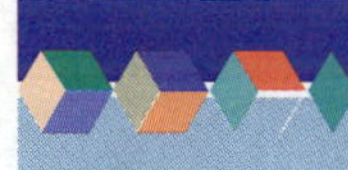

PROCEDURE 43-2

Catheterizing the Female Urinary Bladder (Straight and Indwelling)

Equipment

Sterile catheterization kit that contains:
- Sterile gloves
- Sterile drapes (one of which is fenestrated)
- Antiseptic solution
- Lubricant
- Cotton balls or gauze squares
- Forceps
- Straight or indwelling catheter (size must be appropriate for client)
- Prefilled syringe
- Basin (base of kit usually serves as this)

Specimen container
Flashlight or lamp
Urine collection bag and drainage tubing (may be connected to sterile indwelling catheter if a closed drainage system is used)
Velcro leg strap or tape
Disposal bag
Waterproof pad or Chux

Action	Rationale
1. Assemble equipment. Wash your hands. Explain the procedure and its purpose to the client.	Organization facilitates performance of the task. Handwashing deters spread of microorganisms. An explanation encourages client cooperation and reduces apprehension.
2. Provide for good light. Artificial light is recommended (use of a flashlight requires an assistant to hold and position it).	Good lighting is necessary to see the meatus clearly.
3. Provide for privacy by closing the curtains or door.	The procedure may be embarassing for the client.
4. Assist the client to the dorsal recumbent position with the knees flexed and the feet about 2 feet apart and drape the client. Or, if preferable, the client can be placed in the side-lying position as shown in Figure 43-8. Slide the waterproof drape under the client.	Good visualization of the meatus is important. Embarrassment, chilliness, and feeling tense can interfere with introducing the catheter. The client's comfort will promote relaxation. The drape will protect bed linens from moisture.
5. Clean the genital and perineal area with warm soap and water. Rinse and dry. Wash your hands again.	Clean technique decreases the possibility of introducing organisms into the bladder.
6. Prepare urine drainage setup if indwelling catheter is to be inserted and separate urine collection system is used. Secure to bed frame according to manufacturer's directions.	This facilitates connection of the catheter to the drainage system and provides for easy access.
7. Open the sterile catheterization tray on overbed table using sterile technique.	Placement of equipment near the work site increases efficiency. Sterile technique protects the client and prevents the spread of microorganisms.
8. Put on sterile gloves. Grasp the upper corners of the drape and unfold the drape without touching unsterile areas. Fold back a cuff over gloved hands. Ask the client to lift her buttocks and slide the sterile drape under her with gloves protected by cuff.	The drape provides a sterile field close to the meatus. Covering the gloved hands will help keep the gloves sterile while placing the drape.
9. A fenestrated sterile drape may be placed over the perineal area, exposing the labia.	The drape expands the sterile field and protects against contamination. Use of a fenestrated drape may limit visualization and is considered optional by some practitioners.
10. Place the sterile tray on the drape between the client's thighs.	This provides easy access to supplies.

(continued)

PROCEDURE 43-2 (continued)

Catheterizing the Female Urinary Bladder (Straight and Indwelling)

Action	Rationale
11. Open all supplies:	
a. *If the catheter is to be indwelling,* test the catheter balloon. Remove the protective cap on the tip of the syringe and attach the syringe prefilled with sterile water to injection port. Inject appropriate amount of fluid. If the balloon inflates properly, withdraw fluid and leave the syringe attached to the port.	A balloon that does not inflate or that leaks needs to be replaced before insertion in the client.
b. Pour antiseptic solution over cotton balls or gauze. Open the specimen container if specimen is to be obtained.	It is necessary to open all supplies and prepare for the procedure while both hands are sterile.
c. Lubricate 1 to 2 inches of the catheter tip.	Lubrication facilitates the insertion of the catheter and reduces trauma to the tissues.

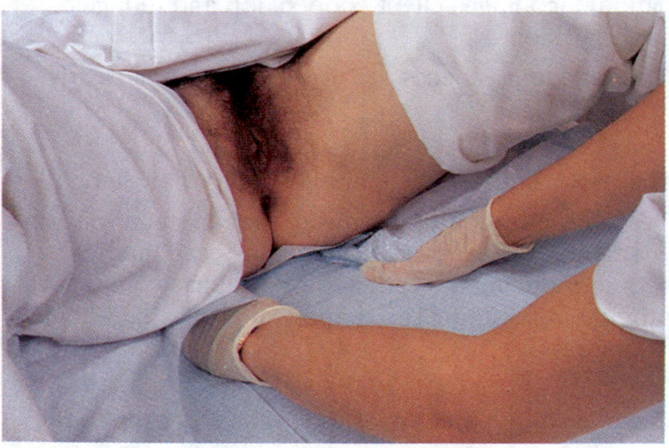

Action 8: Keeping sterile gloves protected while positioning drape under client.

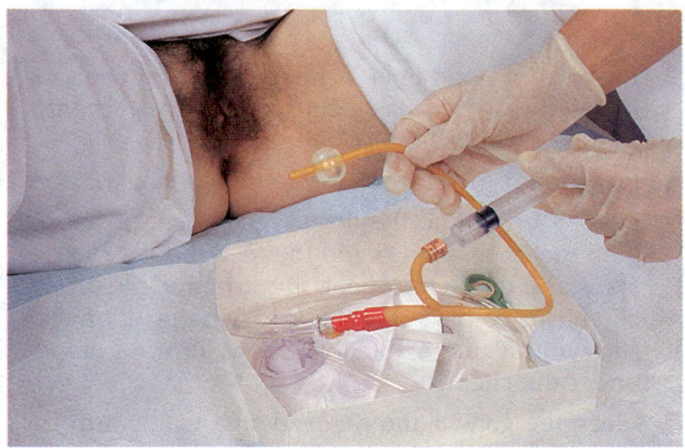

Action 11a: Testing the balloon.

Action	Rationale
12. With the thumb and one finger of your nondominant hand, spread the labia and identify the meatus, as shown in figure. Be prepared to maintain separation of the labia with one hand until urine is flowing well and continuously.	Smoothing the area immediately surrounding the meatus helps to make it visible. Allowing the labia to drop back into position may contaminate the area around the meatus, as well as the catheter. Your nondominant hand is now contaminated.
13. Using cotton balls held with forceps, clean both labial folds and then directly over the meatus. Move the cotton ball from above the meatus down toward the rectum. Discard each cotton ball after one downward stroke.	Moving from an area where there is likely to be less contamination to an area where there is more contamination helps prevent the spread of organisms. Cleaning the meatus last helps reduce the possibility of introducing organisms into the bladder.
14. With the uncontaminated gloved hand, place the drainage end of the catheter in the receptacle. *For insertion of an indwelling catheter* that is preattached to sterile tubing and drainage container (closed drainage system), position the catheter and setup withing easy reach on the sterile field.	This facilitates drainage of urine and minimizes risk of contaminating sterile equipment.

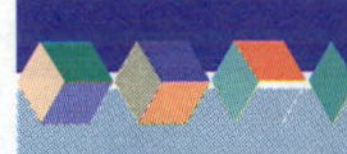

PROCEDURE 43-2 *(continued)*

Catheterizing the Female Urinary Bladder (Straight and Indwelling)

Action | **Rationale**

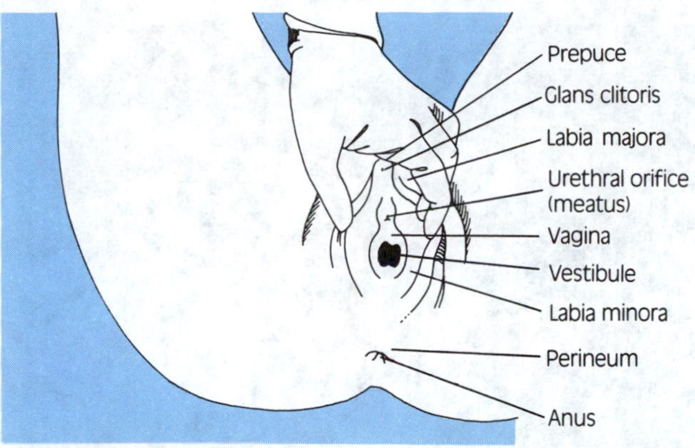

Action 12: Spreading the labia with nondominant hand to identify the meatus.

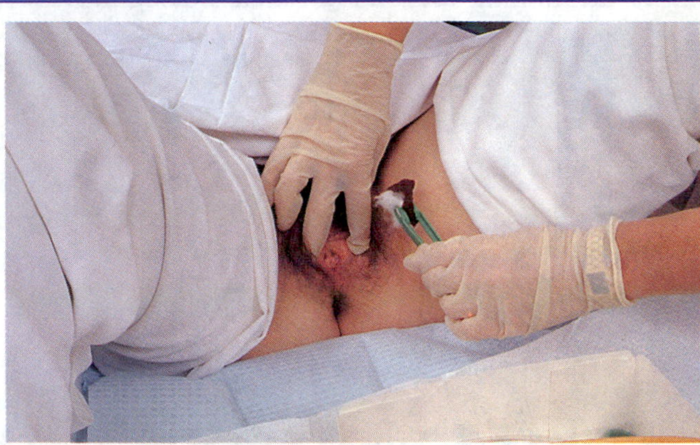

Action 13: Preparing to clean the labial folds.

15. Insert the catheter tip into the meatus 5 to 7.5 cm (2–3 in) or until urine flows. Do not use force to push the catheter through the urethra into the bladder. Ask the client to breathe deeply, and rotate the catheter gently if slight resistance is met as the catheter reaches the external sphincter. *For an indwelling catheter*, once urine drains, advance the catheter another 2.5 to 5.0 cm (1–2 in).

The female urethra is about 3.7 to 6.2 cm (1½–2½ in) long. Applying force on the catheter is likely to injure mucous membranes. The sphincter relaxes and the catheter can enter the bladder easily when the client relaxes. Advancing an indwelling catheter an additional 1.3 to 2.5 cm (½ to 1 in) ensures placement in the bladder and facilitates inflation of the balloon without damaging the urethra.

16. Hold the catheter securely with the nondominant hand while the bladder empties. Collect a specimen if required. Continue drainage according to agency policy.

Withdrawing and reinserting the catheter increases the chances of contaminating it. In general, no more than 750 mL of urine should be removed at one time. Pelvic floor blood vessels may become engorged from the sudden release of pressure leading to possible hypotensive episode.

17. Remove the catheter smoothly and slowly if a straight catheterization was ordered.

This causes less discomfort to the client.

18. *If the catheter is to be indwelling:*
    a. Inflate the balloon according to the manufacturer's recommendations. Inject the entire volume supplied in the prefilled syringe.

    The balloon anchors the catheter in place in the bladder. Sterile water is used to inflate the balloon as a precaution in case the balloon ruptures.

    b. Tug gently on the catheter after the balloon is inflated to feel resistance.

    Improper inflation can cause client discomfort and malpositioning of catheter.

    c. Attach the catheter to the drainage system if necessary.

    Closed drainage system minimizes the risk of organisms being introduced into the bladder.

    d. Secure to the upper thigh with a Velcro leg strap or tape. Leave some slack in the catheter to allow for leg movement.

    Proper attachment prevents trauma to the urethra and meatus from tension on the tubing.

    e. Check that the drainage tubing is not kinked and that movement of side rails does not interfere with catheter or drainage bag.

    This facilitates drainage of urine and prevents the backflow of urine.

(continued)

PROCEDURE 43-2 *(continued)*

Catheterizing the Female Urinary Bladder (Straight and Indwelling)

Action | **Rationale**

Action 15: Inserting the tip of the catheter into the meatus, using the uncontaminated gloved hand.

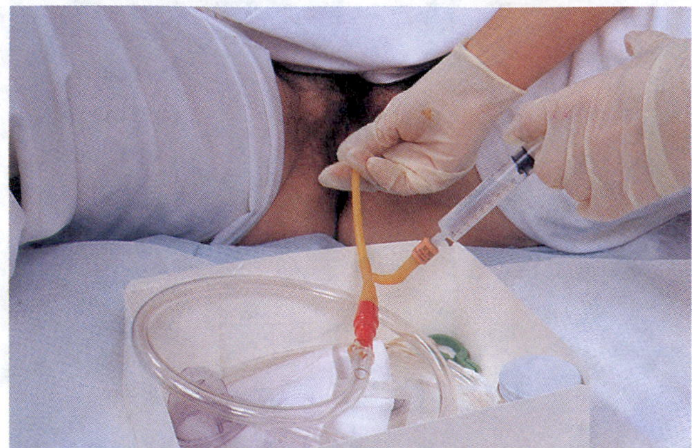

Action 18a: Injecting sterile water to inflate balloon.

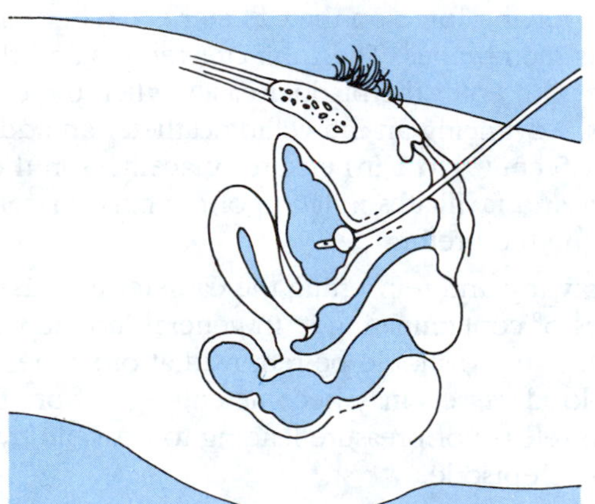

Action 18b: Tugging gently on catheter after balloon is in place to feel resistance.

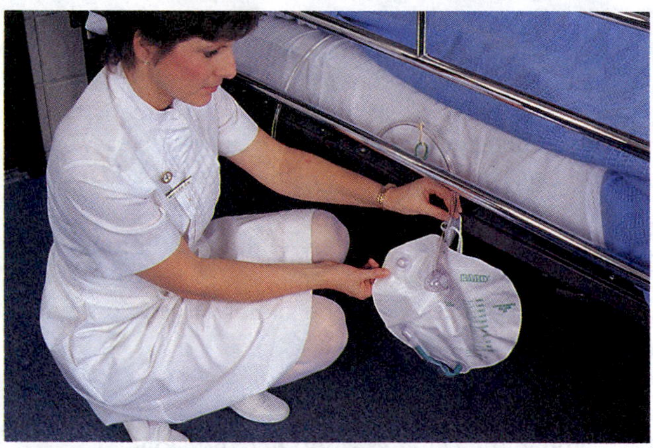

Action 18e: Checking position of drainage setup.

19. Remove the equipment and make the client comfortable in bed. Clean and dry the perineal area, if necessary. Care for the equipment according to agency policy. Send the urine specimen to the laboratory promptly or refrigerate it.

    Urine kept at room temperature may cause organisms, if present, to grow and distort laboratory findings.

20. Wash your hands.

    Handwashing deters the spread of microorganisms.

21. Record the time of the catheterization, the amount of urine removed, a description of the urine, the client's reaction to the procedure, and your name.

    A careful record is important for planning the client's care.

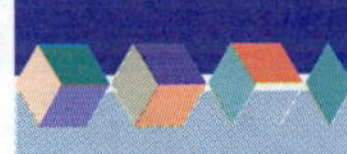

PROCEDURE 43-2 *(continued)*

Catheterizing the Female Urinary Bladder (Straight and Indwelling)

Age Considerations

If the client is a child, the size of the catheter must be adapted accordingly.

Elderly women may be uncomfortable in the lithotomy position, and require variable positions for catheterization. If the client is able to remain on her back, another nurse can assist her to flex her knees and hips, thus bringing the knees closer to the abdomen and allowing visualization of the urinary meatus. Catheterization also is possible with the client on her side in a modified Sims' position as discussed and shown in Figure 43-8.

Home Care Considerations

If self-catheterization must be performed in the home, clean technique is appropriate. The bladder's natural resistance to microorganisms normally found in the home makes sterile technique unnecessary. Rubber catheters must be washed thoroughly before boiling for 20 minutes. Dry and store properly for next usage.

A shower rather than a tub bath is recommended for clients with an indwelling catheter. Sitting in the bathtub may allow for easier access of bacteria into the urinary tract.

Special Considerations

If there is not an immediate flow of urine after the catheter has been inserted, several measures may prove helpful:

- Have the client take a deep breath, which helps to relax the perineal and abdominal muscles.
- Rotate the catheter slightly because a drainage hole may be resting against the bladder wall.
- Raise the head of the client's bed to increase pressure in the bladder area.
- Placed a gloved finger in the vagina to feel digitally for the position of the catheter through the anterior vaginal wall.
- Temporarily leave a catheter that has inadvertently been placed in the vagina in place as a guide while the nurse regloves and inserts another sterile catheter directly above it into the urinary meatus.

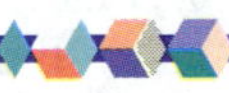

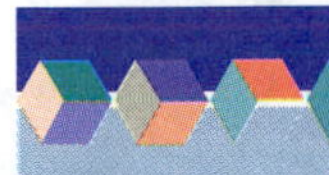

PROCEDURE 43-3

Catheterizing the Male Urinary Bladder (Straight and Indwelling)

Equipment

Sterile catheterization kit that contains:
- Sterile gloves
- Sterile drapes (one of which is fenestrated)
- Antiseptic solution
- Lubricant
- Cotton balls or gauze squares

Forceps
Straight or indwelling catheter
Prefilled syringe
Basin (base of kit usually serves as this)
Specimen container
Flashlight or lamp

Urine collection bag and drainage tubing (may be connected to sterile indwelling catheter if a closed drainage system is used)
Velcro leg strap or tape
Disposal bag
Waterproof pad or Chux

Action	Rationale
1. Assemble the equipment and follow actions 1 through 3 for female catheterization in Procedure 43-2.	

(continued)

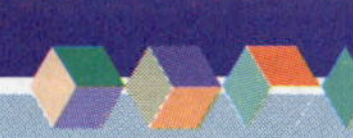

PROCEDURE 43-3 *(continued)*

Catheterizing the Male Urinary Bladder (Straight and Indwelling)

Action	Rationale
2. Position the client on his back with the thighs slightly apart. Drape the client so that only the area around the penis is exposed.	This prevents unnecessary exposure.
3. Follow actions 5 to 7 for female catheterization in Procedure 43-2.	

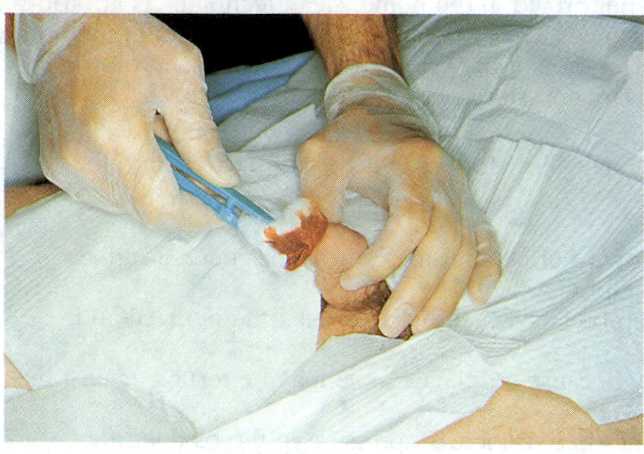

Action 3: Clean the area of the meatus.

Action	Rationale
4. Put on sterile gloves. Open the sterile drape and place on the client's thighs. Place the fenestrated drape with the opening over the penis.	This maintains a sterile working area.
5. Place the catheter set on or next to the client's legs on the sterile drape.	The sterile setup should be arranged so that the nurse's back is not turned to it, nor should it be out of the nurse's range of vision.
6. Open all supplies:	
a. *If the catheter is to be indwelling,* test the catheter balloon. Remove the protective cap on the tip of the syringe and attach the syringe prefilled with sterile water to the injection port. Inject appropriate amount of fluid. If balloon inflates properly, withdraw fluid and leave syringe attached to port.	A balloon that does not inflate or that leaks must be replaced before insertion in the client.
b. Pour antiseptic solution over cotton balls or gauze. Open the specimen container if specimen is to be obtained.	It is necessary to open all supplies and prepare for the procedure while both hands are sterile.
7. *Generously* lubricate the catheter for about 15 to 18 cm (6 to 7 inches).	Generous lubrication is especially important because of the length and tortuousness of the male urethra. The lubricant decreases friction.
8. Lift the penis with your nondominant hand, which is then considered contaminated. Retract the foreskin in the uncircumcised male client. Clean the area at the meatus with a cotton ball held with a forceps. Use a circular motion, moving from the meatus toward the base of the penis for three cleansings.	The hand touching the penis becomes contaminated. Cleansing the area around the meatus and under the foreskin in the uncircumcised male client helps prevent infection. Moving from the meatus toward the base of the penis prevents bringing organisms to the meatus.

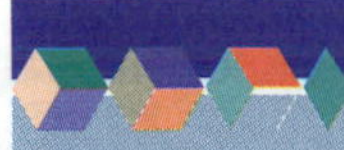

PROCEDURE 43-3 *(continued)*

Catheterizing the Male Urinary Bladder (Straight and Indwelling)

Action	Rationale
9. Hold the penis with slight upward tension and perpendicular to the client's body. Ask the client to bear down as if voiding. With your dominant hand, place the drainage end of the catheter in the receptacle. *For insertion of an indwelling catheter* that is preattached to sterile tubing and a drainage container (closed drainage system), position the catheter and setup withing easy reach on the sterile field.	Holding the penis up with slight traction helps straighten the urethra.
10. Insert the tip into the meatus. Advance the catheter 15 to 20 cm (6–8 in) or until urine flows. Do not use force to introduce the catheter. If the catheter resists entry, ask the client to breathe deeply and rotate the catheter slightly. *For an indwelling catheter,* once urine drains, advance the catheter to the bifurcation of the catheter. Once the balloon is inflated, the catheter may be gently pulled back into place. Lower the penis.	The male urethra is about 20 cm long. Deep breaths or slight twisting of the catheter may ease the catheter past resistance at the sphincters. Advancing an indwelling catheter to the bifurcation ensures its placement in the bladder and facilitates inflation of the balloon without damaging the urethra.
11. Follow Actions 16 through 21 for female catheterization in Procedure 43-2 except that the catheter may be secured to the upper thigh or lower abdomen with the penis directed toward the client's chest. Slack should be left in the catheter to prevent tension.	This is done to prevent irritation at the angle of the penis and scrotum. Slack left in the catheter allows for penile erection, which can occur naturally during sleep.

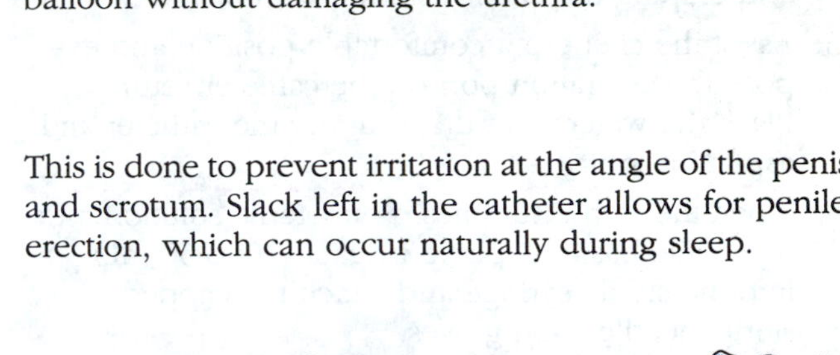

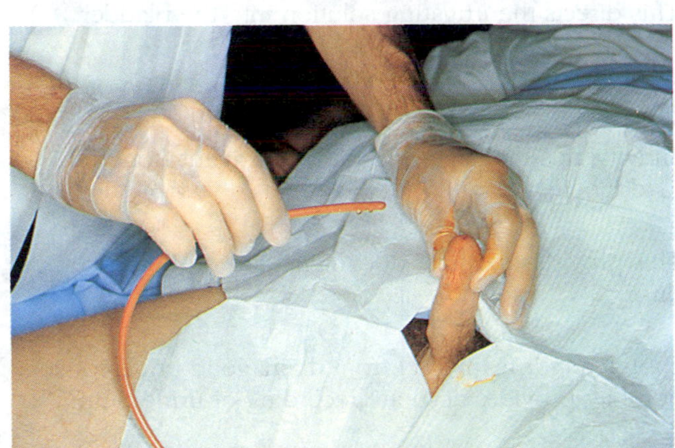

Action 9: Preparing to insert the catheter.

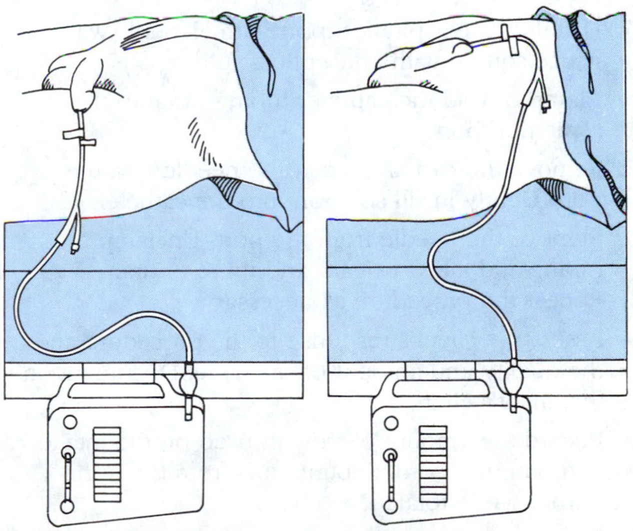

Action 11: Secure the catheter to the upper thigh or lower abdomen, allowing slack to prevent tension.

Age Considerations If the client is a child, the size of the catheter must be adapted accordingly.

Home Care Considerations If self-catheterization must be performed in the home, clean technique is appropriate. The bladder's natural resistance to microorganisms normally found in the home makes sterile technique unnecessary. Rubber catheters must be washed thoroughly before boiling for 20 minutes. Dry and store properly for next usage.

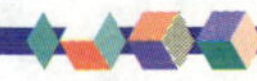

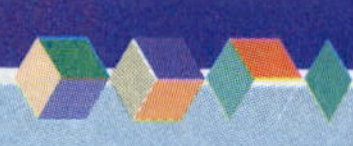

PROCEDURE 43-4

Irrigating the Catheter Using the Closed System

Equipment

Sterile basin or container
Gauze squares or cotton balls with disinfectant or alcohol swabs
Waterproof drape
30- to 50-mL syringe with 18- or 19-gauge needle
Sterile irrigating solution (at room temperature or warmed to body temperature)
Bath blanket
Disposable gloves

Action	Rationale
1. Assemble equipment. Wash your hands. Explain the procedure and its purpose to the client.	Organization facilitates performance of task. Handwashing deters spread of microorganisms. An explanation encourages client cooperation and reduces apprehension.
2. Provide for privacy by closing the curtains or door and draping the client with the bath blanket.	The procedure may be embarrassing for the client.
3. Assist the client to a comfortable position and expose the aspiration port on the catheter setup. Place the waterproof drape under the catheter and aspiration port.	This provides for adequate visualization. The drape protects the client and the bed from leakage.
4. Open the sterile supplies. Pour sterile solution into the sterile basin. Aspirate irrigant (30 to 50 mL) into the sterile syringe and attach the capped sterile needle. Don gloves.	This prevents the spread of microorganisms and contact with blood or body substances.
5. Disinfect the aspiration port with alcohol swabs or gauze square with antiseptic solution.	This prevents the spread of microorganisms.
6. Clamp or fold the catheter tubing distal to the aspiration port.	This directs the irrigating solution into the bladder.
7. Remove the cap and insert the needle into the port. Gently instill solution into the catheter.	Gentle irrigation prevents damage to the lining of the bladder.
8. Remove the needle from the port. Unclamp the tubing and allow irrigant and urine to drain. Repeat the procedure as necessary.	Gravity aids drainage of urine and irrigant from the bladder.
9. Assess the client's response to the procedure and the quality and amount of drainage. Document on the client's chart.	This provides accurate documentation of the procedure.
10. Record the amount of irrigant used on the intake and output record. Subtract this from the urine output when totaled.	Subtracting irrigant total from drainage in urine collection bag provides accurate recording of urine output.
11. Remove equipment and discard uncapped needle and syringe in appropriate receptacle. Remove gloves and wash your hands. Make client comfortable.	Handwashing deters the spread of microorganisms. Proper disposal of needle prevents the nurse accidentally puncturing self.

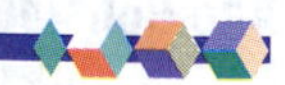

this is another means of introducing pathogens, it is now recommended that only the closed system is used. Natural irrigation of the catheter through increased fluid intake by the client is the preferred technique.

Preferably, the client who needs frequent irrigation so that the catheter and tubing remain patent will have a triple-lumen catheter with continuous irrigation. Procedure 43-5 describes continuous bladder irrigation.

Caring for the Client. The following are nursing measures used when caring for a client with an indwelling catheter:

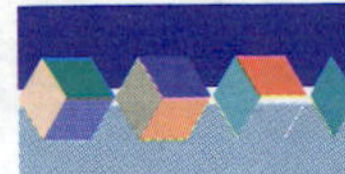

PROCEDURE 43-5

Giving a Continuous Bladder Irrigation

Equipment

Sterile irrigating solution (at room temperature or warmed to body temperature), usually 2000-mL bags
Sterile tubing with drip chamber and clamp for connection to irrigating solution
IV pole
Three-way Foley catheter in place in client's bladder
Foley drainage setup (tubing and collection bag)
Bath blanket
Disposable gloves (optional)

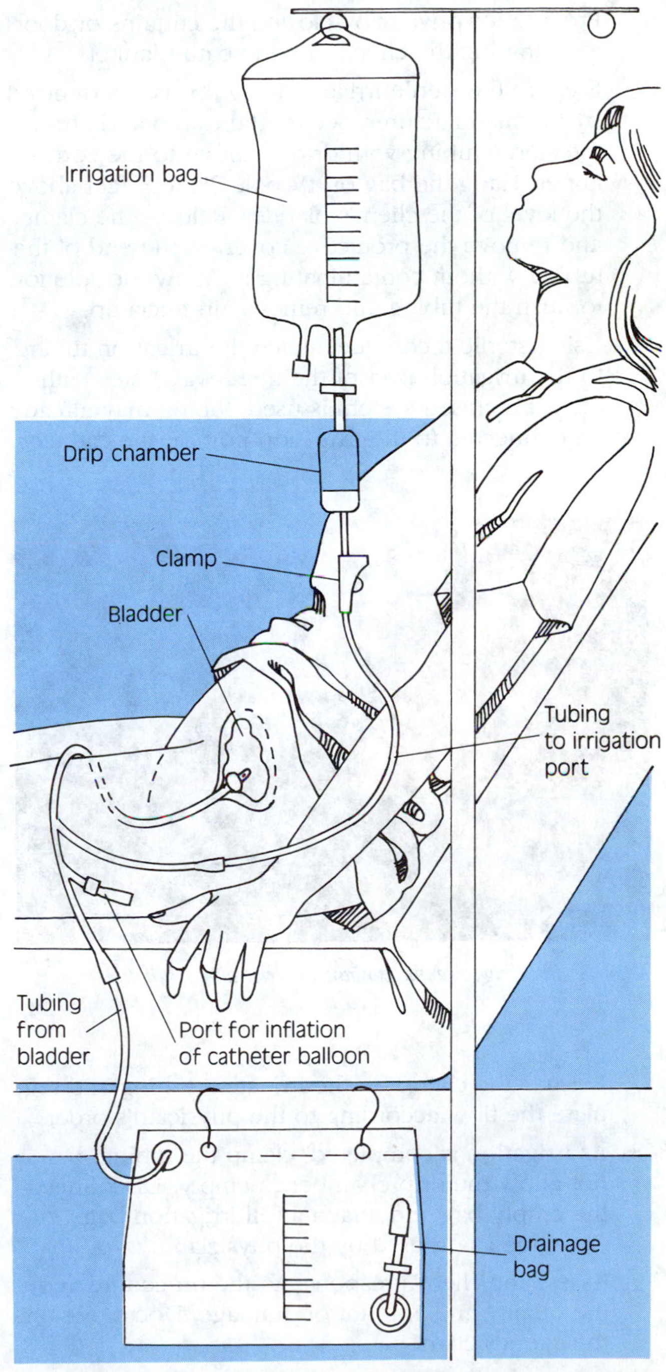

Continuous irrigation.

(continued)

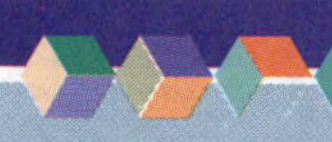

PROCEDURE 43-5 *(continued)*

Giving a Continuous Bladder Irrigation

Action	Rationale
1. Explain the procedure and its purpose to the client.	An explanation encourages client cooperation and reduces apprehension.
2. Assemble the equipment.	Organization facilitates performance of tasks.
3. Wash your hands.	Handwashing deters the spread of microorganisms.
4. Provide for privacy by closing the curtains or door and draping the client with the bath blanket.	The procedure may be embarrassing for the client.
5. Prepare the sterile irrigation bag for use as directed by the manufacturer. Secure the clamp and attach the sterile tubing with drip chamber to the container. Hang the bag on IV pole 2½ to 3 feet above the level of the client's bladder. Release the clamp and remove the protective cover on the end of the tubing without contaminating it. Allow the solution to flush the tubing and remove air. Reclamp.	Irrigation solution continuously bathes the lining of the bladder and keeps the catheter patent. Flushing the tubing before irrigation clears air from the tubing that might cause bladder distention.
6. Using sterile technique, attach the irrigation tubing to the irrigation port of the three-way Foley catheter. If a closed system is used, tubing may already be connected to the irrigation port on the catheter.	Sterile technique prevents the spread of microorganisms into the bladder.

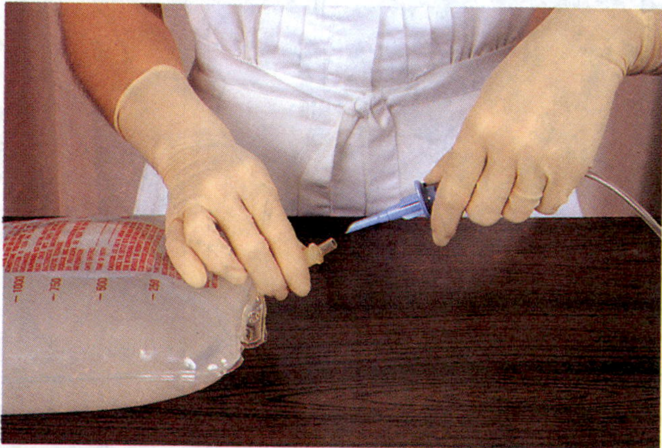

Action 5: Inserting spike into container of irrigating solution.

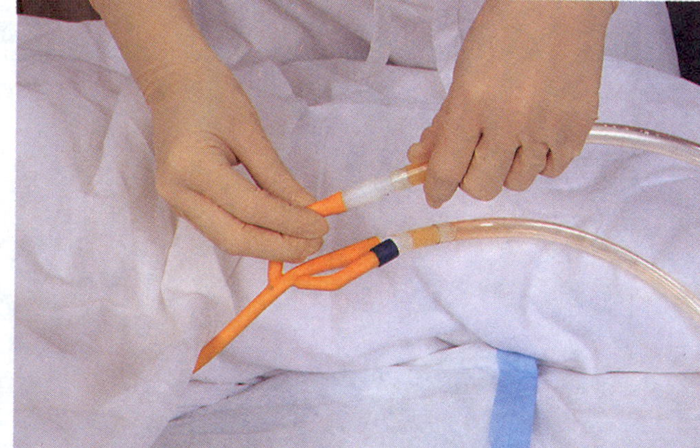

Action 6: Attaching irrigation tubing to irrigation port of three-way Foley catheter using sterile technique.

Action	Rationale
7. Release the clamp on the irrigation tubing and regulate the flow according to the physician's order.	This allows for continual gentle irrigation without causing discomfort to the client.
8. As irrigation is completed, clamp the tubing. Do not allow the drip chamber to empty. Disconnect the empty bag and attach a full irrigation bag. Continue as ordered by the physician.	This eliminates the need to separate tubing from the catheter and clear air from the tubing. Opening the drainage system provides access for introduction of microorganisms.
9. Assess the client's response to the procedure and the quality and amount of drainage. Document on the client's chart.	This provides accurate documentation of the procedure.

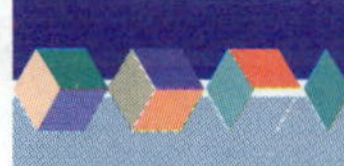

PROCEDURE 43-5 *(continued)*

Giving a Continuous Bladder Irrigation

Action	Rationale
10. Record the amount of irrigant used on the intake and output record. Don gloves and empty the drainage collection bag as each new container is hung and record.	This ensures accurate recording of urine output. Gloves protect against exposure to blood, body substances, and microorganisms.
11. Wash your hands.	Handwashing deters the spread of microorganisms.

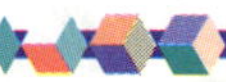

- Be sure to wash hands before and after caring for a client with an indwelling catheter. Wear gloves to protect against possible exposure to blood and body substances.
- Clean the perineal area thoroughly, especially around the meatus, twice a day and after each bowel movement.
- Use soap or detergent and water to clean the perineal area, and rinse the area well. Do not use powders and lotions after cleaning.
- Apply a topical antibiotic ointment at the meatus, as ordered.
- Make sure that the client maintains a generous fluid intake. This helps prevent infection and irrigates the catheter naturally by increasing urine output.
- Encourage the client to be up and about, as ordered.
- Note the volume and character of urine, and record observations carefully. The urine can be observed through the drainage tubing and in the collecting container. The usual procedure is to note and record the amount of urine on the client's intake-and-output record every 8 hours. The collecting container is calibrated, but the volume markings are only approximations. The urine should be emptied into a graduated container that is accurately calibrated for correct determination of output.
- Do not open the drainage system to obtain urine specimens or to measure urine. If the tubing becomes disconnected, wipe the ends of both tubes with antiseptic solution before reconnecting. When emptying the drainage bag, make sure the drainage spout does not touch a contaminated surface.
- Teach the client the importance of personal hygiene, especially the importance of careful cleaning after having a bowel movement and thorough washing of hands frequently.
- Promptly report any signs of infection. These include a burning sensation and irritation at the meatus, cloudy urine, a strong odor to the urine, an elevated temperature, and chills.
- Help keep the urine acid in character, since acidity retards bacterial growth. Plain water in increased amounts, cranberry juice, prune juice, and ascorbic acid are helpful in acidifying urine. Regular use of cranberry juice cocktail reduced the bacterial and white blood cell count in a population of older women (Avorn et al., 1994).
- Help the client take a tub or shower bath when permitted. The catheter should be clamped temporarily if the collecting container is higher than the bladder at any time. In a tub, with the catheter clamped, the container can be hung over the side of the tub. Care should be taken so that the catheter does not remain clamped after the bath. In a shower, the container can be attached to the client's leg, in which case clamping the tube usually is unnecessary.
- Plan to change indwelling catheters only as necessary. If rolling the drainage tubing between the hands frees the tubing of sandy particles, it is time to change the catheter. The usual interval between catheter changes varies from 5 days to 2 weeks. The less often a catheter is changed, the less the likelihood that an infection will develop.

Home Healthcare Alert

When a client at home has an indwelling catheter, it is important that the client and caregivers know the signs and symptoms of infection, follow aseptic technique, and be aware that prompt treatment is essential.

Teaching the Client

Clients who have indwelling catheters should be taught how the system functions and how they can assist with their care. Teaching points include keeping the tubing free of kinks, maintaining a constant downward flow of

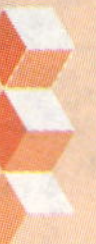

Helpscan

The following are resources for clients and health-care professionals:

- For information on incontinence and bladder training programs:
  Alliance for Aging Research
  2021 K Street, N.W., Suite 305
  Washington, DC 20006
  (202) 293-2856
- For information that can be used to educate the public about urinary incontinence:
  HIP, Help for Incontinent People
  P.O. Box 544
  Union, SC 29379
  (800) BLADDER
- For information from a support group for incontinence:
  The Simon Foundation for Continence
  P.O. Box 835
  Wilmette, IL 60091
  (800) 23-SIMON (for patient information)
  (708) 864-3913 (for professional information)

the urine, maintaining an adequate fluid intake, and promptly reporting any unusual symptoms.

Removing the Indwelling Catheter. The removal of an indwelling catheter and the aftercare of the client should include the following nursing measures:

- Don disposable gloves.
- *Be sure the balloon is deflated before attempting to remove the catheter.* This is done by inserting a syringe into the balloon valve and aspirating the fluid initially used to inflate the balloon. Carefully check the size of the balloon so you know how much fluid to remove before proceeding. Do *not* cut the tubing with scissors.
- Have the client take several deep breaths to relax while gently removing the catheter. Wrap the catheter in a towel or disposable, waterproof drape.
- Clean the perineal area after the catheter is removed.
- See to it that the client's fluid intake is generous, and record the client's intake as well as time and amount of output for at least 24 hours or according to agency policy. Instruct the client to void into the bedpan or urinal.
- Inform the client that it may take a little while for the bladder to reestablish voluntary control and that an accident is not unusual.
- Tell the client that there may be a slight burning sensation the first time or two the client voids after the catheter is removed.
- Observe the urine carefully for any abnormalities.
- Record and report any unusual signs, such as discomfort, a burning sensation when voiding, bleeding, and changes in vital signs, especially the client's temperature. Be alert to any signs of infection, and report them *promptly*.

Teaching Self-Catheterization

Medical asepsis practices are used by clients who self-catheterize. There is less danger of nosocomial urinary tract infection when the procedure is done at home rather than in a hospital. Research has shown that the technique is safe. The procedure for self-catheterization is essentially the same as that used by the nurse to catheterize a client. The following are some differences, which should be emphasized when teaching self-catheterization:

- The client voids first and then inserts the catheter for residual urine.
- The male client uses a comfortable position in bed or a sitting or standing position. The female client may sit on a toilet or lie in bed in a comfortable position.
- A good light is important, especially for the female client.
- The female client can locate the meatus with the use of a mirror but should learn to insert the catheter using the touch technique. She more easily locates the urinary meatus by developing an awareness of the different sensations when the clitoris, urinary meatus, and vagina are touched. The fingers on the nondominant hand locate the meatus by placing the index finger on the clitoris and the third and fourth fingers at the vagina.
- The client should press down with the abdominal muscles to remove as much urine from the bladder as possible before removing the catheter.
- The interval between catheterizations will vary. At first, catheterization may be necessary every 2 to 3

hours, but the interval can gradually be increased. According to Webber-Jones (1991), an oral intake greater than 2 qt (about 2000 mL) daily and catheterized amounts greater than 450 mL (about 1 pint) usually indicate the need to catheterize five times a day.
- The client must wash reusable plastic equipment well in soap or detergent and water, and rinse, dry, and store it in a clean, covered container.
- A minimum of 1500 mL (1.6 quart) of fluid a day is recommended for adults.

Applying a Condom Catheter

When voluntary control of urination is not possible for male clients, an alternative to an indwelling catheter is the **condom catheter**. This soft, pliable device made of plastic or rubberized material is applied externally to the penis. It is connected to tubing and a leg bag during the day and a drainage bag at night, and thus allows the client to be dressed and to participate in activities without problem. Instructions for applying a condom catheter are given in Procedure 43-6.

Nursing care includes vigilant skin care to prevent excoriation. The condom should be removed daily and the penis washed with soap and water, carefully dried, and inspected for irritation. The manufacturer's instructions for applying the condom should be followed because there are several variations. In all cases, care must be taken to fasten the condom securely enough to prevent leakage, yet not so tightly as to constrict the blood vessels in the area. Self-adhesive condom catheters are now available. The tip of the tubing should be kept 2.5 to 5 cm (1–2 in) beyond the tip of the penis to prevent irritation to the sensitive glans. Maintaining free urinary drainage is another nursing priority because tubing may become kinked. To prevent urine from excoriating the glans, the tubing that collects urine from the condom should be positioned to draw urine away from the penis.

Assisting With Urinary Diversions

Obstructions or tumors in the urinary tract may require some clients to have the urinary flow diverted surgically. An **ileal conduit** is a surgical diversion of the ureters to the ileum rather than the bladder. This separated section of the small intestine is then brought to the abdominal wall, where urine is excreted through a stoma or artificial opening on the body surface created surgically. Figure 43-9 shows how the ureters are diverted in an ileal conduit. Other types of surgery for urinary diversion also are performed, and except for the location of the stoma, the nursing care is similar. Such diversions usually are permanent, and the client wears an external appliance to collect the urine since voluntary control over elimination of the urine from the stoma is not possible.

The client who has an ileal conduit must adapt to an altered body image and usually needs assistance in coping. The time required for adaptation varies, and the adjustment often can be promoted by numerous sources of support, such as family, friends, nurses, physicians, and people with a similar health problem. Most of all, the client needs to understand that an active, useful life is compatible with a urinary diversion.

Appliances to Collect Urine. Typically, the external appliance is a soft rubber or plastic pouch that is either reusable or disposable. The upper part of the pouch has a firm faceplate several inches in diameter that has an opening the size of the stoma. Some faceplates are detachable from the pouch. The plate surface is firmly secured around the stoma opening with a moisture-proof adherent so that no urine leakage can occur. Many clients also use an elasticized belt worn around the waist for added support. The lower end of the pouch may have a drainage valve, which is used for emptying the pouch.

The pouch should be emptied before it becomes heavy with the weight of urine and causes the seal to loosen. For most people, this means emptying the appliance several times a day. Urine-collection receptacles designed to be placed under the bed are available for attachment to the appliance at night.

Changing the Urinary Appliance. The frequency of changing the appliance varies with the type being used. The appliance should be changed after a time of low fluid intake, such as early morning. Urine production will be less at this time, which makes changing the appliance easier. Procedure 43-7 describes how to change an appliance worn over an ileal conduit.

Teaching the Client. Nursing care is directed toward client education and the achievement of optimal self-care. As responsibility for self-care is assumed, the client should be taught to make the necessary observations, to be aware of indications of problems, and to recognize when to seek assistance. For these goals to be met, the client needs to be able to do the following:
- Explain the cause for the urinary diversion and the rationale for treatment
- Demonstrate self-care behaviors that effectively manage the diversion
- Describe follow-up care and existing support resources
- Report where supplies may be obtained in the community
- Verbalize related fears and concerns
- Demonstrate positive body image

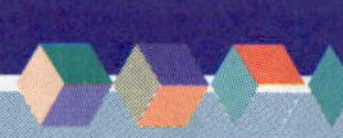

PROCEDURE 43-6

Applying a Condom Catheter

Equipment

Condom sheath in appropriate size
Basin of warm water and soap
Washcloth and towel
Bath blanket
Disposable gloves (optional)
Elastic strip or Velcro strap (optional)
Reusable leg bag with drainage tubing or urinary drainage setup

Action	Rationale
1. Explain the procedure to the client. Ask if the client is aware of any allergy to latex.	This provides reassurance and promotes client cooperation. If the client is allergic to latex, a latex-free condom catheter must be used.
2. Assemble the equipment. Prepare urinary drainage setup or reusable leg bag for attachment to the condom sheath.	This provides for an organized approach to the task.
3. Wash your hands.	Handwashing deters the spread of microorganisms.
4. Assist the client to the supine position. Close the curtain or door. Use the bath blanket and sheet to expose only the client's genital area.	This provides privacy for the client.
5. Don disposable gloves. Wash the genital area with soap and water, rinse, and dry thoroughly.	Washing removes urine, secretions, and microorganisms. The penis must be clean and dry to minimize skin irritation.
6. Roll the condom sheath outward onto itself. Grasp the penis firmly with your nondominant hand. Apply the condom sheath by rolling it onto the penis with your dominant hand. Leave 2.5- to 5-cm (1 to 2-inch) space between the tip of the penis and the end of the condom sheath.	Rolling the condom sheath outward allows for easier application. The space prevents irritation to the tip of the penis and allows for free drainage of urine.
7. Apply the elastic or Velcro strap in a snug but not tight manner. Do not allow the elastic or Velcro to come in contact with the skin.	The elastic or Velcro strap should secure the condom sheath but not interfere with blood circulation to the penis.

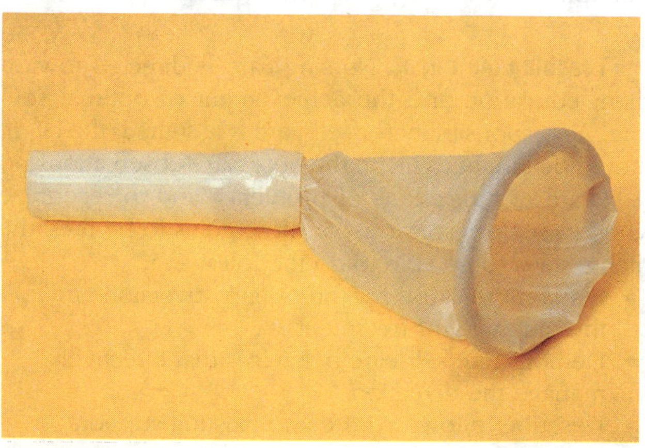

Condom sheath.

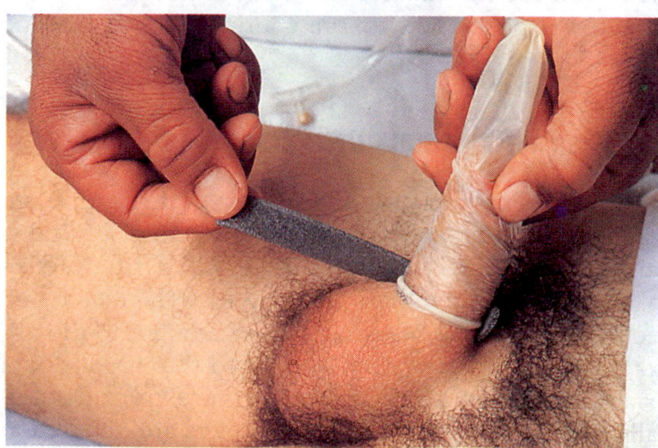

Action 7: Application of a Velcro strap at the base of the condom sheath.

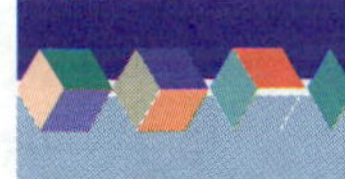

PROCEDURE 43-6 *(continued)*

Applying a Condom Catheter

Action	Rationale
8. Connect the condom sheath to the drainage setup. Avoid kinking or twisting of the drainage tubing.	The collection device keeps the client dry. Kinked tubing encourages backflow of urine.

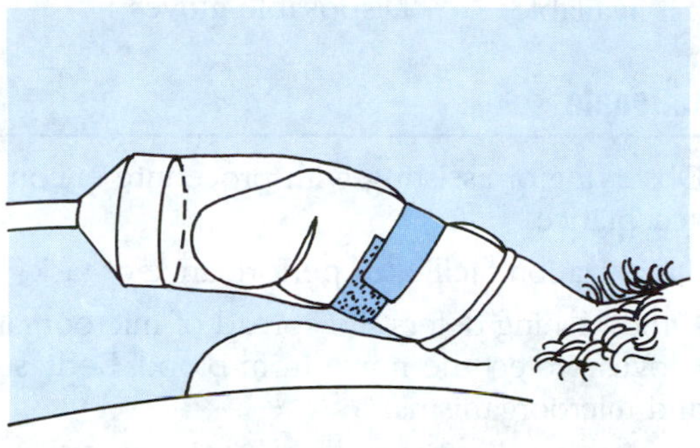

Action 8: Drawing of extra space at end of sheath and smoothing tubing to drainage unit.

Action	Rationale
9. Remove the equipment. Place the client in a comfortable, safe position. Wash your hands.	This provides a safe, comfortable setting for the client. Handwashing deters the spread of microorganisms.
10. Assess the client's response and record observations on the client's chart.	This provides accurate documentation and observation of urine output.

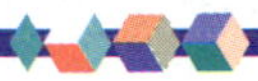

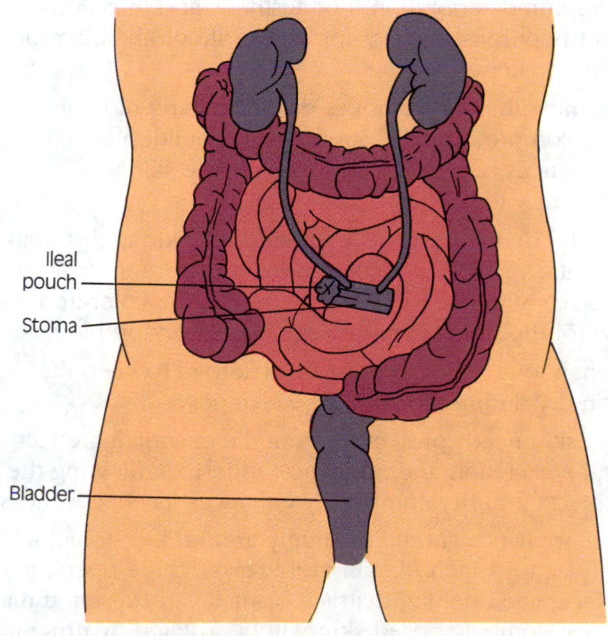

Figure 43-9
Location of an ileal conduit. The ureters are brought to the ileum of the small intestine and a stoma is made where the urine is excreted. (Redrawn after Types of Ostomies. Copyright 1979. Hollister Inc. All rights reserved.)

The assistance of an enterostomal therapist can be invaluable in helping the client to achieve these outcomes. The client may be referred to the United Ostomy Association for further information and helpful periodicals. Detailed discussion of other aspects of caring for a client with a urinary diversion can be found in clinical texts.

EVALUATING

The nurse evaluates the effectiveness of a plan of care to promote healthy urinary functioning by checking whether the client has met the individualized client goals specified in the plan. Nursing care is considered effective if the client expresses satisfaction with the regular voiding pattern and is able to:

- Produce a sufficient quantity of urine to maintain fluid, electrolyte, and acid–base balance
- Empty the bladder completely at regular intervals without discomfort
- Develop a plan to modify any factors that contribute to current urinary problems or that might adversely affect urinary functioning in the future
- Correct unhealthy urinary habits, such as delaying voiding, drinking insufficient water, and abusing diuretics

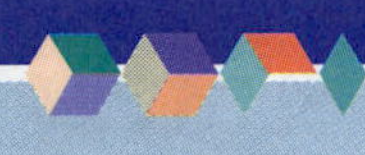

PROCEDURE 43-7

Changing a Stoma Appliance on an Ileal Conduit

Equipment

Basin with warm water, soap, towel, washcloth or cotton balls
Graduated container
Skin protectant or barrier
Sterile 2 × 2 gauze squares
Ostomy bag cut to the correct stomal size (with adhesive-backed faceplate, if available)
Ostomy belt (optional)
Adhesive cement (optional for reusable pouches)
Disposable gloves

Action	Rationale
1. Explain the procedure and encourage the client to observe or participate if possible. Provide for privacy.	Observing or assisting with procedure encourages self-acceptance.
2. Assemble the equipment.	Organization facilitates performance of task.
3. Wash your hands and don disposable gloves.	Handwashing deters the spread of microorganisms. Gloves protect the nurse from blood, body substances, and microorganisms.
4. Have the client sit or stand if able to assist with procedure or assume supine position in bed.	These positions result in less abdominal folds and facilitate removal and application of the device.
5. Empty the pouch being worn into the graduated container (before removing if it is reusable and not attached to straight drainage).	Having the pouch empty before handling it reduces the likelihood of spilling the excretions. The physician may have ordered recording of intake and output.
6. Gently remove the pouch faceplate from the skin.	The seal between the surface of the faceplate and the skin must be broken before the faceplate can be removed. Harsh handling of the appliance can damage the skin and impair the development of a secure seal in the future.
7. Discard the pouch appropriately if disposable, or wash reusable pouch in lukewarm soap and water and allow to air dry.	Thorough cleaning and airing of the appliance reduce odor and deterioration. For aesthetic and infection-control purposes, used appliances should be discarded appropriately.
8. Clean the skin around the stoma with soap and water or a commercial cleaner using washcloth or cotton balls. Make sure you remove all of old adhesive from the skin.	Cleaning the skin removes excretions and old adhesive and skin protectant. Excretions or a buildup of other substances can irritate and damage the skin.
9. Gently pat dry. Make sure the skin around the stoma is thoroughly dry. Assess the stoma and the condition of the surrounding skin.	Careful drying prevents trauma to the skin and stoma. An intact, properly applied urinary collection device protects skin integrity. Any change in the color and size of the stoma may indicate circulatory problems.
10. Place a gauze square or two over the stoma opening.	Continuous drainage must be absorbed to keep the skin dry during the appliance change.
11. Apply a skin protectant to a 5-cm (2-in) radius around the stoma, and allow it to dry completely, which takes about 30 seconds.	The skin needs protection from the excoriating effect of the excretion and appliance adhesive. Allowing the protectant to dry completely enhances its effectiveness.
12. If necessary, enlarge the size of the faceplate opening to fit the stoma.	The appliance should fit snugly around the stoma, with only $\frac{1}{16}$ to $\frac{1}{8}$ inch of skin visible around the opening. A faceplate opening that is too small can cause trauma to the stoma. Exposed skin will be irritated by urine if the opening is too large.

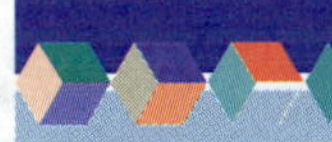

PROCEDURE 43-7 *(continued)*

Changing a Stoma Appliance on an Ileal Conduit

Action	Rationale
13. Apply adhesive to the faceplate or remove the protective covering from the disposable faceplate, carefully position the appliance, and press it in place, moving from the center outward. Remove the gauze squares from the stoma before applying the pouch.	The appliance is effective only if it is properly positioned and securely adhered. Commercial deodorants may be used if odor is a problem.
14. Secure the optional belt to the appliance and around the client.	An elasticized belt helps support the appliance for some people.
15. Remove or discard the equipment and assess the client's response to the procedure. Wash your hands and remove gloves.	The client's response may indicate acceptance of the ostomy as well as the need for health teaching. Handwashing deters the spread of microorganisms.
16. Record the appearance of the stoma and the surrounding skin as well as the client's reaction to the procedure.	A careful record is important for planning the client's care.

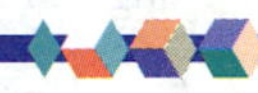

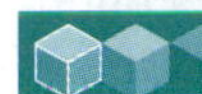

Nursing Process in Clinical Practice

After a urinary problem is detected, the nurse implements each phase of the nursing process to ensure correct identification and treatment of the problem. To identify and manage the urinary problem correctly, the nurse must possess the knowledge and clinical skills described earlier in this chapter. Following in outline format are the focused assessment priorities, expected outcomes, and nursing interventions for common nursing diagnoses.

Altered Urinary Elimination related to dysuria
Altered Urinary Elimination related to maturational enuresis
Urinary Retention related to varying causes
Risk for Infection related to indwelling catheter

Altered Urinary Elimination Related to Dysuria

> The state in which the individual experiences or is at risk of experiencing a disturbance in urine elimination (NANDA, 1994)

Dysuria, or difficult urination, is most often associated with a sensation of pain or burning. Clients report feeling the need to void but having great difficulty and pain in starting the stream. Common in women, dysuria is associated with lower urinary tract infections and irritation of the urethral meatus after sexual intercourse or caused by use of bath and feminine hygiene products.

Assessment Priorities

- Interview the client for report of painful or burning sensation while voiding and presence of fever, chills, nausea, or flank pain.
- Identify potential causative factors:
  - Infection
  - Sexual activity 1 to 2 days before symptoms
  - Liquid detergent or bubble bath in bath water
- Examine urine for cloudiness, foul odor, hematuria, and proteinuria.

Expected Outcomes

The client will:

- Report absence of pain and burning during urination
- Describe appropriate self-care measures to prevent recurrence

Interventions

- Instruct the client about the probable cause of the dysuria, and reassure the client that the distressing symptoms will be relieved with treatment.
- Teach perineal care to include wiping from front to back after voiding and the need to clean the perianal region with soap and water after defecation and intercourse. Female clients also should be instructed to void before and after intercourse to

flush the lower urinary tract of bacteria. Because the urethra in the female is short and close to the vagina and anus, bacteria from these areas can easily migrate to the urethral meatus and ascend the urinary tract.

- Encourage a fluid intake of 2000 to 3000 mL to dilute infected urine and flush the system.
- If indicated, assist the client to alter urinary pH by dietary manipulation. Large quantities of water and cranberry juice may acidify the urine and be helpful in reducing bacterial growth. If urine alkalization is warranted to soothe an irritated bladder, eating more vegetables and fruits may be helpful.
- Sitz baths promote relaxation of tense muscles and facilitate healing of an irritated urethral meatus.
- Administer prescribed medications to treat the pathology underlying dysuria.

Altered Urinary Elimination Related to Maturational Enuresis

The state in which a child experiences involuntary voiding during sleep which is not pathophysiologic in origin (Carpenito, 1995)

Enuresis is involuntary urination after an age when continence should be present. *Nocturnal enuresis* is bed wetting that occurs while a person is sleeping, and *diurnal enuresis* occurs when a person is awake. In *primary enuresis*, the child has never had a long period of dryness; in *secondary enuresis*, the pattern of bed wetting follows a period of dryness of weeks or months. An identifiable stress, such as the birth of a sibling or parental divorce, often precedes the onset of secondary enuresis. It is helpful for parents to understand that enuresis is primarily a maturational problem that usually ceases between ages 6 and 8.

Assessment Priorities

- Interview the child and parents to determine:
  - Pattern of bed wetting and precipitating factors (if present)
  - Response of family members to the child
  - History of toilet training
  - Familial history of enuresis
- Assess bladder capacity by measuring voided specimen after the child has been instructed to delay voiding as long as possible. Use at least three recordings. Small bladder capacity is less than 300 mL.

Expected Outcomes

- Child will develop day and nighttime control over urination
- Parents will respond constructively to child

Interventions

- Instruct the parents that enuresis usually is a maturational problem that the child will outgrow with assistance, and that punishing or shaming the child can have harmful effects.
- Share with the child that many other children bed-wet and that this problem will be outgrown.
- If both the parents and the child are motivated, use responsibility and reinforcement therapy. The child can keep a calendar of dry days and nights and contract for rewards.
- If the child has a small bladder capacity, encourage daytime bladder-stretching by helping the child to postpone voiding after drinking fluids.
- If the child is a sound sleeper, limit fluids at bedtime and have the child void immediately before retiring.
- If the child gets too absorbed in daytime play to respond to a full bladder, teach the child how to sense a full bladder and the importance of stopping to void. Reinforce dry days.
- Explore with the family various laundry aids.
- Assist the family to evaluate the pros and cons of a conditioning therapy that involves an alarm system, as well as other therapies.

Urinary Retention Related to Varying Etiologies

The state in which an individual experiences incomplete emptying of the bladder (NANDA, 1994)

Retention occurs when urine is produced normally but not excreted from the bladder. The bladder continues to fill, and may distend to hold 3000 to 4000 mL of urine. In adults, the micturition reflex normally is triggered when the bladder holds 250 to 450 mL of urine. Retention is suspected when clients report:

- Difficulty voiding despite urge to void
- Frequent small voidings (less than 50 mL)
- Discomfort in the pubic area
- Urine output that is much less than fluid intake

Palpation and percussion above the symphysis pubis are used to assess bladder distention. The abdomen swells as the bladder rises above the level of the symphysis pubis. The height of the bladder can be determined by palpating with light pressure on the abdomen. Physicians may order a client catheterized for residual urine to determine if urine is being retained in the bladder after voiding. All but 1 to 3 mL of urine normally is excreted from the bladder with each voiding. The client is catheterized after voiding, and both the amount of urine voided and that collected by catheterization are recorded.

Retention often is temporary, commonly after surgery that involves the lower abdomen, pelvis, bladder, or urethra, especially if ambulation is delayed or fluid intake is minimal. Any mechanical obstruction, such as swelling at the meatus, which often occurs after childbirth, or an enlarged prostate in men, may cause retention. The underlying cause of urinary retention for men is likely to be an enlarged prostate gland; there is no clear etiology for women (Williams, Wallhagen, &

Dowling, 1993). The cause also may be psychic or due to certain disease conditions. Injuries to the spinal cord may cause permanent retention. Urine that pools in the bladder predisposes the client to urinary tract infection.

Assessment Priorities

- Establish strict fluid intake and output and record time and amount of voidings.
- Note complaints of pain in the pubic area, swelling, urgency, frequency, dysuria.
- Palpate and percuss above the symphysis pubis.
- Catheterize for residual urine if indicated (ordered).

Expected Outcomes

The client will:

- Verbalize the importance of emptying the bladder as soon as possible
- Empty the bladder completely as evidenced by:
  - Quantity of urine voided (24-hour output about equal to fluid intake)
  - Normal pattern of voiding reestablished (each voiding more than 50 mL)
  - Flattened pubic area
  - Absence of complaints
- Demonstrate no signs of urinary tract infection

Interventions

- Use nursing measures to stimulate micturition:
  - Provide privacy.
  - Help client to assume natural position.
  - Offer warm fluids to drink.
  - Warm the bedpan.
  - Run tap water within client's hearing.
  - Pour warm water over the perineal area.
  - Place client's hands in warm water.
  - Manually press on the client's abdomen.
- Administer prescribed analgesics, if appropriate, to promote comfort.
- If independent nursing measures fail to produce bladder emptying, contact a physician.
- If prescribed, administer bethanechol chloride (Urecholine), a parasympathomimetic agent that stimulates micturition.
- Catheterization may be ordered. Nursing measures should be exhausted before resorting to catheterizing clients with retention because of the danger of urinary tract infection.

Risk for Infection Related to Indwelling Catheter

The state in which an individual is at increased risk for being invaded by pathogenic organisms (NANDA, 1994)

Urinary tract infections are second only to respiratory tract infections in frequency of occurrence. Of special importance to nurses is that urinary tract infections account for 50% of hospital-acquired (nosocomial) infections and urinary catheters have been implicated in 80% of these urinary tract infections (Pinkerman, 1994).

Catheterization predisposes to urinary tract infection for the following reasons:

- The introduction of the catheter through the urethra provides a direct route for microorganisms to travel up the urinary tract to the bladder.
- Catheter-induced local irritation to the urethra or bladder predisposes to infection.
- The catheter interferes with the most important defense against bacterial urinary tract infection, the unobstructed flow of urine throughout the urinary tract and regular, complete evacuation of the bladder.
- Clients who require catheterization often have diseases or other conditions that interfere with the body's immune system, thereby decreasing the efficiency of the urinary tract's reaction to bacteriuria.

In summary, clients being catheterized are a highly vulnerable population and demand vigilant nursing care to prevent urinary tract infection. Breaks in aseptic technique may result in serious and even fatal consequences.

Assessment Priorities

- Note client complaints of frequency, urgency, dysuria, and nocturia.
- Palpate the suprapubic area for tenderness.
- Urinalysis: Urine may be dark yellow or pinkish red, and cloudy with or without sediment, bacteriuria, and hematuria.
- Urine culture and sensitivity: More than 100,000/mL bacterial colonies; sensitivity disks indicate bacterial sensitivity, intermediate sensitivity, or resistance to a given antibiotic agent.
- With worsening urinary tract infections, fever, chills, nausea, vomiting, and malaise may be present.
- Note that about half of clients with significant bacteriuria are asymptomatic. This is especially true for older clients.

Expected Outcomes

The client will:

- Have a negative urine culture
- Demonstrate no signs of urinary tract infection

Interventions

Prevention

- Force fluids to 2500 to 3000 mL/day.
- Teach client appropriate hygiene (careful cleaning of perineal area after each voiding and bowel movement; wiping front to back).
- Observe urine for color, odor, amount, and frequency.
- Use strict asepsis with catheter insertion and maintenance unless clean technique is indicated. (Intermittent clean catheterization is recommended for long-term maintenance at home when a catheter is required for bladder emptying. The

reduced number and types of bacteria present in the home environment decrease the likelihood of nosocomial infection.)

Treatment

- Obtain urine for urinalysis and for urine culture and sensitivity.
- Administer antimicrobial medication as ordered. Encourage client to continue medication for the entire period prescribed (usually 10 days).
- Ensure adequate hydration by oral or intravenous route.
- Monitor intake and output.
- Maintain thorough perineal hygiene.

Client Care Study

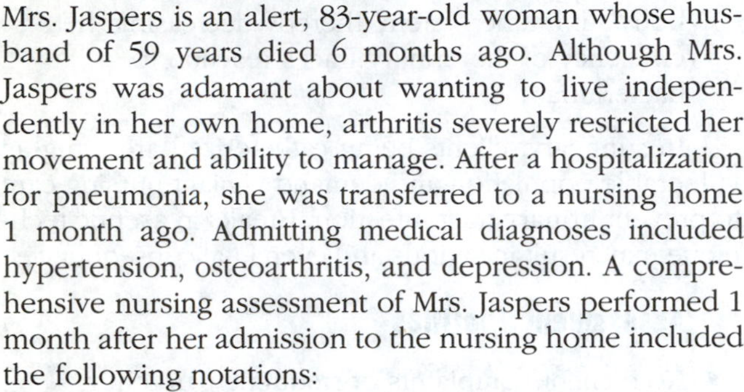

Mrs. Jaspers is an alert, 83-year-old woman whose husband of 59 years died 6 months ago. Although Mrs. Jaspers was adamant about wanting to live independently in her own home, arthritis severely restricted her movement and ability to manage. After a hospitalization for pneumonia, she was transferred to a nursing home 1 month ago. Admitting medical diagnoses included hypertension, osteoarthritis, and depression. A comprehensive nursing assessment of Mrs. Jaspers performed 1 month after her admission to the nursing home included the following notations:

- Continent of urine on admission
- At present, incontinent of urine one or two times a day; often found wet in the morning; states it is "too much bother to get into the bathroom"
- Sits in chair in room unless encouraged and assisted to walk, although capable of independent ambulation with care; progressive muscle atrophy and joint stiffness
- No identifiable pathology underlying incontinence
- Medications include a diuretic for hypertension and a tricyclic antidepressant
- Reddened skin in the perineal area

Essential Nursing Skills

In order to implement this plan of care, the nurse needs the following specialized abilities:

Cognitive Skills: Critical Thinking

- Knowledge of pathologic and nonpathologic basis for urinary incontinence and successful treatment strategies
- Teaching skills to empower Mrs. Jaspers to value and reestablish urinary continence
- Ability to develop nursing diagnoses that reflect Mrs. Jaspers' unique urinary elimination problems
- Conviction that nursing can make a difference in the quality of Mrs. Jaspers' present life
- Knowledge of behavioral techniques that have potential to decrease the frequency of Mrs. Jaspers' urinary incontinence

Technical Skills

- Strong assessment skills (interviewing and physical assessment) to carefully identify the problem and its cause
- Caregiver skills directed toward maintaining urinary continence for Mrs. Jaspers and providing positive reinforcement for effort and progress

Interpersonal Skills

- Interpersonal skills to communicate to Mrs. Jaspers empathy for her situation and the hope that with help, better outcomes are a real possibility
- Interpersonal and leadership skills to motivate the nursing staff to help Mrs. Jaspers reestablish urinary continence
- Ability to establish a trusting nurse–client relationship grounded in responsible caring

Ethical/Legal Skills

- Accountability and willingness to use competence to help Mrs. Jaspers regain maximal control of urinary elimination
- Competence in documenting nursing interventions
- Ability to serve as a trusted and effective client advocate

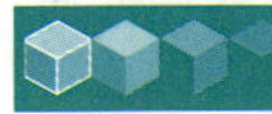

Nursing Plan of Care

for Mrs. Jaspers

Nursing Diagnosis: **Functional Incontinence related to difficult transition to nursing home and mobility deficit as manifested by incontinence of urine one or two times a day; feeling toileting is too much bother; mobility deficits secondary to osteoarthritis; taking a diuretic and antidepressant.**

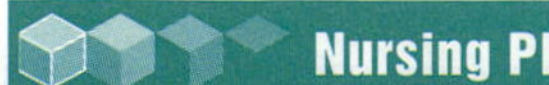

Nursing Plan of Care

for Mrs. Jaspers

Expected Outcome: By the next monthly assessment, 5/1/98, the client will:

- Verbalize the importance of getting to bathroom or toilet when she first feels the need to void.

Nursing Interventions	Rationale	Evaluative Statement
Assess the value the client attaches to voluntary control of urination and urinary continence; counsel appropriately.	Unless the client is committed to the plan of care, goal achievement is impossible.	5/1/98 Goal partially met. Client has commented on the importance of regular toileting but still finds this "too much trouble" some days. *Revision:* Reinforce value. *D. Mora, RN*
Teach the importance of complete bladder emptying at regular intervals and the harmful effects of ignoring the urge to void.	Client understanding of the causes and harmful effects of urinary incontinence may motivate desire for reestablishment of voluntary control.	
Assess client's normal voiding habits at home and assist her to reestablish these. Initial reminders to toilet herself may be necessary.	Respect for the client's normal voiding schedule and patterns communicates nursing's sincere concern for the individual and encourages client achievement of goals.	

Expected Outcome: By the next monthly assessment, 5/1/98, the client will:

- Demonstrate the ability to walk independently to the bathroom (using cane) to toilet herself.

Nursing Interventions	Rationale	Evaluative Statement
Assess the client's ability to toilet herself independently. Work consistently with her to increase activity tolerance: encourage short walks throughout the day to increase mobility.	One response to experiencing the multiple losses associated with aging is to surrender all control and become increasingly dependent. Non-pathology-based incontinence is less likely to occur if the daily living of the person keeps her more mobile, flexible, oriented, and motivated. An older person who seeks to take control and has a positive self-image is more continent.	5/1/98 Goal met. Client can safely walk to bathroom using cane and toilet herself when she wants to. *D. Mora, RN*
Refer client to occupational therapy for assistance with diagnosis and treatment if necessary.	The specialized skills of the occupational therapist may facilitate relearning toileting skills.	
Communicate clearly that the client is expected to use the toilet to urinate. Refrain from using incontinent briefs or pads. Talk with family about client's having sufficient undergarments to allow changes as needed until control is reestablished.	Understanding that the staff *expects* continence and is committed to working with the client to achieve it is a powerful client motivator.	

Expected Outcome: By the next monthly assessment, 5/1/98, the client will:

- Demonstrate satisfactory perineal hygiene

(continued)

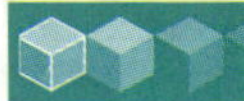

Nursing Plan of Care *(continued)*

for Mrs. Jaspers

Nursing Interventions	Rationale	Evaluative Statement
Assess client's motivation and ability to be clean, dry, and comfortable.	Client may not understand how easily skin irritation can occur and danger of pressure ulcers.	5/1/98 Goal not met. Client repeatedly neglects AM perineal care.
Teach perineal hygiene.	Keeping the perineal area clean and dry promotes intact skin around the urinary meatus and the perineal area. Proper hygiene measures also decrease the possibility of bacteria or organisms migrating into the bladder.	*Revision:* Reteach both the importance and procedure of perineal care. Assess each AM. *D. Mora, RN*

Expected Outcome: By the next monthly assessment, 5/1/98, the client will:

- Decrease urinary incontinent episodes to less than three or four per week

Nursing Interventions	Rationale	Evaluative Statement
Communicate to client that the nurses *care* about her reestablishing urinary continence and believe she can do this. Use verbal reinforcement to reward "dry" days.	A common feeling of recently institutionalized elderly people is *abandonment* and the sense that no one cares; response: "Why should I?" Communicating that the client's progress toward goal achievement is valued by the nurses is an excellent encouragement to continue progress.	5/1/98 Goal met. Client in last week was completely dry for 4 of 7 days. Recorded four incontinent episodes. *D. Mora, RN*
Chart incontinent episodes and monitor progress; discuss this with client.	This records progress with incontinent episodes and provides positive reinforcement.	

Nursing Diagnosis: Impaired Skin Integrity related to functional incontinence as manifested by reddened perineal area (skin still intact)

Expected Outcome: By next monthly assessment, 5/1/98, the client will:

- Demonstrate healing of reddened perineal area

Nursing Interventions	Rationale	Evaluative Statement
Assess skin for breakdown each AM and PM and after each incontinent episode.	Perineal care is often neglected or assigned to the least trained personnel in care settings. Skin irritation not detected and treated early may progress to serious pressure ulcers.	5/1/98 Goal partially met. Perineal area is less inflamed. *Revision:* Continue to monitor perineal hygiene. No need for protective ointment. *D. Mora, RN*
Teach the client the importance of washing this area carefully with soap and water each AM and after incontinent episodes. Teach the importance of always cleaning and wiping the perineum from front to back to prevent autoinfection. Until incontinent episodes are eliminated, a protective waterproof ointment may be indicated.	The woman who is doing self-care may neglect it entirely or use incorrect technique.	

(continued)

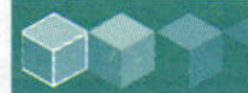

Nursing Plan of Care *(continued)*

for Mrs. Jaspers

Nursing Interventions	Rationale	Evaluative Statement
Cotton underwear should be worn. Nylon pantyhose, girdles, tight-fitting pants should be avoided.	Nylon products tend to hold moisture and may minimize airflow to the perineal area.	

Sample Documentation: 4/3/98, Nursing

This AM, after an incontinent episode, Mrs. Jaspers began to talk about how hard it is to get adjusted to living here, and commented, "I feel like just giving up." We talked about the importance of being as independent as possible and the dangers of becoming passively dependent. Nursing teaching and counseling included values of independently adhering to usual toileting schedule and importance of perineal hygiene. Two hours later, after lunch, Mrs. Jaspers walked to bathroom and toileted herself. Progress with urinary incontinence will continue to be monitored. Ability definitely present but encouragement needed.

D. Mora, RN

Key Points

- Urinary elimination, a natural process in which the body excretes waste products and material that exceed bodily needs, usually is taken for granted. When urinary problems arise, the nurse realizes that many clients consider urination a private act and may become embarrassed when they need to discuss urination or require assistance with elimination. The nurse implements nursing interventions accordingly.
- Healthy urinary elimination presupposes well-functioning kidneys, ureters, urinary bladder, and urethra. Problems in any of these areas can affect both the amount and the quality of the urine formed and the manner in which it is expelled from the body.
- Other factors that affect urination include growth and development, food and fluid intake, lifestyle variables, psychologic variables, activity and muscle tone, pathologic conditions, and medications.
- A comprehensive assessment of the urinary system includes the collection of data about voiding patterns and urinary problems and the physical assessment of the kidneys, bladder, urethral meatus, skin integrity, and urine. These findings may need to be correlated with the results of diagnostic tests and procedures for examining urine and the urinary tract.
- Identification of client health problems often is aided by the nurse's careful monitoring of fluid intake and output, collection of urine specimens, and testing of urine specimens for abnormalities.
- Nursing diagnoses may be written specifically addressing problems in urinary functioning (incontinence, pattern alteration, and retention) and identifying the effect urinary problems have on other areas of human functioning (eg, anxiety, comfort, skin integrity).
- Nursing attention to the client's usual voiding schedule, need for privacy, natural position while voiding, and hygiene habits will help ensure the client's comfort and satisfactory urine output. Other measures facilitating normal urination include promoting an optimal fluid intake, strengthening tone in the perineal and abdominal muscles, and using specific measures (eg, running tap water) to initiate voiding.
- The client with cognitive, sensory, motor, neurologic, or endurance deficits may need nursing assistance with the toilet, bedpan, commode, or urinal. Family members also may need to be taught how to assist the client with elimination needs.
- Urinary catheterization may be indicated to relieve urinary retention, obtain select urine specimens, measure residual urine, or empty the bladder before and during surgery and before certain diagnostic procedures. Catheterization is consid-

ered the most prominent cause of nosocomial infections, and should be avoided whenever possible.

- Obstructions or tumors in the urinary tract may require some people to have the urinary flow diverted surgically. In the ileal conduit, the ureters are connected to the ileum, and a stoma is created on the abdominal wall. Nursing care is directed toward client education and the achievement of optimal self-care.

Study Questions

1. The nurse collects a urine specimen for routine urinalysis from a client. She is aware that
   a. a sterile specimen is required
   b. standing at room temperature for a prolonged period may alter the urine chemistry
   c. the external meatus should be cleaned with antiseptic soap and water before voiding
   d. a clean-catch midstream specimen is required
2. Which statement would be correct to teach the client in regard to healthy urinary functioning?
   a. Drinking more than 2000 mL of fluid per day will cause fluid retention.
   b. The healthy adult should drink four to six 8-oz glasses of water per day.
   c. Because of greater thirst sensitivity, children will drink required amounts of fluid without being reminded.
   d. Caffeine-containing beverages should be monitored to prevent excess intake.
3. When a person has a fever or diaphoresis, the urine output will be which of the following?
   a. decreased and highly concentrated
   b. decreased and highly dilute
   c. increased and concentrated
   d. increased and dilute
4. The physician has ordered an indwelling catheter inserted in a hospitalized male client. The nurse is aware that
   a. the male urethra is more vulnerable to injury during insertion
   b. normally a clean technique is required
   c. the catheter is inserted 2 to 3 inches into the meatus
   d. usually smaller catheters are necessary because of the size of the urethra
5. Nursing care for a client with an indwelling catheter includes
   a. irrigation of the catheter with 30 mL of normal saline solution every 4 hours
   b. disconnecting and reconnecting the drainage system quickly to obtain a urine specimen
   c. encouraging a generous fluid intake if permitted
   d. informing the client that burning and irritation at the meatus are normal and should subside within a few days
6. After surgery, Ms. Young is having difficulty voiding. Which nursing action will cause increased difficulty with voiding rather than stimulation of voiding?
   a. pouring warm water over Ms. Young's fingers
   b. having Ms. Young ignore the urge to void until her bladder is full
   c. using a warm bedpan when Ms. Young feels the urge to void
   d. stroking Ms. Young's leg or thigh
7. Mrs. Chang has a neurologic condition that requires her to do self-catheterization at home. The visiting nurse teaches her that
   a. she should limit fluids to decrease the amount of times necessary to self-catheterize.
   b. sterile technique is required to prevent a nosocomial infection.
   c. dorsal recumbent position should be used consistently.
   d. the plastic catheter should be washed thoroughly, dried, and stored for reuse.
8. The inability to void although the kidneys are producing urine and it enters the bladder is known as
   a. urgency
   b. retention
   c. oliguria
   d. dysuria
9. Mrs. D'Ambrosia, an alert, ambulatory, older nursing home resident, voids frequently and has difficulty making it to the bathroom on time. As the nurse plans her care, she is aware that
   a. incontinence is to be expected in a woman Mrs. D'Ambrosia's age.
   b. 1 of every 10 nursing home residents is incontinent.
   c. Kegel exercises at regular intervals throughout the day may be helpful.
   d. an indwelling catheter should be inserted as soon as possible.
10. The priority treatment option for Mrs. D'Ambrosia would most likely involve
    a. behavioral techniques
    b. pharmacologic measures
    c. surgical intervention
    d. use of absorbent products

11. A client taking Pyridium (a urinary tract analgesic) should be cautioned that her urine color may change to
    a. pale yellow
    b. green
    c. orange-red
    d. brown
12. Mr. Bales is 60 years old and alert. He is timid and reluctant to talk about his urinary retention problem. Which part of this plan could create stress for Mr. Bales and possibly increase his inability to urinate?
    a. assisting client in assuming his normal voiding position
    b. pulling curtains around client to provide privacy during voiding
    c. staying with client while voiding
    d. offering the urinal on a regular schedule
13. Which of the following is a nursing priority when caring for a male client with a condom catheter?
    a. preventing the tubing from kinking to maintain free urinary drainage
    b. not removing the catheter for any reason
    c. fastening the condom securely to prevent the possibility of leakage
    d. maintaining bed rest at all times to prevent the catheter from slipping off
14. If you read the nursing diagnosis, Altered Urinary Elimination related to maturational enuresis, you would recognize that your client is which of the following?
    a. an adult over age 65 who is incontinent
    b. a child over age 4 who has involuntary urination
    c. a 12-month-old child who has involuntary urination
    d. a client with neurologic damage resulting in bladder dysfunction
15. Data must be collected to evaluate the effectiveness of a plan to reduce urinary incontinence in the older adult client. Of the data below, which is least necessary for the evaluation process?
    a. the incontinence pattern
    b. state of physical mobility
    c. medications being taken
    d. age of the client

Answers With Rationale

1. The correct response is *b.* For a routine urinalysis, a clean specimen is adequate. The external meatus does not need to be cleaned with an antiseptic, as is required for a clean-catch midstream specimen.
2. The correct response is *d.* Caffeine intake should be limited because it is irritating to the bladder mucosa. It is recommended that a healthy adult drink 8 to 10 8-oz glasses of fluid daily. Unless a disease process is present, this will not cause fluid retention. Children frequently need to be reminded to drink fluids.
3. The correct response is *a.* Fever and diaphoresis cause the kidneys to conserve body fluids. Thus, the urine is concentrated and decreased in amount.
4. The correct response is *a.* Because of its length, the male urethra is more prone to injury and requires that the catheter be inserted 6 to 8 inches or until urine flows. This procedure requires surgical asepsis to prevent introducing bacteria into the urinary tract. Larger catheters are used for male catheterization.
5. The correct response is *c.* A generous fluid intake promotes healthy urinary tract functioning. Irrigation may introduce bacteria into the urinary tract and is not routinely ordered. The drainage system should never be disconnected to obtain a specimen, since this may provide the opportunity for bacteria to enter the urinary tract. Burning and irritation may indicate that an infection is present and should never be disregarded.
6. The correct response is *b.* Ignoring the urge to void makes urination even more difficult and should be avoided. The other activities are all recommended nursing activities to promote voiding.
7. The correct response is *d.* For self-catheterization at home, the catheter may be reused as long as it is cleaned and dried properly. Fluids should be encouraged, not limited, and clean technique and varied positions to insert the catheter are appropriate when the client is at home.
8. The correct response is *b.* Urgency is a strong desire to void. Oliguria is scanty or greatly diminished amount of urine voided in a given time. Dysuria is difficulty urinating.
9. The correct response is *c.* Kegel exercises may help a client regain better control of the micturition process. Incontinence is not a normal consequence of aging, and at least half of nursing home residents may be incontinent. An indwelling catheter is the last choice of treatment.
10. The correct response is *a.* The least invasive interventions should be attempted first. Pharmacologic and surgical interventions are not recommended until behavioral techniques have been attempted. Using absorbent products may remove motivation on the client's and caregiver's part to seek evaluation and treatment of the incontinence. They should be used only after careful evaluation by a healthcare provider.

11. The correct response is *c.* Pyridium is noted for turning the urine orange-red, and the client needs to be aware of this.
12. The correct response is *c.* Mr. Bales will be embarrassed if the nurse remains with him as he attempts to void and is more likely to have difficulty voiding.
13. The correct response is *a.* The catheter should be removed daily to prevent skin excoriation, and should not be fastened too tightly or restriction of blood vessels in the area is likely. Confining a client to bed rest increases the risk of other hazards related to immobility.
14. The correct response is *b.* Maturational enuresis is involuntary urination after an age when continence should be present. The 12-month-old child is not expected to be continent, and incontinence and neurologic damage are not maturational problems.
15. The correct response is *d.* Incontinence is not a natural consequence of the aging process. All the other factors are necessary information for the plan of care.

Bibliography

Agency for Health Care Policy and Research, Public Health Service, Urinary Incontinence Guideline Panel. (1992). *Urinary Incontinence in Adults: Clinical Practice Guideline* (AHCPR Pub. No. 92-0038). Rockville, MD: U. S. Department of Health and Human Services.

Andrews, M., & Boyle, J. (1995). *Transcultural concepts in nursing care* (2nd ed.). Philadelphia: Lippincott.

Avorn, J., Monane, M., Gurwitz, J., Glynn, R., Choodnovskiy, I., & Lipsitz, L. (1994). Reduction of bacteriuria and pyuria after ingestion of cranberry juice. *Journal of the American Medical Association, 271*(10), 751–754.

Brooks, M. (1993). Urinary incontinence: Assessment, treatment, and reimbursement. *Home Healthcare Nurse, 11*(4), 41–46.

Carpenito, L. (1995). *Nursing diagnosis: Application to clinical practice* (6th ed.). Philadelphia: Lippincott.

Colling, J., Owen, T., & McCreedy, M. (1994). Urine volumes and voiding patterns among incontinent nursing home residents. *Geriatric Nursing, 15*(4), 188–192.

DeGroot-Kosolcharoen, J. (1995). 13 ways to protect your patient from bacteriuria: How to keep catheters from causing harm. *Nursing, 25*(4), 30.

Dunne, D. (1994). Understanding urological stents. *Nursing, 24*(11), 32C–32F.

Enberg, S., McDowell, B., Burgio, K., Watson, J., & Belle, S. (1995). Self-care behaviors of older women with urinary incontinence. *Journal of Gerontological Nursing, 21*(8), 7–14.

Fischbach, F. (1996). *A manual of laboratory and diagnostic tests* (5th ed.). Philadelphia: Lippincott.

Flynn, L., Cell, P., & Luisi, E. (1994). Effectiveness of pelvic muscle exercises in reducing urge incontinence among community residing elders. *Journal of Gerontological Nursing, 20*(5), 23–27.

Gerhard, C., Nichols, A., & Smith, D. (1995). Nurse practitioner-directed continence management. *Nursing Spectrum, 4*(1), 9.

Lukaz, K. (1995). Urinary incontinence: Suffering in isolation. *Canadian Nurse, 91*(5), 23–26.

McConnell, E. (1994). How to apply a self-adhesive condom catheter. *Nursing, 24*(11), 26.

McConnell, E. (1995). How to remove an indwelling urinary catheter. *Nursing, 25*(1), 22.

McCormick, K., Newman, D., Colling, J., & Pearson, B. (1992). Urinary incontinence in adults. *American Journal of Nursing, 92*(10), 75–88.

McDowell, B., Engberg, S., Weber, E., Brodak, I., & Engberg, R. (1994). Successful treatment using behavioral interventions of urinary incontinence in homebound older adults. *Geriatric Nursing, 15*(6), 303–307.

Mondoux, L. (1994). Patients won't ask. *RN, 57*(2), 35–40.

Neskey, K., & Loehner, D. (1994). Urinary diversion with an Indiana pouch. *Nursing, 24*(1), 32C–32H.

Newman, D., Brannan, P., Blackwood, N., Spencer, C., & Wallace, J. (1995). Managing urinary incontinence: An independent NP model. *NP News, 3*(3), 7–8.

North American Nursing Diagnosis Association. (1994). *NANDA nursing diagnoses: Definitions and classification 1995–1996.* Philadelphia: NANDA.

Pinkerman, M. (1994). Indwelling urinary catheters: Reducing infection risks. *Nursing, 24*(9), 66–68.

Resnick, B. (1993). Retraining the bladder after catheterization. *American Journal of Nursing, 93*(11), 46–49.

Rice, R. (1995). *Handbook of home health nursing procedures.* St. Louis: Mosby.

Thayer, D. (1994). How to assess and control urinary incontinence. *American Journal of Nursing, 94*(10), 42–47.

Trout, S., Dattolo, J., & Hansbrough, J. (1993). Catheterization: How far should you go? *RN, 56*(8), 52–54.

Webber-Jones, J. (1991). Performing clean, intermittent self-catheterization. *Nursing, 21*(8), 56–59.

Williams, M., Wallhagen, M., & Dowling, G. (1993). Urinary retention in hospitalized elderly women. *Journal of Gerontological Nursing, 19*(2), 7–13.

Winslow, E. (1993a). Myth of the clean catch. *American Journal of Nursing, 93*(8), 20.

Winslow, E. (1993b). Continence cues. *American Journal of Nursing, 93*(5), 20.

Woodtli, M. (1993). Assessing urge incontinence in elderly women. *Geriatric Nursing, 14*(1), 19–22.

Chapter 44

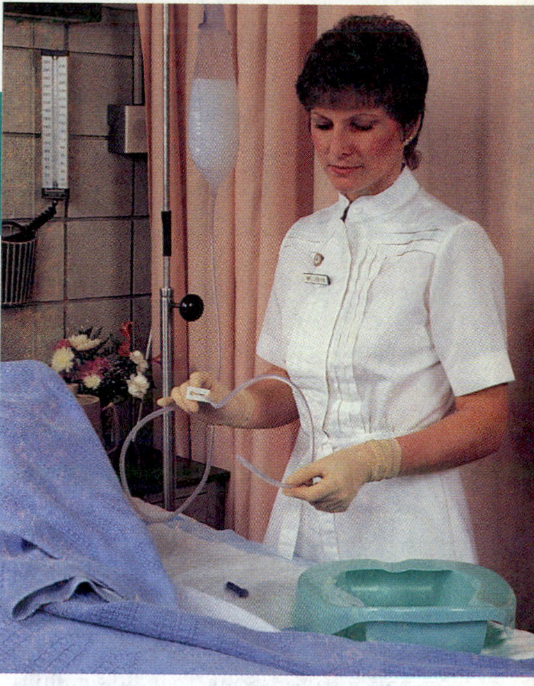

Bowel Elimination

Objectives

After studying this chapter, the learner should be able to:

Define key terms used in the chapter.

Describe the physiology of bowel elimination.

Identify 10 variables that influence bowel elimination.

Assess bowel elimination using appropriate interview questions and physical assessment skills.

Assist with the following diagnostic measures: stool collection for laboratory analysis and direct and indirect visualization studies of the gastrointestinal tract.

Develop nursing diagnoses that correctly identify bowel elimination problems amenable to nursing therapy.

Demonstrate how to (1) promote regular bowel habits (timing, positioning, privacy, nutrition, exercise); (2) use cathartics, laxatives, and antidiarrheals; (3) empty the colon of feces (enemas, rectal suppositories, rectal catheters, digital removal of stool); (4) design and implement bowel training programs; and (5) use comfort measures to ease defecation.

Describe nursing care for a client with an ostomy.

Plan, implement, and evaluate nursing care related to select nursing diagnoses that involve bowel problems.

Key Terms

bowel movement

bowel training program

cathartic

chyme

colostomy

constipation

diarrhea

endoscopy

enema

fecal impaction

feces

flatulence

flatus

hemorrhoids

ileostomy

incontinence (bowel)

laxative

occult blood

ostomy

peristalsis

stoma

stool

suppository

Valsalva maneuver

Elimination of the waste products of digestion is a natural process critical to human functioning. Clients differ widely in their expectations regarding bowel elimination, their usual pattern of defecation, and the ease with which they can and do speak of bowel problems. Although most people have experienced minor acute bouts of diarrhea or constipation, some clients experience severe or chronic bowel elimination alterations that affect fluid and electrolyte balance, hydration, nutritional status, skin integrity, comfort, and, particularly, self-concept. Because many of the clients that nurses encounter are experiencing illnesses that affect bowel elimination or undergoing diagnostic testing and pharmacologic or surgical treatment that affects functioning, nurses need to be knowledgeable in both preventing and treating bowel problems.

Study of this chapter will provide the student with knowledge of the physiology of bowel elimination and the multiple factors that influence this process. A practical guide to assess bowel elimination is presented that includes a description of nursing responsibilities related to diagnostic studies of the gastrointestinal tract. Numerous examples of nursing diagnoses are offered.

Goals are suggested for both the nurse and the client, and nursing strategies are described in detail. In the section titled Nursing Process in Clinical Practice, focused assessment, planning, implementation, and evaluation guides are offered for select nursing diagnoses of common bowel elimination problems—constipation, bowel incontinence, and diarrhea. These guides and the concluding client care study illustrate how the nurse's knowledge of bowel elimination may be combined with specific nursing interventions and caring to successfully resolve bowel elimination problems.

Physiology

The anatomy of the gastrointestinal tract is shown in Figure 44-1.

Large Intestine

The large intestine, the primary organ of bowel elimination, is the lower or distal part of the alimentary tract. It extends from the ileocecal valve to the anus. Waste products of digestion, termed **chyme**, are received by the large intestine from the small intestine. About 1500 mL of chyme is processed daily by the large intestine and most is absorbed in the proximal portion of the colon, except for about 100 mL of fluid that is eliminated in the feces. Functions of the large intestine include the completion of absorption, the manufacture of certain vitamins, the formation of feces, and the expulsion of feces from the body.

The length of the large intestine in adults is about 1.5 m (about 59 inches), but variations have been observed in normal people. The width of the colon varies. At its narrowest point, the colon is about 2.5 cm (1 inch) wide; at its widest point, it is about 7.5 cm (3 inches). Its diameter decreases from the cecum to the anus.

The barrier between the large intestine and the ileum of the small intestine is the ileocecal, or ileocolic, valve. This valve normally prevents contents from entering the large intestine prematurely and prevents waste products from returning to the small intestine.

The waste contents pass through the ileocecal valve and enter the cecum, which is the first part of the large intestine. It is situated on the right side of the body, and to it is attached the vermiform process or appendix. When waste products enter the large intestine, the contents are liquid or watery. While passing through the large intestine, water is absorbed. About 800 to 1000 mL of liquid is absorbed daily by the intestinal tract. This absorption of water accounts for the formed, semisolid consistency of the normal stool. When absorption does not occur properly—as when the waste products pass through the large intestine at a rapid rate—the stool is soft and watery. If the stool remains in the colon too long, or if too much water is absorbed, the stool becomes dry and hardened.

From the cecum, the contents enter the colon, which is divided into several parts. The ascending colon extends from the cecum upward, toward the liver, where it turns to cross the abdomen. This turn is the hepatic flexure. The transverse colon crosses the abdomen from right to left. The turn from the transverse colon to form the descending colon is the splenic flexure. The descending colon passes down the left side of the body, from the splenic flexure to the sigmoid or pelvic colon. When the waste products reach the distal end of the

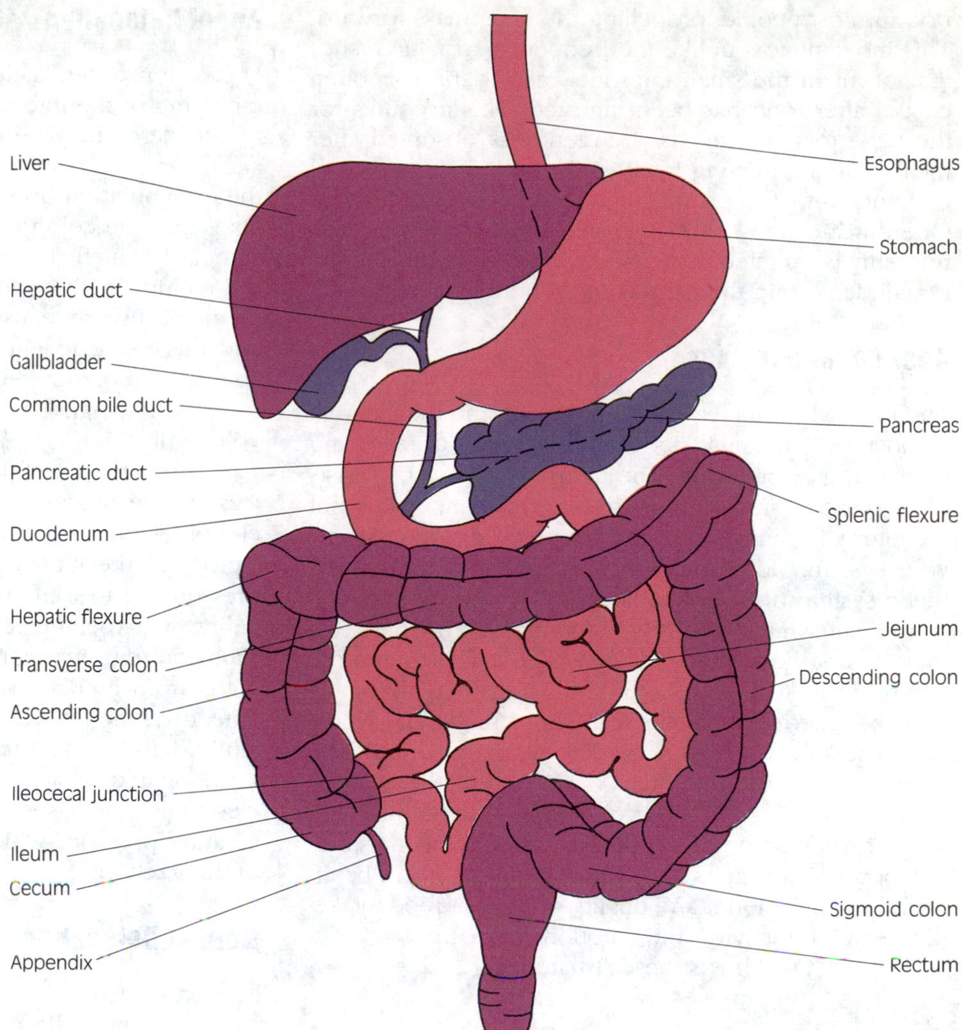

Figure 44-1
Organs of the gastrointestinal system.

colon, they are called **feces**, and when excreted, feces are called the **stool**.

The sigmoid colon contains feces ready for excretion, and empties into the rectum, which is the last part of the large intestine. The rectum is about 12 cm (about 5 inches) long, 2.5 cm (1 inch) of which is the anal canal. Three transverse folds of tissue normally are present in the rectum. These folds may help to hold the fecal material in the rectum temporarily. In addition, there are vertical folds, each of which contains an artery and a vein. Abnormally distended veins are called **hemorrhoids**.

The rectum is empty except during and immediately before defecation. Feces are excreted from the rectum through the anal canal and the anus, which is about 2.5 to 3.8 cm (1 to 1.5 inches) long.

The muscles of the colon are innervated by the autonomic nervous system. The parasympathetic system stimulates movement, and the sympathetic system inhibits movement. Contractions of the circular and longitudinal muscles of the intestine (**peristalsis**) occur every 3 to 12 minutes and continually move waste products along the length of the intestine (Fig. 44-2). Mass peristaltic sweeps occur one to four times each 24-hour pe-

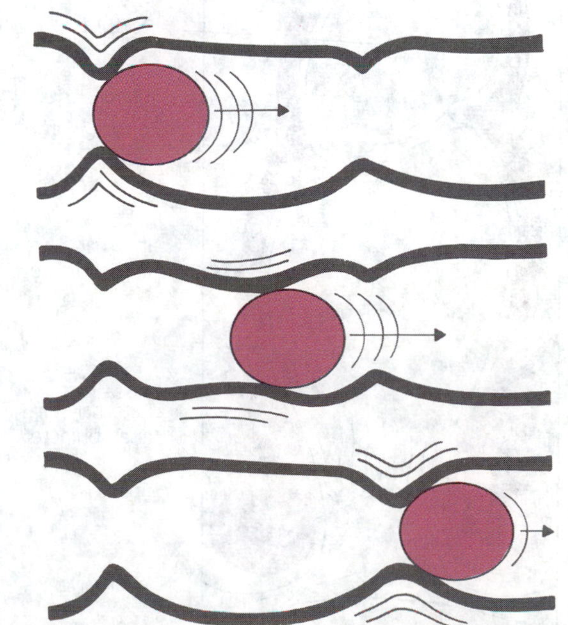

Figure 44-2
Peristaltic movements in the intestine.

riod in most people, propelling the fecal mass forward. This movement is unlike the frequent peristaltic rushes that occur in the small intestine. Mass peristalsis often occurs after food has been ingested. This accounts for the urge to defecate that frequently is observed after meals. Timing nursing interventions to evacuate bowel contents with this natural urge to defecate is helpful. One-third to one-half of ingested food waste products normally is excreted in the stool within 24 hours and the remainder within the next 24 to 48 hours.

Anal Canal and Anus

The internal sphincter in the anal canal and the external sphincter at the anus control the discharge of feces and intestinal gas, or **flatus**. The internal sphincter consists of involuntary smooth muscle tissue. The innervation of the internal sphincter occurs through the autonomic nervous system. Motor impulses are carried by the sympathetic system (thoracolumbar), and inhibitory impulses by the parasympathetic system (craniosacral). These two divisions of the autonomic nervous system function antagonistically to each other in a dynamic equilibrium.

The external sphincter at the anus has striated muscle tissue and is, therefore, under voluntary control. The levator ani muscle reinforces the action of the external sphincter and is controlled voluntarily. Interference with the normal functioning of elimination from the intestines can occur in health as it can during illness. It can be affected by the amount and quality of fluid or food intake, the degree of activity, and emotional states.

Figure 44-3 shows these structures.

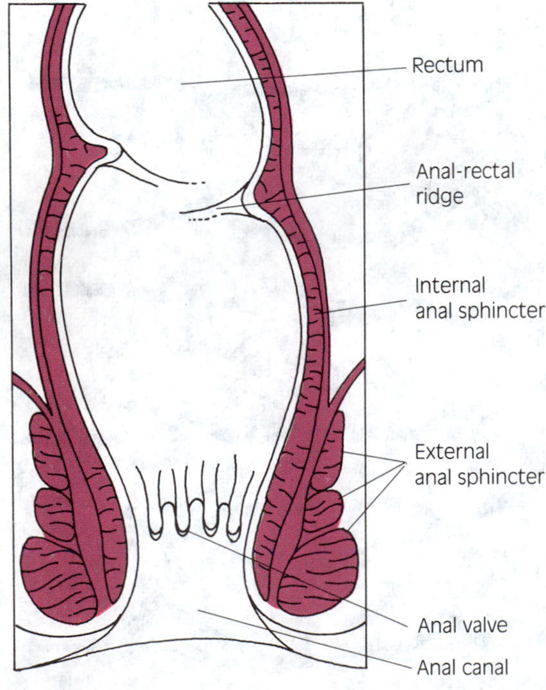

Figure 43-3
Interior view of the rectum and the anal canal.

Act of Defecation

Defecation, often called a **bowel movement**, is the emptying of the intestines. Two centers govern the reflex to defecate. One is situated in the medulla, and a subsidiary one is in the spinal cord. When parasympathetic stimulation occurs, the internal anal sphincter relaxes and the colon contracts. The defecation reflex is stimulated chiefly by the fecal mass in the rectum. When the rectum is distended, the intrarectal pressure rises, the defecation reflex is stimulated by the muscle stretch, and the desire to eliminate results. The external anal sphincter is constricted or relaxed at will. If the desire to defecate is ignored, defecation often can be delayed voluntarily.

During the act of defecation, several additional muscles aid the process. Voluntary contraction of the muscles of the abdominal wall, fixing of the diaphragm, and closing of the glottis aid in increasing intraabdominal pressure up to four or five times the normal pressure, aiding in expelling feces. This technique, termed the **Valsalva maneuver**, may be contraindicated in people with cardiovascular problems and other illnesses. Simultaneously, the muscles on the pelvic floor contract and aid in drawing the anus over the fecal mass.

Ease in defecation is aided by flexing the thigh muscles, which increases abdominal pressure, and assuming a sitting position, which increases downward pressure on the rectum.

Normal Defecation

The act of defecation usually is painless. Normally, it is associated with the regularity and type of stool. If the bowels move at regular intervals and the stools are formed and soft, functional problems of frequency of elimination seldom occur. Nurses find that many people show concern if they do not have a daily bowel movement. The normal frequency of bowel movements cannot be stated arbitrarily. Although many adults pass one stool each day, healthy people have been observed to have more frequent or less frequent bowel movements. Some people have a bowel movement two or three times a week; others, as often as two or three times a day.

Factors Affecting Bowel Elimination

Developmental Considerations

Age affects what a person eats and the body's ability to digest nutrients and eliminate wastes. There is a marked difference between the stools of an infant and those of an older person. Because clients often are reluctant to discuss bowel habits and stool characteristics, nurses need to be familiar with bowel concerns pertinent to each developmental group. These are highlighted in Table 44-1 with related nursing interventions.

Table 44-1
Developmental Variations in Bowel Elimination With Related Nursing Interventions

	Developmental Variations	Related Nursing Interventions
Infant	Stool characteristics depend on whether the infant is being fed breast milk or cow's milk. Breastfed babies have frequent, yellow to golden stools of salvelike consistency. With cow's milk feedings, the stools vary from yellow to brown, are firmer, and have a stronger fecal odor because of the decomposition of protein. Both stools may have curds and mucus. Infants have no voluntary control over bowel elimination.	Parents should be advised that the number of stools an infant passes can vary greatly. In the first 4 months, breastfed infants average two to four stools daily and bottle-fed infants one or two stools daily. By the time the infant is 1 year old, he or she may only have one stool daily. Parents may mistake the infant's liquid stool for diarrhea. Loose stools may be related to overfeeding or too much corn syrup in the formula. Real diarrhea requires evaluation. The initial treatment for constipation is dietary manipulation; consistent use of suppositories and laxatives is to be discouraged. Infants with persistent constipation should be evaluated for structural defects.
Toddler	Between ages 18 and 24 months, the nerve fibers innervating the anal sphincter become fully developed and voluntary control of defecation becomes possible. Voluntary defecation requires intact muscular, sensory, and nervous structures. Successful bowel training includes: 1. Toddler demonstrates awareness of the need to defecate and communicates this (grunting, tugging at diaper, special word). 2. Toddler wants to avoid the discomfort of involuntary defecation and wishes to please the significant person managing bowel training. 3. Significant person has clearly and consistently communicated expectations, praises and reinforces successful behavior, does not punish accidents. Daytime bowel control is normally attained by 30 months.	The parents' approach to toilet training and understanding of the need for physiologic maturity should be assessed. Guidance may be offered to ensure that the process of toilet training strengthens the parent–child relationship. It is critical for parents to understand that a child should never be punished or shamed for elimination accidents or for a lack of readiness to become toilet-trained. Toddlers who are toilet-trained may regress when hospitalized until they become comfortable in their new environment. Children who feel hostile to parents or staff may retaliate by soiling. Scolding or disgust only reinforces this behavior, and the only constructive approach is to seek out the underlying cause, which is most often some form of emotional turmoil.
Child or adolescent, adult	Defecation patterns vary in quantity, frequency, and rhythmicity.	Each comprehensive nursing assessment should include questions about the client's bowel habits. Many people may not understand the significance of changes in bowel habits or may worry needlessly about normal stool characteristics or bowel habits. The use of over-the-counter laxatives and enemas should be evaluated.
Older adult	Decreased physical activity, decreased gastrointestinal motility, and changes in nutritional habits make constipation a chronic problem for many elderly people. Abuse of laxatives and enemas may cause rebound diarrhea and negatively affect other body systems.	Strenuous teaching of the importance of nonpharmacologic remedies for constipation is needed. These include regular exercise, increased fiber in the diet, decreased animal fat and refined sugar, and increased fluid intake.

Daily Patterns

Most people have regular patterns of bowel elimination that include frequency, timing considerations, position, and place. Changes in any of these may upset a person's routine and lead to constipation. For example, many people defecate after breakfast, when the gastrocolic and duodenocolic reflexes cause mass propulsive movements in the large intestine. If this urge to defecate is ignored because the person finds the time inconvenient, the feces remains in the rectum until the defecation reflex is again initiated. Meanwhile, water continues to be absorbed from the unexpelled feces, which makes it dry, hard, and painful to pass.

The position most people assume for defecation is squatting or sitting slightly forward with the thighs flexed. In this position, increased pressure is placed on the abdomen as well as downward pressure on the rectum; both facilitate defecation. It is difficult to obtain the same results when seated on a bedpan, and embarrassment may further inhibit defecation.

Lastly, for many people, defecation is a private affair that can be done easily only in the comfort of one's own bathroom. Defecation in a shared hospital room with only a curtain separating one from a roommate or other people may be difficult.

Food and Fluid

Both the type and the amount of foods eaten and the amount of fluids ingested affect elimination. Healthy elimination is facilitated by a high-fiber diet and a daily fluid intake of 2000 to 3000 mL. High-fiber foods increase the bulk in fecal material. As the bulk of feces expands, it places pressure on the intestinal wall, which serves as a stimulus for peristalsis. When fecal material moves quickly through the intestine, there is less time for water to be reabsorbed, and the resultant stool is soft and easily passed. There also is less time for toxins to be absorbed from feces by the colon. Many believe that these toxins play an important role in colon cancer.

People digest and tolerate food very differently. This variation is determined in part by one's culture. Traveling to a different country and eating the native foods may result in severe indigestion and elimination problems. Differences in water also may affect elimination when traveling. People who lack the enzyme lactase, which helps to break down the simple sugar lactose found in milk and milk products, cannot digest milk. This is called lactose intolerance. Food intolerances may result in diarrhea, gaseous distention, and cramping.

In addition to high-fiber, bulk-producing foods, other general food classifications that influence bowel elimination include the following:

Constipating foods—processed cheese, lean meat, eggs, and pasta

Foods with laxative effect—certain fruits and vegetables (eg, prunes), bran, chocolate, spicy foods, alcohol, and coffee

Gas-producing foods—onions, cabbage, beans, cauliflower

Activity and Muscle Tone

Regular exercise improves gastrointestinal motility and muscle tone, whereas inactivity decreases both. Adequate tone in the abdominal muscles, the diaphragm, and the perineal muscles is essential to ease in defecation. Clients who are on prolonged bed rest are prime candidates for constipation.

Lifestyle

Many individual, family, and sociocultural variables influence a person's usual elimination habits. The long-term effects of bowel training may result in a person's (1) acceptance of bowel elimination as a normal life process, (2) preoccupation with bowel elimination, or (3) feeling that bowel elimination is a "dirty" process. Rituals associated with bowel elimination, cleanliness considerations, the language used to talk about bowel elimination or reluctance to discuss it, individual responses to involuntary passage of flatus (gas), and so forth vary widely among individuals. A person's daily schedule, occupation, and leisure activities may contribute to a habit of defecating at regular times or to an irregular pattern.

Psychologic Variables

Emotional stress affects the body in many ways. In some people, anxiety seems to have a direct effect on gastrointestinal motility, and diarrhea can be expected to accompany periods of high anxiety. During the fight-or-flight response, when the body mobilizes itself for intense action, blood is shunted away from the stomach, and intestines and gastrointestinal motility slow. Chronic worriers and certain personality types who tend to hold on to problems and feelings may experience frequent constipation.

Pathologic Conditions

Numerous pathologic processes may result in changes in a person's usual bowel elimination. When a client reports that his or her stool is now narrower or ribbonlike, it is important for the nurse to consider the possibility of a tumor in the colon forming an obstruction to normal stool passage and to report this finding to the physician. Similarly, if a parent reports that a child's stools are frequent, bulky, greasy, and foul smelling, one possible explanation is cystic fibrosis; this would need to be ruled out if other clinical manifestations are present. Changes in stool characteristics or frequency may, therefore, be one of the first clinical manifestations of a disease, and their evaluation may lead to the diagnosis of the disease.

Pathologic conditions that may result in diarrhea include diverticulitis, infection, malabsorption syndromes, neoplastic diseases, diabetic neuropathy, hyperthyroidism, and uremia. Conditions that predispose to constipation include diseases within the colon or rectum, injury to or degeneration of the spinal cord, and megacolon. Conditions that traumatize the stomach or intestines or that interfere with normal digestion may change the color, contents, odor, and appearance of the stool, making stool assessment an important diagnostic task for nursing.

Medications

Medications are available to either promote peristalsis (cathartics and laxatives) or inhibit peristalsis (antidiarrheal medications). These are discussed later in the chapter.

Other types of medications may affect bowel elimination and stool characteristics. Narcotic analgesics (opioids), antacids containing aluminum, and anticholinergic medications all have the potential to cause constipation by decreasing gastrointestinal motility. Many medications have diarrhea as an adverse effect. Twenty percent of the time, antibiotic use is accompanied

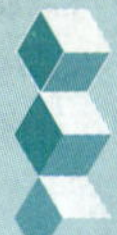

Research in Nursing: Making a Difference

Bowel Elimination

Normal bowel elimination is an ongoing, expected client outcome for nurses. Nursing assessment provides for early identification of bowel alterations and aids in the development of an individualized plan of care. Changes in bowel elimination patterns are distressing to clients and caregivers. Nursing interventions help alleviate the hopelessness and stress associated with constipation and promote the emotional as well as the physical well-being of the client.

Related Research

Neal, L. (1995). Power pudding: Natural laxative therapy for the elderly who are homebound. ***Home Healthcare Nurse, 13*****(3), 66–71.**
Constipation among the older adult population is a common problem. "Power pudding" (applesauce, wheat bran flakes, prunes, and Cool Whip), when given to a group of older homebound clients, resulted in an acceptable stool consistency and elimination pattern. Nurses working in the community need to consider this nonpharmacologic nursing intervention when constipation is reported by the older person. Before implementing this remedy, the nurse should obtain a physician's order and take a bowel history.

Gibson, C., Opalka, P., Moore, C., Brady, R., & Mion, L. (1995). Effectiveness of bran supplement on the bowel management of elderly rehabilitation patients. ***Journal of Gerontological Nursing, 21*****(10), 21–30.**
Constipation in the geriatric population is a common and costly problem. When a group of older clients in geriatric rehabilitation received a fiber supplement of applesauce, bran, and prune juice, the number of bowel agents they used per day also decreased. The additional fiber did, however, cause adverse effects such as gas, cramps, and loose stools in some of the population. Nurses giving fiber supplements to the older adult need to add them gradually and continually assess for any signs of adverse effects.

Day, R., & Monsma, M. (1995). Fruitlax: Management of constipation in children with disabilities. ***Clinical Nursing Research, 4*****(3), 306–322.**
Constipation can be a lifelong problem in children with disabilities. A group of physically challenged children who suffered from chronic constipation were treated with fruitlax, a mixture of raisins, currants, dates, figs, prunes, and prune juice. This natural laxative was found to have a positive effect on the bowel problems of these children. Nurses who treat constipation with a natural remedy need to assess not only the child's response but also the consistency of the stool.

Summary

Nursing journals contain increasingly more research on bowel elimination. This is valuable because studies by other health professionals do not provide enough information to help in making nursing care decisions. Problems in bowel elimination are commonly identified and treated by nurses, supporting the need for ongoing research on normal and altered patterns of bowel elimination.

by diarrhea (Abrams, 1995). The use of antidiarrheal drugs in this situation is not recommended, since it further prolongs the exposure of the intestinal mucosa to the irritating effect of the antibiotics or toxins. The diarrhea may be severe enough to warrant cessation of the drug.

Medications may influence the appearance of the stool for a variety of reasons. Any drug with the potential to cause gastrointestinal bleeding (eg, anticoagulants, aspirin products) may result in the stool appearing pink to red to black; iron salts result in a black stool from the oxidation of iron; antacids may cause a white discoloration or speckling in the stool; and antibiotics may cause a green-gray color because of impaired digestion.

Diagnostic Tests

Clients may need to fast for diagnostic studies. Additionally, the stress of hospitalization and waiting for the results of the study combined with changes in food intake can severely alter usual elimination patterns. Bowel cleansing by use of cathartics or enemas is a prerequisite for certain diagnostic studies of the gastrointestinal tract (refer to Table 44-3 later in this chapter).

Surgery and Anesthesia

Direct manipulation of the bowel during abdominal surgery inhibits peristalsis, causing a condition termed paralytic ileus. This temporary stoppage of peristalsis normally lasts 24 to 48 hours, and during this time, food and fluids are withheld. If this condition persists, it may cause distention and symptoms of acute obstruction and may require surgical intervention. General anesthetic agents that are inhaled also inhibit peristalsis by blocking the parasympathetic impulses to the intestinal musculature. Local and regional anesthetics have little effect on peristalsis.

The Nurse as Role Model

Before intervening to help clients develop healthy bowel elimination patterns, it is important for nurses to assess the adequacy of their own bowel elimination habits and patterns. If you are unable to meet the following goals, you may want to take the time now to revise your own health practices, so that you will be an effective role model for clients. Use the assessment checklist to see how well you are meeting bowel elimination needs. The nurse:

- Has a normal bowel elimination pattern without discomfort
- Responds to the normal urge to defecate
- Includes in each day's nutritional intake sufficient high-fiber foods and fluid to promote peristalsis and reduce stool retention
- Identifies many ways to increase fiber and fluid in different types of diets
- Exercises vigorously for 15 to 30 minutes three or four times a week
- Responds to changes in stool characteristics (or frequency) by seeking their cause and getting medical assistance when necessary

ASSESSING

Nursing History

Because many clients are reluctant to initiate a discussion of their bowel status, nurses should include pertinent bowel elimination questions in each comprehensive nursing history (see the accompanying box).

If the client is experiencing any disturbance in bowel elimination, a more detailed assessment is conducted with attention directed to each of the factors that may influence bowel elimination (described earlier).

Clients who are critically ill or who have impaired cognition may be incapable of reporting their bowel status accurately. In this instance, nurses need to record the client's daily bowel status to be alert to impending problems. While making daily rounds, the nurse asks the client who is a reliable historian, "Did you move your bowels yesterday or today?" and charts the response. If the client cannot offer this information, the nurse who is assisting with bowel elimination records daily stools.

Physical Assessment

Assessment of bowel elimination includes physical assessment of the abdomen, anus, and rectum. (This is discussed in Chapter 26.) Described below are examination techniques that may be helpful when assessing the functioning of the gastrointestinal tract.

Abdomen

The sequence for abdominal assessment proceeds from inspection, auscultation, and percussion to palpation. Auscultation is done before palpation because palpation may disturb normal peristalsis. The client is comfortably positioned in the supine position with the abdomen exposed and the chest and pubic area draped. The bladder should be emptied.

Inspection. The nurse first observes the contour of the abdomen, noting any masses or areas of distention. Peristalsis is not visible except in very thin clients and

Promoting Wellness

Bowel Elimination

Use the assessment checklist to determine how well you are meeting your need for bowel elimination. Then develop a prescription for self-care by choosing appropriate behaviors from the list of suggestions.

Assessment Checklist

almost always	sometimes	almost never	
☐	☐	☐	1. I have a regular bowel elimination pattern, satisfactory to support comfort and activities of daily living.
☐	☐	☐	2. I eat a diet high in fiber.
☐	☐	☐	3. I exercise regularly.
☐	☐	☐	4. I have an adequate intake of fluids.

Self-Care Behaviors

1. Accept individual patterns of defecation as normal.
2. Eat a balanced diet, including high-fiber foods, such as fruits, vegetables, and nuts.
3. Follow a regular exercise program with 30 to 45 minutes of activity three to four times a week.
4. Do not ignore the urge to defecate.
5. Establish a routine, if needed (1 hour after meals is usually best).
6. Avoid prolonged use of over-the-counter medications or enemas to treat constipation.

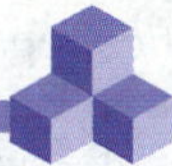

Focused Assessment Guide

Bowel Elimination

Factors to Assess	Questions and Approaches
Usual patterns of bowel elimination	How often do you move your bowels? Any special time of the day? What does your stool look like? • Frequency • Time of day • Description of usual stool characteristics (amount, consistency, shape, color, odor)
Recent changes in bowel elimination	Have you noticed any changes in your stool recently? Have you noticed any blood in your stool? Have you noted a difference in the appearance of your stool (narrowing, presence of mucus)?
Aids to elimination	Do you use anything to help move your bowels? • Natural aids (liquids, food) • Pharmacologic aids (laxatives) • Enemas
Problems with bowel elimination	Are your bowels causing you any problem now? • Nature of disturbance • Onset and frequency • Causes (*physical:* food and fluid intake, exercise status, history of surgery or illnesses influencing GI tract; *psychosocial*; *medicine related*) • Severity • Symptoms • Interventions attempted and results
Presence of artificial orifices	What is your usual routine with your colostomy or ileostomy? Do you have any problems with it?

when observed (visible waves) may indicate an intestinal obstruction.

Auscultation. The nurse uses a warmed stethoscope to listen for bowel sounds in a systematic, clockwise manner in all abdominal quadrants. If the client has a nasogastric tube in place, it should be disconnected from suction during this assessment to allow for accurate interpretation of sounds. The presence of a full bladder or the timing of the client's most recent meal may also impact on the examination (McConnell, 1994). The frequency and character of bowel sounds are noted. Bowel sounds are audible clicks and gurgles produced by the movement of air and flatus in the gastrointestinal tract. They usually are high-pitched, gurgling, and soft. Their frequency may range from 5 to 34 bowel sounds per minute, depending on the rate of peristalsis. Of significance are absent or infrequent bowel sounds, indicating hypoperistalsis or paralytic ileus (no decision should be made until the nurse has listened for 5 minutes), or abnormally intense and frequent bowel sounds (borborygmus), indicating hyperperistalsis. Bowel sounds usually are described as being audible, hyperactive, hypoactive, or inaudible.

Percussion. The nurse next percusses all quadrants of the abdomen in a systematic, clockwise manner to identify any masses, fluid, or air in the abdomen. A resonant sound or tympany is expected over the abdomen and stomach because these are hollow organs. With practice, the nurse can distinguish normal resonance from the hyperresonance that occurs when excess flatus is trapped in the intestines. An intestinal obstruction sounds dull on percussion. Areas of increased dullness may be caused by fluid, a mass, or a tumor.

Palpation. Both light and deep palpation in each quadrant are next performed by the skilled nurse, noting muscular resistance, tenderness, enlargement of organs, and masses. The beginning nurse quickly learns the feel of a distended abdomen. If the client is in pain, medication should be administered before proceeding with the palpation.

Anus and Rectum

The skill of the nurse examiner determines the extent of the rectal examination. A superficial examination is performed each time a nurse washes a client's anal area or assists with bowel evacuation. The client is most often positioned in left Sims' position.

Inspection and Palpation. The nurse first examines the anal area for cracks, nodules, distended veins (hemorrhoids), masses, or polyps. A fecal mass may be observed distending the anus. A gloved and lubricated finger is next inserted through the anus into the rectum to assess sphincter tone and smoothness of mucosal lining, and to note the presence of masses, polyps, hardened stool, bleeding, or abnormal discharge. The perineal area also is inspected for areas of skin irritation or breakdown secondary to diarrhea or fecal incontinence.

Stool Characteristics

Nurses are responsible for observing and recording information about the client's stool. Table 44-2 describes characteristics of a normal stool and presents special considerations to take into account when observing a stool. Anything unusual should be reported and recorded. Passing little or no gas or unusual amounts also should be recorded and reported.

The frequency with which the client has bowel movements is noted and recorded. Frequency is recorded as I, II, III, or i, ii, iii, and so on. The frequency of the client's bowel movements as well as specific information about the amount and characteristics of stool is usually appropriately recorded on a bedside flow sheet. Any additional unusual observations are described in the nurses' notes on the client's permanent record. When auxiliary personnel or the client assumes this responsibility, the nurse should check at regular intervals to see that it is being done correctly.

Ideally, populations at high risk for bowel elimination problems will be identified, and such problems will be prevented or minimized through vigilant nursing care. The nurse also must be aware of clinical manifestations of colon cancer, since early detection significantly improves survival statistics (see the accompanying box). To perform these assessments accurately, the nurse needs a thorough knowledge of the factors that contribute to these problems and of pertinent assessment priorities. These may be found later in the chapter, in the section titled Nursing Process in Clinical Practice.

Assisting With Diagnostic Studies

The nurse often is responsible for caring for clients with elimination problems who are undergoing diagnostic testing. Following are specific guidelines for nursing's role with stool collection and direct and indirect visualization studies.

Stool Collection. The nurse is responsible for obtaining the specimen according to agency procedure, labeling the specimen, and ensuring that the specimen is transported to the laboratory in a timely manner. The institution's policy and procedure manual or laboratory manual must be checked to determine specifics regarding the amount of stool needed, the time frame during which stool is to be collected, and the type of specimen container to use.

Medical aseptic techniques are imperative. Disposable gloves should be worn when any contact or handling of a stool specimen is likely. Handwashing before and after glove use is essential. Care also must be taken not to contaminate the outside of the specimen container with stool. Specimens should be packaged, labeled, and transported to the laboratory according to the specific agency policy in a manner that guarantees that there is no leakage of the specimen.

Specific instructions the nurse needs to give the client when collecting a stool specimen may include the following:

- Void first because the laboratory study may be inaccurate if the stool contains urine.
- Use a clean or sterile bedpan or the bedside commode, depending on the specific specimen required.
- Defecate into the required container rather than the toilet bowl because the laboratory study may be hindered by the water in the bowl.
- Do not place toilet tissue in the bedpan or specimen container because contents in the paper may influence laboratory results.
- Notify the nurse when the specimen is available, so that it may be collected and transported to the laboratory in the required manner.

To place a specimen in a laboratory container, the nurse should use two clean tongue blades and gloved hands. Usually 1 inch (2.5 cm) of formed stool or 15 to 30 mL of liquid stool is sufficient. If portions of the stool include visible blood, mucus, or pus, include these with the specimen. The specimen also should be free of barium and enema solution. Because a fresh specimen produces the most accurate results, the specimen should be sent to the laboratory immediately. If this is not possible, it should be refrigerated, unless contraindicated.

If testing the stool for pH or blood, use commercial tapes, dipsticks, and solutions according to manufacturer's directions. **Occult blood** in the stool—that is, blood that is hidden in the specimen or cannot be seen on gross examination—can be detected by simple screening tests. Certain disease conditions, such as ulcer disease, inflammatory bowel disorders, and colon cancer, place the client at high risk for intestinal bleeding. The color of the stool may reflect the source of the bleeding. Generally, black stools reflect a reaction between hemoglobin and gastric acid and indicate upper GI bleeding (eg, peptic ulcer). Lower GI bleeding (eg, hemorrhoids) may produce bright red blood in the stool. It is also important to remember that certain foods and medications can cause a black or reddish-colored stool.

Tests for occult blood in the stool may be done quickly by the nurse in the clinical area or by the client at home. These are simply done and rely on reagent substances to detect the presence of the enzyme perox-

Table 44-2
The Stool: Normal Characteristics and Special Considerations for Observation

Characteristic	Normal Finding	Special Considerations for Observation
Volume	Variable	The volume of the stool depends on the amount the person eats and the nature of the diet. For example, a diet high in roughage produces more feces than a soft, bland diet. Consistently large diarrheal stools suggest a disorder in the small bowel or proximal colon; small, frequent stools with urgency to pass them suggest a disorder of the left colon or rectum.
Color	Infant: Yellow Adult: Brown	The brown color of the stool is due to stercobilin, a bile pigment derivative. The rapid rate of peristalsis in the infant causes the stool to be yellow. The color of the stool is influenced by diet. For example, the stool will be almost black if the person eats red meat and dark green vegetables, such as spinach. The stool will be light brown if the diet is high in milk and milk products and low in meat. The absence of bile may cause the stool to appear white or clay-colored. Certain drugs influence the color of the stool. For example, iron salts cause the stool to be black. Antacids cause it to be whitish. Bleeding high in the intestinal tract causes a stool to be black owing to the digestion of the blood. Bleeding low in the intestinal tract will result in fresh blood in the stool. The stool darkens with standing.
Odor	Aromatic; may be affected by foods ingested	The characteristic odor of the stool is due to indole and skatole, caused by putrefaction and fermentation in the lower intestinal tract. The odor of the stool is influenced by its pH value, which normally is neutral or slightly alkaline. Excessive putrefaction causes a strong odor. The presence of blood in the stool causes a unique odor.
Consistency	Soft, semisolid, and formed	The consistency of the stool is influenced by fluid and food intake and gastric motility. The less time stool spends in the intestine (or the shorter the intestine), the more liquid the stool. Many pathologic conditions influence consistency.
Shape	Formed stool is usually about 1 inch (2.5 cm) in diameter and has the tubular shape of the colon, but may be larger or smaller, depending on the condition of the colon.	A gastrointestinal obstruction may result in a narrow, pencil-shaped stool. Rapid peristalsis thins the stool. Increased time spent in the large intestine may result in a hard, marblelike fecal mass.
Constituents	Waste residues of digestion: bile, intestinal secretions, shedded epithelial cells, bacteria, and inorganic material (chiefly calcium and phosphates); seeds, meat fibers, and fat may be present in small amounts.	Internal bleeding, infection, inflammation, and other pathologic conditions may result in abnormal constituents. These include blood, pus, excessive fat, parasites, ova, and mucus. Foreign bodies also may be found in the stool.

idase in the hemoglobin molecule. A diet high in red meat, other food substances such as horseradish, raw fruits and raw vegetables, and certain medications (eg, salicylates, steroids, iron preparations, and anticoagulants) may result in a false-positive reading. In contrast, ingestion of vitamin C can produce false-negative results even if bleeding is present. For home testing, recommendations usually include restricting food and drugs that may alter test results for 3 days prior to the stool testing. In the clinical setting, these restrictions are usually not practical (Watson & Jaffe, 1995). A Hematest and guaiac test are types of chemical tests used to determine occult blood in the stool. The accompanying box gives additional nursing considerations for fecal occult blood

Warning Signs of Colon Cancer

- Change in the bowel elimination pattern
- Blood in the stools
- Rectal or abdominal pain
- Change in the character of the stool
- Sensation of incomplete emptying after bowel movement

testing, and Figure 44-4 demonstrates the procedure for a hemoccult test.

Timed Specimens. Consider the first stool passed by the client as the start of the collection period. Collect a specimen of *every* stool passed within the designated period (the test may require saving the entire stool passed or only a sample). Follow instructions for sending stools to the laboratory.

Pinworms. Use clear cellophane tape for collecting a specimen for pinworms (frosted tape makes examination difficult). The tape is placed directly over the client's anal area, removed immediately, and then placed on a slide. Collect this specimen in the morning, immediately after the client awakens and before the client has a bowel movement or bath. Pinworms tend to come to the anal area during the night and retreat into the anal canal during the day. For accurate results, this test may need to be repeated on consecutive days.

Direct Visualization Studies. Endoscopy is the direct visualization of the lining of a hollow body organ using a fiber-optic endoscope (ie, a long flexible tube filled with glass fibers that transmits light into the organ and returns an image to the scope's optical head). Pincers may be inserted through the tube for the biopsy of tissues. An endoscope enables the physician to view the integrity of the mucosa, blood vessels, and specific organ parts, and is helpful in diagnosing inflammatory, ulcerative, and infectious diseases; benign and malignant neoplasms; and other lesions of the esophageal, gastric, and intestinal mucosa. Studies include the following:

Esophagogastroduodenoscopy—visual examination of the lining of the esophagus, the stomach, and the upper duodenum with a flexible, fiber-optic endoscope

Colonoscopy—visual examination of the lining of the large intestine with a flexible, fiber-optic endoscope

Sigmoidoscopy—visual examination of the lining of the distal sigmoid colon, the rectum, and the anal canal using either a flexible or rigid instrument. The tube has an attached light source and is equipped to allow biopsy. The rigid sigmoidoscope may produce greater client discomfort, especially in the client who is not relaxed.

Nursing responsibilities for these studies are highlighted in Table 44-3.

Indirect Visualization Studies. Indirect visualization of the gastrointestinal tract is commonly achieved by radiography. The passage of x-rays through the client creates a radiograph or film that depicts body structures. This technique is useful in detecting obstruction, strictures, inflammatory disease, tumors, ulcers, and other lesions, and in diagnosing hiatal hernia and other structural changes in the gastrointestinal tract. Use of a radiopaque contrast medium, such as barium sulfate, accentuates the body structures being visualized. In the *upper gastrointestinal examination* and *small-bowel se-*

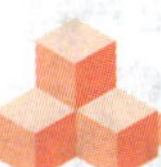

Guidelines for Nursing Care

Testing for Fecal Occult Blood

- Instruct the client about food and drug restrictions for at least 2 to 3 days prior to the test, if they apply.
- Review manufacturer's directions for collecting the specimen. Equipment may include a specimen card, collection tissues, or test paper.
- Avoid mixing the specimen with urine or water.
- Inform the client that multiple or serial specimens are usually collected from different bowel movements to verify results.
- Collect the amount recommended for the articular test (usually only a small amount is required).
- Wear gloves and wash hands thoroughly if collecting a specimen from a bedpan, commode, or plastic receptacle.
- Use tongue blades to transfer the stool to the test tape or folder.
- Follow instructions based on type of test. Hemoccult slide test requires placing 2 drops of developer solution on the opposite side of specimen paper. The tablet test directions include placing 2 to 3 drops of tap water on the tablet, which is centered on the stool specimen.
- Document the test results according to agency policy. *A blue color is a positive result and needs to be reported.*
- Inform the client of the test results.

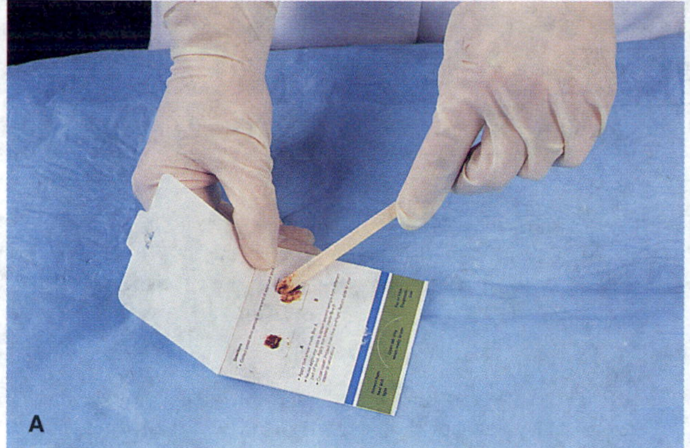
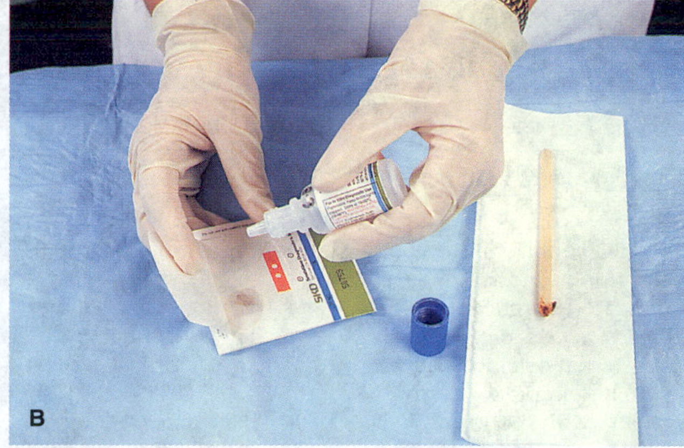
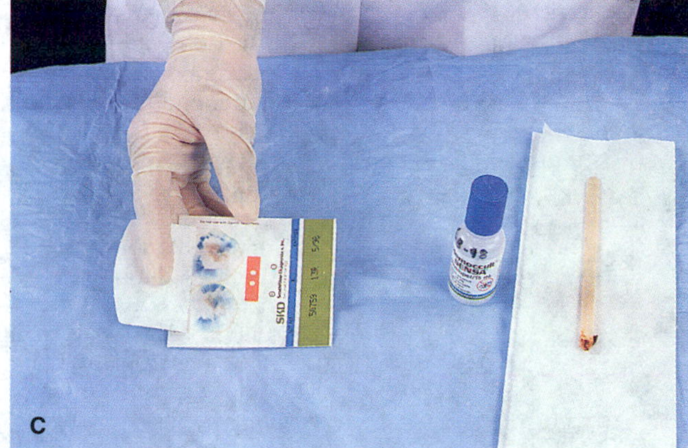

Figure 44-4
Testing a stool specimen for occult blood. (**A**) Applying a stool specimen to the test paper; (**B**) adding developing solution to the opposite side according to directions; (**C**) blue coloration indicating positive results. (Copyright © B. Proud.)

ries, the client drinks the barium sulfate like a milk shake and the esophagus, stomach, and small intestine are coated and visualized. In the *barium enema* or *lower gastrointestinal examination,* barium sulfate is instilled into the large intestine by means of a rectal tube inserted through the anus. Fluoroscopy projects the x-ray films onto a screen and permits continuous observation of the flow of the barium. Specific nursing responsibilities are included in Table 44-3.

Scheduling Diagnostic Studies. Because nurses commonly are involved in the scheduling of diagnostic studies when multiple orders are written, it is helpful to remember certain guidelines for scheduling studies of the gastrointestinal tract.

1. The following is a logical sequence when more than one test is required for accurate diagnosis:
   - *Fecal occult blood test*—to detect gastrointestinal bleeding
   - *Barium studies*—to visualize gastrointestinal structures and, possibly, reveal inflammation or ulcers, tumors, strictures, or other lesions
   - *Endoscopic examinations*—to directly visualize an abnormality, locate a source of bleeding, and, if necessary, provide a channel for biopsy
2. The barium enema and routine radiography should precede the upper gastrointestinal series because retained barium from the latter may take several days to pass through the gastrointestinal tract and may cloud anatomic detail on the barium enema studies.
3. Noninvasive procedures usually take precedence over invasive procedures, such as endoscopic studies, when sufficient diagnostic data can be obtained. (In some instances, endoscopic studies may be done before barium studies to ensure visualization.)

DIAGNOSING

Bowel Elimination as the Problem. When analysis of assessment data points to a bowel elimination problem that can be prevented or resolved by independent nursing intervention, a nursing diagnosis is developed. Common alterations in bowel elimination for which a nursing diagnosis may be identified include the following:

Constipation
Colonic Constipation
Perceived Constipation
Diarrhea
Bowel Incontinence

Whenever alterations in bowel elimination require new self-care behaviors (eg, colostomy management), Knowledge Deficit may be an appropriate nursing diagnosis. Examples of specific causes and defining charac-

(text continues on page 1282)

Table 44-3
Diagnostic Studies of the Gastrointestinal Tract

Test and Purpose	Client Preparation	Nursing Care During Test	Client Aftercare
Esophagogastroduodenoscopy			
• Allows visual examination of the esophagus, stomach, and upper duodenum • Indicated for clients with hematemesis, melena, or substernal or epigastric pain and in postoperative clients with recurrent or new symptoms • Assists in the diagnosis of inflammatory, ulcerative, and infectious diseases; tumors; and structural abnormalities • Allows biopsy, removal of foreign objects, and coagulation of bleeding	1. Explain to the client: • Nature and purpose of the test • Directions for fasting (6 to 12 hours before the test; check guidelines) • That the test requires about 30 minutes and involves the passage of a flexible tube through the mouth (client may experience gagging or sense of fullness; cannot speak during this time) • Dentures need to be removed; mouth guard often used to protect natural teeth • Client will be awake, although a sedative (and sometimes an anticholinergic drug to decrease GI secretions) is administered • A bitter-tasting local anesthetic is sprayed into the mouth and throat to decrease sensation (tongue will feel swollen temporarily—difficulty swallowing) 2. Ensure that informed consent is signed. 3. Assist client into hospital gown and complete agency protocol for testing (empty bladder, remove jewelry, and so forth). 4. Administer prescribed sedative, anticholinergic, and, if ordered, an analgesic.	• Position client in left lateral or left Sims' position. • Provide emotional support. • Obtain baseline vital signs. • Check that IV is in place; administer prescribed medications. • Place any tissue or cell specimens in properly labeled containers with preservatives and send to laboratory. • Observe for untoward responses; have emergency resuscitative equipment available.	• Check vital signs according to agency protocol. • Withhold food and fluids until the gag reflex returns. • Observe for signs of perforation: pain, persistent difficulty swallowing, vomiting blood, or black stools. • Explain to the client that it is normal to sense throat soreness and hoarseness for several days; warm saline gargles and lozenges may help.
Colonoscopy			
• Allows visual examination of the large intestine • Indicated for clients with histories of constipation and diarrhea, persistent rectal bleeding, or lower abdominal pain when results of proctosigmoidoscopy and barium enema are negative or inconclusive	1. Explain to the client: • Nature and purpose of the test • Directions for dietary and bowel preparation (clear liquid diet for 48 hours before test; laxative evening before test; and tap water or sodium biphosphate enema 3 to 4 hours before test)	• Position client on left side with knees flexed; drape to avoid embarrassment. • Provide emotional support. • Assist in positioning client (client may need to assume supine position to aid scope's advance).	• Check vital signs according to agency protocol. • Resume usual diet after client recovers from sedation. • Observe for signs of bowel perforation: rectal bleeding, abdominal pain and distention, fever, malaise.

Table 44-3 *(continued)*
Diagnostic Studies of the Gastrointestinal Tract

Test and Purpose	Client Preparation	Nursing Care During Test	Client Aftercare
Colonoscopy			
• Assists in the diagnosis of inflammatory and ulcerative bowel disease, colonic stricture, and tumors • Allows biopsy, removal of polyps by electrocautery	• Test involves passage of a well-lubricated, flexible tube through the anus; air is used to distend the intestine during the procedure; urge to defecate and to pass gas are to be expected • Relaxation is important; breathe deeply and exhale through mouth • Sedative may be administered 2. Ensure that informed consent is signed. 3. If client is unable to complete bowel preparation, administer the prescribed laxative and enema. 4. Assist client into hospital gown and complete agency protocol for testing (empty bladder, remove jewelry, and so forth). 5. Administer sedative if prescribed.	• Place any tissue or cell specimens in properly labeled containers with preservatives and send to laboratory. • Watch closely for untoward responses; have emergency resuscitative equipment available.	• If polyp was removed, inform client it is normal to see some blood in stool. • Inform client it is helpful and usual to expel large amounts of flatus—urge not to withhold.
Sigmoidoscopy			
• Allows visual examination of the lining of the distal sigmoid colon, the rectum, and the anal canal • Indicated for clients with recent changes in bowel habits, lower abdominal and perineal pain, prolapse on defecation, and passage of mucus, blood, or pus in stool • Assists in the diagnosis of inflammatory, infectious, and ulcerative bowel disease and tumors; and in detection of hemorrhoids, polyps, fissures, fistulas, and abscesses within the rectum and canal	1. Explain to the client: • Nature and purpose of the test • That the client may be positioned on the left side or assisted into the knee-chest position • That a rigid or flexible tube is placed into the rectum and advanced to its maximal point • Sedation is usually not required; discomfort is minimal. • Biopsy and removal of polyps can be performed during the test. • Directions for dietary and bowel preparation vary according to agency; usually involve light meal prior to test with instruction to avoid caffeine and give two Fleet enemas	• Position client in knee-chest or left lateral position and drape to avoid embarrassment. • Provide emotional support. • Instruct client to bear down as scope is passed through the anal sphincter. • Place any tissue or all specimens in properly labeled container with preservatives and send to laboratory.	See client aftercare for colonoscopy.

(continued)

Table 44-3 *(continued)*
Diagnostic Studies of the Gastrointestinal Tract

Test and Purpose	Client Preparation	Nursing Care During Test	Client Aftercare
Sigmoidoscopy			
	• Both the examiner's finger and the scopes are well lubricated; they may feel cool and stimulate urge to defecate; air is used to distend the intestine and client may feel urge to pass gas • Relaxation is important and eases discomfort; breathe deeply and exhale through mouth 2. Ensure the informed consent is signed. 3. If the client is unable to complete the bowel preparation, administer any prescribed laxatives or enemas. 4. Administer local anesthetic if prescribed to minimize discomfort of rectal inflammation.		
Upper Gastrointestinal (UGI) and Small-Bowel Series			
• Fluoroscopic examination of the esophagus, stomach, and small intestine after ingestion of barium sulfate • Indicated for clients with upper GI symptoms (difficulty swallowing, regurgitation, burning, or epigastric pain), signs of small-bowel disease (diarrhea, weight loss), and signs of GI bleeding (hematemesis, melena) • Assists in the diagnosis of strictures, ulcers, tumors, regional enteritis, and malabsorption syndrome, and in the detection of hiatal hernia, diverticula, varices, and motility disorders	1. Explain to the client: • Nature and purpose of the test • Need to maintain a low-residue diet for 2 to 3 days before the test and to fast and avoid smoking after midnight the day of the test • That the UGI with the small-bowel series can take up to 6 hours to complete • That he or she will be on a rotating x-ray table and will need to assume different positions • That a chalky-tasting barium contrast mixture (16 to 20 oz) will be given to drink before the test 2. Ensure that an informed consent is signed. 3. Assist client to get into hospital gown and to remove jewelry or any objects that would interfere with the x-ray.	• A technician in the radiology department cares for the client during the test.	• Before allowing the client to resume food and fluids, check to be sure that additional x-rays have not been ordered. • Encourage fluids to prevent dehydration. • Administer the posttest cathartic prescribed by agency policy; if there is any question about its advisability for a particular client check with the physician. • Explain to the client the necessity of his or her eliminating the barium and that it will lighten the color of the stool the next few days. • If the cathartic and increased fluid intake do not result in the elimination of the barium within 2 to 3 days, notify the physician. • Encourage extra rest because this test is fatiguing.

Table 44-3 *(continued)*
Diagnostic Studies of the Gastrointestinal Tract

Test and Purpose	Client Preparation	Nursing Care During Test	Client Aftercare
Barium Enema			
• Radiographic examination of the large intestine after rectal instillation of barium sulfate (single-contrast technique) or barium sulfate and air (double-contrast technique) • Indicated for clients with altered bowel habits, lower abdominal pain, or the passage of blood, mucus, or pus in the stool • Assists in the diagnosis of colorectal cancer and inflammatory disease and in the detection of polyps, diverticula, and structural changes in the larger intestine	1. *Nursing alert:* Review the client's history for any evidence of ulcerative colitis or active GI bleeding, which would prohibit the use of the standard bowel preparation procedure of laxatives and enemas. Consult with the physician to determine a safe bowel preparation program. 2. Explain to the client: • Nature and purpose of the test (test takes 30 to 45 minutes) • Importance of following the prescribed dietary and bowel preparation because residual fecal material interferes with accurate test results a. Dietary modifications may include a low-residue diet for 1 to 3 days before the test, clear liquids the evening before the test, and increased water and clear liquid intake for 12 to 24 hours before the test. b. A cathartic is usually administered the afternoon or evening before the test and cleansing enemas (tap water) until clear (not to exceed three) the evening before the test or that morning. • That he or she will be on a tilting x-ray table and will need to assume different positions • That he or she may experience cramping pains or the urge to defecate as the barium (500 to 1500 mL) is instilled in the rectum; relaxation and deep breathing may ease this discomfort	• A technician in the radiology department cares for the client during the test.	• Before allowing the client to resume food and fluids, check to be sure that additional x-rays have not been ordered. • Encourage fluids to prevent dehydration. • Encourage rest because this test and the preceding bowel preparation exhaust most clients. • Administer the prescribed cathartic or cleansing enema to promote elimination of the barium and to prevent fecal impaction and bowel obstruction; instruct the client that barium will lighten the color of the stool. • If the barium is not eliminated within 2 to 3 days, notify the physician.

(continued)

Table 44-3 *(continued)*
Diagnostic Studies of the Gastrointestinal Tract

Test and Purpose	Client Preparation	Nursing Care During Test	Client Aftercare
Barium Enema			
	• That it is important to retain the entire barium enema to get good visualization (keeping the anal sphincter tightly contracted against the rectal tube helps) 3. Ensure that an informed consent is signed. 4. Assist the client into a hospital gown and prepare for transport to radiology following agency protocol.		

(Adapted from Fischbach, F. [1992]. *A manual of laboratory diagnostic tests* [4th ed., pp. 647-653, 734-736, 745-751]. Philadelphia: Lippincott.)

teristics for these problems are given in the accompanying box.

Bowel Elimination as the Etiology. Problems of bowel elimination also may affect other areas of human functioning. In the nursing diagnoses that follow, problems of bowel elimination are the etiology for other problems:

Altered Growth and Development related to parents' misconceptions about bowel and bladder training

Altered Nutrition: Less Than Body Requirements, related to loss of appetite from flatulence or impaction

Anxiety related to lack of voluntary control of fecal elimination and significant others' response to ostomy

Body Image Disturbance related to ostomy, need to wear disposable adult briefs

Fluid Volume Deficit related to prolonged diarrhea

Impaired Skin Integrity related to prolonged diarrhea, fecal incontinence

Ineffective Individual Coping related to inability to accept permanent ostomy

Knowledge Deficit: Bowel Training, related to no previous experience

Pain related to intestinal distention, prolonged constipation or impaction, fecal incontinence, hemorrhoids

Self-Care Deficit: Toileting, related to mobility deficit, weakness, confusion

Self-Esteem Disturbance related to need for assistance with toileting, fecal incontinence

Sexual Dysfunction related to perceived change in body image, lack of interest, loss of self-esteem

PLANNING: EXPECTED OUTCOMES

Nursing measures for clients without specific bowel elimination problems are directed toward the client's achievement of the following goals. The client will:

- Have a soft, formed bowel movement every 1 to 3 days without discomfort
- Explain the relation between bowel elimination and dietary fiber, fluid intake, and exercise
- Relate the importance of seeking medical evaluation if changes in stool color or consistency persist

Specific expected client outcomes for common bowel elimination problems are presented later in the chapter.

IMPLEMENTING

Promoting Regular Bowel Habits

Regular bowel habits can be promoted in both well and ill clients by attention to timing, positioning, privacy, nutrition, and exercise.

Timing. Once the nurse knows when a client usually experiences the urge to defecate (this occurs most often about an hour after meals when mass colonic peristalsis occurs), the nurse offers whatever assistance is needed to help the client to the bathroom, commode, or bedpan at this time. It is important not to schedule nursing care or treatments during this time. Many clients feel uncomfortable about requesting time for elimination. It is helpful for the nurse to communicate to all clients the importance to heed this natural urge and that postponing it only results in constipation and other problems..

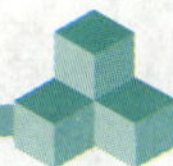

Nursing Diagnoses for Common Problems

Bowel Elimination

Problem	Related Factors	Sample Defining Characteristics
Constipation	• Decreased fiber in diet • Decreased fluid intake • Inactivity • Delaying defecation when urge is present • Abuse of laxatives • Use of constipating medications (antacids, narcotic analgesics [opioids], anticholinergics) • Change in routine • Pain associated with defecation	• "I feel bloated and know I have to move my bowels but I can't." • "Whenever I'm constipated I feel lethargic and lose my appetite." • Reports straining during defecation with little result • Passes small "marbles" of dry, hard stool • Decreased frequency • Decreased frequency of bowel sounds or changes in abdominal growling • Straining often results in small amount of bleeding from swollen external hemorrhoids • Reports feeling rectal fullness or pressure in rectum • Headache
Colonic Constipation	• Decreased fiber intake • Decreased fluid intake • Inactivity • Immobility • Lack of privacy • Abuse of laxatives • Stress • Change in routine • Metabolic alterations	• Decreased frequency • Passed small, hard, dry stool • Reports straining at stool • "I have pain when I move my bowels." • Reports feeling bloated • Palpable mass • Reports feeling rectal pressure
Perceived Constipation	• Culture • Family health beliefs • Faulty appraisal • Impaired thought processes	• Expectation of daily bowel movement with resulting abuse of laxatives, enemas, suppositories • Expected passage of stool at the same time every day
Diarrhea	• Food intolerance (coarse, greasy, or spicy foods) • Food or drug allergies • Abuse of laxatives • Alteration in normal bacterial flora of the intestine (antibiotic therapy) • Emotional stress • Intestinal infection • Colon disease and other diseases • Surgical alterations	• Loose liquid stools, increased frequency • Urgency with soiling • Reports of abdominal pain and cramping • Increased frequency of bowel sounds
Bowel Incontinence	• Gross constipation with impaction and subsequent overflow • Organic changes in neural innervation of the rectum • Local causes (inflammation, cancer of rectum, prolapsed anus, semifluid stool) • Extreme debilitation • Cognitive impairment	• Involuntary passage of stool (stool characteristics vary) • "I'm sorry, I couldn't get into the bathroom (or onto the bedpan) quickly enough." • "It came so fast I couldn't hold it back." • History of constipation with sudden development of oozing diarrhea stool

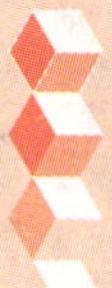

Helpscan

The following are resources for clients and health-care professionals:

- For information about ostomies and locations of support groups:
  United Ostomy Association
  36 Executive Park
  Suite 120
  Irvine, CA 92714-6744
  (800) 826-0826
- For information about cancer, its treatment, and local chapters:
  American Cancer Society
  777 Third Avenue
  New York, NY 10017
  (212) 371-2900

  Canadian Cancer Society
  10 Alcorn Avenue, Suite 200
  Toronto, ON M4V3B1
  (416) 961-7223

Positioning. The squatting position best facilitates defecation, but most clients routinely use a sitting position while leaning a bit forward. Most clients who are able to use the bedside commode or bathroom toilet have little difficulty assuming this posture, although they may need support. An elevated toilet seat may be ordered for clients with orthopedic problems who cannot lower themselves to a toilet seat.

Clients who need to use the bedpan in bed benefit from having the head of the bed elevated 30 degrees, unless this is contraindicated. This eliminates the hyperextension of the back that occurs when a client who is lying flat attempts to lift the hips onto the pan. Once the head of the bed is elevated, the client raises the hips by bending the knees, digging in the heels, and lifting the hips upward. An overhead trapeze may be helpful to clients with weak lower extremities. The head of the bed should not be raised more than 45 degrees because this makes it harder to lift the hips straight up. Positioning a client with a bedpan is described in Procedure 43-1. Many clients on bed rest appreciate having moistened hand-wipes at the bedside to substitute for handwashing after toileting. Bedpans should be emptied, cleaned, and returned to the client's bedside stand promptly.

Privacy. Because elimination is considered a private act by most people, nurses must respect the client's need to be alone while defecating, unless the client's weakness makes this impossible. Bedside drapes should be pulled around the client using a bedside commode or bedpan. Well clients who cannot defecate in a public restroom or strange environment may need assistance in developing a workable schedule of defecation that makes use of private toilet facilities.

Nutrition. Clients with elimination problems may need a dietary analysis to determine which foods and fluids are contributing to their problem and which may help in its treatment. General dietary recommendations to promote regular defecation include a fluid intake of 2000 to 3000 mL and a high-fiber intake. Water is recommended as the fluid of choice because other fluids (ie, coffee, tea, and juice) may have a diuretic effect instead (Stanley & Beare, 1995). Increasing fiber intake without sufficient fluid intake can result in severe gastrointestinal problems, including fecal impaction. Specific recommendations are as follows:

Constipation. Increase high-fiber foods (fruits, vegetables, whole-grain cereals and bread) and fluid intake (fruit juices, especially prune, and hot liquids). Research has demonstrated that bran and fluids are more effective than medications in reducing constipation (Beverley & Travis, 1992). Specific recommendations for bowel problems that affect older adults are included in the accompanying box.

Diarrhea. Prepare and store food properly. Avoid highly spiced foods or laxative-type foods such as raw fruits and vegetables. Encourage foods with low fiber content. Replace lost fluids and electrolytes with weak tea, water, bouillon, clear soup, gelatin; if diarrhea is severe, intravenous therapy may be needed.

Flatulence. Excessive formation of gases in the stomach or intestines is known as **flatulence**. When the gas is not expelled and accumulates in the intestinal tract, the condition is referred to as *intestinal distention* or *tympanites*. Gas-producing foods, such as beans, cabbage, onions, cauliflower, and beer, often predispose to flatulence and distention. Avoiding these foods may be helpful for people with ostomies who are concerned about odor.

Ostomies. Clients with ostomies need to experiment with their diets to see which foods result in the regular evacuation of a moderate amount of stool. A low-fiber diet usually is recommended. High-fiber foods, which could block the passage to the stoma, should be avoided; these include foods with skins, seeds, and shells (eg, raw fruits, popcorn, sunflower seeds, and nuts).

Exercise. Regular exercise improves gastrointestinal motility and aids in defecation. Well clients should be encouraged to incorporate three to five periods of regular exercise into each week's schedule. Ill clients should be ambulated as soon as possible and should be instructed about the relation between inactivity and constipation, distention, and impaction. Bedside exercises may be helpful for the immobilized client.

Focus on the Older Adult

Nursing Strategies for Bowel Elimination Problems Affecting Older Adults

Constipation

- Determine normal bowel pattern.
- Encourage drinking of six to eight glasses of water per day if medical condition permits.
- Implement regular physical exercise routine, even if bedridden.
- Discourage laxative use (particularly mineral oil, cascara, and castor oil) and recommend use of bulk-forming agents (ie, Metamucil) instead.
- Increase fiber in diet moderately and gradually.
- Evaluate drug regimen for medications that constipate (ie, iron, calcium supplements, antacids, and antidepressants).
- Teach client to avoid straining and the Valsalva maneuver.
- Encourage client to eat regular meals and avoid highly processed foods.
- Encourage remaining on the toilet or commode for 20-minute periods.
- Emphasize that bowel pattern may change and lack of a daily bowel movement does not always indicate constipation.

Diarrhea

- Carefully document the occurrence of diarrhea episodes.
- Assess for fecal impaction.
- Monitor for dehydration and fluid and electrolyte imbalance.
- Evaluate diet for possible cause:
  - Lactase deficiency
  - Food poisoning
  - Foods with high sorbitol content
  - Foods high in sugar
  - Raw seafood
  - Improperly cooked or refrigerated food
- Encourage use of yogurt or buttermilk if diet permits to restore normal intestinal flora.

Flatulence

- Avoid foods known to produce gas.
- Encourage slower eating and thorough chewing of food.
- Increase physical activity.

Clients with weak abdominal and perineal muscles who are using a bedpan may be helped by the following exercises:

Abdominal Settings: The client, lying in a supine position, tightens and holds the abdominal muscles for 6 seconds and then relaxes them. This should be repeated several times each waking hour.

Thigh Strengthening: The thigh muscles are flexed and contracted by slowly bringing the knees up to the chest—one at a time—and then lowering them to the bed. This also should be performed several times for each knee each waking hour.

Teaching About Cathartics, Laxatives, and Antidiarrheals

Constipation and diarrhea are further discussed in the Nursing Process in Clinical Practice section at the end of the chapter.

Cathartics and Laxatives

Cathartics and **laxatives** are drugs that induce emptying of the intestinal tract. Sometimes used interchangeably, cathartics exert a stronger effect on the intestines than laxatives. Some of these drugs, such as castor oil, cascara, senna, phenolphthalein, and bisacodyl (Dulcolax), act chemically by stimulating peristalsis. Others, such as magnesium sulfate and psyllium hydrophilic mucilloid (Metamucil), act by increasing the intestinal bulk, which promotes additional mechanical stimulation on the intestine. Still others, such as mineral oil and dioctyl sodium sulfosuccinate (Colace), act on the fecal material itself by softening it. Another frequently used laxative is milk of magnesia. It has antacid properties in small dosages and laxative properties when taken in larger doses (see Table 44-4 for a summary of the types of laxatives).

Laxatives have their rightful place in healthcare. They are necessary at times for people whose activity is limited or whose food intake is poor. They also are used for emptying the intestinal tract in preparation for surgical or diagnostic exploration. Their occasional use is not harmful for most people, but all efforts should be taken to prevent a person from becoming dependent on this means of stimulating defecation. Because many laxatives are available as nonprescription drugs, and because modern advertising promotes their use, many people take them frequently on their own initiative, whether they need them or not.

Most people are aware that laxatives have a chemical action and, therefore, should not be taken when there is abdominal pain because of the danger of intestinal pathology and subsequent harm from increased peristalsis. Although many people take laxatives because they believe they are constipated, most are unaware that habitual use of laxatives is the most common cause of chronic constipation.

Nurses often are in a position to help clients who abuse laxatives. Breaking the laxative habit, from both a physical and a psychologic viewpoint, is not easy for a person who has come to depend on laxatives. It often

Table 44-4
Classification of Laxatives

Type	Action	Advantages	Caution
Bulk-forming (eg, Metamucil)	Psyllium, grain, or synthetic product that causes stool to absorb water and swell, thus stimulating peristalsis	Usually acts within 24 hours	May interfere with absorption of calcium and iron and certain drugs Should not be given to bedridden clients or those with intestinal strictures May be expensive
Emollient/stool softener (eg, Colace)	Agents with detergent activity that allow water and fat to penetrate and lubricate the stool	Recommended for those who must avoid straining	Lubricant component of drug may interfere with absorption of fat-soluble vitamins
Lubricant (eg, mineral oil)	Lubricant absorbed from intestinal tract and softens stool, making it easier to pass	Usually effective within 8 hours	May interfere with absorption of fat-soluble vitamins Aspiration of drug may result in a lipid pneumonia
Stimulant (eg, Dulcolax)	Promotes peristalsis by irritating the intestinal mucosa or stimulating nerve endings in intestinal wall	Works more quickly than bulking agents	Most abused laxatives on the market Cause lazy bowel syndrome May affect absorption of vitamin D and calcium Not recommended for elderly clients due to prolonged action Alters electrolyte transport
Saline-osmotic (eg, Fleets)	Draws water into intestine and stimulates peristalsis	Use when rapid cleansing desired	Should not be used by elderly people Can produce dehydration Not recommended in clients with kidney disease or heart failure

requires a great deal of patience, support, and teaching by the nurse. The person also frequently needs to be helped with diet, fluid intake, activity, and regularity of habits.

Antidiarrheals

Antidiarrheal medications usually are reserved for treatment of chronic diarrhea and not recommended initially for acute episodes of diarrhea. Acute diarrhea may occur as the result of a viral or bacterial infection, reactions to medications, or alterations in diet, and is characterized by its sudden onset and a duration of several hours to several days. The duration of chronic diarrhea (more than 3 to 4 weeks) and the many possible causative agents (secondary disease states, surgery, laxative and alcohol abuse, and radiation and chemotherapeutic agents) usually necessitate pharmacologic intervention in addition to fluid and electrolyte replacement. Whatever the type of diarrhea, every effort should be made to identify and eliminate its underlying cause. The most effective nonspecific antidiarrheal medications are the opiates (eg, opium tincture [paregoric]) and related opiate derivatives (eg, loperamide [Imodium]), which act systemically to reduce intestinal hypermotility and slow peristalsis.

Abrams (1995) reviews some implications for use of the various antidiarrheal agents:

- Using opiates to treat diarrhea that is caused by poisons, toxins, or infections may actually prolong the diarrhea because it slows peristalsis and results in additional exposure of the intestinal mucosa to the causative agent. They may occasionally be used for acute, severe diarrhea.
- Dose requirements of opiates used for treatment of diarrhea usually are smaller than those for analgesia.
- The over-the-counter availability of loperamide (Imodium) requires client awareness of possible adverse effects and dependence with long-term use.
- Some antidiarrheal medications may cause drowsiness, and clients need to be cautioned about the hazards of driving or performing certain tasks when using these drugs.

- Kaolin–pectin preparations (Kaopectate) are available over-the-counter but their effectiveness for diarrhea is questionable. They may absorb nutrients and other antidiarrheal agents if given with them.

It is important for the nurse to focus on eliminating the cause of the diarrhea and replacing lost fluid as well as treating the symptoms. Some commercially available products, such as Gatorade, may prove helpful. Pillitteri (1995) suggests the BRAT routine (*b*ananas, *r*ice, *a*pplesauce, and *t*oast) as one protocol for providing a bland diet while replacing fluids and electrolytes during acute episodes of diarrhea in children. The Centers for Disease Control and Prevention also recommends oral rehydration therapy (ORT) for management of severe diarrhea in children. A cereal-based ORT has proven effective not only in rehydrating children but also in decreasing the duration of the diarrhea (Pediatric Update, 1994). Oral rehydration therapy for adults is cost-effective and replaces fluid loss. It is particularly important that fluid balance be maintained in older clients.

Decreasing Flatulence

In addition to avoiding irritating foods, other nursing interventions are helpful in decreasing flatus. Having the client move about in bed and walk promotes peristalsis and the escape of flatus. Reclining after meals should be avoided.

A rectal tube also may be used to help gas escape when ambulation has proven ineffective. The introduction of the tube helps to stimulate peristalsis and provides a passageway for the escape of flatus. The procedure for inserting a rectal tube is as follows:

- Use a 22 to 34 French tube for adults; smaller sizes are used for children.
- Position the client on his or her side, and drape the client properly when preparing to insert a rectal tube.
- Lubricate the rectal tube to reduce irritation to mucous membranes when inserting it.
- Separate the buttocks well so that the anus is in plain view, and introduce the rectal tube beyond the anal canal into the rectum for about 10 cm (about 4 inches). It may be inserted a bit further if it is noted that no flatus is being removed.
- Secure a dressing or waterproof pad to the end of the rectal tube. Or, place the end of the tube in a specimen container or urinal placed between the client's legs. These techniques allow any discharge that empties through the rectal tube to be caught.
- Leave the rectal tube in place for a short period—no longer than about 20 minutes; the tube no longer acts as a stimulant for peristalsis if left in place longer. If distention is not relieved, use the rectal tube intermittently every 2 to 3 hours, as necessary.
- Have the client assume various positions to help move flatus along the intestinal tract toward the anus. Gas is lighter than fluids and solids, and it will rise. Positions that help gas rise include lying on the abdomen, assuming the knee–chest position, and positioning the upper part of the body over the edge of the bed while the lower part rests across the bed. Do not use these positions if they are contraindicated or unsafe for the client.
- Confer with the physician if these measures bring no relief. An enema, a suppository, or a medication may be prescribed to help bring relief.

Emptying the Colon of Feces

Several methods are used to help promote elimination of feces—enemas, suppositories, oral intestinal lavage, and digital removal of stool.

Enemas

An **enema** is the introduction of a solution into the large intestine, usually for the purpose of removing feces. The instilled solution distends the intestine, may irritate intestinal mucosa, and thus increases peristalsis.

Types of Enemas. Enemas are classified as cleansing, retention, or return-flow enemas.

Cleansing Enemas. Cleansing enemas are given to remove feces from the colon. They are used for four common purposes:

- To relieve constipation or fecal impaction
- To prevent involuntary escape of fecal material during surgical procedures
- To promote visualization of the intestinal tract by x-ray film or instrument examination
- To help establish regular bowel function during a bowel training program

The most frequent types of solutions used for cleansing enemas are tap water, normal saline solution, soap solution, and hypertonic solution. These are described in Table 44-5. Hypotonic (tap water) and isotonic (normal saline solution) enemas are large-volume enemas that result in rapid colonic emptying. The large volumes of solution (adults, 500 to 1000 mL; infants, 150 to 250 mL) may present a danger to clients with weakened intestinal walls. These solutions often require special preparation and equipment. Hypertonic solution preparations are available commercially and are administered in smaller volumes (adult, 70 to 130 mL). These solutions draw water into the colon, which stimulates the defecation reflex. They may be contraindicated in clients for whom sodium retention is a problem.

Retention Enemas. Retention enemas are retained in the bowel for a prolonged period for different reasons.

Oil-retention enemas—lubricate the stool and intestinal mucosa, making defecation easier. About 150 to 200 mL of solution is administered to adults.

Carminative enemas—help to expel flatus from the rectum and provide relief from gaseous distention. Common solutions include the milk-and-molasses enema (equal parts) and the MGW enema (30 mL

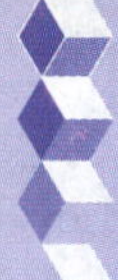

Through the Eyes of a Student

"Administer soapsuds enema." Oh please, not *my* patient, not *me*. Oh what that word meant, what I would have to do . . . and could I really do it? Oh sure I could . . . I just kept telling myself that, like the little train that could. I kept saying, "I think I can, I think I can."

I read up on how to correctly administer an enema. I was to give a soapsuds enema that I needed to prepare myself in a bag with long tubing attached; it resembled an IV bag. It was obvious that I needed some assistance—oh no, that meant my instructor would be in the room also. I didn't know what was worse.

I went through the procedure first with my instructor. Later I ventured into the patient's room and explained to him what I was going to do, thus preparing him for the ordeal.

I rolled the tip of the tubing in KY jelly and inserted it into the rectum. The patient moaned and groaned while my instructor lent her support. Then suddenly something went haywire: the patient started to get up, the tubing started to come out, and my instructor was yelling, "Clamp the tubing." By that time, it was too late. The tubing was out and squirting like a fountain, wetting the patient and giving me a bath. I eventually dragged myself out of the room after cleaning up the mess, not knowing whether to laugh or cry.

I really thought that was the worst day of my life, but I got over it and I look back and laugh, and so does my instructor.

—Frances Faries, Holy Family College, Philadelphia

of magnesium sulfate, 60 mL of glycerin, and 90 mL of warm water).

Medicated enema—used to administer medications that are absorbed through the rectal mucosa

Anthelmintic enemas—administered to destroy intestinal parasites

Nutritive enemas—administer fluids and nutrition rectally

Return-Flow Enemas. *Return-flow*, or *Harris flush, enemas* are occasionally prescribed to expel flatus. For an adult, 100 to 200 mL of a solution is instilled into the rectum and sigmoid colon and then the solution container is lowered so that the solution flows back into the container. This process is repeated five or six times, and the alternating flow of solution stimulates peristalsis and aids in the expelling of flatus. The procedure is terminated when abdominal distention is relieved. If the return solution becomes thick with feces, it is replaced by fresh solution.

Equipment. Commercially prepared enema kits include a flexible bottle containing hypertonic solution with an attached prelubricated firm tip about 5 to 7.5 cm (2 to 3 inches) in length. Its ease of use makes it particularly convenient in the home setting. Clients can readily administer their own enema in many instances.

For the tap water, saline solution, or soap solution enema, a container, rubber or plastic tubing with side openings near its distal end, a tubing clamp, lubricant, and the solution are necessary. Although the commercially prepared equipment is sterile, and any reusable equipment is sterilized between clients in a health agency, the procedure for administering an enema requires clean or medical asepsis technique, not sterile

Table 44-5
Commonly Used Enema Solutions

Solution	Amount	Action	Time to Take Effect	Adverse Effects
Tap water (hypotonic)	500–1000 mL	Distends intestine, increases peristalsis, softens stool	15 min	Fluid and electrolyte imbalance, water intoxication
Normal saline (isotonic)	500–1000 mL	Distends intestine, increases peristalsis, softens stool	15 min	Fluid and electrolyte imbalance, sodium retention
Soap	500–1000 mL (concentrate at 3–5 mL/1000 mL)	Distends intestine, irritates intestinal mucosa, softens stool	10–15 min	Rectal mucosa irritation or damage
Hypertonic	70–130 mL	Distends intestine, irritates intestinal mucosa	5–10 min	Sodium retention
Oil (mineral, olive, or cottonseed oil)	150–200 mL	Lubricates stool and intestinal mucosa	30 min	

technique. Disposable gloves protect the caregiver from exposure to blood, body substances, and microorganisms.

Client Preparation. Because the enema is a common procedure, many clients understand its use and how it is administered. Other clients who have not experienced an enema before need an explanation of its purpose, what they can expect, and how they can participate. The procedure offers an excellent opportunity for health teaching because many people are not familiar with the functioning of the intestinal tract. Failure to observe one or more of these principles may be responsible for the clients' considering the procedure a disagreeable one.

A reclining position during the enema is recommended, however, a client with a respiratory disorder may need the head of the bed elevated slightly. Results are usually ineffective when an enema is given to a person in Fowler's position. The solution remains in the rectum and results in distention and rapid expulsion with minimal cleansing effect (Shollenberger, 1994).

Most clients think that solutions are to be expelled as soon as possible. When a solution is to be retained, care should be taken to have the client understand this.

Administering an Enema Using a Large Volume of Solution. The procedure for administering a cleansing enema using either a large volume of solution or a commercially prepared solution is described in Procedure 44-1.

Administering an Enema Using a Hypertonic Solution. Administering a cleansing enema using a hypertonic solution differs somewhat from the procedure described in Procedure 44-1.

- The equipment is included in the commercially prepared sets. The only additional equipment needed is the bedpan for the bedridden client and a disposable waterproof pad to protect bed linens.
- It is unnecessary to warm the hypertonic solution. Administer it at room temperature, and warm it only if it is very cold.
- The side-lying position usually is used. The knee–chest position helps to distribute the solution throughout the lower intestinal tract and is recommended if the client is able to assume it. Lubrication of the rectal tips is recommended, even though they are prelubricated.
- The solution is forced into the rectum by applying gentle pressure on the collapsible solution container. It should take 1 to 2 minutes to administer the enema.
- The hypertonic enema solution (Fleet enema) should be administered cautiously to a client with hemorrhoids. The rigid tip may tear fragile rectal mucosa that is enlarged and inflamed, causing pain, torn rectal tissue, and necrosis. A rectal exam and generous lubrication are recommended before inserting the enema tip. A tap water or saline enema may be a better choice for this client (Schmelzer & Wright, 1993).

Administering an Oil-Retention Enema. The procedure for giving an oil enema differs from that of giving a cleansing enema in certain respects:

- A small rectal tube is used. The small size helps to reduce intestinal contractions so that the client can retain the oil more easily. Oil enemas are available in commercial kits similar to those for the hypertonic-solution enema. The kits contain a small rectal tube.
- Oil is given at body temperature to minimize muscle contractions caused by a warmer or cooler solution.
- The client should be instructed to retain the oil for at least 30 minutes for best cleansing results.

Rectal Suppositories

A **suppository** is a conical or oval solid substance shaped for easy insertion into a body cavity and designed to melt at body temperature. Various rectal suppositories are available. Some act as fecal softeners, others have direct action on the nerve endings in the rectal mucosa, and some liberate carbon dioxide when moistened. Fecal softeners are useful when the stool is very hard; substances that stimulate the rectal nerves are helpful for people with weak muscle tone or poor innervation. The carbon dioxide suppositories liberate about 200 mL of gas, which causes distention, thus producing stimulation and elimination impulses (see the accompanying box).

Oral Intestinal Lavage

An oral solution such as GoLYTELY or Colyte can be used to cleanse the intestine of feces. This solution can be administered prior to diagnostic tests that require a clear bowel for visualization purposes or as a "bowel prep" before intestinal surgery. Tap water is added to the powder in a 4-L container and mixed thoroughly. Recommended intake is one glass every 10 to 15 minutes until finished. Evacuation of feces usually begins within 1 hour after the first glass and is completed within 4 to 6 hours. As with an enema, a clear return is an indication that the bowel preparation is complete. A clear diet for 24 hours prior to taking this solution lessens the time needed for completion of the bowel prep, but potassium replacement may be required before surgery because of the limited potassium in a clear diet. The solution has a slightly salty taste and is easier to tolerate if it is cold and consumed quickly. Older clients require careful assessment because they are more prone to electrolyte imbalances (Murray, Preuss, & Schultz, 1992).

Digital Removal of Stool

A **fecal impaction** is prolonged retention or an accumulation of fecal material that forms a hardened mass in the rectum. It is common for a fecal impaction to prevent the passage of normal stools. Small amounts of fluid may go around the impacted mass. In fact, liquid fecal

(text continues on page 1294)

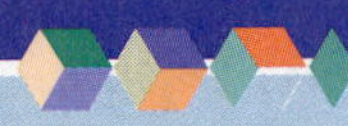

PROCEDURE 44-1

Administering a Cleansing Enema

Equipment

Disposable enema set
Water-soluble lubricant
Solution as ordered by physician:
Temperature:
For adult—105°–110°F (40°–43°C)
For children—100°F (37.7°C)
Amount: Will vary, depending on type of solution, age of the person, and the client's ability to retain the solution. Average cleansing enema for an adult may range from 750 to 1000 mL.
Necessary additives (soap, salt, and so forth)
Bath thermometer
Waterproof pad
Bath blanket
Bedpan and toilet tissue
IV pole
Disposable gloves
Paper towel
Washcloth, soap, and towel, or Handi-wipes

Action	Rationale
1. Assemble the necessary equipment. Warm solution in amount ordered, and check temperature with a bath thermometer if available. If tap water is used, adjust temperature as it flows from faucet.	Organization facilitates performance of task. If bath thermometer is not available, warm to room temperature or slightly higher, and test on inner wrist.
2. Explain the procedure to the client and plan where he or she will defecate. Have a bedpan, commode, or nearby bathroom ready for his use.	The client is better able to relax and cooperate if he or she is familiar with the procedure and knows everything is in readiness when the urge to defecate is felt. Defecation usually occurs within 5 to 15 minutes.
3. Wash your hands.	Handwashing deters the spread of microorganisms.
4. Add enema solution to container. Release the clamp and allow fluid to progress through tube before reclamping.	This causes any air to be expelled from the tubing. Although allowing air to enter the intestine is not harmful, it may further distend the intestine.
5. Position waterproof pad under the client.	This protects bed linen.
6. Provide for client's privacy. Position and drape the client on the left side (Sims' position) with anus exposed or on the back, as dictated by client comfort and condition.	The client's comfort and warmth help him or her relax. The exact position of the reclining person has not been found to alter results of an enema significantly.
7. Put on disposable gloves.	This protects the nurse from microorganisms in the feces.
8. Elevate the solution so that it is 45 cm (18 inches) above the level of the client's anus. Plan to give the solution slowly over a period of 5 to 10 minutes. The container may be hung on an IV pole or held in the nurse's hands at the proper height.	Gravity forces the solution to enter the intestine. The amount of pressure determines the rate of flow and pressure exerted on the intestinal wall. Giving the solution too quickly causes rapid distention and pressure in the intestine, resulting in too rapid expulsion of the solution, poor defecation, or damage to the mucous membrane.
9. Generously lubricate the end of the rectal tube for 5 to 7 cm (2–3 inches). A disposable enema set may have a prelubricated rectal tube.	This facilitates passage of the rectal tube through the anal sphincter and prevents injury to the mucosa.
10. Lift the buttock to expose the anus. Slowly and gently insert the rectal tube 7 to 10 cm (3–4 inches). Direct it at an angle pointing toward the umbilicus.	Good visualization of the anus helps prevent injury to tissues. The anal canal is about 2.5 to 5 cm (1–2 inches) in length. The tube should be inserted past the internal sphincter. Further insertion may damage intestinal mucous membrane. The suggested angle follows the normal intestinal contour. Slow insertion of the tube minimizes spasms of the intestinal wall and sphincters.

PROCEDURE 44-1 *(continued)*

Administering a Cleansing Enema

Action	Rationale

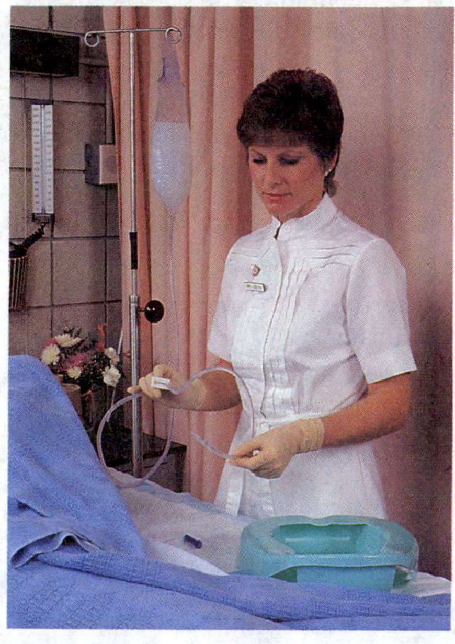

Action 8: Preparing to administer the enema.

Action	Rationale
11. If the tube meets resistance while inserting it, permit a small amount of solution to enter, withdraw the tube slightly and then continue to insert it. Do not force entry of the tube. Ask the client to take several deep breaths.	Resistance may be due to spasms of the intestine or failure of the internal sphincter to open. The solution may help to reduce spasms and relax the sphincter, thus making continued insertion of the tube safe. Forcing a tube may injure the intestinal wall. Taking deep breaths helps relax the anal sphincter.
12. Introduce the solution slowly over a period of 5 to 10 minutes. Hold tubing all the time that solution is being instilled. Commercial preparations may be administered by compressing container with hands, according to package directions.	Introducing the solution slowly helps prevent rapid distention of the intestine and a desire to defecate.

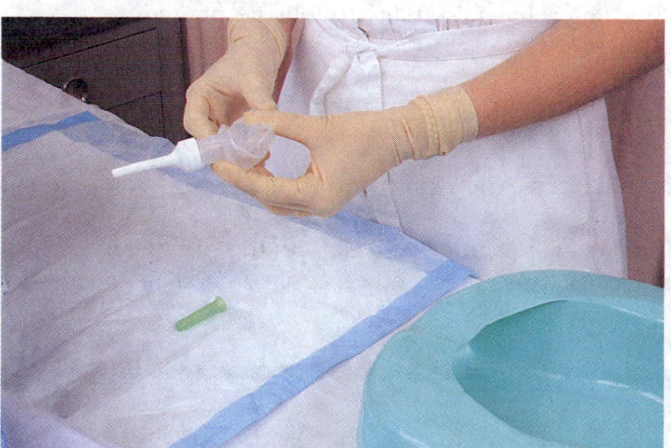

Action 12: Technique for compressing Fleets enema container.

(continued)

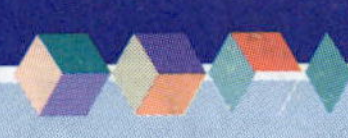

PROCEDURE 44-1 *(continued)*

Administering a Cleansing Enema

Action	Rationale
13. Clamp the tubing or lower the container if the client has the desire to defecate or cramping occurs. Client also may be instructed to take small, fast breaths or to pant.	These techniques help relax muscles and prevent the expulsion of the solution prematurely.
14. After solution has been given, clamp the tubing and remove the tube. Have paper towel ready to receive tube as it is withdrawn. Have the client retain the solution until the urge to defecate becomes strong, usually in about 5 to 15 minutes.	This amount of time usually allows muscle contractions to become sufficient to produce good results.
15. Remove disposable gloves from inside out and discard.	This protects the nurse from contact with any microorganisms.
16. When the client has a strong urge to defecate, place him or her in a sitting position on a bedpan or assist to a commode or to the bathroom.	The sitting position is most natural and facilitates the act of defecation.
17. Record the character of the stool and the client's reaction to the enema. Remind the client not to flush commode before nurse inspects results of enema.	The nurse needs to observe and record the results. Additional enemas may be necessary if physician has ordered enemas "until clear."
18. Assist client if necessary with cleaning of anal area. Offer washcloth, soap, and water to wash client's hands.	Deters spread of microorganisms.
19. Leave the client clean and comfortable. Care for the equipment properly.	There is abundant growth of bacteria in the intestine, which can be spread to others when equipment is not properly cared for.
20. Wash your hands.	Handwashing deters the spread of microorganisms.

Age Considerations

Infirm or elderly clients who are unable to retain the enema solution should receive the enema while on the bedpan in the supine position. For comfort, the head of the bed can be elevated 30 degrees if necessary and pillows used appropriately. Disposable gloves protect the hands as the enema is being expelled.

Parents should be encouraged to assist in relieving anxiety and encouraging cooperation when young children require enemas.

Modify amount of solution according to client's ability to tolerate procedure and size of client.

Home Care Considerations

Give enema in area that is as close to bathroom as possible. If using bedpan or commode, have it readily accessible.

Inform client about availability of commercially prepared solutions and equipment.

Special Considerations

The limit for "enemas until clear" usually is three. Check with the physician before continuing with additional enemas because fluid and electrolyte imbalance can occur.

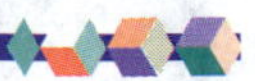

seepage and no passage of normal feces are symptomatic of the existence of an impaction.

If a client with a fecal impaction is unable to expel the fecal mass voluntarily, and oil and cleansing enemas fail to break up the mass, it is necessary to break up the impaction manually. A physician's order is required. This procedure may cause great discomfort to the client and cause irritation of the rectal mucosa and bleeding. The nurse also needs to be aware that digital removal of a fecal mass can stimulate the vagus nerve,

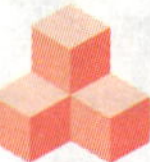

Guidelines for Nursing Care

Inserting a Rectal Suppository

- Use a glove for protection while inserting the suppository.
- Have the client lie on either side, and pie-fold top linens over him or her.
- Lubricate the suppository and fingertips to reduce irritation on intestinal mucosa while inserting the suppository.
- Separate the buttocks and then have the client relax by breathing through the mouth while the suppository is inserted.
- Introduce the suppository well beyond the internal sphincter (4 inches for adults and 2 inches for children and infants) so that the suppository is in the rectum, where its effect is desired.
- Avoid embedding the suppository in the fecal mass. Correct placement when there is stool in the rectum is between the stool and the rectal mucosa.
- Be sure the client understands that he or she is to retain the suppository, usually for 30 to 45 minutes after insertion.
- Encourage the client to walk about if ambulatory; this often helps promote peristalsis.

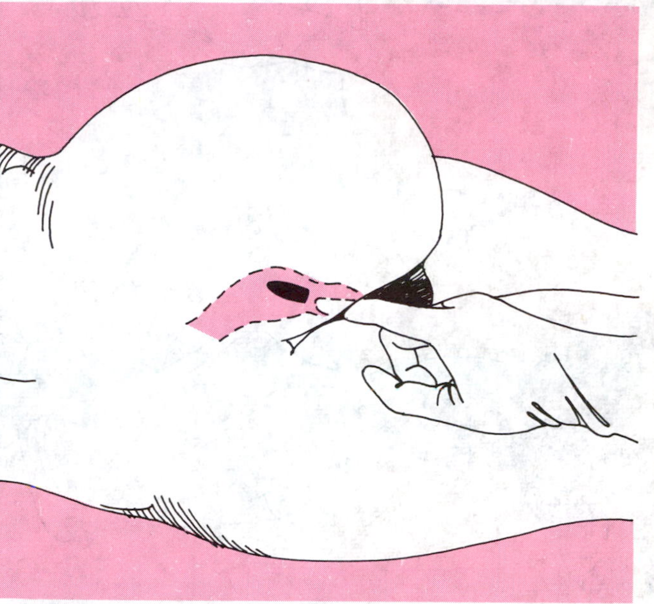

resulting in a slowed heart rate. If this occurs, the procedure should be terminated immediately and the physician notified. The following techniques are recommended:

- Have a second person assist with the procedure. The second person can assure and comfort the client while the first person works to break up the mass.
- Place the client in a side-lying position for the convenience of the nurses.
- Place a bedpan in the bed so that pieces of removed feces can be deposited into it.
- Drape the client to preserve privacy yet provide easy access.
- Use clean gloves for the procedure; the intestinal tract is not sterile.
- Lubricate the forefinger generously to reduce irritating the rectum, and insert the finger *gently* into the anal canal. The presence of the finger added to the mass tends to cause discomfort for the client when work is not done slowly and gently. Instruct the client to bear down, if possible, while extracting feces to ease in removal. To minimize discomfort, a local anesthetic may be used. Weidner (1992) reports the following technique:
  - Place 1 to 2 mL of lidocaine on the gloved forefinger into the rectum as far as possible, remove immediately, and wait 5 minutes before proceeding with the digital removal. This should not be attempted without a physician's order.
- Work the finger around and into the hardened mass to break it up and then remove pieces of it.
- Remove the impaction at intervals if it is severe. This helps to avoid discomfort as well as irritation, which can injure intestinal mucosa.
- Use an oil-retention enema as necessary. The enema may be given before attempts are made to break up and remove an impaction digitally. Or, it may be ordered after digital attempts fail. A cleansing enema often is ordered after an oil-retention enema.

Figure 44-5 demonstrates the procedure for removal of fecal impaction. Many clients find that a sitz bath or tub bath after this procedure soothes the irritated perineal area.

Managing Fecal Incontinence

Caring for a client who is incontinent of feces poses a nursing challenge. Not only is it embarrassing for the client, it also places him or her at risk for skin breakdown. Refer to the Nursing Process in Clinical Practice section for additional information on fecal incontinence.

Fecal Incontinence Pouch

In many healthcare agencies, the rectal indwelling catheter has been used for clients with uncontrollable diarrhea. Relatively little research supports the safety of this procedure. Some nurses claim that the rectal in-

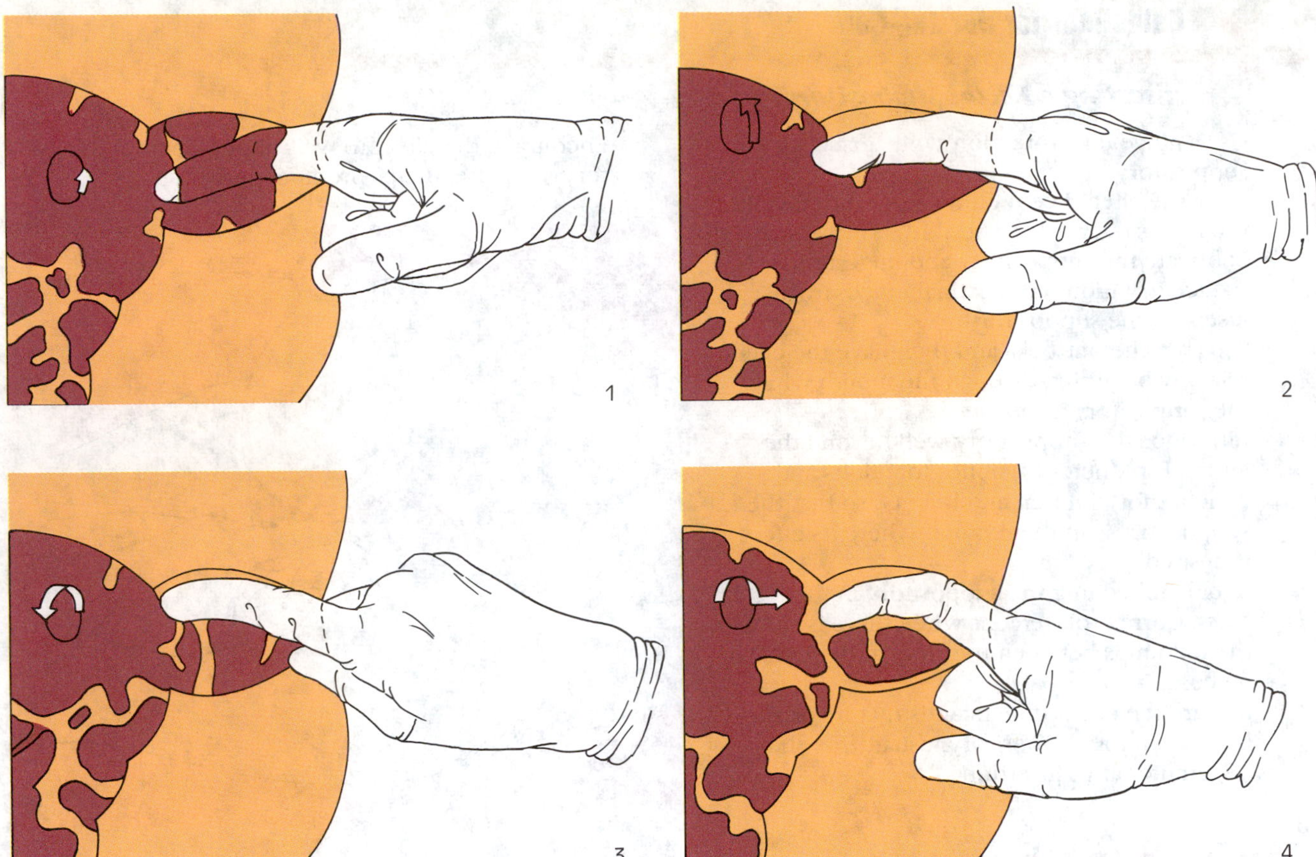

Figure 44-5
Digital removal of fecal impaction.

dwelling catheter stimulates sensory nerve fibers in the rectum, thus increasing peristalsis and worsening diarrhea. Others are concerned about the danger of rectal perforation and the development of mucosal necrosis. Most experts agree that indwelling rectal catheters should not be used to manage large volumes of diarrhea.

An alternative measure to protect perianal skin from repeated episodes of fecal incontinence is the fecal incontinence pouch. This device can be secured around the anal opening and attached to gravity drainage, allowing liquid stool to accumulate in a collection bag. It is best applied before the perianal area becomes excoriated, but a skin barrier is effective if this has already occurred. Wolf (1995) summarizes a protocol for managing this challenging problem that entails use of a fecal incontinence pouch and a nasopharyngeal airway or nasal trumpet. These soft, thin, pliable airways can be safely inserted into the rectum and a fecal incontinence pouch is applied to the area to collect the liquid feces.

Nursing responsibilities include careful assessment and documentation of the perianal skin condition on a regular basis and attentive management of the drainage system. The pouch should be changed at least every 72 hours, or sooner if it is not intact or leakage has occurred. Families, particularly, may need explanation and support to understand the benefits of this system.

Designing and Implementing Bowel Training Programs

Clients with a history of chronic constipation and impaction and those who are incontinent of stool may benefit from a **bowel training program**. The purpose of this program is to manipulate factors within the person's control (food and fluid intake, exercise, time for defecation) to produce the elimination of a soft, formed stool at regular intervals without laxative support. This effort to regain bowel control may be initiated in the health-care setting or implemented in the client's home. Steps in a bowel training program include the following:

- Explain the program and its aim to the client in an effort to enlist the client's full participation.
- Assess the client's bowel elimination patterns and identifying factors that promote or hinder defecation.
- Design a plan to modify contributing lifestyle variables: (1) increase fluid intake to 2500 to 3000 mL—include hot drinks or fruit juices known to promote peristalsis for the client; (2) increase the fiber content of the diet; and (3) increase exercise if possible.
- Start the program with a clean bowel (rectal examination for impaction—remove if present).
- Maintain a daily training routine for 14 to 21 days until a regular pattern of defecation without laxatives is established:

- Administer a cathartic suppository (eg, Dulcolax) to stimulate peristalsis 30 minutes before the client's usual defecation time (note this in plan).
- Assist the client to the bathroom or commode or onto a bedpan. Note the time it usually takes for the suppository to work and when the client has an urge to evacuate (usually 15 minutes to an hour).
- Allow the client privacy and ample time for evacuation (usually 20 to 30 minutes is adequate); avoid both rushing the client and abandoning the client on the bedpan or commode for prolonged periods.
- Share the client's success and offer positive verbal reinforcement and encouragement; refrain from criticizing the client who is unsuccessful.

- Communicate that patience may be necessary before regular elimination patterns resume—project a "can do" mentality.

When the client has established a pattern of regular defecation, continue to offer assistance with toileting at the successful time but discontinue use of the laxative.

A protocol developed by students and staff members at a long-term care facility to implement a bowel management program for residents (Karam & Nies, 1994) emphasized an increase in the intake of fiber and fluids coupled with additional exercise, ambulation, and toileting measures. Results of the research indicated that laxative use decreased and the number of spontaneous bowel movements increased.

Meeting Needs of Clients With Bowel Diversions

Sometimes surgical procedures are required to create an opening into the abdominal wall for fecal elimination. The intestinal mucosa is brought out to the abdominal wall, and a **stoma** is formed by suturing the mucosa to the skin. The word **ostomy** is a general term for an opening into the body; it usually is used to refer to an opening created for the excretion of body wastes. An **ileostomy** allows liquid fecal content from the ileum of the small intestine to be eliminated through the stoma. A **colostomy** permits formed feces from the colon to exit through the stoma. Figure 44-6 shows the location of an ileostomy and variously placed colostomies. A *continent ileostomy* is an alternative to the traditional surgical procedure. An internal pouch is created that the client accesses through a nipple-like valve constructed from the ileum on the abdominal wall. An advantage is that the client is not required to wear an external collection device, but malfunctions with the valve occur frequently and use of this type of procedure is limited at this time.

An ileostomy or a colostomy may be either temporary or permanent. Temporary ostomies are done to allow the intestine to repair itself after inflammatory disease, some types of intestinal surgery, or injury. Permanent ostomies are done as the result of debilitating intestinal diseases or cancer of the colon or rectum. Clinical texts further discuss pathophysiologic conditions for which ostomies are required.

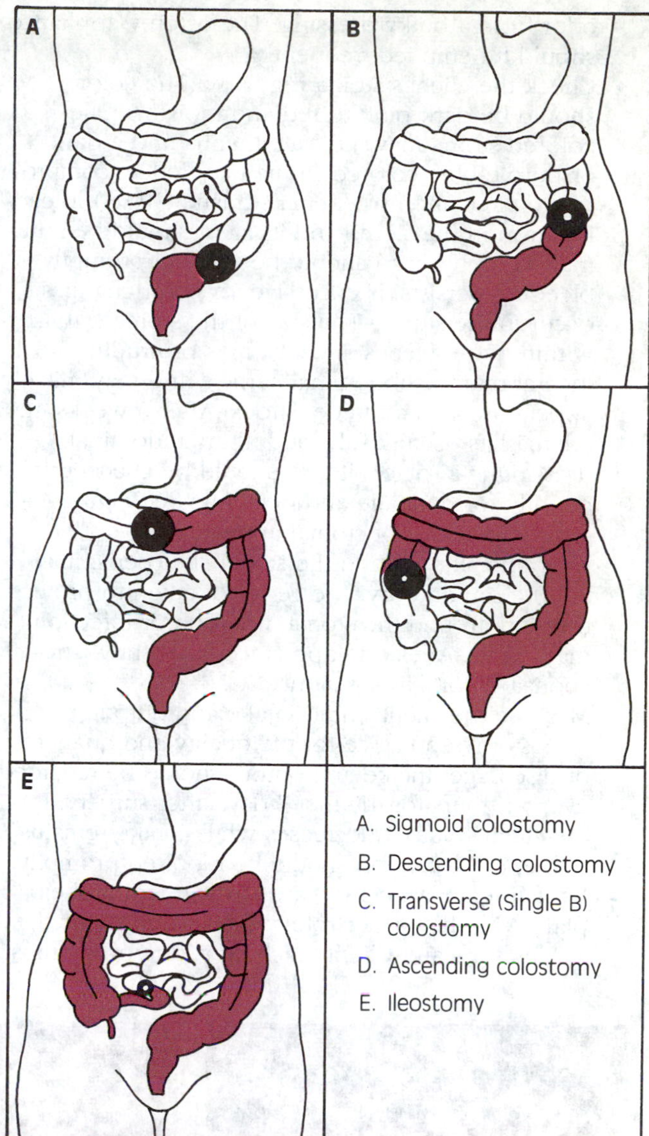

Figure 44-6
Location of various colostomies and the location of an ileostomy.

Colostomy and Ileostomy Care. The client with an ostomy needs physical and psychologic support both preoperatively and postoperatively. This support can come from people who are close to the client as well as from members of the health team and from people who have had similar experiences. The ostomy requires specific physical care for which the nurse is initially responsible. The following guidelines help to promote physical and psychologic comfort for the ostomy client:

- Keep the client as free of odors as possible. The application of a temporary appliance after surgery or during the time of the first dressing change postoperatively can eliminate much of the fecal odor from a bulky dressing. The ostomy appliance should be emptied frequently.

- Check the client's stoma regularly. The color should be dark pink to red and moist. A pale-colored stoma may indicate anemia and a dark or purple-blue colored stoma may reflect compromised circulation or edema (Krasner, 1993). Bleeding around the stoma and its stem should be minimal. The physician should be notified promptly if bleeding persists, is excessive, or color changes occur in the stoma. The size of the stoma stabilizes within 4 to 6 weeks. Most stomas protrude ½ to 1 inch above the abdominal surface and may initially appear swollen and edematous. After 6 weeks, the edema has usually subsided. If an abdominal dressing is in place, it also should be checked frequently for drainage and bleeding. See Figure 44-7 for comparisons of stomal appearance.
- Keep the skin around the stoma site (peristomal area) clean and dry. If care is not taken to protect the skin around the stoma, irritation or infection may occur. A leaking appliance frequently is responsible for skin erosion.
- Measure the client's fluid intake and output. Check the ostomy appliance for the quality and quantity of discharge. Intake and output should be recorded every 4 hours for the first 3 days after surgery. If the client's output decreases while intake remains stable, the condition should be reported promptly.
- Explain each aspect of care to the client and explain what his or her role will be when he or she begins self-care. Client teaching is one of the most important aspects of colostomy care and should include family members when appropriate.
- Encourage the client to participate in care and to look at the ostomy. It is expected that the client will experience emotional depression during the early postoperative period. The nurse can help the client to cope by listening, explaining, and being available and supportive. A visit from a representative of the local ostomy support group may be helpful. The client usually begins to accept his or her altered body image when he or she is willing to look at the stoma, makes neutral or positive statements concerning the ostomy, and expresses interest in learning self-care.

Changing the Ostomy Appliance. The ostomy appliance should protect the skin, collect the fecal discharge, and control odor. For the first few days after surgery, most clients wear an open-ended appliance that allows for drainage of fecal material without removing the appliance. It is unusual to see any output from a colostomy until normal peristalsis returns (2 to 5 days). An ileostomy drains within 24 to 48 hours because of the liquid contents in the small intestine. A pouch that can be drained should be emptied when it is one-third to one-half full and replaced every 3 to 7 days. Nondrainable pouches require removal and changing when they are one-half full. The drainable pouch is cleansed by rinsing the inside with tepid water and wiping the lower 2 inches of the pouch with tissue to remove any fecal material. Types of ostomy equipment are illustrated in

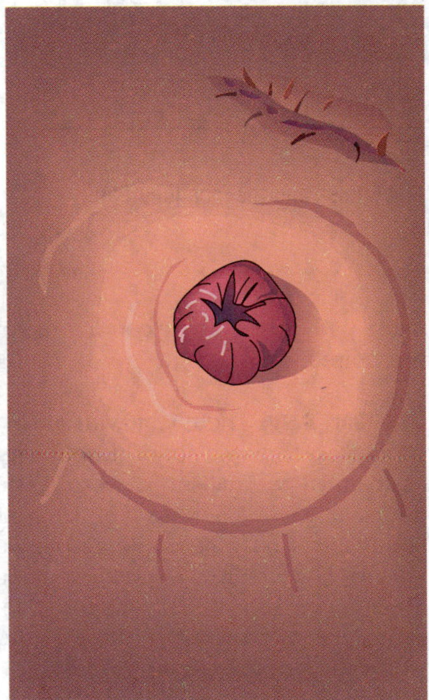

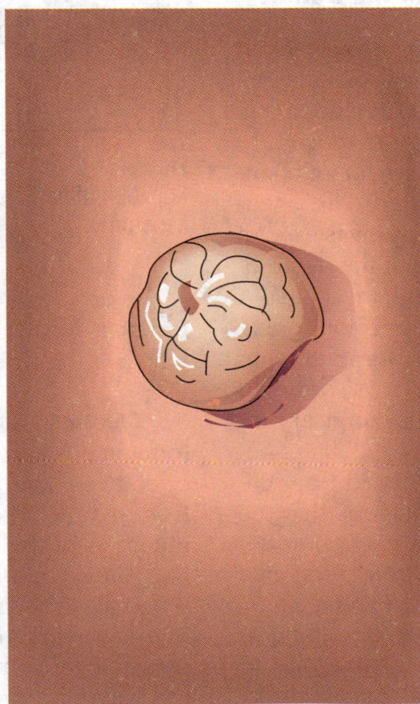

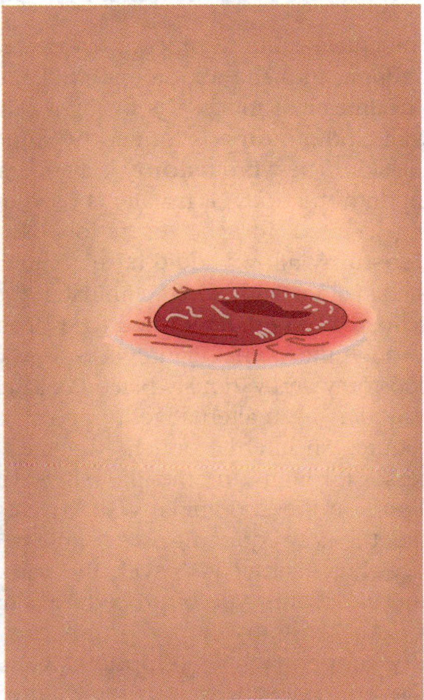

Figure 44-7
Comparisons of stomal appearance. (**A**) Normal-appearing stoma is bright red, moist, and perfectly round. (**B**) A pale stoma indicates severe anemia in this colostomy client. (**C**) Eroded skin around the area may lead to a flush stoma.

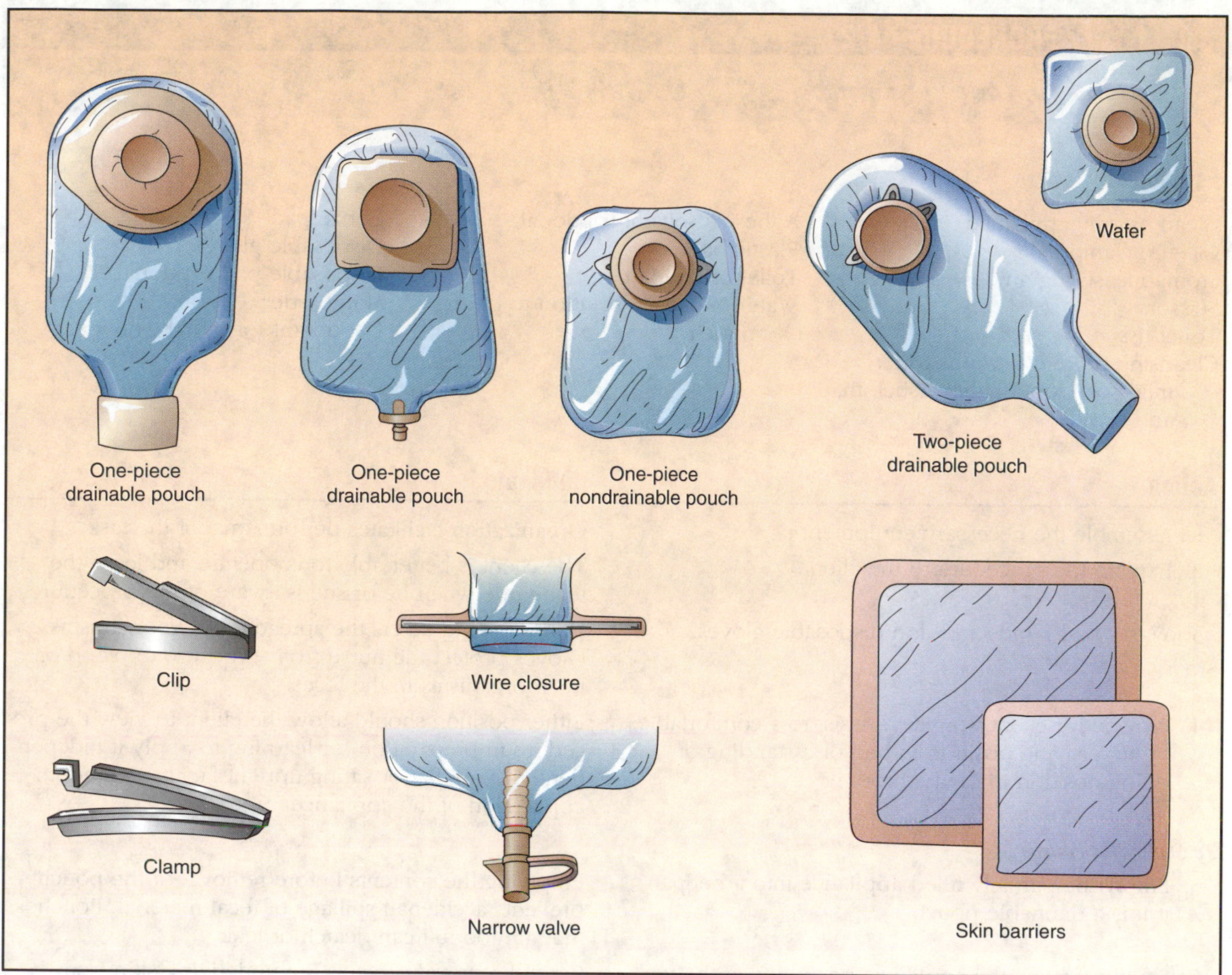

Figure 44-8
Examples of types of ostomy pouches, closures, and skin barriers. This equipment comes in various models and sizes. Convex pouches, belts, and other devices to prevent leaks and irritation are also available.

Figure 44-8, while changing or emptying an ostomy appliance is shown in Procedure 44-2.

Colostomy Irrigation. Ileostomies are not irrigated because the fecal content of the ileum is liquid, and cannot be controlled. Irrigations may be used to help regulate some colostomies, typically those in the lower right portion of the colon. Various factors, such as the site of the colostomy in the colon and the client's and physician's preferences, determine whether or not a colostomy is irrigated.

If an irrigation is to be done, the nurse should familiarize the client with the technique to be used. The nurse should explain the procedure, demonstrate the equipment, and explain how the return fluid can be directed into a bedpan, commode, or toilet bowl. It also may be helpful to have a family member learn the irrigation techniques in case there are times when the client cannot do the irrigation. The procedure for irrigating a colostomy is similar to that for administering an enema, except that the irrigating catheter is inserted into an abdominal stoma instead of into the anus. A commercially obtained irrigation set usually has all the equipment needed and comes with explicit directions.

In many health agencies, ostomy care, colostomy irrigations, and client teaching are done by specially trained enterostomal therapists.

Long-Term Ostomy Care. The client can live an active and useful life with an ostomy. He or she should be aware of community resources available for assistance, such as home healthcare nurses, special clinics, and ostomy support groups. The client should be encouraged to seek medical follow-up care on a regular basis.

Ostomy clients are encouraged to avoid foods high in fiber content initially, as well as any other foods that cause them to have diarrhea or excessive amounts of fla-

(text continues on page 1301)

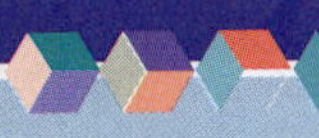

PROCEDURE 44-2

Changing or Emptying an Ostomy Appliance

Equipment

Clean ostomy appliance
Closure clamp
Stoma measuring guide
Scissors
Toilet tissue
Cleansing products (warm water, mild soap [optional], washcloth, and towel)
Adhesive solvent (optional)
Plastic bag
Toilet or bedpan
Water or special solution to clean pouch
Gauze pad
Disposable gloves
Disposable pad (optional)
Skin barrier (optional)
Deodorant for pouch (optional)

Action	Rationale
1. Assemble the necessary equipment.	Organization facilitates performance of the task.
2. Explain the procedure to the client.	The client is better able to cooperate and learn the technique when he or she is aware of the procedure.
3. Wash your hands and don disposable gloves.	Handwashing deters the spread of microorganisms. Gloves protect the nurse from exposure to blood or microorganisms in the feces.
4. Provide for client's privacy. Assist to a comfortable sitting or lying position in bed or a standing or sitting position in the bathroom.	Either position should allow the client to view the procedure in preparation for learning to apply it independently. Lying flat or sitting upright facilitates smooth application of the appliance.
To Change the Pouch	
5. Empty the partially filled appliance into a bedpan if it is a drainable pouch.	Emptying the contents before removal of the pouch prevents accidental spillage of fecal material. Pouches that are too full can detach or leak.
6. Slowly remove the appliance beginning at the top while keeping the abdominal skin taut. If any resistance is felt, use warm water or the adhesive solvent to facilitate removal. Discard the disposable pouch in the plastic bag.	Careful removal protects the underlying skin from damage and minimizes discomfort for the client. Solvent is rarely necessary to ease removal of the pouch.
7. Use toilet tissue to remove any excess stool from the stoma. Cover stoma with a gauze pad. Gently wash and pat dry the peristomal skin. Mild soap or a cleansing agent may be used according to agency policy.	Soap may not be recommended because it may be irritating to the peristomal skin. Toilet tissue, used gently, will not damage the stoma. The gauze absorbs any drainage from the stoma while the skin is being prepared.
8. Assess the appearance of the peristomal skin and stoma. A moist, reddish-pink stoma is considered normal.	Any change in normal appearance may indicate either anemia (pale stoma) or altered circulation (bluish-purple color) and the physician should be notified.
9. Apply the skin barrier and appliance together (wafer or disc style): • Select size for stoma opening by using the measurement guide (Fig. 44-9). • Trace same size circle on the back and center of the skin barrier. • Use scissors to cut an opening ¼- to ⅛-inch larger than stoma.	Placing both the skin barrier disc and the appliance together over the stoma makes application easier for the client. The opening is cut slightly larger to prevent irritation to the stoma as peristalsis occurs. Smooth application of the pouch prevents escape of odor and feces. The warmth from the nurse's hands facilitates a tight seal.

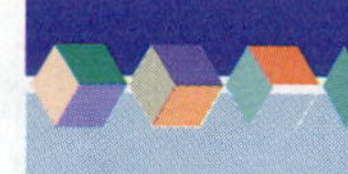

PROCEDURE 44-2 *(continued)*

Changing or Emptying an Ostomy Appliance

Action	Rationale
• Remove the backing to expose sticky side. • Remove gauze pad covering stoma. • Ease barrier and pouch over the stoma and gently press onto skin while smoothing out creases or wrinkles. Hold the pouch in place for 5 minutes.	
10. Close the pouch if it is drainable by folding the end upward and using a clamp or clip (see manufacturer's directions).	A tightly sealed appliance will not leak and cause embarrassment and discomfort for the client.
To Empty the Pouch	
11. Plan to drain the pouch when it is ⅓ to ½ full. Remove clamp and fold the end of the pouch upward like a cuff.	Allowing the pouch to fill more than half-way increases its weight and makes it more likely to separate or loosen from the skin. Creating a cuff before emptying prevents additional soilage and odor.
12. Empty contents into bedpan or toilet. Rinse pouch with tepid water or water mixed with a drop of mouthwash administered via a squeeze bottle.	Rinsing the inside of the pouch provides a cleaner appearance and minimizes odor.
13. Wipe the lower 2 inches of the pouch with toilet tissue.	Drying the lower section of the pouch removes any additional fecal material.
14. Uncuff the edge of the pouch and apply the clip or clamp.	The edge of the pouch should remain clean. The clamp secures closure of the appliance.
15. Dispose of used equipment according to agency policy. Remove gloves and wash hands.	Proper disposal of equipment and handwashing prevent contamination from microorganisms.
16. Document appearance of stoma, condition of peristomal skin, characteristics of drainage (amount, color, consistency, unusual odor), and client's reaction to the procedure.	Careful documentation facilitates continuity of care.

Special Considerations

Many different types of appliances are available; the nurse should always read manufacturer's instructions or check with the enterostomal therapist before handling unfamiliar equipment.

Flatus may cause a pouch to balloon out. This requires immediate attention because if flatus is not released, the pouch may separate from the skin barrier causing seepage of fecal contents or release of fecal odor. Open the clamp and release the flatus. Never puncture a hole in the appliance.

Age Considerations

A one-piece appliance makes application easier for an older client, particularly if impaired vision or compromised mobility from arthritis is present.

Home Care Considerations

Written directions should always be sent home with the client.

Encourage client to participate in a support group.

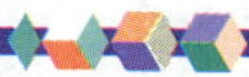

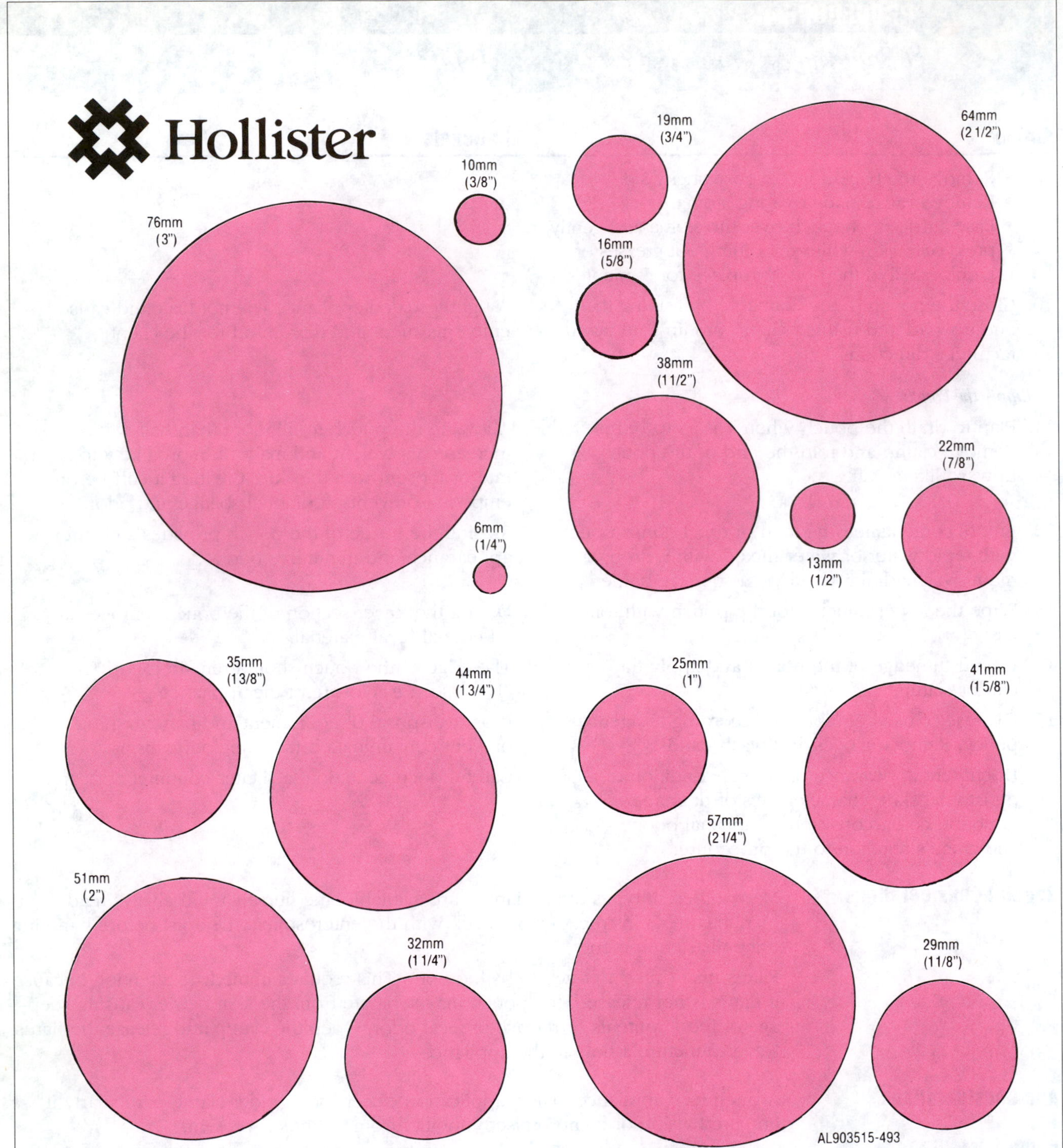

Figure 44-9
Measuring card. (Courtesy Hollister, Inc., Libertyville, IL.)

tus. By gradually adding new foods, the ostomy client can build up to a normal diet. He or she may choose to avoid some foods that are bothersome.

Health teaching about medication use frequently is overlooked for the client with an ostomy. Madda (1991) offers the following helpful guidelines:

- Remind the client that some medications discolor the stool and cause unusual odors.
- Encourage the client to check the ostomy pouch after starting on new medication to make sure the medication has been completely dissolved.
- Review the common drugs that cause constipation.
- Ileostomy clients need to be particularly alert about drug absorption problems, since the small bowel is where most absorption occurs. They should use liquid, chewable, or injectable forms rather than long-acting, enteric-coated, or sustained-release medications. Laxatives and enemas are dangerous because they may cause severe fluid and electrolyte imbalance.

Clients with ostomies should be taught various methods of odor control. The chlorophyll content in dark green vegetables helps to deodorize the feces when these vegetables are included in the diet. Bismuth subgallots, which can be purchased at drug stores and taken with meals, help to lessen fecal odor. Charcoal filter discs are available with some appliances or a deodorizer can be placed in the pouch. The enterostomal therapist can aid in the selection of odor control strategies.

Some clients can achieve control over fecal elimination from a colostomy by regular irrigations and by habitual emptying of the colon at a certain time each day. Few clients with an ileostomy gain any degree of control of the excretion of wastes and seldom may dispense with the use of an appliance, except for short periods.

Normal activity, including work, can be resumed. Direct physical contact sports and heavy lifting should be avoided. The client can go swimming and needs to wear only gauze or a large adhesive bandage over the stoma. Whenever travel is required, advise the client to carry a 1 to 2 day supply of equipment in a carry-on bag in case luggage that has been checked should get lost.

Providing Comfort Measures

Comfort measures related to defecation include working with the client to develop a bowel elimination routine that results in the easy passage of a soft, formed stool, being attentive to perineal hygiene and the maintenance of skin integrity, and using warm moist heat (sitz bath or tub bath) to soothe the perineal area. Clients with hemorrhoids may require special comfort measures, such as the application of topical medications to reduce inflammation and the administration of stool softeners.

EVALUATING

The nurse evaluates the effectiveness of a plan of care to promote regular bowel elimination by checking to see if the client has met the individualized client goals specified in the plan. Nursing care is considered effective if the client expresses satisfaction with his or her regular pattern of defecation and the ability to comfortably pass a soft, formed stool without the use of medications or laxatives. The plan of care is most successful when the client is able to:

- Verbalize the relation between bowel elimination and nutrition, fluid intake, exercise, and stress management
- Develop a plan to modify any factors that contribute to current bowel problems or that might adversely affect bowel functioning in the future
- Correct unhealthy bowel habits, such as ignoring the urge to defecate and abusing laxatives and enemas

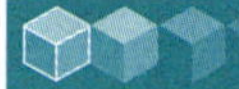

Nursing Process in Clinical Practice

Once a bowel elimination problem is detected, the nurse implements each phase of the nursing process to ensure its correct identification and treatment. The nurse who wants to identify and manage the bowel elimination problem correctly must possess the knowledge and clinical skills described earlier in this chapter. What follows in outline format are focused assessment priorities, expected outcomes, and nursing interventions for the nursing diagnoses:

Constipation
Bowel Incontinence
Diarrhea

In the client care study that follows, a plan of care is developed to address the elimination needs of a pediatric client with severe diarrhea.

Constipation

> A state in which an individual experiences a change in normal bowel habits characterized by a decrease in frequency and/or passage of hard, dry stools (NANDA, 1994)

Constipation is the passage of dry, hard stools. Decreased gastric motility slows the passage of feces through the large intestine, resulting in increased fluid absorption from the fecal mass and the dry, hard stool. Straining often accompanies defecation. Some people may be constipated and yet have a daily bowel movement, whereas others who regularly defecate no more than three times a week are not constipated. The habits of elimination vary greatly among healthy people.

Assessment Priorities

- Assess bowel elimination patterns noting (1) decrease in the usual number of bowel movements; (2) dry, hard stools; (3) straining and difficult evacuation; (4) abdominal distention; (5) swollen hemorrhoids; and (6) complaints of headache, lassitude, anorexia, low back pain, or irritability.
- Identify contributing factors: insufficient fluid intake, low-fiber diet, lack of exercise, environmental changes, delaying defecation when urge is present, abuse of enemas or laxatives, use of constipating drugs, mental stress or depression, neurologic degeneration.
- Identify high-risk populations: (1) clients on bed rest who take constipating medications (narcotic analgesics [opioids], anticholinergics), (2) clients who reduce fluids or bulk in their diet, (3) depressed people, and (4) clients with central nervous system disease or local lesions that cause pain.

Expected Outcomes

The client will:

- Have a soft, formed bowel movement every 1 to 3 days without straining or discomfort
- Modify lifestyle variables that contribute to constipation (specify, eg, increase fluid intake to 2000 to 2800 mL, increase fiber in diet, incorporate three to five periods of regular exercise into week's routine)

Interventions

- Encourage the client to respond to the urge to defecate and to establish a routine for having a bowel movement when the urge is most likely to be present. Ignoring the urge is a common cause of constipation. Most people experience an urge after a meal, especially breakfast.
- Provide privacy, and allow sufficient time to defecate when stress is at a minimum. Lack of privacy, being under stress, and rushing usually will quickly eliminate the urge to defecate. Emotions tend to cause spasticity, producing *hypertonic* or *spastic constipation.*
- See to it that the client's food and fluid intake are conducive to having a bowel movement. Balanced food content and varied bulk are important to produce fecal matter and promote its movement in the intestinal tract. Fresh fruits, vegetables, and bran cereals increase intestinal bulk, whereas such foods as lean meats, rice, and eggs leave little residue. Ingesting sufficient fluids is important to help prevent a dry, hard stool. Many people find that drinking such fluids as hot water or prune juice on awakening promotes elimination. Adequate hot meals rather than small cold meals stimulate peristalsis.
- Teach the client the importance of exercise and activity. Studies clearly have shown that lack of activity leads to poor muscle tone, a poor appetite, and sluggish intestinal activity.
- Position the client so that defecation is promoted. The squatting position, which allows maximum use of abdominal muscles, is best, but few people find this position comfortable. The sitting position, or semisitting position for bedridden clients, is most often used.
- Encourage the client to seek medical attention when minor rectal or anal problems, such as hemorrhoids or small linear ulcers called *anal fissures,* affect elimination. They cause discomfort, which causes the person to ignore the urge to defecate as long as possible.
- Teach the client to minimize the use of over-the-counter constipating drugs and to consult with the physician about limiting the use of constipating drugs when possible.
- Use laxatives, enemas, and suppositories as a last resort or temporary treatment. Various measures to stimulate defecation are presented earlier in the chapter.

Bowel Incontinence

> A state in which an individual experiences a change in normal bowel habits characterized by involuntary passage of stool (NANDA, 1994)

Bowel incontinence is the inability of the anal sphincter to control the discharge of fecal and gaseous material. The cause of incontinence usually is an organic disease, resulting either in a mechanical condition that hinders the proper functioning of the anal sphincter or in an impairment in the nerve supply to the anal sphincter. Mental illnesses also may be responsible for the client's indifference to the passage of stool. Although bowel incontinence seldom is a threat to life, incontinent clients suffer embarrassment and may become emotionally disturbed.

Assessment Priorities

- Assess bowel elimination pattern, noting onset of bowel incontinence and regularity and number of incontinent episodes. Note stool characteristics. Rule out impaction by rectal examination.
- Identify contributing factors: gross constipation with impaction and subsequent overflow, organic changes in neural innervation of the rectum, local causes (cancer of rectum, prolapsed anus, semifluid stool), mental illnesses resulting in indifference to passage of stool, extreme debilitation.
- Assess effects of incontinence on self-concept.
- Examine perineal area for skin breakdown.

Expected Outcomes

The client will:

- Eliminate incontinent episodes (or reduce their number) if this is realistic
- Demonstrate appropriate self-care measures (or receive related nursing measures): perineal hygiene,

use of absorbent pads or waterproof briefs, and so forth
- Demonstrate no signs of perineal excoriation
- Participate in bowel training program to time defecation and reduce the risk of accidents

Interventions

- Take into account that the client suffers embarrassment. The client requires emotional support and understanding.
- Note when incontinence is most likely to occur, and place the client on a bedpan at those times. If there is no pattern, offer a bedpan at regular intervals, such as every few hours.
- Keep the skin clean and dry by using proper hygienic measures. Pressure ulcers may develop when such measures are overlooked.
- Change bed linens and clothing as necessary to avoid odor, skin irritation, and embarrassment. Disposable bed pads and moisture-proof undergarments are a consideration but should not be used until other measures have been attempted.
- Confer with the physician about the use of a suppository or a daily cleansing enema. These measures empty the lower colon regularly and often help to decrease incontinence. Bowel training programs may be helpful.

The nurse should keep in mind that emotional problems of clients with diarrhea and bowel incontinence are as important for the nurse to manage as the physical problems.

Diarrhea

> A state in which an individual experiences a change in normal bowel habits characterized by the frequent passage of loose, fluid, unformed stools (NANDA, 1994)

Diarrhea is the passage of excessively liquid and unformed stools. Frequent bowel movements do not necessarily mean that diarrhea is present, although clients with diarrhea usually pass stools at frequent intervals. Diarrhea often is associated with intestinal cramps. Nausea and vomiting may be present as well as blood in the stools. Diarrhea is protective in nature when its cause is the presence of irritants in the intestinal tract.

Diarrhea may have a functional basis. The client may have allergies to ingested food or drugs. The abuse of cathartics as well as certain dietary indiscretions may cause diarrhea. Diseases in parts of the body other than the intestinal tract may be at the root of the trouble. Examples include uremia and certain cardiovascular and neurologic disorders.

Diarrhea may be caused by certain intrinsic conditions that exist in the intestine itself. These include viral, bacteriologic, fungal, protozoan, and metazoan invasions; alterations in the normal bacterial flora of the intestine; antimicrobial therapy; fistulas; inflammatory conditions, such as ulcerative colitis; and tumors in the intestinal tract.

If the cause of the diarrhea is psychologic, the nurse may be able to play an important part in assisting the client to understand the cause. Situations in daily living may be disturbing to the client. Diarrhea, however, may be associated with deep-seated emotional problems that require psychologic counseling.

Large amounts of fluids and electrolytes may be lost relatively quickly in the presence of diarrhea. This is especially true with infants and young children; if neglected, such loss may easily place a youngster's life in jeopardy. Giving fluids other than by mouth may be necessary when diarrhea is present. If oral intake is possible, cold fluids and rich foods, especially sweets, should be avoided.

Assessment Priorities

- Assess bowel elimination patterns, noting (1) increased frequency or intensity of bowel movements; (2) increased fluid content in stool, greenish color, mucus, or blood; (3) increased bowel sounds; (4) whether diarrhea is acute, chronic, or recurrent; (5) fecal soiling; (6) being awakened at night to defecate; (7) complaints of abdominal pain and cramping, generalized weakness and fatigue, nausea and vomiting, fever.
- Assess anal and perineal area for excoriation.
- Identify contributing factors: recent travel, food intolerance, food or drug allergies (new medication), emotional stress, abuse of laxatives, alteration in the normal bacterial flora of the intestine (after antibiotic therapy), colon disease and other diseases, intestinal infection, surgical alterations.
- For clients with chronic diarrhea, assess effect on person's self-image and physiologic and social functioning. Note problems with hydration, nutritional status, skin integrity, sleep, performance of usual self-care activities, and social interactions. Note abnormal laboratory values (electrolyte levels and hematocrit).

Expected Outcomes

The client will:
- Reestablish usual defecation patterns (soft, formed stool) or experience less diarrhea
- Modify contributing factors when possible (specify, eg, eliminate certain foods from diet, practice stress management techniques)
- Maintain skin integrity in anal and perineal areas
- Demonstrate signs of adequate hydration and nutritional status

Interventions

- Recognize that diarrhea is an embarrassing problem. The client is in need of emotional support and needs to know that the nurse is there to help.
- Answer the client's call signal promptly. The client with diarrhea often cannot control the urge to

defecate. It may be necessary to place a bedpan within easy reach but out of sight to prevent embarrassment.

- Whenever possible, remove the cause of diarrhea. Discontinuation of medications that cause diarrhea usually results in a return to normal defecation within 1 to 3 days.
- If there is any indication of an impaction, a rectal examination should be performed before using antidiarrheal medications.
- Maintain the client's fluid and electrolyte balance. A nonirritating diet is important until symptoms subside. Cold fluids and rich foods aggravate the problem.
- Give special care to the region around the anus, where skin irritation is common. Keep the area clean and dry. Use skin creams, ointments, or powders as necessary. Avoid toilet tissue when it irritates, and use something softer, such as cotton balls, to clean and dry the area.
- Fecal incontinence pouches are now being used in some instances for clients with uncontrollable diarrhea after chemotherapy, antibiotic therapy, and tube feedings.
- Once diarrhea stops, it is important to promote a return to normal bowel flora. Fermented dairy products, such as buttermilk or yogurt, aid this process.
- When diarrhea is a regular or intermittent phenomenon that interferes with daily living, clients need additional counseling regarding judicious use of medications, individualized dietary modifications, fluid balance, skin protection, special clothing, and strategies to permit social interactions (eg, preplanning seating on a plane or in a theater or restaurant to be near a bathroom).

Client Care Study

Jeremy Green, aged 4, height 45 inches (114.3 cm), weight 36 lb (16.3 kg), was placed in day care when his mother returned to work 6 months ago. He presents at the hospital with a diagnosis of viral gastroenteritis. A comprehensive nursing assessment included the following notations:

- Admitted with complaints of diarrhea beginning three days ago
- Seen today by pediatrician who recommended admission and work-up to rule out causes other than viral
- Mother reports liquid stools (no observable blood, pus, or mucus) six to seven times daily beginning 3 days ago with amounts of "one to two cups"
- Urgency results in soiling of pants
- Child has sipped boiled skim milk and Coke and ate a small amount of broth and a few pretzels but has no appetite
- Complained of nausea and vomited twice 3 days ago
- Child is pale and eyes are sunken
- Skin warm and dry with decreased turgor; dry mucous membranes
- Hyperactive bowel sounds
- Ht—45 in, weight—36 lbs, T—99.8°F (rectally), P—88, R—18
- Mother reported several other children in same day care center are out sick with diarrhea

Core Competencies

Cognitive Competencies

- Knowledge of child development, normal bowel elimination, causes and manifestations of diarrhea and related problems, and successful treatment strategies
- Teaching and counseling skills to meet the child's and parents' needs
- Ability to develop nursing diagnoses that reflect Jeremy's unique problem of diarrhea
- Knowledge of which nursing interventions are most likely to yield desired outcomes

Technical Competencies

- Strong assessment skills (interviewing and physical assessment) to carefully identify and label Jeremy's problems and their cause
- Ability to provide safe physical care to Jeremy aimed at promoting optimal functioning of all body systems
- Ability to create a secure, comfortable, and developmentally stimulating environment for Jeremy

Interpersonal Competencies

- Strong interpersonal skills to work effectively with children and their families
- Interpersonal and leadership skills to work with the nursing staff and healthcare team to implement the plan of care
- Ability to establish a trusting nurse–client relationship grounded in responsible caring

Ethical/Legal Competencies

- Accountability and willingness to use competence to help Jeremy and his parents regain maximal control of his diarrhea
- Competence in documenting nursing interventions
- Ability to serve as a trusted and effective client advocate

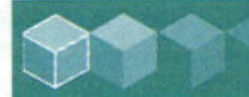

Nursing Plan of Care

for Jeremy Green

Nursing Diagnosis: Diarrhea related to unknown cause (possibly viral, rule out malabsorption of lactose and other causes) as manifested by passage of liquid stools (1–2 cups) for 3 days; urgency with fecal soiling; anorexia, nausea, vomiting twice on day 1; signs of dehydration: decreased skin turgor, dry mucous membranes, sunken eyeballs

Expected Outcome: At the time of discharge, the client will:

- Voluntarily pass a formed stool of usual consistency (experience less or no diarrhea)

Nursing Interventions	Rationale	Evaluative Statement
Assess and chart frequency and amount of diarrhea, stool characteristics, precipitating factors, and accompanying manifestations (gastrointestinal symptoms, hyperactive bowel sounds).	This assists in identifying the cause of the diarrhea.	5/8/98 Goal partially met. No recurrence of liquid stools for 24 hours. *Revision:* Continue to monitor. *D. Lentsky, RN*

Expected Outcome: At the time of discharge, the client will:

- Exhibit decreased bowel sounds

Nursing Interventions	Rationale	Evaluative Statement
Work collaboratively with the physician to identify the cause of the diarrhea. Obtain stool specimens and send to laboratory.	Correct treatment depends on identification of the cause of the diarrhea. Viral diarrhea is usually self-limiting and lasts 24 to 72 hours. Prolonged diarrhea after acute viral illness may be from temporary malabsorption of lactose or other simple sugars.	5/8/98 Goal met. Bowel sounds are normal. *D. Lentsky, RN*
Instruct Jeremy and his parents (if they want to participate in care) on correct enteric precautions for handling stool.	Prevents transmissions of infectious diarrhea to others.	
Increase frequency and length of rest periods and discourage strenuous activity.	Exercise and activity stimulate peristalsis.	
Administer prescribed antidiarrheal medication and observe for adverse effects.	Antidiarrheal medications may cause drowsiness and dizziness.	

Expected Outcome: At the time of discharge, the client will:

- Demonstrate signs of fluid and electrolyte balance: (1) improved skin turgor, (2) moist mucous membranes, and (3) normal eyeballs

Nursing Interventions	Rationale	Evaluative Statement
Continue to assess hydration status and be alert to signs of electrolyte imbalance.	Reestablishing normal fluid and electrolyte balance by replacing ongoing fluid losses and providing maintenance fluids is a priority for the child with severe and prolonged diarrhea. Diarrhea stools contain large amounts of water and often are relatively low in sodium and high in potassium.	5/8/98 Goal partially met. Skin turgor improved, eyeballs normal, mucous membranes still dry.

(continued)

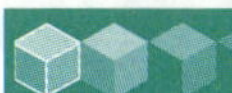

Nursing Plan of Care *(continued)*

for Jeremy Green

Nursing Interventions	Rationale	Evaluative Statement
Administer prescribed intravenous therapy and clear liquids—note client response as new fluids and foods are added to the diet.	There is no ideal oral replacement fluid. Some may cause diarrhea or provide inappropriate amounts of electrolytes.	*Revision:* Continue to encourage PO fluids. Enjoys clear chicken broth and half-strength gelatin products. *D. Lentsky, RN*
Chart daily weight.	Daily weights are the most accurate indicator of fluid balance.	
Monitor intake and output. Note concentration of urine.	Urine becomes more concentrated when a person is dehydrated.	

Expected Outcome: At the time of discharge, the client will:

- Demonstrate signs of improved nutritional status: (1) eats low-fiber diet without abdominal cramping, nausea, or vomiting; and (2) maintains or increases admission weight

Nursing Interventions	Rationale	Evaluative Statement
Discontinue milk products and solid foods. Until the diarrhea resolves, offer a combination of clear liquids (half-strength apple juice or gelatin products; commercial products: Lytren, Pedialyte, 5% glucose water): 30 mL/hr for first 8 hours, then 60 to 90 mL every 1 to 2 hours if number of stools lessens.	If one fluid is used exclusively, inappropriate amounts of electrolytes may be provided. Commercial preparations tend to be expensive. Objective is to provide the necessary water, electrolytes, and minimal calories in a milk-free and solid-free diet—until the diarrhea resolves.	5/8/98 Goal met. Tolerating rice cereal and bananas. Gained 1 lb since admission. *D. Lentsky, RN*
As gastrointestinal symptoms subside, advance to other liquids and solids (bananas, applesauce, and rice cereal solidify stool)—milk should be the last liquid added.	Adding new fluids and foods slowly enables intolerances to be quickly detected.	

Expected Outcome: At the time of discharge, the client will:

- Show no signs of skin breakdown in the perianal area

Nursing Interventions	Rationale	Evaluative Statement
Assess the perianal area after each passage of stool and note any irritation.	Perianal irritation is a common problem with severe diarrhea. The goal of treatment is prevention.	5/8/98 Goal partially met. Small area of excoriation remains around anus. Continue plan. *D. Lentsky, RN*
Wash and dry the area carefully after each episode of diarrhea and apply protective ointment (as ordered or per agency protocol).	Keeping the skin clean and dry and protected with a waterproof ointment or skin barrier may prevent breakdown.	

Sample Documentation

5/7/98 Nursing

Liquid stools have decreased to two in the past 24 hours. Negative report on stool culture. Normal bowel sounds auscultated in all four quadrants. Skin turgor normal and mucous membranes pink in color with moist appearance. Urine clear and light amber in color. Has gained 1 lb since admission. Jeremy stated this AM, "My stomach doesn't hurt so much anymore." Rice cereal and bananas will be added to diet tomorrow. Milk and milk products will be last items added to diet. Parents instructed to monitor child for manifestations of lactose intolerance.

D. Lentsky, RN

Key Points

- Bowel elimination, a natural process in which the body excretes the waste products of digestion, is an essential component of healthy body functioning.
- Problems with bowel elimination may affect fluid and electrolyte balance, nutritional status, skin integrity, and self-concept.
- Healthy bowel elimination presupposes a well-functioning gastrointestinal tract. The large intestine is the primary organ of bowel elimination.
- *Defecation* and *bowel movement* are the terms used to describe the emptying of the intestines. People vary in the frequency of their bowel movements. The aim is to have the bowels move regularly and for the stools to be formed, soft, and passed without discomfort.
- Factors that affect bowel elimination include growth and development, daily patterns, food and fluid intake, activity and muscle tone, lifestyle variables, psychologic variables, pathologic conditions, medications, diagnostic tests, surgery, and anesthesia.
- A comprehensive assessment of bowel elimination includes the collection of data about usual patterns of elimination; recent changes in these patterns; aids to elimination; elimination problems; physical assessment of the abdomen, anus, and rectum; and stool characteristics. These findings may need to be correlated with the results of diagnostic studies of the stool and gastrointestinal tract.
- When caring for a debilitated, confused, or unconscious client, the nurse needs to monitor bowel status daily to identify and treat bowel elimination problems early. Nursing care is directed to the prevention of bowel problems.
- Endoscopic examinations using a lighted tube allow the direct visualization of the gastrointestinal tract and are helpful in the diagnosis of inflammatory, ulcerative, and infectious diseases; neoplastic diseases; and lesions of the esophageal, gastric, and intestinal mucosa.
- Indirect visualization of the gastrointestinal tract is achieved through radiography. Important nursing responsibilities are assisting the client to complete a safe and effective dietary and bowel preparation program and ensuring that the client eliminates the contrast medium (barium sulfate) used in the study. Standard bowel preparation agents may be contraindicated for some clients.
- Nursing diagnoses may be written to address specifically problems in bowel elimination (constipation, diarrhea, bowel incontinence) and to identify the effect bowel elimination problems have on other areas of human functioning (anxiety, comfort, self-concept, skin integrity).
- Regular bowel elimination may be promoted in both well and ill clients by attention to timing, positioning, privacy, nutrition, and exercise. Clients need to understand the importance of heeding the urge to defecate and the relation between bowel elimination and nutrition and exercise.
- Specific nursing strategies for bowel elimination include use of cathartics, laxatives, and antidiarrheals; techniques for emptying the colon of feces (enemas, rectal suppositories, oral intestinal lavage, and digital removal of stool); bowel training programs; and comfort measures.
- Although laxatives have valid uses, they frequently are abused. Many people who take laxatives for what they think is constipation do not realize that the habitual use of laxatives is the most common cause of chronic constipation.
- A physician's order may be needed before the nurse digitally removes a fecal impaction because this may result in irritation of the rectal mucosa and bleeding, and because vagal stimulation can decrease the heart rate.
- The purpose of a bowel training program is to manipulate factors within the person's control (food and fluid intake, exercise, time of defecation) and to achieve the elimination of a soft, formed stool at regular intervals without laxative support.
- The client with a bowel diversion needs physical and psychologic support both preoperatively and postoperatively. The nurse works collaboratively with the physician and enterostomal therapist to ensure that the client and family can manage the care of the bowel diversion after discharge.
- Clients with acute or chronic constipation, impaction, diarrhea, incontinence, or flatulence require special nursing care. These problems, if uncorrected, may seriously affect the client's comfort, self-concept, and other areas of physical functioning.

Study Questions

1. The nurse encourages Mr. Brown to avoid foods that have a laxative effect. He is instructed to avoid
   a. cheese
   b. alcohol
   c. eggs
   d. pasta
2. Which of the following is a true statement about the effects of medication on bowel elimination?
   a. Diarrhea occurs with antibiotic use about 20% of the time.
   b. Anticoagulants cause a white discoloration of the stool.

c. Narcotic analgesics increase gastrointestinal motility.
d. Iron salts impair digestion and cause a green stool.

3. Mr. Jones has a fecal impaction. The nurse correctly administers an oil-retention enema by
   a. administering a large volume of solution (500 to 1000 mL)
   b. mixing milk and molasses in equal parts for an enema
   c. instructing the client to retain the enema for at least 30 minutes
   d. following the return-flow or Harris flush procedure
4. As the nurse prepares to assist Mrs. Perez with her newly created ileostomy, she is aware that
   a. an appliance will not be required on a continual basis
   b. the size of the stoma stabilizes within 2 weeks
   c. irrigation is necessary for regulation
   d. fecal drainage will be liquid
5. The class of laxative that acts by causing stool to absorb water and swell is
   a. bulk forming
   b. emollient
   c. lubricant
   d. stimulant
6. Mr. Toney is nervous about a colonoscopy scheduled for tomorrow. The nurse describes the test by explaining that
   a. it allows visual examination of the esophagus and stomach
   b. it allows visual examination of the large intestine
   c. it is a radiographic examination of the large intestine
   d. it is a fluoroscopic examination of the small intestine
7. A bowel training program includes
   a. a 1 week trial period
   b. decreasing fluid intake to 1000 mL
   c. administering an enema once a day to stimulate peristalsis
   d. allowing ample time for evacuation
8. Your client complains of excessive flatulence. Which food, if eaten regularly, may be responsible for this?
   a. meat
   b. cauliflower
   c. potatoes
   d. ice cream
9. The barium enema should be done before the upper gastrointestinal series because of which of the following?
   a. Retained barium may cloud the colon.
   b. Barium can cause lower gastrointestinal bleeding.
   c. The physician orders in that sequence.
   d. Barium is absorbed readily in the lower intestine.
10. Nurses should recommend to their clients the avoidance of habitual use of laxatives. Which of the following is the rationale for this?
    a. They will cause a fecal impaction.
    b. They will cause chronic constipation.
    c. They change the pH of the gastrointestinal tract.
    d. They inhibit the intestinal enzymes.
11. Which of the following is the physiology behind a hypertonic solution enema?
    a. bowel mucosa irritation
    b. diffusion of water out of colon
    c. osmosis of water into colon
    d. softening of fecal contents
12. Which of the following is the rationale for discouraging use of rectal Foley catheters?
    a. decrease peristalsis
    b. require a physician's order
    c. cause rectal necrosis
    d. prevent the liquid stool from draining
13. During removal of a fecal impaction, which of the following could occur because of vagal stimulation?
    a. bradycardia
    b. atelectasis
    c. tachycardia
    d. cardiac tamponade
14. Which of the following would be a common nursing diagnosis for the client with an ileostomy?
    a. Body Image Disturbance
    b. Constipation
    c. Altered Growth and Development
    d. Fluid Volume Excess
15. Your client who is experiencing flatulence would be helped if he were placed in which of the following positions?
    a. Trendelenburg position
    b. knee–chest position
    c. semi-Fowler's position
    d. Fowler's position

Answers With Rationale

1. The correct response is *b.* All the foods listed except alcohol have a constipating effect.
2. The correct response is *a.* Anticoagulants may result in the stool having a pink, to red, to black appearance, whereas iron salts also cause a black stool. Narcotic analgesics decrease gastric motility.
3. The correct response is *c.* The usual amount of solution administered with a retention enema is 150 to 200 mL for an adult. The milk-and-molasses mixture is a carminative enema that helps to expel flatus, as does the Harris flush procedure.

4. The correct response is *d.* An appliance usually is required on a continual basis because the fecal drainage is liquid. Stoma size usually stabilizes within 4 to 6 weeks, and irrigation is not necessary because fecal matter is liquid.
5. The correct response is *a.* Emollients lubricate the stool; lubricants soften the stool, making it easier to pass; and stimulants promote peristalsis by irritating the intestinal mucosa or stimulating nerve endings in the intestinal wall.
6. The correct response is *b.* An esophagogastroduodenoscopy allows visual examination of the esophagus and stomach. The radiographic examination of the large intestine is a barium enema, and a fluoroscopic examination of the small intestine is an upper gastrointestinal series.
7. The correct response is *d.* For a bowel training program to be effective, the client must have ample time for evacuation (usually 20 to 30 minutes). Fluid intake is increased to 2500 to 3000 mL; it usually requires 14 to 21 days to establish this routine; and a daily enema is not administered in a bowel training program. A cathartic suppository is used 30 minutes before the client's usual defecation time to stimulate peristalsis.
8. The correct response is *b.* Cauliflower is a gas-producing food that results in flatulence.
9. The correct response is *a.* The barium enema should always precede the upper gastrointestinal series because retained barium from the latter may take several days to pass through the gastrointestinal tract and cloud anatomic detail on the barium enema studies.
10. The correct response is *b.* Habitual use of laxatives is the most common cause of chronic constipation.
11. The correct response is *c.* Hypertonic solutions draw water into the colon by osmosis, thus stimulating the defecation reflex. Oil solutions soften fecal contents, and soap solutions distend the intestine and irritate the bowel mucosa.
12. The correct response is *c.* Concern for mucosal necrosis is one of the main reasons why the use of rectal Foley catheters is being discouraged. Nurses also feel that the catheter stimulates sensory nerve fibers in the rectum, thus worsening diarrhea. The catheter allows liquid feces to drain and the necessity of obtaining a physician's order is not a factor in determining the safety of the rectal catheter.
13. The correct response is *a.* Removing a fecal impaction manually may result in stimulation of the vagal nerve and a resulting bradycardia.
14. The correct response is *a.* Constipation will not occur with an ileostomy, since the drainage is liquid. Growth and development are not affected by the formation of an ileostomy. Fluid volume excess is unlikely to occur because the drainage is liquid and probably continual.
15. The correct response is *b.* Because gas rises, the knee–chest position facilitates the passage of flatus.

Bibliography

Abrams, A. (1995). *Clinical drug therapy* (4th ed.). Philadelphia: Lippincott.

Anastasi, J. (1993). AIDS update: Caring for patients with diarrhea. *Nursing, 23*(8), 68–70.

Beverley, L., & Travis, I. (1992). Constipation: Proposed natural laxative mixtures. *Journal of Gerontological Nursing, 18*(10), 5–12.

Carpenito, L. (1995). *Nursing diagnosis: Application to clinical practice* (6th ed.). Philadelphia: Lippincott.

Fischbach, F. (1995). *A manual of laboratory diagnostic tests* (5th ed.). Philadelphia: Lippincott.

Fuller, J., & Schaller-Ayers, J. (1994). *Health assessment: A nursing approach* (2nd ed.). Philadelphia: Lippincott.

Gurevich, I. (1994). Your patients don't need diarrhea, too! *RN, 57*(4), 52–55.

Hammerhofer-Jereb, K. (1996). Laparoscopic bowel resection? *RN, 59*(3), 22–25.

Hampton, B. & Bryant, R. (1992). *Ostomies and continent diversions*. St. Louis: Mosby.

Hogstel, M. & Nelson, M. (1992). Anticipation and early detection can reduce bowel elimination complications. *Geriatric Nursing, 13*(1), 28–33.

Jess, L. (1993). Acute abdominal pain. *Nursing, 23*(9), 34–42.

Karam, S., & Nies, D. (1994). Student/staff collaboration: A pilot bowel management program. *Journal of Gerontological Nursing, 20*(3), 32–40.

Krasner, D. (1993). Six steps to successful stoma care. *RN, 56*(7), 32–37.

Madda, M. (1991). Helping ostomy patients manage medications. *Nursing, 21*(3), 47–49.

McConnell, E. (1994). Auscultating bowel sounds. *Nursing, 24*(6), 20.

Mehler, E. (1994). Preparing your patient to use a fecal occult blood test. *Nursing, 24*(5), 32R.

Mihalopoulos, N., Trunnell, E., Ball, K. & Moncur, C. (1994). The psychologic impact of ostomy surgery on persons 50 years and older. *Journal of Wound, Ostomy and Continence Nursing, 21*(4), 149–155.

Murray, S., Preuss, M., & Schultz, F. (1992). How do you prep the bowel without enemas? *American Journal of Nursing, 92*(8), 66–67.

North American Nursing Diagnosis Association. (1994). *NANDA nursing diagnoses: Definitions and classification 1995–1996.* Philadelphia: NANDA.

Pagana, K., & Pagana, T. (1995). *Diagnostic and laboratory test reference* (2nd ed.). St. Louis: Mosby.

Paulford-Lecher, N. (1993). Teaching your patient stoma care. *Nursing, 23*(9), 47–49.

Paulford-Lecher, N. (1995). Getting your patient started with an ostomy pouch. *Nursing, 25*(4), 32L.

Pediatric Update. (1994). Acute diarrhea: Managing dehydration, *Nursing, 24*(8), 45–46.

Pillitteri, A. (1995). *Maternal & child health nursing: Care of the childbearing and childrearing family* (2nd ed.). Philadelphia: Lippincott.

Rice, R. (1995). *Home health nursing procedures.* St. Louis: Mosby.

Schmelzer, M., & Wright, K. (1993). Risky enemas: What's the ideal solution? *American Journal of Nursing, 93*(7), 16.

Shollenberger, D. (1994). Giving enemas safely. *Nursing, 24*(9), 32X–32Z.

Stanley, M., & Beare, P. (1995). *Gerontological Nursing.* Philadelphia: Davis.

Watson, J., & Jaffe, M. (1995). *Nurse's manual of laboratory and diagnostic tests* (2nd ed.). Philadelphia: Davis.

Weidner, B. (1992). Constipation: Removing an impaction. *Nursing, 22*(4), 78.

Wolf, Z. (1995). Fecal incontinence bags help handle a challenging problem. *Nursing Spectrum, 4*(10), 9.

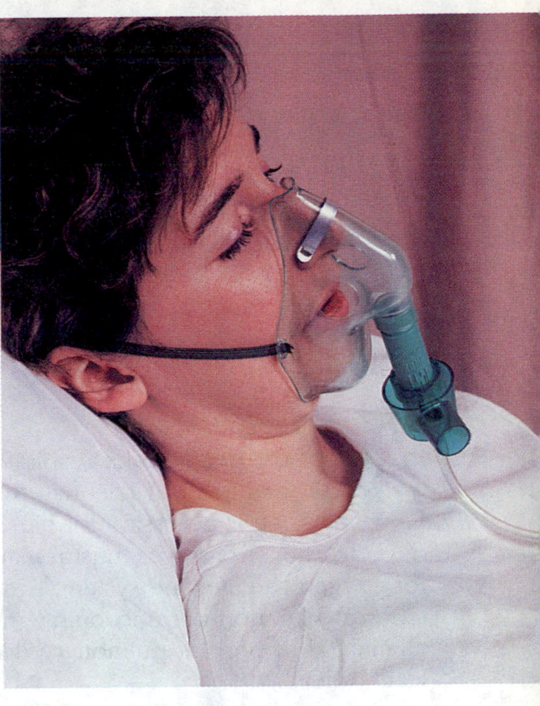

Chapter 45

Oxygenation

Objectives

After studying this chapter, the learner should be able to:

Define key terms used in the chapter.

Describe the principles of respiratory physiology.

Describe age-related differences that influence care of the client with respiratory problems.

Identify six factors that influence respiratory function.

Perform a comprehensive respiratory assessment using appropriate interview questions and physical assessment skills.

Develop nursing diagnoses that correctly identify problems that may be treated by independent nursing interventions.

Describe 11 nursing strategies to promote adequate respiratory functioning, identifying their rationale.

Plan, implement, and evaluate nursing care related to select nursing diagnoses involving respiratory problems.

Key Terms

alveoli
atelectasis
bronchodilator
crackles
endotracheal tube
expiration
gurgles
hemoptysis
hyperventilation
hypoventilation
hypoxia
inspiration
nasal cannula
perfusion
pulse oximetry
spirometer
thoracentesis
tracheostomy tube
ventilation
wheezes

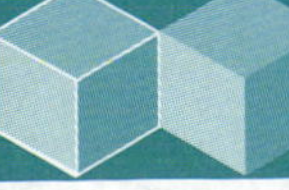

Most people take respiratory functioning for granted, but adequate respiratory functioning is necessary for life. Living cells require oxygen. The air passages must remain patent (ie, open) for oxygen to enter the system. Any condition that interferes with normal functioning must be reduced or eliminated to prevent pulmonary distress, which could lead to death.

Normal functioning depends on essentially three factors:

- The integrity of the airway system to transport air to and from the lungs
- A properly functioning alveolar system in the lungs to oxygenate venous blood and to remove carbon dioxide from the blood
- A properly functioning cardiovascular system to carry nutrients and wastes to and from body cells

Study of this chapter will provide the nurse with knowledge of the physiology, general purpose, and general factors affecting respiratory functioning. Practical suggestions for performing a comprehensive respiratory assessment are given. Sample interview questions for both a general and focused respiratory history are presented along with information and data collected from the nursing examination. The incorporation of results from laboratory and radiology studies is addressed in the assessment. After analyzing the data, it is important to decide whether the respiratory data lead to the problem statement, indicate another problem, or are the possible cause of a problem. Numerous examples of nursing diagnoses are given. Expected client outcomes and specific nursing strategies for implementation are described. In the section entitled Nursing Process in Clinical Practice, assessment priorities, expected outcomes, and nursing interventions are offered for selected nursing diagnoses related to alteration in respiratory functioning—Impaired Gas Exchange, Ineffective Breathing Pattern, and Ineffective Airway Clearance. These guides and the concluding client care study illustrate how the nurse's knowledge of respiratory functioning is combined with skilled nursing interventions to resolve respiratory problems successfully.

Physiology of Respiration

A brief review of basic anatomy and physiology will aid the reader in understanding assessment findings and rationale for nursing interventions.

The Respiratory System

The airway system provides a pathway for the transport and exchange of oxygen and carbon dioxide. The upper airway comprises the nose, pharynx, larynx, and epiglottis. Its main function is to warm, filter, and humidify inspired air. The lower airway, known as the tracheobronchial tree, includes the trachea, right and left main-stem bronchus, segmental bronchi, and terminal bronchioles. The major functions are conduction of air, mucociliary clearance, and production of pulmonary surfactant. *Cilia*, microscopic hairlike projections, propel sheets of mucus toward the upper airway so the mucus can be removed (by cough) after it has trapped cells, particles, and infectious debris. Fluid is necessary for the production of watery mucus normally present in the respiratory tract and for ciliary action. This covering of mucus also protects the underlying tissues from irritation and infection. A few milliliters of fluid between the pleural surfaces allow the lungs to move easily along the chest wall as they expand and contract. In its absence, filling and emptying of the lungs are difficult. *Surfactant*, a detergent-like phospholipid, reduces surface tension of the fluid lining the alveoli. When surfactant production is reduced, the lung becomes stiff and the alveoli collapse.

The main organs of respiration, the lungs, are located within the thoracic cavity (Fig. 45-1). The right lung has three lobes, and the left has two lobes. Each lobe is further subdivided into segments or lobules. The right lung has 10 bronchopulmonary segments; the left has 8. The lungs extend from the base at the level of the diaphragm to the apex (top), which is above the first rib. The heart lies between the right and left lung. The lungs comprise elastic tissue that is capable of stretching or recoiling. Normally, the elastic fibers are partially stretched at all times, partially filling the thoracic cavity. The actual lung is composed of **alveoli**, small air sacs at the

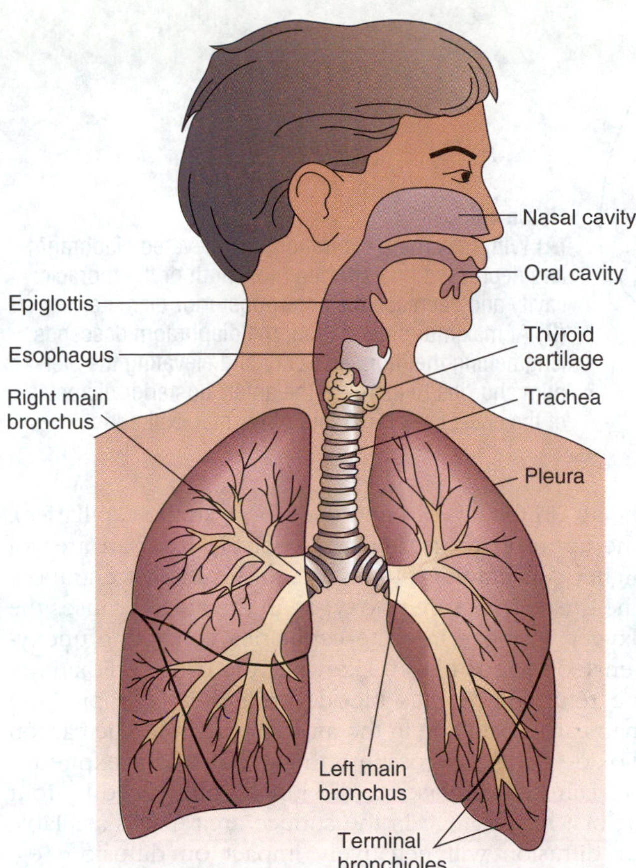

Figure 45-1
The organs of the respiratory tract.

end of the terminal bronchioles (Fig. 45-2). These structures are the site of gas exchange. The average adult has more than 300 million alveoli.

The *pleurae* are two-layered membranes: the visceral pleura covers the lungs, and the parietal pleura lines the thoracic cavity. These two are continuous with one another and form a closed sac. There is normally a potential space between them, not an actual space. Pleural fluid between the membranes acts as a lubricant and as an adhesive agent to hold the lungs in an expanded position. Pressure within the pleural space (intrapleural pressure) is always subatmospheric (ie, negative). This constant intrapleural negative pressure is essential for normal ventilation.

Pulmonary Ventilation

Ventilation is the movement of air in and out of the lungs. The process of ventilation has two phases: inspiration, or inhalation, and expiration, or exhalation. **Inspiration**, the active phase, involves movement of muscles and thorax to bring air into the lungs. **Expiration**, the passive phase, is the movement of air out of the lungs. The diaphragm and the intercostal muscles are responsible for normal inspiration and expiration.

Immediately prior to inspiration, the air pressure in the lungs is equal to that of the surrounding atmospheric pressure. According to *Boyle's law,* the volume of a gas at a constant temperature varies inversely with the pressure. Simply stated, this means that less pressure in the lungs facilitates the movement of an increased volume of air into the lungs. The pressure within the lungs (intrapulmonic pressure) will decrease as the volume of the lungs increases. During inspiration the following events occur: the diaphragm contracts and descends, lengthening the thoracic cavity; the external intercostal muscles contract, lifting the ribs upward and outward; and the sternum is pushed forward, enlarging the chest from front to back. This combination of an increased lung volume and decreased intrapulmonic pressure allows atmospheric air to move from greater pressure to lesser pressure and rush into the lungs. The relaxation or recoil of the structures involved in inspiration results in expiration. The diaphragm relaxes and moves up, the ribs move down, and the sternum drops back into position. This causes a decreased volume in the lungs and an increase in intrapulmonic pressure, and the air in the lungs moves from greater to lesser pressure and is expired (Fig. 45-3).

Accessory muscles of the abdomen, neck, and back are used to maintain respiratory movements at times when breathing is difficult. The condition of the body's

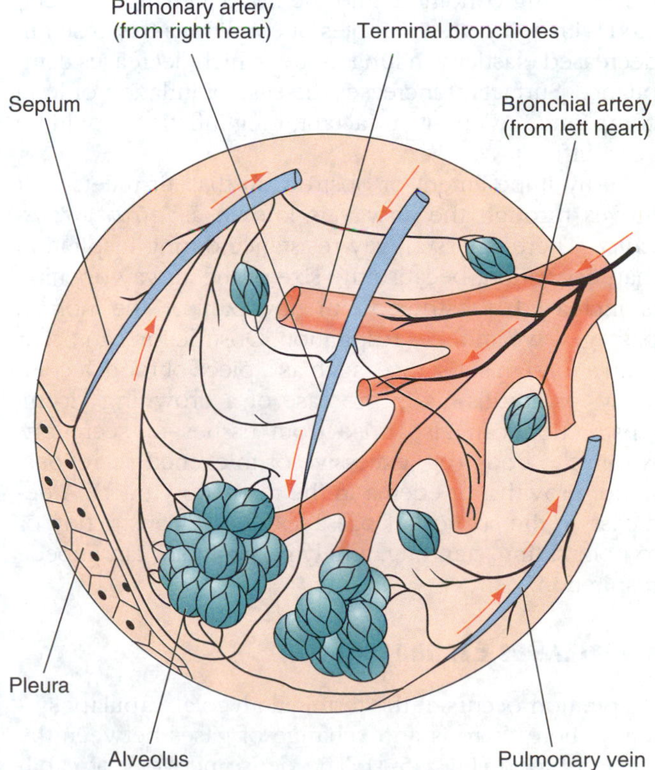

Figure 45-2
Alveoli and the intrapulmonary circulatory system where gas exchange takes place.

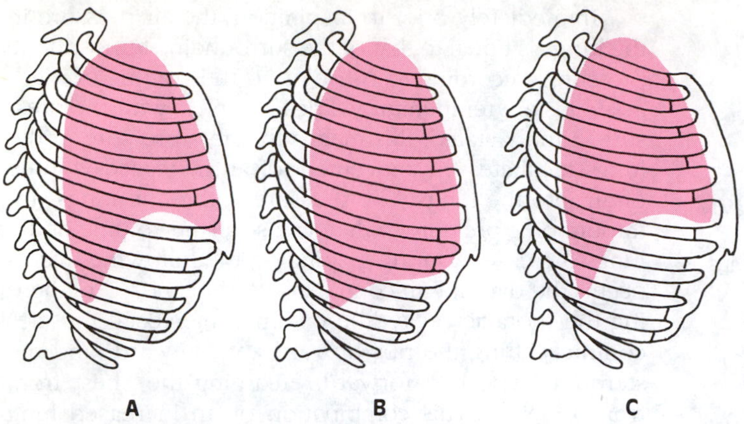

Figure 45-3
(**A**) With maximum expiration, the elevated diaphragm and depressed ribs shorten the length of the thoracic cavity and decrease the anteroposterior diameter. (**B**) At maximum inspiration, the diaphragm descends, lengthening the thoracic cavity and elevating the sternum and ribs to increase the anteroposterior diameter of the chest cavity. (**C**) End of normal expiration.

musculature can affect the process of respiration. For example, a depression of the respiratory center and pulmonary congestion with inadequate respiratory efforts are conditions that interfere with the normal movement of air into and out of the lungs.

The compliance of lung tissue also affects lung volume. *Lung compliance* refers to the stretchability of the lungs or the ease with which lungs can be inflated. Porth (1994) contrasts the varying changes in lung pressure and resulting lung compliance to the difference in blowing up a new and noncompliant balloon compared to one that has previously been inflated. A stiff, noncompliant lung (like a new balloon) requires a greater inspiratory effort to inflate it. Emphysema, a chronic lung condition, and the normal changes associated with aging are examples of conditions that result in decreased elasticity in lung tissue, which decreases compliance. Surfactant increases the ease of inflation or lung compliance. Without surfactant, lung inflation would be very difficult.

Any impediment or obstruction that air meets as it moves through the airway is known as *airway resistance.* There is less airway resistance during inspiration than expiration, because the size of the airway opening is increased. Obstruction in any part of the normal passageways impedes respiration. Obstruction can occur from a foreign substance, such as a piece of food, a coin, a toy, or liquids, as in the case of a drowning victim. Obstruction can also arise from tissues or secretions within the body (eg, excessive or thickened secretions, tumor growths, or edema in the respiratory tract). A decrease in the size of air passages due to constriction or to poor sitting, standing, and lying positions can impede respiration.

Alveolar Gas Exchange

Respiration occurs at the terminal alveolar capillary system, where there is an exchange of gases between the air and blood (Fig. 45-4). The dense network of capillaries in the respiratory portion of the lungs and the thin alveolar walls facilitate gas exchange. *Diffusion* refers to the movement of oxygen and carbon dioxide between the air (in the alveoli) and the blood (in the capillaries). The appropriate gas moves passively from an area of higher concentration to an area of lesser concentration. The greater pressure of oxygen in the alveoli causes the oxygen to move into the capillaries containing unoxygenated venous blood. Likewise, the carbon dioxide in the returning venous blood exerts a greater pressure than carbon dioxide in the air in the alveoli. The carbon dioxide diffuses across into the alveoli and is expired.

Diffusion of gases in the lung is influenced by four factors. Any change in the surface area that is available for diffusion will negatively impact on diffusion (eg, removal of a lung or the presence of a disease that destroys lung tissue). Incomplete lung expansion or lung collapse, known as **atelectasis**, prevents the pressure changes and the exchange of gas by diffusion in the lungs. Atelectatic areas of the lung cannot fulfill a function of respiration. Examples of conditions that predispose to atelectasis include obstructions of the airway by foreign bodies, mucus, constricted airways, external compression by tumors or enlarged blood vessels, and immobility. Any disease or condition that results in thickening of the alveolar–capillary membrane makes

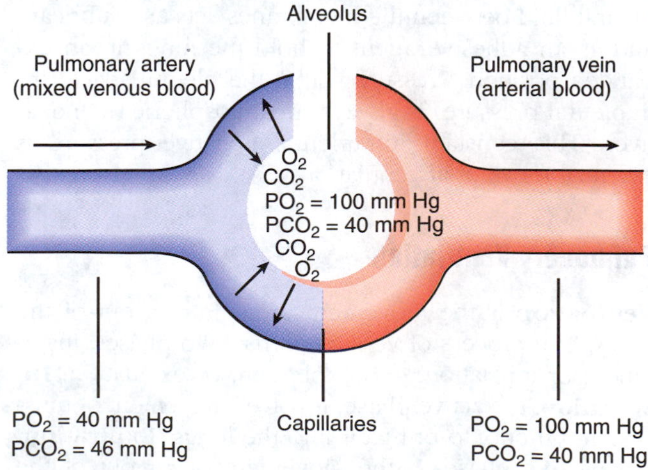

Figure 45-4
Diagram of gas exchange in the alveolus.

diffusion more difficult (eg, pneumonia or pulmonary edema). The *partial pressure,* or pressure resulting from any gas in a mixture depending on its concentration, can also affect diffusion. If environmental oxygen is in short supply (eg, at higher altitudes and in the presence of toxic fumes), less is available for diffusion. When oxygen is administered therapeutically, the increased amount that is available results in greater diffusion across capillary membranes. Finally, the solubility and molecular weight of the gas are factors in diffusion (eg, carbon dioxide has greater solubility in the respiratory membranes and diffuses more rapidly than oxygen).

This oxygenated capillary blood passes through tissue in the process known as **perfusion.** The amount of blood flow through the lungs is a factor in the amount of oxygen and other gases that are exchanged. The amount of blood present in any given area of lung tissue depends partially on whether the person is sitting, standing, or lying down. The perfusion of lung tissue also depends on activity. Greater activity results in increased cellular oxygen need and cardiac output and, consequently, in increased blood return to the lungs. In addition, perfusion depends on an adequate blood supply and proper cardiovascular functioning to carry oxygen and carbon dioxide to and from the lung tissues. Cardiovascular function is discussed in relation to vital signs in Chapter 25.

Transport of Respiratory Gases

Oxygen and carbon dioxide must move through the alveoli and be carried to and from body cells by the blood. Oxygen is carried two ways in the body. It is dissolved in plasma, but because oxygen is insoluble in liquids, little oxygen is carried in this way. The hemoglobin in red blood cells has a strong affinity for oxygen, and, therefore, most oxygen (97%) is carried in the body by red blood cells in the form of oxyhemoglobin. Hemoglobin also carries carbon dioxide easily. Any abnormality in the alveoli or in the blood's constituents influences proper internal respirations. A decrease in cardiac output (eg, hemorrhage or loss of blood) means a reduction in the amount of circulating blood that is available to deliver oxygen to the tissues. Any decrease in the amount of red blood cells or erythrocytes results in insufficient hemoglobin that is available to transport oxygen. Anemia exists when the hemoglobin content of the blood is inadequate to meet the body's oxygen demands. Exercise can have a positive effect on the transport of oxygen because the heart pumps more effectively and cells are better able to utilize oxygen.

If a problem exists in any part of the respiratory process, **hypoxia**, an inadequate amount of oxygen available to cells, may occur. The most common symptoms of hypoxia are *dyspnea* (difficulty breathing), an elevated blood pressure with a small pulse pressure, increased respiratory and pulse rates, paleness, and cyanosis. Anxiety and restlessness are also common signs of hypoxia. Hypoxia is often caused by **hypoventilation**, a decreased rate or depth of air movement into the lungs. The effects of chronic hypoxia are detected in all body systems and include altered thought processes, headaches, chest pain, enlarged heart, anorexia, constipation, decreased urinary output, decreased libido, weakness of extremity muscles, and muscle pain. At the other extreme is **hyperventilation**, the increased rate and depth of ventilation above the body's normal metabolic requirements. This is discussed in more detail in the section entitled Diagnosing.

Control of Respirations

The medulla in the brain stem immediately above the spinal cord is the respiratory center. It is stimulated by the increased concentration of carbon dioxide and hydrogen ions and, to a lesser degree, by the decreased amount of oxygen in the arterial blood. Chemoreceptors in the aortic arch and carotid bodies are also sensitive to the same arterial blood gas levels and can activate the medulla. Stimulation of the medulla increases the rate and depth of ventilation so carbon dioxide and hydrogen are blown off and oxygen levels are increased. The medulla sends an impulse down the spinal cord to the respiratory muscles to stimulate a contraction leading to inhalation. If the system is intact, the diaphragm, the major respiratory muscle, contracts and descends into the abdomen. The thoracic cavity enlarges. Lungs expand in response to pressure changes in the intrapleural space and the lung. Inhalation ceases when atmospheric air pressure and pulmonary air pressure are equal. Exhalation occurs, and the lungs return to their resting position. The accompanying box summarizes the general principles of respiration.

General Principles of Respiration

- All living cells require oxygen, which the body cannot store.
- The air passageways must remain patent for respiration to occur.
- Muscle movements provide the physical force essential for respiration.
- The pressure changes resulting from expansion and contraction of the thoracic cavity produce pulmonary gas exchange.
- Adequate fluid intake is essential to respiratory functioning.
- Ventilation depends on the extent of perfusion in the area.
- Oxygen and carbon dioxide must move through the alveoli and be carried to and from body cells by the blood.
- There must be an exchange of oxygen and carbon dioxide between the blood and body cells.

Table 45-1
Respiratory Variations in the Life Cycle

	Infant (Birth–1 year)	Early Childhood (1–5 years)	Late Childhood (6–12 years)	Aged Adult (65+ years)
Respiratory rate	30–60/min	20–40/min	15–25/min	16–20/min
Respiratory pattern	Abdominal breathing, irregular in rate and depth	Abdominal breathing, irregular	Thoracic breathing, regular	Thoracic, regular
Chest wall	Thin, little muscle, ribs and sternum easily seen	Same as infant's but with more subcutaneous fat	Further subcutaneous fat deposited, structures less prominent	Thin, structures prominent
Breath sounds	Loud, harsh crackles at end of deep inspiration	Loud, harsh expiration longer than inspiration	Clear inspiration is longer than expiration	Clear
Shape of thorax	Round	Elliptical	Elliptical	Barrel shaped or elliptical

Developmental Variations

Birth necessitates many adaptations in the newborn. The most blatant of these changes occur in the lungs, which are transformed from fluid-filled structures to air-filled organs. The normal infant's chest is small, the airways are short, and aspiration is a potential problem. The respiratory rate is more rapid in the infant than in any other age group (Table 45-1). As alveoli increase in number and size, adequate oxygenation is accomplished at lower respiratory rates. Respiratory rates stabilize in young adulthood.

Respiratory activity is abdominal in the infant. The infant's chest wall is so thin, with so little musculature, that ribs, sternum, and xiphoid process are easily noted. The infant has a rounded chest wall where anteroposterior diameter (ie, the measurement from the front to back of the thorax) equals transverse diameter. Occasional fine crackles at the end of deep inspiration noted on auscultation in the infant's thorax are normal.

In the preschool and school-age child, some subcutaneous fat is deposited on the chest wall so landmarks are less prominent than in the infant. Muscular development is also more noticeable. Transverse diameter and anteroposterior diameter ratio reaches adult configurations of 1:2 by age 6 years. The preschool child's eustachian tubes, bronchi, and bronchioles are elongated and less angular, so the number of routine colds and infections decreases until they enter school. Also, young children usually have not had the opportunity to develop antibodies for the variety of viruses and bacteria encountered. Good handwashing techniques and tissue etiquette are practices to be encouraged. Most children at this age experience colds or upper respiratory infections, but some have more serious problems of otitis media, bronchitis, and pneumonia. At the end of late childhood and during adulthood, the immune system is sufficiently seasoned to protect the person from most infections.

There are specific physical changes in older people that are unrelated to any pathology. Bony landmarks are more prominent because of the loss of subcutaneous fat. Kyphosis (curvature of the spine) contributes to the older person's appearance of leaning forward. Barrel chest deformity may result in a widening of the anterior–posterior diameter. In the absence of any abnormal findings with the physical examination, this is known as senile emphysema. The tissues and airways of the respiratory tract (including alveoli) become more rigid with age. Power of respiratory and abdominal muscles is reduced so the diaphragm moves less efficiently. These alterations increase the risk of disease, especially pneumonia.

Factors Affecting Respiratory Functioning

A variety of factors affect adequate respiratory functioning. Six important factors are included here.

Levels of Health

People with renal or cardiac disorders often demonstrate a compromise in respiratory functioning due to fluid overload. People with chronic illnesses often have muscle wasting and poor muscle tone, including muscles of the respiratory system.

Development

Developmental variations were discussed previously in this chapter. Physical changes such as scoliosis (curvature of the spine) influence breathing patterns so that air trapping occurs. There is a statistically significant correlation between obesity and chronic bronchitis. Obese people are often short of breath with activity and thus participate in little exercise. The alveoli at the base of the lungs are rarely stimulated to expand fully.

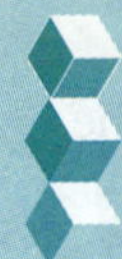

Research in Nursing: Making a Difference

Oxygenation

All body cells require oxygen to function, and supplying the body with oxygen is fundamental to life. The following studies have important implications for tailoring client care to promote efficient gas exchange. Nursing is challenged with meeting the unique needs and enhancing the quality of life for clients of all ages who are experiencing the sense of helplessness that usually accompanies an oxygen deficit.

Related Research

Marino, B., O'Brien, P., & Lore, H. (1995). Oxygen saturations during breast and bottle feedings in infants with congenital heart disease. *Journal of Pediatric Nursing, 10*(6), 360–364.
It has long been the belief that breast feeding is more strenuous than bottle feeding in children with congenital heart disease (CHD). In a group of infants with CHD, oxygen saturation decreased during bottle feeding and remained below baseline for the first 10 minutes after feeding ended. Four of the seven infants experienced oxygen saturation of less than 90% during these feedings. In the breast-fed infant, oxygen saturation remained above 90%. Nurses caring for infants with CHD need to assess oxygen saturation during bottle feeding to see if supplemental oxygen is needed. Based on the results of this study, breast feeding should be considered as an option for infants with CHD.

Waldo, M., Ide, B., & Thomas, D. (1995). Postcardiac-event elderly: Effect of exercise on cardiopulmonary function. *Journal of Gerontological Nursing, 21*(2), 12–19.
This study evaluated oxygen saturation, blood pressure, and heart rate in response to physical conditioning exercises in a sample of older individuals recovering from an acute cardiac event. Following a 6-week conditioning program, significantly lower blood pressures and heart rates during exercise indicated that myocardial oxygen consumption decreased in this population. This beneficial response to a conditioning exercise program appears to provide cardioprotective benefits and allows the postcardiac-event client to function more effectively.

Shiao, S., Youngblut, J., Anderson, G., DiFiore, J., & Martin, R. (1995). Nasogastric tube placement: Effects on breathing and sucking in very-low-birth-weight infants. *Nursing Research, 44*(2), 82–88.
Eighteen very-low-birth-weight (VLBW) infants were observed during routinely scheduled feedings with and without a nasogastric tube in place. This study indicated that the presence of the NG tube had negative effects on sucking and breathing for these infants. Whether to leave the NG tube in place or reinsert it before tube feedings has not been resolved. In the meantime, nurses responsible for oral feedings of VLBW infants with NG tubes need to monitor for compromised breathing, oxygen desaturation, and bradycardia.

Summary

Interference with oxygen requirements necessitates a comprehensive approach by the nurse that involves monitoring respiratory status, recognizing deviations from normal, and meeting the unique needs of individual clients. Besides being life threatening, oxygen deficits frequently result in alteration in lifestyle and body image. By recognizing physiologic and psychologic concerns, the nurse facilitates the client's ability to cope with alterations in oxygen needs.

Opioids (Narcotic Analgesics)

These chemical agents depress the medullary respiratory center so that the rate and depth of respirations are decreased. This is especially noted with the use of morphine and meperidine (Demerol). One must be alert to the potential of respiratory arrest when administering any narcotic or sedative.

Lifestyle

Sedentary activity patterns do not encourage the expansion of alveoli and the development of pulmonary exercise patterns (deep breathing). People who exercise routinely three to six times per week (eg, aerobics, walking, swimming) are better able to respond to stressors to respiratory health. Cigarette smoking (active and passive) is a major contributor to lung disease and respiratory distress.

Environment

It is impossible to pinpoint all effects of air pollution, but researchers have demonstrated a statistically high correlation between air pollution and cancer and lung diseases. A person with adequate respiratory functioning who is exposed to air pollution experiences stinging of eyes, coughing, choking, headache, and dizziness. People who have experienced an alteration in respiratory functioning in the past are often unable to continue self-care activities in a polluted environment.

Psychologic Health

Individuals responding to stress might demonstrate excessive sighing or hyperventilation breathing patterns. Generalized anxiety has been implicated by some scientists in establishing enough bronchospasm to produce an episode of bronchial asthma. Those experiencing an alteration in respiratory functioning develop some anxiety as a result of a physical disorder.

The Nurse as Role Model

Nurses working with clients to initiate changes in health habits that affect respiration must also examine themselves as a factor in the success of the plan. Clients use nurses as role models in achieving healthy lifestyles. Nurses dealing with stresses from professional and personal aspects of their own lives sometimes channel their energies into destructive behaviors. If the nurse wishes to encourage optimal respiratory functioning, he or she must demonstrate behaviors that support a healthy lifestyle (see the accompanying box). With this goal in mind, the nurse will do the following:

- Maintain adequate fluid intake and proper nutrition.
- Use deep breathing exercises.
- Evaluate his or her own use of nicotine.
- Incorporate a plan to reduce smoking and then stop smoking on a specific target date.
- Reduce activity patterns (ie, rest at home) in the presence of infection.
- Create a pollution-reduced environment by avoiding use of strong perfumes, aftershaves, or other scents.
- Arrange to have a tuberculin test (PPD) done annually.
- Schedule three to four periods of exercise per week.

ASSESSING RESPIRATORY FUNCTIONING

The health history is an essential component of assessing respiratory functioning. Either the client or the accompanying person can provide information. The nursing examination combined with laboratory findings can provide information to identify a client's strengths, the nature of the problem, its course, related signs and symptoms, onset, frequency, and effect on activities of daily living. The nurse decides, based on the findings, what problems can be treated independently by nursing. Other problems are referred to the physician for decisions on treatment.

Nursing History

The nursing history, an important clinical tool in the early steps of the nursing process, always includes a respiratory component. The information gained provides

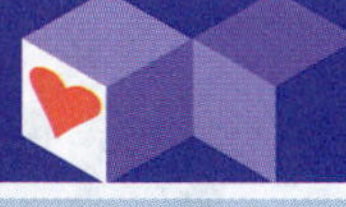

Promoting Wellness

Oxygenation

Use the assessment checklist to determine how well you are meeting oxygenation needs. Then develop a prescription for self-care by choosing appropriate behaviors from the list of suggestions.

Assessment Checklist

almost always	sometimes	almost never	
☐	☐	☐	1. I breathe easily, without discomfort and without feeling short of breath.
☐	☐	☐	2. I exercise regularly.
☐	☐	☐	3. I maintain normal weight for my height and body frame.
☐	☐	☐	4. I live in an environment free of pollution.
☐	☐	☐	5. I avoid substances (tobacco, chemicals) that cause respiratory problems.

Self-Care Behaviors

1. Follow a regular exercise program with 30 to 45 minutes of moderate activity three or four times a week.
2. Maintain normal body weight.
3. Obtain medical evaluation for chest pain, problems with breathing, chronic cough with sputum or blood.
4. Avoid smoking cigarettes, cigars, or pipes.
5. Avoid chemical substances that cause respiratory depression.
6. Maintain a pollution-free environment (as much as possible).
7. Support federal and community efforts to keep the air free of pollution.
8. Avoid exposure to second-hand smoke (from another's cigarette) when possible.

data on why a client needs nursing care and what kind of care is required to maintain a sufficient intake of air. Interview questions are used to identify current or potential health deviations, client actions for meeting this need and their effects, contributing factors, use of aids to improve intake of air, and effect on current lifestyle and relationships with others.

Before starting the interview, the nurse ascertains that the client and accompanying people are comfortable. If the client is in any respiratory distress, appropriate actions should be initiated to relieve symptoms. The accompanying people can answer questions to provide a data base. The nurse can expand this when the client is able to provide information. If the clinical condition of the client indicates that no emergency interventions are necessary, a comprehensive history can be obtained.

When a health deviation is noted during the data collection, the nurse needs to collect as much descriptive information as possible, verifying whether the status of the problem changed suddenly or slowly. Sample questions are given in the accompanying box.

Physical Assessment

The basic examination of the lungs and respiratory status are discussed in Chapter 26. The nurse proceeds in a well-organized manner with a sequence of inspection, palpation, percussion, and auscultation.

Inspection. Observation of the chest normally shows that the contour is slightly convex with no sternal depression. The anteroposterior diameter should be less than the transverse diameter. Any abnormalities in thoracic structure should be described or sketched (see Fig. 26-31 for examples). The contour of the intercostal spaces should be flat or depressed. Movement of the chest should be symmetric. The skin at the thorax should be warm and dry and exhibit even distribution of color with no cyanosis or pallor. Note any scars; origin would have been recorded in the history under previous surgery or accidents. Observe the respiratory rate and rhythm for 1 full minute. Normally, respirations are quiet and nonlabored. Any flaring of nostrils, intercostal restriction, tachypnea, or bradypnea suggests a health deviation that necessitates further evaluation.

The nurse must always be alert for common clinical manifestations that may indicate an airway emergency (see the accompanying box). Specific disease processes and conditions leading to acute respiratory failure, as well as specific clinical manifestations, are discussed in a medical–surgical textbook.

Palpation. The trachea should be equidistant from each clavicle. Skin temperature should be the same as the rest of the body. Respiratory excursion is measured by placing one's hand on the client's posterior thorax at the tenth rib with both thumbs almost touching the vertebrae. While the client takes a few deep breaths, the nurse's thumbs should move 5 to 8 cm symmetrically at maximal inspiration (see Fig. 26-33). To assess vocal *fremitus* (the capacity to feel sound on the chest wall), the nurse should place his or her palm surface to the client's chest wall, avoiding bony areas (eg, scapulae); the nurse should detect equal vibrations as the client says some multisyllable word (eg, "ninety-nine"). Bilaterally equal mild fremitus should be detected, with the greatest intensity noted at the anterior and posterior base of the neck and along the trachea and large bronchi. Increased fremitus is noted in clients with pneumonia, because solid tissue conducts sound well. Conversely, clients with chronic obstructive pulmonary disease (COPD) have decreased fremitus, because air does not conduct sound well. The presence or absence of crepitation, masses, edema, or tenderness should be noted.

Percussion. Percussion is performed posteriorly as the client pulls shoulders forward; examination proceeds down the client's back, comparing one side to the other. The anterior and lateral thorax can be examined with the client in a supine position. The nurse must listen to the intensity and quality of each sound as the chest wall and underlying structures are set in motion. Resonance, a loud, hollow, low-pitched sound, is heard over the normal lung. Emphysematous lungs produce a loud, low, booming sound called hyperresonance. A flat sound is detected over bone or heavy muscle. A dull sound with medium pitch and intensity is percussed on the liver (fifth intercostal space at the right midclavicular line). Tympany is a high-pitched, loud, drumlike sound produced over the stomach. Dullness over the lung field occurs when fluid or solid tissue replaces normal lung tissue in the pleural space; this finding requires further investigation.

Auscultation. The nurse should move from apex to base with the stethoscope, comparing one side with the other side. Normal breath sounds are of three types: *vesicular* (low pitch, soft expiration, and heard over most of lung); *bronchial* (high pitch and longer and heard over the trachea); and *bronchovesicular* (medium pitch and medium expiration and heard over the upper anterior chest and intercostal area; see Fig. 26-35). The client should breathe through the opened mouth slowly. Nasal breathing produces false abnormal breath sounds. Hyperventilation is conducive to syncope and client distress. If any abnormal breath sound is detected, the nurse should instruct the client to cough and should auscultate again for at least two breaths. A recording of location, change in breath sounds after coughing, and phase of respiration (eg, expiration) in which abnormal sound was heard is imperative.

Adventitious sounds can be divided into four categories: (1) crackles (formerly called rales); (2) gurgles (formerly called rhonchi); (3) wheezes; and (4) rubs. **Crackles** are discontinuous (intermittent) sounds that occur when air moves through airways that contain fluid. They are produced by a delayed reopening of deflated airways. Crackles can be further classified as fine or

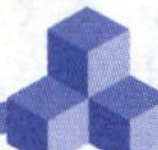

Focused Assessment Guide

Respiration

Factors to Assess	Questions and Approaches
Usual patterns of respiration	How would you describe your breathing patterns? Do you have allergies? Do you smoke? Do you live with a smoker or are there smokers in your workplace?
Recent changes	Have you noticed any changes in your breathing pattern (out of breath, cough, pain)? Do you have chest pain?
Cough	How much and how often do you cough? Is the cough related to the time of day or any activity? What is it like (dry, bubbly, hoarse)? Do you have a history of allergies? Do you ever wheeze? Are you exposed to dust? Fumes? Where do you work? What kind of work? How are you treating the cough?
Sputum	Do you ever cough up and spit out mucus? How much do you spit out and do you associate it with anything (time of day, environment)? What color is it? Is it ever blood tinged? What is its odor?
Chest pain	On a scale of 0 to 5 (5 being very painful), how severe is the pain? Where is the pain? Is the pain worse with inspiration? Expiration? Cough? Does the pain radiate? What measures are you using to relieve the pain?
Dyspnea	Is it constant or remittent or related to any activity? How do different positions affect it? How does it affect your daily activities? Is any part of your body bluish during the breathing problem? What do you do during and after the breathing attack? Have you ever been told that you have asthma? Emphysema? Tuberculosis? Heart disease? Do you think the problem is getting worse or staying the same?
Fever	Have you had pneumonia recently? Do you have any contact with people who have tuberculosis? Do you have night sweats? Are others in your household well or ill? Have you traveled anywhere recently? What medications are you using? Have you been exposed to any pollutants?
Fatigue	Have you noticed you feel more tired lately? Are you getting your normal amount of sleep at night? Has your sleep at night been affected by any difficulty breathing? Do you become easily fatigued when you climb stairs? Has your pattern of daily activity changed lately?

Recognizing Airway Emergencies

Common Clinical Manifestations

Universal distress signal (clutching throat with both hands)

and

Inability to speak or cough
Pain with respiration
Hemoptysis
Frothy white or pink sputum
Presence of adventitious breath sounds
Dyspnea

coarse. Fine crackles, high-pitched sounds heard toward the end of inspiration, indicate congestion in small air passages and alveoli. Rubbing strands of hair between your fingers creates a sound similar to fine crackles. They are usually first detected in the lung bases, usually cannot be cleared with coughing, and may be auscultated in a client who has pneumonia. Coarse crackles are somewhat louder, bubbly noises heard during inspiration and possibly expiration and not cleared by coughing. They result when air passes through fluid in the larger airways and indicate increasing pulmonary congestion. **Gurgles** are continuous, musical sounds that are more pronounced during expiration. Gurgles (also called rhonchi, and more recently, sonorous wheezes) reflect obstruction in large upper airways due to secretions or edema. They can sometimes be cleared with coughing and sound like snoring. **Wheezes** are continuous, high-pitched, squeaky sounds heard on expiration and sometimes on inspiration. They originate in smaller bronchi or bronchioles and are often detected in asthmatics. A *pleural friction rub* is a dry grating sound caused by inflammation of pleural surfaces. It is more often heard on inspiration than expiration, is unaltered by coughing, and resembles the sound made by rubbing two leather surfaces together. A pleural friction rub is easily confused with a pericardial friction rub. Stiesmeyer (1993) recommends an easy way to differentiate between the two: ask the client to hold his or her breath, and if the sound continues it is pericardial in nature because the sound occurs with each heart beat.

Common Methods to Assess Respiratory Functioning

Diagnostic Procedures

In addition to the nursing history and physical examination, various laboratory and radiologic tests described in Table 45-2 provide further assessment data that can aid in the formation of nursing diagnoses. These tests are not distinctive of a particular disease but they do reflect how well the respiratory system is functioning. Figure 45-5 demonstrates a pulse oximetry unit used for measuring oxygen saturation (SaO_2) of arterial blood, and Procedure 45-1 outlines nursing responsibilities when using a pulse oximetry unit.

Thoracentesis

A **thoracentesis** is the entering and aspirating of fluid from the pleural cavity. The pleural cavity is a potential cavity since it normally is not distended with fluid or air. The physician usually performs thoracentesis at the bedside with the nurse assisting. The client is required to sign a permit for this procedure. A thoracentesis may be performed to obtain and analyze a specimen for diagnostic purposes or to remove fluid that has accumulated in the pleural cavity and is causing respiratory difficulty and discomfort. Because the cavity being entered is sterile, surgical asepsis is used. Body substance precautions must be used.

One way to remove fluid or air from the pleural cavity is to aspirate it with a syringe. Another method for removing fluid is to drain the fluid into a bottle in which a partial vacuum has been created. A small plastic catheter may be threaded through the needle, allowing the needle to be withdrawn. This catheter reduces the possibility of puncturing the lung. When this method is used, the tubing connecting the needle and the bottle should be sterile. It is convenient to use a calibrated bottle for the drainage to determine readily the amount of fluid that has been removed. The upper limit usually is 1000 mL.

The skin is prepared over the area where the physician indicates the needle will be inserted. The exact location depends on the area in which fluid is present and where the physician can best aspirate it. After a local anesthetic is administered, the needle is inserted between the ribs through the intercostal muscles and fascia and into the pleura. When the procedure is completed, the needle or plastic catheter is removed and a small sterile dressing is placed over the entry site.

Nursing Responsibilities. The nurse is responsible for the collection of baseline data before the examination. The client must be instructed not to cough or breathe deeply during the test. It is imperative that the client remain as still as possible to diminish the risk of accidental injury to the lung.

This procedure usually is carried out when the client is sitting on a chair or on the edge of the bed with the feet supported on a chair. Figure 45-6 shows this position. If unable to sit up, the client may lie on the affected side with the hand of that side resting on the opposite shoulder.

During the procedure, the nurse observes the client for reactions. The client's color, pulse, and respiratory rates are observed, and any deviation from the norm is reported to the physician immediately. Fainting, nausea, and vomiting may occur. After the procedure, the client should be observed for changes in respirations. If a large

(text continues on page 1324)

Table 45-2
Common Methods to Assess Respiratory Functioning

Definition and Purpose	Normal Values	Nursing Implications
Spirometry measures lung capacity, volumes, and flow rates with the use of an instrument called a **spirometer**.		
Spirometry helps evaluate the pulmonary status and the efficacy of treatment. Corrections are made for age, sex, weight, and height. Common measurements are included.	*Tidal volume* (TV): The amount of air inspired and expired in a normal respiration. Normal is 500 mL. *Inspiratory reserve volume* (IRV): The amount of air that can be inspired beyond tidal volume. Normal is 3100 mL. *Expiratory reserve volume* (ERV): The amount of air that can be exhaled beyond tidal volume. Normal is 1200 mL. *Residual volume* (RV): The amount of air remaining in the lungs after a maximal expiration. Normal is 1200 mL. *Vital capacity* (VC): The maximal amount of air that can be exhaled following a maximal inhalation. Normal is 4800 mL. *Inspiratory capacity* (IC): The largest amount of air that can be inhaled following a normal quiet exhalation. Normal is 3600 mL. *Functional residual capacity* (FRC): FRC is equal to the expiratory reserve volume plus the residual volume. Normal is 2400 mL. A normal range is 75% to 125% of normal FRC. *Total lung capacity* (TLC): The sum of the TV + IRV + ERV + RV. Normal is 6000 mL.	The client's understanding and cooperation are important to successful study. Explanations should include teaching the client to wear a nose clip and a mouthpiece for breathing. Suffocation will not occur. The examination is not painful but it is fatiguing. The client should wear comfortable clothing. Tight clothing, such as a girdle or belt, may restrict breathing. Drugs affecting the respiratory tract, such as bronchodilators, are withheld before the examination so that test results reflect the client's present status. There is no special aftercare, but the client may need extra rest.
Arterial blood gas and pH analysis examine arterial blood to determine the pressure exerted by oxygen and carbon dioxide in the blood and the blood pH.		The procedure for obtaining arterial blood is uncomfortable, more so than an injection into a vein, muscle, or subcutaneous tissue, and the client should be prepared for this. The arm is usually used to obtain a blood sample. The radial artery or an artery in the inner aspect of the elbow is used. Occasionally, the femoral artery is entered. A pressure dressing is applied at the entry site for 3 minutes and watched for evidence of bleeding.
A blood sample is used to measure gas components in arterial blood and the pH of blood. It reflects quality of ventilation and perfusion.	The pressure of carbon dioxide ($PaCO_2$) is normally 35 to 45 mm Hg. The pressure of oxygen (PaO_2) is normally 80 to 100 mm Hg. The pH is normally between 7.35 and 7.45.	
Pulse oximetry is a noninvasive technique that measures the oxygen saturation (SaO_2) of arterial blood.		
Pulse oximetry is useful for monitoring people on oxygen, those at risk for hypoxia, and postoperative clients, and effectively records trends in oxygen saturation (SaO_2). It is not a replacement for arterial blood gas analysis but can be used selectively as adjunct therapy.	A range of 95% to 98% is considered normal oxygen saturation (SaO_2).	Movement, low perfusion (eg, peripheral vascular disease), and cigarette smoking can affect the SaO_2 value. Always check that the alarms are turned on before leaving the room. It is important to be aware of the client's hemoglobin level before evaluating oxygen saturation because this test measures only the percentage of oxygen carried by the available hemoglobin. Even a client with a low hemoglobin could appear to have a normal SaO_2 because most of that hemoglobin is saturated yet may not have enough oxygen to meet body needs.

Table 45-2 *(continued)*
Common Methods to Assess Respiratory Functioning

Definition and Purpose	Normal Values	Nursing Implications
Cytologic study of respiratory secretions involves a study of sputum and cells it contains.		
A *cytologic study* is done primarily to study cells that may be malignant, determine organisms causing infection, and identify blood or pus in the sputum.	Sputum is free of abnormal cells and of pus, blood, and bacteria.	Sputum is best obtained in the morning, before breakfast, after secretions have accumulated in the respiratory tract during the night. Usually, specimens are collected on 3 successive days. It is best to have the client brush his or her teeth and rinse the mouth so that saliva and oral debris do not contaminate the specimen. The client should be taught that sputum is matter ejected from the lower respiratory tract through the mouth and that saliva is an unsatisfactory specimen. The client should be instructed to inhale deeply and cough deeply on exhalation. About 1 teaspoon of sputum is needed for a specimen. The sputum should be coughed directly into a sterile specimen container, which is then covered with a sterile lid, properly labeled, and sent to the laboratory. A note should be made on the client's record about the character of the sputum, including amount, appearance, and odor. If a specimen cannot be obtained, an induced sputum specimen may be required.
Endoscopy is the direct visualization of a body cavity. A *bronchoscope* is used to examine the bronchi and a *laryngoscope* is used to examine the larynx. These are lighted, tubular instruments.		
Respiratory endoscopy is used to view lesions, obtain a biopsy, improve drainage, remove foreign substances, and drain abscesses.	No obstructions are normally found in respiratory passageways, and tissues appear normal.	An informed consent is necessary for endoscopy. Endoscopic examinations are uncomfortable for most clients, especially the bronchoscopy, and the client should be prepared for this. The client should be without food or fluid for 4 to 6 hours before endoscopy to avoid the risk of aspirating stomach contents. An analgesic, sedative, or tranquilizer is generally given about 30 minutes before endoscopy. The client should be taught that there may be gagging when local anesthesia is applied to the throat and there is a feeling that one cannot swallow or breathe. However, the airway remains open. Aftercare includes withholding fluids and food, usually for 1 or 2 hours, until the client can swallow and cough. Vital signs should be checked for signs of atelectasis and pneumonitis. Warm gargles may be used to relieve irritation in the pharynx once the gag reflex has returned.

(continued)

Table 45-2 *(continued)*
Common Methods to Assess Respiratory Functioning

Definition and Purpose	Normal Values	Nursing Implications
		The client should be observed for **hemoptysis,** which is sputum containing blood, and for excessive bleeding, especially if a biopsy has been obtained. If contrast media were used during the examination, the client should be helped and encouraged to cough to rid the bronchial tree of the material.
Skin tests determine antigen–antibody reactions.		
In intradermal tests, antigens, those to which the client may have been previously exposed, are injected into the superficial layer of skin with a needle and syringe or a sterile four-pronged lancet to evaluate immune response. Patch and scratch tests, applied to hairless portions of the client's body, are used to evaluate the immune system's ability to respond to known allergens.	Negative reactions indicate a lack of sensitivity. Positive reactions, which indicate a positive antigen–antibody reaction, are discussed in clinical texts.	Check the client's history for hypersensitivity to any of the test antigens. If positive, notify physician before performing tests. These skin tests are not usually performed with infants because of their immature immune system. If the client is an outpatient, instruct him or her to return at the appropriate time to have the test results read. Do not perform tests in areas with acne, dermatitis, or excessive hair. On the chart, record the test, time, date, method, and site of administration. After reading the results, document the reaction noting amount of erythema or induration.
Radiography is an x-ray examination of the lungs and thoracic cavity.		
X-ray examinations of the lungs are done to help diagnose pulmonary diseases and to determine the progress of development of disease.	The bony thoracic and soft tissues have normal positions, symmetry, and shape.	There is no special preparation for flat films of the chest, and the examinations are without discomfort. The client should be taught that clothing and jewelry from the waist up must be removed and that the client will be asked to hold his or her breath when the x-ray film is taken.
Lung scan is the recording on a photographic plate of the emissions of radioactive waves from a substance injected into a vein as it circulates through the lung.		
A *perfusion scan* (Q scan) is done to measure integrity of pulmonary blood vessels and evaluate blood flow abnormalities (eg, pulmonary emboli). A *ventilation scan* (V scan) is done to detect ventilation abnormalities (especially in clients with emphysema). Both scans used together provide greater and more accurate diagnostic information than either test used solely.	Q scan shows no increased uptake of radioactive drug. V scan shows no abnormalities.	Explain procedure to client. In a Q scan, the radiologist injects radiopharmaceutical into a peripheral vein. Scan of chest is done in x-ray department. Client lies under the camera for 20 to 40 minutes. Ventilation scan is done after the perfusion scan. Scan is completed in x-ray department after client inhales radioactive gas by mask and then exhales it out of the lungs to room air. In 8 hours, the radioactive isotope disintegrates and is cleared from the circulation.

amount of fluid is removed, respirations usually are eased. If the lung has been punctured inadvertently, respiratory distress becomes acute. If blood appears in the sputum or the client has severe coughing, the physician should be notified promptly. A chest x-ray usually is done following the procedure to verify the absence of complications.

DIAGNOSING

Alterations in Respiratory Function as the Problem. After the assessment is completed and the data are examined, the nurse concludes either that there is no problem at this time or that there is an actual or potential respiratory problem that is amenable to independent or inter-

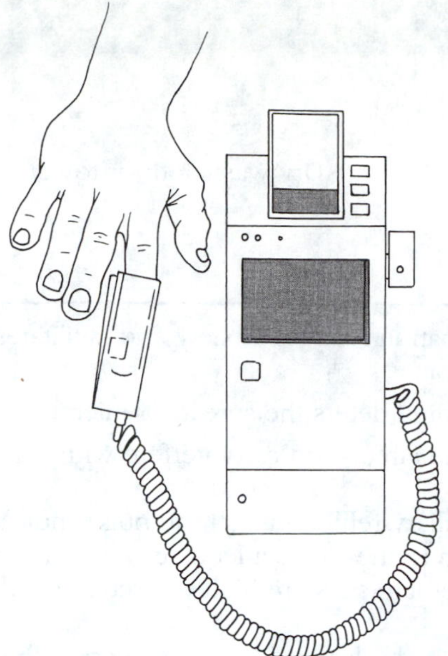

Figure 45-5
Portable pulse oximetry unit used to measure oxygen saturation (SaO_2) of arterial blood.

dependent nursing action. Nursing diagnoses indicating alterations in respiratory function are as follows:

Ineffective Airway Clearance
Ineffective Breathing Pattern
Impaired Gas Exchange

These three nursing diagnoses are discussed in detail at the end of this chapter in the section entitled Nursing Process in Clinical Practice.

Common etiologies for these diagnoses are inability to maintain proper position, pain or fear of pain, viscous secretions, fatigue, decreased level of consciousness, lack of knowledge, smoking, allergy, mechanical obstruction, medications, and decreased elasticity of lungs.

Examples of these diagnoses, etiologic factors, and defining characteristics are given in the accompanying box.

Alterations in Respiratory Function as the Etiology. Alteration in respiratory functioning may affect other areas of human functioning. Examples of other nursing diagnoses resulting from alterations in respiratory functioning are the following:

Activity Intolerance related to shortness of breath
Anxiety related to feeling of suffocation
Pain related to pleurisy
Impaired Verbal Communication related to endotracheal intubation
Ineffective Individual Coping related to frequent hospitalization due to acute symptoms of COPD
Diversional Activity Deficit related to loss of ability to perform specific activities due to shortness of breath
Fatigue related to impaired oxygen transport system
Fear related to disabling respiratory illness
Dysfunctional Grieving related to loss of normal respiratory functioning
Altered Health Maintenance related to smoking
Noncompliance With [eg, Performance of Daily Respiratory Exercises] related to side effects of therapy
Altered Nutrition: Less Than Body Requirements, related to difficulty breathing
Altered Oral Mucous Membrane related to presence of endotracheal tube
Powerlessness related to inability for self-care due to COPD
Self-Esteem Disturbance related to loss of normal respiratory function
Sleep Pattern Disturbance related to orthopnea and bronchodilators
Social Isolation related to inability to walk to usual "people places"
Risk for Suffocation related to child playing with a plastic bag
Risk for Aspiration related to reduced level of consciousness

Important Distinctions. Each nursing statement identifies what is wrong with the client and suggests expected client outcomes. The etiology of the problem directs nursing interventions. The nurse, in analyzing the assessment data, must decide if the alteration in respiratory functioning:

- Is the problem
- Is contributing to a different problem
- Is a sign or symptom of a problem

Altered respiratory functioning can fit into all three categories. This can be illustrated by examining how ineffective airway clearance in a 17-year-old asthmatic baseball player who is waiting to hear from the college of his choice plays a role in three different nursing diagnoses:

Ineffective Airway Clearance related to pollen exposure, exercise, and stress of questionable college admission. The airway clearance is the problem statement. Nursing interventions are directed to reducing exposure to pollens, specific stressors, and timing or degree of exercise. The outcome will be that the client achieves effective airway clearance.

Activity Intolerance related to ineffective airway clearance during and after baseball games, fatigue, and stress. Here, the activity intolerance is the problem statement and ineffective airway clearance is just one of the many factors contributing to the problem. All the nursing interventions are directed to improving the tolerance for activity.

Ineffective Individual Coping related to stress of career choices and stress of performance during baseball games as demonstrated by recent increase in episodes of asthmatic attacks. In this case, the ineffective airway clearance is a symptom of the client's real problem—ineffective coping. Nursing interventions are directed to reducing stressors. When the client is able to improve the use of his coping skills, the expected outcome is that the number of asthma attacks will decrease.

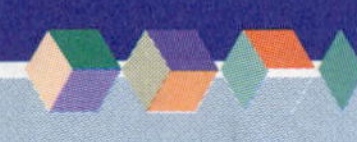

PROCEDURE 45-1

Using a Pulse Oximeter

Equipment

Pulse oximeter
Alcohol swab
Dry washcloth or towel
Nail polish remover (if necessary)

Action	Rationale
1. Explain procedure to client.	An explanation relieves anxiety and facilitates client cooperation.
2. Wash your hands.	Handwashing deters the spread of microorganisms.
3. Select an adequate site for application of the sensor:	Inadequate circulation can interfere with the SaO_2 reading.
a. Use the client's index, middle, or ring finger.	
b. Check the proximal pulse and capillary refill at the pulse closest to the site.	Brisk capillary refill and a strong pulse indicate that circulation to the site is adequate.
c. If circulation at site is inadequate, the earlobe, forehead, or bridge of nose may be considered.	These alternate sites are highly vascular alternatives.
d. Use a toe only if lower extremity circulation is not compromised.	Peripheral vascular disease is common in lower extremities.
4. Use the proper equipment:	Inaccurate readings can result if probe or sensor is not attached correctly.
a. If one finger is too large for the probe, use a smaller one. A pediatric probe may be used for a small adult.	
b. Use probes appropriate for client's age and size.	
c. Check if client is allergic to adhesive. A nonadhesive finger clip or reflectance sensor is available.	A reaction may occur if client is allergic to adhesive substance.
5. Prepare the monitoring site:	Skin oils, dirt, or grime on site; polish; and artificial nails can interfere with the passage of light waves. Newer oximeters can read through red and pink nail polish and some artificial nails. Blue, green, gold, black, and brown polish should always be removed.
a. Cleanse the selected area with an alcohol prep. Allow site to dry.	
b. Remove nail polish and artificial nails after checking manufacturer's instructions.	
6. Apply the probe securely to the skin. Make sure that the light-emitting sensor and the light-receiving sensor are aligned opposite each other (not necessary to check if placed on the forehead or bridge of the nose).	Secure attachments and proper alignment of the markings for the light-emitting and light-receiving sensor promote satisfactory operation of the equipment and accurate recording of the SaO_2.
7. Connect the sensor probe to the pulse oximeter and check operation of the equipment (presence of audible beep and fluctuation of bar of light or waveform on the face of the oximeter).	Audible beep represents the arterial pulse and fluctuating waveform indicates strength of the pulse. A weak signal will produce an inaccurate recording of the SaO_2.
8. Set the alarms on the pulse oximeter. Check manufacturer's alarm limits for high and low pulse rate settings.	Alarm provides additional safeguard for client and signals when high or low limits have been surpassed.
9. Check oxygen saturation at regular intervals as ordered by physician and necessitated by alarms. Monitor client's hemoglobin level.	Monitoring SaO_2 provides ongoing assessment of client's condition. A low hemoglobin level may be satisfactorily saturated yet not be adequate to meet a client's oxygen needs.
10. Remove sensor on a regular basis and check for skin irritation or signs of pressure (every 2 hr for spring-tension sensor or every 4 hr for adhesive finger or toe sensor).	Prolonged pressure may lead to tissue necrosis and adhesive sensor may cause skin irritation.

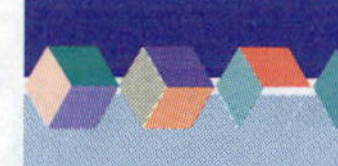

PROCEDURE 45-1 *(continued)*

Using a Pulse Oximeter

Action	Rationale
11. Evaluate any malfunctions or problems with equipment.	
a. For absent or weak signal check the client's vital signs and condition. If satisfactory, check connections and circulation to site.	Hypotension makes an accurate recording difficult. Equipment (restraint, BP cuff) may compromise circulation to site and cause venous blood to pulsate, giving an inaccurate reading.
b. For inaccurate reading check prescribed medications and history of circulatory disorders. Try device on a healthy person to see if problem is equipment-related or client-related.	Drugs that cause vasoconstriction interfere with accurate recording of oxygen saturation.
c. If bright light (sunlight or fluorescent light) is suspected of causing equipment malfunction, cover probe with a dry washcloth.	Bright light can interfere with operation of light sensors and cause unreliable report.
12. Document and report SaO_2 appropriately.	Ensures continuity of care and ongoing assessment record.

Home Care Consideration Portable units are available for use in the home or an outpatient setting.

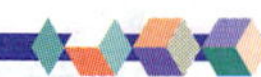

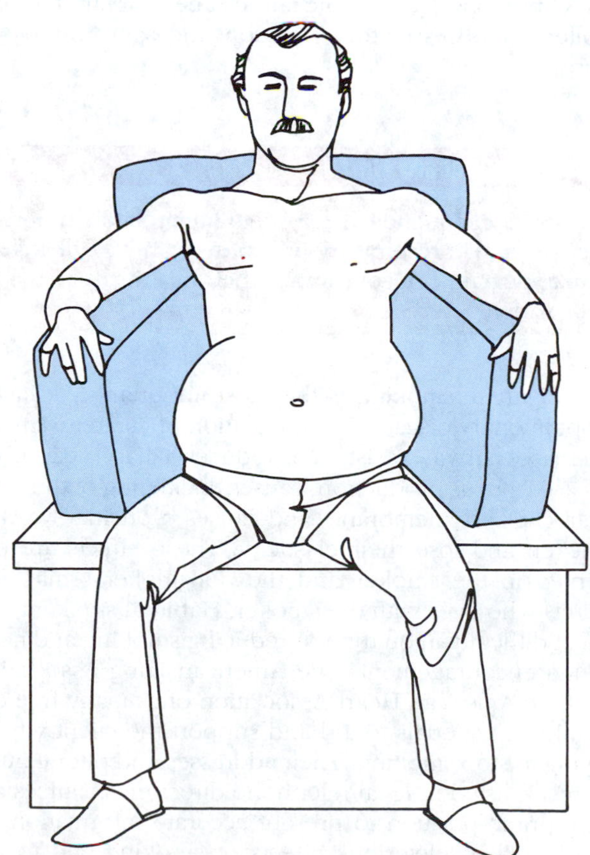

Figure 45-6
Position of the client for thoracentesis.

Each nursing diagnosis is unique to the situation, and the etiology varies with each client. The nurse, with the client, decides which problem is the priority. With creativity and patience, the nurse arrives at a nursing diagnosis that clearly directs nursing interventions and expected outcomes. However, there might be interventions initiated by another member of the healthcare team for the nurse to follow (eg, the prescription for administering medications). This would be the dependent aspect of nursing practice. The interdependent aspect refers to problems in which the nurse and other healthcare team members collaborate to treat (eg, nurses monitoring side effects of prescribed medications).

PLANNING: EXPECTED OUTCOMES

Whenever nurses care for clients with an alteration in respiratory functioning, nursing measures are supportive of the following general expected outcomes. The client will:

- Demonstrate improved gas exchange in his or her lungs by an absence of cyanosis or chest pain
- Relate causative factors, if known, and relate adaptive method of coping with the factors
- Preserve pulmonary function by maintaining optimal level of activity
- Demonstrate self-care behaviors that provide relief from symptoms and prevent further pulmonary problems

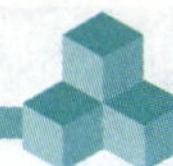

Nursing Diagnoses for Common Problems

Respiration

Problem	Related Factors	Sample Defining Characteristics
Ineffective Airway Clearance	Thick yellow secretions, fever, fatigue, dehydration, poor nutrition	"I never feel as though I am getting enough air." Seventy-year-old man with a 20-year history of COPD, recent development of pneumonia. He is pale with circumoral cyanosis. His respiratory rate is 40 per minute and shallow. Rhonchi are auscultated bilaterally. He does not sit quietly in chair or on bed. He cannot walk length of room without coughing episode, which produces little sputum.
Impaired Gas Exchange	Smokes one pack per day; works with asbestos in auto factory; has had a cold for 7 days	Cyanotic 50-year-old man. Using pursed-lip breathing while sitting on emergency room stretcher. Sitting hunched forward with overbed table supporting arms. Altered blood gases show respiratory acidosis. Admits to shortness of breath, nausea, and ankle edema for 1 week.
Ineffective Breathing Pattern	Anxious about results of cardiac catheterization and possible cardiac surgery	Hyperventilating, tachypneic (40 minutes). "I have a tingling feeling in my fingers."

When the client's physical, psychosocial, and spiritual conditions contribute to alterations in respiratory function, individualized expected outcomes are developed with the client's input. For example: "By March 15, the client will be able to walk up one flight of steps at home without dyspnea."

IMPLEMENTING

Teaching About Pollution-Free Environments

A pollution-free environment is particularly important for individuals with respiratory problems. The nurse needs to teach the client to assess the environment and make adjustments, where possible, to factors that impair respiratory functioning. The client must actively plan to prevent exposure to pollutants. This might involve a job change, use of protective equipment, enforcement of existing laws by government agencies, or subcontracting jobs. Dusting and vacuuming of office and home must be done minimally twice per week. If it is the client who must perform the tasks, a mask prevents some symptoms of respiratory distress. Exposure to industrial or occupational hazards (eg, paint, varnish, gaseous fumes, and asbestos) must be restricted.

In the United States and Canada, fine pollutants that pose a hazard to health are monitored closely. They are carbon monoxide, sulfur dioxide, total suspended particulates, ozone, and nitrogen dioxide. On days when pollutant levels are significantly elevated, morbidity and mortality rates among people with preexisting pulmonary disease are greatly increased. Thus, on those days when pollution alerts are announced, the nurse instructs the client with an alteration in respiratory function to decrease activity level, stay indoors, and use an air conditioner, electronic air cleaner, or air filter. If pollen alters respiratory function, the same principles apply.

Home Healthcare Alert

Instruct client and caregivers to immediately report any sign of a respiratory infection (eg, fever, change in appearance of sputum) to their healthcare provider.

Cigarette smoking is the most important risk factor in pulmonary disease. The inhalation of cigarette smoke increases airway resistance, reduces ciliary action, increases mucus production, causes thickening of the alveolar–capillary membrane, and causes bronchial walls to thicken and lose their elasticity. These effects are observed in the smoker and the nonsmoker (child and adult) who lives with the smoker. Habitual smokers find great difficulty in quitting or reducing smoking and need much encouragement. The American Lung Association and the American Heart Association offer many free educational materials to aid and support the client who is trying to stop smoking. Their addresses and phone numbers are listed in local telephone directories. Nurses are in a prime position to present accurate information regarding the deleterious effects of smoking and to encourage the decision to stop smoking or never to start smoking.

Establishing a Trusting Nurse–Client Relationship

Most people with a deviation in respiratory functioning experience anxiety as a result of symptoms and an actual or potential loss of independence. Oxygen deficits, particularly in older people, negatively affect all aspects of their daily living. The accompanying box focuses on oxygen problems and nursing education strategies for this particular group.

The nurse needs to create an environment that is likely to reduce anxiety. Immediate discomfort should be treated. Use of effective listening skills and accurate observation validate a caring attitude. Nurses must seek to understand clients' life experiences and habits without prejudging them. Clients often bring a fear of stigma into a professional relationship (especially with detrimental health habits), and this impedes the application of nursing interventions. The client who believes the nurse is genuinely concerned about him or her and the family is more willing to work toward achieving mutually desirable outcomes.

Promoting Proper Breathing

Breathing exercises are designed to aid the client to achieve more efficient and controlled ventilations, to decrease the work of breathing, and to correct respiratory defects.

Deep Breathing

Habits of breathing that are not conducive to maximal respiratory functioning are common in well and ill people. Some people develop a pattern of shallow breathing or walk with a caved-in–appearing chest wall. Ill people, for any number of reasons, may limit respiratory efforts. Hypoventilation occurs when there is a decreased amount of air entering and leaving the lungs. Deep-breathing exercises to produce hyperventilation are often used to overcome hypoventilation.

The nurse instructs the client to make each breath deep enough to move the bottom ribs. Unless there is a nasal condition that prohibits or prevents normal breathing, the client should start slow, deep ventilations nasally and expire slowly through the mouth. Breathing through the nose warms, filters, and humidifies the air. Respiratory status, motivation, and general clinical condition dictate the timing of this exercise, done hourly while awake or four times daily.

Using Incentive Spirometry

In incentive spirometry, the client takes a deep breath and observes the results of his or her efforts registered on the spirometry equipment as the client sustains that maximal inspiration. Incentive spirometry keeps the alveoli from collapsing so that gas exchange can occur and secretions can be cleared and expectorated. Instructions are necessary before using incentive spirometry equipment and also effectively validate correct use of this equipment in the home environment. This intervention offers immediate positive reinforcement to the client for his or her breathing efforts. See the accompanying box for additional suggestions when teaching the client to use this device.

Abdominal or Diaphragmatic Breathing

Many people with COPD have a tendency to breathe in a shallow, rapid, and exhausting pattern. This type of upper chest breathing can be changed to diaphragmatic breathing, reducing the rate, increasing the tidal volume, and reducing the functional residual capacity. The client

Focus on the Older Adult

Nursing Strategies for Oxygen Problems Affecting Older Adults

Decreased Gas Exchange and Increased Work of Breathing

- Encourage rest periods as necessary.
- Teach stair-climbing techniques.
- Encourage cessation or moderation of smoking.
- Teach breathing exercises.
- Remind about avoiding air pollutants.
- Caution about effect of extreme weather conditions.
- Instruct to avoid narcotics and sleeping pills.
- Discuss home management with client and family.
- Teach avoidance of infection and preventive measures (ie, flu vaccination).
- Use pillows as necessary to sleep.
- Encourage moderate exercise as tolerated.
- Encourage smaller, more frequent meals.

Decreased Ventilation and Ineffective Cough

- Encourage increased fluid intake, especially water, as allowed.
- Use cool-mist humidifier.
- Encourage attendance at pulmonary exercise rehabilitation program.
- Discourage use of over-the-counter medications.
- Teach how to splint thorax and cough effectively.
- Instruct in use of supplemental oxygen.
- Teach avoidance of milk products if they are troublesome.

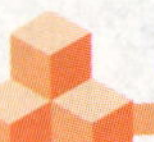

Guidelines for Nursing Care

Using an Incentive Spirometer

- Assist client to upright position if possible.
- Remove dentures if they fit poorly.
- Demonstrate how to steady device with one hand and hold mouthpiece with other hand.
- Instruct the client to exhale normally and place lips securely around mouthpiece.
- Instruct client not to breathe through his or her nose. Use a nose clip if necessary.
- Instruct the client to inhale slowly and as deeply as possible through the mouthpiece.
- Tell client to hold breath and count to three. Check position of gauge to determine progress and level attained.
- Instruct client to remove lips from mouthpiece and exhale normally.
- Tell client to complete breathing exercises approximately 10 times every hour if possible. Rest in between breaths as necessary.

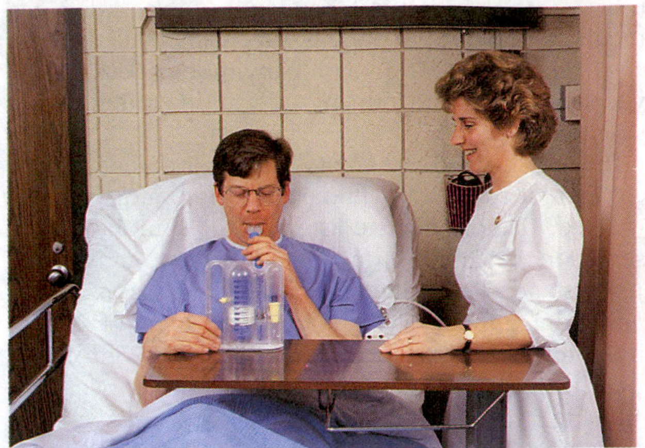

is instructed to place one hand on the stomach and the other on the middle of the chest. The client then should breathe in slowly through the nose, letting the abdomen protrude as far as it will go. Next, he or she should breathe out through pursed lips while contracting the abdominal muscles. One hand should be pressing inward and upward on the abdomen. These steps should be repeated for 1 minute followed by rest for 2 minutes. The breathing pattern should be practiced several times during the day. Eventually it will become automatic.

Pursed-Lip Breathing. Clients who experience dyspnea and feelings of panic often obtain control of the respiration by using pursed-lip breathing. This exercise trains the muscles to prolong exhalation, increasing airway pressure during expiration and loosening the amount of airway trapping and resistance. To do this, the client inhales through the nose while counting to three and exhales slowly and evenly against pursed lips while tightening the abdominal muscles. During exhalation, the client counts to seven. To purse the lips, the client should position the lips as though he or she were sucking through a straw or whistling. While walking, the client should inhale while walking two steps and then exhale through pursed lips while taking the next four steps and then repeat the cycle. Before teaching these techniques, the nurse should practice them alone and then with a partner.

Managing Chest Tubes

Clients who develop fluid (*pleural effusion*), blood (*hemothorax*), or air (*pneumothorax*) in the pleural space require the assistance of a chest tube to drain these substances and allow the compressed lung to reexpand. A chest tube is a firm plastic tube with drainage holes in the proximal end that is placed in the pleural space, secured with a suture and tape, covered with an air-tight dressing, and attached to a drainage system that may or may not include suction. Other components of the system may include an air seal to prevent air from reentering the chest once it has escaped and a suction control chamber that protects against excess suction pressure in the pleural cavity (Smith, Fallentine, & Kessel, 1995). Most healthcare agencies currently use molded plastic, three-compartment disposable chest drainage units in place of the one-, two-, or three-bottle system. Placement of the chest tubes in the chest cavity is determined by the type of drainage. To drain air, the tube is placed higher in the chest, whereas gravity forces fluids to settle at the base of the lung, thus requiring a lower tube.

Nursing responsibilities include assisting with insertion and removal of a chest tube and, once the tube is in place, monitoring the client's respiratory status and vital signs, checking the dressing, and maintaining the patency and integrity of the drainage system. Sterile gauze and a padded clamp should be kept at the bedside for emergency use if the tube is accidentally dislodged or disconnected from the drainage system. The drainage unit should always be maintained below the client's chest level. Drainage assessment (amount and type) requires assessment every hour postoperatively for 24 hours, followed by subsequent checks every eight hours. Drainage for a certain time period may be indicated on the collection chamber but is never emptied from the chest tube drainage set-up. The physician should be notified if drainage exceeds 100 mL/h. Figure 45-7 illustrates a chest drainage system.

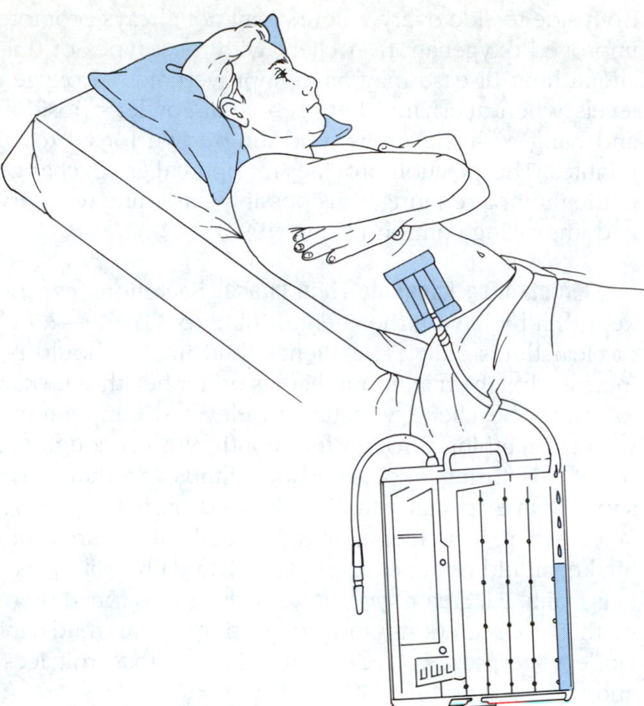

Figure 45-7
A chest drainage system attached to a client.

Promoting and Controlling Coughing

The presence of excessive fluids or secretions in an organ or body tissue is called *congestion*, and a person with secretions or fluid in the lungs is said to have congested lungs. If the cough is dry, the client is said to be congested with a *nonproductive cough*. If the cough produces respiratory tract secretions, the client is referred to as being congested with a *productive cough*. Thick respiratory secretions are sometimes called *phlegm*. A client who is coughing with no congestion or secretions produced is described as being noncongested with a nonproductive cough.

Cough Mechanism. The cough mechanism (Fig. 45-8) consists of an initial irritation; a deep inspiration; a quick, tight closure of the glottis together with a forceful contraction of the expiratory intercostal muscles; and the upward push of the diaphragm. This causes an explosive movement of air from the lower to the upper respiratory tract. To be effective, a cough should have enough muscle contraction to force air to be expelled and to propel a liquid or a solid on its way out of the respiratory tract. This is most effective when the client is sitting upright with feet flat on the floor. A cough is a cleaning mechanism of the body. It is a means of helping to keep the airway clear of secretions and other debris.

Voluntary Coughing. When a cough does not occur as a result of reflex stimulation of the cough-sensitive areas, it can be induced voluntarily. Teaching the client to cough voluntarily is an important aspect of preoperative and postoperative care. Although the teaching of deep breathing and coughing is relatively easy, experience has shown that it is difficult to have the client follow through and do them on his or her own. Frequent reminders throughout the day are necessary for many clients. Having a specific schedule on the nursing plan of care is advised. Coughing early in the morning after rising removes phlegm that accumulated during the night. Coughing before meals improves the taste of food and oxygenation. At bedtime, coughing removes any buildup of phlegm and improves sleep patterns. For a client who is unable to cough voluntarily, manual stimulation over the trachea and prolonged exhalation can be helpful. If neither of these methods is successful, mechanical endotracheal suctioning with a catheter is used sometimes.

Involuntary Coughing. Involuntary coughing often accompanies respiratory tract infections and irritations. It helps clear the airway if it is productive, but it is fatiguing and irritating when it is nonproductive. Medication may control involuntary coughing. Observations of the characteristics of breathing and coughing are necessary to determine the appropriate type of medication.

Cough Suppressants. *Suppressants* are drugs that depress a body function, in this case, the cough reflex. Codeine, which is present in many cough preparations, is generally considered the preferred cough suppressant ingredient. However, codeine can be addictive. Because of possible abuse, many states require a physician's prescription for its use. Dextromethorphan hydrobromide (Benylin DM, Balminil DM) is considered by some authorities to be as effective as codeine, and it is not addictive. Diphenhydramine hydrochloride (Benadryl), a potent antihistamine, is an effective cough suppressant. However, drowsiness (also common in other antihistamines) is a side effect of its use. Therefore, it may not be

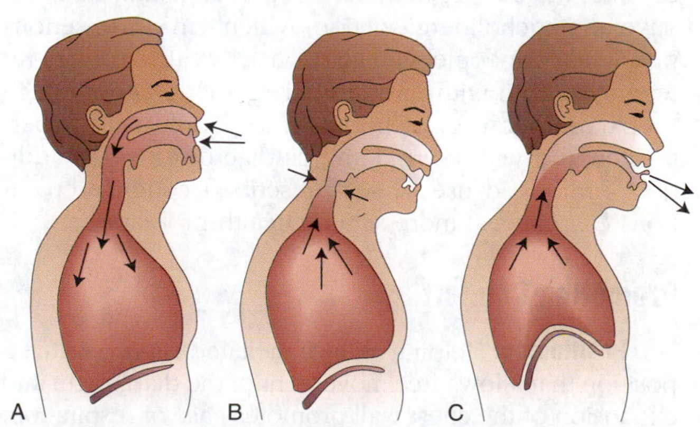

Figure 45-8
(**A**) A cough begins with a deep inspiration, distending the trachea and hyperinflating the lungs. (**B**) After inspiration, the glottis closes while intercostal and abdominal muscles contract forcibly. (**C**) When intrathoracic pressure reaches a high level, the glottis opens slightly, the diaphragm is pushed up, producing an explosive movement of air.

safe to use when the person must remain alert, as when driving a car.

An irritating nonproductive cough in people without congestion may be appropriately treated with suppressants. Inappropriate suppression of the cough in a person with respiratory congestion can result in harmful retention of the secretions.

Expectorants. *Expectorants* are drugs that facilitate the removal of respiratory tract secretions by reducing the secretion viscosity. Clients with extremely tenacious secretions may need the secretions liquefied so the cough can be effective. In that way, the nonproductive cough of a person with lung congestion can become productive. An expectorant used by a person who does not have congestion is inappropriate. Guaifenesin (Robitussin) is widely used as an expectorant in cough preparations. Adequate fluid intake and air humidification are considered effective expectorants by some authorities.

Lozenges. Mild nonproductive coughs in people without congestion can often be relieved by lozenges. A *lozenge* is a small, solid medication intended to be held in the mouth until it dissolves. Lozenges generally control coughs by the local anesthetic effect of benzocaine. The local anesthetic can act on sensory and motor nerves by controlling the primary irritation and by inhibiting afferent and efferent impulses.

Teaching About Cough Preparations. Because cough preparations are so readily available and people who purchase them are usually eager for relief, the consumer sometimes takes excessive amounts of more than one type. The nurse can offer health teaching about the appropriate choice of expectorants and suppressants. Also, the nurse should teach other misuses of cough mixtures. For example, cough syrups with a high sugar or alcohol content can disturb the metabolic balance of people with diabetes mellitus. Preparations containing antihistamines have an anticholinergic action, which can cause serious problems for people with glaucoma, or cause urinary retention in men with prostate enlargement. Other cough preparations can be detrimental to people with hypertension and with thyroid and cardiac diseases. In addition, prolonged use of self-prescribed cough preparations can conceal more serious health problems.

Promoting Comfort

Positioning. Helping an incapacitated client assume a position that allows free movement of the diaphragm and expansion of the chest wall promotes ease of respiration. For example, sitting in a slumped position, which permits the abdominal contents to push upward on the diaphragm, results in less lung expansion during inspiration. People with dyspnea and orthopnea are most comfortable in a high Fowler's position because the accessory muscle can then be used easily to promote respiration. Research has demonstrated that turning bedridden clients from side to side every 2 hours may not always promote improved oxygenation. A client with most types of unilateral lung disease may have improved arterial oxygen levels when alternated between semi-Fowler's position and lying with the undiseased lung down for 60 to 90 minutes. This position provides for optimal gas exchange in the unimpaired lung, thus possibly hastening recovery and improving comfort (Yeaw, 1992).

Maintaining Adequate Fluid Intake. Secretions can be kept thin by having the client drink 2 to 3 qt (1.9–2.9 L) of clear fluids daily. The client's fluid intake should be increased to the maximum that his or her health state can tolerate. The client who has an elevated temperature, who is breathing through the mouth, who is coughing, or who is losing excessive body fluids in other ways should have special attention focused on his or her intake. If there is incidence of right side heart failure, fluid intake should not exceed 1½ qt (1.4 L) daily. Milk products (milk, ice cream, yogurt, cheese, and so forth) work to thicken secretions and congestion. Clear fluids include water, tea, coffee, apple juice, broths, fruit ices, and flavored gelatin.

Providing Humidified Air. When air humidity is low, artificial means for humidifying inspired air may be advisable. The inspiration of dry air removes the normal moisture in the respiratory passages, which is essential for protection from irritation and infection. Room humidifiers may be helpful for some clients. Electric vaporizers that produce steam or cool mist are available. Authorities believe the therapeutic value of one over the other has not been demonstrated. A cool-mist vaporizer does not present dangers with burns because it does not generate heat or hot water. However, it can provide the medium for pathogen growth if inadequately cleaned. The steam vaporizer does not present this problem.

Percussing. *Cupping* (Fig. 45-9) is the manual percussion of lung areas to loosen pulmonary secretions so that they can be expectorated with greater ease. Percussion by cupping with the client supine or prone is carried out as follows:

1. Cup the hand by holding it in a rigid, dome-shaped position.
2. Strike rhythmically over the lobes of the lungs to be drained while keeping your wrists, elbows, and shoulders relaxed. Move the cupped hands from the client's lower ribs to the shoulders in back, and from the lower ribs to the top of the chest in front.
3. Listen for a hollow sound while percussing. The client should experience no pain. If the sound is not hollow and the client is uncomfortable, you are probably not cupping the hand enough and are slapping the client's skin.
4. Do not percuss on bare skin. The client may wear a gown or underclothing.
5. Do not percuss below the ribs or over the spine or breasts because of the danger of tissue damage.

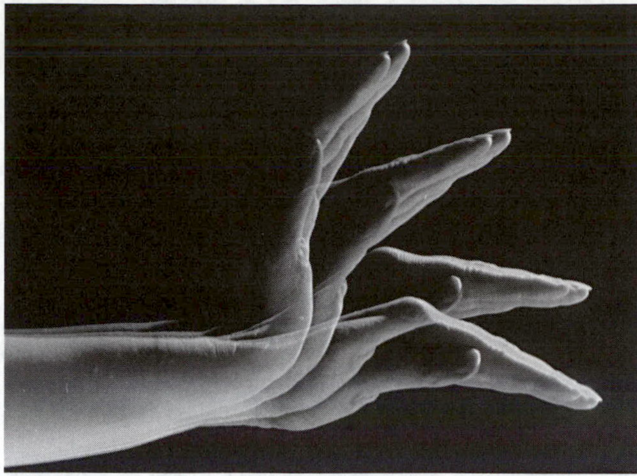

Figure 45-9
The cupping position and action of the hand in manual percussion of lung area.

6. Use percussion for 30 to 60 seconds over an area several times a day, but up to 3 to 5 minutes for clients with tenacious secretions.

The client may learn to percuss anterior surfaces of his or her chest wall. Family members are often taught to percuss posterior surfaces. Also, mechanical devices are available for percussion on the chest wall.

Vibrating. *Vibration* involves the nurse's rhythmic contraction and relaxation of the arm and shoulder muscles while holding the hands flat on the client's chest wall. The purpose is to help loosen respiratory secretions so that they can be expectorated with ease. Vibration (Fig. 45-10) is carried out as follows:

1. Place your hands flat on the client's chest wall, where vibration is desired, and hold the hands side by side with the fingers extended and together. Some authorities prefer placing one hand on top of the other.

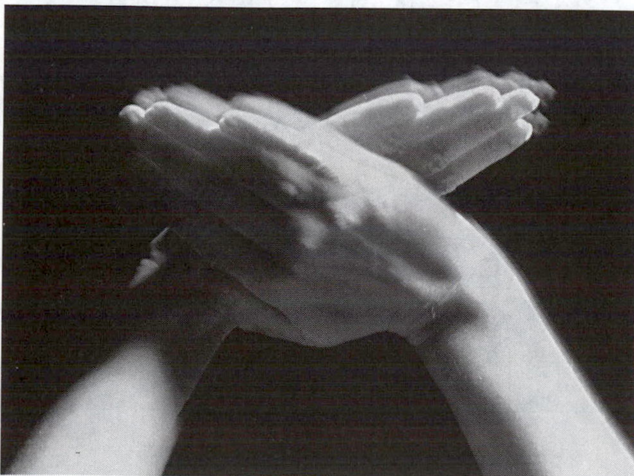

Figure 45-10
The position and action of the hands to use vibration to loosen respiratory secretions in the lungs.

2. Ask the client to inhale deeply and then exhale slowly.
3. While the client exhales, vibrate the chest wall by contracting and relaxing your arm and shoulder muscles rhythmically and quickly.
4. Stop vibration on the client's inhalations.
5. Do not vibrate over the client's breasts, spine, sternum, and lower rib cage.
6. Use vibration for several minutes several times a day.
7. Plan to deliver a vibration frequency of about 200 per minute.

Family members can be taught to use vibration on the client's chest wall. Also, mechanical devices are available for vibrating the chest wall.

Providing Postural Drainage. In *postural drainage*, gravity is used to drain secretions from the lungs. The person is positioned in a way that promotes the drainage of secretions from smaller pulmonary branches into larger ones, where they can be removed by drainage or coughing (Fig. 45-11). Postural drainage is often preceded by vibration, percussion, or both. Postural drainage is carried out as follows:

1. Have tissues and an emesis basin close at hand for the client to use when coughing and expectorating secretions.
2. Place the client in an appropriate position to promote drainage from the lobes of the lungs, as follows:
   - Use a high Fowler's position to drain the apical sections of the upper lobes of the lungs.
   - Place the client in a lying position, half on the abdomen and half on the side, right and left, to drain the posterior sections of the upper lobes of the lungs.
   - Place the client lying on the left side with a pillow under the chest wall to drain the right lobe of the lung.
   - Place the client in Trendelenburg's position to drain the lower lobes of the lungs.
3. Carry out postural drainage two to four times a day for 20 to 30 minutes. Discontinue the drainage if the client begins to feel weak or faint.
4. Delay postural drainage after meals for 1 to 2 hours to avoid vomiting.

Maintaining Good Nutrition. People who are working hard at breathing often do not have energy for eating. Assessment of nutritional status is determined by measuring client's height, weight, upper arm circumference, serum protein levels, and nitrogen balance. Special attention and deliberate planning should be directed to adequate intake of proteins, vitamins, and minerals. Six small meals should be distributed over the course of the day instead of the usual three meals. Meals should be arranged 1 to 2 hours after breathing treatments and exercises.

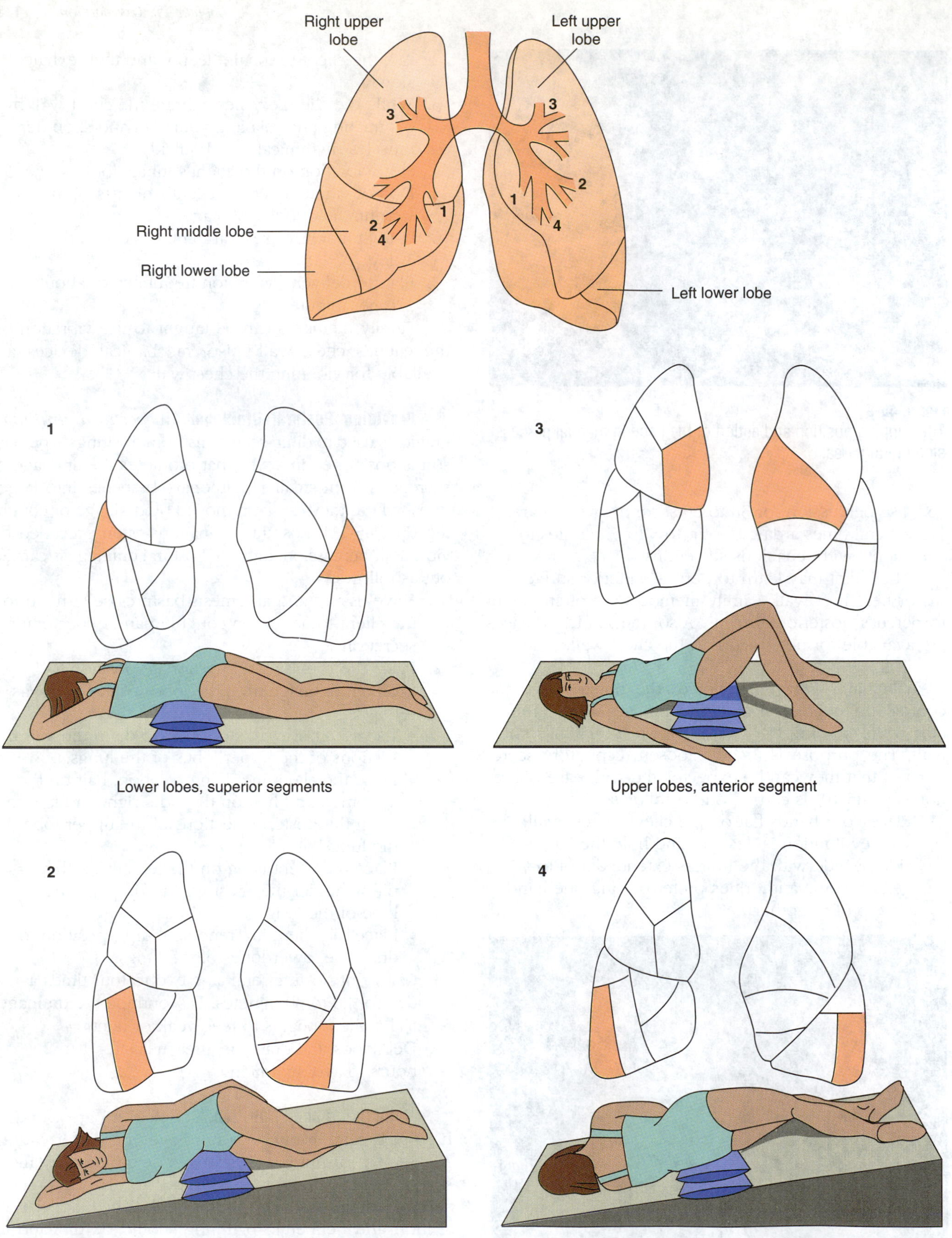

Figure 45-11
Postural drainage. Shown are four positions that use the force of gravity to assist the drainage of secretions from the smaller bronchial airways into the main bronchi and trachea so the client is able to cough them up.

Home Healthcare Alert

Nutritional intake can be improved by providing frequent oral hygiene and rest periods before small, frequent meals.

Meeting Respiratory Needs With Medications. Although treating clients with medications is a dependent nursing intervention, monitoring client response and side effects to medication is an independent nursing action. Table 45-3 shows some common medications for respiratory functioning, side effects, and nursing implications.

Home Healthcare Alert

Remind clients and caregivers that caffeine may potentiate the side effects of drugs commonly used to dilate bronchial airways.

Using Nebulizers

Clients use nebulizers to disperse fine particles of medication into the deeper passages of the respiratory tract where absorption occurs. Inhaled medications may be administered to open narrowed airways (bronchodilators), to liquefy or loosen thick secretions (mucolytic agents), or to reduce inflammation in airways (corticosteroids). A metered-dose inhaler (MDI) delivers a controlled dose of medication with each compression of the canister while a small-volume nebulizer is used until all the medication in the nebulizer cup has been inhaled. Clients need instruction to use inhalers and nebulizers effectively and safely. Overuse may result in serious side effects and eventual ineffectiveness of the medication. Nurses need to be aware of the common mistakes that clients make when using a metered-dose inhaler. They include:

- Failing to shake the canister
- Holding the inhaler upside down
- Inhaling through the nose rather than the mouth
- Inhaling too rapidly
- Stopping the inhalation when the cold propellant is felt in the throat
- Failing to hold their breath after inhalation
- Inhaling two sprays with one breath

For some clients, a spacing or extender device is necessary to aid in delivery of medication by the inhalation route. Using a metered-dose inhaler requires that the client activate the device while continuing to inhale. Young children and older clients are candidates for the addition of a spacer if inhalation therapy is prescribed. The spacer acts as a reservoir. When the MDI is compressed, the medication is deposited in the reservoir of the spacer and the client then inhales the medication from the spacer device making administration less complicated and the administered dose more predictable. To ensure correct use, slow deep inspirations are still necessary; some spacers are equipped with a whistle device that sounds if inhalation is too rapid. A spacer is also recommended for clients using steroid inhalers because it reduces the risk of developing an oral fungal infection. Refer to the accompanying box to instruct clients in the proper use of metered-dose inhalers and small-volume nebulizers. Package inserts accompanying medication also reinforce correct technique for using inhalers.

Providing Supplemental Oxygen

The amount of oxygen the client uses for inspiration can be increased by providing a supplemental supply. The provision of therapeutic oxygen is called oxygen therapy, and is usually prescribed by the physician. Oxygen therapy can frighten clients. Explanations from the nurse regarding procedures and purpose play a major role in reducing this fear. The client should be encouraged to discuss anxieties. If oxygen is given in an emergency, explanations concurrent with administration are appropriate.

Sources of Oxygen

Therapeutic oxygen is supplied from a wall outlet or a portable cylinder. The wall outlet source can be prepared for use quickly. The oxygen is supplied from a central source through a pipeline, usually at 50 to 60 pounds per square inch (psi) of pressure. A specially designed flowmeter is attached to the outlet and opens it (see Procedure 45-2 for an illustration of a flowmeter). A valve makes regulation of oxygen flow possible.

Oxygen can also be dispersed under pressure in steel cylinders or tanks. The tank is delivered with a protective cap to prevent accidental force against the cylinder outlet. When a standard, large-sized cylinder is full, its contents are under more than 2000 psi of pressure. The force behind an accidentally partially opened outlet could cause the tank to take off like an uncontrolled, dangerous jet. Smaller cylinders are available for emergency, ambulatory, and home use. The principles and precautions are the same for all size cylinders.

To release oxygen safely and at a desirable rate, a regulator is used. The regulator has two gauges. The one nearest the tank shows the pressure or amount of oxygen in the tank. The other gauge indicates the number of liters per minute of oxygen being released.

The oxygen cylinder and the regulator must be handled cautiously. The oxygen cylinder should be transported carefully, preferably strapped onto a wheeled carrier to avoid possible falling and breaking the outlet. The cylinder should be stabilized securely in a properly fitting stand.

Because of the possibility of dust and other particles becoming lodged in the outlet of the tank and being forced in the regulator, the tank is primed with two hands before a regulator is applied. The handle of the tank is turned slightly counterclockwise. This releases a

(text continues on page 1338)

Table 45-3
Medications Used to Improve Respiratory Functioning

Medication	Activity	Route	Side Effects	Nursing Implications
Epinephrine	Relaxes muscles that line bronchi and bronchioles	IV, SQ	Tremors, anxiety, insomnia, headache, palpitations, elevated blood pressure, vomiting	Position client upright to prevent aspiration if vomiting occurs. Monitor heart rate, respirations, breath sounds, and blood pressure every 15 minutes. May repeat medication within 15 minutes with an order.
Isoproterenol (Isuprel)	Bronchodilator	Inhaler	Same as with epinephrine but milder	Monitor heart rate. Demonstrate proper use of inhaler. Warn client not to exceed prescribed frequency of doses.
Metaproterenol (Alupent)	Bronchodilator	PO, inhalation	Same as with epinephrine	Same as with epinephrine
Theophylline (aminophylline)	Bronchodilator	PO, IV, rectally	Nausea, vomiting, rapid heart rate, diuresis, irritability, vertigo, convulsions	Monitor vital signs closely. Force fluids as clinical status allows. Monitor serum theophylline levels, especially if client does not respond to drug or severe side effects develop.
Corticosteroids (ACTH, prednisone, dexamethasone)	Reduces inflammation	PO, IV	Fluid retention, hypertension, mood swings, weight gain, gastritis, hyperglycemia	Reduce sodium intake. Make client and family aware of potential for labile emotions. Weigh daily in morning. Monitor blood pressure and blood sugar. Warn client to follow administration directions accurately. Instruct client about correct use of inhaler.
Antihistamines	Blocks histamine and relieves congestion of an allergic origin	PO	Drowsiness, anorexia, constipation, dry mouth, blurred vision, urinary retention	Warn client to use only with physician's advice in presence of bronchial asthma. Do not mix with alcohol, tranquilizers, or sedatives. Client should avoid driving or using machinery. Observe clients for prolonged bleeding if they are using warfarin anticoagulants.
Cromolyn sodium (Intal)	Prevents the release of histamines, serotonin, prostaglandin by the mast cell in an antigen–antibody reaction in asthma	Inhaler	Cough	Remind client this is used to prevent asthma attacks, not to treat acute episodes. This drug contains lactose and will cause diarrhea in lactose-deficient clients. Inform client that this is effective only if taken routinely (two to four times per day).

IV, intravenous; SQ, subcutaneous; PO, oral.

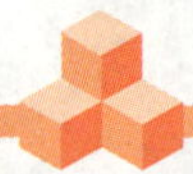

Guidelines for Nursing Care

Using a Nebulizer Device

- Assess the client's ability to manage a metered-dose inhaler or small-volume nebulizer.
- Explain, demonstrate, and encourage the client to manipulate the inhaler or nebulizer apparatus.
- Encourage client to wash hands thoroughly before using device.

Instructions for the client:

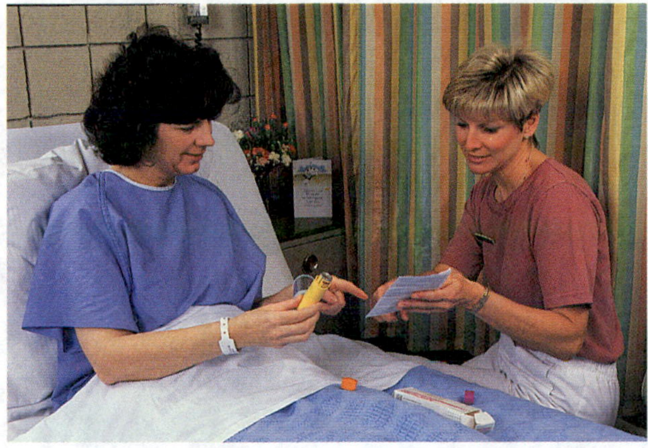

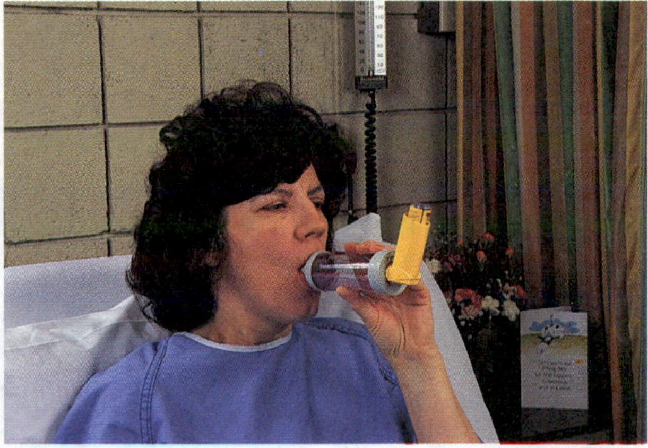

The Metered-Dose Inhaler

- Remove the mouthpiece cover and shake inhaler well.
- Follow caregiver's or manufacturer's recommendations for placement of the mouthpiece. Two methods are possible:
  - Hold the inhaler 1–2 inches in front of open mouth; or
  - Place mouthpiece into mouth grasping securely with teeth and lips (an MDI coupled with a spacer or extender is always placed in the mouth)
- Take a deep breath and exhale.
- Inhale slowly and deeply through the mouth. Press down on the medication canister while continuing to inhale a full breath (when using a spacer or extender, depress the canister about one-quarter or one-third through the inspiration).
- Hold your breath for 5 to 10 seconds or as long as possible.
- Exhale slowly through pursed lips.
- If another puff is prescribed, wait 1 to 5 minutes before the next inhalation.
- If desired, gargle with tap water and blow nose into a tissue to remove any remaining trace of medication.
- Use mild soap and water to clean the mouthpiece, rinse it, and let it dry before replacing it.
- Follow physician's order regarding frequency of inhaler use.

The Small-Volume Nebulizer

- Remove the nebulizer cup from the device, open it, and place it on a flat working surface.
- Place premeasured unit dose medication in the bottom section of the cup or use a dropper to place concentrated dose of medication in cup and add prescribed fluid to dilute it.

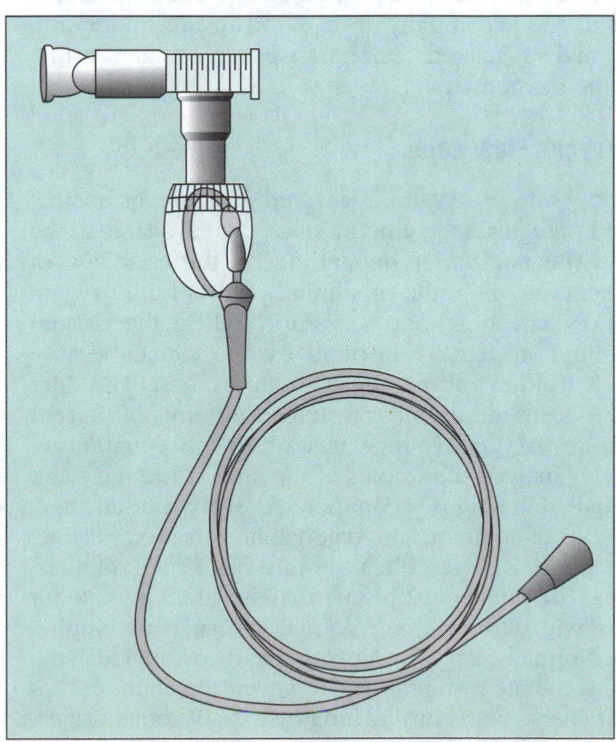

(continued)

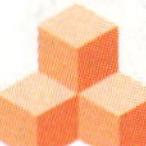

Guidelines for Nursing Care *(continued)*

Using a Nebulizer Device

- Screw the top portion of nebulizer cup back in place and attach the cup to the nebulizer.
- Attach one end of tubing to the stem on the bottom of the nebulizer cuff and the other end to the air compressor or oxygen source (if valve to control airflow is not available, a Y-tube can be added to the tubing so that one branch of the Y-tube connects to the nebulizer cup and the other branch is left open).
- Turn on the air compressor or oxygen.
- Check that a fine medication mist is produced by opening valve or placing thumb over open branch of Y-tube.
- Place mouthpiece into mouth and grasp securely with teeth and lips.
- Inhale slowly through the mouth (a nose clip may be necessary if client is also breathing through the nose).
- Hold each breath for 5 to 10 seconds or as long as possible before exhaling.
- Continue this inhalation technique until all medication in the nebulizer cup has been aerosolized (usually approximately 15 minutes).
- If desired, gargle with tap water after using nebulizer.
- Rinse the equipment in warm water and allow to air dry on a clean towel.

Special Considerations

- Instructions above are not meant for use with a breath-activated MDI.

Home Considerations

- Once a week, MDI mouthpiece, spacer or extender, or nebulizer parts should be soaked in a vinegar solution (1 pint of water to 2 oz. of vinegar) for 20 minutes. Rinse with clean water and allow to air dry.

small amount of oxygen and flushes out the outlet. The cylinder is closed again by turning the handle clockwise. The force with which the oxygen is released from this opening causes a loud, hissing sound that startles most people. Thus, clients and visitors need to be prepared for the noise with an appropriate explanation. It is recommended that tanks be primed away from the bedside. Refer to the accompanying box for an illustration and additional suggestions when transporting a client with a portable oxygen tank.

Oxygen Flow Rate

The flow rate of oxygen, measured in liters per minute, is used to regulate the amount of oxygen available to the client. The rate varies depending on the condition of the client and the route of administration of the oxygen. The flow rate does not necessarily reflect the oxygen concentration actually inspired by the client, because there is leaking and mixing with atmospheric air. More precise doses are usually prescribed in terms of percent of inspired oxygen. To regulate oxygen concentration accurately, analysis of samples of the air mixture the client is actually inhaling is recommended every 4 hours. Several types of commercial oxygen analyzers are available.

A physician prescribes the rate of oxygen administration. The nurse must monitor closely the flow rate for clients with chronic lung conditions, such as emphysema. Normally, excessive levels of carbon dioxide in the blood stimulate respirations. However, the chemoreceptors of clients with chronic lung disease become insensitive to carbon dioxide and respond to hypoxia to stimulate breathing. If excessive oxygen is given, the stimulus to breathe is removed and the client may stop breathing completely. Most clients with chronic lung disease can tolerate oxygen with a nasal cannula at 2 L/min but arterial blood gas analysis should be monitored closely.

Humidifying Oxygen

Controversy exists about the benefits of humidifying oxygen before delivering it to the client by way of a nasal cannula. Research has indicated that in very low flow oxygen (2 L/min or less) delivered by nasal cannula, humidification is unnecessary. Since oxygen drys and dehydrates the respiratory mucous membranes, humidifying devices are commonly used for delivery of oxygen at higher flow rates. These supply 20% to 40% humidity.

Distilled or sterile water is commonly used to humidify oxygen. Cahill and Heath (1990) suggest that tap water may be safely used instead to humidify low-flow oxygen therapy. They recommend that local tap water initially be cultured to determine the presence of bacterial contamination and approved by the hospital infection control committee before widespread use. Using tap water instead of sterile water is viewed as a reasonable method of reducing hospital costs.

Precautions for Oxygen Administration

Oxygen, which constitutes 20% of normal air, is a tasteless, odorless, colorless gas. It supports combustion. To prevent fires and injuries, the following precautions must be taken:

- Avoid open flames in the client's room.
- Place No Smoking signs in conspicuous places in the client's room or home setting. Instruct client

Guidelines for Nursing Care

Transporting a Client With a Portable Oxygen Cylinder

Before the Transfer:

- Check that the oxygen cylinder contains oxygen.
- Check that additional oxygen source is available where client is being transferred.
- Check amount of oxygen in cylinder (place cylinder key or wrench on valve stem and turn fully counterclockwise until needle on gauge indicates amount of available oxygen; turn the key back a half turn; use cylinder only if gauge indicates more than 500 psi).
- Connect oxygen tubing or humidifier bottle with tubing to the flowmeter adapter and attach other end to client's oxygen cannula.
- Adjust the flow-control dial to the prescribed setting.
- Ensure that the cylinder is secured in holder before transporting client (it is a dangerous practice to place the cylinder between the client's legs or next to the client during transfer because injury to the client may result).
- Place coiled tubing under pillow or attach to linen or client's gown.

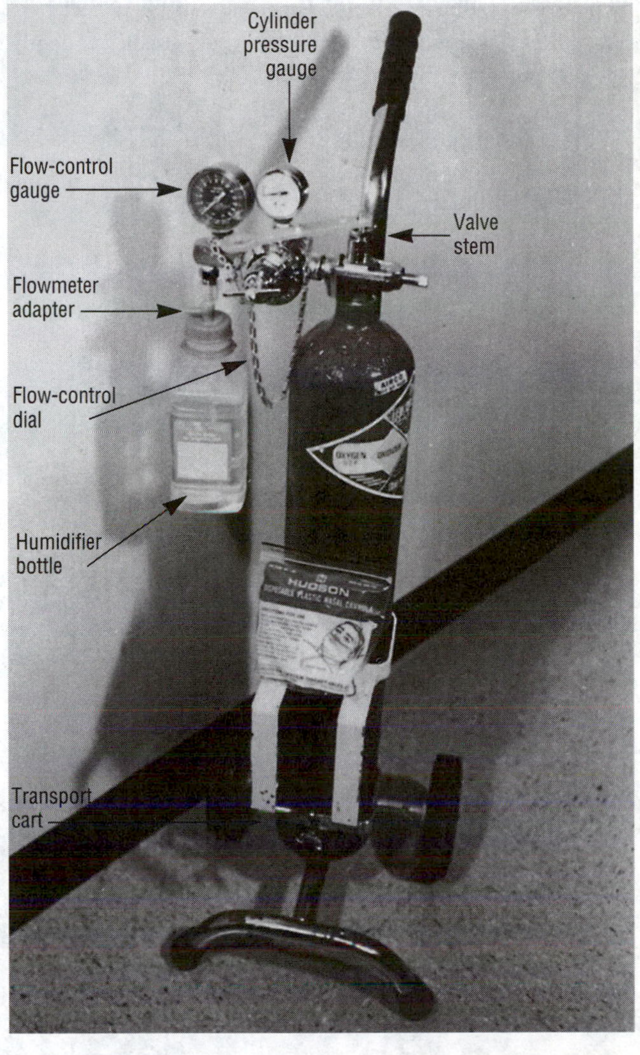

After the Transfer:

- Attach client to wall oxygen.
- Turn off the oxygen flow from the cylinder by turning the cylinder key clockwise until it is tight.
- Remove any excess oxygen in the pressure gauge by "bleeding" it. Turn the flow-control dial back on until hissing sound stops and needle on gauge has fallen to zero. Turn flow-control dial off.

(Source: Mathews, P. [1995]. Safely delivering a breath of fresh air. *Nursing, 25*(5), 66–69)

and visitors on the hazard of smoking with oxygen in use.

- Check to see that electric equipment used in the room, such as electric bell cords, razors, radios, and suctioning equipment, is in good working order and emits no sparks.
- Avoid wearing and using synthetic fabrics that build up static electricity.
- Avoid using oils in the area. Oil can ignite spontaneously in the presence of oxygen.

Oxygen Administration

Oxygen can be administered by nasal cannula, nasal catheter, transtracheal catheter, simple mask, partial rebreather mask, nonrebreather mask, Venturi mask, and tent. Refer to Table 45-4 for comparison of oxygen delivery systems.

Nasal Cannula. A **nasal cannula**, also called nasal prongs, is probably the most commonly used aid to breathing. The cannula is a disposable, plastic device with two protruding prongs for insertion into the nostrils; the cannula is connected to an oxygen source with a humidifier and flowmeter. The cannula does not impede eating or speaking. Procedure 45-2 explains oxygen administration by nasal cannula.

Nasal Catheter. A nasal, or oropharyngeal, catheter is another efficient means for administering oxygen, but it

Table 45-4
Oxygen Delivery Systems

Method	Amount Delivered FiO_2 (Fraction Inspired Oxygen)	Priority Nursing Interventions	Advantages	Disadvantages
Nasal Cannula	*Low Flow* 1 L/min = 24% 2 L/min = 28% 3 L/min = 32% 4 L/min = 36% 5 L/min = 40% 6 L/min = 44%	Check frequently that both prongs are in client's nares. Never deliver more than 2–3 L/min to client with chronic lung disease.	Client able to talk and eat with oxygen in place Easily used in home setting	Can easily be dislodged Can cause dryness of nasal mucosa
Simple Mask	*Low Flow* 5–10 L/min = 40%–60% (5 L/min is minimum setting)	Monitor client frequently to check placement of the mask. Support client if claustrophobia is a concern. Secure physician's order to replace mask with nasal cannula during meal time.	Can provide increased delivery of oxygen for short period of time	Tight seal required to deliver higher concentration Difficult to keep mask in position over nose and mouth Potential for skin breakdown (pressure, moisture) Difficult to eat and talk
Partial Rebreather Mask	*Low Flow* 6–15 L/min = 70%–90%	Set flow rate so mask remains two-thirds full during inspiration. Keep reservoir bag free of twists or kinks.	Client can inhale room air through openings in mask if oxygen supply is briefly interrupted	Requires tight seal (eating and talking difficult, uncomfortable) Potential for skin breakdown
Nonrebreather Mask	*Low Flow* 6–15 L/min = 60%–100%	Maintain flow rate so reservoir bag collapses only slightly during inspiration. Check that valves and rubber flaps are functioning properly (open during expiration and closed during inhalation). Monitor SaO_2 with pulse oximeter.	Delivers the highest possible oxygen concentration (except for intubation and mechanical ventilation) Not as drying to mucous membranes	Impractical for long-term therapy Malfunction can cause CO_2 buildup and suffocation Requires tight seal (eating and talking difficult, uncomfortable)
Venturi Mask	*High Flow* 4–10 L/min = 24%–55%	Requires careful monitoring to verify FiO_2 at flow rate ordered. Check that air intake valves are not blocked.	Delivers most precise oxygen concentration despite client's respiratory pattern Doesn't dry mucous membranes (humidity or aerosol can be added)	Requires tight seal (eating and talking difficult, uncomfortable) Risk for skin irritation

is infrequently used because it is uncomfortable for the client and may cause trauma to respiratory mucous membranes. It is inserted into the throat through one nostril and must be changed to the other nostril every 8 hours. Gastric distention often occurs because the gas flow can be misdirected into the stomach.

Face Masks. Disposable and reusable face masks are available in plastic and rubber. The mask should be fitted carefully to the client's face to avoid leakage of oxygen. It should be comfortably snug but not tight against the client's face. The most commonly used types of masks include the simple face mask, the partial rebreather mask, the nonrebreather mask, and the Venturi mask. Procedure 45-3 describes actions and rationale in using face masks.

The *simple oxygen mask* connects to oxygen tubing, a humidifier, and a flowmeter, just as the nasal cannula does. At a flow rate of 6 to 10 L/min, the mask delivers 35% to 60% oxygen. This mask has vents on its sides that

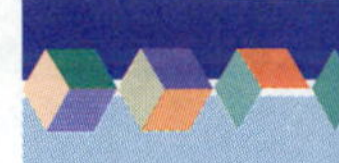

PROCEDURE 45-2

Administering Oxygen by Nasal Cannula

Equipment

Flowmeter connected to oxygen supply

Humidifier with sterile distilled water (optional with low-flow system)

Nasal cannula and tubing

Gauze to pad tubing over ears (optional)

Action	**Rationale**
1. Explain procedure to client and review safety precautions necessary when oxygen is in use. Place NO SMOKING signs in appropriate areas.	Oxygen supports combustion.
2. Wash your hands.	Handwashing deters the spread of microorganisms.
3. Connect the nasal cannula to the oxygen setup with humidification, if one is in use. Adjust the flow rate as ordered by physician. Check that oxygen is flowing out of prongs.	Oxygen forced through a water reservoir is humidified before it is delivered to the client, thus preventing dehydration of the mucous membranes. Recent research has questioned the necessity of humidification with low-flow oxygen delivery by way of cannula.

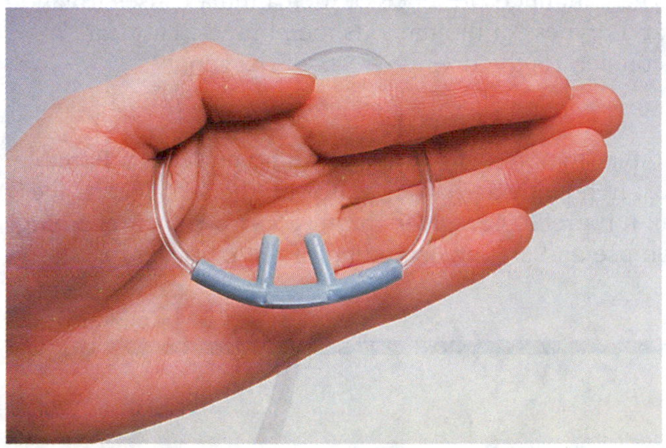

Nasal cannula.

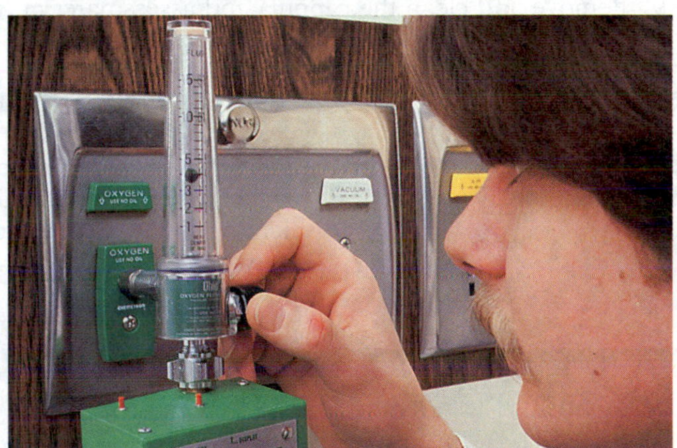

Action 3: Adjusting flow rate.

Action	**Rationale**
4. Place the prongs in the client's nostrils. Adjust according to type of equipment. a. Over and behind each ear with adjuster comfortably under chin; *or* b. Around the client's head	Correct placement of the prongs and fastener facilitates oxygen administration and comfort for the client.
5. Use gauze pads at ear beneath the tubing as necessary.	Pads reduce irritation and pressure and protect the skin.
6. Encourage client to breathe through his or her nose with mouth closed.	Provides for optimal delivery of oxygen to client.
7. Wash your hands.	Handwashing deters the spread of microorganisms.
8. Assess and chart client's response to therapy.	Client's respirations, color, breathing pattern, and chest movements indicate effectiveness of oxygen therapy.

(continued)

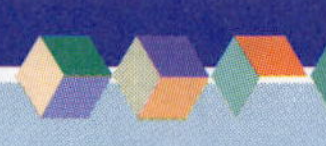

PROCEDURE 45-2 *(continued)*

Administering Oxygen by Nasal Cannula

Action	Rationale

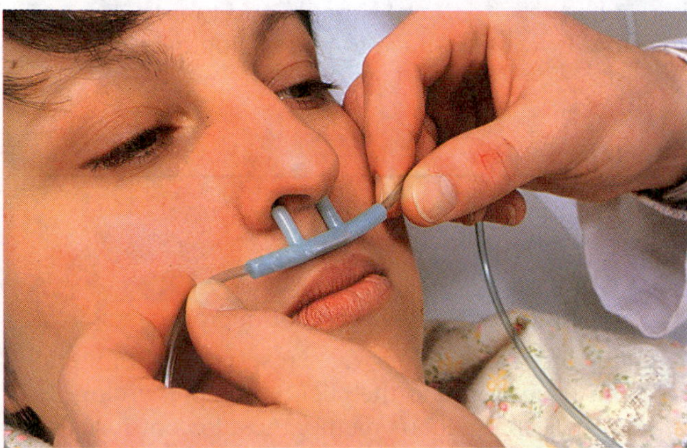

Action 4: Placing cannula prongs in nostrils.

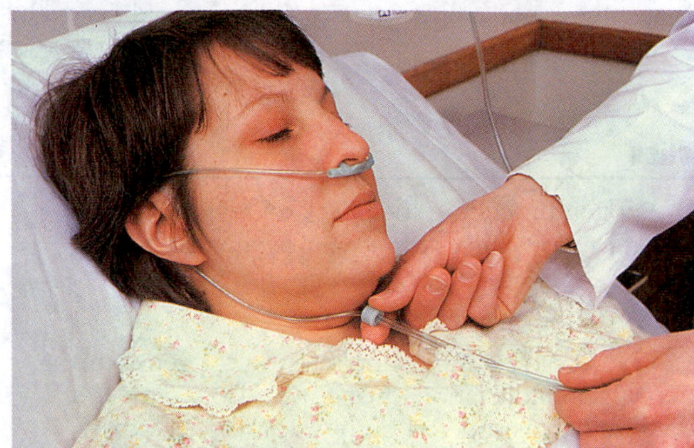

Action 4: Adjusting for comfort.

Action	Rationale
9. Remove and clean the cannula and assess nares at least every 8 hours or according to agency recommendations. Check nares for evidence of irritation or bleeding.	The continued presence of the cannula causes irritation and dryness of the mucous membranes. Lubricant counteracts the drying effects of oxygen.

Home Care Considerations

Clients may require oxygen administration to continue in the home setting. Portable oxygen cylinders are used most frequently and an indicator on the setup alerts the client or family member to call for a refill. Caregivers require instruction concerning safety precautions with oxygen use and an understanding of the rationale for the specific liter flow of oxygen.

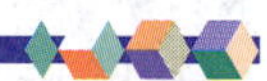

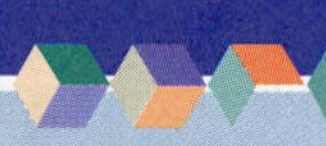

PROCEDURE 45-3

Administering Oxygen by Mask

Equipment

- Flowmeter connected to oxygen supply
- Humidifier with sterile distilled water
- Face mask specified by physician
- Gauze to pad elastic band (optional)

Action	Rationale
1. Explain procedure to client and review safety precautions necessary when oxygen is in use. Place NO SMOKING signs in appropriate areas.	Oxygen supports combustion. Explanation alleviates anxiety.
2. Wash your hands.	Handwashing deters the spread of microorganisms.

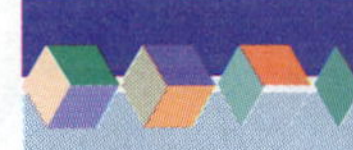

PROCEDURE 45-3

Administering Oxygen by Mask

Action	Rationale
3. Attach the face mask to the oxygen setup with humidification. Start the flow of oxygen at the specified rate.	Oxygen forced through a water reservoir is humidified before it is delivered to the client, thus preventing dehydration of the mucous membranes.
4. Position the face mask over the client's nose and mouth. Adjust it with the elastic strap so that the mask fits snugly but comfortably on the face.	A loose or poorly fitting mask will result in oxygen loss and decreased therapeutic value. Masks may cause feeling of suffocation, and client needs frequent attention and reassurance.
5. Use gauze pads to reduce irritation on the client's ears and scalp.	Pads reduce irritation and pressure and protect the skin.
6. Wash your hands.	Handwashing deters the spread of microorganisms.
7. Remove the mask and dry the skin every 2 to 3 hours if the oxygen is running continuously. Do not powder around the mask.	The tight-fitting mask and moisture from condensation can irritate the skin on the face. There is danger of inhaling powder if it is placed on the mask.
8. Assess and chart client's response to therapy.	Client's respiratory rate and pattern, color, and so forth, indicate effectiveness of oxygen therapy.

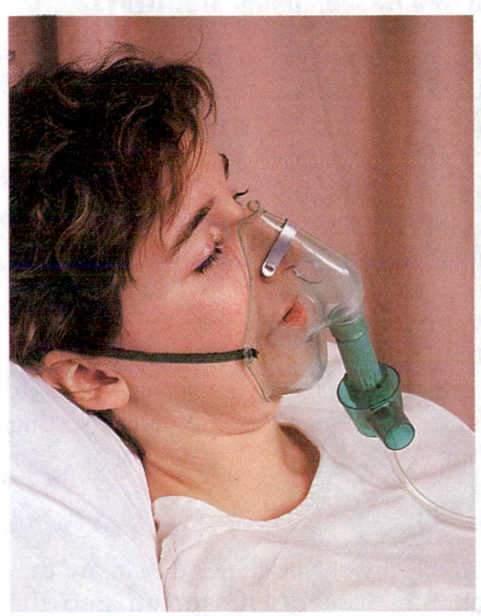

Venturi mask.
(Photos © 1987 Ken Kasper.)

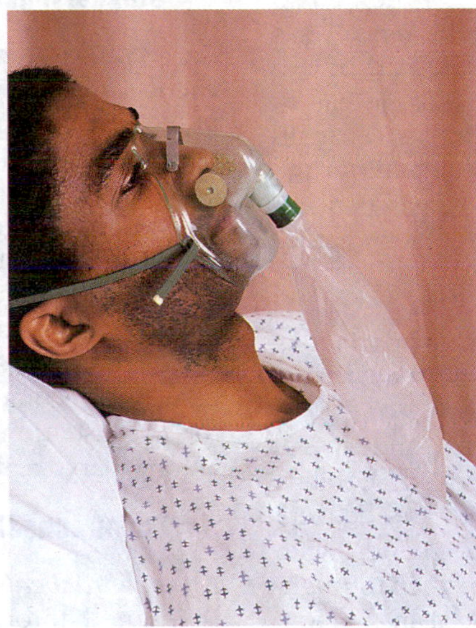

Nonrebreather mask.

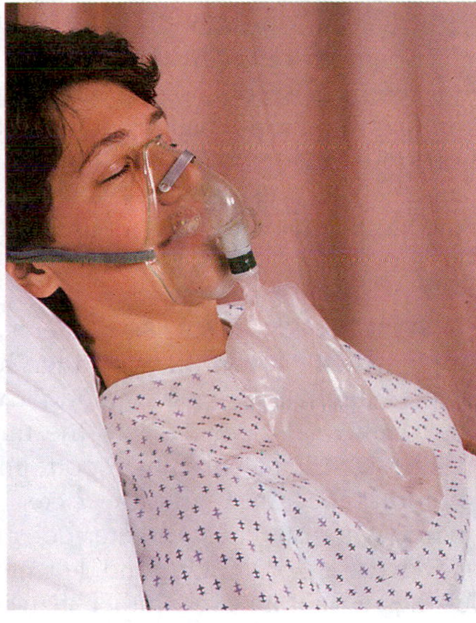

Partial rebreather mask.

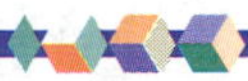

allow room air to leak in at many places, thereby diluting the source oxygen. Often it is used when an increased delivery of oxygen is needed for short periods (eg, less than 12 hours). This mask should cover the nose and the mouth if the client breathes through the mouth.

The *partial rebreather mask* is equipped with a reservoir bag for the collection of the first parts of the client's exhaled air. The air is mixed with 100% oxygen for the next inhalation. The client rebreathes about one third of the expired air from the reservoir bag. The remaining exhaled air exits through vents. The use of this type of mask permits the conservation of oxygen. This bag should deflate slightly with inspiration. If it deflates completely, the flow rate should be increased until only a slight deflation is noted.

The *nonrebreather mask* provides the highest concentration of oxygen with a mask to a spontaneously breathing client. It is similar to the partial rebreather mask except two one-way valves prevent conservation of exhaled air. The reservoir bag is filled with oxygen that enters the mask on inspiration. Exhaled air escapes through side vents. This mask can also be used to administer other gases.

The *Venturi mask* gets its name from the Venturi effect, which allows the mask to deliver the most precise concentrations of oxygen. This mask has a large tube with an oxygen inlet. As the tube narrows, the pressure drops, causing air to be sucked in through side ports. These ports are adjusted according to the prescription for oxygen concentration. It is a nursing responsibility to make sure the ports are always open. If these are occluded by linens, clothing, or a client rolling on it, the oxygen delivered might be at an unsafe concentration.

Oxygen Tent. Oxygen also can be administered by way of a tent, a light, portable structure made of clear plastic and attached to a motor-driven unit. The motor helps to circulate and cool the air in the tent. The cooling device functions on the same principles as an electric refrigeration unit. A thermostat in the unit keeps the tent at the temperature considered most comfortable for the client. The tent fits over the top part of the bed so that the client's head and thorax are in the tent. It has side openings through which nursing care can be administered. It is commonly used with pediatric clients who need a cool and highly humidified air flow (eg, children with pneumonia). The tent does not allow the maintenance of a satisfactory or precise oxygen concentration and, thus, is usually not used outside of pediatrics (see Procedure 45-4).

Oxygen Therapy in the Home. Clients using continuous supplemental oxygen therapy in the home setting have another alternative—*transtracheal oxygen delivery.* A small catheter is inserted into the trachea under local anesthesia. Clients usually report improved mobility, comfort, appearance, and lower cost with this delivery system. A transtracheal catheter does not interfere with talking, eating, or drinking and delivers oxygen throughout the respiratory cycle rather than just at inspiration. This system does require that the client or family assume responsibility for daily catheter care. A transtracheal oxygen setup is illustrated in Figure 45-12.

Clients using oxygen at home need instruction regarding safety precautions. The following items must be reviewed and stressed:

- No smoking or open flames within 10 feet of the oxygen source.
- Do not use electrical equipment near the oxygen administration set-up (eg, space heaters).
- Remove oxygen when client uses an electric razor.
- Use caution with gas or electric appliances when client is receiving oxygen therapy.
- Follow physician's prescription for oxygen flow rate (using too little or too much oxygen can prove life-threatening).
- Secure oxygen tank in holder and away from direct sunlight or heat.
- Allow adequate air flow around oxygen concentrator (avoid placing concentrator flush against wall).
- Ground oxygen concentrators.
- Have physician's and nurse's telephone numbers readily available.
- Review with client directions for reaching oxygen equipment vendor and reasons for contacting vendor.
- Discuss signs and symptoms that indicate the need to call for emergency assistance or visit the local emergency room (Rice, 1995).

Home Healthcare Alert

When oxygen is in use in the home, emphasize the importance of also instructing visitors to avoid smoking in the home.

Using Artificial Airways

Oropharyngeal and Nasopharyngeal Airways

An *oropharyngeal* or *nasopharyngeal airway* is a semicircular tube of plastic or rubber inserted into the back of the pharynx through the mouth or nose in the spontaneously breathing client. It is used to keep the tongue clear of the airway and to permit suctioning of secretions. It is often used for postoperative clients until they regain consciousness. According to McConnell (1994a), it is vital for the nurse to insert an airway that is the correct size and to avoid using tape to hold the airway in place. The client should be able to expel the airway once he or she becomes alert. Refer to the accompanying box for an illustration and techniques to use when inserting an oropharyngeal airway.

Endotracheal Tube

An *endotracheal tube* is a polyvinylchloride airway that is inserted through the nose or the mouth into the trachea using a laryngoscope as a guide. It is used to administer oxygen by mechanical ventilator, to suction secretions easily, or to bypass upper airway obstructions (eg, tongue or tracheal edema). Though uncomfortable and easier to manipulate with the tongue, orotracheal insertion is often the method of choice, especially in an emergency, because insertion is easier and a larger size tube can be used making breathing easier. Placement of the tube by way of the nasotracheal route, though tolerated better by clients, is more difficult and requires the use of a narrower tube. Most commonly, a cuffed endotracheal tube is used that prevents air leakage and bronchial aspiration of foreign material, and allows more precise control of oxygen and mechanical ventilation (Fig. 45-13). Careful monitoring of endotracheal cuff pressure decreases the risk of tracheal necrosis. The

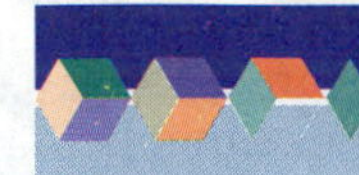

PROCEDURE 45-4

Administering Oxygen by Tent

Equipment

Oxygen tent with tubing, flow regulator, and oxygen analyzer
Oxygen source
Humidifier
Sterile distilled water
Bath blankets
Ice

Action	Rationale
1. Explain procedure to client and family.	This reassures client and facilitates cooperation.
2. Gather equipment.	This provides for organized approach to task.
3. Wash your hands.	Handwashing deters the spread of microorganisms.
4. Use bath blanket to cover plastic mattress. Place second bath blanket over bottom sheet.	Bath blanket minimizes potential for static electricity from plastic mattress. Additional bath blanket is used to provide warmth and absorb moisture.
5. Prepare tent and position over bed. Attach to oxygen source.	Tent allows oxygen to be delivered in a confined environment.
6. Fill ice trough or start refrigeration component.	Ice or refrigeration unit cools the air in the tent.
7. Fill nebulizer or humidifier to recommended level with sterile distilled water. Turn on flowmeter and adjust oxygen flow to deliver required amount. Use oxygen analyzer now and recheck at least every 4 hours.	Humidification of oxygen prevents excessive drying of the respiratory tract. Oxygen analyzer measures oxygen concentration.
8. Place client in tent. Observe all safety precautions.	Oxygen supports combustion.
9. Secure tent between folded top sheet and under mattress.	Oxygen is heavier than air. If tent is not secure, oxygen content may be decreased.
10. Wash your hands.	Handwashing deters the spread of microorganisms.
11. Open tent as little as possible by organizing nursing care.	This maintains oxygen content in tent.
12. Assess client at frequent intervals (vital signs, color, response to therapy). Monitor equipment on a frequent basis.	Oxygen toxicity may develop in response to exposure to a high concentration of oxygen.
13. Change gown and linens as necessary. Edges of tent may be loosened, and tent may be secured with bath blanket under client's chin when performing hygienic care or other procedures.	This provides warmth and comfort.
14. Record type of therapy and client's response.	Keeping records provides accurate documentation of procedure.

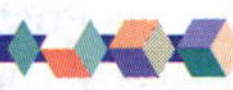

smallest amount of air that results in an airtight seal between the trachea and the tube is desirable and less likely to result in complications.

Tracheostomy

A *tracheostomy* is an artificial opening made into the trachea. The curved **tracheostomy tube** inserted into this opening is made of semiflexible plastic, rigid plastic, or metal and comes in multiple sizes with varied angles. A tracheostomy tube consists of an outer cannula or main shaft, the inner cannula, and an obturator. An obturator guides the direction of the outer cannula and is inserted into the tube during placement. It is removed once the outer cannula of the tube is in place (Fig. 45-14) but must remain at the bedside in addition to a replacement tracheostomy tube of the same size. Many tubes also have inner cannulas which may or may not be dispos-

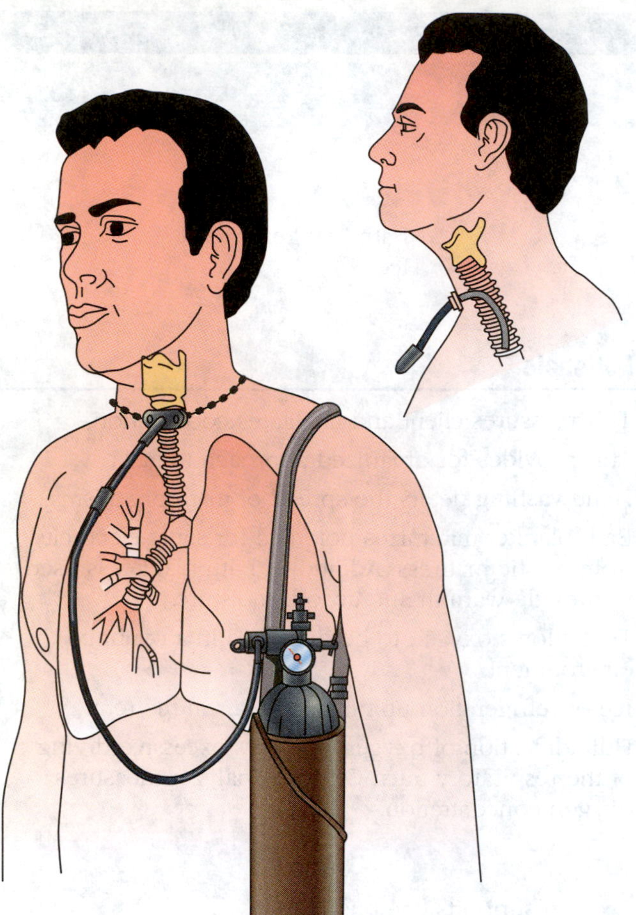

Figure 45-12
A transtracheal oxygen setup.

able. The outer cannula remains in place in the trachea while the inner cannula is removed for cleaning or replaced with a new one. A tube with an inner cannula is necessary when clients have excessive secretions or have difficulty clearing their secretions and may also be recommended for a client discharged with a tracheostomy tube in place. The condition and needs of the client determine the selection of either a metal or plastic tracheostomy tube. While metal tubes are more cost-effective for long-term use, only plastic tubes have an adaptor at the neckplate that permits connection to respiratory therapy equipment (eg, an oxygen delivery system, Ambu bag, or mechanical ventilator). A *fenestrated* tracheostomy tube has one large or several small openings or windows on its outer curve, has an inner cannula, and can be cuffed or cuffless. When the client is being mechanically ventilated, the inner cannula is in place blocking the small openings. Once the client is no longer connected to the ventilator, the inner cannula can be removed, the cuff deflated, and the tube plugged, allowing the client to speak. Since the tube has these openings, it is not recommended for use if a client has a history of aspiration (Weilitz and Dettenmeier, 1994).

Tracheostomy tubes may be either cuffed or cuffless (see Fig. 45-14). The inflated cuff seals the opening around the tube against air leakage, prevents aspiration, and permits mechanical ventilation. Newer tracheal cuffs are low pressure, do not require deflating for short intervals every few hours, and can be maintained at lower than tracheal capillary pressure. A cuffed tube should be deflated before oral feeding unless the

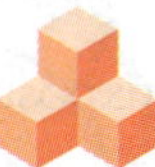

Guidelines for Nursing Care

Inserting an Oropharyngeal Airway

- Use an airway that is the correct size (size 4 or 5 is appropriate for the average adult).
- Explain what you are doing to the client even though the client appears unconscious.
- Wash your hands and don gloves (if client is coughing, wear mask and goggles or face shield).
- Remove dentures if they are present.
- Position client on his or her back with neck hyperextended (unless this is inappropriate).
- Open client's mouth by using your thumb and index finger to gently pry teeth apart.
- Insert the airway with the curved tip pointing up toward the roof of the mouth.
- Slide the airway across the tongue to the back of the mouth.
- Rotate the airway 180 degrees as it passes the uvula (a flashlight can confirm the position of the airway with the curve fitting over the tongue).
- Ensure adequate ventilation by auscultating breath sounds.
- Position client on his or her side when airway is in place.
- Remove airway for a brief period every 4 hours. Provide mouth care and rinse airway before reinserting it.

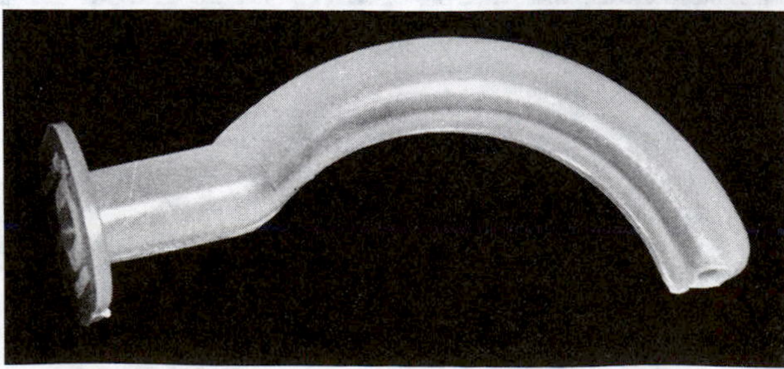

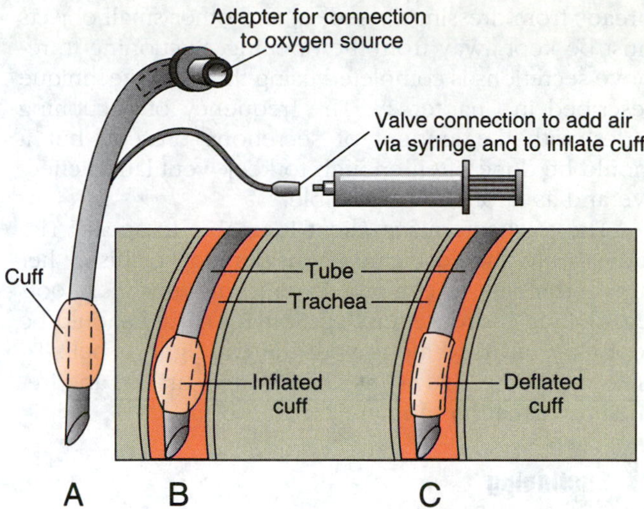

Figure 45-13
(**A**) Parts of a cuffed endotracheal tube. (**B**) Tube in place with the cuff inflated. (**C**) Tube in place with the cuff deflated.

client is at high risk for aspiration. If left cuffed, the balloon can cause pressure that extends through the trachea and onto the esophagus, possibly impeding swallowing.

A tracheostomy tube is inserted for a variety of reasons (eg, to replace an endotracheal tube, to provide a method to mechanically ventilate, to bypass an upper airway obstruction, or to remove tracheobronchial secretions). It is inserted in the operating room or intensive care unit under sterile conditions using local anesthesia. The tracheostomy tube is held in place by twill tapes or a Velcro strip fastened around the client's neck. Usually, a sterile, square gauze pad that has been precut by the manufacturer is placed between the skin and outer wings of the tube before the tube is tied. This tracheostomy dressing must be kept dry to prevent infection and skin irritation. The tracheostomy can be temporary or permanent.

Nursing responsibilities may include regularly checking cuff pressure, although some tubes have a pressure-release valve that prevents pressure from increasing to damaging levels. Also, because the tracheostomy tube bypasses the natural humidifying and heating mechanisms in the nose and mouth, the oxygen must be heated and humidified to prevent secretions from becoming dry.

The tracheostomy tube must remain free from foreign objects and nonsterile materials. Cotton balls, loose

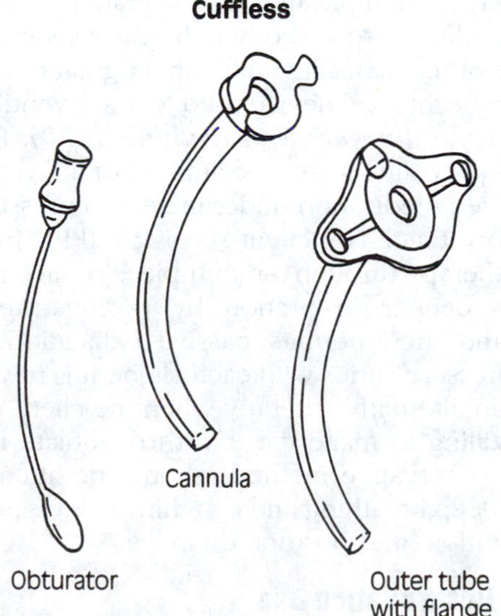

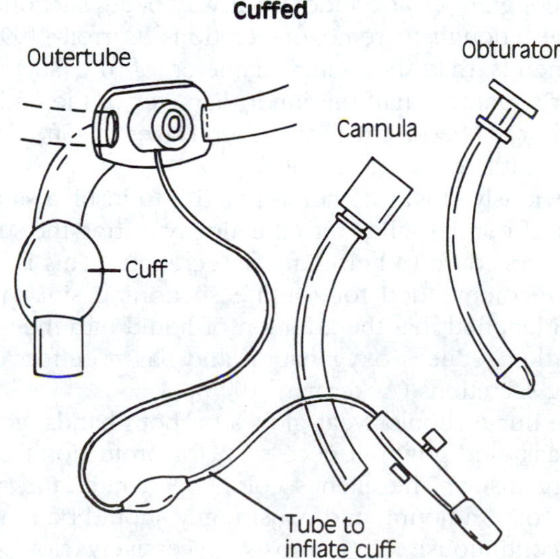

Figure 45-14
Two types of tracheostomy sets—cuffless and cuffed.

threads from dressings, needles, and other small objects must be kept away from the opening. Suctioning to remove secretions is completed using the sterile technique described in Chapter 28. The frequency of suctioning varies with the amount of secretions present, but it should be done often enough to keep ventilation effective and as effortless as possible.

The tracheotomized client is unable to speak. The client's care should include consideration of his or her impaired ability to communicate. Communication tools (eg, writing board, letters, vocabulary cards) should be kept close at hand along with the call light or bell. To prevent anxiety, this client requires reassurance and frequent explanations and anticipation of needs.

Suctioning

If the client is unable to remove secretions with coughing after the application of artificial airways, secretions can be aspirated with a suctioning device (Procedure 45-5). Suctioning irritates the mucosa and removes oxygen from the respiratory tract, possibly causing *hypoxemia* (insufficient oxygen in the blood). Thus, the client must be hyperoxygenated before suctioning. Tracheal suctioning may be performed by passing a sterile catheter through the mouth (orotracheal), through the nose (nasotracheal), through an endotracheal tube, or through a tracheostomy tube. Procedure 45-6 describes suctioning the tracheostomy. When performed correctly, suctioning provides comfort by relieving respiratory distress. It is normally painless; however, a postoperative or trauma client should receive analgesic medication prior to suctioning since the cough reflex will be stimulated. When performed incorrectly, it can increase anxiety and pain and cause respiratory arrest. Possible complications include infection, cardiac arrhythmias, hypoxia, mucosa trauma, and death. The suctioning catheter should be small enough not to occlude the airway being suctioned but large enough to remove secretions. Carroll (1994) recommends that the outer diameter of the suction catheter should be half the inner diameter of the endotracheal or tracheostomy tube. Several sizes of soft, plastic, clear catheters are available.

Previously, it was common practice to instill a small amount of normal saline into the airway during the suctioning procedure to help liquefy secretions. This is no longer recommended for routine suctioning since research identified that the addition of liquid into the airway further reduces oxygenation and has no effect on thinning secretions (Ackerman, 1993).

The nurse should wear gloves on both hands, goggles, mask, and gown, if necessary, for protection from microorganisms. The client's color; heart rate; and secretion color, amount, and consistency should be monitored continuously. If cyanosis, excessively slow or rapid heart rate, or suddenly bloody secretions are noted, the nurse should stop suctioning immediately. The client should be ventilated with oxygen, and the physician should be notified.

Providing Tracheostomy Care

In addition to suctioning the tracheostomy, the nurse is responsible for either cleaning a nondisposable inner cannula or replacing a disposable one. The inner cannula requires cleaning or replacement to prevent accumulation of secretions that can interfere with respiration and occlude the airway. Because soiled tracheostomy dressings place the client at risk for development of skin breakdown and infection, the nurse changes dressings and ties on a regular basis. Non–cotton-filled gauze dressings are used to prevent aspiration of foreign bodies (eg, lint or cotton fibers) into the trachea. Care must be exercised when changing the tracheostomy ties to prevent accidental extubation or expulsion of the tube. It is recommended either that an assistant holds the tube in place during the change or that the soiled tie is left in place until a clean one is securely attached. Agency policy determines specific procedures and schedules; however, a newly inserted tracheostomy may require attention every 1 to 2 hours. Procedure 45-7 outlines care of a client's tracheostomy.

Assisting Ventilation

Mechanical ventilators are used to assist or completely control ventilation. These machines are used with critically ill clients in conjunction with endotracheal or tracheostomy tubes, in acute care facilities, extended care settings, and in the home. Mechanical ventilation improves oxygenation and ventilation and supports the client's breathing function during emergency or acute care episodes as well as in selected long-term situations. Many types of ventilators are available and the nurse must address both physical and psychologic concerns of the client and family. The nurse has responsibility for evaluating the client's response to ventilation therapy, using safe practice and techniques, and monitoring the client carefully for complications. (The reader is referred to the general literature and other clinical texts that discuss the use of mechanical ventilators in great detail.)

Another mechanical device used to assist ventilation is *intermittent positive-pressure breathing (IPPB)*. This is a method of providing a specific amount of air, oxygen, and aerosolized medication under increased pressure to the respiratory tract. The client receiving IPPB inhales the aerosol therapy through a mouthpiece or face mask. IPPB forces deeper inspiration by positive-pressure inhalation and then permits passive exhalation. The amount of pressure varies with each client. It is now recognized as an alternative therapy when the client is unable or unwilling to make the effort to ventilate his or her lungs. Conservative methods should be attempted first such as deep breathing and coughing exercises, percussion, vibration, and postural drainage.

Manual Resuscitation Bag

In emergency situations, the manual resuscitation bag can be used to assist ventilation for clients whose respirations have ceased. With the client's head tilted back,

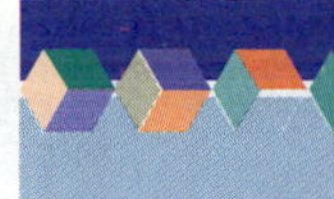

PROCEDURE 45-5

Suctioning the Nasopharyngeal and Oropharyngeal Areas

Equipment

Portable or wall suction unit with tubing
Sterile suction catheter with Y-port
Sterile water or saline
Sterile disposable container
Sterile gloves
Towel or waterproof pad

Action	Rationale
1. Determine the need for suctioning. Administer pain medication before suctioning to postoperative client.	Suctioning should be done only when secretions have accumulated or adventitious breath sounds are audible. This minimizes trauma to airway mucosa. Suctioning stimulates coughing which is painful for clients with surgical incisions.
2. Explain procedure to client.	This provides reassurance and promotes cooperation.
3. Assemble equipment.	This provides for organized approach.
4. Wash your hands.	Handwashing deters spread of microorganisms.
5. Adjust bed to comfortable working position. Lower side rail closer to you. Place the client in a semi-Fowler's position if conscious. An unconscious client should be placed in the lateral position facing you.	Having the client in a sitting position helps him or her to cough and makes breathing easier. Gravity also facilitates the insertion of the catheter. Lateral position prevents the airway from becoming obstructed and promotes drainage of secretions.
6. Place towel or waterproof pad across client's chest.	This protects bed linens.
7. Turn suction to appropriate pressure: a. Wall unit Adult: 100 to 120 mm Hg Child: 95 to 110 mm Hg Infant: 50 to 95 mm Hg b. Portable unit Adult: 10 to 15 mm Hg Child: 5 to 10 mm Hg Infant: 2 to 5 mm Hg	Negative pressure must be at a safe level or pneumothorax may occur.
8. Open sterile suction package. Set up sterile container touching only the outside surface, and pour sterile saline or water into it.	Sterile normal saline or water is used to lubricate the outside of the catheter, thus minimizing irritation of mucosa as it is being introduced.
9. Don sterile gloves. The dominant hand that will handle the catheter must remain sterile while the nondominant hand is considered clean rather than sterile.	Handling the sterile catheter with a hand wearing a sterile glove helps prevent introducing organisms into the respiratory tract and the clean glove protects the nurse from microorganisms.
10. With sterile gloved hand, pick up sterile catheter and connect to suction tubing that is held with unsterile hand.	Sterilization can be maintained.
11. Moisten the catheter by dipping it into the container of sterile saline. Occlude Y-tube to check suction.	Lubricating the inside of the catheter with saline helps move secretions in the catheter.
12. Estimate the distance from the earlobe to the nostril, and place thumb and forefinger of gloved hand at that point on the catheter.	Ensures that catheter remains in pharynx rather than trachea.

(continued)

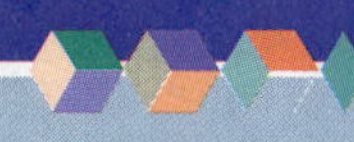

PROCEDURE 45-5 *(continued)*

Suctioning the Nasopharyngeal and Oropharyngeal Areas

Action	Rationale

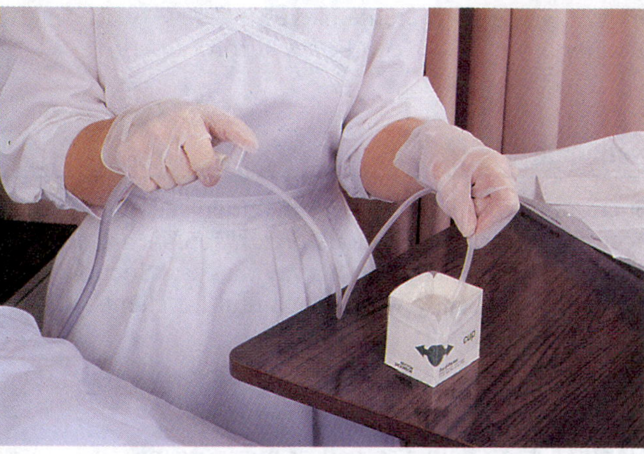

Action 11: Moisten the catheter by dipping it into the sterile saline container and occlude Y-tube to check suction.

13. Gently insert the catheter with the suction off by leaving the vent on the Y-connector open. Slip the catheter gently along the floor of an unobstructed nostril toward the trachea to suction the nasopharynx. Or, insert the catheter along the side of the mouth toward the trachea to suction the oropharynx. Never apply suction as the catheter is introduced.

Using suction while inserting the catheter can cause trauma to the mucosa and removes oxygen from the respiratory tract. Coughing is induced when the trachea is touched. This helps the client raise secretions.

14. Apply suction by occluding the suctioning port with your thumb and gently rotate the catheter as it is being withdrawn. Do not allow the suctioning to continue for more than 10 to 15 seconds at a time.

Turning the catheter as it is withdrawn helps clean all surfaces of the respiratory passageways. Suctioning the client for longer than 10 to 15 seconds robs the respiratory tract of oxygen, which may result in hypoxia.

15. Flush the catheter with saline and repeat suctioning as needed and according to client's toleration of procedure.

Flushing cleans and clears catheter and lubricates it for next insertion.

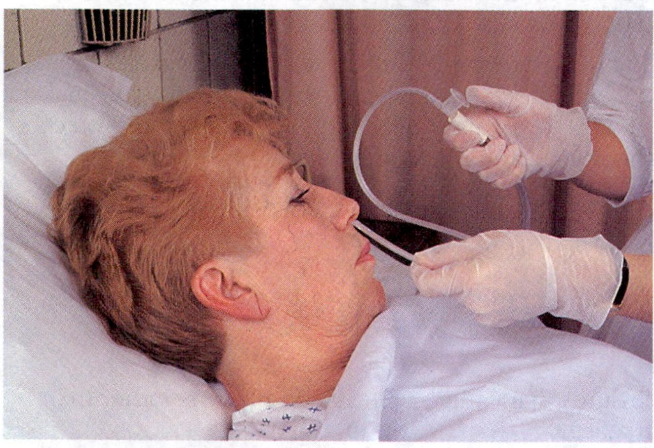

Action 13: Inserting the catheter.

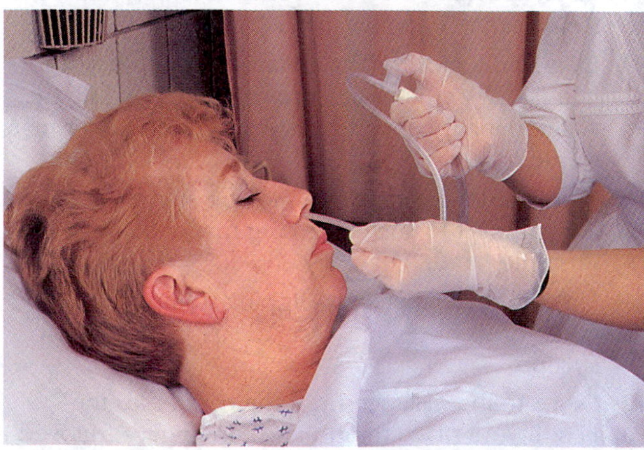

Action 14: Occluding port and rotating catheter while withdrawing.

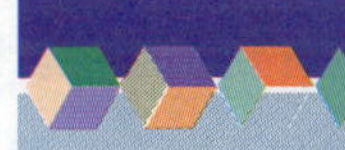

PROCEDURE 45-5 *(continued)*

Suctioning the Nasopharyngeal and Oropharyngeal Areas

Action	Rationale
16. Allow at least 20- to 30-second interval if additional suctioning is needed. The nares should be alternated when repeated suctioning is required. Do not force catheter through the nares. Encourage client to cough and deep breathe between suctionings.	Normal breathing between suctioning helps compensate for any hypoxia induced by the previous suctioning.
17. When suctioning is completed, remove gloves inside out and dispose of gloves, catheter, and container with solution in proper receptacle. Wash your hands.	Handwashing prevents transmission of microorganisms.
18. Use auscultation to listen to chest and breathing sounds to assess the effectiveness of suctioning.	Listening to chest and breathing sounds helps determine whether the respiratory passageways are clear of secretions.

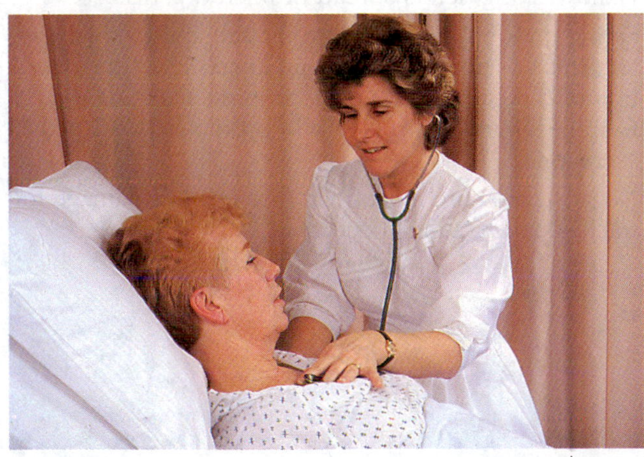

Action 18: Assessing effectiveness of suctioning. (Photos © 1992 B. Proud.)

Action	Rationale
19. Record the time of suctioning and the nature and amount of secretions. Also note the character of the client's respirations before and after the suctioning.	Records of nursing measures used help assess, evaluate, and coordinate care.
20. Offer oral hygiene after suctionings.	Respiratory secretions that are allowed to accumulate in the mouth are irritating to mucous membranes and unpleasant for the client.

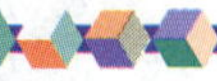

jaw pulled forward, and airway cleared, the mask is held tightly over the client's nose and mouth. The operator's other hand compresses the bag at a rate that approximates normal respiratory rate (eg, 16 to 20 breaths per minute in the adult). The one-way valve in the mask allows exhaled air to escape. Artificial ventilation can be sustained until spontaneous breathing starts, until other mechanical assistance is available, or until death is confirmed. The bag is self-inflating.

The manual resuscitation bag has also been the conventional method of hyperoxygenating a client prior to a suctioning procedure. Researchers have discovered that using this device for this purpose is unpredictable

(text continues on page 1354)

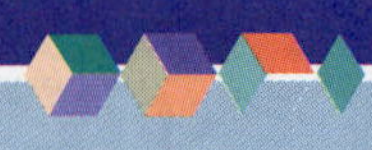

PROCEDURE 45-6

Suctioning the Tracheostomy

Equipment

Portable or wall suction device with connecting tubing
Sterile suction kit containing the following or gather separately:
- Sterile suction catheter of appropriate size with Y-port
  - Infants: 6–8 F
  - Children: 8–10 F
  - Adults: 12–16 F
- Sterile container
- Sterile glove
- Sterile normal saline

Clean towel or sterile drape (optional)
Goggles (or glasses) and mask
Gown (optional)
Resuscitation bag connected to 100% oxygen

Action	Rationale
1. Explain procedure to client and reassure him or her that you will interrupt procedure if the client indicates respiratory difficulty. Administer pain medication before suctioning to postoperative client.	Explanation facilitates cooperation and provides reassurance for client. Any procedure that compromises respiration is frightening for the client. Suctioning stimulates coughing which is painful for clients with surgical incisions.
2. Gather equipment and provide privacy for client.	This provides for organized approach to task.
3. Wash your hands.	Handwashing deters spread of microorganisms.
4. Assist the client to a semi-Fowler's or Fowler's position if conscious. An unconscious client should be placed in the lateral position facing you.	Sitting position helps client to cough and breathe easier. This position also uses gravity to aid in the insertion of catheter. Lateral position prevents the airway from becoming obstructed and promotes drainage of secretions.
5. Turn suction to appropriate pressure: a. Wall unit Adult: 100 to 120 mm Hg Child: 95 to 110 mm Hg Infant: 50 mm Hg b. Portable unit Adult: 10 to 15 mm Hg Child: 5 to 10 mm Hg Infant: 2 to 5 mm Hg	Negative pressure must be at safe level or damage to tracheal mucosa may occur.
6. Place clean towel, if being used, across client's chest. Don goggles, mask, and gown, if necessary.	Towel protects client and bed linens. Wearing protective equipment prevents contamination of the caregiver's mucous membranes.
7. Open sterile kit or set up equipment, and prepare to suction:	
a. Place sterile drape, if available, across client's chest.	Drape protects client and bed linens.
b. Open sterile container and place on bedside table or overbed table without contaminating inner surface. Pour sterile saline into it.	This maintains sterile setup.
c. Hyperoxygenate client using manual resuscitation bag or sigh mechanism on mechanical ventilator.	This prevents hypoxemia that can occur during suctioning.
d. Don sterile gloves or one sterile glove on dominant hand and clean glove on nondominant hand.	Gloves maintain sterility of procedure and protect the nurse from microorganisms.
e. Connect sterile suction catheter to suction tubing that is held with unsterile gloved hand.	Sterile technique helps prevent introducing organisms into the respiratory tract.

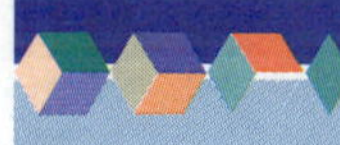

PROCEDURE 45-6 *(continued)*

Suctioning the Tracheostomy

Action	**Rationale**

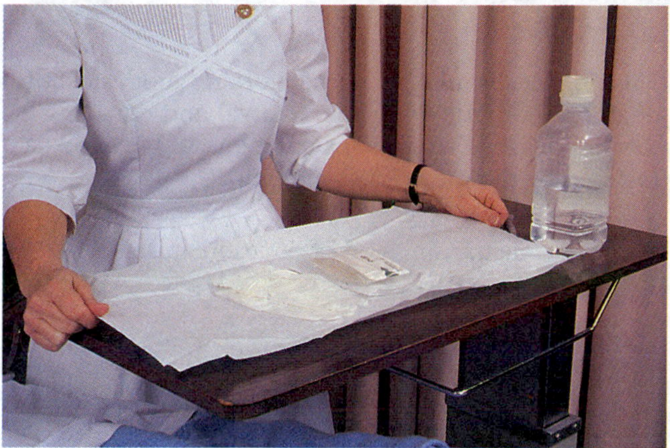

Action 7: Opening the sterile kit.

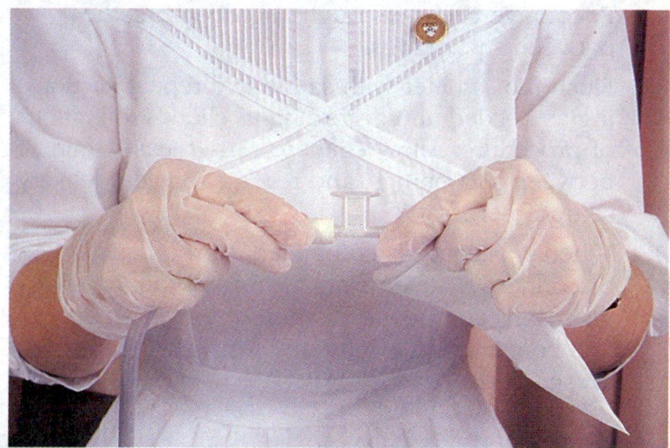

Action 7e: Connecting catheter to suction tube.

Action	Rationale
8. Moisten the catheter by dipping it into the container of sterile saline unless it is one of the newer silicone catheters that do not require lubrication.	Lubricating the inside of catheter with saline helps move secretions in the catheter. Silicone catheters do not require lubrication.
9. Remove oxygen delivery setup with unsterile gloved hand if it is still in place.	This exposes tracheostomy tube.
10. Using sterile gloved hand, gently and quickly insert catheter into the trachea. Advance about 10 to 12.5 cm (4 to 5 inches) or until client coughs. *Do not occlude Y-port when inserting catheter.*	Using suction when inserting catheter can cause trauma to mucosa and removes oxygen from the respiratory tract.

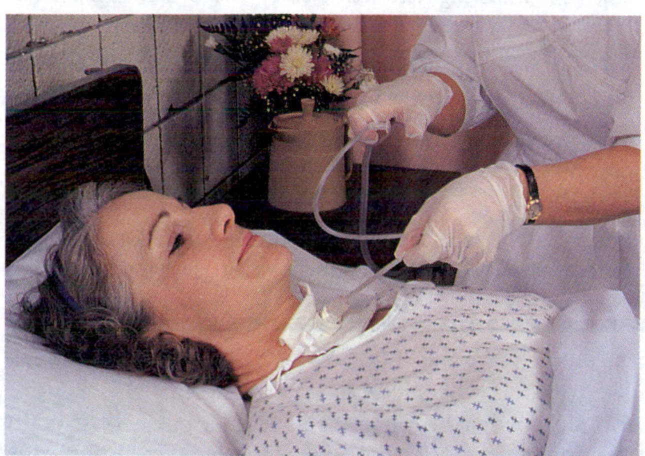

Action 10: Inserting catheter with Y-port open.

Action	Rationale
11. Apply intermittent suction by occluding Y-port with thumb of unsterile gloved hand. Gently rotate catheter with thumb and index finger of sterile gloved hand as catheter is being withdrawn. Do not allow suctioning to continue for more than 10 seconds.	Turning the catheter while withdrawing it helps clean surfaces of respiratory tract and prevents injury to tracheal mucosa. Suctioning for longer than 10 seconds may result in hypoxia.

(continued)

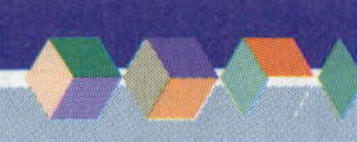

PROCEDURE 45-6 (continued)

Suctioning the Tracheostomy

Action	Rationale
Encourage client to cough and deep breathe between suctionings.	
12. Flush the catheter with saline and repeat suctioning as needed and according to client's toleration of procedure. Allow client to rest at least 1 minute between suctionings, and replace oxygen delivery setup if necessary.	Flushing cleans and clears catheter and lubricates it for next insertion. Allowing time interval and replacing oxygen delivery setup helps compensate for hypoxia induced by the previous suctioning.
13. When procedure is completed, turn off suction and disconnect catheter from suction tubing. Remove gloves inside out and dispose of gloves, catheter, and container with solution in proper receptacle. Wash hands.	This prevents transmission of microorganisms.

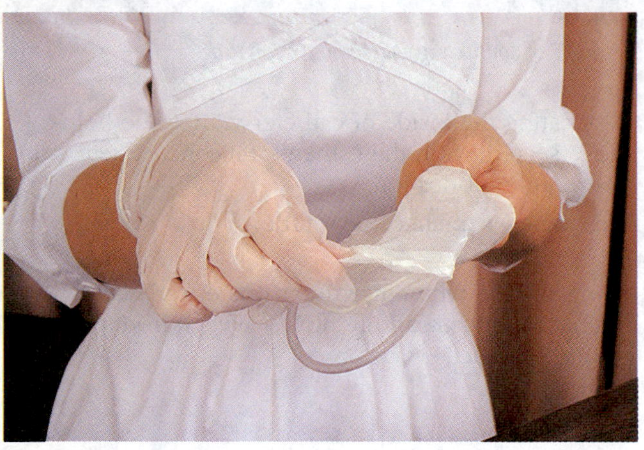

Action 13: Removing glove over catheter. (Photos © 1992 B. Proud.)

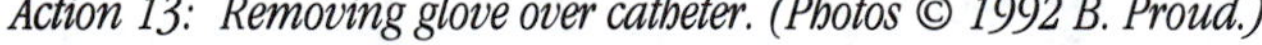

Action	Rationale
14. Adjust client's position. Auscultate chest to evaluate breath sounds.	Auscultation helps determine if respiratory passageways are cleared of secretions.
15. Record the time of suctioning and the nature and amount of secretions. Also note the character of client's respirations before and after suctioning.	This provides accurate documentation and provides for comprehensive care.
16. Offer oral hygiene.	Respiratory secretions that accumulate are irritating to mucous membranes and unpleasant for the client.

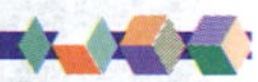

because it is difficult to compress the bag thoroughly and the concentration of oxygen delivered to the client is unreliable (Carroll, 1994).

Clearing an Obstructed Airway

Foreign body obstruction of the airway usually occurs during eating. In adults, meat is the most common cause. In children, any variety of foods or objects have obstructed the upper airway. A semiconscious or unconscious client can develop airway obstruction because the tongue covers the pharynx as it falls back, obstructing the upper airway. The tongue is the most common cause of airway obstruction.

Foreign bodies can cause either partial airway obstruction or complete airway obstruction. In partial airway obstruction with good air exchange, the client can cough forcefully. This person should be allowed and encouraged to cough and breathe spontaneously. At this time, the nurse should not interfere with the client's efforts to expel the object. Good air exchange can progress to poor air exchange, indicated by weak, ineffective

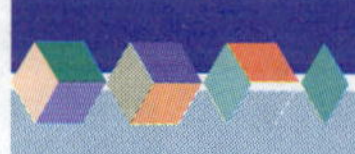

PROCEDURE 45-7

Providing Tracheostomy Care

Equipment

Disposable gloves
Sterile gloves
Goggles or face shield (optional)
Sterile tracheostomy cleaning kit (if available) *or*
Sterile basins (2)
Sterile brush/pipe cleaners
Sterile cotton-tipped applicators
Sterile cleaning solutions:
Hydrogen peroxide
Normal saline solution
Replacement inner cannula (if available)
Commercially prepared tracheostomy dressing or sterile non–cotton-filled 4 × 4 gauze pad
Tracheostomy ties (twill tape or Velcro)
Scissors
Plastic disposal bag

Action	Rationale
1. Explain procedure to client.	Explanation facilitates cooperation and provides reassurance for client.
2. If tracheostomy tube has just been suctioned, remove soiled dressing from around tube and discard with gloves when they are removed.	Suctioning prevents secretions from accumulating in inner cannula and occluding airway.
3. Wash your hands and open necessary supplies.	Handwashing deters spread of microorganisms.
Cleaning a Nondisposable Inner Cannula	
4. Prepare supplies prior to cleaning inner cannula:	
a. Open tracheostomy care kit and separate basins touching only the edges. If kit is not available, open two sterile basins.	Basins are sterile receptacles for cleaning solutions.
b. Fill one basin ½ in (1.25 cm) deep with hydrogen peroxide.	Hydrogen peroxide facilitates removal of dry, encrusted secretions.
c. Fill other basin ½ in (1.25 cm) deep with saline.	Saline rinses and removes hydrogen peroxide and lubricates the outer surface of the inner cannula for easier reinsertion.
d. Open sterile brush or pipe cleaners if they are not already available in a cleaning kit.	Sterile brush or pipe cleaner provides friction to clean inner surface of cannula.
5. Don disposable gloves.	Gloves protect from exposure to blood and body substances.
6. Remove the oxygen source if one is present. Rotate the lock on the inner cannula in a counterclockwise motion to release it.	Releasing the lock permits removal of the inner cannula.
7. Gently remove the inner cannula and carefully drop it in the basin with hydrogen peroxide. Remove gloves and discard.	Soaking in hydrogen peroxide loosens dry, hardened secretions.
8. Clean the inner cannula:	
a. Don sterile gloves.	Sterile gloves maintain surgical asepsis.
b. Remove inner cannula from soaking solution. Moisten brush or pipe cleaners in saline and insert into tube, using back-and-forth motion.	Movement of brush creates friction and aids in removal of accumulated secretions.
c. Agitate cannula in saline solution. Remove and tap against inner surface of basin.	Saline rinses inner cannula. Tapping tube against basin removes excess saline in inner tube.
9. Replace inner cannula into outer cannula. Turn lock clockwise and check that inner cannula is secure. Reapply oxygen source if needed.	Clockwise motion secures inner cannula in place.

(continued)

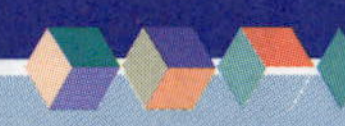

PROCEDURE 45-7 (continued)

Providing Tracheostomy Care

Action	Rationale
Replacing a Disposable Inner Cannula	
1. Release lock. Gently remove inner cannula and place in disposal bag. Replace with appropriately sized new cannula. Engage lock on inner cannula.	Disposable cannulas, although more costly, ensure that airway is clean and patent.

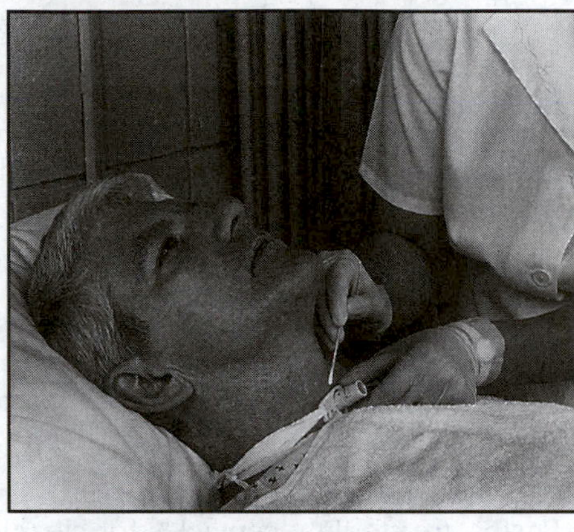

Action 1: Cleaning underneath the faceplate.

Action	Rationale
Applying Clean Dressing and Tape	
1. Dip cotton-tipped applicator in saline and clean stoma under faceplate. Use each applicator only once, moving from stoma site outward.	Saline is nonirritating to tissue. Cleansing from stoma outward and using each applicator only once promotes aseptic technique.
2. Apply hydrogen peroxide to area around stoma, faceplate, and outer cannula if secretions prove difficult to remove. Rinse area with saline.	Hydrogen peroxide may cause tissue damage and needs to be removed from skin and surrounding area.
3. Pat skin gently with dry 4 × 4 gauze.	Gauze removes excess moisture.
4. Slide commercially prepared tracheostomy dressing or prefolded non–cotton-filled 4 × 4 dressing under faceplate.	Lint or fiber from cotton-filled gauze pad can be aspirated into the trachea and cause irritation.

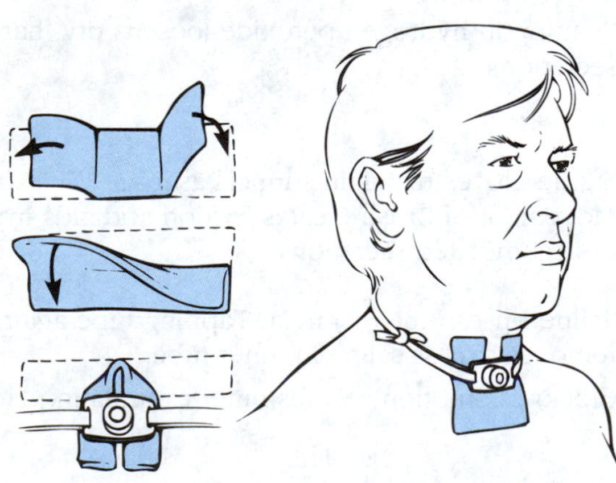

Action 4: Folding gauze square or placing commercially prepared dressing under faceplate of tracheostomy tube.

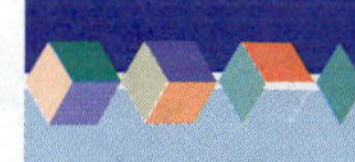

PROCEDURE 45-7 *(continued)*

Providing Tracheostomy Care

Action	Rationale
5. Change the tracheostomy tape:	
a. Leave soiled tape in place until new one is applied.	Ensures that tracheostomy will not be expelled if client coughs or moves.
b. Cut piece of tape that is twice the neck circumference plus 4 in (10 cm). Trim ends of tape on the diagonal.	Provides for secure attachment with knot in front at neckplate. Diagonal cut facilitates insertion of tape into openings on faceplate.
c. Insert one end of tape through faceplate opening alongside old tape. Pull through until both ends are even.	Provides attachment for one side of faceplate.

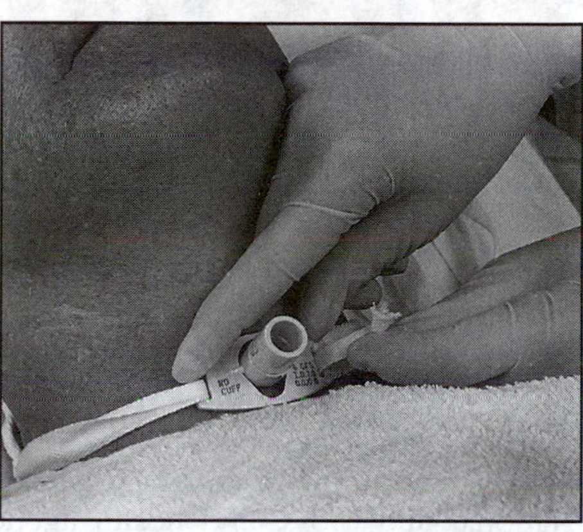

Action 5d: Inserting the tracheostomy tape through the opening and pulling through. (Photos © B. Proud.)

Action	Rationale
d. Slide both tapes under client's neck and insert one end through remaining opening on other side of faceplate. Pull snugly and tie ends in double square knot. Check that client can flex neck comfortably.	A secure tape prevents accidental expulsion of the tracheostomy tube. Neck flexion that is comfortable assures that tape will not compromise circulation to the area.
e. Carefully remove old tape. Reapply oxygen source if necessary.	New tape provides for secure attachment.
6. Remove gloves and discard. Wash hands. Assess the client's respirations. Document assessments and completion of procedure.	Assessment and accurate documentation provide for comprehensive care.

Home Care Considerations

The client and home caregiver are given instructions on how to perform tracheostomy care. The nurse also observes the return demonstration and provides feedback. Clean rather than sterile technique can be used in the home setting. Sterile saline can be made by mixing 1 teaspoon of table salt in 1 quart of water and boiling for 15 minutes. The solution is cooled and stored in a clean dry container. Saline is discarded at the end of each day to prevent growth of bacteria. If the client is performing self-care, the nurse recommends the use of a mirror to view the steps in the procedure.

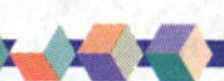

cough, high-pitched noises while inhaling, increased breathing difficulties, and cyanosis. This should be managed the same way as complete airway obstruction.

With complete airway obstruction, the victim is unable to speak or cough. The client may demonstrate the universal distress signal (ie, clutching his or her throat with both hands). Immediate action is necessary or the client will become unconscious as the brain becomes hypoxic. Once complete airway obstruction has been established, the Heimlich maneuver (abdominal thrusts) should be provided. The American Heart Association has developed and continually updates its protocols for cardiopulmonary resuscitation and obstructed airways.

Administering Cardiopulmonary Resuscitation

CPR is the combination of mouth-to-mouth breathing, which supplies oxygen to the lungs, and chest compressions, which circulate blood. It is often described as the ABCs of basic life support:

*A*irway: Tip the head and check for breathing. The respiratory tract must be opened so air can enter.

*B*reathing: If the victim does not start to breathe spontaneously after the airway is opened, give two slow, full breaths.

*C*irculation: Check the pulse. If the victim has no pulse, artificial circulation must be started with breathing.

CPR should be started for any situation in which either breathing alone or breathing and heart beat are absent. The brain is sensitive to hypoxia and will sustain irreversible damage after 4 to 6 minutes of no oxygen. The faster CPR is initiated, the greater the chance of survival.

At regular intervals, the American Heart Association revises CPR protocols. In 1992, changes the AHA recommended included (1) early activation if a person is found unconscious and breathless rather than 1 minute of CPR and then telephoning for help and (2) the initial two breaths are slower and more deliberate (1.5 to 2 seconds each). Blood and body substance precautions should be followed even though there may not be contact with a client's blood or body fluids during CPR. OSHA standards require healthcare facilities to provide an ample supply of ventilation masks along with other protective barriers for staff to use during resuscitation efforts. A recent survey indicated that only 4 of 10 nurses would perform mouth-to-mouth resuscitation in a trauma situation because of fear of contracting AIDS or other infectious diseases (Brenner & Kauffman, 1993). When ventilation masks are available, most nurses stated they would never refuse to resuscitate any client.

The automated external defibrillator (AED) has also proved effective in reducing deaths attributed to cardiac arrest. This computer-based device is easy to use and designed to quickly deliver a shock to the heart muscle to interrupt ventricular fibrillation, a frequent cause of cardiac arrest. The AED has the ability to analyze the heart's rhythm, direct the operator to deliver a shock when appropriate, and then reanalyze the rhythm to determine if it has returned to normal. The American Heart Association promotes the use of AEDs for use by trained laypersons and emergency medical technicians (EMTs) for prehospital cardiac arrests (see placement of AED electrode pads in Fig. 45-15). It is required as part of advanced cardiac life support training, and awareness training concerning AEDs is also included in basic cardiac life support instructions (Angelini & Boecklen, 1994).

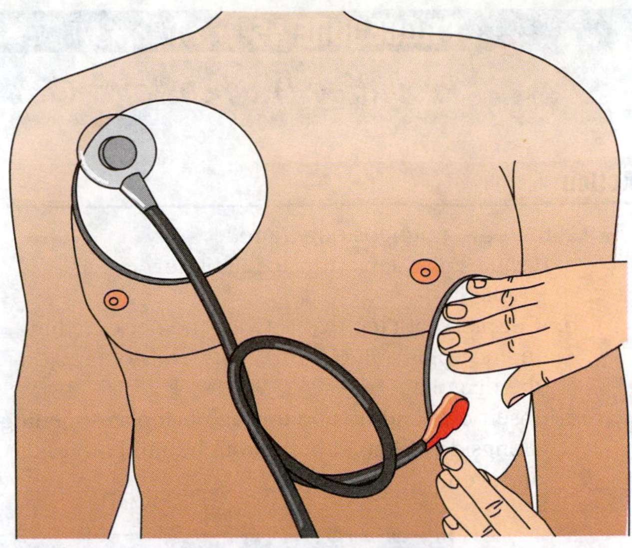

Figure 45-15
Place the AED pad attached to the red cable connector to the left of the heart apex. To help remember where to place the pads, think "white right, red ribs." (Placement for both electrode pads is the same as for manual defibrillation/cardioversion.)

Most professional organizations recommend and support widespread efforts to teach CPR to laypeople and all health professionals. Mannequins for practice can be obtained from the American Heart Association, the National Red Cross, and health agencies. It is a professional responsibility to maintain proficiency in CPR skills. This necessitates periodic practice with mannequins (adult and infant). CPR should be administered quickly and accurately, without hesitation, when an emergency arises.

Hyperbaric Oxygen Therapy

Studies are ongoing evaluating the effectiveness of hyperbaric oxygen therapy (HBOT). Many remember this technique as the treatment for the decompression sickness or "bends" suffered by deep-sea divers. Today, wound healing is the most common indication for using hyperbaric oxygen therapy (Collison, 1993). HBOT's therapeutic effects result from exposure to oxygen under greatly increased pressure. Various types of sealed enclosures or chambers are available. When in the chamber, the tissues are flooded with more than the usual supply of oxygen. The client receiving this therapy requires careful monitoring because various complications can occur related to the delivery of oxygen under pressure. Other conditions that respond to hyperbaric oxygen therapy include carbon monoxide poisoning, tetanus, gas gangrene, and certain infections caused by bacteria that are resistant to antibiotics but vulnerable to oxygen. As more information becomes available, this adjunctive therapy is gaining widespread recognition and respect.

Helpscan

The following are resources for clients and healthcare professionals:

- For information related to respiratory concerns and conditions:
  American Lung Association
  1740 Broadway
  New York, NY 10019
  (212) 315-8700

  Canadian Lung Association
  75 Albert St., Suite 908
  Ottawa, ON KIP 5E7
  (613) 237-1208
- For information about asthma and allergies:
  Asthma and Allergy Foundation of America
  1125 15th Street NW, Suite 502
  Washington, DC 20005
  (202) 466-7643
- For more information about hyperbaric oxygen therapy:
  Baramedical Nurses Association
  P.O. Box 2727
  Palm Desert, CA 92261
  (619) 770-3676

EVALUATING

Evaluation is an ongoing and deliberate part of the nursing process that involves the nurse, client, family, and other healthcare team members. It includes a comparison of the client's health status and the previously defined expected outcomes and an examination of the client's projected progress in meeting those outcomes. All involved in the evaluation process need to identify effective interventions and reasons for any failures in achieving these expected outcomes. Adjustments in the nursing plan of care must be made accordingly.

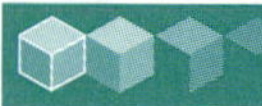

Nursing Process in Clinical Practice

The nurse uses all phases of the nursing process when identifying and treating alterations in respiratory functioning. The nurse's knowledge and application of clinical skills described in this chapter play a major role in treating respiratory problems. This section addresses assessment priorities, expected outcomes, and nursing interventions for those common types of respiratory problems treated by nurses:

Impaired Gas Exchange
Ineffective Breathing Pattern
Ineffective Airway Clearance

In the client care study that follows, nursing care is described for a young child with an alteration in respiratory functioning.

Impaired Gas Exchange

The state in which the individual experiences a decreased passage of oxygen and/or carbon dioxide between the alveoli of the lungs and the vascular system (NANDA, 1994)

Assessment Priorities

- Use interview questions directed to the client and significant others to determine exactly what is the problem.
- Determine if the client's perception of the impaired gas exchange corresponds to actual physiologic changes.
- Explore the client's lifestyle and physical and mental health for contributing factors.
- Examine the client for signs of impaired gas exchange (eg, tachypnea, abnormal breath sounds, cough, neck vein distention, or barrel chest).
- Check lab and radiology data for more information (chest x-ray, pulse oximetry readings, arterial blood gas results, hemoglobin, protein levels, and so forth).
- Observe client's technique when dealing with actual or perceived impaired gas exchange.
- Assess client's effectiveness in dealing with impaired gas exchange.

Expected Outcomes

The client will:

- Identify causes of the impaired gas exchange
- Incorporate adequate pulmonary hygiene techniques into the daily routine
- Institute lifestyle changes to eliminate factors contributing to impaired gas exchange
- Seek treatment for early signs of infection
- Use breathing techniques with ease to decrease the work of breathing

Interventions

- Instruct client to cough properly and deep breathe four times a day (30 minutes before meals and at bedtime).

- Demonstrate and encourage client use of diaphragmatic breathing and pursed-lip breathing.
- Encourage good oral hygiene.
- Arrange (or encourage home manager to arrange) four or five small meals per day.
- Assist client to drink 2 to 3 qt of clear fluid each day. Keep a container of favorite juice at client's side.
- Incorporate a period of regular exercise into each day.
- Encourage client to socialize with others (friends, respiratory support group, church, and so forth).
- Use simple explanations (written and verbal) on medications, their actions, dose, timing, and side effects.
- Explore with client and others who live with him or her methods to reduce pollution in home or work environment.
- Use air conditioner on high pollution days.
- Avoid using respiratory irritants.
- If the client smokes, discuss the idea of reducing smoking with the goal of stopping the smoking habit.

Ineffective Breathing Pattern

The state in which an individual's inhalation and/or exhalation pattern does not enable adequate pulmonary inflation or emptying (NANDA, 1994)

Assessment Priorities

- Use interview questions directed to the client and significant others to determine the nature of the problem, its probable cause, and its effect on lifestyle.
- Examine client and assess respiratory rate, rhythm, and symptoms of anxiety or pain.

Expected Outcomes

The client will:

- Demonstrate effective respiratory rate and rhythm
- Identify possible contributing factors
- Evaluate adaptive coping mechanisms when dealing with stress or anxiety

Interventions

- Demonstrate conscious controlled breathing and encourage client to use it during periods of anxiety or activity.
- Maintain a safe environment. Same nurses always work with this client. Maintain eye contact during conversation.
- If fear is the cause, encourage client to verbalize concerns. Reduce cause of fear, if feasible.
- If there is a strong emotional component, discuss with client the development of effective coping skills with professional counseling.
- If pain is present, use appropriate methods for comfort (eg, position, analgesics, blankets, and so forth).

Ineffective Airway Clearance

A state in which an individual is unable to clear secretions or obstructions from the respiratory tract to maintain airway patency (NANDA, 1994)

Assessment Priorities

- Use interview questions directed to client or significant others to determine nature of the problem and its suspected cause.
- Examine the client and assess for signs of airway obstruction (eg, abnormal or absent breath sounds, inability to move secretions, cyanosis, restlessness, ineffective cough, nasal flaring).
- Evaluate laboratory studies (eg, arterial blood gases, pulse oximetry, tidal volume, vital capacity).
- Assess client's coughing techniques and other pulmonary hygiene practices.
- Verify client's ability to maintain a position that prevents aspiration and allows for complete opening of the airway.

Expected Outcomes

The client will:

- Maintain good body alignment to ensure effective air exchange
- Maintain fluid intake so secretions are thin
- Demonstrate appropriate use of controlled coughing and diaphragmatic breathing techniques
- Follow medication regimen accurately and be able to state drug actions, dose, and side effects

Interventions

- Auscultate client's breath sounds every 4 hours.
- Encourage client to cough effectively or suction every 2 to 4 hours.
- Keep client's head elevated at least 45 degrees or maintain side-lying position to maintain an open airway.
- Splint incisions (if any) for support. Treat pain with analgesics as needed.
- Force favorite fluids (2 to 3 qt) unless cardiac or renal disturbances prevent this intake.
- Arrange periods of rest around activity (eg, 8 AM: After the walk down the hall, the client can sleep for 1 hour).
- Use praise liberally to encourage efforts and work.
- Review (orally and in writing) medications, their dose, actions, side effects, and possible interactions.
- Let the client and caregiver know about support groups in the area.
- Encourage family to contact the American Lung Association for free pamphlets.

Client Care Study

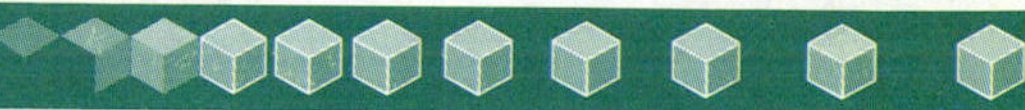

Freddie is a 1-year-old alert, well-developed child who has been a client on the pediatric unit for 3 days with status asthmaticus. He has had two other admissions for acute asthma during which he responded quickly to intravenous and inhalation bronchodilators. During this hospitalization, either his mother, a teacher, or his father, a psychologist, has stayed with him. Other relatives are caring for Freddie's 9-year-old sister and 5-year-old brother.

Freddie interacts happily with staff as long as a parent is within sight. Gross and fine motor coordination are appropriate for his age. His vocabulary consists of 25 words. History is from his mother, who is a reliable source. Child has had a clear nasal discharge with slight, intermittent, nonproductive cough for 3 days with no change in appetite or activity pattern.

On day of admission, he attended the daycare center as usual. After being there for 3 hours, his cough became more frequent and respirations became more labored. The caregivers were not alarmed because he continued to eat, drink, nap, and play in usual pattern. Mother states that when she arrived in the afternoon to pick up the boys, she discovered this child to be using his intercostal and neck muscles excessively with every breath. His respirations were 50 per minute, labored, and accompanied by a grunt. By the time she arrived home, he was pale and fitful and was crying weakly. Respirations were 60 per minute and circumoral, and peripheral cyanosis was noted. The pediatrician advised lung evaluation in the emergency department. While there, three subcutaneous injections of epinephrine were administered 5 minutes apart. The child did not respond satisfactorily, so he was admitted for intravenous aminophylline and steroid administration.

In addition to the history of asthma, Freddie is allergic to eggs and peanuts and has eczema on his face, arms, legs, and upper back. His current medications include metaproterenol sulfate (Alupent) every 8 hours; a topical steroid (Lidex Cream); and a multivitamin and mineral supplement (Poly-Vi-Sol Chewable Tabs), 0.5 mL daily. No one in the family smokes. The caregivers at the daycare center smoke outside the building. The day-care center is clean and had the rugs shampooed the night before this child's illness. This child had no sputum production or fever. Immunizations are current. A comprehensive assessment revealed the following findings:

Respiratory rate, 44 breaths/min
Irregular rhythm
Excessive use of accessory muscles
Nonproductive, frequent cough
Gurgles and expiratory wheezes noted
Pale, no cyanosis
Blood pressure, 100/60; heart rate, 120 beats/min
Restless child who naps for only 20 to 30 minutes at intervals day and night
Arterial blood gases: normal values
Chest x-ray: normal
Poor appetite, vomiting one or two times daily
Up early in morning
Sweat test: negative for cystic fibrosis

Core Competencies

Cognitive Competencies

- Knowledge of multiple factors that contribute to pulmonary distress
- Knowledge of which nursing interventions are most likely to improve respiratory functioning
- Teaching skills to help the family understand the relationship between environment (dust, stuffed animals, pets, pollution, etc.) and the development of Freddie's respiratory difficulties and to initiate the necessary changes
- Ability to develop nursing diagnoses that reflect Freddie's unique respiratory problems
- Conviction that nursing can make a difference in the quality of life for Freddie and his family

Technical Competencies

- Strong assessment skills (interviewing and physical assessment) to carefully identify the problem and its cause
- Caregiver skills directed toward promoting healthy respiratory functioning for Freddie and providing positive reinforcement for effort and progress

Interpersonal Competencies

- Interpersonal skills necessary to communicate with Freddie and his family
- Ability to establish a trusting nurse–client relationship grounded in responsible caring
- Leadership skills to motivate the nursing staff to value the family's expected outcomes and to work with the entire healthcare team (physicians, dietary, respiratory therapy)

Ethical/Legal Competencies

- Accountability and willingness to use competence to help Freddie and his family promote optimal respiratory functioning
- Competence in documenting nursing interventions
- Ability to serve as a trusted and effective client advocate

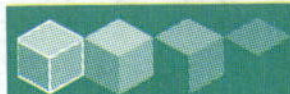

Nursing Plan of Care

for Freddie

Nursing Diagnosis: Ineffective Airway Clearance related to exposure to allergens, viral infection, bronchospasm, overproduction of mucus as manifested by: nonproductive frequent cough, presence of gurgles (rhonchi) and expiratory wheeze, restlessness, interrupted sleep.

Expected Outcome: By 12/5/98, the client will:

- Have rare episodes of coughing and no vomiting

Nursing Interventions	Rationale	Evaluative Statement
Hold meals until inhalation treatments are done.	Bronchodilators stimulate coughing and often cause vomiting if given after meals.	12/4/98 Goal met. Freddie has not vomited in 2 days and has 2-hour intervals between coughing episodes. *Mary Jones, RN*
Avoid milk products.	Milk accelerates the production of mucus.	
Offer clear juices every 3 hours in a bottle or cup.	Clear liquids help to liquefy secretions and prevent dehydration.	
Perform percussion during morning and evening bath.	Percussion loosens pulmonary secretions so they are more easily expectorated.	

Expected Outcome: By 12/5/98, the client's parents will:

- Remove dust-collecting toys

Nursing Interventions	Rationale	Evaluative Statement
Give parents allergy pamphlets from American Lung Association.	Adequate information reinforces instruction given by healthcare providers.	12/2/98 Goal met. Parents removed furry toys from hospital room. *Mary Jones, RN*
Review with both parents methods to reduce exposure to possible allergens at home.	Constant exposure to allergens (dust, mold, mildew, and so forth) and irritants (perfume, smog, cleaners, and so forth) produces bronchospasm and stimulates copious mucus production. Medications are most effective when allergens are removed.	
Encourage parents to examine daycare environment. Explore options with them.	Environment in daycare may contain allergens. The least irritating setting is desirable.	

Sample Documentation

12/1/98, nursing

Family and staff conference to discuss Freddie's respiratory disturbance initiated by primary nurse's concern. Present were Freddie's mother; MJ (primary nurse); TK (clinical coordinator); TR (head of respiratory department); and MM and LQ (staff nurses). Primary nurse presented findings from assessment and nursing examination. Discussion centered on strategies to control airway edema and reduce wheezes, reduce coughing episodes and control vomiting, and prevent further bronchospasms and edema resulting from exposure to allergens in environment. See plan of care. Client progress will be evaluated in 4 days during nursing grand rounds, 12/5/98.

Mary Jones, RN

Key Points

- The functioning units of the respiratory system are the alveoli, where the actual exchange of oxygen and carbon dioxide between the lung and circulation occurs. Airways conduct available gases during inspiratory and expiratory phases of ventilation.
- There are normal variations in respiratory functioning unique to specific ages that allow appropriate oxygenation to meet cellular needs. These differences involve chest shape, breath sounds, and presence of landmarks. In addition to age, other factors affect adequate respiratory functioning—level of health, growth and development, environment, and psychologic health. Persons with health deviations in respiratory functioning can initiate changes to improve the work of breathing.
- The health history is an essential component of respiratory function assessment. The client's physical examination and laboratory findings can provide information to identify the nature of the problem, its course, related signs and symptoms, onset and frequency, and effect on everyday living.
- Nursing diagnoses can be written to address inadequate breathing patterns, ineffective airway clearance, and impaired gas exchange. Nursing diagnoses also can be written to address how altered respiratory functioning has an effect on other areas of human functioning (eg, anxiety).
- Nursing interventions to promote adequate respiratory functioning include educating clients to maintain a pollution-free environment, promoting effective breathing and coughing exercises, maintaining adequate fluid intake, maintaining good nutrition, promoting comfort by positioning, providing supplemental oxygen, and using medications to promote adequate respiratory functioning.
- Evaluation is ongoing. The healthcare team and the client examine progress toward achieving the established outcomes. The plan is modified based on the client's response to nursing actions.

Study Questions

1. A client has a fractured rib and is breathing less often and with less depth because of the pain. This is best described as
   a. fremitus
   b. hyperventilation
   c. pleural friction rub
   d. hypoventilation
2. When auscultating Mr. Chang's breath sounds, the nurse detects a high-pitched, squeaky sound heard on expiration. She assesses this as
   a. crackles or rales
   b. wheezes
   c. gurgles or rhonchi
   d. pleural friction rub
3. Air that develops in the pleural space is referred to as
   a. pneumothorax
   b. pleural effusion
   c. hemothorax
   d. atelectasis
4. When planning care for a client with chronic lung disease who is receiving oxygen by way of a nasal cannula, the nurse expects that
   a. the oxygen must always be humidified
   b. the rate will be 2 L/min or less
   c. arterial blood gases must be drawn every 4 hours to determine flow rate
   d. the rate will be 6 L/min or more
5. The highest concentration of oxygen is provided by the
   a. partial rebreather mask
   b. nonrebreather mask
   c. simple mask
   d. Venturi mask
6. Which of the following is a correct statement about pulse oximetry measurement?
   a. A range of 95% to 98% is considered normal oxygen saturation.
   b. Oximetry measurement measures oxygen saturation of venous blood.
   c. Fasting is required for 12 hours prior to the test.
   d. Pulse oximetry is a replacement for arterial blood gas analysis.
7. The nurse correctly performs oropharyngeal suctioning on a client by
   a. using clean technique
   b. applying suction as the catheter is introduced
   c. flushing the catheter with saline between catheter insertions
   d. limiting suctioning to 25- to 30-second intervals at one time
8. Effective use of a metered-dose inhaler requires that the client
   a. breathe in through the nose
   b. inhale two sprays with one breath
   c. hold his or her breath after inspiration for 5 to 10 seconds
   d. exhale quickly through an open mouth
9. Mr. Parks has chronic obstructive pulmonary disease. The nurse has taught him pursed-lip breathing that helps him by
   a. increasing carbon dioxide, which stimulates breathing
   b. teaching him to prolong inspiration and shorten expiration

c. helping liquefy his secretions
d. decreasing the amount of air trapping and resistance

10. A client has suddenly had a cardiac arrest. What is the critical time that the nurse must keep in mind before irreversible brain damage occurs?
 a. 1 to 3 minutes
 b. 2 to 4 minutes
 c. 4 to 6 minutes
 d. 8 to 10 minutes
11. David White is in the hospital with a medical diagnosis of viral pneumonia. He is getting oxygen by way of a simple face mask. Why must the mask fit snugly over the client's face?
 a. It prevents mask movement and consequent skin breakdown.
 b. It helps the client feel secure.
 c. It maintains carbon dioxide retention.
 d. It aids in maintaining expected oxygen delivery.
12. When suctioning her client through a tracheostomy tube, the nurse was careful not to occlude the Y-port when inserting the suction catheter because it would
 a. prevent suctioning from occurring
 b. cause trauma to the tracheal mucosa
 c. break the sterile technique
 d. suction out all the carbon dioxide
13. The nurse follows safe technique when using a portable oxygen cylinder by
 a. checking the amount of oxygen in the cylinder before using it
 b. using a cylinder for a client transfer that indicates available oxygen is 500 psi
 c. placing the oxygen cylinder on the stretcher next to the client
 d. discontinuing the oxygen flow by turning the cylinder key counterclockwise until it is tight
14. Which of the following blood gas values are considered within the normal range?
 a. pH, 7.25 to 7.35; $PaCO_2$, 25 to 35 mm Hg; PaO_2, 50 to 100 mm Hg
 b. pH, 7.35 to 7.45; $PaCO_2$, 45 to 50 mm Hg; PaO_2, 90 to 100 mm Hg
 c. pH, 7.35 to 7.45; $PaCO_2$, 35 to 45 mm Hg; PaO_2, 80 to 100 mm Hg
 d. pH, 7.30 to 7.40; $PaCO_2$, 30 to 45 mm Hg; PaO_2, 70 to 100 mm Hg
15. Abdominal breathing at 30 to 60 breaths/min with an irregular pattern of rate and depth would closely describe the breathing patterns of what age group?
 a. aged adult
 b. infant
 c. early childhood
 d. late childhood

Answers With Rationale

1. The correct response is *d.* Hypoventilation is a decreased rate or depth of air movement into the lungs. Hyperventilation is an increased rate and depth of ventilation, whereas fremitus is the vibration of the chest wall that can be palpated. A pleural friction rub is a dry grating sound caused by inflammation of pleural surfaces.
2. The correct response is *b.* Crackles and gurgles are not described as squeaky and the pleural friction rub is a dry, grating sound.
3. The correct response is *a.* Fluid in the pleural space is referred to as a pleural effusion and blood in the pleural space is called hemothorax. Atelectasis is an incomplete expansion or collapse of the lungs.
4. The correct response is *b.* A rate higher than 2 L/min may destroy the hypoxic drive that stimulates respirations in the medulla in a client with chronic lung disease. Oxygen delivered at low rates does not necessarily have to be humidified, and arterial blood gases are not required at regular intervals to determine flow rate.
5. The correct response is *b.* The nonrebreather mask provides the highest concentration of oxygen to a spontaneously breathing client.
6. The correct response is *a.* Pulse oximetry measures oxygen saturation levels of arterial blood, fasting is not required prior to the test, and pulse oximetry is an adjunct therapy, not a replacement for arterial blood gas analysis.
7. The correct response is *c.* The nurse should use sterile technique, should not apply suction as the catheter is being introduced, and suctioning should be limited to 10- to 15-second intervals to avoid causing hypoxia.
8. The correct response is *c.* Holding one's breath for 5 to 10 seconds after inspiration of the medication allows the drug to reach the alveoli. Correct technique for using an MDI includes breathing in through the mouth so that all the medication is properly delivered to the lungs, using one spray of medication for each breath to receive the correct dose, and exhaling slowly through pursed lips to minimize airway trapping and resistance.
9. The correct response is *d.* Pursed-lip breathing prolongs expiration, increases airway pressure, and loosens the amount of airway trapping and resistance. Doing pursed-lip breathing correctly diminishes carbon dioxide retention.
10. The correct response is *c.* After 4 to 6 minutes without oxygen, irreversible brain damage can occur.
11. The correct response is *d.* A snug-fitting mask is necessary to deliver expected rates of oxygen. A

simple face mask does not trap carbon dioxide or cause retention.

12. The correct response is *b.* Occluding the Y-port causes suction and may traumatize the tracheal mucosa if applied when the catheter is inserted.
13. The correct response is *a.* The cylinder must always be checked prior to use to ensure that enough oxygen is available for the client. It is unsafe to use a cylinder that reads 500 psi or less since not enough oxygen remains for a client transfer. A cylinder that is not secured properly may result in injury to the client. Oxygen flow is discontinued by turning the valve clockwise until it is tight.
14. The correct response is *c.* These are the normal arterial blood gas ranges for pH, carbon dioxide, and oxygen.
15. The correct response is *b.* Respirations in the infant are more rapid and have not stabilized. As alveoli increase in number and size, the respiratory rate is lower.

Bibliography

Ackerman, M. (1993). The effect of saline lavage prior to suctioning. *American Journal of Critical Care, 2*(4), 326.

Angelini, K., & Boecklen, S. (1994). Take it to heart: How to operate an automated external defibrillator. *Nursing, 24*(3), 50–53.

Braun, A. (1993). Emergency cardiac care: Fine-tuning for the '90s. *RN, 56*(9), 50–55.

Brenner, B., & Kauffman, J. (1993). Reluctance of internists and medical nurses to perform mouth-to-mouth resuscitation. *Archives of Internal Medicine, 153*(15), 1763.

Cahill, K., & Heath, J. (1990). Sterile water used for humidification in low-flow oxygen therapy: Is it necessary? *American Journal of Infection Control, 18*(1), 13–17.

Calianno, C., Clifford, D., & Titano, K. (1995). Oxygen therapy: Giving your patient breathing room. *Nursing, 25*(12), 33–38.

Carpenito, L. (1995). *Nursing diagnosis: Application to clinical practice* (6th ed.). Philadelphia: Lippincott.

Carroll, P. (1994). Safe suctioning. *RN, 57*(5), 32–36.

Coleman, S. (1992). Cardiac issues in CPR: What the future might hold. *Nursing, 22*(4), 54–57.

Collison, L. (1993). Hyperbarics: When pressuring patients helps. *RN, 56*(3), 44–48.

Ehrhardt, B., & Daleiden, J. (1994). Pulse oximeters. *Nursing, 24*(8), 32V–32X.

Finesilver, C. (1992). Perfecting the art: Respiratory assessment. *RN, 55*(2), 22–29.

Fischbach, F. (1995). *A manual of laboratory tests* (5th ed.). Philadelphia: Lippincott.

Foyt, M. (1992). Impaired gas exchange in the elderly. *Geriatric Nursing, 13*(5), 262–268.

Fuller, J., & Schaller-Ayers, J. (1994). *Health assessment* (2nd ed.). Philadelphia: Lippincott.

Haydon, R. (1992). What keeps oxygenation on track? *American Journal of Nursing, 92*(12), 32–40.

How to use a volume incentive spirometer. (1994). *Nursing, 24*(11), 32T.

Karper, W., & Boschen, M. (1993). Effects of exercise on acute respiratory tract infections and related symptoms. *Geriatric Nursing, 14*(1), 15–18.

Mathews, P. (1994). 6 Steps for safe suctioning. *Nursing, 24*(2), 18.

Mathews, P. (1995). Safely delivering a breath of fresh air. *Nursing, 25*(5), 66–69.

McConnell, E. (1992). Using a metered-dose nebulizer correctly. *Nursing, 22*(2), 18.

McConnell, E. (1994a). Inserting an oropharyngeal airway properly. *Nursing, 24*(12), 20.

McConnell, E. (1994b). Performing pulse oximetry. *Nursing, 24*(10), 23.

McGaffigan, P. (1996). Hazards of hypoxemia: How to protect your patient from low oxygen levels. *Nursing, 26*(5), 41–46.

Meyer, C. (1992). Doing the CPR two-step. *American Journal of Nursing, 92*(3), 15.

Miracle, V. (1994). Occluded airway. *Nursing, 24*(11), 33.

Morgan, S. (1993). Effects of age on cardiovascular functioning. *Geriatric Nursing, 14*(5), 249–251.

North American Nursing Diagnosis Association. (1994). *NANDA nursing diagnoses: Definitions and classification 1995–1996.* Philadelphia: NANDA.

Osborne, E. (1993). Administering aerosol therapy. *Nursing, 23*(12), 24C–24H.

Porth, C. (1994). *Pathophysiology: Concepts of altered health states* (4th ed.). Philadelphia: Lippincott.

Rice, R. (1995). *Home health nursing procedures.* St. Louis: Mosby.

Smith, R., Fallentine, J., & Kessel, S. (1995). Underwater chest drainage. *Nursing, 25*(2), 60–63.

Sommers, M. (1992). The shattering consequences of CPR. *Nursing, 22*(7), 34–41.

Stiesmeyer, J. (1993). A four-step approach to pulmonary assessment. *American Journal of Nursing, 93*(8), 22–28.

Using nebulizers correctly. (1995). *Nursing, 25*(4), 22–23.

Weilitz, P., & Dettenmeier, P. (1994). Test your knowledge of tracheostomy tubes. *American Journal of Nursing, 94*(2), 46–50.

Weixler, D. (1994). Correcting metered-dose inhaler misuse. *Nursing, 24*(7), 62–64.

Willens, J. (1993). Strengthen your life-support skills. *Nursing, 23*(4), 54–58.

Yeaw, E. (1992). How position affects oxygenation: Good lung down? *American Journal of Nursing, 92*(3), 26–29.

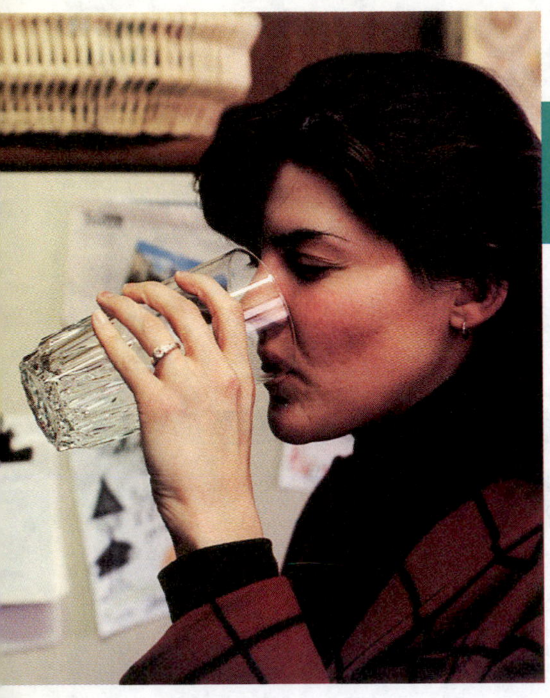

Chapter 46

Fluid, Electrolyte, and Acid–Base Balance

Objectives

After studying this chapter, the learner should be able to:

Define key terms used in the chapter.

Describe the location and functions of body fluids and factors that affect variations in fluid compartments.

Describe the functions, regulation, sources, and losses of the main electrolytes of the body.

Explain the principles of osmosis, diffusion, active transport, and filtration.

Describe how thirst and the organs of homeostasis (kidneys, heart and blood vessels, lungs, adrenal glands, pituitary gland, and parathyroid glands) function to maintain fluid homeostasis.

Describe the role of buffer systems and respiratory and renal mechanisms in achieving acid–base balance.

Identify the etiologies, defining characteristics, and treatment modalities for common fluid, electrolyte, and acid–base disturbances.

Perform a fluid, electrolyte, and acid–base balance assessment.

Describe the role of dietary modification, modification of fluid intake, medication administration, intravenous therapy, blood replacement, and total parenteral nutrition in resolving fluid, electrolyte, and acid–base imbalances.

Plan, implement, and evaluate nursing care related to select nursing diagnoses involving fluid, electrolyte, and acid–base imbalances.

Key Terms

acid
acidosis
active transport
alkalosis
anion
base
buffer
cation
colloid osmotic pressure
diffusion
electrolyte
filtration
hydrostatic pressure
ion
oncotic pressure
osmolarity
osmosis
pH
solute
solvent

The human body is composed of between 50% and 60% of water by weight. Because fluid is the main constituent of the body, the importance of the body's fluid balance is readily apparent. Body fluids contain other dissolved substances in the form of electrolytes, gases, and nonelectrolytes. The balance or homeostasis of water and the dissolved substances is maintained through functions of almost every organ of the body. Nurses routinely care for clients with serious and even life-threatening fluid, electrolyte, and acid–base disturbances. One of nursing's most important roles is the prevention of these disturbances in high-risk populations such as infants, older individuals, and clients with cardiac and renal disorders.

Information in this chapter provides basic knowledge about the principles of fluid, electrolyte, and acid–base balance and the etiologies, defining characteristics, and nursing interventions for common disturbances. Sample interview questions for performing a fluid balance assessment are presented, along with information on specific physical assessment measures and laboratory studies. Numerous examples of nursing diagnoses are provided. Expected outcomes and specific nursing interventions to promote fluid and electrolyte balance are included. These interventions include modifying dietary and fluid intake; administering medications; and assisting with intravenous (IV) therapy, blood replacement, and total parenteral nutrition (TPN). In the section entitled Nursing Process in Clinical Practice, focused assessment, expected outcomes, and implementation guides are offered for surgical and oncology clients with fluid balance nursing diagnoses. These guides and the concluding client care study illustrate how the nurse's knowledge of fluid, electrolyte, and acid–base balance is combined with skilled nursing interventions and caring to successfully resolve alterations in health status and improve client outcome.

Physiology

Body Fluids

As the primary body fluid, water is the most important nutrient of life. Whereas life can be sustained for many days without food, it can be sustained for only a few days without water. The following are the primary functions of water in the body:

- Provides a medium for transporting nutrients to cells and wastes from cells, and for transporting such substances as hormones, enzymes, blood platelets, and red and white blood cells
- Facilitates cellular metabolism and proper cellular chemical functioning
- Acts as a solvent for electrolytes and nonelectrolytes
- Helps maintain normal body temperature
- Facilitates digestion and promotes elimination
- Acts as a tissue lubricant

Body Fluid Compartments

The two main compartments, or spaces, in which fluids are located in the body are the *intracellular fluid* (ICF) and *extracellular fluid* (ECF). ICF is the fluid within the cell. It constitutes about 40% of an adult's body weight, or 70% of the total body water. ECF is all the fluid outside of cell walls. It constitutes about 20% of an adult's body weight, or 30% of total body water (Metheny, 1992). ECF includes intravascular and interstitial fluids. *Intravascular fluid* or plasma is the liquid constituent of blood (ie, fluid found within the vascular system). *Interstitial fluid* is the fluid in which tissue cells are bathed and includes lymph. The term *total body water* or fluid (TBW or TBF) refers to the total amount of water in the body expressed as a percentage of body weight. Figure 46-1 illustrates a breakdown of total body fluid; Figure 46-2 provides a microscopic visualization of body fluid distribution.

Variations in Fluid Content

In a healthy person, total body water constitutes about 55% to 75% of the body's weight. Variations depend on such factors as the person's age, lean body mass, and sex. Table 46-1 illustrates age-related changes in total body water and in the various water compartments of the body. An infant has considerably more body fluid and ECF than an adult. Because ECF is more easily lost from the body than ICF, infants are more prone to fluid volume deficits (FVDs).

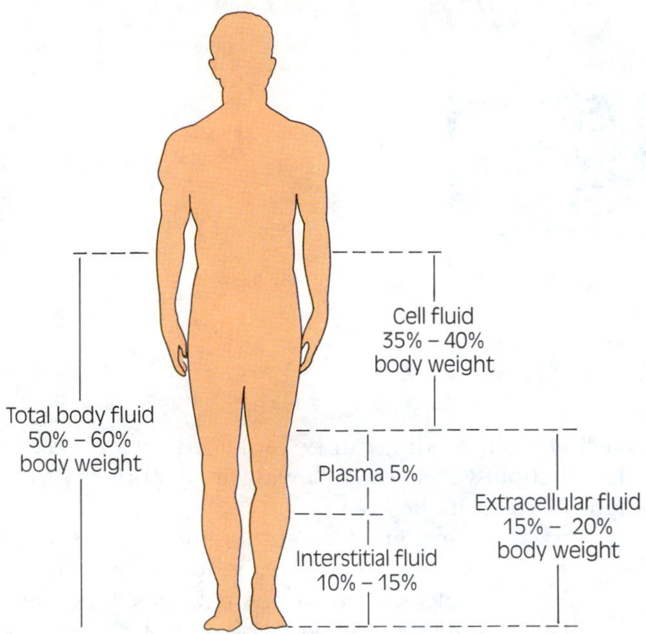

Figure 46-1
Total body fluid represents 50% to 60% of body weight of a normal adult.

Total body water also differs by gender and amount of fat cells. Because fat cells contain little water whereas lean tissue is rich in water, the more obese the person, the smaller the percentage of total body water when compared with body weight. Because females tend to have proportionally more body fat than males, they also have less body fluid than males. Similarly, the decreasing percentage of body fluid in older people is related to an increase in fat cells.

Electrolytes

Certain compounds dissociate in solution or separate into simpler molecules to form ions. An **ion** is an atom or molecule carrying an electric charge. Substances capable of breaking into electrically charged ions when dissolved in a solution are called **electrolytes**. Some ions develop a positive charge and are called **cations**. Others develop a negative charge and are called **anions**.

If molecules in the body's chemical compounds remain intact, they are called nonelectrolytes. In the human body, urea and glucose are nonelectrolytes. **Solvents** are liquids that hold a substance in solution; **solutes** are substances that are dissolved in a solution. Water is the solvent in the body that makes up solutions with solutes. The solutes are electrolytes and nonelectrolytes.

Fluids in various compartments of the body differ from one another in terms of their constituents. For example, ICF has higher concentrations of certain electrolytes than ECF. Figure 46-3 illustrates differences in the electrolyte composition of body fluids according to the compartments in which the fluids are found.

Measurement of Electrolytes

The unit of measure used to describe electrolytes is expressed in terms of their chemical combining power, or chemical activity. The milliequivalent (mEq) is used in the United States as the unit of measure to describe the chemical activity of an electrolyte. One milliequivalent is

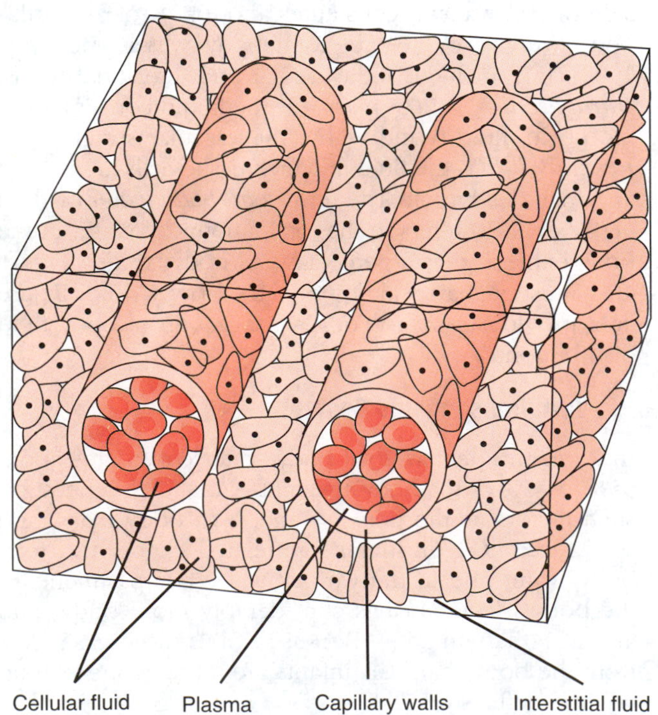

Figure 46-2
Microscopic visualization of body fluid distribution.

Table 46-1
Average Percentages of Water in Relation to Body Weight in People of Different Ages in the Various Water Compartments of the Body

Water Compartment	Infant (%)	Adult (%) Man	Adult (%) Woman	Elderly Person (%)
Extracellular				
Intravascular	4	4	5	5
Interstitial	25	11	10	15
Intracellular	48	45	35	25
Total body water	77	60	50	45

chemically equivalent to the activity of 1 mg of hydrogen. This is true whether the comparison with hydrogen is made with a cation or an anion. Hence, 1 mEq of any cation is equivalent to 1 mEq of any anion.

Using the mEq system, the total cations in the body are normally equal to the total anions. In healthy people, the milliequivalents per liter for electrolytes in the body vary within a relatively narrow range. When electrolytes are not in normal balance, the person is in a state of risk for alterations in health.

Regulation of Electrolytes

Electrolytes regulate water distribution, regulate acid–base balance, and maintain a balanced degree of neuromuscular excitability (Porth, 1994). There are many different kinds of electrolytes in the body. This section summarizes information about the most prevalent ones. Electrolyte disturbances are discussed later in the chapter.

Sodium (Na^+). Sodium is the chief electrolyte of ECF. It moves easily between intravascular and interstitial spaces and moves across cell membranes by active transport. Many chemical reactions in the body are influenced by sodium, particularly in nervous tissue cells and muscle tissue cells.

Functions

- Controls and regulates the volume of body fluids
  - Maintains water balance throughout the body
  - Is the primary regulator of ECF volume
  - Influences intracellular fluid volume
- Participates in the generation and transmission of nerve impulses
- Is an essential electrolyte in the sodium–potassium pump

Sources and Losses

- Average daily requirements for sodium are not known precisely, but in North America, the average adult intake is estimated to be between 6 and 15 g, and the RDA for sodium for adults is approximately 500 mg or 0.5 g (Dudek, 1993).
- Sodium is found in many foods, particularly bacon, ham, sausage, catsup, mustard, relish, processed cheese, canned vegetables, bread, cereal, and salted snack food. It is found in table salt (sodium chloride), which is about 46% sodium. For example, 3 slices of bacon provide approximately 300 mg of sodium, 1 tbsp of catsup equals 150 mg of sodium, and 1 oz of processed cheese supplies 400 mg of sodium.
- Sodium excesses are eliminated primarily by the kidneys; small amounts are lost in feces and perspiration.

Regulation

- Sodium normally is maintained in the body within a relatively narrow range, and deviations quickly result in a serious health problem.
- Salt intake regulates sodium concentrations.
- Sodium is conserved through reabsorption in the kidneys, a process stimulated by aldosterone.

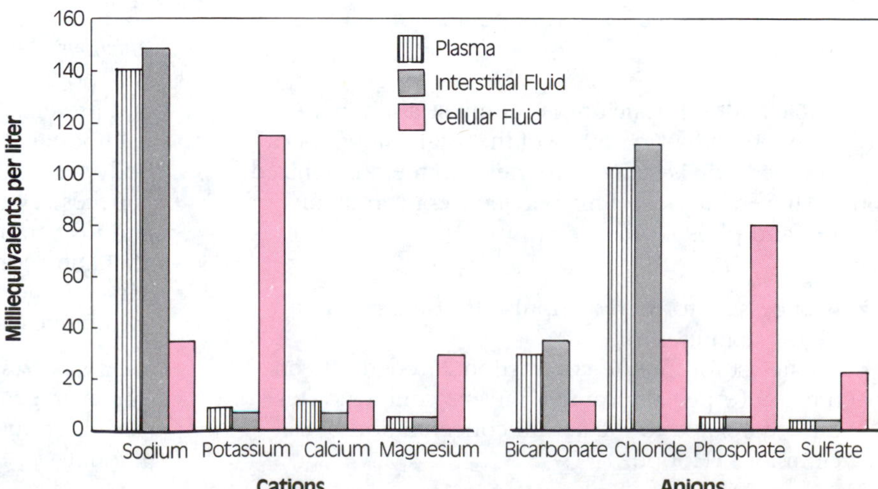

Figure 46-3
Total body fluid represents 50% to 60% of body weight of a normal adult.

- The normal extracellular concentration of sodium is 135 to 145 mEq/L (mmol/L).

Potassium (K^+). Potassium is the major cation of ICF. Potassium and sodium work reciprocally. For example, an excessive intake of sodium results in an excretion of potassium, and vice versa.

Functions

- Is the chief regulator of cellular enzyme activity and cellular water content
- Plays a vital role in such processes as the transmission of electric impulses, particularly in nerve, heart, skeletal, intestinal, and lung tissue; protein and carbohydrate metabolism; and cellular building
- Assists in regulation of acid–base balance by cellular exchange with H^+

Sources/Losses

- Average daily requirements for potassium are not known precisely, but an intake of 50 to 100 mEq daily maintains K^+ balance.
- A well-balanced diet contains adequate quantities of potassium. Leading food sources include bananas, peaches, kiwi, figs, dates, apricots, oranges, prunes, melons, raisins, broccoli, and potatoes. Meat and dairy products also provide adequate amounts of potassium.
- Potassium is excreted primarily by the kidneys. The kidneys have no effective method of conserving potassium. Therefore, deficits develop readily if excreted in excess without being replaced simultaneously.
- Gastrointestinal (GI) secretions contain potassium in large quantities. Some is also found in perspiration and saliva.

Regulation

- Cellular K^+ is conserved by the sodium pump (described later in the chapter) when Na^+ is excluded.
- The kidneys conserve K^+ when cellular K^+ is decreased.
- Aldosterone secretion triggers K^+ excretion in urine.
- The normal range for serum potassium is 3.5 to 5 mEq/L.

Calcium (Ca^{++}). Calcium is the most abundant electrolyte in the body. Up to 99% of the total amount of calcium in the body is found in bones and teeth in ionized form. There is a close link between concentrations of calcium and phosphorus.

Functions

- Is necessary for nerve impulse transmission and blood clotting
- Is catalyst for muscle contraction. Strength of contraction (especially cardiac muscle contraction) is directly related to the serum concentration of calcium ions (Hoppe, 1995)
- Is needed for vitamin B_{12} absorption and for its use by body cells
- Acts as a catalyst for many cell chemical activities
- Is necessary for strong bones and teeth
- Establishes thickness and strength of cell membranes

Sources/Losses

- The average daily requirement for calcium is about 1 g for adults. Higher amounts are required, according to body weight, for children, for pregnant and lactating women, and postmenopausal women.
- It is found in milk, cheese, and dried beans. Some calcium is present in meats and vegetables.
- Use of calcium is stimulated by vitamin D. The most active form of vitamin D (calcitriol) promotes calcium absorption and limits calcium excretion when levels are inadequate.
- It leaves bones and teeth to maintain normal blood calcium levels, if necessary.
- It is excreted in urine, feces, bile, digestive secretions, and perspiration.

Regulation

- When ECF calcium levels decrease, the parathyroid glands increase the secretion of parathyroid hormone (PTH), which acts on bones to increase the release of calcium into the blood, and acts on the kidney tubules and the intestinal mucosa to increase the reabsorption of calcium from the kidneys and the intestine.
- A high serum phosphate concentration increases serum calcium; a low serum phosphate concentration decreases serum calcium.
- Calcitonin, a hormone secreted by the thyroid gland, has an opposite effect on calcium than PTH. Increases in calcitonin reduce serum calcium concentration primarily by opposing osteoclast bone resorption.

Magnesium (Mg^{2+}). Most of the cation magnesium is found within body cells. It is present in heart, bone, nerve, and muscle tissues. Magnesium is the second most important cation of ICF.

Functions

- Is important for the metabolism of carbohydrates and proteins
- Is important for many vital reactions related to the body's enzymes
- Is necessary for protein and DNA synthesis, DNA and RNA transcription, and translation of RNA
- Maintains normal intracellular levels of potassium
- Serves to help maintain electric activity in nervous membranes and muscle membranes

Sources and Losses

- The average daily adult requirement for magnesium is about 18 to 30 mEq; children require larger amounts.

- Magnesium is found in most foods but especially in vegetables, nuts, fish, whole grains, peas, and beans.

Regulation

- Magnesium is absorbed by the intestines and excreted by the kidneys.
- Plasma concentrations of magnesium range from 1.3 to 2.1 mEq/L with about one-third of that amount bound to plasma proteins.

Chloride (Cl^-). Chloride, the chief extracellular anion, is found in blood, interstitial fluid, and lymph, and in minute amounts in ICF.

Functions

- Acts with sodium to maintain the osmotic pressure of the blood
- Plays a role in the body's acid–base balance
- Is important in buffering action when oxygen and carbon dioxide exchange in red blood cells (RBCs)
- Is essential for the production of hydrochloric acid in gastric juices

Sources/Losses

- Average daily requirements of chloride are unknown.
- It is found in foods high in sodium, in dairy products, and meat.

Regulation

- It is normally paired with sodium, and excreted and conserved with sodium by the kidneys.
- Chloride deficits lead to potassium deficits, and vice versa.
- Normal serum chloride levels range from 95 to 105 mEq/L (mmol/L).

Bicarbonate (HCO_3^-). The bicarbonate molecule is an anion. It is the major chemical base buffer within the body and is found in both ECF and ICF.

Function

- Is essential for acid–base balance; bicarbonate and carbonic acid constitute the body's primary buffer system

Regulation

- Bicarbonate levels are regulated primarily by the kidneys.
- Bicarbonate is readily available as a result of carbon dioxide formation during metabolism.
- Normal bicarbonate levels range between 25 and 29 mEq/L (mmol/L).

Phosphate (PO_4^-). The phosphate ion is the major anion in body cells. It is a buffer anion in both ICF and ECF.

Functions

- Helps maintain acid–base balance
- Is involved in important chemical reactions in the body; for example, phosphorus is necessary for many B vitamins to be effective, helps promote nerve and muscle action, and plays a role in carbohydrate metabolism
- Is important for cell division and for the transmission of hereditary traits

Sources/Losses

- Average daily requirements for phosphorus are similar to those for calcium.
- It is found in most foods but especially in beef, pork, and dried peas and beans.
- It is metabolized in the same manner as calcium.

Regulation

- Phosphate is regulated by PTH and by activated vitamin D.
- Calcium and phosphate are inversely proportional; an increase in one results in a decrease in the other.
- The normal range of phosphate is 2.5 to 4.5 mEq/L (mmol/L).

Additional Electrolytes. The anion sulfate is found primarily within cells and is associated with cellular protein. Excesses are excreted by the kidneys. The organic acid anions are normally intermediary in cell metabolism. A major one in the body is lactic acid. The protein anion functions in the process of diffusion to move substances to and from the capillaries. Plasma proteins include albumin, globulin, and fibrinogen.

Other electrolytes are required for proper cell functioning, but they are found only in traces in the body. One example is chromium. A well-balanced diet ordinarily ensures an adequate supply of trace substances in the body.

Fluid and Electrolyte Movement

ECF takes nourishment to each body cell and receives each cell's waste products. These exchanges, which normally result in fluid balance and homeostasis, are essential to life. The most common routes for transporting materials to and from intracellular compartments are osmosis, diffusion, active transport, and filtration.

Osmosis

The membranes of the body's cells are semipermeable. This makes it possible for water, a pure solvent, to be transported through cell walls. **Osmosis** is the major method of transporting body fluids. Water shifts and, hence, fluid balance depend heavily on this mode of transport.

Through the process of osmosis, the solvent water passes from an area of lesser solute concentration to an area of greater solute concentration until equilibrium is established. As a result, the volume of more concentrated solution increases, and the volume of the weaker solution decreases. The greater the difference in the concentration of the two solutions on each side of a semipermeable membrane, the greater the osmotic pressure.

The concentration of particles in a solution, or its pulling power, is referred to as the **osmolarity** of a solution. A solution that has about the same concentration of particles, or osmolarity, as plasma (between 275 and 295 mOsm/L) is considered an *isotonic* solution. An isotonic fluid remains in the intravascular compartment without any net flow across the semipermeable membrane. In contrast, a *hypertonic* solution has a greater osmolarity than plasma (>295 mOsm/L), while a *hypotonic* solution has less osmolarity than plasma (<275 mOsm/L). Because a hypertonic solution has more concentration of particles in solution, water moves out of the cells and into the intravascular compartment toward the hypertonic fluid, causing the cells to shrink. A hypotonic solution, with a lower osmolarity, moves out of the intravascular space into intracellular fluid, causing the cell to swell and possibly burst (Vonfrolio, 1995). Figure 46-4 illustrates the process of osmosis.

Diffusion. Diffusion is the tendency of solutes to move freely throughout a solvent. The solute moves from an area of higher concentration to an area of lower concentration (ie, "downhill") until equilibrium is established. Gases move about by diffusion. Oxygen and carbon dioxide exchange in the lung's alveoli and capillaries occurs by diffusion.

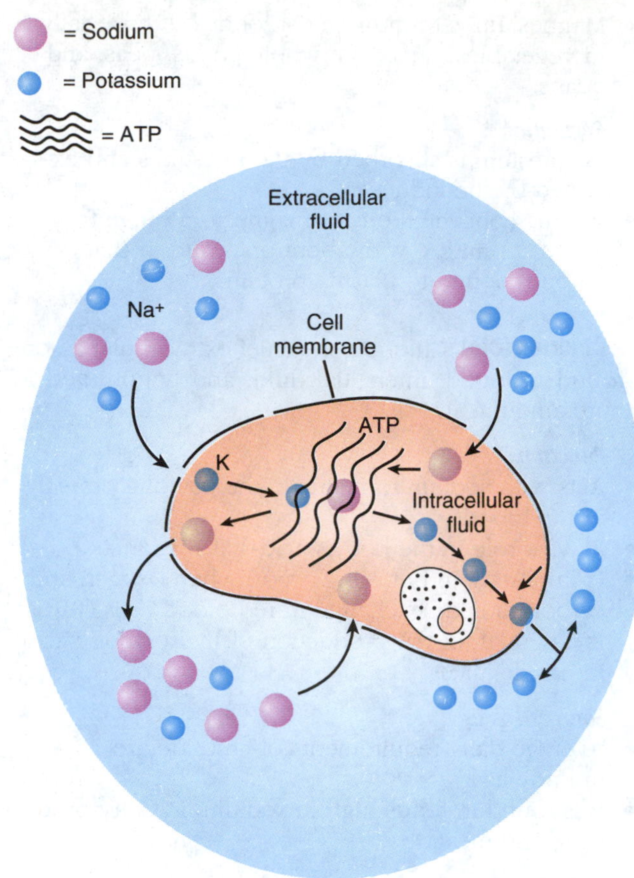

Figure 46-5
Active transport. Sodium that diffuses into the cell through a pore in the cell membrane is actively pumped out of the cell by a carrier system (*wavy lines*). Similarly, potassium that diffuses out of the cell is actively replaced by the carrier system.

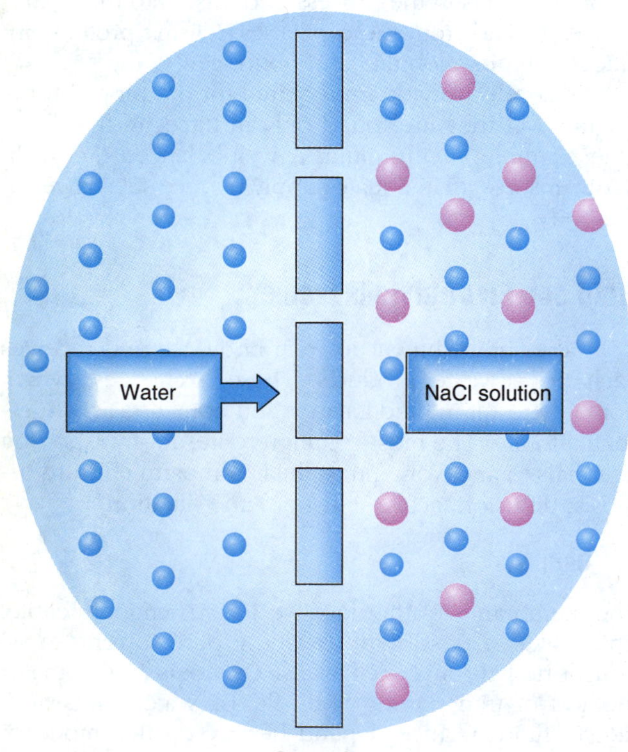

Figure 46-4
Through the process of osmosis, body fluids are transported through cell membranes. The solvent water moves from an area of lesser solute concentration to one of greater solute concentration until equilibrium is established.

Active Transport. Active transport is a process that requires energy for the movement of substances through a cell membrane from an area of lesser concentration to an area of higher concentration. Adenosine triphosphate (ATP), released from a cell, makes it possible for certain substances to acquire energy needed to pass through a cell membrane. Although the process is not entirely understood, the energy requirements are affected by characteristics of the cell membrane, specific enzymes, and concentrations of ions. This process explains the so-called pump mechanism and is illustrated in Figure 46-5 using sodium and potassium as examples. If diffusion can be called "coasting downhill," active transport can be called "pumping uphill." Substances believed to use active transport are amino acids; glucose (but in certain places only, such as in the kidneys and intestines); and ions of sodium, chloride, potassium, hydrogen, phosphate, calcium, and magnesium.

Filtration. Filtration is the passage of a fluid through a permeable membrane. Passage is from an area of high pressure to one of lower pressure.

Certain substances, such as plasma proteins, which have high molecular weights, exert **colloid osmotic pressure**, or **oncotic pressure** on permeable membranes in the body. **Hydrostatic pressure** is force exerted by a fluid against the container wall. Blood hydrostatic pressure is the pressure of plasma and blood cells in the capillaries: it depends primarily on arterial blood pressure on the arteriolar side of capillaries, and on venous blood pressure on the venular side of capillaries. *Filtration pressure* is the difference between colloid osmotic pressure and blood hydrostatic pressure.

These pressures are important in understanding how fluid leaves arterioles, enters the interstitial compartment, and eventually returns to the venules. The filtration pressure is positive in the arterioles, helping to force or filter fluids into interstitial spaces; it is negative in the venules and so helps fluid enter at the venules. This is illustrated in Figure 46-6. Filtration is also involved in the proper functioning of the glomeruli of the kidneys.

Fluid Balance

The desirable amount of fluid intake and loss in adults ranges from 1500 to 3500 mL each 24 hours, with most people averaging 2500 mL per day. Although these figures are helpful guidelines, a person's balance between actual intake and loss must be considered when assessing nursing needs. A person's intake should normally be approximately balanced by output or fluid loss. A general rule is that in the healthy adult, the output of urine normally approximates the ingestion of liquids; and the water from food and oxidation is balanced by the water loss through the feces, the skin, and the respiratory process. The intake–output balance may not always exist in a single 24-hour period but should normally be achieved within 2 to 3 days.

Fluid Sources

Water for the body is derived from several sources, including ingested liquids, food, and metabolism.

Ingested Liquids. This source makes up the largest amount of water normally taken into the body. Fluid intake is primarily regulated by the thirst mechanism. Located within the hypothalamus, the thirst control center is stimulated by intracellular dehydration and decreased blood volume.

Water in Food. This is the second largest source of water for the body. The amount ingested depends on dietary items. For example, melons and citrus fruit are high in water content, whereas cereal and dried fruits have a relatively low water content.

Water from Metabolic Oxidation. Water is an end product of the oxidation that occurs during the metabolism of food substances. This source also varies with dif-

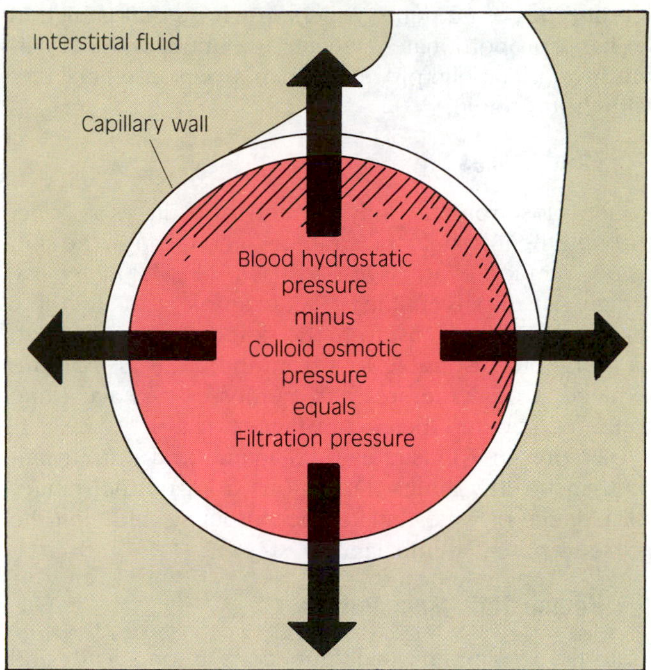

Arteriole: The pressure within the arteriole is **positive** and hence, fluid is forced into interstitial fluid.

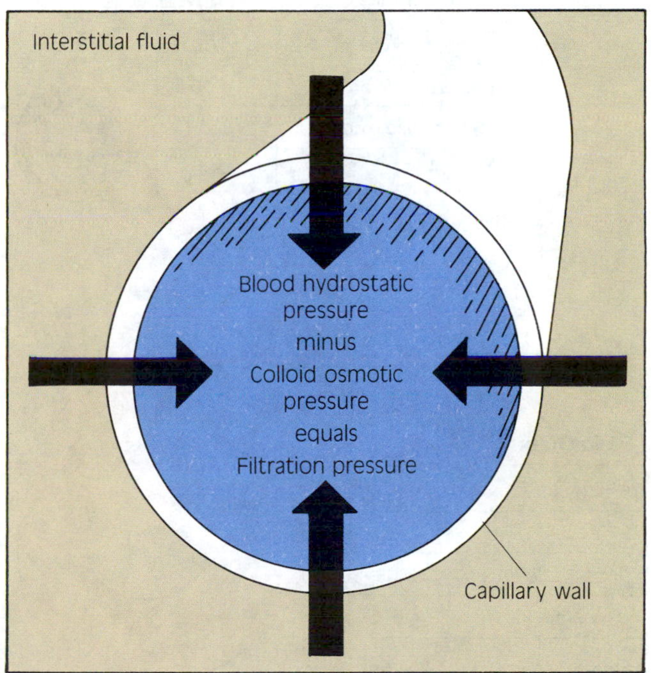

Venule: The pressure within the venule is **negative** and hence, fluid is forced into the venule.

Figure 46-6
Filtration, which is the tendency of solutes to move from an area of higher pressure to an area of lower pressure. (*Top*) *Arteriole:* The pressure within the arteriole is positive and, hence, fluid is forced into interstitial fluid. (*Bottom*) *Venule:* The pressure within the venules is negative and, hence, fluid is forced into the venule.

ferent types of nutrients. A person whose diet is high in fat has a proportionately greater amount of water resulting from metabolic processes than a person whose diet is high in protein.

Fluid Losses

Water is lost from the body through the kidneys as urine, through the intestinal tract in feces, and through the skin as perspiration. Water is also lost as *insensible water loss*, which is unperceptible. For example, an invisible amount of water is lost from the skin constantly through evaporation. Insensible loss from the lungs is moisture exhaled through the breath. Water losses vary according to the person and the circumstances.

Figure 46-7 illustrates fluid intake and output balance in healthy adults. Deviations from normal ranges for balance of water intake and output should alert the nurse to potential imbalances.

Homeostatic Mechanisms

Fluid homeostasis normally functions automatically and effectively. Almost every organ and system in the body helps in some way to maintain fluid homeostasis. The following are the primary organs of homeostasis. Functions are highlighted in Table 46-2. Fluid balance is threatened when any organ fails to function properly.

Kidneys. The kidneys are frequently referred to as the master chemists of the body. They normally filter 170 L of plasma daily in the adult while excreting only 1.5 L of urine. They selectively retain electrolytes and water and excrete wastes and excesses. Renal failure results in serious fluid and electrolyte problems.

Cardiovascular System. The cardiovascular system is responsible for pumping and carrying nutrients and water throughout the body.

Lungs. The lungs regulate oxygen and carbon dioxide levels of the blood. The regulation of the carbon dioxide level is especially crucial in maintaining acid–base balance, and is explained later in this chapter.

Adrenal Glands. The adrenal glands secrete aldosterone, a hormone that conserves sodium. The hormone also helps save chloride and water, and causes potassium to be excreted.

Thyroid Gland. Thyroxine, released by the thyroid gland, increases blood flow in the body. This in turn increases renal circulation, which results in increased glomerular filtration and urinary output.

Parathyroid Glands. The parathyroid glands secrete parathyroid hormone, which regulates the level of calcium in ECF.

Gastrointestinal Tract. The GI tract absorbs water and nutrients that enter the body through this route.

Nervous System. The nervous system acts as a switchboard and inhibits and stimulates mechanisms that influence fluid balance. It functions chiefly as the regulator of sodium and water intake and excretion. The thirst center is located in the hypothalamus. The posterior lobe of the pituitary gland stores ADH, a hormone manufactured in the hypothalamus. Neurons called *osmoreceptors* are sensitive to changes in the concentration of ECF and send appropriate impulses to the pituitary to release ADH or inhibit its release.

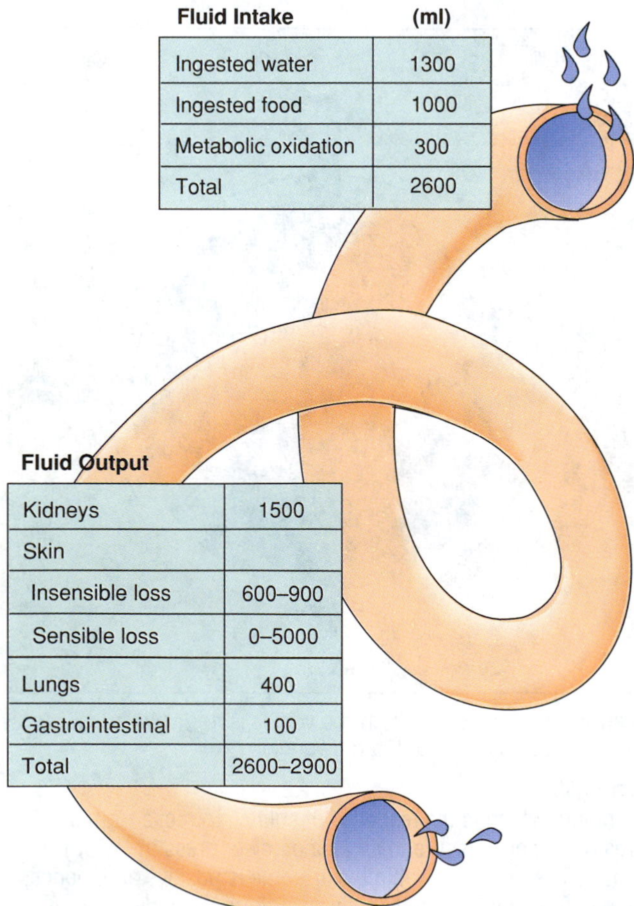

Fluid Intake	(ml)
Ingested water	1300
Ingested food	1000
Metabolic oxidation	300
Total	2600

Fluid Output	
Kidneys	1500
Skin	
Insensible loss	600–900
Sensible loss	0–5000
Lungs	400
Gastrointestinal	100
Total	2600–2900

Figure 46-7
In health, fluid intake and fluid losses are about equal. The amounts indicated are average adult daily fluid sources and losses.

Acid–Base Balance

Body fluids must maintain a normal acid–base balance to sustain health and life. Acidity or alkalinity of a solution is determined by its concentration of hydrogen ions (H^-). An **acid** is a substance containing hydrogen ions that can be liberated or released. An *alkali,* or **base**, is a substance that can accept or trap hydrogen ions. The following equations illustrate:

Table 46-2
Homeostatic Mechanisms That Maintain the Composition and Volume of Body Fluid Within Narrow Limits of Normal

Organs of Homeostasis	Functions
Kidneys	• Regulate extracellular fluid (ECF) volume and osmolality by selective retention and excretion of body fluids • Regulate electrolyte levels in the ECF by selective retention of needed substances and excretion of unneeded substances • Regulate pH of ECF by excretion or retention of hydrogen ions • Excrete metabolic wastes (primarily acids) and toxic substances
Heart and blood vessels	• Circulate blood through the kidneys under sufficient pressure for urine to form (pumping action of the heart) • React to hypovolemia by stimulating fluid retention (stretch receptors in the atria and blood vessels)
Lungs	• Eliminate about 13,000 mEq of hydrogen ions (H^+) daily, as opposed to only 40 to 80 mEq excreted daily by the kidneys • Act promptly to correct metabolic acid-base disturbances; regulate H^+ concentration (pH) by controlling the level of carbon dioxide (CO_2) in the extracellular fluid as follows: 1. Metabolic alkalosis causes compensatory hypoventilation, resulting in CO_2 retention (increases acidity of the extracellular fluid). 2. Metabolic acidosis causes compensatory hyperventilation, resulting in CO_2 excretion (decreases acidity of the extracellular fluid). • Remove approximately 300 mL of water daily through exhalation (insensible water loss) in the normal adult
Adrenal glands	• Regulate blood volume and sodium and potassium balance by secreting aldosterone, a mineral corticoid secreted by the adrenal cortex 1. The primary regulator of aldosterone appears to be angiotensin II, which is produced by the renin–angiotensin system. A decrease in blood volume triggers this system and increases aldosterone secretion, which causes sodium retention (and thus water retention) and potassium loss. 2. Decreased secretion of aldosterone causes sodium and water loss and potassium retention. • Cortisol, another adrenocortical hormone, has only a fraction of the potency of aldosterone. • However, secretion of cortisol in large quantities can produce sodium and water retention and potassium deficit.
Pituitary gland	• Stores and releases the antidiuretic hormone (ADH), which makes the body retain water; functions of ADH include: 1. Maintains osmotic pressure of the cells by controlling renal water retention or excretion a. When osmotic pressure of the ECF is greater than that of the cells (as in hypernatremia—excess sodium—or hyperglycemia), ADH secretion is increased, causing renal retention of water. b. When osmotic pressure of the ECF is less than that of the cells (as in hyponatremia), ADH secretion is decreased, causing renal excretion of water. 2. Controls blood volume (less influential than aldosterone) a. When blood volume is decreased, an increased secretion of ADH results in water conservation. b. When blood volume is increased, a decreased secretion of ADH results in water loss.
Parathyroid glands	• Regulate calcium (Ca^{2+}) and phosphate (HPO_4^{2-}) balance by means of PTH; PTH influences bone reabsorption, calcium absorption from the intestines, and calcium reabsorption from the renal tubules. 1. Increased secretion of PTH causes: a. Elevated serum calcium concentration b. Lowered serum phosphate concentration 2. Conversely, decreased secretion of PTH causes: a. Lowered serum calcium concentration b. Elevated serum phosphate concentration

(Data from Metheny, N. M. [1992]. *Fluid and electrolyte balance* [2nd ed.]. Philadelphia: Lippincott.)

Equation: An acid releases hydrogen, as follows:

$$H_2CO_3 \rightarrow H^+ + HCO_3^-$$

Carbonic acid releases hydrogen ion to form bicarbonate base

Equation: A base traps hydrogen, as follows:

$$HCO_3^- + H^+ \rightarrow H_2CO_3$$

Bicarbonate base traps hydrogen ion to form carbonic acid

An acid that is strong dissociates (separates) completely in solution and releases all of its hydrogen ions while a weak acid releases only a small number of the hydrogen ions. A base that binds or accepts hydrogen ions easily is considered a strong base, while one that accepts hydrogen ions less readily is considered weak.

The unit of measure used to describe acid–base balance is **pH**, which is an expression of hydrogen ion concentration and the resulting acidity or alkalinity of a substance. The pH scale ranges from 1 to 14. A neutral solution measures 7; an example is pure water. Because pH is based on a negative logarithm, as the hydrogen ions increase and a solution becomes more acid, the pH becomes less than 7. When the concentration of hydrogen ions in a solution is reduced or accepted by another substance, the solution is alkaline and the pH is greater than 7. Gastric secretions that are strongly acidic have an approximate pH of 1 to 1.3, whereas strongly alkaline pancreatic secretions have an approximate pH of 10 (Metheny, 1992).

Normal blood plasma is slightly alkaline and has a normal pH range of 7.35 to 7.45. When the normal pH range is exceeded in either direction, the person develops signs and symptoms of illness, and if the condition goes on unabated, death results. **Acidosis** is the condition characterized by a proportionate excess of hydrogen ions in ECF in which the pH falls below 7.35. **Alkalosis** occurs when there is a proportionate lack of hydrogen ions and the pH exceeds 7.45. Figure 46-8 illustrates normal pH, acidosis, and alkalosis, and also the points at which death can be expected to occur.

The narrow range of normal pH is achieved by three major homeostatic regulators of hydrogen ions: (1) buffer systems, (2) respiratory mechanisms, and (3) renal mechanisms. A **buffer** is a substance that prevents body fluids from becoming overly acidic or alkaline. The body has three buffer systems: (1) the carbonic acid–sodium bicarbonate buffer system, (2) the phosphate buffer system, and (3) the protein buffer system.

Buffer Systems

Carbonic Acid–Sodium Bicarbonate Buffer System. The most important buffer system of the body is the carbonic acid–sodium bicarbonate system. This system buffers up to 90% of the H^- of ECF. Ignatavicius, Workman, & Mishler (1995) refer to buffers as hydrogen ion "sponges." They either act like a base and bind or soak up free hydrogen ions or act like an acid and release hydrogen ions when too few are present in a solution. Buffers attempt to bring a body fluid as close as possible to the pH of normal body fluid (7.35 to 7.45).

The ratio of carbonic acid (H_2CO_3), the most common acid in human body fluid, to the body's most common base, bicarbonate (HCO_3^-), is important for acid–base balance. Normal ECF has a ratio of 20 parts bicarbonate to 1 part carbonic acid. The exact quantities are unimportant for acid–base balance as long as they remain in a 20:1 ratio. Carbonic acid and bicarbonate must be carefully controlled to maintain this ratio; if either is increased or decreased, the 20:1 ratio is no longer in effect.

Phosphate Buffer System. This chemical buffer system is active in intracellular fluids and converts alkaline sodium phosphate (Na_2HPO_4), a weak base, to acid sodium phosphate (NaH_2PO_4) in the kidneys.

Protein Buffer System. The third buffer system is a mixture of plasma proteins and the globin portion of hemoglobin in RBCs. Because plasma proteins and hemoglobin possess groups that can combine with or liberate hydrogen ions, they tend to minimize changes in pH and serve as excellent buffering agents over a wide range of pH values. For example, excess hydrogen ions in the blood cross over the plasma membrane of RBCs and bind to the hemoglobin molecules that are plentiful in each RBC.

Respiratory Control of H^- Balance

The lungs are the primary controller of the body's carbonic acid supply. They have a huge surface area from which CO_2 can readily diffuse and they can bring about rapid changes in H^- when needed. Carbon dioxide is constantly produced by cellular metabolism (carbonic acid [H_2CO_3] yields CO_2 and H_2O) and is excreted by exhalation. When the amount of CO_2 in the blood in-

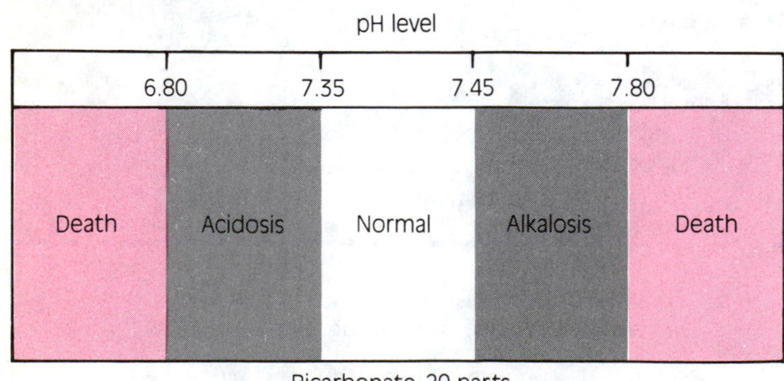

Figure 46-8
Acid–base balance. Note that *acidosis* is used to describe the condition when pH is between 6.80 and 7.35. When the fluid acidity falls below 7, the person is gravely ill or dying.

creases, the sensitive respiratory center in the medulla is stimulated and increases the rate and depth of respirations to eliminate more CO_2. As more CO_2 is exhaled, the H_2CO_3 level in the blood decreases and the pH of the blood becomes more alkaline. When the blood level of CO_2 decreases, the respiratory center decreases the rate and depth of respirations to retain the CO_2 so that carbonic acid can be formed and the delicate balance maintained. This total respiratory process occurs almost as rapidly as the buffering action in the carbonic acid–sodium bicarbonate system.

Renal Control of H^- Balance

The concentration of bicarbonate in the plasma is regulated by the kidneys. Essentially, the kidneys excrete or retain hydrogen ions and form or excrete bicarbonate ions in response to the pH of the blood. In the presence of acidosis, the kidneys excrete hydrogen ions and form and conserve bicarbonate ions, thus raising the pH to the normal range. If alkalosis is present, the kidneys retain hydrogen ions and excrete bicarbonate ions in an effort to return to a balanced state.

Acid–base regulation by the kidneys occurs more slowly than by the carbonic acid–sodium bicarbonate system or by respiratory regulation. It may take up to 3 days for fluid pH to be restored by the kidneys. The pH of urine varies, depending on the ions that are being excreted, but generally it is in the 4.5 to 8.2 range.

Disturbances in Fluid, Electrolyte, and Acid–Base Balance

Nurses commonly encounter disturbances in fluid, electrolyte, and acid–base balance while caring for acutely or chronically ill clients. Although many of these disturbances are interrelated and may occur together, they are presented singly for the purpose of study.

Fluid Imbalances

Fluid imbalances occur when the body's compensatory mechanisms are unable to maintain a homeostatic state. Fluid imbalances may relate to either volume or distribution of water or electrolytes.

Fluid Volume Deficit. *Fluid volume deficit* (FVD) can be caused by a deficiency in the amount of both water and electrolytes in ECF, but the water and electrolyte proportions remain near normal. The state is commonly known as *hypovolemia.* Both osmotic and hydrostatic pressure changes force the interstitial fluid into the intravascular space. As the interstitial space is depleted, its fluid becomes hypertonic, and cellular fluid is then drawn into the interstitial space, leaving cells without adequate fluid to function properly.

Dehydration is sometimes used as a synonym for hypovolemia, but this is technically inaccurate. *Dehydration* refers only to a decreased volume of water, but water is not decreased without electrolyte changes also. *Hydration* is the union of a substance with water and is often used to indicate that there is normal water volume in the body.

FVDs result from the loss of body fluids, especially if fluid intake is simultaneously decreased. Table 46-3 summarizes FVD, common problems, and general nursing interventions. Specific interventions are presented later in this chapter.

The very young, older persons, and people who are ill are especially at risk for hypovolemia. A weight loss of 5% for adults and 10% for infants can occur rapidly. A 5% weight loss is considered to be pronounced fluid deficit, and an 8% loss or more is considered severe. A 15% weight loss owing to fluid deficiency usually threatens life.

Third-space fluid shift refers to a distributional shift of body fluids into potential body spaces such as the pleural, peritoneal, pericardial, or joint cavities; the bowel; or the interstitial space (plasma-to-interstitial shift). Once trapped in these spaces, the fluid is not easily exchanged with ECF. With third-space fluid shift, there is a deficit in ECF volume. The fluid has not been lost but is trapped in another body space for a period of time and essentially unavailable for use. A third-space shift may occur as a result of a severe burn, a bowel obstruction, or pancreatitis. Decreased body weight does not occur as with an ECF volume deficit (vomiting or diarrhea), nor can the fluid loss be measured (Bove, 1994; Metheny, 1992). Treatment is directed toward correction of the cause of the third-space shift, or third-spacing, as it is also commonly called.

Fluid Volume Excess. Excessive retention of water and sodium in ECF in near-normal proportions results in a condition termed *fluid volume excess.* It is also called *hypervolemia.* Overhydration is commonly used as a synonym for hypervolemia, but strictly speaking, this is inaccurate. *Overhydration* refers only to above-normal amounts of water in extracellular spaces. Malfunction of the kidneys, causing an inability to excrete the excesses, and failure of the heart to function as a pump, resulting in accumulation of fluid in the lungs and dependent parts of the body, are common causes. When water is retained in excessive amounts, so is sodium.

Because of the increased extracellular osmotic pressure from the retained sodium, fluid is pulled from the cells to equalize the tonicity. By the time the intracellular and extracellular spaces are isotonic to each other, an excess of both water and sodium are in ECF, while the cells are nearly depleted. The excessive ECF may accumulate in tissue spaces; this is known as *edema.* Edema can be observed around the eyes, fingers, ankles, and sacral space (Fig. 46-9) and also accumulate in or around body organs. It may result in a weight gain in excess of 5%. When the excess fluid remains in the intravascular space, the concentration of solids in the blood is decreased.

Table 46-3
Fluid Volume Disturbances: Related Factors, Defining Characteristics, and Nursing Interventions

Related Factors	Defining Characteristics	Nursing Interventions
Summary of Fluid Volume Deficit		
Loss of water and electrolytes, as in • Vomiting • Diarrhea • Excessive laxative use • Fistulas • GI suction • Polyuria • Fever • Excessive sweating • Third-space fluid shifts Decreased intake, as in: • Anorexia • Nausea • Inability to gain access to fluids • Inability to swallow fluids • Depression	Weight loss over short period (except in third-space losses) Decreased skin and tongue turgor Dry mucous membranes Urine output less than 30 mL/hr in adult Postural hypotension (systolic pressure drops by more than 15 mm Hg when client moves from lying to standing or sitting position) Weak, rapid pulse Slow-filling peripheral veins Decreased body temperature, such as 95° to 98°F (35° to 36.7°C) unless infection is present CVP less than 4 cm H_2O BUN elevated out of proportion to serum creatinine Specific gravity (SG) high (urine) Hematocrit elevated Flat neck veins in supine position Marked oliguria, late Altered sensorium	1. Assess for presence or worsening of FVD (see defining characteristics). 2. Administer oral fluids if indicated. • Consider the client's likes and dislikes when offering fluids. • If the client is reluctant to drink because of oral discomfort, select fluids that are nonirritating to the mucosa, and provide frequent mouth care (offer saline gargles and apply lubricant to lips). • Offer fluids at frequent intervals. • Explain the need for fluid replacement to the client. • Administer prn medications if nausea is present to provide relief before fluids are offered. 3. Consider the following interventions for clients with impaired swallowing: • Assess gag reflex and ability to swallow water before offering solid foods; have a suction apparatus on hand. • Position the client in an upright position with head and neck flexed slightly forward during feeding (tilting the head backward during swallowing predisposes to aspiration because this position opens the airway). • Provide thick fluids or semisolid foods (such as puddings or gelatin). These are more easily swallowed because of their consistency and weight than are thin liquids. 4. If the client is unable to eat and drink, discuss possibility of tube feedings or TPN with the physician. 5. Monitor response to fluid intake, either orally or parenterally. 6. Monitor clients with tendency for abnormal fluid retention (such as renal or cardiac problems) for signs of overload during aggressive fluid replacement. 7. Turn client frequently; apply moisturizing agents to skin.

Table 46-3 *(continued)*
Fluid Volume Disturbances: Related Factors, Defining Characteristics, and Nursing Interventions

Related Factors	Defining Characteristics	Nursing Interventions
Summary of Fluid Volume Excess		
Compromised regulatory mechanisms: • Renal failure • Congestive heart failure • Cirrhosis of liver • Cushing's syndrome Overzealous administration of sodium-containing IV fluids Excessive ingestion of sodium-containing substances in diet or sodium-containing medications	Weight gain over short period Peripheral edema (excess of fluid in interstitial space) Distended neck veins Distended peripheral veins Slow-emptying peripheral veins CVP over 11 cm H_2O Crackles and wheezes in lungs Polyuria (if renal function is normal) Ascites, pleural effusion (when FVE is severe, fluid transudates into body cavities) Decreased BUN (Due to plasma dilution) Decreased hematocrit (also due to plasma dilution) Bounding, full pulse Pulmonary edema, if severe	1. Assess for the presence or worsening of fluid volume excess (FVE). 2. Encourage adherence to sodium-restricted diet, if prescribed. 3. Teach clients requiring sodium restriction to avoid over-the-counter drugs without first checking with the healthcare adviser. 4. When fluid retention persists despite adherence to dietary sodium intake, consider hidden sources of sodium, such as water supply or use of water softeners. 5. When indicated, encourage rest periods. Lying down favors diuresis of edema fluid. 6. Monitor the client's response to diuretics. Discuss significant findings with physician. 7. Monitor rate of parenteral fluids and the client's response. Discuss significant findings with physician. 8. Teach self-monitoring of weight and intake and output measurements to clients with chronic fluid retention (such as those with congestive heart failure, renal disease, or cirrhosis of liver). 9. If dyspnea and orthopnea are present, position the client in semi-Fowler's position to facilitate lung expansion. 10. Turn and position the client frequently; be aware that edematous tissue is more prone to skin breakdown than is normal tissue.

(Data from Metheny, N. M. [1992]. *Fluid and electrolyte balance* [2nd ed.]. Philadelphia: Lippincott.)

Interstitial-to-plasma shift is the movement of fluid from the space surrounding the cells to the blood. This shift, also called hypervolemia, is a compensatory response to volume or osmotic-pressure changes of the intravascular fluid. Although the body attempts to maintain normal balance in all fluid spaces, the intravascular fluid is usually protected at the expense of interstitial fluid and ICF.

Table 46-3 summarizes fluid volume excesses, examples of common problems likely to produce them, and common nursing interventions. Specific nursing interventions for these problems are presented later in this chapter.

Electrolyte Imbalances

When clients present with deficits or excesses of sodium, potassium, calcium, magnesium, or phosphate, special nursing care is required. Table 46-4 highlights etiologic factors, defining characteristics, and nursing interventions for common electrolyte imbalances.

Hyponatremia and Hypernatremia. *Hyponatremia* refers to a sodium deficit in ECF caused by a loss of sodium or a gain of water. Osmotic pressure changes result in ECF moving into the cells. When this occurs, an examiner's fingerprints tend to remain on the client's

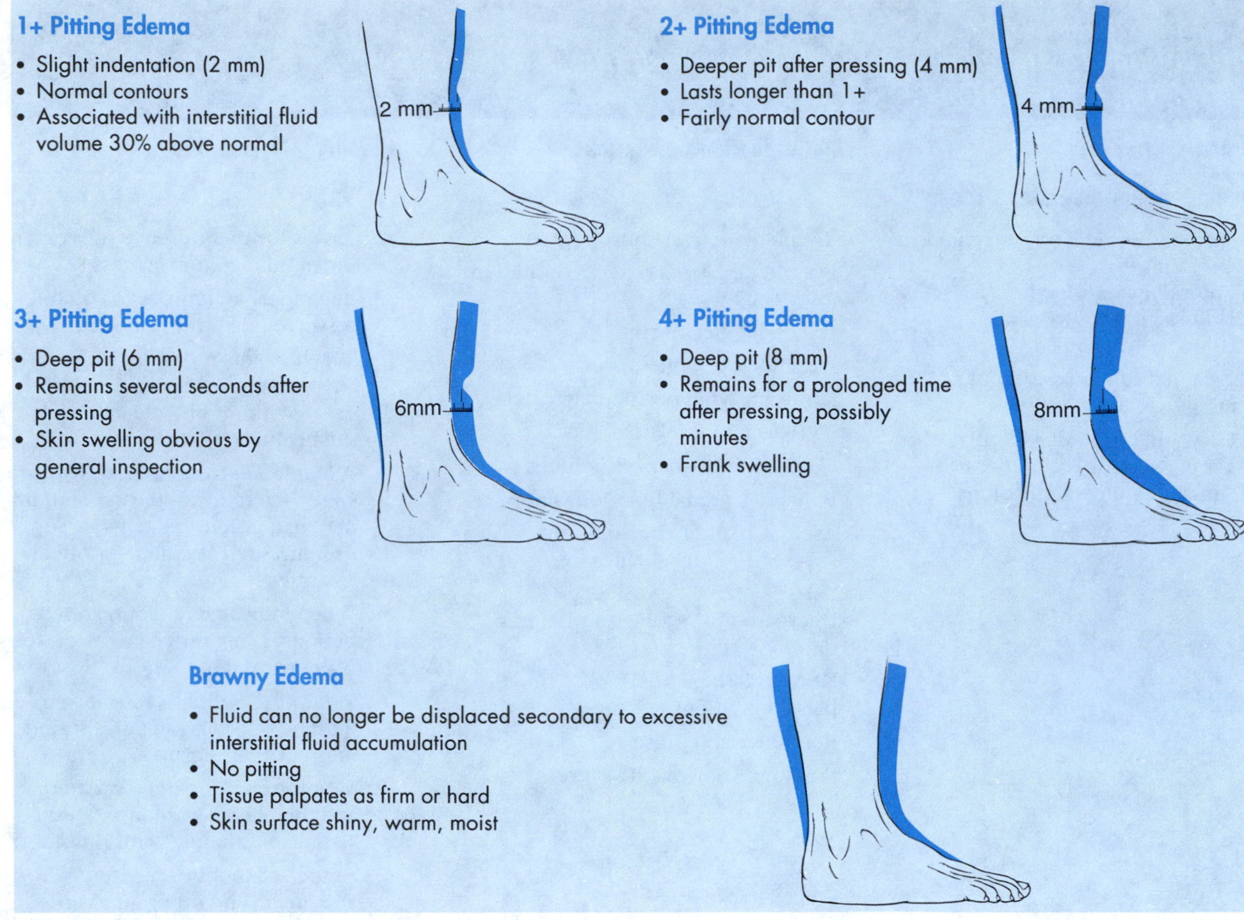

Figure 46-9
System for grading edema. (Fuller, J., & Schaller-Ayers, J. [1994]. *Health assessment: a nursing approach* [2nd ed.]. Philadelphia, Lippincott.)

skin over the sternum when pressure is applied with the fingers. The phenomenon results from tissue plasticity as fluid moves into cells in excess amounts. *Hypernatremia* refers to a surplus of sodium in ECF that can result from excess water loss or an overall excess of sodium. Because of the increased extracellular osmotic pressure, fluids move from the cells, leaving them without sufficient fluid.

Hypokalemia and Hyperkalemia. *Hypokalemia* refers to a potassium deficit in ECF. When the extracellular potassium level falls, potassium moves from the cell, creating an intracellular potassium deficiency. Sodium and hydrogen ions are then retained by the cells to maintain isotonic fluids. These electrolyte shifts influence normal cellular functioning, the pH of ECF, and the functions of most body systems. Skeletal muscles are generally the first to demonstrate a potassium deficiency. Typical signs of hypokalemia include muscle weakness and leg cramps. *Hyperkalemia* refers to an excess of potassium in ECF. Although this condition occurs less frequently than hypokalemia, it can be hazardous. The transmission of stimuli through heart muscle is slowed or prevented, and cardiac arrest eventually occurs if hyperkalemia is not corrected.

Hypocalcemia and Hypercalcemia. *Hypocalcemia* refers to a calcium deficit in ECF. If the condition is prolonged, calcium is taken from the bones. This results in *osteomalacia*, which is characterized by soft and pliable bones. Common signs of hypocalcemia include numbness and tingling of fingers, muscle cramps, and tetany. *Hypercalcemia* refers to an excess of calcium in ECF. Hypercalcemia presents an emergency situation because the condition often leads to cardiac arrest.

Hypomagnesemia and Hypermagnesemia. *Hypomagnesemia* refers to a magnesium deficit. The body's potassium level also drops because the kidneys tend to excrete more potassium when magnesium supplies are poor. As a result, hypomagnesemia and hypokalemia often occur together. According to Cerrato (1992), hypomagnesemia may be the most underdiagnosed electrolyte deficiency in hospital practice. *Hypermagnesemia* refers to a magnesium excess. It can occur especially in end-stage renal

(text continues on page 1386)

Table 46-4
Electrolyte Disturbances: Related Factors, Defining Characteristics, and Nursing Interventions

Related Factors	Defining Characteristics	Nursing Interventions
Hyponatremia		
Loss of sodium, as in: • Loss of GI fluids • Use of diuretics • Adrenal insufficiency Gains of water, as in: • Excessive administration of D_5W Disease states associated with SIADH (a form of hyponatremia) Pharmacologic agents that may impair renal water excretion	Anorexia Nausea and vomiting Lethargy Confusion Muscle cramps Fingerprinting over sternum Muscular twitching Seizures Coma Serum Na below 135 mEq/L	1. Identify clients at risk for hyponatremia. 2. Monitor fluid losses and gains. Look for loss of sodium-containing fluids, particularly in conjunction with low-sodium intake. 3. Monitor for presence of gastrointestinal symptoms, such as anorexia, nausea, vomiting, and abdominal cramping. 4. Monitor for central nervous system changes, such as lethargy, confusion, muscular twitching, and convulsions. 5. Monitor laboratory data for serum sodium levels less than normal. 6. Check specific gravity of urine. 7. With clients able to consume a general diet, encourage foods and fluids with a high sodium content. 8. Be familiar with the sodium content of commonly used parenteral fluids. Monitor clients with cardiovascular disease receiving sodium-containing fluids closely for signs of circulatory overload, such as moist rales in the lungs. 9. Use extreme caution when administering hypertonic saline solutions (3% or 5% NaCl). Be aware that these fluids can be *lethal* if infused carelessly. 10. Avoid giving large water supplements to clients receiving isotonic tube feedings, particularly if routes of abnormal sodium loss are present or water is being retained abnormally.
Hypernatremia		
Deprivation of water, most common in those unable to perceive or respond to thirst Hypertonic tube feedings with inadequate water supplements Increased insensible water loss (as in hyperventilation) Ingestion of salt in unusual amounts Excessive parenteral administration of sodium-containing solutions: • Hypertonic saline (3% or 5% NaCl) • 7.5% sodium bicarbonate • Isotonic saline Profuse sweating Diabetes insipidus Heatstroke Drowning in sea water	Thirst Elevated body temperature Tongue dry and swollen, sticky mucous membranes Severe hypernatremia • Disorientation • Hallucinations • Lethargy when undisturbed • Irritable and hyperreactive when stimulated • Focal or grand mal seizures, coma Serum Na above 145 mEq/L Urinary SG greater than 1.015, provided water loss from nonrenal route	1. Identify clients at risk of hypernatremia. 2. Monitor fluid losses and gains. Look for abnormal losses of water or low water intake, and for large gains of sodium as might occur with ingestion of proprietary drugs with a high sodium content (such as Alka-Seltzer, an effervescent antacid). Also, consider that prescription drugs may have a high sodium content. Of course, one should look for excessive intake of high-sodium foods. 3. Monitor for changes in behavior, such as restlessness, disorientation, and lethargy. 4. Look for excessive thirst and elevated body temperature. If present, evaluate in relation to other signs. 5. Monitor serum sodium levels. 6. Prevent hypernatremia in debilitated clients unable to perceive or respond to thirst by offering them fluids at regular intervals. If fluid intake remains inadequate, consult with the physician to plan an alternate route for intake, either by tube feedings or by the parenteral route. 7. If tube feedings are used, give sufficient water to keep the serum sodium and the BUN levels within normal limits. Be aware that the higher the osmolality of the feeding, the greater the need for water supplements.

(continued)

Table 46-4 *(continued)*

Electrolyte Disturbances: Related Factors, Defining Characteristics, and Nursing Interventions

Related Factors	Defining Characteristics	Nursing Interventions
Hypokalemia		
Diarrhea Vomiting or gastric suction Potassium-losing diuretics (such as furosemide and thiazides) Steroid administration Carbenicillin, sodium penicillin, amphotericin B Hyperaldosteronism Hyperalimentation Poor intake, as in anorexia nervosa, alcoholism, potassium-free parenteral fluids Osmotic diuresis (as occurs in uncontrolled diabetes mellitus or mannitol administration)	Fatigue Anorexia, nausea, and vomiting Muscle weakness Decreased bowel motility (intestinal ileus) Cardiac arrhythmias Increased sensitivity to digitalis Polyuria, nocturia, dilute urine (if hypokalemia is prolonged) Mild hyperglycemia Postural hypotension Serum K below 3.5 mEq/L Paresthesias or tender muscles ECG changes: Flattened T waves ST segment depression	1. Be aware of clients at risk for hypokalemia and monitor for its occurrence. 2. Assess digitalized clients at risk for hypokalemia especially closely for symptoms of digitalis toxicity because hypokalemia potentiates the action of digitalis. Be aware that the physician usually prefers to keep the serum potassium level above 3.5 mEq/L in digitalized clients. 3. Take measures to prevent hypokalemia when possible. a. Prevention may take the form of encouraging extra potassium intake for at-risk client (when the diet allows). b. When hypokalemia is due to abuse of laxatives or diuretics, education of the client may help alleviate the problem. 4. Administer oral potassium supplements when prescribed. 5. Be aware that clients may not need potassium supplements if they are using salt substitutes because these substances usually contain sizable amounts of potassium. 6. Be thoroughly familiar with the critical facts related to administering potassium intravenously.
Hyperkalemia		
Decreased potassium excretion: • Oliguric renal failure • Potassium-conserving diuretics • Hypoaldosteronism High potassium intake, especially in presence of renal insufficiency: • Improper use of oral potassium supplements • Rapid or excessive administration of IV potassium • Rapid transfusion of aged blood • High-dose potassium penicillin • Foods high in potassium (such as dried apricots) Shift of potassium out of cells: • Acidosis • Tissue trauma • Malignant cell lysis	Vague muscular weakness is usually first sign Cardiac arrhythmias, bradycardia, and heart block can occur Paresthesias of face, tongue, feet, and hands Flaccid muscle paralysis (spreads from legs to trunk and arms; respiratory muscles may be affected) GI symptoms such as nausea, intermittent intestinal colic, or diarrhea may occur ECG changes: tall, peaked T waves, absent P waves, widened QRS complex. Serum K above 5.0 mEq/L (mmol/L)	1. Be aware of clients at risk for hyperkalemia and monitor for its occurrence. Hyperkalemia is life-threatening; it is imperative to detect it early. 2. Take measures to prevent hyperkalemia when possible by following guidelines for administering potassium safely, both intravenously and orally. a. Follow rules for safe administration of potassium. b. Avoid administration of potassium-conserving diuretics, potassium supplements, or salt substitutes to clients with renal insufficiency. c. Caution clients to use salt substitutes sparingly if they are taking other supplementary forms of potassium or are taking potassium-conserving diuretics (eg, spironolactone, triamterene, and amiloride). d. Caution hyperkalemic clients to avoid foods high in potassium content. Some of these are coffee, cocoa, tea, dried fruits, dried beans, whole-grain breads.
Hypocalcemia		
Surgical hypoparathyroidism (may follow thyroid surgery or radical neck surgery for cancer) Malabsorption Vitamin D deficiency Acute pancreatitis	Numbness, tingling of fingers, circumoral region, and toes Cramps in muscles of extremities Hyperactive deep-tendon reflexes (such as patellar and triceps)	1. Be aware of clients at risk for hypocalcemia and monitor for its occurrence. 2. Be prepared to take seizure precautions when hypocalcemia is severe. 3. Monitor condition of airway closely because laryngeal stridor can occur. 4. Take safety precautions if confusion is present.

Table 46-4 *(continued)*
Electrolyte Disturbances: Related Factors, Defining Characteristics, and Nursing Interventions

Related Factors	Defining Characteristics	Nursing Interventions
Hypocalcemia		
Excessive administration of citrated blood Primary hypoparathyroidism Alkalotic states (decreased ionized calcium) Hyperphosphatemia Medullary carcinoma of thyroid Hypoalbuminemia (as in cirrhosis, nephrotic syndrome, and starvation) Hypomagnesemia Decreased ultraviolet exposure	Trousseau's sign Chvostek's sign Mental changes, such as confusion and alterations in mood and memory Convulsions (usually generalized but may be focal) Spasm of laryngeal muscles EKG shows prolonged QT interval Spasms of muscles in abdomen (can simulate acute abdominal emergency) Total serum calcium level below 8.5 mg/dL or ionized level below normal (below 50%)	5. Be aware of factors related to the safe administration of calcium replacement salts. 6. Educate people in high-risk groups for osteoporosis (especially postmenopausal women not on estrogen therapy) as to the need for dietary calcium intake. If adequate amounts are not consumed in the diet (as is often the case), calcium supplements should be considered. 7. Educate people at risk for osteoporosis about the value of regular physical exercise in decreasing bone loss. 8. To prevent osteoporosis in later years, educate young women about the need for a normal diet to ensure adequate calcium intake. Also, discuss the calcium-losing aspects of alcohol and nicotine use.
Hypercalcemia		
Hyperparathyroidism Malignant neoplastic disease Prolonged immobilization Large doses of vitamin D Overuse of calcium-containing antacids or calcium supplements Thiazide diuretics	Muscular weakness Tiredness, listlessness, lethargy Constipation Anorexia, nausea, and vomiting Decreased memory span, decreased attention span, and confusion Polyuria and polydipsia Renal stones Neurotic behavior progressing to frank psychoses may occur (reversible with correction of hypercalcemia) Cardiac arrest may occur in hypercalcemic crisis ECG shows shortened QT interval Serum calcium over 10.5 mg/dL	1. Be aware of clients at risk for hypercalcemia and monitor for its presence. 2. Increase client mobilization when feasible. 3. Encourage the oral intake of sufficient fluids to keep the client well hydrated. 4. Discourage excessive consumption of milk products and other high-calcium foods. 5. Encourage adequate bulk in the diet to offset the tendency for constipation. 6. Take safety precautions if confusion or other mental symptoms of hypercalcemia are present. 7. Be aware that cardiac arrest can occur in clients with severe hypercalcemia; be prepared to deal with this emergency. 8. Be aware that bones may fracture more easily in clients with chronic hypercalcemia because bone resorption has been excessive, weakening the bony structure. Transfer clients cautiously. 9. Educate home-bound oncology clients with a predisposition for hypercalcemia, and their families, to be alert for symptoms that occur with this condition and to report them to the healthcare providers before they become severe. 10. Be alert for signs of digitalis toxicity when hypercalcemia occurs in digitalized clients. 11. Help prevent formation of calcium renal stones in clients with long-standing hypercalcemia or immobilization by: a. Forcing fluids to maintain a dilute urine, thus avoiding supersaturation of precipitates b. Encouraging fluids that yield an acid ash (such as prune or cranberry juice) because a urinary pH less than 6.5 favors calcium deposits c. Preventing urinary stasis by turning the immobilized client frequently, elevating the head of the bed, and having the client sit up if this can be tolerated

(continued)

Table 46-4 *(continued)*
Electrolyte Disturbances: Related Factors, Defining Characteristics, and Nursing Interventions

Related Factors	Defining Characteristics	Nursing Interventions
Hypomagnesemia		
Chronic alcoholism Intestinal malabsorption syndromes Diarrhea Nasogastric suction Aggressive refeeding after starvation (as in TPN) Prolonged administration of magnesium-free maintenance IV fluids Diabetic ketoacidosis Hyperaldosteronism Drugs: • Diuretics • Aminoglycoside antibiotics (such as gentamicin) • Cisplatin • Excessive doses of vitamin D or calcium supplements • Citrate preservative in blood products Pancreatitis Thyrotoxicosis Hyperparathyroidism	Neuromuscular irritability • Increased reflexes • Coarse tremors • Positive Chvostek's and Trousseau's signs • Convulsions Cardiac manifestations • Tachyarrhythmias • Increased susceptibility to digitalis toxicity • ECG changes in severe cases: PR and QT interval prolongation, widened QRS complex, ST segment depression, and T-wave inversion Mental changes • Disorientation in memory • Mood changes • Intense confusion • Hallucinations Serum magnesium level below 1.3 mEq/L	1. Be aware of clients at risk for hypomagnesemia and monitor for its presence. 2. Assess digitalized clients at risk for hypomagnesemia especially closely for symptoms of digitalis toxicity because a deficit of magnesium predisposes to toxicity. 3. Be prepared to take seizure precautions when hypomagnesemia is severe. 4. Monitor condition of airway, because laryngeal stridor can occur. 5. Take safety precautions if confusion is present. 6. Be familiar with magnesium replacement salts and factors related to their safe administration. 7. Be aware that magnesium-depleted clients may experience difficulty in swallowing. 8. When magnesium deficit is due to abuse of diuretics or laxatives, educating the client may help alleviate the problem. 9. Be aware that most commonly used IV fluids have either no magnesium or a relatively small amount. When indicated, discuss need for magnesium replacement with physician. 10. For clients experiencing abnormal magnesium losses, but able to consume a general diet, encourage the intake of magnesium-rich foods (such as green vegetables, nuts and legumes, and fruits such as bananas, oranges, and grapefruits).
Hypermagnesemia		
Renal failure (particularly when magnesium-containing medications are administered) Adrenal insufficiency Excessive magnesium administration during treatment of eclampsia Hemodialysis with excessively hard water or with a dialysate inadvertently high in magnesium content	Early signs (serum magnesium level of 3 to 5 mEq/L) • Flushing and a sense of skin warmth (due to peripheral vasodilation) • Hypotension (due to blockage of sympathetic ganglia as well as to a direct effect on smooth muscle) Depressed respirations Drowsiness, hypoactive reflexes, and muscular weakness Cardiac abnormalities Weak or absent cry in newborn	1. Be aware of clients at risk for hypermagnesemia and assess for its presence. When hypermagnesemia is suspected, assess the following parameters: • Vital signs: Look for low blood pressure and shallow respirations with periods of apnea. • Level of consciousness: Look for drowsiness, lethargy, and coma. 2. Do not give magnesium-containing medications to client with renal failure or compromised renal function. (Be particularly careful in following "standing orders" for bowel preparation for x-ray because some of these include the use of magnesium citrate.) 3. Caution clients with renal disease to check with their healthcare providers before taking over-the-counter medications. 4. Be aware of factors related to safe parenteral administration of magnesium salts.
Hypophosphatemia		
Glucose administration Refeeding after starvation Hyperalimentation Alcohol withdrawal Diabetic ketoacidosis	Paresthesias Muscle weakness Muscle pain and tenderness Mental changes, such as apprehension, confusion, delirium, and coma	1. Identify clients at risk for hypophosphatemia. • Severely malnourished clients • Alcoholic clients • Clients with diabetic ketoacidosis 2. Monitor clients at risk for the presence of hypophosphatemia.

Table 46-4 *(continued)*
Electrolyte Disturbances: Related Factors, Defining Characteristics, and Nursing Interventions

Related Factors	Defining Characteristics	Nursing Interventions
Hypophosphatemia		
Respiratory alkalosis Phosphate-binding antacids Recovery phase after severe burns	Cardiomyopathy Acute respiratory failure Seizures Decreased tissue oxygenation Joint stiffness Serum phosphate below 2.5 mg/dL	3. Be aware that severely hypophosphatemic clients are thought to be at greater risk for infection because of changes in white blood cells. 4. Administer IV phosphate products cautiously. 5. Be aware that in adults the usual maintenance dose of phosphorus is 10 to 15 mmol/L of TPN solution. 6. Be aware of the need to introduce hyperalimentation *gradually* in clients who are malnourished. 7. Be aware that sudden increase in the serum phosphorus level can cause hypocalcemia. 8. Because it is possible to give too much phosphorus when administering phosphate solutions, monitor for signs of hyperphosphatemia and of the salt in which it is administered. 9. Monitor for diarrhea in clients taking oral phosphorus supplements; consult with physician if it persists or becomes severe. 10. Mix powdered oral phosphorus supplements with chilled or iced water to make them more palatable.
Hyperphosphatemia		
Renal failure Chemotherapy, particularly for acute lymphoblastic leukemia and lymphoma Large intake of milk Use of cow's milk in infants Excessive intake of phosphate-containing laxatives Overzealous administration of phosphorus supplements, orally or intravenously Excessive use of Fleet's phosphosoda as enema solution, particularly in children and people with slow bowel elimination Large vitamin D intake Hypoparathyroidism Hyperthyroidism	Short-term consequences: symptoms of tetany, such as tingling of fingertips and around mouth, numbness, and muscle spasms Long-term consequences: precipitation of calcium phosphate in nonosseous sites, such as the kidney, joints, arteries, skin, or cornea. Serum phosphate above 4.5 mg/dL	1. Identify clients at risk for hyperphosphatemia. 2. Monitor for signs of tetany, such as tingling sensations in the fingertips and around the mouth, and presence of muscle cramps or positive Chvostek's and Trousseau's signs in at-risk clients. Be aware that these symptoms are probably due to hypocalcemia induced by the high phosphate level and are most likely to occur in clients who have taken in a high phosphate load. 3. Be aware that soft-tissue calcification can be a long-term complication of a chronically elevated serum phosphate level. Calcification may occur in sites such as the kidney, arteries, joints, and cornea. Monitor for signs of these complications. 4. Administer prescribed oral and IV phosphate supplements cautiously and monitor serum phosphorus levels periodically during their use. 5. When appropriate, instruct clients that use of phosphate-containing laxatives may result in acute phosphate poisoning. 6. Be aware that phosphate-containing enemas can result in hyperphosphatemia if used injudiciously, particularly in children and those with slow bowel emptying. Instruct clients accordingly. 7. When a low-phosphorus diet is prescribed, instruct clients to avoid foods high in phosphorus content. Such foods include hard cheese or cream, nuts and nut products; whole grain cereals (eg, bran and oatmeal); dried fruits, dried vegetables; special meats such as kidneys, sardines, and sweetbreads; and desserts made with milk.

(Data from Metheny, N. M. [1992]. *Fluid and electrolyte balance* [2nd ed.]. Philadelphia: Lippincott.)

failure when the kidneys fail to excrete magnesium and excessive amounts are administered therapeutically.

Hypophosphatemia and Hyperphosphatemia. *Hypophosphatemia* refers to a below-normal serum concentration of inorganic phosphorus. Although this may indicate phosphorus deficiency, multiple factors may lower serum phosphate levels while total body phosphorus stores are normal. *Hyperphosphatemia* refers to above-normal serum concentrations of inorganic phosphorus.

Acid–Base Imbalances

Arterial blood gases (ABGs) are most commonly used to assess and treat acid–base imbalances. Results from venous blood are only specific for the particular extremity or area where the blood was sampled and do not provide information on how well the lungs are oxygenating the blood. The pH of plasma indicates balance or impending acidosis or alkalosis. In addition, however, a study of the blood's oxygen and carbon dioxide gases is important. The partial pressures (indicated by "P") of these gases, or their tensions, are determined by the use of a nomogram, which reflects the chemical and physical activities of the two gases. The partial pressure of carbon dioxide is abbreviated $PaCO_2$; for oxygen, it is PaO_2. The "a" indicates an arterial specimen. When the PaO_2 is low, hemoglobin carries less than normal amounts of oxygen; when the PaO_2 is high, the hemoglobin carries more oxygen. Oxygen saturation readings (SaO_2) reveal the percentage of oxygen in the blood that combines with hemoglobin. The $PaCO_2$ is influenced almost entirely by respiratory activity. When $PaCO_2$ is low, carbonic acid leaves the body in excessive amounts; when the $PaCO_2$ is high, there are excessive amounts of carbonic acid in the body. Laboratory levels for ABGs are given later in the chapter.

Acid–base imbalances occur when the carbonic acid or bicarbonate levels become disproportionate. When there is a single primary cause, these disturbances are known as respiratory acidosis or alkalosis and metabolic acidosis or alkalosis, which are defined and described in the sections that follow. These disturbances are a result of an upset in acid–base balance, as follows:

- A respiratory disturbance alters the carbonic acid portion:
  - Respiratory acidosis and alkalosis are the results of respiratory disturbances.
  - Compensation occurs to restore balance in the kidneys by either conserving or excreting more bicarbonate.
- A metabolic disturbance alters the bicarbonate portion:
  - Metabolic acidosis and alkalosis are almost entirely the result of metabolic processes.
  - The primary organs for compensation to restore balance are the lungs, which either try to conserve or excrete more carbon dioxide, which is available in weakly ionized carbonic acid.

Table 46-5 summarizes acid–base imbalances. Complicated clinical situations may occur when respiratory and metabolic imbalances coexist.

Respiratory Acidosis. *Respiratory acidosis* is a primary excess of carbonic acid in ECF. Any decrease in alveolar ventilation that results in retention of carbon dioxide can cause respiratory acidosis. Because the lungs are the source of the problem, they are unable to participate in compensation. As the carbonic acid content increases, the kidneys attempt to retain more bicarbonate and increase their hydrogen excretion. Thus,

respiratory acidosis = high $PaCO_2$ because of alveolar hypoventilation

Respiratory Alkalosis. *Respiratory alkalosis* is a primary deficit of carbonic acid in ECF. It is the result of increased alveolar ventilation and, therefore, a decrease in carbon dioxide. An increase in respiratory rate and depth causes the carbon dioxide loss because the carbon dioxide is excreted faster than normal.

Because of the deficit of carbon dioxide, which is a respiratory stimulant sensed in the medulla of the brain, depression or cessation of respirations eventually can occur. Because the lungs are the source of the problem, they are unable to participate in compensation. Therefore, the kidneys attempt to alleviate the imbalance by increasing the bicarbonate excretion and by retaining more hydrogen. Thus,

respiratory alkalosis = low $PaCO_2$ because of alveolar hyperventilation

Metabolic Acidosis. *Metabolic acidosis* is a proportionate deficit of bicarbonate in ECF. The deficit can occur as the result of an increase in acid components or an excessive loss of bicarbonate. The lungs attempt to increase the carbon dioxide excretion by increasing the rate and depth of respirations. The kidneys attempt to compensate by retaining bicarbonate and by excreting more hydrogen. If the body is unable to achieve normal balance, the person may lose consciousness as metabolic acidosis increases, and death eventually results. Thus,

metabolic acidosis = low bicarbonate. Nonvolatile acid is present to use up HCO_3^- in disproportionate amounts, or HCO_3^- is lost in disproportionate amounts

Metabolic Alkalosis. *Metabolic alkalosis* is a primary excess of bicarbonate in ECF. This may be the result of excessive acid losses or increased base ingestion or retention. The body attempts to compensate by retaining carbon dioxide. The respirations become slow and shallow, and periods of no breathing may occur. The kidneys attempt to excrete potassium and sodium with the excessive bicarbonate, and retain hydrogen in carbonic acid. Thus,

Table 46-5
Acid–Base Disturbances: Related Factors, Defining Characteristics, and Nursing Interventions

Related Factors	Defining Characteristics	Nursing Interventions
Respiratory Acidosis (Carbonic Acid Excess)		

Acute respiratory acidosis:
• Acute pulmonary edema
• Aspiration of a foreign body
• Atelectasis
• Pneumothorax, hemothorax
• Overdosage of sedatives or anesthetic
• Position on operating room table that interferes with respirations
• Cardiac arrest
• Severe pneumonia
• Laryngospasm
• Mechanical ventilation improperly regulated
Chronic respiratory acidosis:
• Emphysema
• Cystic fibrosis
• Advanced multiple sclerosis
• Bronchiectasis
• Bronchial asthma
Factors favoring hypoventilation:
• Obesity
• Tight abdominal binders or dressings
• Postoperative pain (as in high abdominal or chest incisions)
• Abdominal distention from cirrhosis or bowel obstruction
	Acute respiratory acidosis
	• Mental cloudiness
	• Dizziness
	• Palpitations
	• Muscular twitching
	• Convulsions
	• Warm, flushed skin
	• Unconsciousness
	• Ventricular fibrillation may be first sign in anesthetized patient (related to hyperkalemia)
	• Arterial blood gases (ABGs)
	  • pH below 7.35
	  • $PaCO_2$ over 45 mm Hg (primary)
	  • HCO_3^- normal or only slightly elevated
	Chronic respiratory acidosis
	• Weakness
	• Dull headache
	• Symptoms of underlying disease process
	• ABGs
	  • pH below 7.35 or within lower limits of normal
	  • $PaCO_2$ over 45 mm Hg (primary)
	  • HCO_3^- over 26 mEq/L (compensatory)
		Treatment is directed at improving ventilation; exact measures vary with the cause of inadequate ventilation. Pharmacologic agents are used as indicated. For example, bronchodilators help reduce bronchial spasm; antibiotics are used for respiratory infections. Pulmonary hygiene measures are used, when necessary, to rid the respiratory tract of mucus and purulent drainage. Adequate hydration (2 to 3 L/day) is indicated to keep the mucous membranes moist and thereby facilitate removal of secretions. Supplemental oxygen is used as necessary.
		A mechanical respirator, used cautiously, may improve pulmonary ventilation. One must remember that overzealous use of a mechanical respirator may cause such rapid excretion of carbon dioxide that the kidneys will be unable to eliminate excess bicarbonate with sufficient rapidity to prevent alkalosis and convulsions. For this reason, the elevated $PaCO_2$ must be decreased slowly.

Respiratory Alkalosis (Carbonic Acid Deficit)		
Extreme anxiety (most common cause) Hypoxemia High fever Early salicylate intoxication (stimulates respiratory center) Gram-negative bacteremia Central nervous system lesions involving respiratory center Pulmonary emboli Thyrotoxicosis Excessive ventilation by mechanical ventilators Pregnancy (high progesterone level sensitizes the respiratory center to CO_2: physiologic)	Lightheadedness (a low $PaCO_2$ causes cerebral vasoconstriction and thus decreased cerebral blood flow) Inability to concentrate Hyperventilation syndrome • Tinnitus • Palpitations • Sweating • Dry mouth • Tremulousness • Precordial pain (tightness) • Nausea and vomiting • Epigastric pain • Blurred vision • Convulsions and loss of consciousness ABGs • pH over 7.45 • $PaCO_2$ below 35 mm Hg (primary) • HCO_3^- under 22 mEq/L (mmol/L) (compensatory)	If the cause of respiratory alkalosis is anxiety, the client should be made aware that the abnormal breathing practice is responsible for the symptoms accompanying this condition. Instruct the client to breathe more slowly (to cause accumulation of carbon dioxide) or to breathe in a closed system (such as a paper bag). Usually a sedative is required to relieve ventilation in very anxious patients. (If alkalosis is severe enough to cause fainting, the increased ventilation ceases and respirations revert to normal.) Treatment for other causes of respiratory alkalosis is directed at correcting the underlying problem.
Metabolic Acidosis (Base Bicarbonate Deficit)		
Normal anion gap: • Diarrhea • Intestinal fistulas • Ureterosigmoidostomy • Hyperalimentation	Headache Confusion Drowsiness	Treatment is directed toward correcting the metabolic defect. If the cause of the problem is excessive intake of chloride, treatment obviously focuses on eliminating the source. When necessary, bicarbonate is administered.

(continued)

Table 46-5 *(continued)*
Acid–Base Disturbances: Related Factors, Defining Characteristics, and Nursing Interventions

Related Factors	Defining Characteristics	Nursing Interventions
Metabolic Acidosis (Base Bicarbonate Deficit)		
• Acidifying drugs (such as ammonium chloride) • Renal tubular acidosis (RTA) High anion gap: • Diabetic ketoacidosis • Starvational ketoacidosis • Lactic acidosis • Renal failure • Ingestion of toxins (such as salicylates, ethylene glycol, and methanol)	Increased respiratory rate and depth (may not become clinically evident until HCO_3^- is quite low) Nausea and vomiting Peripheral vasodilation (may be present, causing warm, flushed skin) Decreased cardiac output when pH falls below 7; bradycardia may develop ABGs • Fall in pH to below 7.35 • HCO_3^- under 22 mEq/L (mmol/L) (primary) • $PaCO_2$ under 35 mm Hg (compensation by lungs) • Base excess always negative Hyperkalemia is frequently present	
Metabolic Alkalosis (Base Bicarbonate Excess)		
Vomiting or gastric suction Hypokalemia Hyperaldosteronism Cushing's syndrome Potassium-losing diuretics (eg, thiazides, furosemide, ethacrynic acid) Alkali ingestion (bicarbonate-containing antacids) Parenteral $NaHCO_3$ administration for cardiopulmonary resuscitation Abrupt relief of chronic respiratory acidosis	Those related to decreased calcium ionization, such as: • Dizziness • Tingling of fingers and toes • Circumoral paresthesia • Carpopedal spasm • Hypertonic muscles Depressed respiration (compensatory action by lungs) ABGs • pH above 7.45 • Bicarbonate over 26 mEq/L (mmol/L) (primary) • $PaCO_2$ over 45 mm Hg (compensatory) • Base excess always positive Hypokalemia often present Serum Cl relatively lower than Na	Treatment is aimed at reversal of the underlying disorder. Sufficient chloride must be supplied for the kidney to absorb sodium with chloride (allowing the excretion of excess bicarbonate). Treatment also includes restoration of normal fluid volume by administration of sodium chloride fluids (because continued volume depletion serves to maintain the alkalosis).

(Data from Metheny, N. M. [1992]. *Fluid and electrolyte balance* [2nd ed.]. Philadelphia: Lippincott.)

metabolic alkalosis = high bicarbonate. Nonvolatile acid is lost and is not using up HCO_3^-, or HCO_3^- is gained in disproportionate amounts

The Nurse as Role Model

Nurses wishing to be a role model of self-care behaviors that promote fluid, electrolyte, and acid–base balance should meet the following goals. The nurse will:

- Daily ingest the quantity and type of fluids (to include six to eight glasses of water) that promote healthy hydration and urinary functioning
- Evaluate use of fad diets, diuretics, laxatives, and alcohol, identifying potential risks to health
- Identify situations of high risk for fluid and electrolyte imbalance and intervene appropriately

ASSESSING

The pathophysiology underlying both acute and chronic illness, trauma, and select therapeutic interventions may

Promoting Wellness

Fluid and Electrolyte Balance

Use the assessment checklist to determine how well you are meeting fluid and electrolyte needs. Then develop a prescription for self-care by choosing appropriate behaviors from the list of suggestions.

Assessment Checklist

almost always	sometimes	almost never	
☐	☐	☐	1. I drink six to eight glasses of water every day.
☐	☐	☐	2. I am aware of early signs of dehydration or fluid retention.
☐	☐	☐	3. I limit sugar, alcohol, and caffeine in my diet.
☐	☐	☐	4. I am alert for any sudden variations in my weight.
☐	☐	☐	5. I am aware of fluid and electrolyte imbalances that may be associated with intake of certain medications.
☐	☐	☐	6. I diet sensibly when I need to lose weight.

Self-Care Behaviors

1. Consume approximately 1½ quarts of water daily.
2. Maintain normal body weight.
3. Avoid consuming excess amounts of products high in salt, sugar, and caffeine.
4. Limit alcohol intake because of its diuretic effect.
5. Obtain medical evaluation for any ongoing indications of fluid imbalance.
6. Monitor side effects of medications, especially diuresis and diarrhea.

place a client at high risk for fluid, electrolyte, and acid–base imbalances. Once present, these imbalances can seriously compromise the client's health status and may prove life-threatening. Nursing assessment is directed toward the following:

- Identifying clients at high risk for fluid, electrolyte, and acid–base imbalance
- Determining that a specific imbalance is present, identifying the nature of imbalance, severity, etiology, and defining characteristics
- Determining the effectiveness of the plan of care

Important assessment parameters include the nursing history and nursing examination, record of fluid intake and output, daily weight, and laboratory studies.

Nursing History

A comprehensive nursing history includes questions about the client's fluid, electrolyte, and acid–base balance. The accompanying box includes interview questions helpful in identifying the client's usual pattern of fluid intake and elimination and the client's evaluation of his or her hydration status and awareness of particular problems. Interview questions are also directed toward identifying clients at high risk for imbalances. Risk factors include the following:

- The pathophysiology underlying both acute and chronic illness (eg, diabetes mellitus, congestive heart failure, renal failure)
- Abnormal losses of body fluids (eg, prolonged or severe vomiting and diarrhea, draining wounds, fistulas). Table 46-6 lists imbalances that result from fluid loss of specific body fluids.
- Burns and trauma
- Therapies with the potential to disrupt fluid and electrolyte balance (eg, medications such as diuretics and steroids, treatments such as IV therapy and TPN)

Physical Assessment

Metheny (1992) recommends that the nurse pay attention to certain parameters when assessing a client's fluid and electrolyte status:

- Comparison of total intake and output of fluids
- Urine volume and concentration
- Skin and tongue turgor
- Degree of moisture in oral cavity
- Body weight
- Thirst
- Tearing and salivation
- Appearance and temperature of skin
- Facial appearance
- Edema
- Vital signs
- Neck and hand vein filling

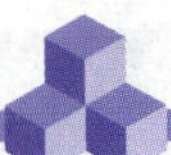

Focused Assessment Guide

Fluid, Electrolyte, and Acid–Base Balance

Factors to Assess	Questions and Approaches
Usual pattern of fluid intake	Describe the amount and types of fluids you usually drink in a 24-hour period. Have there been any recent changes?
Usual pattern of fluid elimination	Describe your usual voiding/urination habits. Any recent changes in frequency or amount? Is your body losing fluids in any other major way? • Vomiting • Diarrhea • Excessive perspiration • Fistula
Client's evaluation of hydration status	Do you think there is an approximate balance between your fluid intake and output? Have you noticed any signs that your body is experiencing too much or too little hydration (difficulty breathing, edema, dry skin and mucous membranes, thirst)?
History of disease process	Is there any history of disease process or injury that might disrupt fluid and electrolyte balance (eg, diabetes mellitus, cancer, burns)?
Medication history	Do you take any medications or treatments that might disrupt fluid and electrolyte balance (eg, steroids, diuretics, total parenteral nutrition, dialysis)?
Fluid, electrolyte, and acid-base imbalances, and contributing factors	Are you aware of any specific fluid, electrolyte, or acid-base problems you may be experiencing? • Nature • Onset of problem and frequency • Causes • Severity • Symptoms • Intervention attempted and results

Table 46-6
Imbalances Resulting From Fluid Loss of Specific Body Fluid

Fluid Lost	Imbalances Likely to Occur	Fluid Lost	Imbalances Likely to Occur
Gastric juice	Extracellular fluid volume deficit Metabolic alkalosis Sodium deficit Potassium deficit Tetany (if metabolic alkalosis is present) Ketosis of starvation Magnesium deficit	Pancreatic juice	Metabolic acidosis Sodium deficit Calcium deficit Extracellular fluid volume deficit
		Sensible perspiration	Extracellular fluid volume deficit Sodium deficit
		Insensible water loss	Water deficit (dehydration) Sodium excess
Intestinal juice	Extracellular fluid volume deficit Metabolic acidosis Sodium deficit Potassium deficit	Wound exudate	Protein deficit Sodium deficit Extracellular fluid volume deficit
Bile	Sodium deficit Metabolic acidosis	Ascites	Protein deficit Sodium deficit Plasma-to-interstitial fluid shift Extracellular fluid volume deficit

- Results of hemodynamic monitoring (eg, CVP [central venous pressure] and PAP [pulmonary artery pressure])
- Neuromuscular irritability

When suspecting imbalance of particular electrolytes, knowledge of their defining characteristics should guide the assessment (see Table 46-4). Table 46-7 presents select nursing considerations for each of these parameters, findings in a healthy adult, and significant findings.

Measuring Fluid Intake and Output

When either the physician or nurse orders that a client's fluid intake and output be continuously measured, the client, his or her family, and all caregivers should be alert to the need to measure all fluids entering and leaving the body—to the extent that this is possible. The client's condition dictates the strictness of the intake and output measurement. Adherence to the guidelines in the accompanying box helps eliminate common errors in measuring fluid intake and output.

Daily Weights

Because of the numerous sources of inaccuracies in fluid intake and output measurement, the recording of a client's daily weight may provide a more accurate depiction of fluid balance status. Guidelines for accurate weight measurement include weighing the client at the same time each day, preferably in the morning before breakfast and after the first morning voiding; with the same or similar clothing; and on the same scale.

Laboratory Studies

Laboratory tests are helpful in determining whether fluid, electrolyte, and acid–base balance exist. Standard tests include the following (tables of normal values are given in Appendix B).

Complete Blood Count. This basic screening test provides a determination of the total number of RBCs and values for hemoglobin and hematocrit. Significant values include the following:

- Increased hematocrit values: Found in severe dehydration and shock (when hemoconcentration rises considerably)
- Decreased hematocrit: Found with acute, massive blood loss, and with hemolytic reaction following transfusion of incompatible blood
- Increased levels of hemoglobin: Found in hemoconcentration of the blood
- Decreased levels of hemoglobin: Found with anemia states, severe hemorrhage, and following a hemolytic reaction

Home Healthcare Alert

As a safety precaution and in compliance with CDC guidelines, the nurse needs to apply a "Biohazard" label to any blood specimen collected from the client at home. The specimen should be transported to the laboratory as soon as possible or refrigerated if a delay of more than 1 hour is expected.

Serum Electrolytes. This screening test provides information on plasma levels of select electrolytes. Commonly determined are plasma levels of sodium, potassium, chloride, and bicarbonate ions.

Urine pH and Specific Gravity. Both the urine pH and specific gravity (SG) may be obtained by dipstick measurement on a fresh voided specimen or through laboratory analysis. Specific gravity is a measure of the kidney's ability to concentrate urine. The range depends on the state of hydration and varies with urine volume and the load of solutes to be excreted. Normal values range from 1.003 to 1.035 (concentrated urine—1.025 to 1.030 or more; dilute urine—1.001 to 1.010).

Arterial Blood Gases. ABGs are obtained to determine the adequacy of oxygenation and ventilation and to assess acid–base status. Refer to Table 46-8 to review the primary laboratory values used to determine acid–base balance. Additional ABG values have not been included in this basic discussion in an attempt to simplify the interpretation of acid–base imbalances. Partial pressure of oxygen ($PaCO_2$) and oxygen saturation (SaO_2) results also directly reflect the adequacy of oxygenation and ventilation. When interpreting blood gases:

1. Determine whether the pH is alkalotic or acidotic.
2. Check for the cause of the change in pH. Is it respiratory ($PaCO_2$) or metabolic (HCO_3)?
   In respiratory acid–base imbalances, the pH and $PaCO_2$ values are inversely abnormal (move in opposite directions):
   Respiratory acidosis:
   ↓pH <7.35 ↑$PaCO_2$ Normal HCO_3^-
   Respiratory alkalosis:
   ↑pH >7.45 ↓$PaCO_2$ Normal HCO_3^-
   In metabolic acid–base imbalances, the pH and HCO_3 values are both high or both low:
   Metabolic acidosis:
   ↓pH <7.35 ↓HCO_3^- Normal $PaCO_2$
   Metabolic alkalosis:
   ↑pH >7.45 ↑HCO_3^- Normal $PaCO_2$
3. Determine whether the body is compensating for the pH change.
   When the problem is respiratory, the renal system attempts to compensate either by ↑HCO_3^- or ↓HCO_3^-. In contrast, the respiratory system com-

(text continues on page 1396)

Table 46-7
Parameters to Be Considered in Clinical Assessment for Fluid, Electrolyte, and Acid–Base Balance

Assessment Parameters	Nursing Considerations	Findings in Healthy Adult	Significant Findings
Comparison of total intake and output of fluids	• Records may be initiated by the nurse for any client with a real or potential water or electrolyte problem. • Intake should include all fluids taken into the body. • Output should include urine, vomitus, diarrhea, drainage from fistulas, and drainage from suction apparatus. Perspiration and drainage from lesions should be noted and estimated. Prolonged hyperventilation should also be noted because it is an important route of water vapor loss.	• Fluid intake about equals fluid output—when averaged over 2 or 3 days. • Range of 1500 to 3500 mL fluid intake and loss; 2000 mL is average adult intake and loss per day. • Output of urine normally approximates the ingestion of liquids; water from food and oxidation is balanced by the water loss through feces, the skin, and the respiratory process.	• When the total intake is substantially less than the total output, the client is in danger of fluid volume deficit. • When the total intake is substantially more than the total output, the client is in danger of fluid volume excess.
Urine volume and concentration	• Measure all fluid losses according to routes. • Use a device calibrated for small volumes of urine when hourly urine volumes need to be measured. • Account for factors that can alter urinary output: 1. Amount of fluid intake 2. Losses from skin, lungs, and GI tract 3. Amount of waste products for excretions 4. Renal concentrating ability 5. Blood volume 6. Hormonal influences (primarily aldosterone and ADH)	• Normal urinary output is about 1 mL/kg of body weight per hour (for the average adult: 1500 mL/24 hr, which is equivalent to about 40 to 80 mL/hr). • Stress may diminish the 24-hour urine volume in the adult to 750 to 1000 mL (or 30 to 50 mL/hr) because of increased aldosterone and ADH secretion. • The range of specific gravity is from 1.003 to 1.035. Urine osmolality ranges between 500 mOsm and 800 mOsm/kg (mmol/kg).	• A low urine volume with a high specific gravity indicates fluid volume deficit. • A low urine volume with a low specific gravity indicates renal disease. • A high urine volume suggests fluid volume excess. • Urine volume is increased in conditions with high solute loads, such as diabetes mellitus. • Hypovolemia causes decreased renal perfusion and thus oliguria; hypervolemia causes increased urinary volume if the kidneys are functioning normally.
Body weight	• Because of the common inaccuracies in recording intake and output, body weight is believed to be a more accurate indicator of fluid gained and lost. • Guidelines for weighing clients: 1. Use the same scale each time. 2. Measure weight at the same time each day: in the morning before breakfast and after voiding. 3. Be sure the client is wearing the same, or similar clothing (clothing should be dry). 4. If the client is unable to stand on a small, portable scale, use a bed scale. • A client may have a severe fluid volume deficit even though body weight is essentially unchanged when there is a third-space loss of body fluid.	• A client's dry weight should remain relatively stable.	• Rapid variations in weight closely reflect changes in body fluid volume. • A rapid loss of body weight occurs when the total fluid intake is less than the total fluid output. 1. Rapid loss of 2% total body weight (TBW) indicates mild fluid volume deficit. 2. Rapid loss of 5% TBW indicates moderate fluid volume deficit. 3. Rapid loss of 8% or more of TBW indicates severe fluid volume deficit. • A rapid gain of body weight occurs when the total fluid intake is greater than the total fluid output. 1. Rapid gain of 2% TBW indicates mild fluid volume excess.

Table 46-7 *(continued)*
Parameters to Be Considered in Clinical Assessment for Fluid, Electrolyte, and Acid–Base Balance

Assessment Parameters	Nursing Considerations	Findings in Healthy Adult	Significant Findings
Body weight *(continued)*			2. Rapid gain of 5% TBW indicates moderate fluid volume excess. 3. Rapid gain of 8% or more of TBW indicates severe fluid volume excess. • A rapid gain or loss of 1 kg (2.2 lb) of body weight is about equal to the gain or loss of 1 L of fluid.
Skin turgor (elasticity)	• Pinch the client's skin over the sternum, inner aspect of the thighs, or forehead. • Some prefer to test skin turgor in children over the abdominal area and on the medial aspect of the thighs. • Skin turgor can vary with age, nutritional state, and even race and complexion.	• Pinched skin immediately falls back to its normal position when released. • Reduced skin turgor is common in older clients (those more than 55 to 60 years of age) because of a primary decrease in skin elasticity.	• In a person with a fluid volume deficit, the skin flattens more slowly after the pinch is released; the skin may remain elevated for many seconds. • Severe malnutrition, particularly in infants, can cause depressed skin turgor even in the absence of fluid depletion.
Tongue turgor	• Unlike skin turgor, tongue turgor is not affected appreciably by age and thus is a useful assessment for all age groups. (In an arid climate, this may not be a reliable parameter.)	• Tongue has one longitudinal furrow.	• In the person with fluid volume deficit there are additional longitudinal furrows and the tongue is smaller. • Sodium excess causes the tongue to look red and swollen.
Moisture and oral cavity	• A dry mouth may be the result of fluid volume deficit or of mouth breathing. (Exposure to an arid climate may result in a dry mouth.)	• Mucous membranes in oral cavity are moist.	• Dryness of the membrane where the cheek and gum meet indicates fluid volume deficit. • Dry sticky mucous membranes are noted in sodium excess. (The oral cavity feels like flypaper.)
Tearing and salivation		• Tearing and salivation decrease normally with age.	• The absence of tearing and salivation in a child is a sign of fluid volume deficit; it becomes obvious with a fluid loss of 5% of TBW.
Appearance of skin and skin temperature			• Metabolic acidosis can cause warm, flushed skin (due to peripheral vasodilation).
Facial appearance			• A person with a severe fluid volume deficit has a pinched and drawn facial expression. • A fluid volume deficit of 10% of body weight causes decreased intraocular pressure, causing the eyes to appear sunken and to feel soft to the touch.
Edema (excessive accumulation of interstitial fluid)	• Pitting edema (see Fig. 46-9) • Measurement of an extremity or body part with a millimeter tape, in the same area each day, is a more exact method of measurement.	• No edema	• Clinically edema is not usually apparent in the adult until the retention of 5 to 10 lb of excess fluid occurs.

(continued)

Table 46-7 *(continued)*
Parameters to Be Considered in Clinical Assessment for Fluid, Electrolyte, and Acid–Base Balance

Assessment Parameters	Nursing Considerations	Findings in Healthy Adult	Significant Findings
Edema *(continued)*	• An excess of interstitial fluid may accumulate predominantly in the lower extremities of ambulatory clients and in the presacral region of bedridden clients. • The presence of periorbital (around the eyes) edema or pedal edema should prompt one to look for edema in other parts of the body.		• Pitting edema is not evident until at least a 10% increase in weight has occurred. • Formation of edema may be localized (as in thrombophlebitis) or generalized (as in heart failure, cirrhosis of liver, or nephrotic syndrome). Edema of congestive heart failure, liver cirrhosis, or nephrotic syndrome is the result of sodium retention.
Body temperature	• Because fever increases the loss of body fluids it is important that temperature elevations be detected early and appropriate interventions be taken. • Body temperature and other vital signs should be assessed at the nurse's discretion.	• Baseline temperature: diurnal variations	• There is an elevation of body temperature in hypernatremia (dehydration) probably related to lack of available fluid for sweating. • There is a decrease in body temperature in fluid volume deficit, when uncomplicated by infection. • Fever increases the loss of body fluids. • A temperature elevation between 101°F (38.3°C) and 103°F (39.4°C) increases the 24-hour fluid requirement by at least 500 mL, and a temperature above 103°F increases it by at least 1000 mL.
Pulse		• Baseline pulse rate, rhythm, and volume	• Tachycardia is usually the earliest sign of the decreased vascular volume associated with fluid volume deficit. • Irregular pulse rates also occur with potassium imbalances and magnesium deficit. • Pulse volume is decreased in fluid volume deficit and increased in fluid volume excess.
Respirations		• Baseline respiratory rate, rhythm, and qualities	• Deep, rapid respirations may be a compensatory mechanism for metabolic acidosis or a primary disorder causing respiratory alkalosis. • Slow, shallow respirations may be a compensatory mechanism for metabolic alkalosis or a primary disorder causing respiratory acidosis. • Moist crackles, in the absence of cardiopulmonary disease, indicate fluid volume excess.

Table 46-7 *(continued)*
Parameters to Be Considered in Clinical Assessment for Fluid, Electrolyte, and Acid–Base Balance

Assessment Parameters	Nursing Considerations	Findings in Healthy Adult	Significant Findings
Blood pressure	• Whenever a fluid imbalance is suspected, check the client's blood pressure while he or she is lying down, sitting, and standing.	• Baseline blood pressure	• A fall in systolic pressure greater than 15 mm Hg from the lying to the sitting or standing position (postural hypotension) usually indicates fluid volume deficit.
Neck veins and central venous pressure (CVP)	• The jugular veins provide a built-in manometer for following changes in CVP. • To estimate CVP, the nurse: 1. Positions the client in a semi-Fowler's position (head of bed elevated to a 30- to 45-degree angle), keeping the neck straight 2. Removes any of the client's clothing that could constrict the neck or upper chest 3. Provides adequate lighting to visualize effectively the external jugular veins on each side of the neck 4. Measures the levels to which the veins are distended on the neck or above the level of the manubrium • More accurate assessments of blood volume are obtained by measuring CVP by hemodynamic monitoring.	• Normally, when the client is supine, the external jugular veins fill to the anterior border of the sternocleidomastoid muscle. With the client positioned sitting at a 45-degree angle, the venous distensions normally should not extend higher than 2 cm above the sternal angle. • Pressure in the right atrium is usually 0 to 4 cm H_2O; pressure in the vena cava is about 4 to 11 cm H_2O.	• A low CVP may indicate: 1. Decreased blood volume 2. Drug-induced vasodilation (causing pooling of blood in peripheral veins) • A high CVP may indicate: 1. Increased blood volume 2. Heart failure 3. Vasoconstriction
Neuromuscular irritability	• When imbalances in calcium, magnesium, and sodium are suspected it is important to assess clients for increased or decreased neuromuscular irritability		
	• To test for *Chvostek's sign,* the facial nerve should be percussed about 2 cm anterior to the earlobe.	• Negative response	• Clients with hypocalcemia or hypomagnesemia respond positively with a unilateral twitching of the facial muscles, including the eyelid and lips.
	• To test for *Trousseau's sign,* place a blood pressure cuff on the arm and inflate above systolic pressure for 3 minutes.	• Negative response	• A positive response is the development of carpal spasm.
	• A deep tendon reflex is elicited by briskly tapping a partially stretched tendon with a rubber percussion hammer, preferably over the tendon insertion of the muscle.	• The response in the prospective muscle is a sudden contraction (2+).	• Deep tendon reflexes may be hyperactive in the presence of hypocalcemia, hypomagnesemia, hypernatremia, and alkalosis.

(continued)

Table 46-7 *(continued)*
Parameters to Be Considered in Clinical Assessment for Fluid, Electrolyte, and Acid–Base Balance

Assessment Parameters	Nursing Considerations	Findings in Healthy Adult	Significant Findings
Neuromuscular irritability *(continued)*	• The muscle being tested should be slightly stretched and the client should be relaxed. • Reflexes usually graded on a 0 to 4+ scale 0 = no response 1+ = somewhat diminished, but present 2+ = normal 3+ = brisker than average and possibly but not necessarily indicative of disease 4+ = hyperactive		• Deep tendon reflexes may be hypoactive in the presence of hypercalcemia, hypermagnesemia, hyponatremia, hypokalemia, and acidosis.
• Behavior • Sensation • Fatigue Level	• Because these changes are often vague, they are best evaluated in context with specific imbalances.		

(Data from Metheny, N. M. [1992]. *Fluid and electrolyte balance* [2nd ed.]. Philadelphia: Lippincott.)

pensates for a metabolic acid–base imbalance by regulating CO_2 levels. When compensation occurs,the $PaCO_2$ and the HCO_3^- will always point in the same direction. The focus of compensation efforts is to return the pH to the normal range.

Respiratory acidosis:
$\downarrow$pH <7.35 $\uparrow PaCO_2$ $\uparrow HCO_3^-$ (compensation attempt)

Respiratory alkalosis:
$\uparrow$pH >7.45 $\downarrow PaCO_2$ $\downarrow HCO_3^-$ (compensation attempt)

Metabolic acidosis:
$\downarrow$pH <7.35 $\downarrow HCO_3^-$ $\downarrow PaCO_2$ (compensation attempt)

Metabolic alkalosis:
$\uparrow$pH >7.45 $\uparrow HCO_3^-$ $\uparrow PaCO_2$ (compensation attempt)

4. Look at the total picture and determine if compensation has occurred. Compensation is classified as follows:

Absent if:
pH abnormal
One component abnormal
Second component within normal range

Partial if:
pH abnormal
One component abnormal
Second component beginning to change

Complete if:
pH within normal range
One component abnormal
Second changed to move pH within normal range

DIAGNOSING

Fluid and Electrolyte Disturbances as the Problem. When assessment data point to fluid and electrolyte problems amenable to nursing therapy, they receive one of three diagnostic labels:

Fluid Volume Excess
Fluid Volume Deficit
Risk for Fluid Volume Deficit

Excess fluid volume may result from greatly increased fluid intake, or more frequently from decreased excretion such as occurs in progressive renal disease and with certain cancers. FVDs may result from decreased intake; increased excretion of fluids; fluid shifts; and the special need for fluids and electrolytes created by strenuous exercise, extreme heat or dryness, and conditions (eg, fever) that increase the metabolic rate. The accompanying box presents contributing factors and defining characteristics for these diagnoses.

The nurse's analysis of assessment data may also lead to the diagnosis of specific electrolyte or acid–base disturbances that are termed collaborative problems because they require joint intervention by nursing and medicine (see Tables 46-4 and 46-5).

Fluid and Electrolyte Disturbances as the Etiology. Disturbances in fluid, electrolyte, and acid–base balance may affect many other areas of human functioning. Sample diagnoses follow:

Activity Intolerance related to dyspnea on exertion
Anxiety related to pulmonary edema

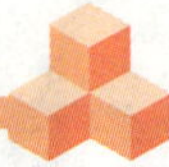

Guidelines for Nursing Care

Measuring Fluid Intake and Output

As soon as measured intake and output is ordered for the client, the client and family are instructed that the nurse needs a record of all fluids entering the body and all fluid output. A simple explanation of why this is being done is offered as well as specific instructions as to how the client can help to keep his or her record accurate. Some clients may need to be reminded during nursing rounds each morning that this measurement will continue.

The client's plan of care and nursing Kardex are used to communicate to nursing personnel the need to measure fluid intake and output. A sign posted in the client's room and bedside form for recording intake and output are helpful reminders for both the client and nurses.

The client's fluid intake includes the following:

- All fluids and foods that are liquid at room temperature (ice cream, gelatin dessert [Jell-O], and so forth)
  Use the agency's designation of specific volumes for common food containers (eg, juice glass = 90 mL; milk carton = 240 mL).
  Remind the client that sips of water or other fluids in between meals need to be recorded; small disposable calibrated cups at the bedside facilitate accurate measurement.
  Remember that liquid medications or water taken with pills may significantly increase the fluid intake of some clients.
- All parenteral fluids
- Other fluids taken into the body: subcutaneous fluids, fluids instilled into drainage tubes, enema solutions

The client's fluid output includes the following:

- Urine; vomitus; diarrhea; drainage from fistulas, wounds, and ulcers; and drainage from suctioning devices. Calibrated measuring devices should be readily available for accurate measurement. Disposable, calibrated urine collection containers that fit under the toilet seat are available for ambulatory clients. Urine or liquid feces in diapers or bed clothes, vomitus on clothing or bed linens, wound drainage saturating dressings, and so forth, need to be estimated.
- Heavy perspiration should be noted on the output record especially when the client's clothing or bed linens are soaked.
- Hyperventilation (water vapor loss) should also be noted on the output record. Record rate and depth of respirations.

Both intake and output should be measured whenever possible, rather than estimated. Output measurement is described in Chapter 43. Failure to record intake or output when it is measured may result in its being forgotten.

Intake and output totals are generally recorded for each 8-hour shift and totaled each 24 hours. At the conclusion of each shift, the alert client should be questioned about his or her intake and output.

Ineffective Breathing Pattern related to compensatory mechanism by lungs (hypoventilation or hyperventilation)
Decreased Cardiac Output related to decreased blood volume, shock
Risk for Injury related to neuromuscular irritability, cardiac arrhythmia
Knowledge Deficit: Harmful Effects of Abuses of Dieting, Alcohol, Diuretics, Laxatives, and Enemas, related to no previous experience
Altered Oral Mucous Membrane related to dehydration
Impaired Skin Integrity related to dehydration, edema
Altered Thought Processes related to cerebral edema, mental confusion or disorientation, convulsions
Altered Tissue Perfusion: [specify type] related to decreased cardiac output
Altered Urinary Elimination related to decreased kidney perfusion secondary to decreased plasma volume

Table 46-8
Acid–Base Parameters

	Normal	Acid	Base
pH	7.35–7.45	<7.35	>7.45
$PaCO_2$	35–45	>45	<35
HCO_3^-	22–26	<22	>26

PLANNING: EXPECTED OUTCOMES

Nursing care for any client supports the following expected outcomes. The healthy adult client will:

- Maintain an approximate balance between fluid intake and fluid output (average about 2500 mL fluid intake and output over 3 days)
- Maintain a urine SG within normal range (1.010 to 1.025)
- Practice self-care behaviors to promote fluid, electrolyte, and acid–base balance—maintain adequate intake of fluid and electrolytes; respond appropri-

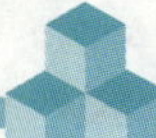

Nursing Diagnoses for Common Problems

Fluid and Electrolyte Balance

Problem	Related Factors	Sample Defining Characteristics
Fluid Volume Excess	Pathophysiologic factors: renal failure, decreased cardiac output, liver disease, abnormal fluid accumulations, hormonal problems	• "I've noticed that my wedding ring is tight . . . also my clothes don't fit as well as they used to. I guess I've gained some weight." • Reports dyspnea with exertion, feeling weak and fatigued • Pitting edema in feet, ankles, lower legs • Taut, shiny skin • Jugular venous distention
	Situational factors: excessive IV infusion	• Bounding pulse, increased from baseline • Shallow, rapid respirations, rales • Increased blood pressure
	Nutritional factors: excessive sodium intake, low protein intake	• 10-lb (4.5-kg) weight gain over past month • Fluid intake greater than output • "Sometimes I can't catch my breath and I feel like my heart is pounding away." • "I feel bloated."
Fluid Volume Deficit Risk for Fluid Volume Deficit	Decreased fluid intake: imposed fluid restrictions, inability to obtain or swallow fluids (debilitation, oral pain), depression	• "After I got the flu I got so weak I couldn't get out of bed. . . . I think I was out of it for a couple of days." • Increased pulse and respirations • Dry oral mucosa, cracked lips, furrowed tongue • Scanty urine output
	Abnormal fluid loss: vomiting; diarrhea; abnormal drainage; excessive use of laxative, enemas, diuretics; blood loss; diaphoresis; burns	• "I'm thirsty all the time." • "I've been vomiting and I have diarrhea—several times a day." • Weight loss: 5 lb (2–3 kg) • Urine is concentrated (specific gravity, 1.035). • Fluid output greater than fluid intake • Neck veins collapsed when lying flat • Decreased skin turgor
	Increased need for fluids: strenuous exercise, extreme heat or dryness, fever (increased metabolic rate)	• Skin is warm to touch, moist, and flushed • Increased temperature, pulse, respirations • Decreased blood pressure

ately to body's signals of impending fluid, electrolyte, or acid–base imbalance

When an imbalance exists, the client will:

- Relate relief of symptoms (specify) after implementation of treatment regimen (eg, 1 month after decreasing sodium intake client reports 4 lb [1.8 kg] weight loss)

IMPLEMENTING

Nursing interventions to prevent or correct fluid, electrolyte, and acid–base imbalances include dietary modification, modification of fluid intake, medication administration, IV therapy, blood and blood products replacement, and TPN.

Preventing Fluid Imbalances

An adequate fluid intake and a well-balanced, nutritious diet with appropriate adjustments throughout the life cycle are essential to promote fluid balance. The following are some of the basic items the nurse needs to consider to help prevent fluid imbalances:

- Be familiar with common events in life that lead to fluid imbalances, and observe the client carefully. Infants are particularly vulnerable to fluid imbalances because body water accounts for a greater percentage of their weight and fluid fluctuations are more common. Loss of fluid due to an illness can cause serious and life-threatening problems in infants.
- Note the client's present fluid and food intake, and learn what his or her previous eating and drinking patterns have been. Learn whether the client has used fad diets, which may lead to imbalances.
- Note whether thirst is excessive or whether the client experiences little or no thirst. Thirst is a subjective sensation and an important factor in determining water intake and, eventually, output through the kidneys. Thirst is poorly understood, although both psychologic and physiologic factors appear to be involved.
- Be aware of excessive losses of fluids from the body, and attempt to prevent losses when possible. Vomiting, pronounced perspiration, diarrhea, draining wounds, and excessive urinary output, for example, may cause excessive losses.
- Consider ways in which the client's medical regimen may lead to imbalances. For example, diuretics which stimulate urine formation may increase the elimination of potassium. If food supplements high in potassium are not included in the diet or if drug therapy is not started, hypokalemia often follows (refer to Table 46-4 for clinical manifestations). Corticosteroids may lead to sodium and water retention and to excessive potassium excretion.
- Learn whether the client has been "treating" himself or herself and, as a result, threatening fluid balance. Common practices that threaten fluid balance include the indiscriminate use of enemas, laxatives, antacids, and over-the-counter drugs to promote urination.
- Consider conditions that induce destructive effects on the body as threats to fluid balance. Examples include immobilization, trauma, burns, surgical procedures, and exposure to toxic agents.
- Teach clients to observe for fluid imbalances and to report them promptly. Examples include rapid weight gains and losses; swollen fingers, feet, and ankles; puffy eyelids; muscle weakness; change in skin sensations; and scanty or profuse urine production.
- Help clients and their families understand the significance of maintaining fluid balance and preventing imbalances.
- Be aware that normal physiologic changes associated with aging impact on the elder client's ability to maintain fluid balance. Dehydration is a common fluid and electrolyte disorder in this population. The accompanying box suggests specific nursing strategies to prevent and correct fluid and electrolyte imbalance.

Developing a Dietary Plan

Simple dietary changes may help to resolve fluid and electrolyte disturbances. After doing a nutritional assessment to identify actual or potential imbalances and food

Focus on the Older Adult

Nursing Strategies for Ensuring Fluid Balance in Older Adults

Decrease in Total Body Weight

- Ensure that oral intake is at least 1500 mL for 24 hours.
- Assess for signs of dehydration or fluid retention.
- Assess 24-hour intake and output for consistency and balance.
- Teach family to notify physician when persistent diarrhea or vomiting occur.
- Assess skin turgor and mucous membranes.
- Be aware of schedule for diagnostic tests (and associated dietary and fluid restrictions).
- Assess medication history for drugs that have a diuretic action or require additional fluid intake.

Altered Sense of Thirst

- Offer fluids at regular intervals.
- Replace fluids as necessary either orally or IV.
- Investigate individual fluid preferences.
- Provide assistance or assistive devices for encouraging fluid intake.

Loss of Nephrons and Decreased Renal Blood Flow

- Record output accurately.
- Note appearance and specific gravity of urine.
- Check laboratory values for abnormal levels.

preferences, the nurse can initiate teaching. It is important to involve both the client and the person who prepares the meals in the development of the nutritional plan. The plan should include foods that both help to resolve the fluid or electrolyte imbalance and are acceptable to the client. For example, for FVD, increase foods with high water content (eg, citrus fruit, melons, celery); for hypokalemia, increase foods with high potassium content (eg, bananas, citrus fruits, apricots, melons, broccoli, potatoes); for hypernatremia, avoid foods high in sodium (eg, processed cheese, lunch meats, canned soups and vegetables, salted snack foods) and eliminate use of table salt.

When given a list of foods, the client should be able to identify those that can be eaten freely or moderately as well as those that should be avoided. Both the client and person responsible for food preparation should be able to describe a 24-hour diet plan compatible with the recommended modifications.

Modifying Fluid Intake

Depending on the nature of the fluid or electrolyte imbalance, a client's fluids may need to be increased, decreased, or modified in terms of types of fluids ingested. The nurse is responsible for:

- Identifying the appropriate fluid modification (with certain illnesses, the physician may order fluid directives [eg, "Restrict fluids to 1000 mL/d"])
- Determining if the client understands the rationale for the fluid modification, is motivated to comply with the modification, and is capable of compliance (eg, a bedridden client who needs to increase fluid intake cannot do this independently)
- Developing and implementing a plan of care based on the preceding information. For example, three clients with the same tendency to retain fluids may need different nursing care. One has never learned that the high-sodium beverages she frequently drinks are contributing to her problem. One teaching session may be sufficient to resolve her fluid imbalance. A second client has a history of poor self-care behaviors. Intelligent and the recipient of much health education in the past, this client has no need for further teaching. Nursing time is best invested in counseling and exploring why the client fails to value his health sufficiently to comply with the treatment regimen. Until the client values the proposed fluid modification, compliance will probably be poor. The third client is a frail older woman with pneumonia and a history of congestive heart failure who depends on the nursing staff for care. Her fluid intake will be determined by the fluids offered her by the nursing staff. This client's fluid retention may also be affected by diuretic medication which has most likely been prescribed for her and places her at risk for fluid deficits and potassium imbalances.

Increasing Fluids

An above-average intake of fluids is prescribed for certain clients. The usual order reads, "Force fluids," and indicates the amount of fluid the client is to have in each 24-hour period. The plan of care should specify the amount of fluid to be ingested in 24 hours (for hospitalized clients shift totals are helpful [eg, 7 to 3, 1200 mL; 3 to 11, 900 mL; 11 to 7, 300 mL]) and the client's food preferences. Fluids should be chosen that best provide the calories and electrolytes needed by the client.

A variety of techniques is recommended to help the client take more than average amounts of fluids:

- Explain to the client in understandable terms the specific goal of taking the daily amount of fluid prescribed for the client. This helps promote motivation and is more meaningful than simply telling the client to increase fluid intake.
- Mutually establish short-term goals with the client. Examples include a glass of water every hour, a particular beverage by the time a television program is finished, or a pitcher of water by lunch. Most clients try to reach goals that they help to set, even when they do not feel thirsty.
- Plan to offer a proportionately larger amount of fluid during the early hours of the client's waking day. The client is usually able to take fluids relatively easily after having few or no fluids during sleeping hours.
- Try to avoid making it necessary to offer large amounts of fluid before sleep. This helps prevent disturbing rest because the client needs to urinate.
- Encourage as wide a variety of liquids as possible to make larger intake more interesting and palatable. If clients dislike taking fluids (a common problem with children) or have swallowing difficulties, offering a gelatin dessert (Jell-O), flavored frozen water (Popsicles), water ice, and so forth may meet with more success.
- Keep fluids readily available for the client. It is distressing to see people who are unable to secure their own fluids left with an unfilled water pitcher, an empty glass, a full pitcher out of reach, or a pitcher too heavy to lift.
- Serve fluids at the appropriate temperature. For example, the client is likely to drink more when iced liquids are iced and cold, and coffee and tea when they are hot but not so hot that the client is likely to be burned.
- Use attractive, clean, and easily handled cups and glasses, a practice that helps to encourage the client's desire to take fluids.
- Have the client assist in keeping a record of his or her intake when this is possible. This often serves as a motivating factor to increase fluid intake.
- Provide support, understanding, and encouragement because forcing fluid intake for the person experiencing no thirst can be uncomfortable.

Increasing the fluid intake of clients is among the most common nursing care objectives. Often, creativity and considerable patience by the nurse are necessary to reach desired goals. The box indicates nursing interventions that focus on maintaining fluid balance. Fluids may also be replaced through nasogastric, gastrostomy, or jejunostomy tubes and any irrigations of these tubes also need to be included in the fluid balance summary (see Chapter 42).

Restricting Fluids

Restricting the client's fluid intake is sometimes necessary. The usual order reads, "Restrict fluids," and indicates the amount of fluid the client is to have in each 24-hour period.

A variety of techniques is recommended to help the client restrict the intake of fluids:

- Explain to the client in understandable terms the specific goal of taking the daily amount of fluid prescribed. This often helps promote motivation and is more meaningful to the client than simply telling him or her to restrict fluid intake.
- Discuss with the client the time intervals at which fluids will be served. Usually, it is best to offer fluids between meals because food often helps to relieve some feelings of thirst.
- Mutually establish short-term or interim goals for offering small amounts of fluids at 1- or 2-hour intervals when this seems helpful and when the client can cooperate.
- Serve ice chips instead of water from time to time. When they melt, the water is about one half of its volume when frozen.
- Use small glasses or cups so that the container appears to contain more fluid than it actually does. Large containers partially full make the amount of fluid seem smaller than it actually is.
- Provide oral hygiene at regular intervals so that the client's mouth remains clean. Lubricate the lips and mucous membranes as indicated.
- Allow the cooperative client to rinse the mouth with water without swallowing the fluid and exceeding the intake limit.
- Avoid offering the client dry, salty, or sweet foods and fluids, because they tend to increase thirst.
- Avoid offering the client hard candy or gum. They were often thought to relieve thirst by stimulating salivation. The sugar content increases oral tonicity

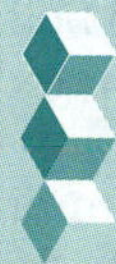

Research in Nursing: Making a Difference

Fluid and Electrolyte Balance

Monitoring and maintaining fluid and electrolyte balance in clients is a major component of nursing care. The older population is particularly at risk for life-threatening imbalances. Unfortunately, little research has been carried out by nurses with respect to fluid and electrolyte status.

Related Research

Pals, J., Weinberg, A., Beal, L., Levesque, P., Cunningham, T., & Minaker, K. (1995). Clinical triggers for detection of fever and dehydration: Implications for long-term care nursing. *Journal of Gerontological Nursing, 21*(4), 13–19.

Fever among long-term care residents is a common problem. In a group of 130 residents studied over a 4-month period, 48 febrile episodes (FEs) were detected with the majority of temperature checks initiated by the staff. An FE was defined as a temperature greater than 100.0°F orally or 101.0°F rectally. Only one elevated temperature was found through the routine monthly monitoring. During FEs, either an elevated serum sodium or BUN/creatinine ratio was reported when oral intake declined. Because the symptoms of fever, infection, and dehydration displayed by the residents may be vague and nonspecific, nurses need to assess older residents continually in order to initiate early intervention.

Knox, D., & Martof, M. (1995). Effects of drug therapy on renal function of healthy older adults. *Journal of Gerontological Nursing, 21*(4), 35–40.

Physiologic changes associated with aging can affect the maintenance of fluid balance in the older person. Drug use, both prescription and over-the-counter, increases the risk of developing renal insufficiency in this population. NSAIDs, diuretics, anti-hypertensives, and estrogen therapy are particularly nephrotoxic. This study reported that nurses should encourage increased oral intake and accurately record intake and output to identify any imbalance or inadequacy in hospitalized older persons. Nurses also need to assess an older client's OTC drug intake carefully and focus on collecting information for the nursing history that will aid in early recognition of the development of renal insufficiency.

Summary

Routine nursing interventions that focus on fluid and electrolyte status include daily maintenance of intake and output records and monitoring client's weight, temperature, and laboratory values. Additional research is needed to determine more effective ways nurses can help clients of all ages maintain fluid and electrolyte balance.

and temporarily draws fluids to the mouth membranes. After about 15 to 30 minutes, the membranes are even more dry than before. Sugarless gum may be offered to some clients.
- Divert the client's attention from thirst by involving him or her in various activities to the degree that he or she is able to participate.
- Keep fluids not intended for the client out of sight.
- Have the client assist in keeping an intake record when possible. This may serve as a motivating factor to limit fluid intake.
- Provide understanding, support, and encouragement because limiting fluid intake for the person experiencing thirst is uncomfortable.

Administering Medications

Clients with fluid, electrolyte, and acid–base imbalances are often prescribed medications as part of the therapeutic regimen. Nurses need to be knowledgeable about the therapeutic effects of mineral–electrolyte preparations and diuretics as well as alert for adverse effects of other medications such as steroids and hormone replacements.

Mineral–Electrolyte Preparations. Mineral–electrolyte preparations are frequently prescribed to correct electrolyte imbalances. Nursing responsibilities include:
- Accurately administering the medications, following manufacturer's guidelines (eg, dilute oral potassium supplements to disguise the unpleasant taste and decrease gastric irritation; monitor ABGs for increased pH after each 50 to 100 mEq of sodium bicarbonate to avoid overtreatment and metabolic alkalosis). There are more fatal medication errors with potassium chloride for injection concentrate than with any other medication (Davis, 1995). Efforts continue to work toward the withdrawal of IV potassium chloride concentrate from client-care areas since it may be mistaken for sodium chloride flush solutions and accidentally used to flush a catheter with fatal results (Cohen, 1996).
- Knowing and evaluating the intended therapeutic effect (eg, with magnesium sulfate, look for decreased restlessness and irritability, decreased muscle tremors, and control of convulsions)
- Assessing for adverse effects (eg, with sodium chloride injection, observe for hypernatremia and circulatory overload)
- Assessing for drug interactions (eg, drugs that increase the effects of minerals and electrolytes include acidifying agents, alkalinizing agents, cation exchange resin, iron salts, and potassium salts)
- Teaching the clients appropriate self-care behaviors

Diuretics. Diuretics are drugs that increase renal excretion of water, sodium, and other electrolytes. Although helpful in treating clients with FVE, they increase the risk of dehydration and serious electrolyte deficiencies. Clients need careful monitoring (eg, check urine output and serum K^+ level) and education while on diuretic therapy.

Administering Intravenous Therapy

A relatively common form of therapy for handling fluid disturbances is the use of various solutions infused by vein (IV). IV therapy is delivered annually to millions of clients in homes and hospitals. Eight of ten hospitalized clients are on intravenous therapy (Hastings-Tolsma & Yucha, 1994). The physician is responsible for prescribing the kind and amount of solution to be used. The nurse is responsible for initiating, monitoring, and discontinuing the therapy. As is true with other therapeutic agents, the nurse should understand the client's need for IV therapy, the type of solution being used, its desired effect, and untoward reactions that may occur. Contents of selected water and electrolyte solutions with comments about their use are presented in Table 46-9.

Equipment

Sterile technique is observed when a vein is entered. Disposable infusion tubing and needles are used to help eliminate many possible sources of contamination and to reduce the cost of equipment aftercare.

Equipment varies according to the manufacturer. The nurse is responsible for being familiar with the equipment used in the agency or home setting. Typically, the majority of solutions for infusions are dispensed in 1-L or 500-mL flexible or rigid plastic containers. Currently, the glass system is used infrequently. Plastic bags collapse under atmospheric pressure as the solution enters the client's vein and do not require air to replace fluid flowing from the container. Rigid containers, such as glass bottles, cannot collapse. Therefore, they have an air vent that allows air to replace fluid as it enters the client's vein. Small 50- and 100-mL solution bags are available to administer intermittent IV medications (such as antibiotics given IV piggyback).

Many options are available for the IV tubing that is attached to the solution container. A basic administration set is illustrated in Figure 46-10. A spike or piercing pin is inserted into the container usually with a twisting motion. The rate of flow is manually controlled by a clamp or constricting device on the tubing. A device called a dripmeter or dripchamber connects the solution bottle and tubing and permits the number of drops per minute of solution to be determined.

There are a variety of needles and catheters commonly used for the IV infusion. IV catheters are plastic tubes that have been mounted on a needle or are threaded through a needle for insertion. Once inserted, the needle is withdrawn and the flexible catheter remains in the vein. The over-the-needle catheter is easy

Table 46-9
Selected IV Solutions With Comments About Their Use

Solution	Comments
Isotonic Solutions	
5% dextrose in water (D_5W)	Supplies about 170 cal/L and free water to aid in renal excretion of solutes Should not be used in excessive volumes in clients with increased ADH activity or to replace fluids in hypovolemic patients
0.9% NaCl (normal saline)	Not desirable as a routine maintenance solution because it provides only Na^+ and Cl^-, which are provided in excessive amounts
Lactated Ringer's solution	A roughly isotonic solution that contains multiple electrolytes in approximately the same concentrations as found in plasma (note that this solution is lacking in Mg and PO_4) Used in the treatment of hypovolemia, burns, and fluid lost as bile or diarrhea Useful in treating mild metabolic acidosis
Hypotonic Solutions	
0.33% NaCl (⅓-strength saline)	A hypotonic solution that provides Na^+, Cl^-, and free water Na^+ and Cl^- allows kidneys to select and retain needed amounts Free water desirable as aid to kidneys in elimination of solutes
0.45% NaCl (½-strength saline)	A hypotonic solution that provides Na^+, Cl^- and free water Often used to treat hypernatremia (because this solution contains a small amount of Na^+, it dilutes the plasma sodium while not allowing it to drop too rapidly)
Hypertonic Solutions	
5% dextrose in 0.45% NaCl	A common hypertonic solution used to treat hypovolemia; used to maintain fluid intake
10% dextrose in water ($D_{10}W$)	Supplies 340 cal/L Used for peripheral parenteral nutrition (PPN)
5% dextrose in 0.9% NaCl (normal saline)	Replaces nutrients and electrolytes Can temporarily be used to treat hypovolemia if plasma expander is not available

(Data from Metheny, N. M. [1992]. *Fluid and electrolyte balance* [2nd ed.]. Philadelphia: Lippincott.)

to insert and stable, and its placement is easily detected with x-ray. Infiltration is rare with this device. Inside-the-needle catheters are rarely used because the potential exists for the needle to shear off the catheter during insertion. Single- or double-winged infusion needles (butterflies) are short-beveled, thin-walled needles with plastic flaps. They are used in pediatric settings and when short-term therapy is expected. Butterfly or scalp vein needles are not flexible and, thus, more likely to infiltrate. Other equipment necessary to start an IV infusion is listed in Procedure 46-1.

The nurse is the healthcare provider most at risk for a needlestick injury. Many devices are available that minimize potential for injury and promote safety when connecting, accessing, or disposing of IV equipment. Needleless systems and needle-housing systems where the needle is recessed and protected are becoming increasingly common. Refer to Chapters 28 and 29 for additional information about these protective measures.

Other Venous Access Devices

The *central venous catheter* (*CVC*) is usually introduced into the subclavian or internal jugular veins and passed to the superior vena cava just above the right atrium. In the United States, its use is becoming more common; some 3 million CVCs are inserted annually (Viall, 1990). Traditionally only used in critical care situations, CVCs are now common on medical–surgical units and in home care. They provide access for a variety of IV fluids and medications as well as a means for hemodynamic monitoring. CVCs may be used for short (up to 4 weeks) or long-term periods and have a single, double, or triple lumen or entry port. An example of CVC placement is illustrated in Figure 46-11. Long-term CVCs are made of flexible silicone rubber rather than the polyurethane used for short-term access and are less likely to result in thrombus formation. The Groshong long-term CVC is unique because pressure-sensitive valves seal off each lumen, further reducing the risk of complications and simplifying routine catheter maintenance. A short-term CVC may be inserted at the bedside under sterile conditions, whereas a long-term catheter is surgically inserted in the operating room and the proximal portion of the catheter is tunneled through subcutaneous fascia to an exit point on the chest wall below the nipple line. Both types of catheter require a chest x-ray to confirm proper placement before infusion of IV solutions begins. Discussion continues regarding the ideal dressing for the IV site. An occlusive dressing protects the insertion site. Transparent dressings have become more common in clinical practice because they allow easy inspection of

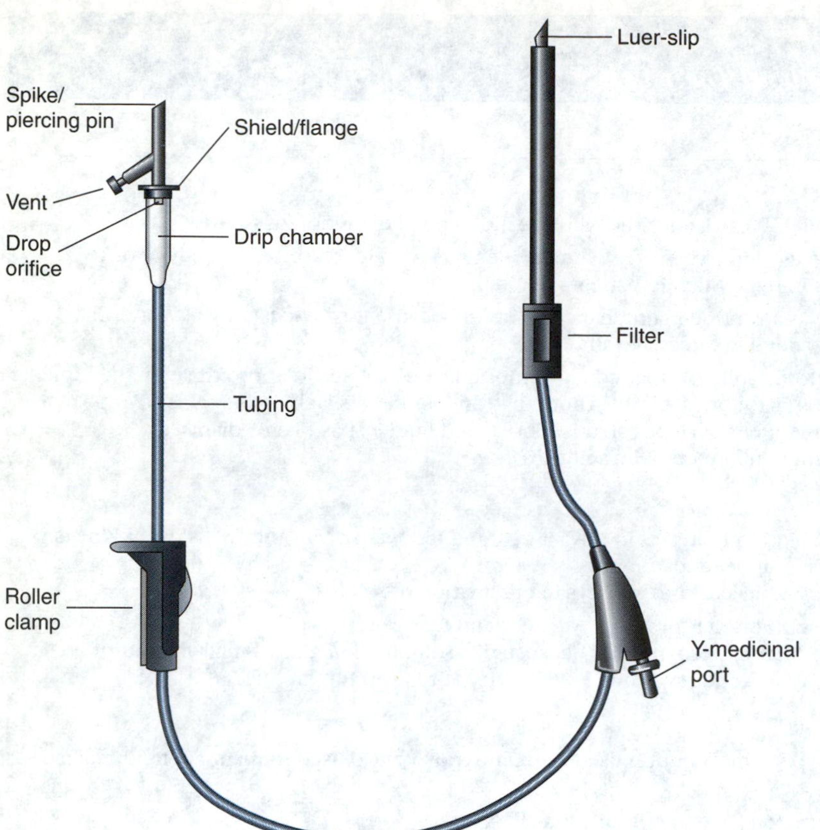

Figure 46-10
Basic administration set for intravenous therapy.

the IV site. Recent information indicates that the rate of bacterial colonization at the insertion site is higher with this type of dressing. Gauze and tape dressings are less likely to support growth of bacteria and are less expensive, but a view of the IV site is limited unless the dressing is removed or lifted. The tape can be irritating to client's skin and the dressing needs to be covered when the client showers or bathes. A newer transparent dressing is available that allows the nurse to see the site without removing the dressing and has small squares of gauze to absorb drainage. Agency policy generally determines the type of dressing and the intervals for dressing changes. The Intravenous Nurses Society recommends an IV dressing change every 48 hours while the CDC suggests changing them every 48 to 72 hours (Sheldon, 1994). (See Procedure 46-1 for additional information about IV dressing changes.)

Nursing responsibilities with CVCs include using sterile technique, changing the dressing according to agency policy, carefully assessing for any sign of infection, changing injection caps on the lumens, and flushing with a prescribed solution (usually saline and heparin) to prevent clotting and blockage of the lumen. Many agencies have a policy to discard the injection cap once it is removed (eg, when blood is drawn) and replace it with a sterile cap since contaminated caps have been implicated as a cause of systemic infections.

Peripherally inserted central catheters (*PICCs*) are a type of central venous access that can be introduced into a peripheral vein (usually the basilic or cephalic veins) ideally above or below the antecubital space and advanced as far as the superior vena cava (Fig. 46-12). X-ray verification is always required if the tip of the catheter is advanced beyond the axillary vein. They may be single- or multiple-lumen catheters. In many areas of the country, specially trained registered nurses are permitted by their state boards of nursing to insert these catheters (Sansivero, 1995; Green & Gerlach, 1994). PICCs are used extensively in the home for IV therapy and have become an increasingly popular venous access device in acute care settings. Indications for use of PICCs include administration of IV antibiotics for an extended period (2 to 6 weeks), infusion of parenteral nutrition, chemotherapy, continuous narcotic infusions, blood components, other specific medications (eg, vasopressors, anticoagulants), and long-term rehydration (Sansivero, 1995). Advantages of this type of IV access include a decreased risk of pneumothorax because of peripheral insertion, cost effectiveness, less pain and discomfort because multiple venipunctures are unnecessary, and reliability (Phillips, 1993).

Nursing responsibilities include sterile dressing changes per agency schedule and protocol, routine heparin or saline flushes to maintain patency, and careful observation for any complications of PICC therapy such as phlebitis, cellulitis, infiltration, and infection or sepsis. The decreased risk of complications as well as the other

(text continues on page 1409)

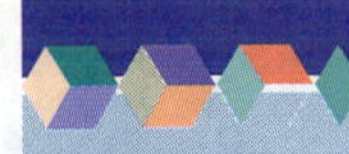

PROCEDURE 46-1

Starting an Intravenous Infusion

Equipment

- IV solution
- IV infusion set
- IV tubing
- IV catheter (over-the-needle, angiocath) or butterfly needle
- Tourniquet
- Cleansing swabs (alcohol, povidone-iodine)
- Towel or disposable pad
- Gauze or transparent dressing (according to agency policy)
- Antiseptic ointment (optional)
- Time tape or label (for IV container)
- Tape
- Electronic infusion device (if ordered)
- Armboard, if needed
- Clean gloves
- IV pole

Action	Rationale
1. Gather all equipment and bring to bedside. Check IV solution and medication additives with physician's order.	Having equipment available saves time and facilitates accomplishment of task. Ensures that client receives the correct IV solution and medication as ordered by physician.
2. Explain procedure to client.	Explanation allays client's anxiety.
3. Wash your hands.	Handwashing deters the spread of microorganisms.
4. Prepare IV solution and tubing:	
a. Maintain aseptic technique when opening sterile packages and IV solution	This prevents spread of microorganisms.
b. Clamp tubing, uncap spike, and insert into entry site on bag or bottle as manufacturer directs.	This punctures the seal in the IV bag or bottle.
c. Squeeze drip chamber and allow it to fill at least half way.	Suction effect causes fluid to move into drip chamber. Also prevents air from moving down the tubing.

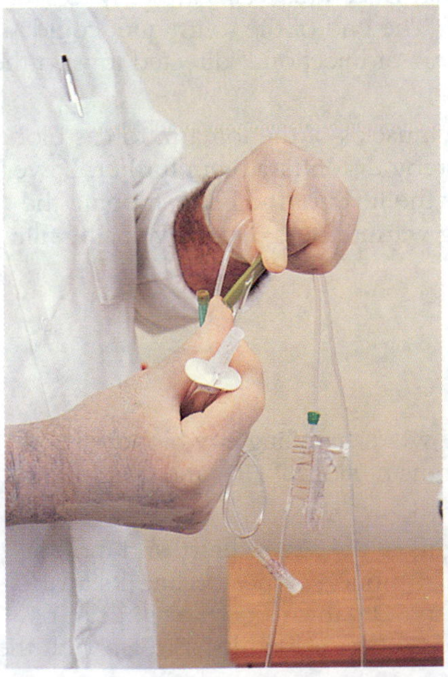

Action 4b: Clamping tubing.

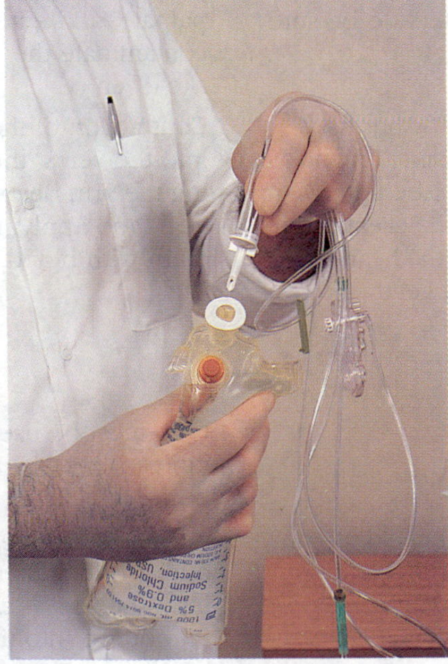

Action 4b: Inserting spike.

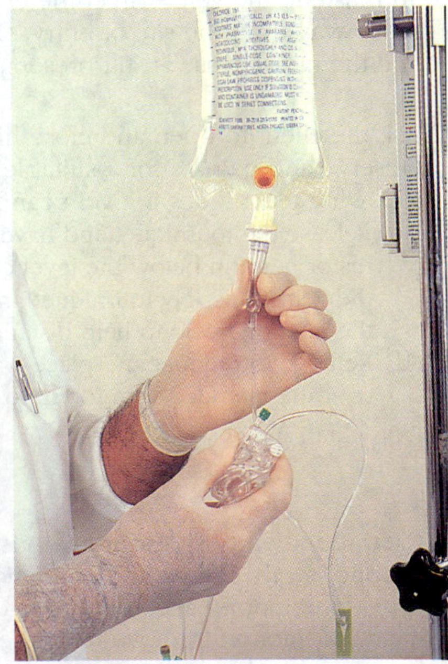

Action 4c: Squeezing drip chamber.

(continued)

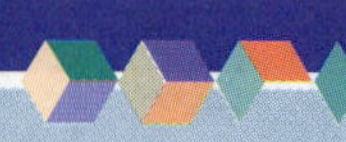

PROCEDURE 46-1 *(continued)*

Starting an Intravenous Infusion

Action	Rationale
d. Remove cap at end of tubing, release clamp, and allow fluid to move through tubing. Allow fluid to flow until all air bubbles have disappeared. Close clamp and recap end of tubing, maintaining sterility of setup.	This removes air from tubing that can, in larger amounts, act as an air embolus.
e. If an electronic device is to be used, follow manufacturer's instructions for inserting tubing and setting infusion rate.	This ensures correct flow rate and proper use of equipment.
f. Apply label if medication was added to container (pharmacy may have added medication and applied label).	Provides for administration of correct solution with prescribed medication or additive.
g. Place time-tape on container.	Permits immediate evaluation of IV according to schedule.
5. Have the client in a low Fowler's position in bed. Place protective towel or pad under client's arm.	The supine position permits either arm to be used and allows for good body alignment. The low Fowler's position is usually most comfortable for the client.
6. Select an appropriate site and palpate accessible veins.	The selection of an appropriate site decreases discomfort for the client and possible damage to body tissues.
7. If the site is hairy and agency policy permits, shave or clip a 2-inch area around the intended site of entry.	It is difficult to clean the site of entry in the presence of hair because hair can harbor microorganisms. Adhesive tape will adhere better and may be removed more easily if hair is removed from site.
8. Apply a tourniquet 5 to 6 inches above the venipuncture site to obstruct venous blood flow and distend the vein. Direct the ends of the tourniquet away from the site of entry. Check to be sure that the radial pulse is still present.	Interrupting the blood flow to the heart causes the vein to distend. Interruption of the arterial flow impedes venous filling. Distended veins are easy to see, palpate, and enter. The end of the tourniquet could contaminate the area of injection if directed toward the site of entry.
9. Ask the client to open and close his or her fist. Observe and palpate for a suitable vein. Try the following techniques if a vein cannot be felt: a. Release the tourniquet and have the client lower his or her arm below the level of the heart to fill the veins. Reapply tourniquet and gently tap over the intended vein to help distend it. b. Remove tourniquet and place warm compresses over the intended vein for 10 to 15 minutes.	Contraction of the muscles of the forearm forces blood into the veins, thereby distending them further. Lowering the arm below the level of the heart, tapping the vein, and applying warmth help distend veins by filling them with blood.
10. Don clean gloves.	Care must be used when handling any blood or body fluids to prevent transmission of HIV and other bloodborne infections.
11. Cleanse the entry site with an antiseptic solution (alcohol swab) followed by antimicrobial solution (povidone-iodine) according to agency policy. Use a circular motion to move from the center outward for several inches.	Cleansing that begins at the site of entry and moves outward in a circular motion carries organisms away from the site of entry. Organisms on the skin can be introduced into the tissues or the bloodstream with the needle.
12. Use the nondominant hand, placed about 1 inch or 2 inches below entry site, to hold the skin taut against the vein.	Pressure on the vein and surrounding tissues helps prevent movement of the vein as the needle or catheter is being inserted.

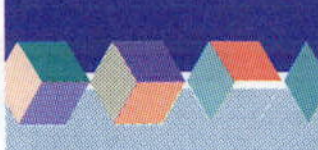

PROCEDURE 46-1 *(continued)*

Starting an Intravenous Infusion

Action	Rationale
13. Enter the skin gently with the catheter held by the hub in the dominant hand, bevel side up, at a 25- to 45-degree angle. The catheter may be inserted from either directly over the vein or the side of the vein. While following the course of the vein, advance the needle or catheter into the vein. A sensation of "give" can be felt when the needle enters the vein.	This allows needle or catheter to enter the vein with minimal trauma and deters passage of the needle through the vein.

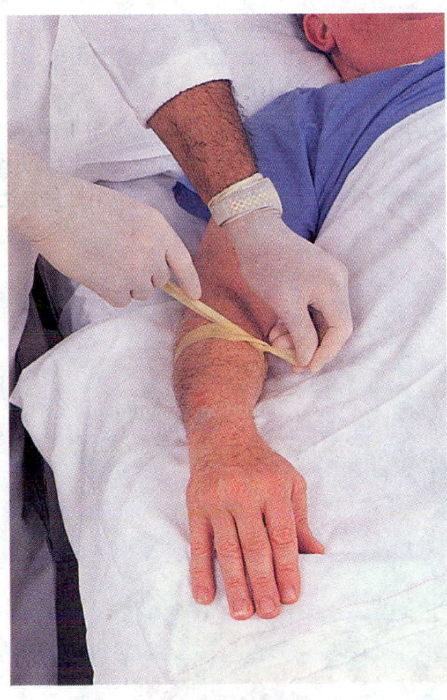

Action 8: Applying tourniquet.

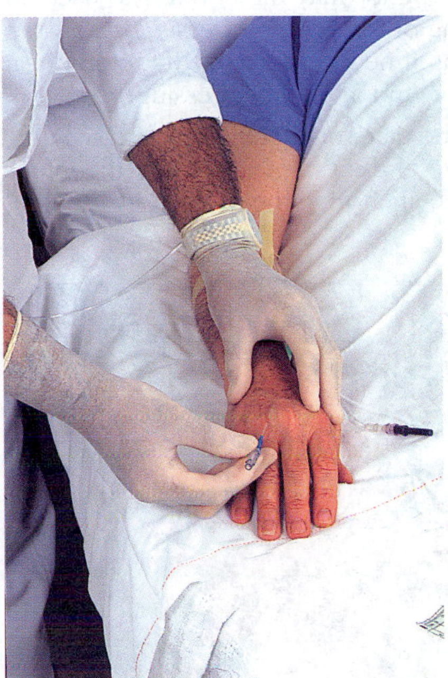

Action 13: Entering vein.

Action	Rationale
14. When blood returns through the lumen of the needle or the flashback chamber of the catheter, advance either device farther into the vein. A catheter needs to be advanced until the hub is at the venipuncture site but the exact technique depends on the type of device used.	The tourniquet causes increased venous pressure resulting in automatic backflow. Having the catheter placed well into the vein helps to prevent dislodgement.
15. Quickly remove protective cap from the IV tubing and attach the tubing to the catheter or needle. Stabilize the catheter or needle with nondominant hand and release the tourniquet with your other hand.	Bleeding is minimized and patency of the vein is maintained if the connection is made smoothly between the catheter and tubing.
16. Start the flow of solution promptly by releasing the clamp on the tubing. Examine the tissue around the entry site for signs of infiltration.	Blood clots readily if intravenous flow is not maintained. If catheter accidentally slips out of vein, solution will accumulate and infiltrate into surrounding tissue.
17. Support the catheter with small piece of gauze under the hub.	This helps to maintain the catheter in proper position in the vein.

(continued)

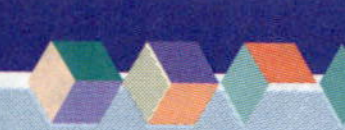

PROCEDURE 46-1 *(continued)*

Starting an Intravenous Infusion

Action	Rationale
18. Secure the catheter with narrow tape (½ in) placed sticky side up under the hub and crossed over the top of the hub.	The smooth structure of the vein does not offer resistance to the movement of the catheter. The weight of the tubing is sufficient to pull it out of the vein if it is not well anchored.
19. An antiseptic ointment may be applied to the catheter's site of entry if a gauze dressing will be applied.	Antiseptic ointment reduces skin contamination and protects against infection.
20. Place sterile dressing over venipuncture site. Agency policy may direct nurse to use gauze dressing or transparent dressing. Apply tape to dressing if necessary. Loop the tubing near the site of entry, and anchor to dressing.	Transparent dressing allows easy visualization of site but may place client at increased risk of infection. Gauze dressing absorbs drainage and may have a decreased infection rate. Discussion continues about effectiveness of types of dressings.
21. Mark the date, time, venipuncture site and type and size of the catheter used for the infusion on the tape anchoring the tubing.	Personnel working with the infusion will know what type of device is being used, the site, and when it was inserted. Protects client and IV site from infection.

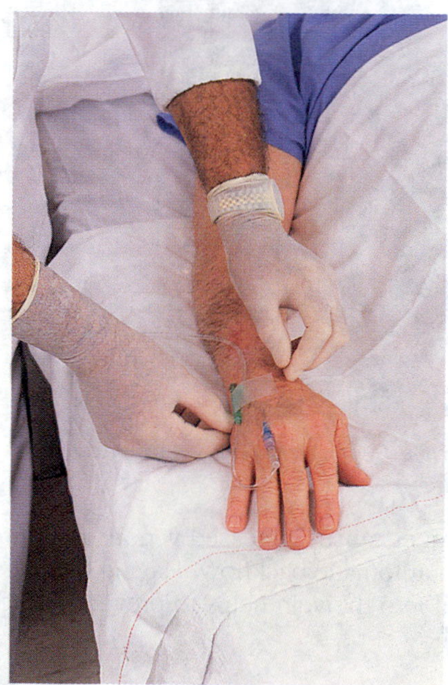

Action 20: Looping and anchoring tubing.

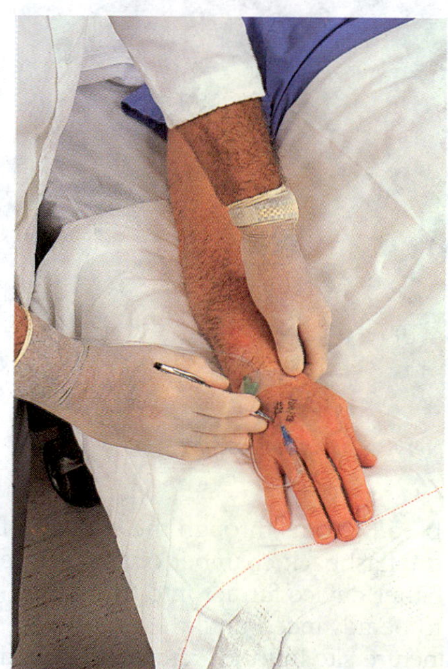

Action 21: Marking pertinent information on tape. (Photos © B. Proud.)

Action	Rationale
22. Anchor arm to an armboard for support, if necessary.	An armboard protects against change in the position of the vein and acts as a reminder to the client to minimize movements of his or her arm.
23. Adjust the rate of solution flow according to the amount prescribed or follow manufacturer's directions for adjusting flow rate on infusion pump.	The physician prescribes the rate of flow.

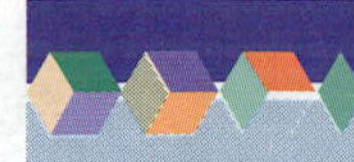

PROCEDURE 46-1 *(continued)*

Starting an Intravenous Infusion

Action	Rationale
24. Remove all equipment and dispose in proper manner. Remove gloves and wash hands.	Handwashing deters the spread of microorganisms.
25. Document the procedure and client's response. Chart time, site, device used, and solution.	This provides accurate documentation and ensures continuity of care.
26. Return to check flow rate and observe for infiltration 30 minutes after starting infusion.	This documents client's response to infusion.

Age Considerations

Tape is more likely to tear the thinner, more fragile skin of an older client. Special skin preparations (eg, Skin Prep) can be applied to the skin before taping.

In older clients, it may be necessary to delay rotating peripheral IV sites after a certain amount of days due to limited availability of locations.

Special Considerations

The Landry Vein Light Venoscope is a device developed to locate veins that are not easily seen or palpated. It consists of two fiber-optic probes that are placed on the skin several inches apart and shine an intense light into the client's subcutaneous tissue. The veins appear as dark lines under the skin. The venoscope can be used on any age or size client but requires a dimly lit or dark environment (Gonsoulin & Broussard, 1991).

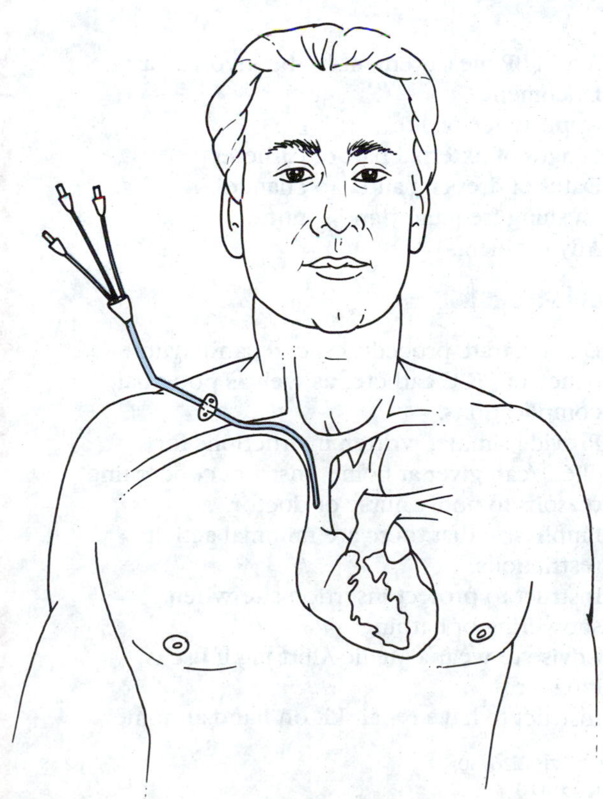

Figure 46-11
Placement of triple-lumen central venous catheter (CVC).

benefits of comfort, simplicity of insertion, and length of dwell time make PICCs an excellent alternative for many clients. Refer to the accompanying box for additional information related to nursing care of the client with a PICC catheter.

Another type of long-term CVC is an *implanted port.* The catheter tip is again placed in the subclavian or internal jugular vein but the proximal end or port is implanted in a subcutaneous pocket of the upper chest wall, abdomen, or thigh so that no external parts of the system are visible. Newer implanted ports are currently available for placement in the antecubital area of the arm and are referred to as peripheral access system ports or PAS ports. Initially, implanted ports were intended for chemotherapy but recently have also been used in home care clients as a route for TPN or IV antibiotics. A special angled needle is inserted through the skin and rubber septum and into the port reservoir (Fig. 46-13). Strict aseptic technique is necessary to prevent infection when an implanted venous port is accessed. Agency policy may require that the client as well as the nurse wear a mask when accessing the port. Care is minimal and involves a heparin flush before and after use or at least every 8 weeks (Christianson, 1994). Nurses have many opportunities for health teaching about medical and surgical asepsis and meticulous skin care as they care for clients with implanted ports.

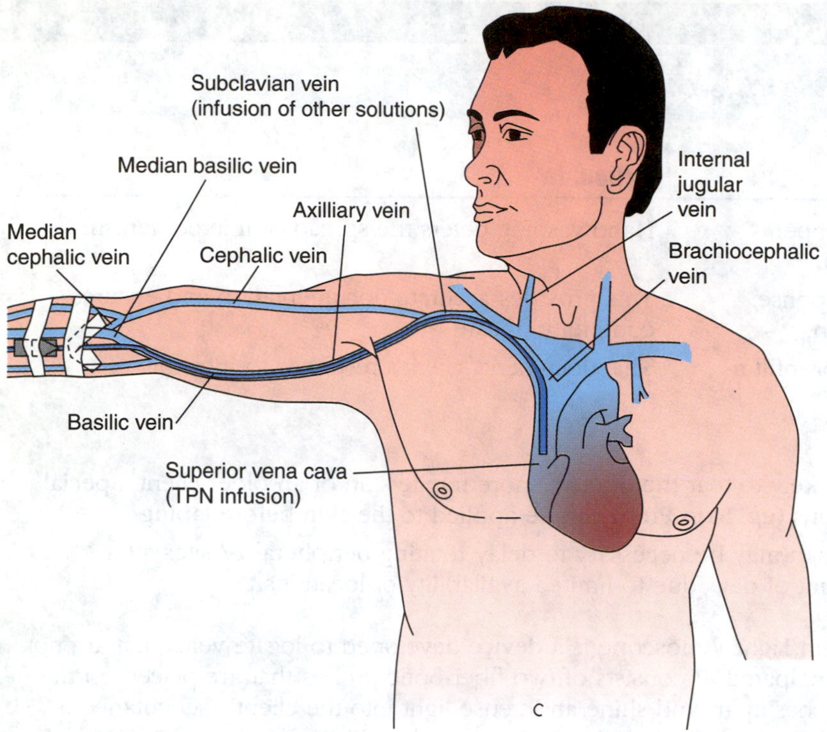

Figure 46-12
Placement of peripherally inserted central catheter (PICC).

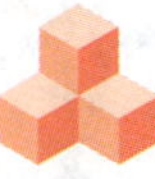

Guidelines for Nursing Care

Caring for a Client With a PICC

Maintenance

Always check agency policy for specific guidelines.

- Use sterile technique when changing dressings (24 hours after insertion and once a week thereafter). Also change dressing if soiled or loose.
- When accessing port or changing dressing, many agencies require nurse and client to wear a mask.
- Keep external portion of catheter coiled under dressing.
- Change catheter caps every 3 to 7 days depending on frequency of access and agency policy. Many agencies have a policy to replace caps once they have been removed (eg, when blood is drawn).
- Flush: Using a 10cc syringe, flush *open-ended catheter* with heparin solution after intermittent use or every 12 hours if catheter is not currently in use. Using a 10cc syringe, flush a *close-ended catheter* with saline after each intermittent use or once a week if not in use.
- Avoid BP measurement in the involved arm.
- Document:
  Appearance of site
  Length of external part of catheter
  Dates of dressing and cap change
  Flushing frequency and routine
  Any problems

Client Instruction

- Demonstrate procedures, care, and maintenance of PICC catheter as well as potential complications.
- Provide simple, written instructions for client/caregiver at home. Instruct concerning reasons to notify nurse or doctor.
- Emphasize that there are minimal activity restrictions.
- Instruct to protect insertion site when showering or bathing.
- Advise to wear a Medic-Alert tag if use is long-term.
- Instruct to have repair kit on hand at home.

(Source: Greene, L., & Gerlach, C. [1994]. Central lines have moved out. *RN, 57*[5], 26–30; Sansivero, G. [1995]. Why pick a PICC: What you need to know. *RN, 58*[7], 35–41.)

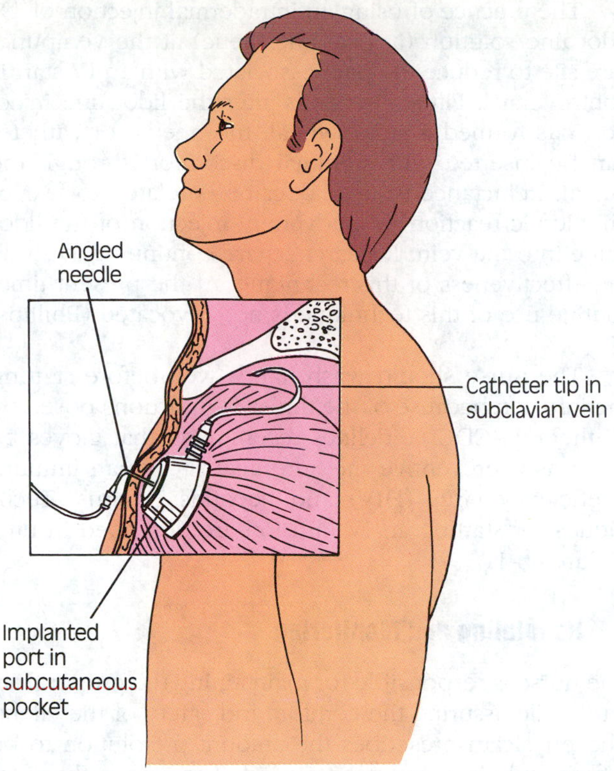

Figure 46-13
Placement of an implanted port with the tip in the subclavian vein. Angled needle is inserted through skin and rubber septum into port.

Site Selection

Suitability of veins for IV infusions varies with individual circumstances. Selection should be determined after considering several factors.

Accessibility of a Vein

- Determine the most desirable accessible vein. The lower cephalic vein, accessory cephalic vein, and the basilic vein are good sites for infusion. The superficial veins on the dorsal aspect of the hand can also be used successfully for some people. Figure 46-14 illustrates common infusion sites on the arm and hand. Either arm may be used for IV therapy. If the client is right-handed and both arms appear to be equally usable, usually the left arm is selected to free the right arm for the client's use.
- Determine accessibility based on the client's condition. For example, a person with severe burns on both forearms does not have vessels available in these areas.
- Avoid the antecubital veins for long-term infusions. They are not a good choice for infusion because flexion of the client's arm can displace the needle or catheter over an extended period. These vessels are quite satisfactory for blood withdrawal or for small amounts of IV medication administration.
- Avoid veins in the leg, unless other sites are inaccessible, because of the danger of stagnation of peripheral circulation and possible serious complications.
- Avoid veins in surgical areas. For example, infusions in the arm should not be given on the same side as recent extensive breast surgery, because of vascular disturbances in the area, or in an arm with a dialysis access device (eg, fistula or shunt).
- Select scalp veins for infants because of their accessibility and because of relative ease of preventing dislocation of the needle.

Condition of the Vein

- Determine the condition of the vein. Thin-walled and scarred veins, especially in some older clients,

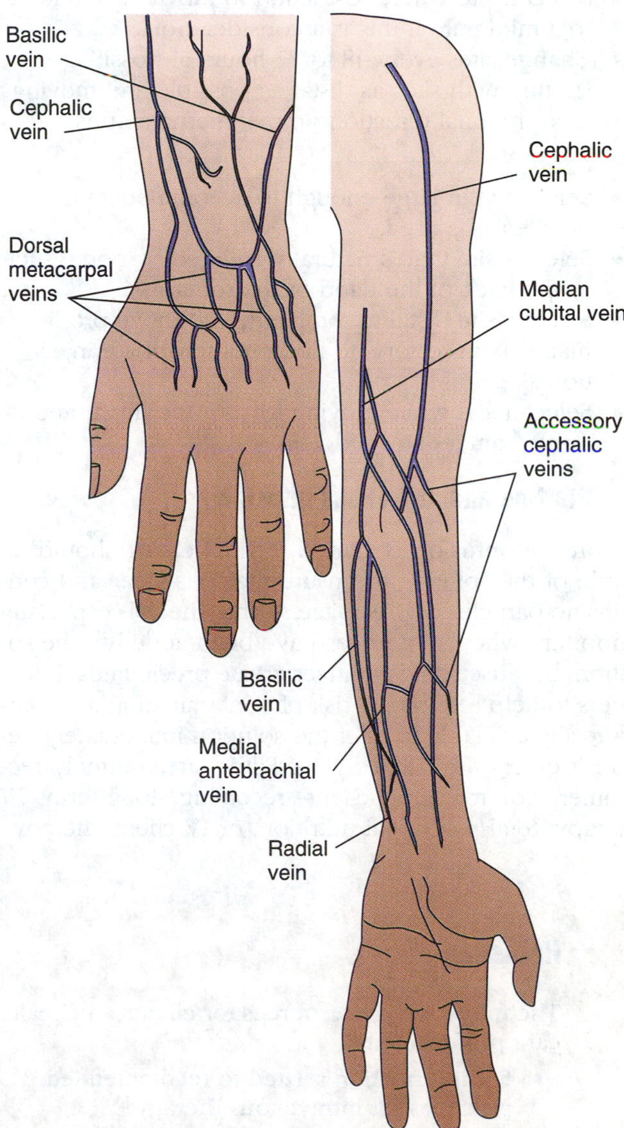

Figure 46-14
Infusion sites on the ventral and dorsal aspects of the lower arm and hand.

make continued infusion a problem. Experience helps the nurse acquire skill in palpating veins to determine their general condition.

Type of Fluid to Be Infused

- Select a vein appropriate for the solution. Hypertonic solutions, those containing irritating medications, those administered at a rapid rate, and those with a high viscosity should be given in a large vein to minimize vessel trauma and to facilitate the rate of flow.
- Advise the client that some medications administered intravenously in a peripheral vein may cause irritation and pain (eg, potassium chloride and certain antibiotics) and the nurse should be notified if this occurs.

Anticipated Duration of Infusion

- Select a site where restriction in movement is kept to a minimum if this is a consideration.
- Change sites every 48 to 72 hours, if possible, starting with sites as distal as possible and moving in a proximal direction on the alternate arms.

Other

- Select a vein large enough to accommodate the needle to be used.
- Select a site that is naturally splinted by bone, such as the back of the hand or the forearm.
- Select a site distal to the heart, and move proximally, as necessary, to find an appropriate injection site.
- Select a site while moving toward the heart, and away from a damaged vein.

Starting an Intravenous Infusion

Before the infusion is started, a final check should be made of the solution to ensure that it is clear and contains no particles or precipitates. This check is especially important when substances have been added to the solution, because some additives create precipitates. Inline filters to help reduce the risk of contamination are commercially available to filter the solution immediately before it enters the client's vein. Filters are routinely recommended for any client receiving long-term IV therapy, total parenteral nutrition, or IV chemotherapy.

The practice of using an intradermal injection of 1% lidocaine solution (a local anesthetic) at the venipuncture site to reduce the pain associated with an IV start is controversial. Fifteen seconds after the lidocaine injection has formed a small wheal, the needle or catheter can be inserted with minimal discomfort through the wheal. Reluctance to use lidocaine is related to fear of an allergic reaction or inadvertent injection of the lidocaine into the vein. Researchers are continuing to study the effectiveness of this technique. At the present time, routine use of this technique is not advocated (Phillips, 1993).

The nurse should wash hands well before starting the infusion because of the threat of infections posed by IV therapy. CDC guidelines recommend that gloves be worn as a preventive measure against human immunodeficiency virus (HIV) and hepatitis B virus. Techniques for starting an IV infusion are described in Procedure 46-1.

Regulating and Monitoring

The nurse is responsible for maintaining the proper flow rate while assuring the comfort and safety of the client. The physician prescribes the amount of solution to be infused within a specified period. The rate is then determined on the basis of the amount of solution to be infused over 1 hour. This is called the drip rate.

The drop factor, or drops per milliliter of solution, is determined by the size of the opening in the infusion apparatus. It varies with the company producing the product. Most health agencies use the products of a single company. The most common drop factors are macrodrop systems (10, 15, 20 drops per mL), a microdrip or pediatric setup (60 drops per mL), and a blood administration set (10 drops per mL). Sixty drops per milliliter is used most often when small fluid volumes are important, such as with infants and small children. A buretrol or volume control device can also be used to reduce the risk of fluid overload or medication overdose. Adapters may be added to common infusion tubings to reduce the size of the drops. A method for determining flow rate is given in Procedure 46-2.

A time tape can be placed on the container of solution to provide a quick reference for the nurse to moni-

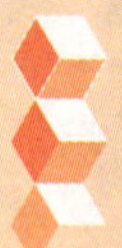

Helpscan

The following are resources for clients and healthcare professionals:

- For information related to recommended practices for intravenous therapy:
  Intravenous Nurses Society (INS)
  2 Brighton Street, Suite 200
  Belmont, MA 02178
  (617) 489-5205

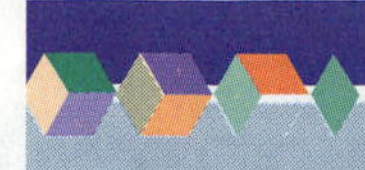

PROCEDURE 46-2

Regulating IV Flow Rate

Action	Rationale
1. Check physician's order for IV solution.	This ensures that correct solution is being given with the correct medications and determines the exact time period for administration of IV.
2. Check patency of IV line and needle.	Any interference with patency influences IV flow rate.
3. Verify drop factor (number of drops in 1 mL) of the equipment in use.	Drop factor of the equipment varies according to manufacturer and will be displayed on outer package. Equipment labeled *microdrop* or *minidrip* is standard and delivers 60 gtt/mL, but macrodrip delivery systems vary. Some of the more common types of equipment according to manufacturer are: Travenol Macrodrip 10 gtt/mL Abbott Macrodrip 15 gtt/mL McGaw Macrodrip 15 gtt/mL
4. Calculate the flow rate:	
a. *Standard formula* $\text{gtt/min} = \dfrac{\text{volume (mL)} \times \text{drop factor (gtt/mL)}}{\text{time (in minutes)}}$ EXAMPLE—Administer 1000 mL 5% D/W over 10 hours (set delivers 60 gtt/1 mL). $\text{gtt/min} = \dfrac{1000 \text{ mL} \times 60}{600 \text{ (60 min} \times \text{10 h)}}$ $= \dfrac{60{,}000}{600}$ $= 100 \text{ gtt/min}$	Standard formula for calculating IV flow rate produces the correct number of gtt/min.
b. *Short formula using milliliters per hour* $\text{gtt/min} = \dfrac{\text{milliliters per hour} \times \text{drop factor (gtt/mL)}}{\text{time (60 min)}}$ EXAMPLE—Administer 1000 mL 5% D/W over 10 hours (set delivers 60 gtt/1 mL). Find milliliters per hour by dividing 1000 mL by 10 hours: $\dfrac{1000}{10} = 100 \text{ mL/hr}$ $\text{gtt/min} = \dfrac{100 \text{ mL} \times 60}{60 \text{ min}}$ $= \dfrac{6{,}000}{600}$ $= 100 \text{ gtt/min}$	Short formula results in calculations using smaller numbers by using milliliters per hour. This is particularly useful for calculating drip rates when infusing piggyback IV medication.
5. Count drops per minute in drip chamber (number of gtt/15-sec interval × 4 = gtt/min). Hold watch beside drip chamber.	Holding watch next to drip chamber allows eyes to focus on drops and second hand on watch to provide accurate count.

(continued)

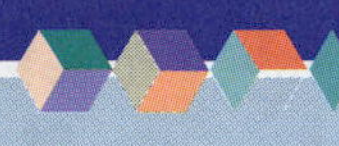

PROCEDURE 46-2 *(continued)*

Regulating IV Flow Rate

Action	Rationale
6. Adjust IV clamp as needed and recount drops per minute.	Clamp regulates flow rate into drip chamber.
7. Mark IV container according to agency policy and manufacturer's recommendations. Use a time tape or label to measure amount to be infused at timed intervals.	This allows for comparison of volume actually infused with scheduled infusion rate.
8. Monitor IV flow rate at frequent intervals. Document client's response to infusion at prescribed rate.	This provides for observation of IV infusion and ensures accurate documentation of client's response to IV infusion.

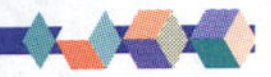

tor the rate at which the solution is entering the client. The tape gives an hourly indication of where the fluid level should be, based on the nurse's calculation of the drip rate. A time tape is illustrated in Figure 46-15.

Many factors can alter the rate of flow of an IV infusion, such as the height of the container in relation to the client, the client's blood pressure, the client's position, the patency of the IV needle or catheter, infiltration, and a knot or kink in the tubing. The nurse periodically checks the infusion and determines quickly by glancing at the time tape if the solution is being infused at the proper hourly rate. If it is not, the nurse again regulates the flow. Because the client's movements, disturbances of the regulation mechanism, or change in the height of the infusion bottle or bed can alter the flow rate, even after it is regulated, the nurse needs to continue to check on the infusion at regular intervals. It has been reported that standard IV administration sets lose up to one half of their initial flow rate during the first hour of infusion because of tubing flexibility, and therefore the rate needs adjustment.

Maintenance of the flow rate is important because of the implications relative to the client's fluid balance. Too slow a flow may result in either the occurrence of deficits because the input is not balancing the loss, or in delaying the restoration of the balance. Infusing IV fluid too rapidly can overtax the body's capacities to adjust to the increase in the water volume or the electrolytes it contains. Nurses who allow infusions to get behind schedule and increase the rate to catch up may be seriously insulting the client's compensatory mechanisms and jeopardizing the client's well-being.

Electronic infusion devices (EIDs) limit the amount of fluid to be infused at any one time and in some healthcare facilities are used to regulate all IV infusions. They can automatically regulate the flow rate at preset limits and notify the nurse by an alarm system when air is in the tubing, the flow is obstructed, or the solution level of the bottle or bag is getting low. Either a pump or controller may be used, but many healthcare facilities select pumps because their accuracy is greater, alarms are triggered less easily, and there are fewer IV-related problems (LaRocca & Otto, 1993). Pumps totally control the delivery rate by exerting positive pressure based on preset limits when resistance develops. Controllers do not rely on pressure to control solution flow but rely on the height of the IV container in relation to the IV site to affect flow rate over time.

An infiltrated IV with a pump EID may not recognize an infusion problem if pressure build-up from the leaking solution in subcutaneous tissues is not significant enough to trigger the alarm. In addition, problems with free-flow may occur if unprotected EIDs are used. If a pump door is opened or IV tubing is removed from a pump that is not equipped with free-flow protection, the IV solution can flow at an uncontrolled rate into the client, possibly causing fluid overload and/or drug toxicity. To prevent this problem *the gravity control clamp should always be closed before opening the door or removing an IV set from a pump* (Cohen & Davis, 1993).

Syringe pumps are also available. They deliver small amounts of fluid, 100 mL or less, and are particularly useful with infants and children. There are portable models on the market also, which are handy for the ambulatory or home-care setting. Clients can receive insulin infusions, pain medication, antibiotic therapy, cancer

Home Healthcare Alert

Candidates for infusion pump IV therapy in the home should meet certain criteria. They should be medically stable, have a full- or part-time caregiver, have access to a telephone, and have a refrigerator available for storage of prefilled medication cassettes.

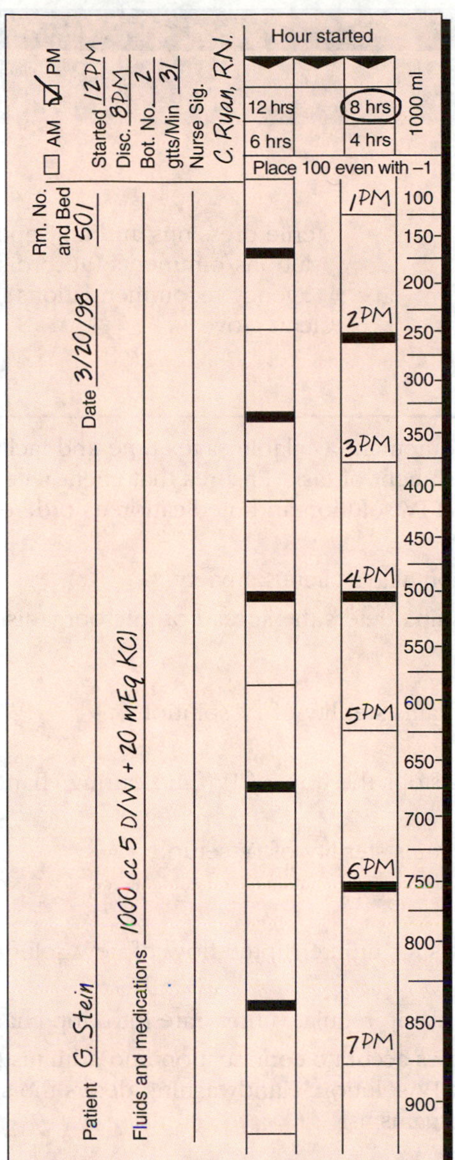

Figure 46-15
A time tape enables the nurse to quickly evaluate if the IV solution is infusing according to schedule and to regulate the drip rate if needed.

chemotherapy, and total parenteral nutrition via portable infusion pumps at home. See Procedure 46-4 for an illustration of an infusion pump.

Changing Solutions and Tubing

If more than one bottle of solution is ordered for the client, the nurse attaches the additional bottles. The method by which this is done depends on the procedure of the agency. Some IV equipment is designed to simplify the procedure by making it possible to attach additional bottles with a tandemlike arrangement. Because infusions often are continued after the responsibility for a client's care changes from one nurse to another, it is a good practice to agree on one common method for managing infusions. Without such uniformity, serious errors can occur, or valuable time is lost in checking and rechecking. One method for changing the solution and tubing is presented in Procedure 46-3.

Caring for the Infusion Site

Scrupulous care of the infusion site should be observed to help control contamination and to help prevent the introduction of microorganisms into the bloodstream. Regular dressing changes and tubing replacements are important means of preventing infection. As mentioned earlier in the chapter, studies have shown that insertion sites covered with gauze and tape have a much lower bacterial count than do those under transparent dressings (Sheldon, 1994). Agency policy should be followed in relation to changing dressings and tubing.

It is best to change the needle or catheter and the site of entry to a vein every 48 to 72 hours. The longer the needle remains in place, the greater the chances of complications, such as infection and phlebitis. Under certain circumstances, the nurse must use discretion in deciding how often to change the infusion site. For example, the client who is receiving long-term chemotherapy quickly runs out of suitable veins. Procedures 46-4 and 46-5 explain how to monitor an IV site and how to change an IV dressing.

A controversial aspect of the care of the insertion site concerns irrigation of the needle. An irrigation is sometimes used when the needle begins to clog with blood and the client does not have other good sites for starting another infusion. *The procedure should not be used unless agency policy recommends it.*

Complications

The client can be an important source of information regarding the possibility of complications associated with IV therapy. If the client is uncomfortable, the nurse should check to see that the infusion is entering the vein as intended, that the flow rate is not too rapid, and that the client's position is satisfactory. Anxiety over the implications of an infusion can also cause discomfort for the client.

Local complications such as infiltration, phlebitis, and thrombophlebitis occur more frequently than systemic complications. Systemic complications (eg, fluid overload, embolus, infection), however, are more serious and may be life-threatening. Table 46-10 defines these complications, noting common causes, signs and symptoms, and pertinent nursing considerations.

Converting a Primary Line to a Heparin or Saline Lock

When a continuous IV is no longer necessary, the primary IV line can be converted to a heparin lock, which provides venous access for intermittent or emergency medications. A heparin or saline lock consists of a plastic tube with a sealed injection port on the end that is connected to an indwelling needle or catheter. Periodic injection with heparin or saline according to agency pol-

(text continues on page 1423)

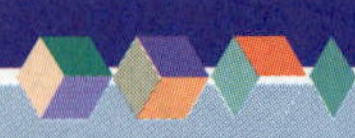

PROCEDURE 46-3

Changing IV Solution and Tubing

Equipment

For solution change:
- IV solution as ordered by physician

For tubing change:
- Administration set
- Sterile gauze
- Timing tape or label

Sterile dressings and antiseptic solutions/ointments (according to agency recommendations)

Clean gloves

Action	Rationale
1. Gather all equipment and bring to bedside. Check IV solution and medication additives with physician's order.	Having equipment available saves time and facilitates accomplishment of task. Ensures that client receives the correct IV solution and medication as ordered by physician.
2. Explain procedure to client.	Explanation allays client's anxiety.
3. Wash your hands.	Handwashing deters the spread of microorganisms.
To Change IV Solution	
4. Carefully remove protective cover from new solution container and expose entry site.	This maintains sterility of IV solution.
5. Close clamp on tubing.	Clamping stops the flow of IV fluid during change of solution.
6. Lift container off IV pole and invert it. Quickly remove the spike from the old IV container, being careful not to contaminate it.	This maintains sterility of IV setup.
7. Steady new container and insert spike. Hang on IV pole.	This allows for uninterrupted flow of new solution.
8. Reopen clamp on tubing and adjust flow.	Opening clamp regulates flow rate into drip chamber.
9. Label container according to agency policy. Record on intake and output record and document on chart according to agency policy. Discard used equipment in proper manner. Wash your hands.	This ensures accurate continuation and administration of correct IV solution. Handwashing deters the spread of microorganisms.
To Change IV Tubing and Solution	
10. Follow actions 1 through 4.	This maintains sterility of IV setup.
11. Open the administration set and remove protective covering from infusion spike. Using sterile technique, insert into new container.	
12. Close clamp on new tubing. Hang IV container on pole and squeeze drip chamber to fill at least halfway.	Gravity and suction effect cause fluid to move into drip chamber. This action also prevents air from moving down the tubing.
13. Remove cap at end of tubing, release clamp, and allow fluid to move through tubing until all air bubbles have disappeared. Close clamp and recap end of tubing maintaining sterility of setup.	This removes air from tubing that can, in larger amounts, act as an air embolus.

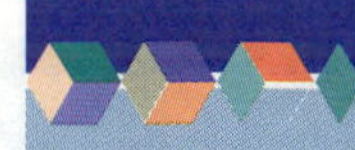

PROCEDURE 46-3 *(continued)*

Changing IV Solution and Tubing

Action	Rationale

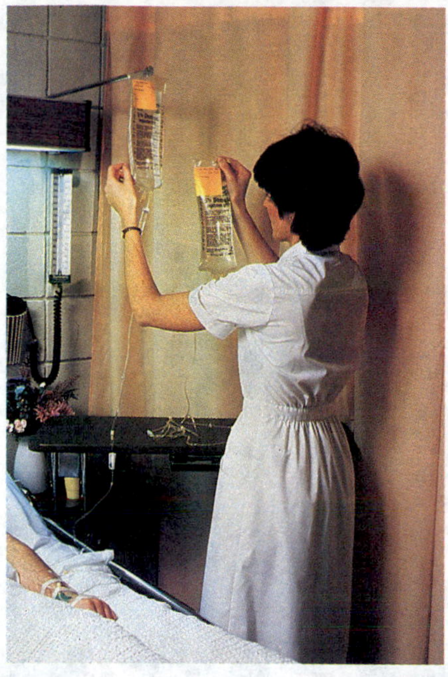

Action 12: Hanging new bag and tubing.

Action	Rationale
14. Loosen tape at IV insertion site. Don clean gloves. Carefully remove dressing and tape.	Care must be used when blood contact is possible. This prevents transmission of HIV and other blood-borne infections. Removing dressing provides access to needle hub necessary for tubing change.
15. Place sterile gauze square under needle hub.	Gauze absorbs any leakage when tubing is disconnected from needle.
16. Place new IV tubing close to client's IV site and slightly loosen protective cap.	This facilitates removal of cap and attachment to needle hub.
17. Clamp the old IV tubing. Steady the needle hub with nondominant hand until change is completed. Remove tubing with dominant hand using a twisting motion.	This stabilizes needle and prevents inadvertently dislodging it.
18. Set old tubing aside. While maintaining sterility, carefully remove cap and insert sterile end of tubing into the needle hub. Twist to secure it. Remove soiled gloves.	This maintains sterility of IV setup.
19. Open the clamp.	Opening clamp allows solution to flow to client.
20. Reapply sterile dressing to site according to agency protocol (see Procedure 46-5).	This deters entry of microorganisms at site.
21. Regulate the IV flow according to physician's order (see Procedure 46-2).	This ensures that client receives IV solution at the prescribed rate.

(continued)

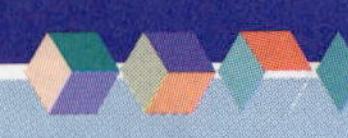

PROCEDURE 46-3 *(continued)*

Changing IV Solution and Tubing

Action	Rationale
22. Attach to IV tubing tape or label that states date, time, and your initials. Label container and record procedure according to agency policy. Discard used equipment in proper manner and wash hands.	This documents IV tubing change. Handwashing deters the spread of microorganisms.
23. Record client's response to IV infusion.	This ensures accurate documentation of client's response.

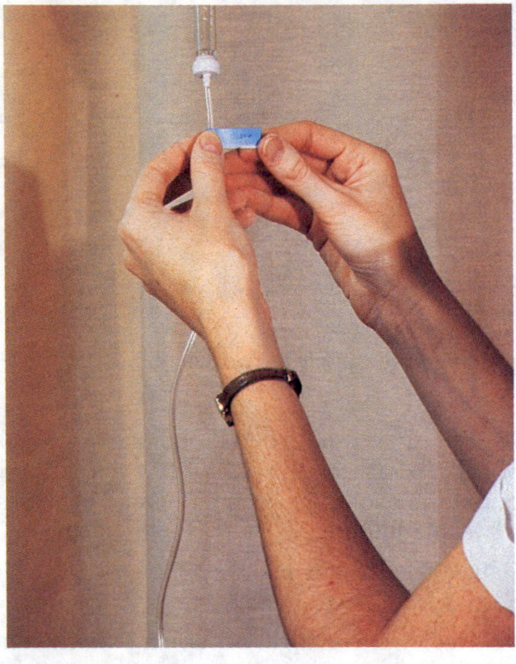

Action 22: Labeling IV tubing.

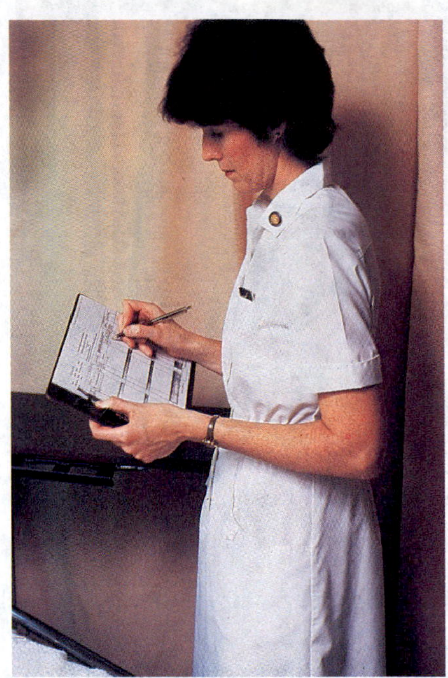

Action 23: Recording client's response to infusion.

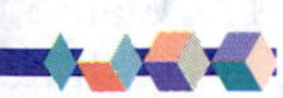

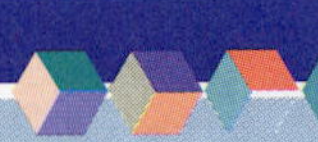

PROCEDURE 46-4

Monitoring an IV Site and Infusion

Action	Rationale
1. Monitor IV infusion at least once every hour. More frequent checks may be necessary if medication is being infused:	Promotes safe administration of IV fluids and medication. Too rapid administration of medications can result in the development of speed shock.
a. Check physician's order for IV solution.	This ensures that correct solution is being given at the correct rate and in the proper sequence with the correct medications.

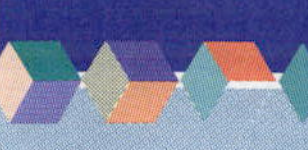

PROCEDURE 46-4 *(continued)*

Monitoring an IV Site and Infusion

Action	Rationale
b. Check drip chamber and time drops if IV is not regulated by an infusion control device.	This ensures that flow rate is correct.
c. Check tubing for anything that might interfere with flow. Be sure that clamp is in the open position. Observe dressing for leakage of IV solution.	Any kink or pressure on tubing may interfere with flow. Leakage may occur at connection of tubing with hub of needle or catheter and allow for loss of IV solution.

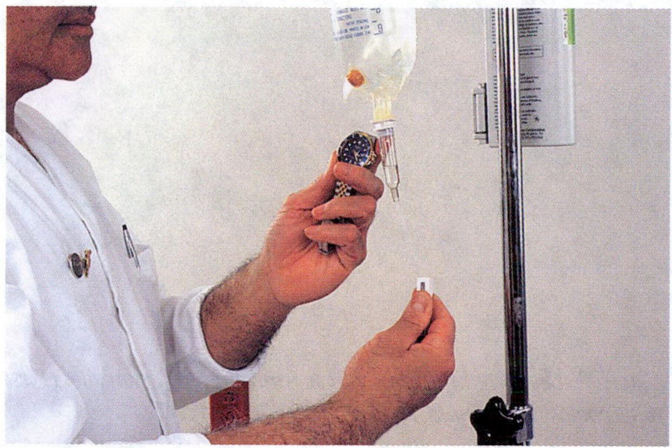

Action 1b: Timing drops.

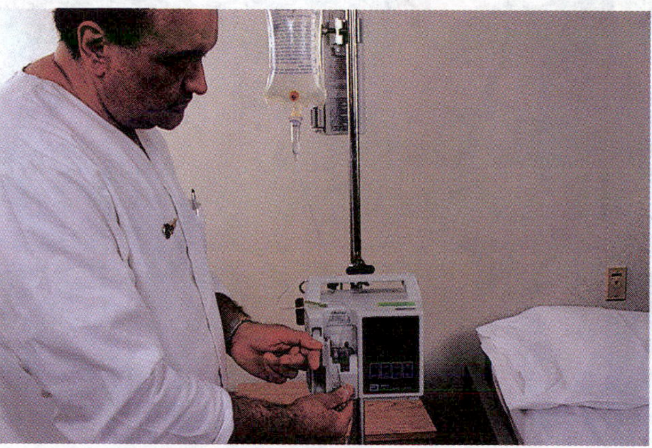

Action 1d: Setting up the pump.

Action	Rationale
d. Observe settings, alarm, and indicator lights on infusion control device if one is being used.	Observation ensures that infusion control device is functioning and that alarm is in ON position.

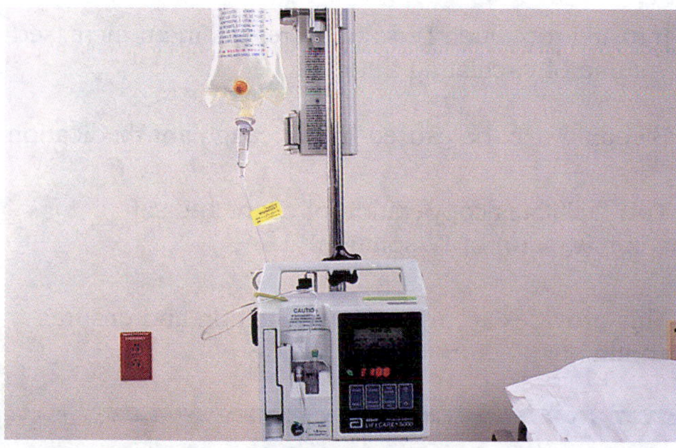

Action 1d: Checking pump setting and alarms.

Action	Rationale
2. Inspect site for swelling, pain, coolness, or pallor at site of insertion, which may indicate infiltration of IV. This necessitates removing IV and restarting at another site.	Needle may become dislodged from vein, and IV solution may flow into subcutaneous tissue.

(continued)

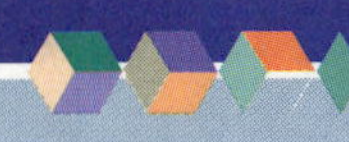

PROCEDURE 46-4 *(continued)*

Monitoring an IV Site and Infusion

Action	Rationale
3. Inspect site for redness, swelling, heat, and pain at the IV site, which may indicate phlebitis is present. IV will need to be discontinued and restarted at another site. Notify physician if you suspect that phlebitis may have occurred.	Chemical irritation or mechanical trauma cause injury to the vein and can lead to the development of phlebitis.

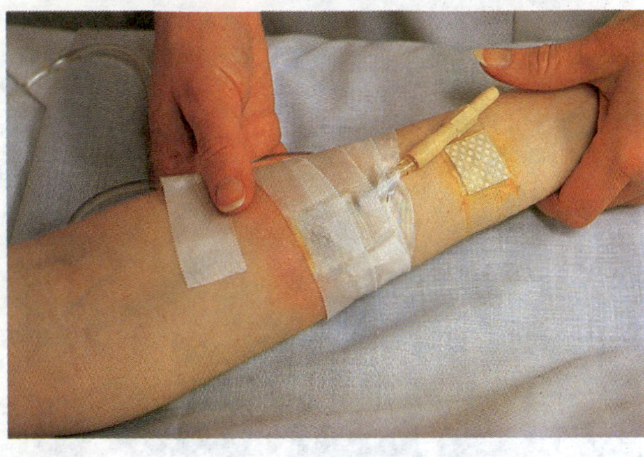

Action 3: Checking inflammation surrounding infusion site. (First three photos © B. Proud.)

Action	Rationale
4. Check for local or systemic manifestations that indicate an infection is present at the site. IV will be discontinued and physician notified. Never disconnect IV tubing when putting on client's hospital gown.	Poor aseptic technique may allow bacteria to enter the needle or catheter insertion site or tubing connection.
5. Be alert for additional complications of IV therapy.	
a. Circulatory overload can result in signs of cardiac failure and pulmonary edema. Monitor intake and output during IV therapy.	Infusing too much IV solution results in an increased volume of circulating fluid.
b. Bleeding at the site is most likely to occur when the IV is discontinued.	Bleeding may be caused by anticoagulant medication.
6. If possible, instruct client to call for assistance if any discomfort is noted at site, solution container is nearly empty, or flow has changed in any way.	This facilitates cooperation of client and safe administration of IV solution.
7. Document IV infusion, any complications of therapy, and client's reaction to therapy.	This provides accurate documentation and ensures continuity of care.

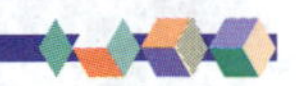

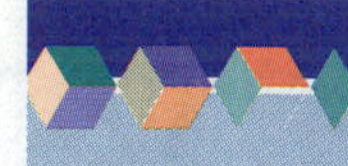

PROCEDURE 46-5

Changing an IV Dressing

Equipment

Sterile gauze (2 × 2 or 4 × 4) or transparent polyurethane dressing
Povidone-iodine (Betadine) solution or swabs
Adhesive remover
Povidone-iodine ointment (or other antiseptic ointment recommended by agency)
Alcohol swabs
Tape
Clean gloves
Towel or disposable pad

Action	Rationale
1. Assess client's need for dressing change.	Agency policy determines interval for dressing change (every 24 to 72 hours). The presence of moisture or a nonadhering dressing increases risk of bacterial contamination at the site.
2. Gather equipment and bring to bedside. Place towel or disposable pad under extremity.	Having equipment available saves time and facilitates the performance of the task.
3. Explain procedure to client.	Explanation allays client's anxiety.
4. Wash your hands. Don clean gloves.	Handwashing deters the spread of microorganisms. Gloves prevent transmission of HIV and other blood-borne infections.
5. Carefully remove old dressing but leave tape that anchors IV needle or catheter in place. Discard in proper manner.	This prevents dislodging of IV needle or catheter.
6. Assess IV site for presence of inflammation or infiltration. Discontinue and relocate the IV if noted.	Inflammation or infiltration causes trauma to tissues and necessitates removal of the IV needle or catheter.
7. Loosen tape and gently remove, being careful to steady catheter or needle hub with one hand.	Tape stabilizes needle and prevents inadvertently dislodging it.
8. Use adhesive remover to initiate cleansing procedure at site.	Process removes adhesive residue and facilitates attachment of new dressing.
9. Cleanse the entry site with povidone-iodine solution. Use a circular motion to move from the center outward. Follow with alcohol cleansing according to agency policy.	Cleansing in a circular motion while moving outward carries organisms away from the entry site. Use of antiseptic solutions reduces the number of microorganisms on the skin surface.
10. Reapply tape strip to needle or catheter at entry site.	Tape anchors needle or catheter to prevent dislodgement.
11. Apply povidone-iodine ointment to the entry site if agency policy recommends this.	Antiseptic ointment reduces skin contamination and protects against infection.
12. Apply sterile gauze or transparent polyurethane dressing over entry site. Remove gloves and dispose of properly.	Dressing protects site and deters contamination with microorganisms.
13. Secure IV tubing with additional tape if necessary. Label dressing with date, time of change, and initials. Check that IV flow is accurate and system is patent.	Label documents IV dressing change.
14. Discard equipment properly and wash hands.	Handwashing protects against spread of microorganisms.
15. Record client's response to dressing change and observation of site.	This provides accurate documentation and ensures continuity of care.

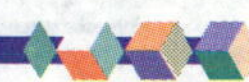

Table 46-10
Complications Associated With Intravenous Infusions

Name and Definition	Causes	Signs and Symptoms	Nursing Considerations
Infiltration: The escape of fluid into the subcutaneous tissue	• Dislodged needle • Penetrated vessel wall	Swelling, pallor, coldness, or pain around the infusion site; significant decrease in the flow rate	• Check the infusion site often for symptoms. • Discontinue the infusion if symptoms occur. • Restart the infusion at a different site. • Limit the movement of the extremity with the IV.
Phlebitis: An inflammation of a vein	• Mechanical trauma from needle or catheter • Chemical trauma from solution • Septic (due to contamination)	Local, acute tenderness; redness, warmth, and slight edema of the vein above the insertion site	• Discontinue the infusion immediately. • Apply warm, moist compresses to the affected site. • Avoid further use of the vein. • Restart the infusion in another vein.
Thrombus: A blood clot	• Tissue trauma from needle or catheter	Symptoms similar to phlebitis IV fluid flow may cease if clot obstructs needle	• Stop the infusion immediately. • Apply warm compresses as ordered by the physician. • Restart the IV at another site. • *Do not rub or massage the affected area.*
Speed shock: The body's reaction to a substance that is injected into the circulatory system too rapidly	• Too rapid a rate of fluid infusion into circulation	Pounding headache, fainting, rapid pulse rate, apprehension, chills, back pains, and dyspnea	• If symptoms develop, discontinue the infusion immediately. • Report symptoms of speed shock to the physician immediately. • Monitor vital signs if symptoms develop. • Use the proper IV tubing. A microdrip (60 gtt/mL) should be used on all pediatric clients. • Carefully monitor the rate of fluid flow. • Check the rate frequently for accuracy. A time tape is useful for this purpose.
Fluid overload: The condition caused when too large a volume of fluid infuses into the circulatory system	• Too large a volume of fluid infused into circulation	Engorged neck veins, increased blood pressure, and difficulty in breathing (dyspnea)	• If symptoms develop, slow the rate of infusion. • Notify the physician immediately. • Monitor vital signs. • Carefully monitor the rate of fluid flow. • Check the rate frequently for accuracy.
Embolus: A foreign body or air in the circulatory system	• Thrombus dislodges and circulates in the blood • Air enters the vein through the infusion line	Dependent on whether the embolism causes an obstruction or infarction in the circulatory system	• Check the site regularly to identify signs of phlebitis. • Do not allow air to enter the infusion line. • Treat phlebitis with the utmost caution.

Table 46-10 *(continued)*
Complications Associated With Intravenous Infusions

Name and Definition	Causes	Signs and Symptoms	Nursing Considerations
			• Report any sudden pain or breathing difficulty immediately.
Infection: An invasion of pathogenic organisms into the body	• Nonsterile technique used in starting infusion • Improper care of infusion site • Contaminated IV solution	Fever; malaise; and pain, swelling, inflammation, or discharge at IV insertion site	• Use scrupulous aseptic technique when starting an infusion. • Change the dressing over the site regularly. • Change IV tubing every 24 hours if agency policy permits. • Always wash hands before working with the IV.

icy is required to keep the catheter patent. Procedure 46-6 describes this technique.

Discontinuing the Infusion

When the amount of solution the physician has ordered has been infused, the nurse assumes responsibility for discontinuing the infusion. If the needle or catheter are to be removed, the adhesive strips and sterile dressing are removed, the needle or catheter is removed in line with the vein, and pressure is immediately applied to the site. A dry sterile gauze pad is preferable to an alcohol preparation to apply pressure to the site because alcohol tends to burn and does not stop blood flow from the puncture wound. If the client is able to do so, he or she may be asked to hold the pressure for a minute or more.

If the client's extremity has been immobilized for several hours or longer, the nurse should manipulate it carefully in an attempt to put the joint through range of motion and passively move the muscles of the area.

The following information is recorded when the infusion has been completed:

- The date and time the infusion was completed
- The kind and amount of solution infused
- The name of the person discontinuing the infusion
- Symptoms of any adverse reactions
- Signs of the desired effects of the infusion

Teaching About Home Infusion

Many clients return to their home from a healthcare facility with intravenous infusions. Portable infusion pumps and the availability of home care nurses have made this an acceptable alternative. Once a client has been identified as a candidate for home infusion therapy, the nurse needs to begin assessment and education to assure a successful outcome. The client and any caregivers must be able to perform necessary skills independently prior to discharge from the healthcare facility.

Home Healthcare Alert

Emphasis on good handwashing technique provides the starting point for health teaching about maintaining an intravenous infusion at home.

Important points that need to be addressed include handling all equipment, performing dressing changes, assessing for any indications of infection or other complications, and maintaining the supplies necessary to continue home infusion. The nurse ensures that the client understands the physician's orders and is familiar with when and how to contact the physician or nurses should questions or concerns arise. Prior to initiating this therapy, the nurse and the infusion service consider the home environment, ability of the client or caregiver to maintain the IV infusion, and any other potential considerations necessary to promote a smooth transition.

Replacing Blood and Blood Products

A *blood transfusion* is the infusion of whole blood or a blood component such as plasma, RBCs, or platelets into the venous circulation. Whole blood is infrequently used because the various components can be easily separated and used for replacement therapy. The person receiving the blood is the *recipient.* The person giving the blood is the *donor.* Steps in administering blood transfusions are given in Procedure 46-7.

Typing and Crossmatching

Before blood can be given to a person, it must be determined that the blood of the donor and that of the recipient are compatible. If incompatible, clumping and hemolysis of the recipient's blood cells results and death can occur. The laboratory examination to determine a

(text continues on page 1427

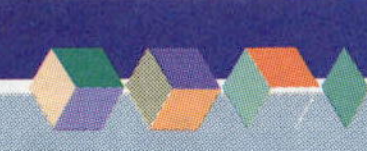

PROCEDURE 46-6

Converting a Primary Intravenous Access to a Heparin or Saline Lock

Equipment

Lock device (also called male adaptor or Luer-Lok)
Clean gloves
4 × 4 gauze pad
Saline, Nonpreservative saline, or heparin flush (1 mL) prepared in a syringe with a 25-gauge needle or according to agency policy
Alcohol wipe
Tape
Plastic clamp or hemostat

Action	Rationale
1. Gather equipment and verify physician's order.	Having equipment available saves time and facilitates the task; ensures that the procedure has been ordered by the physician.
2. Explain the procedure to the client.	Explanation allays the client's anxiety.
3. Wash your hands.	Handwashing deters the spread of microorganisms.
4. Assess the IV site.	Complications such as infiltration or phlebitis necessitate discontinuation of the IV infusion at that site.
5. Use a plastic clamp or hemostat to close off primary line.	Protects client and nurse from inadvertent blood loss when IV and tubing are disconnected.
6. Don clean gloves.	Gloves protect the nurse from contact with the client's blood.
7. Place gauze 4 × 4 sponge underneath IV connection hub between IV catheter and tubing.	Gauze absorbs any blood leakage when IV and tubing are disconnected.
8. Stabilize hub of IV catheter with nondominant hand. Use dominant hand to quickly twist and disconnect IV tubing from the catheter, discard it, and attach heparin device to hub without contaminating the tips of the catheter and the lock.	This maintain sterility of IV setup.

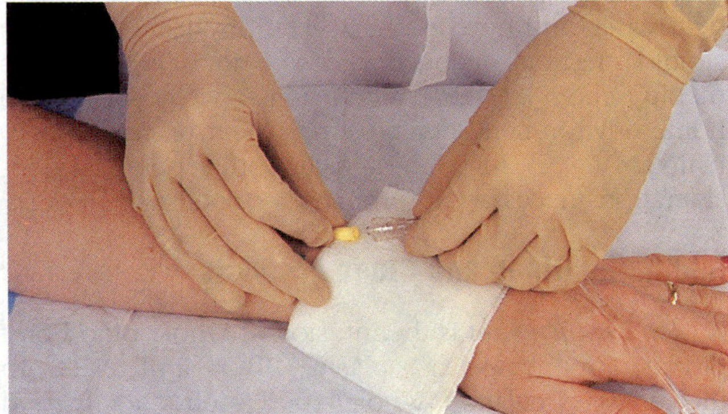

Action 8: Disconnecting tubing from IV catheter.

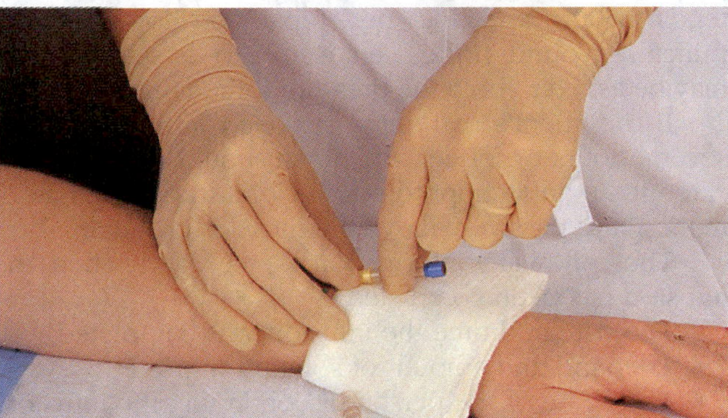

Action 8: Attaching heparin lock to IV catheter hub.

Action	Rationale
9. Cleanse lock entry with an alcohol wipe.	Cleansing removes surface bacteria at the heparin lock entry site.
10. Insert the syringe needle into the heparin lock port and gently flush catheter with saline, nonpreservative saline, or heparin flush as per agency policy. Remove syringe carefully.	This maintains patency of the IV access line. Clinical evidence has demonstrated that a saline flush is as effective as heparin for peripheral IVs and avoids the adverse effects of heparin, is less expensive, and prevents drug incompatibilities.
11. Tape heparin lock securely in place.	Tape secures the heparin lock and IV in place.
12. Chart on IV administration record or medication Kardex per institutional policy.	Accurate documentation is necessary to prevent error.

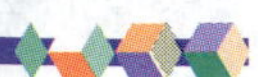

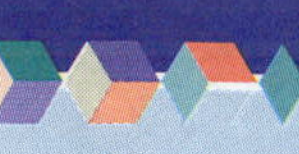

PROCEDURE 46-7

Administering a Blood Transfusion

Equipment

- Blood product
- Blood administration set (tubing with in-line filter and Y for saline administration)
- 0.9% Normal saline
- IV pole
- Intravenous line with a #18 or #19 needle or catheter
- Disposable gloves
- Tape

Action	Rationale
1. Determine if client knows reason for transfusion. Ask if the client has had a transfusion or transfusion reaction in the past.	This directs teaching before beginning transfusion.
2. Explain procedure to client. Check for signed consent for transfusion if required by agency. Advise client to report any chills, itching, rash, or unusual symptoms.	Explanation provides reassurance and facilitates cooperation. Prompt reporting of any reaction to transfusion necessitates stopping immediately.
3. Wash your hands and put on clean gloves.	Handwashing deters the spread of microorganisms. Gloves protect against accidental exposure to the client's blood.
4. Hang container of 0.9% normal saline with blood administration set to initiate IV infusion and follow administration of blood.	Dextrose may lead to clumping of red blood cells and hemolysis. Filter in blood administration set removes particulate material formed during storage of blood.

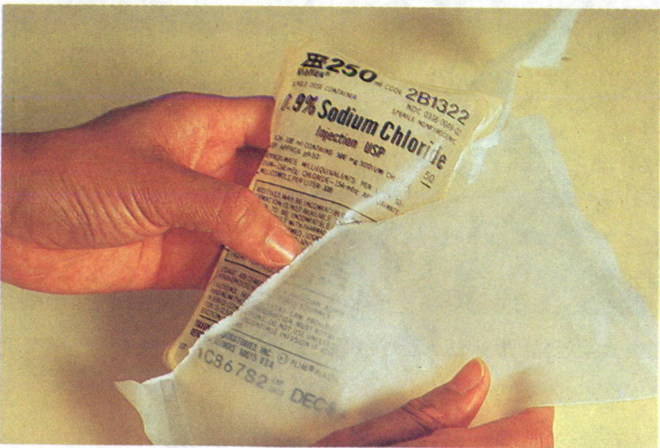

Normal saline container.

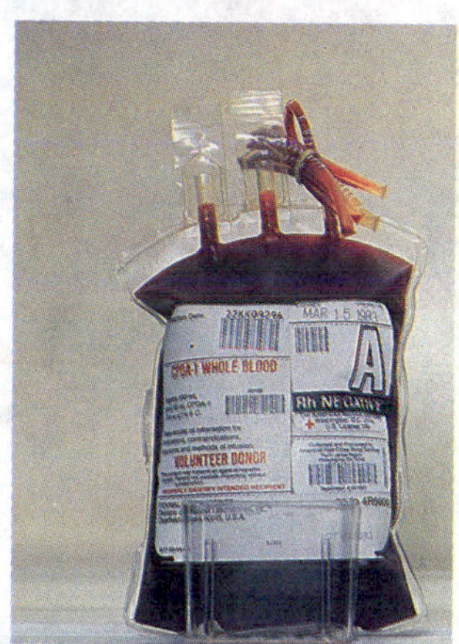

Unit of packed red blood cells.

Action	Rationale
5. Start intravenous with #18 or #19 catheter if not already present (see Procedure 46-1). Keep IV open by starting flow of normal saline.	Large-bore needle or catheter is necessary for infusion of blood products. The lumen must be large enough not to cause damage to red blood cells.
6. Obtain blood product from blood bank according to agency policy.	Blood must be stored in refrigerated unit at carefully controlled temperature (4°C).
7. Complete identification and checks as required by agency:	Some agencies require two registered nurses to verify information:
a. Identification number	Verifies that unit numbers match
b. Blood group and type	Verifies that ABO group and Rh type are the same

(continued)

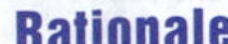

Administering a Blood Transfusion

Action	Rationale
c. Expiration date	Safe storage of blood is limited to 35 days before red blood cells begin to deteriorate.
d. Client's name	Never administer blood to a client without a name band.
e. Inspect blood for clots	If clots are present, blood should be returned to blood bank.
8. Take baseline set of vital signs prior to beginning transfusion.	Any change in vital signs during the transfusion may indicate a reaction.
9. Start infusion of the blood product:	
a. Prime in-line filter with blood.	Priming is necessary if blood is to flow properly.
b. Start administration slowly (no more than 10–25 mL for the first 15 minutes). Stay with the client for the first 15 minutes of transfusion.	Transfusion reactions typically occur during this period, and a slow rate will minimize the volume of red blood cells infused. If there have been no adverse effects during this time, the infusion rate is increased.
c. Check vital signs at least every 15 minutes for the first half hour after the start of the transfusion and then every half hour or hour after the transfusion depending on agency policy.	If complications occur, they can be observed, and the blood can be stopped immediately.

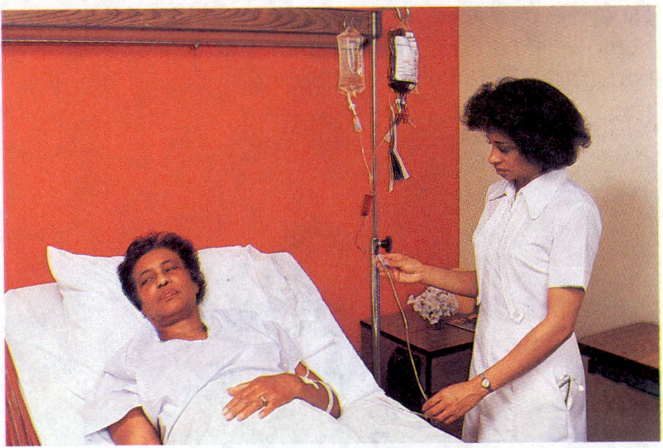

Action 9a: Priming the in-line filter.

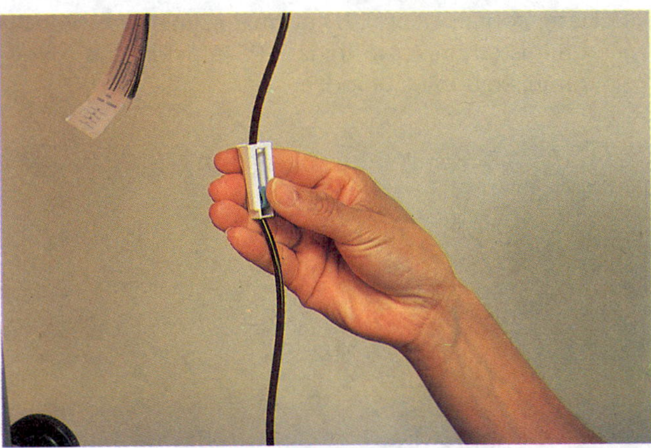

Action 9b: Starting infusion of blood slowly.

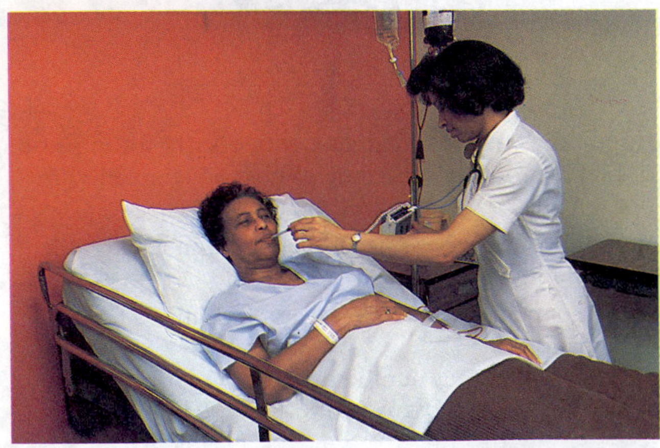

Action 9c: Checking vital signs.

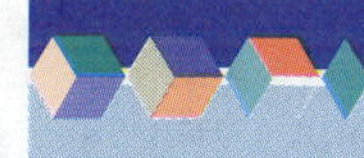

PROCEDURE 46-7 *(continued)*

Administering a Blood Transfusion

Action	Rationale
d. Observe client for flushing, dyspnea, itching, hives, or rash.	These symptoms may be early indication of a transfusion reaction.
e. Use a blood warming device, if indicated, especially with rapid transfusions through a CVP catheter.	Rapid administration of cold blood can result in cardiac arrhythmias.
10. Maintain the prescribed flow rate as ordered and assess frequently for transfusion reaction. Stop blood transfusion and allow saline to flow if you suspect a reaction. Notify physician and blood bank.	Rate must be carefully controlled, and client's reaction must be monitored on a frequent basis.
11. When transfusion is complete, infuse 0.9% normal saline.	Saline prevents hemolysis of red blood cells and clears remainder of blood in IV line.
12. Record administration of blood and client's reaction as ordered by agency. Return blood transfusion bag to blood bank according to agency policy.	This provides for accurate documentation of client's response to blood transfusion.

Special Considerations

Electronic infusion devices may be used to maintain prescribed rate but must be specifically designed for use with blood transfusions.

Home Care Considerations

Home care agencies evaluate clients who are candidates for a blood transfusion at home. Home transfusion is not appropriate for clients who are actively bleeding, require more than 4 hours for the transfusion, or recently had a reaction to a blood transfusion. Written consent must be obtained from the client and the physician. The nurse transports the blood product to the client's home in a special cooler. The nurse and client's caregiver check serial number and other identification information together.

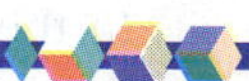

person's blood type is called *typing*. The process of determining compatibility between blood specimens is *crossmatching*.

Blood Types. The four main blood groups in the ABO system of blood typing are A, B, AB, and O. Some of these groups are broken down into still more subgroups.

Blood type is an inherited trait and is determined by the type of antigens and antibodies present in the blood. An *antigen* is a substance that causes the formation of antibodies. An *antibody* is a protein substance developed in the body in response to the presence of an antigen that has in some way gained access to the body. An *agglutinin* is an antibody that causes a clumping of specific antigens. People who have type A blood have an A antigen in their RBCs; those with type B blood have B antigens in their cells; those in the AB group have A and B antigens; and people with type O blood have neither A nor B antigens in their RBCs. People in each blood group have the agglutinins to the red cell antigens that they lack. Group A people have the agglutinin for B; group AB people have no agglutinins for A and B, whereas group O people have both A and B agglutinins in their blood serum. Assume a person with type O blood is transfused with blood from either a person with group A or group B blood. There would be destruction of the recipient's red cells because his or her anti-A or anti-B agglutinins would react with the A or B antigens in the donor's red cells. From this example, it can be seen why group AB people are often called universal recipients (because people in this blood group have no agglutinins for either A or B antigens), and group O people are often called universal donors (because they have neither A nor B antigens).

Rh Factor. The Rh factor is an inherited antigen in human blood. There are five antigens in the Rh system, but the one designated D is of first concern. A person whose blood contains a D antigen is called Rh positive; an Rh-negative person lacks D. It is important that an Rh-negative person receive blood from another Rh-negative person. If Rh-positive blood is injected into an Rh-negative person, the recipient develops anti-Rh agglutinins. Subsequent transfusion with Rh-positive blood may cause serious reactions with clumping and hemolysis of RBCs.

The Rh factor is of special importance during pregnancy because Rh incompatibility between mother and fetus is often the problem when an infant has hemolytic disease. An Rh-negative mother who gives birth to an Rh-positive child is given RhoGam (an anti-Rh gamma globulin) within 72 hours after birth to prevent the development of permanent active immunity to the Rh antigen.

Selection of Blood Donors

The selection of blood donors must be done with care. Not only must the donor's blood be accurately typed, but it is also important to determine whether the donor is free from diseases. Their blood will be tested for human immunodeficiency virus (HIV) and hepatitis B virus (HBV). These viruses can be transmitted to the recipient. Blood donated from people who have allergies or those with a history of a chronic disease, such as tuberculosis, certain types of cancer, and hemophilia, is usually not used. As a further precaution, some blood banks do not accept blood from a donor who has been immunized recently because of a possible allergic reaction to the blood by a recipient.

The donor is examined carefully at the time of donation and receives specific information about eligibility as well as a confidential method to allow or disallow the distribution of their donated blood. Prospective donors are questioned about high risk behaviors such as unsafe sex, IV drug abuse, and the presence of any of the signs and symptoms of AIDS. Individuals may give blood only if blood count, temperature, pulse, respiration, and blood pressure are within normal range.

In the early 1980s, a number of people contracted HIV after receiving contaminated blood. Although careful screening of both donors and donated blood has greatly decreased the likelihood of this happening, both blood donors and recipients continue to have many questions regarding safety. *There is no way that donors may contract HIV or any other disease by giving blood* because single-use sterile setups are used for each donor. Some clients who know in advance that they will need blood request to give their own blood (autologous transfusion) or to have family members donate the blood. Autotransfusion eliminates the danger of transmitting cross-infection from donor to recipient but requires advance planning. This practice is growing in popularity.

Blood Extracts

Whole blood is rarely used unless blood loss has been massive. With current technology, whole blood can be easily separated into its components and clients receive only the blood product they need. For example, one may need RBCs but not the blood plasma and its constituents. RBCs in concentrated form are called packed RBCs and may be used in the following situations:

- Client with anemia suffering with a low RBC count
- Client with cardiovascular failure, to increase blood volume and RBCs while avoiding cardiovascular overload
- Client with GI bleeding, to maintain adequate hemoglobin levels without increasing blood pressure, which would likely lead to more bleeding

In other situations, only plasma is required, such as when plasma protein or the blood's clotting factor is in low supply. Fresh frozen plasma is particularly useful in emergencies for immediate restoration of fluid because serum presents no compatibility problems and time need not be lost seeking donors and matching blood. It is also an excellent blood-volume expander when time is of essence, an example being for the person who is severely burned and losing plasma rapidly from burn areas. Components of plasma that are used therapeutically include human albumin (hypovolemic shock, albuminemia, liver failure); cryoprecipitates (bleeding due to hemophilia or disseminated intravascular coagulation); and gamma globulins—the antibody-containing part of plasma (gamma globulin deficiencies).

Platelet infusion is indicated for treatment or prevention of bleeding associated with deficiencies in the number or function of a client's platelets. The demand for platelets has noticeably risen over the past several decades and specialized products and preparation methods have been developed to reduce the risk of complications and improve the client's response to platelet therapy.

Initiating the Transfusion

The procedure for starting a blood transfusion (Procedure 46-7) is basically the same as for an IV solution. If possible, larger veins should be selected because no smaller needle or catheter than a No. 19 gauge should be used. This size is necessary because of the viscosity of blood. Vital signs should be taken and recorded just prior to starting the transfusion. If the client's temperature is 100°F (37.8°C) or higher, the physician should be notified. Blood that has not been used within 30 minutes after its arrival from the blood bank must be returned. The temperature will exceed 50°F (10°C) after that time frame and the blood may not be safe for use (Harovas & Anthony, 1993b).

Transfusion Reactions

When preparing and administering the transfusion, the nurse should take every precaution to prevent the occurrence of transfusion reactions through scrupulous technique. Table 46-11 describes some potential transfusion reactions. A nurse should try to stay with the client for the first 15 minutes after starting a blood transfusion and then check the client's vital signs at least every 15 minutes for the first half hour and then every half hour or hour, as the agency recommends, until the transfusion is completed. A transfusion reaction can be serious.

Table 46-11
Transfusion Reactions

Reaction	Signs and Symptoms	Nursing Activity
Allergic reaction: Allergy to transfused blood	Hives, itching Anaphylaxis	• Stop transfusion immediately and keep vein open with normal saline. • Notify physician stat. • Administer antihistamine parenterally as necessary.
Febrile reaction: Fever develops during infusion	Fever and chills Headache Malaise	• Stop transfusion immediately and keep vein open with normal saline. • Notify physician. • Treat symptoms.
Hemolytic transfusion reaction: Incompatibility of blood product	Immediate onset Facial flushing Fever, chills Headache Low back pain Shock	• Stop infusion immediately and keep vein open with normal saline. • Notify physician stat. • Obtain blood samples from site. • Obtain first voided urine. • Treat shock if present. • Send unit, tubing, and filter to lab. • Draw blood sample for serologic testing and send urine specimen to the lab.
Circulatory overload: Too much blood administered	Dyspnea Dry cough Pulmonary edema	• Slow or stop infusion. • Monitor vital signs. • Notify physician. • Place in upright position with feet dependent.
Bacterial reaction: Bacteria present in blood	Fever Hypertension Dry, flushed skin Abdominal pain	• Stop infusion immediately. • Obtain culture of client's blood and return blood bag to lab. • Monitor vital signs. • Notify physician. • Administer antibiotics stat.

Giving Total Parenteral Nutrition

Hypertonic solutions consisting of dextrose, amino acids, and select electrolytes and minerals may be infused using a central vein by a procedure known as *total parenteral nutrition.* Used in cases of severe malnutrition, TPN is directed to:

- Reestablish and maintain positive nitrogen balance
- Increase or maintain weight
- Correct metabolic complications

This procedure and related nursing responsibilities are described in Chapter 42.

EVALUATING

When evaluating the effectiveness of the plan of care aimed at promoting healthy fluid, electrolyte, and acid–base balance, the nurse pays attention to the following parameters:

- Are the client's drinking and eating patterns supplying the needed fluid and electrolytes? Are food and fluid likes and dislikes interfering with the implementation of the care plan? Is the client having any difficulties with oral fluids, tube feedings, IV therapy, or TPN?
- Is the client's urine output approximately equal to the fluid intake? Does the client void at least once each shift (except when sleeping)? Do urine characteristics (color, odor, SG) indicate healthy functioning of the kidneys and excretion of fluids?
- Are abnormal sources of fluid loss (vomiting, diarrhea, draining wounds, fistula, and so forth) responding to treatment? Are these losses effectively being replaced by the designated therapy? Are the signs of FVD improving?
- Do the client's weight and record of fluid intake and output indicate fluid balance?
- Are the signs and symptoms that initially manifested fluid, electrolyte, or acid–base imbalances absent or improved? Has therapy created any troublesome new signs or symptoms?
- Is the client now able to practice self-care behaviors to maintain fluid, electrolyte, and acid–base balance? Can the client describe appropriate responses to potential future problems?

This evaluation should be ongoing as the plan of care is implemented. As the client achieves expected outcomes, these should be noted and reinforced. Before nursing care is terminated, the client (and family) should be able to independently promote fluid, electrolyte, and acid–base balance.

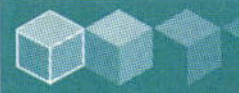

Nursing Process in Clinical Practice

When identifying and treating fluid, electrolyte, and acid–base balance problems categorized as nursing diagnoses, the nurse uses each phase of the nursing process. Quality care depends on the nurse's possession of the knowledge and clinical skills described earlier in this chapter. In this section, the special fluid, electrolyte, and acid–base balance needs of two target populations are explored—surgical clients and oncology clients. What follows are the assessment priorities, expected outcomes, and nursing interventions for common types of fluid, electrolyte, and acid–base balance problems treated by nurses.

Fluid Volume Deficit
Fluid Volume Excess

In the client care study that follows, nursing care is described for a client with an FVD related to prolonged diarrhea.

The Surgical Client

Fluid Volume Deficit

The state in which an individual experiences vascular, cellular, or intracellular dehydration (NANDA, 1994)

Clients undergoing surgery are at high risk for fluid, electrolyte, and acid–base balance problems preoperatively, intraoperatively, and postoperatively for many reasons:

- The pathology that underlies the need for surgery
- Aggressive diagnostic testing
- The stress of anesthesia and surgery
- Postoperative treatment
- Effects of surgery

Preoperatively, the fluid deficit can be related to fluid restrictions for diagnostic tests or pathology that results in decreased fluid intake (anorexia, intestinal obstruction) or abnormal fluid losses (vomiting, draining fistula).

Intraoperatively, severe bleeding may cause shock and acute renal failure or actual fluid loss and third-space fluid shift during surgical procedure.

Postoperatively, the fluid deficit can be related to vomiting, gastric suction, or oral fluid restriction secondary to ileus following abdominal surgery.

Fluid Volume Excess

The state in which an individual experiences increased fluid retention and edema (NANDA, 1994)

Postoperatively, the client can experience manifestations of fluid volume excess due to increased antidiuretic hormone secondary to surgery and anesthesia, aldosterone secretion, or overadministration of isotonic solutions.

Assessment Priorities

Preoperative

- Obtain baseline vital signs, body weight.
- Review laboratory data to ensure normal electrolytes and a hematocrit at 33% or higher (because transport of oxygen to cells depends on an adequate hemoglobin level). Notify physicians of any abnormalities so these can be corrected before surgery.
- Use intake and output records (and daily weights if fluid balance problems are suspected) and assessment of urine characteristics to assess fluid balance.
- Check for malnutrition (muscles with a wasted appearance—decreased strength, pale skin that breaks down easily, listlessness and apathy, dull, dry hair that falls out easily).

Postoperative

- Monitor vital signs according to agency policy and client's condition. Tachycardia and hypotension may indicate severe FVD. Changes in respirations and abnormal breath sounds are key indicators of acid–base and fluid volume disturbances.
- Maintain accurate intake and output record that includes intraoperative fluid intake and output. Ensure in adults an hourly urine output of 30 to 50 mL. Factors that contribute to decreased urinary volume in the postoperative period include the following:
  - Stress reaction (healthy physiologic response to surgery)
  - Hypovolemia resulting from fluid loss incurred in surgery
  - Preoperative dehydration
  - Subtle accumulation of fluid at the surgical site
  - Disturbance in myocardial function causing decreased blood flow to the kidneys
  - Renal failure, a serious cause of postoperative oliguria (Metheny, 1992)
- Assess for signs of electrolyte imbalance (see Table 40-4).

Expected Outcomes

Preoperative. The client will:

- Enter surgery in fluid balance as evidenced by the following:
  - Stable body weight
  - Urine output of 30 to 50 mL/hr
  - Urine SG of 1.010 to 1.025
- Enter surgery in electrolyte balance as evidenced by normal laboratory values for sodium, chloride, potassium, and bicarbonate

Postoperative. The client will:

- Maintain approximately equal fluid intake and output
- Maintain urine output of 30 to 50 mL/hr
- Maintain stable body weight
- Maintain stable vital signs
- Be free of signs indicating fluid, electrolyte, or acid–base disturbance

Interventions. The best intervention for fluid, electrolyte, and acid–base disturbances is *prevention.*

- Before client's surgery, offer oral foods and fluids that the client likes and that are most likely to result in fluid, electrolyte, and nutritional balance.
- Bring any suspected abnormality to the physician's attention and execute orders for fluid or electrolyte replacement, strategies to reduce excesses, and so forth.
- Assist in identifying contributing factors and reduce or eliminate these factors, if possible.
- Administer IV fluids as prescribed and maintain accurate drip rates to prevent underinfusion or overinfusion.
- As soon as the client is able to tolerate oral fluids (check for swallowing reflex and bowel sounds), begin oral fluid replacement with fluids the client prefers.
- In clients with severe fluid imbalances, an indwelling Foley catheter may need to be inserted so that hourly urine outputs can be monitored.

The Oncology Client

Fluid Volume Deficit

Most clients with cancer experience problems with fluid and electrolyte regulation during their illness. These problems are related to the following:

- Faulty regulation or availability of calcium, uric acid, sodium, potassium, phosphate
- Altered hormonal regulation (malignant tumors may produce hormones that interfere with water and electrolyte balance: ADH, PTH, osteoclastic activating factor, adrenocorticotropic hormone)
- Third-space fluid accumulation related to malignant effusions into the peritoneal, pericardial, or pleural compartments, or to edema resulting from blocked lymphatic drainage or venous return
- Treatment-related imbalances (Metheny, 1992)

The fluid volume deficit may be related to anorexia and vomiting that is secondary to chemotherapy or radiation therapy. Prolonged gastric suction or third-space fluid shifts into the peritoneal, pericardial, or pleural compartment can lead to manifestations of fluid deficit.

Fluid Volume Excess

The edema related to obstruction of lymphatic drainage or venous return secondary to tumor pressure can cause manifestations of fluid volume excess.

Assessment Priorities

- Assess for the signs and symptoms that accompany electrolyte disturbances associated with specific tumors and treatment modalities.
- Weigh clients daily or weekly for signs of fluid deficit or excess. FVD is characterized by decreased skin turgor, decreased urinary output, concentrated urine, and postural hypotension. Clients with third-space fluid shifts have an *increase* in total body fluid, and thus no decrease in weight, although clinically their condition is described as FVD.
- Be alert for signs of third-space fluid shifts:
  - Peritoneal—increased abdominal girth
  - Pleural—difficulty breathing
- Assess for signs of dependent edema; check the feet and ankles of people who sit or stand for long periods and the back and sacral area of the bedridden client.
- Assess for the development of weeping edema (leakage of fluid through the pores).

Expected Outcomes. The client will:

- Take in sufficient fluids (oral if possible) to maintain fluid balance as evidenced by the following:
  - Normal skin turgor
  - Moist mucous membranes
  - Stable body weight
  - Baseline blood pressure
- Report (demonstrate) relief of symptoms of dehydration, third-space fluid shifts, edema, or other electrolyte disturbances
- Exhibit decreased dependent edema
- Describe self-care behaviors to prevent future fluid and electrolyte disturbances

Interventions. Interventions vary according to the nature of the fluid, electrolyte, or acid–base disturbance. To prevent problems, the client should be encouraged to drink sufficient fluids (about 2500 mL for the adult) and to eat nutritious meals.

- Clients with anorexia may need to be taught how to choose times when their systems will best tolerate food and fluids and to ingest high-calorie liquids with key electrolytes.
- Clients with abnormal fluid losses may need to be taught the importance of fluid replacement.
- Clients with FVDs resulting from third-space fluid shifts may require IV fluid replacement; however, this also increases the volume of fluids trapped in the third space (eg, pleural cavity) and may increase the client's discomfort. The client needs to be monitored carefully for signs of fluid overload during the administration of IV fluids.
- Clients with dependent edema require frequent position changes and a skin care program to prevent skin breakdown. Special mattresses are helpful. Refer to Chapter 38 for nursing interventions to maintain skin integrity.
- See Tables 46-3 through 46-5 for nursing interventions to treat specific fluid, electrolyte, and acid–base balance disturbances.

Client Care Study

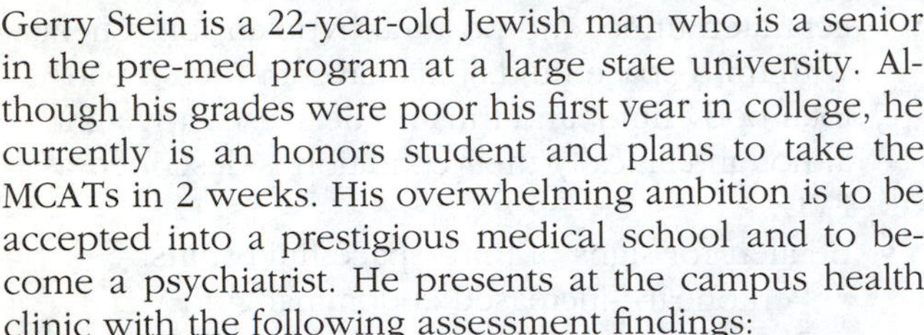

Gerry Stein is a 22-year-old Jewish man who is a senior in the pre-med program at a large state university. Although his grades were poor his first year in college, he currently is an honors student and plans to take the MCATs in 2 weeks. His overwhelming ambition is to be accepted into a prestigious medical school and to become a psychiatrist. He presents at the campus health clinic with the following assessment findings:

- History of problems with diarrhea since his junior year in high school; treatment—kaolin and pectin (Kaopectate) and limiting his food and fluid intake; believes diarrhea is stress related; no medical evaluation to date
- Has had two or three loose bowel movements per day for the past week with urgency and occasional incontinence; believes this is related to anxiety about performance on MCATs and need for good grades; always thirsty but afraid to drink much; urine output is decreased and he noted it is darker in color and has a stronger odor
- Nursing examination: Temperature, 99.8°F (37.6°C); pulse, 92 beats per minute; respirations, 18; blood pressure, 100/60; skin and mucous membranes are pale and dry; weight is 4 lb less than usual (current weight 170 lb)

Core Competencies

Cognitive Competencies

- Knowledge of basic theory related to fluid and electrolyte balance and the factors and variables that affect it
- Knowledge of effective stress management techniques
- Ability to develop nursing diagnoses that reflect Mr. Stein's unique health problem
- Knowledge of which nursing interventions are most likely to yield desired outcomes
- Teaching skills to help Mr. Stein understand the need for lifestyle modifications

Technical Competencies

- Strong assessment skills to determine how stress has placed Mr. Stein at risk for fluid and electrolyte imbalances
- Caregiver skills directed toward stress reduction and maintenance of adequate fluid and electrolyte balance
- Ability to competently document nursing interventions and evaluations pertinent to Mr. Stein's plan of care

Interpersonal Competencies

- Interpersonal skills to communicate to Mr. Stein the realistic hope that his situation can be improved
- Ability to establish a trusting nurse–client relationship grounded in responsible caring
- Counseling skills that will enable Mr. Stein to live with his chronic condition with minimal discomfort and complications

Ethical/Legal Competencies

- Competence in documenting nursing interventions
- Willingness to assume responsibility for ensuring that the plan of care successfully assists Mr. Stein to cope with a chronic condition
- Ability to serve as a trusted and effective client advocate

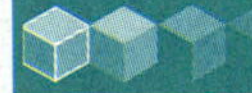

Nursing Plan of Care

for Mr. Stein

Nursing Diagnosis: Fluid Volume Deficit related to prolonged diarrhea and decreased fluid intake as evidenced by 4-lb weight loss, dry skin and mucous membranes, and report of decreased urine output and concentrated urine

Expected Outcome: By next week's visit, 3/24/98, the client will:

- Describe two effective means he has used to cope with stress

Nursing Interventions	Rationale	Evaluative Statement
Explore with the client (1) what he finds most stressing at present, (2) the control he believes he has over these stressors, and (3) the adequacy of his past and present stress management strategies.	Assisting the client to eliminate and reduce stress where possible and learn to cope better with unavoidable stress (identify and eliminate causative factors) is critical in controlling stress-related diarrhea.	3/24/98 Goal not met. Client reports little progress in coping with stress. With MCATs 1 week away, he feels more tense than ever before. Reports no time to explore stress management techniques.

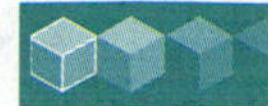

Nursing Plan of Care *(continued)*
for Mr. Stein

Nursing Interventions	Rationale	Evaluative Statement
Assess for other factors contributing to diarrhea and fluid volume deficit.	Diarrhea may have a functional basis.	*Revision:* Goal is appropriate. Encourage visit to counseling center if not before MCATs then as soon as possible afterward. *C. Ryan, RN*
Teach relation between stress and bouts of diarrhea.	Stress may result in increased intestinal mobility.	
Refer to counseling center on campus for assistance with stress management.	Professional assistance may facilitate identification and management of stressful situation.	

Expected Outcome: By the next week's visit, 3/24/98, the client will:

- Report that his diarrhea is eliminated or decreased to one or two episodes per day

Nursing Interventions	Rationale	Evaluative Statement
Teach client to link causative factors with diarrhea and to note anything that brings relief or assists in establishment of usual pattern of defecation.	Being able to make these connections helps client to assume charge of own condition and to reinforce preventive strategies and successful relief measures.	3/24/98 Goal met. Client reports diarrhea decreased to one or two episodes per day. *Recommendation:* Advise client that it is important to keep appointment with gastroenterologist because relief may only be temporary. *C. Ryan, RN*
Make sure client understands diet: chemically and mechanically nonirritating diet high in calories, protein, and minerals; exclude foods such as cocoa, chocolate, alcohol, cold or carbonated beverages, citrus juices; try frequent, small meals.	Some clients fear eating because it stimulates the gastrocolic reflex and may result in a stool. Eating the proper diet actually reduces bowel irritation and decreases peristalsis.	
Teach client proper use of prescribed medications.	Loperamide hydrochloride controls diarrhea, and methylcellulose increases consistency of stool.	

Expected Outcome: By next week's visit, 3/24/98, the client will:

- Demonstrate improved fluid and electrolyte balance as evidenced by (1) maintenance of present weight (170 lb), (2) moist mucous membranes, and (3) report of increased urinary output

Nursing Actions	Rationale	Evaluative Statement
Explore with client workable plan for oral replacement of fluids.	Collaboration with client to determine acceptable sources of fluid intake may allay his fear that fluid intake causes diarrheal episodes.	3/24/98 Goal partially met. Client reports diarrhea decreased to once or twice a day. Two days there was no diarrhea. Weight, 169 lb. Mucous membranes are moist. Urine output is increased. *C. Ryan, RN*
Have client note which calorie- and electrolyte- (sodium and potassium) rich fluids he can tolerate. Increase fluid intake to maintain a normal urine specific gravity.	Increased fluid intake is necessary to compensate for excessive loss in diarrhea and to reestablish fluid balance.	

(continued)

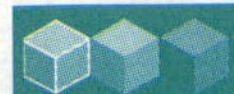

Nursing Plan of Care *(continued)*

for Mr. Stein

Nursing Actions	Rationale	Evaluative Statement
Instruct client to weigh himself every other day and to note changes in the volume or appearance of his urine.	All other things being equal, weight loss is a good indicator of continued fluid volume deficit. Other signs include decreased urinary output and high specific gravity.	
Teach client defining characteristics of electrolyte imbalances associated with prolonged diarrhea—hyponatremia and hypokalemia.	Excreted stool pulls electrolytes with it, especially sodium and potassium.	

Sample Documentation

3/24/98, nursing

Mr. Stein returned to the clinic reporting that his diarrhea is decreased to one to two episodes per day and that he has an appointment with a gastroenterologist. He believes that modifying his diet, increasing rest periods, and medications (loperamide hydrochloride to control diarrhea and methylcellulose to increase the consistency of stool) were of great help. He still does not know how he can reduce his stress level. Nursing examination revealed temperature, 98.9°F (37.1°C); pulse, 88 beats/min; respirations, 18; blood pressure, 110/60; weight, 169 lb; skin and mucous membranes less dry than on previous visit. States he has not noted much change in urine output but possibly less concentrated.

C. Ryan, RN

Key Points

- Whereas life can be sustained for many days without food, it can be sustained for only a few days without water.
- There are two major compartments for body fluids: (1) intracellular fluid, which is the fluid within cells, and (2) extracellular fluid, located outside of body cells, which includes intravascular fluid (plasma) and interstitial fluid (fluid in which tissue cells are bathed).
- A person's age, lean body mass, and sex can all influence the distribution of body fluids in the different compartments. Because lean tissue has higher water content than fat, thin people, males, and younger people tend to have higher percentages of total body water in relation to body weight than obese, female, and older people because of their increased lean body mass.
- Sodium and chloride are the principal ions of ECF; potassium and phosphate are principal ions of ICF.
- The most common routes for transporting fluid and electrolytes among the body compartments are osmosis, diffusion, active transport, and filtration.
- In a healthy adult, fluid intake and loss should average about 2500 mL over 2 to 3 days. The output of urine generally approximates the ingestion of liquids; water from food and oxidation is balanced by water loss through the feces, the skin, and the respiratory process.
- Deficiencies in the amount of both water and electrolytes in ECF in near-normal proportions are termed *fluid volume deficits*. Excessive retention of water and electrolytes in ECF is termed *fluid volume excess*.
- To prevent the serious complications that can result from untreated electrolyte imbalances, nurses must be familiar with the etiologies, defining characteristics, and treatment of imbalances of sodium, potassium, calcium, magnesium, and phosphate.
- Normal blood plasma is slightly alkaline and has a normal pH range from 7.35 to 7.45. Slight deviations in either direction (acid-base imbalances), if untreated, may result in death.
- The narrow range of normal pH is achieved by complex buffer systems (bicarbonate, phosphate, protein) and specific respiratory and renal mechanisms.

- Failure of acid-base regulating mechanisms may result in respiratory or metabolic disturbances, which can be acidosis or alkalosis.
- Risk factors for fluid, electrolyte, and acid-base imbalances include pathologies involving homeostatic regulators of fluid balance (eg, diabetes mellitus, congestive heart failure, renal failure); abnormal losses of body fluids; burns and trauma; and therapies with the potential to disrupt fluid and electrolyte balance (eg, medications such as diuretics and steroids, IV therapy, TPN).
- Pertinent assessment measures include maintaining accurate intake and output records, recording daily weights, observing for the signs and symptoms that characterize specific imbalances, and monitoring results of laboratory studies.
- Nursing diagnoses may be developed in which the fluid imbalance is the problem statement (Fluid Volume Deficit or Fluid Volume Excess), or the etiology (Pain related to edema, Impaired Oral Mucous Membrane related to dehydration).
- Nursing interventions are directed to maintaining a client's fluid, electrolyte, and acid-base balance; to preventing disturbances; and to correcting imbalances.
- When fluids are being encouraged or restricted, it is important that both the nursing staff and client understand the target amount of fluid to be taken each shift and that the client's fluid preferences be respected.
- Nurses administering IV fluids should accurately prepare the prescribed solution; understand the desired effect of treatment and possible adverse responses; and assume responsibility for initiating, monitoring, and, when ordered, discontinuing the therapy.
- Complications associated with IV infusions include infiltration, phlebitis, thrombus, speed shock, fluid overload, embolus, and infection.
- Administering blood transfusions requires a careful pretransfusion assessment of the client, accurate identification and matching of the blood to be transfused with its intended recipient, and ongoing monitoring of the client throughout the transfusion for transfusion reactions. These include hemolytic, febrile, allergic, and hypervolemic reactions.
- In TPN, hypertonic solutions of dextrose, amino acids, and select electrolytes and minerals—capable of reestablishing positive nitrogen balance and weight gain—are infused using a central vein.

Study Questions

1. Plasma, the liquid constituent of blood, is correctly identified as
   a. interstitial fluid
   b. intravascular fluid
   c. intracellular fluid
   d. 40% of total body fluid
2. Potassium functions as
   a. the chief electrolyte of extracellular fluid
   b. the most abundant electrolyte in the body
   c. the major cation of intracellular fluid
   d. the chief extracellular anion
3. The movement of the solvent water from an area of lesser solute concentration to an area of greater solute concentration until equilibrium is established is known as
   a. osmosis
   b. diffusion
   c. active transport
   d. filtration
4. The most accurate indication of fluid balance status is
   a. intake and output
   b. skin turgor
   c. complete blood count
   d. daily weight
5. After assessing the following arterial blood gas values (pH, 7.30; $PaCO_2$, 32; HCO_3^-, 14), the nurse correctly identifies
   a. respiratory acidosis
   b. respiratory alkalosis
   c. metabolic acidosis
   d. metabolic alkalosis
6. Mrs. Podralski, a client in the hospital, has been encouraged to increase her fluid intake. The nurse can best facilitate this by
   a. explaining the mechanisms involved in transporting fluids to and from intracellular compartments
   b. keeping fluids readily available for the client
   c. emphasizing the long-term goal of increasing fluids when she returns home
   d. planning to offer the larger amount of fluids in the evening
7. As the nurse prepares to assist the physician with insertion of a short-term CVC, she is aware that
   a. this catheter usually remains in place for 2 to 3 months
   b. the catheter is introduced by way of the basilic or cephalic veins in the antecubital space
   c. nursing responsibility includes changing the CVC dressing at least once weekly
   d. a chest x-ray is required to confirm placement
8. The nurse alertly assesses the acid–base balance of a client because she is aware that the client will be unable to effectively control his carbonic acid supply. This is most likely a client with badly damaged
   a. kidneys
   b. lungs
   c. adrenal glands
   d. blood vessels

9. Having the client focus on breathing more slowly would be the most helpful intervention for the problem of
   a. respiratory acidosis (carbonic acid excess)
   b. respiratory alkalosis (carbonic acid deficit)
   c. metabolic acidosis (base bicarbonate deficit)
   d. metabolic alkalosis (base bicarbonate excess)
10. Which of the following is the most common etiologic factor related to the nursing diagnosis of fluid volume excess?
   a. increased need for fluids secondary to fever
   b. abnormal fluid loss from vomiting
   c. excessive IV infusion
   d. decreased fluid intake secondary to depression
11. In evaluating for complications of IV therapy, which of the following is evidence that the IV has infiltrated?
   a. In the past hour, only 50 mL of fluid has infused.
   b. The insertion site is red, hot, and swollen.
   c. The client's temperature has risen to 101°F (38.3°C).
   d. The site is pale, cool, swollen, and painful.
12. For a client at risk for hyperkalemia, it is important to teach the client to avoid certain foods. Included in the foods to avoid would be
   a. carrots and squash
   b. canned soups and potato chips
   c. bananas, apricots, broccoli
   d. whole grain cereals
13. Your client has multiple injuries after an automobile accident and you are to start IV therapy. His right arm is in a cast. Which site would you choose for venipuncture?
   a. left antecubital
   b. dorsal aspect of either foot
   c. right hand
   d. left forearm
14. For clients who are receiving IV therapy, the nurse should
   a. change the IV catheter and entry site daily
   b. change the tubing every 8 hours
   c. increase the rate to catch up if the correct amount has not been infused at the end of the shift
   d. monitor the flow rate at least every hour
15. While a client is receiving blood, the nurse should evaluate for transfusion reaction
   a. 15 minutes after the infusion is started
   b. after the blood is all infused
   c. every hour
   d. every 15 minutes

Answers With Rationale

1. The correct response is *b.* Intravascular fluid or plasma is extracellular fluid and composes 5% of total body fluid.
2. The correct response is *c.* Sodium is the chief electrolyte of extracellular fluid, calcium is the most abundant electrolyte in the body, and chloride is the chief extracellular anion.
3. The correct response is *a.* Gases move about by diffusion. Active transport is a process that requires energy for the movement of substances through a cell membrane from an area of lesser to higher concentration. Filtration is the passage of fluids through a permeable membrane from an area of high pressure to one of low pressure.
4. The correct response is *d.* Intake and output are not always as accurate and may involve a subjective component. Measurement of skin turgor is subjective and the complete blood count does not necessarily reflect fluid balance.
5. The correct response is *c.* Metabolic acidosis equals low bicarbonate. Acidosis equals low pH. Decreased $PaCO_2$ represents a respiratory compensatory attempt.
6. The correct response is *b.* Explanation of the fluid transportation mechanisms is inappropriate and it does not focus on the immediate problem of increasing fluid intake. Meeting short-term goals provides further reinforcement and additional fluids should be taken earlier in the day.
7. The correct response is *d.* Short-term CVCs remain in place up to 4 weeks, they are introduced into the subclavian or internal jugular vein, and dressings should be changed according to agency policy but at least every 72 hours.
8. The correct response is *b.* The lungs are the primary controller of the body's carbonic acid supply.
9. The correct response is *b.* Breathing more slowly causes accumulation of carbon dioxide to reverse carbonic acid deficit.
10. The correct response is *c.* The other alternatives are related to fluid volume deficit.
11. The correct response is *d.* A decrease in flow rate may indicate an infiltration but is not as significant as the other signs of a pale, cool, swollen, and painful site. Phlebitis is an inflammatory process and results in redness, warmth, and possibly a temperature elevation.
12. The correct response is *c.* Hyperkalemia is an elevated serum potassium level: bananas, apricots, and broccoli are foods high in potassium and should be avoided in this situation.

13. The correct response is *d.* Based on the condition of the right arm, this is not a choice. The left forearm is preferable to the antecubital space of the left arm or the lower extremities.
14. The correct response is *d.* IV catheter and entry site should be changed every 48 to 72 hours in most circumstances. Tubing is changed according to agency policy but not at the frequency of every 8 hours. Increasing the rate may lead to fluid overload.
15. The correct response is *d.* The nurse should closely observe a client for the first 15 minutes and then check the client thereafter every 15 minutes while he or she is receiving the blood transfusion.

Bibliography

American Association of Critical-Care Nurses. (1992). Evaluation of the effects of heparinized flush solutions on the patency of arterial pressure monitoring lines: The AACN Thunder Project. *American Journal of Critical Care, 2*(1), 3.

Angelucci, D., & Todaro, A. (1993). Reversing acute dehydration. *Nursing, 23*(6), 33.

Bohony, J. (1993). 9 common IV complications and what to do about them. *American Journal of Nursing, 93*(10), 45–49.

Bove, L. (1994). How fluids and electrolytes shift. *Nursing, 24*(8), 34–39.

Carpenito, L. (1995). *Nursing diagnosis: Application to clinical practice* (6th ed.). Philadelphia: Lippincott.

Cerrato, P. (1992). Don't overlook this mineral deficiency. *RN, 55*(7), 61–62.

Choosing a venipuncture site. (1995). *Nursing, 25*(3), 32L.

Christianson, D. (1994). Caring for a patient who has an implanted venous port. *American Journal of Nursing, 94*(11), 40–44.

Cirolia, B. (1996). Understanding edema. *Nursing, 26*(2), 66–70.

Cohen, M. (1996). Medication errors. *Nursing, 26*(2), 16.

Cohen, M., & Davis, N. (1993). Recognizing the dangers of free flow from an EID. *Nursing, 23*(6), 56–59.

Davis, N. (1995). Potassium perils. *American Journal of Nursing, 95*(3), 14.

Dudek, S. (1993). *Nutrition handbook for nursing practice* (2nd ed.). Philadelphia: Lippincott.

Fischbach, F. (1995). *A manual of laboratory tests* (5th ed.). Philadelphia: Lippincott.

Gonsoulin, S., & Broussard, P. (1991). Shedding light on IV therapy. *Nursing, 21*(12), 62–64.

Green, L., & Gerlach, C. (1994). Central lines have moved out. *RN, 57*(5), 26–30.

Harovas, J., & Anthony, H. (1993a). Managing transfusion reactions. *RN, 56*(12), 32–36.

Harovas, J., & Anthony, H. (1993b). Your guide to trouble-free transfusions. *RN, 56*(11), 26–35.

Hastings-Tolsma, M., & Yucha, C. (1994). IV infiltration: No clear signs, no clear treatment? *RN, 57*(12), 34–38.

Hoppe, B. (1995). Taking the confusion out of calcium levels. *Nursing, 25*(7), 32KK–32MM.

Ignatavicius, D., Workman, M., & Mishler, M. (1995). *Medical–surgical nursing: A nursing process approach* (2nd ed.). Philadelphia: Saunders.

Kirton, C. (1996). Assessing for ascites. *Nursing, 26*(4), 53.

LaRocca, J., & Otto, S. (1993). *Pocket guide: Intravenous therapy.* St. Louis: Mosby.

Masoorli, S. (1995). When IV practice spells malpractice. *RN, 58*(8), 53–55.

Mathews, L. (1994). Preparing your patient for home infusion. *Nursing, 24*(10), 28.

Mays, D. (1995). Turn ABGs into child's play. *RN, 58*(1), 36–39.

Metheny, N. (1992). *Fluid and electrolyte balance: Nursing considerations* (2nd ed.). Philadelphia: Lippincott.

Meyer, C. (1992). Transparent dressings' clear disadvantage. *American Journal of Nursing, 92*(6), 14.

Millam, D. (1992). Starting I.V.s: How to develop your venipuncture expertise. *Nursing, 22*(9), 33–46.

Millam, D. (1993). How to teach good venipuncture technique. *American Journal of Nursing, 93*(7), 38–41.

Millam, D. (1993). I.V. technology helps you stay out of harm's way. *Nursing, 23*(10), 62–63.

Murray, E. (1993). Probing the safety of central venous catheters. *American Journal of Nursing, 93*(5), 72–76.

North American Nursing Diagnosis Association. (1994). *NANDA nursing diagnoses: Definitions and classification 1995–1996.* Philadelphia: NANDA.

Owens, M. (1993). Keeping an eye on magnesium. *American Journal of Nursing, 93*(2), 66–67.

Phillips, L. (1993). *Manual of I.V. therapeutics.* Philadelphia: Davis.

Porth, C. (1994). *Pathophysiology: Concepts of altered health states* (4th ed.). Philadelphia: Lippincott.

Questions and answers about blood transfusions. (1995). *Nursing, 25*(2), 32C–32G.

Rice, R. (1995). *Handbook of home health nursing procedures.* St. Louis: Mosby.

Sansivero, G. (1995). Why pick a PICC: What you need to know. *Nursing, 25*(7), 34–41.

Sheldon, J. (1994). What you should know about I.V. dressings. *Nursing, 24*(8), 32.

Sieh, A., & Brentin, L. (1993). A little light makes venipuncture easier. *RN, 56*(3), 40–43.

Smith, R. (1993). A nurse's guide to implanted ports. *RN, 56*(4), 48–52.

Stringfield, Y. (1993). Back to basics: Acidosis, alkalosis, and ABG's. *American Journal of Nursing, 93*(11), 43–44.

Tasoda, F., & Weismiller, S. (1994). Assessing ABGs: Maintaining the delicate balance. *Nursing, 24*(5), 34–35.

Taylor, D. (1990a). Respiratory acidosis: Pathophysiology, signs, and symptoms. *Nursing, 19*(9), 52–53.

Taylor, D. (1990b). Respiratory alkalosis: Pathophysiology, signs, and symptoms. *Nursing, 20*(8), 60–61.

Viall, C. (1990). Your complete guide to central venous catheters. *Nursing, 20*(2), 34–41.

Vonfrolio, L. (1995). Would you hang these IV solutions? *American Journal of Nursing, 95*(6), 37–39.

Woodtli, A. (1990). Thirst: A critical care nursing challenge. *Dimensions of Critical Care Nursing, 9*(1), 6–15.

Yarnell, R., & Craig, M. (1991). Detecting hypomagnesemia: The most overlooked electrolyte imbalance. *Nursing, 21*(7), 55–57.

Appendices

Equivalents

Metric Units

The metric system, developed by the French, uses the *meter* as the basic unit. The metric system is a decimal system, with prefixes that designate the various multiples or divisibles of 10. The most commonly used prefixes in medicine are:

Milli, which means one one-thousandth (0.001)
Centi, which means one one-hundredth (0.01)
Kilo, which means one thousand (1000)

These prefixes may be affixed to any of the three basic units of measurements, which are

Meter (m), the unit of length
Gram (g), the unit of weight
Liter (L), the unit of volume

Therefore

1 millimeter (mm) = 0.001 m
1 milligram (mg) = 0.001 g
1 milliliter (mL) = 0.001 L
1 kilometer (km) = 1000 m
1 kilogram (kg) = 1000 g
1 kiloliter (kl) = 1000 L

Length

The meter (a little longer than a yard) and the kilometer (about 0.6 mile) seldom are used in medicine or nursing. The commonly used measure of length is 1 centimeter (cm) = 0.01 m = about 0.4 inch.

Volume

The most frequently used measures of volume are the *liter* and the *milliliter*. Some useful equivalents to know are

1000 milliliters (mL) = 1 liter (L)
1000 cubic centimeters (cc) = 1 liter (L)
1 milliliter (mL) = 1 cc

Weight

The gram designates the weight of 1 mL of distilled water at 4°C. The most frequently used units of weight are

1,000,000 micrograms (mcg or µg) = 1 gram (g)
1000 micrograms (mcg) = 1 milligram (mg)
1000 milligrams (mg) = 1 gram (g)
1000 grams (g) = 1 kilogram (kg) = 2.2 pounds (lb)

Table A-1
Metric and Household Equivalents

Metric Unit	Household Unit
5 mL	1 tsp
15 mL	1 Tbs
180 mL	1 full teacup
240 ml	1 full glass

Metric Units and Their Household Equivalents

Household measurement is inaccurate, with wide variations in the size of teaspoons, teacups, and so forth. The generally accepted household measures are:

60 drops (gtt) = 1 teaspoon (tsp or t)
3 tsp = 1 tablespoon (Tbs or T)
12 Tbs = 1 teacup
16 Tbs = 1 glass (or a standard measuring cup)

Apothecary Units

In the apothecary system
The unit of weight is the *grain.*
The unit of volume is the *minim.*

Of the many units of measure in the apothecary system, you should know the following units, abbreviations, and equivalents.

Weight

60 grains (gr) = 1 dram (dr or ʒ)
8 drams (dr or ʒ) = 1 ounce (oz or ℥)

Volume

60 minims (min) = 1 fluid dram (fl dr or fʒ)
8 fl dr = 1 fluid ounce (fl oz or f℥)
16 fl oz = 1 pint (pt)
2 pt = 1 quart (qt)
4 qt = 1 gallon (gal)

In the apothecary system, when the symbol or abbreviation is used, the quantity is written in lowercase Roman numerals and follows the symbol. Arabic numerals are used, however, in preference to large Roman numerals. For example

5 gr = gr v
8 dr = ʒ viii

The quantity one-half may be indicated by the symbol ss.

1½ gr = gr iss
7½ gr = gr viiss

Other fractional parts are expressed as common fractions, for example, gr 1/250, gr 1/10.

When pint, quart, and gallon are written, the quantity is expressed in Arabic numerals, (eg, 1½ pints or 7½ quarts).

Apothecary Units and Their Household Equivalents

1 drop = 1 minim (m i)
1 tsp = 1 dr (ʒ i)
1 Tbs = ½ oz (℥ ss)
2 Tbs = 1 oz (℥ i)
1 teacup = 6 oz (℥ vi)
1 glass or measuring cup = 8 oz (℥ viii)
2 measuring cups = 1 pt

Table A-2
Most Commonly Used Approximate Equivalents*

Metric	Apothecary	Household
0.06 g	gr i	
0.06 mL	min i	1 drop
1.0 g	gr xv	
1.0 mL	min xv	⅕ tsp
5 mL	(1 dr) ʒ i	1 tsp
15 mL	(½ oz) ʒ ss	1 Tbs
30 mL	(1 oz) ℥ i	2 Tbs
500 mL	(16 oz) ℥ 16	1 pt
1000 mL	(32 oz) ℥ 32	1 qt

* There are many discrepancies among these approximate equivalents. For example, 30 mL is the accepted equivalent for 1 oz (29.57 mL is the exact equivalent). Such discrepancies are inevitable when two systems are used whose equivalents are not exact. If the discrepancies are within a 10% margin of error, they usually are acceptable in pharmacology.

Table A-3
Commonly Used Metric Units and Their Approximate Apothecary Equivalents

Metric		Apothecary
1 g	1000 mg	gr xv
0.6 g	600 mg	gr x
0.5 g	500 mg	gr viiss
0.3 g	300 mg	gr v
0.2 g	200 mg	gr iii
0.1 g	100 mg	gr iss
0.06 g	60 mg	gr i
0.05 g	50 mg	gr 3/4
0.03 g	30 mg	gr 1/2 or gr ss
0.02 g	20 mg	gr 1/3
0.015 g	15 mg	gr 1/4
0.016 g	16 mg	gr 1/4
0.010 g	10 mg	gr 1/6
0.008 g	8 mg	gr 1/8
0.006 g	6 mg	gr 1/10
0.005 g	5 mg	gr 1/12
0.003 g	3 mg	gr 1/20
0.002 g	2 mg	gr 1/30
0.001 g	1 mg	gr 1/60
	0.6 mg	gr 1/100
	0.5 mg	gr 1/120
	0.4 mg	gr 1/150
	0.3 mg	gr 1/200

Appendix B

Normal Adult Laboratory Values*

Commonly Used Abbreviations

kg = kilogram
g = gram
mg = milligram
μg = microgram
μμg = micromicrogram
ng = nanogram
mEq = milliequivalent
L = liter
dl = 100 milliliters
mL = milliliter
cu mm (mm^3) = cubic millimeter
nM = nanomolar
mIU = milliInternational Unit
pg = picogram
mm = millimeter
μ = micron or micrometer
mm Hg = millimeters of mercury
mU = milliunit
μU = microunit
IU = International Unit

* Laboratory values may vary according to techniques used in different laboratories.

Table B-1
Hematologic Values—Reference Ranges

Determination	Conventional	SI
Coagulation Factors		
Factor I (fibrinogen)	0.15–0.35 g/100 mL	4.0–10.0 μmol/L
Factor II (prothrombin)	60%–140%	0.60–1.40 μmol/L
Factor V (accelerator globulin)	60%–140%	0.60–1.40 μmol/L
Factors VII to X (proconvertin to Stuart factor)	70%–130%	0.70–1.30 μmol/L
Factor X (Stuart factor)	60%–140%	0.70–1.30 μmol/L
Factor VIII (antihemophilic globulin)	50%–200%	0.50–2.0 μmol/L
Factor IX (plasma thromboplastic cofactor)	60%–140%	0.60–1.40 μmol/L
Factor XI (plasma thromboplastic antecedent)	60%–140%	0.60–1.40 μmol/L
Factor XII (Hageman factor)	60%–140%	0.60–1.40 μmol/L
Coagulation Screening Tests		
Bleeding time (Simplate)	2–8 min	180–540 sec
Prothrombin time	9.5–12 sec	Less than 2 sec from control
Partial thromboplastin time (activated)	20–45 sec	25–37 sec
Whole blood clot lysis	No clot lysis in 24 hr	0/day
Fibrinolytic Studies		
Euglobin lysis	No lysis in 2 hr	0 (in 2 hr)
Thrombin time		Control +5 sec
Complete Blood Count		
Hematocrit	Male: 42%–50% Female: 40%–48%	Male: 0.42–0.52 Female: 0.37–0.48
Hemoglobin	Male: 13–18 g/dL Female: 12–16 g/dL	Male: 8.1–11.2 mmol/L Female: 7.4–9.9 mmol/L
Leukocyte count	5000–10,000/mm^3	4.3–10.8 × 10^9/L
Erythrocyte count	4.2 million–5.9 million/mm^3	4.2–5.9 × 10^{12}/L
Mean corpuscular volume (MCV)	80–94 $μm^3$	80–94 fl
Mean corpuscular hemoglobin (MCH)	27–32 pg	1.7–2.0 fmol
Mean corpuscular hemoglobin concentration (MCHC)	33%–38%	19–22.8 mmol/L
Erythrocyte sedimentation rate (Zeta Centrifuge)	41%–54%	Male: 1–13 mm/h Female: 1–20 mm/h

(continued)

Table B-1 *(continued)*
Hematologic Values—Reference Ranges

Determination	Conventional	SI
Erythrocyte Enzymes		
Glucose-6-phosphate dehydrogenase	5–15 U/g Hb	5–15 U/g
Pyruvate kinase	13–17 U/g Hb	13–17 U/g
Ferritin (serum)	Females: 5–100 ng/mL Males: 10–270 ng/mL	
Folic acid, RIA	4–16 ng/mL	
Haptoglobin	50–250 mg/dL	1.0 g–3.0 g/L
Hemoglobin Studies		
Electrophoresis for A_2 hemoglobin	1.5%–3.5%	0.015–0.035
Hemoglobin, met- and sulf-	0	0
Serum hemoglobin	2–3 mg/100 mL	1.2–1.9 μmol/L
Lupus erythematosus (LE) preparation		
Heparin as anticoagulant	0	0
Defibrinated blood	0	0
Muramidase	Serum, 3–7 μg/mL Urine, 0–2 μg/mL	3–7 mg/L 0–2 mg/L
Osmotic fragility of erythrocyte	Increased if hemolysis occurs in over 0.5% NaCl; decreased if hemolysis is incomplete in 0.3% NaCl	
Peroxide hemolysis	Less than 10%	<0.10
Platelet count	100,000–400,000/mm^3	150–350 × 10^9/L
Platelet Function Tests		
Clot retraction	50%–100%/2 hr	0.50–1.00/2 hr
Platelet aggregation	Full response to ADP, epinephrine and collagen	1.0
Platelet factor 3	33–57 sec	33–57 sec
Reticulocyte count	0.5%–1.5% red cells	0.005–0.15
Vitamin B_{12}	90–280 pg/mL (borderline: 70–90)	66–207 pmol/L (borderline: 52–66)

Table B-2
Blood, Plasma or Serum Values—Reference Ranges

Determination	Conventional	SI
Acetoacetate plus acetone	0.3–2.0 mg/dL	3–20 mg/L
Aldolase	1.3–8.2 mU/mL	12–75 nmol sec^{-1}/L
Alpha amino nitrogen	3.0–5.5 mg/100 mL	2.1–3.9 mmol/L
Ammonia	80–110 μg/100 mL	47–65 μmol/L
Ascorbic acid	0.4–1.5 mg/100 mL	23–85 μmol/L
Bilirubin (van den Bergh test)	1 minute: 0.4 mg/100 mL	Up to 7 μmol/L
	Direct: 0.1–0.2 mg/dL	Up to 17 μmol/L
	Total: 1.0 mg/100 mL	
	Indirect: 0.1–1.0 mg/dL	
Blood volume	8.5%–9.0% of body weight in kg	80–85 mL/kg
	Toxic level: 17 mEq/L	
Bromsulphalein (BSP)	Less than 5% retention 45 min after 5 mg/kg IV	<0.05 L
Calcium	8.5–10.5 mg/100 mL	2.1–2.5 mmol/L
Carbon dioxide content	24 mEq–32 mEq/L	24–30 mmol/L
Carcinoembryonic antigen (CEA)	0.25 mg/mL	0–2.5 μg/L
Carotenoids	0.8–4.0 μg/mL	1.5–7.4 μmol/L
Ceruloplasmin	27–37 mg/100 mL	1.8–2.4 μmol/L
Chloride	95–105 mEq/L	100–106 mmol/L
Cholesterol	<200 mg/dL	
Cholinesterase (pseudocholinesterase)	0.5 pH U or more/hr	0.5 arb unit or more
	0.7 pH U or more/hr for packed cells	
Copper	Total: 100–200 μg/100 mL	16–31 μmol/L
Creatine phosphokinase (CPK)	Female: 50–250 mU/mL	0.08–0.58 μmol sec^{-1}/L
	Male: 50–325 mU/mL	
Creatinine	0.7–1.4 mg/100 mL	60–130 μmol/L
Ethanol	0.3%–0.4%, marked intoxication;	65–87 mmol/L
	0.4%–0.5%, alcoholic stupor;	87–109 mmol/L
	0.5% or over, alcoholic coma	>109 mmol/L
Glucose	Fasting: 60–110 mg/100 mL	3.9–5.6 mmol/L
Iron	65–170 μg/100 mL (higher in males)	9.0–26.9 μmol/L
Iron-binding capacity	250–410 μg/100 mL	44.8–73.4 μmol/L
Lactic acid	0.6–1.8 mEq/L	0.6–1.8 mmol/L
Lactic dehydrogenase isoenzymes	100–225 mU/mL	1.00–2.00 μmol sec^{-1}/L
Lead	50 μg/100 mL or less	Up to 2.4 μmol/L
Lipase	2 U/mL or less	Up to 2 arb units
Lipids, total	400–1000 mg/dL	3.10–5.69 mmol/L
Magnesium	0.33–2.4 mEq/L	0.8–1.3 mmol/L
5′ Nucleotidase	0.3–3.2 Bodansky U	30–290 nmol sec^{-1}/L
Osmolality	280–300 mOsm/kg water	285–295 mmol/kg
Oxygen saturation (arterial)	95%–100%	0.96–1.00 L
Pco_2	35–45 mm Hg	4.7–6.0 kPg
pH	7.35–7.45	Same
Po_2	95–100 mm Hg (dependent on age while breathing room air)	10.0–13.3 kPa
	Above 500 mm Hg while on 100% O_2	
Phenylalanine	0–2 mg/100 mL	0–120 μmol/L
Phosphorus (inorganic)	3.0–4.5 mg/100 mL	1.0–1.5 mmol/L
Potassium	3.8–5.0 mEq/L	3.5–5.0 mmol/L

(continued)

Table B-2 *(continued)*
Blood, Plasma or Serum Values—Reference Ranges

Primidone (Mysoline)	Therapeutic level, 4–12 μg/mL	18–55 μmol/L
Protein, total	6.0–8.0 g/100 mL	60–84 g/L
Albumin	3.5–5.0 g/100 mL	33–50 g/L
Globulin	1.5–3.0 g/100 mL	23–35 g/L
Electrophoresis	% of total protein	% of total protein
Albumin	3.3–5.0 g/dL	0.52–0.68
Globulin		
$Alpha_1$	0.2–0.4 g/dL	0.042–0.072
$Alpha_2$	0.6–1.0 g/dL	0.068–0.12
Beta	0.6–1.2 g/dL	0.093–0.15
Gamma	0.7–1.5 g/dL	0.13–0.23
	0.3–0.7 mg/dL	0–0.11 mmol/L
Sodium	135–145 mEq/L	135–145 mmol/L
Sulfate	0.5–1.5 mg/100 mL	0.05–1.2 mmol/L
Transaminase (SGOT) (aspartate aminotransferase)	7–40 U/mL	0.08–0.32 μmol sec^{-1}/L
Urea nitrogen (BUN)	10–20 mg/100 mL	2.9–8.9 mmol/L
Uric acid	2.5–8.0 mg/100 mL	0.13–0.42 mmol/L
Vitamin A	50–220 μg/dL	0.5–2.1 μmol/L

Table B-3
Urine Values—Reference Ranges

Determination		Conventional		SI	
Acetone plus acetoacetate (quantitative)		0		0 mg/L	
Alpha amino nitrogen		64–199 mg/day; not over 1.5% of total nitrogen		4.6–14.2 mmol/day	
Amylase		35–260 U/mL		24–76 arb units	
Calcium		150 mg/day or less		3.8 mmol/day or less	
Catecholamines		Epinephrine, 10%–40%		<55 nmol/day	
		Norepinephrine, 60%–90%		<590 nmol/day	
Copper		20–70 µg/day		0–1.6 µmol/day	
Coproporphyrin		50–300 µg/day		80–380 nmol/day	
Creatine		0–200 mg/24 hr		<0.75 mmol/day	
Cystine or cysteine		0		0	
Follicle-stimulating hormone					
Follicular phase		5–20 IU/day		Same	
Midcycle		15–60 IU/day			
Luteal phase		5–15 IU/day			
Menopausal		50–100 IU/day			
Men		5–25 IU/day			
Hemoglobin and myoglobin		0			
5-Hydroxyindole acetic acid		2–9 mg/day (women lower than men)		10–45 µmol/day	
Phenolsulfonphthalein (PSP)		At least 25% excreted by 15 min; 40% by 30 min; 60% by 120 min		0.25 L	
Phosphorus (inorganic)		Varies with intake; average 1 g/day		32 mmol/day	
Porphobilinogen		0		0	
Protein, quantitative		<150 mg/24 hr		<0.15 g/day	
Steroids					
17-Ketosteroids (per day)	Age (yr)	Male (mg)	Female (mg)	Male (µmol/day)	Female (µmol/day)
	10	1–4	1–4	3–14	3–14
	20	6–21	4–16	21–73	14–56
	30	8–26	4–14	28–90	14–49
	50	5–18	3–9	17–62	10–31
	70	2–10	1–7	7–35	3–24
17-Hydroxysteroids		3–8 mg/day (women lower than men)		8–22 µmol/day as hydrocortisone	
Sugar					
Quantitative glucose		0		0 mmol/L	
Identification of reducing substances					
Fructose		0		0 mmol/L	
Pentose		0		0 mmol/L	
Titratable acidity		20–40 mEq/day		20–40 mmol/day	
Urobilinogen		<0.25 mg/dL		To 1.0 arb unit	
Uroporphyrin		Up to 50 µg in 24 hr		0 nmol/day	
Vanilmandelic acid (VMA)		0.7–6.8 mg/24 hr		Up to 45 µmol/day	

Table B-4
Cerebrospinal Fluid Values—Reference Ranges

Determination	Conventional	SI
Bilirubin	0	0 μmol/L
Chloride	100–130 mEq/L	
Albumin	15.5–32.0 mg/dL	0.295 g/L ± 2 SD (0.11–0.48)
IgG	0–6.6 mg/dL	0.043 g/L ± 2 SD (0–0.086)
Glucose	50–75 mg/100 mL (30%–50% less than blood)	2.8–4.2 mmol/L
Pressure (initial)	70–180 mm H_2O	70–80 arb units
Protein		
Lumbar	15–45 mg/100 mL	0.15–0.45 g/L
Cisternal	15–25 mg/100 mL	0.15–0.25 g/L
Ventricular	5–15 mg/100 mL	0.05–0.15 g/L

Table B-5
Special Endocrine Tests—Reference Ranges

Steroid Hormones		
Aldosterone	Excretion: 5–19 μg/24 hr	14–53 nmol/day
Fasting, at rest, 210 mEq sodium diet	Supine: 48 ± 29 pg/mL	133 ± 80 pmol/L
	Upright: (2h) 65± 23 pg/mL	180 ± 64 pmol/L
Fasting, at rest, 110 mEq sodium diet	Supine: 107 ± 45 pg/mL	279 ± 125 pmol/L
	Upright: (2h) 239 ± 123 pg/mL	663 ± 341 pmol/L
Fasting, at rest, 10 mEq sodium diet	Supine: 175 ± 75 pg/mL	485 ± 208 pmol/L
	Upright: (2h) 532 ± 228 pg/mL	1476 ± 632 pmol/L

(continued)

Table B-5 *(continued)*
Special Endocrine Tests—Reference Ranges

Steroid Hormones		
Cortisol		
Fasting	8 AM: 5–25 μg/100 mL	0.14–0.69 μmol/L
At rest	8 PM: below 10 μg/100 mL	0–0.28 μmol/L
20 U ACTH	4-hour ACTH test: 30–45 μg/100 mL	0.83–1.24 μmol/L
Dexamethasone at midnight	Overnight suppression test: below 5 μg/100 mL	<0.14 nmol/L
	Excretion: 20–70 μg/24 hr	55–193 nmol/day
11-Deoxycortisol	Responsive: over 7.5 μg/100 mL (after metrapone)	>0.22 μmol/L
Testosterone	Adult male: 300–1100 ng/100 mL	10.4–38.1 nmol/L
	Adolescent male: over 100 ng/100 mL	>3.5 nmol/L
	Females: 25–90 ng/100 mL	0.87–3.12 nmol/L
Unbound testosterone	Adult male: 3.06–24.0 ng/100 mL	106–832 pmol/L
	Adult female: 0.09–1.28 ng/100 mL	3.1–44.4 pmol/L
Polypeptide Hormones		
Adrenocorticotrophin (ACTH)	15–70 pg/mL	3.3–15.4 pmol/L
Calcitonin	Undetectable in normals	0
	>100 pg/mL in medullary carcinoma	>29.3 pmol/L
Growth hormone		
Fasting, at rest	Below 5 ng/mL	<233 pmol/L
After exercise	Children: over 10 ng/mL	>465 pmol/L
	Male: below 5 ng/mL	<233 pmol/L
	Female: up to 30 ng/mL	0–1395 pmol/L
After glucose	Male: below 5 ng/mL	<233 pmol/L
	Female: below 10 mg/mL	0–465 pmol/L
Insulin		
Fasting	6–26 μU/mL	43–187 pmol/L
During hypoglycemia	Below 20 μU/mL	<144 pmol/L
After glucose	Up to 150 μU/mL	0–1078 pmol/L
Luteinizing hormone	Male: 6–18 mU/mL	6–18 U/L
Preovulatory or postovulatory	Female: 5–22 mU/mL	5–22 U/L
Midcycle peak	30–250 mU/mL	30–250 U/L
Parathyroid hormone	<10 μl equiv/mL	<10 mL equiv/L
Prolactin	2–15 ng/mL	0.08–6.0 nmol/L
Renin activity		
Normal diet	Supine: 1.1 ± 0.8 ng/mL/hr	0.9 ± 0.6 nmol/L/hr
	Upright: 1.9 ± 1.7 ng/mL/hr	1.5 ± 1.3 nmol/L/hr
Low-sodium diet	Supine: 2.7 ± 1.8 ng/mL/hr	2.1 ± 1.4 nmol/L/hr
	Upright: 6.6 ± 2.5 ng/mL/hr	5.1 ± 1.9 nmol/L/hr
High-sodium diet	Diuretics: 10.0 ± 3.7 ng/mL/hr	7.7 ± 2.9 nmol/L/hr
Thyroid Hormones		
Thyroid-stimulating hormone (TSH)	0.5–3.5 μU/mL	0.5–3.5 mU/L
Thyroxine-binding globulin capacity	15–25 μg T_4/100 mL	193–322 mU/L
Total triiodothyronine by radioimmunoassay (T_3)	70–190 ng/100 mL	1.08–2.92 nmol/L
Total thyroxine (T_4) by RIA	4–12 μg/100 mL	52–154 nmol/L
T_3 resin uptake	25%–35%	0.25–0.35
Free thyroxine index (FT_4I)	1–4 ng/100 mL	12.8–51.2 pmol/L

Appendix C

U.S. Nutritional Tables

Table C-1
U.S. Recommended Daily Allowances

Category	Age (yr) or Condition	Weight† (kg)	Weight† (lb)	Height† (cm)	Height† (in)	Protein (g)	Fat-Soluble Vitamins: *Vitamin A (μg RE)‡*	Fat-Soluble Vitamins: *Vitamin D (μg)§*	Fat-Soluble Vitamins: *Vitamin E (mg α-TE)¶*	Fat-Soluble Vitamins: *Vitamin K (μg)*	*Vitamin C (mg)*
Infants	0.0–0.5	6	13	60	24	13	375	7.5	3	5	30
	0.5–1.0	9	20	71	28	14	375	10	4	10	35
Children	1–3	13	29	90	35	16	400	10	6	15	40
	4–6	20	44	112	44	24	500	10	7	20	45
	7–10	28	62	132	52	28	700	10	7	30	45
Males	11–14	45	99	157	62	45	1000	10	10	45	50
	15–18	66	145	176	69	59	1000	10	10	65	60
	19–24	72	160	177	70	58	1000	10	10	70	60
	25–50	79	174	176	70	63	1000	5	10	80	60
	51+	77	170	173	68	63	1000	5	10	80	60
Females	11–14	46	101	157	62	46	800	10	8	45	50
	15–18	55	120	163	64	44	800	10	8	55	60
	19–24	58	128	164	65	46	800	10	8	60	60
	25–50	63	138	163	64	50	800	5	8	65	60
	51+	65	143	160	63	50	800	5	8	65	60
	Pregnant					60	800	10	10	65	70
	Lactating										
	1st 6 mo				65		1300	10	12	65	95
	2nd 6 mo				62		1200	10	11	65	90

* Designed for the maintenance of good nutrition of practically all healthy people in the United States. The allowances, expressed as average daily intakes over time are intended to provide for individual variations among most normal people as they live in the United States under usual environmental stresses. Diets should be based on a variety of common foods to provide other nutrients for which human requirements have been less well defined.

† Weights and heights of reference adults are actual medians for the U.S. population of the designated age, as reported by NHANES II. The use of these figures does not imply that the height-to-weight ratios are ideal.

‡ Retinol equivalents. 1 RE = 1 μg retinol or 6 μg beta-carotene.

§ As cholecalciferol. 10 μg cholecalciferol = 400 IU of vitamin D.

¶ α-Tocopherol equivalents. 1 mg d-α-tocopherol = 1 a-TE.

‖1 NE (niacin equivalent) is equal to 1 mg of niacin or 60 mg of dietary tryptophan.

(Food and Nutrition Board. [1989]. *National Research Council recommended dietary allowances* [10th ed.]. Washington, D.C.: National Academy Press.)

Table C-1 *(continued)*
U.S. Recommended Daily Allowances

Water-Soluble Vitamins						Minerals						
Thiamin (mg)	Riboflavin (mg)	Niacin (mg NE)‖	Vitamin B_6 (mg)	Folate (μg)	Vitamin B_{12} (μg)	Calcium (mg)	Phosphorus (mg)	Magnesium (mg)	Iron (mg)	Zinc (mg)	Iodine (μg)	Selenium (μg)
0.3	0.4	5	0.3	25	0.3	400	300	40	6	5	40	10
0.4	0.5	6	0.6	35	0.5	600	500	60	10	5	50	15
0.7	0.8	9	1.0	50	0.7	800	800	80	10	10	70	20
0.9	1.1	12	1.1	75	1.0	800	800	120	10	10	90	20
1.0	1.2	13	1.4	100	1.4	800	800	170	10	10	120	30
1.3	1.5	17	1.7	150	2.0	1200	1200	270	12	15	150	40
1.5	1.8	20	2.0	200	2.0	1200	1200	400	12	15	150	50
1.5	1.7	19	2.0	200	2.0	1200	1200	350	10	15	150	70
1.5	1.7	19	2.0	200	2.0	800	800	350	10	15	150	70
1.2	1.4	15	2.0	200	2.0	800	800	350	10	15	150	70
1.1	1.3	15	1.4	150	2.0	1200	1200	280	15	12	150	45
1.1	1.3	15	1.5	180	2.0	1200	1200	300	15	12	150	50
1.1	1.3	15	1.6	180	2.0	1200	1200	280	15	12	150	55
1.1	1.3	15	1.6	180	2.0	800	800	280	15	12	150	55
1.0	1.2	13	1.6	180	2.0	800	800	280	10	12	150	55
1.5	1.6	17	2.2	400	2.2	1200	1200	320	30	15	175	65
1.6	1.8	20	2.1	280	2.6	1200	1200	355	15	19	200	75
1.6	1.7	20	2.1	260	2.6	1200	1200	340	15	16	200	75

Appendix D

Canadian Recommended Nutrient Intake Based on Age and Body Weight Expressed as Daily Rates

Age	Sex	Weight (kg)	Protein (g)	Vitamin A (RE*)	Vitamin D (μg)	Vitamin E (mg)	Vitamin C (mg)	Folate (μg)	Vitamin B_{12} (μg)	Calcium (mg)	Phosphorus (mg)	Magnesium (mg)	Iron (mg)	Iodine (μg)	Zinc (mg)
Months															
0–4	Both	6.0	12†	400	10	3	20	25	0.3	250‡	150	20	0.3§	30	2§
5–12	Both	9.0	12	400	10	3	20	40	0.4	400	200	32	7	40	3
Years															
1	Both	11	13	400	10	3	20	40	0.5	500	300	40	6	55	4
2–3	Both	14	16	400	5	4	20	50	0.6	550	350	50	6	65	4
4–6	Both	18	19	500	5	5	25	70	0.8	600	400	65	8	85	5
7–9	M	25	26	700	2.5	7	25	90	1.0	700	500	100	8	110	7
	F	25	26	700	2.5	6	25	90	1.0	700	500	100	8	95	7
10–12	M	34	34	800	2.5	8	25	120	1.0	900	700	130	8	125	9
	F	36	36	800	2.5	7	25	130	1.0	1100	800	135	8	110	9
13–15	M	50	49	900	2.5	9	30‖	175	1.0	1100	900	185	10	160	12
	F	48	46	800	2.5	7	30‖	170	1.0	1000	850	180	13	160	9
16–18	M	62	58	1000	2.5	10	40‖	220	1.0	900	1000	230	10	160	12
	F	53	47	800	2.5	7	30‖	190	1.0	700	850	200	12	160	9
19–24	M	71	61	1000	2.5	10	40‖	220	1.0	800	1000	240	9	160	12
	F	58	50	800	2.5	7	30‖	180	1.0	700	850	200	13	160	9
25–49	M	74	64	1000	2.5	9	40‖	230	1.0	800	1000	250	9	160	12
	F	59	51	800	2.5	6	30‖	185	1.0	700	850	200	13	160	9
50–74	M	73	63	1000	5	7	40‖	230	1.0	800	1000	250	9	160	12
	F	63	54	800	5	6	30‖	195	1.0	800	850	210	8	160	9
75+	M	69	59	1000	5	6	40‖	215	1.0	800	1000	230	9	160	12
	F	64	55	800	5	5	30‖	200	1.0	800	850	210	8	160	9
Pregnancy (additional)															
1st trimester			5	0	2.5	2	0	200	0.2	500	200	15	0	25	6
2nd trimester			15	0	2.5	2	10	200	0.2	500	200	45	5	25	6
3rd trimester			24	0	2.5	2	10	200	0.2	500	200	45	10	25	6
Lactation (additional)			20	400	2.5	3	25	100	0.2	500	200	65	0	50	6

* Retinol equivalents

† Protein is assumed to be from breast milk and must be adjusted for infant formula.

‡ Infant formula with high phosphorus should contain 375 mg calcium.

§ Breast milk is assumed to be the source of the mineral.

‖ Smokers should increase vitamin C by 50%.

(Minister of National Health and Welfare. [1990]. *Nutrition recommendations: Report of the Scientific Review Committee* [p. 204]. Ottawa: Author.)

Glossary

Abduction: lateral movement of the body part away from the midline of the body

Absorption: process by which drugs are transferred from the site of entry into the body to the bloodstream

Accommodation: (1) ability to adjust the eye to see at various distances; (2) process by which intellectual acts are changed to handle increasingly complex information

Accreditation: process by which an educational program is evaluated and then recognized as having met certain predetermined standards of education

Acid: substance containing a hydrogen ion that can be liberated or released

Acidosis: condition characterized by a proportionate excess of hydrogen ions in the extracellular fluid, in which the pH falls below 7.35

Acquired immunodeficiency syndrome (AIDS): fatal condition in which the body's immune system is rendered ineffective as a result of infection by the retrovirus HIV

Active exercise: joint movement activated by the person

Active euthanasia: someone other than the client commits an action with the intent to end the client's life, for example, injecting him or her with a lethal dose

Active immunity: antibodies against harmful effects of microorganisms or toxins that are self-produced

Active transport: movement of ions or molecules across cell membranes, usually against a pressure gradient and with the expenditure of metabolic energy

Acute illness: rapidly occurring illness that runs its course, allowing the person to return to his or her previous level of functioning

Acute pain: episode of pain that lasts for seconds to less than 6 months

Adaptation: adjustment of living to other living things and environmental conditions

Addictive: substance to which a person develops a psychological and physiologic dependency

Adduction: movement of a body part toward the midline of the body

Adolescence: the period of time between childhood and adulthood; a time of rapid physical change, reproductive maturity, and emotional development

Advance directive: written directive that allows people to state in advance what their choices for health care would be if certain circumstances should develop

Adventitious breath sounds: abnormal breath sound heard over the lungs

Advocacy: protection and support of another's rights

Aerobic bacteria: bacteria that require oxygen to live and grow

Aerobic exercise: exercise that promotes cardiovascular fitness; it increases blood flow, heart rate, and the metabolic demand for oxygen over a period of time

Afebrile: a condition in which the body temperature is not elevated

Affective learning: changes in attitudes, values, and feelings

Ageism: attitudes that stereotype the older adult on the basis of chronologic age

Agency for Health Care Policy and Research (AHCPR): a group of multidisciplinary experts who utilize research as well as a broad range of input from professional and consumer organizations and individuals to develop clinical practice guidelines; established by the Omnibus Budget Reconciliation Act of 1989

Agnostic: person who holds that nothing can be known about the existence of a god

Albuminuria: albumin in the urine; indication of kidney disease

Alkali: substance that can accept or trap a hydrogen ion; synonym for base

Alkalosis: condition, characterized by a proportionate lack of hydrogen ions in the extracellular fluid concentration, in which the pH exceeds 7.45

Alopecia: baldness

Alternative care: general term used to identify various methods of non-hospital health care, including residential housing, day-care, respite care, hospice, and extended-care facilities

Alveoli: small air sacs at the end of the terminal bronchioles that are the site of gas exchange

Alzheimer's disease: type of dementia in which discrete patches of brain tissue degenerate; this devastating disease eventually affects all body systems

Ambulatory care: healthcare settings located in areas that are convenient for people to walk into and receive care; may be provided in hospitals, clinics, or centers

Amino acid: basic building blocks used to manufacture protein and the end products of protein digestion

Ampule: glass flask containing a single dose of medication for parenteral administration

Anaerobic bacteria: bacteria that can live without oxygen

Anaerobic exercise: exercise in which the supply of oxygen is less than the demand created by contracting muscles; oxygen debt results

Analgesic drug: pharmaceutical agent used to relieve pain

Anaphylactic reaction: severe reaction occurring immediately after exposure to a drug; characterized by respiratory distress and vascular collapse

Anion: ion that carries a negative electric charge

Ankylosis: fixation or immobilization of a joint

Anorexia: lack or loss of appetite for food

Anorexia nervosa: eating disorder characterized by the denial of appetite and bizarre eating habits

Anoxia: absence of oxygen

Antagonistic effect: combined effect of two or more drugs that produces less than the effect of each drug alone

Anthropometric: measurements of the body and body parts

Antibacterial: agent that kills bacteria or suppresses their growth

Antibody: immunoglobin produced by the body in response to a specific antigen

Antigen: foreign material capable of inducing a specific immune response

Antimicrobial: antibacterial agent that kills bacteria or suppresses their growth

Antipyretic: agent that reduces fever

Antiseptic: substance that inhibits the growth of bacteria

Anuria: technically, no urine voided; 24-hour urine output is less than 100 mL; synonyms are *complete kidney shutdown* and *renal failure*

Anxiety: vague sense of impending doom or apprehension precipitated by new and unknown experiences

Apnea: absence of breathing

Arousal: condition in which the cortical area of the brain receives and responds appropriately to stimuli

Ascites: accumulation of fluid in the peritoneal cavity

Asepsis: absence of disease-producing microorganisms; being free of infection

Asphyxiation: stoppage of breathing or the lack of air reaching the lungs; synonym for suffocation

Assault: threat or an attempt to make bodily contact with another person without that person's permission

Assertiveness: ability to stand up for oneself and others using open, honest, and direct communication

Assessing: systematic and continuous collection, validation, and communication of client data

Assimilation: process by which a person interprets information to fit the current level of cognition

Assisted suicide: the act of making a means of suicide (eg, providing pills or a weapon) available to a client with knowledge of his or her intention; in assisted suicide, someone makes the means of death available but does not act as the direct agent of death

Atelectasis: incomplete expansion or collapse of a part of the lungs

Atheist: person who denies the existence of a god

Atrophy: decrease in the size of a body structure

Attachment: active, affectionate, reciprocal relationship between two persons

Attitude: feeling or emotion, generally including a positive or negative judgment toward people, objects, or ideas

Auditory: pertaining to hearing

Auscultation: listening for sounds within the body

Authoritative knowledge: knowledge that comes from an expert and is accepted as truth based on a perceived level of expertise

Autocratic leadership: leadership style in which the leader assumes complete control over the decisions and activities of the group

Autonomy: self-determination; being independent and self-governing

Bacteria: the most significant and most commonly observed infection-causing agents

Bacteriuria: an asymptomatic condition that occurs when bacteria enter the bladder during catheterization or when organisms migrate up the catheter lumen or the urethra into the bladder

Bandage: piece of gauze or other material used to cover a wound

Basal metabolism: amount of energy required to carry out involuntary activities of the body at rest

Base: substance that can accept or trap a hydrogen ion; synonym for *alkali*

Base of support: foundation that provides stability for an object

Basic human needs: something essential to the health and survival of humans; common to all people

Battery: assault that is carried out

Beliefs: special class of intellectual attitudes based primarily on faith as opposed to fact

Beneficence: principle of doing good

Bereavement: state of grieving or going through the grief process

Bilateral: pertaining to two sides of the body

Binder: type of bandage, usually designed to fit a large body area

Biologic gender: the term used to denote chromosomal sexual development: male (XY) or female (XX)

Biopsy: removal of a piece of tissue for microscopic examination

Bisexuality: having sexual feelings for people of both sexes

Blended family: two single-parent families joined together to form a new family unit

Blood pressure: force of blood against arterial walls

Body image: how a person experiences his or her body

Body language: nonverbal communication

Body mechanics: efficient use of the body as a machine and as a means of locomotion

Body substance isolation (BSI): type of isolation that considers all body substances as potentially infective regardless of a person's diagnosis

Bolus: single injection of a concentrated solution administered intravenously

Bonding: a process of initial fusing of the mother and infant that occurs most often in the first few hours after birth and is necessary for later attachment

Bowel movement: emptying of the intestinal tract; synonym for *defecation*

Bowel training program: program that manipulates factors within a person's control (timing of defecation, exercise, diet) to produce a regular pattern of comfortable defecation without medication or enemas

Bradycardia: slow heart rate

Bradypnea: abnormally slow rate of breathing

Bronchial sounds: those heard over the trachea; high in pitch and intensity with expiration being longer than inspiration

Bronchodilator: medication that relaxes contractions of smooth muscles of the bronchioles

Bronchoscopy: visual examination of the trachea and bronchi

Bronchovesicular: normal breath sounds heard over the upper anterior chest and intercostal area

Bruit: unusual sound, usually abnormal, heard in auscultation

Buffer: substance that prevents body fluid from becoming overly acid or alkaline

Bulimia: eating disorder characterized by episodes of gorging followed by purging; often occurs in conjunction with anorexia nervosa

Burnout: behaviors exhibited as the result of prolonged occupational stress

Calorie: measure of heat, or energy; *kilocalorie,* commonly referred to as a calorie, defined as the amount of heat required to raise 1 kg of water 1°C

Carbohydrate: organic compounds (commonly known as sugars and starches) that are composed of carbon, hydrogen, and oxygen; the most abundant and least expensive source of calories in the diet worldwide

Cardiac output: volume of blood pumped from the left ventricle per minute

Cardinal signs: body temperature, pulse and respiratory rates, and blood pressure; synonym for *vital signs*

Caregiver burden: stress responses experienced during prolonged periods of home care by family caregivers

Caries: cavitation of the teeth

Case management: the process of coordinating an individual's healthcare for the purpose of maximizing positive outcomes and containing costs

Cathartic: medication that strongly increases gastrointestinal motility and promotes defecation

Catheter: tube for injecting or removing fluids

Cation: ion that carries a positive electric charge

Center of gravity: point at which the mass of an object is centered

Centers for Disease Control (CDC): U.S. government agency whose responsibilities include investigation, identification, prevention, and control of disease

Central venous catheter: venous access device usually introduced into the subclavian or internal jugular veins and passed to the superior vena cava just above the right atrium

Certification: process by which a person who has met certain criteria established by a nongovernmental association is granted recognition

Ceruminal gland: gland found in the external auditory canal that secretes a substance called *cerumen*

Change: process of transforming, altering, or modifying something

Change agent: person who purposefully and systematically implements change

Change of shift report: communication method used by nurses completing care for a client to transmit client information to nurses about to assume responsibility for continuing care; may be exchanged verbally in a meeting or audiotaped

Channel: a term used in communication theory to denote the medium selected to convey the message; the channel may target any of the receiver's senses

Charting by exception: shorthand method for documenting client data that is based on well-defined standards of practice; only exceptions to these standards are documented in narrative notes

Chemical name: precise description of a drug's chemical composition

Cheyne-Stokes respirations: gradual increase and then gradual decrease in depth of respirations followed by a period of apnea

Child abuse: intentional, nonaccidental physical or mental abuse of a child by a parent or other caregiver

Cholesterol: fat-like substance found only in animal tissues; it is important for cell membrane structure, a precursor of steroid hormones, and a constituent of bile; high serum cholesterol levels are a risk factor in the development of atherosclerosis

Chronic illness: irreversible illness that causes permanent physical impairment and requires long-term health care

Chronic pain: episode of pain that lasts for 6 months or longer; may be intermittent or continuous

Chyme: semifluid state that food is in when it leaves the stomach

Circadian rhythm: rhythm that completes a full cycle every 24 hours; synonym for *diurnal rhythm*

Circumduction: moving the distal part of the limb to trace a complete circle while the proximal end of the bone remains fixed

Civil law: rule that regulates relationships among people; synonym for *private law*

Client: the person receiving care

Client goal: statement describing an expected client outcome

Client record: a compilation of a client's health information; the client record is the only permanent legal document that details the nurse's interactions with the client

Clinical pathway/critical path: case management tools used to communicate the standardized, interdisciplinary plan of care for a particular group of clients; care guidelines and outcomes are specified for each day of the client's stay

Clubbing: rounding and swelling of nailbeds

Cognition: cerebral functioning; process of perceiving and understanding one's world

Cognitive competency: enables nurses to reason about the nature of things sufficiently to "make sense" of their world and to conceptually grasp what is necessary to achieve valued goals

Cognitive learning: storing and recalling of new knowledge in the brain

Coitus: sexual activity in which the penis is placed in the vagina; synonym for *sexual intercourse*

Colic: acute abdominal pain caused by spasmodic contractions of the intestine during the first 3 months of life

Collaborative problem: actual or potential health problem that may occur from complications of disease, diagnostic studies, or the treatment regimen; the nurse works together with other members of the health care team toward its resolution

Colloid osmotic pressure: pressure exerted by plasma proteins on permeable membranes in the body; synonym for *oncotic pressure*

Colon: section of the large intestine from the cecum to the rectum

Colostomy: an opening into the colon that permits feces from the colon to exit through the stoma

Comfort measures only: an order written to indicate that the goal of treatment is a comfortable, dignified death and that further life-sustaining measures are no longer indicated

Common law: law resulting from court decisions that is then followed when other cases involving similar circumstances and facts arise; common law is as binding as civil law

Communication: process of sharing information; process of generating and transmitting meanings

Community-based healthcare: healthcare that is provided to people who live within a defined geographic region or who have common needs; designed to meet the needs of people as they move between and among healthcare settings

Complaint: legal statement of the plaintiff's claim; once filed, it initiates legal proceedings

Compliance: act of completing what is expected of one

Computerized nursing care plan: plan of client care developed by computer software programs that enable the nurse to call up screens listing causes, goals, and related nursing interventions for nursing diagnoses and medical diagnoses

Concept: abstract images that are formed as impressions from the environment and organized into symbols of reality

Conceptual framework/model: set of concepts, along with the statements that arrange the concepts into an understandable pattern

Concurrent audit: evaluation of nursing care and client outcomes conducted while the client is receiving care; may use direct observation of nursing care, client interview, and chart review

Condom catheter: tube for draining urine; it connects a device applied externally to the penis to a collection bag

Confidentiality: respecting privileged information

Congestion: presence of excessive fluids or secretions in an organ or body tissue

Constipation: passage of dry, hard, fecal material

Consultation: a process in which two or more individuals with varying degrees of experience and expertise deliberate about a problem and its solution

Consumer: the person who uses healthcare services (the client)

Continuity of care: coordination of services provided to clients before they enter a health care setting, during the time they are in the setting, and after they leave the setting

Continuum: graduated scale

Contraception: prevention of conception or pregnancy; also used to describe methods used for birth control

Contractual agreement: pact made between two persons for the achievement of mutually set goals

Contracture: permanent contraction state of a muscle

Convalescent period: stage of an infection that represents recovery from the infection

Coping mechanism: patterns of behavior used to neutralize, deny, or counteract anxiety

Counseling: giving guidance, assisting with problem solving

Crackles: fine crackling sounds made as air moves through wet secretions in the lungs

Credentialing: general term that refers to ways in which professional competence is maintained

Crime: offense against people or property; the act is considered to be against the government, referred to in a lawsuit as "the people," and the accused is prosecuted by the state

Crisis: (1) point at which body temperature drops rapidly to normal; (2) occurs when coping and defense mechanisms are no longer effective, resulting in high levels of anxiety, disorganized behavior, and the inability to function normally

Crisis intervention: five-step problem-solving technique to promote adaptation and improve future coping

Criteria: specified behavior; for example, the measurable criteria in a client goal specifies how the client must perform the desired behavior

Critical thinking: thought that is disciplined, comprehensive, based on intellectual standards, and, as a result, well-reasoned; a systematic way to form and shape one's thinking that functions purposefully and exactingly

Crossmatching: act of determining the compatibility of two blood specimens

Cue: significant data that is helpful in making decisions

Cultural assimilation: process that occurs when a minority group, living as part of a dominant group within a culture, loses the cultural characteristics that made it different

Cultural blindness: the process of ignoring differences in people and proceeding as though the differences do not exist

Cultural care deprivation: a lack of culturally assistive, supportive, or facilitative acts in the health care setting

Cultural imposition: tendency of some to impose their beliefs, practices, and values on another culture because they believe that their ideas are superior to those of another person or group

Culture: sum total of human behavior or social characteristics peculiar to a specific group and passed from generation to generation or from one to another within the group

Culture shock: those feelings, usually negative, a person experiences when placed in a different culture

Cumulative effect: occurs when the body cannot metabolize a drug before additional doses are administered

Cutaneous pain: superficial pain usually involving the skin or subcutaneous tissue

Cyanosis: bluish coloring of the skin and mucous membranes

Cystoscopy: direct visual examination of the bladder, ureteral orifices, and urethra with a cystoscope

Cytologic study: study of cells and fluids from the body

Data: information

Data base: all the pertinent client information that enables a comprehensive and effective plan of care to be designed and implemented for the client

Data cluster: grouping of client data or cues that points to the existence of a client health problem

Day-care center: centers that provide care for infants, children, elderly people, and people with special health care needs

Death: termination of life and its related clinical signs

Débridement: cleaning away of devitalized tissue and foreign matter from a wound; can be accomplished by various methods

Deductive reasoning: a cognitive process in which one examines a general idea and then considers specific actions or ideas

Defamation: wrongs of slander and libel; making derogatory remarks about one person to another

Defecation: emptying of the intestinal tract; synonym for *bowel movement*

Defense mechanisms: forms of self-deception; unconscious process the self uses to protect itself from anxiety or threats to self-esteem

Dehiscence: separation of the layers of a surgical wound; may be partial, superficial, or a complete disruption of the surgical wound

Dehydration: decreased water volume

Delta sleep: deep sleep, occurring during stage III and especially stage IV in NREM sleep

Dementia: organic impairment of intellectual functioning, gradually leading to interference with social or occupational functioning, memory, and often personality integration

Democratic leadership: leadership style characterized by a sense of equality between the leader and followers

Deontologic: ethical system in which actions are right or wrong independent of the consequences they produce

Dependent action: nursing action carried out at the instruction or order of an authorized health care professional other than a nurse; synonym for *physician-initiated* or *physician-prescribed intervention*

Dermis: underlying portion of the skin

Development: increase in the complexity of function and progression to skill advancement

Development theory: theory to describe the orderly and predictable process of the growth and development of humans, individualized by social, biologic, and environmental factors

Developmental crisis: predictable patterns of behavior and change occurring throughout the lifespan

Developmental delay: measure of development that lags behind the normal range for a given age

Developmental task: successful achievement of psychomotor, psychosocial, or cognitive skills at certain periods in life; failure to obtain the developmental task can lead to unhappiness and difficulty with later tasks

Diagnosis (nursing): analysis of client data to identify client strengths and health problems that independent nursing intervention can prevent or resolve

Diagnosis related groups (DRGs): classification of clients by major medical diagnosis for the purpose of standardizing health care costs (see *prospective payment*)

Diarrhea: passage of liquid and unformed stools

Diastolic pressure: least amount of pressure exerted on arterial walls, which occurs when the heart is at rest between ventricular contractions

Dietary Guidelines: recommendations for choosing a healthy diet made by the U.S. Department of Agriculture and the U.S. Department of Health and Human Services

Diffuse pain: pain that covers a large area

Diffusion: tendency of solutes to move freely throughout a solvent from an area of higher concentration to an area of lower concentration until equilibrium is established

Direct transfusion: infusion of blood while it is being taken from the donor

Discharge planning: systematic process of preparing the client to leave the health care facility and for maintaining continuity of care

Discharge summary: description of where the client stands in relation to problems identified in the record at discharge; documents any special teaching or counseling the client received, including referrals

Discipline: specific and unique body of knowledge that uses existing and new knowledge to creatively solve problems and meet human needs within ever-changing boundaries

Disease: pathologic change in the structure or function of the body or mind

Distribution: movement of drugs by the circulatory system to the site of action

Documentation: written, legal record of all pertinent interventions with the client—assessments, diagnoses, plans, interventions, and evaluations

Dominant group: group within a culture that has the authority to control the value system and determine the rewards of the system; usually the largest group in a society

Donor: person who donates blood to be given to another person

Do-not-hospitalize: an order specifying that a client, usually one who is terminally ill and anticipating death, not be admitted to the hospital in the event of a worsening of condition

Do-not-resuscitate: An order specifying that there be no attempt to resuscitate a client in the event of cardiopulmonary arrest

Dressing: protective covering placed over a wound

Drug: substance that modifies body functions when taken into the living organism; synonym for *medication*

Drug allergy: hypersensitivity caused by previous exposure to a medication; may occur immediately or be delayed; manifestations range from mild to severe

Drug tolerance: tendency of the body to become accustomed to a drug over time; larger doses are required to produce the desired effects

Dysrhythmia: an abnormal cardiac rhythm; synonym for *arrhythmia*

Dysuria: difficulty in voiding; may or may not be associated with pain; a feeling of warm local irritation occurring during voiding is called *burning*

Ecchymosis: collection of blood in subcutaneous tissues that causes a purplish discoloration

Edema: accumulation of fluid in extracellular spaces

Elective surgery: surgery that is recommended but can be omitted or delayed without catastrophe

Electrocardiogram (ECG; EKG): graphic record produced by the electrocardiograph

Electroencephalograph: instrument that measures and records electric impulses of the brain

Electrolyte: substance capable of breaking into ions and developing an electric charge when dissolved in solution

Electromyograph (EMG): instrument that records muscle tone

Electrooculogram: recording of the electric current or potential produced by eye movements

Embolism: blocking of an artery by a blood clot or by other foreign matter brought to the site by the blood flow

Embolus: foreign body or air in the circulatory system; plural form is *emboli*

Emergency surgery: surgery that must be performed immediately to save the person's life or a body organ

Empathy: intellectually identifying with the way another person feels

Endogenous: infection in which the causative organism comes from microbial life the person himself or herself harbors

Endorphins: morphine-like substances released by the body that appear to alter the perception of pain

Endoscopy: direct visualization of hollow organs of the body using an endoscope or flexible, lighted tube

Endotracheal tube: polyvinylchloride airway that is inserted through the nose or the mouth into the trachea using a laryngoscope as a guide

Enema: introduction of solution into the lower intestinal tract

Enkephalins: opioids that are widespread throughout the brain and dorsal horn of the spinal cord and are believed to reduce pain sensation by inhibiting the release of substance P

Enteral nutrition: alternate form of feeding that involves passing a tube into the gastrointestinal tract to allow instillation of the appropriate formula

Entry phase: the phase of the home visit in which the nurse develops rapport with the client and family members, mutually determines outcomes, makes assessments, plans and implements prescribed care, and provides teaching

Enuresis: involuntary urination; most often used to refer to a child who involuntarily urinates during the night

Epidermis: a superficial portion of the skin

Epidural analgesia: means of providing pain relief with an opioid injection delivered by way of a catheter inserted in the midlumbar region into the epidural space

Epithelialization: stage of wound healing in which epithelial cells move across the surface of a wound; tissue color ranges from the color of "ground glass" to pink

Erection: condition that results when erectile tissue of the penis fills with blood as a result of stimulation

Erogenous zones: areas of the body that produce sexual desire and arousal when stimulated

Erythema: redness of the skin

Eschar: a thick, leathery scab or dry crust that is necrotic and must be removed for adequate pressure ulcer staging to occur

Ethical/legal competencies: enable nurses to live life in a manner that is consistent with their personal moral code and role responsibilities

Ethics: system dealing with standards of character and behavior related to what is right and wrong

Ethnicity: sense of identification that a cultural group collectively has; the sharing of common and unique cultural and social beliefs and behavior patterns, including language and dialect, religious practices, literature, folklore, music, political interests, food preferences, and employment patterns

Ethnocentrism: judgment of other people based on the standards and practices of one's own culture

Euphoria: unrealistic sense of well-being

Eupnea: normal respirations

Euthanasia: mercy killing; the deliberate termination of the life of a person

Evaluating: measurement of the extent to which the client has achieved the goals specified in the plan of care; factors that positively or negatively influence goal achievement are identified, and the plan of care is terminated or revised

Evisceration: protrusion of viscera through an incisional area

Excretion: removal of a drug from the body

Exercise: active exertion of muscles involving the contraction and relaxation of muscle groups

Exogenous: infection in which the causative organism is acquired from outside the host

Expected outcome: the specific, measurable criteria used to evaluate whether the client goal has been met

Expectorant: drug that facilitates the removal of respiratory secretions

Expert witness: nurse who explains to the judge and jury what happened based on the client's record and who offers an opinion as to whether the nursing care met acceptable standards of practice

Expiration: act of breathing out; synonym is *exhalation*

Extended-care facility: type of care given after hospitalization of acute illness; includes residential care and intermediate or skilled nursing home care

Extended family: nuclear family and other related people

Extracellular fluid (ECF): fluid outside the cells; includes intravascular and interstitial fluids

Exudate: fluid that accumulates in a wound; may contain serum, cellular debris, bacteria, and white blood cells

Fact witness: nurse who has knowledge of the actual incident prompting a legal case; bases testimony on firsthand knowledge of the incident not on assumptions

Failure to thrive (FTT): physical and developmental retardation of infants or children resulting from physical or emotional neglect

Faith: (1) spiritual dimensions of a person's life regardless of religious affiliation; (2) confident belief in something for which there is no proof or material evidence

Family: any group of two or more people who live together and are emotionally involved with each other

Febrile: a condition in which the body temperature is elevated

Fasting state: abstinence from food and fluids

Fecal impaction: collection in the rectum of hardened feces that cannot be passed

Feces: intestinal waste products

Feedback: verbal and nonverbal evidence that the message is received and understood

Felony: (1) crime punishable by imprisonment in a state or federal penitentiary for more than 1 year; (2) crime of greater offense than a misdemeanor

Fever: elevation above the upper limit of normal body temperature; synonym for *pyrexia*

Fiber: all dietary plant material that is not digestible by gastrointestinal tract, enzymes, and secretions

Fidelity: keeping promises and commitments made to others

Fight-or-flight response: the body prepares itself against threat, to either resist (fight) or evade (flight) the danger

Filtration: passage of a fluid through a permeable membrane whose spaces do not allow certain solutes to pass; passage is from an area of higher pressure to one of lower pressure

Flaccidity: decreased muscle tone; synonym for *hypotonicity*

Flatulence: excessive formation of gases in the gastrointestinal tract

Flatus: intestinal gas

Flexibility: ability to use a muscle through its entire range of motion

Flexion: state of being bent

Flowsheets: graphic record of abbreviated aspects of client's condition (eg, vital signs, routine aspects of care)

Fluid balance: state in which water and its solutes in the body are in normal proportions and concentrations and are in appropriate body compartments

Fluid imbalance: state in which water and its solutes in the body are in improper proportions and concentrations or are improperly located in body compartments

Fluid volume deficit: deficiency in the amount of both water and electrolytes in extracellular fluid; water and electrolyte proportions remain near normal

Fluid volume excess: excessive retention of water and sodium in extracellular fluid in near-normal proportions

Flushing: red appearance of the skin

Focus charting: a documentation system that replaces the problem list with a focus column that incorporates many aspects of a client and client care; the focus may be a client strength or a problem or need; the narrative portion of focus charting uses the data (D), action (A), response (R) format

Foley catheter: indwelling or retention catheter that remains in place to drain urine

Footdrop: complication resulting from extended plantar flexion

Formal teaching: planned teaching based on learner objectives

Frail-old: term for people over age 75; the fastest-growing segment of the population

Fraud: willful and purposeful misrepresentation that could cause, or has caused, loss or harm to people or property

Fremitus: vibration of the chest wall that can be palpated during the physical examination

Frequency: increased incidence of voiding

Friction: occurs when two surfaces rub against each other; the resulting injury resembles an abrasion and can also damage superficial blood vessels directly under the skin

Friction rub: crackling sounds heard in the chest cavity caused by inflamed pleura rubbing against the chest wall

Functional health: level of health defined by one's ability to carry out usual and desired daily activities

Functional incontinence: state in which a person experiences an involuntary, unpredictable passage of urine

Fungi: plant-like organisms (molds and yeasts) that also can cause infection

Gate control theory: theory that explains that excitatory pain stimuli carried by small-diameter nerve fibers can be blocked by inhibiting signals carried by large-diameter nerve fibers

Gender identity: the inner sense a person has of being male or female, which may be the same as or different from biologic gender; synonym is *sexual identity*

Gender role behavior: the behavior a person conveys about being male or female, which may or may not be the same as biologic gender or gender identity (Pilliteri, 1995)

General adaptation syndrome (GAS): biochemical model of stress describing the body's general response to stress

General anesthesia: anesthetic drugs that produce narcosis, relaxation of skeletal muscles, and reduced or absent reflex action

Generic name: name assigned by the manufacturer who first develops a drug; it is often derived from the chemical name

Gerontologic nursing: nursing specialty concerned with the care of both the well and the ill older adult

Gerontology: study of all aspects of the aging process and their consequences

Gingivitis: inflammation of the gingivae or gums

Glycosuria: presence of sugar in the urine; if due to an unusually large intake of sugar or to marked emotional disturbances and is temporary, there is little cause for alarm

Good Samaritan law: law that holds certain health practitioners blameless when undertaking to aid a person in an emergency

Gram-negative bacteria: bacteria with chemically more complex cell walls that can be decolorized by alcohol

Gram-positive bacteria: bacteria with a thick cell wall that resists decolorization (loss of color) and are stained violet

Granulation tissue: new tissue that is pink/red in color and composed of fibroblasts and small blood vessels that fill an open wound when it starts to heal

Graphic sheet: a form used to record specific client variables

Grief: emotional response to loss. *Dysfunctional grief:* distorted or abnormal grief response, including *inhibited grief* (suppression of grief reaction) and *unresolved grief* (lengthy or denied grief reaction). *Abbreviated grief:* short but genuine grief reaction. *Anticipatory grief:* grief reaction before actual loss.

Ground: conducting connection between a source of electricity and the earth

Group dynamics: study of a group's characteristics and ways of functioning

Gurgles: continuous musical sounds that are audible in expiration or inspiration, or both; formerly called *rhonchi*

Gustatory: pertaining to taste

Halitosis: offensive breath

Health: state of optimal functioning or well-being

Health-belief model: what people believe to be true about themselves in relation to health

Health maintenance organization (HMO): broad term encompassing various health care delivery systems that use group practice and provide an incentive to use a prepaid comprehensive health care system

Health problem: condition related to health requiring intervention if disease or illness is to be prevented or resolved and coping and wellness are to be promoted

Helping relationship: interaction that sets the climate of movement of the participants toward common goals

Hematuria: blood in the urine; if present in large enough quantities, urine may be bright red or reddish brown

Hemolysis: process of freeing a red blood cell of its hemoglobin by destruction of the cell membrane

Hemoptysis: sputum containing blood

Hemorrhage: excessive blood loss due to the escape of blood from blood vessels

Hemorrhoids: abnormally distended rectal veins

Heparin lock: intravenous needle or catheter with an injection pad attached at the end

Hesitancy: delay or difficulty in initiating voiding

Heterosexuality: having sexual feelings for a person of the opposite sex

Hierarchy of needs: as defined by Maslow, certain needs are more basic than others; a person strives to at least minimally meet certain needs before attending to others

High-level wellness: functioning to one's maximum potential while maintaining balance and purposeful direction in the environment

Holistic health care: health care that takes into account the whole person interacting in the environment

Home health agency: agency, eligible to receive federal funds, that provides home-based care; may be independent, hospital operated, or health department managed

Home healthcare: healthcare services provided in a client's home

Homeostasis: various physiologic and psychological mechanisms respond to changes in the internal and external environment to maintain a balanced state

Homosexuality: having sexual feelings for a person of the same sex

Hospice: a type of end-of-life care for persons who are terminally ill, characterized by the following: (1) clients are kept as free of pain as possible so that they may die comfortably and with dignity; (2) clients receive continuity of care, are not abandoned, and do not lose personal identity; (3) clients retain as much control as possible over decisions regarding their care and are allowed to refuse further life-prolonging technologic interventions; and (4) clients are viewed as individuals with personal fears, thoughts, feelings, values, and hopes

Hospitals: acute-care settings that provide various healthcare services, such as emergency care, inpatient care, surgery, diagnostic tests, and client education

Host: animal or person on or within which microorganisms live

Hydration: union of a substance with water; term often is used as the opposite of dehydration, in which case it means that there is normal intracellular and extracellular water volume

Hydrometer: instrument used to determine the specific gravity of urine

Hydrostatic pressure: force exerted by a fluid against the container wall

Hypercalcemia: excess of calcium in the extracellular fluid

Hyperkalemia: excess of potassium in the extracellular fluid
Hypermagnesemia: excess of magnesium in the extracellular fluid
Hypernatremia: excess of sodium in the extracellular fluid
Hyperphosphatemia: above normal serum concentration of inorganic phosphorus
Hyperpyrexia: high fever, above 41°C (105.8°F)
Hypersomnia: condition characterized by excessive sleeping, especially daytime sleeping
Hypertension: blood pressure elevated above the upper limit of normal
Hypertonic: having a greater concentration than the solution with which it is being compared
Hyperventilation: condition in which there is more than the normal amount of air entering and leaving lungs
Hypervolemia: excess of plasma
Hypnotic: pharmaceutical agent used to induce sleep
Hypocalcemia: insufficient amount of calcium in the extracellular fluid
Hypokalemia: insufficient amount of potassium in the extracellular fluid
Hypomagnesemia: insufficient amount of magnesium in the extracellular fluid
Hyponatremia: insufficient amount of sodium in the extracellular fluid
Hypophosphatemia: below normal serum concentration of inorganic phosphorus
Hypoproteinemia: insufficient amount of protein substances in the extracellular fluid
Hypotension: blood pressure below the lower limit of normal
Hypotonic: having a lesser concentration than the solution with which it is being compared
Hypoventilation: a decreased rate or depth of air movement into the lungs
Hypovolemia: deficiency of plasma
Hypovolemic shock: shock due to a decrease in blood volume
Hypoxemia: deficient oxygenation of blood
Hypoxia: inadequate amount of oxygen available to the cells

Iatrogenic infection: infection that occurs as a result of a treatment or diagnostic procedure
Ideal self: self a person would like to be or thinks he or she should be; includes aspirations, moral ideas, and values
Idiosyncratic effect: unusual, unexpected response to a drug that may manifest itself by overresponse, underresponse, or response different from the expected outcome
Ileal conduit: urinary diversion in which the ureters are connected to the ileum with a stoma created on the abdominal wall
Ileostomy: allows fecal content from the ileum to be eliminated through the stoma
Illness: abnormal process in which any aspect of the person's functioning is altered (in comparison to the previous condition of health)
Immunization: process of rendering a person immune or resistant to particular antigenic agents or bacteria
Implementing: carrying out the plan of care
Impotence: condition in which a man is unable to attain or maintain an erection to such an extent that he cannot have satisfactory sexual intercourse; synonym for *erectile failure*
Incentive spirometer: equipment to help maximize lung inflation
Incident report: documentation that describes any injury or potential for injury suffered by a client in a health care agency
Incision: wound made with a sharp, cutting instrument
Incontinence: inability to voluntarily control the discharge of urine or feces
Independent action: (1) nursing action carried out at the instruction or order of a nurse; (2) actions within the legal scope of nursing's independent domain; synonym for *nurse-initiated* or *nurse-prescribed intervention*
Inductive reasoning: a cognitive process in which one identifies a specific idea or action and then makes conclusions about general ideas
Indwelling urethral catheter: catheter that remains in place for continuous urine drainage; synonym for *Foley catheter*
Infancy: period from 1 month to 1 year of age
Infection: disease state resulting from pathogens in or on the body
Infiltration: escape of fluid into subcutaneous tissue
Inflammatory response: localized response of the body to injury or infection; protective mechanism that eliminates invading pathogens and allows for tissue repair to occur
Informal teaching: unplanned teaching sessions dealing with the client's immediate learning needs and concerns
Informed consent: knowledgeable, voluntary permission obtained from a client to perform a specific test or procedure
Inhalation: (1) act of breathing in; synonym for *inspiration;* (2) administration of a drug in solution by way of the respiratory tract
Injection: introduction of medication into the body by a syringe attached to a needle
Inpatient: person who enters a health care setting for a stay ranging from 24 hours to many years
Insomnia: difficulty in falling asleep, intermittent sleep, or early awakening from sleep
Inspection: purposeful and systematic observation
Inspiration: act of breathing in; synonym is *inhalation*
Integument: skin
Integumentary system: skin and its appendages (ie, hair, glands in the skin, and nails)
Interdependent action: nursing action performed by the nurse in collaboration with other members of the health care team
Intermittent fever: body temperature that alternates between fever and normal or subnormal temperature
Intermittent pulse: normal pulse rhythm broken by periods of irregular rhythm
Interpersonal competency: skills that enable a nurse to establish and maintain caring relationships that facilitate the achievement of valued goals while simultaneously affirming the worth of participants in the relationship
Interstitial fluid: fluid between the cells
Interview: planned communication for a specific purpose (eg, data collection)

Interviewing techniques: communication skills specifically designed to gather and validate information

Intracellular fluid (ICF): fluid within the cell; synonym for *cellular fluid*

Intractable pain: severe pain that is extremely resistant to relief measures

Intradermal injection: injection placed just below the epidermis

Intramuscular injection: an injection into deep muscle tissue, usually of the buttock, thigh, or upper arm

Intraoperative phase: period lasting from admission to the operating room area to transfer to the postanesthesia recovery area after surgery is completed

Intravascular fluid: fluid within the vascular system; synonym for *plasma*

Intravenous infusion: injection of relatively large quantities of solution into a vein

Intravenous route: injection of a solution into the vein

Intuitive problem solving: direct understanding of a situation based on a background of experience, knowledge, and skill that makes expert decision making possible

Ion: atom or molecule carrying an electric charge in solution

Irrigation: flushing of a tube, canal, or area with solution

Ischemia: deficiency of blood in a particular area

Isokinetic exercise: exercise involving muscle contractions with resistance varying at a constant rate

Isolation: protective procedure designed to prevent the transmission of specific microorganisms; also called *protective aseptic techniques* and *barrier techniques*

Isometric exercise: exercise in which muscle tension occurs without a significant change in muscle length

Isotonic: (1) having about the same concentration as the solution with which it is being compared; (2) exercise in which muscles shorten (contract) and move

Jaundice: yellow appearance of the skin

Justice: process that distributes benefits, risks, and costs fairly

Kardex nursing care plan: trade name for a care plan documentation system that encompasses (1) prescriptions for nursing care related to activities of daily living; (2) nursing diagnoses and related client goals and nursing orders; and (3) the nursing care related to diagnostic measures and the medical regimen

Kegel exercises: repetitious contraction and relaxation of the pubococcygeal muscle to improve vaginal tone and urinary continence

Kinesthesia: awareness of positioning of body parts and body movement

Korotkoff sounds: series of sounds that correspond to changes in blood flow through an artery as pressure is released

Kussmaul's respiration breathing: an extreme rate and depth of breathing

Laissez-faire leadership: leadership style in which the leader relinquishes all power to the group

Language: prescribed way of using words; a means to express thoughts and feelings

Law: rule of conduct established and enforced by the government of a society

Lawsuit: legal action in a court of law

Laxative: drug used to induce emptying of the intestinal tract

Leadership: ability to direct or motivate others toward the achievement of predetermined goals

Learning: increasing one's knowledge; having one's behavior changed in a measurable way as a result of an experience

Liability: legal responsibility for one's acts (and failure to act); includes responsibility for financial restitution of harms resulting from negligent acts

Licensure: to be given a license to practice nursing in a state or province after successfully meeting requirements

Life review/reminiscence: universal phenomenon identified by Butler as a review of one's life through one's recollections

Line of gravity: vertical line that passes through the center of gravity

Lipid: group name for fatty substances, including fats, oils, waxes, and related compounds

Literacy: ability to read and write

Litigation: process of lawsuit

Living will: advance directive specifying the medical care a person would want or refuse should he or she lack the capacity to consent to or refuse treatment himself or herself

Local adaptation syndrome (LAS): localized response of the body to stress, precipitated by trauma or pathology

Localized symptoms: symptoms that are limited or restricted to a discrete area

Long-term care: facilities for long-term care provide healthcare and help with activities of daily living for people of any age who are physically or mentally unable to independently care for themselves

Loss: inaccessibility or change in a valued person, object, or situation. *Actual loss:* loss tangible to both the person sustaining the loss and to others. *Perceived loss:* loss tangible only to the person sustaining it. *Physical loss:* loss of life, limb, an object, person, pet, or job. *Psychological loss:* loss that affects a person's self-image. *Anticipatory loss:* loss behaviors displayed before the actual loss occurs

Love and belonging needs: understanding and acceptance of others in giving and receiving love

Macromineral: mineral that is needed by the body in amount greater than 100 mg/day

Macronutrient: essential nutrient that supplies energy and builds tissue, such as carbohydrate, fat, and protein

Macroshock: electric current passing through a relatively large area of a person

Malpractice: act of negligence as applied to a professional person such as a physician, nurse, or dentist

Managed care: an organized, high-quality; cost-effective system of healthcare that influences the selection and use of healthcare services of a population

Management: process of directing others toward goal achievement

Masturbation: self-stimulation for sexual satisfaction

Medicaid: Title XIX (Social Security Act, 1965) to make health care available to those people with less than the minimum income who do not qualify for Medicare

Medical asepsis: practices designed to reduce the number and transfer of pathogens; synonym for *clean technique*

Medical diagnosis: statement about a specific disease process using terminology from a well-developed classification system accepted by the medical profession

Medicare: Title XVIII (Social Security Act, 1965) to provide a measure of health coverage to all Social Security recipients

Medication: substance that modifies body functions when taken into the living organisms; synonym for *drug*

Medication record: record documenting all medications administered to the client, the nurse administering the drugs, and sometimes the reason the drug was administered and its effectiveness

Menarche: initiation of the menstrual cycle

Meniscus: curved surface at the top of a column of liquid in a tube

Menopause: decrease of cyclic hormonal production and cessation of menses in females, usually between ages 45 and 60 years

Menstruation: a cycle of about 20 days during which the female body prepares for the presence of a fertilized ovum

Mentorship: relationship in which an experienced person (the mentor) advises and assists a less experienced person

Message: term used in communication theory to denote the actual physical product of the source or encoder (eg, a speech, interview, phone conversation, chart)

Metabolic acidosis: proportionate deficiency of bicarbonate ions in the extracellular fluid

Metabolic alkalosis: proportionate excess of bicarbonate ions in the extracellular fluid

Metabolism: (1) chemical changes in the body by which energy is provided; (2) breakdown of a drug to an inactive form; also referred to as *biotransformation*

Micromineral: mineral or trace element that is needed by the body in an amount less than 100 mg/day

Micronutrient: vitamin or mineral needed in much smaller amount to regulate and control body processes

Microshock: electric current passing through a relatively small area of a person, usually part of the heart

Micturition: process of emptying the bladder; urination; voiding

Middle adult: the adult between the ages of 40 and 60 years; also called *middle adulthood*

Midlife crisis: realization that the halfway point in life has been reached and youthful goals may not have been achieved

Minerals: inorganic elements found in nature

Minority group: group having some physical or cultural characteristic that identifies the people within the group as different from the dominant culture

Misdemeanor: crime of lesser offense than a felony and punishable by fines, imprisonment (usually for less than 1 year) or both

Morals: like ethics, concerned with what constitutes right action; more informal and personal than the term ethics

Mourning: period during which a person learns to accept grief

Narcolepsy: condition characterized by an uncontrolled desire to sleep

Narrative: descriptive record of the client's condition; includes client's response to interventions by health professionals and client's progress toward goal achievement

Nasal cannula: disposable, plastic device that delivers oxygen with two protruding prongs for insertion into the nostrils

Nasogastric tube: a tube inserted through the nose and into the stomach

Nasointestinal tube: a tube inserted through the nose and into the upper portion of the small intestine

National Medical Care: healthcare services in Canada, funded by taxes and provided to every Canadian citizen

Necrosis: death of cells

Negative reinforcement: an ineffective teaching strategy that uses criticism or punishment

Negativism: negative verbalizations and behaviors

Negligence: performing an act that a reasonably prudent person under similar circumstances would not do, or failing to perform an act that a reasonably prudent person under similar circumstances would do

Neonate: period from birth to 1 month of age

Neuromodulator: endogenous opioid chemical regulators that appear to have analgesic activity and alter pain perception

Neurotransmitters: substances that either excite or inhibit target nerve cells

Nociceptors: pain receptors

Nocturia: frequency of urination during the night

Nocturnal myoclonus: condition characterized by marked muscle contraction that results in the jerking of one or both legs during sleep

Noncompliance: nonadherence to a therapeutic recommendation

Nonmaleficence: principle of avoiding evil

Nonproductive cough: forceful expiratory effort without production of mucus; also called a *dry cough*

Nonverbal communication: exchange of information without the use of words

Normal flora: microorganisms that normally inhabit various body sites and are part of the body's natural defense system

Nosocomial infection: hospital-acquired infection

NREM: non–rapid eye movement that characterizes four stages of sleep

Nuclear family: family unit, family of marriage, parenthood, or procreation, and their immediate children

Nurse practice act: law established to regulate nursing practice

Nursing: profession focusing on the holistic person receiving health care services and providing a unique contribution to the prevention of illness and maintenance of health

Nursing actions: any action performed by a nurse to assist clients to meet health goals: promote wellness, prevent disease or illness, restore health, facilitate coping with altered functioning

Nursing audit: method of evaluating the outcomes of nursing care or the process by which these outcomes are achieved using a review of client records

Nursing care conference: formal meeting of nurses to discuss some aspect of client's care

Nursing care rounds: procedure in which a group of nurses visit clients individually at bedside to gather information that helps to plan and evaluate nursing care

Nursing diagnosis: actual or potential health problem that independent nursing intervention can prevent or resolve. *Actual problem* is present. *Possible problem* may be present, but more data are needed to confirm or disconfirm the problem. *Potential problem* may occur; defining characteristics are present as risk factors

Nursing history: assessment of the client by interview to identify the client's health status, strengths, health problems, health risks, and need for nursing

Nursing order: prescribes the nursing care to be given to assist clients to meet health goals

Nursing plan of care: written guide to direct the efforts of the nursing team as they work with clients to meet health goals; specifies prioritized nursing diagnoses, client goals, and nursing orders

Nursing process: five-step systematic method for giving client care; involves assessing, diagnosing, planning, implementing, and evaluating

Nutrient: specific biochemical substance used by the body for growth, development, activity, reproduction, lactation, health maintenance, and recovery from illness or injury

Nutrition: study of the nutrients and how they are handled by the body, as well as the impact of human behavior and environment on the process of nourishment

Obesity: weight greater than 20% above ideal body weight

Objective data: information perceptible to the senses; may be verified by another person

Observation: conscious and deliberate use of the five senses to gather data

Occult blood: blood present in such minute quantities that it cannot be detected with the unassisted eye

Occupational Safety and Health Administration (OSHA): government agency that establishes minimum health and safety standards for workers

Official name: name by which a drug is identified in official publications

Old-old: term used to describe older adults over age 75; sometimes referred to as frail-old

Older adult: after middle age; refers to adults over age of 65

Olfactory: pertaining to smell

Oliguria: scanty or greatly diminished amount of urine voided in a given time; 24-hour urine output is 100 to 400 mL

Oncotic pressure: pressure exerted by plasma proteins on permeable membranes in the body; synonym for *colloid osmotic pressure*

Opioid: more correct term for narcotic analgesics, since these drugs act by binding to opiate receptor sites in the central nervous system

Opportunist: bacteria that may potentially be harmful

Organism: a living being

Orgasm: apex of sexual activity in which rhythmic contractions of the genital organs and many other physiologic changes occur

Orthopnea: type of dyspnea in which breathing is easier when the client sits or stands

Orthostatic hypotension: temporary fall in blood pressure associated with assuming an upright position; synonym for *postural hypotension*

Osmolarity: the concentration of particles in a solution, or a solution's pulling power

Osmosis: passage of a solvent through a semipermeable membrane from an area of lesser concentration to an area of greater concentration until equilibrium is established

Osmotic pressure: drawing power for water or the attraction for water exerted by solute particles

Osteoporosis: condition characterized by loss of calcium from bone tissue

Ostomy: general term referring to an artificial opening; usually used to refer to an opening created for the excretion of body wastes

Outcome: end product of nursing care; client outcomes are measurable changes in client behavior or state of health

Outpatient: a person who requires healthcare services but does not need to stay in an institution for those services

Overflow incontinence: the involuntary loss of urine associated with overdistention and overflow of the bladder

Ovulation: discharge of ovum from the female ovary at about the midpoint of each menstrual cycle

Ovum: female reproductive cell, often called an *egg*

Pain: sensation of physical or mental suffering or hurt that usually causes distress or agony to the one experiencing it

Pain threshold: amount of stimulation required before a person experiences the sensation of pain

Pain tolerance: point beyond which a person is no longer willing to endure pain (ie, pain of greater duration or intensity)

Pallor: paleness of the skin

Palpation: method of examining by feeling a part with the fingers or hand

Palpitation: perception of one's own heartbeat

Paracentesis: withdrawal of fluid from a body cavity, usually from the abdominal cavity

Parasomnia: patterns of waking behavior that appear during sleep (eg, sleep walking, sleep talking, nocturnal erections)

Paralytic ileus: paralysis of intestinal peristalsis

Paraplegia: paralysis of the legs

Parenteral: outside of intestines or alimentary canal; popularly used to refer to injection routes

Paresthesia: numbness and tingling

Passive exercise: manual or mechanical means of moving the joints

Paternalism: an action that is based on what a parent would do

Pathogen: disease-producing microorganism

Patient-controlled analgesia (PCA): method of controlling pain that involves an infusion pump that holds a vial of an intravenous analgesic that the client controls and self-administers in small doses

Pediculosis: infestation with lice

Perception: conscious process of organizing and interpreting data from the senses into meaningful information

Percussion: the act of striking one object against another for the purpose of producing a sound; used to assess the location, shape, size, and density of body tissues

Percutaneous endoscopic gastrostomy tube (PEG): a surgically or laparoscopically placed gastrostomy tube

Perfusion: passing of fluid through body tissue

Perioperative nursing: wide variety of nursing activities carried out before, during, and after surgery

Peripheral resistance: restraint to blood flow created by arteriole walls in a partial state of contraction

Peripherally inserted central catheter (PICC): a type of venous access device that can be introduced into a peripheral vein and advanced as far as the superior vena cava

Peristalsis: involuntary, progressive wavelike movement of the musculature of the gastrointestinal tract

Personal identity: an individual's conscious sense of who he or she is

Personal space: external environment surrounding a person that is regarded as being part of that person

Petechiae: small, purplish hemorrhagic spots on the skin that do not blanch with applied pressure

pH: expression of hydrogen ion concentration and resulting acidity of a substance

Phagocytosis: engulfing of microorganisms, foreign particles, or other cells by phagocytes

Phantom pain: sensation of pain without demonstrable physiologic or pathologic substance; commonly observed after the amputation of a limb

Pharmacology: study of actions of chemicals on living organisms

Phlebitis: inflammation of a vein

Phlegm: thick, respiratory secretions

Physical assessment: systematic examination of the client for objective data to better define the client's condition and help the nurse in planning care; usually performed in a head-to-toe format

Physiologic needs: need for oxygen, food, water, temperature, elimination, sexuality, activity, and rest; these needs have the highest priority and are essential for survival

PIE charting: a documentation system that is unique in that it does not develop a separate care plan; the care plan is incorporated into the progress notes in which problems are identified by number, worked up using the problem (P), intervention (I), evaluation (E) format, and evaluated each shift

Piggyback infusion: intermittent intravenous administration of medications through a primary intravenous line with the additive container positioned higher than the primary intravenous solution

Placebo: Latin word meaning "I shall please"; an inactive substance that gives satisfaction to the person using it

Plaintiff: person or government bringing a lawsuit against another

Planning: establishment of client goals to prevent, reduce, or resolve the problems identified in the nursing diagnoses and determination of related nursing interventions

Plaque: transparent, adhesive coating on teeth consisting of mucin, carbohydrate, and bacteria

Plasma: liquid constituent of blood; synonym for *intravascular fluid*

Pneumonia: inflammation or infection of the lungs

Podiatrist: one who treats foot disorders; synonym for *chiropodist*

Polyp: tumor on a stem that bleeds easily and may become malignant

Polysomnography: sleep study consisting of an electroencephalographic recording of the stages of sleep and any episodes of apnea, continuous monitoring of arterial oxygen saturation, and an electrocardiographic recording to detect any cardiac dysrhythmias

Polyuria: excessive output of urine (diuresis)

Positive reinforcement: affirmation of the efforts of clients

Postoperative: period lasting from admission to the postanesthesia recovery area through recovery and convalescence

Postural hypotension: temporary fall in blood pressure associated with assuming an upright position; synonym for *orthostatic hypotension*

Post-void residual (PVR): urine that remains in the bladder after the act of micturition; a synonym for *residual urine*

Power: ability to influence others to achieve a desired effect

Preceptorship: process by which an experienced person facilitates an orientee's introduction to new responsibilities by way of teaching and guidance

Precordium: anterior surface of the chest wall overlying the heart and its related structures

Pre-entry phase: the phase of the home visit in which the nurse collects information about the client's healthcare needs, gathers needed supplies, and evaluates safety factors

Preferred provider organization (PPO): any arrangement whereby clients are channeled to specific organizations as providers of health plans

Premenstrual (tension) syndrome (PMS): menstrual cycle–related distress; occurs a few days before the onset of menstruation

Preoperative: period lasting from the decision that surgery is necessary until the client is transferred to the operating room area

Presbycusis: age-related hearing loss in which there is decreased ability to distinguish higher frequencies

Presbyopia: condition of aging in which decreased elasticity of the eye lens hinders accommodation to close vision

Preschooler: period from ages 3 to 6 years

Prescription: used by physician to convey medication plans for a client

Pressure ulcer: any lesion caused by unrelieved pressure that results in damage to underlying tissue

Primary healthcare: essential healthcare based on practical, scientifically sound, and socially acceptable methods and technology, made universally accessible through the community's full participation and at a cost the community can afford

Primary preventive care: care directed toward health promotion and specific protection against illness

Principle-based approach: an approach to bioethics that offers specific action guides

Problem-oriented record (POR): documentation system organized according to the person's specific health problems; includes data base, problem list, plan of care, and progress notes

Process: series of actions, changes, or functions to bring about a result

Productive cough: cough that produces respiratory tract secretions

Progress notes: any of a variety of methods of notes that relate how a client is progressing toward expected outcomes

Protein: vital component of every living cell; composed of carbon, hydrogen, oxygen, and nitrogen

Proteinuria: albumin in the urine; indication of kidney disease

Protocol: written plan that details the nursing activities to be executed in specific situations

Psychogenic pain: pain for which no physical cause can be identified

Psychomotor learning: acquisition of physical skills

Psychosomatic disorder: physiologic alterations and illness believed to be due to psychological influences

Puberty: period during which primary and secondary sexual characteristics develop and the capability of sexual reproduction is attained

Public health agencies: local, state, provincial, or federal agencies that provide public health services to members of communities

Pulse: wave produced in the wall of an artery with each beat of the heart

Pulse deficit: difference between the apical and radial pulse rates

Pulse oximetry: noninvasive technique that measures the oxygen saturation (SaO_2) of arterial blood

Pulse pressure: difference between systolic and diastolic pressures

Purulent: containing pus

Pyorrhea: extensive inflammation of the gums and alveolar tissues; synonym for *periodontitis*

Pyrexia: elevation above the upper limit of normal body temperature; synonym for *fever*

Pyuria: pus in the urine; urine appears cloudy

Quality assurance program: ongoing evaluation program designed and implemented to secure the excellence of health care; may involve an assessment of structure, process, and outcome standards

Quality improvement: the commitment and approach used to continuously improve every process in every part of an organization, with the intent of meeting and exceeding customer expectations and outcomes (also known as continuous quality improvement [CQI] or total quality management [TQM])

Race: division of human beings based on distinct physical characteristics

Radiography: examination by x-ray film

Range of motion: complete extent of movement of which a joint is normally capable

Rape: sexual violation of a person by someone who uses force, threats, and abuse

Rapid eye movement sleep: stage that constitutes 20% to 25% of a person's nightly sleep; person is difficult to arouse during this stage

Rapport: feeling of mutual trust experienced by people in a satisfactory relationship

Reactive hyperemia: the body's flooding of an area with blood after it has suffered from poor circulation for a period; the occurrence of a blanchable reddening of the skin when pressure is removed

Reality orientation: method of care used to promote awareness of reality in confused or disoriented clients

Receiver (decoder): term used in communication theory that specifies the person or object to which the message is directed

Reception: process of receiving data about the internal or external environment through the senses

Recommended dietary allowance (RDA): recommendations for average daily amounts of essential nutrients that healthy population groups should consume over time

Referral: process of sending or guiding someone to another source for assistance

Referred pain: pain in an area removed from that in which stimulation has its origin

Reflex pain response: automatic response of the central nervous system to the stimulus of pain

Regional anesthesia: anesthetic drug is injected or applied topically to inhibit transmission of sensory stimuli

Regression: behavior that is more characteristic of an earlier age

Rehabilitation: process of restoring a person's highest level of possible wellness and returning that person's ability to live and work as normally as possible after a disabling illness or injury

Rehabilitation centers: centers specializing in services for clients requiring physical or emotional rehabilitation and for treatment of any type of drug dependency

Relationship: interaction of people over time

Religion: organized system of beliefs about a higher power; often includes set forms of worship, spiritual practices, and codes of conduct

REM: rapid eye movement that characterizes the dream state of sleep

Report: oral, written, or computer-based communication of client data with the purpose of informing others

Repression: exclusion of an anxiety-producing event from conscious awareness

Reservoir: natural habitat for the growth and multiplication of microorganisms

Residual urine: urine that remains in the bladder after the act of micturition

Respiration: act of breathing and using oxygen in body cells

Respiratory acidosis: proportionate excess of carbonic acid in the extracellular fluid

Respiratory alkalosis: proportionate deficiency of carbonic acid in the extracellular fluid

Rest: condition in which the body is in a decreased state of activity with the consequent feeling of being refreshed

Restraint: device used to limit movement or immobilize a client

Retention: inability to void although urine is produced by the kidneys and enters the bladder; excessive storage of urine in the bladder

Retention sutures: sutures used to provide extra support in wounds in obese clients or in wounds with increased risk of dehiscence

Reticular activating system: network of neurons in the core of the brain stem with ascending and descending tracts to other areas of the brain that monitors and regulates incoming sensory stimuli and level of arousal

Retrospective audit: evaluation of nursing care and client outcomes after the client has been discharged (may use postdischarge questionnaires, client interviews, or chart review)

Risk factor: something that increases a person's chance for illness or injury

Role performance: ability to successfully execute societal expectations regarding role-specific behaviors

Safety and security needs: person's need to be protected from actual or potential harm and to have freedom from fear

Sanguineous: containing or mixed with blood

Scar: connective tissue that fills a wound area

School-age: period from ages 6 to 12 years

Scientific knowledge: knowledge arrived at by applying scientific methods

Scientific problem solving: systematic problem-solving process that involves (1) problem identification, (2) data collection, (3) hypothesis formulation, (4) plan of action, (5) hypothesis testing, (6) interpretation of results, and (7) evaluation resulting in conclusion or revision of the study

Scrub nurse: nurse who assists the surgeon during surgery, maintaining surgical asepsis while draping, handling instruments, and handling supplies

Scultetus binder: type of bandage with multiple tails; synonym for *many-tailed binder*

Sebaceous gland: gland found in the skin that secretes an oily substance called sebum

Secondary preventive care: care directed to health maintenance for clients experiencing health problems or to prevention of complications or disabilities

Self-actualization needs: need to reach one's potential through full development of one's unique capabilities; highest level need

Self-concept: mental image or picture of self; includes body image, subjective self, ideal self, and social self

Self-esteem: person's perception of his or her total being, including self-worth and body image

Self-esteem needs: need to feel good about oneself and to believe others hold one in high regard

Semantics: study of the meaning of words

Semen: seminal plasma containing sperm

Semipermeable membrane: selectively permeable membrane that allows water to pass through it but is either impermeable or selectively permeable to solutes

Sensoristasis: arousal state of the reticular activating system; general drive state

Sensory deficit: impaired or absent functioning of one or more senses

Sensory deprivation: condition resulting from decreased sensory input or input that is monotonous, unpatterned, or meaningless

Sensory overload: condition resulting from excessive sensory input to which the brain is unable to meaningfully respond

Sensory/perceptual alteration: disturbance in the body's ability to receive or process data from its internal or external environment. NANDA-approved nursing diagnosis

Separation anxiety: condition that occurs when a child is afraid of being sent away from caregivers who are loved and provide security

Serous: resembling blood serum; clear and watery in appearance

Set point: level at which the hypothalamus attempts to maintain body temperature

Sexual dysfunction: condition that prevents a person or couple from engaging in or obtaining satisfaction from sexual activity

Sexual harassment: unwelcome verbal or physical advance or sexually explicit statement (eg, leers, pats, grabs, jokes, requests for dates, and even rape) that interferes with one's ability to do one's job by making one feel humiliated, intimidated, or uncomfortable

Sexuality: degree to which a person exhibits and experiences maleness and femaleness physically, emotionally, and mentally

Sexually transmitted disease: a disease that spreads from one person to another through intimate sexual contact

Shearing force: force created when layers of tissue move on one another

Shock: body's reaction to acute peripheral circulatory failure due to an abnormality of circulatory control or to a loss of circulating fluid

Situational crisis: change that results when a person faces an event or situation that causes a disruption in his life

Sitz bath: special type of bath that applies heated water to the pelvic or rectal area

Skin sutures: used to approximate wound tissues and skin; may be silk, synthetic, wire, or metal staples

Skin tests: tests to determine antigen–antibody reaction

Sleep: state of altered consciousness throughout which varying degrees of stimuli preclude wakefulness

Sleep apnea: periods of no breathing during sleep that may last from 15 seconds to 2 minutes

Sleep cycle: passage through the four states of NREM sleep (I, II, III, IV), then reversal (IV, III, II), and finally, instead of reentering stage I and awakening, entering REM sleep and returning to stage II

Sleep deprivation: a decrease in the amount, consistency, and quality of sleep; results from decreased REM or NREM sleep

SOAP format: method of charting narrative progress notes; organizes data according to subjective information (S), objective information (O), assessment (A), and plan (P)

Social isolation: sense of aloneness because of decreasing relationships with others, resulting from attitudinal, geographic, financial, or illness-related factors

Social self: way a person believes that others see him or her

Solute: substance dissolved in a solution

Solvent: liquid holding a substance in solution

Somatic pain: pain originating in structures in the body's external wall

Somnambulism: sleep walking

Sordes: accumulation of mucus and crust formation on the teeth and around the lips

Source (encoder): term used in communication theory to specify the one who prepares and sends a message to the receiver

Source-oriented record: documentation system in which each health care group records data on its own separate form

Spasticity: increased muscle tone

Sperm: male reproductive cell; synonym for *spermatozoan*

Spermicide: chemical agent used to destroy sperm

Sphincter: circular muscle that constricts a passage or closes a natural orifice

Spiritual distress: nursing diagnosis describing an alteration in spiritual health (eg, spiritual pain, alienation, anxiety, guilt, anger, loss, despair)

Spiritual need: lack of anything necessary for spiritual health (eg, meaning and purpose, love and relatedness, forgiveness)

Spirituality: anything that pertains to a person's relationship with a nonmaterial life force or higher power

Spirometer: instrument used to measure lung capacities and volumes; one type is used to encourage deep breathing (incentive spirometry)

Standard: acceptable, expected, level of performance established by authority, custom, or consent

Standardized plan of care: prepared plan of care that identifies the nursing diagnoses, client goals, and related nursing orders common to a specific population (eg, normal neonates) or problem

Standard Precautions: new CDC precautions used in the care of all clients regardless of their diagnosis or possible infection status; this category combines universal and body substance precautions

Standing order: document that details the nursing care to be implemented in specific nursing situations, frequently when a physician is not present; may expand scope of nursing responsibilities

Statutory law: law enacted by a legislative body

Stereognosis: the sense that perceives the solidity of objects, their size, shape, and texture

Stereotyping: assigning characteristics to a group of people without considering specific individuality

Sterilization: (1) the process by which all microorganisms, including spores, are destroyed; (2) surgical procedure performed to render a person infertile

Stertorous breathing: noisy respirations

Stimulus: agent, act, or other influence capable of initiating a response by the nervous system

Stoma: artificial opening for waste excretion located on the body surface

Stool: excreted feces

Strength (muscle): ability of the muscle to move actively against resistance

Stress: condition in which the human system responds to change in its normal balanced state

Stress incontinence: state in which the person experiences a loss of urine of less than 50 mL that occurs with increased abdominal pressure

Stressor: anything causing a person to experience stress; change in the balanced state

Stridor: harsh, high-pitched sound usually heard on inspiration when upper airways become narrowed

Subculture: group of people with different interests or goals than the primary culture

Subcutaneous injection: injection into the subcutaneous tissue that lies between the epidermis and the muscle

Subjective data (symptoms, covert data): information perceived only by the affected person

Subjective self: how one sees oneself; who one thinks one is

Sublingual: area in the mouth under the tongue

Sudden infant death syndrome (SIDS): sudden death of any infant or young child without demonstrated cause

Sundowning syndrome: describes a phenomenon when a person habitually becomes confused or disoriented with darkness

Suppository: oval- or cone-shaped substance that is inserted into a body cavity and that melts at body temperature

Suprapubic catheter: catheter inserted into the bladder through a small abdominal incision above the pubic area

Surgical asepsis: practices that render and keep objects and areas free from microorganisms; synonym for *sterile technique*

Susceptibility: degree of resistance of a host to a pathogen

Symptom: abnormality indicative of illness as experienced by the client; synonym for *subjective data*

Synergistic effect: combined effect of two or more drugs is greater than the effect of each drug alone

Systemic symptoms: symptoms manifested throughout the entire body

Systolic pressure: highest point of pressure on arterial walls when the ventricles contract

Tachycardia: rapid heart rate

Tachypnea: abnormally rapid rate of breathing

Tactile: pertaining to touch

Tartar: hard deposit on the teeth near the gum line formed by plaque buildup and dead bacteria

Teaching: planned method or series of methods used to help someone learn

Technical competencies: skills that enable a nurse to skillfully manipulate equipment in a manner conducive to achieving a desired goal

Temperament: person's style of approaching people, situations, or events

Temperature: refers to the hotness or coldness of a substance

Terminal illness: illness from which there is no reasonable expectation of recovery or cure

Terminal wean: the withdrawal of life-sustaining therapy with the understanding that death may result, generally after a decision is made that the therapy in question is medically futile or disproportionately burdensome

Tertiary preventive care: care directed at helping rehabilitate clients and restore them to a maximum level of functioning after an illness

Therapeutic touch: an alternative therapy that involves using one's hands to consciously direct an energy exchange from the practitioner to the client to facilitate healing or pain relief

Third-space fluid shift: distributional shift and trapping of body fluids into body spaces such as the pleural, peritoneal, or pericardial, or into the interstitial space (plasma-to-interstitial shift)

Thoracentesis: aspiration of fluid or air from the pleural space

Thrill: abnormal tremor accompanying a vascular or cardiac murmur felt on palpation

Thrombophlebitis: inflammation in a vein associated with thrombus formation

Thrombus: blood clot; plural is *thrombi*

Toddler: period from ages 1 to 3 years

Tonus: normal, partially steady state of muscle contraction

Topical application: application of a substance directly to a body site

Tort: wrong committed by a person against another person or his property

Total body water (TBW): total amount of water in the body, expressed as a percentage of body weight. The term *total body fluid* also is used; fluids usually are considered to include water and electrolytes

Total parenteral nutrition (TPN): nutritional therapy that bypasses the gastrointestinal tract for clients who are unable to take food orally; meets the client's nutritional needs by way of nutrient-filled solutions administered intravenously through a central vein

Trace elements: minerals found in the body in quantities less than 5 g and needed in only small amounts (18 mg or less)

Tracheostomy tube: curved tube inserted into an artificial opening made into the trachea that comes with varied angles and in multiple sizes

Trade name: drug name selected and trademarked by the company selling the drug to market the drug; also called *brand name* or *proprietary name*

Traditional family: composed of a husband, wife, and their children, who live together in one house

Traditional knowledge: knowledge passed down from generation to generation

Transcultural nursing: providing nursing care that is planned and implemented in a way that is sensitive to the needs of individuals, families, and groups representing the diverse cultural populations within our society

Transformational leadership: type of leadership in which the person creates revolutionary change and commits to the personal and professional growth of self and others

Transmission-based precautions: new CDC precautions used in clients known or suspected to be infected with pathogens that can be transmitted by airborne, droplet, or contact routes; used in addition to Standard Precautions

Trauma: injury

Tremor: involuntary muscular movements

Trial: hearing of evidence in a legal case before a judge (and jury) with the intent of reaching a decision or verdict

Triglycerides: predominant form of fat in food and the major storage form of fat in the body; composed of one glyceride molecule and three fatty acids

Turgor: tension of a cell determined by its hydration

Typing: determining a person's blood type

Unilateral: affecting or occurring on one side only

Universal precautions: isolation system that considers blood, body fluids containing blood, semen, and vaginal secretions of all clients as potentially infective

Urge incontinence: state in which a person experiences involuntary passage of urine that occurs soon after a strong sense of urgency to void

Urgency: strong desire to void

Urinary retention: inability to void although urine is produced by the kidneys and enters the bladder; excessive storage of urine in the bladder

Urination: process of emptying the bladder; micturition; voiding

Utilitarianism: ethical theory that states that those acts that produce the greatest overall balance of good for the greatest number of people are right

Validation: act of confirming or verifying

Valsalva maneuver: forcible exhalation against a closed glottis, resulting in increased intrathoracic pressure

Value system: organization of values ranked along a continuum of importance

Values: set of beliefs that are meaningful in life and that influence relationships with others

Values clarification: process by which people come to understand their own values and value system

Variables: factors in a research study

Variance charting: documentation method in case management that records unexpected events, the cause for the event, actions taken in response to the event, and discharge planning when appropriate

Varicosity: swollen, twisted vein

Ventilation: exchange of gases

Veracity: truth telling

Verbal communication: exchange of information using words

Vesicular breath sounds: normal sound of respirations heard on auscultation over peripheral lung areas

Vial: glass bottle with self-sealing stopper through which medication is removed; may be single or multiple dose

Virulence: ability to produce disease

Virus: smallest of all microorganisms that can be seen only by using an electron microscope

Visceral: pertaining to inner organs

Visceral pain: pain originating in the internal organs in the thorax, cranium, or abdomen

Visual: pertaining to sight

Vital signs: body temperature, pulse and respiratory rates, and blood pressure; synonym for *cardinal signs*

Vitamins: organic substances needed by the body in small amounts to help regulate body processes; are susceptible to oxidation and destruction

Voiding: process of emptying the bladder; also called *micturition* or *urination*

Voluntary agencies: community agencies that are often funded by private donations, grants, or fund-raising and that provide a wide variety of direct services and education

Wellness: an active process in which an individual progresses toward the maximum possible potential, regardless of his or her current state of health

Wellness diagnosis: clinical judgment about an individual, family, or community in transition from a specific level of wellness to a higher level of wellness

Wheeze: a continuous, high-pitched squeak or musical sound made as air moves through narrowed or partially obstructed airway passages

Whistleblowing: term generally used to refer to employees who report their employers' violation of the law to appropriate law enforcement agencies outside the employers' facilities

Wound: injury that results in a disruption in the normal continuity of a body structure

X-ray: high-energy electromagnetic wave capable of penetrating solid matter and acting on photographic film; synonym for *roentgen ray*

Yin-yang: energy forces in Chinese teaching that must be in balance for good health; expression of strong emotions results in disharmony and imbalance between these forces

Young adult: the adult between the ages of 20 and 40 years; also called *early adulthood*

Z-track: zigzag technique used to administer medications intramuscularly

Photo Credits

Photos in Table of Contents, Unit and Chapter Opener Photos

Courtesy of Brett Ainsworth: Chapters 38, 40, 46; Unit III; TOC xxxiv

Courtesy of Susan Blaker: Chapter 9

Courtesy of Sandy Gilmour, photo by Paul Jonson: TOC xxx

Courtesy of Laurie K. Glass, University of Wisconsin: Chapter 29; TOC xxvii

Courtesy of John Harkins: Chapter 35

© Ken Kasper: Chapters 26, 45

Courtesy of Maryann Keneally: Chapter 10

Dave Macklem, University of Wisconsin Photo Services: Chapters 14, 20

© B. Proud: Chapters 28, 29; Unit VIII; TOC xxiv, xxv

© Gates Rhodes, courtesy of the School of Nursing, University of Pennsylvania: Chapters 2, 19

Courtesy of Bill Rowe, Rockford Health System, Rockford, IL: Unit I

© Kathy Sloane: Chapters 1, 7, 8, 11, 16, 27, 31, 32, 41; TOC xix

Courtesy of Nursing Spectrum: Chapter 23; Units IV, V, VI
  Children's Seashore House: Unit VII
  Daniel Hagan, Mercy Catholic Memorial Center: Chapter 15
  Montgomery ICU, Photo by Linda Hadly: Chapter 30; Unit II; TOC xxvi
  Shore Memorial Hospital, Einrosia Photography: Chapters 4, 13; TOC xxi

Courtesy of Ed Woods: Chapter 36

Index

Numbers followed by *f* indicate a figure; *t* following a page number indicates tabular material.

Abbreviated grief, 782
Abbreviations
  in documentation, 332, 344t–345t
  for drug dosage, 603, 603t
  for drug prescription, 603–604, 603t–605t
  for laboratory values, 1441
Abdomen
  examination of, 503–507, 505f–506f, 1272–1273
  organs of, 505f
  quadrants of, 504, 506f
Abdominal breathing, 1329–1330
Abdominal reflex, assessment of, 516t
Abdominal setting exercises, in bowel elimination, 1285
Abdominal thrust, for airway clearance, procedure for, 1357–1358
Abducens nerve, assessment of, 513, 513t
Abduction, definition of, 1000t, 1001f–1002f
ABO blood groups, 1427
Abrasion
  definition of, 699t
  emergency care of, 705
Absorption, of drugs, 596
  from skin, 642, 646
Absorptive dressings, 722, 989t
Abstinence, sexual, 848
Acceptance stage, in dying, 782
Accessory nerve, assessment of, 513t, 514, 514f
Accidents
  in adolescents, 146, 147t, 526
  causes of, 525
  in children, 526
  deaths caused by, 526t
    reactions to, 793
  in elderly persons, 167, 526
  infectious agent exposure in, reporting of, 588
  prevention of. *See* Safety
  in young adults, 152
Accommodation, in intellectual growth, 119
Accommodation (visual), assessment of, 487, 488f
Accountability
  development of, 241–243
  in documentation, 332
  in home healthcare, 210–211, 211t
Accreditation, for nursing educational program, 98
Acculturation, cultural, 34
Achilles tendon (ankle) reflex, assessment of, 516t, 517
Achondroplasia, mobility in, 1007
Acid, definition of, 1374–1376
Acid-base balance, 1374–1377
  assessment of, 1391, 1396, 1397t
  buffer systems in, 1376–1377
  planning in, 1378–1379
  regulation of, 1375t
    renal, 1377
    respiratory, 1376–1377
Acid-base imbalance, 1386, 1387t–1388t, 1388. *See also specific disorder, e.g.,* Acidosis
  respiration in, 1387t
Acidosis
  definition of, 1376, 1376f
  metabolic
    blood gas analysis in, 1391, 1396
    causes of, 1387t–1388t
    characteristics of, 1387t–1388t
    definition of, 1386
    treatment of, 1387t–1388t
  respiratory
    blood gas analysis in, 1391, 1396
    causes of, 1387t
    characteristics of, 1387t
    definition of, 1386
    treatment of, 1387t
Acne, care of, 941
Acoustic nerve, assessment of, 513t, 514
Acquired immunodeficiency syndrome. *See* Human immunodeficiency virus infection
ACTH (adrenocorticotropic hormone), in respiratory disorders, 1336t
Acting, in value clarification, 81–82
Active-assistive exercise, range-of-motion, 1037
Active exercise, range-of-motion, 1037
Active transport, of electrolytes, 1372, 1372f
Activity. *See also* Exercise; Movement
  calorie requirements for, 1152
  daily
    as exercise, 1017, 1051
    preoperative assessment of, 676
    stress and, 768–769
  intolerance of
    causes of, 1030
    characteristics of, 1030
    in immobility, 1011t
  sleep and, 1076
Activity flowsheet, in client record, 335t
Activity theory, older adults and, 160
Actual loss, definition of, 781
Acumassage, 43, 47t
Acupressure, 43, 47t, 1125
Acupuncture, 43, 47t, 1125–1126
Acute illness, definition of, 59–60
Acyclovir, in herpes infection, 854t
Adaptation. *See also* Coping mechanisms
  to body image changes, 736
  to constant stimulus, 815
  definition of, 755
  by elderly persons, 163–165, 164f
  failure of, 763
  general adaptation syndrome in, 758–759, 759f
  to illness, 761–762
  inflammatory response in, 758
  local adaptation syndrome in, 758
  mind-body interaction in, 757–758
  to pain, 1107–1108
  physiologic, 758–759, 759f
  psychosocial, 759–760
  reflex pain response in, 758
  of skin pigmentation, 38
Adaptation model of nursing (Roy), 71t, 74–75
Adaptation theory, 67
Addiction, definition of, 1129

Adduction, definition of, 100t, 1001f–1002f
A delta fibers, in pain transmission, 1104
Adjustable bed, body alignment and, 1032
Administration (executive function), nurse role in, 11t
Administration (medications). *See under* Drugs/medications
Administrative law, 96
Admission
  to ambulatory facility, 194
  to healthcare unit, procedure for, 192–194
  to hospital, 194–195
    client arrival on unit and, 195, 200t
    data base form for, 198–199
    documentation of, 335t
    procedure for, 196–197
    room preparation in, 194–195, 195f
Adolescents
  body alignment in, 1009t
  bowel elimination in, 1269t
  developmental tasks in, 120
  growth and development of
    cognitive, 143
    moral, 146
    physiologic, 142–143, 144f–145f, 146t
    psychosocial, 143, 146
    spiritual, 146
  health problems in, 146–147
  identity development in, 118
  mobility in, 1009t
  nutrition in, 1163, 1167t, 1169
  poisoning in, 530
  safety considerations for, 526, 537t, 538
  self-concept in, 732t
  self-esteem in, development of, 742
  sexuality in, 117, 850t
  skin condition in, 913
  sleep in, 1078t
  wellness promotion in, 147–148, 147t–148t
Adrenal gland, fluid/electrolyte homeostasis and, 1374, 1375t
Adrenocorticotropic hormone (ACTH), in respiratory disorders, 1336t
Advance directives, 426–427, 785, 786f–788f, 789
Adventists, 886t
Adventitious breath sounds, definition of, 497, 500f, 1319
Advocacy, 84, 424–427
  assertiveness in, 426
  bill of rights in, 425
  ethics and, 424–427
  in home healthcare, 211
  as nursing function, 10t
  persons requiring, 425–426, 425f
  political action and, 427
  for sexual needs, 869–870
Aerobic bacteria, 556
Aerobic exercise, 1017
Afebrile, definition of, 435
Affective behavior, in sensory deprivation, 816t
Affective goals, 285
  evaluation of, 315
Affective learning, 388, 395
Afferent system, in pain transmission, 1106
African-American people
  cultural characteristics of, 46t–47t
  drug action in, 599
  nutrition in, 1169, 1170t
  physiologic characteristics of, 38–39
Afternoon care, 918
Age. *See also* Developmental level
  blood pressure and, 458, 459t
  body temperature and, 435
  vs. body water distribution, 1367, 1369t
  pain attitudes and, 1111–1112
  pulse rate and, 449t
  skin changes in, 977, 979f
Ageism, 165–166, 165t, 166f
Agencies, healthcare, 181–182, 181f–182f
Agent-host-environment model, of health and illness, 54–55, 55f
Agglutinin, definition of, 1427
Aging. *See also* Elderly persons
  physiology of, 157
  self-concept and, 733, 733f, 742–743
  surgical risks in, 675
  theories on, 157
Agnostic, definition of, 883
AIDS. *See* Human immunodeficiency virus infection
Air
  humidification of, in respiratory disorders, 1332
  in infectious agent transmission, 557, 558t
  pollution of, respiratory disorders and, 1317–1318
Airborne precautions, 580, 582
Air mattresses and beds, in pressure ulcer prevention, 987t
Airway
  artificial, 1344–1348, 1347f
  clearance of, ineffective, 1328, 1360–1361
    in immobility, 1012t
  obstruction of
    clearance of, 1354, 1357–1358
    clinical manifestations of, 1321
  patency of, in respiration, 1314
  resistance in, 1314
Alarm reaction, in general adaptation syndrome, 758, 759f
Albumin
  as electrolyte, 1371
  measurement of, in nutritional assessment, 1175
Albuminuria, orthostatic, definition of, 1219
Alcohol (ingested)
  nutrition requirements and, 1168
  sexual function effects of, 869–870
  sleep and, 1080
  as surgical risk, 676
Alcoholics Anonymous, 181
Aldosterone, function of, 1375t
Alienation, spiritual, 890, 893
Alignment of body. *See* Body alignment
Alkali, definition of, 1374
Alkalosis
  definition of, 1376, 1376f
  metabolic
    blood gas analysis in, 1391, 1396
    causes of, 1388t
    characteristics of, 1388t
    definition of, 1386, 1388
    treatment of, 1388t
  respiratory
    blood gas analysis in, 1391, 1396
    causes of, 1387t
    characteristics of, 1387t
    definition of, 1386
    treatment of, 1387t
Allergy
  in blood transfusion, 1429t
  to drugs, 600
  in respiratory disorders, testing for, 1324t
  skin testing for, 1324t
Alma-Ata declaration, 183
Alopecia, definition of, 485, 955
Altered function, coping with, 11
Alternative healing systems, 41, 43
Altruism, as essential value, 80
Alupent (metaproterenol), in respiratory disorders, 1336t
Alveoli
  function of, 1312–1313
  gas exchange in, 1314–1315, 1314f
Alzheimer's disease, 157, 160
AMA (against medical advice), discharging client and, 201
Ambulation
  assistance with, 1048–1056
    client fainting during, 1051
    mechanical aids for, 1052–1056, 1054f–1058f
    with one nurse, 1052, 1053f
    physical conditioning for, 1048, 1050–1051
    preparation for, 1048, 1050–1051
    with two nurses, 1052, 1053f
  developmental level and, 1008t–1009t
Ambulatory facilities
  admission to, 194
  nursing activities in, 178
  surgery in
    postoperative care in, 697
    preparation for, 672–673, 674f
AM care (morning care), 918
American Hospital Association, patient's bill of rights, 84, 87–88
American Muslim Mission, 887
American Nurses Association, 15

code of ethics of, 85
nursing defined by, 7–9
nursing practice standards of, 16
quality assurance program of, 323
Americans with Disabilities Act, 110
Amino acids, from protein metabolism, 1153, 1155, 1156f
Aminophylline, in respiratory disorders, 1336t
Ampules
drug packaging in, 617, 617f
drug removal from, procedure for, 618–619
Amputation, accidental, emergency care of, 705
Amyl nitrite, sexual function effects of, 856t
ANA. *See* American Nurses Association
Anaerobic bacteria, 556
Anal canal, function of, 1268, 1268f
Analgesics
adjuvant, 1129
administration of
in acute pain, 1130, 1132f
in children, 1130, 1132
in chronic pain, 1130, 1133f–1134f
in elderly persons, 1132–1133, 1135
epidural, 1133, 1135–1136, 1135f
in home care, 1137
patient-controlled, 1133, 1135f
principles of, 1129–1130
regimens for, 1130, 1132f–1134f
timing of, 1130, 1131f
classes of, 1128
respiratory function and, 1317
urinary elimination and, 1216
Anal intercourse, 848
Anal stage, in Freudian theory, 117, 117t
toddlerhood as, 136
Anaphylactic reaction, to drugs, 600
Andragogy, definition of, 389
Andropause, 154
Anemia
iron deficiency, 1201–1202
sickle cell, ethnic differences in, 39
Aneroid manometer, in blood pressure equipment, 460–461, 461f
Anesthesia, 671–672
bowel elimination and, 1271
general, 672
local, in pain management, 1136–1137
recovery from, 688
regional, 672
Anesthetist, nurse, 11t
Anger
in dying, 782
spiritual, 890, 893
Animals, as pathogen reservoirs, 557
Anion, definition of, 1368
Anion gap, in metabolic acidosis, 1388t
Ankle, range of motion of, 1002f
Ankle reflex, assessment of, 516t, 517
Ankylosis, of joint, in immobility, 1019
Anorexia
appetite stimulation in, 1179–1180
definition of, 1169
Anorexia nervosa, 147, 1169
Antagonistic effects, of drugs, 600
Antebrachial vein, intravenous therapy in, 1411f
Anthropometric data, in nutritional status assessment, 1173–1174, 1176f
Antibiotics, resistance to, 561–562
Antibodies
blood types and, 1427
definition of, 558
Anticholinergics, preoperative, 686
Anticipatory grief, 782
Anticipatory guidance, in stress management, 770
Anticipatory loss, definition of, 781
Anticonvulsants, sexual function effects of, 856t
Antidepressants, sexual function effects of, 856t
Antidiarrheal medications, 1286–1287
Antidiuretic hormone, in fluid/electrolyte homeostasis, 1374, 1375t
Antiembolism stockings, assistance with, 927, 930
procedure for, 928–929
Antigens
blood types and, 1427
definition of, 558
Antihelmintic enema, 1288
Antihistamines
in respiratory disorders, 1336t
sexual function effects of, 856t
Antimicrobial agents, in asepsis, 563
Antiperspirants, in skin care, 940–941
Antipsychotic drugs, sexual function effects of, 856t
Antipyretic drugs, 436–437
Anuria, definition of, 1219
Anus, examination of, 508, 1273–1274
Anxiety
coping mechanisms for, 773–774
in interview, 253t
levels of, 759–760
pain aggravated by, 1112
release of, 762
respiratory function and, 1318
responses to, 765
separation, in toddlers, 137
spiritual, 890, 893
from wounds, 704
Aortic area, pulse at, 499, 501f
Apgar Rating Scale, for neonates, 130, 130t
Aphasia, 380, 512
Apical impulse, 499, 501f
Apical pulse rate, assessment of, 449
procedure for, 455–456
Apical-radial pulse rate, 452
Apnea
definition of, 456
sleep, 1081, 1082t, 1084f
Apothecary system, 607, 1439, 1439t–1440t
Appalachian people, cultural characteristics of, 50t
Appearance, general, assessment of, 481
Appellate court, 97
Appetite
disorders of, 1169
stimulation of, 1179–1180
Appliance, ostomy, changing of, 1296–1297, 1297f
Aquathermia therapy, skin alterations from, 917t
Areola, examination of, 503
Arm, injection into, 631f, 632
Arousal mechanism, in sensation, 814–815
Arrhythmia, cardiac, definition of, 449, 450t
Arterial blood gases, 1322t
in acid-base balance/imbalance, 1386, 1387t–1388t, 1388
measurement of, 1391, 1396, 1397t
Arterioles, 457
filtration through, 1373f
Arthritis
mobility in, 1007
pain in, 1105t
Articulations. *See* Joints
Artificial airway, 1344–1348, 1347f
Ascites, imbalances resulting from, 1390t
Ascorbic acid (vitamin C), 1159t
Asepsis. *See also* Surgical asepsis
definition of, 560
medical, 560, 562–565
Asian people
cultural characteristics of, 47t–48t
drug action in, 599
nutrition in, 1170t
psychological characteristics of, 42
religions of, 887, 893
As needed (prn) care, 918–919
As needed (prn) order, for medications, 602
Asphyxiation
accidental, causes of, 530–531, 533
prevention of, 530–531
Aspiration
from nasogastric tube, 1186
from pleural cavity (thoracentesis), 1321, 1321f, 1324
procedures for, 520t
into respiratory tract in tube feeding, 1191
Assault, legal aspects of, 99
Assertiveness
in advocacy, 426
in communication, 377, 377t–378t
Assessing, 225, 227t, 248–265. *See also specific types of care e.g.,* Bowel elimination; Movement; Oral care

Assessing *(continued)*
  communication in, 364–365
  components of, 474
  core competencies, 244–245
  cultural, 44
  data collection in
    comprehensive vs. focused, 260
    data characteristics in, 248–249, 250t
    focused, 260
    interview in, 250–252, 253t
    methods of, 249–254, 252f, 253t
    observation in, 249–250
    physical assessment in. *See* Physical assessment
    planning for, 261–262
    priorities in, 261–262
    problems in, 262, 263t
    sample form for, 255–259
    sources for, 254, 260f
    structure for, 262
  data communication in, 263–264, 264f
  data validation in, 262–263
  definition of, 248, 249f
  documentation of, 264, 337
  evaluation of, problems in, 320t
  focus of, 248
  health history in, 474
  in home healthcare, 214
  illustration of, 228
  legal issues in, 263
  medical vs. nursing, 248
  potential liability in, 103t
  in teaching-learning process, 392, 393f
Assimilation
  cultural, 34
  of experiences, 119
Assurance, false, 371
Asthma, case study of, 1361–1362
Ataque, as reactive behavior, 41, 48t
Ataxia
  cerebellar, 1028f
  sensory, 1028f
Atelectasis
  definition of, 1314–1315
  from immobility, 1019
  postoperative, 696
Atheist, definition of, 883
Athetosis, definition of, 1025
Athlete's foot, 960
ATP, in active transport, 1372, 1372f
Atrioventricular valves, 500f
Atrophy
  of muscle, 509, 1003, 1027, 1029
    in immobility, 1019
  of skin, 484t
Attachment vs. bonding, 133
Attack behavior, as coping mechanism, 760
Attitude
  definition of, 79
  toward exercise, 1015
Attorney, durable power of, 785, 787f, 789
Audiologist, 379
Audiotaped message, in communication, 340t
Audiovisual materials, in teaching, 396
Auditory sensation. *See* Hearing
Auscultation, 480–481
  of abdomen, 506–507, 1273
  definition of, 449
  of precordium, 501–502, 502f, 502t
  of respiratory system, 1319, 1321
  of thorax, 496–497, 499f–500f
Authoritative knowledge, 422
Autocratic leadership, 414
Automated external defibrillator, in CPR, 1358, 1358f
Automated temperature monitoring, 438–439
Autonomic bladder, 1219
Autonomic nervous system, in homeostasis, 756, 757t
Autonomy
  development of, 118
    in toddler, 137
  in ethical code, 83
  in nursing practice, 18–19, 69
  vs. shame and doubt in toddlers, 118, 137
Autopsy, 791–792
Awareness
  as grief reaction, 781
  states of, 815
Axilla, examination of, 502–503, 503f–504f
Axillary temperature
  assessment of, 445–446
    procedure for, 447–448
  normal, 437t
Azithromycin, in sexually transmitted diseases, 854t

Babies. *See* Infants; Neonates
Babinski reflex, assessment of, 516t
Back
  injury of, in nursing activities, 1023
  massage of, 930
    procedure for, 1126
  pain in, 1123t
Bacteremia, in blood transfusion, 1429t
Bacteria
  on hands, 563
  as infectious agents, 556
Bag, resuscitation, 1348, 1351, 1354
"Bag bath," 927, 927f
Bag technique, for infection control, in home healthcare, 213–214
Balance
  assessment of, 514
  in body alignment, 1004, 1004f
Baldness, 955
Ball-and-socket joint, 1000
Bandages, 709, 712
  roller, 713, 714f–715f
Bar, trapeze, on bed, 1033, 1034f
Barbiturates, sexual function effects of, 856t
Bargaining, in dying, 782
Barium enema, 1277, 1281t–1282t
Barium studies, of gastrointestinal system, 1276–1277, 1280t–1282t
Barrel chest, 496, 496f
Barrier methods, of contraception, 866–867
Barriers, in isolation, 571, 576f, 586f
Barton, Clara, 7f
Basal body temperature method, of contraception, 866
Basal ganglia, mobility control and, 1010
Basal metabolism, 1150–1151
Base. *See also* Acid-base balance; Acid-base imbalance
  deficit of. *See* Acidosis, metabolic
  definition of, 1374–1376
  excess of. *See* Alkalosis, metabolic
Base of support, in body alignment, 1004, 1004f
Basic human needs. *See* Human needs
Basilic vein, intravenous therapy in, 1411–1412
Bathing
  "bag" technique in, 927, 927f
  in bed, 920, 927, 927f
    procedure for, 921–926
  with indwelling catheter, 1249
  with lotion, 920, 927
  purposes of, 919
  shower, 919–920, 920f
  sitz bath in, 963
  towel, 920, 927
  tub, 919–920, 920f
Bathroom, assistance in, 1229
Battery, legal aspects of, 99
Beard, care of, 957
Beau's lines, in nails, 485, 485f
Bed
  adjustable, 1032
  circular, 1032
  comfort of, 940, 940f
  making of, 930
    procedure for
      occupied, 935–939
      unoccupied, 931–935
  movement in, pressure ulcer formation and, 973–974, 975f
  movement of client in/from. *See* Movement, of client by nurse
  pressure ulcer prevention and, 985, 987t
  safety of, 939–940
  shampooing in, 956–957, 957f
  side rails on, 539, 541f, 1033
  Stryker frame type, 1032
  support surfaces for, in pressure ulcer prevention, 987t
  therapeutic, 940, 940f
  turning of client in, 1037
    postoperative, 684
    procedure for, 1038

Bed bath, 920, 927, 927f
  procedure for, 921–926
Bed board, body alignment and, 1032
Bedpan
  handling of, 1284
  specialized, for fracture patients, 1231
  use of, 1230
    procedure for, 1231–1232
Bed rest
  passive exercise in, 1037
  skin alteration risks and, 917t
Bedside unit, environmental conditions in, 930, 939–940, 940f
Bedsore. *See* Pressure ulcers
Behavior
  in coping, 760
  in illness, 60–61
  modification of, in obesity management, 1200–1201
  in sensory deprivation/overload, 815, 816t, 822, 832
Behavioral response, to pain, 1108–1109, 1110t
Behavioral systems model of nursing (Johnson), 70t, 72
Beliefs
  cultural differences in, 46t–50t
  definition of, 79
  in health and illness model, 55, 56f
  spiritual, 884–885
Bell, of stethoscope, 449, 451f
Belonging, as human need, 23–24, 23f
Belt, walking, 1051, 1052f
Beneficence, in ethical code, 83
Beneficiary, of will, 110
Bereavement
  definition of, 781
  support systems for, 800
Beverages, urine production and, 1214
Bicarbonate, 1369f, 1371
  in buffer system, 1376
  deficit of. *See* Acidosis, metabolic
  excess of. *See* Alkalosis, metabolic
  regulation of, by kidney, 1377
Biceps reflex, assessment of, 515, 515t
Bigeminal pulse, 450t
Bile loss, imbalances resulting from, 1390t
Billing's method, of contraception, 866
Bill of rights, patient, 84, 87–88
  advocacy in, 425
  in death and dying, 783
  in pain management, 1138
Binders, application of, 709, 712–713, 716
Biofeedback
  in pain management, 1127
  in stress management, 772
  in urinary incontinence, 1234
Biomechanics. *See* Body mechanics
Biotin, 1159t
Biot's respiration, definition of, 458t
Birth control, 864, 866–868
Bisacodyl (Dulcolax), as laxative, 1285, 1286t
Bisexuality, definition of, 847
Black Muslim sect, 887
Black persons. *See* African-American people
Bladder
  autonomic, 1214
  characteristics of, catheterization and, 1236
  compression of, in Credé maneuver, 1229
  cystoscopy of, 1224, 1226t
  examination of, 1217
  irrigation of
    continuous, 1247–1249
    with indwelling catheter, 1238
      procedure for, 1246–1247
  physiology of, 1212–1213, 1213f
  post-void residual in, measurement of, 1234
Bladder training program, 1234
Bleeding. *See* Hemorrhage
Blended family, 25
Blindness, cultural, 35
Blood
  crossmatching of, 1423, 1427
  occult, testing for, 1274–1276, 1277f
  pH of, 1376
  role of, in tissue healing, 700
  testing of
    in fluid balance assessment, 1386
    reference ranges for, 1442t–1444t
  types of, 1427
  typing of, 1423, 1427
  viscosity of, blood pressure and, 458
  volume of
    blood pressure and, 457
    regulation of, 1375t
Blood-body fluid precautions, in dressing change, 722
Blood-borne pathogens, transmission of, prevention of, 572, 577t
Blood extracts, transfusion of, 1428
Blood gases. *See* Arterial blood gases
Blood groups, definition of, 1427
Blood pressure, 456–469
  abnormal, 459–460
  assessment of, 460–468
    at brachial artery, 463–466, 467t
    Doppler ultrasound in, 467
    electronic meters in, 467, 467f
    equipment care in, 467–468
    in home care, 469
    intra-arterial (direct), 467
    manometer in, 460–461, 461f
    by palpation, 467
    at popliteal artery, 462
    procedure for, 463–466
    sphygmomanometer in, 460–461, 460f–461f, 460t
    stethoscope in, 461
  diastolic
    definition of, 457
    in Korotkoff sounds, 461–462, 462t
  in elderly persons, 434
  elevated, 459
  factors affecting, 456–458
  fluid and electrolyte balance and, 1395t
  normal, 458–459, 459t
  physiology of, 456–457
  regulation of, 457–458
  salt intake and, 1369
  subnormal, 459–460
  systolic
    definition of, 456–457
    in Korotkoff sounds, 461–462, 462t
Blood transfusions
  administration of, 1428
    procedure for, 1425–1427
  blood extracts in, 1428
  donor selection for, 1428
  initiation of, 1428
  reactions to, 1428, 1429t
  typing for, 1423, 1427–1428
Blood vessels, elasticity of, blood pressure and, 458
Board of nursing, state/province, authority of, 16–17
Body alignment. *See also* Posture
  assessment of, 1008t–1009t, 1027, 1029f, 1036t
  attitude and, 1015
  correct, 1004, 1004f
    devices aiding, 1031–1032, 1032f–1034f
  developmental considerations and, 1006, 1008t–1009t
  health status and, 1006–1007, 1010
  lifestyle and, 1010–1015
  mental status and, 1010
  stress and, 1016
  in work situation, 1005–1006, 1005f–1007f
Body-fluid precautions, 572, 576–578, 577t
Body fluids. *See under* Fluid(s)
Body image
  definition of, 729
  disturbances of
    in mastectomy, 853, 873–874
    nursing diagnosis of, 738
    postoperative, 697
    responses to, 736
  positive, development of, 742
  preoperative anxiety about, 677
  in self-concept assessment, 736
  sexuality and, 851, 853
Body language (nonverbal communication), 360, 361f–362f
Body lice, 955–956
Body mass index, 1151, 1152f
Body mechanics, 1003–1006
  application of, to work situation, 1005–1006, 1005f–1007f
  balance and, 1004, 1004f
  body alignment and, 1004
  coordination and, 1004–1005
  postural reflexes and, 1005
  posture and, 1004
Body substance isolation, 578–580

Body surface area formula, for drug dosage calculations, 608, 608f
Body temperature, 433–446
assessment of
automatic monitoring in, 438–439
axillary method in, 445–446
procedures for, 447–448
disposable thermometer in, 438
electronic thermometer in, 437
procedure for, 442–443
equipment cleaning after, 446
glass thermometer in, 437, 439f, 439t
procedures for, 440–441, 443–445
in home care, 468
oral method in, 439
procedures for, 440–443
rectal method in, 439
procedures for, 443–445
sites for, 437t, 439
temperature-sensitive tape in, 438
tympanic membrane thermometer in, 437–438, 445, 445f
circadian rhythm in, 434
contraceptive method based on, 866
core (esophageal), 433–434, 436t
in elderly persons, 434
elevated, 435–437, 438t
factors affecting, 434–435, 436t
normal, 435, 437f, 437t
regulation of, 434–435, 435t–436t, 913t
set point of, 433
subnormal, 436t, 437, 439t
Body weight. *See* Weight
Boiling water, in sterilization/disinfection, 567t
Bolus, of medication in intravenous therapy, 637
procedure for, 640–641
Bonding, vs. attachment, 132f, 133
Bones. *See also* Skeletal system
demineralization of, in immobility, 1019
examination of, 509
malformation of, mobility and, 1007
muscle relationship to, 1003, 1003f
types of, 999
Bounding pulse, 451t
Bowel diversion, ostomy care in, 1295–1301, 1295f–1297f, 1300f
Bowel elimination, 1265–1310
activity and, 1270
anesthesia affecting, 1271
assessment of
diagnostic studies in, 1274–1277, 1277f, 1278t–1282t
history in, 1272
physical assessment in, 1272–1274
stool characteristics in, 1274, 1275t
daily patterns of, 1269–1270
developmental level and, 1268, 1269t
diagnostic tests and, 1271
diet and, 1270, 1302
in elderly persons, 1269t, 1285
enemas in, 1287–1292
exercise and, 1270, 1274–1275
factors affecting, 1268–1271, 1269t
flatulence control and, 1287
implementing in, 1282–1301
in bowel diversion, 1295–1297, 1295f–1297f, 1301
procedure for, 1298–1299
bowel training programs, 1294–1295
drugs for control of, 1285–1287, 1286t
feces emptying methods, 1287–1289, 1288t, 1292–1293, 1294f
procedures for, 1290–1292
in incontinence, 1293–1294
regular habits promotion, 1282, 1284–1285
incontinence pouch in, 1293–1294
indwelling catheter in, 1293–1294
lifestyle and, 1270
medications affecting, 1270–1271
muscle tone and, 1270
nurse as role model in, 1270
nutrition and, 1270, 1284
pathologic conditions affecting, 1270
patterns of, 1269–1270
physiology of, 1266–1268, 1267f–1268f
positioning for, 1284
postoperative, 696
preoperative, 685
privacy in, 1284
problems of. *See also* Constipation; Diarrhea; Flatulence/flatus
case study in, 1304–1306
fecal impaction, 1289, 1292–1293, 1294f
incontinence, 1283, 1293–1295, 1302–1303
nursing diagnosis of, 1277, 1282–1283
planning in, 1282
psychologic variables and, 1270
surgery affecting, 1271
teaching about, 1285–1287, 1286t
timing of, 1282
Bowel movement, definition of, 1268
Bowel sounds, 506–507, 1273
Bowel training program, 1294–1295
Boyle's law, 1313
Braces, as walking aid, 1055
Brachial artery, blood pressure assessment at, 462, 467t
procedure for, 463–464
Brachial pulse, 452f
assessment of, 502
Brachioradialis reflex, assessment of, 517
Braden scale, for pressure ulcer assessment, 982, 983f
Bradycardia, definition of, 448, 450t
Bradykinin, in pain response, 1104, 1106f
Bradypnea, 458t, 498f
Brain
disorders of, mobility and, 1010
function of, assessment of, 509, 512, 512t
respiratory control center in, 1315
BRAT regime, in diarrhea, 1287
Brawny edema, 1380f
Breach of duty, definition of, 101, 102t
Breast
anatomy of, 498f, 500f, 503f
examination of, 502–503, 503f–504f, 864, 866f
male, 845
physiology of, 843
removal of, sexual dysfunction in, 853, 873–874
Breastfeeding, immunity transmitted by, 131
Breathing. *See also* Respiration
abdominal, 1329–1330
deep
exercises for, postoperative, 683
promotion of, 1329
in stress management, 770
diaphragmatic, 1329–1330
exercises for, 683, 1329–1330
mouth-to-mouth, 1358
patterns of
developmental level and, 1316, 1316t
ineffective, 1012t, 1328, 1360
proper, 1329–1330
pursed lip, 1330
relaxation, patient education on, 396
Breath sounds, 456–457, 458t, 496–497, 499f–500f, 1319, 1321
bronchial, 497, 499f, 1319
bronchovesicular, 497, 498f, 1319
developmental level and, 1316, 1316t
vesicular, 497, 499f, 1319
Bronchial breath sounds, 497, 499f, 1319
Bronchodilators
inhalation of, 655–656
in respiratory disorders, 1335
Bronchoscopy, 1323t
Bronchovesicular breath sounds, 497, 499f, 1319
Bruits, in arteries, 502
Bruxism, 1081, 1083t
Buddhism, 888t
Buffer, definition of, 1376
Buffer systems, in acid-base balance, 1376–1377
Bulimia, 147, 1169
Bulk-forming laxatives, 1285, 1286t
Bulla, definition of, 484t
Buried bumper syndrome, in enteral nutrition, 1191
Burnout, in nurses, 772
Buttock, injection into, 631f, 632

Caffeine
sleep and, 1080
urine production and, 1214

Calcium
dietary, 1160t, 1370
as electrolyte, 1369f, 1370
imbalance in, 1380, 1382t–1383t
regulation of, 1375t
Calendar method, of contraception, 866
Calories
definition of, 1150
requirements of, 1152
Canada
healthcare financing in, 185
healthcare system of, 177–178
recommended nutrient intake tables, 1449t–1450t
Canadian Food and Drug Act, 594
Canadian Health Act, 185
Canadian Narcotic Control Act, 594
Canadian Nurses Association, 15
code of ethics of, 85–86
nursing defined by, 9
nursing practice standards of, 17
Canadian Nurses Association Testing Service examination, 12
Canadian Student Nurses Association, 15
Cancer
cervical, 854t
colorectal, warning signs of, 1276
fluid and electrolyte imbalance in, 1431–1432
information resources for, 1284
oral, 944
pain in, 1105t, 1130, 1133f–1134f
Canes, 1054–1055, 1054f
Capsule, definition of, 596t
Caput succedaneum, 132
Carbohydrates
classification of, 1153, 1154t
functions of, 1153, 1154t
metabolism of, 1153, 1155f
recommended allowance of, 1153
significance of, 1152–1153, 1154t
sources of, 1154t
Carbon dioxide
excretion of, in lungs, 1376–1377
partial pressure of, 1386, 1397t
in acid-base imbalance, 1391, 1396, 1397t
in alveolar gas exchange, 1314f, 1315
transport of, 1314
Carbonic acid
deficit of. *See* Alkalosis, respiratory
excess of. *See* Acidosis, respiratory
production/breakdown of, in lungs, 1376–1377
Carbonic acid-sodium bicarbonate buffer system, 1376
Carbon monoxide poisoning, 530, 547
Cardiac arrhythmia, definition of, 449, 450t
Cardiac cycle, heart sounds in, 502f
Cardinal signs. *See* Vital signs
Cardiopulmonary resuscitation, 1358, 1358f
legal aspects of, 790–791
Cardiovascular system
disorders of
exercise and, 1023
sexuality and, 851
as surgical risk, 675
of elderly person, 159
exercise effects on, 1017, 1018f
fluid/electrolyte homeostasis and, 1374, 1375t
immobility effects on, 1011t–1012t, 1017–1018
postoperative complications in, 694–695
postoperative status of, in recovery room, 689
Care, continuity of. *See* Continuity of care
Caregivers, 10t
needs of, 216–217
self-concept disturbances in, 740
stress in, 763
Caries, dental, 943
Caring
cultural considerations in, 44
development of, 238–241, 240f
Caring model of nursing (Watson), 71t, 75
Carminative enema, 1287–1288
Carotid pulse, 452f
Carriers, of infectious agents, 577
Cart, for drug administration, 605, 607f
Cartilage, definition of, 1000
Cartridge, prefilled, drug packaging in, 617, 617f
Case management, 182–183
nursing care plans for, 291–293
Case management model, in documentation, 334–336, 338t, 350f–353f
Cast, skin alteration risks and, 917t
Castor oil, as laxative, 1285
Catabolism, 1020
Cataplexy, 1082t
Categorizing, faulty, in self-concept disturbances, 745
Cathartics, 1285–1286, 1286t
Catheter(ization) (nasal), oxygen administration by, 1339–1340
Catheter(ization) (rectal), for incontinence, 1283–1294
Catheter(ization) (urinary), 1235–1251
client preparation for, 1237
closed drainage system for, 1237–1238
condom-type, 1251
application of, procedure for, 1252–1253
equipment for, 1237
of female, procedure for, 1238f, 1239–1243
hazards of, 1236–1237
indwelling (Foley or retention)
client care in, 1246, 1249
components of, 1235, 1235f
connection to drainage system, 1236
infection in, 1236–1237, 1257–1258
irrigation of, 1238, 1246
procedures for, 1246–1249
removal of, 1250
in specimen collection, 1223
procedure for, 1239–1245
infection considerations and, 1236–1237, 1257–1258
intermittent (straight), 1235
of male, procedure for, 1243–1245
perineal care with, 964
preoperative, 685
reasons for, 1236
retention. *See subhead*: indwelling
self-catheterization in, 1250–1251
specimen collection and, 1223, 1224f
procedure for, 1238–1245
suprapubic, 1235
teaching of, 1249–1251
triple-lumen, 1235, 1235f
types of, 1235–1246, 1235f
urine output measurement in, 1219
Catheter(ization) (vascular)
complications with, in parenteral nutrition, 1196
for intravenous therapy, 1402–1404
Cation, definition of, 1368
Causalgia, description of, 1105t
Causation, legal definition of, 101, 102t
Ceftriaxone, in sexually transmitted disease, 854t
Celibacy, 848
Cellulose, dietary, 1154t
Center of gravity, of body, 1004, 1004f
Centers for Disease Control, 182
recommendations of
airborne precautions, 580, 582
contact precautions, 580, 582
droplet precautions, 580, 582
for isolation, 580–582
standard precautions, 580
for sterilization and disinfection, 566
transmission-based precautions, 580, 582
universal precautions, 572, 576–578
for vancomycin-resistant enterococci transmission control, 578
Centigrade scale, on thermometer, 437, 439f, 439t
Central nervous system. *See also* Brain; Spinal cord
disorders of, mobility and, 1010
postoperative status of, in recovery room, 689
Central venous catheter, for intravenous therapy, 1403–1404, 1409–1410, 1409f, 1411f
Central venous pressure, fluid balance and, 1395t
Cephalic vein, intravenous therapy in, 1411–1412, 1411f
Cerebellar ataxia, 1028f
Cerebellum, mobility control and, 1010
Cerebral cortex, mobility control and, 1010

Cerebrospinal fluid, laboratory tests of, reference ranges for, 1445t
Cerebrovascular accident, exercise program after, case study of, 1062–1068
Certification, for nursing practice, 98
Cerumen
  function of, 911
  removal of, 954
Cervical cap, as contraceptive method, 867
Cervix
  cancer of, 854t
  intraepithelial neoplasia of, 854t
  physiology of, 842, 842f
C fibers, in pain transmission, 1104
Chair, movement of client to/from, 1040
  procedure for, 1045–1049
Change
  leadership role in, 416–418
  resistance to, 416–417
Change-of-shift report, 340, 341f
Channel, in communication, 359, 360f
Chaplain, services of, 184
Character, defamation of, 99–100
Charting. *See also* Client record
  by exception, 334, 338t, 349f
  focus, 334, 338t, 348f
  PIE system for, 334, 338t, 348f
  variance, 336
Cheilosis, 944
Chemical name, of drug, 594
Chemicals, in sterilization/disinfection, 567t
Chest pain, in respiratory disease, 1320
Chest tubes, management of, 1330, 1331f
Chest wall, developmental variations in, 1316, 1316t
Cheyne-Stokes respiration, 458t, 498f
Child abuse, 134–135
  obligation to report, 109
Children. *See also* Toddlers
  accident prevention and, 526, 537t, 538
  analgesic administration in, 1130, 1132
  blood pressure of, 459t
  body alignment of, 1008t–1009t
  bowel elimination in, 1269t
  calorie requirements of, 1152
  death of, family reactions to, 792
  diarrhea in, oral rehydration in, 1287
  drug action in, 598
  drug administration in, 610, 614–615
  drug dosage calculation for, 608, 609f
  grief reactions of, 792
  growth and development of. *See* Developmental theory; Growth and development
  mobility of, 1008t–1009t
  pain assessment in, 1115, 1120f
  pain attitudes of, 1112
  poisoning of, 530
    prevention of, 549
  preschool
    growth and development of
      cognitive, 138–139
      moral, 140
      physiologic, 138
      psychosocial, 139–140
      spiritual, 140
    health problems of, 140
    nutrition in, 1166t
    respiratory function in, 1316, 1316t
    safety considerations for, 537t, 538
    sexuality of, 850t
    sleep in, 1077t–1078t
    wellness promotion in, 140, 141t
  pulse rate of, 449t
  recommended daily allowances for, 1447t–1450t
  recommended nutrient intake for, 1449t–1450t
  respiratory function of, 1316, 1316t
  school-age
    growth and development of
      cognitive, 140
      moral, 141
      physiologic, 140
      psychosocial, 140–141
      spiritual, 141
    health problems of, 141
    nutrition in, 1166t
    respiratory function in, 1316, 1316t
    safety considerations for, 537t, 538
    sexuality of, 850t
    sleep in, 1078t
    wellness promotion in, 141, 143t
  self-concept of, 732t, 742
  self-esteem in, development of, 731
  sensory deprivation in, 818
  sensory stimulation of, 818
  sexual acts with, 848
  sexuality of, 117, 117t, 850t
  skin condition of, 913
  sleep in, 1077t–1078t
  spirituality of, 889
  suffocation of, 530–531, 533
  urination in, 1214
  urine specimen collection from, 1219–1220, 1223f
Chlamydia trachomatis infection, 854t
Chloride
  dietary, 1160t, 1371
  as electrolyte, 1369f, 1371
Choice in Dying, 785
Choking, on foreign body, 530
Cholecalciferol (vitamin D), 1159t
Cholesterol, dietary, 1157
Cholinergic drugs, urinary elimination and, 1216
Choosing, in value clarification, 81–82
Chorea, definition of, 1024–1025
Christianity, 886–887
Christian Science, 886t
Chromium
  dietary, 1160t
  as electrolyte, 1371
Chronic illness, definition of, 61
Chronotherapeutics, 1080
Church of Jesus Christ of Latter Day Saints, 886t
Chvostek's sign, of neuromuscular irritability, 1395t
Chyme, definition of, 1266
Cilia, in respiratory system, 1312
Circadian rhythm
  in body temperature, 434
  sleep and, 1074
Circular bed, body alignment and, 1032
Circular turn, in bandage application, 713, 714f
Circulating nurse, functions of, 687
Circulation
  impairment of, by bandage/binder, 712
  tissue healing and, 701–702
Circumduction, definition of, 1000t
Civil law, definition of, 96
Clean-catch urine specimen, collection of, 1220, 1222–1223
Clean-contaminated wound, 699t
Cleaning
  of dentures, 945, 950f
  of equipment, before sterilization, 566
  of eye, 952–953
  of eyeglasses, 953
  of pressure ulcers, 985–986
  of thermometers, 446
  of wound, procedure for, 710–712
Cleansing agents, for wound, 708
Cleansing enema, 1287, 1288t
  procedure for, 1290–1292
Clean technique (medical asepsis), 560, 562–565
Clean wound, 699t
Clergy, referral to, 896
Cliches, avoidance of, in communication, 370
Client goals. *See* Goals
Client record
  accountability in, 332
  case management model for, 334–336, 338t, 350f–353f
  charting by exception in, 334, 338t, 349f
  computerized, 336–337
  confidentiality of, 332
  content of, 332
  definition of, 330
  focus charting in, 334, 338t, 348f
  formats for, 332, 337, 338t, 339, 344t–345t, 354f–356f
  guidelines for, 332
  JCAHO standards on, 331
  legal issues in, 339
  PIE charting system in, 334, 338t, 348f
  policies for, 330, 333
  preparation of, timing of, 332
  problem-oriented, 334, 336t, 347f
  purposes of, 333
  source-oriented, 333–334, 335t, 346f
  variance charting in, 336

Clinical nurse specialist, 11t
Clinical pathways, in nursing care plan, 291–293
Clitoris, anatomy of, 841, 842f
Clonidine, sexual function effects of, 856t
Closed wound, 699
Clothing
 in infection control, 582, 585–587, 586f
 as nonverbal communication, 362
Clubbing, of nails, 485f
CNA. *See* Canadian Nurses Association
Coagulation factors, reference ranges for, 1441t
Cobalamin (vitamin B_{12}), 1159t
Cobalt, dietary, 1160t
Cocaine, sexual function effects of, 856t
Codeine, as cough suppressant, 1331
Codes of ethics, 84–86
Cognition
 definition of, 157
 in elderly persons, 157, 160, 169t
Cognitive core competencies. *See under* Core competencies
Cognitive development theory of Piaget. *See under* Developmental theory
Cognitive dysfunction
 pain assessment in, 1115
 in sensory deprivation, 816t
Cognitive goals, 285
 evaluation of, 315
Cognitive learning, 388, 395, 401
Cognitive response, in sensory deprivation, 817
Cohabiting family, 26
Coitus, 844, 848
Coitus interruptus, 866
Colace (dioctyl sodium sulfosuccinate), as stool softener, 1285, 1286t
Cold sores, 854t
Colic, in infants, 134
Collaborative care, 183–184, 183f
 documentation of, 337, 350f–355f
Collaborative interventions, 19, 301
Collaborative problem, definition of, 267–268, 269f–270f
Colloid osmotic pressure, definition of, 1373
Colon
 cancer of, warning signs of, 1276
 physiology of, 1266–1268, 1267f
Colonoscopy, 1276, 1278t–1279t
Color
 of skin, 482–483, 483t
 of urine, 1214, 1216, 1216t, 1220t
Colostomy
 care of, 1295–1301, 1206f–1207f, 1300f
 definition of, 1295, 1295f
 irrigation of, 1297
Colyte, in oral intestinal lavage, 1291
Coma, definition of, 512
Comedo, definition of, 484t
Comfort measures. *See also* Pain, management of
 bed and, 940, 940f
 in communication, 371
 devices aiding, 1031–1033, 1032f–1034f
 in dressing change, 716
 in enteral nutrition, 1192
 in injections, 636–637
 postoperative, 690, 697
 in respiratory disorders, 1332–1333, 1333f–1334f, 1335, 1336t
 before sleep, 1091
 during withholding of food, 1181
Comfort measures only order, 791
Commode, use of, 1230
Common law, 96
Communicable disease, obligation to report, 96
Communication, 359–385. *See also* Documentation; Reporting
 advice in, 371
 assertive skills in, 377, 377t–378t
 of assessment findings, 263–264, 264f
 assessment of, 512
 blocks to, 370–371
 changing subject during, 371
 characteristics of, 360f, 361
 cliches in, 370
 client focus in, 369
 client record in, 333
 comfort in, 364
 computers in, 382
 conferences in, 341–343
 confidentiality in, 369, 371–372
 in confusion, 828–829
 conversational skills in, 371–372
 core competencies in, 375–377, 377t–378t
 cultural factors in, 363, 376
 definition of, 359, 360f
 in dementia, 381
 developmental considerations in, 362–363
 disorders of, 377–380
  in elderly persons, 380
 documentation of, 365
 with dying patient, 797, 800
 empathy in, 375
 with endotracheal tube, 381
 environment for, 364, 368
 eye contact in, 361, 361f
 factors influencing, 362–364
 factors promoting, 368–370, 369f
 false assurance and, 371
 with family, 341
 with foreign-language speaking client, 35–36, 381
 forms of, 359–362, 361f–362f
 gender differences in, 363
 gossip in, 371
 in groups, 359–360, 379, 382–384, 383t
 with hearing-impaired client, 381, 828, 954
 humor in, 375
 impaired, safety and, 528
 during implementation. *See under* Implementing
 inappropriate comments in, 370
 interviewing techniques in, 373–374. *See also* Interview
 intrapersonal skills in, 375–377
 judgmental comments in, 371
 in laryngectomy, 381
 in leadership, 412
 listening skills in, 370, 372–373, 373f
 methods for, among healthcare workers, 340t
 nonverbal, 360–362, 361f–362f
 as nursing function, 10t
 in nursing process, 364–365
 nursing theory concepts and, 69
 objectives in, 368
 observation during, 369
 one-to-one, 359
 openness in, 375
 pacing of conversation in, 369
 personal space during, 364, 369–370
 preoperative psychological needs and, 681–682
 privacy in, 369
 question use in, 370–371, 373–374
 rumor in, 371
 silence during, 362, 373
 sociocultural differences in, 363
 touch used in, 360–361, 374–375, 375f
 with tracheostomy, 1348
 with unconscious client, 381, 829
 validation in, 374
 values in, 364
 verbal, 360
  impaired, 377, 379
 with visually impaired person, 381, 826
Community
 definition of, 29
 healthcare in. *See also* Healthcare, settings for
  agencies for, 181–182, 181f–182f
  client care needs and, 188
  collaborative, 183–184, 183f
  cost containment in, 188
  ethical aspects of, 189
  financial aspects of, 184–186, 185t
  fragmentation of, 188
  frameworks for, 182–183
  reforms in, 175
  trends in, 186–189, 186f, 188f
 health risk factors and, 29–30
 influence of, on health, 29–30
 need for, 884
 nursing in, 30. *See also* Home healthcare
Compadrazgo, in Hispanic families, 48t
Compendium of Pharmaceutical Specialties, 603
Compensation, as defense mechanism, 760

Competence, in self-esteem, 737
Competency, core. *See* Core competencies
Competent practice, as legal safeguard, 104, 106f
Complete blood count
 in fluid balance assessment, 1391
 reference ranges for, 1441t
Complete care, in personal hygiene, 918
Complete protein, definition of, 1153, 1155
Compliance
 of blood vessel walls, blood pressure and, 458
 in discharge planning, 203
 lung, 1314
Comprehensive Drug Abuse Prevention and Control Act, 594
Compromise behavior, as defense mechanism, 760
Computed tomography, in urinary tract evaluation, 1224–1225, 1226t
Computers
 in communication, 340t, 382
 in documentation, 336–337, 342
  confidentiality issues in, 101
 in ethical analysis, 91
 in implementing, 311
 in instruction, 397–398
 in licensure examination, 12
 in nursing care plan generation, 291
 in nursing process, 230
 point-of-care applications of, 324
 in research literature reviews, 424
Conception, 129
Concepts, in nursing, 66
Conceptual models, for nursing theory, definition of, 66
Concrete operational stage, in cognitive development, 119
Concurrent evaluation, 324
Condom, as contraceptive method, 867
Condom catheter, 1251
 application of, procedure for, 1252–1253
Conduction, as heat transfer mechanism, 434, 435t
Conductive hearing loss, 491, 826
Condyloid joint, 1000
Condylomata acuminata, 855t
Conferences, 341–343
Confidentiality
 in communication, 369
 in documentation, 332
 ethical aspects of, 84, 86
Conflict
 cultural, 35
 between religious beliefs and treatment, 885, 896
Confucianism, 888t
Confusion
 communication in, 828–829
 sensory stimulation in, 828–829
Congenital malformations
 mobility and, 1006
 in neonates, 131–132
Congestion, definition of, 1331
Consciousness, levels of, 815
 assessment of, 509, 512, 512t
Consensual reflex, of pupil, 487
Consent, informed. *See* Informed consent
Conservation principles, in Levine theory of nursing, 73
Constant fever, 438t
Constipation
 causes of, 1283
 characteristics of, 1283
 colonic, 1283
 definition of, 1301
 diet and, 1270, 1284, 1302
 in elderly persons, 1285
 in immobility, 1014t, 1021
 management of, 1302
 perceived, 1283
Constitutional law, 96
Consultation, 341–342
 for nursing care plan, 289
Consumerism
 in healthcare, 187–188
 impact of, on research, 423
Contact, in infectious agent transmission, 557, 558t
Contact isolation, specifications for, 577t
Contact lenses, care/removal of, 953–954
Contact precautions, 580–582
Contaminated wound, 699t
Continent ileostomy, 1295
Continuing education, 14
Continuity of care, 192–206
 in admission to healthcare setting, 192–195
  ambulatory, 194
  hospital, 194–197, 195f, 200t
 definition of, 192
 in discharge from healthcare setting, 200–206, 202f
 nurse-client relationship in, 193
 nurse's role in, 192
 in transfer within and between settings, 195, 197, 200
Contraception, 864, 866–868
 coerced, 868
Contract
 definition of, 104
 in teaching-learning, 398
Contracture, muscular, in immobility, 1019
Controlled substances
 regulation of, 109–110
 safety with, 609, 609f
Contusion, definition of, 699t
Convalescence, 558
Convection, as heat transfer mechanism, 434, 435t
Conventionality, self-concept and, 745
Conventional level, in Kohlberg moral development theory, 120, 121t
Convergence, visual, assessment of, 487, 488f
Conversational skills, 371–372
Coordination
 assessment of, 514
 in movement, 1004–1005
Coping mechanisms
 in death and dying. *See* Death and dying; Grief; Loss
 defense mechanisms in, 760
 definition of, 760
 in elderly persons, 169t
 facilitation of
  as nursing aim, 11
  as teaching aim, 387
 ineffective, in immobility, 1015t
 for pain, 1109–1112
 for postoperative body image alterations, 697
 preoperative assessment of, 676–677
 task-oriented reactions in, 760
 types of, 760
Copper, dietary, 1160t
Cordotomy, in pain management, 1137
Core competencies, 233–246
 assessment of, 244–245
 cognitive, 233, 234t
  development of, 235–236
  in planning, 284
 ethical/legal, 235
  development of, 241–243
  in planning, 284
 for evaluating, 316
 for implementing, 304, 306
 interpersonal, 233, 235
  in communication, 375–377, 377t–378t
  development of, 238–241, 240f
  in planning, 284
 in planning, 284
 for self-concept changes, 746–747
 for sensory alterations, 832–833
 for sleep promotion, 1096
 for spirituality, 900
 technical, 233
  development of, 236, 238
  in planning, 284
Core (esophageal) temperature, 433–434, 436t
Corpus luteum, 843, 843f
Corticosteroids, in respiratory disorders, 1336t
Cosmetics, use of, 941
Cost containment, 188
Costovertebral angle, tenderness at, 1217
Coughing, 1331–1332
 assessment of, 1320
 ineffective
  in elderly persons, 1329
  in immobility, 1014t
 as postoperative exercise, 684
Counseling, 404–409
 examples of, 405t–406t
 for HIV testing, 399–400

in implementing, 307
long-term, 407
motivational, 407–408
of noncompliant client, 408
nursing diagnosis in, 408–409
as nursing function, 10t
purposes of, 387
in sexual dysfunction, 870
short-term, 387
in spirituality, 895–896
topics for, 388
Countershock phase, in general adaptation syndrome, 759
Court actions, 97
CPR (cardiopulmonary resuscitation), 1358, 1358f
legal aspects of, 790–791
CPS (Compendium of Pharmaceutical Specialties), 603
Crab lice, 955–956
"Crack babies," 132
Crackles (rales), 456, 497, 1319, 1321
Cradle, for protection of lower extremities, 1033
Cradling, in joint exercise, 1033, 1037
Cramps, heat, 436t
Cranial nerve function, assessment of, 512–514
Creams
application of, 646
in skin care, 940
vaginal, 653, 655–656
Credé maneuver, 1229
Credentialing, for nursing practice, 98. *See also* Licensure
Crepitation, in joints, 509
Crime
legal aspects of, 98–99
obligation to report, 109
Crisis
developmental, 117, 118t, 763
fever, 438t
intervention in, techniques for, 770, 772
in stress response, 763
Criteria
for goal writing, 286
for nursing evaluation, 314
Critical thinking
affective dimensions of, 234t
building blocks of, 234t
decision-making in, 236, 238
definition of, 233
domains of, 234t
illustration of, 237–238
intellectual standards for, 234t
knowledge adequacy in, 236–237
potential problems and, 236–237
purpose of, 235–236
resources for, 236–237
skills for, 234t
Cromolyn sodium, in respiratory disorders, 1336t
Crossmatching, of blood, 1423, 1427
Crust, on skin, 484t
Crutches, 1055–1056, 1055f–1058f
Cubital vein, intravenous therapy in, 1411f
Cuff, for blood pressure equipment, 460, 460f, 460t
Cuffed tracheostomy tube, 1346–1347, 1347f
Cultural assimilation, 23
Cultural blindness, 35
Cultural care deprivation, 818
Cultural imposition, 34
Cultural needs, health-illness status and, 57
Culture (wound), collection of, 716
procedure for, 717–718
Culture and ethnicity, 33–51. *See also* Transcultural nursing
African American characteristics in, 38–39, 46t–47t
alternative healing systems and, 41, 43
Asian characteristics in, 42, 47t–48t
assessment of, 44
communication and, 35–36, 363, 376
conflict in, 35
cultural assimilation in, 34
definitions related to, 33–34
diversity promotion in, 36
dominant group in, 33
drug action and, 599
drug administration and, 599
economic status and. *See* Socioeconomic factors
exercise and, 1010, 1015
family support in, 38
gender roles in, 35
grief reactions and, 792
health-illness status and, 57
Hispanic characteristics in, 48t
home healthcare and, 216
imposition of, 44
language in, 35–36
Leininger nursing theory model and, 70t, 72–73
minority group in, 33
Native American characteristics in, 49t
nursing diagnosis of, 39
in nursing practice, 68, 72–73
nutrition in, 37, 1169, 1170t
pain expression and, 1109–1112
personal hygiene and, 913
physiologic characteristics in, 38–40
poverty and, 37–38
psychological characteristics in, 41
self-concept and, 731
sensory function and, 818–819
sexuality and, 849
sleep and, 1076, 1080
socioeconomic factors in. *See* Socioeconomic factors
spatial orientation in, 36–37
spirituality and. *See* Spirituality
stereotyping and, 34–35, 35f
subcultures in, 33
surgery and, 678
temporal orientation in, 36–37
white middle class characteristics in, 43–44, 46t
Culture shock, 41
Cumulative effect, of drugs, 600
Cunnilingus, definition of, 848
Cupping
in joint exercise, 1037, 1039f
as treatment in respiratory disorders, 1332–1333, 1333f
Curanderas(os), in Hispanic families, 48t
Cutaneous pain, definition of, 1103
Cyanosis, of skin, 483, 483t
Cystoscopy, 1224, 1226t
Cytology, in respiratory function assessment, 1323t
Cytomegalovirus, sexually transmitted, 854t

Daily activities
as exercise, 1017, 1051
preoperative assessment of, 676
stress and, 768–769
Damages, legal definition of, 101, 102t
Dandruff, 955
Dangling, assistance with, 1050–1051
Daoism, 888t
DAR (data, action, response) system, for focus charting, 334, 338t, 348f
Data
accuracy of, in assessing, 248–249
analysis of, in diagnosing, 272–273, 272t
comparison of, to standards, in diagnosing, 269
completeness of, in assessing, 248
definition of, 248
interpretation of, in diagnosing, 269–273, 272t
objective, in assessing, 248, 250t
relevance of, in assessing, 249
subjective, in assessing, 248, 250t
validation of, in assessing, 262–263
Data base
in client record, 336
definition of, 248
Data cluster, in diagnosing, 269–270, 272t
Data collection
in assessing. *See under* Assessing
dietary, 1171–1173, 1173f
in evaluation, 314–318
in implementing step, 311
Day-care centers, 178–179
Deaconess, duties of, 6
Death and dying. *See also* Grief; Loss; Hospice care; Suicide
accidental, grief reactions to, 793
assessment of, 794–795
autopsy in, 791–792

Death and dying *(continued)*
bill of rights for, 783
care of body after, 801–802
case study of, 805–808
cause of, grief reactions and, 792–793
of child, family reactions to, 792
client needs in, assessment of, 794–795
clinical signs of, 784
communication and, 797, 800
cultural factors in, 792
death certificate requirements in, 791
decisional conflicts in, 804–805
definition of, 784, 784t
developmental considerations in, 792
ethical dimensions of, 784–785, 786f–788f, 789
euthanasia and, 789–790
family needs/care in, 792, 794, 800–801
in home care, 794, 799
impending, signs of, 784
interventions for, 797, 799–803
legal aspects of, 110, 784–785, 786f–788f, 789
living will in, 426–427, 785, 787f–788f, 789–790
nurse's feelings and needs and, 793–794
nursing diagnosis in, 794, 796–797
organ donation and, 791, 791f
other clients affected by, 803
physiologic needs in, 799
preoperative anxiety about, 676
psychologic needs in, 799–800
reactions to, stages of, 782–783
religious influences on, 792
self-care promotion in, 799
self-esteem maintenance in, 799
sexuality and, 869
socioeconomic factors and, 792
spiritual needs in, 800
stages of, 782–783
sudden
family care after, 802
in infants, 134
terminal illness and, 783
violent, grief reactions to, 793
web site concerning, 785
Death certificate, 791
Debridement, of pressure ulcer, 986, 988
Deception, ethical problems with, 86
Decision analysis, client record in, 333
Decision-making
in critical thinking, 236
at end of life, 804–805
ethical, 86
Decoder, in communication, 359, 360f
Decongestants, inhalation of, 655–656
Decubitus ulcers. *See* Pressure ulcers
Deductive reasoning, 66
Deep breathing. *See under* Breathing
Defamation of character, 99–100
Defecation
normal patterns of, 1268
physiology of, 1269–1270
position for, 1284
privacy for, 1284
Defendant, in litigation, 97
nurse as, 102
Defense mechanisms
in coping, 760
in Freudian theory, 117
Defibrillation, in CPR, 1358, 1358f
Degenerative joint disease, mobility in, 1007
Dehiscence, of wound, 703, 703f
Dehydration
definition of, 483, 1377
skin condition in, 913, 917t
Delano, Jane, 7f
Delegation, of implementing, 304, 306–307
Delta sleep, 1074, 1075t
Deltoid muscle site, for injections, 631f, 632
Dementia
communication in, 381
in older adults, 157, 160
Demineralization, of bones in immobility, 1019
Democratic leadership, 414
Demonstration, as teaching strategy, 395
Denial
as defense mechanism, 760
in dying, 782
in self-concept disturbances, 745
Dental care. *See also* Oral care
for preschool children, 141t
for toddlers, 138t
Dental caries, 943
Dentifrices, 950
Dentition
care of. *See* Oral care
of elderly person, 159
Dentures, care of, 945, 950f
procedure for, 947
Denver Developmental Screening Test for infants and children, 133
Deodorants
for sanitary napkins, 964
for skin care, 940–941
Deontologic theory, of ethics, 83
Dependence, on drugs, definition of, 1129
Dependency
of patient, 60
response to, 736
Dependent interventions, 301
Dependent nursing actions, definition of, 19
Dependent variables, in research, 423
Depression
in dying, 782
posture in, 1010
safety affected by, 528
Dermal application, of drugs. *See* Topical medications
Dermis, definition of, 911, 912f
Despair, spiritual, 890, 894, 896
Detergents
for handwashing, 563
for skin care, 940
Detrusor muscle, function of, 1212–1213
Developmental crisis, 763
counseling in, 407
in Erikson theory, 117, 118t, 150, 151t
in middle adults, 150, 151t
in young adults, 150, 151t
Developmental level
accident prevention and, 536, 536t–537t, 538
bowel elimination and, 1268, 1269t
communication and, 362–363
drug action and, 598
infection risks and, 559
mobility and, 1006, 1008t–1009t
nutrition requirements and, 1163, 1165, 1166t, 1168t
personal hygiene and, 914
respiratory function and, 1316, 1316t
self-concept and, 731, 732t
sensory stimulation and, 818
sexuality and, 849, 850t–851t
skin condition and, 913
sleep and, 1076, 1076f, 1077t–1079t
spirituality and, 889
surgery and, 673, 676
tissue healing and, 701
urinary elimination and, 1214
Developmental stress, 763
Developmental tasks, 119–120
in adults, 150, 151t
consideration of, in meeting client goals, 307–308
of family, 27, 28t
Developmental task theory of Havighurst. *See under* Developmental theory
Developmental theory, 67. *See also* Growth and development
adults and, 150–151, 151t
clinical applications of, 124–126
Erikson psychosocial development theory, 67, 117–118, 118f–119f, 118t, 143, 146
elderly persons and, 160–161, 161f
infants and, 133
preschool children and, 139–140
school-age children and, 140–141
toddlers and, 136–137
Fowler faith development theory, 122–123, 123f, 123t
adolescents and, 146
middle adults and, 156
preschool children and, 140
school-age children and, 141
young adults and, 152
Freud psychoanalytic development theory, 117, 117t
adolescents and, 143
infants and, 133

preschool children and, 139
school-age children and, 141
toddlers and, 136, 137
Gilligan moral development, 121–122
Havighurst developmental task theory, 119–120
adolescents and, 143, 146
elderly persons and, 161–163, 162f
infants and, 133
preschool children and, 139
school-age children and, 141
toddlers and, 137
Kohlberg moral development theory, 119–121
adolescents and, 146
in middle adults, 155–156
preschool children and, 140
school-age children and, 141
young adults and, 152
Piaget cognitive development theory, 119, 121f–122f, 121t
adolescents and, 143
infants and, 133
learning process and, 388–389, 391
preschool children and, 138–139
school-age children and, 140
toddlers and, 136
Dexamethasone, in respiratory disorders, 1336t
Dextromethorphan, as cough suppressant, 1331
Dextrose solutions, for intravenous therapy, 1403t
Diabetes mellitus
foot care in, 960
sexuality and, 849
skin alteration risks and, 917t
Diagnosing. *See* Nursing diagnosis
Diagnosis-related groups, 184–185
Diagnostic procedures, 202. *See also specific procedure*
endoscopic. *See* Endoscopy
of gastrointestinal tract, stool collection for, 1274–1276, 1277f
laboratory tests. *See* Laboratory tests
nursing responsibilities in, 517–521
types of, 520t–521t
of urinary system, 1224–1225, 1226t
Diaphoresis
definition of, 483
personal hygiene in, 919
Diaphragm
as contraceptive method, 867
of stethoscope, 449, 451f
Diaphragmatic breathing, 1329–1330
Diarrhea
case studies of, 1304–1306, 1432–1434
causes of, 1283, 1303
characteristics of, 1283
definition of, 1303
diet and, 1284
in elderly persons, 1285
fluid and electrolyte imbalance with, 1432–1434
management of, 1303–1304
medications for, 1286–1287
from tube feeding, 1191
Diarthrotic joints, movement at, 1000
Diary
food, 1172
sleep, 1084, 1086
Diastolic blood pressure, 457, 461–462, 462t
Diet. *See also* Food; Nutrition
bowel elimination and, 1270, 1284, 1302
clear liquid, 1171–1172
in discharge planning, 203
in electrolyte imbalance, 1399–1400
electrolytes in, 1369–1371
in fluid imbalance, 1399–1400
fluids in, 1373, 1374f
full liquid, 1181
high-fiber, 1202
liquid, 1181
mobility and, 1007
in obesity, 1200
for ostomy patients, 1297, 1301
recommended allowances for. *See* Recommended dietary allowances
sleep and, 1080
soft, 1181
types of, 1181
urine production and, 1214
vegetarian, 1181
for weight loss, 1200
in young adults, 152
Dietitian, services of, 184
Diffusion
of fluids and electrolytes, 1372
of gases in respiration, 1314–1315, 1314f
Dignity, human
as essential value, 80
promotion of, 238–240
Dilemma, moral, 86
Diluent, definition of, 622
Dimpling, of breast skin, 503
Dioctyl sodium sulfosuccinate, as stool softener, 1285, 1286t
Diphenhydramine, as cough suppressant, 1331–1332
Diphtheria, immunization for, 136t
Diploma program, in nursing, 13
Disabilities, legal aspects of, 110
Disaccharides, definition of, 1153
Disbelief, as grief reaction, 781
Disc, medication, for eye administration, 652
Discharge planning, 200–206, 202f, 284
assessing in, 202–203
client goals in, 202–203
for client leaving against medical advice, 201
components of, 202
definition of, 201
documentation of, 331, 336t, 339, 341
evaluation of, 206
implementation of, 205–206, 205f
indications for, 202
nursing diagnosis in, 202
procedure for, 201
purpose of, 192
summary form for, 204
Discipline, nursing as, 9
Discovery, as teaching strategy, 395
Discrimination, legal aspects of, 110
Discussion, as teaching strategy, 395
Disease
causes of, 59
definition of, 53
Disease-specific category isolation, 572
Disengagement theory, older adults and, 160
Disinfection
of glass thermometer, 446
methods for, 563, 566, 567t
Dislocation, of joint, mobility in, 1007
Displacement, as defense mechanism, 760
Distortion, in self-concept disturbances, 745
Distraction, in pain relief, 1123–1124
Distribution, of drugs in body, 596–597
Disuse osteoporosis, in immobility, 1019
Diuretics
action of, 1216
in fluid and electrolyte imbalance, 1402
Diversity, cultural, promotion of, 36
DNR (do not resuscitate orders), legal aspects of, 790
Documentation, 330–339
of accidental exposure to infectious agents, 588
accountability for, 332
of assessment findings, 264, 517
case management model in, 334–336, 338t, 350f–353f
charting by exception in, 334, 338t, 349f
client record in. *See* Client record
communication in, 365
computers in, 336–337, 342
confidentiality in, 101, 332
content of, 332
definition of, 330
of diagnostic procedures, 520
focus charting in, 334, 338t, 348f
formats for, 332, 337, 338t, 339, 344t–345t, 354f–355f
guidelines for, 330, 332–333, 344t–345t
historic, 333
of home healthcare, 339
incident report, 107–108
intraoperative, 688
JCAHO standards on, 331
legal aspects of, 106–107, 106f, 339
of medication administration, 656, 657f–658f, 659
methods for, 333–337, 335t–336t, 346f–353f

Documentation *(continued)*
minimum data set in, 333
of nursing evaluation, 316
of nursing process, 226
PIE charting system in, 334, 338t, 348f
policies on, 330, 333
problem-oriented records in, 334, 336t, 347f
in reporting care, 339–340, 340t
of sexual harassment, 856
source-oriented records in, 333–334, 335t, 346f
in teaching, 404
timing of, 332
of wound care, 716
Dominant group, in culture, 33
Donor, for blood transfusion, 1428
Do not resuscitate orders (DNR), legal aspects of, 790
Doppler ultrasound, in blood pressure assessment, 451–452
Dorsalis pedis pulse, 452f
assessment of, 502
Dorsal recumbent position, 476, 477f
protective, 1034, 1035t
Dorsiflexion, definition of, 1000t
Dorsogluteal site, for injections, 631f, 632
Dosage, of drug
abbreviations for, 603, 603t
calculations for, 605, 607–608, 608f
Douche, vaginal, 964
DPT vaccine, 136t
Drainage
postural, in respiratory disorders, 1333, 1334f
from wound
assessment of, 704–705
dressing change and, 716, 721, 721f
Drainage-secretion precautions, specifications for, 577t
Drains, for wounds, 705–706, 707f, 708t
Draping
for physical assessment, 478
sterile, 568, 571, 576f
during surgery, 688
Dress/clothing
in infection control, 582, 585–587, 586f
as nonverbal communication, 362
Dressings
absorptive, 722
for pressure ulcers, 989t
advantages of, 707–708
bandages for, 709, 712–716, 714f–715f
binders for, 709, 712–713, 716
for central venous catheter site, 1404
changing of, 709
for draining wound, 716, 721, 721f
for infected wound, 722
procedure for, 710–712
definition of, 707
disadvantages of, 707
gauze, 989t
hydrocolloid, 722, 989f, 989t
hydrogel, 989t
moisture-retentive, 988, 989t
occlusive, 988, 989t
for pressure ulcers, 986, 988, 989f, 989t
purposes of, 707
supplies for, 708, 709t
transparent, 708, 722, 989t
DRGs (diagnostic-related groups), 184–185
Drinking, urine production and, 1228
Dripmeter, in intravenous therapy, 1402, 1404f
Drop factor, in intravenous therapy, 1412
Droplet precautions, 580, 582
Drops, installation of
in ear, 652–653
in eye, 646, 650
in nose, 652–653, 655
Drowning, causes of, 530–531
Drowsiness, 1077t
Drugs/medications, 593–668. *See also specific drug*
absorption of, 596
abuse of. *See* Substance abuse
in acid-base imbalance, 1402
action of
factors affecting, 598–599
mechanisms of, 595–597
administration of
to child, 608, 608f, 610, 614–615
client identification before, 609
cultural factors in, 599
documentation of, 656, 657f–658f, 659
to elderly person, 614
errors in, 106, 650–661
five rights in, 608
frequency of, 603–604, 605t
with gastrointestinal tube, 615
by inhalation, 655–656
nursing responsibilities in, 610
omission of, 659
oral, 610–615
procedure for, 611–614
orders for, 601–605, 605t, 606f
parenteral. *See* Parenteral medications
by patient, 605
pharmacokinetics of, 596–597
rectal, 655
refusal of
by client, 659
by nurse, 605
routes for, 603, 604t
safety in, 608–609, 609f
site conditions at, 596
sublingual, 615
three checks in, 608
timing of, 599
topical, 642
to ear, 652, 654–655
to eye, 646, 650–652
to nose, 652–653, 655
to skin, 642, 646
vaginal, 653, 655–656
adverse effects of, 600
allergy to, 600
antagonistic effects of, 600
bowel elimination and, 1270–1271
cart for handling of, 605, 607f
classification of, 595
controlled, safe handling of, 609, 609f
cumulative effects of, 600
definition of, 594
in discharge planning, 203
distribution of, 596–597
documentation of, 335t, 339
dosage of
abbreviations used in, 603, 603t
calculations for, 605, 607–608, 608f
pharmacokinetics and, 596
in electrolyte imbalance, 1402
excretion of, 597
in fluid imbalance, 1402
vs. herbs in folk medicine, 41, 43
history of, assessment of, 600–601
idiosyncratic effects of, 600
interaction of, 600
legislation concerning, 594
measurement systems for, 605, 607
metabolism of, 597
nomenclature of, 594–595
reference sources for, 603
nutrition requirements and, 1168
orders for, 601–605
checking of, 604, 606f
parts of, 602–605, 603t–605t
questioning of, 604–605
types of, 602
parenteral. *See* Parenteral medications
pharmacodynamics of, 595–596
pharmacokinetics of, 596–597
pH of, 596
poisoning by, 530, 533t
powdered, reconstitution of, 622
preoperative, 686
preoperative evaluation of, 675–676
preparation of, safety measures for, 608–610, 609f
preparations (formulations) of, types of, 594–595, 596t
reference books on, 603
refusal of, 659
in respiratory disorders, 1335, 1336t
response to
in elderly persons, 598
evaluation of, 662
self-administration of, 605
sensory stimulation and, 819
sexuality and, 853, 855, 856t
skin alteration risks and, 917t
for sleep promotion, 1091
sleep quality and, 1080–1081
solubility of, 596
supply systems for, 605, 607f

synergistic effects of, 600
teaching about, 661
tolerance to, 600
urinary elimination and, 1216
Dry mouth, 944, 1343t
Dry shampoo, 957
Dry skin, care of, 941
Due process, in license revocation, 98
Dulcolax (bisacodyl), as laxative, 1285, 1286t
Dullness, in percussion, 481t, 496
"Dumping syndrome," in tube feeding, 1181
Dunn high-level wellness model, 54
Durable power of attorney, 785, 787f, 789
Duration, of sound in auscultation, 481, 481t
Duty, definition of, 101, 102t
Dying. *See* Death and dying
Dysarthria, 380
Dysfunctional grief, 782
Dyskinesia, orofacial, definition of, 1025
Dyspareunia, 859, 860t, 862
Dyspnea, 456, 1320
Dysrhythmia, cardiac, 449, 450t
Dystonia, definition of, 1025
Dysuria, 1219, 1253–1254

Ear
anatomy of, 490f–491f
care of, 826, 952, 954, 955f
examination of, 489–491, 490f–491f, 950
instruments for, 475–476, 475f, 490, 491f
instillations in, 652–653
irrigation of, 652
procedure for, 654–655
physical assessment of, 489–491, 490f–491f
Early morning care, 918
Eastern Orthodox Church, 887
Eastern philosophies, 887, 888t
Eating
assistance with, 1180
disorders of, 1169
Ecchymosis, definition of, 483
ECG (electrocardiography), 449, 451f
Economic factors
in healthcare, 184–186
client records and, 333
in nutrition, 1169
Economic status. *See also* Socioeconomic factors
healthcare and, 37–38
Ectoderm, development of, 129
Edema
definition of, 484, 1377, 1380t
of face, 486
fluid balance and, 1393t–1394t
types of, 1380f
Education. *See also* Counseling; Learning; Teaching
nursing
accreditation of schools and, 98
associate degree program in, 13–14
baccalaureate program in, 13–14
client record in, 333
continuing, 14
in leadership training, 421
diploma program in, 13
educational influences on, 68–69
graduate programs in, 14–15
history of, 6–7, 7f, 68–69
in-service, 15
levels of, 11–15
nursing theory and, 68–69
for practical/vocational nurse, 12
for registered nurse, 12–14
patient
on accident prevention, 535–536, 535f, 536t–537t, 538
of adults vs. children, 388–389, 391
on catheterization technique, 1249–1251
on contraception, 864, 866–868
on coping with special sexual needs, 868–869
on cough preparations, 1332
guidelines for, 104–105
health-belief model in, 55, 56f
on home healthcare, 212–213, 216
on infant care, 134, 135t
on infection control, 560–561
on medications, 661–662
as nursing function, 10t, 11t
on nutrition, 1178–1179
on pain, 1138
preoperative, 682–684, 684f
on pressure ulcer prevention, 985
on responsible sexual expression, 869
on sensory stimulation, 826
on sex, for adolescents, 148t
on sexuality, 863–864, 866f–867f
on sleep promotion, 1091
on toddler care, 137, 138t
on urinary diversion care, 1251, 1253
on vital sign assessment, 468–469
EEG (electroencephalography), in sleep study, 1074, 1074f
Efferent system, in pain transmission, 1104
Ego, in Freudian theory, 117
Ego-integrity, vs. despair in elderly persons, 118, 160–161
Ejaculation, 844–845
premature, 859, 860t
retarded, 859, 860t
Elastic stockings, assistance with, 927, 930
procedure for, 928–929
Elbow, range of motion of, 1001f
Elderly persons (older adults), 156–163
accident prevention and, 60, 526. *See also* Falls
adaptation by, 163–165, 164f
ageism and, 165–166, 165t, 166f
analgesic administration in, 1132–1133, 1135
body alignment in, 1009t
body fluids in, variations in, 1367, 1369t
bowel elimination in, 1269t, 1285
chronic illness in, 167
communication disorders in, 380
day-care centers for, 178–179
demographics of, 163
despair in, 160–161
developmental tasks of, 118, 120
drug action in, 598
drug administration to, 614
elimination in, 168t
exercise in, 168t, 1009t, 1022, 1058
family of, 165
fluid balance maintenance in, 1399
frail-old classification of, 163
functional status of, 157, 160f
growth and development of
cognitive, 157, 160
developmental theories and, 160
physiologic status of, 157, 159
physiologic theories of, 157, 160f
healthcare needs of, 166–168, 168t–169t
healthcare trends and, 188
illness risk factors in, 59
increasing population of, 18
infections in, 559
injuries in, 167
lifetime social changes experienced by, 163, 164f
living arrangements for, 162–163
long-term care facilities for, 180
mobility of, 1007
nutrition in, 1163, 1165, 1168t
assessment of, 1172
old-old classification of, 163
pain in
assessment of, 1115, 1119
attitudes toward, 1112
physical assessment of, normal alterations in, 482
physiologic status of, 157, 159
poisoning of, 530, 549
in poverty culture, 38
pressure ulcer formation in, 977, 979f
recommended nutrient intake for, 1447t–1450t
respiratory function of, 1316, 1316t, 1329
retirement adjustments by, 161–162
safety considerations for, 526, 538
self-concept of, 160, 169t, 732t, 733, 733f
self-esteem of, development of, 742–744
sensory deprivation in, 829, 831–832
sensory stimulation in, 819
sexuality of, 162, 169t, 851t
discussion with, 859

Elderly persons *(continued)*
skin condition of, 913–914
sleep in, 169t, 1079t
social organizations for, 162
social roles of, 162
spouse's health status and, 162
stereotypic view of, 165–166, 165t, 166f
surgery risk and, 673, 675
teaching-learning process in, 391
tissue healing in, 701
urination in, 1214
problems with, 1229–1230
vital signs in, 434
Electra complex, 117
Electrical stimulation
of nerves in pain management, 1125, 1127f
in urinary incontinence, 1234
Electric shock, from equipment, prevention of, 549–550
Electrocardiography, 449, 451f, 520t
Electroencephalography, 520t
in sleep study, 1074, 1074f
Electrolytes. *See also specific electrolyte*; Fluids and electrolytes
in body fluid compartments, 1368, 1369f
definition of, 1368
functions of, in body, 1369–1371
imbalance of, 1379–1380
in cancer patient, 1431–1432
characteristics of, 1381t–1385t, 1386
in diarrhea, case study of, 1432–1434
intravenous therapy for. *See* Intravenous therapy
medications in, 1402
losses of, 1369–1371
measurement of, 1368–1369
movement of, in body, 1371–1373, 1372f–1373f
physiology of, 1368–1371, 1369f
postoperative, 689
regulation of, in body, 1369–1371
sources of, 1369–1371
terminology of, 1368
Electromyogram (EMG), in sleep study, 1074, 1074f
Electronic devices
blood pressure meters, 457
for infusion, in intravenous therapy, 1414
thermometer, 437, 442–443
Electrooculogram (EOG), in sleep study, 1074, 1074f
Elimination. *See also* Bowel elimination; Toilet training; Urinary elimination
in dying patient, 799
in older adults, 168t
as physiologic need, 22
postoperative, 696
preoperative, 685
Elixir, definition of, 596t
Embolism
in intravenous therapy, 1422t–1423t
postoperative, 695
Embryo, development of, 129–130
Emergency care
good Samaritan laws and, 108
of wounds, 704–705
EMG (electromyogram), in sleep study, 1074, 1074f
Emollient, in dry skin care, 941
Emotional dimension, in health-illness status, 56
Emotional needs, 23
health-illness status and, 58
Emotional response, to sensory deprivation, 818, 822
Empathy, in communication, 375
"Empty-nest syndrome," 155
Encoder, in communication, 359, 360f
Endocrine system, in homeostasis, 756, 757t
Endoderm, development of, 129
Endogenous infection, definition of, 561
Endometrium, definition of, 842
Endorphins, pain perception and, 1108
Endoscopy, 521t
of bladder (cystoscopy), 1224, 1226t
definition of, 1276
of gastrointestinal system, 1276, 1278t–1280t
of respiratory system, 1323t–1324t
Endotracheal tube, 1344–1345, 1347f
communication with, 381
Endurance
assessment of, 1026t, 1029
exercises for, 1017
Enema, 1287–1290
barium, 1277, 1281t–1282t
carminative, 1287–1288
cleansing, 685, 1287, 1288t
client preparation for, 1289
equipment for, 1288–1289
hypertonic, 1289
large-volume, 1289–1292
oil-retention, 1287, 1289
preoperative, 685
procedure for, 1290–1292
return-flow, 1288
types of, 1287–1288, 1288t
Energy balance, of diet, 1150–1152, 1151t, 1152f
Engel's stages, of grief reactions, 781–782
Enkephalins, in pain perception, 1108
Enteral nutrition, 1181–1193
administration of, 1186–1187
procedure for, 1188–1190
complications from, 1191–1192
continuous, 1186–1187, 1190
cyclic, 1187
discharge planning for, 1192
formulas for, 1187
intermittent, 1187–1189
long-term, 1181–1182, 1186f
with nasogastric tube, insertion of, 1181
procedure for, 1183–1186
nursing responsibilities in, 1187, 1191–1193
pumps in, 1187
scheduling of, 1186–1187
short-term, 1181
tube irrigation in, 1191–1192
procedure for, 1194
tube placement in, confirmation of, 1182, 1186
tube removal in, 1193
Enteric precautions, specifications for, 577t
Enterococci, vancomycin resistant, transmission of, prevention of, 561–562, 578
Entrepreneur, nurse, 11t
Entry, portal of, for infectious agents, 557, 557f
Entry phase, of home visit, 213–214, 216
Enuresis, 1219, 1256
nocturnal, 1083t
Environment
of bedside unit, 930, 939–940, 940f
drug action and, 599
for effective communication, 364, 368
exercise and, 1016
growth and development affected by, 129
in health and illness model, 54–55, 55f
in health-illness status, 56–57
in pain management, 1112
for physical assessment, 478
respiratory function and, 1317–1318, 1328
risks of, in young adults, 153
for sleep, 1080, 1089
temperature of, body temperature and, 435, 436t
Environmental needs, health-illness status and, 58
Environmental safety. *See* Safety
EOG (electrooculogram), in sleep study, 1074, 1074f
Epidermis, definition of, 911, 912f
Epididymis, anatomy of, 844
Epidural analgesia, 1133, 1135–1136, 1135f
Epinephrine, in respiratory disorders, 1336t
Epithelialization, of pressure ulcer, 980, 982f
Equality, as essential value, 80
Equipment
accident prevention and, 549–550
cleaning of, before sterilization, 566
for physical assessment, 474–476, 475f
protective, in infection control, 582, 585–587, 586f
sterilization of, 563, 566, 567t

Erection, penile, 844–845
  failure of, 849, 859, 860t, 862
Erect position, 477f, 478
Ergosterol (vitamin D), 1159t
Erikson developmental theory for adulthood, 150, 151t
Erikson psychosocial development theory, 67, 117–118, 118f–119f, 118t, 123t
  adolescents and, 143, 146
  elderly persons and, 160–161, 161f
  infants and, 133
  preschool children and, 139
  school-age children and, 139–140
  toddlers and, 136–137
Erogenous zones, definition of, 846
Erosion of skin surface, definition of, 484t
ERV (expiratory reserve volume), definition of, 1322t
Erythema, 483, 483t
  in acne, 941
Erythromycin, in sexually transmitted diseases, 854t
Eschar, in pressure ulcer, 975
Esophageal (core) temperature, 433–434, 436t
Esophagogastroduodenoscopy, 1276, 1278t
Essential hypertension, 459
Ethical problems
  in client-nurse interactions, 86, 88
  core competencies for, 235, 241–243
  institutional policy and, 92
  in nurse-nurse interactions, 91–92
  physician incompetence and, 91
  in physician-nurse interactions, 91
  resolution of
    case study of, 89–90
    computer-aided, 91
Ethics, 83–93
  advocacy in, 84, 427–428
  of care, in Gilligan moral development theory, 121–122
  care-based approach to, 83–84
  client goals and, 308
  codes of, 84–86
    American Nurses Association, 85
    Canadian Nurses Association, 85–86
    International Council of Nurses, 85
  committees for, 92
  death and, 784–785, 786f–788f, 789
  definition of, 83
  development of, Kohlberg theory of, 118–119
  of healthcare allocation, 88, 92, 189
  of infection control, 587–588
  nursing, 84
  in pain management, 1137–1138
  patient bill of rights and, 84
  principles of, 83
  problems with. *See* Ethical problems
  religious beliefs and, 889
  sexuality and, 849
  theories of, 83–84
Ethnicity. *See also* Culture and ethnicity
  definition of, 33–34
Ethnocentrism, 44
Ethylene oxide, in sterilization/disinfection, 567t
Eupnea, definition of, 458t
Euthanasia, direct voluntary, 789–790
Evaluating, 225–226, 227t, 313–328. *See also type of care, e.g.,* Oral care
  care plan modification after, 318, 320t–322t
  checklist for, 325
  communication in, 365
  concurrent, 324
  core competencies for, 316
  criteria for, 314
  data collection in, 314–318
  definition of, 314, 315f
  documentation in, 316
  evaluation of, checklist of, 325
  factors influencing goal achievement and, 316–318, 319t
  illustration of, 228
  nursing audit in, 324
  outcome of, 323
  overview of, 326f
  in planning step, 287
  problems in, 320t–322t
  programs in, 322–324
  quality assurance and, 322–324
  retrospective, 324
  of safety precautions, 551
  of self, 324–327
  standards for, 314
  in teaching-learning process, 402–404, 403f
Evaluation, potential liability in, 104t
Evaporation, as heat transfer mechanism, 434, 435t
Eversion, definition of, 1000, 1001f–1002f
Evisceration, through wound, 703, 703f
Exacerbation, of chronic illness, 61
Examination
  for licensure, 12
  nursing. *See* Physical assessment
Exception, charting by, 334, 338t, 349f
Excitement, sexual, 845f, 846
Excoriation, of skin, 484t
Excretion, of drugs, 597
Excretory urography, 1224, 1226t
Exercise, 1016–1023
  active, range-of-motion, 1037
  active-assistive, range-of-motion, 1037
  aerobic, 1017
  before ambulation, 1048, 1050–1051
  attitudes toward, 1015
  avoidance of, 1023
  bowel elimination and, 1284
  breathing, 1329–1330
    postoperative, 683
  cardiovascular effects of, 1017, 1018f, 1019
  coughing, postoperative, 684
  before crutch walking, 1055–1056
  daily activities as, 1017, 1051
  definition of, 1016
  effects of
    on cardiovascular system, 1017, 1018f, 1019
    on gastrointestinal system, 1018f, 1021
    on metabolism, 1018f, 1020–1021
    on musculoskeletal system, 1018f, 1019–1020
    psychosocial, 1021–1022
    on respiratory system, 1018f, 1019
    on skin, 1018f, 1021
    on urinary system, 1018f, 1021
  in elderly persons, 168t, 1009t, 1022, 1058
  for endurance, 1017
  fatigue and, 1016
  gastrointestinal effects of, 1018f, 1021
  in illness prevention, 1022
  injuries from, 1023
  isokinetic, 1016f, 1017
  isometric, 1016, 1016f
  isotonic, 1016, 1016f
  Kegel, 863–864, 1228
  lack of, reasons for, 1061–1062
  for legs, postoperative, 684, 684f
  metabolic effects of, 1018f, 1020–1021
  musculoskeletal effects of, 1018f, 1019–1020
  passive, range-of-motion, 1037
  as physiologic need, 23
  postoperative, 684, 684f
  program for, 1056, 1058
  psychosocial effects of, 1021–1022
  push-ups, 1050
  quadriceps drills, 1048, 1050
  range-of-motion, 1037, 1039, 1039f
  respiratory effects of, 1018f, 1019
  risks of, 1022–1023
  skin effects of, 1018f, 1021
  strengthening, 1017
  stress and, 768–769, 1016
  stretching, 1017
  target heart rate in, 1058
  teaching about, 1058–1059
  trapeze bar in, 1033, 1034f
  types of, 1016, 1016f
  urinary elimination and, 1018f, 1021, 1215–1216
  in wellness promotion, 1022
  in young adults, 152
Exhalation, 455, 1313
Exhaustion, heat, 436t
Exhaustion phase, in general adaptation syndrome, 759, 759f
Exit, portal of, for infectious agents, 557, 557f
Exogenous infection, definition of, 561
Expected outcome, of planning, 282
Expectorants, 1332

Expert witness, in malpractice litigation, nurse as, 102
Expiration (exhalation), definition of, 455, 1313
Expiratory reserve volume (ERV), definition of, 1322t
Expressive aphasia, definition of, 512
Extended-care. *See* Long-term care
Extended family, 26
Extended-release drugs, 596t
Extension, definition of, 1000t, 1001f–1002f
Extensor reflexes, 1005
External resources, self-concept and, 731
External rotation, definition of, 1000t, 1001f–1002f
Extracellular fluid, 1367, 1368f, 1369t
  electrolyte composition of, 1368, 1369t
  regulation of, 1375t
Extraneous variables, in research, 423
Extraocular movements, assessment of, 488–489, 490f
Extubation, unplanned, in enteral nutrition, 1191
Exudate
  in pressure ulcer, 980
  from wound, 701
Eye
  anatomy of, 486f
  artificial, care of, 954
  care of, 826, 952–954
    cleaning in, 952–953
    planning in, 952
    in unconscious client, 953
  examination of, 486–489, 486f–490f, 950
    cranial nerve function and, 513, 513t
    instruments for, 474–475, 475f, 487–489, 488f–489f
  instillations in, 646, 650
  irrigation of, 650
    procedure for, 651–652
  medication disc for, 652
Eyebrow, examination of, 486
Eye chart, for examination, 475f, 476, 488
Eye contact
  cultural differences in, 36
  as nonverbal communication, 361, 361f
Eyedrops, installation of, 646, 650
Eyeglasses, care of, 953
Eyelid, examination of, 486
Eyewear, protective, 586

Face
  appearance of, in fluid balance assessment, 1393t
  examination of, 486
  expression of, as nonverbal communication, 361f, 362
  mask for. *See* Mask
Face-to-face meeting, communication in, 340t
Facial nerve, assessment of, 513t, 514
Fact witness, in malpractice litigation, nurse as, 102
Fahrenheit scale, on thermometer, 437, 439f, 439t
Failure, self-concept and, 731–732
Failure to thrive, in infants, 134
Faith
  definition of, 122–123, 883
  growth in, 884
Faith development theory of Fowler. *See under* Developmental theory
Fallopian tubes
  ligation of, 868
  physiology of, 842
Falls
  in older adults, 167
  prevention of, 539–541, 541f–542f, 544f
  risk of, 529–530
False imprisonment, 101
Family
  blended, 25
  changes in, during middle adulthood, 154–155, 155f
  cohabiting, 26
  communication with, 341
  cultural differences in, 46t–50t
  definitions of, 24
  developmental tasks of, 27, 28t
  dominant member of, 35
  of dying/dead patient
    grief reactions in, 792
    impacts on, 783
    needs of, 794, 802–803
  of elderly person, 165
  ethnic differences in, 46t–50t
  extended, 26
  in family-centered nursing, 26
  functions of, 27
  growth and development and, 123–124
  health promotion in, interventions for, 28–29, 30t
  health risk factors and, 27–29
  illness effects on, 27–28, 61, 763
  inadequate stimulation from, sensory deprivation in, 830–831
  as information source, 254
  nuclear, 25–26, 26f
  nursing care performed by, for dying patient, 799
  pain attitudes of, 1111–1112
  poverty in, 37–38
  preoperative information for, 686
  relationships with, 302t
  single adult as, 27
  single-parent, 26
  spirituality and, 889
  stages of, vs. developmental tasks, 28t
  step, 25
  structures of, 24–27
  as support system, cultural differences in, 38
  terminal illness impacts on, 783
  traditional, 24–26, 26f
  two-career, 26
  values of
    conflict in, 82–83
    development of, 79
Family planning, natural, 866
Fantasies, in preschool children, 138
Fasciculations, definition of, 1025
Fat
  dietary, 1154t, 1156–1157, 1157f
  in emulsions, for parenteral nutrition, 1193
Fatigue
  exercise and, 1016
  in respiratory disorders, 1320
Fatty acids
  essential, 1157
  saturation of, 1156
Faulty categorizing, in self-concept disturbances, 745
Fear
  vs. anxiety, 759
  in dying patient, 797, 801
  preoperative, causes of, 676–677
  in preschool children, 139
  of wounds, 704
Febrile, definition of, 435
Fecal incontinence. *See under* Incontinence
Feces. *See also* Defecation
  definition of, 1267
  formation of, 1266–1267
  impaction of, removal of, 1289, 1292–1293, 1294f
Federal Food, Drug and Cosmetic Act, 594
Feedback, in communication, 359, 360f
Feeding, tube. *See* Enteral nutrition
Fellatio, definition of, 848
Felony, definition of, 99
Female
  genitalia of
    examination of, 507–508, 507f, 860–861
    physiology of, 841–844, 842f–843f
  sexual dysfunction in, 859–860, 860t
  sexual response pattern in, 845–846, 845f
  urinary catheterization of, procedure for, 1238f, 1239–1243
  urine specimen collection from, 1220, 1222
Feminine hygiene
  case study in, 966–968
  after urination, 1228, 1230
Femoral pulse, 452f
  assessment of, 502
Fenestrated tracheostomy tube, 1346
Fertilization, of ovum, 129
Fetal alcohol syndrome, 132
Fetishism, definition of, 848

Fetus
  development of, 130
  safety considerations for, 526, 536, 536t
Fever, 435–437, 438t
  in blood transfusion, 1429t
  course of, 438t
  fluid balance and, 1394t
  in respiratory disorders, 1320
Fiber, dietary, 1153, 1154t
  bowel elimination and, 1270
Fibrinogen, as electrolyte, 1371
Fibrinolytic studies, reference ranges for, 1441t
Fidelity, in ethical code, 84
"Fight-or-flight" response, 757
Figure-of-eight turn, in bandage application, 713, 714f
Filtration, of fluids and electrolytes, 1373, 1373f
Filtration pressure, definition of, 1373, 1373f
Financing, of healthcare. *See under* Healthcare
Fingers, range of motion of, 1001f
Firearms injury, prevention of, 533, 548–549
Fires
  causes of, 530
  prevention of, 543–544, 548f
    checklist for, 531–532
  procedures during, 530
First intention, healing by, 701, 702f
Fissure, skin, definition of, 484t
Fitness. *See* Exercise
Five rights, in drug administration, 608
Flaccidity, muscular, 509, 1029
Flagyl (metronidazole), in sexually transmitted disease, 854t–855t
Flat affect, in depression, 1010
Flatness, in percussion, 481t, 496
Flatulence/flatus
  definition of, 1268
  diet and, 1284
  in elderly persons, 1285
  reduction of, 1287
Flexion, definition of, 1000t, 1001f–1002f
Flossing, of teeth, 945, 951f
Flotation bed, in pressure ulcer prevention, 987t
Flowsheets, in client record, 336t, 337, 339, 346f, 352f–356f
Fluid(s). *See also* Water
  balance of, 1373–1374
    documentation of, 337, 339
    in elderly persons, maintenance of, 1399
    homeostatic mechanisms for, 1374, 1375t
    postoperative assessment of, in recovery room, 689
  in body compartments, 1367, 1368f
  body variations in, 1367–1368, 1369t
  imbalance of, 1377, 1378t–1379t, 1379
    in cancer patient, 1431–1432
    in diarrhea, case study of, 1432–1434
    intravenous therapy for. *See* Intravenous therapy
    medications in, 1402
    prevention of, 1399
    in surgical client, 1430–1431
  intake of
    modification of, 1400–1402
    promotion of, 1228, 1400–1401
    requirements for, 1373
    in respiratory disorders, 1332
  intake-output measurement of, 1391, 1392t, 1397
    forms for, 337, 339
  loss of, 1374, 1374f
    imbalances resulting from, 1389, 1390t
  movement of, among body compartments, 1371–1373, 1372f–1373f
  as physiologic need, 23
  physiology of, 1367–1368, 1368f, 1369t
  postoperative, 696–697
  preoperative, 685
  restriction of, 1401–1402
  sources of, 1373–1374, 1374f
  third-space shift of, 1377
  urine production and, 1214
Fluidized bed, in pressure ulcer prevention, 987t
Fluid overload
  in blood transfusion, 1429t
  in intravenous therapy, 1422t
Fluids and electrolytes. *See also* Electrolytes; Fluid(s)
  balance of, planning in, 1397–1398
  imbalance of
    assessment in, 1389–1391, 1392t–1396t
    blood and blood products in. *See* Blood transfusions
    diet in, 1399–1400
    fluid intake control in, 1399–1400
    intravenous therapy in, 1402–1429
      blood transfusions in. *See* Blood transfusions
      changing solutions and tubings in, 1415–1418
      complications of, 1415, 1422t–1423t
      discontinuing, 1423
      equipment for, 1402–1403, 1404f
      heparin lock in, 1415, 1424
      procedure for, 1405–1409
      regulation of, 1412–1415, 1415f, 1418–1420
      site care in, 1415, 1421
      sites for, 1411–1412, 1411f
      solutions for, 1403t
      starting, 1412, 1405–1409
      teaching about, 1423
      venous access devices for, 1403–1404, 1409, 1409f, 1411f
    medications for, 1402
    nursing diagnosis of, 1396–1398
    in parenteral nutrition, 1196
    physical assessment in, 1389, 1391, 1392t–1396t
    surgery and, 1430–1431
  nurse as role model concerning, 1388–1389
  status of, assessment of, 1389, 1390t, 1391, 1392t, 1396, 1397t
Fluid volume deficit, 1377, 1378t
  in cancer, 1431
  case study of, 1432–1434
  causes of, 1398
  characteristics of, 1398
  in surgery, 1432–1434
Fluid volume excess, 1377, 1379t, 1380
  in blood transfusions, 1429t
  in cancer, 1431
  causes of, 1398
  characteristics of, 1398
  in intravenous therapy, 1422t
  in surgery, 1430–1431
Fluoride, dietary, 1160t
Flushing, of skin, 483, 483t
Foam overlay, in pressure ulcer prevention, 987t
Focus charting, 334, 338t, 348f
Foley catheter
  rectal use of, 1293–1294
  urinary. *See under* Catheter(ization) (urinary)
Folic acid, 1159t
Folk healers, 41
Folk medicine, 41, 43, 46t–50t
Follicular phase, of ovarian cycle, 843, 843f
Food. *See also* Diet; Nutrition
  decreased intake of, 1169
  drug action and, 599
  as physiologic need, 23
  withholding of, 1181
    preoperative, 685
Food and Drug Administration, 594
Food diary, 1172
Food guide pyramid, 1161–1162, 1162f
Food labeling, 1163, 1164f
Footboard, body alignment and, 1032–1033, 1032f
Foot care, 958–960
Footdrop, footboard for, 1032–1033, 1032f
"Force fluid" order, 1400–1401
Forceps, in sterile procedures, 568, 571f
Forearm, range of motion of, 1001f
Forehead temperature, normal, 437t
Foreign body
  in airway, choking on, 530
  wound healing and, 700
Foreign-language-speaking clients, communication with, 35–36, 381
Foreplay, 846
Foreskin, 844
Formal operational stage, in cognitive development, 119, 122f

Four-point gait, in crutch walking, 1056, 1057f
Fowler faith development theory, 122–123, 123f, 123t
  adolescents and, 136
  preschool children and, 140
  school-age children and, 141
Fowler's position, 1034, 1035t
  in postural drainage, 1333
Fracture(s)
  mobility and, 1010
  pathologic, in immobility, 1013t
"Fracture" bedpan, 1231
Frail-old classification, of older adults, 163
Fraud, 101
FRC (functional residual capacity), definition of, 1322t
Freedom, as essential value, 80
Fremitus
  definition of, 496
  in respiratory disorders, 1319
Frequency, of urination
  definition of, 1219
  in older adults, 1229
Freud psychoanalytic theory, 117, 117t
  adolescents and, 143
  infants and, 133
  preschool children and, 139
  school-age children and, 141
  toddlers and, 136
Friction, in pressure ulcer formation, 974, 975f
Friction rub, pleural, 497, 500f, 1321
Frontal sinuses, physical assessment of, 492, 492f
Full stage, of illness, 558
Functional health
  definition of, 164–165
  patterns in, 262
Functional incontinence
  characteristics of, 1232
  definition of, 1227
Functional residual capacity (FRC), definition of, 1322t
Fungi, as infectious agents, 556

Gait
  abnormal, 1026, 1028f
  assessment of, 514, 1024–1026, 1026t, 1027f–1028f
  crutch, 1056, 1057f–1058f
  as nonverbal communication, 362
  normal, 1027, 1027f
  parkinsonian, 1028f
  scissors, 1028f
  steppage, 1028f
Gardnerella vaginalis infection, 854t
Gas exchange, 1314–1315, 1314f
  impaired, 1359–1360
    causes of, 1328
    characteristics of, 1328
    in elderly persons, 1329
    in immobility, 1013t
  physiology of, 1314–1315, 1314f
Gas sterilization, of equipment, 567t
Gastric fluid loss, imbalances resulting from, 1390t
Gastrointestinal series, 1276–1277, 1280t–1282t
  skin alteration risks and, 917t
Gastrointestinal system
  anatomy of, 1267f
  diagnostic procedures for, 1274–1277, 1278t–1282t
    multiple, sequence of, 1277
  of elderly person, 159
  endoscopy of, 1276, 1278t–1280t
  exercise effects on, 1018f, 1021
  fluid/electrolyte homeostasis and, 1374, 1374f
  immobility effects on, 1014t, 1018f, 1021
  radiography of, 1276, 1280t–1282t
Gastrostomy
  percutaneous endoscopic, 1182
  in tube feeding, 1181–1182
Gate control theory of pain, 1106–1107, 1108f
Gatorade, in diarrhea, 1287
Gauze dressings, 708, 708t, 989t
Gay, definition of, 847
Gender. *See also* Female; Male
  body temperature and, 435
  body water distribution and, 1368, 1369t
  communication and, 363
  definition of, 841
  drug action and, 598–599
  nutrition requirements and, 1163
  pain attitudes and, 1111–1112
  roles of, cultural differences in, 35
Gender role, definition of, 841
General adaptation syndrome, 758–759, 759f
General anesthesia, 672
General appearance, assessment of, 481
General systems theory, 67
Generativity, vs. stagnation in middle adult, 118
Generic name, of drug, 595
Genetic factors, drug action and, 599
Genetic theory, of aging, 157
Genitalia/genital system
  of adolescent, 142–143, 144f–145f
  care of, 960–965, 963f
  of elderly person, 159
  female
    examination of, 507–508, 507f, 860–861
    physiology of, 841–844, 842f–843f
  male
    examination of, 508, 508f, 860–861
    physiology of, 844–845
  oral stimulation of, 848
  warts of, 855t
Genital stage, in Freudian theory, 117, 117t
  adolescent in, 143
Gerontologic nursing, 166, 166f
Gerontology, definition of, 166
Gestures, as nonverbal communication, 362
Gilligan moral development theory, 121–122
Gingivitis, 943
Glasgow Coma Scale, 512, 512t
Glass thermometer. *See under* Thermometer
Gliding joint, 1000
Global self, definition of, 729
Globulin, as electrolyte, 1371
Glossitis, 944
Glossopharyngeal nerve, assessment of, 513t, 514
Gloves
  allergy to, 582, 584
  in care of isolated client, 582, 585
  sterile
    procedure for donning and removing of, 573–575
    in surgical asepsis, 586
Gluconeogenesis, 1153, 1155f
Glucose
  formation of, in carbohydrate metabolism, 1153, 1155f
  for intravenous therapy, solutions for, 1403t
  monitoring of, in parenteral nutrition, 1193
    procedure for, 1197–1198
Glucose-6-phosphate dehydrogenase deficiency, ethnic differences in, 39
Glycogenesis, 1153, 1155f
Glycogenolysis, 1153, 1155f
Glycosuria, definition of, 1219
Goals, client
  achievement of, factors affecting, 316–318, 319t
  affective, 285, 315
  assistance in meeting of, 307
  attainment of, King's theory of, 70t, 72
  cognitive, 285, 315
  definition of, 282, 285
  derivation of, 285, 285t
  in discharge planning, 202–203
  evaluation of. *See* Evaluating
  in helping relationship, 366
  long-term vs. short-term, 285–286
  physical changes and, 315
  psychomotor, 285, 315
  types of, 20–286, 286f
  writing of, 286–287
God, relationships with. *See* Spirituality
Goggles, protective, 586
GoLYTELY, in oral intestinal lavage, 1289
Gonorrhea, 854t
Goodness, in Gilligan moral development theory, 122
Good Samaritan laws, 108
Gossip, 371

Gould transformation theory, 150–151
Gout, ethnic differences in, 40
Government, healthcare financing by, 184–185, 185t
Government agencies, healthcare services of, 181–182, 182f
Gowns
in isolation care, 585
removal of, for bathing, with intravenous line, 926
Gram-negative bacteria, 556
Gram-positive bacteria, 556
Granulation tissue
in healing, 701
in pressure ulcer, 980, 982f
Graphic sheet, in client record, 335t, 337, 354f–356f
Gravity
center of, in body alignment, 1004, 1004f
in postural drainage, 1333, 1334f
Grief, 781–782. *See also* Death and dying; Loss
dysfunctional, 782
nursing process in, 803–804
Grooming, as nonverbal communication, 362
Groshong central venous catheter, 1403
Ground, electrical, in accident prevention, 550
Group(s)
communication in, 379, 382–384, 383t
efficacy of, 383t
member roles in, 382–384, 383t
purposes of, 382
as support systems, 383
types of, 379, 382
Group dynamics, communication and, 379, 382–384, 383t
Group healthcare plans, 185–186
Growth and development, 115–127. *See also* Developmental theory
in adolescence. *See under* Adolescents
of adults, theories for, 150–151, 151t
cephalocaudal trend in, 115, 116f
of children. *See under* Children
differentiation in, 115
of elderly persons. *See under* Elderly persons
environmental factors and, 129
family influences on, 123–124
individuality in, 116
of infants. *See under* Infants
integration in, 115–116
of middle adults
cognitive, 155
moral, 155–156
physiologic, 154
psychosocial, 154–155, 155f
spiritual, 155–156
of neonates, 130–132, 130t, 131f
nursing applications of, 124–126
nutritional factors and, 129
orderly nature of, 115
prenatal, 129–130
of preschool child, 130–140, 139f, 141t
principles of, 115–116, 116f
proximodistal, 115
of school-age child, 140–141, 142f, 143t
specificity of, 116
teaching-learning process and, 388–389, 391
theories on. *See* Developmental theory
of toddlers. *See under* Toddlers
of young adults
physiologic, 151, 152t
psychosocial, 151
Guaifenesin, as expectorant, 1332
Guided imagery, in stress management, 770
Guilt, spiritual, 890, 893
Gums
disease of, 943–944
examination of, 492–493
Gurgles (rhonchi), 456, 497, 500f, 1321
Gustatory sensation. *See* Taste

Habit training program, for incontinence, 1234
Haemophilus influenzae, immunization for, 136t
Hair
care of, 954–958
facial, 957–958, 958f
dandruff in, 955
examination of, 485
grooming of, 956
lice in, 955
loss of, 955
problems with, 955–956
pubic, 841
shampooing of, 956–957, 957f
shaving of, 957–958, 958f
transplantation of, 955
Halitosis, in periodontal disease, 944
Hallucinations, hypnagogic, 1082t
Hammer, in physical assessment, 475f, 476
Hand
intravenous therapy infusions in, 1411–1412, 1411f
splint for, body alignment and, 1033
Handwashing
bacteria and, 563
cleansing agents for, 563
importance of, 562–563
procedure for, 564–565
techniques for, 563
Harris flush enema, 1288
Havighurst developmental task theory, 119–120
adolescents and, 143, 146
elderly persons and, 161–163, 162f
infants and, 133
preschool children and, 140
school-age children and, 141
toddlers and, 137
Hawaiian people, cultural characteristics of, 49t–50t
Hazards
assessment of, 529–533, 533t
control of. *See* Safety
Headache, 1105t
Head and neck
anatomy of, 492f, 494f
examination of. *See under* Physical assessment
Healers, folk, 41
Healing (concept), spirituality and, 884–885
Healing (tissue)
blood transport in, 700
body response in, 702
of draining wound, 721, 721f
factors affecting, 701–702
foreign bodies and, 700
health status and, 702
microorganism defenses in, 700
phases of, 700–701
primary intention, 701, 702f
principles of, 700
secondary intention (granulation), 701, 702f
tertiary intention, 701, 702f
Health
definition of, 53
promotion of, in discharge planning, 203
restoration of
as nursing aim, 10–11
as teaching aim, 387
vs. wellness, 53
Health assessment. *See also* Health history; Physical assessment
components of, 474
Health-belief model, 55, 56f
Healthcare
access to, poverty effects on, 37–38
agencies providing, 181–182, 181f–182f
allocation of, ethical problems in, 88, 92
in Canada, funding of, 185
case management in, 182–183
collaborative, 183–184, 183f
community-based, 175
competencies for, 176
consumerism in, 187–188
as culture, 43–44
delivery of, models for, 416
federally funded, 184–185, 185t
financial aspects of, 184–186
client records and, 333
fragmentation of, 188, 188f
frameworks for, 182–183
goals of, 175–176
group plans for, 185–186
health maintenance organizations in, 186

Healthcare *(continued)*
  of infants, 134, 135t–136t
  inpatient, 176
  insurance in, 186
  managed care systems, 182
  outpatient, 176
  preferred provider organizations for, 186
  primary, vs. primary care, 183
  reform of, 175
  settings for, 175–176, 175f, 179f
    ambulatory facilities. *See* Ambulatory facilities
    continuity of care in. *See* Continuity of care
    day-care centers, 178–179
    home. *See* Home healthcare
    homeless shelters, 180
    hospice. *See* Hospice care
    hospitals. *See* Hospitals
    industry, 180
    long-term care facilities, 180
    mental health centers, 179
    nursing activities in, 178
    primary care centers, 178
    rehabilitation centers, 180
    rural health centers, 179
    schools, 179–180
  trends in, 186–189, 186f, 188f
Health-care systems model of nursing (Neuman), 71t, 73
Health history, 250–251
  in acid-base balance, 1389, 1390t
  bowel elimination in, 1272
  diet in, 1172
  documentation of, 335t
  in electrolyte imbalance, 1389, 1390t
  medications in, 600
  mobility in, 1023–1024
  oral care in, 942
  personal hygiene in, 915–916
  in physical assessment, 474
  preoperative, 673, 674f, 675–678
  respiratory function in, 1318–1319
  sexuality in, 857–859
  sleep patterns in, 1083–1084
  urinary elimination in, 1216–1217
Health-illness continuum, 54, 54f
  stress in, 761–762
Health-illness models, 54–55, 54f–56f
Health-illness status
  factors affecting, 55–59
    basic human needs, 57–58
    emotional, 56
    environmental, 56–57
    intellectual, 56
    physical, 55–56
    self-concept, 58–59
    sociocultural, 57
    spiritual, 57
  mobility and, 1006
  nutrition requirements and, 1168
  personal hygiene and, 913–914, 917t
  respiratory function and, 1316
  safety and, 528
  sexuality and, 849, 851, 854t–855t
  tissue healing and, 700
Health maintenance organizations, 186
Health problems, in nursing diagnosis, 267, 273, 275t
Health-risk appraisal, forms for, 62–63
Healthy People 2000, 175–176
Hearing (auditory sensation)
  assessment of, 490–491, 821
    cranial nerve function and, 513t, 514
  impairment/loss of, 491
    characteristics of, 823
    communication in, 378–381, 954
    conductive, 491, 826
    needs in, 826, 828
    prevention of, 826, 828
    sensorineural, 491, 826
  stimulation of, 816t, 827
Hearing aid, care of, 954, 955f
Heart
  anatomy of, 500f
  examination of, 498–502, 500f–502f, 502t
  pumping action of, blood pressure and, 457
Heart murmurs, 502, 502t
Heart rate
  factors affecting, 446, 448
  target, in exercise, 1058
Heart sounds, 501–502, 502f
Heat, in sterilization/disinfection, 563, 567t
Heat application, skin alteration risks and, 917t
Heat cramps, 436t
Heat exhaustion, 436t
Heatstroke, 436t
Heat syncope, 436t
Heat transfer, body temperature and, 434, 435t
Heaves, with heartbeat, 499
Height
  nutritional status and, 1174
  in physical assessment, 481
Height-weight tables, 1151, 1151t
Heimlich maneuver, for airway clearance, 1357–1358
Helping relationship
  characteristics of, 366
  in communication, 366–371, 366f, 369f
  definition of, 366, 366f
  goals of, 366
  phases of, 366–368, 367f
  vs. social relationship, 366
Hematocrit, in nutritional assessment, 1175
Hematologic tests, reference ranges for, 1441t–1442t
Hematuria, definition of, 1216, 1219
Hemiparesis
  definition of, 1029
  spastic, gait in, 1028f
Hemiplegia, definition of, 1029
Hemoglobin
  in acid-base balance regulation, 1376
  in nutritional assessment, 1175
  in oxygen transport, 1315
  reference ranges for, 1442t
Hemolytic reaction, in blood transfusion, 1429t
Hemorrhage
  postoperative, 694
  subconjunctival, in neonates, 132
  wound, 703
Hemorrhoids, definition of, 1267
Hemostasis, in healing, 701
Hemovac tube, 708t
Heparin lock, 1415, 1424
  in intravenous therapy, 637, 641–642
    procedure for, 647–649
Hepatitis, from blood transfusion, 1415, 1423–1424
Hepatitis B
  immunization for, 136t
  testing for, in blood transfusion, 1428
  transmission of, 558t
    prevention of, 577
Herbalism, 41, 43
Herpes simplex virus infection, 854t
  neuralgia after, 1105t
Hesitancy, in urination, definition of, 1219, 1228–1229
Heterosexuality, 847
Hiccups, postoperative, 697
Hierarchy of needs. *See* Maslow's hierarchy of needs
High-level wellness model, 54
Hinduism, 888t
Hinge joint, 1000
Hip
  injection into, 631–632, 631f
  range of motion of, 1002f
Hirsutism, definition of, 485
Hispanic people
  cultural characteristics of, 48t
  nutrition in, 1170t
Histamine-2-receptor antagonists, preoperative, 686
History
  health. *See* Health history
  of nursing, 5–6, 7f, 8t
HIV infection. *See* Human immunodeficiency virus infection
HMOs (health maintenance organizations), 186
Holding area, surgical, skin preparation in, 685
Holistic healthcare
  cultural considerations in, 44
  interdependent parts of person in, 54, 55f
  wellness model in, 54
Homan's sign, 929
Home healthcare, 176–177, 208–218
  analgesic administration in, 1137
  caregiver needs in, 216–217
  culture and ethnicity in, 216
  definition of, 208, 209t

documentation of, 339
of dying person, 801
future of, 217
history of, 208–209
importance of, 177
intravenous therapy in, 1423
legal issues in, 210–211, 211t
nursing in, 178, 209–213, 209f
accountability in, 210–211, 211t
characteristics of, 210–211, 210f, 211t
coordination of services in, 211–212
hospice, 217
independence in, 210
roles of, 211–213
skills for, 210, 210f
unique role of, 210
oxygen administration in, 1344, 1346f
self-concept disturbances in, 740
teaching in, 212–213, 216
team for, 208, 209t
in urinary incontinence, 1234–1235
visit in, 213–216
entry phase of, 213–214, 216
pre-entry phase of, 213
vital sign assessment in, 468–469
of wound, 722–723
Homeless shelters, healthcare in, 180
Homeostasis
of body fluids, 1374, 1375t, 1415, 1423–1424
definition of, 756
physiologic, 756, 757t
psychologic, 756
Homosexuality, 847
Hormones
in contraception, 868
laboratory tests for, reference ranges for, 1445t–1446t
Hospice care
characteristics of, 782
in home, 217
services provided by, 180
Hospitals
admission to. *See under* Admission
functions of, 177–178, 179f
nursing activities in, 178
nursing education in, 6–7, 7f
types of, 177–178, 179f
Host, for infectious agents, 557, 557f
Host factors, in health and illness model, 54–55, 55f
Hot-cold balance, treatments based on, 48t
Hour of sleep care (hs care), 918
Household measurements, 607, 1439, 1439t
Hoyer hydraulic lift, 1048, 1050f
hs care (hour of sleep care), 918
Human dignity
as essential value, 80
promotion of, 238–240
Human immunodeficiency virus infection
accidental exposure to, 588
in adolescents, 147
blood transfusions and, 1428
challenges in, 588
human reservoirs of, 557
infection control in, ethics of, 588
legal aspects of, 107
symptoms of, 854t
testing for, counseling in, 399–400
transmission of, 558t
prevention of, 577
treatment of, 854t
Human needs, 22–31. *See also specific need*
of community, 29–30
consideration of, in meeting client goals, 307
in dying, 799–800
of family, 27–28, 28t
health-illness status and, 57–58
of individual, 22–23, 23f
levels of, 22
love and belonging as, 23–24, 23f
nursing diagnosis and, 278
nursing theory and, 67
physiologic, 22–23, 23f
in dying patient, 799
in physical assessment, 478, 478f
stress effects on, 761
psychologic
in dying patient, 799–800
of isolated client, 587
in physical assessment, 478, 478f
before surgery, 679, 681–682
safety and security as, 23, 23f, 525
self-actualization as, 23f, 24
self-esteem as, 23f, 24
spiritual, 58, 883–884
in dying patient, 800
stress effects on, 761
Human papillomavirus infection, 855t
Humidification
of air, in respiratory disorders, 1332
of oxygen, 1338
Humor, in communication, 375
Humoral immunity, 558
Humors, body, treatments based on, 48t
Hydration
definition of, 1377
status of, pressure ulcer formation and, 975
urinary problems affecting, 1218
Hydraulic lift, 1048, 1050f
Hydrocolloid dressings, 722, 989f, 989t
Hydrogel dressings, 722, 989t
Hydrogen ions, vs. pH, 1376
Hydrometer, in urine specific gravity determination, 1224, 1225f
Hydrostatic pressure, definition of, 1373, 1373f
Hygiene, 910–971
of ears, 954, 955f
of eyes, 950–954
of feet, 958–960
feminine, 960–965, 963f
case study in, 966–968
after urination, 1228, 1230
of hair. *See under* Hair
of nails, 958–959
oral. *See* Oral care
perineal, 960–965, 963f
personal. *See* Personal hygiene
preoperative, 685
pressure ulcer prevention and. *See* Pressure ulcers
for toddlers, 135t, 138t
vaginal, 960–965, 963f
Hymen, anatomy of, 841
Hyperalimentation. *See* Parenteral nutrition
Hyperbaric oxygen therapy, 1358
Hypercalcemia, 1380, 1383t
Hyperchloremia, 1160t
Hyperemia, reactive, in pressure ulcer formation, 975, 976t
Hyperextension, definition of, 1000t, 1001f
Hyperkalemia, 1160t, 1380, 1382t
Hypermagnesemia, 1160t, 1380, 1384t
Hypernatremia, 1379–1380, 1381t
Hyperphosphatemia, 1160t, 1385t, 1386
Hyperpyrexia, definition of, 435
Hyperresonance, in percussion, 481t, 496
Hypersomnia, 1081
Hypertension, 459
drugs for, sexuality and, 851, 856t
Hyperthermia, 435, 436t
Hypertonic solutions
definition of, 1372
for enema, 1289
for intravenous therapy, 1403t
Hypertrophy, muscular, definition of, 1029
Hyperventilation, definition of, 1315
Hypervolemia, 1377, 1379t, 1380
Hypnagogic hallucinations, 1082t
Hypnosis, in pain management, 1126–1127
Hypocalcemia, 1380, 1382t–1383t
Hypochloremia, 1160t
Hypoglossal nerve, assessment of, 513t, 514
Hypokalemia, 1160t, 1380, 1382t
Hypomagnesemia, 1380, 1384t
Hyponatremia, 1160t, 1379–1380, 1381t
Hypophosphatemia, 1160t, 1384t–1385t, 1386
Hypostatic pneumonia, from immobility, 1019
Hypotension, 459–460
orthostatic, in immobility, 1011t, 1017
Hypothalamus
body temperature regulation by, 433
sleep control by, 1073
Hypothermia, 435, 436t, 437, 439f
Hypothyroidism, nutrition and, 1178
Hypotonic solutions
definition of, 1372
for intravenous therapy, 1403t

Hypoventilation
  causes of, 1387t
  definition of, 1315
Hypovolemia, definition of, 1377
Hypovolemic shock, postoperative, 694
Hypoxia, definition of, 1315

Iatrogenic disease/infection, definition of, 561, 600
IC (inspiratory capacity), definition of, 1322t
ICN (International Council of Nurses), 15
Id, in Freudian theory, 117
Idealization, as grief reaction, 782
Ideal self
  definition of, 729
  vs. real self, 736, 736f
Identification
  of client, before drug administration, 609
  of personal strength, 735–736, 741, 741f
Identity. *See also* Personal identity
  vs. role confusion in adolescence, 118
Identity-continuity theory, older adults and, 160
Idiosyncratic effect, of drugs, 600
Ileal conduit, for urinary diversion, 1251, 1253, 1253f
  changing appliance on, procedure for, 1254–1255
Ileocecal valve, 1266
Ileostomy
  care of, 1295–1301, 1296f–1297f, 1300f
  definition of, 1295, 1295f
Illiteracy, teaching and, 391
Illness. *See also* Health-illness status
  acute, definition of, 59–60
  adaptation to, 761–762
  behavior stages in, 60–61
  chronic, definition of, 61
  definition of, 53
  family affected by, 27–28, 61, 763
  full stage of, 558
  mobility and, 1023–1024
  prevention of, 59–61, 59t. *See also* Preventive care
    exercise in, 1022
    as nursing aim, 10
    risk factors in, 59, 59t
  risk factors in, prevention and, 59, 59t
  self-concept and, 732t, 733, 733f
  sensory stimulation in, 819
  skin condition in, 913–914, 917t
  sleep quality and, 1080
  urine production and, 1216
Imagery, in pain relief, 1124
Immobility
  in bed rest
    passive exercise in, 1037
    skin alteration risks and, 917t
  effects of
    on cardiovascular system, 1011t–1012t, 1017, 1018f, 1019
    on gastrointestinal system, 1014t, 1018f, 1021
    on metabolism, 1013t–1014t, 1018f, 1020–1021
    on musculoskeletal system, 1013t, 1018f, 1019–1020
    psychosocial, 1015t, 1021–1022
    on respiratory system, 1012t–1013t, 1018f, 1019
    on skin, 1014t, 1018f, 1021
    on urinary system, 1014t, 1018f, 1021
  pressure ulcer formation and, 975
Immune response, definition of, 558
Immunity, in infants, 131
Immunization
  for hepatitis B, 136t
  of infants, 136t
Immunoglobulins, development of, in infant, 131
Imodium (loperamide), in diarrhea, 1286
Impaction, fecal, removal of, 1289, 1292–1293, 1294f
Impaled object wound, emergency care of, 705
Implanted port, for intravenous therapy, 1409, 1411f
Implementation, potential liability in, 103t
Implementing, 225, 227t, 228, 300–312. *See also specific type of care, e.g.,* Personal hygiene; Interventions; Preoperative care
  client need for assistance and, 307
  communication in, 365
  computers in, 311
  coordination of, 303
  core competencies for, 304, 306
  counseling in, 307
  data collection during, 311
  definition of, 301, 303f
  delegation of, 304, 306–307
  evaluation of, 325
    checklist of, 325
    problems in, 322t
  focus of, 301–303, 304f, 305t
  guidelines for, 307
  illustration of, 228
  in noncompliance, 308, 310
  overview of, 303f
  protocols in, 302–303
  self-care and, 304, 307
  standing orders in, 302–303
  student responsibilities in, 310–311
  taxonomy structure for, 302, 305f
  variables influencing, 303f, 307–308
Imposition, cultural, 34
Impotence, 859, 860t, 862
  in diabetes mellitus, 849
Imprisonment, false, 101
Incentive spirometry, 1329–1330
  postoperative, 684
Incident report, 107–108, 551
Incision, definition of, 699t
Incompetence
  ethical problems with, 91–92
  reporting of, 243–244
Incomplete protein, definition of, 1155
Incontinence, pressure ulcer risk and, 980
Incontinence (fecal)
  causes of, 1283
  characteristics of, 1283
  definition of, 1302
  management of, 1293–1295, 1303
Incontinence (urinary), 1230, 1232, 1234–1235
  case study of, 1258–1261
  causes of, 1227
  characteristics of, 1227
  definition of, 1213, 1219
  diagnosis of, 1232, 1234
  in elderly persons, 1229–1230
  functional, 1227, 1232
  in home care, 1234–1235
  incidence of, 1230
  information resources for, 1250
  overflow, 1230, 1232
  reflex, 1227
  stress, 1227, 1230
  total, 1227
  treatment of, 1234
  types of, 1230, 1232
  urge, 1227, 1230
Incubation period, of pathogen, 558
Independence, in home healthcare, 210
Independent interventions, 301
Independent nursing actions, definition of, 19
Independent variables, in research, 423
Individual supply system, for medications, 605
Inductive reasoning, 66
Industry
  healthcare in, 180
  vs. inferiority in school-age children, 118, 118f, 141
Indwelling catheter. *See under* Catheter(ization) (urinary)
Infants. *See also* Neonates
  accident prevention and, 526
  blood pressure in, 459t
  body alignment of, 1008t
  body fluid variations in, 1367, 1369t
  bowel elimination in, 1269t
  cognitive development in, 119, 121f
  day-care centers for, 178–179
  developmental tasks of, 118, 118f, 118t
  drug action in, 598
  drug administration to, 610, 614
  drug dosage calculations for, 608, 608f
  growth and development of

cognitive, 133
health problems, 133–134
physiologic, 132–133
psychosocial, 133
health problems of, 133–134
immunization of, 136t
mobility of, 1008t
nutrition for, 133, 135t, 1163, 1166t
pain perception of, 1112
pulse rate of, 449t
recommended daily allowances for, 1447t–1448t
recommended nutrient intake for, 1449t–1450t
respiratory function of, 1316, 1316t
safety considerations for, 536, 536t–537t, 538
sexuality of, 117, 117t, 850t
skin condition of, 913
sleep in, 1077t
surgery risk and, 673
trust development in, 118, 118f
urination in, 1214
urine specimen collection from, 1219–1220, 1223f
wellness promotion in, 134, 135t–136t
Infection(s)
body defense against, 558
cycle of, 560–561
definition of, 556
detection of, 556
in elderly persons, 559
risks for, 559
endogenous, 561
exogenous, 561
iatrogenic, 561
in intravenous therapy, 1423t
nosocomial, 561–562
nursing diagnosis of, 560
in parenteral nutrition, 1196
prevention of. *See* Infection control and prevention
risk of, 558–559
stages of, 557–558
of stomal, in enteral nutrition, 1191
transmission of, nosocomial, 561–562
in urinary catheterization, 1236–1237, 1257–1258
of wound, 699t, 702–703
dressing changes in, 722
Infection control and prevention
accidental exposure reports in, 588
assessment of, 559
body defenses in, 558
disinfection in, 563, 566, 567t
in dressing change, 722
ethical issues in, 587–588
handwashing in, 562–565
in home healthcare, 213–214
infection cycle and, 556–557, 557f, 558t
infection risks and, 558–559
infection stages and, 557–558
isolation in, 571, 576–581, 576f, 577t
medical asepsis in, 561–563
nosocomial, 561–562
nurse responsible for, 589
nursing diagnosis of, 560
personal protective equipment for, 582–587, 586f
planning for, 560
in pressure ulcers, 988–990
principles of, 561
sterilization in, 563, 566, 567t
surgical asepsis in, 566–568, 568f, 571f–572f
teaching about, 560–561
Infectious agents, 566–567
accidental exposure to, 588
transmission of, 557, 558t
Infiltration, in intravenous therapy, 1422t
Inflammatory response, 758
definition of, 558
in healing, 700–701
Information management. *See* Documentation; Reporting
Informed consent
checklist for, 100
ethical problems with, 88
legal aspects of, 99, 100f
refusal of, 99
in research, 423
for surgery, 672
Infusion pump, in intravenous therapy, 1414
Inhalation
definition of, 455
medication administration by, 655–656
process of, 1313
Inhalers, for nebulized medications, 1335, 1337–1338
Inhibited grief, 782
Initiative, vs. guilt in preschool children, 118, 139
Injections
drug packaging for, 616–621, 617f
equipment for, 616, 616f–617f
intradermal, administration of, 623
procedure for, 625–626
intramuscular, administration of
discomfort reduction in, 636–637
pain in, 632–635
procedure for, 632–635, 636f
sites for, 627, 631–632, 631f
Z-track technique in, 632, 635–636, 636f
removing medication from packaging for, procedures for, 617–621
subcutaneous, administration of, 626–627, 627f
procedure for, 629–631
surgical asepsis for, 616
Injury. *See also* Wounds
back, in nursing activities, 1023
in elderly persons, 152
in exercise, 1023
fractures in
mobility and, 1010
pathologic, in immobility, 1013t
inflammatory response to, 758
to musculoskeletal system, mobility and, 1010
reflex pain response to, 758
self-concept and, 733
systemic response to, 700
Inner canthus of eye, cleaning of, 952
Inpatient services, 176
Insensible water loss, 1374, 1374f
imbalances resulting from, 1390t
Insertion, of muscle, 1003, 1003f
In-service education, 15
Insomnia, 1081, 1082t, 1093–1094
Inspection
in physical assessment, 478–479
abdomen, 504, 506, 1272–1273
breast, 503
of genitalia, 507–508
peripheral vascular system, 502
precordium, 498–499, 501f
respiratory system, 1319
skin, 482–483, 483f, 483t
thorax, 496, 496f
precordial, 498–499, 501f
of pressure ulcers, 979–980, 982f
Inspiration (inhalation), 455, 1313
Inspiratory capacity (IC), 1322t
Inspiratory reserve volume, 1322t
Instillation
into ear, 652–653
of eyedrops, 646, 650
into nose, 652–653, 655
Institutional care plans, 290–291
Instructor, liability of, 109
Instruments, for physical assessment, 474–476, 475f
Insulins, mixing of, in one syringe, 622
procedure for, 623–624
Insurance
healthcare, 186
professional liability, 108
Intake-output measurement, of fluids, 1391, 1392t, 1397
Intal (cromolyn sodium), in respiratory disorders, 1336t
Integument. *See also* Hair; Nails; Skin
assessment of, 482–485, 483f, 483t–484t, 485f
definition of, 911
Intellectual dimension, in health-illness status, 56
Intellectual needs, health-illness status and, 58
Intelligence, in older adults, 157, 160
Intentional wound, 699
Intention tremor, definition of, 1024
Interchange, mutual, rewards of, 240–241, 240f
Intercourse, sexual, 844, 848
Interdependent interventions, 301
Interdependent nursing actions, 19
Intermittent catheters, 1235

Intermittent fever, 438t
Intermittent medication administration, intravenous, 637, 642f
Intermittent pneumatic compression stockings, 930
Intermittent positive-pressure breathing, 1348
Intermittent pulse, 450f
Internal resources, self-concept and, 731
Internal rotation, definition of, 1000t, 1001f–1002f
International Council of Nurses, 15
  code of ethics of, 85
  nursing defined by, 7
Interpersonal core competencies, 233, 235
  in communication, 375–377, 377t–378t
  development of, 238–241, 240f
Interstitial fluid, 1367, 1368f, 1369t
  electrolyte composition of, 1369f
Interstitial-to-plasma fluid shift, definition of, 1379
Interventions. *See also* Implementing
  derived from nursing diagnosis, 287–289, 288f
  types of, 301
Intervertebral disc syndrome, 1105t
Interview
  in assessing, 250–252, 253t
  questions in, 370–371
  techniques for, 373–374
Intestinal distention, 1284. *See also* Flatulence/flatus
Intestinal juice, loss of, imbalances resulting from, 1390t
Intimacy, vs. isolation in young adult, 118, 119f
Intracellular fluid, 1367, 1368f, 1369t
  electrolyte composition of, 1368, 1369f
Intractable pain, 1109
Intradermal injection, administration of, 625
  procedure for, 625–626
Intramuscular injections. *See under* Injections
Intraoperative care, 687–688
Intraoperative phase, definition of, 670
Intrauterine device, as contraceptive method, 867–868
Intravascular fluid, 1367, 1368f
Intravenous pyelography, 1224, 1226t
Intravenous therapy
  ambulation with, 1051–1052, 1052f
  with blood and blood products. *See* Blood transfusions
  central venous catheter for, 1403, 1409f
  changing solution/tubing, 1415
    procedure for, 1416–1418
  complications of, 1415, 1422t–1423t
  discontinuance of, 1423
  equipment for, 1402–1405, 1404f
  flow rate calculation in, 1412–1413
  gown removal with, 926
  heparin lock in, 1415, 1423
    procedure for, 1424
  in home care, 1423
  implanted port in, 1409, 1411f
  intermittent
    central venous catheter in, 641–642
    medication administration in, piggyback, 637, 642f, 643–644
    tandem, 637, 642f
  medication administration in
    adding to solution containers, procedure for, 638–639
    with bolus, 637
      procedure for, 640–641
    continuous, 637
    with controlled-administration set, 637, 646f
    dangers of, 637
    with heparin lock, 637, 641–642, 1415, 1424
      procedure for, 647–649
    intermittent, 637, 642f
      piggyback, 637, 642f, 643–644
    with volume-administration set, procedure for, 645–646
  microdrip equipment for, 1412
  minidrip equipment for, 1412
  monitoring of, 1412, 1414–1415, 1415f
    procedure for, 1418–1420
  regulation of, 1412, 1414–1415, 1415f
    procedure for, 1413–1414
  sites for
    care of, 1415
      procedure for, 1421
    selection of, 1411–1412, 1411f
  solutions for, 1403t
  starting of, 1412
    procedure for, 1405–1409
  teaching about, 1423
  venous access devices for, 1403–1404, 1409, 1410f–1411f
Introjection, as defense mechanism, 760
Intuitive problem solving, 227–228
Inunction, definition of, 642
Invasion of privacy, 100–101
Inversion, definition of, 1000t, 1002f
Involuntary coughing, 1331
Iodine, dietary, 1160t
Ion, definition of, 1368
Iris, examination of, 487, 487f–488f
Iron, dietary, 1160t
Iron deficiency anemia, 1201–1202
Irrigation
  of colostomy, 1297
  of ear, 652–653
    procedure for, 654–655
  of eye, 650
    procedure for, 651–652
  of indwelling urinary catheter, 1238
    procedure for, 1246–1249
  of nasogastric tube, 1191–1192
    procedure for, 1195–1196
  of needles, in intravenous therapy, 1415
  of pressure ulcer, 988
  of wound, 716
    procedure for, 718–720
IRV (inspiratory reserve volume), definition of, 1322t
Ischemia, in pressure ulcer formation, 975
Islam, 887
Isokinetic exercise, 1016f, 1017
Isolation
  body substance, 578–580
  category-specific, 571, 577t
  Centers for Disease Control recommendations on, 580–587, 586f
  definition of, 571
  disease-specific categories in, 572
  in dying, 782
  protective equipment for, 582–587
  psychologic needs in, 587
  social, in older adults, 162
  transmission barriers in, 571, 576f, 586f
  universal precautions in, 572, 576–577
Isometric exercise, 1016, 1016f
Isoproterenol (Isuprel), in respiratory disorders, 1336t
Isotonic exercise, 1016, 1016f
Isotonic solutions
  definition of, 1372
  for intravenous therapy, 1403t
Isuprel (isoproterenol), in respiratory disorders, 1336t
IUD (intrauterine device), as contraceptive method, 867–868

Jackson-Pratt drain tube, 708t, 721, 721f
Jaundice
  appearance of, 483, 483t
  in neonates, 132
  skin condition in, 913
JCAHO (Joint Commission of Accreditation of Healthcare Organizations), documentation standards of, 330–331
Jehovah's Witnesses, 886t
Jejunostomy, in tube feeding, 1181–1182
Jewelry, removal of, for surgery, 686
Jewish people
  pain attitudes of, 1111
  religious traditions of, 885–886
  Tay-Sachs disease in, 39
Johnson, Dorothy E., behavioral systems model of nursing, 70t, 73
Joint Commission of Accreditation of Healthcare Organizations, documentation standards of, 330–331
Joints
  diseases of, sexuality and, 851

examination of, 509
function of, 1000
mobility of
assessment of, 1026t, 1027
problems affecting, 1007, 1010
range of motion of, 1001f–1002f, 1027
support of, in range-of-motion exercise, 1037, 1039, 1039f
types of, 1000
Judaism, 885–886
Judgmental comments, 371
Jugular vein
central venous catheter in, 1403, 1409f
implanted port in, 1409
Justice
as essential value, 80
in ethical code, 83

Kaopectate, in diarrhea, 1287
Kardex system
for medication records, 604, 607f
for nursing care, 291
Kegel exercises
sexuality and, 863–864
urinary elimination and, 1228
Keloid
definition of, 484t
formation of, ethnic differences in, 39
Kidney
acid-base balance and, 1377
drug toxicity to, 1216
dysfunction of, as surgical risk, 675
examination of, 1217
fluid/electrolyte homeostasis and, 1374, 1374f, 1375t
physiology of, 1212, 1213f
stones in, from immobility, 1021
Kinesthesia
assessment of, 822
definition of, 814
impairment of, characteristics of, 823
Kinesthetic sense, 1005
King, Imogene M., open systems framework model of nursing, 70t, 72
Knee-chest position, 477f, 478
Knee reflex, assessment of, 515t, 517
Knots, for restraints, 546
Knowledge, roots of, in research, 422–423
Knowledge deficit, in sexuality, 872–873
case study of, 874–878
Kohlberg moral development theory, 119–121
adolescents and, 146
preschool children and, 140
school-age children and, 141
Korotkoff sounds, in blood pressure assessment, 461–462, 462t
Kübler-Ross stages of grief and death reactions, 782
Kussmaul respiration, 498f
Kwashiorkor, 1156

Labeling, of food, 1163, 1164f
Labia, minora and majora, 841, 842f
Laboratory tests
abbreviations in, 1441
in fluid balance assessment, 1391
for nutritional status, 1174–1175, 1178
preoperative, 578
reference ranges for
blood, 1442t–1444t
cerebrospinal fluid, 1445t
hematologic studies, 1441t–1442t
hormones, 1445t–1446t
plasma, 1442t–1444t
serum, 1442t–1444t
urine, 1444t–1445t
Labyrinthine sense, 1005
Laceration
definition of, 699t
emergency care of, 705
Lactase deficiency, ethnic differences in, 39
Lactated Ringer's solution, for intravenous therapy, 1403t
Lactation, nutrition in
recommended daily allowances for, 1447t–1448t
recommended nutrient intake for, 1449t–1450t
Lactic acid, as electrolyte, 1371
Laissez-faire leadership, 414–415
Language, 360
assessment of, 512
body (nonverbal communication), 360, 361f–362f
development of
in infants, 133
in preschool children, 139
in toddlers, 136
disorders of, 378–380
interviewing in, 253t
of foreign-born clients, 35–36
Large intestine, physiology of, 1266–1268, 1267f
Laryngectomy, communication in, 381
Laryngoscopy, 1323t
Latency stage, in Freudian theory, 117, 117t
school-age children in, 141
Lateral position, protective, 1034, 1036f
Latex materials, allergy to, 582–583
Lavage, intestinal, oral, 1289
Laws. *See also* Legal issues
administrative, 96
civil, 96
common, 96–97
constitutional, 96
on controlled substances, 109–110, 609
definition of, 96
good Samaritan, 108
Occupational Safety and Health Act, 109
public, 96
on reportable crimes and diseases, 109–110
sources of, 96–97
statutory, 96
on wills, 110
Lawsuit (litigation), 97
malpractice, 101–102, 105f
Laxatives, 1285–1286, 1286t
Leadership, 412–421
areas of, 419–420, 420f
autocratic, 414
change effected through, 416–418
client care delivery models and, 416
definition of, 412
democratic, 414
development of skills for, 413
group dynamics and, 379, 382–383, 383t
laissez-faire, 414–415
management and, 416
nurse role in, 10t
qualities of, 412
skills for, 412, 414, 418
styles of, 414–416, 414f
training for, 420–421, 421f
transformational, 415–416
Learning. *See also* Counseling; Education; Teaching
ability to, 393
in adults, 389, 391
affective, 388, 395
assessment of needs for, 392, 393f
cognitive, 388, 395
definition of, 388
developmental considerations in, 388–389, 391
documentation of, 404
domains of, 388, 395
evaluation of, 402–404, 403f
implementation of teaching plan in, 401–402, 402f
need diagnosis in, 393
nursing diagnosis in, 408–409
planning for, 393–401
content of, 394
contracts in, 398
formal vs. informal teaching in, 403–404
group vs. individual teaching in, 400–401
learner objectives in, 394
sample plan for, 390t
scheduling in, 400
teaching strategies for, 390t, 395–398
time constraints in, 400
principles of, 391–392
psychomotor, 388, 395
readiness for, 392, 393f
reinforcement of, 402–403
strengths in, 393
Leavell-Clark agent-host-environment model, of health and illness, 54–55, 55f
Lectures, as teaching strategy, 395
Legal issues, 95–111
assault and battery, 99

Legal issues *(continued)*
  in assessing, 263
  of client record, 333
  controlled substance use, 109–110
  core competencies in, 235, 241–243
  credentialing, 98
  crimes, 98–99
  in death and dying, 110, 784–786, 786f–788f, 789
  defamation, 99–100
  definitions in, 96–97
  discrimination, 110
  in documentation, 333, 339
  false imprisonment, 101
  fraud, 101
  in home healthcare, 210–211, 211t
  invasion of privacy, 100–101
  laws. *See* Laws
  liability
    elements of, 101, 102t
    potential areas of, 103t–104t
    of students, 109
  litigation, 97
  malpractice, 101–102, 105f
  in meeting client goals, 308
  negligence, 99, 101–104, 102t–104t, 105f
  of nursing practice, 16–17
  nursing practice regulation, 12, 16–17, 97–98, 97f
  occupational regulations, 109
  in pain management, 1137–1138
  persons with disabilities, 110
  religious beliefs and, 889
  reporting obligations, 109–110
  safeguards against malpractice, 104–108, 106f
  sexual harassment, 110
  standards for nursing practice, 102, 103t–104t
  student liability, 109
  torts. *See* Torts
  wills, 110
Legal safeguards
  awareness of potential liability, 103t–104t
  client education guidelines, 104–105
  competent practice, 104, 106f
  contracts, 104
  documentation, 106–107, 339
  execution of physician's orders, guidelines for, 105–106
  Good Samaritan laws, 108
  in home healthcare, 210–211, 211t
  incident reports, 108
  insurance, 108
  interventions to reduce common risks, 106t–107t
  risk management program, 108
  understaffing, avoidance of, 107–108
Leg exercises, postoperative, 684, 684f
Legislation
  drug, 594, 609
  nurse's involvement with, 420, 420f, 427
Leininger, Madeline, transcultural nursing theory of, 43, 70t, 72–73
Lens, contact, care of, 953–954
Lesbian, definition of, 847
Lethargy, definition of, 509
Levine, Myra E., theory of nursing, 70t, 73
Levinson individual life structure theory, 150
Liability
  elements of, 101, 102t
  potential areas of, 103t–104t
  of student nurses, 109
Libel, 100
Libido
  in adolescent, 143
  in Freudian theory, 117
Lice infestation, 955–956
Licensure, for nursing practice, 98
  education for, 16–17
  examinations for, 12
Lichenification, of skin, 484t
Lidocaine, in intravenous therapy, for needle insertion, 1412
Life changes, stress in, 758
Life events, spirituality and, 890
Life review, by elderly persons, 161, 161f
Lifestyle
  accidents caused by, 527
  active vs. sedentary, 1010, 1015
  bowel elimination and, 1270
  changing of, in obesity treatment, 1200
  infection risk and, 559
  respiratory function and, 1317
  sensory function and, 819
  sensory stimulation and, 819
  sexuality and, 849
  skin alteration risks and, 917t
  sleep and, 1080
  as surgical risk, 676
  urination and, 1214–1215
  of young adults, 152
Lifting. *See also* Movement, of client by nurse
  guidelines for, 1039–1040
  with hydraulic lift, 1048, 1050f
Lifts, with heartbeat, 499
Ligaments, 1000
Light, pupillary reaction to, 487, 487f
Lighting, at bedside unit, 939
Line of gravity, in body alignment, 1004, 1004f
Liniment, definition of, 596t
Linoleic acid, as essential fatty acid, 1157
Lip(s)
  examination of, 493
  ulceration of, 944
Lipids, 1154t, 1156–1157, 1157f
  in emulsions, for parenteral nutrition, 1193
Liquids
  diet restricted to, 1181
  sterile, handling of, 568, 572f
Listening
  need for, 884
  skills for, 370, 372–373, 373f
Literacy, learning and, 391
Lithium carbonate, sexual function effects of, 856t
Lithotomy position, 477f, 478, 688
Litigation, 97
Liver, dysfunction of, as surgical risk, 675
Liver spots, on skin, 913
Living will, legal aspects of, 785, 787f–788f, 789–790
Local adaptation syndrome, 758
Local anesthesia, in pain management, 1136–1137
Localized symptoms, definition of, 558
Logrolling, 1048, 1050f
Long-term care
  facilities for, 180
  insurance for, 186
  nursing activities in, 178
  transfer to, 197, 200
Loperamide, in diarrhea, 1286
Loss. *See also* Death and dying; Grief
  as nursing diagnosis, 794
  spiritual, 890, 894
  types of, 781
Lotion
  application of, 646
  bath with, 920, 927
  definition of, 596t
Loudness, in auscultation, 480
Love, as human need, 23–24, 23f
Love and belonging needs, stress effects on, 761
Loyalty, ethical problems with, 92
Lozenge
  cough, 1332
  definition of, 596t
Lung
  acid-base balance and, 1376–1377
  compliance of, 1314
  congestion in, 1331
  examination of, 495–497, 495f–500f
  fluid/electrolyte homeostasis and, 1374, 1374f, 1375t
  function of, 1312–1316, 1313f–1314f
  pressure changes in, 1313
Lung scan, 1324t
Luteal phase, of ovarian cycle, 843, 843f
Lying position, body alignment in, 1027, 1029f
Lyme disease, transmission of, 558t
Lymph nodes
  axillary, palpation of, 503, 504f
  of neck, examination of, 494, 494f
Lysis, in fever resolution, 438t

Macrominerals, 1160t
Macronutrients, definition of, 1150
Macroshock, from electric equipment, 550

Macule, definition of, 484t
Magnesium
  dietary, 1160t, 1371
  as electrolyte, 1369f, 1370–1371
  imbalance of, 1379–1380, 1381t
Magnetic resonance imaging, 521t
Malabsorption, 1178
Maladaptation, to body image disturbance, 736
Male
  breast of, 845
  genitalia of
    examination of, 508, 508f, 860–861
    physiology of, 844–845
  sexual dysfunction in, 859, 860t
  sexual response pattern in, 845–846, 845f
  urinary catheterization of, procedure for, 1243–1245
  urine specimen collection from, 1222–1223
Malnutrition
  clinical signs of, 1174, 1177t
  in immobility, 1020
  in pressure ulcer formation, 975
  protein-calorie, 1156
  risk factors for
    anthropometric, 1174
    dietary, 1172
    socioeconomic, 1173, 1175t
  skin alteration risks and, 917t
Malpractice, 101–102, 105f
  prevention of, 106–107
Managed care systems, 182
Management, leadership and, 416
Managerial responsibility, 416, 419
Manganese, dietary, 1160t
Manometer, in blood pressure equipment, 460–561, 461f
  care of, 468
Many-tailed binders, application of, 713, 715f
Marasmus, 1156
Marijuana, sexual function effects of, 856t
Mask
  in care of isolated client, 586
  oxygen administration by, 1333–1334, 1340, 1340t
    procedure for, 1342–1343
Maslow's hierarchy of needs, 67
  application of, 24
  health-illness status and, 57–58
  levels of, 22, 23f
  nursing diagnosis and, 278
  stress effects on, 761
Masochism, definition of, 848
Massage
  back, 930
  in pain relief, 1125, 1127f
    procedure for, 1126
Mastectomy, sexuality and, 853, 873–874
Masturbation, 848
Mattress
  body alignment and, 1032
  comfort of, 940, 940f
Maturation. *See also* Developmental theory; Growth and development
  developmental tasks and, 120
Maturation phase, of healing, 701
Maxillary sinuses, physical assessment of, 492, 492f
Meals on Wheels, 181
Meaning of life, importance of, 884
Measles, immunization for, 136t
Measurements
  apothecary, 607, 1439, 1440t
  household, 607, 1439, 1439t
  metric, 605, 607, 1438–1439, 1440t
Mechanical ventilation, 1348
  weaning from, in terminal illness, 791
Mechanics, body. *See* Body mechanics
Medicaid, 184–185, 185t
Medical asepsis
  definition of, 560
  handwashing in, 562–563
    procedure for, 564–565
  principles of, 562
Medical diagnosis, vs. nursing diagnosis, 267, 271t
Medical history. *See* Health history
Medical record. *See* Client record
Medicare, 184–185, 185t
  documentation for, 339
Medications. *See* Drugs/medications
Meditation, in stress management, 770
Memory
  assessment of, 512
  in older adults, 157
Menarche, definition of, 843
Meniscus, in manometer reading, 461, 461f
Menopause, 154, 843
Menses, definition of, 843–844, 843f
Menstrual cycle, 843–844, 843f
Mental health, homeostasis in, 757–758
Mental health centers, 179
Mental illness, sexuality and, 853
Mental status
  assessment of, 509, 512, 512t
  cultural considerations in, 41
  of elderly persons, 157, 160
  mobility and, 1010
  pressure ulcer formation and, 977
  in sensory deprivation, 831
Mentorship, in leadership training, 420–421
Mesoderm, development of, 129
Messages, in communication, 340t, 359, 360f
Metabolic acidosis. *See under* Acidosis
Metabolic alkalosis. *See under* Alkalosis
Metabolism
  basal, 1150–1151
  of carbohydrates, 1153, 1155f
  disorders of
    in parenteral nutrition, 1196
    as surgical risk, 675
  of drugs, 597
  exercise effects on, 1010f, 1020
  immobility effects on, 1013t–1014t, 1018f, 1020–1021
  of lipids, 1157, 1157f
  of protein, 1155, 1156f
  water produced in, 1373–1374, 1374f
Metacarpal veins, intravenous therapy in, 1411f
Metamucil (psyllium mucilloid), as laxative, 1285, 1286t
Metaproterenol (Alupent), in respiratory disorders, 1336t
Metered-dose inhaler, 1335, 1337
Methicillin, resistance to, 561
Methyldopa, sexual function effects of, 856t
Metric system, 605, 607, 1438–1439, 1440t
Metronidazole (Flagyl), in sexually transmitted disease, 854t–855t
Microminerals, 1160t–1161t
Micronutrients, definition of, 1150
Microorganisms. *See also* Infection(s)
  as normal inhabitant of body site, 556
  normal population of, 556
Microshock, from electric equipment, 550
Microwave, for "bag bath," 927, 927f
Micturition. *See also* Urination
  definition of, 1213–1214
  factors affecting, 1214–1216
  frequency of, 1214
Midarm circumference, in nutritional assessment, 1174
Midlife transition, 155
Midstream urine specimen, collection of, 1220, 1222–1223
Midwife, nurse, 11t
Military agencies, healthcare services of, 181
Milk, intolerance of, ethnic differences in, 39
Milk of magnesia, as laxative, 1285
Mind-body interaction, in stress, 757–758
Mineral(s)
  dietary, 1160t–1161t
  recommended daily allowances for, 1448t
Mineral-electrolyte preparations, for electrolyte imbalance correction, 1402
Mineral oil, as laxative, 1285, 1286t
Minimum data set, nursing, 333, 342
Minority group, in culture, 33
Miosis, 487
Misdemeanor, definition of, 99
Missionary position, in intercourse, 849
Mittelschmerz, 843
Mobility. *See also* Immobility; Movement
  assessment of, pressure ulcer risk and, 980
  attitudes toward, 1015

Mobility *(continued)*
  developmental considerations and, 1006, 1008t–1009t
  external factors affecting, 1016
  health status and, 1006
  impaired
    case study of, 1062–1068
    causes of, 1030
    characteristics of, 1030
    safety precautions in, 527–528
  lifestyle and, 1010, 1015
  mental status and, 1010
  sensory stimulation and, 831
  stress and, 1016
Models, for nursing theory. *See also under* Nursing theory
  definition of, 66
Moisture, skin, pressure ulcer formation and, 975, 977, 980
Mole (nevus), definition of, 484t
Molybdenum, dietary, 1160t
Monitoring, inadequate, legal aspects of, 106
Monosaccharides, definition of, 1153
Montgomery straps, for frequent dressing change, 721, 721f
Moral development theory of Kohlberg. *See under* Developmental theory
Moral dilemma, 86
Moral distress, 86
Morality, definition of, 83
Moral problems. *See* Ethical problems
Mormons, 886t
Morning care (AM care), 918
Moro reflex, 131f
Morphine, 1128
Motivational counseling, 407–408
Motor skills, assessment of, 514
Mourning, definition of, 781
Mouth
  anatomy of, 493f
  care of. *See* Oral care
  dryness of, 944
    in fluid volume deficit, 1393t
  examination of, 492–493, 493f
Mouth-to-mouth resuscitation, 1358
Mouthwash, in oral care, 950
Movement. *See also* Activity; Exercise; Gait; Immobility; Mobility
  assessment of, 1023–1029, 1026t, 1027f–1029f
  body alignment and. *See* Body alignment
  of client by nurse
    from bed to chair, 1040, 1049
      procedures for, 1045–1049
    from bed to stretcher, 1040
      procedures for, 1042–1045
    coordinated body movement in, 1004
    guidelines for, 1039–1040
    to head of bed, 1040
      procedure for, 1041–1042
    hydraulic lift in, 1048, 1050f
    lifting guidelines, 1039–1040
    logrolling, 1048, 1050f
    up in bed, 1040
      procedure for, 1041–1042
  ease of, 1024–1026, 1026t, 1027f–1029f
  factors affecting, 1006–1016
    attitude, 1015
    developmental, 1006, 1008t–1009t
    external, 1016
    fatigue, 1016
    health status, 1006–1007, 1010, 1011t–1015t
    lifestyle variables, 1010, 1015
    mental health, 1010
    stress, 1016
  implementing strategies and, 1031
    ambulation assistance, 1048–1056
    exercise programs, 1037, 1039, 1039f
    positioning, 1031–1038, 1032f–1034f, 1035t–1036t, 1037f
    range-of-motion exercises, 1037, 1039, 1039f
  involuntary, 1024–1025
  joints and, 1000
  nursing diagnosis of, 1029–1030
  physiology of
    body mechanics in, 1003–1006
    muscular system in, 1003, 1003f
    nervous system in, 1003
    skeletal system in, 999–1000, 1001f–1002f
  planning and, 1031
  problems with, case study in, 1062–1068
  terminology of, 1000t
Mucosal route, for drug application. *See* Topical medications
Mucous membrane, functions of, 912, 913t
Mumps, immunization for, 136t
Murmurs, heart, 502, 502t
Muscles
  atrophy of, 509
    definition of, 1003, 1027, 1029
    in immobility, 1019
  contraction of, in exercise, 1016–1017, 1016f
  of elderly person, 159
  examination of, 509, 510f–511f
  flaccidity of, 1029
  functions of, 1003, 1003f
  hypertrophy of, 1029
  malfunction of, mobility and, 1007
  mass of, assessment of, 1026t, 1027, 1029
  movement of, 999, 1003, 1003f
  relaxation of, in stress management, 770
  in respiration, 1313
  spasticity of, 1029
  strength of, assessment of, 1026t, 1029
  tone of, 1004
    assessment of, 509, 1026t, 1029
    bowel elimination and, 1270
    urinary elimination and, 1215–1216, 1228
  types of, 1003, 1003f
  weakness of, in immobility, 1018f, 1019
Muscular dystrophy, mobility in, 1007
Musculoskeletal system. *See also* Bones; Muscles; Skeletal system
  disorders of, mobility and, 1006–1007, 1010
  examination of, 508–509, 510f–511f
  exercise effects on, 1018f, 1019
  immobility effects on, 1018f, 1019–1020
  pain syndromes involving, 1105t
Mustache, care of, 957
Mutual interchange, rewards of, 240–241, 240f
Mydriasis, 487
Myocardial infarction, sexuality and, 851
Myoclonus, 1025
  nocturnal, 1086
Myofascial pain syndrome, 1105t
Myometrium, definition of, 842

Nails
  abnormalities of, 485, 485f
  care of, 958–959
  examination of, 485, 485f
Naloxone, in opioid reversal, 1129
Names, of drugs, 594–595
NANDA (North American Nursing Diagnosis Association), 224
  diagnosis list of, 273–274
Narcolepsy, 1081, 1082t
Narcotics. *See* Opioids (narcotics)
Narrative notes, in client record, 334, 335t–336t, 338t, 346f
Nasal. *See* Nose
Nasogastric tube
  aspiration from, 1186
  in decompression, 1193
    procedure for, 1195–1196
  in enteral nutrition. *See* Enteral nutrition
  insertion of, procedure for, 1183–1186
  monitoring of, procedure for, 1193
  removal of, 1193
    procedure for, 1194
Nasointestinal tube, for enteral nutrition, 1181
Nasopharyngeal airway, 1344
Nasopharyngeal tube, suctioning with, procedures for, 1349–1354
National Center for Nursing Research, 421–422
National Council Licensure Examination
  for practical nurses (NCLEX-PN), 12
  for registered nurses (NCLEX-RN), 12

National Formulary, 594
National League for Nursing, 15
  accreditation of nursing schools by, 98
National Medical Care Insurance Program, of Canada, 185
National Practitioner Data Bank, 109
National Student Nurses Association, 15
Native Americans
  cultural characteristics of, 49t
  religions of, 887–888
Natural family planning, 866
Nausea and vomiting
  postoperative, 697
  in pregnancy, case study of, 1202–1206
Nebulization
  medication administration by, 655–656
  in respiratory disorders, 1335, 1337–1338
Neck
  anatomy of, 492f, 494f
  examination of, 493–494, 494f. *See* Physical assessment, of head and neck
  range of motion of, 1001f
Neck vein distention, fluid balance and, 1395t
Necrosis, in pressure ulcer formation, 973, 980, 982f
Needleless systems, for drug administration, 616, 617f
Needles
  for injections, 616, 616f
  for intravenous therapy, 1402
  irrigation of, 1415
  safe handling of, 576–578
Needs, human. *See* Human needs
Negative reinforcement, in learning, 403
Negativism, in toddlers, 137, 138t
Negligence, 99
  prevention of, 106–107
  by student nurses, 109
Neonates
  blood pressure of, 459t
  body alignment in, 1008t
  growth and development of, 130–132, 130t
  health problems of, 131–132
  mobility in, 1008t
  physical characteristics of, 131–132
  pulse rate of, 449t
  respiratory function in, 1316
  safety considerations for, 536t
Nephrons, function of, 1212
Nerve block, 672, 1136–1137
Nerves, electrical stimulation of, in pain management, 1125, 1127f
Nervous system. *See also* Brain; Spinal cord
  of elderly person, 159
  examination of, 509–517
    cranial nerve function, 512–514, 514f
    mental status, 509, 512, 512t
    motor abilities, 514
    reflexes, 514–515, 515t–517t
    sensory abilities, 514
  fluid/electrolyte homeostasis and, 1374
  functions of, in movement, 1003
Neuman, Betty, health-care systems model of nursing, 71t, 73
Neuralgia
  postherpetic, 1105t
  trigeminal, 1105t
Neurectomy, in pain management, 1137
Neuroleptics, preoperative, 686
Neurologic hammer, in physical assessment, 475f, 476
Neuromodulators, of pain, 1108
Neuromuscular irritability, in electrolyte imbalance, 1395t–1396t
Neurons, 1003
Neurosurgery, in pain management, 1137
Neurotransmitters, of pain, 1104
Nevus, definition of, 484t
Newborns. *See* Neonates
NF (National Formulary), 594
Niacin, 1159t
Nightingale, Florence, 6, 7f
  nursing theory of, 68, 68f
Night terrors, 1083t
Nipple, examination of, 503
Nitrogen balance, 1155, 1156f
  negative, in immobility, 1020
Nits, 955
Nociceptors, 1104
No-code orders, 790
Nocturia, 1219
  in older adults, 1229
Nocturnal emission, 845
Nocturnal enuresis, 1256
Nocturnal myoclonus, 1086
Nodule, skin, definition of, 484t
Noise, at bedside unit, 939
Noncompliance, implementing in, 308, 310
Nonmaleficence, in ethical code, 83
Nonproductive cough, definition of, 1331
Nonrapid eye movement (NREM) sleep, 1074, 1074f, 1075t
Nonrebreather mask, in oxygen administration, 1340t, 1343–1344
Nonsteroidal anti-inflammatory drugs, in pain management, 1128
Nonverbal communication, 360–362, 361f–362f
Nonviolence, in Gilligan moral development theory, 122
Normal flora, in body sites, 556
Norplant contraceptive, 868
North American Nursing Diagnosis Association, 224
  diagnosis list of, 273–274
Norton scale, for pressure ulcer assessment, 981–982, 982f
Nose. *See also* Nasogastric tube
  anatomy of, 491, 492f
  cannula/catheter in, oxygen administration by, 1339, 1340t
    procedure for, 1341–1342
  care of, 952, 954
  examination of, 491, 492f, 950
  injury of, in enteral nutrition, 1191
  instillation into, 652–653, 655
  speculum for, 491, 492f
Nosocomial infection, 561–562
"No-touch technique," for pressure ulcer treatment, 988–990
NPO (nothing by mouth) orders, 1181
  preoperative, 685
NREM (nonrapid eye movement) sleep, 1074, 1074f, 1075t
Nuclear family, 25–26, 26f
Nuclear scanning, 521t
Nurse, infection-control, responsibilities of, 589
Nurse administrator, 11t
Nurse anesthetist, 11t
Nurse-client relationship
  establishment of, guidelines for, 193
  in pain relief program, 1122
  for sexuality concern discussion, 862–863
Nurse educator, 11t
Nurse entrepreneur, 11t
Nurse midwife, 11t
Nurse practice acts, 16–17
Nurse practitioner, 11t
Nurse researcher, 11t
Nursing, 9
  aims of, 9–10, 10t, 11t
  attitudes toward, 5–6
  client population changes and, 18
  current trends in, 17–19
  definition of, 7–9
    American Nurses Association, 7–9
    as art, 5
    Canadian Nurses Association, 9
    as discipline, 9
    International Council of Nurses, 7
    as profession, 9
  healthcare reform role of, 175
  historical background of, 5–6, 8t
    in home healthcare, 208–209
  personnel shortage in, 18
    ethical problems with, 92
    legal aspects of, 107–108
  as profession, 9
  relationships in, types of, 302t
  role modeling in, 63
    for bowel elimination patterns, 1272
    for exercise habits, 1023
    for fluid and electrolyte management, 1388–1389
    for good nutrition, 1169–1170
    for oxygenation, 1318
    for pain management, 1113
    for self-concept, 733–734
    for sensory function, 819

Nursing, role modeling in *(continued)*
for sexuality, 855–856
for sleep needs, 1081
for spirituality, 890
in teaching, 395
for urinary elimination, 1216
roles in, 10t, 11t
science of, 5
technology impact on, 18
Nursing actions, definitions of, 19
Nursing assessment. *See* Assessing
Nursing audit, 324
Nursing care conference, definition of, 342
Nursing care plan
for case management, 291–293
in client record, 336
computer-generated, 291
definition of, 290
documentation of, 337
implementation of. *See* Implementing
institutional, 290–291
modification of, 318, 320t–322t
purposes of, 290
for spirituality, 900–902
standardized, 283, 292–293
student, 291, 294–296
writing of, 290–291
Nursing care rounds, 342–343
Nursing diagnosis, 225, 227t, 267–280. *See also specific type of care, e.g.,* Nutrition; Urinary elimination
accepted list of, 273–274
actual, 275
client preferences in, 278
vs. collaborative problems, 267–268, 269f–270f, 271t
communication in, 365
conclusions in, 272–273
core competencies in, 270
data clusters in, 269–270, 272t
data interpretation in, 269–273, 272t
defining characteristics in, 273, 275t
definition of, 267, 268f
errors in documentation of, 275, 277t
etiologic factors in, 273
evaluation of, 325
checklist of, 325
problems in, 320t
evolution of, 223–224
focus of, 267
formulation of, 273–275, 277
of future problems, 278
goals derived from, 285, 285t
in home healthcare, 215
human needs and, 278
identification of strengths and problems in, 270–271
illustration of, 228
incorrect use of, 275, 277t
list of, 273–274
vs. medical diagnosis, 267, 271t
nursing interventions derived from, 287–289, 288f
possible, 275
possible problems in, 272
potential, 275
potential liability in, 103t
priorities in, 278
problem areas in, 270–271
problem statement in, 273, 275t
significant data in, 269
in teaching-learning process, 408–409
validation of, 272t, 277
writing of, guidelines for, 273, 275, 276t
Nursing education. *See under* Education
Nursing ethics, 84
Nursing examination. *See* Physical assessment
Nursing history. *See* Health history
Nursing homes, 180
Nursing minimum data set, 333, 342
Nursing orders
standard protocols for, 302–303
writing of, 289–290, 289f
Nursing practice. *See also* Nursing process
competency in, as legal safeguard, 104, 106f
cultural influences on, 68
educational influences on, 68–69
guidelines for, 16–17
illegal, reporting of, 243–244
incompetency in, reporting of, 243–244
legal aspects of, 16–17
regulatory, 97–98, 97f
licensure for, 12, 98
scientific basis for, 69
standards for, 16, 98
unethical, reporting of, 243–244
Nursing process
application of, to teaching-learning process. *See under* Learning
benefits of, 230–231
characteristics of, 228–230, 230f
definition of, 17
description of, 224–225, 225f
documenting, 226
dynamic nature of, 229
goal orientation in, 229–230
historic perspective of, 223–224
intrapersonal considerations in, 229, 230f
overview of, 227t
potential liability in, 103t–104t
purpose of, 224, 225f
steps of, 225–226, 226f, 228. *See also specific step e.g.,* Assessing
systematic nature of, 229
universal applicability of, 230
Nursing theory, 66–77
application of, 69
autonomy and, 69
characteristics of, 69
communication and, 69
components of, 67–68, 68f
concepts in, 67–68, 68f
definition of, 67
derivation of, 67
developmental, 67
educational influences on, 68–69
evolution of, 69
general systems, 67
goals of, 69
historical perspectives of, 68–69, 68f
models for, 69–75
definition of, 66
Johnson behavioral systems model, 70t, 72
King open systems framework, 70t, 72
Leininger transcultural care model, 43, 70t, 72–73
Levine theory of nursing, 70t, 73
Neuman health-care systems model, 71t, 73
Orem self-care model, 71t, 73–74
Rogers science of unitary man, 71t, 74
Roy's adaptation model, 71t, 74–75
Watson caring model, 71t, 75
nursing practice and, 68–69, 68f
philosophy in, 66
process in, 66
publishing effects on, 69
research effects on, 69
scientific basis for, 69
stress/adaptation, 67
value of, 69
Nutrients
essential, 1150
nonessential, 1150
regulator. *See* Mineral(s); Vitamin(s)
Nutrition, 1149–1210. *See also* Diet; Food; Malnutrition
adequate, nurse as role model for, 1169–1170
in adolescents, 147, 147t
alcohol abuse and, 1168
assessment of, 1170–1175, 1173f, 1175t, 1176f, 1177t
bowel elimination and, 1284
carbohydrates in, 1152–1153, 1154t, 1155
cultural factors in, 37, 1169
decreased food intake and, 1169
definition of, 1150
developmental level and, 1163, 1165, 1166t–1168t
dietary recommendations for, 1161–1163
dietary selection in, 1158, 1161–1163, 1162f, 1164f
in dying patient, 799
economics and, 1169
in elderly persons, 168t
energy balance and, 1150–1152, 1151t
enteral. *See* Enteral nutrition
factors affecting, 1163, 1165, 1166t–1168t, 1168–1169
fats in, 1154t, 1156–1157, 1157f

food guide pyramid in, 1161–1162, 1161f
food labeling in, 1163, 1164f
gender and, 1163
growth and development affected by, 129
health status and, 1168
in infants, 133, 135t
information resources for, 1179
medication affecting, 1168
minerals in, 1158, 1160t–1161t
nutrient supplement imbalances and, 1168, 1178
parenteral. *See* Parenteral nutrition
postoperative, 696–697
in pregnancy, 1167, 1167t
preoperative, 676, 685
pressure ulcer formation and, 975
problems of
case study in, 1202–1206
implementing in
appetite stimulation, 1179–1180
assistance with eating, 1180
enteral nutrition in. *See* Enteral nutrition
parenteral nutrition. *See* Parenteral nutrition
special diets, 1180–1181
iron deficiency anemia, 1201–1202
knowledge deficit, 1202
nursing diagnosis of, 1175–1176, 1178
obesity, 1199–1202
planning for, 1176
protein in, 1153, 1154t, 1155–1156
psychological factors in, 1169
religion and, 1169
requirements for
Canadian tables, 1449t–1450t
United States tables, 1447t–1448t
in respiratory disorders, 1333
status of, assessment of, 1170–1175, 1173f, 1175t, 1176f, 1177t
in stress management, 769
in toddlers, 138t
vitamins in, 1157–1158, 1159t
Nutritional status, assessment of, pressure ulcer risk and, 980
Nutritive enema, 1288

Obesity, 1199–1201
causes of, 1199
definition of, 1199
hydraulic lifts for, 1048, 1050f
respiratory function and, 1316
Objective data, in assessing, 248–250, 250t
Oblique position, 1034, 1037f
Observation, during communication, 369
Obstructive apnea, 1081, 1084f, 1082t
Occult blood, in stool, 1274–1276, 1277f
Occupation
accidents related to, 527
air quality in, 1328
body mechanics in, 1005–1006, 1005f–1007f
preoperative assessment of, 676
skin alteration risks in, 917t
Occupational Safety and Health Act/Administration, 109
particulate respirator for tuberculosis, 586, 586f
universal precautions regulations of, 578
Occupational therapist, services of, 184
Occurrence report, 108
Oculomotor nerve, assessment of, 513, 513t
Odor
at bedside unit, 939
of urine, 1220t
Oedipus complex, 117
Official name, of drug, 595
Oil retention enema, 1287, 1288t
Ointment
application of, 646
definition of, 596t
at draining wound, 716
eye, application of, 650
Older adult. *See* Elderly persons
Old-old classification, of older adults, definition of, 163
Olfactory nerve, assessment of, 512–513, 513t
Oliguria, definition of, 1219
Oncotic pressure, definition of, 1373, 1373f
Onycholysis, 485
Open systems framework model of nursing (King), 70t, 72
Open wound, 699
Ophthalmoscope, 474–475, 475f
use of, 487–489, 488f–489f
Opioids (narcotics), 1128–1129
in diarrhea, 1286
preoperative, 686
respiratory function and, 1317
safety measures for, 609, 609f
sexual function effects of, 856t
Opportunistic organisms, 556
Optic nerve, assessment of, 513, 513t
Optic reflexes, 1005
Oral care, 942–950
assessment in, 942–944
denture care in, 945, 947, 950f
flossing in, 945, 951f
implementing of, 944–945, 950f–951f
importance of, 942
mouthwashes in, 950
nursing diagnosis for, 944
planning of, 944
procedure for
for dependent client, 948–950
for partially independent client, 946–947
toothbrushing, 946–947
toothbrushing in, 945–947, 950, 951f
Oral contraceptives, 868
Oral-genital stimulation, 848
Oral hygiene, in enteral nutrition, 1192
Oral intestinal lavage, 1291
Oral medications, administration of, 610–615
to child, 610, 614
contraindications for, 610
to elderly person, 614
by gastrointestinal tube, 615
preparation of, 610
procedure for, 611–614
sublingual, 615
taste disguise in, 610
Oral problems, 943–944
Oral rehydration, in diarrhea, 1287
Oral stage, in Freudian theory, 117, 117t
Oral temperature
assessment of, 439
procedures for, 440–443
normal, 437t
Orders
for medications. *See under* Drugs/medications
nursing
standard protocols for, 302–303
writing of, 289–290, 289f
physician's, execution of, 105–106
telephone, 105–106, 341
Orem, Dorothea E., self-care model of nursing, 70t, 73–74
Organ donation, 791, 791f
Organizations. *See also specific organization*
leadership in, 421, 421f
for leadership training, 421, 421f
professional, 15–16
specialty, 16
for stress management, 758
Orgasm, 845f, 846, 848
dysfunctional, 849, 859, 860t
Orientation
assessment of, 509
to space, cultural differences in, 36–37
to time, cultural differences in, 36–37
Origin of muscle, 1003, 1003f
Orofacial dyskinesia, definition of, 1025
Oropharyngeal airway, 1344, 1346
Orthopedic injury, in exercise, 1023
Orthopedics, definition of, 1004
Orthopnea, definition of, 456
Orthostatic albuminuria, definition of, 1219
Orthostatic hypotension, 459–460
in immobility, 1011t, 1017
OSHA (Occupational Safety and Health Act/Administration), 109
particulate respirator for tuberculosis, 586, 586f
universal precautions regulations of, 578
Osmolarity, definition of, 1372

Osmoreceptors, definition of, 1374
Osmosis, in fluid and electrolyte movement, 1371–1373, 1372f–1373f
Osmotic laxatives, 1285, 1286t
Osmotic pressure, maintenance of, antidiuretic hormone in, 1375t
Osteoarthritis, mobility in, 1007
Osteoporosis
in immobility, 1019
mobility problems in, 1007
Ostomy
appliance for, changing of, 1296–1297, 1297f
procedure for, 1298–1299, 1300f
for bowel diversion, 1295–1301, 1295f–1297f, 1300f
definition of, 1295
diet and, 1284
ileal conduit, for urinary diversion, 1251, 1253, 1253f
changing appliance on, 1254–1255
information resources for, 1284
sexuality and, 853
Otoscope, 475–476, 475f
use of, 490, 491f
Outcome
definition of, 282
evaluation of. *See also* Evaluating
definition of, 323
expected, of planning, 282
as grief reaction, 781
Outer canthus of eye, cleaning of, 952
Outpatient services, 176
Ovary, physiology of, 842–844, 843f
Overflow incontinence, 1230, 1232
Overhydration, definition of, 1377
Overweight. *See also* Obesity
Ovulation, 843–844, 843f
prediction of, 866
Ovum, in menstrual cycle, 842–843, 843f
Oximetry, pulse, 1325, 1325f
procedure for, 1326–1327
Oxygen
administration of
flow rate of, 1338
in home care, 1344, 1346f
humidification in, 1338
hyperbaric, 1358
by mask, 1340, 1343–1344, 1340t
procedure for, 1342–1343
by nasal cannula, 1339, 1340t
procedure for, 1341–1342
by nasal catheter, 1339–1340
precautions for, 1338–1339
sources of, 1336, 1338
by tent, 1344
procedure for, 1345
during transport, 1399
transtracheal, 1344, 1346f
partial pressure of, 1386, 1397t
in acid-base imbalance, 1391, 1396, 1397t
in alveolar gas exchange, 1314f, 1315
as physiologic need, 23
transport of, 1315
Oxygenation. *See also* Respiration; Respiratory function; Respiratory system
tissue healing and, 701–702

Packing, of wound, 716
procedure for, 718–720
Paget disease, mobility in, 1007
Pain, 1102–1148
acute
vs. chronic, 1109
definition of, 1109
management of, 1130, 1132f, 1140
affective response to, 1108–1109, 1110t
age variables and, 1111–1112
anxiety and, 1112
assessment of, 1113–1119, 1114t, 1118f–1120f
back, 1123t
behavioral response to, 1108–1109, 1110t
chronic
vs. acute, 1109
definition of, 1109
in malignancy, 1140–1142
management of, 1130, 1132–1133, 1133f–1134f, 1140–1142
chronic malignant, 1109
chronic nonmalignant, 1109
continuous, definition of, 1109t
coping with, 1109–1112
cultural factors and, 1109–1111
cutaneous, definition of, 1103
definition of, 1103
diffuse, definition of, 1109t
dull, definition of, 1109t
duration of, 1108, 1109t
environment and, 1112
ethnic variables and, 1109–1111
excruciating, definition of, 1109t
factors affecting, 1109–1113
family variables in, 1111–1112
gate control theory of, 1106–1107, 1108f
gender and, 1111–1112
from injection, reduction of, 636–637
intermittent, definition of, 1109t
in interview, 253t
intractable, 1109
management of
acupuncture in, 1125–1126
acute, 1130, 1132f, 1140
analgesic administration in. *See* Analgesics
biofeedback in, 1127
case study of, 1142–1144
cause removal in, 1122
in children, 1130, 1132
chronic, 1130, 1132–1133, 1133f–1134f, 1140–1142
cutaneous stimulation in, 1125, 1126t
distraction in, 1123–1124
in dying patient, 799
in elderly persons, 1132–1133
electrical nerve stimulation in, 1125, 1125f
epidural analgesia in, 1133, 1135–1136, 1135f
ethical considerations in, 1137–1138
family response in, 1139
goals of, 1129–1130, 1132f–1133f
in home care, 1137
hypnosis in, 1126–1127
imagery in, 1129
inadequate, 1128
increasing tolerance in, 1122–1123
legal issues in, 1137–1138
local anesthesia in, 1136–1137
neurectomy in, 1137
neurosurgery in, 1137
nurse as role model in, 1113
patient-controlled, 1133, 1135f
patient education on, 396–398
placebos and, 1137–1138
postoperative, 683
relationship establishment in, 1122
relaxation in, 1125
rhizotomy in, 1137
sympathectomy in, 1137
teaching about, 1138
therapeutic touch in, 1127
transcutaneous electrical nerve stimulation in, 1125, 1127f
mild, definition of, 1109t
misconceptions about, 1114, 1114t
moderate, definition of, 1109t
modulation of, 1108
nursing diagnosis of, 1119–1122
origins of, 1103–1104
past experience with, 1112–1113
perception of, 1107–1108
phantom limb, 1105t
physiologic response to, 1108–1109, 1110t
postoperative, 697, 1140
preoperative anxiety about, 683
psychogenic, definition of, 1104
quality of, 1108, 1109t
referred, 1104–1106, 1107f
reflex response to, 758
religious beliefs and, 1112
responses to, 1108–1109, 1110t
cultural factors in, 41
secondary gain from, 1112
severe, definition of, 1109t
severity of, 1108, 1109t
sexuality and, 849, 862
sharp, definition of, 1109t
shifting, definition of, 1109t
slight, definition of, 1109t
somatic, definition of, 1103–1104
spiritual, 890, 893
stress and, 1112
support persons and, 1112

syndromes of, 1104, 1105t
teaching about, 1138
transient, definition of, 1109t
transmission of, 1104, 1105–1107, 1106f–1108f
undertreatment of, 1128
visceral, definition of, 1104
from wound, 704
Pain threshold, 1107
Pallor, of skin, 483, 483t
Palpation
in blood pressure assessment, 467
in physical assessment, 479–480, 479f, 480t
abdomen, 507, 1273
breast, 503, 504f
neck, 494, 494f
peripheral vascular system, 502
precordium, 499, 501f
respiratory system, 1319
skin, 483–485, 485f
thorax, 496, 497f–498f
Pancreatic juice, loss of, imbalances resulting from, 1390t
Panel discussions, 395
Panic, definition of, 759–760
Pantothenic acid, 1159t
Papilloma virus, 855t
Papule, definition of, 484t
Parallax, in manometer reading, 461, 461f
Paralysis
definition of, 1029
sleep, 1082t
Paralytic ileus, postoperative, 696
Paraplegia, definition of, 1029
Parasomnia, 1081
Parasympathetic nervous system control
of defecation, 1267–1268
of intestine, 1267–1268
Parathormone, function of, 1374, 1375t
Parathyroid gland, fluid/electrolyte homeostasis and, 1374, 1375t
Parenteral medications, 615–642
administration of
intradermal, 623
procedure for, 625–626
intramuscular, 632–635, 636f
discomfort reduction in, 636–637
procedure for, 632–635
intravenous
adding medications to solution container, 638–639
as bolus, 637, 640–641
in continuous infusion, 637
controlled-volume, 637, 646f
heparin lock and flush in, 637, 641–642, 647–649, 1415, 1423
intermittent, 637, 642f
piggyback method in, 637, 642f, 643–644
volume-control set in, 645–646
mixing in one syringe, 617, 622, 622f
procedure for, 623–624
needles for, 616, 616f
removing from containers, 617
procedures for, 618–621
subcutaneous, 626–627, 627f
discomfort reduction in, 636–637
procedure for, 629–631
syringes for, 616, 616f
definition of, 615
needleless systems for, 616, 617f
powdered, reconstitution of, 622
Parenteral nutrition, 1193–1196, 1429
complications of, 1196
formulas for, 1193
glucose monitoring in, 1193
procedure for, 1197–1198
indications for, 1193
nursing considerations in, 1193–1994
partial, 1193
peripheral, 1193
total, 1193
types of, 1193
Parenting, inadequate, sensory deprivation in, 830–831
Paresis, definition of, 1029
Parkinsonian gait, 1028f
Paronychia, 485, 485f
Partial care, in personal hygiene, 918
Partial pressure
in alveolar gas exchange, 1314f, 1315
of carbon dioxide, 1386, 1397t
in acid-base imbalance, 1391, 1396, 1397t
in alveolar gas exchange, 1314f, 1315
of oxygen, 1386, 1397t
in alveolar gas exchange, 1314f, 1315
Partial rebreather mask, in oxygen administration, 1340t, 1343
Particulate respirator, in care of isolated client, 586, 586f
Passive exercise, range-of-motion, 1037
Patch
as skin lesion, 484t
transdermal, 596t, 649
Patellar (knee) reflex, assessment of, 516t, 517
Paternalism, ethical problems with, 86
Pathogen, definition of, 556
Patient-controlled analgesia, 1133, 1135f
Patient rights, 84, 87–88
in dying, 783
in pain management, 1138
Patient Self-Determination Act (1990), 789
Pavor nocturnis, 1083t
pCO_2 (partial pressure of carbon dioxide), 1396, 1397t
in acid-base imbalance, 1391, 1396, 1397t
in alveolar gas exchange, 1314f, 1315
PDR (Physician's Desk Reference), 603
Pedagogy, definition of, 389
Pediatric clients. *See* Children; Infants; Neonates; Toddlers
Pediculocides, 956
Pediculosis, 955–956
Pedophilia, 848
Peer relationships, in school-age children, 141
Penetration, in sexual intercourse, 846
Penicillin, in sexually transmitted disease, 854t–855t
Penis
anatomy of, 844–845
erection of, 844–845
failure of, 849, 859, 860t, 862
Penrose drain, for wound, 707f, 708t, 721
Perceived loss, definition of, 781
Perception
about health, in health and illness model, 55, 56f
alterations of, in sensory deprivation, 816t
in sensory experience, 814, 817
Percussion
in physical assessment, 440, 481, 481t
abdomen, 507, 1273
thorax, 496
as treatment in respiratory disorders, 1332, 1333f
Percussion hammer, in physical assessment, 475f, 476
Percutaneous endoscopic gastrostomy, 1182
Perfectionism, self-concept and, 745
Perfusion, tissue, definition of, 1315
Perfusion scan, in respiratory disorders, 1324t
Perimetrium, definition of, 842
Perineal care, 960–965, 963f
Periodontal disease, 943–944
Perioperative period. *See also* Postoperative care; Preoperative care; Surgery
intraoperative, 687–688
phases of, 670
Peripheral vascular resistance, in blood pressure maintenance, 457
Peripheral vascular system, examination of, 502
Peristalsis, 1267–1268, 1277f
Personal hygiene
assessment of, 915–916, 917t
complete care in, 918
cultural factors in, 913–914
definition of, 911
developmental level and, 914
for dying patient, 799
evaluation of, 942
health state and, 913–914
implementing of. *See also* Bathing; Skin care
assistance with antiembolism stockings, 927, 930
procedure for, 928–929
scheduled care provision, 918–919
nurse as role model in, 914–915
nursing diagnosis in, 916–918

Personal hygiene *(continued)*
  partial care in, 918
  personal preferences in, 914
  planning in, 918
  religion and, 914
  scheduled, 918–919
  self-care in, 918
  skin physiology and, 911–913, 912f, 913t
  socioeconomic class and, 914
  after urination, 1228, 1230
Personal identity
  disturbances of, nursing diagnosis of, 739
  self-concept and, 735–736
Personality
  sensory function and, 819
  sensory stimulation and, 819
Personal protective equipment, in infection control, 582, 585–587, 586f
Personal space
  in communication, 369–370
  cultural differences in, 36–37
Personal strength, identification of, 735–736, 741, 741f
Perspiration, imbalances resulting from, 1390t
Pertussis, immunization for, 136t
Petechiae, definition of, 483
Peyotist religion, 49t
pH. *See also* Acid-base balance; Acid-base imbalance
  definition of, 1376
  of urine, 1220t
    in fluid balance assessment, 1391
Phallic stage, in Freudian theory, 117, 117t
  preschool children in, 139
Phantom limb pain, 1105t
Pharmacist
  definition of, 594
  services of, 184
Pharmaco-anthropology, 599
Pharmacodynamics, definition of, 595–596
Pharmacokinetics, 596
Pharmacology. *See also* Drugs/medications
  definition of, 594
Pharynx, examination of, 492–493, 493f
Philosophy, of nursing, 66
Phlebitis, in intravenous therapy, 1422t
Phlegm, definition of, 1331
Phosphate buffer system, 1376
Phosphate/phosphorus
  dietary, 1160t, 1371
  as electrolyte, 1369f, 1371
  imbalance of, 1384t–1385t, 1386
  regulation of, 1375t
Physical activity, as physiologic need, 23
Physical assessment, 253–254, 254f, 474–517
  of abdomen, 503–507, 505f–506f
  of anus, 508
  of axilla, 502–503, 503f–504f
  of bladder, 1217
  of bones, 509
  of bowel elimination, 1272–1274, 1275t
  of breast, 502–503, 503f–504f
  client preparation for, 478, 478f
  data documentation in, 517
  documentation of, 335t
  draping for, 478
  of ear, 489–491, 490f–491f
  of elderly persons, normal alterations in, 482
  environment preparation for, 478
  of eye, 486–489, 486f–490f
  in fluid and electrolyte imbalance, 1389, 1391, 1392t–1396t
  form for, 255–259
  general appearance assessment in, 481
  of genitalia
    female, 507–508, 507f
    male, 507–508
  of head and neck, 485–494
    ear, 489–491, 490f–491f, 950
    eye, 486–489, 486f–490f, 950
    face, 486
    lymph nodes, 494, 494f
    mouth, 492–493, 493f, 942–943
    neck region, 493–494, 494f
    nose, 491, 492f, 950
    pharynx, 492–493, 493f
    sinuses, 492, 493f
    skull, 486
    thyroid, 493–494, 494f
    trachea, 493
  of heart, 498–502, 500f–502f, 502t
  height measurement in, 481
  instruments for, 474–476, 475f
  of integument, 482–485
    hair/scalp, 485
    nails, 485, 485f
    skin, 483–485, 483f, 483t–484t, 485f
  of joints, 509
  of kidney, 1217
  of lungs, 495–497, 495f–500f
  of mobility, 1024–1029, 1026t, 1027f, 1029f
  of musculoskeletal system, 508–509, 510f–511f
  of neurologic system, 509–517
    cranial nerve function, 512–513, 513t, 514f
    mental status, 509, 512, 512t
    reflexes, 514–515, 515t–517t
  in nutritional assessment, 1174, 1177t
  of peripheral vascular system, 502
  personal hygiene in, 916, 917t
  positions for, 476, 477f, 478
  preoperative, 678, 679t
  of rectum, 508
  of reproductive system, 860–861
  of respiratory system, 1319, 1321
  of skin, 916, 917t
    in urinary problems, 1218
  sleep and, 1086
  in stress, 766
  techniques for, 478–481
    auscultation, 480–481
    inspection, 478–479
    palpation, 479–480, 479f–480f, 480t
    percussion, 480, 481f, 481t
  of thorax, 495–497, 495f–500f
  of urethra, 1217
  of urinary elimination, 1217–1218
  vital signs in, 481
  weight measurement in, 481
Physical dimension, in health-illness status, 55–56
Physical examination. *See* Physical assessment
Physical fitness, in school-age children, 143t
Physical loss, definition of, 781
Physical needs, health-illness status and, 58
Physical therapist, services of, 184
Physicians
  conflict with nurse, 91
  offices of, 178
  orders of, execution of, 105–106
  progress notes of, 335t
  services of, 183
Physician's assistant, services of, 183–184
Physician's Desk Reference, 603
Physiologic homeostasis, 756, 757t
Physiologic needs, 22–23, 23f
  of dying patient, 799
  in physical assessment, 478, 478f
  stress effects on, 761
Physiologic stressors, 758–759, 759f, 764
Piaget cognitive development theory, 119, 121f–122f, 121t
  adolescents and, 143
  infants and, 133
  learning process and, 388–389, 391
  preschool children and, 138–139
  school-age children and, 140
  toddlers and, 136
PIE charting system, in documentation, 334, 338t, 348f
Piggyback method, of medication administration, 637, 642f
  procedure for, 643–644
Pigmentation, of skin, 482–483, 483t
  adaptation of, 38
Pill, definition of, 596t
"The Pill" (oral contraceptive), 868
Pillow
  body alignment and, 1031–1032
  pressure ulcer prevention and, 985
Pinworms, specimen collection of, 1276
Pitch, in auscultation, 480
Pitting edema, 1380f
Pituitary gland, fluid/electrolyte homeostasis and, 1375t
Pivot joint, 1000
Placebo, pain management and, 1137–1138

Rales (crackles), 456, 497, 1319, 1321
Range of motion
  assessment of, 1027
  definition of, 1000, 1000t, 1001f–1002f, 1037
  examination of, 509
  exercise for, 1037, 1039, 1039f
Rape
  obligation to report, 109
  sensory overload in, 824
Rapid eye movement (REM) sleep, 1074–1075, 1075t
Rapport, with client, 368, 369f
Rash, 483
  skin care in, 941–942
Rathbone, William, as visiting nurse originator, 208
Rationalization, as defense mechanism, 760
Razors, 957–958, 958f
Reach to Recovery, 181
Reaction formation, as defense mechanism, 760
Reactive hyperemia, in pressure ulcer formation, 975, 976t
Reality orientation, in confusion, 160
Reasoning
  assessment of, 512
  in nursing theory, 66
Receiver, in communication, 359, 360f
Reception, in sensory experience, 814, 819, 821–822
Receptive aphasia, definition of, 512
Recommended dietary allowances, 1161–1163, 1447t–1448t
  of carbohydrates, 1153
  of fat, 1157
  of protein, 1156
Recommended nutrient intakes, 1161–1162
Reconstitution, of powdered medications, 622
Records. *See* Documentation; Client record
Recovery, from illness, behavior in, 60–61
Recovery room, activities involving, 688
Rectal suppository, 1289, 1293
Rectal temperature
  assessment of, 439
    procedures for, 443–445
  normal, 437t
Rectal tube, in flatulence, 1287
Rectum
  examination of, 508
    in bowel elimination assessment, 1273–1274
  Foley catheter use in, 1293–1294
  instillations into, 655
Rectus femoris site, for injections, 631f, 632
Recurrent bandage, application of, 713, 715f
Red cells, enzymes of, reference ranges for, 1442t
Referrals, 341–342
  in discharge planning, 203
Referred pain, 1104, 1106, 1107f
Reflexes
  assessment of, 514, 515f–516f, 517, 517t
    instruments for, 475f, 476
  deep tendon, in electrolyte imbalance, 1395t–1396t
  extensor, 1005
  in neonates, 131, 131f
  optic, 1005
  postural, 1005
  pupillary, 487
  stretch, 1005
  visual, 1005
Reflex pain response, 758
Refractory period, of sexual cycle, 845f, 846
Regional anesthesia, 672
Registration, for nursing practice, 98
Regressive behavior
  as defense mechanism, 760
  in toddlers, 137
Rehabilitation, behavior in, 60–61
Rehabilitation centers, 180
Relapsing fever, 438t
Relationships
  establishment of, caring, 240
  in nursing, types of, 302t
Relaxation
  in pain relief, 1125
  patient education on, 396
  before sleep, 1090
  in stress management, 770
Religion, definition of, 883
Religious faiths
  Adventists, 886t
  American Muslim Mission, 887
  Christianity, 886–887
  Christian Science, 886t
  common characteristics of, 890
  Eastern Orthodox Church, 887
  Eastern philosophies, 887, 888t
  healthcare services provided by, 181
  Islam, 887
  Jehovah's Witnesses, 886t
  Judaism, 885–886
  Mormons, 886t
  Native Americans, 887–888
  practice of, facilitation of, 894
  Protestantism, 887
  Roman Catholicism, 886–887
  Unification Church, 886t
  Unitarianism, 886t
Religious values. *See also* Spirituality
  nutrition and, 1169
  pain attitudes and, 1112
  personal hygiene and, 914
  sexuality and, 849
Reminiscence, by elderly persons, 161, 161f
Remission, of chronic illness, 61
Remittent fever, 438t
REM (rapid eye movement) sleep, 1074–1075, 1075t
Reporting
  change-of-shift, 340, 341f
  definition of, 339
  to family, 341
  formats for, 339–340, 340t
  of illegal practices, 243–244
  of incompetency, 243–244
  telephone, 340–341
  on transfers, 341
  of unethical practices, 243–244
Reporting obligations, 109
Repression, as defense mechanism, 760
Reproductive system. *See* Genitalia/genital system
Research, 421–424
  in advancement of nursing profession, 422
  client record in, 333
  nurse's role in, 420, 420f
  as nursing function, 10t, 11t
  in nursing practice, 69
  problems for, 423
  protecting subject rights in, 423
  relating to practice, 423
  resources for, 423–425
Reserpine, sexual function effects of, 856t
Reservoirs, for infectious agents, 557, 557f, 558t
Residual volume (RV), definition of, 1322t
Resistance
  airway, 1314
  in general adaptation syndrome, 759, 759f
Resolution phase
  of grief reaction, 782
  of sexual response cycle, 845f, 846
Resonance, in percussion, 481t, 496
Respect
  in communication, 376
  need for, 884
  for persons, promotion of, 238–240
Respiration, 455–456, 1311–1365. *See also* Breathing
  acid-base balance and, 1376–1377
  assessment of, breath sounds in, 456–457, 458t
  control of, 1315
  depth of, 456
  developmental variations in, 1316, 1316t
  external, 455
  fluid and electrolyte balance and, 1394t
  internal, 455
  patterns of, abnormal, 498
  physiology of, 450, 1312–1316, 1313f–1314f
  principles of, 1315
Respirator, particulate, in care of isolated client, 586, 586f
Respiratory acidosis. *See under* Acidosis
Respiratory alkalosis. *See under* Alkalosis

Plaintiff, in litigation, 97
Planned change, leadership role in, 417
Planning, 225, 227t, 281–299. *See also specific type of care, e.g.* Bowel elimination; Infection control
  client record in, 333
  communication in, 365
  comprehensive, 283–284
  consultation in, 289
  discharge. *See* Discharge planning
  elements of, 282, 283f
  errors in, 286–287
  evaluation of, 325
    checklist of, 325
    problems in, 321t–322t
  evaluative strategy in, 287
  focus of, 282–284
  formal, 282
  goals in, 285–287, 285t, 286f
  illustration of, 228
  informal, 282
  initial, 283
  institutional care plans in, 290–291
  for learning. *See under* Learning
  nursing orders derived from, 289–290, 289f
  ongoing, 284
  option identification in, 288–289
  option selection in, 289
  potential liability in, 103t
  priorities in, 284–285
  problem-oriented, 284
  problems in, 296
  selection of nursing interventions in, 287–290, 288f
  student care plan for, 291, 294–296
Plantar flexion, definition of, 1000t, 1002f
Plaque
  dental, 943
    removal of. *See* Oral care
  skin, definition of, 484t
Plasma, laboratory tests of, reference ranges for, 1442t–1444t
Plateau phase, of sexual response cycle, 845f, 846
Platelets, laboratory tests of, reference ranges for, 1442t
Play
  in infants, 133
  in preschool children, 141t
  in school-age children, 143t
  in toddlers, 138t
  types of, 133
Pleura, function of, 1313
Pleural effusion, chest tube in, 1330, 1331f
Pleural fluid, aspiration of (thoracentesis), 1321, 1321f, 1324
Pleural friction rub, 497, 500f, 1321
PLISSIT model, for counseling in sexual dysfunction, 870
PM care (afternoon care), 918
Pneumatic compression devices, postoperative, 695
Pneumatic compression stockings, 930
Pneumaturia, definition of, 1219
Pneumonia
  in elderly persons, 559
  hypostatic, from immobility, 1019
  nosocomial, 561
  postoperative, 695–696
Pneumothorax, chest tube in, 1330, 1331f
pO_2 (partial pressure of oxygen), 1386, 1397t
  in acid-base imbalance, 1391, 1396, 1397t
  in alveolar gas exchange, 1314f, 1315
Podiatrist, 960
Podophyllum, in genital warts, 855t
Poison control center, 547
Poisoning, prevention of, 530, 534, 544, 547, 549
Poliomyelitis, immunization for, 136t
Polypnea, definition of, 458t
Polyps, nasal, 491
Polysaccharides, definition of, 1153
Polysomnography, 1081
Polyuria, definition of, 1219
Popliteal artery, blood pressure assessment at, 462
Popliteal pulse, 452f
  assessment of, 502
Port, implanted, for intravenous therapy, 1409, 1411f
Portal of entry, for infectious agents, 557, 557f
Portal of exit, for infectious agents, 557, 557f
Positions
  for bandage/binder use, 712
  for correct alignment
    devices for, 1031–1034, 1032f–1034f
    protective, 1033–1034, 1035t–1036t, 1036–1038, 1037f
    turning techniques in, 1037
      procedure for, 1038
  for defecation, 1284
  for diagnostic procedures. *See specific procedure*
  operative, 688
  for physical assessment, 476, 477f, 478
  postoperative, 690
  for pressure ulcer prevention, 985
  for respiratory efficiency, 1332
  terminology of, 1000t
  for urinary catheterization, 1237, 1238f
  for urination, 1228
Positive reinforcement, in learning, 403
Postanesthesia recovery room, 688
Postconventional level, in Kohlberg moral development theory, 120–121, 121t
Postherpetic neuralgia, 1105t
Postoperative care, 688–698
  assessment in, 690
  general, procedure for, 691–692
  immediate, 688–690, 693f
    procedure for, 691–692
  implementing of
    preventing complications, 694–696
    promoting return to health, 696–697
  nursing diagnosis in, 690
  planning for, 692–693
  preoperative teaching about, 682–684, 684f
Postoperative phase, definition of, 670
Postural drainage, in respiratory disorders, 1333, 1334f
Postural hypotension, definition of, 459–460
Postural reflexes, 1005
Postural tremor, definition of, 1024
Posture. *See also* Body alignment
  abnormal, mobility and, 1006–1007
  assessment of, 1026t
  body mechanics and, 1004
  as nonverbal communication, 362
Post-void residual, measurement of, 1234
Potassium
  dietary, 1160t, 1370
  as electrolyte, 1369f, 1370
  imbalance of, 1380, 1382t
Potential problems
  in critical thinking, 236–237
  in nursing diagnosis, 275
Pouch
  for fecal incontinence, 1293–1294
  vaginal, as contraceptive, 867
Poverty
  culture of, 37–38
  healthcare and, 37–38
Powdered medications, 596t
  application of, 646
  reconstitution of, 622
Power
  in leadership, 418
  in self-esteem, 737
Powerlessness, in immobility, 1015t
Power of attorney, durable, 785, 787f, 789
PPAs (preferred provider arrangement), 186
PPOs (preferred provider organizations), 186
Practical nursing, education for, 12
Prayer, with client, 895, 898
Precedent, in common law, 97
Preceptorship, in leadership training, 421
Preconventional level, in Kohlberg moral development theory, 119–120, 121t
Precordial thrills, 499
Precordium, assessment of, 498–499, 501f
Prednisone, in respiratory disorders, 1336t
Pre-entry phase, of home visit, 213

Respiratory depression, from opioids, 1129
Respiratory distress syndrome, in neonates, 131
Respiratory function
  assessment of
    diagnostic procedures for, 1322t–1324t, 1324f, 1326–1327
    guidelines for, 1320
    health history in, 1318–1319
    physical, 1319, 1321
    pulse oximetry in, 1325–1326
    thoracentesis in, 1321, 1321f, 1324
  in elderly persons, 1329
  factors affecting, 1316–1318
  nurse as role model in, 1318
  nursing diagnosis in, 1324–1325, 1327
  planning in, 1327–1328
  problems in
    asthma, case study in, 1361–1362
    in dying patient, 799
    impaired gas exchange, 1359–1360
    implementing in
      airway clearance, 1354, 1357–1358
      artificial airways, 1344–1348
      breathing techniques, 1329–1330
      cardiopulmonary resuscitation, 790–791, 1358, 1358f
      chest tube management, 1330, 1331f
      comfort measures, 1332–1336, 1333f–1334f
      coughing, 1331–1332, 1331f
      hyperbaric oxygen therapy in, 1358–1359
      nebulizers in, 1335, 1337
      nurse-client relationship in, 1329
      oxygen supplementation in, 1336, 1338–1339, 1340t, 1344, 1346f
      pollution control, 1328
      suctioning, 1348–1354
      ventilation assistance, 1348, 1354, 357
    ineffective airway clearance, 1360
    ineffective breathing patterns, 1360
    postoperative, 683–684, 695–696
    as surgical risk, 675
Respiratory isolation, specifications for, 571t
Respiratory rate, 456
  assessment of, procedure for, 457
  developmental level and, 1316, 1316t
  in older adults, 434
Respiratory system
  cytologic studies of, 1323t
  endoscopy of, 1323t–1324t
  exercise effects on, 1018f, 1019
  immobility effects on, 1012t–1013t, 1018f, 1019
  physiology of, 1312–1316, 1313f–1314f
  postoperative status of, in recovery room, 688–689
  radiography of, 1324t
Respiratory therapist, services of, 184
Rest. *See also* Sleep
  bed
    passive exercise in, 1037
    skin alteration risks and, 917t
  definition of, 1073
  as physiologic need, 23
  postoperative, 697
  preoperative, 685
  in stress management, 769
Resting tremor, definition of, 1024
Restitution, as grief reaction, 781–782
Restless leg syndrome, in sleep, 1086
Restraints
  alternatives to, 544
  as false imprisonment, 101
  guidelines for, 543
  knots for, 546
  types of, 542
  use of, 539, 541, 542f, 544f
    procedure for, 545–547
"Restrict fluid" order, 1401–1402
Resuscitation, cardiopulmonary, 1358, 1358f
  legal aspects of, 790–791
Resuscitation bag, 1348, 1351, 1354
Retarded ejaculation, 859, 860t
Retention, urinary, 1227
  in immobility, 1014t
Retention catheter. *See* Catheter(ization) (urinary), indwelling
Retention sutures, 705, 706f
Reticular activating system
  in arousal to sensation, 814, 815f
  sleep control by, 1073, 1074f
Retina, examination of, 487–488, 488f
Retinol (vitamin A), 1159t
Retirement, adjustments to, 161–162
Retraction, of breast skin, 503
Retrograde pyelogram, 1224, 1226t
Retrospective evaluation, 324
Return flow enema, 1288
Rh factor, 1427–1428
Rhizotomy, in pain management, 1137
Rhonchi (gurgles), 456, 497, 500f, 1321
Rhythm method, of contraception, 866
Riboflavin (vitamin B_2), 1159t
Rights, patient, 84, 87–88
  advocacy in, 425
  in dying, 783
  in pain management, 1138
Ringer's lactate, for intravenous therapy, 1403t
Rinne's test, for hearing, 491
Risk factors
  for illness, 59, 59t
  in surgery, 670, 671t
Risk management, 108
Rituals, before sleep, 1089–1090
Robitussin (guaifenesin), as expectorant, 1332
Rogers, Martha E., science of unitary man model of nursing, 71t, 74
Role model, nurse as. *See* Nursing, role modeling in
Role performance, disturbances in, nursing diagnosis of, 737–739
Role playing, in teaching, 395–396
Roman Catholicism, 886–887
Romberg's sign, in sensory ataxia, 1028f
Rosenstock health-belief model, 55, 56f
Rotation, definition of, 1000t, 1001f–1002f
Rounds, nursing care, 342–343
Roy, Sister Calista, adaptation model of nursing, 71t, 74–75
Rub, back, 930
Rubella, immunization for, 136t
Rule of thumb method, in ideal weight estimate, 1151
Rumor, 371
Rural health centers, 179
RV (residual volume), definition of, 1322t

Saddle joint, 1000
Sadism, definition of, 848
Sadomasochism, definition of, 848
Safety, 60, 524–554. *See also* Infection control and prevention
  accident-prone behavior and, 527, 529
  in bathing, shower/tub, 919–920, 920f
  of bed, 939–940
  client goals in, 528, 534–535
  in computer charting, 337
  developmental levels and, 536, 536t–537t, 538
  in drug administration, oral, 610
  equipment-related, 549–550
  factors affecting, 525–528, 526t
  fall prevention and, 539–541, 541f–542f, 544f
    procedure for, 545–547
  firearm, 548–549
  fire prevention and, 543–544, 548f
  hazard assessment and, 528–533, 533t
  health state and, 528
  in home healthcare, 213
  as human need, 23, 23f, 525, 761
  incident report in, 551
  in infants, 133–134
  laws concerning, 109
  lifestyle and, 527
  mobility and, 527–528
  in needle handling, 576–578
  nursing diagnoses pertaining to, 533–534
  occupation and, 527
  orientation to surroundings and, 539
  in oxygen administration, 1344
  poisoning prevention and, 534, 544, 547, 549
  postoperative, 690
  in preschool children, 141t
  procedure-related, 550, 550f
  program for, 106

Skin *(continued)*
  of child, 913
  color of, 482–483, 483t
  as defense against microorganisms, 700
  vs. developmental stage, 913
  dry, 941
  of elderly person, 159, 913–914
  examination of, 916, 917t
  exercise effects on, 1018f, 1021
  functions of, 912, 913t
  vs. health status, 913
  immobility effects on, 1014t, 1018f, 1021
  of infant, 913
  infections of, in older adults, 559
  lesions of, 483, 484t
  medication application to, 642, 646
  moisture status of, 483
    pressure ulcer formation and, 975, 977, 980
  physical assessment of, in pressure ulcer prevention and treatment, 977–981, 980f, 982f
  physiology of, 911–913, 912f, 913t
  pigmentation of, 482–483, 483t
    adaptation of, 38
  preoperative preparation of, 685
  rash on, 483, 941–942
  stimulation of, in pain relief, 1125
  structure of, 979f
  sutures in, 705
  temperature of, 483
  texture of, 485
  turgor of, 484, 485f
    in fluid balance assessment, 1393t
  urinary problems affecting, 1218
  vascularity of, 483
Skin care
  cleaning agents for, 940
  with condom catheter, 1251
  cosmetics for, 941
  deodorants for, 940–941
  in diabetic foot, 960
  at draining wound, 716, 720
  of dry skin, 941
  principles of, 912
  of stoma, 1296, 1296f
  teaching about, 940–942
Skin fold measurements, nutritional status and, 1174, 1175f
Skull, examination of, 486
Slander, 100
Sleep, 1072–1101
  activity and, 1076
  in adolescents, 1078t
  alcohol intake and, 1080
  assessment of, 1083–1086
  caffeine and, 1080
  in children, 1077t–1078t
  circadian rhythms and, 1074
  comfort measures for, 1091
  cultural factors in, 1076, 1080
  definition of, 1073
  delta, 1074, 1075t
  deprivation of, 1081, 1083t, 1094–1095
  developmental level and, 1076, 1076f, 1077t–1079t
  diary of, 1084, 1086
  diet and, 1080
  disorders of, 1081, 1082–1083t, 1084f
    case study of, 1095–1098
    developmental stage and, 1076, 1076f, 1077t–1079t
    insomnia, 1081, 1082t, 1093–1094
    nursing diagnosis of, 1086–1089
    in preschool children, 141t
  in elderly persons, 169t, 1079t
  environmental factors and, 1089
  factors affecting, 1076, 1077t–1079t
  functions of, 1073
  history of, 1083–1084
  hygiene care before, 918
  immobility effects on, 1015t
  in infants, 1077t
  irregular, 1077t
  lifestyle and, 1080
  medications for, 1091
  in middle adults, 1079t
  motivation for, 1076
  nocturnal myoclonus in, 1086
  nonrapid eye movement (NREM), 1074, 1074f, 1075t
  in nurses, 1081
  nursing care scheduling and, 1091
  paralysis in, 1082t
  patterns of, 1075–1076
    abnormal, 1086–1088
      case study in, 1095–1098
    circadian rhythm of, 1074
    vs. developmental level, 1076, 1076f, 1077t–1078t
    respect for, 1091
  periodic, 1077t
  physical activity and, 1076
  physical assessment of, 1086
  as physiologic need, 23
  physiology of, 1073–1076, 1074f, 1075t, 1076f
  preoperative, 685
  promotion of, 1089–1091
    core competencies for, 1096
  quality of
    in illness, 1080
    medications and, 1080–1081
  rapid eye movement (REM), 1074–1075, 1075t
  relaxation before, 1090
  requirements for, 1075–1076
  rituals before, 1089–1090
  smoking and, 1080
  snacks before, 1090
  snoring in, 1086
  stages of, 1074–1075, 1074f, 1075t
  stress and, 1076
  in stress management, 769
  teaching about, 1091
  in toddlers, 1077t
  in young adults, 1078t–1079t
Sleep apnea, 1081, 1082t, 1084f
Sleep cycle, 1075, 1076f
Sleep talking, 1081, 1083t
Sleep walking, 1081, 1083t
Sling, 713, 715f
Slow-code orders, 790
Slow-wave (delta) sleep, 1074, 1075t
Small bowel series, 1276–1277, 1280t
Smell (olfactory sensation)
  assessment of, 821
  impairment of, characteristics of, 823
  stimulation of, 816t, 827–828
Smoke detectors, 544
Smoking
  respiratory disease and, 1328
  sleep, 1080
  as surgical risk, 676
Snacks, before sleep, 1090
Snellen eye chart, 475f, 476
Snoring, 1086
Soap
  for handwashing, 563
  in skin care, 940
SOAP method, for documentation, 334, 336t, 347f, 338t
Soapsuds enema, 1288t
Social isolation, in older adults, 162
Socialization, disturbances in, responses to, 736
Social relationship vs. helping relationship, 366
Social Security Administration, Medicare program of, 184, 185t
Social self, definition of, 729
Social worker, services of, 184
Sociocultural dimension
  in communication, 363
  in health-illness status, 57
Sociocultural needs
  health-illness status and, 58
  preoperative assessment of, 678
Socioeconomic factors
  in grief reactions, 792
  in healthcare access, 37–38
  in personal hygiene, 914
Sodium
  dietary, 1160t, 1369
  as electrolyte, 1369–1370, 1369f
  imbalance of, 1379–1380, 1381t
Sodium-potassium pump, in electrolyte movement, 1372, 1372f
Soft diet, 1181
Soil, as pathogen reservoir, 557
Soixante-neuf, 848
Solute, definition of, 1368
Solutions
  definition of, 596t
  for intravenous therapy, 1402, 1403t
    changing of, 1415
      procedure for, 1416–1418
  sterile, handling of, 568, 572f
Solvent, definition of, 1368
Somatic pain, definition of, 1103–1104
Somnambulism, definition of, 1081, 1082t

Sounds
  adventitious, 497, 500f, 1319
  bowel, 506–507, 1273
  breath, 456–457, 458t, 1319, 1321
    developmental level and, 1316, 1316t
  in communication, 362, 373
  heart, 501–502, 502f, 502t
  percussion, 496
Source, in communication, 359, 360f
Source-oriented records, 333–334, 335t, 346f
Space, orientation to, cultural differences in, 36–37
Spastic hemiparesis, gait in, 1028f
Spasticity, of muscle, definition of, 1029
Specialists
  certification of, 98
  nurse, 11t
Specific gravity, of urine, 1220t
  determination of, 1224, 1225f
  in fluid balance assessment, 1391
Specimens, collection and handling of, urine. *See* Urine, specimens of
Speculum
  nasal, 475f, 476, 491, 492f
  vaginal, 475f, 476, 507–508
Speech. *See also* Language
  disorders of, 378–380
Speech-language pathologist, 379
Speech therapist, services of, 184
Speed shock, in intravenous therapy, 1422t
Sperm, production of, 844
Spermicides, 867
Sphincters
  of anal canal, 1268, 1268f
  control of, in toddlers, 136
  of urinary system, 1212–1213
Sphygmomanometer, 460–461, 460f–461f
  care of, 467–468
Spica bandage, application of, 713, 714f
Spinal accessory nerve, assessment of, 513t, 514, 514f
Spinal cord
  injury of, sexuality and, 853
  pain transmission in, 1106–1107, 1106f, 1108f
Spiral-reverse turn, in bandage application, 713, 714f
Spiral turn, in bandage application, 713, 714f
Spiritual alienation, 890, 893
Spiritual anger, 890, 893
Spiritual anxiety, 890, 893
Spiritual beliefs, 884–885
Spiritual despair, 894, 896, 890
Spiritual dimension, in health-illness status, 57
Spiritual distress, 898–899
  case study of, 899–902
  nursing diagnosis of, 891
Spiritual guilt, 890, 893
Spirituality, 882–906. *See also* Religious values
  assessment of, 890–892
  core competencies of, 900
  counseling in, 895–896
  definition of, 883
  development of
    in middle adults, 156
    in preschool children, 140
    in school-age children, 141
    in young adults, 152
  ethics and, 889
  evaluation of, 897
  everyday living and, 883–884
  facilitating religious practice in, 894
  factors affecting, 889–890
  grief and, 792
  health and, 884–885
  illness and, 884–885
  implementing in, 892, 894–896
  legal aspects of, 889
  nurse as role model in, 890
  nursing care plan for, 900–902
  nursing diagnosis of, 891
  nurturing of, 895
  observation of, 890–891
  prayer with client, 895, 898
  preoperative assessment of, 678
  referral to religious counselor, 896
  religious faiths and, 885–888
    Adventists, 886t
    American Muslim Mission, 887
    Christianity, 886–887
    Christian Science, 886t
    Eastern Orthodox Church, 887
    Islam, 887
    Jehovah's Witnesses, 886t
    Judaism, 885–886
    Mormons, 886t
    Native Americans, 887–888
    Protestantism, 887
    Roman Catholicism, 886–887
    Unification Church, 886t
    Unitarianism, 886t
    western philosophies, 885–887
  resolving conflicts in, 896
  resources for, 896
  as source of conflict, 885, 896
  support for, 892, 894, 895f
Spiritual loss, 890, 894
Spiritual needs, 883–884
  of dying patient, 800
  health-illness status and, 58
Spiritual pain, 890, 893
Spirometry
  incentive
    as breathing exercise, 1329–1330
    postoperative, 684
  in respiratory function assessment, 1322t
Splint, hand-wrist, body alignment and, 1033
Sponge, vaginal, as contraceptive method, 867
Spoon nails, 485f
Sprain, joint, mobility in, 1007
Sputum
  analysis of, 1323t
  assessment of, 1320
Stairs, crutch use on, 1056, 1056f
Standard orders, for nursing activities, 302–303
Standard precautions, 580
Standards
  comparison of, to data, in diagnosing, 269
  for documentation, 330–331
  inappropriate, in self-concept disturbances, 745
  for nursing care plan, 283, 292–293
  for nursing education, 98
  for nursing evaluation, 314
  for nursing practice, 16, 98
Standards of care
  in meeting client goals, 308
  in negligence cases, 102, 103t–104t
  student nurses responsibility for, 109
Standing order, for medications, 602
Standing position, 477f, 478
  body alignment in, 1027, 1029f
Staphylococcus aureus, transmission of, 558t
Staples, in wound closure, 705
  removal of, 705, 706f, 707
Stare decisis, in common law, 96–97
Stat order, for medications, 602
Statutory law, 96
Steam, in sterilization/disinfection, 567t
Stent, urologic, 1235–1236
Step family, 25
Steppage gait, 1028f
Stepping reflex, 131f
Stereognosis, definition of, 814
Stereotyping, of cultural and ethnic groups, 34–35, 35f
Sterile field, preparation of, 586, 586f
  procedure for, 569–571
Sterile technique. *See* Surgical asepsis
Sterile urine specimen, collection of, 1223, 1224f, 1239–1245
Sterilization (aseptic procedure), methods for, 563, 566, 567t
Sterilization (contraception), 868
Steroid hormones, reference ranges for, 1445t–1446t
Stertorous breathing, definition of, 456
Stethoscope
  in auscultation, 480
  in blood pressure assessment, 461
  in breath sounds assessment, 456
  in heart examination, 501–502
  in pulse assessment, 449, 451f
  in thorax assessment, 495–497, 499f–500f
Stimulants, as laxatives, 1285, 1286t
Stimulation
  of appetite, 1179–1180
  in pain management
    cutaneous, 1125
    electrical, 1125, 1127f
  sensory. *See* Sensory function
  of urination, 1228–1229

Tetanus, immunization for, 136t
Tetracycline, in sexually transmitted disease, 854t
Thalamic syndrome, 1105t
Thalassemia, ethnic differences in, 39
Theophylline, in respiratory disorders, 1336t
Theory. *See also* Nursing theory
  definition of, 66
Therapeutic touch, 375
  in pain management, 1127
Thermometer
  disposable, 438
  electronic, 437, 442–443
  glass, 437, 439t
    in axillary temperature assessment, 445, 447–448
    cleaning of, 446
    in oral temperature assessment, 439–443
    in rectal temperature assessment, 439, 443–445
  single-use, 438
  tympanic membrane, 437–438
Thermoregulation, as physiologic need, 22
Thiamine (vitamin B_1), 1159t
Thigh
  as injection site, 631f, 632
  strengthening exercise for, in bowel elimination, 1285
Thinking, critical. *See* Critical thinking
Third intention, healing by, 701, 702t
Third-space fluid shift, 1377
Thirst, postoperative, 697
Thoracentesis, 1321, 1321f, 1324
Thorax, examination of, 495–497, 495f–500f
Thready pulse, 451t
Three-carrier lift, 1040
  procedure for, 1044–1045
Three checks, in drug administration, 608
Three-point gait, in crutch walking, 1056, 1057f
Thrills, precordial, 499
Thrombophlebitis, postoperative, 694–695
Thrombosis, in immobility, 1011t, 1017
Thrombus, in intravenous therapy, 1422t
Thumb, range of motion of, 1001f
Thyroid gland
  examination of, 493–494, 494f
  fluid and electrolyte homeostasis and, 1374
  hormones of, reference ranges for, 1446t–1447t
Tibial pulse, 452f
Tic, definition of, 1024
Ticks, removal of, 956
Tidal volume, definition of, 1322t
Time, orientation to, cultural differences in, 36–37
Time criteria, in data collection, 315–316
Time tape, in intravenous infusion monitoring, 1412, 1414, 1415f
Tissue perfusion
  alterations in, in immobility, 1011t
  definition of, 1315
TLC (total lung capacity), definition of, 1322t
Tocopherol (vitamin E), 1159t
Toddlers
  body alignment of, 1008t
  bowel elimination in, 1269t
  growth and development of
    cognitive, 136
    physiologic, 134, 136
    psychosocial, 136–137
  health problems of, 137
  mobility of, 1008t
  nutrition in, 1166t
  respiratory function in, 1316, 1316t
  safety considerations for, 526, 537t, 538
  sexuality of, 850t
  sleep in, 1077t
  urinary elimination in, 1214
  wellness promotion in, 137–138, 138t
Toes, range of motion of, 1002f
Toileting, assistance with, 1229. *See also* Bedpan
Toilet training, 1269t
  psychological aspects of, 136
  as toddler developmental task, 136, 138t
  in urination, 1214–1215
Tolerance
  to drugs, 600
    definition of, 1129
  to pain, 1122–1123
Tone, muscular. *See under* Muscles
Tongue
  drug administration under, 615
  examination of, 492–493
  inflammation of, 944
  turgor of, in fluid balance assessment, 1393t
Tonsils, physical assessment of, 492–493
Tonus, definition of, 1004
Toothbrushing, 945, 950, 951f
Toothpaste, 950
Topical anesthesia, 672
Topical medications, administration of
  to ear, 652–655
  to eye, 646, 650–652
  by inhalation, 655–656
  to nose, 652–653, 655
  to rectum, 655
  to skin, 642
  to vagina, 653, 655–656
Torts
  classified as crime, 98
  definition of, 99
  intentional, 99–100, 100f
  unintentional (negligence), 101–104, 102t–104t, 105f
Total body water
  definition of, 1367, 1368f
  variations in, 1368, 1369t
Total incontinence, urinary, 1227
Total lung capacity (TLC), definition of, 1322t
Total parenteral nutrition, 1429. *See* Parenteral nutrition
Total person approach (Neuman), in nursing theory, 71t, 73
Touch, therapeutic, in pain management, 1127
Touch (action)
  as nonverbal communication, 360–361, 374–375, 375f
  therapeutic, 375, 1127
Touch (tactile sensation)
  assessment of, 821–822
  impairment of, characteristics of, 823
  stimulation of, 816t, 828
Towel bath, 920, 927
TPN (total parenteral nutrition). *See* Parenteral nutrition
Trachea
  examination of, 493
  percutaneous oxygen administration to, 1344, 1346f
Tracheostomy, 1345–1348, 1347f
  care of, 1348
    procedure for, 1355–1357
  suctioning from, 1248
    procedures for, 1352–1354
Trade name, of drug, 595
Traditional family, 24–26, 26f
Traditional knowledge, 422
Training, leadership, 420–421, 421f
Tranquilizers
  preoperative, 686
  urinary elimination and, 1216
Transcultural nursing
  cultural assessment in, 44–45
  cultural imposition and, 44
  definition of, 43
  ethnocentrism and, 44
  factors affecting, 44–46, 46t–50t
  guidelines for, 44–46, 50
  holistic care in, 44
  model for (Leininger), 43, 70t, 72–73
Transcutaneous electrical nerve stimulation, 1125, 1127f
Transdermal patch, 596t, 649
Transfer, in/between healthcare settings, 195, 197, 200
  documentation of, 339, 341
Transformation, in adult years, 150–151
Transformational leadership, 415–416
Transfusion, blood. *See* Blood transfusion
Transmission-based precautions, 580, 582
Transmission-perception-reaction, 822
Transparent dressings, 989t
Transplantation
  hair, 955
  organ, 671t
Transsexuality, 847

Transtracheal oxygen delivery, 1344, 1346f
Transvestism, definition of, 847
Trapeze bar, 1033, 1034f
Trauma. *See* Injury
Treatment
  improper, legal aspects of, 101–104, 102t–104t, 105f
  refusal of, 99, 100f
Tremor, 486, 1024
Trendelenburg position, effects of, 688
Trial-and-error method, of problem solving, 226
Trial court, 97
Triceps reflex, assessment of, 515t, 517
Triceps skin fold measurement, 1174, 1175f
Trichomoniasis, 855t
Tricuspid area, pulse at, 501f
Trigeminal nerve, assessment of, 513, 513t
Trigeminal neuralgia, 1105t
Triglycerides, definition of, 1156
Triple-lumen catheter, in continuous urinary irrigation, 1235–1236, 1235f
Tripod position, in crutch use, 1056, 1056f
Trochanter roll, body alignment and, 1033, 1033f
Troche (lozenge), cough, 1332
Trochlear nerve, assessment of, 513, 513t
Trousseau's sign, of neuromuscular irritability, 1395t
Trust
  development of, 118, 118f
  vs. mistrust, in infants, 118
Truth, as essential value, 80
T-tube, for drainage, 708t
Tubal ligation, 868
Tub bathing, 919–920, 920f
Tube feeding. *See* Enteral nutrition
Tuberculosis
  in elderly persons, 559
  isolation specifications for, 577t
  mask protection in, 586, 586f
  transmission of, 558t
Tube/tubing. *See also* Catheter(ization)
  chest, management of, 1330, 1331f
  endotracheal, 1344–1345, 1347f
  gastrointestinal, drug administration through, 615
  for intravenous therapy, changing of, 1415
    procedure for, 1416–1418
  oropharyngeal, 1344, 1346
  postoperative assessment of, 690
  rectal, in flatulence, 1287
  tracheostomy, 1345, 1348, 1347f
  for wound drainage, 705–706, 707f, 708t
Tumor, skin, definition of, 484t
Tuning fork, in physical assessment, 475f, 476
Tunneling, of pressure ulcer, 979, 991
Turbidity, of urine, 1220t
Turbinates, nasal, 491, 492f
Turgor, of skin in physical assessment, 484, 485f, 1393t
Turning, of client in bed
  by client, 684
  by nurse, 1037
    procedure for, 1038
TV (tidal volume), definition of, 1322t
T wave, in electrocardiography, 449
Twenty-four-hour urine specimen collection, 1223–1224
Two-point gait, in crutch walking, 1056, 1057f
Tympanic membrane, examination of, 490, 491f
Tympanic temperature
  assessment of, thermometer for, 437–438
  normal, 437t
Tympanites, 1284
Tympany, in percussion, 481t, 496
Typing, of blood, 1423, 1427

Ulcers
  pressure. *See* Pressure ulcers
  skin, definition of, 484t
Ulnar deviation, definition of, 1001f
Ultrasonography, 521t
  of urinary system, 1225, 1226t
Ultrasound, Doppler, in pulse assessment, 451–452
Unconscious mind, in Freudian theory, 117
Unconsciousness
  communication in, 381, 829
  definition of, 815
  eye care in, 953
Unction. *See* Ointment
Undermining, of pressure ulcer, 980, 991
Understaffing, 18, 92
  legal aspects of, 107–108
Unification Church, 886t
Unintentional wound, 699
Unitary man model of nursing (Rogers), 71t, 74–75
Unit dose system, for drugs, 605
United States Pharmacopeia, 594
Units
  apothecary, 607, 1439, 1439t–1440t
  household, 607, 1439, 1439t
  metric, 605, 607
Universal precautions, 572, 576–578
  in wound care, 722
Unresolved grief, 782
Upper gastrointestinal series, 1276–1277, 1280t
Urea nitrogen, measurement of, 1175
Ureter
  physiology of, 1212, 1213f
  stent in, 1235–1236
Urethra
  examination of, 1217
  function of, 1213
  stent in, 1235–1236
Urethritis, nongonococcal, 854t
Urge incontinence, 1230
Urgency, urinary
  definition of, 1219
  in older adults, 1229
Uric acid deposition (gout), ethnic differences in, 40
Urinal, use of, 1230
  procedure for, 1231–1232
Urinalysis
  with diagnostic kits, 1224
  reference ranges for, 1444t–1445t
  routine, specimen collection for, 1219–1220, 1222–1224, 1223f–1224f, 1239–1245
Urinary diversion, 1251, 1253, 1253f
  appliance changing in, 1251
    procedure for, 1254–1255
Urinary elimination, 1211–1264
  assessment of, 1216–1225
    diagnostic procedures for, 1224–1225, 1226t
    history in, 1216–1217
    measures for, 1218–1225, 1221f–1225f, 1226t
    physical assessment in, 1217–1218, 1220t
  bedpan use in, 1230
    procedures for, 1231–1232
  factors affecting, 1214–1216, 1216t
  implementing in
    assistance with urinary diversions, 1251, 1253–1255, 1253f
    catheterization. *See* Catheter(ization) (urinary)
    promotion of normal urination, 1228–1232
  nurse as role model in, 1216
  nursing diagnosis of, 1225, 1227
  physiology of, 1212–1214, 1213f
  planning in, 1225
  postoperative, 696
  preoperative, 685
  problems with, 1219. *See also specific problem*
    catheter infection, 1257–1258
    dysuria, 1255–1256
    in elderly persons, 1229
    enuresis, 1256
    incontinence. *See* Incontinence (urinary)
    retention, 1256–1257
    types of, 1227
  safety in, 1230
Urinary tract
  of elderly person, 159
  exercise effects on, 1018f, 1029
  immobility effects on, 1014t, 1018f, 1021
  infections of
    in catheterization, 1236–1237, 1257–1258

Urinary tract, infections of *(continued)*
in elderly persons, 559, 1229
in immobility, 1014t, 1021
nosocomial, 561
Urination
act of, 1213–1214
control of, 1213–1214
developmental level and, 1214
factors affecting, 1214–1216
frequency of, 1214, 1219, 1228–1229
in older adults, 1229
hygiene after, 1228, 1230
involuntary, 1213
position for, 1228
privacy in, 1228
problems with, 1219. *See also* Incontinence (urinary)
promotion of normal habits in, 1228–1232
prompted, 1234
stimulation of, 1228–1229
urgency of
definition of, 1219
in elderly persons, 1229
Urine
characteristics of, 1218, 1220t
color of, 1214, 1216, 1216t, 1220t
concentration of, in fluid balance assessment, 1392t
constituents of, 1220t
formation of, 1212
output of, measurement of, 1218–1219, 1221f–1222f
in fluid balance assessment, 1392t
pH of, in fluid balance assessment, 1391
post-void residual of, measurement of, 1234
retention of, 1256–1257
causes of, 1214
in immobility, 1014t
specific gravity of, 1220t, 1224, 1225f
in fluid balance assessment, 1391
specimen collection of, 1219–1220, 1223f–1224f, 1222–1224
in children, 1219–1220, 1223f
clean-catch (midstream), 1220, 1223–1224
in infants, 1219–1220, 1223f
procedure for, 1239–1245
sterile, 1223, 1239–1245, 1224f
twenty-four hour, 1223–1224
storage of, in bladder, 1212–1213
testing of. *See* Urinalysis
Urinometer, 1224, 1225f
Urography, excretory, 1224, 1226t
USP (United States Pharmacopeia), 594
Uterus, physiology of, 842, 842f
Utilitarianism, 83

Vaccines, contraceptive, 868
Vagina
care of, 960–965, 963f
medication administration into, 653, 655–656
physiology of, 842–843, 842f
Vaginal pouch, as contraceptive, 867
Vaginal speculum, 475f, 476
use of, 507–508
Vaginal sponge, as contraceptive method, 867
Vaginismus, 859–860, 860t
Vaginitis, 854t
Vagus nerve, assessment of, 513t, 514
Validation
in communication, 374
of data, in assessing, 262–263
of nursing diagnosis, 272t, 277
Valsalva maneuver, in defecation, 1268
Values, 79–83
clarification of, 81–83
in clinical situation, 81–83
in communication, 364
conflict of
client-family, 82–83
patient-nurse, 82–83
cultural differences in, 46t–50t
definition of, 79
development of, 79
exercise options and, 1015
neutrality of, 80–81
nonjudgmental attitude toward, 80–81
of nursing profession, 79–81
types of, 79
Value system, definition of, 79
Valves of heart, anatomy of, 500f, 501
Vancomycin, resistance to, 561–562, 578
Variables, in research, 423
Variance charting, 336
Variance report, 108
Vas deferens, anatomy of, 844
Vasectomy, 868
Vastus lateralis site, for injections, 631f, 632
VC (vital capacity), definition of, 1322t
Vectors, of organism transmission, 557, 558t
Vegetarian diet, 1181
Vehicle, of transmission for infectious agents, 557, 558t
Veins, infusion into. *See* Intravenous therapy
Venereal warts, 855t
Venoscope, in vein location, 1409
Venous thrombosis, in immobility, 1011t
Ventilation
assistance with, 1348
at bedside unit, 939
decreased, in older adults, 1329
definition of, 1313
mechanical, 791, 1348
phases of, 1313–1314, 1314f
pulmonary, 455
Ventilation scan, in respiratory disorders, 1324t
Ventrogluteal site, for injection, 631–632, 631f
Venturi mask, in oxygen administration, 1340t, 1344
Venules, filtration through, 1373f
Veracity, in ethical code, 84
Verbal communication. *See also* Language
Vesicle, definition of, 484t
Vesicular breath sounds, 497, 499f, 1319
Veterans Administration, healthcare services of, 181
Vials
drug packaging in, 617, 617f
medication removal from, procedure for, 620–621
Vibration, as treatment in respiratory disorders, 1333, 1333f
Violence, 58
domestic, 526
in home healthcare, 213
Virginity, 841
Virtue, in self-esteem, 737
Virulence, of infectious agents, 556
Visceral pain, definition of, 1104
Visceral sensation, definition of, 814, 822
Vision
assessment of, 488–489, 821
cranial nerve function and, 513, 513t
impairment of
characteristics of, 823
communication in, 381
needs in, 826
stimulation of, 816t, 827
Visits to home. *See* Home healthcare
Visual reflexes, 1005
Vital capacity (VC), definition of, 1322t
Vital signs, 432–472. *See also* Blood pressure; Body temperature; Pulse; Respiration
assessment of
frequency of, 433
responsibility for, 433
definition of, 433
in elderly persons, 434
in physical assessment, 481
postoperative, 690
preoperative, 685
Vitamin(s), 1157–1158, 1159t
deficiencies of, 1157–1158, 1159t
excess of, 1159t
recommended daily allowances for, 1447t–1448t
Vitiligo, 483t
Vocational nursing, education for, 12
Voice problems, 380
Voiding. *See* Urination
Volume-administration set, for intravenous medication, procedure for, 645–646
Voluntary agencies, for healthcare, 181, 181f

Voluntary coughing, 1331
Vomiting and nausea
  postoperative, 697
  in pregnancy, case study of, 1202–1206
von Bertalanffy, Ludwig, general systems theory of, 67
Voyeurism, 848

Wakefulness. *See* Sleep, patterns of
Walkers, 1053–1054, 1054f
Walking. *See* Ambulation; Gait
Warts, venereal, 855t
Waste disposal, of biohazardous substances, 587
Water. *See also* Fluid(s)
  absorption of, in colon, 1266
  function of, in body, 1367
  loss of, 1374, 1374f
  sources of, 1373–1374
Water bed, in pressure ulcer prevention, 987t
Watson, Jean, caring model of nursing, 71t, 75
Weaning, terminal, 791
Wear-and-tear theory of aging, 157
Weber's test, for hearing, 491
Weight
  drug action and, 598
  excess. *See* Obesity
  ideal, 1151, 1151t
  measurement of
    in fluid balance assessment, 1391, 1392t–1393t
    in nutritional assessment, 1174
  in physical assessment, 481
  water as proportion of, 1369t
Wellness
  definition of, 10, 53
  focus on, healthcare delivery trends and, 186–187, 186f
  vs. health, 54
  models of, 54
  promotion of. *See also* Illness, prevention of; Preventive care
    in adolescents, 147–148, 147t–148t
    in discharge planning, 203
    in elderly persons, 168–170, 168t–169t
    exercise in, 1022
    in family, 28–29, 30t
    in infants, 134, 135t–136t
    in middle adults, 156
    as nursing aim, 10
    in preschool children, 140, 141t
    safety in, 529
    in school-age children, 141, 143t
    as teaching aim, 387
    in toddlers, 137–138, 138t
    in young adults, 153–154
Wellness diagnosis, 275, 277
West nomogram, for drug dosage, 608, 608f
Wheal, definition of, 484t
Wheezing, 456, 497, 500f, 1321
Whistleblowing, 243–244
White middle class, cultural characteristics of, 43–44, 46t
Widowhood, 155, 162, 783
Wills
  living, 785, 787f–788f, 789
  witnessing of, 110
Withdrawal behavior, as coping mechanism, 760
Witness
  in malpractice litigation, nurse as, 102
  to will, 110
World Health Organization
  health as defined by, 53
  primary health care concept of, 183
Wounds, 699–723
  anxiety about, 704
  appearance of, in assessment, 704
  care of, 704–706, 706f–707f, 708t
    bandage application in, 709, 712–713, 714f–715f
    binder application in, 709, 712–713, 716
    chronic, 722
    culture collection in, 716–718
    documentation of, 716
    draining, 716, 721, 721f
    emergency, 704–705
    healing promotion in, 721, 721f
    at home, 722–723
    implementing of, dressings in. *See* Dressings
    infected, 722
    irrigation in, 716, 718–720
    open, 722
    staple removal in, 705, 706f, 707
    suture removal in, 705, 706f, 707
    teaching about, 722–723
  clean, 699t
  clean-contaminated, 699t
  cleaning of, 709
    procedure for, 710–712
  closed, 699
  complications of, 702–703
  contaminated, 699t
  culture collection from, 716
    procedure for, 717–718
  definition of, 483, 699
  dehiscence of, 703, 703f
  draining, 704–705, 716, 721, 721f
    assessment of, 704–705
    dressing change for, 716, 721, 721f
  evisceration through, 703, 703f
  fear and, 704
  fluid loss from, imbalances resulting from, 1390t
  healing of, 700–702, 702f
  hemorrhage from, 703
  infected, 702–703
    dressing changes for, 722
  intentional, 699
  irrigation of, 716
    procedure for, 718–720
  open, 699
  pain from, 704–705
  postoperative assessment of, in recovery room, 689–690
  postoperative complications of, 696
  psychologic effects of, 703–704
  self-concept alterations and, 704
  staples in, 705, 706f
  surgical, assessment of, 704–706, 706f–707f, 708t
  sutures in, 705, 706f
  types of, 699–700, 699t
  unintentional, 699
Wrist
  range of motion of, 1001f
  splint for, body alignment and, 1033
Written message, in communication, 340t

Yin and yang, 41

Zinc, dietary, 1160t
Z-track (zig-zag) technique, for injection, 632, 635–636, 636f
Zygote, 129

Fundamentals of Nursing: The Art and Science of Nursing Care

Self-Study Computer Program Instructions

This electronic self-study program has been designed for use with an IBM-compatible computer with an Intel 386 or better processor and requires Windows 3.1 or later. For use in Windows 3.1, 4 megabytes or RAM is the minimum requirement, but 8 MB RAM is recommended. For Windows 95, 8 megabytes or RAM is the minimum requirement, but 12 MB RAM is recommended. 3 megabytes of available hard disk space is also required.

Installation

Installing *Fundamentals* for Windows

1. Start up Windows
2. Insert the *Fundamentals* disk into the floppy disk drive.
3. From the Program Manager's File Menu, choose the Run command.
4. When the Run dialog box appears, type a:\setup (or b:\setup if you're using the B drive) in the Command Line box. Click OK or press the Enter button.
5. The Fundamentals installation process will begin. A dialog proposing the directory "FUNDNSG" on the drive containing Windows will appear. If the name and location are correct, click OK. If you want to change this information, type over the existing data, then click OK.
6. When the *Fundamentals* setup routine is complete, a new group called "*Fundamentals*" will appear on your desktop.
7. Start the program by double-clicking on its icon.

Fundamentals

Fundamentals contains 350 questions that review the content covered in *Fundamentals of Nursing: The Art and Science of Nursing Care*, Third Edition. As in the NCLEX, all questions in this program are multiple choice.

This is not a timed test. Take your time; consider the questions and the possible answers carefully.

To begin the test, choose Start Test from the Main Menu screen. To continue a test that you have already begun, choose Resume Test. To restart the test and erase your results from a previous test, choose Restart Test. To review the answers you have given and compare them with the correct answers, choose Answers.

When you choose Start Test, Resume Test, Restart Test, or Answers, the test and the program's Toolbar will appear.

Fundamentals' *Toolbar*

The Toolbar contains a series of buttons that provide direct access to all test program functions. When you move the cursor over a button, an explanation of its function displays in the Status Bar, which is immediately above the ToolBar.

To get help at any time during the test, choose the Program Help button. Program Help reviews basic functions of the program.

Answer each question by clicking on the oval to the left of an answer selection or by selecting the appropriate letter on the keyboard (e.g., A, B, C, D, etc.). When an answer is selected, its oval will darken. If you change your mind about an answer, simply select that choice, by mouse or keyboard, again.

To register your answer selection and proceed to the next question, click on the Right Arrow button or press Return.

After taking the test and receiving your score, you may review your answers by clicking on the Answers button on the Main Menu screen.

If you are unsure about an answer to a particular question, the program allows you to mark it for later review. Flag the question by clicking on the Mark button. To review all marked questions for a test, click on the Table of Contents button, which is immediately to the right of the Mark button.

The Table of Contents window lists every question included on the test and summarizes whether it has been answered, left unanswered, or marked for later review. Click on an item in the Table of Contents window and the program will move to that test question.

Use the Arrow buttons to move to the first, previous, next, or last question.

At any time during the test or when you are finished taking the test, click on the Stop button. If you wish, you may return to the session at a later time without erasing your existing answers by clicking on the Resume Test button on the Main Menu.